Vascular and Endovascular Surgery

SEVENTH EDITION

Vascular and Endovascular Surgery:

A Comprehensive Review

Wesley S. Moore, MD

Professor and Chief Emeritus
David Geffen School of Medicine
University of California, Los Angeles
Vascular Surgeon
University of California, Los Angeles,
    Center for the Health Sciences
Los Angeles, California

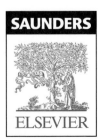

SAUNDERS

ELSEVIER

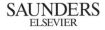

SAUNDERS
ELSEVIER

1600 John F. Kennedy Blvd.
Ste. 1800
Philadelphia, PA 19103-2899

VASCULAR AND ENDOVASCULAR SURGERY: ISBN 13: 978-1-4160-0183-6
A COMPREHENSIVE REVIEW   ISBN 10: 1-4160-0183-2
Copyright © 2006, 2002, 1998, 1993, 1991, 1986, 1983 by Elsevier Inc.

Library of Congress Cataloging-in-Publication Data
Vascular and endovascular surgery: a comprehensive review / [edited by] Wesley S.
  Moore.–7th ed.
    p. ; cm.
  Rev. ed. of: Vascular surgery. 6th ed. c2002.
  Includes bibliographical references and index.
  ISBN 1-4160-0183-2
    1. Blood-vessels–Surgery. I. Moore, Wesley S. II. Vascular surgery.
  [DNLM: 1. Vascular Surgical Procedures. 2. Vascular Diseases–surgery. WG 170
V3283 2006]
  RD598.5.V374 2006
  617.4'13–dc22   2005042847

Acquisitions Editor: Judith Fletcher
Developmental Editor: Denise LeMelledo
Publishing Services Manager: Tina Rebane
Senior Project Manager: Amy Norwitz
Interior Design Direction: Steven Stave
Cover Designer: Steven Stave

Printed in the United States of America

Last digit is the print number: 9 8 7 6 5 4 3 2 1

The seventh edition of this book is dedicated to the next generation of vascular surgeons. The effort that has gone into this book by the editor and chapter contributors is directed primarily to the education of our trainees. The future of our specialty will be in their capable hands.

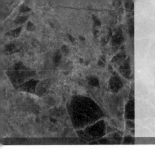

Contributors

William A. Abbott, MD
Professor of Surgery
Harvard Medical School
Massachusetts General Hospital
Boston, Massachusetts
*Vascular Grafts: Characteristics and Rational
Selection*

Samuel S. Ahn, MD
Professor of Surgery and Director of
Endovascular Surgery
David Geffen School of Medicine
University of California, Los Angeles
Attending Surgeon
University of California, Los Angeles,
Medical Center
Los Angeles, California
*Thoracic Outlet Syndrome and Vascular Disease
of the Upper Extremity*

George Andros, MD
Assistant Clinical Professor of Vascular Surgery
University of Southern California
Los Angeles, California
Director, Vascular Laboratory
Providence St. Joseph Medical Center
Burbank, California
*Arterial Access; Guidewires, Catheters,
and Sheaths; and Balloon Angioplasty
Catheters*

Niren Angle, MD, RVT
Assistant Professor of Surgery In Residence
University of California, San Diego,
School of Medicine
Attending Vascular Surgeon
University of California, San Diego,
Medical Center
San Diego, California
*Thrombolytic Therapy for Vascular Disease
Acute Arterial and Graft Occlusion
Prosthetic Graft Infections*

J. Dennis Baker, MD
Division of Vascular Surgery
David Geffen School of Medicine
University of California, Los Angeles
Gonda (Goldschmied) Vascular Center
Los Angeles, California
The Noninvasive Vascular Laboratory

Jeffrey L. Ballard, MD
Clinical Professor of Surgery
University of California, Irvine
School of Medicine
Staff Vascular Surgeon
St. Joseph Hospital
Orange, California
*Anatomy and Surgical Exposure of the
Vascular System*

Wiley F. Barker, MD
Professor Emeritus (Surgery/Vascular Surgery)
University of California, Los Angeles
Los Angeles, California
A History of Vascular Surgery

Michael Belkin, MD
Division of Vascular Surgery
Brigham & Women's Hospital
Boston, Massachusetts
Aortoiliac Occlusive Disease

Robert S. Bennion, MD
Professor of Surgery
David Geffen School of Medicine
University of California, Los Angeles
Los Angeles, California
Attending Surgeon
Los Angeles County Olive View Medical Center
Sylmar, California
Hemodialysis and Vascular Access

John Bergan, MD
Professor of Surgery
University of California, San Diego,
School of Medicine
San Diego, California
Staff Surgeon
Scripps Memorial Hospital
La Jolla, California
Varicose Veins: Chronic Venous Insufficiency

Ramon Berguer, MD, PhD
Professor and Chief
Frankel Professor of Vascular Surgery
University of Michigan Medical Center
Ann Arbor, Michigan
*Surgical Reconstruction of the Supra-aortic Trunks
and Vertebral Arteries*

Frederic S. Bongard, MD
Chief, Division of Trauma and Critical Care
University of California, Los Angeles,
   Harbor View Medical Center
Torrance, California
   Vascular Trauma

Ruth L. Bush, MD
Assistant Professor
Division of Vascular Surgery and
   Endovascular Therapy
Michael E. DeBakey Department
   of Surgery
Baylor College of Medicine
Assistant Professor
Department of Vascular Surgery
Michael E. DeBakey Veterans Affairs
   Medical Center
Houston, Texas
   *Angioplasty and Stenting for Aortoiliac Disease:
      Technique and Results*

Michael T. Caps, MD, MPH
Division of Vascular Therapy
Hawaii Permanente Medical Group
Honolulu, Hawaii
   *Angioplasty and Stenting for Infrainguinal
      Disease: Technique and Results*

Deborah R. Caswell, RN, ANP
Director, Gonda Wound Care Center
David Geffen School of Medicine
University of California, Los Angeles
Los Angeles, California
   *The Wound Care Center and
      Limb Salvage*

Alexander W. Clowes, MD
Professor of Surgery
University of Washington School of Medicine
Seattle, Washington
   *Anatomy, Physiology, and Pharmacology of the
      Vascular Wall*

Sheila M. Coogan, MD
Assistant Professor of Surgery
Stanford University School of Medicine
Chief, Vascular and Endovascular Surgery
Palo Alto VA Hospital
Palo Alto, California
   *Arterial Access; Guidewires, Catheters,
      and Sheaths; and Balloon Angioplasty
      Catheters*

Richard H. Dean, MD
Professor of Surgery
Wake Forest University School of Medicine
President and CEO
Wake Forest University Health Sciences
Winston-Salem, North Carolina
   Management of Renovascular Disease

Ralph G. DePalma, MD
Professor of Surgery
Uniformed Services University of the Health Sciences
Bethesda, Maryland
Consultant in Surgery
National Director of Surgery
Department of Veterans Affairs
District of Columbia Veterans Affairs Medical Center
Washington, DC
   *Atherosclerosis: Pathology, Pathogenesis, and
      Medical Management*
   Vasculogenic Erectile Dysfunction

Magruder C. Donaldson, MD
Associate Professor of Surgery
Harvard Medical School
Staff, Brigham and Women's Hospital
Boston, Massachusetts
   Aortoiliac Occlusive Disease

James M. Edwards, MD
Associate Professor of Surgery
Division of Vascular Surgery
Oregon Health and Science University
Chief of Surgery
Portland Veterans Administration Medical Center
Portland, Oregon
   Nonatherosclerotic Vascular Disease

Cindy L. Felty, RN, MSN, CNP, FCCWS
Assistant Professor of Medicine
Mayo Clinic College of Medicine
Director, Vascular Ulcer/Wound Healing Clinic
Vascular Center
Mayo Clinic
Rochester, Minnesota
   Lymphedema

D. Preston Flanigan, MD
Clinical Professor of Surgery
University of California, Irvine
School of Medicine
Medical Director
St. Joseph's Hospital Vascular Institute
Orange, California
   Aneurysms of the Peripheral Arteries

Julie A. Freischlag, MD
William Stewart Halsted Professor and
   Chairman of Surgery
Johns Hopkins School of Medicine
Surgeon-in-Chief
The Johns Hopkins Hospital
Baltimore, Maryland
   Prosthetic Graft Infections

Brian Funaki, MD
Associate Professor of Radiology
Section Chief, Angiography and Interventional Radiology
University of Chicago
Pritzker School of Medicine
Chicago, Illinois
   Visceral Ischemic Syndromes

Hugh A. Gelabert, MD
Professor of Surgery
David Geffen School of Medicine
University of California, Los Angeles
Attending Staff
University of California, Los Angeles, Medical Center
Los Angeles, California
*Primary Arterial Infections and Antibiotic
Prophylaxis*
Portal Hypertension

Bruce L. Gewertz, MD
Dallas B. Phemister Professor and Chairman,
Department of Surgery
University of Chicago
Pritzker School of Medicine
Chief, Section of Vascular Surgery
University of Chicago Medical Center
Chicago, Illinois
Visceral Ischemic Syndromes

Peter Gloviczki, MD
Professor of Surgery
Mayo Clinic College of Medicine
Chair, Division of Vascular Surgery
Director, Gonda Vascular Center
Mayo Clinic
Rochester, Minnesota
Vascular Malformations
*Thoracic and Lumbar Sympathectomy:
Indications, Technique, and Results*

Jerry Goldstone, MD
Professor of Surgery
Case School of Medicine
Case Western Reserve University
Chief, Division of Vascular Surgery
University Hospitals of Cleveland
Cleveland, Ohio
Aneurysms of the Aorta and Iliac Arteries

Antoinette S. Gomes, MD
Professor of Radiological Sciences and Medicine
Department of Radiological Sciences
David Geffen School of Medicine
University of California, Los Angeles
Los Angeles, California
Principles of Imaging in Vascular Disease

Carlos Gracia, MD
Associate Professor of Surgery
Chief of Minimally Invasive Surgery
David Geffen School of Medicine
University of California, Los Angeles
Los Angeles, California
*Laparoscopic Aortic Surgery for Aneurysms and
Occlusive Disease: Technique and Results*

Lazar J. Greenfield, MD
Professor of Surgery
Chair, Emeritus
University of Michigan Medical School
Ann Arbor, Michigan
Venous Thromboembolic Disease

Kimberley J. Hansen, MD
Professor of Surgery
Head, Section on Vascular Surgery
Wake Forest University School of Medicine
Winston-Salem, North Carolina
Management of Renovascular Disease

Paul B. Haser, MD
Clinical Assistant Professor of Surgery
University of Medicine and Dentistry of New Jersey
Medical School
Newark, New Jersey
*Arterial Access; Guidewires, Catheters,
and Sheaths; and Balloon Angioplasty
Catheters*

Kim J. Hodgson, MD
Professor and Chairman, Division of
Vascular Surgery
Southern Illinois University School of Medicine
Springfield, Illinois
*Endovascular Treatment of
Renovascular Disease*

Larry H. Hollier, MD
Professor of Surgery and Dean
Louisiana State University School of Medicine
New Orleans, Louisiana
Thoracoabdominal Aortic Aneurysms

Douglas B. Hood, MD
Assistant Professor of Surgery and Radiology
Keck School of Medicine
University of Southern California
Los Angeles, California
*Endovascular Treatment of
Renovascular Disease*

Glenn C. Hunter, MD
Professor of Surgery
Chief of Vascular Surgery
University of Texas Medical Branch
Galveston, Texas
Noninfectious Complications in Vascular Surgery

Ted R. Kohler, MD, MSc
Professor of Surgery
University of Washington School of Medicine
Chief, Peripheral Vascular Surgery
Puget Sound Healthcare System
Seattle, Washington
*Anatomy, Physiology, and Pharmacology of the
Vascular Wall*
Myointimal Hyperplasia

Toshifumi Kudo, MD, PhD
Endovascular Research Fellow
Division of Vascular Surgery
David Geffen School of Medicine
University of California, Los Angeles
Los Angeles, California
*Thoracic Outlet Syndrome and Vascular Disease
of the Upper Extremity*

Gregory J. Landry, MD
Associate Professor of Surgery
Division of Vascular Surgery
Dotter Interventional Institute
Oregon Health and Science University
Portland, Oregon
　Nonatherosclerotic Vascular Disease
　Natural History and Nonoperative Treatment of
　　Chronic Lower Extremity Ischemia

Peter F. Lawrence, MD
Bergman Professor and Chief of Vascular Surgery
David Geffen School of Medicine
University of California, Los Angeles
Director, Gonda (Goldschmied) Vascular Center
Los Angeles, California
　The Wound Care Center and Limb Salvage

Timothy K. Liem, MD
Associate Professor of Surgery
Oregon Health and Science University
Attending Surgeon
Oregon Health Science University
Legacy Emanuel Hospital
Portland, Oregon
　Hemostasis and Thrombosis

Peter H. Lin, MD
Assistant Professor
Division of Vascular Surgery and Endovascular Therapy
Michael E. DeBakey Department of Surgery
Baylor College of Medicine
Assistant Professor
Department of Vascular Surgery
Michael E. DeBakey Veterans Affairs Medical Center
Houston, Texas
　Angioplasty and Stenting for Aortoiliac Disease:
　　Technique and Results

Evan C. Lipsitz, MD
Associate Professor of Surgery
Albert Einstein College of Medicine of Yeshiva University
Attending Physician
Montefiore Medical Center
Bronx, New York
　Femoral, Popliteal, and Tibial Occlusive Disease

G. Matthew Longo, MD
Assistant Professor of Vascular Surgery
University of Nebraska Medical Center
Omaha, Nebraska
　Endovascular Repair of Abdominal Aortic
　　Aneurysms: Technique and Results

Alan B. Lumsden, MD
Professor and Division Chief
Division of Vascular and Endovascular Therapy
Michael E. DeBakey Department of Surgery
Baylor College of Medicine
Professor and Chief of Division of Vascular Surgery
Department of Vascular Surgery
Michael E. DeBakey Veterans Affairs Medical Center
Houston, Texas
　Angioplasty and Stenting for Aortoiliac Disease:
　　Technique and Results

James M. Malone, MD
Clinical Professor of Surgery
University of Arizona College of Medicine
Tucson, Arizona
Chief of Vascular Services
Scottsdale Healthcare-Shea
Scottsdale, Arizona
　Lower Extremity Amputation

John A. Mannick, MD
Professor of Surgery
Harvard Medical School
Staff, Brigham and Women's Hospital
Boston, Massachusetts
　Aortoiliac Occlusive Disease

Jon S. Matsumura, MD
Associate Professor of Surgery
Feinberg School of Medicine
Northwestern University
Attending, Northwestern Memorial Hospital
Chicago, Illinois
　Endovascular Repair of Abdominal Aortic
　　Aneurysms: Technique and Results

David S. Maxwell*, MD
Formerly, Professor of Anatomy and Cell Biology
David Geffen School of Medicine
University of California, Los Angeles
Formerly, Professor of Surgery and Anatomy
Charles Drew Medical School
Los Angeles, California
　Embryology of the Vascular System

James F. McKinsey, MD
Associate Professor of Clinical Surgery
Columbia University College of Physicians and Surgeons
Adjunct Associate Professor
Weill Medical College of Cornell University
Site Chief, Division of Vascular Surgery
Columbia University Medical Center
Assistant Attending Surgeon
New York-Presbyterian Hospital
New York, New York
　Visceral Ischemic Syndromes

Louis M. Messina, MD
Professor of Surgery and Chief
Division of Vascular Surgery
University of California, San Francisco
Moffitt Hospital
San Francisco, California
　Splanchnic and Renal Artery Aneurysms

Erica L. Mitchell, MD
University of Colorado
Health Sciences Center
Division of Vascular and Interventional Radiology
Denver, Colorado
　Hemostasis and Thrombosis
　Natural History and Nonoperative
　　Treatment of Chronic Lower Extremity
　　Ischemia

*Deceased

Gregory L. Moneta, MD
Professor of Surgery and Chief of Vascular Surgery
Oregon Health Sciences University
Portland, Oregon
  *Natural History and Nonoperative
    Treatment of Chronic Lower Extremity
    Ischemia*

Wesley S. Moore, MD
Professor and Chief Emeritus
David Geffen School of Medicine
University of California, Los Angeles
Vascular Surgeon
University of California, Los Angeles, Center
  for the Health Sciences
Los Angeles, California
  *Extracranial Cerebrovascular Disease:
    The Carotid Artery
  Myointimal Hyperplasia*

Matthew M. Nalbandian, MD
Assistant Professor of Surgery
New York University School of Medicine
Chief, Vascular and Endovascular Surgery
Bellevue Hospital Center
New York, New York
  *Spine Exposure: Operative Techniques for the
    Vascular Surgeon*

Mark R. Nehler, MD
Vascular Surgery Section
Denver, Colorado
  *Natural History and Nonoperative
    Treatment of Chronic Lower Extremity
    Ischemia*

Takao Ohki, MD, PhD
Associate Professor of Surgery
Albert Einstein College of Medicine of
  Yeshiva University
Chief, Division of Vascular and Endovascular
  Surgery
Montefiore Medical Center
Bronx, New York
  *Technique of Carotid Angioplasty
    and Stenting*

Luigi Pascarella, MD
Postdoctorate Researcher
Department of Bioengineering
Clinical Instructor
Department of Surgery
University of California, San Diego
San Diego, California
  Varicose Veins: Chronic Venous Insufficiency

Malcolm O. Perry, MD
Professor Emeritus, Vascular Surgery
University of Texas Southwestern Medical School
Chairman, Department of Surgery
St. Paul Medical Center
Dallas, Texas
  Vascular Trauma

Charles M. Peterson, MD, MBA
Director, Division of Blood Diseases and Resources
National Heart, Lung, and Blood Institute
National Institutes of Health
Bethesda, Maryland
  *Influence of Diabetes Mellitus on Vascular
    Disease and Its Complications*

K. Todd Piercy, MD
Vascular Fellow
Wake Forest University School of Medicine
Winston-Salem, North Carolina
  Management of Renovascular Disease

William J. Quiñones-Baldrich, MD
Professor of Surgery
David Geffen School of Medicine
University of California, Los Angeles
Attending Vascular Surgeon
University of California, Los Angeles, Center for Health
  Sciences
Los Angeles, California
  *Thrombolytic Therapy for Vascular Disease
  Acute Arterial and Graft Occlusion*

Todd D. Reil, MD
Assistant Professor of Surgery
Division of Vascular Surgery
David Geffen School of Medicine
University of California, Los Angeles
Los Angeles, California
  *Pharmacology of Drugs Used in the Management
    of Vascular Disease*

David A. Rigberg, MD
Assistant Professor of Surgery
David Geffen School of Medicine
University of California, Los Angeles
Gonda (Goldschmied) Vascular Center
Los Angeles, California
  Portal Hypertension

Thom W. Rooke, MD
Krehbiel Professor of Vascular Medicine
Mayo Clinic College of Medicine
Head, Section of Vascular Medicine
Mayo Clinic
Rochester, Minnesota
  Lymphedema

Stephanie S. Saltzberg, MD
Assistant Professor of Surgery
New York University School of Medicine
New York, New York
  *Spine Exposure: Operative Techniques for the
    Vascular Surgeon*

Peter A. Schneider, MD
Hawaii Permanente Medical Group
Honolulu, Hawaii
  *Arterial Access; Guidewires, Catheters, and
    Sheaths; and Balloon Angioplasty Catheters
  Angioplasty and Stenting for Infrainguinal
    Disease: Technique and Results*

Lewis B. Schwartz, MD
Lecturer
University of Chicago
Pritzker School of Medicine
Chicago, Illinois
Divisional Vice President
Drug Fluting Stent Program
Abbott Laboratories
Abbott Park, Illinois
Visceral Ischemic Syndromes

Roger F. J. Shepherd, MB, BCh
Assistant Professor of Medicine
Mayo Clinic College of Medicine
Rochester, Minnesota
Lymphedema

Michael B. Silva, Jr., MD
Texas Tech University Health Sciences Center
Lubbock, Texas
Arterial Access; Guidewires, Catheters, and Sheaths; and Balloon Angioplasty Catheters

James C. Stanley, MD
Professor of Surgery
Section of Vascular Surgery
University of Michigan
Director of Vascular Surgery
Cardiovascular Center
University of Michigan Hospital
Ann Arbor, Michigan
Splanchnic and Renal Artery Aneurysms

Michael C. Stoner, MD
Brody School of Medicine at
East Carolina University
Division of Vascular Surgery
Greenville, North Carolina
Vascular Grafts: Characteristics and Rational Selection

D. Eugene Strandness, Jr., MD*
Formerly, Professor of Surgery
University of Washington School of Medicine
Seattle, Washington
Hemodynamics for the Vascular Surgeon

Carlos H. Timaran, MD
Assistant Professor of Surgery
University of Texas, Southwestern Medical Center
Dallas, Texas
Technique of Carotid Angioplasty and Stenting

Frank J. Veith, MD
Professor of Surgery
Albert Einstein College of Medicine of
Yeshiva University
William von Lebig Chair
Attending Physician
Vice Chairman, Department of Surgery
Montefiore Medical Center
Bronx, New York
Femoral, Popliteal, and Tibial Occlusive Disease

Alex Westerband, MD
Surgeon
St. Mary's Hospital
Tucson, Arizona
Noninfectious Complications in Vascular Surgery

Anthony D. Whittemore, MD
Professor of Surgery
Harvard Medical School
Chief of Vascular Surgery
Brigham and Women's Hospital
Boston, Massachusetts
Aortoiliac Occlusive Disease

Samuel E. Wilson, MD
Professor of Surgery
University of California, Irvine
Irvine, California
Attending Surgeon
University of California, Irvine, Medical Center
Orange, California
Hemodialysis and Vascular Access

Jay Yadav, MD
Director, Vascular Intervention
The Cleveland Clinic Foundation
Cleveland, Ohio
Technique of Carotid Angioplasty and Stenting

Gerald B. Zelenock, MD
Director, Surgical Services
William Beaumont Hospital
Royal Oak, Michigan
Splanchnic and Renal Artery Aneurysms

R. Eugene Zierler, MD
Professor of Surgery
University of Washington School of Medicine
Medical Director, Vascular Diagnostic Service
University of Washington Medical Center
Seattle, Washington
Hemodynamics for the Vascular Surgeon

*Deceased

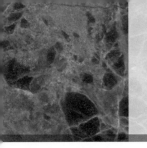

Preface to the Seventh Edition

The seventh edition has been completely revised, beginning with its title. In recognition of the increasing role of endovascular surgery in our specialty, the title has been revised to VASCULAR AND ENDOVASCULAR SURGERY: A COMPREHENSIVE REVIEW. The signature chapters remain, and the authors fully updated their material. The increasing use of drugs in the management of our patients is recognized by a chapter entitled "Pharmacology of Drugs Used in the Management of Vascular Disease." New material covering endovascular surgery includes a chapter on arterial access, guidewires, catheters, sheaths, angioplasty catheters, and stents. Specific anatomic regions with attention to the technical considerations and results of endovascular techniques are included in chapters addressing aortoiliac disease, mesenteric and renal disease, infrainguinal disease, and cerebrovascular disease. A new chapter on stent grafting

for aneurysms of the abdominal aorta brings us up to date on the various devices currently available as well as comparative techniques and results. We have added a new chapter that addresses the emerging field of laparoscopic aortic surgery. A new chapter has been included on wound care, with specific emphasis on limb salvage. Additionally, a new chapter has been included addressing the vascular surgeon's role in spine exposure. Finally, with this new edition comes a DVD-ROM containing video clips of key procedures, case studies and questions and answers (also found in the book) for review and assessment, and references linked to PubMed abstracts.

In summary, we now have a completely revised and up-to-date volume directed to the comprehensive management of patients with vascular disorders.

Wesley S. Moore, MD

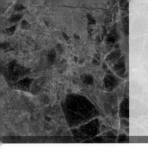

Preface to the First Edition

During the past 20 years of rapid growth and development in vascular surgery, many graduates of general surgery programs found that their training in vascular surgery represented a valuable new resource for their hospital and practice communities. That training in vascular surgery often provided an important edge in establishing a new practice and led to the widespread use of the term *general and vascular surgery* on the community announcements and business cards of new surgeons.

Yet in 1969, a survey conducted by a committee composed of James A. DeWeese, F. William Blaisdell, and John H. Foster discovered that among the 83 residents graduating from the 22 general surgery training programs surveyed, only 19 had performed more than 40 arterial reconstructive procedures during the course of their training, and more than half of the graduating residents had performed fewer than 20 arterial reconstructive procedures. The DeWeese committee, which had been established in 1969 to develop a document on optimal resources in vascular surgery, thus concluded that there was considerable suboptimal vascular surgery being performed in the United States, owing to a combination of both inadequate training and continued deficiencies in vascular surgery experience following training. A survey of the frequency of vascular operations in 1143 hospitals across the United States had revealed that in over 75% of these hospitals, fewer than 10 aneurysm resections and 10 femoropopliteal arterial reconstruction were conducted annually. This discovery led to the unfortunate conclusion that many surgeons were performing only occasional vascular operations, often leading to poor results.

The substance of the DeWeese report was reviewed by the two national vascular societies and their responsible leadership. This paved the way for, among other things, the definition of adequate training in vascular surgery and the recommendation that physicians who wish to practice vascular surgery spend an additional year of training to guarantee adequate experience in the speciality. To ensure prospective candidates that a given fellowship program in vascular surgery would provide a broad and responsible experience, the vascular societies established a committee for program evaluation and endorsements from which program directors could request review. Programs reviewed and found to meet the criteria of appropriate education as established by the committee would be announced annually.

Program evaluation by the joint council of the two national vascular societies was taken on as a temporary responsibility because the role would ultimately become the purview of the Residency Review Committee and the Liaison Committee for Graduate Medical Education. It was recognized that once adequate training programs were developed, the certification of candidates successfully completing training rested with the American Board of Surgery.

After approximately 10 years of experience, debate, and review, the American Board of Medical Specialties approved an application by the American Board of Surgery to grant "Certification of Special Competence in General Vascular Surgery." The first examination for certification was given to qualified members of the American Board of Surgery and Thoracic Surgery in June 1982. The second written examination was held in November 1983 in several centers across the United States.

The intent of this textbook is to provide a comprehensive review of vascular surgery, together with the related medical and basic science disciplines. This edition of the text has been developed to accompany a postgraduate course designed to help candidates prepare for the examination leading to certification in general vascular surgery. Accordingly, a list of questions designed to aid the reader in self-examination completes each chapter. All question sets simply represent the authors' opinion, a fair and adequate survey of the material covered, as none of the chapter authors is a member of the American Board of Surgery (this would be a conflict of interest).

Although chapter outlines were suggested by an editorial committee, the final chapter test represents, in the opinion of its authors, core material in each subject. Particular effort to identify and separate generally accepted concepts from new or controversial material was made. Although this book was designed as a comprehensive review to prepare for an examination, it is also in view of its organization and content, a comprehensive text of vascular surgery.

Wesley S. Moore, MD

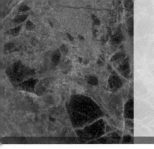

Contents

*Deceased

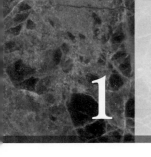

1

Wiley F. Barker

A History of Vascular Surgery

History is not a precise record, for it is only that which has been remembered or written down. Inevitably, there is much personal interpretation of that original material. In addition, interpreting events from the past is often difficult, and "history" sometimes changes as new information becomes available. It is often hard for an observer to see recent events in proper perspective, especially when the observer is close to or even involved with those events.

In the last few years, there have been immense developments in molecular biology and in the techniques of minimally invasive surgery and interventional endovascular procedures. The value of these developments remains difficult to assess, despite their incalculable promise for the future. As Mao Zedong reportedly replied when asked about the effect of the French Revolution on the revolution in China, "It is much too soon to tell."

This chapter is presented in sections that may be thought of as a series of scenes and acts. As with many modern stage plays, different actors appear in different scenes in different roles, and many scenes take place concurrently and must be observed from different points of view, depending on the subject at hand. Ultimately, the whole fits together.

Prologue

Although some might argue that Guy de Chauliac or Ambroise Paré should properly be called the sire of surgery, to me, John Hunter above all others is the prototype of the modern vascular surgeon. He was an unbelievably productive and tireless worker, cut from the same Scottish mold as his brother William, who was 10 years older. John was largely unlettered, whereas William had become sophisticated through his education at Glasgow, yet they shared a frenetic capacity for work and an incurable curiosity.

To place the Hunters in a clear perspective with regard to nonmedical history, one should note that they were contemporaries of George Washington and Benjamin Franklin. William Hunter was born in Scotland in 1718, his brother John 10 years later; William died in 1783, John in 1793.[1,2] John was even made a member of the American Philosophical Society, although he never attended a meeting.

William Hunter preceded John to London, where he soon established a busy medical practice and interested himself in many subjects, including aneurysms. In fact, William proposed the concept that a lancet used carelessly during bloodletting might enter both artery and vein, and after healing, the two channels might be connected. He thus imagined an arteriovenous fistula. He soon found just such a patient and described the clinical manifestations with great accuracy.[3] William's primary activity, however, was focused on obstetrics and on the teaching of anatomy. In this latter project John became his assistant.

John Hunter is remembered for many things, but especially for his studies of the dynamics and efficiency of collateral arterial circulation. This he described in the vessels feeding the antlers of a stag after he had interrupted the major arteries in its neck. More renown came from his ligation of the femoral artery in its subsartorial course at a distance above a popliteal aneurysm—in Hunter's canal.[1,2]

To be sure, others had preceded him in performing proximal ligation of arteries to treat aneurysms. In the third century, a Roman surgeon, Antyllus, had described proximal and distal ligation of the artery, followed by incision of the aneurysm and removal of its contents—a formidable operation without either anesthesia or asepsis.[4] In 1680, Purmann, faced with a large aneurysm in the antecubital space, carried out ligation of the vessels and excision of the aneurysmal mass.[5] In 1714, Anel described an operation in which he placed one ligature on the artery at the proximal extent of the aneurysm. Hunter, however, had found that the ligature would sometimes cut through the artery when it was placed too close to the popliteal aneurysm, so he chose a site that was more remote, but one that was easily reached by the surgeon and would preserve collaterals. Most of Anel's patients suffered from false aneurysms caused by bloodletting in otherwise healthy arteries. The femoropopliteal aneurysms treated by Hunter were due to degenerative processes, probably a mixture of syphilis and trauma.[1,6]

Many other surgeons were ligating aneurysms in various anatomic sites at this time. Cooper, one of John Hunter's students, was soon established as one of the early vascular surgeons when he ligated the carotid artery for an aneurysm in 1805,[7] as well as the aorta for an iliac artery aneurysm.[8] Only these few important events occurred before the latter part of the 19th century.

At the time, ligation was virtually the only procedure available to surgeons for the management of arterial problems, and those problems were limited to the control of hemorrhage and the treatment of aneurysms. Hallowell in Newcastle-on-Tyne carried out one arterial repair of an artery torn during bloodletting. The laceration was a short one, and at the suggestion of Lambert, he placed a short (1/4-inch) steel pin through the edges of the wound and looped a ligature around it in a figure-of-eight pattern, approximating the edges of the wound with apparent success. Hallowell wrote to William Hunter concerning this operation in 1761, foreseeing that if this were a successful technique, "we might be able to cure wounds of some arteries that would otherwise require amputation, or be altogether incurable."[9] That Hallowell wrote to William instead of John is probably due to William's published work on arteriovenous fistulas secondary to inept bloodletting. Twelve years later (1773), Asman reviewed the Newcastle repair, attempted some experiments of his own that were disastrous, and concluded that such a procedure could not work and that Lambert and Hallowell's efforts had probably failed as well.[10] After Asman's criticism, the matter of arterial repair rested quietly for nearly another hundred years.

John Hunter's less widely known contributions are scattered throughout the immense museum he left to the Royal College of Surgeons of England, and they hint at an understanding of arterial pathology that would not be general knowledge for half a century. They include dissections of several atherosclerotic aortic bifurcations (specimens P.1177 and P.1178), showing the atheromatous lesion at the aortic bifurcation that Leriche would describe 150 years later; a carotid bifurcation with an ulcerated atheroma from a patient who died of a ruptured syphilitic thoracic aneurysm (specimen P.1171); and an extracranial internal carotid aneurysm (specimen P.282) in a patient whose neatly described symptoms are almost typical of what today are recognized as classic transient ischemic episodes.[11] Regrettably, most of Hunter's notes did not survive to give us more than this fragmentary view of his understanding of vascular disease. To cap it all, in a postmortem specimen, Hunter had dissected the atheromatous layers (although the term *atheroma* had not yet come into use) from the remaining intact wall of an atherosclerotic terminal aorta (specimen P.1176), foreshadowing dos Santos by a century and a half.

Both Hunter and Cooper seemed to hold with the teleologic belief of the times that when senile or spontaneous gangrene occurred in older persons, thrombosis of the major vessels supervened so that the patient would not bleed to death when the gangrenous part separated.[12] It was Cruveilhier who first clearly stated that the phrase "gangrene due to obstruction of the arteries" by thickening and by thrombosis should replace the terms *spontaneous* and *senile* gangrene,[13] but he attributed the concept to Dupuytren.

The recognition that arterial obstruction causes functional disability that limits the use of the affected part may have arisen in the veterinary world. Bouley described the clinical picture in a horse in 1831.[14]

Four years later (1835), a nearly anonymous physician on the ward of a Professor Louis provided the first clear description of human claudication. Barth's patient was a 51-year-old woman who died of heart failure due to mitral valvular disease. His report described her incidental history of claudication in terms that we would recognize today.[15] In the postmortem report he noted thrombosis of the terminal aorta and included a sketch that suggests that the lesion was a thrombosed hypoplastic terminal aorta, a contracted atherosclerotic lesion, or a combination of both. Barth also repeated Hunter's observation that the obstructing material could easily be separated from the residual intact arterial wall. Barth was never identified further, not even by an initial.

Charcot is often erroneously given credit for recognizing the syndrome of intermittent claudication due to arterial insufficiency in humans.[16] Charcot described, just as Bouley had done, the vanishing pulses, the cold extremity, and what we now recognize as the loss of sympathetic tone in a horse in the throes of a spasm of severe claudication; he reported a human case as well. Homans liked to joke that Charcot observed the former because he spent so much time at the horse races.

As a neurologist, Charcot was familiar with intermittent claudication in humans caused by various neurologic processes. The patient Charcot described, however, suffered claudication in one leg secondary to an old gunshot wound that resulted in occlusion of the iliac artery as well as an aneurysm proximal to the occlusion. The aneurysm, which was adherent to and in communication with the jejunum, gave rise to a series of small gastrointestinal hemorrhages before the final fatal episode. Charcot thus deserves credit for identifying the herald hemorrhages that often presage major bleeding from an aortoenteric fistula. (Charcot credited both Bouley and Barth with their prior observations regarding claudication.)

Successful Arterial Suture

Such information was of little utility to surgeons, however, until arterial repair became a reality. Consistent with the observations of Asman, several German masters had ex cathedra deemed arterial repair (as opposed to ligation) to be impossible. Langenbeck stated in 1825 that because the primary requirement for healing is perfect rest, as long as the pulsatile movements of the arterial wall continued, an arterial incision could never heal.[17] Heinecke was certain that the patient would bleed to death through the suture holes and the apposed edges of the arterial wall.[18]

Repair of small injuries to veins, however, was becoming an established procedure. The lateral ligature, in which a clamp is placed on the defect in the venous wall and a ligature is tied around the puckered wall, had been performed in 1816 (Travers, cited by Jassinowsky).[19] The first lateral suture of a venous defect (an erosion of the common jugular vein from an infected neck wound) was undertaken by Czerny in 1881, but the patient died of sepsis and hemorrhage.[20] Jassinowsky[19] credits Schede[21] with the first *successful* repair of a large venous injury (to the common femoral vein) by lateral sutures.

Going beyond the stage of venous repair, Eck reported the experimental creation of a portocaval fistula in dogs.[22] The original description hints that he had little to confirm his success. Among a series of eight dogs, one died within 24 hours, six lived 2 to 6 days, and the one survivor "tired of life in the laboratory and ran away after two months." The doctoral dissertation of Jassinowsky, written in 1889 and based purely on library research, reviewed the published information on arterial suture and concluded that it could not be successful at that time, but there might be hope in the future.[19]

Only 2 years later, however, Jassinowsky himself succeeded. In 1891, he reported his successful animal experiments involving arterial suture.[23] The suture he described was passed carefully *only two thirds* of the way through the media; he tried to avoid penetrating the intima, except in very thin-walled vessels. This effort should be recognized for its intrinsic difficulty using even the finest milliner's needles, for without sutures swaged onto needles, two pieces of suture have to be dragged through the arterial wall. Dörfler modified Jassinowsky's method and passed the suture through all thicknesses of the arterial wall.[24] He also recognized that the arterial suture exposed in the lumen of the vessel did no harm if uninfected. He observed that it soon became covered with a glistening membrane. Shortly thereafter, in 1896, Jaboulay and Briau described successful end-to-end carotid arterial anastomoses in animals using an everting U-shaped suture.[25]

Jaboulay was one of the surgeons at Lyon under whom Carrel studied. When Sadi Carnot, the president of the Republic of France, was wounded by an assassin and died because no one dared to try to repair his portal vein, Carrel was highly critical, for he believed that blood vessels could be sutured as well as any other tissue.[26] He soon undertook experimental arterial anastomoses. Some of the earliest of these were arteriovenous communications in which the high-flow system ensured patency. Carrel's contributions to technical arterial surgery included methods that vascular surgeons routinely use today.[27,28] He devised the triangulation suture to facilitate end-to-end anastomosis, described the patch technique to anastomose a small vessel to the side of a larger one (as in replantation of an inferior mesenteric artery), and pioneered the use of vessel grafts and organ transplantation. His work, however, was not fully accepted in the United States for many years. In part, this stemmed from disputes that arose between him and Guthrie, who was his coworker for a year.[29]

In contrast, European surgeons not only accepted Carrel's work but also began to follow his lead. In 1906, Goyanes of Madrid resected a popliteal aneurysm, then restored arterial continuity with an in situ venous graft using the popliteal vein, probably the first successful clinical vascular replacement.[30]

Surgeons in America were beginning to perform vascular surgery in their own way. In New Orleans in 1888, Matas described a landmark operation.[31] He stumbled onto the surgical procedure for which he is commonly remembered, endo-aneurysmorrhaphy, when an aneurysm for which he had ligated only the proximal brachial artery, with apparent initial success, began to pulsate again 10 days later. Reportedly, it was a medical student who called this to the professor's attention. He chose to reoperate and to ligate the brachial artery distally. Even after this distal ligation, the aneurysm continued to pulsate, and he was forced to open the aneurysm, clean out the sac (the operation performed by Antyllus), and oversew the other arteries feeding the aneurysm from inside the sac. This foreshadowed the problems with endoleaks that harass vascular surgeons who place endovascular aortic prostheses today.

Matas's operation differed from that of Antyllus, in that he used a suture within the aneurysmal sac to obliterate the feeding vessels instead of ligating them outside the sac. The extensive dissection that would have been required outside might have damaged the collateral circulation and other adherent anatomic structures. It was many years before Matas performed another endoaneurysmorrhaphy, for most patients were treated successfully by simple proximal ligation.[32] Matas ultimately expanded the descriptions of his technique to include "restorative" and "reconstructive" modifications, and he reported an approach to the arteriovenous fistula through the venous component,[33] as had been proposed by Bickham.[34]

Murphy, of Chicago, performed a series of experiments on animals in which he successfully restored continuity by invagination of the proximal into the distal vessel. In 1897, he presented a successful human case.[35] Edwards briefly revived this anastomotic technique of invagination when he recommended the use of the first braided nylon grafts.[36]

Murphy's invagination techniques were reflected in other nonsuture methods of anastomosis: Nitze[37] and Payr[38] used small metal or ivory rings through which the vessel was drawn, everted, and tied in place; this unit was then inserted into the mouth of the distal vessel, and another ligature secured it there. This is substantially the Blakemore tube,[39] used, albeit without signal success, in World War II.[40]

During his tenure at Johns Hopkins Hospital, W. S. Halsted had an abundance of traumatic and syphilitic aneurysms commanding his attention. In the early 1900s, Carrel visited Halsted and described his own technical experiments, including his early arteriovenous anastomoses. As a result, Halsted *almost* made history in 1907 when he faced the dilemma of a patient whose popliteal artery and vein had been sacrificed during an en bloc dissection of a sarcoma of the popliteal space.[41] Halsted went to the other leg, took the saphenous vein, reversed it, and anastomosed the distal saphenous vein to the proximal femoral artery. For his distal anastomosis, however, he chose the popliteal *vein*. Although the graft pulsated for 40 minutes, it soon thrombosed. It is possible that Halsted was pursuing the chimera of reversal of arterial flow through the venous bed. One can only imagine what a dramatic leap forward vascular surgery would have made if Halsted, with his superb supporting cast of talented surgeons, had chosen the popliteal artery for the distal anastomosis and had achieved a truly successful arterial reconstruction in the pattern of the modern vascular surgeon.

There is a considerable literature on attempts to revascularize ischemic extremities via arteriovenous anastomoses. San Martín[42] and A. E. Halsted[43] attempted to improve the distal circulation using arteriovenous anastomoses.

Meanwhile, German surgeons such as Höpfner,[44] Lexer,[45,46] and Jeger[47] had become familiar with the use of short (<10 cm) vein grafts. Höpfner described the bypass procedure, which was illustrated in an encyclopedic book by Jeger. Jeger's book, republished posthumously in 1937, included a foreword that described Jeger's replantation of the completely severed arm of a German soldier, which he had performed in 1914. A year later, Jeger came to an untimely death from typhus while on the Russian front.

Lexer collected and reported on 65 vein transplants, 13 of which were his personal cases.[45] In 8 of these 13 cases, Lexer had obtained a distal pulse. This report prompted a Polish surgeon, Weglowski, to present his own personal series of 51 vein grafts, mostly for trauma, operated on between 1914 and 1921; in 40 patients he could document good distal pulses and normal arterial tracings.[48] Yet all this seemed to be forgotten for the next 25 years as Germany suffered the agonies of the interbellum years, and as the forceful and charismatic personality of Leriche appeared on the scene (Leriche's role is described in a later section).

Abdominal Aortic Aneurysms

Beyond the management of trauma to the arteries, the aneurysm is clearly one of the great surgical challenges. The previous section detailed early attempts to treat peripheral aneurysms, but these were sporadic and lacked a continuing series.

Vesalius is said to have been the first to describe an abdominal aneurysm.[49] The successful management of the abdominal aneurysm is certainly one of vascular surgery's major accomplishments. The technical maneuvers described previously concerning the ligation of aneurysms in various anatomic sites usually involved aneurysms of the peripheral vessels; aneurysms of the trunk were sacrosanct, for proximal control was not feasible. Cooper had continued many of Hunter's studies, including evaluation of collateral arterial supplies. In 1805, he had ligated the common carotid artery for an aneurysm,[7] but he opened the door for even wider surgical applications when, in 1818, he ligated the abdominal aorta to control external hemorrhage from an aneurysm of the external iliac artery that had eroded to the surface of the skin of the flank, bleeding openly at that site.[9]

Interest in the treatment of major vessel aneurysms lagged for almost a century. Eventually Colt, at the end of the 19th century, used wire to pack an aneurysm and then heated the wire.[50] Blakemore and King revived interest in this technique in 1938,[51] and many surgeons undertook modifications of the wiring technique, largely without success. Meanwhile, more direct attempts were being made by the major actors in the next scene: Matas of New Orleans and Halsted of Baltimore. Their interest in the management of vessel trauma, and in the management of late sequelae of such trauma, provided material for the fertile imaginations of the many surgeons who were emboldened to follow in their footsteps. Reid reported the experience of the Johns Hopkins Hospital (headed by Halsted) with aneurysms in 1926.[52] The aneurysms treated included many varieties, both anatomic and etiologic, but treatment of abdominal aneurysms was substantially a failure. These operations were only preparation for the end of ligation as a treatment for aneurysms of the abdominal aorta.

Matas finally accomplished a successful aortic ligation (just below the renal arteries) for an aneurysm at the bifurcation of the aorta. He reported it first in 1925 and then again in 1940.[53,54] In the issue of *Annals of Surgery* that contained Matas's second report was a similar paper by Elkin,[55] as well as a hint of the coming era of vascular reconstruction in a report by Bigger of Virginia.[56] Bigger had ligated the neck of an abdominal aneurysm using fascia that he expected to loosen gradually and allow restoration of flow. With the protection of this temporary control, he performed a plication of the aneurysm, restoring the aorta to its proper caliber. The patient had a protracted survival without recurrence of the aneurysm and also with restoration of femoral pulses.

About this time, however, cardiac surgery began to emerge. The narrative has to step back in time here. During the first decade of the 20th century, Jeger had proposed valved venous grafts between the left pulmonary veins and the left ventricle to bypass mitral stenosis, and a valved venous graft from the left ventricle to the innominate artery to bypass aortic stenosis.[47] In the mid-1920s, Cutler and associates had attempted to treat mitral stenosis surgically, but with minimal success.[57] A valvulotome was used through a ventricular approach.

Nonetheless, the influence of these attempts led Gross to the successful ligation and, 5 years later, division of the patent ductus arteriosus.[58,59] In Baltimore, Blalock and Taussig began their series of pioneering surgical procedures for various cardiac anomalies, the first and most dramatic of which was the

"blue baby" operation—the creation of a systemic shunt from the subclavian artery to the pulmonary artery in patients with congenital pulmonic stenosis.[60]

Crafoord and Nylin[61] reported the successful end-to-end anastomosis of the aorta after resection of an aortic coarctation at the same time that Gross and Hufnagel[62] carried out their first case. This last operation demonstrated that lesions of the thoracic and abdominal segments of the aorta were amenable to a surgical approach.

DEVELOPMENT OF VASCULAR PROSTHESES

Although arterial homografts functioned fairly well in the aorta (discussed later), they were difficult to obtain, harvest, sterilize, and store. Grafts other than those of the aorta fared poorly. Homografts of smaller vessels containing a higher proportion of smooth muscle were even less satisfactory. The development of an artificial arterial substitute would allow the expansion of arterial reconstruction.

Following the experience in the laboratory reported by Abbe,[63] Tuffier had used rigid tubes of metal and of paraffined glass to try to replace small to medium-size arteries during World War I, without success.[64] Similar tubes were used in World War II, but the results were no better than those obtained by immediate ligation of the artery.[40] Hufnagel chose a more inert surface, methylmethacrylate, as well as a tube with a better hemodynamic design.[65] Hufnagel's tubes functioned remarkably well in animal experiments, except for the difficulty in securing them within a major artery such as the aorta without the risk of ultimate erosion. Eventually the use of pliable plastic fabrics virtually eliminated the rigid tube.

In 1947, Hufnagel reported on the use of rapid freezing for the preservation of arterial homografts and suggested their utility in the repair of long aortic coarctations.[66] Gross, who at first feared that frozen vessels could not survive, published a laboratory and clinical report on his experiences with homografts preserved in electrolyte solutions for use in various cardiac operations, but particularly for the management of coarctation of the aorta.[67] Swan soon used a homograft for a thoracic aneurysm associated with a coarctation.[68]

The arterial homograft initially seemed to be a good substitute for the thoracic or abdominal aorta. At first, fresh grafts were used; then they were preserved in Tyrode's solution. Improvements in the preservation of grafts by freezing[69] and then lyophilization[70] facilitated the development of arterial graft banks. Early successes were soon erased by late failures of the homografts, however, and a truly satisfactory aortic substitute was sorely needed.

In 1952, Voorhees and colleagues observed that fabric threads in a chamber of the heart soon became covered with endothelium.[71] Dörfler had made a similar gross observation 60 years earlier but had not carried the observation to its conclusion.[64] Voorhees and his associates at Columbia pursued experiments not only with Vinyon-N but also with parachute silk and other materials. Many fabrics were tried, and most were quickly discarded. Braided and crimped nylon tubes were introduced by Edwards and Tapp,[36] but it was soon discovered that nylon rapidly lost strength and was unsatisfactory.[72] Both Orlon[73] and Teflon[74] were used. Szilagyi and colleagues[75] and Julian and associates[76] introduced various fabrications of Dacron. The transcripts of the vascular surgery meetings of the late 1950s might be mistaken for a textile journal, as various weaves, deniers, calenderizing, and the advantages of braid versus knit versus taffeta weaves were discussed. The summation of the principles of vascular grafting by Wesolowski and coworkers had enunciated the importance of porosity,[77,78] but the substantially nonporous Teflon undercut that thesis.

The knitted Dacron introduced by DeBakey placed a generally successful graft in the hands of every surgeon.[79] Subsequent modifications by the addition of velour to the surface by Sauvage[80] and also by Cooley[81] refined this outstanding contribution. Wesolowski's concept[78] that the fabric tube would become "encapsulated" and might develop a firm new endothelial surface has been pursued as a goal but has not been achieved in humans.

The immediate porosity of the grafts has been troublesome on occasion, especially in patients who require heparinization or in whom even minor blood loss from a weeping graft is intolerable. Impregnation with either collagen[82] or albumin[83] was a useful advance. Teflon in the form of an extruded tube (Gore-Tex) rather than as a woven or knitted fabric was introduced clinically by Soyer,[84] and it has achieved great popularity. Introduced first for use as a venous substitute, it came to be used extensively in arterial reconstructions as a second choice after autologous vein,[85] although Quiñones-Baldrich expressed a preference for Gore-Tex in femoral anastomoses above the knee, preserving the vein for more distal reconstructions if such become necessary.[86]

Biologic substitutes other than the arterial homograft have also been suggested. Rosenberg and associates used bovine carotid arteries that had been subjected to enzymatic treatment to remove all the tissue-specific protein except the basic structural collagen of the bovine artery.[87] Sawyer and colleagues attempted to modify the bovine heterograft by inducing a negatively charged lining in an effort to inhibit thrombosis.[88] Dardik and coworkers used treated umbilical vein grafts supported with a mesh of Dacron as a peripheral arterial substitute.[89]

The world turns, however, and there is currently renewed interest in the use of cryopreserved (frozen but not lyophilized) arterial homografts, especially in infected aortic sites. Experience is limited, and this topic deserves to be in a clinical area rather than a historic one.

MODERN MANAGEMENT OF AORTIC ANEURYSMS

The grave risk posed by abdominal aneurysms was exposed in a timely paper by Estes in 1951.[90] Other experiences with the aorta were preparing the way for present-day management of abdominal aneurysms. Alexander and Byron had resected a thoracic aneurysm associated with coarctation of the aorta and successfully oversewn the ends of the vessel, although the patient ultimately died of renovascular hypertension.[91,92] Swan had used a homograft to replace a thoracic aneurysm.[68]

Various attempts were made to use either reactive cellophane[93] or the tissue-irritating plasticizer dicetyl phosphate[94] as a means of inducing sclerosis that might restrain the dilatation of the aneurysm. These attempts to control the growth of the aneurysm were not rewarding.

Oudot set the stage for other forms of aortic replacement when he used a homograft to restore circulation in a patient with Leriche syndrome.[95] Dubost is recognized as the pioneer who first successfully replaced an abdominal aneurysm with a homograft on March 19, 1951.[96] Schaffer and Hardin actually preceded Dubost by 4 weeks, but their publication appeared considerably later and focused on the use of a polythene shunt to maintain distal circulation during the operation rather than on the priority of resecting the aneurysm itself.[97] It appears that Wylie actually accomplished a successful endarterectomy of an abdominal aneurysm on January 13, 1951. Similarly, Freeman and Leeds treated three patients, two successfully, with inlay grafts of the patient's own iliac veins beginning on February 12, 1951. Wylie's and Freeman's operations were not graft replacements, however, but rather modifications of Bigger's procedure.[56]

Dubost's operation was soon followed by those of Julian,[98] Brock,[99] DeBakey,[100] and Bahnson.[101] It is a curious twist of fate to find that Dubost had left the practice of colorectal surgery to become a cardiac surgeon after he saw Blalock and Bahnson perform dramatic cardiac operations while they were visiting France in the late 1940s. Szilagyi's[102] classic study of the benefits of the operation in 1966 provided confirmation and justification of the thesis Estes had presented in 1950.

The complicated abdominal aneurysm still posed a major problem. Ellis was one of the first to implant the renal arteries into the graft when the aneurysm was found to include their orifices.[103] Etheredge extended this operation to resect a major thoracoabdominal aortic aneurysm.[104] He used a heparinized plastic shunt of the type described in Schaffer's resection and replacement of an abdominal aneurysm with a homograft in March 1951. Etheredge established the shunt, divided the aorta, and performed the proximal anastomosis; he then moved the clamp down the graft after each successive visceral anastomosis was completed and finished with the lower aortic anastomosis to the graft.

DeBakey[105] reported in 1956 a series of complicated abdominal and thoracoabdominal aneurysms that were resected by a technique similar to that later used by Shumacker.[106] In 1973, Stoney and Wylie popularized the long thoracoabdominal incision for the approach to this lesion.[107] The great advance in the management of these complicated lesions was made by Crawford,[108] who introduced a direct approach to the aneurysm in which the aorta is clamped above and below and then opened throughout the length of the aneurysm. A fabric graft is sewn into the proximal aorta; the major groups of arteries, including the lower intercostals when possible, are sewn into the wall of the fabric tube using the expeditious Carrel patch method of anastomosis; then the distal anastomosis is completed. This direct method has greatly simplified the approach to these challenging lesions.

The placement of a graft within the lumen of an aneurysm, whether abdominal, thoracic, or peripheral, was logically extended by a technique that allows one to place the graft within the aneurysm from a distance through a short arteriotomy in either the femoral or the external iliac artery. The evolution of this method stems circuitously from Dotter and coworkers. In 1983, they attempted to improve the results of simple arterial dilatation or to maintain the patency of a graft with small endarterial spiral coils.[109] After several generations of devices that did not gain wide acceptance, Palmaz and associates introduced a metal mesh stent that can be expanded by balloon dilatation, which secures the stent in place.[110] Introduced originally to maintain the patency of a segment of artery that had undergone percutaneous dilatation, this method was at first used in occlusive disease, but Parodi modified the technique to secure a fabric graft that had been placed within an aneurysm.[111] Although initially used as a tube graft, modifications soon allowed the placement of bifurcation grafts.[112,113] The anticipated decrease in morbidity and mortality accompanying this method led to its widespread use, although not all aneurysms are amenable. The need for prolonged follow-up versus the security of a one-time operation has brought up the clinical question of the ultimate role of the endovascular repair of aneurysms. Here the narrative becomes so contemporaneous as to require clinical rather than historical description.

Peripheral Arterial Aneurysms

The peripheral arterial aneurysm was one of the first arterial lesions treated by surgeons, but its importance paled beside the advances made in the management of the aortic neurysm. The early history of treatment by ligation was described earlier.

In 1949, Linton used Leriche's concept of arteriectomy and sympathectomy for the management of 14 patients who had popliteal aneurysms—an ingenious approach that resulted in no amputations in his series.[114] The patients received a preliminary sympathectomy; then shortly afterward, or sometimes at the same operation, the aneurysm was resected, with ligation of the artery above and below it.

The ability to replace vessels of the size of the popliteal artery brought to the fore the concept that the popliteal aneurysm had a risk-benefit pattern similar to that of the abdominal aneurysm; if operations were done electively, the results were excellent, but once thrombosis occurred, the risk to the limb was grave, as Wychulis and associates demonstrated.[115] Wylie (in the discussion of Wychulis[115]) and Edwards[116] introduced the procedure of excluding the aneurysm and restoring flow through a bypass technique.

Occlusive Arterial Disease

As mentioned earlier in this chapter, it was not until the middle of the 19th century that the relationship between arterial occlusion and gangrene was clearly established. Repair of acute injuries had been accomplished, but management of more chronic arterial obstructions had hardly been considered a surgical problem. Recognition of the clinical symptoms of less severe ischemia came to surgery by way of veterinary medicine.[14] The association between the sympathetic nervous system and the arteries was recognized in the early 20th century, especially during World War I.

Leriche, born in 1879, had been educated and trained at Lyon, where he had known Jaboulay and Carrel. Shortly after Leriche completed his training, World War I broke out, and Leriche acquired considerable experience with wounds of the extremities. After he was demobilized, Leriche continued to work in a trauma hospital in Lyon for several years. There he saw many patients with post-traumatic neuralgias, and he developed his concepts of the role of the sympathetic nervous system and the possible treatment by periarterial sympathectomy, about which he had first written in 1917.[117] Then, seeing patients with arterial thrombosis due to *artérite* (a nonspecific term used by French surgeons to describe arterial disease and occlusion in general), Leriche concluded that if the patient was seen before the occluding thrombosis was too

widespread, local resection of the thrombosed artery provided relief. Because many patients did well after this simple procedure and soon developed relatively warm feet, he concluded that the collateral circulation in these patients must have been satisfactory and that the coldness of the extremity was due to vasospasm rather than insufficient arterial flow. He therefore applied the principle of sympathectomy, first as a periarterial operation, then as an arteriectomy (excising the obstructed segment), and then as a division of the sympathetic rami.[118]

Diez, dissatisfied with the results of periarterial sympathectomy, modified that operation into the lumbar ganglionectomy.[119] At nearly the same time, Royle[120] and Hunter[121] introduced the same fruitless operation for the management of spasm in striated muscle. Use of this operation for the management of pain syndromes and ischemic extremities remains controversial.

It seems likely that the forcefulness of Leriche's personality led European surgical thought to diverge from the known techniques of vascular grafting. This is not to say that Leriche actively spoke against the use of grafts; in fact, it was noted by some of his former trainees that he often said that it would be ideal to connect the two ends of a severed artery by a graft, but the risk of infection and the distance to be bridged always seemed too great. Instead, he offered arterial excision and sympathectomy, an approach that seemed to be beneficial and posed less risk.

One of Leriche's most important early observations was the definition of the syndrome that now bears his name, the atherosclerotic obliteration of the terminal aorta and the iliac arteries. He described this in 1923, during the period when he was beginning to evaluate arteriectomy.[122] It would be 17 years, however, before he found a suitable case in which he could perform resection of the aortic bifurcation and lumbar sympathectomy.[123]

Leriche's surgical clinic became famous, and he attracted a long line of surgeons who came to learn: DeBakey, Learmonth, dos Santos, and Kunlin, to name only a few.

The possibility of effective arterial suture anastomosis had been developed through the ideas of Jaboulay[25] and Carrel[27] at Lyon. After World War I, another surgeon from Lyon assumed a major role in vascular surgery.

Here it is necessary to flash back briefly to 1909, for in that year, Murphy removed an embolus from the common iliac artery and restored flow into the femoral system. Although locally successful, distal thrombosis required a distal amputation.[124] Two years later, Labey (as cited by Mosney and Dumont[125]) removed an embolus from the artery of a patient, with complete success. Embolectomy was thereafter performed with occasional success worldwide, but it did not become a fully satisfactory procedure because of the need to operate hastily, before extensive distal thrombosis supervened. After the clinical introduction of heparin by Murray,[126] it became possible to extend the indications for embolectomy and to extend the time limit for undertaking the procedure and thus improve the results.

Surgeons such as João Cid dos Santos and his father, Reynaldo, used heparin to prevent thrombosis after performing the nearly forgotten Matas endoaneurysmorrhaphy.[127] The younger dos Santos believed that with the protection of heparin, he might be able to remove chronically adherent arterial emboli and their associated thrombus and achieve healing without rethrombosis. After finding such a patient with advanced renal disease and a seriously ischemic extremity, dos Santos removed the clot and reestablished flow. He was chided by the pathologist for having removed the intima as well. After another successful case, in which he removed a chronic thrombosis of the subclavian, axillary, and brachial arteries secondary to scalenus anticus syndrome, he sent his report to Leriche. Leriche presented the work in the name of dos Santos to the French Academy of Surgery[128] and introduced endarterectomy to the surgical world. It is interesting to note that neither of these patients suffered primarily from the usual forms of atherosclerotic thrombosis.

Subsequently, Freeman and colleagues,[129,130] Wylie and associates,[131] and others adopted the operation, using the open technique that was championed primarily by Bazy and coworkers.[132] In September 1951, Wylie described endoaneurysmectomy and endarterectomy of the aorta. At the time, my colleagues and I had undertaken six procedures without success, but in the summer of 1951 Wylie had visited us, and in October 1951 we performed the first successful endarterectomy in our series.[133] The operation consisted of a combination of the Matas endoaneurysmorrhaphy and the dos Santos endarterectomy (or, rather, the technique as revised by Reboul): an abdominal aneurysm was endarterectomized, tailored to a proper size, and wrapped with fascia lata, and an endarterectomy in continuity was performed throughout the length of the left iliofemoropopliteal system. In fact, these operations were only extensions of the aneurysm repair performed by Bigger in 1940.[56]

Cannon and Barker later introduced the long, closed endarterectomy using intraluminal strippers,[134] which was a modification of the original method of dos Santos. Several very similar varieties of endarterectomy loops were devised by Butcher[135] and by Vollmar and Laubaeh,[136] among others. A period of early success was followed by disenchantment owing to the difficulty of the operation in comparison with the increasingly popular grafting procedures.

Leriche and his close associate Kunlin had not had great technical success with endarterectomy, especially in the femoral artery system. Kunlin revived the use of the vein graft in the form of a long venous bypass.[137] His first patient had already undergone arteriectomy and sympathectomy, thus justifying the then-unorthodox procedure.

Veins had been used for very short (4 to 8 cm) replacements on rare occasions during the prior 40 years. This technique has persisted as the basic method of arterial reconstruction ever since.

Saphenous vein grafting was useful only in the femoral and iliofemoral systems, however, and it remained for Oudot to perform a comparable reconstructive operation on the aorta using an aortic homograft,[95] which thoracic and cardiac surgeons were already using to replace segments of the thoracic aorta. Oudot was presented with a 51-year-old patient with claudication as a result of proximal iliac and distal aortic occlusion. Oudot's operation is commonly described as a simple bifurcation graft, common iliac to common iliac, but it was actually a much more complicated procedure. He approached the bifurcation extraperitoneally through a left flank incision and resected the bifurcation. The patient's internal iliacs were found to be thrombosed and were ligated. The external iliac arteries of the graft were very small, but the graft's internal iliacs were large; Oudot therefore anastomosed

the graft's internal iliacs to the patient's external iliacs. However, he did the left-sided anastomosis first and then found that the repaired vessel obstructed his view and hindered manipulations of the right-sided anastomosis. This difficult anastomosis thrombosed promptly. Oudot made the best of a bad situation and pointed out that he had done a perfect experiment, as there was still some discussion from Leriche's camp about whether grafting at this level would be worthwhile. On the right side, Oudot had performed substantially nothing more than an arteriectomy; on the left, he had reconstituted the lumen. The right side was warm but pulseless and still fatigued easily, whereas the left side had a pulse and did not tire. Six months later, Oudot reoperated on the patient, who was still complaining of right-sided claudication; he performed an iliac-to-iliac "extra-anatomic" bypass, as had been suggested by Kunlin in 1951.

A few months later, Oudot climbed Annapurna with the French team. Shortly after his return to France he was killed in an automobile accident at the age of 40.

The saga of the treatment of arterial disease continues with the development and then the failure of artery banks and the introduction of the plastic prosthesis, but by 1952 the stage was set for nearly everything that is done today. Linton's espousal of the reversed saphenous vein in 1952 confirmed the approach of Kunlin and established the procedure of choice for peripheral reconstruction for many years.[138]

Endarterectomy did not die out completely; it persists in carotid operations, but only occasionally is it used in the aorta and as part of local tailoring procedures elsewhere. Edwards made one important attempt to use it in the femoral artery by means of a long patch; the procedure worked well unless the patch was so wide it created a stagnant column of blood in the femoral artery.[139] Femoropopliteal endarterectomy fell from favor because of its limited applicability to reconstructions that ended proximal to the distal portion of the popliteal artery. The full open repair was tedious, and most surgeons had limited success in restoring flow.

In recent years, however, closed endarterial procedures have become commonplace. Dotter and Judkins began in 1956 by using a stiff dilator,[140] a procedure that was not widely accepted. Gruntzig and Hopff modified this method by using a balloon that could distend and fracture the stenotic plaque.[141]

Endarterial procedures have been extended to include not only dilatation and placement of emboli of several kinds in bleeding arteries but also removal of atherosclerotic lesions by endarterial manipulations through a percutaneous route. A major requirement for endarterial procedures was believed to be endarterial visualization, beyond that provided by contrast radiography. Visualization began effectively with the work of Greenstone and others.[142]

Actual removal of plaque by several mechanical means followed: Simpson and associates used a side-biting forceps in a catheter,[143] Kensey and coworkers used a catheter through which a rapidly rotating auger-like tip was passed,[144] and Ahn and colleagues advocated a high-speed rotary bur.[145] Others have used various forms of laser energy to destroy plaque.[146] In one procedure, the laser recognizes the difference between plaque and normal arterial wall.[147] In another, the laser-heated probe "melts" the atheroma.[148] Further mechanical dilatation often accompanies these initial coring methods. Appraisal of these methods, however, belongs in the clinical rather than the historical section of this volume; they appear to achieve only limited removal of the atheromatous material and much less satisfactory results than the classic techniques of endarterectomy, albeit without requiring a major operative procedure.

Dotter and others proposed the addition of intraluminal stents to maintain graft patency, as well as the patency of vessels that had been dilated.[109] In the surgical literature, this maneuver was largely ignored until Palmaz and associates introduced balloon-expandable stents,[110] which were first used to maintain patency in dilated arteries. The use of percutaneous arterial dilatation and endarterectomy has suffered from inadequate and inconstant reporting standards in the hands of many nonsurgeons, but the technique appears to have reached a level of acceptance that requires the definition of its historical role.

Parodi and coworkers hybridized the technique of endarterial placement of these stents and added the placement of fabric grafts,[111] a technique described previously in the section on aneurysms.

Two other important extensions of distal femoral reconstruction came on the scene. The first was introduction of the graft to the infrapopliteal artery. In 1960, Palma published descriptions of vein graft insertions into the tibial arteries.[149] Later information from Palma (personal communication, 1990) indicates that these were performed as early as 1956. McCaughan described the exposure of the "distal popliteal artery" (more commonly known as the tibioperoneal trunk) and anastomoses to it in 1958,[150] but his work went unrecognized because of his unconventional terminology. In that paper, McCaughan described a successful graft into the tibial vessels in July 1957, using an exposure in the upper third of the calf. He presented six additional patients with grafts into the tibial segment in 1960.[151] In 1966, McCaughan went one step further when he reported four grafts in which the distal insertion of the graft was into the posterior tibial artery at the ankle.[152] Morris and coworkers[153] and Tyson and DeLaurentis[154] were other contemporary pioneers in the development of various configurations of infrapopliteal procedures.

The second extension of distal femoral reconstruction was application of the in situ vein graft, with destruction of valvular competence within the vein, by Hall.[155] The procedure did not receive much attention until it was revitalized by Leather and associates in 1981.[156] Many variations on the theme of the distal bypass have been introduced, combining free grafts and in situ methods.

Dardik and associates introduced the use of tanned human umbilical vein and then added a distal arteriovenous fistula.[157] The fistula was not a revival of earlier attempts by Carrel and others to revascularize an extremity through the veins but rather an attempt to provide sufficient outflow for a long graft to ensure its patency, with some of the graft flow still directed through the distal arterial tree. DeLaurentis and Friedman introduced a method of sequential multiple bypasses in the extremity,[158] and Veith and associates carried this to extremes with bypasses from one tibial artery to another, and even with bypasses beginning and ending below the malleolus.[159] Nehler's group applied this small vessel bypass technique to the management of small vessel disease in the distal upper extremity.[160]

A different approach to the ischemic lower limb was advocated by Oudot and Cormier when they observed how frequently the superficial femoral artery was occluded but the

profunda femoris remained patent.[161] Martin and coworkers described an extended form of profundaplasty, particularly as the site of insertion of a graft from above.[162]

None of these advances in reconstructive surgery has been helpful in the management of the frustrating syndrome of thromboangiitis obliterans, or Buerger's disease. It is likely that von Winiwarter was describing the pathologic process of thromboangiitis obliterans, but his description and clinical correlation are ambiguous.[163] Certainly, Buerger described the clinical picture,[164] although neither he nor von Winiwarter noted the association with tobacco or the involvement of the upper extremities.

One other major contribution rounds out this section. In 1963, Fogarty and coworkers devised one of the most useful methods for managing occlusive arterial disease—the balloon embolectomy catheter for the extraction of clot in the treatment of embolization.[165] This technique has been modified for use in many other arterial and venous operations and has even been adapted to many general surgical uses.

The development of endarterial stenting and grafting has already been mentioned. These methods have undoubtedly improved the results of arterial dilatation, but the lack of standardized methods of reporting in the nonvascular literature and the overenthusiastic promotion of the method still cloud its value. Further, the application of these techniques has become a point of conflict among radiologists, cardiologists, and surgeons over whose "turf" it should be. Some areas are obviously suitable for treatment by an interventional radiologist or cardiologist, but in many instances, the presence and active participation of a surgeon in the operating room are mandatory. In any event, comparison of methods and results should be made possible by accurate and standardized methods of analysis. Here again, current clinical choices supersede historical interpretation.

Arterial Trauma

Arterial injuries have always been a challenge to surgeons. Trauma was the source of Hallowell's first arterial repair. During the years after the Civil War, Mitchell described the syndrome of burning pain ("causalgia") that followed many arterial injuries[166]; it was this lesion that had intrigued Leriche and led to his interest in the sympathetic nervous system.[118] Halsted had remarked on surgeons' fascination with arterial injuries. During World War I, Makins surveyed the injuries to blood vessels incurred by the British forces.[167] DeBakey and Simeone provided a similar service for U.S. forces after World War II and noted almost no benefit from the vascular surgical techniques then available because of the incidental and associated surgical complications and the problem of delay.[168]

Few arterial injuries were treated definitively, except for ligation of the artery, until the Korean War. Before that time, the main interest in arterial injuries seemed to be estimating the likelihood of survival of the limb and selecting the appropriate level for ligation of the artery. Generations of anatomy students learned the "site of election" for ligation of various arteries.

During the Korean War, however, Jahnke and Howard,[169] Hughes,[170] and Spencer and Grewe[171] participated in a program in which acute vascular injuries were treated with fresh vein grafts. Whelan and coworkers[172] and Rich and Hughes[173] continued using these techniques of arterial repair in Vietnam. The Registry of Vascular Injuries from Vietnam, as maintained at the Walter Reed Army Medical Center under the direction of Rich, has continued to yield a monumental body of information concerning acute vascular repair. Civilian medical centers have continued to apply these techniques to the everyday patterns of vessel injuries.

The arteriovenous fistula is one sequela of trauma to the major vessels that poses a special challenge to surgeons. Its acute effects on the distal circulation, its systemic effects as a major left-to-right shunt, and its local changes, which result in increased blood flow through the feeding arterial supply, are all intriguing examples of the body's adaptability—or lack thereof.

The arteriovenous fistula was first described by William Hunter.[3] The lesion did not become common until the end of the 19th century, as weapons (i.e., high-speed projectiles) and the injuries they caused changed. Volumes have been written in an attempt to interpret the diverse physiologic parameters involved in this lesion, but as early as 1913, Soubbotitich noted that simple ligation of the proximal artery should never be done.[174] Not long after, Lexer introduced the "ideal" operation,[45] consisting of resection of the aneurysmal sac and restoration of flow through the artery with a short venous graft if the ends of the artery could not be brought back together. Reconstruction of the vein was desirable but not mandatory. Bickham suggested approaching the arterial repair through the venous component of the sac, with repair of the vein if possible,[34] a modification of the Matas endoaneurysmorrhaphy.

For the most part, however, until the Korean War era in the 1950s and later, the most common form of surgical management was quadruple ligation and excision of the sac and fistula. Such an operation depended on the development of sufficient collateral circulation to the distal limb to allow the limb to survive after arterial interruption, but it had to be done before the extra load placed on the heart by a left-to-right shunt caused serious cardiac disability; timing was thus a matter of delicate clinical judgment. Holman, whose lifelong interest in the arteriovenous fistula began during his training at Johns Hopkins, was the most eminent contributor to the understanding of the physiology of the arteriovenous fistula.[175] With the advent of prompt exploration and repair of acute arterial injuries, it was anticipated that the number of late arteriovenous fistulas would be greatly reduced, but this has not been the case. The current ability to reconstruct the artery diminishes the need to delay to allow the development of collateral circulation, as was once necessary.

Extracranial Cerebrovascular Arterial Occlusions

The critical nature of the blood flow to the brain through the great arteries of the neck was recognized by the ancient Greeks, who named the carotid artery after the symptoms that followed its occlusion—asphyxia, or stupor. The clinical importance of carotid artery stenosis and obstruction was only slowly accepted by the neurologic community in general, however, despite the fact that eminent neurologists such as Savory,[176] Hunt,[177] and Fisher[178,179] had observed the relationship between arterial lesions and atheroembolic phenomena many years before surgical treatment became accepted.

The first elective attempt to restore flow to the ischemic brain was made by Carrea and associates in 1951 but not reported until 1955.[180] The proximal portion of the diseased internal carotid artery was excised, and flow was restored by an anastomosis of the unusually large proximal external carotid artery to the cut end of the distal internal carotid. A slightly different reconstruction of the carotid bifurcation, necessitated by a gunshot wound, was accomplished by Lefèvre in 1918.[181] He resected the carotid bulb, ligated the common trunk, and anastomosed the distal ends of the internal and external carotid arteries to provide the brain with the arterial supply from the rich anastomoses of the external carotid artery.

The most widely acclaimed early carotid reconstruction and the one that truly began the modern reconstructive era was the resection of the carotid bifurcation and restoration of carotid flow by anastomosis of the common carotid to the internal carotid by Eastcott and colleagues in 1954.[182] It now appears that others, including Cooley and colleagues,[183] Roe,[184] and DeBakey,[185] were among the first to successfully perform true carotid endarterectomies. As was the case with Estes and his paper justifying the approach to abdominal aneurysms, so the report to the National Research Council of Great Britain by Yates and Hutchinson indicated the importance of occlusive disease of the carotid and vertebral arteries.[186]

Whisnant and associates in Rochester, Minnesota, identified the risk of stroke in the presence of transient ischemic attacks and provided the solid basis for operation on the carotid artery to prevent major strokes.[187] Hollenhorst called attention to the bright cholesterol emboli seen in the eye grounds that are pathognomonic of atherosclerotic embolization,[188] but Julian and associates[189] and Moore and Hall[190] clearly demonstrated that embolization was the major cause of transient cerebral ischemic symptoms, rather than simple hemodynamics. Further landmark studies of the morphology of carotid plaque and its evolution were presented by Imparato and coworkers[191] and Lusby and associates.[192] Moore and Hall[193] and others among Wylie's group called attention to the role of carotid back-pressure in identifying patients whose brains needed protection from ischemia during the period of operative occlusion.

Operation for symptomatic patients was soon relatively well accepted, but operation to prevent stroke in asymptomatic patients whose carotid stenosis manifests as a bruit or a measurable change in retinal artery pressure or some other noninvasive laboratory test remains controversial. Work by Thompson and colleagues is the predominant authoritative source, despite criticism concerning its lack of perfect controls.[194] Dixon and associates provided further evidence of the role of large, asymptomatic ulcerations of the carotid bifurcation.[195] Berguer and coworkers showed that many "asymptomatic" patients with carotid lesions actually demonstrate multiple small cerebral infarcts that are not clearly reflected in the patient's symptoms.[196]

In 1992, Moore summarized several early multicenter, randomized trials that were performed to compare carotid endarterectomy with nonsurgical methods.[197] These revealed carotid endarterectomy to be so highly effective that many early criticisms of the operation were quieted. An immense body of controversial literature exists concerning the role of anticoagulant or antiplatelet agents to prevent thrombosis or thromboembolization, but these modalities remain an adjunct to carotid endarterectomy performed by trained surgeons. Continuing comparisons of several different modalities continue to define appropriate clinical measures.

The surgeon's inability to clear the totally occluded bifurcation safely and effectively has been addressed by the use of microsurgical techniques. Yasargil and associates first popularized this technique.[198] Many neurosurgeons have become skillful in the performance of extracranial-to-intracranial bypass. A randomized study cast serious doubts about the value of this technique in preventing strokes,[199] however, and its true role remains to be clarified.

Visceral Vascular Occlusions

One of the most important lesions in relatively small arteries is the occlusive lesion in the coronary arteries. Longmire and colleagues carried out a few successful coronary endarterectomies in 1958.[200] The difficulties associated with endarterectomy in small vessels led others to use the vein graft, first as a replacement by Favoloro[201] in 1968 and then as a bypass by Johnson and associates[202] in 1969.

Renal arterial insufficiency has been treated successfully for many years. Goldblatt and coworkers recognized the importance of renal ischemia as a cause of arterial hypertension,[203] and others explained the details of the deranged physiology. Freeman and associates were among the first to treat this lesion successfully,[129] leading to the surgical management of renovascular hypertension. DeCamp and coworkers,[204] Poutasse,[205] and Foster and associates[206] were leaders in the perfection of these techniques.

Recognition of several forms of fibromuscular hyperplasia in the renal artery was followed by its identification in the internal carotid artery by Connett and Lansche.[207] Ehrenfeld and associates put the surgical management of this lesion on a firm footing.[208]

Occlusive disease is much less common in the mesenteric vessels than in most other visceral beds, but it is frequently lethal when it does occur. It was commonly recognized only when it had reached an advanced stage and caused extensive intestinal necrosis. Dunphy in 1936 related the progression of symptoms of mesenteric ischemia to frank intestinal infarction.[209] Fifteen years later, Klass removed an embolus from the superior mesenteric artery successfully, although the patient died of his primary cardiovascular disease.[210] Barker and Cannon included in their first endarterectomy series a patient who underwent a superior mesenteric endarterectomy at the same time as an aortoiliac procedure.[133] In 1957, Shaw and Rutledge carried out an embolectomy of the superior mesenteric artery without concomitant bowel resection.[211] The following year, Shaw and Maynard identified two patients with both malabsorption and mesenteric ischemia who were treated successfully by endarterectomy.[212] In the meantime, Mikkelsen and Zaro reported similar experiences from California, and they clarified the useful term *intestinal angina*.[213]

The meandering mesenteric collaterals so well described by Kountz and associates provided a radiographic sign suggesting the presence of serious stenosis of the celiac axis and superior mesenteric vessels.[214] Recognition of this sign has become cause for careful evaluation of the mesenteric vessels, whether found in the radiology suite or the operating room.

One of the important nonsurgical lesions that mimics obstructive mesenteric vascular disease is the nonocclusive form of mesenteric vascular insufficiency identified by Heer and associates.[215] This condition occurs in forms of cardiogenic shock in which the cardiac output is low and the mesenteric vascular resistance is high.

The extrinsic compression syndrome of the celiac axis is a subject capable of generating considerable discussion. Marable and associates first described this as compression by the arcuate ligament of the diaphragm.[216] Some authors believe that other anatomic structures, such as the neural components of the celiac ganglion, may also be involved. Many support the existence of this lesion, whatever its anatomic cause, as a source of serious symptoms; others forcefully deny its existence.[217]

Extra-anatomic Bypass and Vascular Infections

There are many technical and mechanical advances that cannot properly be placed in any of the previously described compartments of the history of vascular surgery. One of these is the concept of *extra-anatomic bypass*. The term itself is controversial. It has been suggested that this implies a bypass outside the body instead of outside the classic anatomic routes, but its usage is so well established that it is retained here. It was proposed as a possibility by Kunlin[137] and actually carried out as an ilioiliac bypass by way of the prevesical space by Oudot in 1951. Although rerouting of flow through short shunts had been done by many surgeons for various reasons, the first dramatic step was taken by Blaisdell and colleagues, who led a graft from the thoracic aorta extraperitoneally to the femoral artery.[218] Shortly thereafter, this anatomic arrangement was modified as the axillofemoral and then the axillobifemoral graft in 1963 by Blaisdell and Hall.[219]

The axillofemoral bypass was first advised as a means of establishing flow to the extremity in the presence of an infected aortic reconstruction that had to be removed. Similarly, in 1966, Mahoney and Whelan introduced the obturator bypass to avoid an established infection in the groin.[220] Vetto introduced a slightly different anatomic variant—the femorofemoral bypass—in 1962,[221] 11 years after Oudot's ilioiliac operation. Today the pattern of unusual anatomic configurations seems limited only by the patient's needs and the surgeon's ingenuity.

One of the important indications for replacement of the classic aortic prosthesis is the development of an aortoenteric fistula. These lesions have plagued surgeons since the first aortic grafts were performed. Elliott and coauthors contributed one of the first important papers toward the understanding of this problem.[222] Later, Busuttil and associates defined the common primary role played by the false aneurysm at the aortic suture line and clarified the management.[223]

Venous Surgery

The history of venous surgery is in one sense older and in another sense newer than that of arterial surgery. Venous repairs were undertaken before arterial repairs were generally successful. Most of the first generation of arterial surgeons learned about the vagaries of the venous system as their first experiences in vascular surgery. Varicose veins, venous thrombosis, pulmonary embolism, and the postphlebitic extremity were the four major topics.

Although operations on the veins were the major procedures that "vascular" surgeons were called on to perform in the first half of the 20th century, venous surgery was overshadowed by the more glamorous arterial reconstructions until recently, when the American Venous Forum was established to study the management of problems involving the veins. Phlebology never lost its major role in Europe, and the Venous Forum has returned venous surgery to prominent status in the United States.

The earliest modern operations for varicosities consisted of little more than local excision of the varix, and it was probably Trendelenburg who introduced the physiologically useful ligation of the long saphenous vein in the upper leg.[224,225] Trendelenburg's interruption of the saphenous vein was carried out in the midthigh. Although Trendelenburg's operation introduced and was directed at the concept of reversal of flow in the diseased saphenous system, the collaterals at the saphenous bulb allowed prompt return to a pattern of saphenous flow toward the foot. Homans is generally credited with defining the importance of interrupting the saphenous vein flush with the femoral vein and dividing its major collateral trunks in the first few centimeters below that junction.[226]

Babcock devised techniques to strip or avulse veins by means of extraluminal strippers,[227] and for many years the Mayo external stripper has been a useful instrument to facilitate dissection of the vein.[228]

Radical stripping of the major saphenous trunks has become less common in the last quarter-century, once the importance of preserving a nonvaricose vein for possible later use as an arterial conduit became an important consideration.

Pulmonary embolism has long been a major problem for physicians in all areas of medical practice. In 1908, Trendelenburg introduced the operation of pulmonary embolectomy.[229] This operation was undertaken infrequently and was usually unsuccessful, but its rare successes have continued to challenge surgeons. It is an operation that can be applied more frequently today because of the ability to support the patient's cardiovascular system until the operation can be performed. The role of direct operation may be lessened by the ability to place catheters in the pulmonary artery and dissolve the clot with thrombolytic agents.[230]

In 1934, the true relationship between deep venous thrombosis of the leg veins and pulmonary embolism was clarified by Homans of Boston, who matched the ends of a thrombus taken from the pulmonary artery at autopsy with a residual clot in the popliteal vein, showing that this must have been the source of the embolus.[231,232] Homans recognized that the great venous sinuses in the soleal veins were capable of returning large quantities of blood during exercise, but at rest, blood might be stagnant there. Thus, given the other factors of Virchow's triad (stagnant flow, endothelial injury, and increased coagulability), one might anticipate spontaneous thrombosis at that site. In fact, subsequent studies with radioiodinated fibrinogen showed an alarming rate of thrombosis there. Fortunately, only a very small proportion of these thromboses yields thrombi that propagate into the mainline channels and produce serious clinical problems.

The next step in the management of patients with venous thrombosis was also made by Homans, who introduced ligation of the superficial femoral vein where it joins the deep femoral system in the groin.[233] The introduction of this procedure must be viewed in the context of the times, when there was no practical anticoagulant commonly in use. Allen,[234] Veal,[235] and others quickly took up this operation.

Homans experienced disappointment over the outcome of a patient whose superficial femoral vein he and I had ligated. A clot propagated through the deep femoral system and into the common femoral vein, causing an embolism and the patient's death, despite the interruption of the superficial femoral vein.

The preferred level of venous ligation was moved upward because of other similar failures of superficial femoral vein interruption. First, the common femoral and then the iliac veins were ligated bilaterally. These operations could be performed under local anesthesia through groin incisions, but it was soon recognized that bilateral ligation of the iliac veins was preferred to the common femoral site. Vena caval interruption soon became the procedure of choice. It is hard to identify who first ligated the vena cava for pulmonary embolism, but Northway and Buxton,[236] O'Neill,[237] and Collins and coworkers[238] are all credited with early reports.

It seems unfortunate that once anticoagulants became readily available—first warfarin (Coumadin) and then heparin—their combination with ligation was not common; ligation and anticoagulation were used on an either-or basis by most physicians. Simple ligation without anticoagulant therapy was often associated with extension of thrombosis in the stagnant systems below the ligature, which led to severe postphlebitic symptoms. Anlyan and colleagues,[239] Bowers and Leb,[240] and others seriously criticized interruption, giving rise to a school that treated venous thrombosis primarily with increasingly large doses of heparin.[241] The extent of postphlebitic syndrome, however, seems to be more clearly related to the extent of the inflammatory thrombophlebitic process and its destruction of the valves in the leg than to ligation or the level of ligation.[242] The successful use of large doses of heparin has greatly diminished the need for venous interruption.

Spencer introduced another approach to caval interruption, however, to maintain some flow through the cava but still prevent the passage of emboli to the lungs by plication of the cava with sutures.[243] Other extraluminal occlusive devices were suggested by Moretz and associates,[244] Miles and colleagues,[245] and Adams and DeWeese.[246] Mobin-Uddin's invention of a transvenous umbrella[247] and Greenfield's transvenous wire trap[248] reduced the need for major venous interruption by open surgical methods even further.

The problems of the postphlebitic extremity remain. This syndrome was well described by Homans,[249] but his contributions to its treatment were not particularly fruitful, except that they represent the culmination of the best forms of nonoperative management. Trout,[250] Linton,[251] and Dodd and Cockett[252] separately advocated methods that accomplish subfascial interruption of the communicating veins in the lower leg; this procedure remains a surgical standard.

The re-creation of a venous drainage channel that is protected from regurgitant flow offered a new approach to this old problem. Kistner demonstrated a technique of converting an incompetent valve into a competent one.[253] Venous transposition, redirecting flow through a competent vein and around an area of venous incompetence, is another approach used by Dale[254] and Palma.[255]

Taheri and coworkers published the results of a free graft of a valved segment of the axillary vein into the diseased femoral system.[256] Taheri and others went even further, attempting to develop prosthetic venous valves.[257]

Highlights in Diagnostic Modalities

The diagnosis of both arterial and venous diseases has long depended on the use of contrast radiography. One of the first to use this technique successfully in a living patient was Brooks,[258] who injected sodium iodide to demonstrate the lesions of Buerger's disease in digital vessels. Moniz described "arterial encephalography" for neurologic lesions in 1927.[259] His presentation was not only a seminal paper; it also defined the technical needs of the radiographer in terms that are pertinent nearly 80 years later.

In the audience at Moniz's presentation was dos Santos (the elder). He and his colleagues soon published the basic technical approach to arteriography of the vessels of the abdomen and their branches.[260] Each of these authors foresaw the great advances that would accompany the development of rapid cassette changers and less toxic contrast media, but the techniques of image enhancement and subtraction by electronic means are recent and highly effective contributions.

One of the major technical advances for the angiographer was Seldinger's technique,[261] which, instead of using a single needle to inject contrast material, used a catheter that was passed over a wire that had been introduced through the primary vessel puncture. The guidewire was first advanced to the desired site, then the appropriate catheter was advanced over the wire. Wire and catheter could be alternated so that injections could be made at different sites and at different rates. With this method, a catheter can be placed and injection can be achieved at almost any intravascular site in the body. The culmination of these technical advances is the clarification and modification of the radiographic image by subtraction, digitization, enhancement, and various electronic manipulations.

A totally different field of radiology was signaled by the work of Dotter and Judkins,[140] who used a rigid dilator passed through a large needle under fluoroscopic guidance to dilate narrowed arteries in 1956. Dotter's contributions were followed by those of Gruntzig.[141] This percutaneous intravascular technique evolved into the burgeoning field of *interventional* rather than purely diagnostic radiology.

The growth of vascular surgery in recent years has been almost synonymous with the development of methods of noninvasive diagnosis of peripheral vascular disease. This is an outgrowth of those methods commonly taken for granted, which had their humble beginnings in the stethoscope, the sphygmomanometer,[262] and the ophthalmoscope.

The measurement of many physiologic parameters in the laboratory was extended to the patient by such physicians as Winsor,[263] whose definition of pressure gradients remains a critical basis for the clinical estimation of the severity of arterial obstruction. Combined with a sphygmomanometer and a Doppler sensor, evaluation of segmental arterial pressures became a useful means of evaluating peripheral arterial disease and identifying segmental pressure differences, just as Winsor had done with less accurate sensing methods.

Other common measurements performed in the early vascular diagnostic laboratories included digital and segmental plethysmography and skin temperature and resistance, both before and after sympathetic blockade.

Pachon introduced a modification of the sphygmomanometer and the segmental plethysmograph; the oscillometer provided a very rough measure of the volume of the distensile arterial pulse wave.[264] The values obtained bore no physiologic definition, but comparisons at different levels in one extremity, of comparable levels in opposite extremities, or at one site on successive occasions provided the surgeon with some objective evidence of change. Although the stethoscope is used by all physicians, its role in the evaluation of murmurs over the peripheral arteries was clarified and codified by Edwards and Levine[265] and then by Wylie and McGuiness[266] at a surprisingly late date. The usefulness of inexpensive auscultation has diminished as electronic assessment has become readily available.

One of the interesting early techniques was that of Baillart,[267] who used the ophthalmoscope and concurrent ophthalmodynamometry to evaluate lesions of the eye and thus estimate retinal arterial pressures, which were assumed to reflect pressure and hence flow through the internal carotid artery. Operator sensitivity and reproducibility, critical aspects of many such techniques, were such that the method's utility was not great. Kartchner[268] and Gee[269] and their respective colleagues introduced a recording device to reproduce relative pressure curves within the ocular globe or to compare the peak time of the retinal artery pulse wave, which is reflected in the globe's pressure, with the arrival of the pulse wave in the earlobe; this enabled estimation of the severity of obstruction in the carotid system. Gee and associates developed a method to evaluate the back-pressure in the stenotic carotid artery to predict the necessity of a shunt during operative carotid occlusion. Their method, however, is actually of greater value in evaluating the forward pressure beyond the stenotic carotid artery; it provides more precise measurement of the pressures but does not provide time relationships, as Kartchner's system does. These subtle physiologic evaluations of the intraocular arterial pressure as an indirect reflection of the intracranial carotid flow have been supplanted by more direct physiologic studies of the extracranial arteries in the neck.

Ultrasonography has become one of the most popular modalities in its many ramifications. Leopold and associates used classic ultrasonic imaging (B-mode) techniques to outline the aorta and identify aneurysmal changes there.[270]

Use of the ultrasonic flow detector was soon modified by Brockenbrough to determine the direction of flow through the supraorbital artery,[271] which is reversed in the presence of high-grade obstruction of the ipsilateral carotid artery. Machleder and Barker dramatized the technique,[272] but extreme operator sensitivity limits its use.

Imaging of the crude Doppler signal was introduced by Thomas and coworkers,[273] who simply mounted a Doppler probe on a scanning device. Increased sophistication of these scanning methods ultimately led to duplex scanning techniques.

Ultrasonography in another form (i.e., either the continuous or the gated Doppler mode that measures the shift in frequency of the ultrasonic signal reflected from moving red blood cells) was introduced by Strandness and colleagues[274] and by Sumner and Strandness.[275] Here, ultrasonic B-mode scanning defines the anatomy and obtains a reference point to be combined with pulsed, "gated" Doppler reflections to show blood flow patterns and velocities at the designated site within the lumen. Use of these studies is limited to vessels that can be "reached" by the Doppler signal.[276] This method became widely used to evaluate the carotid bifurcation, but its application has now been extended as a monitor in peripheral arterial sites, vertebral arteries,[277] mesenteric vessels,[278] and at the operating table.[279] Evaluation of the circle of Willis is also possible but is not consistently reliable.[280]

Carotid angiography has been shown to contribute a major proportion of the morbidity and mortality associated with carotid surgery in many randomized trials. As a result, duplex imaging has rapidly replaced it as the primary diagnostic tool for carotid artery disease. It provides highly accurate anatomic as well as physiologic data, although arteriography is still necessary in some patients.

A new twist on computed tomography was introduced by Kalender and associates.[281] Use of this form of spiral computed tomography has become more common, and although its images may lose some of the detail obtained by other methods, it provides a superb overall picture of the course and collaterals of an arterial segment, and its software allows manipulation so that the three-dimensional image can be visualized from many different angles.

Magnetic resonance imaging has become a useful evaluation tool, especially of the aorta, and magnetic resonance angiography also shows promise,[282] but these techniques are at the stage of clinical rather than historical evaluation at the moment.

Evaluation of the venous side of the circulation beyond classic physical examination has not yielded such exact information. Cranley and coworkers introduced "phleborheography," which evaluates changes in venous pulse, outflow, and respiratory excursions to diagnose deep venous disease of the legs.[283] Less sophisticated, easier to handle, but perhaps less informative is Wheeler's impedance plethysmography.[284]

The Doppler velocity probe, despite some drawbacks related to operator sensitivity, remains a useful method for identifying lesions in the major superficial veins, such as in the groin, the popliteal space, and the axilla. It can also be used in the postphlebitic extremity to identify both regurgitant flow in superficial channels and flow from communicating veins. It can be used even in the presence of brawny edema, which otherwise obscures much of the venous system from sight and palpation.

Just as the duplex scan in carotid surgery has become popular, color-assisted duplex imaging is an important part of the evaluation of the venous system,[285] where its use was first popularized.

Vascular Access Surgery

Kolff's introduction of hemodialysis in the mid-1950s revolutionized nephrology,[286] but it also added to the number of difficult procedures that vascular surgeons are asked to perform, including providing and maintaining "access" to the vascular system, often on an emergency basis. Vascular access surgery lacks the glamour of much of the rest of vascular surgery, but it constitutes a significant portion of vascular surgical practice. The construction and maintenance of a well-functioning access site demand both surgical skill and judgment.

The first approaches involved the use of silicone tubing as an external shunt between the arterial and venous systems in the arm.[287] The natural progression by Brescia and his team was to use a direct arteriovenous fistula, usually in the arm.[288] The fistula results in dilated veins suitable for recurrent punctures. The addition of an autologous vein graft to allow a better fistula and better access to the vein[289] was soon followed by the use of other materials as shunts, both biologic and plastic.[290]

Thoracic Outlet Syndromes

The problems and care of the varied thoracic outlet syndromes are shared by vascular surgeons, orthopedists, neurosurgeons, and physiotherapists. Although first treated surgically as an exostosis of the first rib in 1861,[291] clear anatomic understanding was achieved through the works of Murphy,[292] Adson and Coffey,[293] and Ochsner and coworkers.[294] It appeared to early authors that a cervical rib was the offending anatomic structure, but Adson and Coffey introduced the concept of entrapment of the brachial plexus and accompanying artery by the anterior scalene muscle and the highest rib. Naffziger and Grant confirmed the mechanical origins of the syndrome and demonstrated the anterior supraclavicular approach.[295] One of the illustrations, however, taking an anatomist's point of view from inside the chest, showed the anatomy that Roos would subsequently use in his transaxillary approach.[296] Falconer and Li proposed resection of the first rib to relieve the costoclavicular compression of the vessels.[297] Edwards offered a thesis that consolidated the anatomic and evolutionary origins of these syndromes, pointing out that the human is one of the few animals in which there is a descent of the heart and great vessels in relation to the shoulder girdle, which leads to draping of the great vessels over the highest rib, whatever its number might be.[298]

The surgical approaches to this area have been varied: paraspinal and anterior supraclavicular and transaxillary. The latter involves no major muscle division and provides a better cosmetic result. It is especially helpful in muscular athletes, who are prone to symptoms from compression.

The most common form involves pressure on the nerves and arteries, but a slightly different anatomic arrangement is responsible for the variations in Paget-Schroetter syndrome, in which obstruction of the venous system is the major problem. McLeery and coworkers defined the anatomic basis of intermittent venous obstruction from the subclavian and anterior scalene muscles.[299]

KEY REFERENCES

Bigger IA: Surgical treatment of aneurysm of the aorta: Review of the literature and report of two cases, one apparently successful. Ann Surg 112: 879-894, 1940.

Blaisdell FW, Hall AD: Axillary-femoral artery bypass for lower extremity ischemia. Surgery 54:563-568, 1963.

Blalock A, Taussig HB: The surgical treatment of malformations of the heart in which there is pulmonary stenosis or pulmonary atresia. JAMA 128:189-202, 1945.

Buerger L: Thromboangiitis obliterans: A study of the vascular lesions leading to presenile spontaneous gangrene. Am J Med Sci 136:567-580, 1908.

Carrel A: The surgery of blood vessels, etc. Johns Hopkins Hosp Bull 190: 18-28, 1907.

Charcot JM: Obstruction artérielle et claudication intermittente dans le cheval et dans l'homme. Mem Soc Biol 1:225-238, 1858.

Crafoord C, Nylin G: Congenital coarctation of the aorta and its surgical treatment. J Thorac Surg 14:347-361, 1945.

DeBakey ME, Cooley SA, Crawford ES, Morris GC Jr: Clinical application of a new flexible knitted Dacron arterial substitute. Arch Surg 77:713-724, 1958.

DeCamp P, Snyder CH, Bost RB: Severe hypertension due to congenital stenosis of artery to solitary kidney: Correction by splenorenal anastomosis. Arch Surg 75:1026-1030, 1957.

Dobson J: John Hunter. Edinburgh, E & S Livingstone, 1969.

dos Santos JC: Sur la désobstruction des thromboses artérielles anciennes. Mem Acad Chir 73:409-411, 1947.

dos Santos R, Lamas A, Caldas P: L'artériographie des membres, de l'aorte et des ses branches abdominales. Bull Mem Soc Natl Chir 55:587-601, 1929.

Dubost C, Allary M, Oeconomos N: Resection of an aneurysm of the abdominal aorta: Reestablishment of the continuity by a preserved human arterial graft, with result after five months. Arch Surg 64:405-408, 1952.

Dunphy JE: Abdominal pain of vascular origin. Am J Med Sci 92:109-113, 1936.

Eastcott HHG, Pickering GW, Rob C: Reconstruction of internal carotid artery in a patient with intermittent attacks of hemiplegia. Lancet 2:994-996, 1954.

Edwards WS, Tapp JS: Chemically treated nylon tubes as arterial grafts. Surgery 38:61-76, 1955.

Fogarty TJ, Cranley JJ, Krause RJ, et al: A method of extraction of arterial emboli and thrombi. Surg Gynecol Obstet 116:241-244, 1963.

Gross RE: Complete surgical division of the patent ductus arteriosus. Surg Gynecol Obstet 78:36-43, 1944.

Holman E: Clinical and experimental observations on arteriovenous fistulae. Ann Surg 112:840-878, 1940.

Homans J: The late results of femoral thrombophlebitis and their treatment. N Engl J Med 235:249-253, 1946.

Homans J: Thrombosis of the deep veins of the lower leg causing pulmonary embolism. N Engl J Med 211:993-997, 1934.

Jaboulay M, Briau E: Recherches expérimentales sur la suture et la greffe artérielles. Bull Lyon Med 81:97-99, 1896.

Jahnke EJ Jr, Howard JM: Primary repair of major arterial injuries. Arch Surg 66:646-649, 1953.

Jassinowsky A: Die Arteriennaht: Eine experimentelle Studie [dissertation]. Dorpat, Estonia, University of Tartu, 1889.

Julian OC, Dye WS, Javid H, Hunter JA: Ulcerative lesions of the carotid artery bifurcation. Arch Surg 86:803-809, 1963.

Kistner RL: Surgical repair of the incompetent vein valve. Arch Surg 110:1336-1342, 1975.

Kolff WJ: The first clinical experience with the artificial kidney. Ann Intern Med 62:608-619, 1965.

Kunlin J: Le traitement de l'ischemie artéritique par la greffe veineuse longue. Rev Chir 70:207-235, 1951.

Leriche R: Des obliterations artérielles hautes (oblitération de la terminasion de l'aorte) comme causes des insuffisances circulatoires des membres inférieures. Bull Mem Soc Chir (Paris) 49:1404-1406, 1923.

Longmire WP Jr, Cannon JA, Kattus HA: Direct-vision coronary endarterectomy for angina pectoris. N Engl J Med 259:993-999, 1958.

Marrangoni AC, Cecchini LP: Homotransplantation of arterial segments by the freeze-drying method. Ann Surg 134:977-983, 1951.

Matas R: Traumatic aneurysm of the brachial artery. Med News 53:462-466, 1888.

Moore WS, Hall AD: Carotid artery back pressure: A test of cerebral tolerance to temporary carotid artery occlusion. Arch Surg 99:702-710, 1969.

Murphy JB: Resection of arteries and veins injured in continuity... end to end suture... experimental and clinical research. Med Rec 51:73-88, 1897.

Murray GDW: Heparin in thrombosis and embolism. Br J Surg 27:567-576, 1940.

Ochsner A, Gage M, DeBakey ME: Scalenus anticus (Naffziger) syndrome. Am J Surg 28:669-693, 1935.

Parodi J, Palmaz JC, Barone HD: Transfemoral intraluminal graft implantation for abdominal aortic aneurysms. Ann Vasc Surg 5:491-499, 1991.

Strandness DE, Schultz RD, Sumner DS, et al: Ultrasonic flow detection: A useful technique in the evaluation of peripheral vascular disease. Am J Surg 113:311-320, 1967.

Thompson JE, Patman RD, Talkington CM: Asymptomatic carotid bruit. Ann Surg 188:308-316, 1978.

Voorhees AB Jr, Jaretzki A III, Blakemore AH: Use of tubes constructed of Vinyon-"N" cloth in bridging arterial defects. Ann Surg 135:332-336, 1952.

Winsor T: Pressure gradients: Influence of arterial disease on the systolic blood pressure gradients of the extremity. Am J Med Sci 220:117-126, 1950.

REFERENCES

1. Dobson J: John Hunter. Edinburgh, E & S Livingstone, 1969.
2. Gray EA: Portrait of a Surgeon: A Biography of John Hunter. London, Robert Hale, 1952.
3. Hunter WA: History of aneurism of the aorta with some remarks on aneurisms in general. Med Obs Inquiries 1:323, 1757.
4. Cames C: Wörtliche Uebersetzung des Werkes des römischen Arztes Antyllus. Düsseldorf, Germany, Michael Trilitsch Verlag, 1941, p 107.
5. Purmann MG: Chirurgia Curiosa. 1716, p 612.
6. Erichsen JE: Observation on Aneurism (Hunter). London, Sydenham Society, 1844, pp 216, 404.
7. Brock RC: Astley Cooper and carotid artery ligation. Guy's Hosp Rep (special number) 117:219, 1966.
8. Tyrell FG (ed): The Lectures of Sir Astley Cooper, Bart, FRCS, on the Principles and Practice of Surgery, 4th American ed. Philadelphia, EL Carey and A Hart, 1835, pp 212-214.
9. Lambert R: Letter from Mr. Lambert to Dr. Hunter: Giving an account of a new method of treating an aneurism. Med Obs Inquiries 1761.
10. Asman C: Inaugural dissertation. Groningen, Netherlands, University of Groningen, 1773.
11. Blane G: [No title]. Trans Soc Improvement Med Chir Knowledge 2:192, 1800.
12. Cooper A: The Lectures of Sir Astley Cooper, Bart, FRCS, on the Principles and Practice of Surgery, 2nd ed. London, FC Westley, 1830, p 98.
13. Cruveilhier J: Senile gangrene. In Anatomie Pathologique du Corps Humain, sec 27, Malades des Artères. Paris, 1835-1842.
14. Bouley J: Claudication intermittente des membres postérieures par l'oblitération des artères fémorales. Recueil de Médecin Vétérinaire 8:517-518, 1831.
15. Barth: Observation dune oblitération complet de l'aorte abdominale, recuillie dans le service de M. Louis, suivie de reflections. Arch Gen Med (2nd ser) 8:26-53, 1835.
16. Charcot JM: Obstruction artérielle et claudication intermittente dans le cheval et dans l'homme. Mem Soc Biol 1:225-238, 1858.
17. Langenbeck CJM: Pathology and Therapy of Surgical Illnesses, vol 3. Göttingen, Germany, Heimatsverlag, 1825, p 414.
18. Heinecke W: Blutung, Blutstillung, Transfusion nebst Lufteintritt und Infusion. In Billroth T, Luecke H (eds): Deutsche Chirurgie. Stuttgart, Germany, Verlag von Ferdinand Enke, 1885.
19. Jassinowsky A: Die Arteriennaht: Eine experimentelle Studie [dissertation]. Dorpat, Estonia, University of Tartu, 1889.
20. Czerny V: On lateral closure of vein wounds. Langenbecks Arch Chir 28:671, 1881.
21. Schede NI: Einige Bemerkungen über die Naht von Venenwunden. Arch Klin Chir 13:548, 1883.
22. Eck NVK: Voprosu o perevyazkie vorotnois veni. Prevaritelnoye soobshtshjenye. Woen Med J (St. Petersburg) 130:1-2, 1877 (as cited by Child CG III: Eck's fistula. Surg Gynecol Obstet 96:375-376, 1953).
23. Jassinowsky A: Eine Beitrage zur Lehre von der Gefässnaht. Arch Klin Chir 40:816-841, 1891.
24. Dörfler J: Ueber Arteriennaht. Beitr Klin Chir 22:781-825, 1899.
25. Jaboulay M, Briau E: Recherches expérimentales sur la suture et la greffe artérielles. Bull Lyon Med 81:97-99, 1896.
26. Edwards P, Edwards WS: Alexis Carrel: Visionary Surgeon. Springfield, Ill, Charles C Thomas, 1971.
27. Carrel A: Les anastomoses vasculaires et leur technique opératoire. Union Med Can 33:521-527, 1904.
28. Carrel A: The surgery of blood vessels, etc. Johns Hopkins Hosp Bull 190:18-28, 1907.
29. Harbison SP: The origins of vascular surgery: The Carrel-Guthrie letters. Surgery 52:406-418, 1962.
30. Goyanes J: Nuevo trabajos de chirurgia vascular, substitución plastica de los arterios por las venas o arterioplastica venosa, applicada como método nuevo al tratamiento de los aneurismas. El Siglo Med 53:546-561, 1906.
31. Matas R: Traumatic aneurysm of the brachial artery. Med News 53: 462-466, 1888.
32. Cohn I Sr: Rudolf Matas. New York, Doubleday, 1960.
33. Matas R: Some experiences and observations in the treatment of arteriovenous aneurisms by the intrasaccular method of suture (endoaneurismorrhaphy) with special reference to the transvenous route. Ann Surg 71:403-427, 1920.
34. Bickham WS: Arteriovenous aneurisms: A case of arteriovenous aneurism of the common femoral artery and vein unsuccessfully treated by a new method of compression—and finally cured by the proximal ligation of

the external iliac artery—extraperitoneally, with the suggestion that the application to these aneurysms of the Matas method of operation used for ordinary aneurysms—and the mention of some other recent methods of operating. Ann Surg 39:767-775, 1904.

35. Murphy JB: Resection of arteries and veins injured in continuity... end to end suture... experimental and clinical research. Med Rec 51:73-88, 1897.

36. Edwards WS, Tapp JS: Chemically treated nylon tubes as arterial grafts. Surgery 38:61-76, 1955.

37. Nitze F: Kleinere Mittheilungen Kongres im Moskau. Zentralbl Chir 38:1042, 1897.

38. Payr E: Beiträge zur Technik der Blutgefässe und den Nervennaht nebst Mittheilungen der Verwendung eines resorbirbaren Metalles in der Chirurgie. Arch Klin Chir 62:67-93, 1900.

39. Blakemore AH, Lord JW Jr, Stefko PL: The severed primary artery in war wounded: A nonsuture method of bridging arterial defects. Surgery 12:488-508, 1942.

40. Elkin ED, DeBakey ME: Surgery in World War II, vol 4: Vascular Surgery. Washington, DC, Office of the Surgeon General, 1955.

41. Halsted WS: Some of the problems related to surgery of the vascular system: Testing the efficiency of the vascular circulation as a preliminary to the occlusion of the great surgical arteries [discussion of paper by Matas]. Trans Am Surg Assoc 28:49-51, 1910.

42. San Martín y Sastrústegui A: Cirurgia del aparto circulatario. Discurso leido en la session inaugural de la Real Academia de Medicine de Madrid. Madrid, Spain, Jur Méd-farm, 1902, pp 5-71.

43. Halsted AE, Vaughan RT: Arteriovenous anastomoses in treatment of gangrene of the extremities. Surg Gynecol Obstet 14:1-18, 1912.

44. Höpfner E: Ueber Gefässnaht, Gefässtransplantationen und Replantationen von amputierten Extremitäten. Arch Klin Chir 70:417-471, 1903.

45. Lexer E: Die ideale Operation des arteriellen und des arteriellvenösen Aneurysma. Arch Klin Chir 83:459-477, 1907.

46. Lexer E: 20 Jahre Transplantationsforschung in der Chirurgie. Arch Klin Chir 138:251-302, 1925.

47. Jeger E: Die Chirurgie der Blutgefässe und des Herzen [repub, 1913 ed]. Berlin, Springer-Verlag, 1937.

48. Weglowski R: Ueber Gefässtransplantation. Zentralbl Chir 40:2241-2243, 1925.

49. Leonardo RA: History of Surgery. New York, Froben Press, 1943, p 139.

50. Power DA: The palliative treatment of aneurysms by "wiring" with Colt's apparatus. Br J Surg 9:27-36, 1921.

51. Blakemore AH, King BG: Electrothermic coagulation of aortic aneurysms. JAMA 111:1821-1827, 1935.

52. Reid M: Aneurysms in the Johns Hopkins Hospital: All cases treated in the surgical service until 1922. Arch Surg 12:1-74, 1926.

53. Matas R: Ligation of the abdominal aorta: Report of the late result, one year, five months and eight days after ligation of the abdominal aorta for an aneurysm at the bifurcation. Ann Surg 81:457-464, 1925.

54. Matas R: Aneurysm of the aorta at its bifurcation into the iliac arteries; pictorial supplement illustrating the history of Corinne D., previously reported as the first cure of aneurysm by ligation. Ann Surg 112:909-922, 1940.

55. Elkin DC: Aneurysm of the abdominal aorta: Treatment by ligation. Ann Surg 112:895-906, 1940.

56. Bigger IA: Surgical treatment of aneurysm of the aorta: Review of the literature and report of two cases, one apparently successful. Ann Surg 112:879-894, 1940.

57. Cutler EC, Levine SA, Beck CS: The surgical treatment of mitral stenosis. Arch Surg 9:691-821, 1924.

58. Gross RE, Hubbard JD: Surgical ligation of a patent ductus arteriosus: Report of first successful case. JAMA 112:729-731, 1939.

59. Gross RE: Complete surgical division of the patent ductus arteriosus. Surg Gynecol Obstet 78:36-43, 1944.

60. Blalock A, Taussig HB: The surgical treatment of malformations of the heart in which there is pulmonary stenosis or pulmonary atresia. JAMA 128:189-202, 1945.

61. Crafoord C, Nylin G: Congenital coarctation of the aorta and its surgical treatment. J Thorac Surg 14:347-361, 1945.

62. Gross RE, Hufnagel CA: Coarctation of the aorta: Experimental studies regarding its correction. N Engl J Med 233:287-293, 1945.

63. Abbe R: The surgery of the hand. N Y Med J 59:33-40, 1894.

64. Tuffier M: De l'intubation dans le plaies de grosses artères. Bull Acad Med 74:455-460, 1915.

65. Hufnagel CA: Permanent intubation of the thoracic aorta. Arch Surg 54:382-389, 1947.

66. Hufnagel CA: Preserved homologous arterial transplants. Bull Am Coll Surg 32:231, 1947.

67. Gross RE, Bill A, Peirce EC II: Methods for preservation and transplantation of arterial grafts: Observations on arterial grafts in dogs; report of transplantation of preserved arterial grafts in 19 human cases. Surg Gynecol Obstet 88:689-701, 1949.

68. Swan H: Arterial homografts. II. Resection of thoracic aneurysm using a stored human arterial transplant. Arch Surg 61:732-737, 1950.

69. Deterling RA Jr, Coleman CC, Parshley MS: Experimental studies on the frozen homologous aortic graft. Surgery 29:419-440, 1951.

70. Marrangoni AC, Cecchini LP: Homotransplantation of arterial segments by the freeze-drying method. Ann Surg 134:977-983, 1951.

71. Voorhees AB Jr, Jaretzki A III, Blakemore AH: Use of tubes constructed of Vinyon-"N" cloth in bridging arterial defects. Ann Surg 135:332-336, 1952.

72. Deterling RA, Bhonslay SB: An evaluation of synthetic materials and fabrics suitable for blood vessel replacement. Surgery 38:71-89, 1955.

73. Hufnagel CA: The use of rigid and flexible plastic prosthesis for arterial replacement. Surgery 37:165-174, 1955.

74. Girvin CW, Wilhelm MC, Merendino KA: The use of Teflon fabric as arterial grafts: An experimental study in dogs. Am J Surg 92:240-247, 1956.

75. Szilagyi DE, France LC, Smith RF, et al: Clinical use of an elastic Dacron prosthesis. Arch Surg 77:538-551, 1958.

76. Julian OC, Deterling RA, Dye WS, et al: Dacron tube and bifurcation prosthesis produced to specification. Surgery 41:50-61, 1957.

77. Wesolowski SA, Dennis CA (eds): Fundamentals of Vascular Grafting. New York, Blakiston Division, McGraw-Hill, 1963.

78. Wesolowski SA, Fries CC, Karlson KE, et al: Porosity: Primary determinant of ultimate fate of synthetic vascular grafts. Surgery 50:91-96, 105-106, 1961.

79. DeBakey ME, Cooley SA, Crawford ES, Morris GC Jr: Clinical application of a new flexible knitted Dacron arterial substitute. Arch Surg 77:713-724, 1958.

80. Sauvage LR, Berger KE, Wood SJ, et al: An external velour surface for porous arterial prosthesis. Surgery 70:940-953, 1971.

81. Cooley DA, Wukasch DC, Bennet JC, et al: Double velour knitted grafts for aorto-iliac replacement. In Sawyer PN, Kaplitt MJ (eds): Vascular Grafts. New York, Appleton-Century-Crofts, 1978.

82. Quiñones-Baldrich WJ, Moore WS, Ziomek S, Chvapil M: Development of a "leak-proof" knitted Dacron vascular prosthesis. J Vasc Surg 3:895-903, 1986.

83. Guidion R, Snyder B, Martin L, et al: Albumin coating of a knitted polyester arterial prosthesis: An alternative to preclotting: Ann Thorac Surg 37:457-465, 1984.

84. Soyer T, Lempinen M, Cooper P, et al: A new venous prosthesis. Surgery 72:864-872, 1972.

85. Veith FJ, Gupta SK, Ascer E, et al: Six-year prospective multicenter randomized comparison of autologous saphenous vein and expanded polytetrafluoroethylene grafts in infrainguinal arterial reconstructions. J Vasc Surg 3:104-114, 1986.

86. Quiñones-Baldrich WJ, Busuttil RW, Baker JD, et al: Is the preferential use of polytetrafluoroethylene grafts for femoropopliteal bypass justified? J Vasc Surg 8:219-228, 1988.

87. Rosenberg NL, Henderson J, Lord GW, et al: Use of enzyme treated heterografts as arterial substitutes. Arch Surg 85:192-197, 1962.

88. Sawyer PN, Stancezewski B, Lucas TR, et al: Experimental and clinical evaluation of a new negatively charged bovine heterograft for use in peripheral and coronary revascularization. In Sawyer PN, Kaplitt MJ (eds): Vascular Grafts. New York, Appleton-Century-Crofts, 1978.

89. Dardik H, Ibrahim TM, Sprayregan S, et al: Clinical experiences with modified human umbilical cord vein for arterial bypass. Surgery 79:618-624, 1976.

90. Estes JE Jr: Abdominal aortic aneurysm: A study of one hundred and two cases. Circulation 2:258-264, 1950.

91. Alexander J, Byron FX: Aortectomy for thoracic aneurysm. JAMA 1126:1139-1142, 1944.

92. Alexander J, Byron FX: Aortectomy for thoracic aneurysm: A supplemental report. JAMA 132:22, 1946.

93. Pearse HE: Experimental studies on the gradual occlusion of large arteries. Ann Surg 112:923-937, 1940.

94. Yeager G, Cowley RA: Studies on the use of polythene as a fibrous tissue stimulant. Ann Surg 128:509-520, 1940.

95. Oudot J: La greffe vasculaire dans les thromboses du carrefour aortique. Presse Med 59:234-236, 1951.

96. Dubost C, Allary M, Oeconomos N: Resection of an aneurysm of the abdominal aorta: Reestablishment of the continuity by a preserved human arterial graft, with result after five months. Arch Surg 64:405-408, 1952.

97. Schaffer PW, Hardin CW: The use of temporary and polythene shunts to permit occlusion, resection and frozen homologous artery graft replacement of vital vessel segments: A laboratory and clinical study. Surgery 31:186-199, 1952.

98. Julian OC, Grove LVJ, Dye WS, et al: Direct surgery of arteriosclerosis: Resection of abdominal aorta with homologous aortic graft replacement. Ann Surg 138:387-403, 1953.

99. Brock HG: Reconstructive arterial surgery. Proc Soc Med 46:115-130, 1953.

100. DeBakey ME, Cooley DA: Surgical treatment of aneurysm of abdominal aorta by resection and restoration of continuity with homograft. Surg Gynecol Obstet 97:257-266, 1953.

101. Bahnson HT: Considerations in the excision of aortic aneurysms. Ann Surg 138:377-386, 1953.

102. Szilagyi DE, Smith RE, DeRusso FJ, et al: Contribution of abdominal aortic aneurysmectomy to prolongation of life. Ann Surg 164:678-699, 1966.

103. Ellis FH, Helden RA, Hines EA Jr: Aneurysm of the abdominal aorta involving the right renal artery: Report of a case with preservation of renal function after resection and grafting. Ann Surg 142:992-995, 1955.

104. Etheredge SN, Yee JY, Smith JV, et al: Successful resection of a large aneurysm of the upper abdominal aorta and replacement with homograft. Surgery 38:1071-1081, 1955.

105. DeBakey ME, Creech O, Morris GC Jr: Aneurysm of the thoracoabdominal aorta involving the celiac, mesenteric and renal arteries: Report of four cases treated by resection and homograft replacement. Ann Surg 144:549-573, 1956.

106. Shumacker HB Jr: Innovation in the operative management of the thoracoabdominal aortic aneurysm. Surg Gynecol Obstet 136:793-794, 1973.

107. Stoney RJ, Wylie EJ: Surgical management of arterial lesions of the thoracoabdominal aorta. Am J Surg 126:157-164, 1973.

108. Crawford ES: Thoraco-abdominal aortic aneurysms involving renal, superior mesenteric and celiac arteries. Ann Surg 179:763-772, 1974.

109. Dotter CT, Buschman RW, McKinney MK, Rösch J: Transluminal expandable nitinol coil stent grafting: Preliminary report. Radiology 147:259-260, 1983.

110. Palmaz JC, Sibbitt RR, Renter SR, et al: Expandable intraluminal graft: Preliminary study. Radiology 156:73-77, 1985.

111. Parodi J, Palmaz JC, Barone HD: Transfemoral intraluminal graft implantation for abdominal aortic aneurysms. Ann Vasc Surg 5:491-499, 1991.

112. White GH, Yu W, May J, et al: A new nonstented balloon expandable graft for straight or bifurcated endoluminal bypass. J Endovasc Surg 1:16-24, 1994.

113. Moore WS: The role of endovascular grafting technique in the treatment of abdominal aortic aneurysm. Cardiovasc Surg 3:109-114, 1995.

114. Linton RE: The arteriosclerotic popliteal aneurysm: A report of 14 patients treated by preliminary lumbar sympathectomy and aneurysmectomy. Surgery 26:41-58, 1949.

115. Wychulis AR, Spittell JA Jr, Wallace RB: Popliteal aneurysms. Surgery 68:942-952, 1970.

116. Edwards WS: Exclusion and saphenous bypass of popliteal aneurysm. Surg Gynecol Obstet 128:829-830, 1969.

117. Leriche R: De la sympathectomie péri-artèrille et de ses resultats. Presse Med 25:513-515, 1917.

118. Leriche R: Sur une nouvelle opération sympathique (section des rameux comunicantes): Efficace dans les syndrome douloureux des membres. Lyon Med 135:449-452, 1925.

119. Diez J: Le traitement des affections trophiques et gangreneuses des membres inférieurs par la resection du sympathique lumbosacre. Rev Neurol 33:184-192, 1926.

120. Royle N: A new operative procedure in the treatment of spastic paralysis and its experimental basis. Med J Aust 1:77-86, 1924.

121. Hunter JT: The influence of the sympathetic nervous system in the genesis of rigidity in striated muscle in spastic paralysis. Surg Gynecol Obstet 39:721-743, 1924.

122. Leriche R: Des oblitérations artérielles hautes (oblitération de la terminasion de l'aorte) comme causes des insuffisances circulatoires des membres inférieures. Bull Mem Soc Chir (Paris) 49:1404-1406, 1923.

123. Leriche R: De la résèction du carrefour aortico-iliaque avec double sympathectomie lombaire pour thrombose artéritique de l'aorte. Le syndrome de l'oblitération termino-aortique par artérite. Presse Med 54-55:601-604, 1940.

124. Murphy JB: Removal of an embolus from the common iliac artery, with re-establishment of circulation in the femoral. JAMA 52:1661-1663, 1909.

125. Mosny N, Dumont MJ: Embolie fémorale au cours d'un rétrécissement mitral pur artériotomie guérison. Bull Acad Natl Med (Paris) 66:358-361, 1911.

126. Murray GDW: Heparin in thrombosis and embolism. Br J Surg 27:567-576, 1940.

127. dos Santos JC: From embolectomy to endarterectomy or the fall of a myth. Cardiovasc Surg 17:113-126, 1976.

128. dos Santos JC: Sur la désobstruction des thromboses artérielles anciennes. Mem Acad Chir 73:409-411, 1947.

129. Freeman NE, Leeds FH, Elliott WG, Roland SI: Thromboendarterectomy for hypertension due to renal artery occlusion. JAMA 156:1077-1079, 1954.

130. Freeman NE, Leeds FH: Vein inlay graft in treatment of aneurysm and thrombosis of abdominal aorta: Preliminary communication with report of 3 cases. Angiology 2:579-587, 1951.

131. Wylie EJ Jr, Kerr E, Davies O: Experimental and clinical experiences with use of fascia lata applied as a graft about major arteries after thromboendarterectomy and aneurysmorrhaphy. Surg Gynecol Obstet 93:257-272, 1951.

132. Bazy L, Hugier J, Reboul H, et al: Technique des "endartérectomies" pour artérites oblitérantes chroniques des membres inférieures, des iliaques. et de l'aorte abdominale inférieur. J Chir 65:196-210, 1949.

133. Barker WF, Cannon JA: An evaluation of endarterectomy. Arch Surg 66:488-495, 1953.

134. Cannon JA, Barker WF: Successful management of obstructive femoral arteriosclerosis by endarterectomy. Surgery 38:48-60, 1955.

135. Butcher HR Jr: A simple technique for endarterectomy. Surgery 44:984-989, 1956.

136. Vollmar J, Laubaeh K: Chirurgische Behandlung der arterielle Embolie. Ring-desobliteration der Stombahn. Munchen Med Wochenschr 107:756-763, 1965.

137. Kunlin J: Le traitement de l'ischemie artéritique par la greffe veineuse longue. Rev Chir 70:207-235, 1951.

138. Linton RH: Some practical considerations in surgery of blood vessel grafts. Surgery 38:817-834, 1955.

139. Edwards WS: Composite reconstruction of the femoral artery with saphenous vein after endarterectomy. Surg Gynecol Obstet 111:651-653, 1960.

140. Dotter CT, Judkins MP: Percutaneous transluminal treatment of arteriosclerotic obstruction. Radiology 84:631-643, 1965.

141. Gruntzig A, Hopff H: Perkutane Recanalisation chronischer arterieller Arterien-verschlusse mit einem neuen Dilatations-katheter: Modifikation der Dotter-Technik. Dtsch Med Wochenschr 99:2502-2505, 1974.

142. Greenstone SM, Shore JM, Heringman EC, Massel TB: Arterial endoscopy (arterioscopy). Arch Surg 93:811-812, 1966.

143. Simpson JB, Johnson DE, Thapliyal HV, et al: Transluminal atherectomy: A new approach to the treatment of atherosclerotic vascular disease. Circulation 72(Suppl 2):111-146, 1985.

144. Kensey KR, Nash JE, Abrahams C, Zarins CK: Recanalization of obstructed arteries with a flexible, rotating tip catheter. Radiology 165:387-389, 1987.

145. Ahn SS, Auth DC, Marcus DR, Moore SW: Removal of focal atheromatous lesions by angioscopicallv guided high-speed rotary atherectomy: Preliminary experimental observations. J Vasc Surg 7:292-300, 1988.

146. Grundfest WS, Litvack F, Forrester JS, et al: Laser ablation of human atherosclerotic plaque without adjacent tissue injury. J Am Coll Cardiol 5:929-933, 1985.

147. Murphy-Chutorian D, Kosek J, Mok W, et al: Selective absorption of ultraviolet laser energy by human atherosclerotic plaque treated with tetracycline. Am J Cardiol 55:1293-1297, 1985.

148. Abela GS, Fenech A, Crea F, Conti CR: "Hot-tip": Another method of laser vascular recanalization. Lasers Surg Med 5:327-335, 1985.

149. Palma EC: Treatment of arteritis of the lower limbs by autogenous vein grafts. Minerva Cardioangiol Eur 8:36-49, 1960.

150. McCaughan JJ Jr: Surgical exposure of the distal popliteal artery. Surgery 44:536-539, 1958.

151. McCaughan JJ Jr: Study of 100 consecutive bypass grafts of the femoral artery. Memphis Med J 35:227-237, 1960.

152. McCaughan JJ Jr: Bypass graft to the posterior tibial artery at the ankle: Case reports. Am Surg 32:126-130, 1966.
153. Morris GC Jr, DeBakey ME, Cooley DA, Crawford ES: Arterial bypass below the knee. Surg Gynecol Obstet 108:321-332, 1959.
154. Tyson RR, DeLaurentis DA: Femorotibial bypass. Circulation 33 (4 Suppl):I183-I188, 1966.
155. Hall KV: The great saphenous vein used in situ as in arterial shunt after extirpation of the vein valves. Surgery 1:492-495, 1962.
156. Leather RP, Shah DM, Karmody AM: Infrapopliteal bypass for limb salvage: Increased patency and utilization of the saphenous vein "in situ." Surgery 90:1000-1008, 1981.
157. Dardik H, Sussman B, Ibrahim IM, et al: Distal arteriovenous fistula as an adjunct to maintaining arterial graft patency for limb salvage. Surgery 94:478-486, 1983.
158. DeLaurentis DA, Friedman P: Segmental femorotibial bypass: Another approach to the inadequate saphenous vein problem. Surgery 71:400-404, 1972.
159. Veith FJ, Ascer E, Gupta SJ, et al: Tibiotibial vein bypass grafts: A new operation for limb salvage. J Vasc Surg 2:552-557, 1985.
160. Nehler MR, Dalman RL, Harris EJ: Upper extremity arterial bypass distal to the wrist. J Vasc Surg 16:633-642, 1992.
161. Oudot J, Cormier JM: La localization la plus fréquente de l'artérite segmentaire, celle de l'artère fémorale superficielle. Presse Med 61:1361-1364, 1953.
162. Martin P, Renwick S, Stephenson C: On the surgery of the profunda femoris artery: Br J Surg 55:539-542, 1968.
163. von Winiwarter F: Ueber eine eigentümliche Form von Endarteriitis und Endophlebitis mit Gangrän des Fusses. Arch Klin Chir 23:202-225, 1879.
164. Buerger L: Thromboangiitis obliterans: A study of the vascular lesions leading to presenile spontaneous gangrene. Am J Med Sci 136:567-580, 1908.
165. Fogarty TJ, Cranley JJ, Krause RJ, et al: A method of extraction of arterial emboli and thrombi. Surg Gynecol Obstet 116:241-244, 1963.
166. Mitchell SW, Morehouse GR, Keen WW: Gunshot Wounds and Other Injuries of Nerves. Philadelphia, Miller, 1864, pp 100-118.
167. Makins GH: On Gunshot Wounds to the Blood-Vessels. Bristol, England, John Wright and Sons, 1919.
168. DeBakey ME, Simeone FA: Battle injuries of the arteries in World War II. Ann Surg 12:3:534-579, 1946.
169. Jahnke EJ Jr, Howard JM: Primary repair of major arterial injuries. Arch Surg 66:646-649, 1953.
170. Hughes CW: Acute vascular trauma in Korean War casualties: An analysis of 180 cases. Surg Gynecol Obstet 99:91-100, 1954.
171. Spencer FC, Grewe RV: The management of arterial injuries in battle casualties. Ann Surg 141:304-313, 1955.
172. Whelan TJ, Burkhalter WE, Gomez CA: Management of war wounds. Adv Surg 3:227-350, 1968.
173. Rich NL, Hughes CW: Vietnam Vascular Registry: A preliminary report. Surgery 65:218-226, 1969.
174. Soubbotitich V: Military experience of traumatic aneurysms. Lancet 2:720-721, 1913.
175. Holman E: Clinical and experimental observations on arteriovenous fistulae. Ann Surg 112:840-878, 1940.
176. Savory WS: Case of a young woman in whom the main arteries of both upper extremities and of the left side of the neck were throughout completely obliterated. Med Chir Trans Lond 39:205-219, 1856.
177. Hunt JR: The role of the carotid arteries in the causation of vascular lesions of the brain with remarks on certain special features of the symptomatology. Am J Med Sci 147:704-713, 1914.
178. Fisher M: Occlusion of the internal carotid artery. Arch Neurol Pschiatry 65:346-377, 1951.
179. Fisher M: Occlusion of the carotid arteries: Further experiences. Arch Neurol Psychiatry 72:187-204, 1954.
180. Carrea R, Mullins M, Murphy G: Surgical treatment of spontaneous thrombosis of the internal carotid artery in the neck. Carotid-carotideal anastomosis: Report of a case. Acta Neurol Latinoam 1:71-78, 1955.
181. Lefèvre MH: Sur un cas de plaie du bulbe carotidien per balle, traité par la ligature de la carotid primitive et l'anastomose bout à bout de la carotid externe avec la carotid interne. Bull Mem Soc Chir 44:923-928, 1918.
182. Eastcott HHG, Pickering GW, Rob C: Reconstruction of internal carotid artery in a patient with intermittent attacks of hemiplegia. Lancet 2:994-996, 1954.
183. Cooley DA, Al-Naaman YD, Carton CA: Surgical treatment of arteriosclerotic occlusion of common carotid artery. J Neurosurg 13:500-506, 1956.
184. Roe WA: An early successful carotid endarterectomy not previously reported. Paper presented to the Southern California Vascular Surgery Society, Sept 11-12, 1992, Coronado, Calif.
185. DeBakey ME: Successful carotid endarterectomy for cerebrovascular insufficiency: Nineteen year follow-up. JAMA 233:1083-1085, 1975.
186. Yates PO, Hutchinson EC: Cerebral infarction: The role of stenosis of the extracranial arteries. Med Res Council Spec Rep (Lond) 300:1-95, 1961.
187. Whisnant JP, Matsumoto N, Eleback LR: Transient cerebral ischemic attacks in a community: Rochester, Minnesota, 1955 through 1969. Mayo Clin Proc 48:194-198, 1973.
188. Hollenhorst RW: Significance of bright plaques in the retinal arterioles. JAMA 178:23-29, 1961.
189. Julian OC, Dye WS, Javid H, Hunter JA: Ulcerative lesions of the carotid artery bifurcation. Arch Surg 86:803-809, 1963.
190. Moore WS, Hall AD: Ulcerated atheroma of the carotid artery: A cause of transient cerebral ischemia. Am J Surg 116:237-242, 1968.
191. Imparato AM, Riles TJ, Gorstein F: The carotid bifurcation plaque: Pathologic findings associated with cerebral ischemia. Stroke 10:238-245, 1975.
192. Lusby RJ, Ferrell LD, Ehrenfeld WA, et al: Carotid plaque hemorrhage: Its role in production of cerebral ischemia. Arch Surg 117:1479-1488, 1982.
193. Moore WS, Hall AD: Carotid artery back pressure: A test of cerebral tolerance to temporary carotid artery occlusion. Arch Surg 99:702-710, 1969.
194. Thompson JE, Patman RD, Talkington CM: Asymptomatic carotid bruit. Ann Surg 188:308-316, 1978.
195. Dixon S, Pais SO, Raviola C, et al: Natural history of nonstenotic, asymptomatic ulcerations of the carotid artery: A further analysis. Arch Surg 117:1493-1498, 1982.
196. Berguer R, Sieggreen MY, Lazo VA, Hodakowski CT: The silent brain infarct in carotid surgery. J Vasc Surg 3:442-447, 1986.
197. Moore WS: Indications for carotid endarterectomy: Results of randomized trials. Paper presented at the 29th Annual Meeting, "Controversial Areas in General Surgery," UCLA Extension Program, April 2, 1992, Palm Springs, Calif.
198. Yasargil MG, Krayenbuhl HA, Jacobson JH II: Microneurosurgical arterial reconstruction. Surgery 67:221-223, 1970.
199. EC/IC Bypass Group: Failure of extracranial-intracranial bypass to reduce the risk of ischemic stroke: Results of an international randomized trial. N Engl J Med 313:1191-1200, 1985.
200. Longmire WP Jr, Cannon JA, Kattus HA: Direct-vision coronary endarterectomy for angina pectoris. N Engl J Med 259:993-999, 1958.
201. Favoloro RG: Saphenous vein autograft replacement of severe segmental coronary artery occlusion. Ann Thorac Surg 5:334-339, 1968.
202. Johnson WD, Flemma RJ, Lepley D Jr, et al: Extended treatment of severe coronary artery disease: A total surgical approach Ann Surg 170:460-470, 1969.
203. Goldblatt H, Lynch J, Hanzal RF, et al: Studies on experimental hypertension. J Exp Med 59:347-379, 1934.
204. DeCamp P, Snyder CH, Bost RB: Severe hypertension due to congenital stenosis of artery to solitary kidney: Correction by splenorenal anastomosis. Arch Surg 75:1026-1030, 1957.
205. Poutasse EF: Surgical treatment of renal hypertension: Results in patients with occlusive lesions of renal arteries. J Urol 82:403-411, 1959.
206. Foster JH, Dean RH, Pinkerton JA, et al: Ten years' experience with renovascular hypertension Ann Surg 177:755-766, 1973.
207. Connett MC, Lansche JM: Fibromuscular hyperplasia of the internal carotid artery: Report of a case. Ann Surg 162:59-62, 1965.
208. Ehrenfeld WK, Stoney RJ, Wylie EJ: Fibromuscular hyperplasia of the internal carotid artery. Arch Surg 95:284-287, 1967.
209. Dunphy JE: Abdominal pain of vascular origin. Am J Med Sci 92:109-113, 1936.
210. Klass J: Embolectomy in acute mesenteric occlusion. Ann Surg 34:913-917, 1951.
211. Shaw RS, Rutledge RH: Superior-mesenteric-artery embolectomy in treatment of massive mesenteric infarction. N Engl J Med 257:595-598, 1957.

212. Shaw RS, Maynard EP: Acute and chronic thrombosis of the mesenteric arteries associated with malabsorption: Report of two cases successfully treated by thromboendarterectomy. N Engl J Med 258:874-878, 1958.

213. Mikkelsen WP, Zaro JA: Intestinal angina: Report of a case with preoperative diagnosis and surgical relief. N Engl J Med 260:912-914, 1959.

214. Kountz SL, Laub DR, Connolly JE: "Aortoiliac steal" syndrome. Arch Surg 92:490-497, 1966.

215. Heer FW, Silen W, French WS: Intestinal gangrene without apparent vascular occlusion. Am J Surg 110:231-238, 1965.

216. Marable SA, Molnar E, Beman FJ: Abdominal pains secondary to celiac axis compressions. Am J Surg 111:493-495, 1966.

217. Szilagyi DE, Rion RL, Elliott JP, et al: The celiac axis compression syndrome: Does it exist? Surgery 72:849-863, 1972.

218. Blaisdell FW, DeMattei GA, Gauder PJ: Extraperitoneal thoracic aorta to femoral bypass graft as replacement for an infected aortic bifurcation prosthesis. Am J Surg 102:583-585, 1961.

219. Blaisdell FW, Hall AD: Axillary-femoral artery bypass for lower extremity ischemia. Surgery 54:563-568, 1963.

220. Mahoney WD, Whelan TJ: Use of obturator foramen in ileofemoral artery grafting: Case reports. Ann Surg 163:215-220, 1966.

221. Vetto RM: The treatment of unilateral iliac artery obstruction with a transabdominal subcutaneous femorofemoral graft. Surgery 52:342-345, 1962.

222. Elliott JP, Smith RF, Szilagyi DE: Aorto-enteric and paraprosthetic-enteric fistulas: Problems of diagnosis and management. Arch Surg 108:479-490, 1974.

223. Busuttil RW, Rees W, Baker JD, et al: Pathogenesis of aortoduodenal fistula. Surgery 85:1-13, 1979.

224. Trendelenburg F: Beiträge zur klinische Chirurgie, vol 7. Tübingen, Germany, 1890.

225. Trendelenburg F: Ueber die operative Unterbindung der Vena saphena magna bei Unterschenkelvaricen. Beitr Klin Chir 7:195-210, 1890.

226. Homans J: The etiology and treatment of varicose ulcer of the leg. Surg Gynecol Obstet 24:300-311, 1917.

227. Babcock WW: A new operation for the extirpation of varicose veins. N Y Med 86:153-156, 1907.

228. Mayo CH: The surgical treatment of varicose veins. St Paul Med J 6:695-699, 1904.

229. Trendelenburg F: Ueber die operative Behandlung der Embolie der Lungenarterie. Arch Klin Chir 86:686-700, 1908.

230. Greenfield LJ, Proctor MC, Williams DM, et al: Long-term experience with transvenous catheter pulmonary embolectomy. J Vasc Surg 18:450-458, 1993.

231. Homans J: Thrombosis of the deep veins of the lower leg causing pulmonary embolism. N Engl J Med 211:993-997, 1934.

232. Homans J: Venous thrombosis in the lower extremity: Its relation to pulmonary embolism. Am J Surg 38:316-326, 1937.

233. Homans J: Deep quiet thrombosis in the lower limbs: Preferred levels for interruption of the veins: Iliac section or ligation. Surg Gynecol Obstet 79:70-82, 1944.

234. Allen AW: Management of thromboembolic disease in surgical patients. Surg Gynecol Obstet 96:107-114, 1953.

235. Veal JR: Prevention of pulmonary complications in high ligation of the femoral vein. JAMA 121:240-244, 1943.

236. Northway O, Buxton RW: Ligation of the inferior vena cava. Surgery 18:85-94, 1945.

237. O'Neill EE: Ligation of the inferior vena cava in the prevention and treatment of pulmonary embolism. N Engl J Med 232:641-646, 1945.

238. Collins CG, Jones JR, Nelson WE: Surgical treatment of pelvic thrombophlebitis. New Orleans Med Surg J 95:324-329, 1943.

239. Anlyan WG, Campbell FH, Shingleton WW, et al: Pulmonary embolism following venous ligation. Arch Surg 64:200-207, 1952.

240. Bowers RF, Leb SM: Late results of inferior vena cava ligation. Surgery 37:622-628, 1955.

241. Conti S, Daschbach M, Blaisdell FW: A comparison of high-dose versus conventional-dose heparin therapy for deep vein thrombosis. Surgery 92:972-980, 1982.

242. Barker WF, Mandiola S: Postphlebitic syndrome after vena caval interruption. In Foley WT (ed): Advances in the Management of Cardiovascular Disease. Chicago, Year Book, 1980, pp 31-42.

243. Spencer PC: Plication of the inferior vena cava for pulmonary embolism. Surgery 62:388-392, 1967.

244. Moretz WH, Rhode CM, Shepherd MH, et al: Prevention of pulmonary emboli by partial occlusion of the inferior vena cava. Am Surg 25:617-626, 1959.

245. Miles EM, Richardson RR, Wayne L, et al: Long-term results with the serrated Teflon vena cava clip in the prevention of pulmonary embolism. Ann Surg 169:881-891, 1969.

246. Adams JT, DeWeese JA: Partial interruption of the inferior vena cava—a new plastic clip. Surg Gynecol Obstet 124:1087-1088, 1966.

247. Mobin-Uddin K, Smith PE, Martinez ID, et al. A vena cava filter for the prevention of pulmonary embolus. Surg Forum 18:209-211, 1967.

248. Greenfield LJ, Peyton MD, Brown PP, et al: Transvenous management of pulmonary embolic disease. Ann Surg 180:461-468, 1974.

249. Homans J: The late results of femoral thrombophlebitis and their treatment. N Engl J Med 235:249-253, 1946.

250. Trout H: Ulcers due to varicose veins and lymphatic blockage. W V Med J 34:54-60, 1938.

251. Linton RE: The communicating veins of the lower leg and the technique for their ligation. Ann Surg 107:582-593, 1938.

252. Dodd K, Cockett FB: The Pathology and Surgery of the Veins of the Lower Limb. Edinburgh, E & S Livingstone, 1956.

253. Kistner RL: Surgical repair of the incompetent vein valve. Arch Surg 110:1336-1342, 1975.

254. Dale WA: Venous crossover grafts for the relief of iliofemoral venous block. Surgery 57:608-612, 1970.

255. Palma EC, Esperoti R: Vein transplants and grafts in the surgical treatment of the postphlebitic syndrome. J Cardiovasc Surg 1:94-107, 1960.

256. Taheri SA, Lazar L, Elias S, et al: Surgical treatment of postphlebitic syndrome with vein valve transplant. Am J Surg 144:221-224, 1982.

257. Taheri SA, Rigan D, West P, et al: Experimental prosthetic vein valve. Am J Surg 156:111-114, 1988.

258. Brooks B: Intra-arterial injection of sodium iodide. JAMA 82:1016-1019, 1924.

259. Moniz E: L'encéphalographie artérielle, son importance dans la localization des tumeurs cérébrales. Rev Neurol (Paris) 2:72-90, 1927.

260. dos Santos R, Lamas A, Caldas P: L'artériographie des membres, de l'aorte et des ses branches abdominales. Bull Mem Soc Natl Chir 55:587-601, 1929.

261. Seldinger SI: Catheter replacement of the needle in percutaneous angiography. Acta Radiol 39:368-376, 1953.

262. Erlanger J: Blood pressure estimations by indirect methods. I. The mechanisms of the oscillatory criteria. Am J Physiol 40:82-125, 1916.

263. Winsor T: Pressure gradients: Influence of arterial disease on the systolic blood pressure gradients of the extremity. Am J Med Sci 220:117-126, 1950.

264. Pachon V: Sur la méthode des oscillations et les conditons correctes de son emploi en sphygmomanométrie clinique. C R Soc Biol (Paris) 66:733-735, 1909.

265. Edwards EA, Levine HD: Peripheral vascular murmurs: Mechanisms of production and diagnostic significance. Arch Intern Med 90:284-300, 1952.

266. Wylie EJ, McGuiness JS: The recognition and treatment of arteriosclerotic stenosis of major arteries. Surg Gynecol Obstet 97:425-433, 1953.

267. Baillart P: La pression artérielle dans les branches de l'artère centrale de la retine: Nouvelle technique pour la determiner. Ann Occul 154:648-666, 1917.

268. Kartchner MM, McRae LP, Morrison FD: Noninvasive detection and evaluation of carotid occlusive disease. Arch Surg 106:528-535, 1973.

269. Gee WG, Mehigan JI, Wylie EJ: Measurement of collateral cerebral hemispheric blood pressure by ocular pneumoplethysmography. Am J Surg 130:121-127, 1975.

270. Leopold CG, Goldberger LE, Bernstein EF: Ultrasonic detection and evaluation of abdominal aortic aneurysm. Surgery 72:939-945, 1972.

271. Brockenbrough EC: Screening for Prevention of Stroke: Use of a Doppler Flow Meter. Seattle, Washington/Alaska Regional Medical Program, Information and Education Resource Unit, 1969.

272. Machleder HI, Barker WF: The stroke on the wrong side: Use of the Doppler ophthalmic test in cerebrovascular screening. Arch Surg 105:943-947, 1972.

273. Thomas GI, Spencer MD, Jones TW, et al: Non-invasive carotid bifurcation mapping: Its relation to carotid Surgery. Am J Surg 128:168-174, 1974.

274. Strandness DE, Schultz RD, Sumner DS, et al: Ultrasonic flow detection: A useful technique in the evaluation of peripheral vascular disease. Am J Surg 113:311-320, 1967.

275. Sumner DS, Strandness DE Jr: The relationship between calf blood flow and ankle blood pressure in patients with intermittent claudication. Surgery 65:763-771, 1969.

276. Barber FE, Baker DW, Arthur CW, et al: Ultrasonic duplex echo-Doppler scanner. IEEE Trans Biomed Eng 21:109-113, 1974.

277. Bendick PJ, Jackson VP: Evaluation of vertebral arteries by duplex sonography. J Vasc Surg 3:523-530, 1986.

278. Jager K, Bollinger A, Valli C, Amman H: Measurement of mesenteric blood flow by duplex scanning. J Vasc Surg 3:462-469, 1986.

279. Flanigan DP, Douglas DJ, Machi J, et al: Intraoperative ultrasonic imaging of the carotid artery during carotid endarterectomy. Surgery 100:893-899, 1986.

280. Lindegaard KF, Bakke SJ, Grolimund P, et al: Assessment of intracranial hemodynamics in carotid artery by transcranial Doppler ultrasound. J Neurosurg 63:890-898, 1985.

281. Kalender WA, Seissler W, Klotz E, Vock F: Spiral volumetric CT with single-breath-hold technique, continuous transport and continuous scanner rotation. Radiology 176:181-190, 1990.

282. Hoch JR, Tullis MJ, Kennell TW, et al: Use of magnetic resonance angiography for the preoperative evaluation of patients with infrainguinal arterial occlusive disease. J Vasc Surg 23:792-801, 1996.

283. Cranley JJ, Canos JJ, Sull WF, et al: Phleborheographic technique for diagnosing deep venous thrombosis of the lower extremities. Surg Gynecol Obstet 141:331-339, 1975.

284. Wheeler MB, Pearson D, O'Connell D: Impedance plethysmography: Technique, interpretation and results Arch Surg 104:164-169, 1972.

285. Comerota AJ, Katz ML, Greenwald L, et al: Should venous duplex imaging replace hemodynamic tests? J Vasc Surg 11:53-61, 1990.

286. Kolff WJ: First clinical experience with the artificial kidney. Ann Intern Med 62:608-619, 1965.

287. Quinton WE, Dillard DH, Scribner BH: Cannulation of blood vessels for prolonged hemodialysis. Am Soc Artif Int Org 6:104-113, 1960.

288. Brescia MJ, Cimino JE, Appel F, Hurvich BL: Chronic hemodialysis using venipuncture and surgically created arteriovenous fistula. N Engl J Med 275:1089-1092, 1966.

289. May J, Tiller D, Johnson J, Sheil AGR: Saphenous-vein arteriovenous fistula in regular dialysis treatment. N Engl J Med 280:770, 1969.

290. Haimov M, Burrows L, Baez A, et al: Alternatives for vascular access for hemodialysis: Experience with autogenous vein autografts and bovine heterografts. Surgery 75:447-452, 1974.

291. Coote H: Exostosis of the left transverse process of the seventh cervical vertebra, surrounded by blood vessels and nerves; successful removal. Lancet 1:360-361, 1861.

292. Murphy JB: A case of cervical rib with symptoms resembling subclavian aneurysm. Ann Surg 41:399-406, 1905.

293. Adson AW, Coffey JR: Cervical rib: A method of anterior approach for relief of symptoms by division of the scalenus anticus. Ann Surg 85:839-857, 1927.

294. Ochsner A, Gage M, DeBakey ME: Scalenus anticus (Naffziger) syndrome. Am J Surg 28:669-693, 1935.

295. Naffziger HC, Grant WT: Neuritis of the brachial plexus mechanical in origin. Surg Gynecol Obstet 67:722-730, 1938.

296. Roos DB: Transaxillary approach for the first rib resection to relieve thoracic outlet syndrome. Ann Surg 163:354-358, 1966.

297. Falconer MA, Li FWP: Resection of the first rib in costoclavicular compression of the brachial plexus. Lancet 1:59-63, 1962.

298. Edwards E: Anatomic and clinical comments on shoulder girdle syndromes. In Barker WF: Surgical Treatment of Peripheral Vascular Disease. New York, McGraw-Hill, 1962, pp 111-131.

299. McLeery RS, Kesterson JE, Kirtley JA, Love, RB: Subclavius and anterior scalene muscle compression as a cause of intermittent obstruction of the subclavian vein. Ann Surg 133:588-601, 1951.

Questions

1. **Implantation of a small artery into the side of a larger one by the patch technique was described by whom?**
   (a) Linton
   (b) W. Hunter
   (c) DeBakey
   (d) Carrel
   (e) Hufnagel

2. **The first treatment of arterial obstruction in the leg by an endarterial approach was reported by whom?**
   (a) Homans
   (b) Cannon
   (c) Wylie
   (d) Dotter
   (e) Leriche

3. **The chronic burning pain described by Mitchell is known as what?**
   (a) Artérite
   (b) Thromboangiitis
   (c) Causalgia
   (d) Peripheral neuritis
   (e) Postherpetic neuralgia

4. **The first successful coronary artery reconstruction for angina was performed by whom?**
   (a) May
   (b) DeBakey and Cooley
   (c) Cooley and Morris
   (d) Edwards and Lyons
   (e) Longmire and Cannon

5. **Who is commonly credited with interrupting major draining veins in the leg to treat deep venous thrombosis?**
   (a) Holman
   (b) Hall
   (c) Homans
   (d) Allen
   (e) Trendelenburg

6. **The duplex scan was introduced to evaluate what?**
   (a) Flow in the venous system
   (b) Carotid stenosis
   (c) Size and progression of abdominal aneurysms
   (d) Raynaud's syndrome
   (e) Pulmonary embolism

7. **The possibility of an "extra-anatomic" bypass of an obstructed artery was first proposed by _____ and carried out by _____.**
   (a) J. Hunter and Cooper
   (b) Wylie and Moore
   (c) DeBakey and Morris
   (d) Kunlin and Oudot
   (e) Linton and Darling

8. **John Hunter's famous operation to cure popliteal aneurysm consisted of what?**
   (a) Ligation of the popliteal artery above and below the aneurysm
   (b) Sympathectomy and excision of the aneurysm
   (c) Sympathectomy and ligation of the common femoral artery
   (d) Sympathectomy and external compression (using the Massachusetts General compressor) of the popliteal artery
   (e) Ligation of the "superficial" femoral artery in the subsartorial region

9. **Murray's introduction of heparin to clinical use led which surgeon to attempt delayed arterial embolectomy?**
   (a) Homans
   (b) Osler
   (c) Kunlin
   (d) J. dos Santos
   (e) Matas

10. **Although not described in the exact words, the principle behind the concept of "endoleaks" following operation for aneurysm was described by whom?**
   (a) Vesalius
   (b) J. Hunter
   (c) Holman
   (d) Matas
   (e) Parodi

Answers

1. d	2. d	3. c	4. e	5. c
6. a	7. d	8. e	9. d	10. d

2

David S. Maxwell*

Embryology of the Vascular System

It is quite evident that the vascular apparatus does not independently and by itself "unfold" into the adult pattern. On the contrary, it reacts continuously in a most sensitive way to the factors of its environment, the pattern in the adult being the result of the sum of the environmental influences that have played upon it throughout the embryonic period. We thus find that this apparatus is continuously adequate and complete for the structures as they exist at any particular stage as the environmental structures progressively change; the vascular apparatus also changes and thereby is always adapted to the newer conditions. Furthermore, there are no apparent ulterior preparations at any time for the supply and drainage of other structures which have not yet made their appearance. For each stage it is an efficient and complete going-mechanism, apparently uninfluenced by the nature of its subsequent morphology.

GEORGE L. STREETER (1918)

This observation made more than 80 years ago exemplifies the finest tradition of the working scientist: years of attention to the most minute details of a subject, which eventuate in the broadest and most comprehensive view of the fundamental issues. In this statement, Streeter summarizes all that needs to be said and virtually all that can be said about the development of the vascular system, save for some specific details that would only embellish the theme he has laid out.

The story of the development of the vascular system encompasses the life span of the organism. This system retains the ability to grow, change, regenerate, and add on in response to the changing needs of the tissues, from the earliest stages of embryonic life to the final breath. Thus, it supports normal growth, wound healing, and revascularization of tissues endangered by restricted flow in existing vessels, just as it supports the new growth of tumors and transiently develops a highly efficient transport and exchange system through the uteroplacental circulation during pregnancy. All this is accomplished by the opening and enlargement of preexisting vessels and the budding of new vascular growth from preexisting

stem vessels. That it may eventually fail to respond to adequately supply the myocardium or the central nervous system is not as remarkable as the fact that it responds so well for so long. It seems likely that in the embryonic and fetal history of the vascular system there would be clues to the mysteries that surround this responsiveness throughout life. Further, in the prenatal unfolding of the vascular system lie the origins of the various cardiovascular malformations to which the human organism is subject. We do not yet know whether the mechanisms of growth and the stimuli to vascularization of the embryo and fetus are the same as those that encourage and sustain the responsiveness of the vasculature in the postnatal organism.

In this chapter, I do not attempt to review the enormous literature on the subject, and I omit many exciting details in the interest of providing a simple narrative exposition of the high points. The organizational scheme takes us first to a short history of the heart, which is simply a greatly modified blood vessel, followed by descriptions of the development of the large arteries and veins. I conclude with some comments on the growth of small vessels, which, like acorns, must appear and flourish first to produce the mighty trunk and branches of the vascular tree.

Early History

An organism of a cubic millimeter or so in volume (depending on the surface area and other factors related to the effectiveness of diffusion) may thrive without a vascular system. The human embryo enjoys the elaboration of a vascular system from its earliest stages, almost as if it can anticipate that its bulk will soon require a highly sophisticated transport system. As the embryonic disk becomes recognizable, blood islands rapidly accumulate around the periphery of the disk. These isolated "puddles" begin to coalesce and communicate with one another until the embryo resembles a bloody sponge. Most prominent is the precephalic region, where the seemingly random coalescence of blood islands forms a network in the region soon to be identified as the *cardiogenic plate* (Fig. 2-1A).

In these earliest stages of development, the vascular system manifests some of its greatest mysteries: to what extent is the developmental pattern dictated by tissue needs and demands (possibly through the release of angiogenic factors

*Deceased

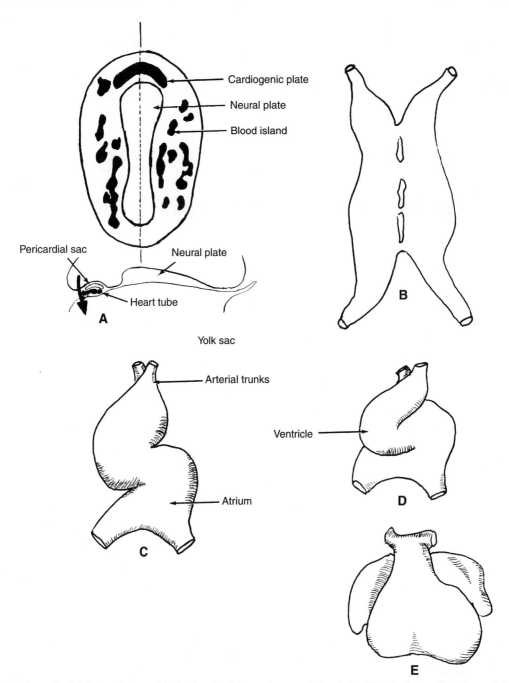

FIGURE 2-1 • *A*, Embryonic disk from above, with the head of the embryo up. The *dotted line* indicates the plane of the longitudinal section below, with the cranial end to the left. In the section, the pericardial sac is above the heart tube, but as the head folds under the forebrain (direction of the *large arrow*), the positions of the heart and sac will be reversed, with the heart invaginating from above the pericardial sac. *B,* The two parallel primitive heart tubes (dorsal view) fuse in the midline to form a single heart tube and a single-chambered heart. *C* to *E,* Successive stages of the folding of the heart tube, viewed from the front. The venous end of the tube swings posteriorly to form the atria, whereas the arterial end (ventricles) remains anterior. This represents the loop stage.[1] (Adapted from Moore KL: The Developing Human, 3rd ed. Philadelphia, WB Saunders, 1982; and Rushmer RF: Cardiovascular Dynamics, 2nd ed. Philadelphia, WB Saunders, 1961.)

or through stimuli provided by metabolic products), and to what extent is it dictated by factors such as extravascular pressures restricting flow in one set of possible blood channels and forcing the enlargement of adjacent alternative routes of blood flow? To what extent is the overall pattern dictated genetically? The *similarity* of the vascular tree from one individual to another favors the speculation that there is a detailed genetic code. The *variability* from one to another—each

pattern seemingly equally efficient in supporting tissues and organs—argues for development according to need and use and based on mechanical and other adventitious factors.

In the case of the heart, a detailed genetic code is surely the guiding factor. Here, curiously, we begin with a parallel pair of cardiac tubes that fuse into one large tube; the latter then divides internally into the right and left hearts. At first glance, this seems inefficient; why not simply have each original tube of the pair form a right or left heart? The reason is clear when we examine the details of internal division of the heart, in which the single outflow tract is divided in such a way as to connect the right heart to the primitive vessels supplying the pulmonary circuit and to connect the remaining members of the branchial arch arteries to the left heart.

Heart

Our interest in the development of the heart in this chapter is restricted to its bearing on the origins of the great vessels. The heart is simply a highly modified artery from both histologic and embryologic viewpoints. Histologically, it resembles a muscular artery because it has three layers to its walls: adventitia (epicardium), tunica media (myocardium), and tunica intima (endocardium). At the beginning, the heart tubes are simply a parallel pair of vessels, seemingly little different from the other components of the random network of primitive blood vessels. Nonetheless, the fusion of these two tubes and the development of a feeble myocardial investment around the endothelium quickly lead to irregular contractions of the musculature, with feeble and inefficient ejection of blood. Subsequent events include the development of septa, dividing the single-chambered heart into right and left halves, and the appearance of valves that dictate unidirectional flow. The heart is beating with increasing regularity and with an efficiency-improving peristalsis and force as the myocardial element thickens and cytodifferentiates. Presumably from these first feeble, sporadic beats there is a stirring of the blood contents of the primitive vessels, perhaps providing some benefit to the growing tissues around them and perhaps beginning to stimulate the enlargement of those channels that will survive into later embryonic stages. Beginning to channel blood through preferred pathways leads to closure and disappearance of less satisfactory routes and enlargement of the more successful channels into definitive blood vessels that are soon worthy of names recognizable in terms of the adult circulatory pattern. Channel formation from blood islands might be influenced simply by the choice of the lowest resistance among the available pathways.

The now-fused heart tube (Fig. 2-1B) begins to invaginate the presumptive pericardial cavity, acquiring its visceral and parietal layers of pericardium while still a single-chambered heart configured as a simple, relatively straight tube. As the somites begin to appear in the neck and trunk region, the heart tube begins to fold on itself, first bulging ventrally, further invaginating the pericardial sac. The heart that is now swinging ventrocaudally comes to lie in front of the head and will continue its descent down the front of the neck and into the anterior chest. The ventrally directed bulge created by the U-shaped fold of the heart characterizes the loop stage.[1] The ventral limb of the U is the arterial outflow path, and the dorsal limb of the U will become the venous inflow tract (Fig. 2-1C through E). By the 10-somite stage, approximately 3 weeks' ovulation age, the heart has begun to fold in a coronal plane as well, directing the ventricular region to the left and forming a recognizable outflow tract, now termed the bulbus cordis, whose distal part is called the truncus arteriosus (see Fig. 2-1C). At this stage, the heart is still a single-chambered structure innocent of valves but completely enclosed in a pericardial sac and demonstrably beating, albeit irregularly. There is no single primordium, no segment of the primitive heart tube, that can be identified as leading to a specific cardiac cavity in the early postloop stage. Instead, there are microscopically and experimentally identifiable zones, each of which gives rise to a specific anatomic region of a definitive "cardiac cavity." These primordia are most accurately termed *primitive cardiac regions;* thus, referring to segments of the heart tube as forerunners of the chambers of the fully formed heart is misleading.[1] The folds in the heart tube and the peristaltic nature of myocardial contraction lead to a predetermined direction of flow out through the bulbus cordis, the folds acting as inefficient "valves" to direct the flow. Such early vitality is not surprising, because the cardiovascular system is the earliest to attain form and function among the organ systems of the body. The heart is disproportionately large for the size of the embryo at this stage, and this disproportion remains until birth, with only a modest decline in heart-body ratio toward birth. Obviously, this is due to the fact that the heart must support not only the growing tissue of the organism but also the embryo's share of the enormous placental circulation.

It is worth digressing here to emphasize the functional problems faced by the developing heart. It is required to form and to function in such a way as to maintain and support the growth of the developing organism in an intrauterine (aquatic) environment; that is, it must support an organism incapable of independent gas exchange and dependent on the placenta for oxygen and nutriments and for other metabolic exchange. The lungs are developed rather late and require only to be supplied with enough blood to support their growth. To perfuse the embryonic lungs with a rate of blood flow commensurate with an air-breathing existence would be energetically inefficient and perhaps an impediment to their growth and development, but during the early stages of development of the cardiovascular system, the lungs are simply not sufficiently developed to be called anything other than buds, volumetrically incapable of containing any significant quantity of blood. So the heart must develop a mechanism whereby it can support the organism in an aquatic environment with extensive exchange across the placenta and provide adequate distribution of blood throughout the growing body of the embryo; yet it must simultaneously develop a configuration that will enable it to shift its mode of function instantly at birth to support the organism by way of pulmonary gas exchange. Simply put, in fetal and embryonic life, the two sides of the heart function as two pumps operating "in parallel," with the output of both ventricles distributed to the placenta and to the growing tissues of the body, and with no interdependence of the output. Yet the two hearts must have the means to shift from functioning "in parallel" to functioning "in tandem" at birth, wherein the outflow of one heart becomes the inflow of the other, and blood is obligated to perfuse the pulmonary circuit, return to the heart, and then perfuse the systemic circuit, and so on. One emphasis of this chapter is to focus on the development of features that render the heart capable of these sequential and different modes of function.

Arteries

During the early folding of the heart, and with identification of a bulbus cordis and truncus arteriosus as an outflow tract, the aortic arches are beginning to form. The truncus arteriosus is continuous with a ventral aorta. This large, single-channeled artery is connected to a pair of dorsal aortas through a series of branchial (pharyngeal) arch arteries. The developing pharynx passes through a period in its development when it is said to mimic the development of the gill apparatus of fish. Outpouchings of the pharyngeal wall grow as pockets toward the surface, where they are met or at least approached by corresponding infoldings of the ectodermal surface. Normally, these outpouchings and infoldings neither meet nor coalesce to form gill slits or fistulas. The supporting tissue on both sides of the pouches is endowed with a cartilaginous supporting bar, a nerve, and a blood vessel, respectively known as the branchial arch (pharyngeal) cartilage, branchial arch nerve, and branchial arch artery. The first such cartilaginous bar is Meckel's cartilage, in front of the first pharyngeal pouch; the second, Reichert's cartilage, lies between the first and second pouches, and so on. The pharynx is supported by six arch complexes, surrounding and intervening between the pharyngeal pouches. The arteries of these arches are the connectives from the ventral aorta to the dorsal aortas, and they appear in sequence from cranial to caudal. Rarely are more than three such arch arteries identifiable at one time; in this case, as elsewhere in the embryo, the cranial development leads or precedes that occurring more caudally. As the fourth arch artery appears, the first is being transformed into its successor structures and ceases to be identifiable as an arch artery. In humans, there are five such arch arteries, numbered 1, 2, 3, 4, and 6, in recognition of the dropping out in phylogeny of the fifth arch artery, which plays no significant role in human development (the fifth pharyngeal pouch fuses with the fourth at its opening into the pharynx; its rudimentary arch between the fourth and fifth pouches contributes to the formation of the larynx). In contrast to the constancy of innervation of the derivatives of the pharyngeal arches, the vascular supply to the arches is subject to later, often extensive modification. The motor nerve to an arch persists throughout phylogeny and throughout ontogenetic development in supplying the derivatives of that arch (first arch, mandibular nerve; second arch, facial nerve; third arch, glossopharyngeal nerve; fourth through sixth arches, recurrent and superior laryngeal nerves and vagal pharyngeal nerve). The geometric representation of the arch artery pattern and the fate of those arteries are summarized in Figure 2-2. The paired dorsal aortas sweep posteriorly and fuse in the midline to form a single dorsal aorta (see Fig. 2-2 inset) posterior to entry points of the arch arteries.

The lungs begin their development as a ventrally directed outgrowth from the pharynx, and the single tube that will become the trachea descends into the presumptive chest cavity, where it branches into a pair of lung buds. These buds from the beginning receive a small blood supply from branches of the sixth aortic arch arteries (see Fig. 2-2A). Clearly, the sixth arch arteries will play a role in the development of the pulmonary arterial tree. The developmental problem posed here is that the sixth arch arteries are initially part of the systemic circulation, simply representing the caudalmost of the branchial arch arteries springing from the truncus arteriosus and uniting with the dorsal aortas. In the division of the heart tube into right and left hearts, some provision must be made for joining the right ventricular outflow tract to the sixth arch arteries and joining the remainder of the great branchial arch system and aortas with

the left ventricle. The rationale for fusion of the primitive heart tubes into a single channel and subsequent division is now clarified by this need to divide the bulbus cordis and truncus arteriosus into a pulmonary artery and an aortic artery. The manner of that division solves the problem of connecting the right ventricle and the developing pulmonary artery to the lungs and connecting the remainder of the arch arteries to the systemic circulation and the left ventricle. The interested reader is encouraged to examine the beautifully illustrated paper of Congdon[2] for further clarification of this point.

We now turn to the division of the heart into four chambers that make up two separate hearts, with provision for a parallel mode of function before birth and a tandem mode after birth. The umbilical veins (after the sixth week, a single left umbilical vein) return blood to the fetal heart by their union with the inferior vena cava. This return route sees the umbilical vein enter the liver, where a shunt, the ductus venosus, bypasses the complex hepatic circulation and shunts the blood directly into the inferior vena cava. Thus, the right atrium receives a supply of freshly oxygenated blood, in contrast to the adult condition. Before separation of the right and left atria, that placental return is into the single atrial chamber, which is diagrammatically depicted in Figure 2-3A. The single chamber undergoes a constriction in the plane of the atrioventricular orifices (and the atrioventricular sulcus on the exterior of the heart). From the margins of this constriction, endocardial cushions grow inward to begin the formation of the tricuspid and mitral valves. The single atrium begins its separation into two halves by downgrowth from the dorsocranial wall of a filmy crescentic curtain, the septum primum (Fig. 2-3B). The leading invaginated edge of the crescent grows down toward the floor of the single atrium; that floor forms by virtue of the growth of the atrioventricular valve primordia. Figure 2-3B shows the septum primum from the right side as it progresses toward complete closure of the single atrial chamber in its midline, and we see that just before the foramen primum closes, a group of perforations forms in the dorsocranial part of the partition (see Fig. 2-3B) and then coalesces into a foramen secundum (Fig. 2-3C). This is necessary because throughout this developmental sequence, the heart is pumping blood to and returning it from the placenta, and the returning blood must be shunted from the right side of the heart into the left atrium in large volume to sustain the systemic circulation. *Thus, at no point in fetal life may the right and left atria be functionally separate.* During the time the placental circulation is intact, the pressure in the right atrium exceeds that in the left atrium, and a right-to-left shunt will be operative. Thus, the foramen secundum opens just in time to continue that shunt as the foramen primum closes. Now, on the right side of the septum primum, a much more robust and rigid septum secundum begins its downgrowth, following the same pattern as that of the septum primum (see Fig. 2-3C); a crescent-shaped leading edge grows down from above toward the endocardial cushions that will finally separate the atria from the ventricles. This downgrowth of the septum secundum comes to overlie the orifice of the foramen secundum. Fortunately, the septum secundum is sturdy and relatively unyielding, whereas the septum primum is thin and curtain-like. As long as the free lower edge of the septum secundum fails to reach the floor of the atrium, thus forming the foramen ovale, the elevated pressure in the right

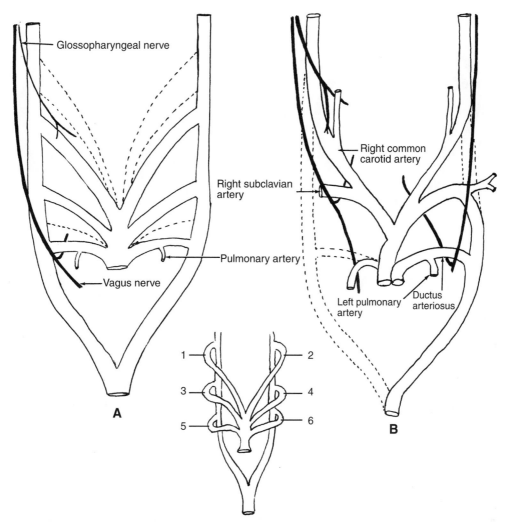

FIGURE 2–2 • Fate of the branchial arch arteries. *A,* Primitive arrangement of six arch arteries. Arches 1 and 2 have formed and have been accommodated into the vessels of the head (*dotted lines* indicate arteries that are no longer arches—that is, 1, 2, and 5). Arches 3, 4, and 6 connect the ventral aorta (aortic sac and truncus arteriosus) with the paired dorsal aortas. The latter fuse posteriorly to form a single dorsal aorta. *B,* Subsequent disposition of these vessels. The *dotted lines* indicate vessels that normally disappear, including the right sixth arch beyond the right pulmonary artery. The glossopharyngeal nerve (motor to the third arch) and the recurrent laryngeal nerve (motor to the sixth arch derivatives) are shown. The recurrent laryngeal nerve is a branch of the vagus "recurring" around the sixth arch in *A;* in *B,* these nerves recur around the ductus arteriosus and around the right subclavian. *Inset,* The first three aortic arch arteries from the front (ventral) view during the branchial period (at no time are all arch arteries evident at the same time). The paired dorsal aortas unite into a single dorsal aorta posterior to the entry of the arch arteries. The postbranchial period, when the heart descends from the branchial region into the chest, is characterized by modification of the arch system into the adult disposition of the derived arteries.

atrium pushes blood through the ovale, deflecting the septum primum and allowing blood to pass through the foramen secundum into the left atrium and permitting continuation of the obligatory right-to-left shunt. Inasmuch as the downgrowth of the septum secundum is arrested, leaving a fixed foramen ovale, such a shunt operates throughout the intrauterine life of the organism. The orifice of the foramen ovale is just above and medial to the orifice of the inferior vena cava (Fig. 2-3D), so inferior caval (i.e., placental) blood is preferentially directed into that foramen, and then into the left atrium, with remarkably little mixing of this oxygenated blood with the oxygen-poor blood returning via the superior vena cava.

The division of the ventricles and the single aortic outflow path are both simpler to understand and more critically complex. The ventricle begins to divide by the upward growth of a

muscular partition of myocardium from the cardiac apex toward the truncus arteriosus (Fig. 2-4A). This will form the muscular part of the interventricular septum. At the same time, a pair of ridges, the spiral ridges, grow toward each other as outgrowths of the walls of the truncus arteriosus. These will fuse to form a spiral septum, dividing the septum from above downward. The lower ends of the spiral ridges contribute to the formation of the final septal closure (Fig. 2-4B). This is an extraordinarily complex phenomenon involving early histologic changes and probably initiated by hemodynamic influences and subsequently controlled by genetic factors (see the careful analysis by Fanapazir and Kaufman[3]). Where the three cushions meet, the membranous interventricular septum is formed. Figure 2-4C and D schematically depict the spiral arrangement of the division of the truncus arteriosus

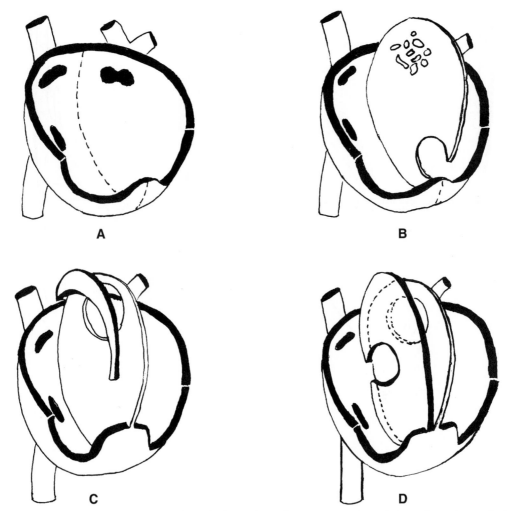

A

B

C

D

FIGURE 2–3 • The single early atrium is represented as a hollow sphere, from an anterolateral view. The atrioventricular canals are the lower part of the cutaway sphere. *A,* The *dotted line* indicates the plane of division into right and left atria. The entry of the superior and inferior venae cavae (right atrial segment of the sphere) and the pulmonary arteries (left segment of the sphere) is indicated by entering tubes. *B to D,* Successive stages in development of the interatrial septum. In *B,* the septum primum grows down, leaving a free margin as the ostium primum. As this ostium prepares to close, holes appear in the upper posterior part of the septum, which in *C* have coalesced into an ostium secundum. In *C,* the septum secundum begins to grow down to the right of the septum primum, covering the ostium secundum on that side. The free margin of the septum secundum does not close over in *D,* leaving the foramen ovale open. The right atrial contents flow into the left atrium via the foramen ovale and ostium secundum. (Adapted from Tuchmann-Duplessis H, David HG, Haegel P: Illustrated Human Embryology. New York, Springer-Verlag, 1972.)

whereby the single outflow tract is divided into pulmonary and aortic tubes, each connected to its corresponding ventricular cavity. The complexity of the closure lies in the precise pitch of the spiral septum; its lower end must be aligned with the upthrusting muscular cushion so as to meet accurately in a single plane. Interference in the fusion of these cushions into a complete membranous septum will lead to a membranous interventricular septal defect. Misalignment of the spiral ridges may result in failure of the great arteries to form and function independently through the accident of a pulmonary aortic fistula. Misalignment of the lower end of the dividing arteries and asymmetry in the positioning of the spiral ridges could lead to such errors as an overriding aorta, with the right ventricular contents partially ejected into the aorta. The features of the tetralogy of Fallot can be readily interpreted as a result of such misalignment in the truncus division. The tetralogy

consists of an overriding aorta, pulmonary stenosis, membranous septal defect (presumably due to asymmetrical division of the proximal truncus arteriosus), and right ventricular hypertrophy (secondary to the right-to-left shunt through the overriding aorta and to the stenotic pulmonary artery).

A superbly illustrated and truly classic account of early experimental findings, as well as an excellent historical review of the anatomy and physiology of fetal circulation, can be found in the book by Barclay and associates.[4] More recent summaries can be obtained in standard works by Arey,[5] Clemente,[6] Hamilton and Mossman,[7] Moore,[8] Sabin,[9] and Tuchmann-Duplessis and associates.[10]

The original plan of five pairs of aortic arch arteries (see Fig. 2-2) becomes modified by incorporation of the first two arch arteries into the internal carotid system, dropping out of the paired dorsal aortas between the third and fourth arches,

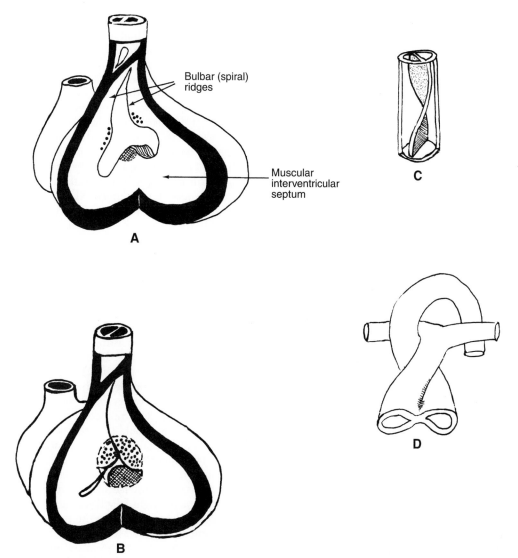

FIGURE 2–4 • Stages in the division of the ventricle and formation of the great arteries from the truncus arteriosus and bulbus cordis. *A,* The ventricle has begun to divide, with formation of the muscular part of the interventricular septum by means of growth of the ventricular wall musculature. The bulbus cordis is dividing into two vessels, beginning with the growing together of two spiral ridges. *B,* The two spiral ridges meet and fuse to divide the bulbus cordis into two outflow tracts: the pulmonary artery and the ascending aorta. The ridges at their lower extremities (*stippled* cushions) meet a muscular cushion derived from the muscular interventricular septum (*hatched*) to form the membranous part of the interventricular septum (outlined by *dotted lines*). The spiral character of the arterial division connects the sixth arch arteries to the right ventricle and connects the left ventricle to the other arch arteries and their derivatives. *C,* Spiral septum shown diagrammatically, in a cutaway cylinder representing the single bulbus cordis. The *hatched* surface of the septum represents the aortic side of the division, and the *stippled* side represents the pulmonary surface of the septum. The two resulting arteries must spiral around each other, as in *D.* Derived from a single tube, they are constrained to remain wrapped in a single pericardial sleeve. (Adapted from Tuchmann-Duplessis H, David HG, Haegel P: Illustrated Human Embryology. New York, Springer-Verlag, 1972; and Moore KL: The Developing Human. Philadelphia, WB Saunders, 1982.)

and participation in the formation of the common carotid arteries by the third arches. Caudal to the lost segments of dorsal aortas, the fourth arches become the roots of the subclavian arteries; the right sixth arch is lost distal to its pulmonary branch, and the left sixth arch becomes the left pulmonary artery, with the segment distal to the pulmonary "branch" serving as the ductus arteriosus (see Fig. 2-2B). This arterial shunt vessel develops specialized muscle in its tunica media, which is stimulated to contract and shut down the shunt vessel after birth. It is believed that abnormal migration of some of this specialized smooth muscle into the aortic wall accounts for aortic stenosis, the stricture developing

in the aorta at the site of this ectopic ductus muscle after birth.

The closure of this right-to-left shunt on the arterial side at birth results in a great increase in pulmonary blood flow (the resistance of pulmonary vessels drops dramatically with inflation of the lungs and elongation of helicine arteries). On the venous side, the rise in left atrial pressure and loss of umbilical venous return arrest the interatrial right-to-left shunt. Elevated left atrial pressure results in the two interatrial septa operating as a flap valve, closing the foramen ovale by applying the curtain-like septum primum against the left one (see Fig. 2-3D).

Certainty in the derivation of the arteries of the head is not easy to achieve. They form from a loose network of interconnected vessels in which it is often impossible to distinguish between arteries and veins.[11] The artery of the first arch becomes a part of the internal carotid artery, which also forms in part from persistence of the rostral parts of the dorsal aortas. The second arch artery appears in the form of the stapedial artery. This artery of the tympanic cavity passes through the annulus (obturator foramen) in the stapes, and in some mammals it persists in this form. In humans, this form of stapedial artery may remain into adulthood as a surgically troublesome vascular anomaly. This artery of the second arch for a time supplies three branches (supraorbital, infraorbital, and mandibular), distributed with the divisions of the trigeminal nerve. An anastomosis between the infraorbital and mandibular branches of the stapedial artery and the external carotid artery is said to give rise to the maxillary artery and its middle meningeal branch. It is further argued that the orbital anastomotic branch of the middle meningeal artery is the remnant of the original supraorbital branch of the stapedial artery. Some information is indicated in the phylogenetic history of the artery. In most mammals, the originally small external carotid artery, as it grows forward, taps the origin of the stapedial artery and appropriates its branches, which at one stroke reduces the size and causes the disappearance of the original stapedial artery and extends the distribution of the external carotid. As Romer colorfully put it, "the process is analogous to 'stream piracy,' whereby one river taps the headwaters of another."[12] Padget offers a detailed discussion and critical appraisal of the literature of the general mammalian stapedial artery and of the human artery, and her discussion is recommended to the interested reader.[13]

The third arch artery forms the common carotid arteries and the first segments of the internal carotid arteries. Thus, it is probable that portions of the first three arches all contribute to the external carotid arteries. The left fourth arch forms the arch of the aorta, and the left dorsal aorta distal to the point of union of this arch forms the descending aorta, along with the single dorsal aorta more caudally (see Fig. 2-2B). The entirety of the right dorsal aorta is lost. The right horn of the aortic sac forms the brachiocephalic artery, from which the right common carotid and subclavian arteries spring.

The sixth arches are associated with the pulmonary blood supply, first as the source of the small twigs to the lung buds. Those twigs and their parent stems from the truncus arteriosus become the definitive pulmonary arteries. Now it should be clear why the complex twist of the spiral septum dividing the truncus arteriosus is necessary. In dividing the truncus, it is essential to connect the right ventricle to the origins of the sixth arches from the truncus, leaving the more rostral arch arteries connected to the part of the truncus connected to the left ventricle. The arch arteries spring from a single vessel, the truncus, and must end as arteries arising from separate arteries—the sixth arising from the pulmonary artery, and the first through fourth from the aortic component of the truncus. The twisting division of the truncus also accounts for the intertwined course of the pulmonary artery and the ascending aorta; their derivation from a single vessel, the truncus, accounts for these great arteries being wrapped in a single pericardial sleeve (see Fig. 2-4D).

The branchial arches develop nerve supplies along with their vascular supplies, and it is an axiom of anatomy that once nerve supply is established, it is never lost. The motor nerves of the branchial arches supply the structures derived from those arches, no matter what developmental events ensue. In Figure 2-2, the position of the glossopharyngeal nerve as the motor nerve of the third arch, and the recurrent laryngeal branch of the vagus as the motor nerve of the sixth arch, can be seen as these nerves are drawn caudally by the descent of the heart and growth of the branchial arch system. The "recurrent" branch of the vagus is in fact the motor nerve derived from the nucleus ambiguus of the brainstem, which happens to distribute by way of the vagus, having emerged from the brainstem as the cranial root of the spinal accessory nerve (cranial nerve XI). The recurring course of the nerve is accounted for by its inherited requirement of lying caudal to the sixth arch artery. The distal part of the left sixth arch artery becomes the ductus arteriosus (the ligamentum arteriosum after birth). Thus arises the asymmetry in the courses of the two recurrent laryngeal nerves. The left nerve is constrained to maintain its original relationship to its arch artery as that artery is drawn down into the chest by the descent of the heart. The right nerve loses that constraint as the sixth arch drops out distal to the origin of the pulmonary artery. The only persisting arch to prevent the nerve's remaining in the neck as the heart descends is the fourth arch on the right side (the right subclavian artery), around which we find the nerve "recurring" in the adult human (see Fig. 2-2B). If, during thyroid surgery, the surgeon finds that the right recurrent nerve does not come up around the subclavian artery, he or she should take that as a warning that a developmental abnormality in the formation of the right subclavian artery might be expected (e.g., a retroesophageal right subclavian). In that event, the right subclavian forms from the right seventh intersegmental artery and part of the right dorsal aorta, the right fourth arch artery and right dorsal aorta having involuted cranial to the origin of the seventh intersegmental artery (see Moore[8] and other embryology texts).

The developing embryo in its earliest stages is supported by a yolk sac of nutriment, sustaining growth until the placenta is sufficiently developed to assume those duties. The embryo lies on the surface of the yolk sac, with the interior of the latter in continuity with the developing gastrointestinal tract. The digestive tract cranial to the yolk sac is termed the foregut, that caudal to the yolk sac is termed the hindgut, and that directly connected to the yolk sac is termed the midgut. Three aortic branches, midline and unpaired, arise to supply each of these segments of the digestive tract, and these arteries remain the source of arterial blood for those portions of the tract and their derivatives. Thus, the celiac artery is the artery of the foregut and the derivatives of the foregut, including the liver and spleen. The artery of the midgut is the superior mesenteric artery; the artery of the hindgut is the inferior mesenteric artery. During development, the digestive tract outgrows the room available for it in the abdominal cavity and temporarily "herniates" out into the umbilical cord. Its return from this extra-abdominal sojourn is accompanied by a rotation that accounts for the disposition of the stomach, the duodenum, and the bowel in the adult. The axis of rotation around which this reentry into the abdomen occurs is the superior mesenteric artery (see the exquisitely illustrated account of Dott[14]).

The kidneys begin their development in the pelvis and migrate cranially to their final position on the posterior

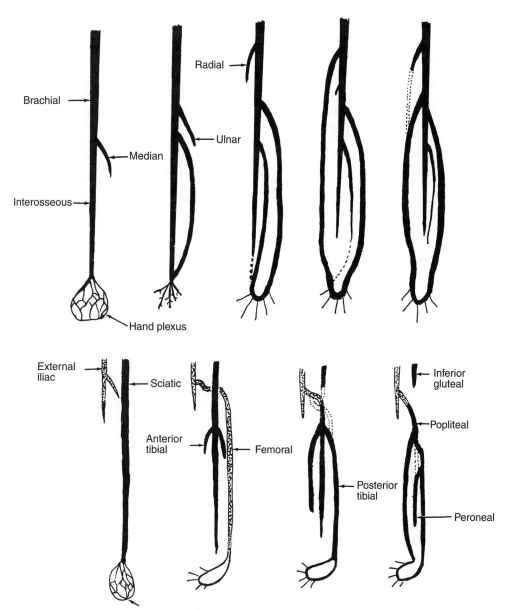

FIGURE 2–5 • Development of the arterial pattern of the limbs. *Top row,* Upper limb. The upper limb is initially organized around a single axial artery—the brachial and its interosseous continuation—terminating in a hand plexus. The hand plexus will develop into the palmar arches. The stem artery gives rise in succession to the median, ulnar, and radial arteries. The median artery normally has an evanescent existence as a major vessel, losing its connection with the hand plexus, which it usurped from the axial vessel. *Bottom row,* Lower limb. The axial vessel for the lower limb is the sciatic, which remains in the adult as the inferior gluteal, and portions of the popliteal and peroneal arteries. The femoral artery arises from the external iliac and appropriates the distal part of the sciatic to dominate the vascular distribution of the limb. The anterior tibial artery arises as a branch of the popliteal; the posterior tibial is developed from the union of the femoral and the popliteal. Notice in the third figure from the left that an upper segment of the femoral artery is lost, allowing the popliteal to become interposed. (Adapted from Arey LB: Developmental Anatomy, 7th ed. Philadelphia, WB Saunders, 1965.)

abdominal wall. The pelvic kidneys derive their arterial blood supply from the iliac system, and as they ascend, the previous arterial supply drops out and new vessels from the aorta are established. The ascent and the history of the previous blood supply can be seen in the sources of small vessels supplying the ureter, their origins indicating the stems of vessels formerly supplying the kidney. Should the ascent of the kidney be arrested, the blood supply at the time remains the supply into adulthood. Thus, the ascent of the horseshoe kidney is arrested by the overhanging inferior mesenteric artery, and the horseshoe kidney has arterial blood supplied from

common iliac vessels or the aorta at a level lower than the origin of the normal renal arteries. So, too, accessory renal arteries usually arise below the renal arteries and enter the inferior pole of the kidney, attesting to a previous source of blood that did not entirely disappear with ascent to the final renal destination.

The limbs seem to be organized around a central arterial stem, so from the beginning, an axial artery is identifiable. Figure 2-5 depicts the changes in circulatory pattern for the two limbs. Generally, the axial artery in large part disappears and certainly ceases to be the principal source of limb blood.

In the upper limb, the axial artery passes down the core of the limb to the hand plexus. It is a continuation of the subclavian and axillary systems, already established in the 5-mm embryo, and is the forerunner of the brachial artery and, more distally, the interosseous artery. The upper limb axial artery sprouts a median branch and an ulnar arterial branch on the medial side of the stem artery. The median temporarily joins with the ulnar in the volar arch. A radial sprout follows on the preaxial side of the limb, and this new branch usurps the median's connection with the volar arch. The distal axial artery persists as the anterior interosseous artery. This pattern is completed before the end of the second month, and the early dominance of the axial and median arteries is permanently lost. The median artery persists as a branch of the anterior interosseous artery, serving as the nutrient artery of the median nerve. It may persist in an enlarged form as an anomaly, accompanying the median nerve into the palm and retaining its connection with and contribution to the palmar arterial arches.

Figure 2-5 shows the steps by which the adult pattern of arterial supply to the lower limb is derived from the axial artery of the limb bud. The axial vessel is the sciatic artery, a direct branch of the umbilical. It is the primary source of the blood for the limb bud in the 9-mm embryo. The major stem artery for the limb becomes the femoral, as the latter continues the course of the external iliac. The femoral annexes the foot plexus of the sciatic and the origin of this axial vessel. The remaining proximal "stump" of the once-dominant sciatic artery persists as the inferior gluteal artery. A branch of the latter, the artery of the sciatic nerve, is all that remains of the former glory of the sciatic artery. The distal parts of the sciatic stem, appropriated by the femoral artery near its origin from the external iliac, give rise to the anterior tibial artery, which connects with the plantar arch distally. The newer, more distal femoral artery establishes a new connection to the distal sciatic so that it and the plantar arch come to branch from the sciatic. The most distal segment of the sciatic shifts its origin to the posterior tibial as the peroneal, and the adult pattern is established. The remnants of the sciatic persist (from above downward) as the inferior gluteal with its small artery of the sciatic nerve, the popliteal artery, and the peroneal artery. In the adult arterial plan, these persisting segments of the original sciatic artery no longer have continuity with one another in any significant way.

The umbilical arteries, carrying blood to the placenta for gas and metabolite exchange, appear as large branches of the internal iliac arteries and persist unmodified throughout gestation. These arteries develop robust branches to the upper surface of the urinary bladder. At birth, the segments of the umbilical arteries distal to the origin of the arteries to the bladder are obliterated and remain as fibrous cords, the medial umbilical ligaments. The stem of these arteries and the branches to the bladder are henceforth known as the superior vesicle arteries.

Veins

As the arterial distribution system develops, appropriate return pathways arise simultaneously. The venous system is extensively interconnected, with a great capacity for collateral routes of venous return, and arteries are generally accompanied by corresponding veins. The short review of the venous system here focuses only on the great systems of veins that arise early in embryonic life and give rise to the major collecting pathways recognizable in the normal adult. Thus, even such important but developmentally simple systems as the pulmonary venous system are not discussed here.

A passing comment on venous valves is appropriate here, to draw attention to a provocative analysis and comparative study of superficial veins in the limbs of primates.[15] The number and spacing of venous valves are dictated genetically and are relevant to the need to maintain optimum pressures within capillary beds to ensure a balanced fluid exchange in tissues. The distance between venous valves in the limbs is just that needed to provide the transcapillary pressure gradients required for an equilibrium in fluid efflux and return to the vascular bed; it is not, as previously supposed, an adaptation to counter the effects of gravity in the bipedal posture.

The veins of the embryo fall into three major groups: vitelline (omphalomesenteric) veins, umbilical veins, and the cardinal system of veins. The coalesced blood islands that give rise to undifferentiated blood networks develop a venous side, as they do an arterial side, as directions of blood flow become established through them. Preferential pathways emerge on the venous side, giving rise to larger and more dominant veins that undergo modification as regional or organ-specific changes occur. Many of the venous channels developed in support of fetal life disappear as the need for them vanishes through subsequent development.

The vitelline veins are the veins of the yolk sac. They pass through the intestinal portal of the umbilical cord, alongside the (at first) wide channel of communication between the sac and the midgut region of the alimentary canal. A vitelline plexus is formed of communicating venous channels between the vitelline veins in the septum transversum, and as the liver develops in the septum, it infringes on the vitelline plexus, breaking it up into hepatic sinusoids. The vitelline pathway from the septum transversum into the heart persists, in spite of this encroachment, as hepaticocardiac channels. The right channel of this return persists as the terminal segment of the inferior vena cava (Fig. 2-6). The vitelline plexus also surrounds the duodenum during the stage of hepatic growth, and the plexus is further distorted when the herniated midgut returns in a spiraling motion into the abdominal cavity. It is this rotation during the return that brings the duodenum into its transverse position and fixes this position by peritonealization. This position forces the blood in the surrounding plexus to shunt from the right to the left vitelline vein, which is the segment of the vitelline system lying just caudal to the transversely oriented duodenum. The left vitelline vein then sends its blood directly across to the liver by way of its dorsal anastomosis with the persistent cranial end of the right vitelline vein.

The portal vein thus formed does not spiral around the duodenum, as is so commonly described and illustrated; instead, it is short and straight, with the duodenum spiraling around it. The ease with which these changes take place can be readily understood if two basic facts are appreciated: (1) the essentially plexiform nature of the embryonic vascular system, and (2) the natural tendency for blood to seek the most direct route of flow because of hydrodynamic factors. (Refer to the clear sequence of illustrations of this development in Hamilton and Mossman,[7] page 274.)

The umbilical veins, entering the abdominal cavity by way of the umbilicus, must also traverse the septum transversum

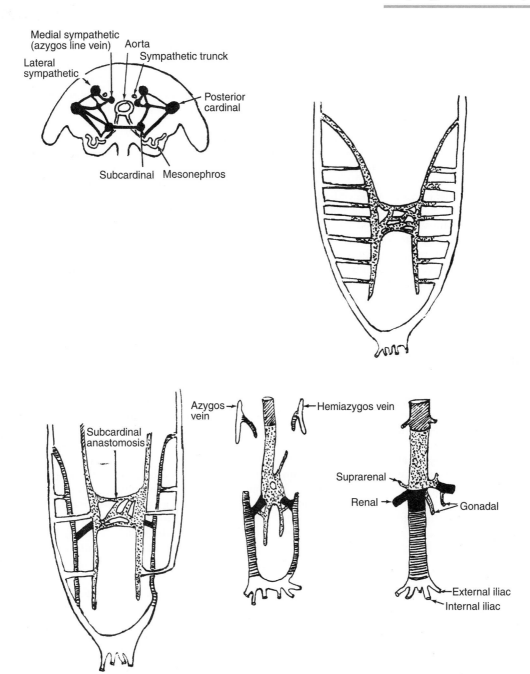

FIGURE 2–6 • Development of the large veins. *Upper left,* Schematic cross section of the embryo shows the relative positions and extensive interconnections of the major body wall veins. *Upper right* and *lower row* (left to right), Succession of stages in the development of the inferior vena cava and the related body wall veins. The key in the lower row identifies the component veins making up the inferior vena cava *(lower right).* For simplicity, the azygos and hemiazygos veins are depicted as if they arise from the lateral sympathetic veins, but in fact they arise as derivatives from the parallel medial sympathetic (azygos line) veins. (Adapted from Williams PL, Wendell-Smith CP, Treadgold S: Basic Human Embryology, 2nd ed. Philadelphia, JB Lippincott, 1969; and Hollinshead WH, Rosse L: Textbook of Anatomy, 4th ed. Philadelphia, Harper & Row, 1985.)

to arrive at the heart, and their septal segments within the septum also become enmeshed with the vitelline veins in the hepatic plexus of sinusoids. In the 5-mm embryo, the umbilical veins communicate extensively with the vitelline plexus in the liver. Two days later, the right umbilical vein undergoes atrophy, and all placental blood returns to the fetal heart via the left vein. The left vein's channel through the liver enlarges to accommodate this enhanced flow and forms the

ductus venosus, a direct channel through the liver between the left umbilical vein and the inferior vena cava. This channel obliterates at birth with cessation of flow through the umbilical system, and the intrahepatic shunt is replaced by the ligamentum venosum. Thus, there is said to be a sphincter in this shunt that regulates umbilical flow, a particularly important feature to prevent overloading the fetal heart during uterine contractions. This sphincter's closure at birth contributes to the prompt obliteration of the shunt. The course of the left umbilical vein caudal to the liver is in the free margin of the ventral mesentery. The obliterated umbilical vein between the umbilicus and liver is the ligamentum teres hepatis of the adult, lying in the free margin of the falciform ligament; the latter is the adult counterpart of the ventral mesentery between the liver and the anterior abdominal wall.

The cardinal veins are the body wall veins of the embryo and fetus. There are several sets designated by distinguishing names, a source of considerable confusion for the student of human anatomy. The anterior cardinal veins (also termed precardinal veins) drain the cranial region of the early embryo. The posterior cardinal veins drain the caudal portion and arise slightly later than the anterior cardinals. The subcardinal veins appear shortly after the posterior cardinal veins and are derived in conjunction with the rapidly growing progenitor of the kidney, the mesonephros. The term *supracardinal veins* is sometimes used to designate lateral sympathetic or thoracolumbar line veins or paraureteric veins. To limit the number of cardinal veins one must attend to, in discussing the veins of the posterior body wall anterior to the segmental vessels, I use the term *lateral sympathetic veins* instead.

The primary head vein of the embryo evolves into the complex system of dural sinuses and venous pathways of the head, and the reader is referred to the classic accounts of Streeter[16] and Padget,[11,13] whose illustrations amply clarify the changes leading to the adult pattern. The anterior and posterior cardinal veins unite behind the heart to form the common cardinal veins, or ducts of Cuvier (right and left). The union of the ducts of Cuvier is the ductus venosus at the venous end of the heart. Part of the ductus venosus becomes incorporated into the walls of the atria, most notably the right atrium.

The posterior cardinal veins are the first of a series of caudal longitudinal body wall veins, which form an interconnected system (see Fig. 2-6), giving rise to the caudal body wall venous drainage and to the inferior vena cava and azygos system of veins.

The subcardinal veins appear soon after the posterior cardinal veins as a pair of veins along the medial side of the urogenital folds. They are associated with the mesonephros and probably arise as a series of longitudinal anastomoses for the plexuses of the mesonephroi. They drain the mesonephroi and the germinal epithelium and terminate cranially and caudally by connecting with the posterior cardinal veins (see Fig. 2-6). The subcardinal veins unite with each other and, along their lengths, with the posterior cardinal veins through anastomoses; the multiple transverse anastomoses of these veins are probably their most distinctive feature. One of these anastomoses is the intersubcardinal anastomosis between the two veins ventral to the aorta. The right subcardinal vein establishes a communication with the liver sinusoids, and that segment becomes the hepatic segment of the inferior vena cava (see Fig. 2-6). The preaortic anastomosis comes into play in the establishment of the vena cava inferior to that segment.

The lateral sympathetic veins appear soon after the hepatic segment of the inferior vena cava, anterior to the segmental vessels. They appear first as a plexus but quickly become a longitudinal trunk, ending cranially in the posterior cardinal vein and anastomosing posteriorly with the subcardinal vein, especially strongly on the right side. The part caudal to that latter anastomosis persists, and most of the remainder of the lateral sympathetic veins regresses; the persisting right caudal segment survives as the infrarenal part of the inferior vena cava (see Fig. 2-6). As the lateral sympathetic veins appear, a medial pair (medial sympathetic or azygos line veins) also arises, but medial to the sympathetic trunk in the abdominal wall. These link across the midline and, with the dropping out of an intermediate segment on the left side, form the azygos system of veins.

The adult pattern is completed by the emerging dominance of the right common cardinal vein. The left upper intercostal spaces drain into the remainder of the left common cardinal vein, which connects with the left brachiocephalic vein after the lateral part of the left common cardinal is lost. The left superior intercostal vein is formed in part by the left posterior and anterior cardinal veins. The potential communication between the two may persist as a left superior vena cava; the latter's position may be identified in the normal adult as the oblique cardiac vein (of Marshall), which may be traced to the left superior intercostal vein as a reminder of that origin.

The inferior vena cava has a complex origin. The hepatic segment, as noted previously, is derived from the cranial segment of the right vitelline vein and the hepatic sinusoids. A prerenal segment forms distal to this as an anastomosis between the hepatic segment and the right subcardinal vein. This latter vein forms the prerenal segment (down to the junction of the renal veins). A renal segment is formed from a renal collar (note the preaortic anastomosis between the subcardinals described previously). The renal collar is an anastomosis involving this preaortic anastomosis and anastomoses between the right subcardinal and lateral sympathetic veins. A postrenal segment forms from the lumbar part of the right lateral sympathetic vein down to the level of the common iliac veins. The common iliacs join with the lower part of the inferior vena cava as the postcardinal veins degenerate, forcing the iliacs to find this secondary route of venous return to the heart. As the kidneys come to rest in the adult position, the definitive renal veins are formed as connections to the inferior vena cava through anastomoses between the subcardinal and lateral lumbar veins. On the left side, the longer path to the inferior vena cava is accomplished through recruitment of this anastomosis between the subcardinal veins. On the right, this anastomosis is incorporated into the formation of the renal segment of the inferior vena cava, and the situation is less complex.

The multiple sources incorporated into the inferior vena cava, including anastomoses across the midline, may lead to some bizarre malformations. Most dramatic of these is the rare retrocaval ureter, which is clearly not a malformation of the ureter or a misguided path of ascent of the kidney; rather, it must be interpreted as incorporation of unusual components of the renal collar into the inferior vena cava. Accounts in the literature agree on this interpretation of a caval rather than a ureteric malformation.[17-19]

Growth of New Vessels

It would be helpful to know whether the development of new blood vessels in the fetus and during postnatal growth is a model for vascular proliferation under other circumstances. It is likely that this is so, although the factors that stimulate and direct such growth might be quite different. The central nervous system (CNS) provides a model that has been studied by a variety of means. The relative maturity of the brain at birth provides an existing and fully functional vascular tree that might be taken as a model of a relatively mature vascular system. The further growth and development of the CNS dictate the need for postnatal neovascularization to support further maturation of the tissue.

Examination of the vascularization of the CNS addresses a fundamental issue in vascular growth during development: To what extent is development of a vascular bed a permissive condition for the subsequent onset of function; that is, to what extent is it anticipatory of and necessary for function? Or, conversely, to what extent is the development of a vasculature the response to the greater metabolic demands of a tissue as it increases or begins to achieve the functional levels expected of it at full maturation?

Studying CNS regions at the time of onset of measurable function (e.g., the auditory system) reveals that vascular sprouting parallels such events in their time courses (Skolnik and Maxwell, unpublished observations). Such observations cannot distinguish cause and effect, and perhaps they must go hand in hand—functional and vascular maturation identically timed or responsive to some common signal from yet another source. Greater temporal resolution would have to be applied than we have been able to achieve to date.

It is possible to describe the manner of new vessel growth in the CNS and to derive some quantitative information

therefrom. Rowan and Maxwell studied the postnatal rat cerebral cortex, which is structurally and cytologically quite immature at birth and undergoes a remarkable degree of maturation in the first 3 weeks after birth.[20] CNS blood vessels are the only CNS tissue elements to display alkaline phosphatase activity. Using a simple histochemical procedure, it is possible to visualize small vessels by light and electron microscopy, relying on the enzyme reaction to label vessels—and those cells in the process of becoming vessels through cytodifferentiation—with no ambiguity whatsoever.[21] It has been widely accepted that new vessels in the CNS and perhaps elsewhere begin as a proliferation of solid cords of cells that later "canalize" (develop lumens). Yet such a mechanism seems improbable on purely mechanistic grounds, and this does not seem to be the case in the CNS. In this tissue, postnatal growth of new vessels seems to occur by budding from preexisting vessels; the buds are recognizable by their enzyme content and by the presence of lumens, although they are collapsed and empty. The lumens are not identifiable by light microscopy, so the interpretation of solid cords of cells is quite understandable. The buds or sprouts have characteristic cytoplasmic protuberances, or fingers, that "explore" in advance of growth of the sprout, seeming to seek the most appropriate path or perhaps sensing the direction where vessel growth will best satisfy the perceived need. Figures 2-7 through 2-10

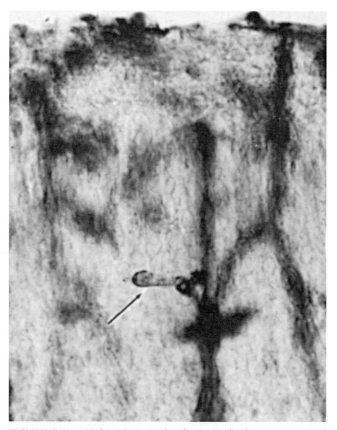

FIGURE 2–7 • Light micrograph of rat cerebral cortex, reacted for alkaline phosphatase. A vascular sprout *(arrow)* is seen in the superficial cortex 2 days after birth. The cortical surface is at the top (×1548). (Courtesy of Dr. R. Rowan.)

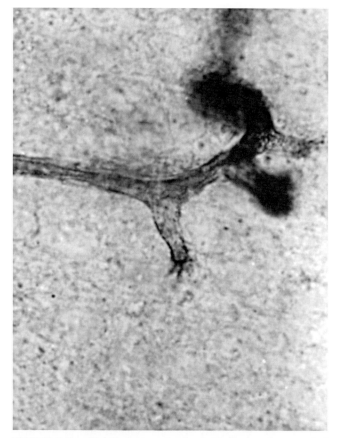

FIGURE 2–8 • Light micrograph of rat cerebral cortex, reacted for alkaline phosphatase. A vascular sprout is seen in the middle third of the rat cortex 7 days after birth. Delicate exploratory fingers, or pseudopodia, are seen at the tip of the sprout (×3148). (Courtesy of Dr. R. Rowan.)

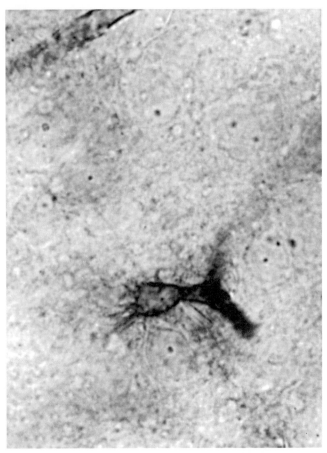

FIGURE 2–9 • Light micrograph of rat cerebral cortex, reacted for alkaline phosphatase. A vascular sprout is seen in the middle third of the cortex 8 days after birth. Pseudopodia are evident at the tip (×3148). (Courtesy of Dr. R. Rowan.)

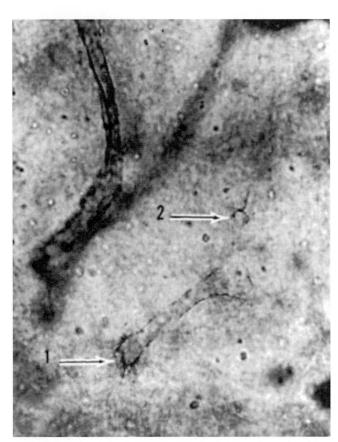

FIGURE 2–10 • Light micrograph of rat cerebral cortex, reacted for alkaline phosphatase. A branched sprout with two tips (arrows) is evident. The larger tip (1) extends down and to the left of the stem vessel; the smaller tip (2) extends upward. The parent sprout and the two sprout tips are much less intensely stained than are the mature vessels dominating the upper and left parts of the micrograph (×3148). (Courtesy of Dr. R. Rowan.)

show a series of such sprouts from the rat cerebral cortex. These sprouts presumably link with a venous channel, establishing hemodynamics, which should serve to open the lumen as a capillary link. Figure 2-11 is an electron micrograph of such a sprout, in which the unopened state of the lumen is evident. Because CNS arteries prominently display alkaline phosphatase activity, and because sprouts at their earliest detectable stages also display this enzyme, we presume that postnatal vascularization proceeds by arteriolar sprouting, with subsequent linkage to the venous bed. An excellent historical review of the study of growth and differentiation of blood vessels and a statement of the status of the field can be found in Eriksson and Zarem's chapter in *Microcirculation*.[22]

The factors that induce an arteriole to sprout may be multiple, possibly legion. An enormous literature on angiogenic factors is available for the CNS and other tissues, including tumors. Attention must be drawn, however, to a series of papers announcing a major achievement by Vallee's group at Harvard.[23-25] These investigators isolated and analyzed an angiogenic factor from human carcinoma cells, marking the first time an angiogenic factor was isolated, its amino acid sequence determined, and its genetic code identified.

Curiously, this factor, angiogenin, is remarkably similar in its amino acid sequence to a ribonuclease, and the unraveling of the biologic meaning of this similarity and possible relationship will be fascinating to watch in the literature. This is not to say that only one angiogenic protein is the cause of neovascularization. There may be many, perhaps different ones, operating in the embryo and fetus, in the adult during wound healing, and in neoplasms. There is abundant evidence that tissue metabolites are capable of stimulating vascular development (e.g., high carbon dioxide and low oxygen content in tissue fluids). A complex list of possibilities will have to be sorted out to determine which factors act to stimulate the production or release of specific angiogenic factors from cells (and which cells) and which are sufficient factors in their own right, acting directly on preexisting vessels.

It may not be satisfying to conclude with a dismaying array of unanswered questions. It is compelling evidence, however, that the questions are there and that the vigorous activity taking place in laboratories around the world will eventually yield some answers. The control of neovascularization, of which the embryo is such a master, may allow us to apply these concepts to a wide spectrum of problems afflicting adults in our clinics and hospitals.

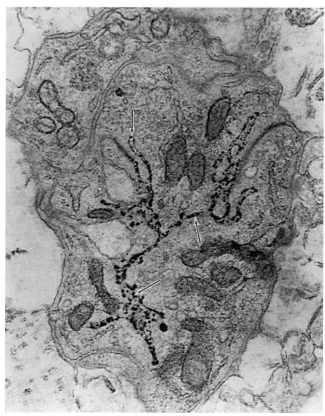

FIGURE 2–11 • Electron micrograph of a sprout in the middle third of the rat cortex 8 days after birth. The unopened lumen *(arrows)* is delicately outlined by the deposition of enzyme (alkaline phosphatase) reaction product (×42,200). (Courtesy of Dr. R. Rowan.)

REFERENCES

1. Delacruz M, Sanchez-Gomez C, Palomino MA: The primitive cardiac regions in the straight tube heart (stage 9) and their anatomical expression in the mature heart: An experimental study in the chick embryo. J Anat 165:121-131, 1989.
2. Congdon ED: Transformation of the aortic-arch system during the development of the human embryo. Carnegie Contr Embryol 14:47-110, 1922.
3. Fanapazir K, Kaufman MH: Observations on the development of the aorticopulmonary spiral septum in the mouse. J Anat 158:157-172, 1988.
4. Barclay AE, Franklin KJ, Prichard MML: The Foetal Circulation. Oxford, Blackwell Scientific, 1946.
5. Arey LB: Developmental Anatomy, 7th ed. Philadelphia, WB Saunders, 1965.
6. Clemente CD: Gray's Anatomy, 30th American ed. Philadelphia, Lea & Febiger, 1985.
7. Hamilton WJ, Mossman HW: Hamilton, Boyd and Mossman's Human Embryology, 4th ed. Baltimore, Williams & Wilkins, 1972.
8. Moore KL: The Developing Human, 3rd ed. Philadelphia, WB Saunders, 1982.
9. Sabin FR: Origin and development of the primitive vessels of the chick and pig. Carnegie Contr Embryol 6:63-124, 1917.
10. Tuchmann-Duplessis H, David HG, Haegel P: Illustrated Human Embryology. New York, Springer-Verlag, 1972.
11. Padget DH: Development of the cranial venous system in man, from the viewpoint of comparative anatomy. Carnegie Contr Embryol 36:79-140, 1957.
12. Romer AS: The Vertebrate Body, 4th ed. Philadelphia, WB Saunders, 1970.
13. Padget DH: The development of the cranial arteries in the human embryo. Carnegie Contr Embryol 32:205-261, 1948.
14. Dott NM: Anomalies of intestinal rotation: Their embryology and surgical aspects: With report of five cases. Br J Surg 11:252-286, 1923.
15. Thiranagama R, Chamberlain AT, Wood BA: Valves in superficial limb veins of humans and nonhuman primates. Clin Anat 2:135-145, 1989.
16. Streeter GL: The developmental alterations in the vascular system of the brain of the human embryo. Carnegie Contr Embryol 9:5-38, 1918.
17. Derbes VJ, Dial WA: Postcaval ureter. J Urol 36:226-233, 1936.
18. Gruenwald P, Surks SN: Pre-ureteric vena cava and its embryological explanation. J Urol 49:195-261, 1943.
19. Randall A, Campbell EW: Anomalous relationship of the right ureter to the vena cava. J Urol 34:565-583, 1935.
20. Rowan RA, Maxwell DS: Patterns of vascular sprouting in the postnatal development of the cerebral cortex of the rat. Am J Anat 160:246-255, 1981.
21. Rowan RA, Maxwell DS: An ultrastructural study of vascular proliferation and vascular alkaline phosphatase activity in the developing cerebral cortex of the rat. Am J Anat 160:257-265, 1981.
22. Eriksson E, Zarem HA: Growth and differentiation of blood vessels. In Kaley G, Altura BM (eds): Microcirculation, vol 1. Baltimore, University Park Press, 1977, pp 393-419.
23. Fett JW, Strydom DJ, Lobb RR, et al: Isolation and characterization of angiogenin, an angiogenic protein from human carcinoma cells. Biochemistry 24:5480-5486, 1985.
24. Kurachi K, Davie CW, Strydom DJ, et al: Sequence of the cDNA and gene for angiogenin, a human angiogenesis factor. Biochemistry 24:5494-5499, 1985.
25. Strydom DJ, Fett JW, Lobb RR, et al: Amino acid sequence of human derived angiogenin. Biochemistry 24:5486-5494, 1985.

Alexander W. Clowes • Ted R. Kohler

Anatomy, Physiology, and Pharmacology of the Vascular Wall

Normal Anatomy

Although the vasculature is a series of tubes whose primary function is to act as nonthrombogenic conduits for blood, it is quite diverse in structure and function. In addition to acting as conduits, the vessels act as capacitors, and they regulate the molecular and cellular traffic between the vascular and extravascular spaces. This latter function is largely a property of small vessels (particularly postcapillary venules). Because the cellular elements (endothelium and smooth muscle cells) in the microvasculature are the same as in the large vessels, one might expect the cells in arteries and veins to have some of the same regulatory properties as those in arterioles and venules. As discussed later in this chapter, the similar properties of the endothelium and smooth muscle cells in large and small vessels may account for some of the abnormal properties of vessels undergoing atherosclerotic change or thickening after transplantation (transplant atherosclerosis).

The vasculature has distinct anatomic and physiologic features. Arteries are divided into three categories: large elastic arteries, medium-size muscular arteries, and small arteries. All arteries possess three layers, or tunics, called the intima, media, and adventitia. The intima, the innermost layer of the wall lying inside the internal elastic lamina and directly adjacent to the flowing blood, is composed of endothelium at the luminal surface and subendothelial extracellular matrix. In some vessels, one or more layers of smooth muscle cells are present; this so-called intimal cushion of smooth muscle cells may in some circumstances be the progenitor of the fibrous intimal plaque. The media, bounded by the internal and external elastic laminae, contains smooth muscle cells embedded in a matrix of collagen, elastin, and proteoglycans. The adventitia lies outside the external elastic lamina and is composed of loose

From Clowes AW: Series of atherosclerosis. In White RA (ed): Atherosclerosis: Human Pathology and Experimental Animal Methods and Models. Boca Raton, Fla, CRC Press, 1989, pp 3-15.

connective tissue, fibroblasts, capillaries, occasional leukocytes (particularly mast cells), and small nerve fibers.

The large elastic arteries include the aorta and its major branches; the medium-size muscular arteries include most of the distributing vessels to the organs. In these two classes of arteries, like in all vessels, all three layers are represented in the wall. They differ principally in the amount of elastic tissue present in the media. The aortic wall is composed of well-defined lamellar units consisting of commonly oriented and elongated smooth muscle cells with their surrounding matrix, including a meshwork of collagen, and a layer of elastin.[1,2] The number of lamellar units in the aortas of various mammalian species, encompassing a wide range of body sizes, is proportional to the radius, regardless of variations in wall thickness.[1] As a result, the average tension per lamellar unit is remarkably constant. This lamellar unit represents the structural and functional unit of the aortic wall. Wall stress, which is pressure multiplied by radius divided by thickness, is fairly constant as a result of the linear relationship between wall thickness and radius and the fact that blood pressure is independent of species and size. This results in a good match between the strength of the wall and the tangential distending force within it. Increases in pressure, as occur in hypertension or in the wall of thin vein grafts placed in the arterial circulation, or increases in vessel diameter that occur when vessels dilate in response to increased flow, result in increased stress and compensatory increases in wall thickness.

In the elastic arteries, the media is composed of layers of smooth muscle cells interspersed with clearly defined lamellae of elastin. The media of muscular arteries is also composed of smooth muscle cells but lacks discrete elastic lamellae, except for the internal and external elastic layers (Fig. 3-1). The elastin is present only as thin fibers. In the largest elastic arteries with more than 28 elastic layers, a microvasculature (vasa vasorum) penetrates the media from the adventitial side and provides a nutrient supply to the deep layers of the wall.[3] The inner layers receive nutrients directly from the lumen.

Wall stress = $\frac{P \times R}{\text{thickness}}$

= $Ct_\$^2$

Unit
SMC
Matrix
Collagen
Elastic fibers

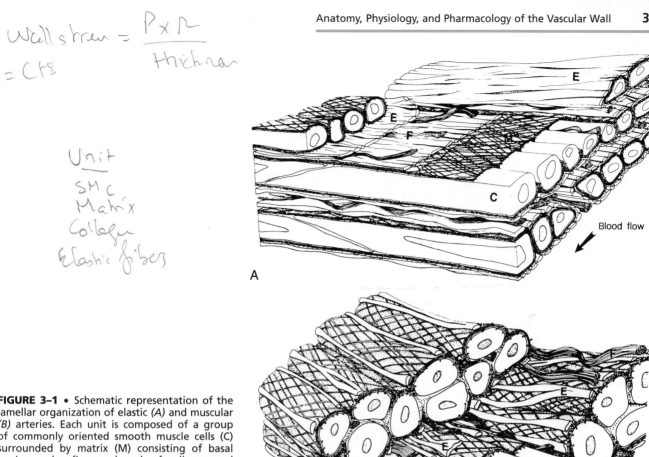

FIGURE 3–1 • Schematic representation of the lamellar organization of elastic *(A)* and muscular *(B)* arteries. Each unit is composed of a group of commonly oriented smooth muscle cells (C) surrounded by matrix (M) consisting of basal lamina and a fine meshwork of collagen and surrounded by elastic fibers (E) oriented in the same direction as the long axes of the cells. Wavy collagen bundles (F) lie between the elastic fibers. The elastic lamellae are much better defined in the elastic arteries *(A)* than in the muscular arteries *(B)*. (From Clark JM, Glagov S: Transmural organization of the arterial media: The lamellar unit revisited. Arteriosclerosis 5:19, 1985.)

As arteries become smaller, there is a progressive loss of elastic tissue; eventually, the internal and external elastic lamellae become discontinuous and fragmented, and the clear distinction between the various layers is lost. At the arteriolar level, the wall is composed of an endothelium, a layer of smooth muscle, and a filamentous collagenous adventitia. Compared with other arteries in the body, the small arteries have a relatively thick media and a large ratio of media to lumen, in keeping with their function as resistance vessels.

As has been pointed out by others,[4] the differentiation of these three types of arteries is of great pathologic significance, because each class of vessels is subject to particular types of disease. Atherosclerosis is confined to elastic and muscular arteries, and medial calcific sclerosis to muscular arteries. Small arteries develop diffuse fibromuscular thickening and hyalinization.

Veins tend to be much larger and more thin walled than arteries. The intima contains only an endothelial layer. The internal elastic layer is clearly evident only in the larger veins, and the media contains relatively few smooth muscle cells, collagen, and little elastin. In the veins of the extremities, there are thin bicuspid valves containing mainly endothelium and connective tissue.

Regulation of Luminal Area

Although a description of the structures of the normal vasculature underscores the point that endothelial and smooth muscle cells are the principal cellular elements, such a description does not provide any insight into the mechanisms that regulate wall structure and function under normal circumstances or during the development of pathologic lesions. Further, such a description provides no clue to how a vessel adjusts its mass and dimensions in response to external stimuli (hypertension, increased blood flow, vascular injury) or to how it maintains a nonthrombogenic state. To understand these physiologic responses, we must consider the functions of the individual cellular elements and the activities of these cells when they exist together as an organ in the fully formed vessel.

Both developing and mature vessels respond to changes in blood flow by adjusting their diameters in a manner that maintains constant shear. A striking example of this change is found in an artery proximal to an arteriovenous fistula.[5] The vessel enlarges and can, over the course of a lifetime, become aneurysmal. Conversely, diameter is reduced when outflow is diminished. This has been observed in mature and developing arteries and in vessels in which flow is reduced by a proximal obstruction.[6-8] Diseased arterial segments also respond to changes in flow. A coronary artery with an enlarging atherosclerotic intima will presumably develop luminal stenosis, and the blood velocity in that stenotic area increases. This increase in blood velocity in turn causes vasodilatation. In fact, a diseased coronary artery can dilate and maintain normal luminal dimensions despite changes in wall structure as long as the intimal lesion does not exceed 40% of the area inside the internal elastic lamina.[9] At that point, pathologic narrowing begins. The endothelium senses changes in blood velocity and shear and translates this biomechanical information into biochemical signals that regulate vessel diameter. Vessels denuded of endothelium do not respond to changes in flow.[10] Acute diameter changes occur by altering vasomotor tone.[6] If the change in flow is chronic, arterial wall structure remodels to the new caliber, and vasomotor tone returns to normal. This is demonstrated in the work of Langille and O'Donnell, who showed that the reduction in lumen that accompanies partial ligation of carotid outflow in rabbits initially is reversible by application of topical vasodilators but later becomes fixed.[6]

Pharmacologic agents regulating vascular wall contraction can be classified as endothelial and nonendothelial dependent.[11] Furchgott and Zawadzki reported in 1980 that the relaxation of isolated rabbit aorta and other arteries induced by acetylcholine and other agonists for muscarinic receptors depends on the presence of endothelial cells.[12] After removal of the endothelial cells, acetylcholine no longer induces relaxation; instead, it causes contraction. A large number of agents, including acetylcholine, arachidonic acid, adenosine triphosphate, adenosine diphosphate, bradykinin, histamine, norepinephrine, serotonin, thrombin, and vasopressin, have been shown to produce an endothelium-dependent relaxation of arteries. Other substances, such as adenosine, adenosine monophosphate, papaverine, isoproterenol, nitrovasodilators (such as sodium nitroprusside), and prostacyclin, do not require the presence of endothelial cells to elicit relaxation. The endothelial-dependent relaxation results from release of nitric oxide, which stimulates guanylate cyclase of the underlying smooth muscle cells and causes an increase in cyclic guanosine monophosphate. Nitric oxide is derived from L-arginine[13] and is present in higher concentrations in small-resistance vessels than in larger conduit arteries.

In addition to expressing a relaxing factor, endothelium can express contracting factors.[11,12] Contracting factors appear to be responsible for contractions in some systemic vessels induced by arachidonic acid and hypoxia and in isolated cerebral vessels by stretch. One of these factors is a peptide, endothelin, which has been isolated from cultured endothelial cells and is a potent vasoconstrictor. Increase in shear stress suppresses the expression of the gene for endothelin and increases the production of nitric oxide synthase (NOS) by endothelial cells. It is likely that these endothelium-derived relaxing and constricting factors contribute to long-term vascular adaptation in response to increased blood flow. As discussed later in the chapter, regulation of wall structure and vessel diameter are closely linked. Nitric oxide inhibits smooth muscle cell growth, whereas endothelin promotes it. Certain pathologic conditions in which endothelium is either missing or abnormal are associated with acute and chronic vasospasm; it is possible that the acute problems of atypical angina (coronary vasospasm) and cerebrovasospasm after cerebral hemorrhage are in part manifestations of abnormal endothelial function and abnormal secretion of these factors.[14]

Regulation of Medial and Intimal Thickening

Arterial wall thickening is a prominent feature of most pathologic processes. In hypertensive animals and humans, arteries exhibit medial thickening, whereas after endothelial denudation or in the presence of hypercholesterolemia, they develop a thick intima.[15-17] Exactly how these responses are regulated is not clear, although it is certain that in each instance, proliferation of smooth muscle cells and accumulation of extracellular matrix are important components. In addition, in hypercholesterolemic subjects, the accumulation of lipid and lipid-filled macrophages contributes to the intimal lesion.

Because smooth muscle accumulation is a central feature of most forms of vascular thickening, it is worth discussing the mechanisms of growth control as we understand them.[18] During growth and development, smooth muscle cells proliferate; they revert spontaneously to a quiescent state in adult vessels. In the adult rat, smooth muscle cells turn over at the rate of 0.06% per day, a number barely detectable with available methods.[19] How the early rapid growth and late quiescence are regulated is not known, but this must be important to the problem of primary hypertension and local susceptibility to atherosclerotic change.

Of the models of smooth muscle growth in vivo, perhaps the best characterized is the balloon injury model.[20] In this model, smooth muscle proliferation is stimulated by the passage of an inflated balloon catheter along an artery. The artery is at once stretched and denuded of its endothelium. Immediately thereafter, platelets begin to adhere to the wall wherever endothelium is missing; they then spread and degranulate.

In most situations, endothelial denudation and platelet adherence are followed 1 to 2 days later by the onset of medial smooth muscle proliferation and migration of these cells across the internal elastic lamina to form a neointima.[19] In the ballooned rat carotid artery, this response can be dramatic, with a marked increase in the thymidine labeling index (a measure of proliferation) (Fig. 3-2). Intimal cells commit to proliferation early after injury. If entry into the cell cycle is blocked by giving the animals heparin during the first few days after injury, the number of dividing cells and the mass of neointima are significantly reduced.[21] Not all smooth muscle cells in the intima respond equally to mitogenic stimuli, probably because there is a mixture of cells derived from either the mesoderm or the ectoderm.[22]

A link between smooth muscle proliferation and earlier platelet granule release has been proposed, based on studies characterizing the proteins within the granules.[16] Among them are several growth factors, including platelet-derived growth factor (PDGF), transforming growth factor-β (TGF-β), and an epidermal growth factor–like protein.[23] Where these granule proteins go after being released from the platelets is not known. One hypothesis suggests that these factors accumulate in the artery wall and stimulate subsequent smooth muscle growth.

The reaction-to-injury hypothesis was first proposed many decades ago as a general mechanism for atherogenesis and

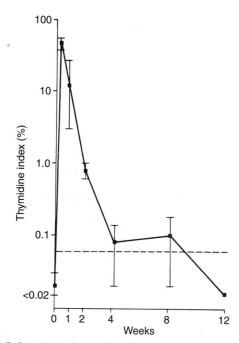

FIGURE 3–2 • Smooth muscle cell proliferation rates following balloon catheter injury of the rat carotid artery, as measured by the percentage of cells that incorporate thymidine. Proliferation is greatest at 48 hours and falls rapidly thereafter. (Adapted from Clowes AW, Reidy MA, Clowes MM: Kinetics of cellular proliferation after arterial injury. I. Smooth muscle growth in the absence of endothelium. Lab Invest 49:327, 1983.)

has been refined in view of more recent information.[16] Although attractive in theory, it is based on rather slim evidence derived mainly from experiments in thrombocytopenic animals. Injured arteries in these animals showed little intimal thickening.[24] Later work using thrombocytopenic rats suggests that platelets may be more important in stimulating migration than in cell proliferation.[25] These animals had reduced intimal thickening even though smooth muscle cell proliferation was not measurably altered. Additional work using anti-PDGF antibodies or infusion of PDGF after balloon injury supports this concept.[26,27]

This early proliferation in the media of the injured artery does not lead to an increase in wall thickness; the wall thickens only after smooth muscle cells migrate from the media and proliferate in the intima. This process persists for a period and subsides spontaneously regardless of whether endothelium reappears at the luminal surface. The intimal mass is further increased by the accumulation of extracellular matrix synthesized by the smooth muscle cells (Fig. 3-3).[28]

Although little is known about what starts or stops the intimal thickening process, there are several interesting and perhaps important observations. The first is that the surface of the injured artery accumulates a single layer of platelets. Fibrin and microthrombi are seen at the luminal surface only when the artery is reinjured after intimal thickening has formed or in small craters in association with adherent macrophages in hypercholesterolemic animals. Thus, active fulminant thrombosis is not a usual feature of injured vessels; when it occurs, it must represent a major aberration of vessel function.[29] Second, in models demonstrating early re-endothelialization or partial de-endothelialization without medial injury, intimal thickening

does not develop, although one or two rounds of medial smooth muscle proliferation can occur. This result suggests that endothelium may play a role in suppressing smooth muscle growth and migration from the media to the intima. We know that smooth muscle growth inhibitors can be extracted from the vessel wall, that endothelium can synthesize a heparin-like molecule that inhibits smooth muscle cell growth in vitro, and that heparin itself can suppress both proliferation and migration of smooth muscle cells in vitro and in vivo.[30] Endothelium also releases nitric oxide, a growth inhibitor whose production is flow dependent (see later). Taken together, these findings suggest that endothelium can inhibit smooth muscle proliferation and that the quiescent state of smooth muscle cells in the normal arteries of adult animals may be an actively maintained state rather than one attributable to the lack of growth factors. Finally, there is the more general concept emerging that the cells of the vascular wall "speak" to one another and regulate one another's function.

The possibility of cell-cell communication has been considered briefly twice: with regard to chronic vasodilatation in response to increased blood velocity, and with regard to control of smooth muscle cell proliferation and migration. Let us examine the kinds of messages and the participants in more detail, particularly as they pertain to growth control and maintenance of the antithrombotic state. At the outset, we can state that, at least in vitro, there is evidence for direct cell-cell communication by means of intercellular junctions; there is also evidence for communication by means of molecules secreted into the extracellular space and acting at a distance.

Direct cell-cell junctional communication has been demonstrated in monolayers of endothelium[31] and in mixed cell populations between endothelium and smooth muscle cells.[32] Gap junctions have been demonstrated morphologically between endothelial cells and between endothelium and smooth muscle cells in vivo and in vitro. The significance of these direct links has not been defined, although in culture, pericytes and smooth muscle cells can inhibit endothelial growth when the cells are in contact with one another.[32] Plasma membrane preparations from confluent large vessel endothelium also actively inhibit growing endothelial cells.[33] In vivo capillary endothelial growth is associated with the absence of pericytes, and cessation of growth is associated with their reappearance. In addition, the intercellular links might help regulate endothelial proliferation and endothelium-mediated vascular relaxation in collateral vessels by propagating signals from one cell to the next upstream from a large vessel occlusion. They would also provide a mechanism for a local response in a vessel without the need for the release and wide dissemination of potent vasoactive or growth-regulating substances.

Cell-cell communication at a distance is likely to be mediated by secreted soluble factors. As mentioned previously, the blood platelet, which in reality is a fragment of a megakaryocyte, carries within it an array of potent mitogens. The notion that platelets are involved in wound-healing processes came from morphologic studies of injured vessels and the observation that whole blood serum contains much more growth-promoting activity than does serum prepared from blood depleted of all cellular elements, including platelets (plasma-derived serum). These findings led to the discovery of PDGF, a basic dimeric protein[34] with a molecular weight of approximately 30,000. It is transported in the blood in the α-granule

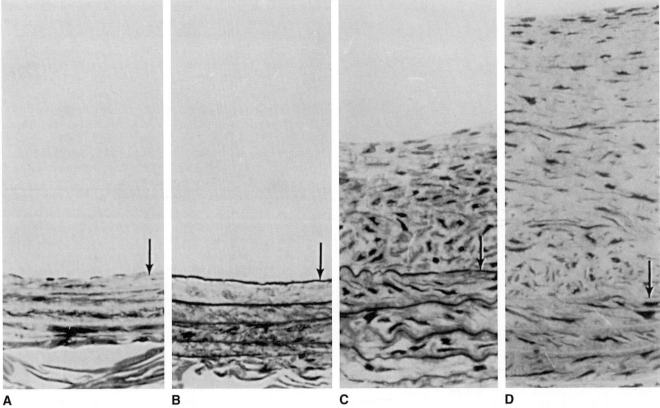

A **B** **C** **D**

FIGURE 3–3 • Histologic cross sections of the region lacking endothelium in injured left carotid arteries. *A,* Normal vessel. Note the single layer of endothelium in the intima. *B,* Denuded vessel at 2 days. Note the loss of endothelium. *C,* Denuded vessel at 2 weeks. The intima is now markedly thickened because of smooth muscle proliferation. *D,* Denuded vessel at 12 weeks. Further intimal thickening has occurred. The internal elastic lamina is indicated by the *arrow.* The lumen is at the top. (From Clowes AW, Reidy MA, Clowes MM: Kinetics of cellular proliferation after arterial injury. I. Smooth muscle growth in the absence of endothelium. Lab Invest 49:327, 1983.)

of the platelet and is released along with other α-granule proteins. PDGF is by itself extremely potent and is active as a smooth muscle mitogen in trace amounts (nanograms per milliliter). It also exhibits a range of other activities (stimulating migration, contraction, and matrix synthesis) on smooth muscle and other types of cells, although it is not a mitogen for endothelium. When placed in a wound chamber in vivo, it induces a granulation tissue response.[35]

The structure of the gene for PDGF is nearly identical to that of the oncogene v-*sis,* a gene associated with cellular transformation by the simian sarcoma virus.[36,37] This discovery, coupled with the finding that a variety of cells (including normal cells) synthesize and secrete active PDGF, raises the possibility that normal wound healing and malignant, unscheduled growth of tumor cells might have striking similarities, with subtle differences in gene regulation. It also led to a search for growth factors in vascular wall cells. We now have solid evidence that endothelium, smooth muscle cells, and leukocytes, including macrophages, can express the PDGF gene (c-*sis*) in vitro and in vivo.[34] What role the gene product, PDGF protein, plays in wall function remains to be resolved. The work mentioned here using anti-PDGF antibodies or infusion of PDGF in animals undergoing carotid injury by balloon catheter suggests that the primary role of PDGF is to stimulate smooth muscle cell migration rather than proliferation.[26,27]

Other work suggests that intracellular mitogens released from injured medial smooth muscle cells are primarily responsible for stimulating cell proliferation. First, smooth muscle cell proliferation occurs when arteries are injured by hydrostatic distention that does not cause significant endothelial injury.[38] In this case, there is very little smooth muscle cell migration, probably because of the lack of platelet factor release.[38] Second, very little smooth muscle cell proliferation is observed when the endothelium is injured by using a fine nylon loop that does not damage the media.[39,40] Basic fibroblast growth factor (bFGF) may be the principal mitogen responsible for smooth muscle cell proliferation after injury. Both bFGF messenger RNA (mRNA) and protein are found in the uninjured vessel wall.[41] Infusion or local administration of bFGF after arterial injury causes a marked increase in smooth muscle cell replication and intimal thickening.[41,42] Conversely, infusion of antibodies to bFGF causes a significant reduction in smooth muscle cell proliferation.[43] Because bFGF does not appear to be mitogenic for cells in uninjured vessels, this suggests that other products of injury are necessary to induce mitogenesis. Cultured smooth muscle cells derived from injured media produce up to five times more PDGF than do cells from uninjured arteries.[44] These injured cells also express mRNA for insulin-like growth factor[45] and TGF-β,[46] both of which are mitogenic for smooth muscle cells in culture. Thus, the smooth muscle cells in the injured

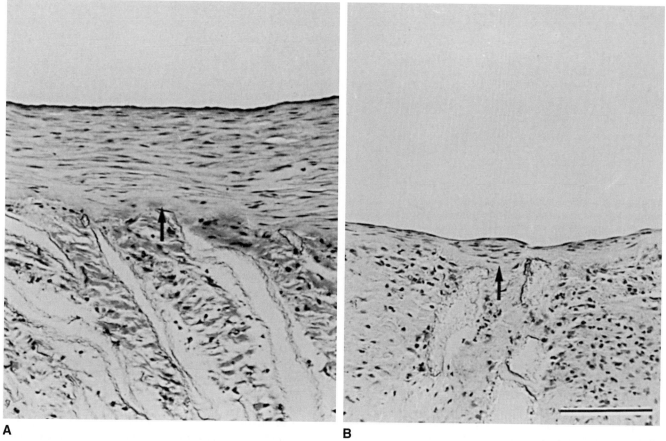

A   **B**

FIGURE 3–4 • Cross sections of polytetrafluoroethylene grafts 3 months after placement in the aortoiliac circulation in baboons. *A,* Control side with normal flow. *B,* Experimental side with a distal arteriovenous fistula causing increased flow. The *arrows* indicate the junction of the graft and neointima. (Bar, 100 μm.) (From Kohler TR, Kirkman TR, Kraiss LW, et al: Increased blood flow inhibits neointimal hyperplasia in endothelialized vascular grafts. Circ Res 69:1557, 1991.)

media may stimulate cell growth in a paracrine fashion by releasing a number of mitogens.

The rate of blood flow, which affects the diameter of developing and mature arteries, also influences intimal hyperplasia in injured vessels and vascular grafts. Wall thickening of vein and synthetic grafts is increased in areas of reduced flow[47,48] and is reduced by high flow (Fig. 3-4).[49,50] Increased flow causes regression of intima in endothelialized baboon polytetrafluoroethylene grafts.[51] As mentioned earlier, the endothelium responds to changes in shear and releases factors that regulate arterial diameter and wall structure in response to flow. For example, reduced flow causes an increase in PDGF expression in rat carotid arteries.[52] High flow upregulates NOS in synthetic grafts. We have found that the suppressive effect of flow on intimal thickening can be blocked by local infusion of an NOS inhibitor. Flow also appears to affect intimal hyperplasia in balloon-injured rat carotid arteries, even though the endothelium is absent in this model.[53] This implies that surface smooth muscle cells can respond to flow in a manner similar to that of endothelium. Finally, restoration of endothelial cell NOS activity in the denuded wall of injured rat carotid arteries by gene transfer suppresses intimal hyperplasia and increases vessel reactivity.[54]

There are several interesting preliminary observations that permit us to outline a theory of growth control in the wall. Endothelial cells in vitro can condition the tissue culture medium with growth-promoting factors for smooth muscle cells; a portion of this activity is due to PDGF-like proteins and perhaps to other characterized factors, such as bFGF. Production of PDGF is increased when the cells are exposed to endotoxin or phorbol esters and decreased when the cells are exposed to oxidized low-density lipoprotein.[55] Smooth muscle cells make PDGF in vitro as well; in particular, cells derived from neonatal as opposed to adult aortas and proliferating cells derived from injury-induced intimal thickening as opposed to quiescent media are prone to do this.[18] Macrophages, when stimulated, increase their production of PDGF. Finally, injured vascular wall cells release intracellular mitogens (e.g., bFGF). These fragmentary results support the concept that "activated" vascular wall cells can amplify the initial stimulus (perhaps an influx of platelet-derived factors) by producing PDGF and other growth-promoting factors that then act on the cells. These factors might also act to regulate the traffic of leukocytes in and out of the wall; the activated leukocytes could then reciprocate by producing factors affecting the function of the vascular wall cells. What emerges here is the notion that there may be a great deal of cross-talk between the cells of the wall and the blood, with many complex feedback loops (Fig. 3-5).[56]

New possibilities for preventing restenosis are emerging from our increasing understanding of cellular and molecular events. A complete listing of therapeutic strategies is beyond

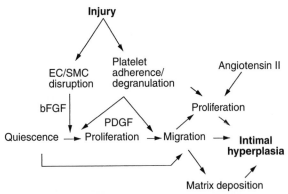

FIGURE 3–5 • Diagram illustrating how injury to the artery might cause endothelial cell (EC) and smooth muscle cell (SMC) disruption and release of intracellular mitogens such as basic fibroblast growth factor (bFGF). The bFGF then stimulates medial smooth muscle proliferation. Factors from platelets (platelet-derived growth factor [PDGF]) regulate movement of the smooth muscle cells from the media to the intima. Angiotensin II also affects the intimal thickening process. (From Clowes AW, Reidy MA: Prevention of stenosis after vascular reconstruction: Pharmacologic control of intimal hyperplasia—a review. J Vasc Surg 13:885, 1991.)

the scope of this chapter, but some other developments are worth noting. For example, our laboratory has found that blockade of the PDGF-β receptor with a chimeric human-murine antibody, in conjunction with heparin, inhibits intimal hyperplasia in a primate arterial injury model.[57] This finding supports the notion that PDGF plays an important role in wall thickening after injury. Platelet glycoprotein IIb/IIIa blockade with the chimeric antibody abciximab inhibits platelet aggregation and reduces the incidence of repeat procedures, death, and myocardial infarction after coronary angioplasty.[58] A single dose of this drug improved clinical results 3 years after the procedure, suggesting either that platelets have a role in initiating intimal hyperplasia or that the drug affects smooth muscle cell proliferation and migration.[59] In this regard, it is interesting to note a clinical trial of ticlopidine showing that 2-year patency rates were improved by the drug in vein grafts of lower extremity arteries.[60]

Many strategies are emerging for local control of smooth muscle cell proliferation following vascular injury. These include antisense oligonucleotides to inhibit cell cycle regulatory proteins and local delivery of radiation.[61-65] Radiation has the potential advantage of affecting adventitial cells. Lumen narrowing after injury results from both the mass of neointima that forms and remodeling of the vessel to a smaller diameter. Adventitial myofibroblasts contribute to each of these processes by forming a fibrotic scar around the injured vessel and by migrating across the wall into the neointima.[66] It is not yet known whether the right dose of radiation can be delivered to halt the restenosis process. So far, trials using ^{32}P radioactive β-emitting stents with low activity levels (0.75 to 3.0 μCi) for coronary angioplasty have shown no beneficial effect. Stents with higher activity levels (>3.0 μCi) have reduced intimal hyperplasia within the stent, but the low doses delivered to the adjacent artery near the end of the stents may actually encourage edge restenosis, particularly if this segment has been overdilated. This creates a "candy wrapper" appearance, with a widely patent stented region flanked on either side by tight stenoses.[67]

Drug-eluting stents are the first major advance in preventing restenosis. These devices provide local delivery of potent cell-cycle inhibitors, such as sirolimus and paclitaxel. They have revolutionized treatment of coronary artery stenosis and have nearly eliminated restenosis.[68] Use of similar devices in other vessels has the great potential to improve the results of percutaneous angioplasty throughout the arterial system.

Regulation of Thrombosis by the Endothelium

Empirical observation clearly demonstrates that a normal endothelium-lined artery is resistant to thrombosis. Even with complete cessation of blood flow for a prolonged period, clotting does not occur, although blood in a damaged vessel clots rather readily. It thus seems that endothelium must make one or more antithrombotic or anticoagulant molecules, and this has proved to be true. What is more striking is that the endothelium expresses an extensive array of procoagulant functions as well. Like the growth factors, these procoagulant-anticoagulant functions are regulated by messages coming from the blood or from neighboring cells.[69]

On the anticoagulant side of the balance, the endothelium synthesizes a membrane-associated heparan sulfate that, like heparin, increases the affinity of antithrombin III for thrombin.[70] Because this interaction requires the binding of heparan sulfate to antithrombin III, the complex must be active at the level of the endothelial surface. Heparan–antithrombin III then rapidly inactivates circulating thrombin and other activated serine proteases in the clotting cascade, including factors VII, IX, and X. Thus, endothelium-derived heparan sulfate can act to impede two aspects of the injury response: activation of the clotting cascade and stimulation of smooth muscle proliferation (referred to earlier).[30] In addition, endothelial cells can inhibit clotting by means of the protein C pathway.[71] Endothelium synthesizes and secretes a protein called thrombomodulin, which in turn is bound to a surface receptor. The receptor-thrombomodulin complex binds thrombin and in so doing inactivates the proteolytic activity for fibrinogen. The thrombomodulin-thrombin complex activates protein C, and the activated protein C binds to protein S on the endothelial surface. The protein C–protein S complex then inactivates factor Va, thereby inhibiting the clotting cascade. That this pathway is important is amply demonstrated in homozygous-deficient patients, who develop spontaneous thrombosis. Finally, endothelial cells can inhibit platelet adhesion and aggregation through the synthesis of prostaglandin I_2 and can degrade formed fibrin by activating plasminogen to plasmin.

On the procoagulant side, endothelial cells synthesize and secrete tissue factor, a plasminogen activator inhibitor, and von Willebrand's factor, and they express a number of receptors for factors of the clotting cascade. When the cells are exposed to a variety of inflammatory mediators derived from the blood or from resident macrophages (e.g., endotoxin, interleukin-1, tumor necrosis factor), endothelial cells respond by changing the balance of anticoagulant-procoagulant activities to favor coagulation. Also, the cells synthesize and express interleukin-1, which could affect the underlying smooth muscle cells.[72] At present, these conclusions are largely based on in vitro experiments; although they have relevance mainly to the microvasculature, they also may prove to be important to large vessels, in view of the recent evidence that not only macrophages but also different populations of lymphocytes are present in atherosclerotic plaque. Further, the ability of the vascular wall cells to maintain the anticoagulant state at the luminal surface must have a direct bearing on the thrombotic complications associated with end-stage atherosclerosis.

Thrombin generated during thrombosis may play an important role in regulating smooth muscle cell growth. It is mitogenic for these cells grown in culture. Antithrombin agents block the increase in PDGF gene expression that normally follows injury and can limit smooth muscle cell proliferation following injury.[73] Thrombin may also potentiate cell growth by activating platelets and attracting activated macrophages, which also produce mitogens.

Summary

The normal blood vessel must be viewed not only as a conduit but also as an organ containing endothelial and smooth muscle cells that can respond to physical and chemical stimuli in the blood by adjusting vascular diameter and thickness. Vascular wall cells can communicate among themselves and express factors that can regulate cell proliferation and coagulation, as well as allow the cells to participate in local inflammatory reactions.

REFERENCES

1. Wolinsky H, Glagov S: A lamellar unit of aortic medial structure and function in mammals. Circ Res 20:99, 1967.
2. Clark JM, Glagov S: Transmural organization of the arterial media: The lamellar unit revisited. Arteriosclerosis 5:19, 1985.
3. Wolinsky H, Glagov S: Nature of species differences in the medial distribution of aortic vasa vasorum in mammals. Circ Res 20:409, 1967.
4. Cotran RS, Kumar V, Robbins SL: Pathologic Basis of Disease. Philadelphia, WB Saunders, 1989, p 553.
5. Zarins CK, Zatina MA, Giddens DP, et al: Shear stress regulation of artery lumen diameter in experimental atherogenesis. J Vasc Surg 5:413, 1987.
6. Langille BL, O'Donnell F: Reductions in arterial diameter produced by chronic decreases in blood flow are endothelium-dependent. Science 231:405, 1986.
7. Guyton JR, Hartley CJ: Flow restriction of one carotid artery in juvenile rats inhibits growth of arterial diameter. Am J Physiol 248:H540, 1985.
8. Brownlee RD, Langille BL: Arterial adaptations to altered blood flow. Can J Physiol Pharmacol 69:978, 1991.
9. Glagov S, Weisenberg E, Zarins CK, et al: Compensatory enlargement of human atherosclerotic coronary arteries. N Engl J Med 316:1371, 1987.
10. Frangos JA, Eskin SG, McIntire LV, Ives CL: Flow effect on prostacyclin production by cultured human endothelial cells. Science 227:1477, 1985.
11. Furchgott RF, Vanhoutte PM: Endothelium-derived relaxing and contracting factors. FASEB J 3:2007, 1989.
12. Furchgott RF, Zawadzki JV: The obligatory role of endothelial cells in the relaxation of arterial smooth muscle by acetylcholine. Nature 288:373, 1980.
13. Moncada S, Higgs EA, Hodson HF, et al: EDRF and EDRF-related substances: The L-arginine:nitric oxide pathway. J Cardiovasc Pharmacol 17(Suppl 3):S1, 1991.
14. Freiman PC, Mitchell GG, Heistad DD, et al: Atherosclerosis impairs endothelium-dependent vascular relaxation to acetylcholine and thrombin in primates. Circ Res 58:783, 1986.
15. Wolinsky H: Long-term effects of hypertension on the rat aortic wall and their relation to concurrent aging changes: Morphological and chemical studies. Circ Res 30:301, 1972.
16. Ross R: Pathogenesis of atherosclerosis—an update. N Engl J Med 314:488, 1986.
17. Steinberg D: Lipoproteins and the pathogenesis of atherosclerosis. Circulation 76:508, 1987.
18. Schwartz SM, Campbell GR, Campbell JH: Replication of smooth muscle cells in vascular disease. Circ Res 58:427, 1986.
19. Clowes AW, Reidy MA, Clowes MM: Kinetics of cellular proliferation after arterial injury. 1.Smooth muscle growth in the absence of endothelium. Lab Invest 49:327, 1983.
20. Baumgartner HR, Studer A: Consequences of vessel catheterization in normal and hypercholesterolemic rabbits [in German]. Pathol Microbiol 29:393, 1966.
21. Clowes AW, Clowes MM: Kinetics of cellular proliferation after arterial injury: IV heparin inhibits rat smooth muscle mitogenesis and migration. Circ Res 58:839, 1986.
22. Topouzis S, Majesky MW: Smooth muscle lineage diversity in the chick embryo: Two types of aortic smooth muscle cell differ in growth and receptor-mediated transcriptional responses to transforming growth factor-beta. Dev Biol 178:430, 1996.
23. Bowen-Pope DF, Ross R, Seifert RA: Locally acting growth factors for vascular smooth muscle cells: Endogenous synthesis and release from platelets. Circulation 72:735, 1985.
24. Friedman RJ, Stemerman MB, Wenz B, et al: The effect of thrombocytopenia on experimental arteriosclerotic lesion formation in rabbits, smooth muscle cell proliferation and re-endothelialization. J Clin Invest 60:1191, 1977.
25. Fingerle J, Johnson R, Clowes AW, et al: Role of platelets in smooth muscle cell proliferation and migration after vascular injury in rat carotid artery. Proc Natl Acad Sci U S A 86:8412, 1989.
26. Ferns GAA, Raines EW, Sprugel KH, et al: Inhibition of neointimal smooth muscle accumulation after angioplasty by an antibody to PDGF. Science 253:1129, 1991.
27. Jawien A, Bowen-Pope DF, Lindner V, et al: Platelet-derived growth factor promotes smooth muscle migration and intimal thickening in a rat model of balloon angioplasty. J Clin Invest 89:507, 1992.
28. Clowes AW, Reidy MA, Clowes MM: Mechanisms of stenosis after arterial injury. Lab Invest 49:208, 1983.
29. Reidy MA: A reassessment of endothelial injury and arterial lesion formation. Lab Invest 53:513, 1985.
30. Clowes AW, Clowes MM: Regulation of smooth muscle proliferation by heparin in vitro and in vivo. Int Angiol 6:45, 1987.
31. Larson DM, Carson MP, Haudenschild CC: Junctional transfer of small molecules in cultured bovine brain microvascular endothelial cells and pericytes. Microvasc Res 34:184, 1987.
32. Orlidge A, D'Amore PA: Inhibition of capillary endothelial cell growth by pericytes and smooth muscle cells. J Cell Biol 105:1455, 1987.
33. Heimark RL, Schwartz SM: The role of membrane-membrane interactions in the regulation of endothelial cell growth. J Cell Biol 100:1934, 1985.
34. Ross R, Raines EW, Bowen-Pope DF: The biology of PDGF. Cell 46:155, 1986.
35. Sprugel KH, McPherson JM, Clowes AW, Ross R: Effects of growth factors in vivo. I. Cell ingrowth into porous subcutaneous chambers. Am J Pathol 129:601, 1987.
36. Doolittle RF, Hunkapillar MW, Hood LE, et al: Simian sarcoma virus oncogene, v-sis, is derived from the gene (or genes) encoding a platelet-derived growth factor. Science 221:275, 1983.
37. Waterfield MD, Scrace GT, Whittle N, et al: Platelet-derived growth factor is structurally related to the putative transforming protein p28-sis of simian sarcoma virus. Nature 304:35, 1983.
38. Clowes AW, Clowes MM, Fingerle J, Reidy MA: Kinetics of cellular proliferation after arterial injury. V. Role of acute distention in the induction of smooth muscle proliferation. Lab Invest 60:360, 1989.
39. Tada T, Reidy MA: Endothelial regeneration. IX. Arterial injury followed by rapid endothelial repair induces smooth-muscle-cell proliferation but not intimal thickening. Am J Pathol 129:429, 1987.
40. Fingerle J, Au YPT, Clowes AW, Reidy MA: Intimal lesion formation in rat carotid arteries after endothelial denudation in absence of medial injury. Arteriosclerosis 10:1082, 1990.
41. Lindner V, Lappi DA, Baird A, et al: Role of basic fibroblast growth factor in vascular lesion formation. Circ Res 68:106, 1991.
42. Edelman ER, Nugent MA, Smith LT, Karnovsky MJ: Basic fibroblast growth factor enhances the coupling of intimal hyperplasia and proliferation of vasa vasorum in injured rat arteries. J Clin Invest 89:465, 1992.
43. Lindner V, Reidy MA: Proliferation of smooth muscle cells after vascular injury is inhibited by an antibody against basic fibroblast growth factor. Proc Natl Acad Sci U S A 88:3739, 1991.

44. Walker LN, Bowen-Pope DF, Reidy MA: Production of platelet-derived growth factor–like molecules by cultured arterial smooth muscle cells accompanies proliferation after arterial injury. Proc Natl Acad Sci U S A 83:7311, 1986.

45. Cercek B, Fishbein MC, Forrester JS, et al: Induction of insulin-like growth factor I messenger RNA in rat aorta after balloon denudation. Circ Res 66:1755, 1990.

46. Majesky MW, Lindner V, Twardzik DR, et al: Production of transforming growth factor β_1 during repair of arterial injury. J Clin Invest 88:904, 1991.

47. Berguer R, Higgins RF, Reddy DJ: Intimal hyperplasia. Arch Surg 115:332, 1980.

48. Rittgers SE, Karayannacos PE, Guy JF: Velocity distribution and intimal proliferation in autologous vein grafts in dogs. Circ Res 42:792, 1978.

49. Kohler TR, Kirkman TR, Kraiss LW, et al: Increased blood flow inhibits neointimal hyperplasia in endothelialized vascular grafts. Circ Res 69:1557, 1991.

50. Kraiss LW, Kirkman TR, Kohler TR, et al: Shear stress regulates smooth muscle proliferation and neointimal thickening in porous polytetrafluoroethylene grafts. Arterioscler Thromb Vasc Biol 11:1844, 1991.

51. Mattsson EJ, Kohler TR, Vergel SM, Clowes AW: Increased blood flow induces regression of intimal hyperplasia. Arterioscler Thromb Vasc Biol 17:2245, 1997.

52. Mondy JS, Lindner V, Miyashiro JK, et al: Platelet-derived growth factor ligand and receptor expression in response to altered blood flow in vivo. Circ Res 81:320, 1997.

53. Kohler TR, Jawien A: Flow affects development of intimal hyperplasia following arterial injury in rats. Arterioscler Thromb Vasc Biol 12:963, 1992.

54. von der Leyen HE, Gibbons GH, Morishita R, et al: Gene therapy inhibiting neointimal vascular lesion: In vivo transfer of endothelial cell nitric oxide synthase gene. Proc Natl Acad Sci U S A 92:1137, 1995.

55. DiCorleto PE, Bowen-Pope DF: Cultured endothelial cells produce a platelet-derived growth factor–like protein. Proc Natl Acad Sci U S A 80:1919, 1983.

56. Libby P, Salomon RN, Payne DO, et al: Functions of vascular wall cells related to development of transplantation-associated coronary arteriosclerosis. Transplant Proc 21:1, 1989.

57. Hart CE, Kraiss LW, Vergel S, et al: PDGF-beta receptor blockade inhibits intimal hyperplasia in the baboon. Circulation 99:564, 1999.

58. EPISTENT Investigators: Randomised placebo-controlled and balloon-angioplasty-controlled trial to assess safety of coronary stenting with use of platelet glycoprotein-IIb/IIIa blockade: Evaluation of platelet IIb/IIIa inhibitor for stenting [see comments]. Lancet 352:87, 1998.

59. Topol EJ, Ferguson JJ, Weisman HF, et al: Long-term protection from myocardial ischemic events in a randomized trial of brief integrin beta3 blockade with percutaneous coronary intervention. EPIC Investigator Group. Evaluation of platelet IIb/IIIa inhibition for prevention of ischemic complication [see comments]. JAMA 278:479, 1997.

60. Schomig A, Neumann FJ, Kastrati A, et al: A randomized comparison of antiplatelet and anticoagulant therapy after the placement of coronary-artery stents [see comments]. N Engl J Med 334:1084, 1996.

61. Mann MJ, Gibbons GH, Kernoff RS, et al: Genetic engineering of vein grafts resistant to atherosclerosis. Proc Natl Acad Sci U S A 92:4502, 1995.

62. Wilcox JN, Waksman R, King SB, Scott NA: The role of the adventitia in the arterial response to angioplasty: The effect of intravascular radiation. Int J Radiat Oncol Biol Phys 36:789, 1996.

63. Meerkin D, Bonan R, Crocker IR, et al: Efficacy of beta radiation in prevention of post-angioplasty restenosis: An interim report from the Beta Energy Restenosis Trial. Herz 23:356, 1998.

64. Waksman R, Robinson KA, Crocker IR, et al: Endovascular low-dose irradiation inhibits neointima formation after coronary artery balloon injury in swine: A possible role for radiation therapy in restenosis prevention. Circulation 91:1533, 1995.

65. Teirstein PS, Massullo V, Jani S, et al: Three-year clinical and angiographic follow-up after intracoronary radiation: Results of a randomized clinical trial. Circulation 101:360, 2000.

66. Wilcox JN, Waksman R, King SB, Scott NA: The role of the adventitia in the arterial response to angioplasty: The effect of intravascular radiation [review]. Int J Radiat Oncol Biol Phys 36:789, 1996.

67. Albiero R, Adamian M, Kobayashi N, et al: Short- and intermediate-term results of ^{32}P radioactive beta-emitting stent implantation in patients with coronary artery disease: The Milan dose-response study. Circulation 101:18, 2000.

68. Dobesh PP, Stacy ZA, Ansara AJ, Enders JM: Drug-eluting stents: A mechanical and pharmacologic approach to coronary artery disease. Pharmacotherapy 24:1554, 2004.

69. Hawiger JJ: Hemostasis, bleeding, and thromboembolic complications of trauma and infection. In Clowes GHA Jr (ed): Trauma, Sepsis and Shock: The Physiological Basis of Therapy. New York, Marcel Dekker, 1988, p 123.

70. Marcum J, McKenney J, Rosenberg R: The acceleration of thrombin-antithrombin III complex formation in rat hind quarters via heparin-like molecules bound to endothelium. J Clin Invest 74:341, 1984.

71. Esmon CT: Protein C. Prog Hemost Thromb 7:25, 1984.

72. Libby P, Ordovas JM, Auger KH, et al: Endotoxin and tumor necrosis factor induce interleukin-1 beta gene expression in adult human vascular endothelial cells. Am J Pathol 124:179, 1986.

73. Harker LA, Hanson SR, Runge MS: Thrombin hypothesis of thrombus generation and vascular lesion formation. Am J Cardiol 75:12B, 1995.

Questions

1. **In normal arteries, most of the smooth muscle cells are found in which area?**
   (a) Intima
   (b) Media
   (c) Adventitia
   (d) None of the above

2. **Arteries respond to an increase in blood flow by doing which of the following?**
   (a) Contracting
   (b) Dilating
   (c) Intermittently contracting
   (d) Intermittently dilating

3. **Endothelial cells synthesize and secrete substances that cause what?**
   (a) Vasodilatation
   (b) Vasoconstriction
   (c) Both vasodilatation and vasoconstriction
   (d) None of the above

4. **What causes injured arteries to thicken?**
   (a) Medial smooth muscle hyperplasia
   (b) Intimal smooth muscle hyperplasia
   (c) Intimal endothelial hyperplasia
   (d) None of the above

5. **The reaction-to-injury hypothesis was proposed to explain the initial stages of atherosclerosis. Which element of this hypothesis has not been proved?**
   (a) Smooth muscle cells are important components of plaque
   (b) Thrombus can accumulate on atherosclerotic lesions
   (c) Platelets contain potent growth factors
   (d) Growth factors released from platelets stimulate smooth muscle growth in vivo

6. **Platelet-derived growth factor (PDGF) is found in which cells?**
   (a) Platelets
   (b) Smooth muscle cells
   (c) Endothelium
   (d) All of the above

7. Smooth muscle cells respond to PDGF by doing which of the following?
   (a) Proliferating
   (b) Synthesizing matrix
   (c) Migrating
   (d) All of the above

8. Based on in vitro studies, endothelial cells appear to express molecules that regulate the behavior of the blood at the luminal surface. Which of the following endothelium-derived molecules act to sustain the anticoagulant state? (There may be more than one correct answer.)
   (a) Heparan sulfate
   (b) Von Willebrand's factor
   (c) Plasminogen activator inhibitor
   (d) Thrombomodulin
   (e) Prostacyclin

9. Which of the following molecules are procoagulants? (There may be more than one correct answer.)
   (a) Heparan sulfate
   (b) Von Willebrand's factor
   (c) Plasminogen activator inhibitor
   (d) Thrombomodulin
   (e) Prostacyclin

10. In general, inflammatory mediators (e.g., interleukin-1) cause endothelial cells to express which of the following?
    (a) Increased procoagulant activities
    (b) Increased anticoagulant activities
    (c) Increased endothelium-derived relaxing factor
    (d) None of the above

Answers

1. b	2. b	3. c	4. b	5. d
6. d	7. d	8. a, d, e	9. b, c	10. a

IL-1 : procoagulant

4

Jeffrey L. Ballard

Anatomy and Surgical Exposure of the Vascular System

A well-planned surgical exposure facilitates even the most difficult operative procedure. Awareness of the relationship between surface anatomy and the underlying vascular structure allows precise incision placement as well as percutaneous access. This minimizes tissue trauma and reduces the likelihood of wound infection. Detailed knowledge of vascular anatomy helps prevent injury to adjacent vital structures within the operative field. In this chapter, anatomic relationships and variations that may be encountered during common vascular exposures are highlighted. Several alternative surgical approaches are also described. Exposure of the carotid bifurcation is discussed first. This is followed by a systematic discussion of the anatomy and surgical exposure of the peripheral vascular system, ending with commonly used approaches for the arterial circulation in the leg and foot.

Exposure of the Carotid Bifurcation

The common carotid artery bifurcates approximately 2.5 cm below the angle of the mandible. Normally, the sternocleidomastoid muscle, the posterior belly of the digastric muscle, and the omohyoid muscle bound the carotid bifurcation. Thus, a skin incision placed along the anterior border of the sternocleidomastoid muscle facilitates exposure of the carotid sheath.

The surgeon must be aware of the location of important cranial and somatic nerves during carotid endarterectomy. The mandibular ramus of the facial nerve is vulnerable to injury during this operation. Nerve damage by retraction or surgical dissection can cause temporary or permanent dysfunction. Turning the head toward the opposite side draws the mandibular ramus well below the mandible and increases the possibility of facial nerve injury.

The great auricular nerve (C-2 and C-3 dermatomes) should be protected in its location on the sternocleidomastoid muscle just anterior to and below the ear. Damage to this nerve results in numbness of the posterior aspect of the auricle and may cause distressing ipsilateral occipital headaches.

The common facial vein comes into view as the incision is deepened. This vessel courses superficial to the carotid bifurcation to join the internal jugular vein. It serves as an important landmark during the dissection. Several small vessels coursing toward the sternocleidomastoid muscle are nutrient branches from the superior thyroid artery and vein. These vessels should be ligated and divided to avoid troublesome postoperative bleeding. In the typical carotid dissection, the common carotid artery should be exposed above the level of the omohyoid muscle. Once this vessel is isolated, further distal dissection along its medial aspect facilitates exposure of the superior thyroid and external carotid arteries. Dissection in the V of the carotid bifurcation should be avoided, because this area is extremely vascular. It is wise to encircle the internal carotid artery well above the level of gross atherosclerotic disease. This dissection is usually 1 to 2 cm above the bifurcation and thereby avoids the highly vascular carotid sinus tissue.

The descending branch of the hypoglossal nerve (ansa cervicalis) is located anterior and parallel to the sternocleidomastoid muscle. If this branch is followed upward, the main hypoglossal nerve trunk can be located. Division of the descending branch of the hypoglossal nerve near its origin allows the main nerve trunk to be displaced upward and forward, thus providing higher exposure of the internal carotid artery. A nutrient vein and artery associated with the sternocleidomastoid muscle course in immediate relation to this nerve at this level. Care should be taken to avoid injury to the underlying hypoglossal nerve when these vessels are ligated and divided. This maneuver allows the nerve to retract superomedially and out of harm's way. Division of this artery-vein "sling" about the hypoglossal nerve facilitates exposure of the internal carotid artery under the posterior belly of the digastric muscle.

The surgeon must also maintain an awareness of the location of the vagus nerve and its branches. It lies within the carotid sheath between the common carotid artery and the internal jugular vein. Normally, it is directly behind the internal carotid artery at its origin. Care must be taken to prevent injury to the nerve at this vulnerable location.

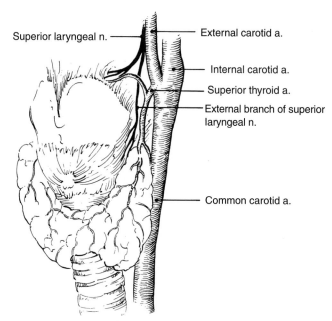

Superior laryngeal n.

External carotid a.

Internal carotid a.

Superior thyroid a.

External branch of superior laryngeal n.

Common carotid a.

FIGURE 4–1 • Note the vulnerable location of the external branch of the superior laryngeal nerve to the superior thyroid artery.

passes behind the internal carotid artery, and descends medial to the superior thyroid artery. Care must be taken during mobilization of this vessel not to injure the superior laryngeal nerve or its external branch (Fig. 4-1). The external branch of the superior laryngeal nerve sometimes passes between the branches of the superior thyroid artery or is adherent to it. Table 4-1 lists the locations and the tests for function of the important nerves encountered during exposure of the carotid bifurcation.

A carotid arteriotomy should be created proximal to the carotid bulb and lateral to the carotid flow divider in the typical endarterectomy scenario. This incision is then lengthened distally through the diseased internal carotid artery under direct vision to a point where there is normal-appearing intima. It is critical not to make this arteriotomy on the anterior aspect of the internal carotid artery near the carotid sinus, because this is a relatively fixed area that is difficult to reapproximate without creating a focal narrowing that is at risk for restenosis. It is wise to find the correct endarterectomy plane at the level of the carotid bulb. Endarterectomy then proceeds proximally first, and the specimen is excised sharply with Potts scissors at the level of the common carotid artery. Everting the external carotid artery into the carotid bulb facilitates endarterectomy at this level. Then, the transition point between the atherosclerotic plaque to be removed and the remaining nondiseased internal carotid artery is located. This is the critical step in the performance of a technically sound carotid endarterectomy, and if it is done correctly, tacking sutures are rarely required. Meticulous care is then taken to ensure that no loose areas of

Additional care is required to prevent vagus nerve injury during redo carotid exposure, owing to the fact that the nerve, which may be encased in scar tissue, frequently courses anterior to the carotid bifurcation. The superior laryngeal nerve arises from the vagus nerve above the carotid bifurcation,

TABLE 4–1   Regional Nerves Encountered during Exposure of the Carotid Bifurcation

Nerve Branch	Location Encountered	Test for Function	Remarks
Mandibular ramus of facial nerve (cranial nerve VII)	Deep to platysma muscle; can be 5-10 mm below inferior margin of mandible	Ask patient to show teeth—check for paralysis of lower lip	Use gentle retraction on mandible; nerve is pulled down when head is rotated to opposite side for operative exposure
Great auricular nerve (C-2 and C-3)	Anteromedial surface of SCM muscle anterior to and below ear	Anesthesia of ear and adjacent scalp	May cause disturbing ipsilateral occipital headache when damaged
Cutaneous cervical nerve (C-2 and C-3)	Subcutaneous on deep fascia	Anesthesia of skin below mandible	Warn patient preoperatively about possible sensory loss
Glossopharyngeal nerve branch (cranial nerve IX)	Between external and internal carotid arteries (branch is the carotid sinus nerve, also known as nerve of Hering)	Loss of ability to swallow	Manipulation of nerve may cause bradycardia or hypotension; IV atropine or local infiltration of the nerve with lidocaine relieves circulatory changes
Vagus nerve (cranial nerve X)	Within carotid sheath; between internal jugular vein and common carotid artery; directly behind proximal internal carotid artery	Indirect laryngoscopy for vocal cord function	Dissect "right on" distal common and internal carotid arteries and avoid "past-pointing" with vascular occluding clamps
External branch of superior laryngeal nerve (branch of cranial nerve X)	Adjacent and medial to superior thyroid artery	Loss of function of cricothyroid muscle	Inability to reproduce high tones
Hypoglossal nerve (cranial nerve XII)	Main nerve trunk crosses internal and external carotid arteries 1-2 cm above carotid bifurcation; SCM artery and vein branches sling around nerve	Extended tongue deviates to side of injured nerve	Visualize descending branch first and follow it to main nerve trunk; carefully ligate SCM arterial and venous branches to preserve dry operative field

IV, intravenous; SCM, sternocleidomastoid.

media remain through the endarterectomized surface. In my practice, Dacron patch angioplasty reapproximates the arteriotomy, and intraoperative duplex ultrasound scanning completes the procedure. The reader is referred to *Wylie's Atlas of Vascular Surgery* for color illustrations of the steps used to perform a classic carotid endarterectomy.[1]

For eversion endarterectomy, the carotid artery is obliquely transected at the transition between the proximal internal carotid artery and the carotid bulb. Plaque control with forceps and gentle eversion of the internal carotid artery enable one to establish an appropriate endarterectomy plane of dissection, as well as a distal break point that will allow the plaque to feather away without the need for tacking sutures. Proximally, angled Potts scissors can be used to extend the arteriotomy, which facilitates endarterectomy at the level of the carotid bulb and external carotid artery. The transected internal carotid artery can be shortened if necessary and then reattached using a continuous Prolene suture. Appropriate suturing of the internal carotid artery to the carotid bulb frequently requires one to further incise the medial aspect of the artery with Potts scissors.

The value of cranial nerve protection during carotid surgery is emphasized by the classic reports of Evans and associates[2] and Hertzer and colleagues.[3] Evans's group prospectively studied the incidence of cranial nerve injury during carotid surgery. Before and after carotid endarterectomy, surgeons and a speech pathologist made observations regarding cranial nerve function. The surgeons reported a 4% incidence of preoperative vagus nerve dysfunction, whereas the speech pathologist found a 30% incidence. Two days after the endarterectomy, the surgeons reported a 14.6% incidence of vagus nerve deficit, whereas the speech pathologist noted a 35% incidence of superior laryngeal or recurrent nerve dysfunction. These data emphasize the wisdom of a thorough vocal cord evaluation before reoperation or when operating on the second side soon after the first, when paresis of cord function may still persist.

In 1999, Ballotta and colleagues reviewed 200 consecutive carotid endarterectomies in Italy.[4] There were 25 cranial nerve injuries (12.5%) in 24 patients, distributed as follows: hypoglossal (11), recurrent laryngeal (8), superior laryngeal (2), marginal mandibular (2), greater auricular (2). Fortunately, the deficits were transient, with all but 4 resolving by 6 months. The mean recovery time was 5.8 months, with a range of 1 week to 37 months. Forssell and associates reviewed 663 consecutive carotid endarterectomy patients in Malmö, Sweden, who were examined pre- and postoperatively at the Department of Phoniatrics to determine cranial nerve function.[5] Seventy-five carotid operations (11.4%) resulted in one or more cranial nerve injuries. These included 70 hypoglossal, 8 recurrent laryngeal, 2 glossopharyngeal, and 2 superior laryngeal injuries. Only two nerve injuries (0.30%) were permanent. The frequency of injury increased with a junior surgeon, shunt use, and patch closure.

In summary, cranial nerve injuries are usually caused by direct trauma such as stretch, retraction, clamping, or transection. Nerve transection should be rare in experienced hands. Reapproximating the epineurium primarily with fine suture at the time of injury is the best way to repair a transected cranial nerve. Most cranial nerve injuries are transient, with full recovery within 6 months, on average.

Exposure of the High Internal Carotid Artery

One of the most difficult vascular surgical exposures is that of the high internal carotid artery. The surgeon must contend with many vital structures within a confined space. This is frequently made more difficult by the presence of a space-occupying vascular lesion or a vascular injury with hemorrhagic staining and displacement of the tissues. Structures that overlie the high internal carotid artery in the neck include the facial nerve, parotid gland, ramus of the mandible, and mastoid and styloid processes. The hypoglossal nerve, glossopharyngeal nerve, digastric and stylohyoid muscles, and occipital and posterior auricular arteries cross it. The distal cervical internal carotid artery courses progressively deeper to enter the petrous canal of the temporal bone.

Exposure routinely begins at the level of the common carotid artery proximal to the carotid bifurcation. The omohyoid muscle serves as a landmark for the proximal extent of this exposure. The dissection continues distally, protecting the vagus nerve, which lies immediately behind the internal carotid artery. The hypoglossal nerve is exposed, and the descending branch is divided to displace the hypoglossal nerve forward. The digastric and stylohyoid muscles are divided to facilitate this exposure. In addition, the styloid process and the stylohyoid ligament are excised. The glossopharyngeal and superior laryngeal nerves must be identified and preserved. One is now working in a progressively narrowing triangle, with inadequate space to perform any major vascular reconstructive procedure.

Anatomic dissection in human cadaver specimens demonstrates that division of the posterior belly of the digastric muscle facilitates exposure of the internal carotid artery to the middle of the first cervical vertebra. Anterior subluxation of the mandible improves exposure to the superior border of the first cervical vertebra. The addition of styloidectomy to the maneuvers described here extends the exposure cephalad approximately 0.5 cm.[6]

Fisher and associates described a unique technique of wire fixation of the mandible to hold its subluxed position during the operative procedure.[7] The 12 to 15 mm of space obtained converts the triangle described earlier into a narrow rectangle (Fig. 4-2). It is important to avoid dislocation of the mandible, because serious injury can occur to the temporomandibular joint and even to the contralateral internal carotid artery. In the discussion of Fisher and associates' paper, Stanley suggested that a towel clip placed on the angle of the mandible through two small stab incisions would allow the subluxation to be fixed by minimal retraction. Dossa and associates also suggested that temporary mandibular subluxation can be accomplished in a safe and expeditious manner using diagonal, interdental Steinmann pin wiring.[8] Figure 4-3 shows a diagram of the relationship of the mandibular condyle to the auricular eminence and infratemporal fossa.

In situations requiring more room for vascular reconstruction, transection of the mandibular ramus with either translocation or temporary removal of the condyle and ramus fragment affords wider exposure. Wylie and associates described this approach and provided detailed color illustrations of the involved anatomy.[9]

Following induction of anesthesia, arch bars and wires immobilize the mandible. The usual carotid endarterectomy

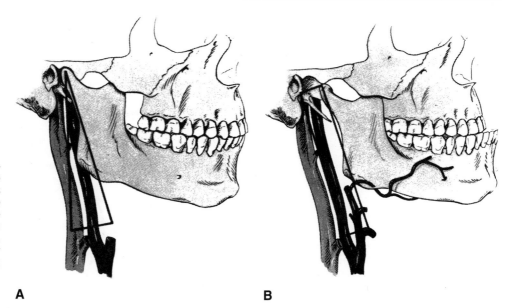

A   **B**

incision is extended posteriorly to a point behind the ear. The carotid bifurcation and internal carotid artery are exposed as described previously. The mandibular ramus of the facial nerve is protected. The angle of the mandible is exposed, and the periosteum is elevated toward the mandibular notch anteriorly and posteriorly. The mandibular ramus is divided vertically using a power saw posterior to the foramen of the inferior alveolar artery and nerve. The posterior bone fragment is gently rotated out and upward as the pterygoid muscles are divided, allowing the fragment's removal. The bone fragment is preserved in chilled lactated Ringer's solution until it is replaced after arterial reconstruction.

Once the mandibular ramus is removed, the digastric and stylohyoid muscles are divided, and the dissection is continued to the skull base. Care should be taken to protect the hypoglossal, glossopharyngeal, and vagus nerves, which are in immediate relation to the high internal carotid artery. The mandibular fragment is returned to its anatomic location after completion of the internal carotid artery reconstruction, and interrupted nonabsorbable sutures close the temporomandibular joint capsule. A thin titanium plate is used to fix

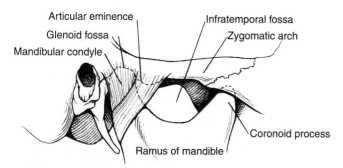

Articular eminence
Glenoid fossa
Mandibular condyle
Infratemporal fossa
Zygomatic arch
Coronoid process
Ramus of mandible

FIGURE 4–3 • Anterior subluxation moves the condyle of the mandible to the articular eminence but not to the infratemporal fossa, as would occur with dislocation of the mandible. (From Fisher DF Jr, Clagett GP, Parker JI, et al: Mandibular subluxation for high carotid exposure. J Vasc Surg 1:727, 1984.)

the mandibular fragment in place. The cervical fascia and platysma muscle are closed in layers, followed by routine skin closure.

Exposure of Aortic Arch Branches and Associated Veins

The most widely accepted direct route for the surgical exposure of the innominate and proximal left common carotid arteries, as well as the superior vena cava and its confluent brachiocephalic veins, is through a full median sternotomy. However, a less invasive surgical exposure for the direct treatment of these aortic arch branch vessels and associated major veins has been described in detail.[10] Similar to a median sternotomy, this surgical approach provides excellent exposure of the aortic arch branch vessels, with the exception of the left subclavian artery. Because the aortic arch passes obliquely posterior and to the left after its origin from the base of the heart, the first portion of the left subclavian artery is inaccessible from this anterior approach.

Mini-sternotomy is performed by first making a limited skin incision measuring 7 to 8 cm in the midline. This should extend from the sternal notch to just past the angle of Louis. The manubrium and upper sternum are divided in the midline down to the third intercostal space with a narrow blade mounted on a redo sternotomy oscillating saw (Stryker, Kalamazoo, Mich.). The sternum is then transected transversely at the third intercostal space, creating an upsidedown **T** incision (Fig. 4-4). Care is taken not to injure the internal mammary arteries, which are adjacent to the sternum. After accurate hemostasis along the periosteal edges, a Rienhoff or similar pediatric sternal retractor is placed to open the upper sternum. The skin incision can be extended upward along the anterior border of either sternocleidomastoid muscle, with division of the strap muscles to expose the proximal right common carotid artery or the more distal left common carotid artery. This extension can also be used to expose the carotid bifurcation.

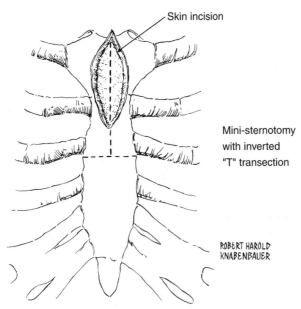

FIGURE 4–4 • Skin incision and mini-sternotomy sternal division. (From Sakopoulos AG, Ballard JL, Gundry SR: Minimally invasive approach for aortic branch vessel reconstruction. J Vasc Surg 31:200, 2000.)

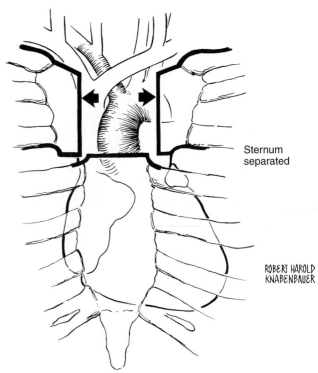

FIGURE 4–5 • The upper sternum is divided and separated, exposing the ascending aorta and arch vessels. (From Sakopoulos AG, Ballard JL, Gundry SR: Minimally invasive approach for aortic branch vessel reconstruction. J Vasc Surg 31:200, 2000.)

The two lobes of the thymus gland are separated in the midline, and if the surgeon carefully observes the pleural bulge during positive-pressure inspiration, entry into either pleural space can be avoided. Nutrient vessels to the thymus gland are carefully ligated and divided, keeping a dry field for visibility. These vessels arise from the internal thoracic artery and drain into the internal thoracic or brachiocephalic veins. The upper pericardium is then opened vertically, and the edges are sewn to the skin with silk suture.

The left brachiocephalic vein can be visualized in the upper portion of the wound. A thymic vein may join this vessel inferiorly, and an inferior thyroid vein may require ligation and division as it joins the brachiocephalic vein superiorly. After complete mobilization of the left brachiocephalic vein, the anterior surface of the aortic arch can be visualized, as well as the origin of the innominate artery. The base of the heart and the innominate and left common carotid arteries are thus exposed (Fig. 4-5). The recurrent laryngeal nerve must be protected during exposure of the distal innominate artery. It courses from the vagus nerve anteriorly around the origin of the subclavian artery to return in the tracheoesophageal groove to its termination in the larynx.

Innominate or left common carotid artery endarterectomy, patch angioplasty, or bypass can then be performed in the usual fashion (Fig. 4-6). After the procedure, a 19 French Blake drain (Johnson & Johnson, Cincinnati, Ohio) is placed in the mediastinum and brought out laterally through one of the intercostal spaces. This is connected to a Heimlich valve grenade suction device. Chest tubes are not used. Two wires are used to bring the upper and lower sternal edges of the T together, and two more are placed in the manubrium. If necessary, another wire placed as a "figure of eight" at the level of the second intercostal space completely rejoins the divided upper sternum. After approximating the muscular and subcutaneous planes in two layers, the skin is closed in a subcuticular fashion.

Exposure of the Origin of the Right Subclavian Artery and Vein

The origin of the right subclavian artery is exposed through a sternotomy incision with extension above and parallel to the clavicle. The right sternohyoid and sternothyroid muscles are divided, followed by exposure of the scalene fat pad. Branches of the thyrocervical trunk are divided, and the dissection is deepened to expose the anterior scalene muscle. The phrenic nerve should be identified and protected as it courses from lateral to medial across the surface of the anterior scalene muscle to pass into the superior mediastinum. The proximal right subclavian artery comes into view with division of the anterior scalene muscle just above its insertion on the first rib.

Traumatic vascular injury at the confluence of the subclavian artery and internal jugular and subclavian veins is difficult to manage solely through a supraclavicular approach. Ideally, sternotomy for proximal vascular control should be followed by supraclavicular extension of the incision. However, in the event that the injury is exposed without proximal control, the incision should be promptly extended via a sternotomy while an assistant maintains compression of the vessels against the undersurface of the sternum to temporarily control hemorrhage (Fig. 4-7). Alternatively, temporary percutaneous balloon occlusion of the distal innominate artery from a femoral or brachial artery approach can be lifesaving and greatly facilitates this exposure.

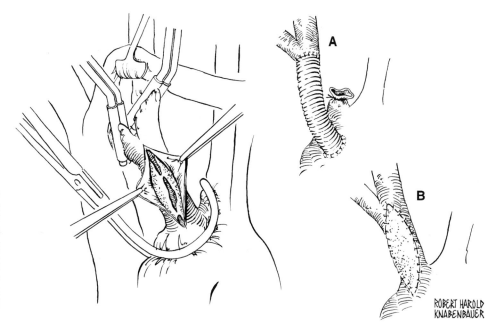

FIGURE 4–6 • Surgical exposure of an innominate artery with visible atherosclerotic stenosis. *A*, Repair by proximal exclusion and ascending aorta–to–innominate artery bypass. *B*, Repair by endarterectomy and patch angioplasty. (From Sakopoulos AG, Ballard JL, Gundry SR: Minimally invasive approach for aortic branch vessel reconstruction. J Vasc Surg 31:200, 2000.)

ROBERT HAROLD KNABENBAUER

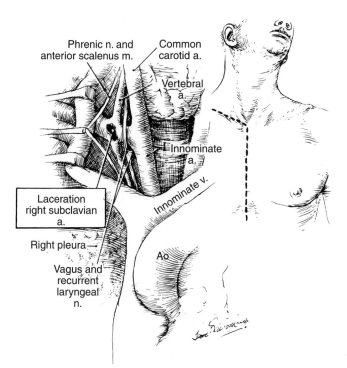

FIGURE 4–7 • Exposure of the anterior aortic arch branches through a median sternotomy incision. Note the location of the phrenic, vagus, and recurrent laryngeal nerves, which must be identified and protected. Ao, aorta. (From Ernst C: Exposure of the subclavian arteries. Semin Vasc Surg 2:202, 1989.)

Exposure of the Origin of the Left Subclavian Artery

The left subclavian artery arises from the aortic arch posteriorly and from the left side of the mediastinum. Therefore, it cannot be adequately exposed for vascular reconstruction through a sternotomy incision. Traumatic injuries and aneurysms of the proximal left subclavian artery should be approached through the left side of the chest. The preferred exposure is an anterolateral thoracotomy through the fourth intercostal space or the bed of the resected fourth rib.

If the vascular injury or aneurysm is extensive, it is wise to prepare the left upper extremity for inclusion in the operative field so that it can be positioned for a second supraclavicular incision. This allows ready access to the second portion of the subclavian artery to gain distal vascular control. Anterolateral exposure of the left side of the chest also facilitates partial occlusion of the aortic arch for lesions involving the origin of the subclavian artery. The phrenic and vagus nerves must be identified and preserved after the pleura is opened and before the dissection of the first portion of the subclavian artery.

In situations in which there is exigent bleeding into the pleural space from a traumatic injury of the proximal left subclavian artery, prompt vascular control can be obtained by an anterior thoracotomy in the third or fourth intercostal space. This exposure facilitates placement of a vascular clamp across the origin of the bleeding subclavian artery (Fig. 4-8). An inframammary incision is preferred in women, with the breast mobilized superiorly for the exposure just described.

Exposure of the Subclavian and Vertebral Arteries

Exposure of the second portion of the subclavian artery is accomplished through a supraclavicular incision beginning over the tendon of the sternocleidomastoid muscle and extending laterally for 8 to 10 cm. The platysma muscle is divided, and the scalene fat pad is mobilized superolaterally. Thyrocervical vessels are ligated and divided as encountered, with exposure of the anterior surface of the anterior scalene muscle. The phrenic nerve can be seen coursing in a lateral to medial direction over this muscle and should be gently mobilized and preserved. The thoracic duct must also be protected at its termination with the confluence of the internal jugular, brachiocephalic, and subclavian veins. Unrecognized injury may result in a lymphocele or lymphocutaneous fistula.

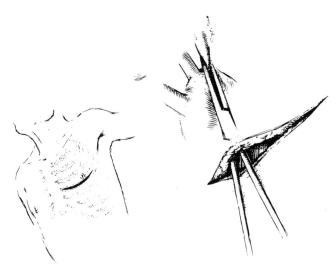

FIGURE 4–8 • Anterior thoracotomy with placement of an occluding vascular clamp for control of exigent bleeding from the proximal left subclavian artery. (From Trunkey D: Great vessel injury. In Blaisdell F, Trunkey D [eds]: Trauma Management, vol 3: Cervicothoracic Trauma. New York, Thieme, 1986, p 255.)

The anterior scalene muscle is divided just above its point of insertion on the first rib to facilitate exposure of the subclavian artery. Division of this muscle should be done under direct vision and without cautery, because the brachial plexus is immediately adjacent to the lateral aspect of the anterior scalene muscle. The origin of the left vertebral artery arises from the medial surface of the subclavian artery medial to the anterior scalene muscle and behind the sternoclavicular joint. The internal thoracic artery, which originates from the inferior surface of the subclavian artery opposite the thyrocervical trunk, should be protected as the subclavian artery is dissected free of surrounding tissue. Figure 4-9 depicts the essential anatomy of this exposure.

Resection of subclavian artery aneurysms and emergency exposure for vascular injury involving the second and third portions of this vessel require wide exposure. This can be accomplished by resecting the clavicle, including the periosteum.

The latter structure, when preserved, results in reossification of a deformed clavicle.

The surgical exposure of the vertebral artery is described in detail in Chapter 36 of this text and in the surgical literature.[11] Injury to the intraosseous portion of the vertebral artery with associated hemorrhage is best managed by embolic occlusion proximal and, if possible, distal to the area of injury.

Exposure of the Axillary Artery

The proximal axillary artery is exposed by a short incision made between the clavicular and sternal portions of the pectoralis major muscle. Branches of the thoracoacromial vessels are divided to expose the axillary vein first and then the axillary artery above and posterior to the vein. Dissection medial to the pectoralis minor muscle provides appropriate exposure of the axillary artery for axillofemoral bypass graft origin. If additional exposure is required laterally, a portion of the pectoralis minor muscle can be divided near its insertion into the coracoid process of the scapula.

The second portion of the axillary artery is more difficult to expose because it lies directly behind the pectoralis major muscle. Extension of the previously mentioned incision continues across the distal portion of the pectoralis major muscle at the anterior axillary fold and out onto the midline of the proximal medial surface of the arm (Fig. 4-10). The tendinous portion of the muscle is divided near its insertion to expose the axillary contents. The pectoralis minor muscle can also be divided if more medial exposure is desired.

Exposure of the Thoracic Outlet

Either a supraclavicular or a transaxillary approach facilitates decompression of the thoracic outlet. Roos described the

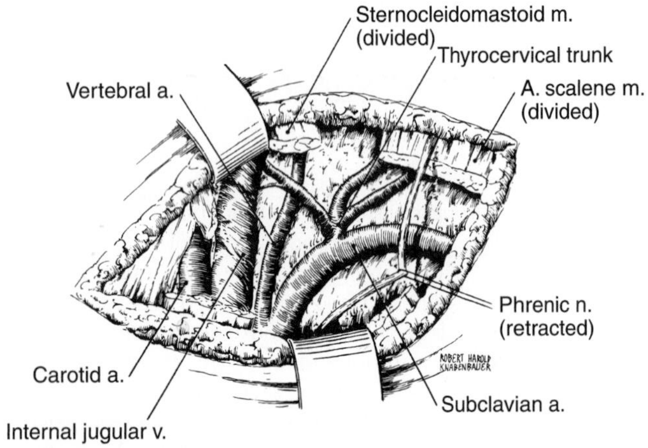

Sternocleidomastoid m.
(divided)
Thyrocervical trunk
Vertebral a.
A. scalene m.
(divided)
Phrenic n.
(retracted)
Carotid a.
Subclavian a.
Internal jugular v.

FIGURE 4–9 • Exposure of the second portion of the left subclavian artery via a supraclavicular incision. Note that both the lateral head of the sternocleidomastoid muscle and the anterior scalene muscle are divided for this exposure.

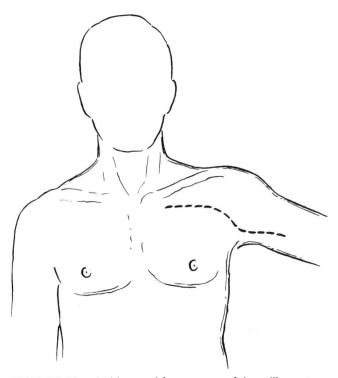

FIGURE 4–10 • Incision used for exposure of the axillary artery.

transaxillary approach for first rib resection in the management of thoracic outlet syndrome.[12] However, current treatment approaches for thoracic outlet syndrome favor supraclavicular exposure of the superior thoracic aperture. Essential anatomic elements of this approach have been detailed in *Wylie's Atlas of Vascular Surgery*.[13]

A transverse supraclavicular incision based 1.5 cm above the medial half of the clavicle is deepened to develop subplatysmal flaps and expose the scalene fat pad. Reflection of the fat pad superolaterally facilitates exposure of the anterior scalene muscle. This exposure also requires ligation and division of the transverse cervical artery and vein and resection of the omohyoid muscle.

Identification and careful manipulation of the phrenic nerve are essential to avoid excessive traction or injury. Complete removal of the anterior scalene muscle begins at the level of the first rib and ends at the transverse processes of the cervical vertebrae. Subtotal removal of the middle scalene muscle in a plane parallel and just inferior to the long thoracic nerve exposes all five roots and three trunks of the brachial plexus.

This unencumbered exposure of the brachial plexus facilitates neurolysis and complete mobilization of the nerve roots. Additional myofibrous bands or bony anomalies are removed at this time. If the course of the lower trunk and C-8 to T-1 nerve roots are deviated by the first rib, the rib should be partially or totally removed to free the path.

Incision of Sibson's fascia and displacement of the dome of the pleura inferiorly help to fully expose the inner aspect of the first rib. Gentle anteromedial retraction of the plexus ensures adequate posterior division of the first rib. Anteriorly, the rib is transected distal to the scalene tubercle. A counterincision just below the clavicle can be used to facilitate anterior transection of the first rib. This approach is useful for rib resection in association with axillosubclavian vein thrombosis. Final removal of the first rib requires division of intercostal muscle attachments to the second rib and division of any other soft tissue.

The scalene fat pad can be wrapped around the plexus if split in a sagittal plane. Repositioning of the fat pad decreases dead space and may help prevent incorporation of the brachial plexus into the healing scar tissue. The wound is closed in layers after secure hemostasis and reapproximation of the lateral head of the sternocleidomastoid muscle.

Exposure of the Descending Thoracic and Proximal Abdominal Aorta

No single approach is better for extensive exposure of the thoracic and abdominal aorta than a properly positioned thoracoabdominal incision. After pulmonary artery and radial artery line placement and dual-lumen tracheal intubation, the patient is placed in a modified right lateral decubitus position, with the hips rotated 45 degrees from horizontal. This allows exposure of both groins. A beanbag device is helpful to support the patient's position on the operating table. The free left upper extremity should be passed across the upper chest and supported on a cushioned Mayo stand. In this way, thoracoabdominal aortic exposure is gained by unwinding the torso, as described by Stoney and Wylie.[14]

Which rib interspace to enter depends primarily on the extent of thoracic aorta to be exposed. The fourth or fifth intercostal space is used when the entire thoracoabdominal aorta from the subclavian artery origin through the abdominal aorta is to be exposed, whereas the seventh or eighth intercostal space allows mid to terminal thoracic aortic exposure plus wide abdominal aortic visualization. Dividing the respective lower rib posteriorly facilitates this exposure. On occasion, two interspaces (e.g., fourth and ninth) may be entered under one thoracoabdominal incision to facilitate proximal descending thoracic and abdominal aortic exposure. The thoracic incision is continued across the costal margin in a paramedian plane to the level of the umbilicus (Fig. 4-11). If the terminal aorta and iliac vessels are to be exposed, the incision is extended to the left lower quadrant.

With the left lung deflated, the origin of the left subclavian artery and proximal descending thoracic aorta can be gently dissected free of surrounding tissue to facilitate cross-clamping. The vagus and recurrent laryngeal nerves are densely adherent to the aorta just proximal to the subclavian artery, and meticulous care should be taken not to injure these structures. Division of the inferior pulmonary ligament exposes the middle and distal descending thoracic aorta. The diaphragm is radially incised toward the aortic hiatus, and the left diaphragmatic crus is divided to expose the terminal descending thoracic aorta. Alternatively, just the central tendinous portion of the diaphragm can be divided, or it can be incised circumferentially at a distance of approximately 2.5 cm from the chest wall.

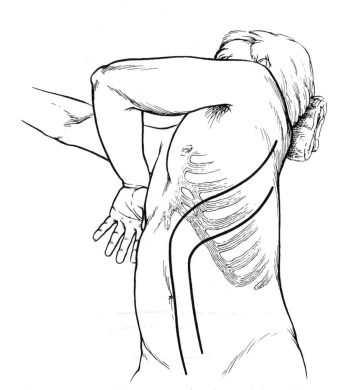

FIGURE 4-11 • Incision options for thoracoabdominal aortic procedures are based on the extent of thoracic aorta to be exposed and the desire to stay in an extraperitoneal plane. (From Rutherford RB: Thoracoabdominal aortic exposures. In Rutherford RB [ed]: Atlas of Vascular Surgery: Basic Techniques and Exposures. Philadelphia, WB Saunders, 1993, p 223.)

The left retroperitoneal space is developed in a retronephric extraperitoneal plane, because surgical exposure of the thoracoabdominal aorta is greatly facilitated by forward mobilization of the left kidney. Division of the median arcuate ligament and lumbar tributary to the left renal vein allows further medial rotation of the abdominal viscera and left kidney. Clearing the posterolateral surface of the thoracoabdominal aorta facilitates aortotomy. With this exposure, the origins of the left renal, celiac, and superior mesenteric arteries can then be visualized and dissected free, as indicated by the disease process present (Fig. 4-12).

Preservation of the blood supply to the spinal cord is critical in this extensive operation. Brockstein and associates stressed the importance of the arteria radicularis magna (artery of Adamkiewicz) in providing circulation to the anterior spinal artery (Fig. 4-13).[15] This vessel is a branch of either a distal intercostal or a proximal lumbar artery. It has been identified as proximally as T-5 and as distally as L-4. However, the artery generally arises at the T-8 to L-1 level. Therefore, it is unwise to ligate any large intercostal or proximal lumbar artery until the aorta has been opened so that an assessment of arterial back-bleeding can be made under direct vision. This important topic is further discussed in Chapter 27.

Closure of this extensive aortic exposure begins by reapproximating the diaphragm with 2-0 Prolene suture. A posterior

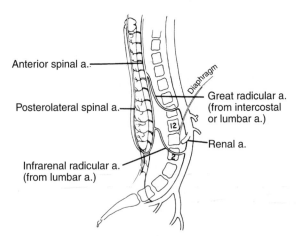

FIGURE 4–13 • Diagram of the great and infrarenal radicular arteries supplying the anterior spinal artery. (From Szilagy DG, Hageman JH, Smith RF, et al: Spinal damage in surgery of the abdominal aorta. Surgery 83:38, 1979.)

(28 or 32 French) chest tube is placed under direct vision, and the ribs are reapproximated with interrupted No. 1 Vicryl suture. Occasionally, a segment of the cartilaginous costal arch is excised to provide stable rib approximation. Thoracic musculature is reapproximated in layers with 1-0 Vicryl suture. In the abdomen, the posterior rectus sheath is reapproximated, and then the anterior rectus sheath is closed with a running No. 1 PDS suture. Finally, the skin is reapproximated with a running 3-0 subcuticular suture.

Retroperitoneal Exposure of the Abdominal Aorta and Its Branches

Transperitoneal exposure is generally regarded as the standard operative approach to the abdominal aorta. However, retroperitoneal exposure has gained wider acceptance among vascular surgeons because it affords a more direct route to the aorta and facilitates complex aortic reconstruction above the level of the renal arteries. Several investigators have demonstrated that in comparison to transperitoneal aortic exposure, the retroperitoneal approach is associated with decreased perioperative morbidity, earlier return of bowel function, fewer respiratory complications, shorter intensive care and hospital stay, and lower overall cost.[16-18]

For this aortic exposure, the patient is positioned on the operating table with the kidney rest at waist level. After pulmonary artery and radial artery line placement and tracheal intubation, the patient is turned to the right lateral decubitus position, with the pelvis rotated posteriorly to allow exposure of both groins. Although not necessary, the kidney rest can be elevated and the operating table gently flexed to open the space between the left anterior superior iliac spine and the costal margin (Fig. 4-14). The free left upper extremity is positioned as described earlier.

The incision begins over the lateral border of the rectus muscle approximately 2 cm below the level of the umbilicus and is carried laterally over the tip of the 12th rib. This decreases the chance of injury to the main trunk of the intercostal nerve within the 11th intercostal space. In males, resection of a significant portion of this rib facilitates retroperitoneal aortic exposure. However, in females, 12th rib resection is

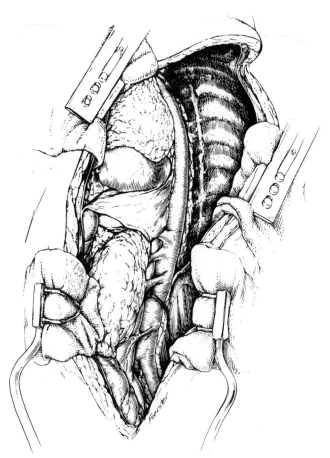

FIGURE 4–12 • Thoracoabdominal aortic exposure from the origin of the left subclavian artery to the common iliac arteries. (From Rutherford RB: Thoracoabdominal aortic exposures. In Rutherford RB [ed]: Atlas of Vascular Surgery: Basic Techniques and Exposures. Philadelphia, WB Saunders, 1993, p 233.)

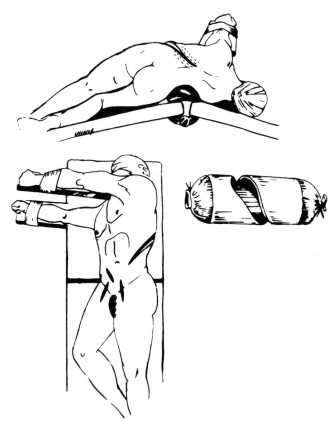

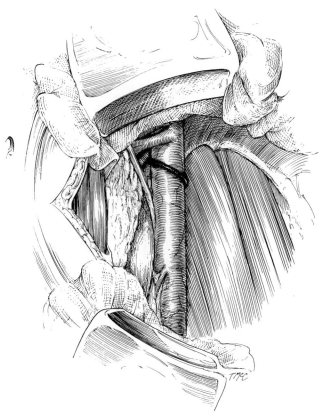

FIGURE 4–14 • Positioning for exposure of the retroperitoneal aorta. *Top,* Flexion of the table increases exposure. *Bottom left,* The hips are positioned at a 45-degree angle with the table, and the left arm is passed across the chest. *Bottom right,* This position unwinds the torso, for greater exposure. Incisions for exposure of the right iliac and common femoral arteries are shown in the *bottom left.* (From Shepard A, Scott G, Mackey W, et al: Retroperitoneal approach to high-risk abdominal aortic aneurysms. Arch Surg 126:157, 1973.)

FIGURE 4–15 • The left renal artery serves as a landmark for this dissection. Note the iliolumbar venous tributary just distal to the left renal artery. (From Rutherford RB: Thoracoabdominal aortic exposures. In Rutherford RB [ed]: Atlas of Vascular Surgery: Basic Techniques and Exposures. Philadelphia, WB Saunders, 1993, p 201.)

not always required. The anterior rectus sheath is opened to allow medial retraction of the left rectus abdominis muscle. The incision is carried laterally through the external and internal oblique muscle fibers. Careful incision of the most lateral aspect of the posterior rectus sheath facilitates development of an extraperitoneal plane. The remaining posterior sheath is divided toward the midline, and laterally, transversus abdominis muscle fibers are split toward the 12th rib.

The peritoneum is gently swept off the posterior rectus sheath, the transversus abdominis fibers, and the diaphragm to allow safe entry into the left retroperitoneal space. This space is best entered inferolaterally. The peritoneum and its contents are swept medially off the psoas muscle toward the diaphragm, along with Gerota's fascia and the contained left kidney. With careful manual control of the left kidney and peritoneal contents and countertraction upward on the diaphragm, further medial rotation of the left kidney and viscera exposes the abdominal aorta from the left diaphragmatic crus to its bifurcation. The Omni-Tract retraction system (Omni-Tract Surgical, Minneapolis, Minn.) is critical for maintaining this exposure.

The left renal artery is readily identified and serves as the main landmark for suprarenal as well as infrarenal aortic exposure (Fig. 4-15). Just above this level, division of the median arcuate ligament and left diaphragmatic crus facilitates exposure of the supraceliac aorta (Fig. 4-16). The celiac and superior mesenteric arteries can be dissected free for a significant length after careful incision of the neural tissue that surrounds both vessels. The distal thoracic aorta is readily accessible if the dissection is carried proximally between the crura and in an extrapleural plane. This extended exposure facilitates repair of suprarenal aortic disease and transaortic renal or mesenteric endarterectomy, as well as antegrade bypass to these vessels.

Exposure of the Visceral and Renal Arteries

The left flank approach is ideal for visceral and renal artery exposure. The celiac artery and proximal aspects of its major branches are readily accessible. In addition, the splenic artery can be mobilized off the posterior aspect of the pancreas to facilitate extra-anatomic splenorenal bypass. Hepatorenal bypass requires a right retroperitoneal approach. There are no major branches that emanate from the superior mesenteric artery for a distance of up to 5 cm distal to its origin. Therefore, bypass or endarterectomy of the superior mesenteric artery well beyond its orifice is possible without ever entering the peritoneal space. The first major branch is usually the middle colic artery, which arises from the anterior and right lateral surface of the superior mesenteric artery as it emerges from

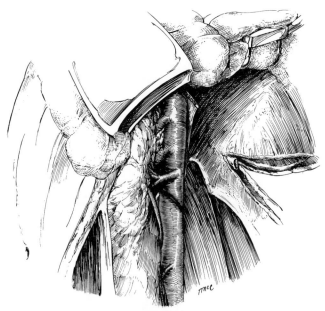

FIGURE 4–16 • Division of the median arcuate ligament and left diaphragmatic crus facilitates suprarenal and supraceliac exposure. (From Rutherford RB: Thoracoabdominal aortic exposures. In Rutherford RB [ed]: Atlas of Vascular Surgery: Basic Techniques and Exposures. Philadelphia, WB Saunders, 1993, p 207.)

the pancreas. This branch is the usual site for an embolus to lodge. It is important to remember that in addition to a possible replaced right hepatic artery, the common hepatic artery occasionally arises from the superior mesenteric artery.[19] In both circumstances, the replaced artery arises from the proximal aspect of the superior mesenteric artery just past its origin and courses back toward the right upper quadrant.

Dissection at the origin of the left renal artery and along the posterolateral aspect of the infrarenal aorta exposes the large communicating vein connecting the renal to the hemiazygos vein. Once this venous tributary (often two tributaries are encountered) is divided, the left renal vein can be elevated off the infrarenal aorta to facilitate cross-clamping. This maneuver facilitates right renal artery exposure as the origin of this vessel comes into view with superolateral retraction of the left renal vein. This retroperitoneal surgical exposure also allows dissection of either renal artery to its branch vessels in preparation for endarterectomy or bypass.

To carry out transaortic renal endarterectomy with direct visualization of a clean end point, it is necessary to dissect the renal arteries well beyond their respective origins. In addition, the segment of aorta to be isolated must be completely mobilized, with control of any adjacent lumbar arteries. This eliminates troublesome back-bleeding that can obscure vision after creation of an aortotomy. Proximal exposure of the suprarenal aorta should include at least the origin of the superior mesenteric artery so that an aortic clamp can be placed above this level. This is particularly important if there is little distance between the origins of the renal arteries and mesenteric vessels. Transaortic endarterectomy is accomplished either by transecting the aorta below the level of the renal arteries or by making a longitudinal aortotomy posterolateral to the left renal artery or superior mesenteric artery.[20] Aortotomy can also be carried to the supraceliac aorta to facilitate visceral endarterectomy. Alternatively, any of these

visceral vessels can be transected well beyond the disease process to facilitate direct end-to-end bypass.[21] The ability to extensively mobilize the renal and mesenteric arteries is a major advantage of this retroperitoneal surgical exposure.

The inferior mesenteric artery is the primary blood supply to the left colon and is located by carrying the infrarenal dissection inferiorly along the posterolateral aspect of the aorta. In some large aneurysms, the thickened wall of the aorta obscures the actual origin of the inferior mesenteric artery. Division of this mesenteric vessel flush with the aorta is generally well tolerated. However, its inadvertent division distal to the left colic branch may result in sigmoid colon infarction. This complication is much more likely to occur when there is atherosclerotic occlusion of the marginal artery of Drummond.[22] In patients with visceral artery occlusive disease, the left colic artery communicates with the left branch of the middle colic artery to become the meandering mesenteric artery (also known as the central anastomotic artery). This artery provides collateral circulation between the superior and inferior mesenteric arteries, and vice versa (Fig. 4-17).[19]

Beyond the pelvic brim, the left common and external iliac arteries are readily accessible for vascular control. Ligation and division of the inferior mesenteric artery flush with the aorta facilitates exposure of the distal anterolateral surface of the infrarenal aorta and the right common and external iliac arteries. It is wise to remember that the common iliac veins and vena cava are adherent to the posteromedial aspect of the left common iliac artery and the posterolateral aspect of the right common iliac artery. Vascular control of these vessels is safest after gently elevating them off their respective underlying major veins. This maneuver also facilitates transection

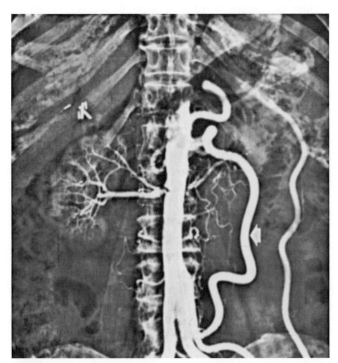

FIGURE 4–17 • Angiogram from a patient with occlusion of the celiac and superior mesenteric arteries. Note the large inferior mesenteric artery with a central anastomotic artery *(arrow)* and a large marginal artery (lateral position) providing collateral circulation.

of the distal common iliac artery under direct vision so that end-to-end aortoiliac reconstruction can be accomplished. If the iliac anastomosis cannot be performed at this level, it is wise to graft end to end to the internal iliac artery and then jump a separate graft to the external iliac artery. With this graft configuration, even an aneurysmal internal iliac artery can be simultaneously excluded (by opening it) and bypassed to the level of its first branch vessel. This helps maintain vital pelvic perfusion.

Wound closure is accomplished in layers using No. 1 Vicryl suture for the posterior rectus sheath, transverse fascia, transversus abdominis, and internal oblique muscle layers. The anterior rectus sheath and external oblique aponeurosis are closed with No. 1 PDS suture. Subcuticular skin closure with 3-0 Vicryl suture completes this multilayer wound closure.

Alternative Exposure of the Renal Artery

The distal right renal artery can be exposed through a right-sided flank incision, which is a "mirror image" of the incision described in the section on retroperitoneal exposure of the aorta. With the patient on the operating table in a modified left lateral decubitus position, the retroperitoneal space is entered laterally after division of the abdominal wall muscles. The peritoneum and contents are gently mobilized anteriorly and medially, including the right kidney enclosed in Gerota's fascia. The renal artery is palpated distally and carefully dissected free of surrounding tissue. The inferior vena cava is also identified and mobilized after ligation of two or three paired lumbar veins. The vena cava can be gently elevated to expose the right posterolateral aspect of the aorta. Partial aortic occlusion with a side-biting vascular clamp is employed for anastomosis of the proximal bypass graft. Thereafter, a distal end-to-end anastomosis completes renal artery revascularization.

Moncure and associates described an extra-anatomic revascularization procedure for the right kidney.[23] This exposure employs a right subcostal incision extending into the right flank. The hepatic flexure of the colon is mobilized and rotated to the left. The duodenum is kocherized toward the midline to expose the right kidney. The renal artery is located behind and just above the right renal vein. Next, the hepatic artery is palpated in the hepatoduodenal ligament, and the gastroduodenal artery is identified. The common hepatic artery proximal to the gastroduodenal artery is dissected free. An end-to-side anastomosis of the bypass graft to the hepatic artery is constructed first. The bypass graft is then routed over the hepatoduodenal ligament and anastomosed to the transected end of the renal artery to revascularize the kidney. Figure 4-18 demonstrates the essential anatomy and a side-to-side distal anastomosis. However, end-to-end reconstruction is recommended and easier to accomplish.

The left renal artery can be exposed peripherally for extra-anatomic bypass by using the same incision described earlier in the section on retroperitoneal exposure of the abdominal aorta. Once the pararenal aorta is exposed, the tail of the pancreas is separated from the left adrenal gland to expose the splenic artery for bypass to the left renal artery (Fig. 4-19).[23] Inflow can also be obtained from the aorta proximal or distal to the renal artery. This bypass can originate from the side of the aorta, with a destination to the transected left renal artery.

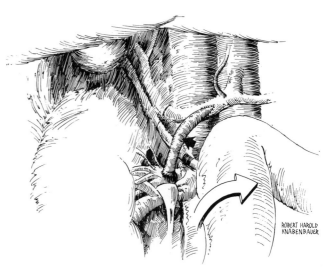

FIGURE 4–18 • Hepatic–to–right renal artery bypass. The duodenum is kocherized *(open arrow)* for exposure. The reverse saphenous vein bypass is identified *(solid arrow)*. Note the retraction of the right renal vein for exposure.

Alternative Exposure of the Abdominal Aorta and Its Branches

A helpful modification of the standard midline abdominal incision that can be used to expose the proximal abdominal aorta without entering the chest is illustrated in Figure 4-20. An inverted hockey-stick incision is used, beginning at the left midcostal margin. The left rectus muscle is transected, and the oblique and transversus muscles are divided in the direction of the skin incision. The incision is continued down the linea alba to the symphysis pubis. The left side of the colon is mobilized by incising the peritoneum along the white line of Toldt from the pelvis to the lateral peritoneal attachments of the spleen. The spleen is gently mobilized and brought forward toward the midline by incising the splenorenal and splenophrenic ligaments.

Dissection is continued by forward mobilization of the spleen, pancreatic tail, and splenic flexure of the colon between the mesocolon and Gerota's fascia, with care not to

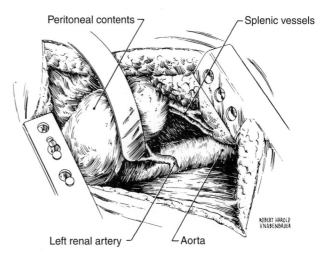

FIGURE 4–19 • Flank exposure of the left renal artery.

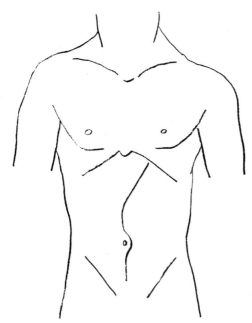

FIGURE 4–20 • Modified abdominal incision for greater left upper quadrant exposure during transperitoneal medial visceral rotation. (From Deiparine MK, Ballard JL: Correspondence re: "Transperitoneal medial visceral rotation." Ann Vasc Surg 9:607, 1995.)

damage the adrenal gland medially or the adrenal vein at its junction with the left renal vein. This left-to-right transperitoneal medial visceral rotation affords excellent exposure of the supraceliac and visceral aorta, including the renal arteries (Fig. 4-21). This exposure is facilitated by forward displacement of the left kidney along with the rest of the mobilized viscera. Division of the median arcuate ligament

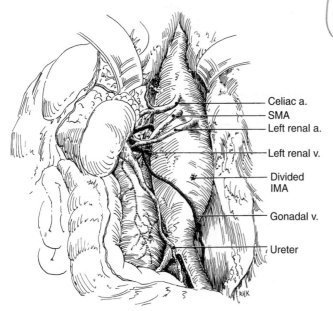

Celiac a.
SMA
Left renal a.
Left renal v.
Divided IMA
Gonadal v.
Ureter

FIGURE 4–21 • Transperitoneal medial visceral rotation, with the left kidney rotated forward, for repair of a supraceliac aortic aneurysm. IMA, inferior mesenteric artery; SMA superior mesenteric artery. (From Ballard JL: Management of renal artery stenosis in conjunction with aortic aneurysm. Semin Vasc Surg 9:221, 1996.)

and diaphragmatic crura exposes the distal thoracic aorta without entering the left chest.

Transperitoneal Exposure of the Abdominal Aorta at the Diaphragmatic Hiatus

Exposure of the supraceliac aorta at the diaphragmatic hiatus is lifesaving for early control of exigent hemorrhage in the case of a ruptured abdominal aortic aneurysm. It is also useful for temporary control of the aorta during repair of aortocaval or aortoenteric fistulas and infected aortic grafts. Less frequently, this exposure is suitable for revascularization of the celiac axis and its proximal branches or the superior mesenteric artery.

This exposure through the lesser sac is facilitated by downward retraction of the stomach and lateral retraction of the esophagus. The aortic pulse is palpated, and the arching fibers of the diaphragm at the aortic hiatus are divided directly over the aorta. The periaortic fascia is opened, and the index and middle fingers are passed medially and laterally to the aorta. Gentle blunt finger dissection between the diaphragmatic fibers and the aorta creates space on either side of the aorta. This maneuver is critical, because any overlying muscle fibers would allow a vascular occluding clamp to slide up and off the aorta. No effort is made to completely encircle the aorta because if an intercostal or proximal lumbar artery or vein is avulsed, troublesome bleeding can result. At this point, a partially opened aortic clamp is advanced over the dorsal hand and fingers that have been appropriately positioned to cross-clamp the aorta and interrupt blood flow. This exposure is illustrated in Figure 4-22.

Celiac artery reconstruction requires more exposure. A generous incision is made in the posterior parietal peritoneum, and the diaphragmatic crura are completely divided. The inferior phrenic arteries should be isolated, ligated, and divided. The aortic branch to the left adrenal gland is also usually visualized and sacrificed. Dissection is continued distally to expose the celiac artery, which can be palpated at its origin from the anterior surface of the aorta. Dense fibers of the median arcuate ligament are divided, along with the neural elements forming the celiac plexus. This tissue is quite vascular; thus, stick ties and cautery are useful for hemostasis. Once the celiac axis has been exposed, the common hepatic artery is dissected free of surrounding tissue as it courses toward the liver hilum. Sympathetic nerve fibers can be seen to entwine on the surface of this vessel. There is usually a 3- to 4-cm segment of the hepatic artery that is free of branches and thus useful as a site for vascular anastomosis. The splenic artery is palpable at the superior border of the pancreas and courses to the left toward the splenic hilum. Here again, there is a 4- to 5-cm segment that is free of branches and can be used for placement of a vascular anastomosis. The left gastric artery is the smallest of the three main branches of the celiac axis. It courses anteriorly to follow the lesser curvature of the stomach and should be protected during this exposure.

The supraceliac aorta can also be used as the bypass origin for superior mesenteric artery reconstruction. The proximal anastomosis is constructed on the anterior surface of the aorta after the aortic hiatus is opened as described earlier. Using careful finger dissection, a tunnel must then be created behind

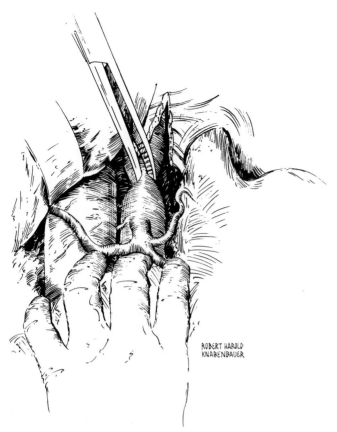

FIGURE 4–22 • Exposure of the abdominal aorta at the diaphragm.

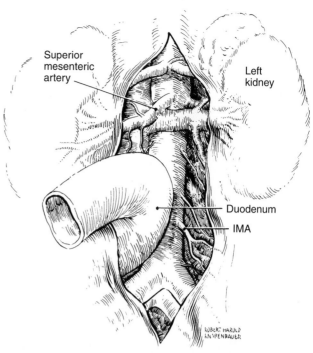

FIGURE 4–23 • Infracolic exposure of the superior mesenteric artery. The pancreas and transverse colon are not shown but are retracted upward and forward. IMA, inferior mesenteric artery.

the pancreas. The bypass graft is passed through the tunnel and anastomosed to the distal patent superior mesenteric artery. Kinking of the bypass, which can occur with retrograde aorta–to–superior mesenteric artery bypass grafts during replacement of bowel, is unlikely in this tunneled position.

Anterior exposure of the superior mesenteric artery inferior to the transverse mesocolon requires opening the posterior parietal peritoneum lateral to the third and fourth portions of the duodenum (Fig. 4-23). The left renal vein is identified and mobilized as described previously for exposure of the renal arteries. The left renal vein is retracted downward, and the dissection is carried upward on the aorta until the superior mesenteric artery origin can be palpated. It usually arises from the left side of the anterior surface of the aorta. The artery is immediately encased by the superior mesenteric sympathetic nerve plexus, which must be incised for exposure. Cautery and suture ligatures are used to control bleeding from the vascular plexus tissue. The overlying transverse mesocolon and pancreas significantly limit this exposure.

Transperitoneal Exposure of the Infrarenal Abdominal Aorta

A midline abdominal incision from the xiphoid to the symphysis pubis is commonly used for anterior exposure of the infrarenal abdominal aorta. One disadvantage of this approach is incomplete visualization of the proximal abdominal aorta or renal artery origins. Proximally extending the midline incision around the xiphoid process and completely mobilizing the third and fourth portions of the duodenum

improve this potential lack of exposure. The dissection continues through the posterior peritoneum just lateral to the duodenum and medial to the inferior mesenteric vein to avoid damaging the circulation to the left or sigmoid colon. This is particularly important in the case of ruptured abdominal aortic aneurysms, when landmarks are frequently obscured by an extensive retroperitoneal hematoma. The duodenum can nearly always be visualized and used as a landmark during this exposure.

It is wise to palpate the aortic bifurcation and expose the common iliac arteries from the midline, thereby avoiding injury to the ureters. Fibers of the sympathetic nerves arch over the left common iliac artery in males, and damage to these sympathetic fibers can result in erectile dysfunction and retrograde ejaculation. Figure 4-24 shows the relationship of the infrarenal sympathetic nerve fibers to the terminal aorta and iliac arteries. Incising along the white line of Toldt and mobilizing the sigmoid or proximal ascending colon toward the midline can readily identify the external iliac arteries. Graft limbs coursing out to this level should be passed under both the colon mesentery and the respective ureter.

Transperitoneal Exposure of the Renal Arteries

The left main renal artery originates from the posterolateral surface of the aorta. Usually, this location is at the level of the upper border of the left renal vein where it crosses over the abdominal aorta. The right renal artery often arises at a slightly lower level. Anterior exposure of either renal artery origin involves incision of the posterior parietal peritoneum just lateral to the fourth portion of the duodenum. Additional exposure is obtained by continuing this incision along the distal third portion of the duodenum.

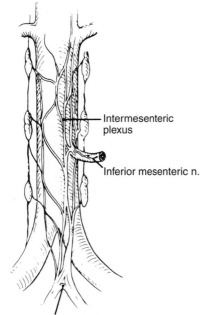

- Intermesenteric plexus
- Inferior mesenteric n.
- Superior hypogastric plexus

FIGURE 4–24 • Relationship of the infrarenal sympathetic nerves to the aorta and iliac arteries. Note the condensation of nerve elements coursing over the left common iliac artery origin. (From Weinstein MH, Machleder HI: Sexual function after aortoiliac surgery. Ann Surg 181:787, 1975.)

The left renal vein is identified and carefully mobilized. Frequently, there is a small parietal vein that terminates in the inferior margin of the left renal vein over the aorta. Otherwise, there are two major venous tributaries to be identified, ligated, and divided. The first is located by following the inferior margin of the left renal vein laterally to the termination of the left gonadal vein. Next, the dissection is carried laterally along the superior surface of the left renal vein until the confluence of the left adrenal vein is identified. This vein should be ligated flush with the renal vein and divided. The entire left renal vein can then be mobilized on a Silastic vascular loop.

Cautious dissection is advisable in this area, as there is an important large communicating vein arising from the posterior surface of the proximal left renal vein. This vein communicates with the adjacent lumbar vein and then to the hemiazygos system and superior vena cava. The presence of this venous collateral allows acute ligation of the left renal vein without impairment of renal function. This lumbar venous communication should be preserved, if possible, during this anterior transperitoneal approach.

Once the left renal vein is mobilized, attention should be directed to exposing the left lateral surface of the aorta above and below the level of the left renal vein. The left renal artery arising from the posterolateral surface of the aorta is thus exposed. Autonomic nerve elements are encountered adjacent to the renal artery but can be divided without concern. Gentle placement of a vein retractor under the left renal vein with upward retraction by an assistant greatly facilitates this exposure. A Silastic loop placed about the renal artery origin aids in the mobilization and dissection of this vessel.

The right renal artery is more difficult to expose because it passes directly behind the inferior vena cava on its course to the renal hilum. The origin of this artery is palpated as it emerges from the right posterolateral aspect of the aorta. Care should be taken not to injure the right adrenal branch, which arises 5 to 10 mm from the origin of the right renal artery. The size of this vessel may be 2 to 3 mm when renal artery stenosis is present because it becomes an important collateral to the distal right renal artery via capsular branches. In the event that the entire right renal artery and its branches must be exposed, the surgeon must completely mobilize the vena cava above and below the artery by carefully ligating and dividing all adjacent lumbar veins.

The subhepatic space is entered, and the duodenum is kocherized to allow exposure of the right renal vein as it joins the inferior vena cava. The renal vein is mobilized on a Silastic loop to aid in identifying the main renal artery lying beneath the vein. Exposure of the right renal artery is complete when this distal dissection joins the medial exposure already described.

Emergency Exposure of the Abdominal Aorta and Vena Cava

Vascular exposure of injured vessels within the abdomen is best carried out through a generous midline abdominal incision. Location of the hematoma determines the exposure to be used. Because the abdominal circulation arises in a retroperitoneal location, the overlying viscera need to be rotated medially or elevated superiorly to expose the aorta and its major branches and the caval and portal venous circulation.

Kudsk and Sheldon divided the retroperitoneal space into three zones (Fig. 4-25).[24] The presence of a central hematoma (zone 1) indicates injury to the aorta, the proximal renal or visceral arteries, the inferior vena cava, or the portal vein. An expanding zone 1 retroperitoneal hematoma with extension to the left indicates a proximal aortic or adjacent major branch vessel injury. Transperitoneal left-to-right medial visceral rotation swiftly and widely exposes the aorta from the diaphragm to its bifurcation. Exposure can be facilitated by division of the left rectus muscle transversely in the left upper quadrant or by the modified abdominal incision described earlier. The splenic flexure is mobilized, including the spleen and the left kidney, with rotation of these viscera to the right. The origins of the celiac, superior mesenteric, and renal arteries are likewise exposed (Fig. 4-26).

The presence of a zone 1 retroperitoneal hematoma with extension into the right flank is indicative of major caval, portal venous, or proximal injury to a major arterial branch in the right upper quadrant. Incising the peritoneum lateral to the ascending colon and reflecting this structure medially, followed by duodenal kocherization, gain exposure. This right-to-left medial visceral rotation exposes the entire vena cava from the iliac confluence to the liver (Fig. 4-27).

Incising the hepatoduodenal ligament above the duodenum exposes the portal vein. The common bile duct is retracted laterally, and the hepatic artery is palpated and isolated for inspection. Thereafter, retracting the hepatic artery toward the midline facilitates examination of the portal vein. The right side of the aorta, as well as the proximal right renal artery, can be inspected if rotation and mobilization of the overlying bowel are continued to the midline.

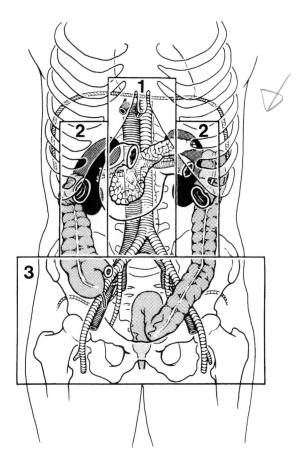

FIGURE 4–25 • Anatomic zones (1, 2, and 3) for exploration of retroperitoneal hematomas. (From Kudsk KA, Sheldon GF: Retroperitoneal hematoma. In Blaisdell FW, Trunkey DD [eds]: Trauma Management, vol 1, 2nd ed. New York, Thieme Medical Publishers, 1993, p 400.)

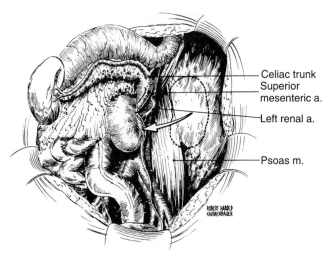

Celiac trunk
Superior
mesenteric a.

Left renal a.

Psoas m.

FIGURE 4–26 • Rotation of the intra-abdominal contents, including the left kidney, to the right for complete visualization of the abdominal aorta. The kidney is rotated forward and to the right *(arrow)* from the renal fossa *(dotted outline)*. (From Smith LL, Catalano RD: Exposure of vascular injuries. In Bongard FS, Wilson SE, Perry MO [eds]: Vascular Injuries in Surgical Practice. Norwalk, Conn, Appleton & Lange, 1991, p 18.)

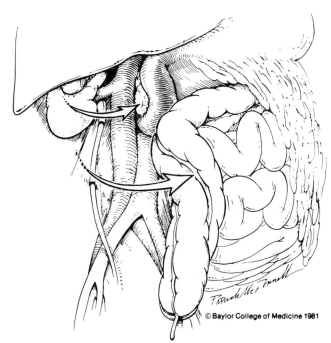

© Baylor College of Medicine 1981

FIGURE 4–27 • Rotation of the intra-abdominal viscera to the left by mobilization of the right colon and kocherization of the duodenum. The right kidney can also be mobilized to inspect the posterior surface of the vena cava if necessary. (Courtesy of M. Dohrmann, the original illustrator.)

Lateral hematomas (zone 2) indicate injury to distal visceral and renal vessels. Despite their lateral location, it is wise not to enter a large hematoma to control exigent hemorrhage until central aortic exposure has been secured for possible cross-clamping. Retroperitoneal pelvic hematomas (zone 3) usually indicate torn branches of the iliac vessels associated with pelvic fractures. These may not require exploration unless the hematoma is expanding or there is evidence of large vessel injury demonstrated by angiography.

Extraperitoneal Exposure of the Iliac Arteries

This exposure begins with an oblique incision in the lower quadrant of the abdomen on the side of involved iliac artery occlusive disease. It is good practice to start the incision near the pubic tubercle, with extension obliquely lateral, staying medial to the anterior superior iliac spine of the pelvis. The external oblique aponeurosis is opened in the direction of its fibers, and the incision is continued into the fleshy portion of this muscle. The internal oblique and transversus abdominis muscles are divided in the direction of the incision to enter the preperitoneal space. The peritoneum is gently rotated medially to expose the external iliac artery. The ureter, which is adherent to the peritoneum and usually retracts with the peritoneal contents, is vulnerable to injury as it courses across the iliac bifurcation. Exposure of the common iliac artery requires extension of the incision proximally and laterally into the flank region.

Care should be taken not to injure the ilioinguinal or genitofemoral nerves during exposure or retraction. Their location on the anterior surface of the psoas muscle is vulnerable. Combination of this incision with a curvilinear incision over

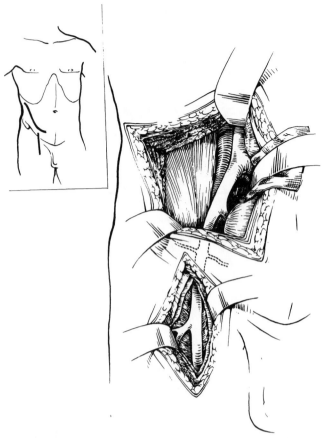

FIGURE 4–28 • Extraperitoneal exposure of the distal common and external iliac arteries. Counterincision at the groin facilitates iliofemoral reconstruction.

the common femoral artery permits exposure from the terminal common iliac artery to the proximal superficial or deep femoral arteries (Fig. 4-28). The iliac artery exposed in this extraperitoneal fashion is particularly appealing as an inflow source in cases in which there is extensive scarring at the groin from previous peripheral vascular procedures.

Exposure of the Common Femoral Artery

A curvilinear incision placed directly over the palpable pulse, with extension above as well as below the groin crease, provides excellent exposure of the common femoral artery and its branches. An incision made just medial to the midpoint of the inguinal ligament suffices in the absence of a palpable pulse. Frequently, the diseased artery can be rolled beneath the index finger, and this guides the plane of deeper dissection. It is important to remember to check for posterior branches, because an aberrant medial femoral circumflex artery can arise anywhere along the posterior surface of the common femoral artery. Failure to control this vessel can result in troublesome bleeding when the common femoral artery is opened.

Gentle dissection about the origin of the deep femoral artery is important. The lateral femoral circumflex artery arises from the lateral side of the deep femoral artery, and this

vessel can be easily injured. Care should also be taken to identify the lateral femoral circumflex vein, which courses from lateral to medial across the origin of the deep femoral artery. Division of this vein facilitates arterial mobilization and distal dissection. This maneuver is paramount if the proximal deep femoral artery is to be used as an inflow source, and it provides excellent exposure for eversion endarterectomy.

Exposure of the Deep Femoral Artery

The deep femoral artery is located 1.5 cm medial to the femur and lies on the pectineus and adductor brevis muscles. In cases in which the deep femoral artery is being exposed as an initial procedure, the dissection is aided by flexion and external rotation of the thigh to relax the involved muscles. Colborn and associates described the surgical anatomy of the deep femoral artery, and the reader is well advised to consult their excellent and well-illustrated article.[25]

The deep femoral artery can be a useful inflow or outflow source in a patient with a hostile groin after previous surgical exposures. Nuñez and associates described a practical approach to the middle and distal thirds of this artery that avoids a scarred femoral bifurcation.[26] This surgical dissection begins lateral to the sartorius muscle. Figure 4-29 demonstrates the incision over the lateral aspect of the sartorius muscle and branches of the lateral femoral circumflex artery. These branches are followed medially to the deep femoral artery after the incision is deepened between the vastus medialis and adductor longus muscles. Complete mobilization of the artery at this level requires division of overlying venous tributaries to the deep femoral vein. This dissection can then be safely extended distally or, if needed, proximally to the femoral bifurcation.

Alternatively, the distal third of the deep femoral artery can be exposed by a surgical plane of dissection that is posterior to the adductor longus muscle in the medial thigh.[27] This exposure is deepened between the gracilis and adductor longus muscles to the medial aspect of the deep femoral artery. Knee flexion relaxes the involved muscles and aids in this exposure.

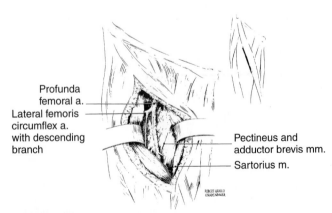

Profunda femoral a.
Lateral femoris circumflex a. with descending branch

Pectineus and adductor brevis mm.
Sartorius m.

FIGURE 4–29 • Lateral approach to the deep femoral artery. *Upper right,* The incision is lateral to the sartorius muscle. *Lower left,* Exposure of the deep femoral vessel.

Exposure of the Popliteal Artery

The popliteal artery is typically exposed from a medial approach, with few exceptions. The proximal and distal portions of this vessel are readily exposed. However, the medial head of the gastrocnemius muscle and the tendinous insertions of the long adductor muscles obscure the midportion of the artery at the joint space of the knee. A posterior approach to the midpopliteal artery is useful for isolated disorders such as popliteal entrapment or cystic adventitial disease and some trauma situations.

The proximal popliteal artery is exposed through an incision placed in the groove between the vastus medialis and sartorius muscles. The greater saphenous vein lies just posterior to this incision, and care must be taken to preserve it during the dissection. The sartorius muscle is retracted posteriorly, and the investing fascia is incised longitudinally, preserving the saphenous nerve, which is usually seen lying on the deep fascial surface. Once the fascia is opened, the popliteal artery can be palpated in its location under the adductor magnus tendon.

Although not usually necessary, additional exposure can be obtained distally by dividing the tendon of the medial head of the gastrocnemius muscle. Gentle insertion of the left index finger behind its tendinous origin aids in isolating this structure and protecting the underlying neurovascular bundle. Should additional distal exposure be necessary, the tendinous insertions of the sartorius, semimembranous, semitendinous, and gracilis muscles can be divided. It is wise to mark these tendons with identifying sutures to aid in their subsequent repair.

The terminal popliteal artery and tibioperoneal trunk are exposed through an incision placed approximately 1.5 cm posterior to the medial margin of the tibia. Once again, the surgeon must be aware of the greater saphenous vein and protect it in its subcutaneous location. The thick muscular fascia overlying the gastrocnemius muscle is incised to enter the popliteal space. The popliteal vein is usually encountered first within the neurovascular sheath. Gentle downward retraction of the vein facilitates dissection of the popliteal artery, which lies superolateral to the vein. The origin of the anterior tibial artery arises anteriorly and laterally from the terminal popliteal artery. Further exposure of the tibioperoneal trunk and proximal peroneal and posterior tibial arteries requires the division of the soleus muscle fibers arising from the medial margin of the tibia. Division of overlying venous tributaries between the often paired popliteal veins facilitates this exposure.

LATERAL EXPOSURE OF THE POPLITEAL ARTERY

A lateral approach to the popliteal artery can be used when previous medial exposure has resulted in dense tissue scarring, making repeat procedures difficult. The incision for the above-knee popliteal artery is placed between the iliotibial tract and the biceps femoris muscle as described by Veith and associates.[28] The dissection is deepened through the fascia lata posterior to the junction of the lateral intramuscular septum and the iliotibial tract to enter the popliteal space. The popliteal vein is encountered first within the vascular sheath. It can be mobilized and retracted posteriorly to allow exposure of the popliteal artery. The tibial and peroneal

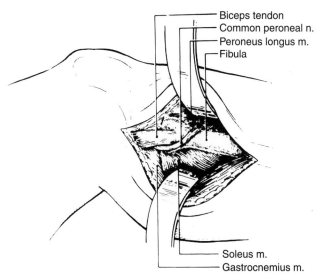

FIGURE 4–30 • Lateral approach to the distal popliteal artery. Note the common peroneal nerve coursing around the neck of the fibula. (From Veith F, Ascer E, Gupta S: Lateral approach to the popliteal artery. J Vasc Surg 6:119, 1987.)

nerves are also posterior and loosely adherent to the hamstrings. They naturally fall out of harm's way with retraction of the biceps femoris, semimembranous, and semitendinous muscles.

The lateral approach to the below-knee popliteal artery begins with an incision over the head and proximal one fourth of the fibula. As the incision is deepened, care must be taken to preserve the common peroneal nerve as it courses around the neck of the fibula (Fig. 4-30). The biceps femoris tendon is divided. The ligamentous attachments to the head of the fibula are also divided, and the proximal fibula is removed. The entire below-knee popliteal artery, anterior tibial artery origin, and tibioperoneal trunk are accessible after removal of the bone fragment (Fig. 4-31). The proximal

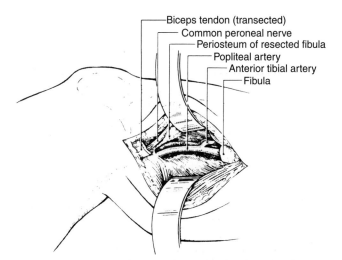

FIGURE 4–31 • Lateral approach to the distal popliteal artery after removal of the proximal fibula. Note the transected tendon of the biceps muscle and the intact common peroneal nerve. (From Veith F, Ascer E, Gupta S: Lateral approach to the popliteal artery. J Vasc Surg 6:119, 1987.)

posterior tibial and peroneal arteries can be exposed if more of the distal fibula is resected.

Exposure of the Tibial and Peroneal Arteries

Management of lower extremity ischemic vascular disease requires accurate knowledge of the arterial and venous circulation of the leg. It is important to keep in mind the relationship of the three major leg arteries to the tibia and fibula as well as the compartments of the leg. Figure 4-32 demonstrates these important relationships. Note the anterior tibial vessels lying on the interosseous membrane in the anterior compartment. The peroneal artery, which is adjacent to the medial margin of the fibula in the deep posterior compartment, lies in close proximity to the transverse crural intermuscular septum. The posterior tibial vessels are medial to the peroneal artery and veins, but also above the intermuscular septum and in the deep posterior compartment of the leg.

Surgical exposure of the crural vessels requires patience and great care. There are numerous small muscular branches, and each artery has two accompanying veins with their respective tributaries to protect. Careless dissection leads to bleeding that obscures the operative field and increases the likelihood of injury to these delicate vascular structures.

ANTERIOR TIBIAL ARTERY

This vessel travels between the anterior tibial and extensor digitorum longus muscles in the proximal portion of the anterior compartment of the leg. The extensor hallucis longus muscle crosses over the artery, laterally to medially, in the distal leg above the level of the flexor retinaculum. Surgical exposure of the anterior tibial artery is best accomplished either in the proximal leg or just above the flexor retinaculum proximal to the ankle.

A skin incision made approximately 2.5 cm lateral to the anterior border of the tibia facilitates proximal exposure of the anterior tibial artery. Deepening the dissection between the two muscle bellies assists this surgical exposure. Dorsiflexion and internal rotation of the foot aid in identifying the groove between these two muscles. The muscles are gently separated down to the anterior tibial artery, which lies between its two accompanying veins and anterior to the deep peroneal nerve on the interosseous membrane.

Alternatively, a dissection course that passes between the extensor hallucis longus and extensor digitorum longus laterally and the anterior tibial muscle medially exposes the artery just above the flexor retinaculum.[27] The upper portion of the flexor retinaculum can be divided to improve distal exposure; however, complete division is not recommended. If the anterior tibial artery is unsuitable for vascular reconstruction at this level, the dissection should skip down to the dorsal pedal artery below the inferior portion of the retinaculum.

POSTERIOR TIBIAL ARTERY

Extending the incision described earlier for medial exposure of the tibioperoneal trunk facilitates proximal exposure of the posterior tibial artery. This requires incising the origin of the

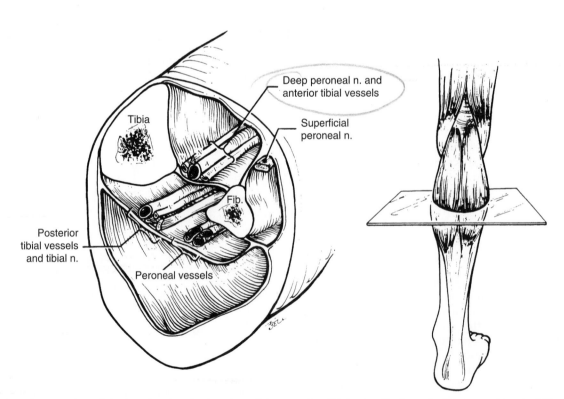

FIGURE 4–32 • Cross section of the leg showing the location of the anterior tibial artery in the anterior compartment of the leg and the posterior tibial and peroneal arteries in the deep posterior compartment. (From Briggs S, Seligson D: Management of extremity trauma. In Richardson D, Polk H, Flint M [eds]: Trauma: Clinical Care and Pathophysiology. Chicago, Year Book Medical, 1987, p 544.)

soleus muscle from the medial border of the tibia. Tributary veins traveling through this muscle origin may cause troublesome bleeding. These should be ligated to keep the operative field dry. Immediately deep to the soleus fibers, the posterior tibial vessels can be observed coursing between the posterior tibial and flexor digitorum longus muscles. The tibial nerve, which crosses the artery posteriorly from medial to lateral, must be protected. This exposure can be challenging, as there is a dense network of venous tributaries overlying the origin of the posterior tibial artery.

Exposure of the middle aspect of the posterior tibial artery is best achieved distal to the lower edge of the soleus muscle fibers in the medial calf.[27] This dissection into the deep posterior compartment of the leg continues above the intermuscular septum to expose the neurovascular bundle. The artery must be carefully dissected free from its accompanying paired veins and tibial nerve.

PERONEAL ARTERY

The proximal and middle aspects of the peroneal artery can be exposed using the same medial leg incisions described for exposure of the posterior tibial artery. Once this latter artery is exposed, the dissection continues on the intermuscular septum to a deeper level. The peroneal artery is located adjacent to the medial border of the fibula. This exposure is quite deep and therefore more difficult in a large leg.

Resecting a short segment of the fibula through a lateral incision over this bone can also expose the peroneal artery. This incision should be placed below the entrance of the peroneal nerve into the anterior compartment of the leg. The peroneal vessels lie just deep to the medial border of the fibula. Once this short segment of bone is removed, the vessels are exposed. Careful division and removal of the fibula are essential, because the accompanying venous plexus that surrounds the peroneal artery is easy to disturb and may cause significant bleeding. Surprisingly little postoperative morbidity is associated with this exposure.

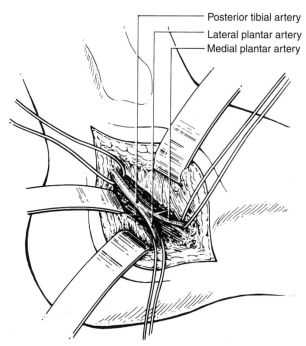

FIGURE 4–34 • Exposure of the terminal left posterior tibial artery using a retromalleolar incision. The terminal branches of this vessel are shown; the larger is the lateral plantar branch. (From Ascer E, Veith F, Gupta S: Bypasses to plantar arteries and other tibial branches: An extended approach to limb salvage. J Vasc Surg 8:436, 1988.)

Exposure of the Pedal Arteries

A detailed understanding of the pedal arterial circulation is important because distal bypass sites in the foot are frequently used for limb-threatening ischemic vascular disease. Ascer and associates described various surgical approaches, as well as the results of these distal lower extremity bypass procedures.[29]

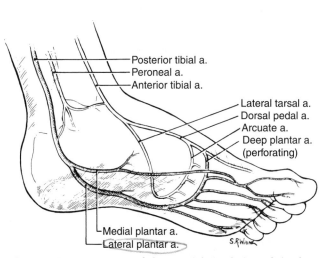

FIGURE 4–33 • Anatomy of the arterial circulation of the foot. (From Ascer E, Veith F, Gupta S: Bypasses to plantar arteries and other tibial branches: An extended approach to limb salvage. J Vasc Surg 8:434, 1988.)

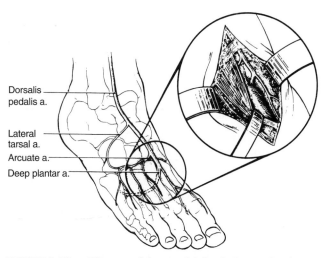

FIGURE 4–35 • Diagram of the arterial circulation on the dorsum of the foot. The *inset* shows the origin of the deep plantar branch as it courses between the two heads of the first dorsal interosseous vessel. (From Ascer E, Veith F, Gupta S: Bypasses to plantar arteries and other tibial branches: An extended approach to limb salvage. J Vasc Surg 8:437, 1988.)

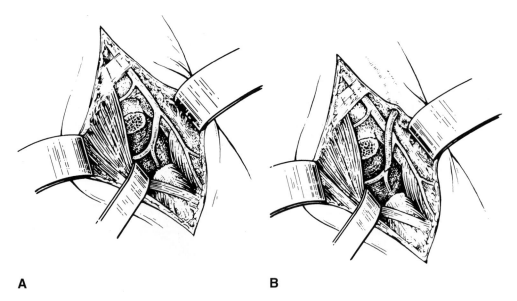

A   **B**

FIGURE 4–36 • *A*, Deep plantar arch branch following resection of a portion of the second metatarsal bone. *B*, Distal anastomosis of a bypass to this vessel. (From Ascer E, Veith F, Gupta S: Bypasses to plantar arteries and other tibial branches: An extended approach to limb salvage. J Vasc Surg 8:437, 1988.)

Figure 4-33 shows the branches and distribution of the distal anterior and posterior tibial arteries in the foot.

DISTAL POSTERIOR TIBIAL ARTERY AND PLANTAR BRANCHES

Exposure of the terminal posterior tibial artery, with its concomitant veins and tibial nerve, is accomplished by a retromalleolar incision. Division of the flexor retinaculum continues the dissection distally. The neurovascular bundle is surrounded by fatty tissue, and the artery is usually superior to the nerve. Further dissection may require sequential incisions to accurately follow the course of the terminal posterior tibial artery into the plantar surface of the foot. Small self-expanding retractors facilitate this exposure, as the plantar tissue is thick and rigid. The plantar aponeurosis and the flexor digitorum brevis muscle can be incised to expose the medial and lateral plantar arteries (Fig. 4-34). This latter vessel continues distally into the foot to form the deep plantar arch.

DORSAL PEDAL ARTERY AND LATERAL TARSAL BRANCH

These vessels are approached through a longitudinal incision lateral to the extensor hallucis longus tendon. The inferior extensor retinaculum is partially incised just distal to the ankle joint to expose the proximal dorsal pedal artery and lateral tarsal branch. The lateral tarsal artery usually arises at the level of the navicular bone and beneath the extensor digitorum brevis muscle. This artery communicates with the arcuate artery in the midfoot. Therefore, it is an important collateral blood supply to the dorsum of the foot. Division of the inferior extensor retinaculum is not required for more distal exposure of the dorsal pedal artery. It is necessary to protect the distal deep peroneal nerve coursing medially to this artery.

DEEP PLANTAR ARTERY

This vessel is the main continuation of the dorsal pedal artery at the level of the metatarsal bones. It is best approached through a curvilinear incision over the dorsum of the foot lateral to the extensor hallucis longus tendon. The artery is followed distally until it divides into the first dorsal metatarsal and deep plantar branches. The latter vessel descends between the two heads of the first dorsal interosseous muscle to collateralize with the lateral plantar branch. This forms the deep plantar arch of the foot (Fig. 4-35). Adequate exposure of the deep plantar branch requires retraction of the extensor hallucis brevis muscle. The periosteum of the second metatarsal bone is then carefully elevated, and a portion of the bone is removed by a rongeur to provide adequate exposure for distal arterial anastomosis (Fig. 4-36). This exposure requires delicate dissection, because injury to adjacent arterial branches and venous tributaries may obscure the operative field or create ischemia to marginally viable tissue.

KEY REFERENCES

Ascer E, Veith F, Gupta S: Bypasses to plantar arteries and other tibial branches: An extended approach to limb salvage. J Vasc Surg 8:434, 1985.

Ballard JL, Abou-Zamzam AM Jr, Teruya TH: Type III and IV thoracoabdominal aortic aneurysm repair: Results of a trifurcated/two-graft technique. J Vasc Surg 36:211, 2002.

Brockstein B, Johns L, Gewertz BL: Blood supply to the spinal cord: Anatomic and physiologic correlations. Ann Vasc Surg 8:394, 1994.

Colborn GL, Mattar SG, Taylor B, et al: The surgical anatomy of the deep femoral artery. Am Surg 61:336, 1995.

Effeney DJ, Stoney RJ: Disorders of the extremities. In Effeney DJ, Stoney RJ (eds): Wylie's Atlas of Vascular Surgery. Philadelphia, JB Lippincott, 1992, p 210.

Mock CN, Lilly MP, McRae RG, Carney WI Jr: Selection of the approach to the distal internal carotid artery from the second cervical vertebra to the base of the skull. J Vasc Surg 13:846, 1991.

Moncure A, Brewster D, Darling R, et al: Use of the splenic and hepatic arteries for renal revascularization. J Vasc Surg 3:196, 1986.

Rutherford RB: Exposure of lower extremity vessels. In Rutherford RB (ed): Atlas of Vascular Surgery: Basic Techniques and Exposures. Philadelphia, WB Saunders, 1993, p 112.

Sakopoulos AG, Ballard JL, Gundry SR: Minimally invasive approach for aortic branch vessel reconstruction. J Vasc Surg 31:200, 2000.

Uflacker R: Abdominal aorta and branches. In Uflacker R (ed): Atlas of Vascular Anatomy: An Angiographic Approach. Baltimore, Williams & Wilkins, 1997, p 405.

REFERENCES

1. Effeney DJ, Stoney RJ: Extracranial cerebrovascular disease. In Effeney DJ, Stoney RJ (eds): Wylie's Atlas of Vascular Surgery. Philadelphia, JB Lippincott, 1992, p 18.
2. Evans W, Mendelowitz D, Liapis C, et al: Motor speech deficit following carotid endarterectomy. Ann Surg 196:461, 1982.
3. Hertzer N, Feldman B, Beven E, et al: A prospective study of the incidence of injury to the cranial nerves during carotid endarterectomy. Surg Gynecol Obstet 151:781, 1980.
4. Ballotta E, Da Giau G, Renon L, et al: Cranial and cervical nerve injuries after carotid endarterectomy: A prospective study. Surgery 125:85, 1999.
5. Forssell C, Kitzing P, Bergqvist D: Cranial nerve injuries after carotid artery surgery: A prospective study of 663 operations. Eur J Vasc Endovasc Surg 10:445, 1995.
6. Mock CN, Lilly MP, McRae RG, Carney WI Jr: Selection of the approach to the distal internal carotid artery from the second cervical vertebra to the base of the skull. J Vasc Surg 13:846, 1991.
7. Fisher D, Clagett G, Parker J, et al: Mandibular subluxation for high carotid exposure. J Vasc Surg 1:727, 1984.
8. Dossa C, Shepard AD, Wolford DG, et al: Distal internal carotid exposure: A simplified technique for temporary mandibular subluxation. J Vasc Surg 12:319, 1990.
9. Wylie E, Stoney R, Ehrenfeld W, Effeney D: Nonatherosclerotic disease of the extracranial carotid arteries. In Egdahl R (ed): Manual of Vascular Surgery, vol 2. New York, Springer-Verlag, 1986.
10. Sakopoulos AG, Ballard JL, Gundry SR: Minimally invasive approach for aortic branch vessel reconstruction. J Vasc Surg 31:200, 2000.
11. Berguer R: Distal vertebral artery bypass: Technique, the "occipital connection," and potential uses. J Vasc Surg 2:621, 1985.
12. Roos D: Surgical treatment of the thoracic outlet syndromes. In Jamison CW (ed): Current Operative Surgery: Vascular Surgery. London, Bailliere & Tindall, 1985.
13. Effeney DJ, Stoney RJ: Disorders of the extremities. In Effeney DJ, Stoney RJ (eds): Wylie's Atlas of Vascular Surgery. Philadelphia, JB Lippincott, 1992, p 210.
14. Stoney R, Wylie E: Surgical management of arterial lesions of the thoracolumbar aorta. Am J Surg 126:157, 1973.
15. Brockstein B, Johns L, Gewertz BL: Blood supply to the spinal cord: Anatomic and physiologic correlations. Ann Vasc Surg 8:394, 1994.
16. Ballard JL, Yonemoto H, Killeen JD: Cost effective aortic exposure: A retroperitoneal experience. Ann Vasc Surg 14:1, 2000.
17. Sicard GA, Reilly JM, Rubin BG, et al: Transabdominal versus retroperitoneal incision for abdominal aortic surgery: Report of a prospective randomized trial. J Vasc Surg 21:174, 1995.
18. Darling RC III, Shah DM, McClellan WR, et al: Decreased morbidity associated with retroperitoneal exclusion treatment for abdominal aortic aneurysm. J Cardiovasc Surg 33:65, 1992.
19. Uflacker R: Abdominal aorta and branches. In Uflacker R (ed): Atlas of Vascular Anatomy: An Angiographic Approach. Baltimore, Williams & Wilkins, 1997, p 405.
20. Ballard JL: Renal artery endarterectomy for treatment of renovascular hypertension combined with infrarenal aortic reconstruction: Analysis of surgical results. Ann Vasc Surg 15:260, 2001.
21. Ballard JL, Abou-Zamzam AM Jr, Teruya TH: Type III and IV thoracoabdominal aortic aneurysm repair: Results of a trifurcated/two-graft technique. J Vasc Surg 36:211, 2002.
22. Tollefson DFJ, Ernst CB: Gastrointestinal and visceral ischemic complications of aortic reconstruction. In Bernhard VM, Towne JB (eds): Complications in Vascular Surgery. St. Louis, Quality Medical Publishing, 1991, p 135.
23. Moncure A, Brewster D, Darling R, et al: Use of the splenic and hepatic arteries for renal revascularization. J Vasc Surg 3:196, 1986.
24. Kudsk KA, Sheldon GF: Retroperitoneal hematoma. In Blaisdell FW, Trunkey DD (eds): Trauma Management: Abdominal Trauma, vol 1. New York, Thieme-Stratton, 1982, p 281.
25. Colborn GL, Mattar SG, Taylor B, et al: The surgical anatomy of the deep femoral artery. Am Surg 61:336, 1995.
26. Nuñez A, Veith F, Gupta S, et al: Direct approaches to the distal portions of the deep femoral artery for limb salvage bypasses. J Vasc Surg 8:576, 1988.
27. Rutherford RB: Exposure of lower extremity vessels. In Rutherford RB (ed): Atlas of Vascular Surgery: Basic Techniques and Exposures. Philadelphia, WB Saunders, 1993, p 112.
28. Veith F, Ascer E, Gupta S: Lateral approach to the popliteal artery. J Vasc Surg 6:119, 1987.
29. Ascer E, Veith F, Gupta S: Bypasses to plantar arteries and other tibial branches: An extended approach to limb salvage. J Vasc Surg 8:434, 1985.

Questions

1. **Which of the following nerves has the highest incidence of injury during carotid endarterectomy?**
   (a) Recurrent laryngeal nerve
   (b) Hypoglossal nerve (cranial nerve XII)
   (c) Superior laryngeal nerve
   (d) Glossopharyngeal nerve (cranial nerve IX)

2. **Structures contributing to thoracic outlet compression syndrome include all of the following except**
   (a) Subclavius muscle
   (b) First rib or congenital cervical rib
   (c) Anterior scanele muscle
   (d) Sternocleidomastoid muscle

3. **Which of the following statements regarding lower extremity circulation is true?**
   (a) The deep femoral artery is accessible only by an approach that is lateral to the sartorius muscle
   (b) It is not possible to expose the popliteal artery above or below the knee by a lateral approach
   (c) The lateral tarsal artery is the largest distal branch of the posterior tibial artery
   (d) The deep plantar arch is formed by the deep plantar artery and the lateral plantar artery

4. **During repair of an infrarenal abdominal aortic aneurysm, all of the following statements are true except**
   (a) Autonomic nerve fibers crossing the left common iliac artery should be protected to preserve erectile function
   (b) A large anastomotic artery appearing on arteriography between the superior and inferior mesenteric arteries indicates satisfactory perfusion of the left colon with little risk of ischemia if the inferior mesenteric artery is ligated
   (c) A large lumbar artery near the renal arteries should be preserved, if possible, because this may represent a significant contribution to the anterior spinal artery
   (d) The left renal vein may be safely ligated and divided to facilitate aortic exposure if the lumbar and adrenal tributaries are maintained for collateral circulation

5. Patients with celiac and superior mesenteric artery occlusive disease would be expected to have all of the following except
   (a) A large central anastomotic artery
   (b) Retrograde filling of the superior mesenteric artery
   (c) A large marginal artery of Drummond
   (d) A low incidence of left colon ischemia following inferior mesenteric artery ligation

6. Which of the following statements about renal artery reconstruction is true?
   (a) It may be performed via a left or right retroperitoneal approach
   (b) It may be difficult in an obese or previously operated patient if an anterior transabdominal approach is used
   (c) It is facilitated in a high-risk patient by using splenic artery–to–left renal artery bypass or hepatic artery–to–right renal artery bypass
   (d) All of the above

7. Regarding carotid artery exposure, all of the following are true except
   (a) The distal internal carotid artery is crossed anteriorly by the hypoglossal nerve (cranial nerve XII)
   (b) The vagus nerve (cranial nerve X) passes posterolateral to the carotid bifurcation
   (c) Distal exposure is safely facilitated by anterior dislocation of the mandible
   (d) Distal exposure may be facilitated by division of the posterior belly of the digastric muscle and the stylohyoid muscle

8. Regarding trauma to the great vessels, which of the following is true?
   (a) Exposure of the proximal left subclavian artery is best accomplished via sternotomy
   (b) Temporary right third interspace thoracotomy can be used to control exigent hemorrhage from the innominate artery

   (c) Exposure of either common carotid artery origin is best accomplished via a sternal splitting incision extended along the anterior border of the appropriate sternocleidomastoid muscle
   (d) Right subclavian exposure via a simple supraclavicular incision is adequate for most traumatic injuries in this area

9. Exposure of the infrapopliteal arteries is best described by which of the following anatomic relationships?
   (a) The anterior tibial artery passes posterior to the interosseous membrane
   (b) Lateral exposure of the peroneal artery requires segmental fibular resection
   (c) The tibial nerve crosses the posterior tibial artery anteriorly
   (d) The posterior tibial artery lies deep to the transverse crural intermuscular septum

10. Which of the following statements regarding the arteria radicularis magna (artery of Adamkiewicz) is true?
    (a) It may provide up to two thirds of the spinal cord blood supply
    (b) It appears as a branch of either a distal intercostal or a proximal lumbar artery
    (c) It is rarely identified preoperatively via standard arteriography
    (d) All of the above

Answers

1. b	2. d	3. d	4. b	5. d
6. d	7. c	8. c	9. b	10. d

5

Erica L. Mitchell • Timothy K. Liem

Hemostasis and Thrombosis

Most of the bleeding that occurs during surgery or in association with trauma is mechanical and usually can be controlled. Occasionally, bleeding is caused or accelerated by congenital or acquired defects of the hemostatic mechanisms. The vascular surgeon must understand the hemostatic system sufficiently to arrest bleeding, restore hemostasis, or both, according to the patient's needs.

There is increasing evidence that a significant number of acute arterial and venous thrombotic disorders are associated with congenital and acquired hypercoagulable states. Therefore, the vascular surgeon should also be able to recognize and manage the common thrombophilic states and restore arterial and venous blood flow by both mechanical and pharmacologic means.

Hemostasis

Hemostasis is the process by which bleeding from injured tissue is controlled.

COMPONENTS OF HEMOSTASIS

Although hemostasis is a dynamic process, it can be divided into four components: vessel response to injury, platelet activation and aggregation, activation of coagulation with clot stabilization, and coagulation inhibition. Each component has numerous modulatory mechanisms.

Vessel Response

When a vessel is injured, the interaction of humoral, neurogenic, and myogenic events leads to temporary vasoconstriction in the muscular arteries and arterioles. Mechanisms for vasoconstriction remain poorly understood, but they may include the release of thromboxane A_2 (TXA_2) by activated platelets, endothelin by endothelial cells, bradykinin, and fibrinopeptide B. Vasoconstriction has less of a role in obtaining hemostasis in veins and venules.

In normal vessels, endothelial cells cover the luminal surface, forming a monolayer with tight cell-cell interaction. The endothelium weighs approximately 1.5 to 2 kg and has a volume equal to that of the liver.[1] Once regarded as a passive barrier between the blood and the underlying thrombogenic subendothelium, the endothelium is now recognized as a biologically active organ that participates in and modulates various physiologic processes, including hemostasis and thrombosis.

In their quiescent state, endothelial cells are actively antithrombotic (Table 5-1). They synthesize and secrete prostacyclin and nitric oxide, potent vasodilators and inhibitors of platelet aggregation. Heparan sulfates are heparin-like mucopolysaccharides that are synthesized and expressed by macrovascular and microvascular endothelial cells. They accelerate the activity of antithrombin III (AT III), thereby inactivating thrombin and several other serine protease coagulation factors. Thrombomodulin (TM), a glycoprotein expressed on the endothelial surface of all organs, with the exception of the brain, also inactivates thrombin.[2]

TABLE 5–1 The Endothelial Cell as Modulator of Hemostasis

Function	Effect
Thrombogenic	
Profound loss of NO and PGI₂ after injury	Loss of vasodilating stimulus
Von Willebrand's factor synthesis	↑ Platelet adhesion
Factor V synthesis	↑ Thrombin
Expression of tissue factor	↑ Thrombin
Binding of factors VIIa and IXa	↑ Thrombin
Surface membrane site for prothrombinase complex	↑ Thrombin
Plasminogen activator inhibitor synthesis	↑ Thrombin
Antithrombotic	
NO and PGI₂ synthesis	Vasodilating stimulus
PGI₂ synthesis and granule release	↓ Platelet aggregation
Thrombomodulin synthesis	↓ Factors Va and VIIIa
Protein S synthesis	↓ Factors Va and VIIIa
Heparan sulfate synthesis	↓ Thrombin
t-PA and urokinase synthesis	↓ Plasmin
Tissue factor pathway inhibitor	↓ Factors IXa and Xa

NO, nitric oxide; PGI₂, prostaglandin I₂; t-PA, tissue plasminogen activator.

The thrombomodulin-thrombin complex in turn is a potent activator of protein C.[3] Protein S is a cofactor for activated protein C and is synthesized by both endothelial cells and the liver.[4,5] Activated protein C inactivates factor Va and factor VIIIa. These factors greatly accelerate the conversion of prothrombin (II) to thrombin (IIa) and factor X to Xa. Tissue factor pathway inhibitor (TFPI) is a potent inhibitor of the external coagulation pathway. TFPI is expressed by megakaryocytes and capillary endothelium, and the majority is bound to the endothelial surface.[6,7] It is released in response to heparin administration and binds to the factor VIIa–tissue factor–factor Xa complex, inhibiting the further conversion of factor X to Xa and factor IX to IXa. The endothelium also synthesizes tissue-type plasminogen activator (t-PA) and urokinase. Both are serine proteases that bind to fibrinogen and remain bound to fibrin. These proteases convert plasminogen to plasmin, the enzyme responsible for fibrinolysis.

The endothelium possesses substantial procoagulant activity and acts as a template for hemostasis when stimulated after vessel injury (see Table 5-1). Tissue factor (thromboplastin, factor III) is a low-molecular-weight lipoprotein that is constitutively expressed by most cells, including vascular adventitia, central nervous system, lung, and placental tissue. It is also expressed in the epithelium of the skin, mucosa, bronchus, and glomeruli. Endothelial cells and blood cells do not express tissue factor on their surfaces unless stimulated by agonists such as interleukin 1, thrombin, or endotoxin. Vessel injury causes endothelial denudation and activation, which result in exposure of blood to tissue factor. Low circulating levels of activated factor VII (VIIa) bind to tissue factor via a calcium ion–dependent interaction that is enhanced by the presence of factor X. This complex catalyzes the conversion of factor IX to IXa and factor X to Xa, leading to thrombin formation.

Endothelial cells and megakaryocytes synthesize and secrete von Willebrand's factor (vWF), which is necessary for platelet adhesion to the vessel wall. This factor has binding sites for collagen, platelet glycoproteins (GPs) Ib and IIb/IIIa, and factor VIII. Factor VIII and vWF circulate together as a complex, although they are the products of two distinct genes. Endothelial cells, in addition to the liver, synthesize factor V. Factors V and VIII are cleaved by thrombin into their activated states (Va and VIIIa) and then become integral components of the membrane-bound prothrombinase and tenase complexes, respectively (mostly on the platelet surface, but also on the endothelium).[8,9] The prothrombinase and tenase complexes accelerate the formation of thrombin (IIa) and factor Xa (Fig. 5-1). Endothelial cells also synthesize a plasminogen activator inhibitor (PAI-1), which rapidly inactivates circulating t-PA. When the plasminogen activator becomes incorporated within a thrombus or hemostatic plug, it is more slowly inactivated by PAI-1.

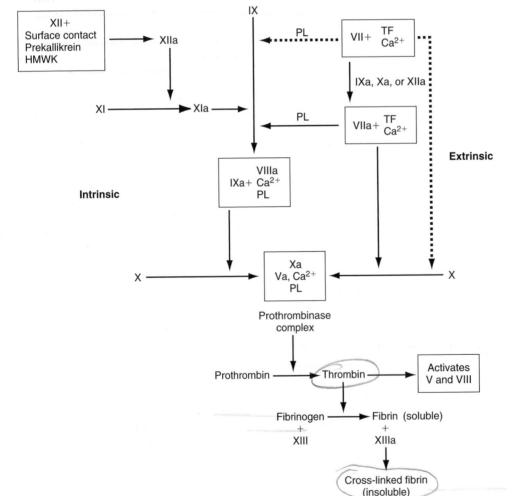

FIGURE 5–1 • The intrinsic and extrinsic pathways of coagulation. The intrinsic pathway is initiated by surface contact; the extrinsic pathway is initiated by the release of tissue factor (TF) from tissues injured during surgery or trauma. Factor VIIa possesses an activity 100 times greater than that of factor VII. The pathways are interrelated and operate in tandem to achieve hemostasis. HMWK, high-molecular-weight kininogen; PL, phospholipid from activated platelet or endothelial membranes.

Platelet Activation

Platelets are small, discoid-shaped, anuclear cells with an average circulatory life span of 8 to 12 days. There are usually 200,000 to 400,000 platelets/mm³ in human blood. Platelets are released as cytoplasmic fragments of megakaryocytes within bone marrow.

The platelet surface membrane is composed of a phospholipid bilayer, glycoproteins, and proteins. Carbohydrate moieties of the glycoproteins make up the outer layer, known as the glycocalyx, with which circulating proteins interact. Surface receptors are known to exist for thrombin, adenosine diphosphate (ADP), epinephrine, TXA_2, fibrinogen, collagen, platelet-activating factor, serotonin, vasopressin, vitronectin, fibronectin, laminin, vWF, and the Fc receptor FcγRIIA.[10] The intercellular adhesion receptors P-selectin, platelet endothelial cell adhesion molecule-1 (PECAM-1), and intercellular adhesion molecule-2 (ICAM-2) most likely mediate the recognition of and attachment to monocytes, neutrophils, and leukocytes.[11,12]

Platelets contain three types of storage granules: (1) amine storage or dense granules, which contain serotonin, ADP, adenosine triphosphate (ATP), and calcium; (2) protein storage or α-granules, which contain coagulation proteins (high-molecular-weight kininogen [HMWK], fibrinogen, fibronectin, factor V, vWF, platelet factor 4), growth factors (platelet-derived growth factor, transforming growth factor-α and -β), and adhesion proteins (fibronectin, thrombospondin, P-selectin); and (3) lysosomes, which contain numerous proteases, glycosidases, and acid hydrolases.

The initial stage of hemostasis, consisting of vasoconstriction and platelet plug formation, is termed primary hemostasis. After vascular injury, platelets adhere within seconds to the subendothelial matrix (via binding to exposed collagen fibrils, vWF, thrombospondin, fibronectin, and laminin). Collagen binds to the platelet via the GP Ia-IIa complex and GP IV, whereas vWF binds primarily to the GP Ib-IX-V complex and, to a lesser degree, the GP IIb-IIIa complex. Collagen-induced platelet activation results in loss of the discoid shape and release of prothrombotic α- and dense granule contents. Shape change occurs when attachments between actin filaments and the cell membrane are severed. Subsequent actin elongation results in the formation of filopods and lamellipodia that allow more efficient platelet-platelet interaction. The granule release reaction further amplifies platelet activation and aggregation via vWF, fibronectin, ADP, serotonin, and the release of fibrinogen, factor V, and platelet factor 4.

Platelet activation is associated with numerous downstream signals that include protein kinase C activation, generation of inositol triphosphate, intracellular calcium mobilization (via phospholipase C), and generation of arachidonic acid (via phospholipase A_2). Arachidonic acid is converted by cyclooxygenase-1 (prostaglandin H synthase-1) to the prostaglandin (PG) endoperoxides PGG_2 and PGH_2. PGG_2 is then converted to TXA_2 by thromboxane synthetase. TXA_2, PGG_2, and PGH_2 stimulate further aggregation and platelet granule release.[13]

The concomitant generation of thrombin via the coagulation cascade and the release of ADP from platelet-dense granules further amplify platelet activation and aggregation. Regardless of the agonist, the final common pathway for platelet aggregation involves a conformational change in the GP IIb-IIIa complex, with the reversible exposure of binding sites for fibrinogen. Circulating fibrinogen and fibrinogen released from α-granules form bridges between adjacent platelets.[14]

Numerous medications inhibit platelet function at several steps in the activation and aggregation pathway. Aspirin irreversibly inhibits platelet cyclooxygenase-1, inhibiting thromboxane-mediated platelet aggregation for the life of the platelet. Ticlopidine and clopidogrel inhibit ADP-mediated platelet activation and aggregation.[15,16] Novel GP IIb-IIIa inhibitors prevent platelet aggregation by blocking the binding of fibrinogen.[17]

Platelets are dynamically involved in the coagulation cascade. Procoagulant phospholipids (platelet factor 3) are exposed on the platelet membrane after stimulation by thrombin and collagen. These phospholipids provide a binding site for the prothrombinase complex. Platelets also release factor V from α-granules. Factor V becomes activated and membrane bound, acting as a receptor for the binding of activated factor X. Additionally, platelets have surface receptors for factors XI, activated XI, and HMWK.

Coagulation Activation

The platelet plug, required for normal hemostasis, deaggregates as its fibrinogen bridges dissociate unless thrombin is generated and fibrin stabilization of the plug occurs (secondary hemostasis). The formation of fibrin requires the interaction of platelet aggregates, endothelial cells, and plasma coagulation proteins.

Thirteen plasma coagulation proteins have been designated by the roman numerals I through XIII (the letter *a* follows the roman numeral when the factor has been activated). Most of these factors are synthesized in the liver. Although factor VIII and vWF circulate together via a tight noncovalent bond, they are the products of two unrelated genes. The nomenclature regarding factor VIII and vWF was clarified by the International Committee on Thrombosis and Haemostasis. Currently, the factor VIII protein, antigenic level, and functional activities are referred to as VIII, VIII:Ag, and VIII:C, respectively. For vWF, the protein and antigenic level are referred to as vWF and vWF:Ag.[18] The hepatic synthesis of factors II, VII, IX, and X is vitamin K dependent. When vitamin K is not available, these factors are synthesized and released, but they are not biologically active.

The sequence of enzymatic events leading to thrombin formation has been termed the coagulation cascade (see Fig. 5-1). The intrinsic pathway is activated when plasma is exposed to a negatively charged surface such as subendothelium, collagen, or endotoxin. Factor XII is activated to XIIa by the interaction of HMWK, prekallikrein, and the negatively charged surface. However, the physiologic significance of factor XII activation is unclear, because deficiencies in factor XII, HMWK, and prekallikrein are not associated with any clinical bleeding diatheses.

The extrinsic pathway to thrombin production is probably the more physiologic route for the generation of thrombin and fibrin. It is initiated by the exposure of tissue factor (TF), which is constitutively expressed in the vascular adventitia and subendothelium. TF binds to low levels of circulating factor VIIa in the presence of calcium (TF-VIIa).[19,20] This complex activates factor X to Xa and factor IX to IXa.[21]

Factor Xa by itself does not generate thrombin efficiently. However, factors Xa and thrombin can activate factor VII to VIIa, factor V to Va, and factor VIII to VIIIa. The latter two active cofactors are critical components of the phospholipid membrane-associated prothrombinase and tenase complexes, respectively (see Fig. 5-1). The prothrombinase (Xa-Va-Ca^{2+}-phospholipid) and tenase (IXa-VIIIa-Ca^{2+}-phospholipid) complexes are 10^5 to 10^6 times more active than their serine protease factors acting independently.[20] The tenase complex is also about 50 times more efficient in activating factor X than is TF-VIIa. The vital role for these complexes is clinically evident. Unlike factor XII deficiency, deficiencies of TF and factors V (parahemophilia), VII, VIII (hemophilia A), IX (hemophilia B), X, and XI may be associated with significant bleeding diatheses. The clinical significance of factor XI deficiency indicates that physiologic amplification of the thrombotic process probably requires additional intrinsic pathway positive feedback that involves activation of factor XI to XIa by thrombin.

Thrombin proteolytically cleaves fibrinopeptides A and B from the fibrinogen molecule. The resulting fibrin monomers polymerize and propagate to form a gel. Thrombin also activates factor XIII to XIIIa in a reaction that is greatly accelerated (>80-fold) by the presence of fibrin.[22] Factor XIIIa covalently cross-links adjacent fibrin monomers, forming a stable clot that is more resistant to lysis by plasmin.

Coagulation Inhibition

Several mechanisms have evolved to control the rate of thrombin and fibrin formation (Fig. 5-2). Antithrombin III is a serine protease inhibitor that is synthesized in the liver and endothelial cells. AT III inhibits numerous coagulation factors, including thrombin (IIa), TF-VIIa, and factors IXa, Xa, XIa, and XIIa, but its most important targets are factors IIa and Xa. AT III activity is enhanced at least 1000-fold whenever it binds to circulating heparin or endothelial-bound heparin-like molecules. After the AT III–heparin complex binds to an activated coagulation factor, the heparin dissociates and continues to act as a catalyst for the formation of other AT III–serine enzyme complexes.

Tissue Factor Pathway Inhibitor

TFPI is a Kunitz-type enzyme inhibitor that is synthesized by the endothelium and megakaryocytes.[23,24] It binds to the TF-VIIa-Xa complex and inhibits the further conversion of factors X to Xa and IX to IXa.[25] TFPI is constitutively expressed on the endothelium, and it circulates bound to plasma lipoproteins (hence the former name lipoprotein-associated coagulation inhibitor). TFPI activity and antigen levels increase severalfold after the administration of heparin.

Thrombomodulin

TM is a proteoglycan expressed on the surface of most endothelial cells, except within the central nervous system.[2] TM readily binds to thrombin, causing a conformational change in the substrate binding site. The thrombin molecule is rendered incapable of binding active coagulation factors but is able to bind and activate circulating protein C. TM also accelerates the inactivation of thrombin by AT III.[26,27] A procoagulant function for TM also has been found: TM

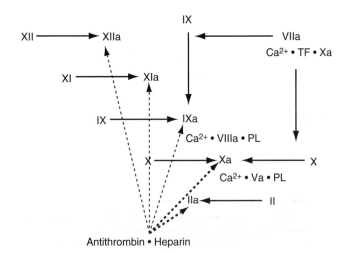

A

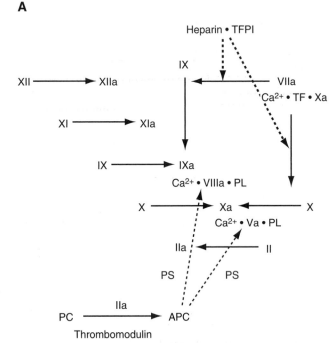

B

FIGURE 5–2 • Sites of activity for natural anticoagulants. *Dotted lines* indicated inhibitory activity. APC, activated protein C; AT, antithrombin; PS, protein S; TF, tissue factor; TFPI, tissue factor pathway inhibitor.

accelerates the activation of thrombin-activatable fibrinolysis inhibitor compared with free thrombin alone.[28]

Protein C and Protein S

Both protein C and protein S are synthesized by the liver, but protein S has also been found in endothelium and platelets.[29,30] Both proteins undergo several post-translational modifications, including the γ-carboxylation of glutamine residues via a vitamin K–dependent reaction. Protein S (a nonenzymatic cofactor for protein C) circulates either free or bound to the C4b binding protein. Activated protein C binds to protein S on the endothelial or platelet surface and cleaves several peptide bonds in factors Va and VIIIa, resulting in decreased formation of the prothrombinase and tenase complexes.

Heparin Cofactor II

Heparin cofactor II is another specific thrombin inhibitor that forms a stable 1:1 complex with thrombin. Heparin, heparan-like molecules, and dermatan sulfate accelerate the activity of heparin cofactor II. Unlike AT III, heparin cofactor II cannot inhibit other coagulation factors. The plasma concentration of heparin cofactor II (70 μg/L) is much lower than that of AT III (150 mg/L), and it is unlikely that heparin cofactor II plays a major role in the regulation of hemostasis.

Fibrinolysis

Plasminogen, an inactive precursor that is synthesized in the liver, can be converted to plasmin by several plasminogen activators. Circulating t-PA (synthesized in the endothelium) does not activate plasminogen efficiently. However, both t-PA and plasminogen have high affinity for fibrin, which acts as a template for accelerated plasminogen activation (>1000-fold).[31,32] Thus, the primary role for t-PA–activated plasmin is the formation of fibrin degradation products. However, exogenously administered t-PA also may activate plasminogen, which is bound to one of the fibrin degradation by-products (the DD[E] complex), resulting in the release of free plasmin.[33,34] This may lead to the limited breakdown of fibrinogen, factor V, and factor VIII and to a systemic fibrinolytic state.

Three types of urokinase plasminogen activator (u-PA) have been studied. The precursor, pro-urokinase (single-chain u-PA), has a low level of enzymatic activity and no affinity for fibrin, but it does demonstrate specificity against fibrin-bound plasminogen. This may be caused by a conformational change in the plasminogen, exposing the critical peptide bond and making it more susceptible to activation by single-chain u-PA.[35] Single-chain u-PA is readily converted by plasmin or kallikrein to the more active two-chain u-PA, which has a high-molecular-weight and a low-molecular-weight form. Commercially produced urokinase is composed primarily of the low-molecular-weight variant. Two-chain u-PA activates circulating plasminogen and fibrin-bound plasminogen equally well, resulting in a more pronounced systemic fibrinolysis.[36] Plasmin activated by u-PA also performs numerous other functions related to cell migration and remodeling, including the activation of matrix metalloproteinases.[37] Monocytes and endothelial cells express the u-PA receptor, which binds to u-PA and localizes plasmin to the cell surface.

Each step within the plasminogen activation system has a known inhibitor. PAI-1 is released by endothelial cells, platelets, and hepatocytes. This inhibitor efficiently inactivates t-PA and two-chain u-PA and performs other functions, including the inhibition of thrombin and smooth muscle cell migration. PAI-2 is a less potent inhibitor of t-PA and two-chain u-PA, but its role in physiologic hemostasis remains uncertain. PAI-2 is released into the circulation during pregnancy, indicating a greater role for hemostasis during pregnancy and delivery. Neither PAI-1 nor PAI-2 inhibits pro-urokinase (single-chain u-PA). α_2-Antiplasmin inactivates circulating plasmin more readily than it does fibrin-bound plasmin, thus decreasing overall systemic fibrinolysis. Other less specific proteases that inhibit fibrinolysis are α_1-protease inhibitor and α_2-macroglobulin.

PREOPERATIVE EVALUATION

A good history and thorough physical examination detect the majority of bleeding disorders preoperatively. Laboratory testing is warranted if a bleeding disorder is present or suspected. Careful questioning should distinguish a congenital bleeding disorder from an acquired one. Determining the pattern of inheritance may further aid in identifying a congenital deficiency. A history of bleeding problems beginning in childhood or at the beginning of menses implies an inherited bleeding disorder. A history of postoperative or spontaneous bleeding in a family member is important, because many patients with inherited disorders do not experience serious bleeding until challenged by an operative procedure or trauma. All patients should be asked about bleeding after tooth extraction, minor trauma, circumcision, and other surgical procedures.

An acquired hemostatic disorder should be suspected in adults who bleed during or after surgery or trauma but who have no previous history of bleeding disorders. However, some patients with congenital disorders, such as von Willebrand's disease, may not demonstrate a bleeding diathesis until challenged. Patients with liver disease are at increased risk for developing a coagulopathy during surgery, after trauma, and after massive transfusion. Patients resuscitated with more than 20 mL/kg of hetastarch in 24 hours are at risk for bleeding from decreased platelet adhesiveness and deficiencies in coagulation proteins. Patients receiving more than 1.5 mg/kg of dextran in 24 hours are also at increased risk for bleeding as a result of impaired platelet function and reduced plasma concentration of vWF. A detailed history of drug use is also important, because many drugs alter platelet function and predispose patients to bleeding complications.

Physical examination should include a thorough inspection for ecchymoses, petechiae, purpura, hemangiomas, jaundice, hematomas, and hemarthroses. Petechiae, ecchymoses, and mucocutaneous bleeding (epistaxis, gastrointestinal or genitourinary bleeding, menorrhagia) are more commonly associated with defects in primary hemostasis. Bleeding into deep tissues (hemarthroses, muscle and retroperitoneal hematomas) tends to occur with defects in coagulation. Splenomegaly may be associated with thrombocytopenia. Signs of hepatic insufficiency should be noted, because these patients may have decreased production of coagulation proteins. Patients suffering from myeloproliferative disorders, some malignant neoplasms, collagen disorders, or renal insufficiency are at increased risk for bleeding complications.

Screening laboratory tests include platelet count and examination of peripheral blood smear; bleeding time; and prothrombin time (PT), activated partial thromboplastin time (aPTT), and thrombin time. The bleeding time, a very sensitive test for hemostasis, is prolonged with qualitative platelet deficiencies, as well as with decreased levels of fibrinogen, factor V, and vWF. The PT assesses the extrinsic pathway and is prolonged by deficiencies of prothrombin, fibrinogen, and factors V, VII, and X. The aPTT is prolonged by deficiencies of factors in the intrinsic pathway, including VIII, IX, XI, and XII. To a lesser extent, aPTT detects factor deficiencies in the common pathway: V, X, prothrombin, and fibrinogen. The aPTT is also prolonged by heparin. The lupus anticoagulant prolongs phospholipid-dependent coagulation reactions in vitro: PT, aPTT, and dilute Russell's viper venom time. However, it does not cause clinical bleeding. The thrombin time is prolonged by hypofibrinogenemia, fibrin abnormalities, and heparin.

PLATELET DISORDERS

Hemorrhagic complications may occur because of quantitative or qualitative platelet disorders that are acquired or congenital in origin. Thrombocytopenia and qualitative platelet defects are among the most common causes of bleeding in surgical patients. Spontaneous bleeding may occur when platelet counts fall below 20,000/mm³. Platelet counts between 30,000 and 50,000/mm³ are adequate to ensure hemostasis, provided that there are no associated functional platelet or coagulation disorders. Platelet counts of 50,000 to 100,000/mm³ are required to restore hemostasis during bleeding.

Thrombocytopenia

Thrombocytopenia may occur from increased platelet destruction, abnormal production, dilution, or temporary sequestration (usually in the spleen). Increased destruction may occur via nonimmune or immune mechanisms. Nonimmune-mediated thrombocytopenia occurs in hemolytic-uremic syndrome, thrombotic thrombocytopenic purpura, disseminated intravascular coagulation (DIC), and some vasculitides. In these syndromes, platelets are stimulated to aggregate within the microcirculation, often affecting the brain, kidneys, heart, lungs, and adrenal glands.[38] Early plasmapheresis and plasma transfusion (platelet-poor fresh frozen plasma, cryoprecipitate-poor plasma), along with high-dose glucocorticoid administration, can reverse most cases of thrombotic thrombocytopenic purpura.[39,40] Platelet transfusions should be used only for intracerebral or other life-threatening hemorrhagic complications. The treatment for hemolytic-uremic syndrome varies considerably but may include hemodialysis, heparin therapy, and plasma exchange, depending on the duration and severity of the illness. GP IIb-IIIa inhibitors may become a useful adjunct in hemolytic-uremic syndrome.[41]

Immune-mediated platelet destruction may occur with certain collagen vascular diseases (lupus erythematosus), immune thrombocytopenic purpura, and lymphoproliferative disorders (chronic lymphocytic leukemia, non-Hodgkin's lymphoma), or it may be drug induced. Acute immune thrombocytopenic purpura is a postinfectious thrombocytopenia that occurs predominantly in children and is usually self-limited. Chronic immune thrombocytopenic purpura is idiopathic and results when autoimmune antibodies are generated against the platelet membrane. Initial therapy for the chronic form consists of corticosteroids (prednisone, methylprednisolone), followed by splenectomy in nonresponders. Severely thrombocytopenic patients with major hemorrhagic complications and patients requiring urgent surgery can be treated with platelet transfusions, intravenous (IV) gamma globulin, and plasmapheresis.

Some drugs (quinidine, quinine, sulfonamides, penicillins, valproic acid, heparin) may induce thrombocytopenia via the formation of antigen-antibody complexes on the platelet surface, increasing platelet destruction. In general, discontinuation of the drug reverses the thrombocytopenia within 2 to 5 days. Adjuvant therapy for active bleeding may include corticosteroids, platelet transfusions, and, in some cases,

IV gamma globulin. Heparin-induced thrombocytopenia is a prothrombotic condition that is discussed later in the section on thrombosis.

Impaired platelet production may be caused by aplastic anemia, megakaryocytic aplasia, radiation, myelosuppressive drugs, viral infections, vitamin B_{12} and folate deficiencies, and several other drugs (ethanol, estrogens, interferon, thiazides). Thrombocytopenia also has been described in association with numerous congenital disorders (Fanconi's aplastic anemia, sex-linked recessive thrombocytopenia, Alport's syndrome).

Thrombocytopenia commonly occurs after massive transfusions of banked blood. Only 10% of platelets remain viable in blood held in cold storage for longer than 24 hours. In general, the replacement of one blood volume decreases the platelet count by one third to one half.[42] Nevertheless, abnormal bleeding is uncommon, and the routine administration of platelets following massive transfusion is not warranted unless hemorrhage is ongoing.[43] Hypothermia (temperature lower than 32°C) also may cause thrombocytopenia, but the mechanism remains unclear. However, sequestration of platelets during hypothermia is well documented. Platelets appear to activate, release α-granule products, aggregate, and sequester in the portal circulation. Rewarming may cause a significant portion to return to the circulation. Cold-induced coagulopathy is best prevented by transfusing warmed blood products and maintaining the core body temperature above 32°C.

The centrifugation of one unit of whole blood yields 8 to 10×10^{10} platelets. Approximately 4 to 8 units of whole blood are required to yield enough platelets for administration in the average adult. Current apheresis techniques can yield 2.5 to 10×10^{11} platelets from a single donor (over 1 to 2 hours). One unit of single-donor platelets usually increases the platelet count by 10,000/mm³ per square meter of body surface area.

Qualitative Disorders of Platelet Function

Qualitative platelet disorders should be suspected when bleeding occurs in patients with normal coagulation studies and platelet counts. Qualitative disorders may be congenital or acquired; acquired disorders are much more common. Disturbances of platelet adherence and aggregation rarely cause bleeding spontaneously but certainly exacerbate bleeding secondary to surgery and trauma. Congenital qualitative disorders of platelet function include von Willebrand's disease, Bernard-Soulier syndrome, Glanzmann's thrombasthenia, storage pool diseases, and diseases of platelet activation.

Von Willebrand's disease is the most common inherited bleeding disorder, characterized by a deficiency or defect in vWF. It has been classified into six subtypes (1, 2A, 2B, 2M, 2N, 3), with type 1 being the most common (70%).[44] Type 1 von Willebrand's disease is usually transmitted as an autosomal dominant trait with incomplete penetrance. In general, patients manifest epistaxis, ecchymoses, menorrhagia, and post-traumatic or postsurgical bleeding. Decreased platelet adherence causes prolongation of the bleeding time. The aPTT also may be elevated, because most patients with this disease have concomitant decreases in factor VIII coagulation activity (VIII:C). Ristocetin agglutination of platelets is impaired but can be corrected with the addition of vWF-rich cryoprecipitate.

Treatment of von Willebrand's disease may consist of replacement (cryoprecipitate, purified factor VIII concentrates, platelet transfusions) or nonreplacement (vasopressin, antifibrinolytic agents) therapy. Approximately 80% of patients with type 1 disease respond to desmopressin acetate (DDAVP) with increased vWF:Ag and VIII:C (within 60 minutes), which may last for 4 to 6 hours. Unfortunately, response to therapy cannot be predicted without trial administration. Repeated administration of DDAVP (every 12 hours) may be required in patients with type 1 disease who undergo surgical procedures. Most type 2 and type 3 patients do not respond to DDAVP. Antifibrinolytic agents (ε-aminocaproic acid, tranexamic acid) have been used for the treatment of mucocutaneous bleeding and for prophylaxis during oral surgical procedures.[45] Patients who are unresponsive to DDAVP may require replacement therapy during the perioperative period. Until recently, cryoprecipitate (rich in vWF, factors VIII and XIII, and fibronectin) was the treatment of choice. More recently, some purified factor VIII concentrates (which contain large quantities of multimeric vWF) and a newly formulated vWF concentrate have been used successfully.[46] There are no clear guidelines regarding the amount and frequency of administration; replacement therapy is largely empirical. The bleeding time and factor VIII levels are used to monitor response to replacement therapy.

Bernard-Soulier syndrome is transmitted as an autosomal recessive trait and is characterized by a deficiency in the GP Ib-IX-V complex (primary binding site for vWF). These patients have prolonged bleeding times (>20 minutes), mild to moderate thrombocytopenia, and absent ristocetin-induced platelet agglutination. Heterozygous patients have half the normal amount of GP Ib-IX-V but demonstrate normal platelet responses. Platelet transfusions are the mainstay of therapy, but they are limited by the development of antibodies to human leukocyte antigens (HLAs) (alloimmunization) and to the GP Ib-IX-V complex. The use of HLA crossmatched and leukocyte-depleted platelets should minimize alloimmunization. Other unproved therapies include DDAVP and corticosteroids.

Glanzmann's thrombasthenia is a rare autosomal recessive trait in which platelet membranes lack GP IIb-IIIa receptors, leading to failure of platelet aggregation regardless of the initial stimulus. These patients have normal platelet counts, markedly prolonged bleeding times, deficient clot retraction, and normal ristocetin-induced agglutination. Patients who are heterozygous exhibit normal platelet aggregation responses. As with Bernard-Soulier syndrome, platelet transfusions are the primary form of therapy. Again, the use of HLA crossmatched and leukocyte-depleted platelets is optimal.

Storage pool diseases are a group of rare hereditary disorders characterized by deficiencies in platelet granules, their contents, or both. These include deficiencies in α-granule contents (gray platelet syndrome), δ-granule storage diseases (Wiskott-Aldrich syndrome, Hermansky-Pudlak syndrome, Chédiak-Higashi syndrome), and αδ-granule storage diseases.[47] Cryoprecipitate and platelet transfusions may be used in the perioperative period. DDAVP also has been used to decrease the requirement for transfusions.

Acquired qualitative platelet abnormalities may be caused by certain drugs, uremia, cirrhosis, myeloproliferative disorders, and dysproteinemias. Aspirin irreversibly acetylates platelet cyclooxygenase-1, inhibiting thromboxane- and endoperoxide-mediated platelet activation for the life of the platelet. The effect of aspirin on the bleeding time is variable and may depend largely on the technique used to perform the test.[48,49] Nonsteroidal anti-inflammatory drugs (indomethacin, phenylbutazone, ibuprofen) reversibly inhibit cyclooxygenase. Numerous antibiotics, including some beta-lactams, cephalosporins, and nitrofurantoin, impair platelet aggregation and prolong the bleeding time. Mechanisms may include inhibition of agonist binding to the membrane receptor and inhibition of intracellular signal transduction. Platelet GP IIb-IIIa inhibitors (abciximab, eptifibatide, tirofiban) block the binding of fibrinogen to the GP IIb-IIIa receptor and effectively prevent platelet aggregation in a dose-dependent fashion. Correction of bleeding may be accomplished with platelet transfusions.

Uremia causes defective platelet adherence and aggregation, resulting in a prolonged bleeding time. Clinical manifestations may include petechiae, ecchymoses, and mucocutaneous bleeding. The pathophysiology remains unclear but may involve impaired thromboxane and calcium metabolism or defective platelet-subendothelial adhesion (via vWF). DDAVP has been shown to shorten bleeding times preoperatively in uremic patients.[50] IV DDAVP, 0.3 to 0.4 μg/kg over 15 to 30 minutes, shortens the bleeding time in most patients within 1 hour. Hemodialysis, peritoneal dialysis, and infusions of cryoprecipitate and conjugated estrogens have been used with some success.[51]

Coagulation factor deficiencies, DIC, dysfibrinogenemias, impaired thrombopoiesis, platelet sequestration, and impaired platelet aggregation all contribute to the hemostatic defects associated with liver failure. Therapy is nonspecific but may include DDAVP and platelet transfusions for severe thrombocytopenia.

COAGULATION DISORDERS

Congenital Disorders

Congenital disorders of coagulation usually involve a single factor. Preoperative transfusion of the appropriate factor is necessary and may be required during surgery and postoperatively as well. Deficiencies of factor XII, HMWK, and prekallikrein cause prolongation of the aPTT but do not cause significant bleeding diatheses. Deficiencies of the remaining factors may result in serious bleeding after surgery or trauma.

Hemophilia A (factor VIII deficiency) is the most common of the inherited coagulation defects, with a prevalence of 1 in 10,000 males. Hemophilia B (Christmas disease, factor IX deficiency) has a prevalence of approximately 1 in 50,000 males. Both are X-linked recessive disorders that are clinically indistinguishable. The severity of these disorders depends on the levels of factor VIII or IX that are present. Severely affected individuals (factor levels <1%) manifest spontaneous hemarthroses and deep tissue hematomas during infancy or early childhood. Patients with mild to moderate hemophilia (factor levels >5%) may develop hemorrhagic complications only after surgery or trauma.

Patients with hemophilia A who require major surgery should receive factor VIII replacement to achieve 100% of normal activity just before the procedure. For each unit per kilogram of body weight infused, the factor VIII level is increased by approximately 0.02 U/mL (normal activity is 1 U/mL).[52] Levels should be monitored postoperatively, and replacement therapy should be repeated every 12 hours to maintain at least 50% of normal activity until all wounds are healed.[53] Factor VIII levels may be restored using donor-directed cryoprecipitate, virus-inactivated factor VIII concentrate, or recombinant factor VIII. DDAVP (which increases factor VIII levels) and ε-aminocaproic acid may be used as adjunctive therapies in patients with mild hemophilia to reduce or avoid the need for replacement therapy during oral or minor surgical procedures.

Patients with hemophilia B should have at least 50% of normal activity before major surgery and for the first 7 to 10 days postoperatively. Factor IX may be replaced with prothrombin complex concentrates (containing factors II, VII, IX, and X), purified factor IX, or recombinant factor IX. Replacement therapy may be limited by several factors. Prothrombin complexes are associated with the development of arterial or venous thromboses in some patients. In addition, therapy with recombinant factor IX may not achieve as much activity as purified factor IX. This may be due to the need for post-translational modifications (γ-carboxylation) that are not present in recombinant factor IX. In addition, replacement therapy for hemophilia A and B is complicated by the development of inhibitors to factors VIII and IX in approximately 15% of patients. Alternative strategies include the use of high-dose factor VIII or recombinant factor VIIa and attempts to induce immune tolerance.

Rare coagulation factor deficiencies of factors II, V, VII, and X occur with a prevalence of 1:500,000 to 1:1,000,000. They are usually transmitted with an autosomal recessive pattern. The most severe complications occur with deficiencies of factors II and X.[54] In general, only low levels of factor activity (10% to 20% of normal) are required for normal hemostasis. Replacement therapy for factors II and X may be accomplished with fresh frozen plasma or factor concentrates. Factor IX concentrates contain significant amounts of factors II and X and may be used for their replacement. The short half-life of factor VII requires a more frequent replacement schedule using factor VII concentrates. Recombinant factor VIIa also may be used for factor VII deficiencies. Factor V deficiencies can be treated with fresh frozen plasma because factor V concentrates are not yet commercially available.

Abnormalities of fibrinogen and fibrinolysis are also heritable. Afibrinogenemia is a rare disorder transmitted as an autosomal recessive trait; hypofibrinogenemia may occur in heterozygous individuals. Clinical manifestations include gastrointestinal and mucous membrane bleeding, hemarthroses, intracranial hemorrhage, and recurrent fetal loss. The PT and aPTT, which are markedly prolonged, usually correct when mixed with normal plasma. Replacement therapy with cryoprecipitate is usually reserved for active bleeding, the perioperative period, and prophylaxis during pregnancy. The level of fibrinogen necessary for hemostasis ranges between 50 and 100 mg/dL. Each unit of cryoprecipitate usually increases the fibrinogen level by approximately 10 mg/dL.[55]

Dysfibrinogenemias are a heterogeneous group of disorders that may cause defective fibrin formation, polymerization, cross-linkage, or impaired fibrinolysis. Patients may manifest mild to moderate bleeding diatheses (30%) or recurrent thromboses (20%).[56] The PT and aPTT usually are prolonged.

Functional assays for fibrinogen are abnormal, whereas antigenic assays are normal. Cryoprecipitate is indicated for hemorrhage but contraindicated for acute thrombotic episodes.

Congenital hyperfibrinolytic states may result in delayed bleeding. The congenital hyperfibrinolytic states include heterozygous and homozygous α_2-antiplasmin deficiencies and functionally abnormal or deficient PAI-1.[57] The whole blood clot lysis time and the euglobulin clot lysis time are characteristically shortened. Antifibrinolytic agents (ε-aminocaproic acid or tranexamic acid) are recommended for the management of active bleeding.[58]

Acquired Disorders

Patients develop coagulation disorders because of deficiencies of coagulation proteins, synthesis of nonfunctioning factors, and consumption or inadequate replacement of coagulation proteins.

Hepatic insufficiency may cause decreased plasma levels of several coagulation factors (including factors II, V, VII, IX, X, XIII, and fibrinogen) because of a decreased synthetic capacity, defective post-translational modification (γ-carboxylation), and increased breakdown of activated factors (because of subclinical DIC). Thrombocytopenia also may occur because of increased splenic sequestration. However, levels of factor VIII and vWF may be elevated because they are synthesized in extrahepatic locations. Correction of the coagulation factor deficits and the thrombocytopenia is accomplished with fresh frozen plasma and platelet transfusions, respectively. Vitamin K administration alone does not completely reverse the coagulopathy.

Vitamin K deficiency may cause a bleeding diathesis as a result of the synthesis of nonfunctional forms of the vitamin K–dependent coagulation factors II, VII, IX, and X. Normal sources of vitamin K include dietary intake (leafy green vegetables, soybean oil) and vitamin K synthesis by normal intestinal flora. Vitamin K deficiency may be caused by poor dietary intake, decreased intestinal absorption of vitamin K, decreased production by the gut flora, and liver failure. This situation more commonly arises in patients receiving antibiotic bowel preparations or long-term parenteral nutrition (without vitamin K supplementation). Vitamin K deficiency also occurs in patients who have a prolonged recovery after intestinal surgery and in those with intrinsic bowel diseases (Crohn's disease, celiac sprue, ulcerative colitis), as well as in patients with obstructive jaundice. Vitamin K should be administered preoperatively to patients with hepatic insufficiency, obstructive jaundice, malabsorption states, or malnutrition. Patients with an intact enterohepatic circulation can receive vitamin K orally (2.5 to 5 mg), with normalization of the PT within 24 to 48 hours. Slow IV administration should be used in patients with biliary obstruction or malabsorption. Patients who require urgent correction of the PT should receive slow IV vitamin K and replacement therapy (fresh frozen plasma or prothrombin concentrates).

DIC is characterized by the systemic generation of fibrin, often resulting in the thrombosis of small and medium-size blood vessels. The consumption of clotting factors and platelets also results in impaired coagulation and hemorrhagic complications. DIC is mediated by several cytokines (including tumor necrosis factor-α and interleukin-6), which result in the systemic generation of TF, thrombin, and fibrin.[59] Fibrinolytic activity, which is initially increased via the release of t-PA, becomes depressed in response to elevated PAI-1.[59,60] DIC may develop in association with bacterial infections (gram-positive and gram-negative infections), trauma, malignancy, obstetric complications, hemolytic transfusion reactions, giant hemangiomas (Kasabach-Merritt syndrome), and aortic aneurysms. A compensated DIC (present in more than 80% of patients who undergo major surgery), in which coagulation factors and platelets are replaced as they are consumed, may be asymptomatic or may appear with ecchymoses and petechiae. Surgery, trauma, hypotension, or transfusion reactions may exacerbate the coagulopathy and hypofibrinolysis, leading to excessive bleeding and intravascular thrombosis.

A combination of laboratory tests may help confirm the clinical diagnosis of DIC. These include detection of thrombocytopenia or a rapidly decreasing platelet count, prolongation of the PT and aPTT, and the presence of fibrin degradation products (D-dimer assay, latex agglutination for fibrous degradation products). Extrinsic pathway coagulation proteins (factors II, V, VII, and X) and physiologic coagulation inhibitors (AT III, protein C) usually are depressed, whereas vWF and factor VIII levels may be increased.[61] The fibrinogen level is variably affected by DIC.

The first goal of management is elimination of the cause of DIC. When this is possible, the intravascular coagulation ceases with the return of normal hemostasis. In severe DIC, with ongoing blood loss, patients are best managed by replacement of deficient blood elements using fresh frozen plasma (up to 6 units per 24 hours) and platelets while the precipitating cause of DIC is eliminated.[59] Administration of AT III and protein C concentrates may retard the consumption of coagulation factors, although this remains to be proved. Some trials have demonstrated a benefit with the administration of heparin or low-molecular-weight heparin (LMWH).[62,63] Given that patients with DIC already have a coagulopathy, heparin should be used cautiously (lower IV dosages of 300 to 500 units/hour), with careful clinical observation and laboratory monitoring. Direct thrombin inhibitors (hirudin, recombinant TM), activated protein C, and extrinsic pathway inhibitors (recombinant TFPI) are under investigation as well.

Thrombosis

In 1856, Virchow suggested that thrombus formation was the result of an interaction among an injured surface, stasis, and the hypercoagulability of blood. One or more components of Virchow's triad can be invoked when determining the cause of an in vivo thrombosis. Hypofibrinolysis is the only major process not recognized by Virchow that contributes to intravascular thrombosis.

Most of the inherited thrombophilic conditions, with the exception of congenital hyperhomocysteinemia, are more closely associated with venous than with arterial thromboembolism. Acquired conditions such as the presence of antiphospholipid antibodies and heparin-associated antibodies have a well-recognized association with both arterial and venous thromboses. The more common inherited and acquired hypercoagulable states are discussed later, as are the indications for testing and the optimal timing for the performance of these assays. The more commonly used antithrombotic agents, as well as alternative agents, are discussed with regard to the management of established thromboses and prophylaxis against thromboembolism.

PROTHROMBOTIC CONDITIONS

Inherited Prothrombotic Conditions

Activated protein C (APC) resistance is most commonly caused by a mutation in the factor V gene, during which Arg506 is replaced with Gln (factor V Leiden), making activated factor V resistant to degradation by APC.[64] It is the most common inherited hypercoagulable condition, occurring in approximately 12% to 33% of patients with venous thromboembolism.[65-68] In contrast, it has a prevalence of 3% to 6% in control populations.[66-68] The white population is affected more commonly than black, Asian, or Native American populations. Individuals who are heterozygous for the factor V mutation have a 2.7- to 7-fold increased risk for venous thromboembolism, whereas homozygous patients may have an 80-fold increased risk.[67,68] A small percentage of patients with APC resistance do not have the Leiden mutation. Other factor V mutations (factor V Cambridge, factor V HR2 haplotype) also may cause APC resistance.[69,70]

Functional APC resistance can be detected by performing the aPTT in the presence and absence of purified APC. In general, an aPTT ratio (aPTT with APC/aPTT without APC) of less than 2.0 is considered a positive study (normal is 2.4 to 4.0). Numerous factors may affect the accuracy of the aPTT ratio, including protein C deficiency, the presence of anticoagulants, and antiphospholipid antibodies. Modifications to this functional assay have improved its sensitivity and specificity.[71] DNA testing using the polymerase chain reaction to amplify the factor V Leiden mutation has already become standardized. The optimal management of patients with APC resistance remains to be defined. APC-resistant individuals in high-risk situations (e.g., pregnancy, surgery) should receive thrombosis prophylaxis. Those patients with prior thrombotic episodes may benefit from long-term warfarin therapy. This is especially true for patients with multiple prior episodes, thromboses in unusual locations, and multiple inherited thrombophilic mutations.

Prothrombin 20210A is a mutation (G to A substitution) in the prothrombin gene at nucleotide 20210, resulting in increased levels of plasma prothrombin.[72] The prothrombin 20210A mutation is present in 18% of selected patients with strong family histories of venous thromboembolism, 6.2% of unselected patients with a first episode of thrombosis, and 2.3% of healthy controls. The prevalence is even higher in southern European whites.[73] A significant number of patients have more than one congenital thrombophilic condition, further increasing their risk for venous thromboembolism.[72,74]

AT III deficiency was the first reported congenital thrombophilic condition.[75] It is transmitted with an autosomal dominant pattern and has a prevalence of 1:5000 in the population.[76] AT III deficiency has been detected in approximately 1% of patients with venous thromboses, conferring a risk that may be as high as 50-fold greater than normal.[77,78] The lifetime risk for developing a thrombotic episode ranges between 17% and 50%.[79] Although thromboembolism may occur spontaneously, it is usually associated with a precipitating event such as surgery, trauma, or pregnancy.

Arterial thromboses, although less common than venous thromboses, also occur. AT III levels may be reduced to less than 80% of normal in other conditions, including hepatic insufficiency, DIC, acute venous thrombosis, sepsis, and nephrotic syndrome, and in patients receiving heparin or estrogen supplementation.

The mainstay of therapy in AT III–deficient patients with venous thromboembolism is still heparin anticoagulation, although supranormal dosages may be required.[80] AT III concentrates may be appropriate in patients who do not achieve adequate anticoagulation with heparin alone. The minimum level of AT III necessary to prevent thrombosis is unknown; however, it is suggested that levels be adjusted to greater than 80% of normal activity. Antithrombin may be replaced with AT III concentrate (1 U/kg increases the AT III activity by 1% to 2%) or fresh frozen plasma. Asymptomatic patients should receive thrombosis prophylaxis during high-risk situations such as prolonged immobilization, surgery, or pregnancy. However, long-term warfarin therapy is usually reserved for AT III–deficient patients who have experienced thrombotic events.

Protein C and protein S deficiencies account for a number of disorders. Congenital protein C deficiency may be transmitted as an autosomal dominant or recessive trait and has a prevalence of 1:200 to 1:500.[81,82] The incidence of thrombosis varies, depending on the population in question. Studies identifying protein C deficiency in healthy blood donors demonstrate a low prevalence of venous thrombosis, whereas studies that screen patients with venous thromboembolism find a higher prevalence of protein C deficiency compared with controls.[77,81-83] Overall, inherited protein C deficiency is associated with approximately a sevenfold increased risk for developing a first venous thromboembolic event.[83] Common sites for venous thromboses include the lower extremities, mesenteric veins, and cerebral venous sinuses. Functional and immunologic assays are available to establish the diagnosis of protein C deficiency. Normal adults have protein C antigen levels ranging from 70% to 140% of normal. Patients with antigen levels less than 55% are likely to have heterozygous protein C deficiency.

Approximately 60% of the total protein S circulates bound to C4b complement-binding protein.[84] Deficiency states may occur with decreased total protein S, decreased free protein S, and decreased functional protein S activity (with total and free protein S concentrations in the normal range). Histories of patients with congenital protein S deficiencies are very similar to those of patients with protein C deficiency, although arterial thromboses also have been described in patients with protein S deficiency. Protein S may be measured with functional assays, assessing the ability to catalyze the inhibition of factor Va by APC, or immunologic assays.

Both protein C and protein S are vitamin K–dependent proteins synthesized in the liver. Consequently, plasma levels may be decreased in patients with hepatic insufficiency. Acquired protein C and protein S deficiencies also may occur with warfarin administration, vitamin K deficiency (malabsorption, biliary obstruction), sepsis, DIC, and acute thromboses and in patients receiving some chemotherapeutic medications. Because C4b is also an acute-phase reactant, inflammatory conditions may increase C4b levels, causing a decrease in free protein S and an increased tendency toward thrombosis.[85]

Heparin is the first line of therapy in the management of acute thromboembolic episodes in patients with known protein C and S deficiencies. Because warfarin-induced skin necrosis is more likely to occur in patients with protein C deficiency, heparin therapy should overlap with the first 4 or 5 days of warfarin therapy, and large loading dosages of warfarin should be avoided. Longer-term treatment with warfarin is effective in the prevention of recurrent venous thromboembolic episodes in patients with protein C and protein S deficiencies. Fresh frozen plasma occasionally may be required to restore functional levels of protein C and protein S.

Abnormalities of fibrinogen and fibrinolysis include dysfibrinogenemias, which may impair any of the steps involved in the generation and cross-linkage of fibrin. They have been reported in association with bleeding diatheses (30%) and venous thromboembolism (20%). Therapeutic alternatives have been described earlier.

Elevated factor XI is a mild risk factor for the development of venous thrombosis.[86] Factor XI levels in the 90th percentile or greater confer a 2.2-fold relative risk for the development of venous thrombosis. Even lower factor XI levels demonstrate a linear dose-response relationship with thrombotic risk. The underlying cause for elevated factor XI levels remains to be determined.

Acquired Prothrombotic Conditions

Many clinical disorders predispose to thrombosis by activating the coagulation system or causing platelet aggregation. Soft tissue trauma, thermal injuries, and operative dissection all predispose to thrombosis through the release of tissue factor and activation of the extrinsic coagulation pathway.

Sepsis predisposes to thrombosis via multiple mechanisms. Gram-positive bacteria may directly cause platelet aggregation and subsequent thrombosis. Gram-negative bacterial endotoxin may stimulate platelet aggregation but may also, through interaction with leukocytes and endothelial cells, cause TF-like activation of the coagulation system. Endotoxin is known to be a major stimulus for the development of DIC.

As many as 11% of patients with malignancies have venous thromboembolic complications.[87] Pancreatic, prostate, gastrointestinal, and lung cancers have a particularly strong association with thrombosis. Conversely, patients with idiopathic venous thromboembolism are more likely to be diagnosed with cancer (up to 7.6%).[88] Aggressive screening for occult malignancies in patients with venous thromboembolism has not yet been shown to be cost-effective or to result in improved long-term survival.

Pregnancy is associated with a fourfold increased risk for venous thromboembolism.[78,89] The risk may be three to five times greater in the immediate postpartum period. Oral contraceptives also are associated with an approximately threefold increased risk, which is conferred immediately and is reversible.[90] Newer preparations with lower dosages of ethinylestradiol may lower the risk. Although the exact mechanism is unclear, these women demonstrate increased levels of thrombin and fibrinogen, with decreased levels of protein S and plasminogen activators.

Antiphospholipid antibodies, including lupus anticoagulants and anticardiolipin antibodies, are IgG, IgM, or IgA immunoglobulins, which are directed against phospholipid-binding proteins (prothrombin and β_2-GP I). These antibodies interfere with in vitro phospholipid-dependent clotting assays, such as aPTT, kaolin clotting time, and the dilute Russell's viper venom time. In vivo, antiphospholipid antibodies may promote thrombosis by interfering with the activation of protein C.[91] The presence of antiphospholipid antibodies is associated with a ninefold increased risk for venous thrombosis. Clinical manifestations of the antiphospholipid syndrome may include venous and arterial thromboses (coronary, cerebral) and recurrent fetal loss. Lupus anticoagulants are also associated with arterial thrombosis. As many as 50% of patients who are positive for lupus anticoagulants and undergo vascular surgical procedures develop thrombotic complications.[92] Patients with thrombotic episodes should receive heparin and warfarin anticoagulation. Long-term warfarin therapy (at higher intensity, international normalized ratio > 3) has been shown to reduce the recurrence of thrombosis.[93] Warfarin may be discontinued when the IgM or IgG immunoglobulins are no longer detectable.

Heparin-associated antibodies (HAAbs) and heparin-induced thrombocytopenia (HIT) are important considerations for patients receiving anticoagulation therapy. HAAbs IgG and IgM target the heparin–platelet factor 4 complex. These immune complexes bind to the Fcγ-RII platelet receptor, causing pathophysiologic platelet activation, aggregation, and thrombocytopenia. The incidence of HAAb formation varies widely, depending on the indications for heparin, the type of heparin used, and the tests used to detect HAAbs. LMWHs are associated with a significantly decreased incidence of HAAb formation and HIT.[94] Up to 20% of patients who undergo vascular surgical procedures develop HAAbs, which are associated with a greater than twofold increased risk for thrombotic complications.[95] The incidence of HIT ranges between 2% and 9%, depending on the type of heparin used, the route of administration, and the definition of thrombocytopenia used.[96,97] Most authors use a platelet count of less than 100,000/mm³ to define HIT-associated thrombocytopenia. However, thrombocytopenia is not a prerequisite for the development of thrombotic complications.

The diagnosis of HIT may be made according to the following criteria:

1. The development of thrombocytopenia or a significantly decreased platelet count while receiving heparin.
2. Resolution of thrombocytopenia after cessation of heparin.
3. Exclusion of other causes for thrombocytopenia.
4. A positive HAAb assay (two-point platelet aggregation assay, serotonin release assay, enzyme-linked immunosorbent assay).

Patients who develop HIT or thrombosis in the setting of a positive HAAb assay should discontinue heparin immediately. Most patients require continued anticoagulation with alternative agents such as recombinant hirudin and danaparoid. Long-term antithrombotic therapy with warfarin remains effective.

Hyperhomocysteinemia may be caused by inborn errors of metabolism (cystathionine β-synthase deficiency, methylene tetrahydrofolate reductase variant) or, more commonly, by acquired deficiencies in vitamin B_6, vitamin B_{12}, and folic acid. Elevated homocysteine is an independent risk factor for myocardial infarction, stroke, and peripheral arterial atherothrombosis.[98] It is also an independent risk factor for venous thrombosis, with an odds ratio of approximately 2 to 2.5.[99-101] The risk may be much higher in patients with combined hyperhomocysteinemia and other thrombophilic conditions.[102,103] Homocysteinemia may be detected using fasting plasma levels or after methionine loading (100 mg/kg). Elevated homocysteine levels may be effectively reduced with folate, vitamin B_6, and vitamin B_{12} supplementation.[104] Whether vitamin supplementation and correction of hyperhomocysteinemia are protective against venous thromboses remains to be determined.

Surgery and trauma are very strong risk factors for the development of venous thrombosis. Venous thromboembolism occurs in up to 25% of patients undergoing general surgical procedures without thrombosis prophylaxis. Orthopedic procedures (hip and knee replacement, hip fracture repair) are associated with an even greater risk for venous thromboembolism (45% to 61%). The incidence of venous thromboembolism in trauma patients depends on the severity of injury. Multisystem trauma is associated with a greater than 50% incidence.[105]

Myeloproliferative diseases (polycythemia vera, chronic myelogenous leukemia, myeloid metaplasia, essential thrombocytosis), hypergammaglobulinemia, and hyperfibrinogenemia may predispose to thrombosis by causing a hyperviscous state. At clinical presentation, patients manifest cerebral (arterial and venous), coronary, pulmonary, and peripheral arterial and venous thromboemboli. Hemolytic-uremic syndrome and thrombotic thrombocytopenic purpura cause microvascular thromboses and thrombocytopenia.

Indications and Timing for Thrombophilia Screening

Before 1993, inherited prothrombotic conditions were detected in less than 10% to 15% of patients with venous thromboembolism. Since the discovery of factor V Leiden and the prothrombin 20210A mutation, the number of patients with detectable thrombophilia has increased significantly. Patients who develop venous thromboembolism at a young age, patients with recurrent thrombosis, and those with a positive family history or thromboses in unusual locations are candidates for screening. Patients who develop warfarin-induced skin necrosis also have a significant chance of having protein C deficiency. Patients with suspected thrombophilia should be screened for APC resistance, prothrombin 20210A mutation, antiphospholipid antibodies, hyperhomocysteinemia, HAAbs, and deficiencies of AT III, protein C, and protein S. Patients with arterial thrombosis who require screening for thrombophilia should be tested for antiphospholipid antibodies (including lupus anticoagulants and anticardiolipin antibodies), HAAbs, and hyperhomocysteinemia.

Because acute thrombosis may be associated with transient depletion of AT III, protein C, and protein S, screening should not be performed during this period. Heparin and warfarin therapy also interfere with screening tests for APC resistance, whereas warfarin decreases functional and antigenic levels of protein C and protein S. Accurate screening is most easily accomplished approximately 2 to 3 weeks after the patient has discontinued warfarin therapy. If the risk of recurrent thromboembolism is deemed too great to discontinue warfarin, the patient may be converted to subcutaneous heparin or LMWH during this 2- to 3-week period. Protein C and S levels should not be affected by heparin administration. Testing for the presence of HAAbs should be performed after heparin has been discontinued, because false-negative results may be obtained for up to 72 hours.

MANAGEMENT OF ESTABLISHED THROMBOSIS

Unfractionated heparin, warfarin, and aspirin are the most commonly used antithrombotic agents. Several newer drugs have been made available by the Food and Drug Administration for limited indications. These include danaparoid, recombinant hirudin, ticlopidine, clopidogrel, and several GP IIb-IIIa receptor antagonists. Although numerous other agents are in development or in clinical trials (recombinant TFPI, GP Ib inhibitors, other factor IIA and Xa inhibitors), they are not discussed in this chapter.

Unfractionated and Low-Molecular-Weight Heparins

Unfractionated bovine lung and porcine intestinal heparin have been the mainstay of therapy for episodes of acute arterial (coronary, cerebral, peripheral arterial) and venous (deep venous) thromboses for the past several decades. Unfractionated heparins are glycosaminoglycans composed of repetitive disaccharide units (uronic acid and glucosamine) with molecular weights ranging from 4000 to 40,000 Da. LMWHs are derived from the enzymatic or alkaline degradation of unfractionated heparin purified from porcine intestinal mucosa. The average molecular weight of the various preparations ranges from 3000 to 6000 Da.[106]

Unfractionated heparin and LMWH bind to AT III via a specific pentasaccharide sequence that is present in only 30% of molecules. This exposes an active site for the neutralization of numerous activated coagulation factors. Factor Xa is inactivated via this mechanism. In contrast, factor IIa (thrombin) inactivation requires the formation of a ternary complex in which thrombin and AT III bind to heparin molecules with at least 18 to 20 saccharide units. Only 25% to 50% of LMWH molecules contain this critical length, thus reducing their anti-IIa activity while maintaining anti-Xa activity. Unfractionated heparin and LMWH also cause a two- to sixfold increase in TFPI, via release from the endothelial surface. TFPI forms a complex with factors VIIa, Xa, and TF, inhibiting the conversion of factor IX to IXa and factor X to Xa.

Unfractionated heparin binds to numerous plasma proteins (platelet factor 4, vitronectin, fibronectin), platelet glycoprotein receptors, and vascular endothelium. This may be responsible for the variable bioavailability and anticoagulant response. Heparin is cleared via the reticuloendothelial cells (saturable) and kidneys (nonsaturable), resulting in a dose-dependent half-life that ranges from 45 to 150 minutes. LMWHs demonstrate less binding to plasma proteins and endothelium, resulting in a greater bioavailability and a more predictable therapeutic response. As a result, weight-adjusted dosages may be administered without therapeutic monitoring. LMWHs are cleared primarily via the kidneys, with plasma half-lives that are twofold to fourfold longer than that of unfractionated heparin.

Unfractionated heparin may be administered as an IV bolus of 80 to 100 U/kg, followed by an infusion of 15 to 18 U/kg per hour. The aPTT is monitored every 6 hours until the dosage and therapeutic response have stabilized. The therapeutic range of 1.5 to 2.5 times control varies from one laboratory to another and should be standardized by protamine titration. Alternatively, direct heparin assays may be used for therapeutic monitoring of patients receiving parenteral unfractionated heparin infusions. Platelet counts should be monitored on a regular basis to allow the early detection of HIT. LMWHs are rapidly absorbed after subcutaneous injection. The dosage varies according to the commercial preparation used. Some preparations with longer half-lives require only once-daily dosing. LMWH is at least as effective as and is perhaps safer than unfractionated heparin for some treatment indications (e.g., venous thromboembolism).[107] The primary advantage of LMWH is the convenience of infrequent subcutaneous dosing without the need for therapeutic monitoring assays, which may allow outpatient treatment in some cases. The lower incidence of HIT is another advantage of LMWH. Disadvantages of LMWH include expense and the need for monitoring in certain patients, including those with advanced renal failure, morbid obesity, and pregnant patients.

Heparinoids

Danaparoid (Organon Inc., West Orange, N.J.) is the most widely tested heparinoid. It is composed of heparan sulfate (83%), dermatan sulfate (12%), and chondroitin sulfate (5%). Like LMWH, danaparoid is derived from animal intestinal mucosa. It has a mean molecular weight of 6000 Da. The heparan sulfate component of danaparoid binds to AT III via the specific pentasaccharide sequence, with preferential inactivation of factor Xa. The dermatan sulfate component of danaparoid also has slight anti-IXa activity through a mechanism involving heparin cofactor II. Rapid anticoagulation may be achieved with an IV bolus of 2250 to 2500 U (adjustment for weight may be required), followed by a continuous infusion with a stepwise decreasing rate (400 U/hour for 2 to 4 hours, then 300 U/hour for 2 to 4 hours, then 150 to 200 U/hour).[108]

Danaparoid has been used successfully as an alternative antithrombotic agent in patients with HIT. However, danaparoid carries a 10% to 20% rate of cross-reactivity with antiheparin antibodies.[108,109] Before using danaparoid in HIT-positive patients, cross-reactivity testing should be performed. Direct thrombin inhibitors have largely supplanted danaparoid in HIT.

Direct Thrombin Inhibitors

Indirect thrombin inhibitors (unfractionated heparin and LMWH) have a limited ability to neutralize fibrin-bound thrombin and are dependent on adequate levels of AT III. In contrast, direct thrombin inhibitors are capable of inhibiting thrombin on established thrombi and do not require the presence of antithrombin in order to exert anticoagulant effects.[110] Direct thombin inhibitors are based on the naturally occurring anticoagulant produced in the salivary gland of the medicinal leech (*Hirudo medicinalis*). Hirudin derivatives (lepirudin and desirudin) and bivalirudin (a hirudin analog) are bivalent direct thrombin inhibitors. Univalent direct thrombin inhibitors include argatroban and ximelagatran.

Hirudin is a 65–amino acid polypeptide derived from the salivary gland of the medicinal leech. It forms a stoichiometric complex with thrombin, blocking the catalytic site, substrate groove, and anion binding site, preventing the formation of fibrin and factors Va, VIIIa, and XIIIa.[111] Hirudin also inhibits thrombin-induced platelet activation and aggregation. Hirudin therapy is initiated with an IV bolus of 0.4 mg/kg, followed by a continuous infusion of 0.15 mg/kg per hour. Therapy may be monitored using the aPTT (therapeutic range, 1.5 to 2.5 times reference) or a more recently developed assay, the ecarin clotting time.[112] After an initial distribution phase, hirudin follows first-order elimination kinetics. It is excreted via the kidneys and has a half-life ranging from 1 to 2 hours. Patients with renal insufficiency or failure and patients weighing more than 110 kg require significant dosage adjustments. Hirudin may also be administered subcutaneously.

Hirudin is currently approved for the management of HIT complicated by thrombosis.[113] However, the rate of adverse events still remains significant (up to 30%), probably reflecting the severity of illness in HIT patients. Numerous clinical trials have compared hirudin with heparin in the treatment of patients undergoing coronary angioplasty and coronary thrombolysis and patients with unstable angina. Hirudin was associated with a decreased risk for ischemic events compared with heparin therapy. Some trials also demonstrated an increased incidence of major hemorrhage, although this complication usually occurred when hirudin was given in conjunction with thrombolytic agents.[114] As with heparin, hirudin has the potential to cause an immunologic reaction with resulting anaphylaxis. Approximately 40% of patients develop detectable antihirudin antibodies. Unlike heparin antibodies, however, these are not associated with the development of any resistance to therapy or with thromboembolic or bleeding complications.[115]

Bivalirudin is a synthetic 20–amino acid polypeptide analog of hirudin that reversibly binds to thrombin. When compared with hirudin, it has several advantages, including the ability to administer the medication intravenously or subcutaneously. Bivalirudin also has a shorter half-life, a nonrenal route of metabolism, and decreased immunogenicity. Currently it is approved in the United States as an anticoagulant in patients with unstable angina who undergo angioplasty.[116]

Argatroban is a synthetic univalent direct thrombin inhibitor that reversibly binds to thrombin.[110] It is approved for use as an anticoagulant for prophylaxis or treatment of thrombosis in patients with HIT. It is also approved as an anticoagulant in patients undergoing percutaneous coronary intervention who are at risk for HIT. Argatroban has a short half-life of 39 to 51 minutes and reaches a steady state with IV infusion at 1 to 3 hours. The level of anticoagulation may be monitored with the aPTT or activated clotting time. Argatroban is metabolized primarily by the liver and is excreted in the feces via biliary secretion. Therefore, doses should be decreased in patients with hepatic impairment.

Ximelagatran is a promising new oral anticoagulant that is in late-phase clinical trials.[117] It is already approved for use in the European Union for the prevention of venous thromboembolism in patients undergoing hip or knee replacement. It can be administered orally without food interactions and has predictable pharmacokinetics. There is also little variability in bioavailability between obese and nonobese individuals. Ximelagatran is a rapidly absorbed prodrug that is converted into its active form melagatran, a reversible direct thrombin inhibitor. Melagatran is excreted renally. Therefore, dosage adjustments should be made in patients with renal insufficiency. In clinical trials, ximelagatran has been as effective as LMWH or warfarin in preventing the progression of deep venous thrombosis.[118] Prolonged administration of ximelagatran is associated with elevated liver enzymes in approximately 2% to 6% of patients.[119] Rare cases of fulminant hepatic failure have been reported.

Warfarin

Coumarin derivatives, including warfarin, block the vitamin K–dependent γ-carboxylation of glutamine residues on factors II, VII, IX, and X and proteins C and S. This results in the production of vitamin K–dependent proteins, which have a decreased number of Gla residues and decreased enzymatic activity. A reduction in the number of Gla residues from the usual 10 to 13 to 6 decreases the coagulation factor biologic activity by more than 95%. An antithrombotic state depends on the replacement of functional coagulation factors present in the circulation with the altered coagulation proteins. Factor VII and protein C have the shortest half-lives—approximately 6 hours each. Factor II and factor X have longer half-lives of approximately 72 and 36 hours, respectively. Although warfarin may prolong the PT within 24 hours, owing to factor VII depletion, an antithrombotic state is usually not attained for 2 to 4 days.

Warfarin is rapidly absorbed and reaches a maximum plasma concentration within 2 to 12 hours. Ninety-seven percent of warfarin circulates bound to albumin, with the unbound portion responsible for the anticoagulant effect. The amount of warfarin required to cause a prolongation of the PT depends on the amount of dietary vitamin K, the age of the patient, and comorbid conditions (liver failure, obstructive jaundice, starvation). Numerous medications have been found to potentiate or interfere with the activity of warfarin (Table 5-2). Patients on long-term oral anticoagulation who begin or stop a medication that may interfere with or potentiate warfarin activity should be monitored with more frequent PT measurements.

Warfarin therapy is initiated by the oral intake of 5 to 7.5 mg once a day. Reduced dosages should be given to elderly patients and patients with liver disease or vitamin K deficiency as a result of malnutrition or long-term parenteral feeding. Because factor II and factor X depletion may not be effective for 2 to 4 days, heparin or an alternative agent should be administered during the first few days of warfarin therapy for patients who require immediate anticoagulation. The PT assay is most commonly used to monitor warfarin therapy. This test is sensitive to changes in activity of factors II, VII, IX, and X. The PT assay is performed by adding thromboplastin and calcium to citrated plasma. Thromboplastins vary according to their ability to activate the external coagulation cascade and are graded by the international sensitivity index (ISI). The international normalized ratio (INR) attempts to standardize PT assays, which use different thromboplastins, according to the following equation:

$$INR = [\text{patient PT (sec)}/\text{population PT (sec)}]^{ISI}$$

TABLE 5–2	Common Drug Interactions with Oral Anticoagulants	
Potentiate		**Antagonize**
Acetaminophen		Barbiturates
Anabolic steroids		Carbamazepine
Cephalosporins		Chlordiazepoxide
Chloral hydrate		Cholestyramine
Cimetidine		Dicloxacillin
Ciprofloxacin		Griseofulvin
Clofibrate		Nafcillin
Cotrimoxazole		Rifampin
Disulfiram		Sucralfate
Erythromycin		Vitamin K
Fluconazole		
Isoniazid		
Itraconazole		
Metronidazole		
Omeprazole		
Phenylbutazone		
Phenytoin		
Piroxicam		
Propafenone		
Propoxyphene		
Propranolol		
Quinidine		
Sulfinpyrazone		
Tamoxifen		
Tetracycline		

From Hirsh J, Dalen JE, Anderson DR, et al: Oral anticoagulants: Mechanism of action, clinical effectiveness, and optimal therapeutic range. Chest 114(Suppl):445S-469S, 1998; and Wells PS, Holbrook AM, Crowther NR, et al: The interaction of warfarin with drugs and food: A critical review of the literature. Ann Intern Med 121:676-683, 1994.

PT should be monitored on a daily basis for the first 4 to 5 days of warfarin therapy. The INR usually achieves the desired range during this period. A longer period of daily monitoring is required in patients resistant to warfarin. Once the therapeutic range is attained, the PT can be monitored two to three times a week and then, when stable, every 4 to 6 weeks. Many patients are receiving heparin at the time that warfarin is initiated. Concomitant administration of heparin prolongs the PT, owing to the inactivation of factors IIa, IXa, and Xa by AT III. It should be expected that the PT will decrease when heparin is discontinued. The effect of heparin on the PT can be reduced by removing the heparin from the test plasma or by stopping the heparin infusion 4 to 6 hours before obtaining blood for the PT.

The primary complication of warfarin therapy is hemorrhage, which occurs in 3% to 12% of patients.[120] Less common complications include alopecia, urticaria, dermatitis, fever, nausea, diarrhea, abdominal cramping, and hypersensitivity reactions. Dermal gangrene is a rare complication (0.01% to 0.1% of patients receiving warfarin) caused by the rapid depletion of protein C before depletion of factors II, IX, and X.[121] This risk increases to approximately 3% in patients with protein C deficiency.[122] Concomitant administration of unfractionated heparin or LMWH should decrease the risk of this complication.

THROMBOEMBOLISM PROPHYLAXIS

Venous Thromboembolism Prophylaxis

The annual incidence of deep venous thombosis (DVT) is between 69 and 139 cases per 100,000 people in the general population.[123] The prevalence of venous thomboembolism (VTE) in hospitalized patients is approximately 350 cases per 100,000 admissions and is a cause of death in approximately 250,000 people per year.[124,125] Pulmonary embolism contributes to or causes up to 12% of all deaths in hospitalized patients.[126] DVT poses an immediate threat to life because of the potential for pulmonary embolism and may also lead to long-term impairment due to resultant venous insufficiency. The 20-year cumulative incidence rate is 26.8% and 3.7% for the development of venous stasis changes and venous ulcers, respectively, after an episode of DVT.[127]

General risk factors for VTE include blood flow stasis, endothelial damage, and hypercoagulability. Relative hypercoagulability appears to be most important in the majority of cases of spontaneous DVT, whereas stasis and endothelial damage are more important in DVT following surgery or trauma. Specific risk factors include prior history of VTE, age, surgery, malignancy, obesity, trauma, varicosities, cardiac disease, hormones, immobilization or paralysis, pregnancy, venous catheterization, and hypercoagulable states.[88,89,126,128-135] In one population-based study, more than 90% of patients hospitalized for VTE had more than one risk factor.[126] In surgical patients, the risk of VTE is dependent on the type of operation and the presence of one or more risk factors.[136] Without prophylaxis, patients undergoing surgery for intraabdominal malignancy have a 25% incidence of DVT; orthopedic patients undergoing hip fracture surgery have a 40% to 50% incidence of DVT in the postoperative period. Those at highest risk are elderly patients undergoing major surgery or those with previous VTE, malignancy, or paralysis.

The incidence of venous thrombosis and pulmonary embolism may be reduced by limiting venous stasis, administering drugs to inhibit coagulation, or a combination of these approaches. Stasis is reduced by ambulation and pneumatic compression of the lower extremities.

Intermittent pneumatic compression (IPC) devices reduce lower extremity venous stasis, enhance fibrinolytic activity, and increase plasma levels of TFPI.[137] Elastic stockings also decrease stasis and increase venous flow velocities. Both devices appear to decrease the incidence of DVT in patients who undergo general, urologic, and gynecologic surgical procedures. The incidence of DVT in control patients ranges from 20% to 27%, whereas the use of IPC is associated with a DVT incidence of 10% to 18%.[129,138] IPC devices also decrease the incidence of DVT in patients undergoing hip or knee replacement. However, mechanical prophylaxis alone is probably not sufficient in patients undergoing total hip replacement and should be supplemented with either LMWH or adjusted-dose unfractionated heparin or warfarin.[105] IPC provides effective thrombosis prophylaxis in patients who undergo neurosurgical procedures (6% incidence with IPC, 23% in controls).[139] The effectiveness of IPC devices is limited by a lack of compliance among patients and nursing staff. Intermittent pneumatic foot compression devices may improve patient acceptance. However, these newer devices are less effective than other forms of DVT prophylaxis, especially in patients undergoing orthopedic procedures.[140]

Subcutaneous heparin is used to decrease the incidence of VTE. Unfractionated heparin (5000 U SC 2 hours preoperatively, followed by 5000 U every 8 to 12 hours postoperatively) decreases the overall incidence of venous thrombosis to approximately 8%.[105] The incidence of pulmonary embolism is reduced as well. This regimen is probably adequate in moderate- and high-risk general surgical patients. Two large meta-analyses have demonstrated that LMWH confers no additional protection in this population and may be associated with an increased risk of hemorrhagic complications.[141,142]

However, fixed low-dose unfractionated heparin prophylaxis is not as effective in patients with hip fractures or in those undergoing total hip or knee replacement. Orthopedic and very high-risk general surgical patients (those with additional risk factors) should receive more effective DVT prophylaxis (LMWH, adjusted-dose warfarin, adjusted-dose unfractionated heparin, or combination prophylaxis with IPC). The aPTT does not require monitoring in patients receiving fixed-dose unfractionated heparin or LMWH prophylaxis. Platelet counts should be monitored for the detection of HIT.

LMWH produces fewer thromboembolic complications than unfractionated heparin does. In a large randomized, double-blinded study comparing low-dose heparin (5000 U SC twice a day) and LMWH (enoxaparin 30 mg SC twice a day) in trauma patients without intracranial hemorrhage, there was a 30% risk reduction ($P = 0.01$) of DVT in patients given LMWH.[143] The overall major bleeding complication rate was 2%, with no statistical difference between the two groups. Early use of LMWH for VTE prophylaxis is contraindicated in patients with intracranial bleeding, spinal hematoma, ongoing and uncontrolled hemorrhage, or uncorrected coagulopathy. Patients who undergo major orthopedic procedures without DVT prophylaxis are at high risk for thromboembolic complications (45% to 61%). Depending on the preparation, LMWH decreases the incidence significantly (15% to 31%) compared with fixed-dose unfractionated heparin (27% to 42%).[105,144] Preoperative initiation of LMWH (vs. beginning postoperatively) may decrease the overall incidence of DVT in patients undergoing hip replacement (10% preoperative vs. 15.3% postoperative) without increasing the incidence of hemorrhage.[145] There is also evidence that longer durations of prophylaxis are more effective. Several randomized trials have found a significantly lower rate of thrombosis with 21 to 35 days of LMWH administration.[146-148] The additional use of IPC devices may decrease the incidence even further.

Numerous randomized trials have compared various LMWH preparations (enoxaparin, certoparin, dalteparin, nadroparin, parnaparin, reviparin, tinzaparin) against unfractionated heparin as DVT prophylaxis in general surgical patients. Only 4 of 29 trials identified a significant improvement with LMWH.[149] Although the dosage regimens varied widely among trials, there was a tendency toward superior prophylaxis with LMWH when higher dosages were used. Very high-risk patients who undergo general surgical procedures (multiple risk factors, malignancy, thrombophilia) may benefit most from LMWH prophylaxis. The optimal timing for the first prophylactic dose of LMWH remains in question. General surgical patients who receive the first dose before surgery do not appear to experience any additional hemorrhagic complications.[149]

Fondaparinux is a chemically synthesized agent that binds and activates antithrombin, which then selectively inhibits factor Xa. It does not act against thrombin (factor IIa). Because it is chemically synthesized, fondaparinux does not contain any animal products. It is specific to antithrombin and does not bind to platelets, therefore minimizing the risk of HIT. The results of a randomized, double-blinded trial comparing fondaparinux and LMWH for the prevention of VTE after elective hip replacement surgery were recently published.[150] There was no statistical difference between the two groups in the incidence of VTE. The incidence of VTE was 6% in the fondaparinux group and 8% in the enoxaparin group. There was also no difference in the incidence of major bleeding complications, with 20 events in the fondaparinux group and 11 events in the LMWH group. Fondaparinux is commercially available but has not been evaluated as prophylactic therapy for VTE in patients other than those undergoing surgery of the hip and knee.

Warfarin has been established in several studies as efficacious prophylaxis against VTE. Sevitt and Gallagher found that the incidence of clinical venous thrombosis in patients with hip fractures decreased from 28.7% in the control group to 2.7% in the group treated with oral anticoagulation. At autopsy, the incidence of thrombosis in the two groups was 83% and 14%, respectively.[151] In other studies, oral anticoagulants with an INR range of 2.0 to 3.0 were effective in preventing venous thrombosis in patients undergoing orthopedic and gynecologic surgery.[152,153] Very high-risk patients, such as those undergoing major orthopedic procedures, should receive either LMWH or adjusted-dose warfarin. LMWH may be more effective than warfarin, but the difference is probably small. If warfarin is selected, it should be started preoperatively or immediately after surgery. The dosage should be adjusted to achieve a target INR between 2.0 and 3.0.[105] With warfarin, the duration of prophylaxis can easily be extended in patients who continue to have risk factors for VTE (immobility, malignancy, a history of previous venous thrombosis).

Current recommendations for VTE prophylaxis in surgical patients vary according to the type of surgical procedure planned and underlying risk factors in a given patient. Table 5-3 summarizes current recommendations from the American College of Chest Physicians' 2004 consensus statement on prophylaxis for surgical patients.[154]

Arterial Thromboembolism Prophylaxis

Arterial thrombosis occurs in regions with disturbed flow or disrupted endothelial coverage (as with plaque rupture or endarterectomy). Subendothelial collagen and vWF initiate platelet adhesion and activation, whereas TF activates the coagulation cascade, leading to the generation of thrombin and fibrin. Arterial thrombi contain relatively higher concentrations of platelets. As a result, most long-term arterial antithrombotic regimens focus on the inhibition of platelet function.

Aspirin acetylates platelet cyclooxygenase-1 (prostaglandin H synthase-1), blocking the conversion of arachidonic acid to the prostaglandin endoperoxides PGH_2 and PGG_2. This effectively inhibits the synthesis of TXA_2 for the life span of the platelet. Aspirin also inhibits prostacyclin

TABLE 5–3	Recommendation for Venous Thromboembolism Prophylaxis in Surgical Patients
Indication	**Prophylaxis Method**
Low-risk general surgery (minor surgery, age < 40 yr, no risk factors)	Early ambulation
Moderate-risk general surgery (minor surgery with risk factors; major surgery, age > 40 yr, no risk factors)	LDH, LMWH, ES, or IPC
High-risk general surgery (minor surgery with risk factors, age > 60 yr; major surgery, age > 40 yr or additional risk factors)	LDH, LMWH, or IPC
Very high risk general surgery (multiple risk factors) Elective hip replacement Elective knee replacement Hip fracture surgery Major trauma Acute spinal cord injury	LMWH, fondaparinux, warfarin (INR 2-3), or IPC/ES + LDH/LMWH

ES, elastic compression stockings; INR, international normalized ratio; IPC, intermittent pneumatic compression; LDH, low-dose heparin; LMWH, low-molecular-weight heparin.

synthesis by endothelial cells. However, endothelial cells have nuclei and can synthesize new prostacyclin synthetase, reversing the effects of aspirin. Noncoated aspirin is rapidly disintegrated and absorbed in the stomach. Enteric-coated aspirin dissolves in the more neutral to alkaline pH within the duodenum. Enteric coating does not significantly delay the bioavailability compared with noncoated aspirin.

Aspirin is the most widely employed antithrombotic agent, and there is considerable evidence supporting its efficacy in reducing the relative risk of serious vascular events (nonfatal myocardial infarction, nonfatal stroke, vascular death) in patients at high risk of these complications. The Antithrombotic Trialists' Collaboration (ATTC) reviewed 287 studies encompassing more than 135,000 patients and noted absolute reductions in serious vascular events in patients with recent or remote myocardial infarction, stroke or transient ischemic attack, stable angina, peripheral arterial disease, and atrial fibrillation.[155] Nonfatal myocardial infarction risk was reduced by 33%, nonfatal stroke was reduced by 25%, and vascular death was reduced by 16%. Aspirin is also efficacious in the primary prevention of stroke and myocardial infarction in patients with known risk factors for these conditions; however, the risk of hemorrhagic complications outweighs the benefits of aspirin therapy in patients at low risk for cardiovascular events.[107,114,156] In general, lower doses of aspirin (75 to 150 mg/day) are effective. The ATTC trialists concluded that aspirin 75 to 150 mg/day is recommended routinely for all patients without contraindications who are at high or intermediate risk of vascular events (>2% per year risk), whether or not they have had a prior vascular event. Aspirin is also efficacious in maintaining vascular graft patency in patients following lower extremity revascularization. The Seventh Antithrombotic Consensus Conference, the American Heart Association, and the American College of Cardiology recommend aspirin 80 to 325 mg/day for prosthetic or saphenous vein peripheral bypass grafts and after carotid endarterectomy.[154,157]

Ticlopidine and clopidogrel are thienopyridine derivatives that irreversibly inhibit ADP-mediated platelet activation. Intact ticlopidine and clopidogrel have no effect on platelets in vitro, suggesting that their metabolites may be the more potent platelet inhibitors. Both are rapidly absorbed after oral administration and are highly bound to plasma proteins (albumin and lipoproteins). Ticlopidine may alter platelet function within 24 to 48 hours, but maximum inhibition is not achieved for 8 to 11 days. Clopidogrel induces a dose-dependent inhibition of platelet aggregation that is more rapid (within 2 hours).

Ticlopidine significantly improves the patency of femoropopliteal and femorotibial saphenous vein grafts (66% vs. 51% at 2 years) compared with placebo.[158] Compared with aspirin, ticlopidine also is associated with a decreased risk of stroke (10% vs. 13%).[159] Other studies have demonstrated a decreased risk of myocardial infarction in patients with unstable angina and improved walking distance in patients with claudication.[160,161] However, no studies have demonstrated that ticlopidine is superior to aspirin in improving lower extremity vascular graft patency. In addition, widespread use of ticlopidine is limited by the potentially severe side effects of pancytopenia and neutropenia.[162]

Clopidogrel has been advocated as an antiplatelet agent with an efficacy superior to that of aspirin. The Clopidogrel versus Aspirin in Patients at Risk of Ischaemic Events (CAPRIE) study evaluated more than 19,000 patients with a history of recent ischemic stroke, recent myocardial infarction, or symptomatic atherosclerotic peripheral vascular disease.[163] Clopidogrel was associated with a relative risk reduction of 8.7% for future ischemic events, representing an absolute reduction of only 0.5% (5.32% with clopidogrel, 5.83% with aspirin). However, subgroup analyses demonstrated that patients with peripheral vascular disease received the greatest degree of risk reduction.

Clopidogrel may be more beneficial as a combination therapy agent, because aspirin and clopidogrel inhibit platelet function via different signal transduction pathways (TXA_2 and ADP inhibition). Some evidence for this comes from the more recent Clopidogrel in Unstable Angina to Prevent Recurrent Events (CURE) trial, involving more than 12,500 patients.[164] Patients receiving clopidogrel and aspirin had a decreased incidence of cardiovascular death, myocardial infarction, or stroke when compared with those receiving aspirin alone (9.3% vs. 11.4%, representing a 20% relative risk reduction). The incidence of neutropenia and pancytopenia with clopidogrel is similar to the incidence with aspirin or placebo.

Glycoprotein IIb-IIIa inhibitors have been evaluated for stroke prevention in clinical trials. Fibrinogen binds to the platelet GP IIb-IIIa receptor via the amino acid sequence Arg-Gly-Asp (RGD), representing the final common pathway for platelet aggregation regardless of the platelet agonist. The first GP IIb-IIIa inhibitor to be developed was c7E3 (abciximab), the antigen-binding fragment (Fab) of a monoclonal anti-GP IIb-IIIa antibody. Subsequently, naturally occurring RGD peptides (trigramin, bitistatin) have been isolated from the venom of several species of vipers. Synthetic RGD peptides (eptifibatide, tirofiban, lamifiban), as well as more potent KGD analogs, have been manufactured and undergone clinical trials.[17] Most trials involved patients who had coronary angioplasty and those with unstable angina or myocardial infarction.[165-167] The primary indication for the use of GP IIb-IIIa receptor antagonists is for acute coronary syndromes. GP IIb-IIIa inhibitors have no role in the long-term prevention of stroke or complications related to peripheral vascular disease.

The major risk of using GP IIb-IIIa receptor antagonists is bleeding. Abciximab has a very short half-life (10 to 30 minutes) caused by rapid binding to the platelet GP IIb-IIIa receptor. Significant platelet function inhibition continues for up to 48 hours after infusions are discontinued.[166] Synthetic RGD peptides (eptifibatide, tirofiban) demonstrate more reversible platelet inhibition. The half-lives of these agents range from 2 to 2.5 hours, with most of the elimination occurring via the kidneys. Platelet function generally returns to near normal within 4 to 8 hours.

Warfarin has an established role in the prevention of thromboembolism in selected patients with atrial fibrillation and prosthetic heart valves. Other possible indications for long-term warfarin therapy include the prevention of myocardial ischemia and the prevention of systemic embolism after acute myocardial infarction.[168]

Several studies also indicate that warfarin may improve the patency of lower extremity bypass grafts. In a randomized trial involving 130 patients who underwent femoropopliteal vein bypass surgery, Kretschmer and coworkers found improved patency, limb salvage, and overall survival in patients receiving phenprocoumon (a coumarin derivative).[169,170] Flinn and colleagues also found that warfarin improved patency in patients with infrageniculate prosthetic grafts.[171] More recent studies involving patients at high risk for failure (suboptimal vein, poor outflow, redo procedures) have confirmed an improved patency with warfarin plus aspirin compared with aspirin alone.[172] Long-term warfarin therapy is a reasonable option for most patients with prosthetic infrainguinal or axillofemoral bypass grafts, suboptimal venous conduit, or poor outflow tracts (e.g., isolated popliteal arteries). Patients who are treated with warfarin should receive overlapping unfractionated heparin, LMWH, or IV heparin until the therapeutic INR is achieved (target INR, 2.0 to 3.0).

KEY REFERENCES

Almeida JI, Coats R, Liem TK, Silver D: Reduced morbidity and mortality of the heparin-induced thrombocytopenia syndrome. J Vasc Surg 27:309-314, 1998.

Antiplatelet Trialists' Collaboration: Collaborative overview of randomised trials of antiplatelet therapy. I. Prevention of death, myocardial infarction, and stroke by prolonged antiplatelet therapy in various categories of patients. BMJ 308:81-106, 1994.

Eriksson H, Wahlander K, Gustafsson D, et al: A randomized, controlled, dose-guiding study of the oral direct thrombin inhibitor ximelagatran compared with standard therapy for the treatment of acute deep vein thrombosis: THRIVE I. J Thromb Haemost 1:41-47, 2003.

Hiatt WR: Preventing atherothrombotic events in peripheral arterial disease: The use of antiplatelet therapy. J Intern Med 251:193-206, 2002.

Hirsh J, Dalen J, Guyatt G: The sixth (2000) ACCP guidelines for antithrombotic therapy for prevention and treatment of thrombosis: American College of Chest Physicians. Chest 119:1S-370S, 2001.

Lowe GDO: State of the art 2003: XIX Congress of the International Society on Thrombosis and Haemostasis. J Thromb Haemost 1, 2003.

Manco-Johnson MJ, Riske B, Kasper CK: Advances in care of children with hemophilia. Semin Thromb Hemost 29:585-594, 2003.

Midathada MV, Mehta P, Waner M, Fink L: Recombinant factor VIIa in the treatment of bleeding. Am J Clin Pathol 121:124-137, 2004.

Ridker PM, Goldhaber SZ, Danielson E, et al: Long-term, low-intensity warfarin therapy for the prevention of recurrent venous thromboembolism. N Engl J Med 348:1425-1434, 2003.

Warkentin TE: Management of heparin-induced thrombocytopenia: A critical comparison of lepirudin and argatroban. Thromb Res 110:73-82, 2003.

REFERENCES

1. Engelberg H: Update on the relationship of heparin to atherosclerosis and its thrombotic complications. Semin Thromb Hemost 14(Suppl):88-105, 1988.
2. Ishii H, Salem HH, Bell CE, et al: Thrombomodulin, an endothelial anticoagulant protein, is absent from the human brain. Blood 67:362-365, 1986.
3. Esmon CT, Owen WG: Identification of an endothelial cell cofactor for thrombin-catalyzed activation of protein C. Proc Natl Acad Sci U S A 78:2249-2252, 1981.
4. Naworth PP, Brett J, Steinberg S: Endothelium and protein S: Synthesis, release and regulation of anticoagulant activity [abstract]. Thromb Haemost 58:49, 1987.
5. Stern D, Brett J, Harris K, et al: Participation of endothelial cells in the protein C-protein S anticoagulant pathway: The synthesis and release of protein S. J Cell Biol 102:1971-1978, 1986.
6. Werling RW, Zacharski LR, Kisiel W, et al: Distribution of tissue factor pathway inhibitor in normal and malignant human tissues. Thromb Haemost 69:366-369, 1993.
7. Osterud B, Bajaj MS, Bajaj SP: Sites of tissue factor pathway inhibitor (TFPI) and tissue factor expression under physiologic and pathologic conditions: On behalf of the Subcommittee on Tissue Factor Pathway Inhibitor (TFPI) of the Scientific and Standardization Committee of the ISTH. Thromb Haemost 73:873-875, 1995.
8. Rodgers GM, Shuman MA: Enhancement of prothrombin activation on platelets by endothelial cells and mechanism of activation of factor V. Thromb Res 45:145-152, 1987.
9. Tracy PB, Eide LL, Mann KG: Human prothrombinase complex assembly and function on isolated peripheral blood cell populations. J Biol Chem 260:2119-2124, 1985.
10. Bennett JS: The molecular biology of platelet membrane proteins. Semin Hematol 27:186-204, 1990.
11. Kansas GS: Selectins and their ligands: Current concepts and controversies. Blood 88:3259-3287, 1996.
12. Diacovo TG, deFougerolles AR, Bainton DF, et al: A functional integrin ligand on the surface of platelets: Intercellular adhesion molecule-2. J Clin Invest 94:1243-1251, 1994.
13. Silver MJ, Smith JB, Ingerman C, et al: Arachidonic acid-induced human platelet aggregation and prostaglandin formation. Prostaglandins 4:863-875, 1973.
14. Nachman RL, Leung LL: Complex formation of platelet membrane glycoproteins IIb and IIIa with fibrinogen. J Clin Invest 69:263-269, 1982.
15. Ito MK, Smith AR, Lee ML: Ticlopidine: A new platelet aggregation inhibitor. Clin Pharm 11:603-617, 1992.
16. Herbert JM FD, Vallee E: Clopidogrel, a novel antiplatelet and antithrombotic agent. Cardiovasc Drug Rev 11:180-198, 1993.
17. Lefkovits J, Plow EF, Topol EJ: Platelet glycoprotein IIb/IIIa receptors in cardiovascular medicine. N Engl J Med 332:1553-1559, 1995.
18. Marder VJ, Mannucci PM, Firkin BG, et al: Standard nomenclature for factor VIII and von Willebrand factor: A recommendation by the International Committee on Thrombosis and Haemostasis. Thromb Haemost 54:871-872, 1985.

19. Morrissey JH, Macik BG, Neuenschwander PF, et al: Quantitation of activated factor VII levels in plasma using a tissue factor mutant selectively deficient in promoting factor VII activation. Blood 81:734-744, 1993.
20. Mann KG: Biochemistry and physiology of blood coagulation. Thromb Haemost 82:165-174, 1999.
21. Osterud B, Rapaport SI: Activation of factor IX by the reaction product of tissue factor and factor VII: Additional pathway for initiating blood coagulation. Proc Natl Acad Sci U S A 74:5260-5264, 1977.
22. Janus TJ, Lewis SD, Lorand L, et al: Promotion of thrombin-catalyzed activation of factor XIII by fibrinogen. Biochemistry 22:6269-6272, 1983.
23. Bajaj MS, Kuppuswamy MN, Saito H, et al: Cultured normal human hepatocytes do not synthesize lipoprotein-associated coagulation inhibitor: Evidence that endothelium is the principal site of its synthesis. Proc Natl Acad Sci U S A 87:8869-8873, 1990.
24. Novotny WF, Girard TJ, Miletich JP, et al: Platelets secrete a coagulation inhibitor functionally and antigenically similar to the lipoprotein associated coagulation inhibitor. Blood 72:2020-2025, 1988.
25. Rapaport SI: The extrinsic pathway inhibitor: A regulator of tissue factor-dependent blood coagulation. Thromb Haemost 66:6-15, 1991.
26. Esmon CT: The regulation of natural anticoagulant pathways. Science 235:1348-1352, 1987.
27. Esmon CT: The roles of protein C and thrombomodulin in the regulation of blood coagulation. J Biol Chem 264:4743-4746, 1989.
28. Nesheim M, Wang W, Boffa M, et al: Thrombin, thrombomodulin and TAFI in the molecular link between coagulation and fibrinolysis. Thromb Haemost 78:386-391, 1997.
29. Fair DS, Marlar RA, Levin EG: Human endothelial cells synthesize protein S. Blood 67:1168-1171, 1986.
30. Schwarz HP, Heeb MJ, Wencel-Drake JD, et al: Identification and quantitation of protein S in human platelets. Blood 66:1452-1455, 1985.
31. Hoylaerts M, Rijken DC, Lijnen HR, et al: Kinetics of the activation of plasminogen by human tissue plasminogen activator: Role of fibrin. J Biol Chem 257:2912-2919, 1982.
32. Horrevoets AJ, Pannekoek H, Nesheim ME: A steady-state template model that describes the kinetics of fibrin-stimulated [Glu1] and [Lys78] plasminogen activation by native tissue-type plasminogen activator and variants that lack either the finger or kringle-2 domain. J Biol Chem 272:2183-2191, 1997.
33. Stewart RJ, Fredenburgh JC, Weitz JI: Characterization of the interactions of plasminogen and tissue and vampire bat plasminogen activators with fibrinogen, fibrin, and the complex of D-dimer noncovalently linked to fragment E. J Biol Chem 273:18292-18299, 1998.
34. Olexa SA, Budzynski AZ: Binding phenomena of isolated unique plasmic degradation products of human cross-linked fibrin. J Biol Chem 254:4925-4932, 1979.
35. Gurewich V, Pannell R, Louie S, et al: Effective and fibrin-specific clot lysis by a zymogen precursor form of urokinase (pro-urokinase): A study in vitro and in two animal species. J Clin Invest 73:1731-1739, 1984.
36. Weitz JI, Stewart RJ, Fredenburgh JC: Mechanism of action of plasminogen activators. Thromb Haemost 82:974-982, 1999.
37. Collen D: The plasminogen (fibrinolytic) system. Thromb Haemost 82:259-270, 1999.
38. Moake JL: Studies on the pathophysiology of thrombotic thrombocytopenic purpura. Semin Hematol 34:83-89, 1997.
39. Bell WR, Braine HG, Ness PM, et al: Improved survival in thrombotic thrombocytopenic purpura–hemolytic uremic syndrome: Clinical experience in 108 patients. N Engl J Med 325:398-403, 1991.
40. Kwaan HC, Soff GA: Management of thrombotic thrombocytopenic purpura and hemolytic uremic syndrome. Semin Hematol 34:159-166, 1997.
41. Taylor FB, Coller BS, Chang AC, et al: 7E3 F(ab')2, a monoclonal antibody to the platelet GPIIb/IIIa receptor, protects against microangiopathic hemolytic anemia and microvascular thrombotic renal failure in baboons treated with C4b binding protein and a sublethal infusion of Escherichia coli. Blood 89:4078-4084, 1997.
42. Murphy S: Platelet transfusion therapy. In Loscalzo J, Shafer AI (eds): Thrombosis and Hemorrhage, 2nd ed. Baltimore, Williams & Wilkins, 1998, pp 1119-1134.
43. Reed RL 2nd, Ciavarella D, Heimbach DM, et al: Prophylactic platelet administration during massive transfusion: A prospective, randomized, double-blind clinical study. Ann Surg 203:40-48, 1986.
44. Sadler JE: A revised classification of von Willebrand disease: For the Subcommittee on von Willebrand Factor of the Scientific and Standardization Committee of the International Society on Thrombosis and Haemostasis. Thromb Haemost 71:520-525, 1994.
45. Logan LJ: Treatment of von Willebrand's disease. Hematol Oncol Clin North Am 6:1079-1094, 1992.
46. Foster PA: A perspective on the use of FVIII concentrates and cryoprecipitate prophylactically in surgery or therapeutically in severe bleeds in patients with von Willebrand disease unresponsive to DDAVP: Results of an international survey. On behalf of the Subcommittee on von Willebrand Factor of the Scientific and Standardization Committee of the ISTH. Thromb Haemost 74:1370-1378, 1995.
47. Nurden AT: Inherited abnormalities of platelets. Thromb Haemost 82:468-480, 1999.
48. Rodgers RP, Levin J: A critical reappraisal of the bleeding time. Semin Thromb Hemost 16:1-20, 1990.
49. Mielke CH Jr: Influence of aspirin on platelets and the bleeding time. Am J Med 74:72-78, 1983.
50. Mannucci PM: Desmopressin (DDAVP) for treatment of disorders of hemostasis. Prog Hemost Thromb 8:19-45, 1986.
51. Shafer AI: Acquired disorders of platelet function. In Loscalzo J, Shafer AI (eds): Thrombosis and Hemorrhage, 2nd ed. Baltimore, Williams & Wilkins, 1998, pp 707-725.
52. Forbes CD: Clinical aspects of the genetic disorders of coagulation. In Ratnoff OD, Forbes CD (eds): Disorders of Hemostasis, 3rd ed. Philadelphia, WB Saunders, 1996, pp 138-185.
53. DiMichele DM, Green D: Hemophilia-factor VIII deficiency. In Loscalzo J, Shafer AI (eds): Thrombosis and Hemorrhage, 2nd ed. Baltimore, Williams & Wilkins, 1998, pp 757-772.
54. Peyvandi F, Mannucci PM: Rare coagulation disorders. Thromb Haemost 82:1207-1214, 1999.
55. Roberts HR, Bingham MD: Other coagulation factor deficiencies. In Loscalzo J, Shafer AI (eds): Thrombosis and Hemorrhage, 2nd ed. Baltimore, Williams & Wilkins, 1998, pp 773-802.
56. Ebert RF: Dysfibrinogenemia: An overview of the field. Thromb Haemost 65:1317, 1991.
57. Schleef RR, Higgins DL, Pillemer E, et al: Bleeding diathesis due to decreased functional activity of type 1 plasminogen activator inhibitor. J Clin Invest 83:1747-1752, 1989.
58. Stump DC, Taylor FB Jr, Nesheim ME, et al: Pathologic fibrinolysis as a cause of clinical bleeding. Semin Thromb Hemost 16:260-273, 1990.
59. Levi M, Ten Cate H: Disseminated intravascular coagulation. N Engl J Med 341:586-592, 1999.
60. Biemond BJ, Levi M, Ten Cate H, et al: Plasminogen activator and plasminogen activator inhibitor I release during experimental endotoxaemia in chimpanzees: Effect of interventions in the cytokine and coagulation cascades. Clin Sci (Lond) 88:587-594, 1995.
61. Spero JA, Lewis JH, Hasiba U: Disseminated intravascular coagulation: Findings in 346 patients. Thromb Haemost 43:28-33, 1980.
62. Feinstein DI: Treatment of disseminated intravascular coagulation. Semin Thromb Hemost 14:351-362, 1988.
63. Sakuragawa N, Hasegawa H, Maki M, et al: Clinical evaluation of low-molecular-weight heparin (FR-860) on disseminated intravascular coagulation (DIC)—a multicenter co-operative double-blind trial in comparison with heparin. Thromb Res 72:475-500, 1993.
64. Bertina RM, Koeleman BP, Koster T, et al: Mutation in blood coagulation factor V associated with resistance to activated protein C. Nature 369:64-67, 1994.
65. Svensson PJ, Dahlback B: Resistance to activated protein C as a basis for venous thrombosis. N Engl J Med 330:517-522, 1994.
66. Koster T, Rosendaal FR, de Ronde H, et al: Venous thrombosis due to poor anticoagulant response to activated protein C: Leiden Thrombophilia Study. Lancet 342:1503-1506, 1993.
67. Rosendaal FR, Koster T, Vandenbroucke JP, et al: High risk of thrombosis in patients homozygous for factor V Leiden (activated protein C resistance). Blood 85:1504-1508, 1995.
68. Ridker PM, Hennekens CH, Lindpaintner K, et al: Mutation in the gene coding for coagulation factor V and the risk of myocardial infarction, stroke, and venous thrombosis in apparently healthy men. N Engl J Med 332:912-917, 1995.
69. Williamson D, Brown K, Luddington R, et al: Factor V Cambridge: A new mutation (Arg306→Thr) associated with resistance to activated protein C. Blood 91:1140-1144, 1998.
70. Bernardi F, Faioni EM, Castoldi E, et al: A factor V genetic component differing from factor V R506Q contributes to the activated protein C resistance phenotype. Blood 90:1552-1557, 1997.
71. Le DT, Griffin JH, Greengard JS, et al: Use of a generally applicable tissue factor–dependent factor V assay to detect activated protein C-resistant factor Va in patients receiving warfarin and in patients with a lupus anticoagulant. Blood 85:1704-1711, 1995.

72. Poort SR, Rosendaal FR, Reitsma PH, et al: A common genetic variation in the 3′-untranslated region of the prothrombin gene is associated with elevated plasma prothrombin levels and an increase in venous thrombosis. Blood 88:3698-3703, 1996.
73. Rosendaal FR, Doggen CJ, Zivelin A, et al: Geographic distribution of the 20210 G to A prothrombin variant. Thromb Haemost 79:706-708, 1998.
74. De Stefano V, Martinelli I, Mannucci PM, et al: The risk of recurrent deep venous thrombosis among heterozygous carriers of both factor V Leiden and the G20210A prothrombin mutation. N Engl J Med 341:801-806, 1999.
75. Egeberg O: Inherited antithrombin deficiency causing thrombophilia. Thromb Diath Haemorrh 13:516-530, 1965.
76. Tait RC, Walker ID, Perry DJ, et al: Prevalence of antithrombin deficiency in the healthy population. Br J Haematol 87:106-112, 1994.
77. Heijboer H, Brandjes DP, Buller HR, et al: Deficiencies of coagulation-inhibiting and fibrinolytic proteins in outpatients with deep-vein thrombosis. N Engl J Med 323:1512-1516, 1990.
78. Rosendaal FR: Risk factors for venous thrombotic disease. Thromb Haemost 82:610-619, 1999.
79. Demers C, Ginsberg JS, Hirsh J, et al: Thrombosis in antithrombin-III-deficient persons: Report of a large kindred and literature review. Ann Intern Med 116:754-761, 1992.
80. Schulman S, Tengborn L: Treatment of venous thromboembolism in patients with congenital deficiency of antithrombin III. Thromb Haemost 68:634-636, 1992.
81. Miletich J, Sherman L, Broze G Jr: Absence of thrombosis in subjects with heterozygous protein C deficiency. N Engl J Med 317:991-996, 1987.
82. Tait RC, Walker ID, Reitsma PH, et al: Prevalence of protein C deficiency in the healthy population. Thromb Haemost 73:87-93, 1995.
83. Koster T, Rosendaal FR, Briet E, et al: Protein C deficiency in a controlled series of unselected outpatients: An infrequent but clear risk factor for venous thrombosis (Leiden Thrombophilia Study). Blood 85:2756-2761, 1995.
84. Dahlback B, Stenflo J: High molecular weight complex in human plasma between vitamin K-dependent protein S and complement component C4b-binding protein. Proc Natl Acad Sci U S A 78:2512-2516, 1981.
85. D'Angelo A, Vigano-D'Angelo S, Esmon CT, et al: Acquired deficiencies of protein S: Protein S activity during oral anticoagulation, in liver disease, and in disseminated intravascular coagulation. J Clin Invest 81:1445-1454, 1988.
86. Meijers JC, Tekelenburg WL, Bouma BN, et al: High levels of coagulation factor XI as a risk factor for venous thrombosis. N Engl J Med 342:696-701, 2000.
87. Sack GH Jr, Levin J, Bell WR: Trousseau's syndrome and other manifestations of chronic disseminated coagulopathy in patients with neoplasms: Clinical, pathophysiologic, and therapeutic features. Medicine (Baltimore) 56:1-37, 1977.
88. Prandoni P, Lensing AW, Buller HR, et al: Deep-vein thrombosis and the incidence of subsequent symptomatic cancer. N Engl J Med 327:1128-1133, 1992.
89. Venous thromboembolic disease and combined oral contraceptives: Results of international multicentre case-control study. World Health Organization Collaborative Study of Cardiovascular Disease and Steroid Hormone Contraception. Lancet 346:1575-1582, 1995.
90. Rosendaal FR, Van Hylckama Vlieg A, Tanis BC, et al: Estrogens, progestogens and thrombosis. J Thromb Haemost 1:1371-1380, 2003.
91. Freyssinet JM, Wiesel ML, Gauchy J, et al: An IgM lupus anticoagulant that neutralizes the enhancing effect of phospholipid on purified endothelial thrombomodulin activity—a mechanism for thrombosis. Thromb Haemost 55:309-313, 1986.
92. Ahn SS, Kalunian K, Rosove M, et al: Postoperative thrombotic complications in patients with lupus anticoagulant: Increased risk after vascular procedures. J Vasc Surg 7:749-756, 1988.
93. Khamashta MA, Cuadrado MJ, Mujic F, et al: The management of thrombosis in the antiphospholipid-antibody syndrome. N Engl J Med 332:993-997, 1995.
94. Warkentin TE, Levine MN, Hirsh J, et al: Heparin-induced thrombocytopenia in patients treated with low-molecular-weight heparin or unfractionated heparin. N Engl J Med 332:1330-1335, 1995.
95. Calaitges JG, Liem TK, Spadone D, et al: The role of heparin-associated antiplatelet antibodies in the outcome of arterial reconstruction. J Vasc Surg 29:779-785, 1999.
96. Schmitt BP, Adelman B: Heparin-associated thrombocytopenia: A critical review and pooled analysis. Am J Med Sci 305:208-215, 1993.
97. Warkentin TE, Kelton JG: Heparin-induced thrombocytopenia. Prog Hemost Thromb 10:1-34, 1991.
98. Guba SC, Fonseca V, Fink LM: Hyperhomocysteinemia and thrombosis. Semin Thromb Hemost 25:291-309, 1999.
99. den Heijer M, Koster T, Blom HJ, et al: Hyperhomocysteinemia as a risk factor for deep-vein thrombosis. N Engl J Med 334:759-762, 1996.
100. Simioni P, Prandoni P, Burlina A, et al: Hyperhomocysteinemia and deep-vein thrombosis: A case-control study. Thromb Haemost 76:883-886, 1996.
101. den Heijer M, Rosendaal FR, Blom HJ, et al: Hyperhomocysteinemia and venous thrombosis: A meta-analysis. Thromb Haemost 80:874-877, 1998.
102. Ridker PM, Hennekens CH, Selhub J, et al: Interrelation of hyperhomocyst(e)inemia, factor V Leiden, and risk of future venous thromboembolism. Circulation 95:1777-1782, 1997.
103. Mandel H, Brenner B, Berant M, et al: Coexistence of hereditary homocystinuria and factor V Leiden—effect on thrombosis. N Engl J Med 334:763-768, 1996.
104. den Heijer M, Brouwer IA, Bos GM, et al: Vitamin supplementation reduces blood homocysteine levels: A controlled trial in patients with venous thrombosis and healthy volunteers. Arterioscler Thromb Vasc Biol 18:356-361, 1998.
105. Clagett GP, Anderson FA Jr, Geerts W, et al: Prevention of venous thromboembolism. Chest 114:531S-560S, 1998.
106. Nader HB, Walenga JM, Berkowitz SD, et al: Preclinical differentiation of low molecular weight heparins. Semin Thromb Hemost 25(Suppl 3):63-72, 1999.
107. Hirsh J, Warkentin TE, Shaughnessy SG, et al: Heparin and low-molecular-weight heparin: Mechanisms of action, pharmacokinetics, dosing, monitoring, efficacy, and safety. Chest 119:64S-94S, 2001.
108. Magnani HN: Heparin-induced thrombocytopenia (HIT): An overview of 230 patients treated with orgaran (Org 10172). Thromb Haemost 70:554-561, 1993.
109. Kikta MJ, Keller MP, Humphrey PW, et al: Can low molecular weight heparins and heparinoids be safely given to patients with heparin-induced thrombocytopenia syndrome? Surgery 114:705-710, 1993.
110. Hirsh J, Weitz JI: New antithrombotic agents. Lancet 353:1431-1436, 1999.
111. Markwardt F: Hirudin and derivatives as anticoagulant agents. Thromb Haemost 66:141-152, 1991.
112. Potzsch B, Madlener K, Seelig C, et al: Monitoring of r-hirudin anticoagulation during cardiopulmonary bypass—assessment of the whole blood ecarin clotting time. Thromb Haemost 77:920-925, 1997.
113. Greinacher A, Volpel H, Janssens U, et al: Recombinant hirudin (lepirudin) provides safe and effective anticoagulation in patients with heparin-induced thrombocytopenia: A prospective study. Circulation 99:73-80, 1999.
114. Superficial Thrombophlebitis Treated By Enoxaparin Study Group: A pilot randomized double-blind comparison of a low-molecular-weight heparin, a nonsteroidal anti-inflammatory agent, and placebo in the treatment of superficial vein thrombosis. Arch Intern Med 163:1657-1663, 2003.
115. Eichler P, Olbrich K, Pötzsch B: Anti-hirudin antibodies in patients treated with recombinant hirudin for more than five days, a prospective study. Thromb Haemost (Suppl):PS2014, 1997.
116. Robson R, White H, Aylward P, et al: Bivalirudin pharmacokinetics and pharmacodynamics: Effect of renal function, dose, and gender. Clin Pharmacol Ther 71:433-439, 2002.
117. Eriksson BI, Bergqvist D, Kalebo P, et al: Ximelagatran and melagatran compared with dalteparin for prevention of venous thromboembolism after total hip or knee replacement: The METHRO II randomised trial. Lancet 360:1441-1447, 2002.
118. Eriksson H, Wahlander K, Gustafsson D, et al: A randomized, controlled, dose-guiding study of the oral direct thrombin inhibitor ximelagatran compared with standard therapy for the treatment of acute deep vein thrombosis: THRIVE I. J Thromb Haemost 1:41-47, 2003.
119. Schulman S, Wahlander K, Lundstrom T, et al: Secondary prevention of venous thromboembolism with the oral direct thrombin inhibitor ximelagatran. N Engl J Med 349:1713-1721, 2003.
120. Liem TK, Silver D: Coumadin: Principles of use. Semin Vasc Surg 9:354-361, 1996.
121. Cole MS, Minifee PK, Wolma FJ: Coumarin necrosis—a review of the literature. Surgery 103:271-277, 1988.

122. Pescatore P, Horellou HM, Conard J, et al: Problems of oral anticoagulation in an adult with homozygous protein C deficiency and late onset of thrombosis. Thromb Haemost 69:311-315, 1993.

123. Bick RL, Kaplan H: Syndromes of thrombosis and hypercoagulability: Congenital and acquired causes of thrombosis. Med Clin North Am 82:409-458, 1998.

124. Silverstein MD, Heit JA, Mohr DN, et al: Trends in the incidence of deep vein thrombosis and pulmonary embolism: A 25-year population-based study. Arch Intern Med 158:585-593, 1998.

125. Proctor MC, Greenfield LJ: Pulmonary embolism: Diagnosis, incidence and implications. Cardiovasc Surg 5:77-81, 1997.

126. Anderson FA Jr, Wheeler HB, Goldberg RJ, et al: A population-based perspective of the hospital incidence and case-fatality rates of deep vein thrombosis and pulmonary embolism: The Worcester DVT Study. Arch Intern Med 151:933-938, 1991.

127. Mohr DN, Silverstein MD, Heit JA, et al: The venous stasis syndrome after deep venous thrombosis or pulmonary embolism: A population-based study. Mayo Clin Proc 75:1249-1256, 2000.

128. Nordstrom M, Lindblad B, Bergqvist D, et al: A prospective study of the incidence of deep-vein thrombosis within a defined urban population. J Intern Med 232:155-160, 1992.

129. Clagett GP, Reisch JS: Prevention of venous thromboembolism in general surgical patients: Results of meta-analysis. Ann Surg 208:227-240, 1988.

130. Geerts WH, Code KI, Jay RM, et al: A prospective study of venous thromboembolism after major trauma. N Engl J Med 331:1601-1606, 1994.

131. Jorgensen JO, Hanel KC, Morgan AM, et al: The incidence of deep venous thrombosis in patients with superficial thrombophlebitis of the lower limbs. J Vasc Surg 18:70-73, 1993.

132. Kotilainen M, Ristola P, Ikkala E, et al: Leg vein thrombosis diagnosed by ^{125}I-fibrinogen test after acute myocardial infarction. Ann Clin Res 5:365-368, 1973.

133. Waring WP, Karunas RS: Acute spinal cord injuries and the incidence of clinically occurring thromboembolic disease. Paraplegia 29:8-16, 1991.

134. Ginsberg JS, Brill-Edwards P, Burrows RF, et al: Venous thrombosis during pregnancy: Leg and trimester of presentation. Thromb Haemost 67:519-520, 1992.

135. Trottier SJ, Veremakis C, O'Brien J, et al: Femoral deep vein thrombosis associated with central venous catheterization: Results from a prospective, randomized trial. Crit Care Med 23:52-59, 1995.

136. Geerts WH, Heit JA, Clagett GP, et al: Prevention of venous thromboembolism. Chest 119:132S-175S, 2001.

137. Chouhan VD, Comerota AJ, Sun L, et al: Inhibition of tissue factor pathway during intermittent pneumatic compression: A possible mechanism for antithrombotic effect. Arterioscler Thromb Vasc Biol 19:2812-2817, 1999.

138. Colditz GA, Tuden RL, Oster G: Rates of venous thrombosis after general surgery: Combined results of randomised clinical trials. Lancet 2:143-146, 1986.

139. Agnelli G: Prevention of venous thromboembolism after neurosurgery. Thromb Haemost 82:925-930, 1999.

140. Bounameaux H: Integrating pharmacologic and mechanical prophylaxis of venous thromboembolism. Thromb Haemost 82:931-937, 1999.

141. Nurmohamed MT, Rosendaal FR, Buller HR, et al: Low-molecular-weight heparin versus standard heparin in general and orthopaedic surgery: A meta-analysis. Lancet 340:152-156, 1992.

142. Koch A, Bouges S, Ziegler S, et al: Low molecular weight heparin and unfractionated heparin in thrombosis prophylaxis after major surgical intervention: Update of previous meta-analyses. Br J Surg 84:750-759, 1997.

143. Geerts WH, Jay RM, Code KI, et al: A comparison of low-dose heparin with low-molecular-weight heparin as prophylaxis against venous thromboembolism after major trauma. N Engl J Med 335:701-707, 1996.

144. Nicolaides AN, Breddin HK, Fareed J, et al: Prevention of venous thromboembolism: International consensus statement. Guidelines compiled in accordance with the scientific evidence. Int Angiol 20:1-37, 2001.

145. Hull RD, Brant RF, Pineo GF, et al: Preoperative vs postoperative initiation of low-molecular-weight heparin prophylaxis against venous thromboembolism in patients undergoing elective hip replacement. Arch Intern Med 159:137-141, 1999.

146. Bergqvist D, Benoni G, Bjorgell O, et al: Low-molecular-weight heparin (enoxaparin) as prophylaxis against venous thromboembolism after total hip replacement. N Engl J Med 335:696-700, 1996.

147. Dahl OE, Andreassen G, Aspelin T, et al: Prolonged thromboprophylaxis following hip replacement surgery—results of a double-blind, prospective, randomised, placebo-controlled study with dalteparin (Fragmin). Thromb Haemost 77:26-31, 1997.

148. Lassen MR, Borris LC, Anderson BS, et al: Efficacy and safety of prolonged thromboprophylaxis with a low molecular weight heparin (dalteparin) after total hip arthroplasty—the Danish Prolonged Prophylaxis (DaPP) Study. Thromb Res 89:281-287, 1998.

149. Breddin HK: Low molecular weight heparins in the prevention of deep-vein thrombosis in general surgery. Semin Thromb Hemost 25 Suppl 3:83-89, 1999.

150. Turpie AG, Bauer KA, Eriksson BI, et al: Postoperative fondaparinux versus postoperative enoxaparin for prevention of venous thromboembolism after elective hip-replacement surgery: A randomised double-blind trial. Lancet 359:1721-1726, 2002.

151. Sevitt S, Gallagher NG: Prevention of venous thrombosis and pulmonary embolism in injured patients: A trial of anticoagulant prophylaxis with phenindione in middle-aged and elderly patients with fractured necks of femur. Lancet 2:981-989, 1959.

152. Powers PJ, Gent M, Jay RM, et al: A randomized trial of less intense postoperative warfarin or aspirin therapy in the prevention of venous thromboembolism after surgery for fractured hip. Arch Intern Med 149:771-774, 1989.

153. Poller L, McKernan A, Thomson JM, et al: Fixed minidose warfarin: A new approach to prophylaxis against venous thrombosis after major surgery. BMJ (Clin Res Ed) 295:1309-1312, 1987.

154. Geerts WH, Pineo GF, Heit JA, et al: Prevention of venous thromboembolism. The seventh ACCP Conference on antithrombotic and thrombolytic therapy. Chest 126:3385-4005, 2004.

155. Antithrombotic Trialists' Collaboration: Collaborative meta-analysis of randomised trials of antiplatelet therapy for prevention of death, myocardial infarction, and stroke in high risk patients. BMJ 324:71-86, 2002.

156. Spinal Cord Injury Thromboprophylaxis Investigators: Prevention of venous thromboembolism in the rehabilitation phase after spinal cord injury: Prophylaxis with low-dose heparin or enoxaparin. J Trauma 54:1111-1115, 2003.

157. Braunwald E, Antman EM, Beasley JW, et al: ACC/AHA guideline update for the management of patients with unstable angina and non-ST-segment elevation myocardial infarction—2002. Summary article: A report of the American College of Cardiology/American Heart Association Task Force on Practice Guidelines (Committee on the Management of Patients with Unstable Angina). Circulation 106:1893-1900, 2002.

158. Becquemin JP: Effect of ticlopidine on the long-term patency of saphenous-vein bypass grafts in the legs: Etude de la Ticlopidine apres Pontage Femoro-Poplite and the Association Universitaire de Recherche en Chirurgie. N Engl J Med 337:1726-1731, 1997.

159. Hass WK, Easton JD, Adams HP Jr, et al: A randomized trial comparing ticlopidine hydrochloride with aspirin for the prevention of stroke in high-risk patients: Ticlopidine Aspirin Stroke Study Group. N Engl J Med 321:501-507, 1989.

160. Balsano F, Rizzon P, Violi F, et al: Antiplatelet treatment with ticlopidine in unstable angina: A controlled multicenter clinical trial. The Studio della Ticlopidina nell'Angina Instabile Group. Circulation 82:17-26, 1990.

161. Arcan JC, Blanchard J, Boissel JP, et al: Multicenter double-blind study of ticlopidine in the treatment of intermittent claudication and the prevention of its complications. Angiology 39:802-811, 1988.

162. Yusuf S, Mehta SR, Zhao F, et al: Early and late effects of clopidogrel in patients with acute coronary syndromes. Circulation 107:966-972, 2003.

163. A randomised, blinded, trial of clopidogrel versus aspirin in patients at risk of ischaemic events (CAPRIE). CAPRIE Steering Committee. Lancet 348:1329-1339, 1996.

164. Yusuf S, Zhao F, Mehta SR, et al: Effects of clopidogrel in addition to aspirin in patients with acute coronary syndromes without ST-segment elevation. N Engl J Med 345:494-502, 2001.

165. Use of a monoclonal antibody directed against the platelet glycoprotein IIb/IIIa receptor in high-risk coronary angioplasty: The EPIC Investigation. N Engl J Med 330:956-961, 1994.

166. Simoons ML, de Boer MJ, van den Brand MJ, et al: Randomized trial of a GPIIb/IIIa platelet receptor blocker in refractory unstable angina: European Cooperative Study Group. Circulation 89:596-603, 1994.

167. Kleiman NS, Ohman EM, Califf RM, et al: Profound inhibition of platelet aggregation with monoclonal antibody 7E3 Fab after thrombolytic therapy: Results of the Thrombolysis and Angioplasty in Myocardial Infarction (TAMI) 8 Pilot Study. J Am Coll Cardiol 22:381-389, 1993.

168. Hirsh J, Dalen JE, Anderson DR, et al: Oral anticoagulants: Mechanism of action, clinical effectiveness, and optimal therapeutic range. Chest 114:445S-469S, 1998.

169. Kretschmer G, Wenzl E, Piza F, et al: The influence of anticoagulant treatment on the probability of function in femoropopliteal vein bypass surgery: Analysis of a clinical series (1970 to 1985) and interim evaluation of a controlled clinical trial. Surgery 102:453-459, 1987.

170. Kretschmer G, Herbst F, Prager M, et al: A decade of oral anticoagulant treatment to maintain autologous vein grafts for femoropopliteal atherosclerosis. Arch Surg 127:1112-1115, 1992.

171. Flinn WR, Rohrer MJ, Yao JS, et al: Improved long-term patency of infragenicular polytetrafluoroethylene grafts. J Vasc Surg 7:685-690, 1988.

172. Sarac TP, Huber TS, Back MR, et al: Warfarin improves the outcome of infrainguinal vein bypass grafting at high risk for failure. J Vasc Surg 28:446-457, 1998.

Questions

1. **Which of the following statements regarding antiplatelet therapy is true?**
   (a) Lower dosages of aspirin (75 to 150 mg/day) are not as effective as higher dosages (325 mg/day) for the prevention of cerebrovascular ischemic events
   (b) Ticlopidine is associated with a small but significant incidence of neutropenia
   (c) When compared with aspirin, clopidogrel is associated with a significantly greater incidence of neutropenia
   (d) For the prevention of ischemic events, combination therapy with clopidogrel and aspirin is no better than aspirin alone

2. **Regarding the management of heparin-induced thrombocytopenia (HIT), which of the following is true?**
   (a) Unfractionated heparin and low-molecular-weight heparin have a similar incidence of heparin-associated antibody formation
   (b) Low-molecular-weight heparin may be safely administered in patients with established HIT
   (c) The platelet count must be <100,000/mm³ to be diagnosed with HIT
   (d) Antihirudin antibodies develop in approximately 40% of patients receiving hirudin, but resistance to therapy is uncommon

3. **Which of the following statements regarding von Willebrand's disease is false?**
   (a) Defects of primary hemostasis commonly cause petechiae and ecchymoses
   (b) Hemophilic disorders commonly cause hemarthroses and deep tissue hematomas
   (c) Von Willebrand's disease is the most common inherited bleeding disorder
   (d) Type 1 von Willebrand's disease is usually unresponsive to DDAVP
   (e) Cryoprecipitate and some factor VIII concentrates are rich in vWF

4. **Which of the following statements regarding thrombophilic conditions is true?**
   (a) Elevated homocysteine levels are associated with arterial and venous thromboses
   (b) The prothrombin 20210A mutation results in resistance to antithrombin III
   (c) Warfarin is ineffective in patients with antiphospholipid syndrome
   (d) Activated protein C resistance may be due to a defect in protein C or protein S
   (e) Antithrombin concentrates are the mainstay of therapy for antithrombin-deficient patients with venous thromboembolism

5. **Following major surgical procedures in patients with hemophilia A, factor VIII:C plasma activity should be at least**
   (a) 5% of normal
   (b) 25% of normal
   (c) 50% of normal
   (d) 75% of normal
   (e) 100% of normal

6. **Which of the following statements regarding low-molecular-weight heparin (LMWH) is false?**
   (a) LMWHs demonstrate less binding to plasma proteins and endothelium
   (b) LMWHs preferentially inactivate factor Xa over factor IIa
   (c) LMWH thrombosis prophylaxis is superior to unfractionated heparin prophylaxis in orthopedic surgery patients
   (d) LMWH is clearly superior to unfractionated heparin for routine general surgical procedures

7. **Which of the following statements regarding danaparoid, hirudin, and argatroban is true?**
   (a) There is no significant cross-reactivity between danaparoid and heparin in patients with heparin-associated antibodies
   (b) Hirudin is a direct thrombin inhibitor, preventing the formation of fibrin
   (c) Hirudin therapy does not have to be adjusted in patients with renal failure
   (d) Argatroban dosing should be adjusted in patients with hepatic insufficiency
   (e) Hirudin therapy may be monitored with the aPTT, and argatroban may be monitored with the PT

8. **Which of the following statements regarding the risk associated with pregnancy and hormonal therapy is false?**
   (a) The risk of venous thrombosis decreases after delivery
   (b) The thrombosis risks associated with oral contraceptives are immediate and reversible
   (c) Oral contraceptives are associated with a two- to fourfold increased risk for venous thrombosis
   (d) LMWHs have been shown to be safe and effective in pregnant patients with venous thromboembolism

9. **Which of the following is not a vitamin K–dependent coagulation factor?**
   (a) Factor II
   (b) Factor V
   (c) Factor VII
   (d) Factor IX
   (e) Factor X

10. **Which of the following is not a major regulator of the coagulation cascade?**
    (a) Antithrombin III
    (b) Protein C
    (c) Protein S
    (d) Tissue factor pathway inhibitor
    (e) Heparin cofactor II

Answers

1. b	2. d	3. d	4. a	5. c
6. d	7. d	8. a	9. b	10. e

6

Ralph G. DePalma

Atherosclerosis: Pathology, Pathogenesis, and Medical Management

Treatment of atherosclerosis and its complications is the most common task for vascular surgeons. Currently, more precise lesion classification, a better understanding of atherogenesis, and innovative medical treatments offer opportunities for improved long-term results. A variety of scientific hypotheses and technical advances provide scientifically based prevention and management strategies. At the beginning of the 21st century, the pivotal role of lipids in the pathogenesis of atherosclerosis has been better delineated, along with the effects of treatment on plaques and the recognition of the role of inflammatory and immune responses affecting the arterial wall. Novel risk factors for late progression, independent of conventional risk factors, have been identified. These include elevated blood levels of inflammatory cytokines, metalloproteinases, and smooth muscle growth factors such as glucose and insulin. Advances in imaging allow the identification of unstable plaques vulnerable to rupture, thrombosis, and downstream embolization. Prospective randomized trials using drugs, micronutrients, and other interventions continue to provide therapeutic guidelines. Practitioners treating vascular disease have long recognized that coronary thrombosis or stroke is the main threat to survival associated with peripheral arterial disease,[1] a point requiring constant reiteration.

Vascular surgeons must be familiar with the location and natural history of individual lesions and, when considering various interventions, they must distinguish primary prevention from secondary treatment. When active intervention is required, vascular surgeons should understand the need for a precise approach geared toward the pathology of a specific vascular lesion in a particular artery. For example, a stenotic lesion composed of smooth muscle and well-organized collagen, although producing some degree of distal ischemia, is a much "safer" lesion than a plaque containing an unstable core of atheromatous debris beneath a tenuous cap. Likewise, the smooth stenosis of an adductor hiatus plaque in the femoral artery, causing stable claudication, is clearly not as threatening as a carotid or coronary plaque with a soft core

and friable cap, causing transient cerebral ischemia and stroke. We now recognize that operative or endovascular treatment of segmental lesions does not prevent the progression of systemic atherosclerosis elsewhere; medical treatment is required to enhance long-term results.

Variations in the patterns and rates of progression of atherosclerosis have critical clinical implications for the timing and choice of treatment.[2,3] Considering the atherosclerotic process as a single disease leads to oversimplification. With the diversity of lesions and their clinical presentations, atherosclerosis should be viewed as a polypathogenic process comprising a group of closely related vascular disorders.[4,5] The multiple risk factors promoting atherosclerosis (including dyslipidemia, smoking, diabetes, hypertension, and, perhaps, hyperhomocysteinemia) make the single-disease view logically invalid. For purposes of this chapter, however, I describe atherosclerosis as if it were a single entity, emphasizing variations in pathogenesis and treatment approaches; I also discuss promising but unproven new concepts and relevant trial data.

Theories of pathogenesis need to be addressed relative to their usefulness for predicting and controlling the disease: some are clearly quite relevant, whereas others appear to be journeys into phenomenology. Yet certain elements of the various theories are applicable when formulating new treatment strategies. For example, direct interventions for certain lesions in specific sites (e.g., unstable carotid atheromas) offer effective definitive approaches, while medical therapy is clearly preferable in other situations (e.g., stable claudication due to infrainguinal atherosclerosis).

Pathology

GENERAL CONCEPTS

The term *atheroma* is derived from the Greek *athere*, meaning "porridge" or "gruel"; *sclerosis* means "induration" or "hardening." A gruel-like color and consistency and induration or

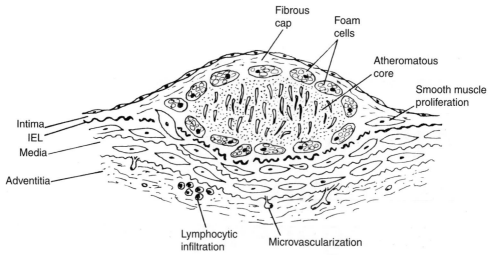

FIGURE 6–1 • Typical atheroma or type IV lesion. Note the central lipid core, fibrous cap, macrophage accumulation, and zone of synthetically active smooth muscle at the "shoulders" of the core. Note too the tendency of the lesion to bulge outward, neovascularization, and adventitial lymphocyte infiltration. IEL, internal elastic lamina. (Modified from DePalma RG: Pathology of atheromas. In Bell PRF, Jamieson CW, Ruckley CV [eds]: Surgical Management of Vascular Disease. London, WB Saunders, 1992, p 21.)

hardening exist to various degrees in different plaques, different disease stages, and different individuals. In 1755, von Haller first applied the term *atheroma* to a common type of plaque that, on sectioning, exuded a yellow, pultaceous content from its core.[6] Figure 6-1 illustrates a typical fibrous plaque containing a central atheromatous core with a fibrous or fibromuscular cap, macrophage accumulation, and round cell adventitial infiltration. Although the classic definition of atherosclerotic plaque is "a variable combination of changes in the *intima* of arteries consisting of focal accumulation of lipids, complex carbohydrates, blood and blood products, fibrous tissue and calcium deposits,"[7] it does not adequately describe the spectrum of atherosclerotic lesions. Advanced plaques invade the media; atheromas at certain stages produce bulging or even enlarged arteries; and round cell infiltration, medial changes, and neovascularization characterize many advanced atherosclerotic lesions. The process involves the entire arterial wall. The descriptions that follow consider progressively severe types of plaque; certain lesions, however, might not evolve in the same way.

The development and expansion of the lipid atherosclerotic core and its relationship to the cap have been recognized as causes of plaque complications. An important fact is the observation that a lipid "core" develops early in atherosclerosis, accumulating in the deep aspects of early lesions before actual fibrous plaque formation begins.[8] Another key insight is the recognition of the role of inflammation and immune reactions in both the early and late stages of atherogenesis.[9,10] The inflammatory cascade in these settings includes the appearance of proinflammatory cytokines such as interleukin-6 (IL-6) and tumor necrosis factor-α (TNF-α) and anti-inflammatory cytokines such as IL-10 within arterial tissue as well as in the bloodstream. Lipid accumulation appears to attract inflammatory cells that produce cytokines locally; these cytokines can also be detected systemically in atherosclerotic subjects. For example, in stable claudicants, plasma levels of inflammatory cytokines TNF-α and IL-6 are elevated, while anti-inflammatory IL-10 levels are reduced.[11] Elevated levels of cytokines such as TNF-α have also been

shown to affect the arterial wall.[12-14] The atherosclerotic plaque contains leukocytes, of which approximately 80% are monocytes or monocyte-derived macrophages. Lymphocytes, predominantly memory T cells,[15] constitute 5% to 20% of this cell population. Inflammation, size, and composition of the lipid core are believed to determine plaque vulnerability, promoting sudden expansion, rupture, release of distal emboli, and vascular occlusion.

FATTY STREAKS

Fatty streaks are gross, minimally raised, yellow lesions found frequently in the aortas of infants and children. These lesions contain lipids deposited intracellularly in macrophages and in smooth muscle cells. A special report by Stary and colleagues[16] defined initial fatty streaks and intermediate lesions of atherosclerosis as follows: Type I lesions in children are the earliest microscopic lesions, consisting of an increase in intimal macrophages and the appearance of foam cells. Type II lesions are grossly visible; in contrast to type I lesions, type II lesions stain with Sudan III or IV. Foam cells and lipid droplets, also found in intimal smooth muscle cells, and heterogeneous droplets of extracellular lipids characterize fatty streaks. Type III lesions are considered intermediate lesions; they are usually the bridge between the fatty streak (Fig. 6-2) and the prototypical atheromatous fibrous plaque, the type IV plaque (see Fig. 6-1).[17] Type III lesions occur in plaque-prone locations in the arterial tree,[18] at sites exposed to forces (particularly low-shear stress) that cause increased low-density lipoprotein (LDL) influx.[19]

The fatty streak type II lipids are chemically similar to those of plasma,[20] although plasma lipids may enter the arterial wall in several ways. As described in a useful review of pathogenesis,[21] LDL accumulation may occur because of (1) alterations in the permeability of the intima, (2) increases in the interstitial space in the intima, (3) poor metabolism of LDL by vascular cells, (4) impeded transport of LDL from the intima to the media, (5) increased plasma LDL concentrations, or (6) specific binding of LDL to connective tissue components,

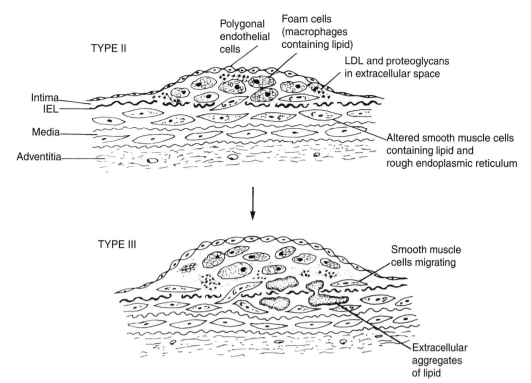

FIGURE 6–2 • Type II fatty streak lesions with foam cells. Note the low-density lipoprotein (LDL) particles in the matrix and altered smooth muscle cells, with developed rough endoplasmic reticulum also containing lipid particles. Note too the evolution to an intermediate, more advanced lesion (type III) containing extracellular aggregates or pools of lipid deep in the intima and extending into the media. IEL, internal elastic lamina. (From DePalma RG: Atherosclerosis: Theories of etiology and pathogenesis. In Sidawy AN, Sumpio BE, DePalma RG [eds]: Basic Science of Vascular Disease. Armonk, NY, Futura Publishing, 1997, pp 319-332.)

particularly proteoglycans in the arterial intima. Experimental studies show that LDL cholesterol accumulates in the intima even before lesions develop and in the presence of intact endothelium. These observations are quite similar to descriptions of lesion formation by Aschoff[22] in the early 20th century and Virchow[23] in the mid-19th century.

A second event in early atherogenesis, as shown in animal experiments, is binding of monocytes to the endothelial lining, with their subsequent diapedesis into the subintimal layer to become tissue macrophages.[24-26] Experimentally, fatty streaks are populated mainly by monocyte-derived macrophages. These lipid-engorged scavenger cells mainly become the foam cells that characterize fatty streaks and other lesions. An important observation is that LDL must be altered in some manner,[27] by oxidation or acetylation, to be taken up by the macrophages to form foam cells. Oxidized LDL is a powerful chemoattractant for monocytes. Another aspect of this theory suggests that the endothelium modifies LDL to promote foam cell formation.

The interactions of plasma LDL with the arterial wall are the subject of intense interest. LDL traverses the endothelium mostly through receptor-independent transport, but also through cell breaks.[28] Endothelial cells,[29] smooth cells,[29] and macrophages[30,31] are each capable of promoting oxidation of LDL. The oxidized LDL, in turn, further attracts monocytes into the intima to promote their transformation into macrophages. Macrophages produce cytokines, including platelet-derived growth factor (PDGF), transforming growth factor-β (TGF-β), and IL-1, which initiates the cytokine cascade. Oxidized LDL

also induces gene products that are ordinarily unexpressed in normal vascular tissue. A notable example is tissue factor, the cellular initiator of the coagulation cascade that is expressed by atheroma monocytes and foam cells.[32] Expression of tissue factor requires the presence of bacterial lipopolysaccharide, suggesting that hypercoagulability in atherosclerosis can be enhanced by endotoxemia.

The large numbers of macrophages and T lymphocytes in the lesion suggest a cellular immune response; oxidized lipoproteins, heat shock proteins, and microorganisms are possible antigens. A study analyzing endarterectomy specimens by immunohistochemistry and reverse transcription polymerase chain reaction showed proinflammatory T-cell cytokines, IL-2, and interferon-7 in a large proportion of plaques, indicating that a helper T-cell 1–type cellular immune response also likely occurs in the atherosclerotic plaque.[33]

ENDOTHELIUM

Animal studies reveal that endothelial cells tend to be oriented away from the direction of flow; these cells show increased stigmata or stomata, increased proliferation, and a decrease in microfilament bundles. In humans and animals, endothelial cells become polyhedral or rounded; in humans, increased formation of multinucleated cells and cilia occurs. Animal studies reveal increased proliferation and cell death, with retraction and exposure of subendothelial foam cells. The endothelium becomes more permeable to macromolecules in experimental models; in humans, it exhibits increased mural thrombus formation and tissue factor expression. Leukocyte adherence increases with the expression of a monocyte adhesion molecule (VCAM-1). Endothelium-derived relaxing factor and prostacyclin release are decreased with enhanced vasoconstriction.

MEDIA

Experimentally, the smooth muscle shows increased proliferation, with increased rough endoplasmic reticulum, phenotypic changes, and increased production of altered intracellular and extracellular matrices. These, in humans, include increased expression of type I and type III collagen, dermatan sulfate, proteoglycan, and stromelysins. The smooth muscle cells produce cytokines, including macrophage colony-stimulating factor, TNF, and monocyte chemoattractant protein-1. Myocytes accumulate native and modified lipoproteins by both native receptor pathways and nonspecific phagocytosis; these cells also express increased lipoprotein lipase activity and experimentally display a scavenger receptor similar to that of foam cells.

MACROPHAGES

Macrophages proliferate and express monocyte chemoattractant protein-1, macrophage colony-stimulating factor, TNF, IL-1 and other interleukins, and PDGF, along with CD immune antigens and tissue factor,[32] as previously described. Plaque macrophages contain increased free and esterified cholesterol and increased acetyl coenzyme A, cholesterol acyltransferase, and acid cholesterol ester hydrolase. Neutral cholesterol ester hydrolase is decreased. These altered cells also express the scavenger receptor 15-lipoxygenase and exhibit increased lipoprotein oxidation products in humans and in animal models. These extensive changes indicate the complexity of the morphologic, functional, biochemical, and genetic expressions of the arterial wall in early atherosclerosis. The reader is referred to an original report for comprehensive details,[17] with references for the cellular alterations given.

GELATINOUS PLAQUES

The intimal gelatinous lesion is another type of early atheroma precursor. Haust described these lesions in 1971,[34] but they were first noted in 1856 by Virchow[23] as potential progenitors of advanced atherosclerosis. Methodical study of these lesions and their evolution has been relatively neglected, although Smith described their identification and composition.[35] Virtually all plasma proteins, particularly their hemostatic components, can enter the arterial intima; these are thought to be mainly responsible for gelatinous lesions. Gelatinous plaques are translucent and neutral in color, with central areas that are grayish or opaque. Most of them are characterized by finely dispersed, perifibrous lipid along with collagen strands around the lesions. Grossly, gelatinous lesions feel soft. With gentle lateral pressure, the plaque "wobbles." Gelatinous plaques can be observed during arterial surgery, and I am struck by the frequency with which these lesions appear in heavy smokers. The gelatinous material separates easily from the underlying arterial wall without entering a conventional endarterectomy plane. Gelatinous plaques

commonly occur in the aorta as extensive areas of flat, translucent thickenings, particularly in the lower abdominal segment. These lesions are characterized by low lipid content and high fluid content. Protein content is variable, but in some plaques, numerous smooth muscle cells are present, and the lesions contain substantial amounts of cross-linked fibrin.

FIBROUS PLAQUES

Figure 6-1 typifies more advanced atherosclerotic lesions, the fibrous or type IV plaque. These are composed of large numbers of smooth muscle cells and connective tissue, which form a fibrous cap over an inner yellow (atheromatous) core. This soft core contains cholesterol esters, mainly cholesteryl oleate, likely derived from disrupted foam cells. A second type of particle contains both free cholesterol and cholesterol linoleates. The early core is associated with vesicular lipids that are rich in free cholesterol.[8] These particles are likely derived directly from LDL, possibly by modification of LDL by specific lipolytic enzymes capable of hydrolyzing LDL cholesterol esters. Lipoprotein aggregation and fusion are thought to be the chief pathway of cholesterol ester accumulation. Fibrous plaques are also composed of large numbers of smooth muscle cells, connective tissue cells, and macrophages. Almost 2 decades ago, the composition and integrity of the atheromatous cap were underscored, as this structure stabilizes the atheroma, preventing intraluminal rupture of its soft core.[36]

Fibrous plaques appear later than fatty streaks, but often in similar locations. Some fibrous plaques evolve from fatty streaks; other precursors, such as gelatinous plaques, injured arterial areas, or thrombi, may also lead to fibrous plaque formation. A mural thrombus can be converted into an atheroma, as demonstrated by chronic intra-arterial catheter implantation.[37]

Fibrous plaques protrude into the arterial lumen in fixed cut sections; however, when arteries are fixed at arterial pressure, they produce an abluminal or external bulge. For example, coronary plaques in vivo must occupy at least 40% of the arterial wall before angiographic detection is possible,[38] and within limits, atheroma growth is compensated by arterial enlargement.[39] Compensatory remodeling of coronary arteries in subhuman primates and humans has been stressed.[40] However, with lesion growth, ulceration, rupture, or overlying thrombosis, the arterial lumen becomes compromised; such change often occurs suddenly to cause a coronary event. A unique adaptive response involving dilatation, with atheromatous involvement of the entire arterial wall and participation of inflammatory cells and immunologically active T lymphocytes, and elastolysis predisposes to aneurysm formation.

During the early stages of evolution from fatty streak to fibrous plaque, cholesterol esters appear in the form of ordered arrays of intracellular lipid crystals. In intermediate type III and fibrous plaques, the lipids assume isotropic forms and occur extracellularly.[41] Cholesterol esters and oxysterols are quite irritating, causing severe inflammatory reactions in the connective tissue[42]; they probably behave similarly within the arterial wall to promote inflammation, fibrosis, and lymphocytic infiltration. Advancing neovascularization from the adventitia characterizes intermediate fibrofatty and fibrous plaque lesions. Atherosclerotic lesions contain IgG in large quantities, as well as other immunoglobulins and complement components. The IgG recognizes epitopes characteristic of oxidized LDL, indicating that immunologic processes characterize more advanced atherosclerotic plaques.[43] This process is associated with systemic effects; for example, patients with carotid atherosclerosis have higher antibody ratios of antioxidized LDL and IgM than do comparable nonatherosclerotic controls.[44]

Experiments in complement-deficient rabbits suggest that the chronic inflammation of atherosclerosis is driven mainly by activation of the complement and monocyte-macrophage systems.[45] In this view, enzymatic degradation, *not oxidation*, becomes a central predisposing process.

COMPLICATED PLAQUES

Fibrous plaques become complicated by calcification, ulceration, intraplaque hemorrhage, or necrosis. These late developments in atherosclerosis cause the clinical complications of stroke, gangrene, and myocardial infarction. Aneurysm formation may represent a unique genetic or immune interaction with atherosclerosis. Alternatively, aneurysms have been viewed as nonspecific or inflammatory, degenerative, or purely mechanical arterial responses. Patients harboring aortic aneurysms have a high prevalence of risk factors for atherosclerosis and concurrent atherosclerotic involvement of other arteries, suggesting a unique response to atherosclerosis involving this arterial segment in certain individuals.[46]

Like the early plaques,[16] advanced atherosclerotic lesions have been described and classified.[17] The type IV lesion, or atheroma, is potentially symptom producing. Extracellular lipid is the precursor of the core that characterizes type IV lesions. Lesions that contain a thick layer of fibrous connective tissue are characterized as type V lesions, whereas those with fissures, hematoma, or thrombus are characterized as type VI lesions. Type V lesions have been further described as largely calcified (type Vc) or consisting mainly of connective tissue with little or no lipid or calcium (type Vb). Atherosclerotic aneurysms have been included in this definition of advanced atherosclerosis.

Theories of Atherogenesis

LIPID HYPOTHESIS

Virchow believed that the cellular changes characterizing atherosclerosis were reactive responses to lipid infiltration.[23] Later, Aschoff remarked, "From plasma of low cholesterin content no deposition of lipids will occur even though mechanical conditions are favorable."[22] As can be seen from fatty streak and fibrous plaque evolution, lipids, particularly LDL cholesterol, play a pivotal role in lesion morphology, composition, and evolution. Early experiments by Anitschkow with cholesterol-fed rabbits appeared to validate the simple "lipid filtration hypothesis."[47] However, the situation is pathogenetically more complex. Atherosclerosis develops in various species in proportion to the ease with which an experimental regimen displaces the normal lipid pattern toward hypercholesterolemia, particularly hyperbetalipoproteinemia. At the same time, arterial susceptibility and inflammatory responses vary among locations, species, and individuals. Unique inflammatory responses, genetically determined, also influence atherogenesis.

Canine and subhuman primate (rhesus and cynomolgus monkey) models develop atherosclerosis in response to dietary manipulation[48-56] and demonstrate plaque regression in response to serum cholesterol lowering. However, lesion production in susceptible species is not a result of simple dietary cholesterol overload. Any diet that causes hypercholesterolemia induces atherosclerosis. The presence of excess, or even any, cholesterol is not necessary in atherogenic diets. In developmental subhuman primate feeding experiments, reduction of cholesterol content to 0.5% combined with sugar and eggs produced rapidly progressive plaques, whereas high cholesterol addition (up to 7% by weight) did not.[49,50] In rabbits, a variety of semipure, purified cholesterol-free diets with various amino acid compositions induced hypercholesterolemia and atherosclerosis.[57]

Epidemiologic observations provide important circumstantial evidence linking hyperlipidemia to atherosclerosis.[58] Compelling evidence that elevated LDL cholesterol is an etiologic factor in atherosclerosis is provided by genetic hyperlipidemias, in spite of Stehbens's objections that highly cellular lipid-laden atheromas may be different lesions in these patients.[59] These metabolic disorders are most often due to a lack or abnormality of LDL receptors on hepatocytes, which causes an ability to internalize and metabolize LDL, an important observation that earned Brown and Goldstein a Nobel Prize.[60] Serum cholesterol levels are markedly elevated early in life; individuals with the homozygous condition die prematurely from atherosclerosis, rarely living beyond age 26 years. Unfortunately, the heterozygous condition is not uncommon, with total cholesterol levels ranging up to 350 mg/dL. These individuals account for 1 in 500 live births,[61] and they suffer from premature atherosclerosis, generally in middle age. The atheromas of these patients appear to be similar in morphology to those seen in individuals with acquired hyperlipidemia or premature atherosclerosis associated with heavy smoking.

This unfortunate natural experiment is powerful evidence that elevated LDL cholesterol is a relentless factor in plaque inception and the rapid progression of atherosclerosis to lethal consequences. Experience with liver transplantation has been successful in retarding the progress of this type of atherosclerosis.[62] Familial hypercholesterolemias are autosomal dominant disorders produced by at least 12 different molecular defects of the LDL receptors. Familial abnormalities of high-density lipoprotein (HDL), a negative risk factor for atherosclerosis, also exist. In addition to LDL and HDL metabolism, surface proteins of the lipoprotein complex or apoproteins appear to be relevant to pathogenesis.

THROMBOGENIC HYPOTHESIS

In the mid-19th century, Rokitansky postulated that fibrinous substances deposited on the arterial intimal surface as a result of abnormal hemostatic elements in the blood could undergo metamorphosis into atheromatous masses containing cholesterol crystals and globules.[63] This theory held that atheromatous lesions resulted mainly from degeneration of blood proteins (i.e., fibrin deposited in the arterial intima). Duguid repopularized this theory in 1946.[64] In experimental models, usually rabbits, indwelling arterial catheters or arterial injury caused cholesterol accumulation and arterial lesions without the necessity of added dietary cholesterol.[65] As mentioned, gelatinous plaques may also evolve in such a manner that accumulation of blood proteins dominates lesion development.

MESENCHYMAL HYPOTHESIS— HEMODYNAMIC EFFECTS

Smooth cells in the intima and subsequent connective tissue production by these cells have been postulated as the primary and even crucial steps in atherogenesis.[66,67] Proteoglycan, an important arterial wall element, can trap infiltrated LDL, even when LDL is not elevated in the blood. Collagen is the other space-filling component of advanced atherosclerotic lesions. Hauss and colleagues proposed that the migration of smooth muscle cells from the media to the intima, with proliferation and production of connective tissue, is a nonspecific arterial reaction to any injury and that atherosclerosis simply reflects a generic arterial response.[68] Chisolm and colleagues called this the "nonspecific" mesenchymal hypothesis.[21] These scenarios are similar to wound-healing responses to injury. In part, this theory attempts to explain why physical factors such as shear stress, vasoactive agents, and repetitive injuries induce similar sequences of events in the vessel wall.

Stehbens, highly skeptical of the lipid hypothesis, stated, "Atherosclerosis constituted the degenerative and reparative process consequent upon the hemodynamically induced engineering fatigue of the blood vessel wall."[59] He postulated that "the vibrations consisting of the pulsations associated with cardiac contractions and the vortex shedding generated in the blood vessels at branchings, unions, curvatures, and fusiform dilatations (carotid sinus) over a lifetime are responsible for fatigue failure after a certain, but individually variable, number of vibrations."[59] In this view, atherosclerosis, a process of wear and tear, becomes an inexorable (and unavoidable) process associated with aging. Hypertension[69] and tachycardia induced in experimental animals through atherogenic feeding caused accelerated plaque development, whereas bradycardia induced by sinoatrial node ablation in monkeys reduced coronary and carotid atherosclerosis.[70,71]

MONOCLONAL HYPOTHESIS—SMOOTH MUSCLE PROLIFERATION

The morphologic similarity of smooth muscle proliferation in some atherosclerotic lesions to uterine smooth muscle myomas led Benditt and Benditt to suggest that atherosclerotic lesions are derived from a singular or, at most, a few mutated smooth muscle cells that, like tumor cells, proliferate in an unregulated fashion.[66] This theory is based on the finding of only one allele for glucose-6-phosphate dehydrogenase in lesions from heterozygotes. A homology exists between the β chain of human PDGF and the protein product of the v-sis oncogene, which is a tumor-causing gene derived from simian sarcoma virus. Tumor-forming cells in culture express the genes for one or both of the PDGF chains and secrete PDGF into the medium.[21] This hypothesis considers events causing smooth muscle cell proliferation to be critical in atherogenesis. Actions of other growth factors, which might either stimulate or inhibit cell proliferation, depend on circumstances as well as on macrophage-derived cytokine activity. For example, the finding of TGF-ß receptors in human atherosclerosis provides evidence of an acquired resistance to apoptosis.[72]

Resistance to apoptosis may lead to proliferation of resistant cell subsets associated with progression of lesions. Multiple factors influence smooth muscle proliferation, transformation, and collagen secretion. Because *all* arterial cells (endothelium, macrophages, and smooth muscle) elaborate chemotactic and growth factors, this hypothesis more likely relates to reactive responses rather than to first causes.

RESPONSE-TO-INJURY HYPOTHESIS

As a result of experimental data and deductive reasoning, Ross and Glomset postulated two pathways for the promotion of atheroma formation.[73] In the first (e.g., in hypercholesterolemia), monocyte and macrophage migration occurs without endothelial denudation. In some instances, endothelial loss might occur, with platelets carpeting bare areas. In this event, platelets would stimulate proliferation of smooth muscle by releasing PDGF.

In the second pathway, the endothelium itself was postulated to release growth factors, stimulating smooth muscle proliferation. Experimental rabbit arterial balloon injury shows that regrowing endothelium induces myointimal proliferation beneath its advancing edges, stimulating accumulation of collagen[74] and glycosaminoglycans.[75] As mentioned, stimulated smooth muscle itself releases growth factors, leading to a continued autocrine proliferative response. In the initial iteration of this theory, the second pathway was postulated to be relevant to atheroma stimulated by diabetes, possibly in relation to insulin-derived growth factors, cigarette smoking, or hypertension. Although hypertension causes endothelial injury, there are striking differences between the behavior of smooth muscle cells in atherosclerosis and in hypertension. Atherosclerosis stimulates an overt smooth muscle proliferative response. In most instances, pure hypertension causes thickening of the arterial wall by virtue of increased protein synthesis, without an increase in cell number.[76]

The reasons for examining atherosclerosis and arterial wall injury should be obvious, particularly to vascular surgeons. Arterial trauma, such as clamping or balloon injury, produces stenoses and vascular injuries (ranging from minor to severe) and initiates both myointimal hyperplasia and atheromas. This view of atherogenesis implies that the process is most often a response to injury. In this scenario, physical or chemical agents cause endothelial denudation, followed by platelet adherence and subsequent release of PDGF,[77] which then triggers smooth muscle migration from the media to the intima, smooth muscle cell proliferation, and lipid accumulation. The sequence applies in specific situations of injury to the arterial wall, particularly with disruption of the internal elastic lamina.

Injury as a global theory of atherogenesis has not been supported by subsequent observations of early atherogenesis, however. Arterial denudation is a *rare event* in early atherogenesis in humans and animals, although endothelial cells can be injured or dysfunctional and remain in place.[78] We now know that systemic endothelial dysfunction exists in atherosclerosis.[79] Such dysfunction exerts profound effects on systemic vasodilatation, and upregulation of endothelial receptors facilitates entry of cells and blood components through intact endothelium. Because all arterial wall cells can secrete growth factors that are very similar if not identical to PDGF and its derivatives, it is not necessary to postulate physical endothelial disruption.

The responses of the arterial wall after injury remain of considerable practical interest in both atherogenesis and intimal hyperplasia. With injury, early medial smooth muscle proliferation is the first step, influenced primarily by basic fibroblast growth factor.[80] Migration and production of an extracellular matrix are the second and third stages of injury. These mechanisms are relevant to trauma-provoked atheromas, which occur as a result of clamping or balloon injuries even with modestly elevated levels of LDL cholesterol.[81] Other mitogens include angiotensin II, which causes smooth muscle to proliferate and induces expression of growth factors.[82,83] One of these growth factors, TGF-β, exerts either stimulatory or inhibitory effects, depending on circumstances. Injury also induces medial angiotensinogen gene expression, along with angiotensin receptor expression.[84] Other smooth muscle antigens include thrombin, catecholamine, and possibly endothelin. Thus, atheromas developing in a setting of injury (mechanical, immunologic, or infectious) are influenced by these trauma-induced growth factors in varying degrees and sequences. In turn, plasma LDL elevation accentuates neointimal hyperplasia[85,86] without actual atheroma formation in the classic sense.

LESION ARREST OR REGRESSION

In considering pathogenesis and treatment, the potential for plaque regression and stabilization of vulnerable plaques are key issues. Regression of atherosclerosis in response to lowered serum cholesterol has been demonstrated in autopsy studies of starved humans dating back to the World War I,[15] in animal models,[87] and in pioneering clinical angiographic trials combining cessation of smoking with lipid reduction.[88] In humans, trials of vascular end points have shown some impressive examples of regression in coronary arteries; more commonly, minimal anatomic regression is seen, along with slowing of progression, but with drastic reductions in coronary events.[89] Importantly, magnetic resonance imaging has documented favorable longitudinal changes in carotid plaque composition, with reduction of the lipid core and increased fibrous tissue.[90]

As atherosclerotic plaques in experimental animals regress, plaque bulk is reduced mainly by lipid egress. This has been shown convincingly in experiments using hypercholesterolemic dogs[48,49] and monkeys.[50-53] The exact mechanisms of lesion regression, particularly the roles of inflammatory and immune responses, are incompletely understood. However, regression has been demonstrated using serial observations of decreased bulk of individual plaques; reduced luminal encroachment, as shown by edge defects on sequential angiography; and decreased plaque lipid and altered fibrous protein content measured histologically and chemically.[53] An important technical aspect of this research was the confirmation of regressive changes using immediate autopsy or surgical observation and biopsy. Grossly or histopathologically, plaque change correlated with observed regressive angiographic changes.[54,55] Stary studied regression of advanced lesions in atherosclerotic rhesus monkeys.[91] He showed disappearance of macrophages, macrophage-derived foam cells, lymphocytes, and extracellular lipids, with drastic reduction of blood cholesterol for 42 months. However, arterial wall calcium deposits did not visibly change, and as might be expected, calcification is clearly a limiting factor in regression.

Correlative observations are not readily obtained in humans, but angiographic and intravascular ultrasonography has been used to assess treatment effects, mainly in coronary arteries. Experimentally, decreased luminal intrusion on sequential angiography coincided with decreased plaque size and reduced lipid content, and this appears to be the case in human observations.[22] In some instances of regression, our laboratory found that fibrous protein increased during regression.[53] Although fibrosis might limit regression, this process converts a soft atheromatous plaque into a more stable lesion. Active lesions, particularly in the coronary arteries, are not necessarily the most occlusive ones, and although angiographic edge changes may be minimal, the reduction in coronary events in response to lipid-lowering treatment appears to be related to plaque stabilization. To produce regression consistently, serum cholesterol must be reduced well below 200 mg/dL. Experimentally, there are serum cholesterol levels above which lesions inevitably progress.[55] In addition, combinations of antiplatelet agents in experimental models cause more rapid progression during hypercholesterolemia.[56] Lipid thresholds in humans approximate a total serum cholesterol level of 150 to 170 mg/dL and an LDL level of 100 mg/dL or less, levels that Roberts cited in populations in which atherosclerosis is virtually absent.[92] In extrapolating such epidemiologic data to secondary treatment, inflammatory responses need to be considered because they might promote instability of plaques, even in the absence of hyperlipidemia.

Medical Management
GENERAL CONSIDERATIONS

The fact that populations free of coronary disease show total cholesterol levels below 150 mg/dL and LDL cholesterol levels below 100 mg/dL led Roberts to question the primacy of other "atherosclerotic risk factors" that are not uncommon in these populations.[92] In examining the usefulness of the lipid hypothesis in treatment rather than prevention, considerable positive evidence has accumulated to support an energetic approach to lipid reduction overall, with qualifications. A recent randomized, placebo-controlled trial with simvastatin in more than 20,000 individuals showed a reduction of adverse cardiovascular events and prolongation of life when this agent was used for primary and secondary prevention, even in individuals without elevated lipid levels.[93] Statins have an anti-inflammatory effect, as shown by decreased C-reactive protein levels,[94] occurring independently of LDL reduction.[95] These results, initially obtained with cerivastatin, which is now off the market due to toxic effects, have also been observed with pravastatin.[96] Overall, many more individuals have become candidates for treatment to reach the recently revised goals of the National Cholesterol Education Project of total cholesterol less than 150 mg/dL and LDL less than 100 mg/dL.[97] These stringent target levels can seldom be achieved with diet alone. Empirically, a statin, along with aspirin (an anti-inflammatory), clopidogrel (an antiplatelet agent), and angiotensin-converting enzyme (ACE) inhibitors now appear to be indicated in patients with peripheral arterial disease.[98]

Clinicians treating atherosclerosis recognize that complications and deleterious clinical events associated with this disease are not singular and univariate but multiple and interactive.

In the late pathogenesis of atheromas, the instability of the fibrous plaques involves more than lipid dynamics. In considering the possible etiologic concepts more than 4 decades ago, Holman and colleagues pointed out that "a sharp line of distinction exists between atherogenesis and the subsequent evolution of lesions that may or may not precipitate *clinical* disease, for the factors involved in the evolution of lesions beyond the stage of fatty streaks may be entirely different from the factors that initiate fatty streaks" (emphasis added).[99] Among these factors, we now know, are inflammatory and immune mechanisms, altered fibrous proteins, accumulation of blood elements, and cap rupture. Among the interventions intended to produce plaque stabilization or regression, lipid manipulation (i.e., decreasing LDL cholesterol or increasing HDL cholesterol) has promoted favorable changes in atheromas and outcomes, although the anti-inflammatory statin effect appears to be a serendipitous benefit. Based on clinical trial data, smoking cessation is required for lipid reduction to achieve the best clinical results.

In angiographic regression trials, the most favorable plaque changes in terms of arrest or regression occur with the degree and duration of blood lipid reduction. Blankenhorn and Hodis reviewed these data in peripheral arteries, noting that regression and stabilization were 1.5 to 2 times more common in treated subjects than in those receiving placebos.[88] Although the angiographic studies show plaque regression trends, wall change is usually small compared with what is believed to be stabilization of vulnerable lesions. Ornish and colleagues reported favorable clinical results using serial coronary angiography among patients randomly assigned to an experimental group consuming a 10% fat, 12-mg cholesterol diet and undergoing smoking cessation, stress management training, and exercise.[100] After 1 year, 82% of the treated group showed regressive changes in coronary artery plaques that depended, in some degree, on the amount of initial lesion encroachment.

Rational treatment aims to improve the arterial lesions, thus affecting outcomes. Increased fibrous protein synthesis produces a stable, fibrotic plaque as opposed to a soft, friable plaque containing an unstable, atheromatous core covered by a tenuous cap. However, a densely sclerotic, highly occlusive lesion can also cause distal ischemia. In evaluating these hypotheses with a view toward better prediction and control, ameliorating the atheroma itself and providing quantifiable evidence of favorable changes has correlated, for the most part, to effective and even drastic blood lipid reduction. Desirable changes include fibrotic, smaller plaques, which might permit enhanced blood flow but are more stable than soft, bulky, friable lesions irrespective of lesion bulk.

Atherosclerosis is often segmental; bypassing or removing symptomatic arterial lesions in selected arterial segments minimizes the deleterious effects of dangerous lesions. These observations, made more than 4 decades ago, were uniquely surgical insights and brought life- and limb-saving interventions to many patients. Arterial interventions, which now include endovascular approaches, are important means of treating patients with advanced, symptomatic atheromas, including specific patterns of coronary involvement, high-grade carotid lesions, and aortic disease. However, surgical or endovascular treatment of one arterial segment does not prevent disease progression in other segments, and life expectancy remains shortened. Continued smoking after reconstruction can make matters worse, particularly after ill-advised infrainguinal reconstruction for stable claudicants. Aspirin, urokinase, and anticoagulants can prevent or minimize superimposed embolic phenomena and clotting, but underlying plaques continue to progress. Modification of inflammatory responses provoked by cytokine-derived or immune-modulating factors has potential and may now be practical, given the current ability to monitor blood levels of inflammatory cytokines and C-reactive protein,[101] which appear to predict and influence coronary events.

Apparently insignificant or small plaques, particularly in coronary or cerebral arteries, can provoke arterial spasm. Atherosclerotic plaques impair the normal effect of endothelium-derived relaxing factor[102,103] and impair vasodilator responses in coronary and cerebral arteries.[104] Dietary treatment of experimental atherosclerosis restores endothelium-dependent relaxation responses within certain limits,[105] whereas long-term inhibition of nitric oxide synthesis by feeding promotes experimental atherosclerosis.[106]

CLINICAL MANAGEMENT

All patients with two or more risk factors or any form of vascular disease require a lipid profile and a fasting blood glucose sample. Fasting blood samples measure HDL cholesterol levels. The LDL cholesterol level is calculated as follows: LDL cholesterol = total cholesterol − HDL cholesterol + (triglycerides/5). This formula holds for fasting patients when triglycerides are below 400 mg/dL. Serum cholesterol levels must be obtained with patients on a regular diet outside the hospital. Acute illnesses cause sudden and inexplicable decrements in total serum cholesterol.

The National Cholesterol Education Program recommends dietary approaches as a first step for patients with atherosclerotic vascular diseases.[97] The patient's age and sex must be considered when choosing a therapy, with routine determination of HDL cholesterol level initially. The initial emphasis is on physical activity and weight loss. I have long supplied hyperlipidemic patients with information on diet and routinely recommend exercise in the form of walking. Drug treatment is delayed in patients with a low risk of coronary heart disease (e.g., no smoking, diabetes, or hypertension) or who are younger than 45 years (men) or 55 years (women). Emphasis has been placed on a high level of HDL cholesterol, as this is a powerful negative risk factor, but selectively increasing HDL levels can be difficult to accomplish.

DRUG THERAPY FOR HYPERLIPIDEMIA

Currently available drugs include cholestyramine and colestipol (bile acid sequestrants), nicotinic acid (a B-complex vitamin), and the widely used statin drugs. Statins are 3-hydroxy-3-methylglutaryl coenzyme A reducing agents that include pravastatin, lovastatin, simvastatin, atorvastatin, and fluvastatin. These agents inhibit hepatic cholesterol biosynthesis. Gemfibrozil is a fibric acid derivative that has an unknown mechanism of action. The drug probucol, along with its monosuccinic ester, is an antioxidant member of a newly emerging class of agents that has been found to be effective in preventing atherosclerosis in animal models and improving coronary artery lumen diameter in the Antioxidant Restenosis Trials.[107] The natural vitamins E and C, considered to be antioxidants, may have an effect in increasing HDL.[108]

Early coronary disease trials examining the use of vitamin E supplements suggested an associated 40% lower risk of coronary disease.[109,110] However, in more recent trials, vitamin C and E supplements had no effect in preventing coronary heart disease events or in improving outcomes in established coronary heart diease.[111,112] Treatment that both lowers LDL cholesterol and raises HDL cholesterol is considered desirable. The dramatic results of intensive LDL lowering in the 2004 REVERSAL trial support the concept of "the lower the better" for treatment of patients with coronary artery disease.[113,114] A higher dose of atorvastatin (80 mg) was more effective than a lower dose of pravastatin (40 mg) in reducing LDL to 79 mg/dL, significantly reducing C-reactive protein while producing a significant reduction in atheroma volume and preventing the progression of coronary lesions. Statin drugs, combined with niacin in nondiabetics, have achieved dramatic reductions in coronary events, possibly related to nonlipid actions affecting endothelial function, inflammatory response, plaque stability, and thrombus formation.[115] The side effects of niacin are difficult to tolerate in many instances, and raising HDL levels remains less practical than lowering LDL levels. A new strategy—administering a new lipid-lowering agent, ezetimibe, along with a statin—has recently proved effective.[116] This agent selectively inhibits intestinal absorption of cholesterol and phytosterols, allowing patients to reach LDL levels less than 100 mg at lower simvastatin doses than with statin monotherapy.

CONTROL OF ASSOCIATED RISK FACTORS

Cigarette Smoking

Cigarette smoking is a powerful risk factor for atherosclerotic disease and promotes its clinical complications even when lipids are normal. This addiction is directly related to limb amputation, high mortality due to ischemic heart disease, and failure of aortic and femoropopliteal grafts.[117-119] The mechanisms by which cigarette smoking promotes atherosclerosis and graft thrombosis are incompletely understood. Carbon monoxidemia possibly predisposes to arterial wall injury, producing increased plasma flux and entry of LDL and other proteins. Cigarette smoking also causes increased platelet reactivity, peripheral vasoconstriction, and lowered HDL levels.[120] From the standpoint of pathogenesis and treatment, lipid abnormalities have received much attention, but from the standpoint of effective clinical interventions, smoking cessation is critical.

At a minimum, clinical practice guidelines should include routine institutional identification of and intervention with all tobacco users at every visit. Clinicians should ask about and record the tobacco use status of every patient All smokers should be offered smoking cessation treatment at every office visit—nicotine replacement therapy short term, and agents such as bupropion long term to treat depression.[121] The latter drug may offer prosexual benefits over other antidepressants. Cessation treatment, even as brief as 3 minutes, may be of some help. Formal clinician-delivered support and life skills training are important treatment components; the more intense the treatment, the more effective it will be in achieving long-term abstinence. To these guidelines I would add another for vascular surgeons: *elective* interventions in smokers for claudication alone should be avoided, because

graft occlusion often occurs and makes eventual amputation more likely.

Hypertension

Control of hypertension prolongs life and reduces coronary mortality.[122] In experimental animals, atherosclerosis associated with hyperlipidemia is accelerated by chronic hypertension.[123] However, as with cigarette smoking, Asian and Caribbean populations may exhibit hypertension with a low incidence of atherosclerotic disease in the absence of hyperlipidemia. In affluent societies, prospective studies show that hypertension is related to the risk of premature atherosclerotic disease independently of the risk factors of hyperlipidemia and cigarette smoking.[124] In older patients, hypertension may be linked with risk factor clustering, including glucose intolerance, hyperinsulinemia, and dyslipidemia promoted by abdominal obesity,[125] the so-called metabolic syndrome, or syndrome X. Here, weight loss, exercise, and drug treatment are needed. Treatment of hypertension with thiazide diuretics was disadvantageous in terms of coronary outcome in a subgroup of men in the Multiple Risk Factor Intervention Trial,[126] likely owing to mediocre control of lipid levels when total cholesterol remained well above 200 mg/dL prior to the availability of statins. The current goal for blood pressure is 120/80 using lifestyle changes, weight loss, and blood pressure medications based on patient age, race, and presence or absence of diabetes. Drugs with specific benefits include ACE inhibitors, diuretics, and beta blockers. Lifestyle alterations include weight reduction, reduced dietary sodium intake, reduced alcohol intake, increased physical activity, and possibly increased calcium intake.[127]

Exercise

Regular exercise decreases total serum cholesterol, LDL, and fasting triglycerides and has variable effects on HDL.[128] The preventive effects of exercise have been well documented; a sedentary lifestyle is an important risk factor for coronary disease.[129] No study, however, has shown that exercise has a direct effect on established atherosclerotic plaques; experimental and clinical data have demonstrated arrest or regression of plaques with lipid reduction. Strenuous unsupervised exercise can be dangerous in the presence of preexisting coronary disease.[130] Exercise does not compensate for persistent uncorrected hyperlipidemia or continued cigarette smoking. This is an important message for patients with vascular disease. Exercise is not sufficient to offset the effects of elevated total cholesterol and LDL, nor should it be considered a replacement for treatment of hypertension. Weight loss and drugs are probably more effective.[131]

Beneficial effects of exercise in peripheral vascular disease (i.e., increased walking distance) relate to improved skeletal muscle oxidative metabolism.[132] Exercise is important secondary therapy. Exercise programs can be more effective for claudication over the long term than surgical or endovascular intervention, particularly in infrainguinal atherosclerosis. In patients with coronary atherosclerosis, exercise prescriptions must be carefully structured. Before prescribing strenuous exercise, stress testing or monitoring to detect silent ischemic heart disease is recommended. Recently, exercise has been shown to reduce C-reactive protein levels, suggesting a favorable effect on this marker or surrogate for inflammation.[133]

Diabetes

Diabetes is one of the most important risk factors or actual pathogenetic factors promoting atherosclerosis. Most patients with peripheral arterial disease who are nonsmokers are diabetic. In its singular form, diabetes is associated with severe infracrural and coronary atherosclerosis. One diabetes control trial showed a reduction in microvascular complications with "tight control" using insulin; unfortunately, this trial was not designed to study end points of macrovascular atherosclerotic complications.[134] Diabetes' effect on atherogenesis has not been studied extensively in animal models of atherosclerosis.

Causes of enhanced atherogenesis in diabetes include abnormalities in apoproteins and lipoprotein particle distribution, particularly elevated levels of lipoprotein(a),[135] an independent thromboatherosclerotic risk factor. In poorly controlled diabetes, a procoagulant state exists. Increased glucose levels are associated with accelerated platelet aggregation in vitro, and the accompanying hypertriglyceridemia enhances thrombogenic factors V, II, and X. Glyco-oxidation and oxidation contribute to LDL entry into macrophages, and glycation of proteins and plasma in the arterial wall contributes to accelerated atherosclerosis. Hormones, growth factors, cytokine-enhanced smooth muscle cell proliferation, and increased foam cell formation are also postulated to be unique aspects of atherogenesis in diabetes mellitus.[136]

Both hyperinsulinemia and insulin resistance are associated with atherosclerosis,[137] and both are associated with type 2 diabetes. Both insulin and glucose stimulate the growth of diabetic infragenicular smooth muscle cells.[138] A possible mechanism accounting for atherogenesis in diabetes is impaired vasoactivity; one study showed that troglitazone, an insulin-action enhancer, corrects impaired brachial artery vasoactivity in patients with occult diabetes (impaired glucose tolerance).[139] This suggests that agents that enhance insulin action may be advantageous. In view of the utility of tight control in preventing microvascular and infectious complications, control of blood glucose on a consistent basis is advisable. For any given level of LDL, coronary heart disease risk is increased three- to fivefold in patients with diabetes compared with nondiabetics,[140] an important consideration in medical management. In diabetic patients, elevated triglyceride levels most commonly accompany severely elevated cholesterol levels; this particular combination greatly increases the risk of adverse coronary events. Diabetics exhibit particular lipid abnormalities, including chylomicronemia, increased very-low-density lipoprotein (VLDL) levels, increased VLDL and chylomicron remnants, and triglyceride-rich LDL and HDL concentrations. Mamo and Proctor emphasized the pathogenicity of these remnants.[141] Glycosylation of lipoproteins and collagen relates directly to levels of glucose, contributing to increased binding of LDL by collagen, and glycosylated lipoproteins are taken up avidly by macrophages to transform these into foam cells. In the morbidly obese, type 2 diabetes can be reversed in early stages by bariatric surgery.[142] Target goals for treatment include fasting glucose below 110 mg/dL, hemoglobin A1c less than 7%, blood pressure below 130/80, LDL less than 100 mg/dL, and triglycerides below 150 mg/dL. The use of an ACE inhibitor along with a statin should be considered in all cases.

ANTIOXIDANTS AND INFLAMMATORY EVENTS

Treatment with antioxidants is based on the theory that "oxidative stress" or reactive oxygen species promote oxidized LDL to form foam cells and activate macrophages, which in turn release inflammatory cytokines and growth factors that stimulate smooth muscle proliferation along with vascular wall remodeling and matrix degradation by locally released metalloproteases. Not all cytokines provoke the inflammatory response; IL-10, an anti-inflammatory cytokine, has been found to prevent atherosclerotic events in vitro and in vivo.[143] Conversely, plaque components such as metalloproteinases, inflammatory cytokines, and high-sensitivity C-reactive protein appear in the systemic circulation, presumably as markers of disease severity.[11,144] Determination of the exact relationship between systemic markers and plaque dynamics requires treatment outcome studies.

As described previously, results of randomized trials with antioxidant vitamins have been disappointing,[145] as recently reiterated by Tardiff and colleagues.[107] In certain circumstances, vitamins C and E might actually function as pro-oxidants. Information has been summarized from angiographic trials using percutaneous coronary interventions to assess restenosis and to examine atherosclerotic progression in uninvolved segments. Briefly, both probucol and an experimental monosuccinic ester of probucol yielded improved lumen dimensions in coronary artery segments (both with and without previous intervention), suggesting a role for antioxidant "vascular protectants" in preventing restenosis in coronary arteries after percutaneous interventions.[146] As in all proposed treatments, survival data from clinical trials are required to provide final answers. After coronary interventions and after myocardial infarction, statins confer long-term survival benefit, paradoxically without much effect on restenosis. Another interesting observation concerns failure of folate to protect against restenosis after coronary catheter-based interventions, despite substantial reductions of blood homocysteine levels.[107]

Related to inflammatory and oxidative hypotheses was the suggestion by Sullivan that elevated total body iron stores, accumulating particularly in men and in women after menopause, cause atherosclerotic events.[147] Iron in its ferrous form is a powerful inflammatory and oxidizing agent. Based on this hypothesis, both iron intake and excess vitamin C intake might be considered undesirable, because vitamin C enhances iron absorption and might promote the formation of reactive oxygen species. Epidemiologic evidence for this thesis is supported by longitudinal data, including those from a study of total body iron stores and stroke risk,[148] although the issue has been hotly debated. Decreased ferritin levels due to blood donation was associated with improvement in atherosclerotic disease, whereas a rising ferritin level was associated with disease complications. Changes in the ferritin level over time were thought to predict fatal and nonfatal vascular events. A Veterans Administration cooperative, prospective, randomized, single-blinded clinical trial (FeAST, Leo R. Zarcharski, principal proponent CSP410) is testing the hypothesis that reducing total body iron stores by phlebotomy to achieve ferritin levels of 25 µg/mL (the level in healthy menstruating women) might reduce mortality by 30% in a patient population with advanced peripheral vascular disease. A preliminary study of cytokine signatures as affected by bleeding suggests an anti-inflammatory effect,[11] but as with all surrogate measures, trial outcomes should be used to accept or reject the idea that lowering iron stores will benefit patients with peripheral arterial disease.

HOMOCYSTEINE AND FOLIC ACID SUPPLEMENTATION

Elevated blood levels of homocysteine have emerged as a risk factor for thromboatherosclerotic disease.[149] Elevated homocysteine can be lowered by increasing folic acid intake. Data from a group in Salt Lake City suggest that individuals developing high homocysteine levels associated with coronary risk generally require higher genetic and environmental exposure.[150] These factors include an individual heat-labile protein genetic mutation along with low folic acid intake. Elevated plasma homocysteine levels in subjects with peripheral vascular disease are associated significantly with death caused by coronary heart disease, likely thrombotic in nature and imposed on an atherosclerotic substrate.[151] It is not known whether therapy with folate or vitamin B_{12} or B_6 might control this process, and benefits from folate therapy have yet to be documented. Folic acid supplementation as a public health initiative is controversial and is no longer widely promoted, as it had been in the past.

ANTIPLATELET AND ANTICOAGULANT THERAPY

Antiplatelet therapy does not produce regressive effects on established lesions, although anti-inflammatory effects probably occur; favorable therapeutic effects may also relate to antithrombotic effects. Smaller rather than larger doses of aspirin may be advantageous. In prevention, 325 mg of aspirin on alternate days was used in the Physicians' Health Study.[152] Current recommendations suggest that 75 to 160 mg of aspirin is as effective as higher doses. Data concerning the possible promotion of intraplaque hemorrhage in carotid lesions in patients receiving aspirin are conflicting.

Results of a long-term study of the effects of clopidogrel indicate a statistical advantage of this therapy over aspirin therapy alone. This population included patients with recent myocardial infarction, recent stroke, or established peripheral arterial disease.[153] The largest relative risk reduction for clopidogrel, compared with aspirin, was in fatal and nonfatal myocardial infarction—19.2%.[154] Antiplatelet therapy and oral anticoagulants appear to reduce the risk of graft occlusion and ischemic events after infrainguinal bypass surgery.[155] Oral anticoagulant therapy is the more effective treatment in high-risk patients. Evidence of the beneficial effect of antiplatelet and oral anticoagulant therapy was based on a small number of trials; there is no proof as to which modality is more effective in preventing graft occlusion and ischemic events. Some clinicians use both agents after infrainguinal bypass.

The end point of epidemiologic and other studies often involves a thrombotic episode,[156] and in a prospective study of hemostatic function and cardiovascular death, elevated levels of factors VIIc and VIIIc and fibrinogen (in addition to elevated plasma cholesterol levels) were found to be salient.[157] Elevated fibrinogen is a major risk factor for coronary artery disease and is highly associated with peripheral arterial disease

in men[158]; leukocyte levels may be elevated in both disease states.[159] Recommended treatment to date involves, in addition to smoking cessation, chronic aspirin therapy.

VASOACTIVE DRUGS

Nonlipid strategies, beyond cholesterol reduction, include the use of β-adrenergic receptor blocking agents to reduce catecholamine release, calcium channel blockers to reduce wall stress and inhibit lipid intake, nitrates to relax vascular smooth muscle by nitric oxide release, and ACE inhibitors to block atherogenic effects on angiotensin II. ACE inhibitors improved the primary end points of myocardial infarction, stroke, and death from cardiovascular causes in the HOPE study.[160] Individuals with cardiac arrhythmias and patients with peripheral arterial disease undergoing cardiac or noncardiac surgery should receive beta blockade, as this has been shown to produce consistent reductions in perioperative mortality,[161,162] although further studies are needed, particularly in the presence of very low cardiac output. Symptomatic medical management of claudication may avert the need for a meddlesome infrainguinal intervention; the drug cilostazol is effective in improving walking distance, thus contributing to enhanced activity.[163]

ATHEROSCLEROSIS AND INFECTION

A relationship appears to exist between atherosclerosis and cytomegalovirus (CMV) and *Chlamydia pneumoniae*. A comprehensive review summarized the evidence in support of this relationship.[164] These data are based on case-control studies and histologic and culture evidence from plaques. In terms of causation, when microorganisms are suggested as risk factors for a chronic disease, Koch's postulates may not be fulfilled, as pointed out in this review.[164] CMV is a ubiquitous virus. A similar virus was reported to induce atherosclerosis in chickens, with cholesterol acting as a cofactor.[165] CMV's role in atherosclerosis was postulated based on the high incidence of restenosis after coronary atherectomy in seropositive patients.[166]

The organism *Chlamydia pneumoniae* or its DNA has been detected in atherosclerotic plaques with varying frequency. The reliability of detecting the organism depends on a careful sampling technique that demands a minimum of 15 sections to ensure a 95% chance of detecting all true positives.[167] Chlamydial heat shock protein colocalizes in plaques with *C. pneumoniae*–specific antigen,[168] leading to the hypothesis that *C. pneumoniae*–infected macrophages, upon entering the intima, mediate inflammatory and autoimmune responses by producing chlamydial heat shock protein 60.[169,170] In addition to *Chlamydia* and CMV, *Helicobacter pylori* and herpesvirus have been proposed to play a role in the pathogenesis of atherosclerotic plaques. The deleterious effects of infection presumably relate to inflammation and bacterial heat shock proteins that produce arterial inflammatory and autoimmune reactions. Antibiotic trials testing these hypotheses are under way; some trials have suggested a benefit,[171,172] others were equivocal,[173] and a secondary prevention trial was negative.[174] In an oblique set of observations, periodontal disease, linked epidemiologically to atherosclerosis,[175] might be biologically related to atherogenesis by increasing circulating cytokine levels, thereby promoting a proatherogenic endothelial cell phenotype, with loss of antithrombotic, growth inhibitory, and vasodilator properties. Subjects with periodontal disease, along with diabetics, show impaired brachial artery dilation.[176] Oral infection in an experimental model with the periodontal pathogen *Porphyromonas gingivalis* has been shown to increase IL-6 levels and accelerate atherosclerosis.[177] A randomized trial of periodontal treatment in individuals with both periodontal disease and atherosclerosis has been proposed.[178]

Summary

Medical therapy for atherosclerosis has been found to induce plaque stabilization, reduce adverse clinical events, and prolong life. Recommendations derive from a broad base of pathologic evidence, imaging observations, and randomized trials. For stable claudicants with infrainguinal atherosclerosis and patients after vascular reconstruction, secondary prevention methods include cessation of smoking; aspirin (preferably 81 mg daily), clopidogrel, or both; lipid reduction of total cholesterol below 150 mg/dL and LDL below 100 mg, best achieved with statins, which also offer anti-inflammatory benefits; walking briskly for 30 to 60 minutes daily; and addition of ACE inhibitors for diabetics even with normal blood pressure. These measures should not substitute for or delay direct arterial interventions in the presence of life- or limb-threatening lesions.

KEY REFERENCES

DeBakey ME, Lawrie GM, Glaeser DH: Patterns of atherosclerosis and their surgical significance. Ann Surg 201:115, 1985.

DePalma RG: Patterns of peripheral atherosclerosis: Implications for treatment. In Shepard J (ed): Atherosclerosis: Developments, Complications and Treatment. New York, Elsevier, 1987, p 161.

DePalma RG, Bellon EM, Manalo PM, Bomberger RA: Failure of antiplatelet treatment in dietary atherosclerosis: A serial intervention study. In Gallo LL, Vahouny GV (eds): Cardiovascular Disease: Molecular and Cellular Mechanisms, Prevention, Treatment. New York, Plenum Press, 1987, p 407.

DePalma RG, Hayes VW, Cafferata HT, et al: Cytokine signatures in atherosclerotic claudicants. J Surg Res 111:215, 2003.

DePalma RG, Hubay CA, Insull W Jr, et al: Progression and regression of experimental atherosclerosis. Surg Gynecol Obstet 131:633, 1970.

Feldman T, Koren M, Insull W Jr, et al: Treatment of high-risk patients with ezetimibe plus simvastatin coadministration versus simvastatin alone to attain NCEP Adult Treatment Panel III low-density lipoprotein cholesterol goals. Am J Cardiol 93:1481, 2004.

Ridker PM, Hennekens CH, Buring JE, et al: C reactive protein and other markers of inflammation in the prediction of cardiovascular disease in women. N Engl J Med 342:836, 1990.

Ross R: Atherosclerosis is an inflammatory disease. Am Heart J 138:S419, 1999.

Stary HC, Chandler AB, Dinsmore RE, et al: A definition of advanced types of atherosclerotic lesions and a histological classification of atherosclerosis. A report from the Committee on Vascular Lesions of the Council on Arteriosclerosis, American Heart Association. Arterioscler Thromb Vasc Biol 15:1512, 1995.

Stary HC, Chandler AB, Glagov S, et al: A definition of initial fatty streak and intermediate lesions of atherosclerosis. A report from the Committee on Vascular Lesions of the Council on Atherosclerosis. Arterioscler Thromb Vasc Biol 14:840, 1994.

REFERENCES

1. Criqui MH, Langer RD, Fronek A, et al: Mortality over a period of 10 years in patients with peripheral arterial disease. N Engl J Med 326:381, 1992.

2. DeBakey ME, Lawrie GM, Glaeser DH: Patterns of atherosclerosis and their surgical significance. Ann Surg 201:115, 1985.

3. DePalma RG: Patterns of peripheral atherosclerosis: Implications for treatment. In Shepard J (ed): Atherosclerosis: Developments, Complications and Treatment. New York, Elsevier, 1987, p 161.

4. McMillan GC: Development of atherosclerosis. Am J Cardiol 31:542, 1973.

5. DeBakey ME: Atherosclerosis: Patterns and rates of progression. In Gotto AM Jr, South LL, Allen B (eds): Atherosclerosis Five: Proceedings of the Fifth International Symposium. New York, Springer-Verlag, 1980, p 3.

6. Haimovici H, DePalma RG: Atherosclerosis: Biologic and surgical considerations. In Haimovici H, Ascer E, Hollier LH, et al (eds): Vascular Surgery: Principles and Techniques, 4th ed. Cambridge, Mass, Blackwell Science, 1996, p 127.

7. Classification of atherosclerotic lesions: Report of study group. World Health Organ Tech Rep Ser 57:1, 1958.

8. Guyton JR, Kemp KF: Development of the lipid-rich core in human atherosclerosis. Arterioscler Thromb Vasc Biol 16:4-11, 1996.

9. Ross R: Atherosclerosis is an inflammatory disease. Am Heart J 138:S419, 1999.

10. Frostegard J, Ulfgren A-K, Nyberg P, et al: Cytokine expression in advanced human atherosclerotic plaques: Dominance of proinflammatory (Th1) and macrophage-stimulating cytokines. Atherosclerosis 145:33, 1999.

11. DePalma RG, Hayes VW, Cafferata HT, et al: Cytokine signatures in atherosclerotic claudicants. J Surg Res 111:215, 2003.

12. Desfaits AC, Serri O, Renier G: Normalization of lipid peroxides, monocyte adhesion, and tumor necrosis factor-alpha production in NIDDM patients after gliclazide treatment. Diabetes Care 21:487, 1998.

13. Winkler G, Lakatos P, Nagy Z, et al: Elevated serum TNF-alpha level as a link between endothelial dysfunction and insulin resistance in normotensive obese patients. Diabet Med 16:207, 1999.

14. Fazio S, Linton MF: The inflamed plaque: Cytokine production and cholesterol balance in the vessel wall. Am J Cardiol 88:122E, 2001.

15. Gerszten RE, Mach F, Sauty A, et al: Chemokines, leukocytes, and atherosclerosis. J Lab Clin Med 136:87, 2000.

16. Stary HC, Chandler AB, Glagov S, et al: A definition of initial fatty streak and intermediate lesions of atherosclerosis. A report from the Committee on Vascular Lesions of the Council on Atherosclerosis. Arterioscler Thromb Vasc Biol 14:840, 1994.

17. Stary HC, Chandler AB, Dinsmore RE, et al: A definition of advanced types of atherosclerotic lesions and a histological classification of atherosclerosis. A report from the Committee on Vascular Lesions of the Council on Arteriosclerosis, American Heart Association. Arterioscler Thromb Vasc Biol 15:1512, 1995.

18. Cornhill JF, Hedrick EE, Stary HC: Topography of human aortic sudanophilic lesions. Monogr Atherosclerosis 15:13, 1990.

19. Glagov S, Zarins C, Giddens DP, et al: Hemodynamics and atherosclerosis: Insights and perspectives gained from studies of human arteries. Arch Pathol Lab Med 112:1018, 1988.

20. Insull W Jr, Bartch GE: Cholesterol, triglyceride and phospholipid content of intima, media and atherosclerotic fatty steak in human thoracic aorta. J Clin Invest 45:513, 1966.

21. Chisolm GM, DiCarleto PE, Erhart LA, et al: Pathogenesis of atherosclerosis. In Young JR, Graor RA, Olin JW, Bartholomew JR (eds): Peripheral Vascular Diseases. St. Louis, Mosby-Year Book, 1991, p 137.

22. Aschoff L: Atherosclerosis. In Lectures on Pathology. New York, Hoeber, 1924, p 131.

23. Virchow R: Gesammelte Abhandlungen zur Wissenschaftlichen Medicin. Frankfurt, Meidinger John, 1856, p 496.

24. Fagiotto A, Ross R, Harker L: Studies of hypercholesterolemia in the nonhuman primate. I. Changes that lead to fatty streak formation. Arterioscler Thromb Vasc Biol 4:323, 1984.

25. Fagiotto A, Ross R: Studies of hypercholesterolemia in the nonhuman primate. II. Fatty streak conversion to fibrous plaque. Arterioscler Thromb Vasc Biol 4:341, 1984.

26. Gerrity RG: The role of monocyte in atherogenesis. I. Transition of blood borne monocytes into foam cells in fatty lesions. Am J Pathol 103:181, 1981.

27. Steinberg D, Parthasarathy S, Carew TE, et al: Beyond cholesterol: Modifications of low density lipoprotein that increase its atherogenicity. N Engl J Med 320:915, 1989.

28. Wiklund O, Carew TF, Steinberg D: Role of the low density lipoprotein receptor in the penetration of low density lipoprotein into the rabbit aortic wall. Arterioscler Thromb Vasc Biol 5:135, 1985.

29. Steinbrecher UP: Role of superoxide in endothelial-cell modification of low-density lipoprotein. Biochim Biophys Acta 959:20, 1988.

30. Heinecke JW, Baker L, Rosen L, Chait A: Superoxide mediates modification of low density lipoprotein by arterial smooth muscle cells. J Clin Invest 77:757, 1986.

31. Parthasarathy S, Printz DJ, Boyd D, et al: Macrophage oxidation of low-density lipoproteins generates a form recognized by the scavenger receptor. Arterioscler Thromb Vasc Biol 6:505, 1986.

32. Brand K, Banka CL, Mackman N, et al: Oxidized LDL enhances lipopolysaccharide induced tissue factor expression in human adherent monocytes. Arterioscler Thromb Vasc Biol 14:790, 1994.

33. Frostegard J, Ulfgren AK, Nyberg P, et al: Cytokine expression in advanced human atherosclerotic plaques: Dominance of inflammatory (Th1) and macrophage stimulating cytokines. Atherosclerosis 145:33, 1999.

34. Haust MD: The morphogenesis and fate of potential and early atherosclerotic lesions in man. Hum Pathol 2:1, 1971.

35. Smith EB: Fibrin in the arterial wall. Atherosclerosis 70:186, 1988.

36. Davies MJ, Thomas A: Thrombosis and acute coronary artery lesions in sudden cardiac ischemic death. N Engl J Med 310:1137, 1984.

37. Moore S: Thromboatherosclerosis in normolipidemic rabbits: A result of continued endothelial damage. Lab Invest 29:478, 1973.

38. Stiel GN, Stiel LSG, Schofer J, et al: Impact of compensatory enlargement of atherosclerotic arteries on angiographic assessment. Circulation 80:1603, 1989.

39. Glagov S, Weisenberg E, Zarins C, et al: Compensatory enlargement of human atherosclerotic coronary arteries. N Engl J Med 316:1371, 1987.

40. Clarkson TB, Prichard RW, Morgan TM, et al: Remodeling of coronary arteries in human and nonhuman primates. JAMA 271:289, 1994.

41. Hata Y, Hower J, Insull W Jr: Cholesterol ester-rich inclusions from human aortic fatty streak and fibrous plaque lesions of atherosclerosis. Am J Pathol 75:423, 1974.

42. Baranowski A, Adams CWM, Bayliss-High OB, et al: Connective tissue responses to oxysterols. Atherosclerosis 41:255, 1982.

43. Yla-Herttuala S, Palinski W, Butler S, et al: Rabbit and human atherosclerotic lesions contain IgG that recognizes epitopes of oxidized LDL. Arterioscler Thromb Vasc Biol 13:32, 1993.

44. Maggi E, Chiesa R, Milissano G, et al: LDL oxidation in patients with severe carotid atherosclerosis: A study of in vitro and in vivo oxidation markers. Arterioscler Thromb Vasc Biol 14:1892, 1994.

45. Schmiedt W, Kinscherf R, Deigner HP, et al: Complement CG deficiency protects against diet-induced atherosclerosis in rabbits. Arterioscler Thromb Vasc Biol 18:1790, 1998.

46. DePalma RG, Sidawy AN, Giordano JM: Associated etiological and atherosclerotic risk factors in abdominal aneurysms. In Greenhalgh RM, Mannick JA (eds): The Cause and Management of Aneurysm. London, WB Saunders, 1990, p 37.

47. Anitschkow R: Experimental atherosclerosis in animals. In Cowdry V (ed): Arteriosclerosis: Review of Problem. New York, Macmillan, 1933.

48. DePalma RG, Hubay CA, Insull W Jr, et al: Progression and regression of experimental atherosclerosis. Surg Gynecol Obstet 131:633, 1970.

49. DePalma RG, Insull W Jr, Bellon EM, et al: Animal models for study of progression and regression of atherosclerosis. Surgery 72:268, 1972.

50. DePalma RG, Bellon EM, Insull W Jr, et al: Studies on progression and regression of experimental atherosclerosis: Techniques and application to the rhesus monkey. Med Primatol 3:313, 1972.

51. DePalma RG, Bellon EM, Klein L, et al: Approaches to evaluating regression of experimental atherosclerosis. In Manning GM, Haust MD (eds): Atherosclerosis: Metabolic, Morphologic and Clinical Aspects. New York, Plenum Press, 1977, p 459.

52. DePalma RG, Bellon EM, Koletsky S, et al: Atherosclerotic plaque regression in a rhesus monkey induced by bile acid sequestrant. Exp Mol Pathol 31:423, 1979.

53. DePalma RG, Klein L, Bellon EM, et al: Regression of atherosclerotic plaques in rhesus monkeys. Arch Surg 115:1268, 1980.

54. DePalma RG: Angiography in experimental atherosclerosis: Advantages and limitations. In Bond JG, Insull W Jr, Glagov S, et al (eds): Clinical Diagnosis of Atherosclerotic Lesions: Quantitative Methods of Evaluation. New York, Springer-Verlag, 1983, p 99.

55. DePalma RG, Koletsky S, Bellon EM, et al: Failure of regression of atherosclerosis in dogs with moderate cholesterolemia. Atherosclerosis 27:297, 1977.

56. DePalma RG, Bellon EM, Manalo PM, Bomberger RA: Failure of antiplatelet treatment in dietary atherosclerosis: A serial intervention study. In Gallo LL, Vahouny GV (eds): Cardiovascular Disease: Molecular and Cellular Mechanisms, Prevention, Treatment. New York, Plenum Press, 1987, p 407.

57. Kritchevsky D: Atherosclerosis and nutrition. Nutrition 2:290, 1986.

58. LaRosa JC: Cholesterol lowering, low cholesterol and mortality. Am J Cardiol 72:776, 1993.

59. Stehbens WE: The Lipid Hypothesis of Atherosclerosis. Austin, Tex, RG Landes, 1993.

60. Brown MS, Goldstein JL: Lipoprotein receptors in the liver: Control signals for plasma cholesterol traffic. J Clin Invest 72:743, 1983.

61. Schonfeld G: Inherited disorders of lipid transport. Endocrinol Metab Clin North Am 19:211, 1990.

62. Hoeg JM: Familial hypercholesterolemia: What the zebra can teach us about the horse. JAMA 271:543, 1994.

63. von Rokitansky C: A Manual of Pathological Anatomy. London, Sydenham Society, 1852.

64. Duguid JB: Thrombosis as a factor in the pathogenesis of coronary atherosclerosis. J Pathol 58:207, 1946.

65. Bjorkerud JS, Bondjers G: Arterial repair and atherosclerosis after mechanical injury. 2. Tissue response after induction of a total necrosis (deep longitudinal injury). Atherosclerosis 14:259, 1971.

66. Benditt EP, Benditt JM: Evidence for a monoclonal origin of human atherosclerotic plaques. Proc Natl Acad Sci U S A 70:1753, 1973.

67. Schwartz SM: Cellular proliferation in atherosclerosis and hypertension. Proc Soc Exp Biol Med 173:1, 1983.

68. Hauss WH, Junge-Hulsing G, Hollanden HJ: Changes in metabolism of connective tissue associated with aging and arterio atherosclerosis. J Atheroscler Res 6:50, 1962.

69. Koletsky S, Roland C, Rivera-Velez JM: Rapid acceleration of atherosclerosis in hypertensive rats on a high fat diet. Exp Mol Pathol 9:322, 1968.

70. Beere PA, Glagov S, Zarins CK: Retarding effects of a lowered heart rate on coronary atherosclerosis. Science 226:180, 1989.

71. Beere PA, Glagov S, Zarins CK: Experimental atherosclerosis at the carotid bifurcation of the cynomolgus monkey: Localization, compensatory enlargement and sparing effect of lowered heart rate. Arterioscler Thromb Vasc Biol 12:1245, 1992.

72. McCaffrey TA, Du B, Fu C, et al: The expressions of TGF-beta receptors in human atherosclerosis: Evidence for acquired resistance to apoptosis due to receptor imbalance J Mol Cell Cardiol 31:1627, 1999.

73. Ross R, Glomset JA: The pathogenesis of atherosclerosis. N Engl J Med 295:369, 1976.

74. Chidi CC, DePalma RG: Collagen formation by transformed smooth muscle after arterial injury. Surg Gynecol Obstet 152:8, 1981.

75. Wight TV, Curwen KD, Litrenta MM, et al: Effect of endothelium on glycosaminoglycan accumulation in the injured rabbit aorta. Am J Pathol 113:156, 1983.

76. Schwartz SM, Ross R: Cellular proliferation in atherosclerosis and hypertension. Prog Cardiovasc Dis 26:355, 1984.

77. Ross R, Glomset F, Kariya B, et al: A platelet dependent factor that stimulates the proliferation of arterial smooth muscle cells in vitro. Proc Natl Acad Sci U S A 71:1207, 1974.

78. Ross R: The pathogenesis of atherosclerosis: A perspective for the 1990s. Nature 362:801, 1993.

79. Anderson TJ, Gerhard MD, Meridith IT, et al: Systemic nature of endothelial dysfunction in atherosclerosis. Am J Cardiol 75:7113, 1995.

80. Lindner V, Lappi DA, Baird A, et al: Role of basic fibroblast growth factor in vascular lesion formation. Circ Res 68:106, 1991.

81. DePalma RG, Chidi CC, Sternfeld WC, Koletsky S: Pathogenesis and prevention of trauma provoked atheromas. Surgery 82:429, 1977.

82. Campbell-Bodwell M, Robertson AL Jr: Effects of angiotensin II and vasopressin on human smooth muscle cells in vitro. Exp Med Pathol 35:265, 1981.

83. Itoh H, Mukuyawa M, Pratt RE, et al: Multiple autocrine growth factors modulate vascular smooth muscle in response to angiotensin II. J Clin Invest 91:2268, 1993.

84. Viswanathan M, Stromberg C, Seltzer A, et al: Balloon angioplasty enhances expression of angiotensin II; ATI receptors in neointima of rat aorta. J Clin Invest 90:1707, 1992.

85. Stevens SL, Hilgarth K, Ryan US, et al: The synergistic effect of hypercholesterolemia and mechanical injury on intimal hyperplasia. Ann Vasc Surg 6:55, 1992.

86. Baumann DS, Doblas M, Dougherty A, et al: The role of cholesterol accumulation in prosthetic vascular graft anastomotic intimal hyperplasia. J Vasc Surg 19:435, 1994.

87. St Clair RSW: Atherosclerosis regression in animal models: Current concepts of cellular and biochemical mechanisms. Prog Cardiovasc Dis 26:109, 1983.

88. Blankenhorn DH, Hodis HN: Arterial imaging and atherosclerosis reversal. Arterioscler Thromb Vasc Biol 14:177, 1994.

89. LaRosa JC: Lipid lowering. In LaRosa JC (ed): Medical Management of Atherosclerosis. New York, Marcel Dekker, 1998, p 1.

90. Zhao XQ, Yuan C, Hattsukami TS, et al: Effects of prolonged intensive lipid lowering therapy on the characteristics of carotid atherosclerotic plaques in vivo by MRI: A case-control study. Arterioscler Thromb Vasc Biol 21:1623, 2001.

91. Stary HC: The development of calcium deposits and their persistence after lipid regression. Am J Cardiol 88:16E, 2001.

92. Roberts WC: Atherosclerotic risk factors: Are there ten or is there only one? Am J Cardiol 64:552, 1989.

93. Heart Protection Study Group: MRC/BHF heart protection study of cholesterol lowering with simvastatin in 20,536 high-risk individuals: A randomized placebo controlled trial. Lancet 360:7, 2002.

94. Ridker PM, Rifai N, Lowenthal SP: Rapid reduction in C-reactive protein with cerivastatin among 785 patients with primary hypercholesterolemia. Circulation 6:1191, 2001

95. Burmudez EA, Ridker PM: C-reactive protein, statins, and the primary prevention of atherosclerotic cardiovascular disease. Prev Cardiol 5:42, 2002.

96. Albert MA, Danielson E, Rifai N, Ridker PM: The pravastatin inflammation/CRP evaluation (PRINCE): A randomized trial and cohort study. JAMA 286:64, 2001.

97. Expert Panel on Detection, Evaluation, and Treatment of High Blood Cholesterol in Adults: Executive Summary of the Third Report of the National Cholesterol Education Program (NCEP) Expert Panel on Detection, Evaluation, and Treatment of High Blood Cholesterol in Adults (Adult Treatment Panel III). JAMA 285:2486, 2001.

98. Hiatt WR: Medical treatment of peripheral arterial disease and claudication. N Engl J Med 344:1608, 2001.

99. Holman RLH, McGill HC Jr, Strong JP, Geer JC: Atherosclerosis—the lesion. Am J Clin Nutr 8:84, 1960.

100. Ornish D, Brown SE, Shewritz LW, et al: Can lifestyle changes reverse coronary heart disease? The Lifestyle Heart Trial. Lancet 336:129, 1990.

101. Ridker PM, Hennekens CH, Buring JE, et al: C reactive protein and other markers of inflammation in the prediction of cardiovascular disease in women. N Engl J Med 342:836, 1990.

102. Chester AH, O'Neill GS, Moncada S, et al: Low basal and stimulated release of nitric oxide in atherosclerotic epicardial coronary arteries. Lancet 336:897, 1990.

103. Forstermann U, Mugge A, Alheid U, et al: Selective attenuation of endothelium-mediated vasodilation in atherosclerotic human coronary arteries. Circ Res 62:185, 1988.

104. Heistad DD, Breese K, Armstrong ML: Cerebral vasoconstrictor response to serotonin after dietary treatment of atherosclerosis: Implications for transient ischemic attacks. Stroke 18:1068, 1987.

105. Harrison DG, Armstrong ML, Freiman DC, Heistad DD: Restoration of endothelium dependent relaxation by dietary treatment of atherosclerosis. J Clin Invest 80:1808, 1987.

106. Naruse K, Shimizu K, Muramatsu M, et al: Long-term inhibition of NO synthesis promotes atherosclerosis in the hypercholesterolemic rabbit thoracic aorta. Arterioscler Thromb Vasc Biol 14:746, 1994.

107. Tardif JC, Gregoire J, Lavoie MA, L'Allier PL: Pharmacologic prevention of both restenosis and atherosclerosis progression: AGI 1067, probucol, statins, folic acid and other therapies. Curr Opin Lipidol 14:615, 2003

108. Muckle TJ, Nazi DJ: Variation in human high-density lipoprotein response to oral vitamin E megadosage. Am J Clin Pathol 91:165, 1989.

109. Rimm EB, Stampfer MJ, Aschenio A, et al: Vitamin E consumption and risk of coronary heart disease in men. N Engl J Med 328:1450, 1993.

110. Stampfer MJ, Hennekens CH, Manson JE: Vitamin E consumption and risk of coronary heart disease in women. N Engl J Med 328:1444, 1993.

111. Muntwyler J, Hennekens CH, Manson JE, et al: Vitamin supplement use in a low-risk population of US male physicians and subsequent cardiovascular events. Arch Intern Med 162:1472, 2002.

112. Heart Protection Study Collaborative Group: MRC/BHF Heart Protection Study of antioxidant vitamin supplementation in 20,536 high-risk individuals: A randomized placebo controlled trial. Lancet 360:23, 2002.

113. Nissen SE, Tuzcu EM, Schoenhagen P, et al: Effect of intensive compared with moderate lipid-lowering therapy on progression of coronary atherosclerosis: A randomized controlled trial. JAMA 291:1071, 2004.

114. Scheen AJ, Kulbertus H: REVERSAL and PROVE-IT: Confirmation of the concept "the lower the better" for cholesterol therapy in patients with coronary heart disease. Rev Med Liege 59:167, 2004.

115. Rosenson RS, Tangney CC: Antiatherothrombotic properties of statins: Implications for cardiovascular event reduction. JAMA 279:1643, 1998.

116. Feldman T, Koren M, Insull W Jr, et al: Treatment of high-risk patients with ezetimibe plus simvastatin coadministration versus simvastatin alone to attain NCEP Adult Treatment Panel III low-density lipoprotein cholesterol goals. Am J Cardiol 93:1481, 2004.

117. Wray R, DePalma RG, Hubay CA: Late occlusion of aortofemoral bypass grafts: Influence of cigarette smoking. Surgery 70:696, 1971.

118. Robiesek F, Daugherty HK, Mullen DC: The effect of continued cigarette smoking on the patency of synthetic vascular grafts in Leriche syndrome. J Thorac Cardiovasc Surg 70:107, 1975.

119. Ameli FM, Stein M, Prosser RJ, et al: Effects of cigarette smoking on outcome of femoropopliteal bypass for limb salvage. J Cardiovasc Surg (Torino) 30:591, 1989.

120. Garrison RJ, Kannel WB, Feinleib M, et al: Cigarette smoking and HDL cholesterol. Atherosclerosis 30:17, 1978.

121. Modell JG, Katholi CR, Modell JG, DePalma RL: Comparative sexual side effects of buproprion, fluoxitine, paraxitine and seratraine. Clin Pharmacol Ther 61:476; 1997.

122. Borhani NO, Blaufox MD, Folk BF: Incidence of coronary heart disease and left ventricular hypertrophy in hypertension detection and follow-up programs. Prog Cardiovasc Dis 29(Suppl):55, 1989.

123. Kolestsky S, Roland C, Rivera-Velez JM: Rapid acceleration of atherosclerosis in hypertensive rats on a high fat diet. Exp Mol Pathol 9:322, 1968.

124. Kannel WB: Hypertension and other risk factors in coronary heart disease. Am Heart J 114:918, 1987.

125. O'Donnell CJ, Kannel WB: Epidemiologic appraisal of hypertension as a risk factor in the elderly. Am J Geriatr Cardiol 11:86, 2002.

126. Multiple Risk Factor Intervention Trial Research Group: Multiple risk factor intervention trial: Risk factor changes and mortality results. JAMA 248:1465, 1982.

127. Stone NJ: Lifestyle interventions in atherosclerosis. In LaRosa JC (ed): Medical Management of Atherosclerosis. New York, Marcel Dekker, 1998, p 91.

128. Beard CM, Barnard RJ, Robbins DC: Effects of diet and exercise on qualitative and quantitative measures of LDL and its susceptibility to oxidation. Arterioscler Thromb Vasc Biol 16:201, 1996.

129. Powell KE, Thompson PD, Caspersen CJ, Kendrick JS: Physical activity and the incidence of coronary heart disease. Annu Rev Public Health 8:253, 1987.

130. Williams LR, Ekers MA, Collins PS, Lee JF: Vascular rehabilitation: Benefits of a structured exercise/risk modification programs. J Vasc Surg 14:320, 1991.

131. Hiatt WR: Medical treatment of peripheral arterial disease and claudication. N Engl J Med 344:1608, 2001.

132. Hiatt WR, Regensteiner JG, Hargarten ME: Benefit of exercise conditioning for patients with peripheral arterial disease. Circulation 81:2, 1990.

133. Ford ES: Does exercise reduce inflammation? Physical activity and C reactive protein among US adults. Epidemiology 13:561, 2002.

134. Diabetes Control and Complication Trial Research Group: The effect of intensive treatment of diabetes on the development and progression of long-term complications in insulin-dependent diabetes mellitus. N Engl J Med 329:977, 1993.

135. Loscalzo J: Lipoprotein (a): A unique risk factor for atherothrombotic disease. Arteriosclerosis 10:672, 1990.

136. Bierman EI: Atherogenesis in diabetes. Arterioscler Thromb Vasc Biol 12:647, 1992.

137. Goldberg RB: Insulin resistance and atherosclerosis. In LaRosa JC (ed): Medical Management of Atherosclerosis. New York, Marcel Dekker, 1998, p 283.

138. Avena R, Mitchell ME, Neville RF, Sidawy AN: The additive effects of glucose and insulin on the proliferation of vascular smooth muscle cells. J Vasc Surg 28:10339, 1998.

139. Avena R, Mitchell ME, Nylen ES, et al: Insulin action enhancement normalizes brachial artery vasoactivity in patients with peripheral vascular disease and occult diabetes. J Vasc Surg 28:1024, 1998.

140. Stamler J, Vaccaro O, Nealon JD, Westworth D: Diabetes and other risk factors and 12 year cardiovascular mortality for men screened for MRFIT. Diabetes Care 16:434, 1993.

141. Mamo CL, Proctor SD: Chylomicron remnants and atherosclerosis. In Barter PJ, Rye KA (eds): Plasma Lipids and Their Role in Disease. Melbourne, Australia, Harwood Academic Publishers, 1999, p 109.

142. Sugarman HJ: Bariatric surgery for severe obesity. J Assoc Acad Minor Phys 12:129, 2001.

143. Pindersky Oslund LJ, Hedrick CC, Olvera T, et al: Interleukin-10 blocks atherosclerotic events in vitro and vivo. Arterioscler Thromb Vasc Biol 19:2847, 1999.

144. Ridker PM, Bassuk SS, Toth PP: C-reactive protein and risk of cardiovascular disease: Evidence and clinical application. Curr Atheroscler Rep 5:341; 2003.

145. Witzum JL: Role of antioxidants in prevention of coronary artery disease. In LaRosa JC (ed): Medical Management of Atherosclerosis. New York, Marcel Dekker, 1998, p 41.

146. Wasserman MA, Sundell CL, Kunsch C, et al: Chemistry and pharmacology of vascular protectants: A novel approach to the treatment of atherosclerosis and coronary artery disease. Am J Cardiol 91:34A, 2003.

147. Sullivan JL: Iron and the sex difference in heart disease risk. Lancet 1:1293, 1981.

148. Kiechl S, Willeit J, Landis M, et al: Body iron stores and the risk of carotid atherosclerosis. Circulation 96:3300, 1997.

149. Taylor LM Jr, Porter JM: Elevated plasma homocysteine as a risk factor for atherosclerosis. Semin Vasc Surg 6:36, 1993.

150. Williams RR, Hopkins PN, Wu L, Hunt SC: Applied genetics now and gene therapy in the future. In LaRosa JC (ed): Medical Management of Atherosclerosis. New York, Marcel Dekker, 1998, p 247.

151. Taylor LM, Moneta GL, Sexton GJ, et al: Prospective blinded study of the relationship between plasma homocysteine and the progression of symptomatic peripheral arterial disease. J Vasc Surg 29:8, 1999.

152. Goldhaber SZ, Manson JE, Stumpfer MJ, et al: Low-dose aspirin and subsequent peripheral arterial surgery in the Physicians' Health Study. Lancet 340:143, 1992.

153. CAPRIE Steering Committee: A randomized blinded trial of clopidogrel in patients at risk for ischemic events. Lancet 348:1329, 1996.

154. Gent M: Benefit of clopidogrel in patients with coronary disease. Circulation 96(Suppl):I-476, 1997.

155. Tangelker MJO, Lawson JA, Algre A, Eikelboom BC: Systematic review of randomized controlled trials of aspirin and oral anticoagulants in the prevention of graft occlusion and ischemic events after infrainguinal bypass surgery. J Vasc Surg 30:701, 1999.

156. Meade TW: Cardiovascular disease, linking pathology and epidemiology. Int J Epidemiol 30:1170, 2001.

157. Stone MC, Thorp JM: Plasma fibrinogen: Major coronary risk factor. J R Coll Gen Prac 35:565, 1985.

158. Kannel WB, Wolf PA, Castelli WP, Dagostino RB: Fibrinogen and the risk of cardiovascular disease: The Framingham Study. JAMA 258:1183, 1987.

159. Ernst E, Hammerschmidt DE, Bagge U, et al: Leukocytes and the risk of ischemic diseases. JAMA 257:2318, 1987.

160. Yusef S, Sleight P, Pogue J, et al: Effects of an angiotensin-converting-enzyme inhibitor, ramipril, on cardiovascular events in high-risk patients: HOPE Study Investigators. N Engl J Med 342:145, 2000.

161. Auerbach AD, Goldman L: Beta-blockers and reduction of cardiac events in noncardiac surgery: Scientific review. J Fam Pract 287:1435, 2002.

162. Ferguson TB Jr, Coombs LP, Peterson ED: Preoperative beta-blocker use and mortality and morbidity following CABAG surgery in North America. JAMA 287:2221, 2002.

163. Creager MA: Medical management of peripheral arterial disease. Cardiol Rev 9:238, 2001.

164. High KP: Atherosclerosis and infection due to *Chlamydia pneumoniae* or cytomegalovirus: Weighing the evidence. Clin Infect Dis 28:746, 1999.

165. Fabricant DG, Fabricant J, Litrenta MM, Minick CR: Virus-induced atherosclerosis. J Exp Med 148:335, 1978.

166. Zhou YF, Leon MB, Waclawiw MA, et al: Association between prior cytomegalovirus infection and re-stenosis after coronary atherectomy. N Engl J Med 335:625, 1996.

167. Cochrane M, Pospichal A, Walker P, et al: Distribution of *Chlamydia pneumoniae* DNA in atherosclerotic carotid arteries: Significance for sampling procedures. J Clin Microbiol 41:1454, 2003.

168. Kuroda S, Kobayashi T, Ishii N, et al: Role of *Chlamydia pneumoniae*-infected macrophages in atherosclerosis developments of the carotid artery. Neuropathology 23:1, 2003.

169. Lamb DJ, El-Sankary W, Ferns GA: Molecular mimicry in atherosclerosis: A role for heat shock proteins in immunisation. Atherosclerosis 167:177, 2003.

170. Lowe GD: The relationship between infection, inflammation and cardiovascular disease: An overview. Ann Periodontol 6:1, 2001.

171. Wiesli P, Czerwenka W, Meniconi A: Roxithromycin treatment prevents progression of peripheral arterial occlusive disease in *Chlamydia pneumoniae* seropositve men: A randomized, double blind, placebo-controlled trial. Circulation 105:2646, 2002.

172. Gurfinkle E, Bozovich G, Darsca A, et al: Randomized trial of roxithromycin in non-Q wave coronary syndromes: ROXIS pilot study. Lancet 350:404, 1997.

173. Brassard P, Bourgault C, Brophy J: Antibiotics in primary prevention of myocardial infarction among elderly patients with hypertension. Am Heart J 145:E20, 2003.

174. Zahn R, Schneider S, Frilling B, et al: Antibiotic therapy after myocardial infarction: A prospective randomized study. Circulation 107:1253, 2003.

175. Pussinen PJ, Jousilahti P, Alfthan G, et al: Antibodies to periodontal pathogens are associated with coronary heart disease. Arterioscler Thromb Vasc Biol 23:1250, 2003.

176. Amar S, Gokce N, Morgan S, et al: Periodontal disease is associated with brachial artery endothelial dysfunction and systemic inflammation. Arterioscler Thromb Vasc Biol 23:1245, 2003.

177. Lalla E, Lamster IB, Hofman MA, et al: Oral infection with a periodontal pathogen accelerates early atherosclerosis in apolipoprotein E-null mice. Arterioscler Thromb Vasc Biol 23:1405, 2003.

178. Haynes WG, Stanford C: Periodontal disease and atherosclerosis: From dental to arterial plaque. Arterioscler. Thromb Vasc Biol 23:1309, 2003.

Questions

1. **Which of the following statements about fibrous plaque is true?**
   (a) It always evolves from fatty streaks
   (b) It is classified as a complicated lesion
   (c) It consists mainly of fibrous tissue
   (d) It is confined to the intima
   (e) It contains a yellow "core"

2. **The earliest lesions of atherosclerosis consist of which of the following?**
   (a) Denuded areas of endothelium
   (b) Increased intimal macrophages containing lipid
   (c) Disruption of the internal elastic lamina
   (d) Focal adventitial lymphocytic infiltration
   (e) Gelatinous plaques

3. **In atherosclerosis, macrophages in plaques produce all of the following except**
   (a) Lipoproteins
   (b) Interleukin-1
   (c) Metalloproteinases
   (d) Growth factors
   (e) Interleukin-10

4. **The "core" of a typical fibrous plaque consists mainly of what?**
   (a) Inflammatory cells
   (b) Fibrin and fibrinogen
   (c) Cholesteryl oleate and free cholesterol
   (d) Lysosomal enzymes
   (e) Proteoglycans

5. **Complicated atherosclerotic plaques usually evolve from which of the following?**
   (a) Mechanical injuries
   (b) Thrombogenesis and fibrin deposition
   (c) Immunologic reactions
   (d) Lipid accumulation in foam cells
   (e) None of the above

6. Consistent experimental production of atherosclerotic plaques requires which of the following?
   (a) Feeding of a high-cholesterol diet
   (b) Hyperbetalipoproteinemia
   (c) Hormonal manipulation
   (d) Balloon injury
   (e) Genetically bred animals

7. Which of the following statements about genetic disorders promoting increased levels of low-density lipoprotein cholesterol and atherosclerosis is true?
   (a) They are exceedingly rare
   (b) They are associated with type 1 diabetes
   (c) They occur in about 1 in 500 live births
   (d) They are related to surface defects in a high-density lipoprotein protein moiety
   (e) They can be treated with diet in most cases

8. Regression or arrest of atherosclerotic lesions occurs under what conditions?
   (a) Only in experimental animals
   (b) By egress of fibrous plaque proteins
   (c) By maintaining cholesterol levels between 200 and 250 mg/dL
   (d) By egress of lipids
   (e) By oxidative stress reduction

9. Changes inducing plaque vulnerability include all of the following except
   (a) Fibrous tissue synthesis
   (b) Macrophage infiltration of the cap
   (c) Increasing lipid accumulation
   (d) Leakage of blood products into the core
   (e) Adventitial lymphocyte infiltration

10. Currently accepted clinical management of peripheral arterial disease includes all of the following except
    (a) ACE inhibitors
    (b) Smoking cessation
    (c) Statins
    (d) Macrolide antibiotics
    (e) Programmed exercise

Answers

1. e	2. b	3. a	4. c	5. e
6. d	7. c	8. d	9. a	10. d

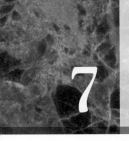

Gregory J. Landry • James M. Edwards

Nonatherosclerotic Vascular Disease

Although the majority of arterial abnormalities of interest to vascular surgeons are caused by atherosclerosis, a significant minority result from inflammatory, acquired, congenital, and developmental abnormalities. This chapter briefly describes the pathogenesis, symptoms, diagnosis, and treatment of a variety of nonatherosclerotic vascular diseases. Topics covered include vasospastic disorders, the vasculitides, heritable arteriopathies, anatomic anomalies, homocystinemia, and a variety of other uncommon disease processes that may be encountered by vascular surgeons.

Vasospastic Disorders

Raynaud's syndrome (RS), variant angina, and migraine headache are the most frequent vasospastic disorders seen in clinical practice. RS is by far the most common vasospastic condition referred to vascular surgeons and is considered in detail here.

RAYNAUD'S SYNDROME

Since the initial description by Maurice Raynaud in 1862, episodic digital ischemia (RS) has remained an enigmatic clinical entity. The digital ischemia in patients with this condition traditionally manifests as tricolor changes—white, blue, and red—although one or more of these color changes may be absent. The affected digits return to normal 10 to 15 minutes after removal of the precipitating stimulus (usually environmental cold or emotional stress), and the fingers remain normal between attacks.

The prevalence of RS in the general population varies with climate and, probably, ethnic origin. In cool, damp climates such as the Pacific Northwest, Scandinavia, and Great Britain, the prevalence approaches 20% to 25%.[1] It is not known whether the lower prevalence in warm, dry climates is due to a decreased occurrence of the syndrome or merely lack of patient complaints. RS occurs most frequently in young women.[2] The median age of onset of RS is 14 years, with only 27% of cases beginning after age 40.[3] Approximately one quarter of patients have a family history of RS in a first-degree relative.[4]

The mechanism of vasoconstriction in RS has been the subject of intense debate for more than a century.

Raynaud speculated that sympathetic nervous system hyperactivity was responsible, a proposition disproved by Lewis in the 1920s when he demonstrated that blockade of digital nerve conduction did not prevent vasospasm.[5] Lewis then proposed the theory of a local vascular fault, the nature of which remains undefined.

In recent years, the focus in RS pathophysiology has been on alterations in peripheral adrenoceptor activity. Increased finger blood flow was noted in patients following α-adrenergic blockade with drugs such as reserpine. Oral and intra-arterial reserpine was the cornerstone of medical management of RS for several years, but it is no longer available.[6] Angiograms of an RS patient before and after cold exposure and before and after intra-arterial reserpine are shown in Figure 7-1.

Research in human vessel models demonstrated increased α_2 receptor sensitivity to cold exposure.[7] α_2 Adrenoceptors appear to play a major role in the production of the symptoms of RS. α_2 Receptors are present in a pure population on human platelets. Receptor levels in circulating cells appear to mirror tissue levels. Owing to the difficulty of obtaining digital arteries from human subjects, we and others have measured levels of platelet α adrenoceptors. An increased level of platelet α_2 adrenoceptors in patients with RS has been demonstrated.[8-10] Increased finger blood flow during body cooling was noted in human controls treated with the α_2-adrenergic antagonist yohimbine,[11] but this finding has not been confirmed by others.[12] Possible mechanisms of α_2-adrenergic–induced RS include an elevation in the number of α_2 receptor sites, receptor hypersensitivity, and alterations in the number of receptors exposed at any one time.

The response of subcutaneous resistance vessels to acetylcholine has been shown to be diminished in patients with RS compared with controls, indicating a possible endothelium-dependent mechanism.[13] The possible roles of the vasoactive peptides endothelin, a potent vasoconstrictor, and calcitonin gene-related peptide (CGRP), a vasodilator, have also been investigated. Serum endothelin levels increased significantly with cold exposure in patients with RS compared with controls.[14,15] Depletion of endogenous CGRP may also contribute, because increased skin blood flow in response to CGRP infusion has been demonstrated in patients with RS compared with that in controls.[16]

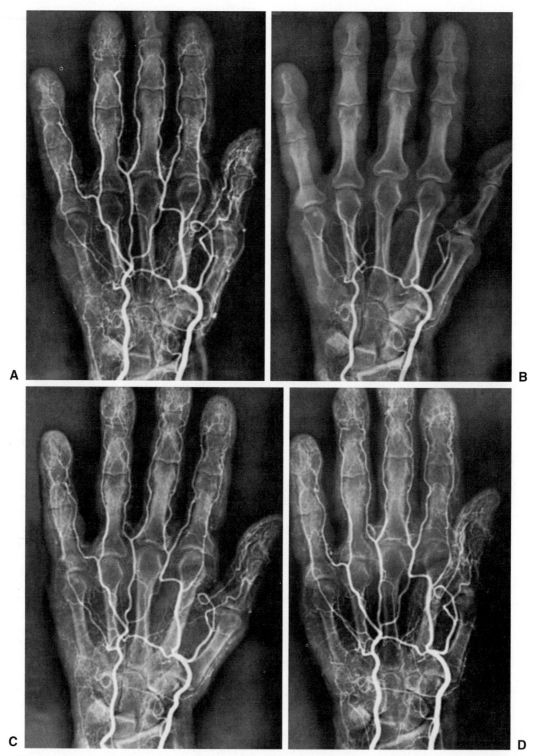

FIGURE 7–1 • Hand angiograms of a Raynaud's syndrome patient before and after cold exposure and before and after administration of intra-arterial reserpine. A marked vasospastic response to cold exposure, which is blocked by reserpine administration, is demonstrated. *A*, Before cold, before reserpine. *B*, After cold, before reserpine. *C*, Before cold, after reserpine. *D*, After cold, after reserpine.

Based on observations primarily at the Mayo Clinic 70 years ago by Allen and Brown,[17] patients with Raynaud's symptoms have traditionally been classified as having either Raynaud's disease or Raynaud's phenomenon, depending on the presence or absence of an associated systemic disease process. However, Raynaud's phenomenon may precede the development of an associated disease by years. In addition, this system does not address the underlying palmar and digital artery disease that may be present. We refer to patients with cold- or stress-induced digital ischemia as having RS, thus avoiding the semantic conflict of "disease" versus "phenomenon."

We have found it useful to subdivide patients with RS into two distinct pathophysiologic groups, obstructive and vasospastic, based on the presence or absence of arterial occlusive disease. Patients with vasospastic RS have patent digital arteries and normal digital artery pressures at room temperature. These patients have an abnormally forceful vasoconstrictive response to cold exposure or emotional stress, leading to digital arterial closure and episodic digital ischemic symptoms. Patients with obstructive RS have significant obstruction of either the palmar and digital arteries or the proximal arm arteries, with a concomitant reduction in resting digital arterial pressure. In these patients, a normal vasoconstrictive response to cold appears to be sufficient to cause digital arterial closure with resultant episodic digital ischemia.

In patients with obstructive RS, the mechanism of the obstructive process is variable. Patients with connective tissue disease typically have an autoimmune vasculitis, which is probably the mechanism underlying the widespread digital and palmar artery occlusions. Patients who work with vibrating tools have a similar process and frequently develop a peculiar fibrotic form of palmar and digital artery obstruction, presumably associated with injury from repeated shear stress.[18] Hypercoagulable states may appear with digital artery occlusions, as can emboli from various sources, including valvular heart disease and subclavian, axillary, and ulnar aneurysms. Atherosclerosis involving the upper extremities is rarely seen in the younger age group but is frequently observed in older patients, especially men.

A number of diseases have been recognized in association with RS, among which the connective tissue diseases are the most frequent; scleroderma is the most common. Associated diseases recognized in our patients with RS are shown in Table 7-1.[19] Estimates of the percentage of patients with RS and an associated disease range from 30% to 80%.[1,20-24] It is important to note that the data from most series come from tertiary care referral centers; therefore, they may not reflect the actual incidence in the general population and may overestimate the actual prevalence of associated diseases. Clearly, most individuals with RS view the condition as a nuisance and do not seek medical advice.

The diagnosis of RS is made by history and physical examination. Noninvasive vascular laboratory testing is used to differentiate obstructive from vasospastic RS. Symptoms are typically described as coldness, numbness, or mild discomfort. Significant pain during attacks is conspicuously absent. Classically, both hands are involved, with frequent sparing of the thumbs. The lower extremities are infrequently involved. Most episodes are induced by cold; however, the cold threshold varies from patient to patient. Emotional stimuli induce attacks in occasional patients. Episodes typically commence with blanching of one or several fingers extending as far as the metacarpophalangeal joint, rarely involving the palm or extending proximally to the wrist. This phase corresponds to vasoconstriction with the absence of blood in digital arteries. After rewarming, the first blood to reach the skin is desaturated, leading to finger cyanosis. Finally, reactive hyperemia leads to digital rubor. Episodes usually last as long as the cold stimulus is present and resolve within 10 to 15 minutes of rewarming. The hands and fingers are normal between attacks.

A history suggestive of an associated connective tissue disease, including arthralgias, dysphagia, sclerodactyly, xerophthalmia, or xerostomia, as well as any prior history of

TABLE 7–1	Associated Diseases in Raynaud's Syndrome Patients: Oregon Health Sciences University Series
Disorder	**Patients (n)**
Autoimmune disease	290
Scleroderma	95
Undifferentiated connective tissue disease	24
Mixed connective tissue disease	23
Systemic lupus erythematosus	17
Sjögren's syndrome	16
Rheumatoid arthritis	9
Positive serology	106
Other diseases or conditions	300
Atherosclerosis	46
Trauma	44
Hematologic abnormalities	42
Carpal tunnel syndrome	35
Frostbite	32
Buerger's disease	28
Vibration	21
Hypersensitivity angiitis	18
Hypothyroidism	13
Cancer	13
Erythromelalgia	8
No associated disease	498
Total	1088

From Landry G, Edwards JM, McLafferty RM, et al: Long-term outcome of Raynaud's syndrome in a prospective analyzed cohort. J Vasc Surg 23:76-86, 1996.

large vessel occlusive disease, malignancy, hypothyroidism, frostbite, trauma, use of vibrating tools, and drug use, should be carefully sought. Carpal tunnel syndrome occurs in approximately 15% of patients with RS.[25] The examiner should carefully evaluate the pulses and assess the digits for evidence of active or healed ulceration, sclerodactyly, telangiectasia, and calcinosis. The optimal serologic evaluation has not been defined. We routinely obtain a complete blood cell count, erythrocyte sedimentation rate, antinuclear antibody titer, and rheumatoid factor. Patients who present with sudden-onset digital ischemia should be evaluated for hypercoagulable states. Tests for specific connective tissue diseases are obtained based on clinical suspicion. Importantly, the physical examination in patients with RS is frequently normal, and the diagnosis relies on history and noninvasive tests.

Routine vascular laboratory testing consists of digital photoplethysmography and digital blood pressures. The digital photoplethysmographic recording provides qualitative information on the character of the arterial waveform.[26] Normal digital blood pressure is within 30 mm Hg of brachial pressure. Patients with obstructive RS have blunted waveforms, whereas patients with vasospastic RS have either normal waveforms or a "peaked pulse." The peaked pulse pattern, first described by Sumner and Strandness,[27] appears to reflect increased vasospastic arterial resistance.

The utility of cold provocation testing remains controversial. Tests involving immersion of patients' hands in ice water are not clinically useful owing to low specificity and reproducibility.[28,29] Of greater clinical utility is a digital hypothermic cold challenge test described by Nielsen and Lassen.[30] This test is performed with a liquid-perfused cuff placed on the proximal phalanx of the target finger. The cuff is inflated to suprasystolic pressure for 5 minutes while it is perfused with cold water. The pressure at which blood flow is detected on deflation of the cuff is recorded. A control finger on the same hand is tested at room temperature. The test is repeated at several temperatures, and the result is expressed as the percentage drop in finger systolic pressure with cooling. In our experience, this test has an overall sensitivity and accuracy of approximately 90%.[31]

Duplex scanning does not appear to have a major role in the diagnosis of RS, although it can be used to search for proximal arterial obstructive or aneurysmal disease. Laser Doppler imaging is a promising new modality that quantifies digital microvascular blood flow and may have future diagnostic applications in RS.[32,33] Angiography was used extensively in the past, particularly in the evaluation of patients with obstructive RS. Patients with an underlying systemic disease process and bilateral palmar and digital arterial obstructive disease documented by vascular laboratory testing do not require angiography to confirm digital artery occlusive disease. Patients with unilateral disease, particularly those who have only one or two digits of one arm involved, should be considered for angiography to determine both the presence of bilateral disease and the presence of any proximal arterial disease.

Avoidance of triggering stimuli, such as cold or emotional stress, is the hallmark of conservative treatment.[34] We advise all patients with RS to avoid tobacco use, although a multicenter epidemiologic study suggested that RS is not strongly influenced by tobacco consumption.[35] Medications that have been associated with the causation of RS symptoms, such as ergot alkaloids and beta blockers, should be avoided if appropriate alternative therapies exist. More than 90% of patients with RS respond adequately to these simple conservative measures and require no additional treatment. The small number of patients who develop digital ulcers in association with obstructive RS can also be managed conservatively. A healing rate of 85% has been achieved with simple treatment consisting of soap and water scrubs, antibiotics as selected by culture, and conservative débridement.[36] Calcium channel blockers are the most widely used pharmacologic agent for the treatment of RS. As a rule, patients with vasospastic RS respond more favorably to medical therapy than do those with occlusive RS. Our current medication of choice for the treatment of RS is extended-release nifedipine (30 mg every night). Approximately two thirds of patients placed on nifedipine experience subjective benefit. Ten percent to 20% of patients are unable to continue the medication because of unacceptable side effects, including headache, ankle swelling, pruritus, and, rarely, severe fatigue.[37,38] The newer, second-generation calcium channel blockers such as amlodipine, isradipine, nicardipine, and felodipine also appear to be effective in patients with RS and may be associated with fewer adverse effects.[39] Our second-line drug is phenoxybenzamine hydrochloride (Dibenzyline), an α-adrenergic blocking agent. A number of our patients take medication only during the cold portion of the year or in anticipation of cold exposure. Low-dose sublingual nifedipine (5 mg) taken 15 to 30 minutes before cold exposure has been shown to be an effective prophylaxis to cold-induced peripheral vasospasm.[40]

Active research continues in the treatment of RS with the prostaglandins: PGE_1, PGE_2, and PGI_2. Intravenous iloprost, a stable analog of PGI_2, has been shown to be effective in the treatment of RS associated with systemic sclerosis.[41,42] In placebo-controlled double-blind studies, intravenous iloprost was associated with both decreased frequency of Raynaud's episodes and increased frequency of ulcer healing.[42,43] Several multicenter clinical trials have examined the efficacy of oral forms of iloprost. Although some groups have detected modest improvements in patients with RS, particularly if associated with systemic sclerosis,[44] others have found no benefit when compared with placebo.[45,46] Clinical trials with other prostaglandins such as oral and intravenous PGE_1 have had less promising results.[47,48] Other pharmacologic agents with potential clinical utility include the angiotensin II receptor inhibitor losartan,[49,50] the selective serotonin reuptake inhibitor fluoxetine,[51] prazosin,[52] and cilostazol.[53]

Temperature biofeedback, in which patients are taught hand warming through behavioral techniques, was initially believed to reduce symptom frequency in patients with vasospastic RS.[54] However, a more recent randomized trial showed no improvement in symptoms after 1 year compared with a control technique.[55] Transcutaneous electrical nerve stimulation, which has been described as causing vasodilatation, resulted in only mild increases in skin temperature; it caused no improvements in digital plethysmography or transcutaneous partial pressure of oxygen in test hands and had a negligible effect on symptoms.[56] Acupuncture has also been suggested as a possible treatment alternative, with a significant reduction in frequency and severity of attacks.[57]

Cervicothoracic sympathectomy has been suggested by some as an effective treatment for RS.[58,59] In our experience, it does not have a lasting benefit, and we do not recommend it for any patient with RS, including those with ischemic ulcerations. In contrast to upper extremity sympathectomy, excellent results have been achieved with lower extremity sympathectomy, with long-term symptomatic relief noted in more than 90% of patients undergoing this procedure.[60] Lumbar sympathectomy remains a viable option in the very rare patient with severely symptomatic lower extremity vasospasm, and it is amenable to minimally invasive laparoscopic techniques.[61]

Periarterial neurectomy is performed by removing the adventitia of the radial, ulnar, palmar, or common digital arteries. Several modifications of this technique have been published, generally characterized by increasing the length of adventitial stripping to facilitate more distal sympathectomy.[62-64] However, digital periarterial sympathectomy has not been proved to be any more effective than cervicothoracic sympathectomy, and its use is generally discouraged.

A minority of patients with RS have an identifiable proximal cause of upper extremity arterial insufficiency demonstrated on angiogram. Patients with subclavian, axillary, or brachial artery obstruction from atherosclerosis, emboli, proximal arterial aneurysms, or other causes are appropriate surgical candidates and can expect excellent results from operative intervention. Restoration of normal hand circulation usually eliminates obstructive RS symptoms. Reconstruction of the palmar arch and direct microvascular bypass of occluded segments of palmar and digital arteries have been successful in a small number of patients.[65,66] Arteriovenous reversal at the wrist has been advocated as a method of providing

TABLE 7–2	Long-Term Outcome of Raynaud's Syndrome Patients Based on Classification at Initial Presentation: Oregon Health Sciences University Series			
Initial Classification	Initial Presence of Connective Tissue Disease (%)	Final Presence of Connective Tissue Disease (%)	Presence of Digital Ulceration (%)	Requirement for Digital or Phalangeal Amputation (%)
Spastic, negative serology	0	2.0	5.2	1.6
Spastic, positive serology	48.6	57.0	15.5	1.4
Obstructive, negative serology	0	8.5	48.2	19.0
Obstructive, positive serology	72.9	81.2	55.6	11.6

From Landry G, Edwards JM, McLafferty RM, et al: Long-term outcome of Raynaud's syndrome in a prospective analyzed cohort. J Vasc Surg 23:76-86, 1996.

retrograde arterial perfusion to ischemic hands for limb salvage.[67] These procedures, however, are applicable to only a few carefully selected patients.

The long-term outcome of patients with RS is not known with certainty. We reviewed our experience with more than 1000 RS patients followed for up to 23 years and found RS to be a relatively benign condition in the majority of patients.[19] We divided the patients into four groups at presentation—vasospastic RS with negative serologies, vasospastic RS with positive serologies, obstructive RS with negative serologies, and obstructive RS with positive serologies—to determine whether this classification scheme provided prognostic information. Patients with no evidence of an associated disease or arterial obstruction did extremely well, with minimal risk of severe finger ischemia or development of an associated disease; those with obstruction and positive serologies were most likely to develop worsening finger ischemia and ulceration. A summary is presented in Table 7-2. Patients without a diagnosable connective tissue disorder but with one or more clinical signs or laboratory tests suggesting such a disease are much more likley to be diagnosed with a connective tissue disorder at a later date. Current estimates of progression range from 2% to 6% in patients with initially negative serologic tests to 30% to 75% in patients with positive serologic tests at presentation.[1,22,23,68] Although fingertip débridement and occasional distal phalanx amputation are required to aid ulcer healing, we have performed major interphalangeal finger amputations in only 2 of the more than 1000 RS patients we have evaluated and treated.

Systemic Vasculitis

Vasculitis has a deceptively simple definition—inflammation, often with necrosis and occlusive changes of the blood vessels—but its clinical manifestations are diverse and complex.[69] The term *arteritis* has been used to describe many of these syndromes, yet *vasculitis* is a more precise term, because many of the entities involve veins as well as arteries. Vasculitis may be generalized or localized. Our knowledge of this condition is incomplete, and the currently used classification systems are chaotic and filled with exceptions and overlapping syndromes. Some classification systems focus on the cause of the vasculitis, with groupings of "idiopathic" and "secondary." Although this is a useful system when considering disease processes, reclassification may be necessary as further knowledge is gained regarding etiology. The most useful classification system is based on the size of the vessels (small, medium, large) involved by the vasculitic process (Table 7-3).[70] Medium and small vessel vasculitis is further subdivided by the presence or absence of antineutrophil cytoplasmic antibodies (ANCAs), a group of autoantibodies formed against enzymes found in primary granules of neutrophils. The most common ANCA-positive vasculitides include Wegener's granulomatosis, microscopic polyangiitis, and Churg-Strauss syndrome, which are rarely encountered by vascular surgeons.[71]

The cause and pathogenesis of most vasculitides are quite complex and are currently either unknown or incompletely understood. Earlier attempts to associate vasculitis with a single mechanism of immune complex-induced injury have not been substantiated in the majority of vasculitides.[72] The basic pathologic mechanism of vasculitis implicates immune-mediated injury, which may include recognition of a vascular structure as antigen, deposition of immune complexes in a vessel wall with complement activation and injury, direct deposition of antigen in a vessel wall, or a delayed hypersensitivity reaction. The inciting antigen has been detected infrequently.

The majority of vasculitides are associated with a cellular immunoreaction involving the production of soluble mediators

TABLE 7–3	Vasculitides with Potential Vascular Surgical Importance

Large Vessel Vasculitis
Giant cell (temporal) arteritis
Takayasu's disease
Radiation-induced arterial damage

Medium Vessel Vasculitis
Polyarteritis nodosa (classic)
Kawasaki disease
Drug abuse arteritis
Behçet's disease
Cogan's syndrome
Vasculitis associated with malignancy

Small Vessel Vasculitis
Hypersensitivity vasculitis
Henoch-Schönlein purpura
Essential cryoglobulinemic vasculitis
Vasculitis of connective tissue diseases

including cytokines, arachidonic acid metabolites, and fibrinolytic and coagulation by-products. The production of cytokines results in neutrophilic, eosinophilic, monocytic, and lymphocytic interactions at the inflammatory site. Endothelial cells express cell membrane receptors specific for many of these inflammatory cells. Binding of inflammatory cells to the endothelial cell triggers intracellular production of additional endothelial cytokines that affect the local inflammatory environment. Complement binding is thought to aid the attachment of leukocytes to endothelial cells. Platelet interactions with both intact and injured endothelium may contribute to the inflammatory process through activation of coagulation pathways and release of cytokines capable of stimulating and modifying immune responses. For a complete description of these cellular, immune, and inflammatory interactions, the interested reader is directed to two excellent summaries.[72,73]

The vascular surgeon attends to the sequelae of vasculitic injury in these diseases. Thrombosis, aneurysm formation, hemorrhage, or arterial occlusion may all follow or accompany transmural damage created by inflammatory reactions on the vascular wall. An abbreviated list of the vasculitides that have potential significance to vascular surgeons is presented in Table 7-3 and is considered in this section.

LARGE VESSEL VASCULITIS

Giant Cell Arteritis Group

The two conditions included in the giant cell arteritis group are systemic giant cell, or temporal, arteritis and Takayasu's disease. Although they have fairly distinctive clinical patterns (Table 7-4), the two entities likely represent different manifestations of the same disease process.[74] The microscopic pathologic findings of the two conditions are similar, and it is often impossible to clearly categorize individual tissue sections as one or the other. Both conditions consist of localized periarteritis with inflammatory mononuclear infiltrates and giant cells, along with disruption and fragmentation of the elastic fibers of the arterial wall. The arterial inflammation begins and is most pronounced in the media. In both conditions, the intensity of the cellular infiltrate and the number of giant cells are variable. Histologically, giant cells are pathognomonic but not essential to make the diagnosis of giant cell arteritis.[75]

Both giant cell arteritis and Takayasu's disease have a propensity for the insidious development of aneurysms of the thoracic and abdominal aorta, which may be accompanied by dissection.[76] Both may be associated with slowly progressive occlusive lesions of the upper extremity, carotid, visceral, and renal arteries. The main differences between these two disease entities are the age and sex of afflicted individuals.[77]

Systemic Giant Cell Arteritis (Temporal Arteritis)

Systemic giant cell arteritis (GCA) is essentially limited to patients older than 55 years; it occurs three times as frequently in women as in men and is more prominent in whites. The annual incidence in white women older than 50 years is about 18 cases per 100,000.[78] A viral cause is suspected but has not been confirmed.[79] Polymyalgia rheumatica, a clinical syndrome of aching and stiffness of the hip and shoulder girdle muscles lasting 4 weeks or longer and associated with an elevated erythrocyte sedimentation rate, is present in 50% to 75% of patients with temporal arteritis.[80,81]

GCA may involve any large artery of the body, although it has a propensity to affect branches of the carotid artery. The clinical history usually begins with a febrile myalgic process involving primarily the back, shoulder, and pelvic regions. Headache, malaise, anorexia, weight loss, and jaw claudication are common. The most characteristic complaint is severe pain along the course of the temporal artery, accompanied by tenderness and nodularity of the artery and overlying skin erythema. The involvement is frequently bilateral. Visual disturbances occur in more than 50% of patients. The mechanism of the visual alterations may be ischemic optic neuritis, retrobulbar neuritis, or occlusion of the central retinal artery. Unilateral blindness occurs in as many as 17% of patients with GCA, followed by contralateral, usually permanent, blindness in one third of these patients within 1 week.[82] Amaurosis fugax is an important warning sign that precedes visual loss in 44% of patients.[83]

GCA is of concern to cardiac and vascular surgeons because it may cause aneurysms or stenoses of the aorta or its main branches. Both true thoracic aortic aneurysms and dissecting aneurysms may occur. Patients with GCA have a 17-fold increased risk of thoracic aortic aneurysms and a 2.4-fold increased risk of abdominal aortic aneurysms compared with age-matched controls.[84] Classic arteriographic findings of GCA include smooth, tapering stenoses of subclavian, axillary, and brachial arteries (Fig. 7-2). Aortic involvement is best visualized with computed tomography (CT) or magnetic resonance angiography (MRA), in which aortic wall thickening is demonstrated.[85] Klein and associates found that 14% of patients with GCA had evidence of symptomatic large artery involvement.[86] Symptomatic subclavian-axillary occlusion is a frequent presenting symptom of GCA.[87] Outside of the head and neck, the areas most commonly involved, in decreasing order, are the upper extremities, the upper and lower extremities, and the lower extremities. Coronary and mesenteric involvement has been described.[88]

Laboratory findings supporting a diagnosis of GCA include an elevated erythrocyte sedimentation rate. The diagnostic criteria of the American College of Rheumatology include an erythrocyte sedimentation rate of at least 50 mm/hour.[89] However, up to 25% of patients with GCA have a normal sedimentation rate at the time of diagnosis,[90] and this finding should not preclude treatment if clinical suspicion

TABLE 7-4	Clinical Patterns in Giant Cell Arteritis	
	Temporal Arteritis	**Takayasu's Disease**
Age, sex	Elderly white women	Young females
Pathology	Inflammatory cellular infiltrates; giant cells	Same
Area of involvement	Usually branches of carotid; may involve any artery	Aortic arch and branches; pulmonary artery
Complications	Blindness	Hypertension, stroke
Response to steroids	Excellent	Unpredictable—unproved

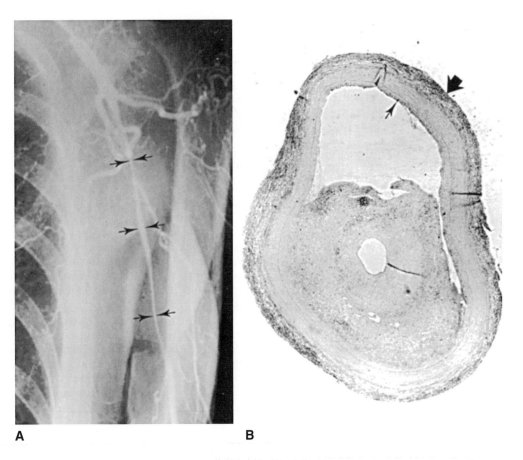

FIGURE 7–2 • *A,* Typical giant cell arteritis with smooth tapering of the axillary artery *(arrows).* *B,* Photomicrograph of an axillary artery involved with giant cell arteritis showing transmural inflammation *(large arrow)* and an inner zone of fibrosis *(small arrow).* (From Rivers SP, Baur GM, Inahara T, Porter JM: Arm ischemia secondary to giant cell arteritis. Am J Surg 143:554-558, 1982.)

A   **B**

is high. C-reactive protein may be a more sensitive indicator of disease activity than the sedimentation rate.[91]

Temporal artery biopsy is indicated in patients suspected of having GCA. When possible, temporal artery biopsy should be performed before corticosteroid treatment; however, histologic evidence of arteritis may be found after up to 2 weeks of treatment.[92] Bilateral sequential temporal artery biopsies are frequently performed if the results of unilateral biopsy are inconclusive, but in 97% of cases, the two specimens show the same findings.[93] Characteristic findings on color-flow duplex scans have been described, and duplex scanning may supplant temporal artery biopsy as the diagnostic procedure of choice.[94]

The importance of a precise and early diagnosis lies in the early initiation of steroid therapy. Prompt steroid therapy frequently results in restoration of pulses and prevention of lasting visual disturbances. Also, vascular reconstructive surgery during the acute phase of GCA is relatively contraindicated. Surgical procedures fail in a high percentage of patients unless accompanied by high-dose steroid administration.[75,87] Although corticosteroids remain the cornerstone of medical therapy, cytotoxic agents (e.g., methotrexate) and other immunosuppressants are occasionally used and are being actively investigated.[95,96] The life expectancy of patients with GCA is the same as that of the general population.[97]

Takayasu's Disease

Takayasu's disease frequently affects the aorta and its major branches and, in contrast to GCA, the pulmonary artery. The majority of patients are Asian, about 85% are female, and the age at onset is between 3 and 35 years.[98,99] The disease has two recognized stages. The first stage is characterized by fever, myalgia, and anorexia in about two thirds of patients. In the second stage, these symptoms may be followed by multiple arterial occlusive symptoms, with manifestations dependent on disease location.

The cardiovascular areas of involvement have been characterized as types I, II, III, and IV and are shown in Figure 7-3. Type I is limited to involvement of the arch and arch vessels and occurs in 8.4% of patients. Type II involves the descending thoracic and abdominal aorta and accounts for 11.2% of cases. Type III involves the arch vessels and the abdominal aorta and its branches and accounts for 65.4% of cases. Type IV consists primarily of pulmonary artery involvement, with or without other vessels, and accounts for 15% of patients.[100] Most of the lesions are stenotic, although localized aneurysms have been reported. Arteriography has traditionally been the imaging modality of choice.[101] However, color-flow duplex scanning,[102,103] CT,[104,105] and magnetic resonance imaging (MRI)[106] have emerged as important alternatives, providing information about both luminal and mural involvement in affected vessels. Involvement of the thoracic aorta predominates in Japan, whereas a predilection for the abdominal aorta predominates in India.[105]

Cardiovascular findings include diminished peripheral arterial pulsations and hypertension. The hypertension may be due to aortic coarctation or renal artery stenosis. The possible relationship of this disease to the middle aortic, or abdominal coarctation, syndrome is described in a subsequent section. Neurologic symptoms may result from hypertension

PA   ?

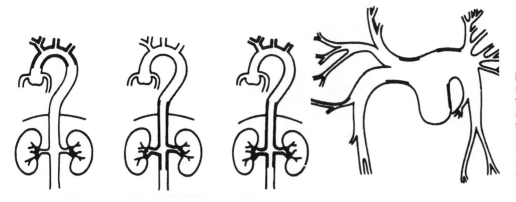

FIGURE 7–3 • Diagrammatic representation of the recognized types of Takayasu's arteritis. The areas of arterial involvement are shown in heavy lines. (From Lupi-Herrera E, Sanchez-Torres G, Marcustiamer J, et al: Takayasu's arteritis: Clinical study of 107 cases. Am Heart J 93:94-103, 1977.)

or central nervous system ischemia associated with large artery occlusion or stenosis. Coronary artery involvement in Takayasu's disease is rare. The cardiac pathologic feature most frequently found is nonspecific and appears to result from heart failure associated with systemic and pulmonary hypertension.

Available information suggests that a conservative surgical approach is best for these patients. A poor long-term outcome is predicted by the presence of major complications (retinopathy, hypertension, aortic insufficiency, aneurysm formation) and a progressive disease course.[107] Surgical intervention is generally reserved to treat symptomatic stenotic or, less commonly, aneurysmal lesions resulting from chronic Takayasu's arteritis. Successful surgical management requires bypass graft implantation into disease-free arterial segments and continuation of corticosteroid therapy.[108,109] Excellent long-term survival rates of up to 75% at 20 years have been reported in large operative series.[110] Owing to its inflammatory nature, endarterectomy has resulted in early failure and is generally not recommended.

Endovascular techniques have been employed, and percutaneous transluminal angioplasty has had mixed success.[111-113] Although initial results of percutaneous angioplasty and stenting have been promising, high rates of in-stent restenosis have been reported.

Radiation-Induced Arterial Damage

Radiation given for the treatment of regional malignancy causes well-recognized changes in arteries within the irradiated field. The primary changes consist of intimal thickening and proliferation, medial hyalinization, and cellular infiltration of the adventitia. Normal endothelium has a very slow rate of turnover, and following irradiation, endothelial cells do not proliferate. Pleomorphic endothelial cells may develop as a result of irradiation, with exposure of the basement membrane leading to thrombosis of small vessels.[114] The effects of radiation on the smooth muscle cell are less well understood. Impairment of nitric oxide–mediated endothelium-dependent relaxation has been suggested.[115] Irradiation also leads to severe inflammation and destruction of the elastic lamellae of small vessels, which can cause aneurysmal dilatation; however, small arteries are most likely to occlude.[116] Postirradiation changes in large arteries often resemble atherosclerosis (Fig. 7-4).[117]

Of considerable importance is the tendency for arteries in an irradiated area to show stenosis years later. There is reportedly an unusually high incidence of carotid artery stenosis in patients years after neck irradiation, along with an increased likelihood of stroke.[118] The lesions vary from diffuse scarring to areas of typical atheromatous narrowing, with a preponderance of the latter. Patients who have had regional irradiation, especially of the cervical region, should have careful vascular follow-up, including noninvasive vascular laboratory examinations. Stenoses of the subclavian and axillary arteries have been demonstrated in patients undergoing radiation therapy for breast cancer and Hodgkin's lymphoma, and aortoiliac involvement has been noted in patients undergoing abdominal or pelvic radiation therapy.

Vascular surgery on irradiated arteries may be performed using standard techniques. Prosthetic and autogenous bypass grafts, as well as endarterectomy, have all been performed satisfactorily.[119] Prudence suggests avoidance of a prosthetic graft in a field in which infection may be expected, such as a radical neck dissection after irradiation, and autologous vein reconstruction is preferred. Late graft infections occurring 2 to 5 years after surgery have been described.[120] The treatment

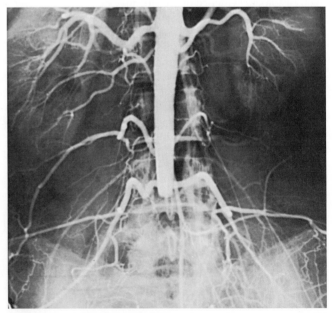

FIGURE 7–4 • Radiation arteritis. Arteriogram in a 40-year-old woman who had received extensive internal and external irradiation for treatment of carcinoma of the cervix. There is a typical absence of atherosclerotic disease of the infrarenal aorta.

of carotid artery stenosis in irradiated areas with percutaneous angioplasty and stenting has been reported, with excellent results.[121,122] Although data are limited, endovascular treatment of other arterial beds appears to be safe and effective in selected cases.[123]

MEDIUM VESSEL VASCULITIS

Polyarteritis Nodosa

Polyarteritis nodosa (PAN) is a disseminated disease characterized by focal necrotizing lesions involving primarily medium-size muscular arteries. This disease has a male-female preponderance of 2:1, with a peak incidence in the 40s. The clinical manifestations of PAN are varied. It may involve only one organ or it may involve multiple organs simultaneously or sequentially over time. The most frequent manifestations of PAN include a characteristic crescent-forming glomerulonephritis, polyarteritis, polymyositis, and abdominal pain.[124]

The essential pathologic feature of PAN is focal transmural arterial inflammatory necrosis. The process begins with medial destruction, followed by a sequential acute inflammatory response, fibroblastic proliferation, and endothelial damage. Immune complexes do not appear to be involved in the endothelial degeneration. The vascular injury is resolved by intimal proliferation, thrombosis, or aneurysm formation, all of which may culminate in luminal occlusion, with consequent organ ischemia and infarction.[125]

The erythrocyte sedimentation rate, C-reactive protein, and factor XIII–related protein, all nonspecific serologic markers of inflammation, are elevated in PAN.[125] Mild anemia and leukocytosis are frequent. ANCAs have been detected in patients with systemic vasculitis, including PAN, Wegener's granulomatosis, Churg-Strauss syndrome, temporal arteritis, and Kawasaki disease.[126] Cytoplasmic (cANCA),

perinuclear (pANCA), and "snow-drift" (xANCA) staining patterns have been recognized. These patterns, however, do not permit stratification of the systemic vasculitides by ANCA patterns, nor do they correlate with disease activity.

The hallmark of PAN is the formation of aneurysms associated with inflammatory destruction of the media, with the most frequently involved organs being the kidney, heart, liver, and gastrointestinal tract. A detailed arteriographic study of 17 patients with PAN reported that 10 of them had multiple arterial aneurysms involving the hepatic, renal, and mesenteric circulations.[127] Another study detected multiple visceral aneurysms in 15 of 26 patients with PAN and made the observation that visceral aneurysms are markers of a more severe clinical course.[128]

Rupture of intra-abdominal PAN aneurysms has been well described and may represent a surgical emergency.[129] Curiously, these aneurysms have been documented to regress on occasion after vigorous steroid and cyclophosphamide therapy, which should be recommended for all asymptomatic visceral aneurysms.[130] An arteriogram of a patient with PAN showing the typical visceral and renal artery aneurysms is shown in Figure 7-5. Visceral PAN lesions may also lead to visceral artery narrowing incident to the inflammatory process, which may progress to occlusion. The visceral ischemia may manifest as cholecystitis, appendicitis, enteric perforation, gastrointestinal hemorrhage, or ischemic stricture formation with bowel obstruction.[129,131]

The routine use of steroid therapy has improved 5-year survival from 15% to the current 50% to 80%.[132] Cyclophosphamide may be added to the steroid regimen in acute, severe cases.[130,133] It has been suggested that prognosis can be determined by the absence or presence of creatinemia, proteinuria, cardiomyopathy, and gastrointestinal or central nervous system involvement at the time of presentation. Five-year mortality with zero, one, or two or more of these signs was 12%, 26%, and 46%, respectively.[134] During the

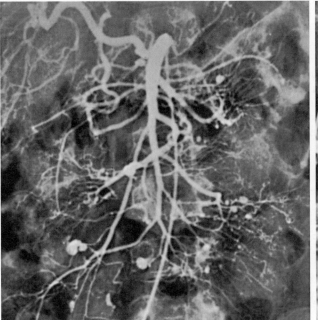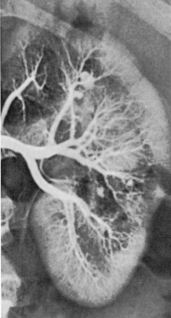

FIGURE 7–5 • *A,* Arteriogram showing multiple visceral aneurysms in a patient with polyarteritis nodosa. *B,* Multiple renal artery aneurysms in the same patient.

A   **B**

acute phase of PAN, renal and gastrointestinal lesions account for the majority of deaths, whereas cardiovascular and cerebral events account for mortality in chronic cases.[132]

To date, little vascular surgical experience with PAN has been reported. The multiplicity of diseased areas renders elective vascular repair of all lesions impossible, and there is no accurate way to recognize the dangerous ones. The role of vascular surgery in intestinal revascularization in PAN is presently undefined.

Kawasaki Disease

In the 1960s, an unusual febrile exanthematous illness swept Japan. Kawasaki observed 50 cases in the Department of Pediatrics at the Japan Red Cross Medical Center and termed the disease the mucocutaneous lymph node syndrome (MCLS).[135,136] Over the next decade, the spread of the disease was noted worldwide, and it became known as Kawasaki disease.[137] During a 2-year period in the early 1990s, more than 11,000 cases were reported in Japan.[138] The disease is not limited to those of Asian descent and occurs in all ethnic groups, although children of Japanese or mixed Japanese ancestry appear to be most susceptible.

As the disease has become better known, strict clinical criteria have evolved for diagnosis: (1) high fever present for 5 or more days; (2) bilateral congestion of ocular conjunctiva; (3) changes in the mucous membranes of the oral cavity, including erythema, dryness, and fissuring of the lips or diffuse reddening of the oropharyngeal mucosa; (4) changes in the peripheral portions of the extremities, including reddening and induration of the hands and feet and periungual desquamation; (5) polymorphous exanthem; and (6) acute nonsuppurative swelling of the cervical lymph nodes. The presence of a prolonged high fever and any four of the five remaining criteria, in the absence of concurrent evidence of bacterial or viral infection, establishes the diagnosis.[139]

Kawasaki disease has a unimodal peak incidence at 1 year of age; it has not been described in neonates and is rarely observed for the first time in those older than 5 years.[138] The acute symptoms may persist for 7 to 14 days before improvement occurs as the fever subsides. Notable laboratory features include elevation of the erythrocyte sedimentation rate and C-reactive protein, thrombocythemia,[140] and elevated levels of von Willebrand's factor.[141] A small proportion of patients with acute Kawasaki disease show exacerbation or recrudescence of symptoms and signs during the convalescent phase, within 1 to 3 weeks after the initial clinical onset. Some believe that this biphasic pattern represents a more severe form of Kawasaki disease with a higher incidence of arterial lesions and a worse prognosis.[142]

An infectious cause has long been assumed, given the self-limited nature of the disease, its seasonal incidence, and geographic outbreaks.[140] However, no single infectious agent has been demonstrated. An immunologic defect has also been postulated, as there appears to be an altered immunoregulatory state in these patients, with decreased numbers of T cells and an increased proportion of activated helper T4 cells. The significance of these changes is not known. The most serious disease manifestation is coronary arteritis, which is likely present in all children with this disease. The spectrum of documented coronary artery pathologic changes consists of active arteritis, thrombosis, calcification, and stenosis, although

the distinguishing feature of Kawasaki disease is the formation of diffuse fusiform and saccular coronary artery aneurysms.

Routine echocardiography in patients with Kawasaki disease has demonstrated coronary artery aneurysms in 25%, with the aneurysms typically appearing in the second week of illness and reaching a maximum size from the third to eighth week after the onset of fever.[143] Echocardiography may show dilatation of the right, left, or anterior descending coronary arteries, while the circumflex coronary artery is rarely involved.[144]

Serial arteriographic studies have shown a considerable capacity for all types of coronary arterial lesions to evolve. The aneurysms may regress, leaving a patent arterial lumen, or the arterial segment may become stenotic. Most stenotic lesions regress, with maintenance of a patent lumen, but a few progress to occlusion. Stenotic lesions demonstrated by coronary angiography are most frequently seen in the left anterior descending artery.[145] Patients older than 2 years with fever lasting longer than 14 days and pericardial effusion and those not treated with anticoagulant agents appear to have a higher incidence of aneurysm formation.[143] Patients treated with immune globulin have shown a decreased incidence of aneurysm formation.[145] New coronary arterial lesions occur infrequently after 2 weeks. Regression of the lesions occurs over a 2-month period, although some lesions remain unchanged for more than a year before regression.[146]

Systemic arteritis also occurs in Kawasaki disease, with iliac arteritis as prevalent as coronary arteritis. Aneurysm formation is far less frequent in the systemic arteries than in the coronary arteries, with one report identifying systemic arterial aneurysms (axillary and iliac) in 3.3% of 662 patients with Kawasaki disease and coronary artery aneurysms.[147] The healing process in the systemic arterial lesions may lead to focal arterial stenosis or aneurysm formation, just as in the coronary arteries. The coexistence of peripheral arterial involvement (subclavian and axillary arteries) and coronary artery aneurysms is shown in Figure 7-6.

Thrombosis of coronary artery aneurysms is the overwhelming cause of death in the early stages of Kawasaki disease, causing acute myocardial infarction or arrhythmia. Coronary aneurysm rupture has also been described. With the initiation of antithrombotic therapy using aspirin and, more recently, immune globulin therapy, the mortality from Kawasaki disease has decreased from 2% to 0.3% over the past 2 decades.[145] Currently, there is a consensus that aspirin and immune globulin therapy should be initiated in the acute phase of the disease for all children younger than 12 months. Immune globulin is given intravenously for 4 days at a dose of 400 mg/kg per day. Aspirin is given orally for 14 days at a dose of 100 mg/kg per day, then continued in low-dose form (3 to 5 mg/kg per day) for an additional 8 weeks.[148,149] Approximately 10% to 15% of patients are refractory to standard therapy,[150] and corticosteroids or newer immunosuppressant agents (e.g., infliximab) are considered in these patients.

Coronary artery bypass grafting was first used in Kawasaki disease in 1976.[151] The first procedure used the saphenous vein as a conduit; however, concerns over its potential to grow with the child have been raised. This led to the use of the internal mammary artery (unilateral or bilateral)[152,153] and the right gastroepiploic artery[154] for coronary revascularization in patients with Kawasaki disease. Internal mammary arterial

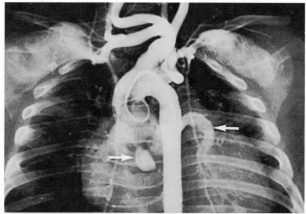

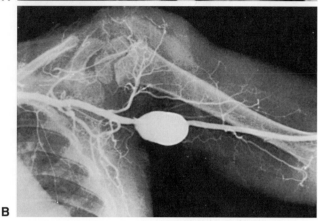

FIGURE 7–6 • *A,* Arteriogram of an infant with Kawasaki disease showing coronary artery aneurysms *(white arrows)* and massive subclavian artery aneurysms. *B,* Arteriogram of a 2-year-old child showing a large axillary artery aneurysm resulting from Kawasaki disease.

grafts had improved patency (77% vs. 46%) and reduced late cardiac death rate (1% vs. 3%) at 7 years compared with saphenous vein grafts in a multicenter study.[155] Cardiac transplantation for severe ischemic heart disease as a sequela of Kawasaki disease is considered in patients who are not candidates for revascularization because of distal coronary stenosis or aneurysms and those with severe irreversible myocardial dysfunction.[156]

Aneurysms of the abdominal aorta and iliac, axillary, brachial, mesenteric, and renal arteries have been observed as late sequelae of systemic vasculitis. When these lesions become symptomatic from occlusion, expansion, or embolization, most surgeons proceed with standard repair techniques using interposition grafting. Although experience is limited, surgical repair of the aneurysms has been accomplished safely.[157]

Drug Abuse Arteritis

Intravenous drug abuse, particularly the use of methamphetamines or cocaine, is associated with a panarteritis similar in presentation and appearance to PAN,[158] with combinations of renal failure, central nervous system dysfunction, and localized intestinal necrosis and perforation. Isolated cerebral angiitis has also been reported in the setting of methamphetamine and cocaine abuse.[159,160] No medical therapy has proved effective for this condition. Necrotizing renal vasculitis

secondary to oral methamphetamines ("ecstasy") has also been described.[161]

A second type of arterial obstruction has been reported in drug abuse patients following the accidental intra-arterial injection of drugs during attempted intravenous injection. The drugs most commonly involved are parenteral barbiturates, in which case arterial injury and thrombosis appear to result from chemical damage, perhaps related to the low pH of the injectant.[162] Another pattern of arterial damage results from the accidental injection of drug preparations intended for oral use. The practice of dissolving tablets in water for intravenous injection is enormously harmful because of the large number of substances (e.g., silica, tragacanth) in tablets. When this material is accidentally injected intra-arterially, significant distal ischemia may result from obstruction of the small arteries by the inert materials (Fig. 7-7).[163]

No convincing evidence has demonstrated the value of any specific treatment in these patients. A number of therapeutic efforts have been tried, including anticoagulation, regional sympathetic block, and the administration of vasodilators, without proof of efficacy. The outcome appears to be determined at the time of injection by the quantity and concentration of injectant reaching the distal arterial bed. Nonetheless, heparin anticoagulation is favored if the patient is seen acutely and has no contraindications to this treatment. Compartment syndrome requiring fasciotomy is an infrequent but reported sequela.[164]

Behçet's Disease

In 1937 Behçet described three patients with iritis and associated oral and genital mucocutaneous ulcerations, an association subsequently termed Behçet's disease.[165] More than half of these patients have joint involvement. The underlying pathologic lesion is a vasculitis, which results in both venous thromboses and specific arterial lesions. Venous thrombosis is the most frequent vascular disorder in Behçet's disease, affecting up to 30% of patients.[166] Arterial lesions are distinctly less frequent and include occlusive and aneurysmal disease; when these lesions are present, mortality is high (up to 20%).[167] This systemic disease largely affects individuals from the Mediterranean area and East Asia.

The pathogenesis of vascular damage in Behçet's disease appears to be an immune-mediated destructive process. A humorally mediated cause has been suggested by the identification of enhanced neutrophil activity and circulating immune complexes in affected patients.[168] Specific T-cell subsets have also been identified in high concentrations at the sites of vascular involvement, indicating a cellular-mediated process.[169] Activation of complement within the vessel wall may lead to destruction of the media and subsequent aneurysm formation. Vasa vasorum occlusion may then lead to transmural necrosis of the large muscular arterial walls, with perforation and pseudoaneurysm formation and injury to adjacent tissues.[170]

Behçet's disease may have a genetic component, because there is an increased incidence of the HLA-B51 allele among patients with the disease.[171] Both viral and bacterial causes have been proposed, although definitive evidence is lacking.[172]

Large artery involvement is an uncommon but serious complication of Behçet's disease. Arterial aneurysms, although distinctly less common than the mucocutaneous, ophthalmic,

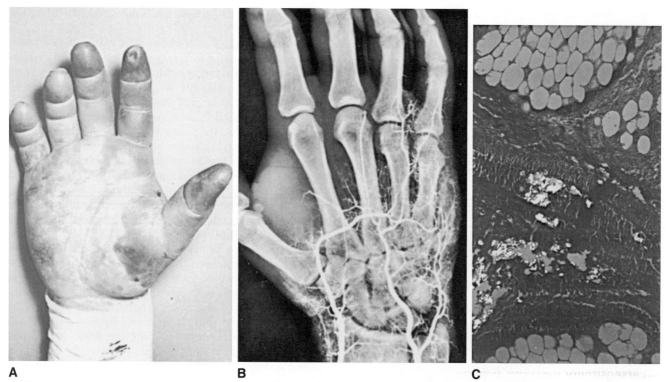

A   **B**   **C**

FIGURE 7–7 • *A*, Photograph of the hand of a 22-year-old man who injected a pentazocine tablet dissolved in tap water into his radial artery. The hand was severely ischemic, with gangrenous changes of the radial side. *B*, Arteriogram showing massive arterial obstruction of the common and proper digital arteries to the thumb, index, and long fingers. *C*, Slide from amputation specimen under polarized light showing bright refractile silica particles in the hand arteries.

or arthritic lesions, are the most frequent cause of death in patients with Behçet's disease.[167] Aneurysms have been described in numerous arteries, including the carotid, popliteal, femoral, iliac, and subclavian, but the aorta is the most frequent site of aneurysm formation in this disease.[173,174] Curiously, the aneurysms frequently appear phlegmonous, suggesting acute bacterial infection, although cultures are invariably negative. The arterial aneurysms are frequently multiple and may be metachronous. Unfortunately, interposition bypass grafts have a high incidence of thrombosis, in addition to the propensity to develop anastomotic pseudoaneurysms; long-term graft patency is the exception rather than the norm. Owing to the recognized difficulties of surgical aneurysm repair in Behçet's disease, endovascular repair is emerging as the treatment of choice. The focal, saccular nature of these lesions makes them ideally suited to endovascular treatment.[175,176]

Venous involvement is prominent, and lower extremity superficial or deep vein thrombosis occurs in 12% to 27% of patients.[166] Thrombosis of the superior or inferior vena cava occurs less frequently but may be fatal. Lifelong anticoagulation is recommended in patients with Behçet's disease who develop venous thrombosis, but the role of prophylactic anticoagulation is uncertain.

Immunosuppressive agents, including azathioprine, corticosteroids, and interferon alfa, have been used with some success for nonarterial symptoms.[170,177] Although corticosteroids may prevent blindness and limit discomfort associated with the mucocutaneous disease, they do not appear to alter the progression or course of the underlying vascular disease.

Currently, no uniformly satisfactory therapy exists for Behçet's disease; however, early diagnosis and meticulous reconstructive management of identified arterial aneurysms have provided long-term limb salvage in some patients, despite the well-recognized propensity for arterial graft complications.[177] Vigilant follow-up is required once large artery disease is recognized. Because this population is at high risk for arteriographic complications, periodic noninvasive imaging and hemodynamic assessment of the arterial system are prudent.[178]

Cogan's Syndrome

Cogan's syndrome is a rare condition consisting of interstitial keratitis and vestibuloauditory symptoms. It is a disease primarily of young adults, with the mean age of onset in the third decade. It is occasionally associated with a systemic vasculitis similar to PAN.[179] Aortitis with subsequent development of clinically significant aortic insufficiency occurs in 10% of patients with Cogan's syndrome. Mesenteric vasculitis and thoracoabdominal aneurysms have also been described in association with Cogan's syndrome.[180,181]

Daily administration of high-dose corticosteroids has been successful in reversing both the visual and the auditory components of Cogan's syndrome, although deafness may be irreversible. The response of the aortitic component to steroids used singly or in combination with cyclosporine is less well established.[182] Surgical therapy, including aortic valve replacement, mesenteric revascularization, and thoracoabdominal aortic aneurysm repair, is occasionally indicated and can be performed safely.

HCL + PAN

Vasculitis Associated with Malignancy

Vasculitis associated with malignancy is infrequent. A strong association has been made between a systemic necrotizing vasculitis resembling PAN and hairy cell leukemia.[183] The vasculitis in this situation presents after the diagnosis of the leukemia and is indistinguishable from classic PAN. An immune-mediated mechanism is postulated. More frequently, vasculitides involving small vessels have been described in association with lymphoproliferative disorders.[184] These have primarily cutaneous manifestations and minimal visceral involvement and are often referred to as paraneoplastic vasculitides.[185]

Vasculitis associated with solid tumors is rare, but resolution with tumor excision has been reported.[186] RS has been reported in association with carcinoma and lymphoproliferative malignancies.[187] These cases were characterized by cold-induced ischemia, which frequently led to digital artery occlusion and ischemic ulcerations. The symptoms of finger ischemia preceded the diagnosis of malignancy, and several of these patients experienced marked improvement of their hand lesions after removal of the tumor.

SMALL VESSEL VASCULITIS

Hypersensitivity Vasculitis Group

The entities in the hypersensitivity vasculitis group include classic hypersensitivity vasculitis, mixed cryoglobulinemic vasculitis, and Henoch-Schönlein purpura. These conditions appear to result from antigen exposure followed by antigen-antibody immune complex deposition in small arteries and arterial damage. Hypersensitivity vasculitis usually has prominent skin involvement. In some conditions, a drug, an environmental chemical, or the hepatitis B virus may be implicated as the inciting antigen, but in more than half of cases, no causative agent is identified. Henoch-Schönlein purpura is a self-limited disease that occurs primarily in children and affects the skin, gastrointestinal tract, and kidneys. The disease course and findings are similar in cryoglobulinemic vasculitis, which may be associated with a hematologic malignancy or hepatitis B infection.[188]

The clinical syndromes typically associated with this group of diseases include skin rash, fever, and evidence of organ dysfunction, none of which specifically concerns vascular surgeons. It is clear, however, that some of these syndromes may present with arteritic involvement substantially limited to the hands and fingers. In these patients, the clinical picture is typically that of severe and widespread palmar and digital arterial occlusions and digital ischemia. The vasculitis may be treated with steroids, with the occasional use of immunosuppressive agents or plasmapheresis. The treatment of hand lesions can otherwise follow the approach outlined later in this chapter for Buerger's disease.[189]

Vasculitis of Connective Tissue Diseases

The connective tissue diseases often are complicated by vasculitis.[74] These diseases have associated immunologic abnormalities, and the occurrence of vasculitis in these patients likely results from immune-mediated damage, as described for other vasculitides.[190] Vasculitis frequently accompanies scleroderma, rheumatoid arthritis, and systemic lupus erythematosus.

Scleroderma is a generalized disorder of connective tissue, microvasculature, and small arteries. It is characterized by progressive scarring and small vessel occlusion in the skin, gastrointestinal tract, kidneys, lungs, and heart. CREST syndrome (calcinosis, Raynaud's syndrome, esophageal dysmotility, sclerodactyly, telangiectases) describes a variant of scleroderma with limited cutaneous involvement. The vasculitis associated with scleroderma results in fibrinoid necrosis and concentric thickening of the intima, with deposition of layers of mucopolysaccharide.

Scleroderma is the most frequent connective tissue disease recognized in our patients with RS, as well as those with digital ulceration (Fig. 7-8).[19] Approximately 80% to 97% of patients with scleroderma have symptoms of RS. In our experience, the RS usually begins as vasospastic and progresses to the obstructive type.

The vasculitis associated with rheumatoid arthritis involves primarily small arteries with a predilection for vasa nervorum and the digital arteries. Intimal proliferation, medial necrosis, and progression to fibrosis with vessel occlusion occur. Symptoms of mononeuritis multiplex are common following involvement of small arteries. Cutaneous lesions are often present and include digital ulcers, nail fold infarcts, and palpable purpura.[191] Rarely, there is coronary, mesenteric, or cerebral artery involvement. Patients with rheumatoid arthritis who have positive ANCAs or higher titers of rheumatoid factor have a more aggressive disease course with a more frequent incidence of rheumatoid vasculitis.[192,193] The presence of vasculitis portends a poor prognosis for patients with rheumatoid arthritis.

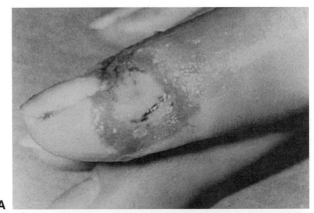

A

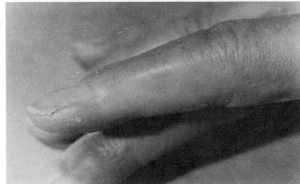

B

FIGURE 7–8 • Photographs of a patient with scleroderma and a digital ulcer. *A,* Digital ulcer. *B,* Healed ulcer following conservative management.

The vasculitis of systemic lupus erythematosus is believed to be due to deposition of immune complexes.[194] The most frequent clinical vascular problem in lupus is RS, which may affect 80% of patients. Other vasculitic manifestations include palpable purpura and mononeuritis multiplex. Thrombotic disorders of the arterial and venous system occur in patients with lupus and appear to be related to the "lupus anticoagulant," not vasculitis. IgA anti–double-stranded DNA antibodies and anti–endothelial cell antibodies are markers of more virulent vasculitic involvement.[195,196] In addition to small vessel vasculitis, patients with systemic lupus erythematosus are clearly prone to premature large vessel atherosclerosis.[197,198]

Management of the vasculitides associated with the connective tissue diseases consists primarily of steroid therapy.[194] Steroids appear to have little or no role in the treatment of the occlusive vascular lesions of scleroderma. Immunosuppressive therapy with cyclophosphamide has also been shown to have modest benefit in selected patients.[199] The treatment of RS associated with lupus or scleroderma is as described earlier.

Buerger's Disease

Buerger's disease, also known as thromboangiitis obliterans, is a clinical syndrome characterized by the occurrence of segmental thrombotic occlusions of small and medium-size arteries in the lower and frequently the upper extremities, accompanied by a prominent arterial wall inflammatory cell infiltration.[200] Buerger's disease is a discrete pathologic entity and is clinically distinct from either atherosclerosis or immune arteritis.[168] Affected patients are predominantly young male smokers (mean age, 34 years); they usually present with distal limb ischemia, frequently accompanied by localized digital gangrene.

Buerger's disease appears to be on the decline in North America, although there has been an increase in the incidence in women. Women currently constitute up to 20% of patients in certain series.[201,202] Whether there is a true decline in incidence or simply more uniform application of strict diagnostic criteria is unclear. The increasing proportion of women has been attributed to the increase in the prevalence of smoking in women.[203] A large volume of patients continue to be reported from East and Southwest Asia. In patients with peripheral vascular disease, the reported incidence of Buerger's disease is 0.75% in North America, 3.3% in Eastern Europe, and 16.6% in Japan.[202]

Approximately 40% to 50% of patients with Buerger's disease have a history of superficial migratory thrombophlebitis, RS, or both.[201] The arterial lesions of Buerger's disease usually occur in the distal portions of both the upper and the lower extremities and may be accompanied by digital gangrene, especially of the toes. Although there have been rare, well-documented reports, both arteriographically and pathologically, of iliac and visceral artery involvement,[204,205] in the overwhelming majority of patients with thromboangiitis obliterans, disease is limited to the arteries distal to the elbow and knee. In North America, about 50% of patients with Buerger's disease have isolated lower extremity involvement, 30% to 40% have upper and lower extremity involvement, and about 10% have isolated upper extremity involvement.[201]

The cause of Buerger's disease remains unknown. Although a strong association with tobacco use has been recognized clinically, a causal relationship has not been conclusively demonstrated.[201] Nonetheless, we have never recognized Buerger's disease in a nonsmoker, with the exception of a single patient who used large amounts of snuff. An increased cellular response to tobacco antigen has been noted in patients with Buerger's disease, as well as in healthy smokers compared with nonsmokers. Tobacco is currently considered at least a permissive factor and likely a causative factor.

The major histocompatibility complex, specifically HLA-A9, -B5, -DR4, and -DRw6, has been implicated in Buerger's disease, but its role is unclear.[201,206] Considerable evidence indicates that an autoimmune process is central to the illness. Several independent investigators have identified elevated levels of anticollagen antibodies[207-209] and antiendothelial antibodies[210] in patients with Buerger's disease. Immunohistochemical analysis of the arterial wall of patients with Buerger's disease demonstrates accumulation of immunoglobulins and complement in the intimal layer, with sparing of the medial and adventitial layers.[211]

The acute lesion of Buerger's disease is a non-necrotizing inflammation of the vascular wall with a prominent component of intraluminal thrombosis. In contrast to both atherosclerosis and immune arteritis, the internal elastic lamina remains intact in Buerger's disease. Therefore, Buerger's disease is not a true vasculitis, because it lacks vascular wall necrosis. Both T- and B-cell–mediated activation of macrophages or dendritic cells in the intima have been implicated in the pathogenesis of Buerger's disease.[211] The chronic phase of Buerger's disease includes a decline in hypercellularity, with the production of perivascular fibrosis and frequent recanalization of the luminal thrombus. Adjacent veins and nerves are frequently involved in the perivascular inflammatory process.

Based on an examination of our patients with Buerger's disease, as well as a review of the published experience, we propose the diagnostic criteria listed in Table 7-5.[212] The major criteria are essential for diagnosis, whereas the minor criteria are supportive. Central to the diagnosis is the onset of symptoms before age 45 years, a uniform exposure to tobacco, and absence of arterial lesions proximal to the knee or elbow. It is essential to exclude other frequent causes of limb ischemia in young adults. In North America, atherosclerosis is much more prevalent than Buerger's disease, and major atherosclerotic risk factors such as hyperlipidemia, diabetes, and hypertension must be absent. Proximal sources of emboli (cardiac, proximal arterial occlusive, or aneurysmal disease), underlying autoimmune disease, hypercoagulable states, trauma, and local lesions (popliteal entrapment, adventitial cystic disease) must also be excluded. We recognize that these criteria are so restrictive that some patients with Buerger's disease will be excluded, but we believe that these strict criteria are essential to eliminate the diagnostic uncertainty obvious in many publications of purported Buerger's disease. Similar clinical diagnostic criteria were reported by Shionoya from Japan: (1) smoking history, (2) onset before age 50 years, (3) infrapopliteal arterial occlusion, (4) either upper limb involvement or phlebitis migrans, and (5) absence of other atherosclerotic risk factors.[213]

After the clinical criteria have been met, objective confirmation of distal occlusive disease limited to small and

TABLE 7–5	Criteria for the Diagnosis of Buerger's Disease

Major Criteria

Onset of distal extremity ischemic symptoms before age 45 yr

Tobacco use

Exclusion of the following:

    Proximal embolic source (cardiac, thoracic outlet syndrome, arteriosclerosis obliterans, aneurysms)

    Trauma and local lesions (entrapment, adventitial cyst)

    Autoimmune disease

    Hypercoagulable states

    Atherosclerosis

    Atherosclerotic risk factors (diabetes, hypertension, hyperlipidemia)

No evidence of arterial disease proximal to popliteal or distal brachial arteries

Objective documentation of distal occlusive disease by one of the following:

    Plethysmography

    Histopathology

    Arteriography

Minor Criteria

Migratory superficial phlebitis

Raynaud's syndrome

Upper extremity involvement

Instep claudication

From Mills JL, Porter JM: Buerger's disease: A review and update. Semin Vasc Surg 6:14-23, 1993.

medium-size vessels is required. This may be satisfied by four-limb digital plethysmography, distinct histopathologic findings when available, or arteriography. The arteriographic findings reveal that the extremity arteries proximal to the popliteal and distal brachial levels are normal, proximal atherosclerosis and vascular calcification are absent, and there is an abrupt transition from a normal, smooth proximal vessel to an area of occlusion.[201] Involvement tends to be segmental rather than diffuse and is commonly symmetrical. In the upper extremity, the ulnar or radial artery is frequently occluded, and extensive digital and palmar arterial occlusion is uniformly present. In the lower extremity, the infragenicu-late vessels are extensively diseased, with diffuse plantar arterial occlusion. Tortuous "corkscrew" collaterals frequently reconstitute patent distal arterial segments and, although not pathognomonic, are suggestive of Buerger's disease (Fig. 7-9).

Arteriography, although desirable, is not essential for the diagnosis of every case of Buerger's disease.[201] Arteriography may be omitted when a patient's history is typical of Buerger's disease, there are no associated atherogenic risk factors, the serologic tests for autoimmune disease and hypercoagulable states are negative, and vascular laboratory examination reveals diffusely abnormal digital plethysmographic tracings in all four extremities accompanied by a conspicuous absence of proximal large artery occlusive disease.

Digital plethysmography frequently provides especially important diagnostic information. In the typical Buerger's patient, obstructive arterial waveforms are present in all digits, providing objective evidence of widespread digital arterial occlusion or stenosis. Patients with unilateral digital

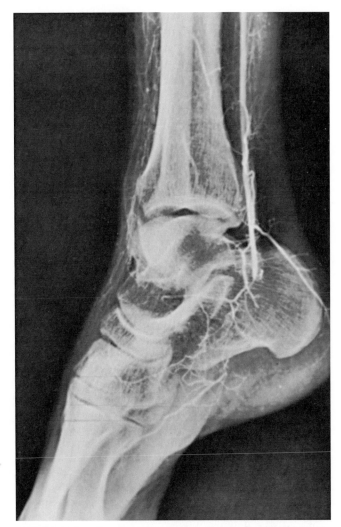

FIGURE 7–9 • Arteriogram of patient with Buerger's disease showing occlusion of the posterior tibial artery at the ankle, total occlusion of the anterior tibial artery, and numerous small collateral vessels.

plethysmographic abnormalities should undergo arteriography to rule out a proximal, potentially correctable arterial lesion causing the digital ischemia. Additionally, patients with symptoms and objective findings localizing their disease to the distal feet and toes and who have normal hand and finger plethysmography should undergo arteriography to rule out a proximal embolic source for the ischemia.

The cornerstone of treatment for patients with Buerger's disease is complete tobacco abstinence. The disease typically undergoes remissions and relapses that correlate closely with the cessation and resumption of cigarette smoking. In our clinical series, no patient sustained further tissue loss following cessation of smoking.[212] Unfortunately, prolonged tobacco abstinence is the exception rather than the norm. Persistent efforts on the part of the physician and family members may ultimately result in smoking cessation. In a report from Japan, an impressive 50% of patients were able to quit smoking.[214]

We use a prolonged, conservative local treatment program for areas of finger ulceration and gangrene, with the primary goal being a clean, dry digit.[215] Ischemic ulcer débridement, often including nail removal, is used frequently, accompanied by minimal rongeur removal of exposed phalangeal bone as needed. Any associated infection is treated with antibiotics. Proximal finger amputations are rarely required, and wrist or forearm amputations have never been necessary in our patients with Buerger's disease. Prolonged conservative management is usually rewarded by healing with preservation of maximal digital length, provided smoking has been discontinued. We have found thoracic sympathectomy ineffectual, and we find no convincing evidence that this procedure is of any significant benefit in these patients.

The course of lower extremity Buerger's disease stands in marked contrast to that observed with upper extremity involvement. Ischemic rest pain can be severe, and narcotic analgesics are frequently required. Several large series reported a 12% to 31% incidence of major leg amputation over a 5- to 10-year period.[216] Our own experience revealed a 31% incidence of major leg amputation.[216] Overall quality of life and the ability to continue working are directly related to limb loss, which is related to continued smoking.[217] Lumbar sympathectomy for refractory Buerger's disease has been advocated by some but is rarely beneficial. Anecdotal reports of improved lower extremity symptoms with the use of an implantable spinal cord stimulator are encouraging,[218] but the device has not yet been subjected to clinical trials.

Arteriography should be performed in all patients with threatened limb loss. If arteriography reveals a patent distal vessel and if autogenous vein is available, a distal arterial bypass may be considered.[219] The use of autogenous vein is mandatory. Distal bypass is seldom feasible because of the diffuse nature of the arterial occlusive disease process. In our experience and that of others, the long-term results of reconstruction are mediocre. However, published Japanese data suggest that acceptable primary (49%) and secondary (63%) 5-year patency rates can be achieved in lower extremity bypasses, including inframalleolar bypasses, in patients with Buerger's disease.[220] A novel operative approach developed in India involves a pedicled omental transfer to the lower extremity for limb-threatening ischemia.[221] In 62 patients treated, 94% experienced relief of pain, and none required amputation.

Many medications have been recommended for the treatment of Buerger's disease, including corticosteroids, PGE_1, vasodilators, hemorheologic agents, antiplatelet agents, and anticoagulants. There is no evidence that any are effective. A randomized European trial comparing the oral prostacyclin analog iloprost with placebo demonstrated improved pain control with iloprost, but no improvement in wound healing.[222] Preliminary results of gene therapy with intramuscular injection of vascular endothelial growth factor have been promising in promoting ulcer healing.[223]

Although lower extremity Buerger's disease portends a significantly worse prognosis for limb salvage than does atherosclerotic occlusive disease, life expectancy for patients with Buerger's disease approaches that of an age-matched population. This is likely due to a lack of coronary artery involvement in the disease process. Reported survival is 97% at 5 years and 94% at 10 years.[216,217]

Heritable Arteriopathies

Hereditary disorders of the arterial wall account for a minute fraction of the problems encountered by vascular surgeons. These disorders affect the structure or stability of collagen or elastin, resulting in weakness of the arterial wall. These patients may possess characteristic phenotypic features, but they are often not recognized until the patient presents with a catastrophic vascular complication. The heritable arteriopathies discussed in this chapter include Marfan's syndrome, Ehlers-Danlos syndrome, cystic medial necrosis, and pseudoxanthoma elasticum. Arteriomegaly is also included in this section, although it is not strictly a heritable disease and there are no distinguishing phenotypic features.

MARFAN'S SYNDROME

Marfan's syndrome is an inherited disorder of connective tissue characterized by abnormalities of the skeletal, ocular, and cardiovascular systems, with variable phenotypic expression. It is serious largely because of its cardiovascular complications.

The pathologic basis of Marfan's syndrome has been uncovered. Hollister and colleagues discovered diminished levels of fibrillin in skin biopsies and cultured fibroblasts in patients with Marfan's syndrome.[224] Fibrillin, a large glycoprotein (350 kD), is one of the structural components of the elastin-associated microfibrils. Subsequently, genetic linkage studies identified an abnormal fibrillin gene on chromosome 15 in a group of patients with Marfan's syndrome.[225,226] Both a reduction in fibrillin formation and abnormalities in the fibrillin molecule have been identified.[227,228]

The incidence of Marfan's syndrome is estimated to be 1 in 10,000, and there has been no identified race or sex preference.[229] Inheritance is by an autosomal dominant pattern, although nearly 25% of all cases are the result of spontaneous genetic mutations. In its classic form, the syndrome is easily recognizable and consists of abnormalities of the eye (subluxation of the lens), skeleton (arachnodactyly, extreme limb length, pectus excavatum or carinatum, and joint laxity), and cardiovascular system (aortic dilatation and aortic valvular incompetence). The diagnosis is established on the basis of clinical manifestations in most cases. However, some patients have only one or a few of the characteristic features. One advance has been the ability to confirm the diagnosis by DNA analysis, whereby quantitative and qualitative defects in fibrillin can be detected.[230] Prenatal diagnosis can be accomplished using chorionic villus sampling.[231]

Patients with Marfan's syndrome develop progressive dilatation of the aortic root, with a resultant ascending aortic aneurysm and aortic valve incompetence (Fig. 7-10). A significant number have mitral valve prolapse and mitral insufficiency. Mild aortic isthmus coarctation may be associated with this syndrome, predisposing the patient to ascending aortic dissection. Less frequently, aneurysmal dilatation and dissection involve the pulmonary, coronary, carotid, and splenic arteries and the infrarenal aorta.

If Marfan's syndrome is untreated, life expectancy is about 40 years, with 95% of deaths related to cardiovascular causes. Progressive aortic root dilatation leading to aortic dissection or aortic valvular insufficiency accounts for 80% of fatal complications. The remainder of deaths are due to congestive heart failure.

Histopathologic evaluation of aortic segments from patients with Marfan's syndrome has revealed cystic medial necrosis, with disruption of collagen fibers and fibrosis of the media.[232] Immunohistochemical analysis has revealed an upregulation of matrix metalloproteinases and abnormalities

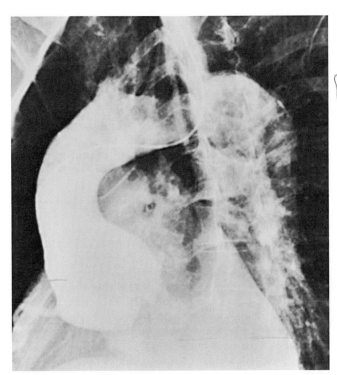

FIGURE 7–10 • Thoracic aortogram of a patient with Marfan's syndrome showing massive aortic dilatation and associated aortic insufficiency.

in elastin synthesis, leading to increased susceptibility to degradation by matrix metalloproteinases.[233] Compared with normal subjects, Marfan's syndrome patients have decreased aortic distensibility and increased aortic stiffness indices in both the ascending and abdominal aortic regions, irrespective of the aortic diameter.[234]

In view of the predictably progressive nature of the aortic dilatation, all patients with Marfan's syndrome should be followed from childhood with annual echocardiograms to detect aortic dilatation.[235] There is some evidence that beta blocker therapy initiated before the development of aortic incompetence may retard the onset of incompetence and perhaps retard aneurysmal degeneration.[236,237]

Elective repair of the aortic valve and ascending aorta should be accomplished prophylactically before severe aortic insufficiency compromises left ventricular function or the ascending aorta exceeds 6 cm in diameter, at which point the risk of dissection and rupture increases. Surgical intervention typically includes graft replacement of the ascending aorta, with concomitant aortic valve replacement. Occasionally, mitral valve replacement is required. As endovascular technology continues to improve, less invasive options for treatment of aneurysmal arch and thoracic aortic aneurysmal disease will surely emerge.[238] Patients should avoid contact sports, isometric exercises, and weightlifting. With modern surgical techniques, the life expectancy of these patients can be improved considerably, as emphasized by reports with low operative mortality, even in severely symptomatic patients.[239,240]

EHLERS-DANLOS SYNDROME

Ehlers-Danlos syndrome refers to a group of diseases first clearly described by van Meekeren in 1682 and later by Ehlers and Danlos, characterized by hyperextensible skin, hypermobile joints, fragile tissues, and a bleeding diathesis primarily related to fragile vessels.[241-243] Ehlers-Danlos syndrome is the most frequent of the heritable connective tissue disorders and occurs in autosomal dominant, autosomal recessive, and sex-linked patterns. Eleven different types of Ehlers-Danlos syndrome have been described, each with variable clinical signs and symptoms. The specific biochemical defects are known in types IV, VI, VII, and XI and involve defects in collagen production.[244,245]

The extreme fragility of tissues in many patients with Ehlers-Danlos syndrome leads to problems of surgical importance. The skin and soft tissues are easily disrupted, tend to fragment and tear with manipulation, and hold sutures and heal poorly. Wound dehiscence is common when surgery is required.[246] In addition to these significant problems incident to any surgery, a number of patients with Ehlers-Danlos syndrome are prone to arterial disorders that may require surgical intervention.

Ehlers-Danlos syndrome types I, III, and IV frequently have arterial complications. Type IV represents only 4% of all cases of Ehlers-Danlos syndrome but causes the most severe arterial complications. These patients produce little or no type III collagen, which is of major structural importance in vessels, viscera, and skin. Patients are prone to spontaneous rupture of major vessels, aneurysm formation, and acute aortic dissections.[247] Other complications include spontaneous lacerations, false aneurysms, and arteriovenous fistulas. Bleeding or easy bruising occurs in two thirds of patients with type IV disease. Hemorrhage can be life threatening despite normal platelet function and coagulation proteins. Defective type III collagen appears to facilitate bleeding by failing to stimulate platelets exposed to subendothelial connective tissue. The media of the arterial wall is thin and disorganized, with fragmented elastic fibers on microscopic examination. There is hyperplasia of the medial cells and increased ground substance in the inner half of the media. Collagen hypoplasia can be seen on skin biopsies, with hypertrophy of elastic fibers.[248]

Treatment of spontaneous arterial rupture in patients with Ehlers-Danlos syndrome should be nonoperative, consisting of compression and transfusion whenever possible. If operation for major arterial disruption is required, the therapeutic objective should be ligation to control bleeding if this procedure can be accomplished without tissue loss. Gentle dissection, proximal vessel control with external tourniquets or internal balloon catheters, and the use of carefully applied heavy ligatures reinforced with fine vascular sutures are the keys to success. Despite the many pitfalls, major arterial reconstruction can be accomplished in patients with Ehlers-Danlos syndrome, including repair of abdominal aortic aneurysms and aortic dissection.[249] Arteriography carries special risks of vessel laceration and hemorrhage in these patients and should be avoided if possible. Prognosis for patients with type IV Ehlers-Danlos syndrome is poor. Forty-four percent of patients with major hemorrhage die before surgical intervention, and there is 20% mortality with operative intervention.[250]

CYSTIC MEDIAL NECROSIS

Cystic medial necrosis is a condition associated with aortic dissection; it manifests pathologically with uniform hyaline degeneration of the media and replacement by a mucoid-appearing basophilic substance. Erdheim believed that the disease was the result of medial replacement by overproduction of mucoid ground substance.[251] Subsequently, numerous studies have shown that the pathologic changes of cystic medial necrosis, with the resultant clinical problems of aortic dissection, spontaneous arterial rupture, and disseminated aneurysm formation, result from a variety of metabolic conditions and syndromes affecting the composition and structure of collagen, elastin, and mucopolysaccharide ground substance. Thus, Marfan's syndrome, Ehlers-Danlos syndrome, any of the mucopolysaccharidoses, and occasionally neurofibromatosis may all present with the typical arterial lesions and pathologic changes identified as cystic medial necrosis. Although the specific biochemical alterations for some of these syndromes have been discovered, others remain obscure.

Although most patients with cystic medial necrosis have an identifiable clinical syndrome, most commonly Marfan's syndrome or Ehlers-Danlos syndrome, a distinct subpopulation of patients with aortic root disease and histologic findings consistent with cystic medial necrosis fail to show the classic phenotypes of either syndrome. These patients often seek treatment at an older age and with more advanced vascular disease. Ninety-four percent of the deaths in this patient group are related to cardiovascular disease, with the majority due to aortic dissection, rupture, or sudden death.[252]

The most frequent arterial condition resulting from cystic medial necrosis is aortic dissection, the treatment of which is discussed elsewhere in this text. Aortic dissection from cystic medial necrosis has been reported as a cause of superior vena cava syndrome.[253] Although unusual, cystic medial necrosis has also been reported to involve the pulmonary arteries and the superficial temporal artery.[254] Cystic medial necrosis has also been implicated as a cause of abdominal aortic aneurysms in children.[255] Rarely, patients have a rapidly progressive syndrome of disseminated arterial dissection, spontaneous arterial rupture, and aneurysm formation in which the only discernible lesion is cystic medial necrosis.[256] The angiograms of such a patient are shown in Figure 7-11.

PSEUDOXANTHOMA ELASTICUM

Pseudoxanthoma elasticum is an inherited disorder of elastic tissue manifested clinically by loose, baggy skin with multiple creases and small yellow-orange cutaneous papules in intertriginous areas. These patients also have changes in the eye (angioid streaks) and distinct vascular abnormalities. The prevalence of pseudoxanthoma elasticum is 1 in 70,000 to 160,000.[257] Studies have demonstrated an autosomal recessive inheritance in the majority, although there is also an autosomally dominant form.[258]

The basic pathologic change is degeneration of medial elastic fibers, with calcification, fragmentation, and secondary proliferation of the intima leading to luminal narrowing and obstruction. This change results in a markedly abnormal

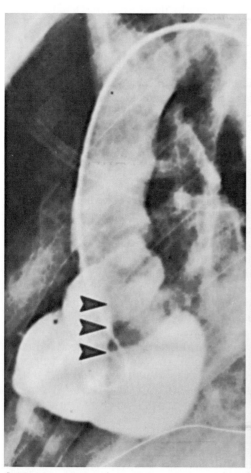

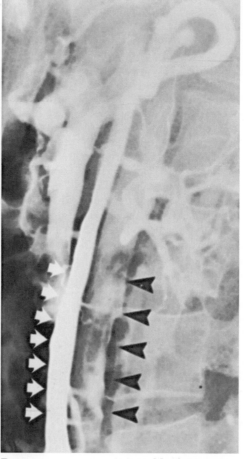

FIGURE 7–11 • *A,* Cystic medial necrosis with aortic root dissection. The junction of the true and false lumen is outlined *(black arrows). B,* Lateral aortogram of the same patient showing the outline of a double-lumen abdominal aorta *(white and black arrows).*

A   **B**

pulse contour due to loss of the elastic recoil and distensibility of vessels and may be demonstrated plethysmographically. Arterial stenoses, occlusions, or both are the end results of this pathologic process and may involve the cerebral, coronary, visceral, and peripheral arteries. Radiography frequently reveals extensive arterial calcification in a young patient without obvious risk factors for atherosclerosis. Arterial occlusive disease occurs at an early age, usually presenting in the 20s or 30s.[259] With careful examination, decreased peripheral pulses and evidence of peripheral arterial occlusive disease can be found in 24% to 80% of these patients.[260] Symptoms include intermittent claudication, periodic abdominal pain, and angina.[261,262] Gastrointestinal hemorrhage is frequent and is believed to originate from the widespread arterial degeneration. Hypertension is common in these patients and is usually ascribed to extensive vascular calcification, although renovascular hypertension has been reported.

Standard techniques of vascular surgery, including autogenous vein bypass and endarterectomy, have been used with success in patients with pseudoxanthoma elasticum.[260] Anecdotal benefit from pentoxifylline for the relief of ischemic pain has been reported.[263] The indications for surgery in these patients are the same as for patients with arteriosclerotic occlusive disease.

ARTERIA MAGNA SYNDROME

Leriche was the first to describe patients with arteria magna syndrome, which is characterized by extreme arterial dilatation, elongation, and tortuosity, which he termed *dolicho et méga-artère*.[264] Since then, many such patients have been recognized, and the terms *arteria magna*, *arteria dolicho et magna*, and *arteriomegaly* have all been used to describe this condition. Pathologic study reveals that the arterial media of these patients has a striking loss of elastic tissue.[265]

Angiography in patients with this syndrome reveals characteristic changes. They have arterial widening and tortuosity (100% of patients), extremely slow arterial flow velocity (100% of patients), and multiple aneurysms (66% of patients) (Fig. 7-12).[266] The slow arterial flow present in patients with this condition makes arteriography difficult. Large amounts of contrast must be used, and visualization of distal vessels may require multiple injections and special timing sequences with delayed filming.

The propensity to form arterial aneurysms at multiple sites results in the frequent need for surgical correction. Because of the generalized arterial dilatation in these patients, standard criteria for determining the size of aneurysms to be repaired may not be useful. All patients with arteria magna should undergo annual examinations of all pertinent sites (aorta and iliac, femoral, and popliteal arteries), together with ultrasound imaging of nonpalpable or questionable areas. Any aneurysm that reaches 2 to 2.5 times the size of the parent vessel or becomes symptomatic should be repaired. Arterial occlusions in these patients are almost always thrombotic or embolic complications of aneurysmal disease.

The relationship of arteria magna to typical atherosclerosis is uncertain. The syndrome occurs, albeit rarely, in young people with no evidence of atherosclerosis, and it has been reported in children. Lawrence and colleagues reported a 36% familial incidence among first-degree relatives.[267] Clinical experience suggests that most patients in the United States

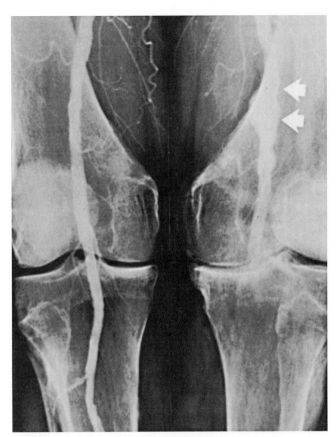

FIGURE 7–12 • Arteriogram of a 68-year-old man showing very dilated popliteal arteries and a left popliteal aneurysm *(arrows)*. This patient's arterial dilatation extended throughout his body, a condition termed *arteria magna syndrome*.

with arteria magna have significant associated atherosclerosis along with the usual risk factors, including tobacco use. In these patients, however, the atherosclerosis is typically nonocclusive, and dilatation predominates.

Congenital Conditions Affecting the Arteries

ABDOMINAL COARCTATION

Coarctation of the aorta below the diaphragm is a rare but well-recognized condition. Quain described a stricture of the abdominal aorta in 1847 that he believed to be congenital in origin.[268] In 1952, Glenn and coworkers reported the first successful surgical repair, which consisted of bypassing the coarctation with a splenic artery graft.[269] Since that time, the surgical treatment and clinical courses of a large number of patients have been reported.[270] Abdominal coarctation is usually discovered during an evaluation for hypertension. Most patients with abdominal coarctation become symptomatic during their teens with complaints associated with hypertension, including headache, fatigue, shortness of breath, and palpitations. The hypertension is mediated through the renin-angiotensin system.[271] Severe leg ischemia is distinctly unusual,[272] but moderate claudication is often present. Involvement of the superior mesenteric artery occurs frequently, although symptoms of visceral ischemia have not been reported.

Physical findings in these patients include reduced or absent lower extremity pulses, with a noticeable radial or femoral pulse delay. All patients have prominent abdominal systolic bruits, and many have systolic bruits in the lumbar region or lower posterior thoracic area. The natural history of untreated abdominal coarctation is severe hypertension, with death from either renal or cardiac failure within a few years of the onset of symptoms.[273]

Multiple variants of abdominal coarctation have been described, with the variable factors being the precise location and length of the aortic involvement and the number of visceral branches affected. The origins of the visceral arteries may be involved even when they originate from an area of relatively uninvolved aorta. Stenosis or occlusion of the visceral arteries usually does not extend beyond a few millimeters from the origin, implicating a process that is primarily aortic.[270]

Two primary pathogenetic theories have been presented. The first proposes a congenital anomaly representing a failure of normal fusion of the two dorsal aortas of the embryo, resulting in aortic narrowing. The existence of multiple renal arteries in a number of these patients supports this theory, because the formation of a single renal artery is a developmental step that coincides in both location and timing with fusion of the dorsal aortas. The congenital origin of abdominal coarctation in some of these patients may be related to intrauterine injury, because the anomaly has been reported in association with the maternal rubella syndrome.[274] In patients in whom the lesion is congenital, the involved vessels are hypoplastic, without gross or microscopic inflammatory reaction.

The second proposed cause of abdominal coarctation is inflammation. In this group of patients, microscopic examination of involved arteries reveals pronounced inflammatory changes. This lesion is sometimes referred to as the "middle aortic syndrome" to emphasize its acquired rather than congenital nature.[275] This inflammatory middle aortic narrowing is probably a variant of Takayasu's arteritis and appears to occur with a frequency reflecting the primarily Asian distribution of that disease.[276] Although this arteritis can be treated successfully with corticosteroids during the acute stage, the diagnosis is usually made later, when the chronic fibrotic and stenotic lesions are amenable only to surgical treatment.

Arteriography is necessary to define the extent of the lesion and to plan treatment (Fig. 7-13). Lateral and oblique views are helpful in detecting the extent of visceral vessel involvement. Renovascular hypertension is assumed, and renin studies or split renal function studies are not necessary unless the potential viability of a poorly visualized kidney is questionable (to determine the need for nephrectomy vs. revascularization).

Many authors have reported successful surgical treatment of abdominal coarctation by a variety of methods, including aortoaortic bypass, iliac or femoral bypass, prosthetic patch aortoplasty, and splenoaortic anastomosis.[270,277,278] In contrast to thoracic coarctation, prosthetic bypass grafting from the descending thoracic aorta to an uninvolved area of the infrarenal aorta or the iliac or femoral arteries has traditionally been the procedure of choice, although some recommend autologous repair with extensive aortic patching.[270,273] When possible, a single abdominal operative incision is preferable, employing medial visceral rotation to allow optimal exposure

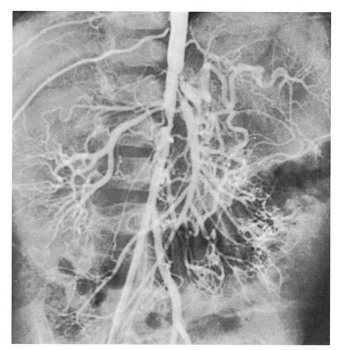

FIGURE 7–13 • Abdominal aortic coarctation in a 2-year-old child with infrarenal aortic narrowing and high-grade stenoses at the origins of the celiac, superior mesenteric, and right renal arteries and nearly total occlusion of the left renal artery.

of the supraceliac aorta. Alternatively, this operation may be performed through a thoracoabdominal incision or through separate laparotomy and thoracotomy incisions. Complete revascularization has been reported as a staged procedure.[278] However, single-stage repair is recommended because most of these patients are young and tolerate extensive procedures well.[279] Successful repair of middle aortic coarctation with stent implantation has been reported, although long-term durability is unknown.[280,281] Restenosis in young patients is a potential problem.[282] In very small children, operation may be delayed until age 5 to 6 years, at which time increased vessel size allows a greater chance of successful repair, as long as cardiac and renal function can be preserved by medical management of hypertension.

Results of surgical treatment of abdominal coarctation have been good. Stanley and associates reviewed the results of 73 reported cases and found an 8% operative mortality and 80% excellent or good results.[273] Renal revascularization is most often performed by bypass grafts originating from the thoracoabdominal graft. Autogenous vein and artery and prosthetic grafts have all been used successfully.[270] Unsuspected proximal stenosis of a visceral (splenic) artery used for renal revascularization has been reported as a cause of failure.[273]

PERSISTENT SCIATIC ARTERY

In the embryo, the axial sciatic artery arises from the umbilical artery and supplies blood to the lower limb, following a dorsal course to the popliteal area and then proceeding through the midcalf to the ankle. As development proceeds, this artery is replaced in its upper part by the femoral artery developing from the external iliac artery. By the third month of gestation, the femoral artery predominates, and the vestiges of the sciatic artery remain only as the inferior gluteal artery, the distal popliteal artery, and the peroneal artery.[283]

Rarely, all or part of the sciatic artery persists into postnatal life as a large artery originating from the internal iliac artery, exiting the pelvis through the sciatic notch near the sciatic nerve, and following a course through the buttock and posterior thigh to join the popliteal artery in the popliteal fossa. The artery may coexist with a normal superficial femoral artery, or the superficial femoral artery may be hypoplastic. In some patients, the entire superficial femoral artery is absent, with the sciatic artery being the only vessel in the limb in continuity with the popliteal artery. The incidence of persistent sciatic artery is reportedly 0.03% to 0.06% in large series of femoral arteriograms, with one third of all cases being bilateral.[284]

The anomalous lower extremity blood supply usually remains undetected until later life (mean age of detection, 51 years). Patients eventually present with claudication or more severe lower extremity ischemic symptoms, pulsatile buttock masses, or, rarely, sciatic neuropathy.[285,286] The anomalous artery has a proclivity for aneurysmal degeneration; more than 25% of detected sciatic arteries have been found to be aneurysmal.[287] The necessity for complete angiographic evaluation of these lesions is obvious. Vascular surgeons are involved in treating both the aneurysmal and the ischemic manifestations of popliteal entrapment. Although the traditional treatment is surgical ligation, endovascular coiling of persistent sciatic artery aneurysms is emerging as the procedure of choice. Arterial reconstruction for lower extremity ischemia is typically performed with either femoropopliteal or iliopopliteal bypass.[287-289]

POPLITEAL ENTRAPMENT SYNDROMES

Stuart in 1879 was the first to describe the anatomic abnormality associated with popliteal entrapment,[290] and Hamming in 1959 reported the first successful treatment of the condition.[291] Love and Whelan coined the term *popliteal artery entrapment syndrome* in 1965.[292] The anatomic basis of this syndrome lies in the anomalous embryonic development of two independent structures, the popliteal artery and the gastrocnemius muscle.[293] Below the knee, the embryonic sciatic artery gives rise to the popliteal and tibial vessels. The femoral artery arises later as the amalgamation of a capillary plexus connecting branches of the external iliac artery proximally and branches of the sciatic artery distally. Both the femoral and sciatic arteries contribute to the popliteal artery. The femoral artery becomes dominant as the proximal sciatic artery regresses.

During this period of femoral maturation and sciatic regression, the heads of the gastrocnemius muscles develop. The anlage of the gastrocnemius muscle develops as a single muscle migrating cephalad from its origin on the calcaneus. As the gastrocnemius matures, it divides into larger medial and smaller lateral heads that gain their final attachments on the femoral epicondyles. The medial head of the gastrocnemius migrates from its lateral origin toward the medial epicondyle at the same developmental stage at which the mature popliteal artery is developing from the femoral and sciatic arteries.

A simplified classification system of popliteal entrapment recognizes four main variants based on the anomalous relationship of the popliteal artery and surrounding musculature (Fig. 7-14).[294,295] In type 1, accounting for about 50% of

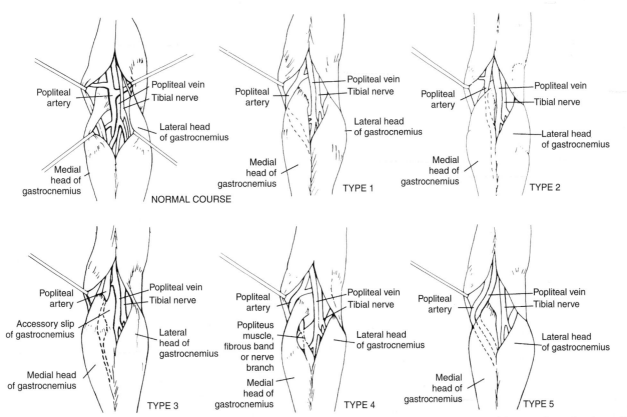

FIGURE 7–14 • Diagram of the types of popliteal artery entrapment. (From Rich NM, Collins G Jr, McDonald PT, et al: Popliteal vascular entrapment: Its increasing interest. Arch Surg 114:1377-1384, 1979.)

all cases, the popliteal artery deviates medial to the normally placed medial head of the gastrocnemius muscle. Type 2 lesions (25% of cases) involve an abnormal attachment of the medial head of the gastrocnemius, with the popliteal artery passing medially but with less deviation than in type 1. In type 3 (6% of cases), the normally situated popliteal artery is compressed by muscle slips of the medial head of the gastrocnemius. Type 4 lesions have associated fibrous bands of the popliteal or plantar muscles compressing the popliteal artery. Type 5 lesions, in which the popliteal vein accompanies the artery in its abnormal course, and type 6 or "functional entrapment," which occurs in symptomatic patients without identifiable anatomic abnormalities, have also been described.[296] The true incidence of popliteal artery entrapment syndrome is unknown. The reported incidence is increasing coincidentally with the development of more sophisticated diagnostic tests. A review of 20,000 patients screened with routine vascular laboratory testing identified verifiable popliteal artery entrapment syndrome in less than 1%.[294] However, in an autopsy series, Gibson and colleagues found an incidence of 3.5% in 86 postmortem examinations.[297] Interestingly, all the patients were older than 60 years when they died, and the popliteal arteries showed no histologic abnormalities. Clearly, not all entrapped popliteal arteries become symptomatic. About 90% of reported cases have occurred in men; more than half these patients became symptomatic before age 30 years. The defect is bilateral in 20% of patients.[293]

Symptoms are due to obstruction of the popliteal artery with gastrocnemius contraction. Histopathologic changes distinct from typical atherosclerosis have been identified.[298] Repeated microtrauma leads to inflammatory cell infiltration and vessel wall disruption, which ultimately causes fibrosis and collagen scar formation. Thrombosis, embolism, or aneurysm formation may ensue. Symptomatic patients may have acute ischemia due to popliteal artery occlusion (10%) or progressive intermittent claudication. Calf claudication in patients younger than 40 years is sufficiently infrequent that its presence should suggest the possibility of popliteal artery entrapment.

Diagnosis of popliteal artery entrapment syndrome is difficult, because most patients are asymptomatic at rest. Symptomatic patients may have normal, reduced, or absent pulses of the lower leg. Ankle dorsiflexion or plantar flexion or knee extension may diminish or occlude distal pulses. Continuous-wave Doppler, photoplethysmography, and arterial duplex scanning have been used with these leg maneuvers to provide objective confirmation of popliteal artery entrapment.[299] Others have used progressively more challenging treadmill exercise regimens to elicit symptoms and an objective decline in the ankle-brachial index in patients suspected of having popliteal artery entrapment syndrome.[300] However, these noninvasive tests and physical findings are nonspecific, as maneuver-induced pulse diminution may occur in normal individuals.

Arteriography demonstrating midpopliteal artery compression or medial deviation with the leg in a position of stress had been the gold standard for the diagnosis of popliteal artery entrapment syndrome, but it is being replaced by noninvasive techniques. CT and MRI have proved useful in precisely defining anomalous anatomic relationships between the popliteal artery and adjacent muscle groups, as well as assessing the patency of the artery.[301] Although both CT and

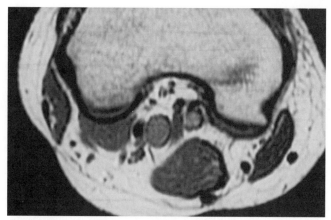

FIGURE 7–15 • Magnetic resonance imaging scan showing the abnormal insertion of the medial head of the gastrocnemius muscle between the popliteal artery and vein. The popliteal artery ends up medial to the medial head of the gastrocnemius muscle.

MRI can define the entrapment, MRI provides better soft tissue definition and does not require the use of intravenous contrast to localize the vascular structures or define their patency status (Fig. 7-15).[302]

Treatment of this condition is surgical. Identifying the specific type of entrapment preoperatively is both difficult and unnecessary, as the surgical management is influenced only by the patency of the popliteal artery. If the syndrome is diagnosed early and if minimal arterial changes are present, sectioning the medial gastrocnemius head may be sufficient. Bypass grafting is required in patients with significant arterial stenosis, occlusion, or aneurysm formation.[303] Autogenous vein is the favored conduit for grafts across the knee. The original descriptions of the surgical technique for this condition favored a posterior approach to the popliteal fossa.[291] Later, a medial approach was emphasized to expose the entire length of the popliteal artery, ensure total division of the medial head of the gastrocnemius, and act as a safeguard against iatrogenic popliteal artery entrapment. To date, similar results have been obtained with both techniques.[304,305]

Fibromuscular Dysplasia

Fibromuscular dysplasia (FMD) is a nonatherosclerotic, noninflammatory vascular disease most frequently involving the renal arteries of young white women.[306] Detailed histologic studies have resulted in the recognition of at least four distinct pathologic types: intimal fibroplasia, medial fibroplasia, medial hyperplasia, and perimedial dysplasia.[307]

The first report of FMD by Leadbetter and Burkland in 1938 described a patient with renal artery involvement.[308] The majority of cases involve the renal artery, with the carotid and iliac arteries representing distant second and third areas of involvement.[309] Rarely, femoral, popliteal, mesenteric, subclavian, axillary, forearm, vertebral, and coronary arteries may be involved. Ninety percent of adult patients with FMD are women. With renal involvement, 70% of patients display bilateral disease. The more severe disease almost always occurs on the right. Lesions affecting the left renal artery alone occur in less than 10% of these patients. The lesions of medial fibroplasia have the classic "string of beads" morphology on angiography (Fig. 7-16).

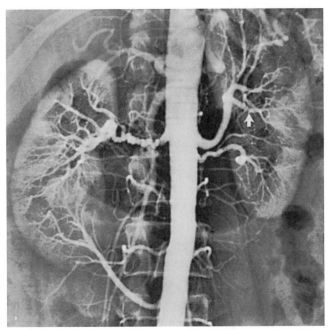

FIGURE 7–16 • Fibromuscular dysplasia (FMD). The superior right renal artery shows typical involvement extending beyond the primary branching. Moderate left kidney segmental artery FMD is present *(white arrow)*.

Medial fibroplasia accounts for 85% of FMD, perimedial dysplasia for 10%, and intimal fibroplasia for 5%. The types are distinguished from one another by which vessel wall layer is primarily affected and by the tissue components that predominate. An increase of fibrous connective tissue, collagen, and ground substance within the media is characteristic of medial fibroplasia. The smooth muscle cell is multipotential and appears to be the source of the proliferative changes in FMD. The cause of FMD is unknown. Several theories have been advanced, including (1) arterial stretching, (2) mural ischemia secondary to an abnormal distribution of vasa vasorum, (3) estrogenic (or other hormonal) effects on the arterial wall, (4) immunologic insult, and (5) anomalous embryologic development.[310] A familial prevalence of 11% has been noted,[311] and an association with the angiotensin-converting enzyme allele ACE-I has also been reported.[312]

Symptoms produced by FMD are generally secondary to the associated arterial stenoses and are indistinguishable from those caused by atherosclerosis. The two most frequently seen clinical syndromes are renovascular hypertension and transient cerebral ischemic attacks. Duplex scanning of the renal arteries has proved useful in the diagnosis of renovascular FMD. As opposed to atherosclerotic renal artery stenosis, which typically involves the orifice or proximal renal artery, FMD lesions have a predilection for the middle and distal renal artery.[313] Duplex scanning not only identifies the lesions but also provides useful information about parenchymal resistance, which has predictive value in determining response to treatment.[314] MRA and CT angiography are also emerging as imaging modalities, although they have not been systematically compared with contrast arteriography, which remains the gold standard for diagnosis.[315]

Treatment is recommended for arterial stenotic lesions only when they produce significant symptoms. Renovascular hypertension caused by FMD has responded more favorably to surgery than has that caused by atherosclerosis.[316-318] Technical success of surgical procedures ranges from 89% to 97%, with cured or improved hypertension in 67% to 93%.[316-318] Results of surgical management of children with renovascular FMD have been particularly encouraging, with cured or improved hypertension in 96% after up to 16 years' follow-up.[319] Percutaneous transluminal angioplasty has emerged as the primary treatment modality, however, with technical success rates of 94% to 100% and cured or improved hypertension in 74% to 88%,[320-322] although the duration of follow-up has not been as long as that of surgical series. Using logistic regression, factors found to independently predict a good response of hypertension to angioplasty included systolic blood pressure before intervention, duration of hypertension, and patient age.[323] FMD of the renal artery may be associated with the formation of renal artery aneurysms and renal artery dissection.

Cerebrovascular FMD causes symptoms identical to atherosclerotic lesions. Unlike atherosclerotic disease, fibromuscular disease typically involves the distal extracranial internal carotid artery and stops before the internal carotid artery enters the base of the skull. Duplex ultrasonography, CT, MRA, and contrast arteriography all play a role in diagnosis. Less than 1% of patients undergoing carotid arteriography have FMD.[310] Ten percent to 51% of patients with FMD of the internal carotid artery harbor intracranial aneurysms.[324]

Treatment of cerebrovascular FMD is generally reserved for symptomatic patients. Before the widespread application of percutaneous revascularization, surgical repair was the favored approach. Multiple techniques, including open graduated internal dilatation, patch angioplasty, and interposition grafting, have been described, depending on the location and extent of involvement.[325] However, percutaneous angioplasty has become the preferred treatment.

Adventitial Cystic Disease

Adventitial cystic disease is a rare condition that must always be considered in the differential diagnosis of claudication in a young patient. Single or multiple synovial-like cysts in the subadventitial layer of the arterial wall compressing the arterial lumen cause arterial stenosis. The cysts typically contain mucinous degenerative debris or clear, gelatinous material similar to that found in ganglia. Eighty percent of patients with this condition are men, and the median age at presentation is 42 years.[326] The first case report describing operative management was in 1954.[327] The popliteal artery is by far the most commonly involved artery, with the femoral and iliac arteries being the next most frequent areas of involvement.

The cause of adventitial cystic disease is unknown. The once-popular theory that it was caused by repeated arterial microtrauma has largely been abandoned. A direct communication with the adjacent knee joint, similar to a true ganglion, has been demonstrated in selected cases.[328] Currently, the most widely accepted theory is that the cysts result from the presence within the arterial wall of mucin-secreting cell rests derived embryologically from the synovial anlage of the knee joint.[329] On examination, the finding of a popliteal bruit and the absence of palpable pulses with knee flexion have been noted in a number of patients with adventitial cystic disease involving the popliteal artery. Diagnosis is possible using ultrasonography, CT, and MRI.[330] Intravascular ultrasonography has also emerged as a helpful imaging modality.[331] Arteriography may demonstrate segmental popliteal arterial occlusion or may show a "scimitar" sign of luminal encroachment by the cyst in a normally placed vessel that has no other signs of occlusive disease.[332]

Several methods of treatment have been described. Although spontaneous resolution has been reported,[333] for most patients, percutaneous or surgical treatment is required. Arteries with a small cyst have been successfully treated with CT- or ultrasound-guided needle aspiration or cyst enucleation,[334] although approximately 10% recur following this treatment. In more severely affected patients, segmental arterial replacement may be required. Patients with popliteal occlusion require bypass grafting with an autogenous conduit. Treatment has been successful in more than 90% of reported cases.[326]

Compartment Syndrome

Compartment syndrome occurs whenever tissue pressure within a confined space becomes sufficiently elevated to impair perfusion. If untreated, diminished nutritive blood flow results in limb dysfunction secondary to ischemic muscle contracture.[335] The first clinical description of this syndrome was by von Volkmann more than a century ago in a report on contracture involving the arm following trauma. He attributed the deformity to a prolonged interruption of the vascular supply to the muscle.[336] In 1926, Jepson reported successful experimental reproduction of the syndrome and demonstrated that early compartment decompression may prevent ischemic muscle paralysis and contracture.[337]

The multiple clinical causes of compartment syndrome have been well described by Matsen and are listed in Table 7-6.[338] Any loss of vascular integrity, such as occurs following prolonged ischemia or reperfusion injury, leads to increased edema within a compartment. This edema then compromises venous outflow and increases venous and capillary pressures, leading to increased compartment pressure and decreased perfusion pressure. Pivotal to the development of the syndrome, whether from external compression or internal tissue swelling, is the production of sufficient intracompartment pressure to impair blood flow to the tissues.

The capillary leak following ischemia and reperfusion is believed to be mediated through inflammatory mediators and oxygen-derived free radicals.[339] The return of oxygenated blood to the microcirculation of ischemic tissue causes activation of inflammatory mediators locally and systemically. Neutrophil adherence to endothelium leads to oxidant release (H_2O_2, O_2, and OH^-), which damages the endothelium. Animal models suggest that treatment with free radical scavengers may mitigate the damage in compartment syndrome.[340] Experimentally blocking neutrophil adherence has also been shown to decrease reperfusion injury.[341]

There is no absolute pressure above which compartment syndrome invariably occurs, although tissue blood flow diminishes rapidly as intracompartment pressure approaches the level of the diastolic blood pressure. Additionally, conditions such as hypotension or vasoconstriction may lead to the syndrome's occurrence at lower intracompartment pressures. In addition to the absolute and relative intracompartment pressures, the duration of ischemia is an important factor. Nerve tissue appears to be most susceptible to ischemia, with

TABLE 7–6	Causes of Compartment Syndrome

Decreased Compartment Volume
Closure of fascial defects
Application of excessive traction to fractured limbs

Increased Compartment Content
Bleeding
Major vascular injury
Coagulation defect
   Bleeding disorder
   Anticoagulant therapy
Increased capillary filtration
Increased capillary permeability
   Reperfusion after arterial revascularization
   Trauma
   Fracture
   Contusion (crush)
   Intensive use of muscles
   Exercise
   Seizures
   Burns
   Intra-arterial drug injection
   Cold
   Orthopedic surgery
   Snakebite
Increased capillary pressure
   Intensive use of muscles (exertional compartment syndrome)
   Venous obstruction
Diminished serum osmolarity—nephrotic syndrome

Externally Applied Pressure
Tight casts, dressings, or splints
Lying on limb

symptoms occurring within minutes and permanent damage at 2 hours or less. Muscle death begins at approximately 4 hours. Maximal muscle contracture appears to require about 12 hours of ischemia.[338] Skin and subcutaneous tissues are capable of tolerating periods of ischemia that are not tolerated by skeletal muscle or peripheral nerves.[342]

In patients with acute interruption of arterial blood flow, the incidence of compartment syndrome averages 8%.[343] The need for fasciotomy following revascularization is increased if the duration of ischemia was more than 6 hours or if there was a substantial period of shock in association with the arterial injury. Other circumstances increasing the need for fasciotomy include the occurrence of a tight swelling of the extremity preoperatively or intraoperatively, the combination of arterial and venous injury, and the presence of concomitant soft tissue crush injury. Compartment syndrome may develop in up to 30% of all extremities after combined fracture and arterial injury. Thrombolytic therapy for acute arterial occlusion must be recognized as a possible mode of reperfusion injury. Acute compartment syndrome following thrombolysis has been observed in our practice and reported in the literature.[344]

In the lower leg, compartment syndrome most frequently occurs in the anterior compartment, followed by the lateral, deep posterior, and superficial posterior compartments. The quadriceps compartment in the thigh and the gluteal compartment in the buttock may be involved. In the upper extremity, the volar forearm compartment is most frequently involved, but involvement of the dorsal forearm, biceps, deltoid, and hand interosseous muscle compartments has also been reported.

The accurate diagnosis of compartment syndrome leading to successful treatment is based on recognition of the early signs and symptoms of increased compartment pressure. Diminished function of the extremity precedes nerve and muscle necrosis by several hours. Clinical signs include fullness and tenderness of the compartment, pain disproportionate to the physical findings, paresthesias of the compartment nerves, and weakness of the involved muscles. The palpable pulse status and Doppler pressures are unreliable reflections of intracompartment pressure. With compression of postcapillary venules and a continued fall in the arteriovenous perfusion gradient, tissue damage may occur despite continued arterial inflow and palpable pulses.[345]

In questionable clinical situations or when the patient is unable to communicate adequately, objective data reflecting either intracompartment pressure or nerve function may be monitored. Continuous or intermittent pressure determinations may be made by the Wick catheter technique, in which a plastic catheter is placed percutaneously into the compartment and connected to a pressure transducer.[346] A solid-state transducer that fits within a catheter tip in a hand-held unit, the "solid-state transducer in catheter" monitor, eliminates the artifacts inherent to pressure lines.[347] Surgical decompression is generally recommended for patients who have a compartment pressure of 40 mm Hg or greater or for those whose compartment pressure is greater than 30 mm Hg for 4 hours.

Others argue that intervention based on fixed pressure is inappropriate and that critical intracompartment pressures occur within 30 mm Hg of the mean arterial pressure or 20 mm Hg of the diastolic pressure.[348]

Once compartment syndrome occurs, the time delay before treatment becomes the critical factor in determining outcome. Twelve hours appears to be the point beyond which significant residual dysfunction will likely occur despite adequate surgical decompression.[349] All circumferential bandages or casts should be removed at the first suspicion of increased compartment pressure to allow a complete examination of the extremity. The extremity should be placed at the level of the heart and not elevated, because elevation may further jeopardize ischemic compartment components. If physical examination, pressure measurements, or nerve conduction studies suggest a compartment syndrome, immediate surgical decompression is indicated. A frequently used decompressive technique is shown in Figure 7-17.

Untreated compartment syndrome results in direct neurologic dysfunction or the development of contractures following fibrous replacement of myonecrosis. Symptomatic severity ranges from mild to critical, and amputation may be required. Frequent examination of the blood from patients with compartment syndrome may reveal elevated levels of creatinine phosphokinase as well as hyperkalemia. Subsequently, there may be myoglobinuria and renal failure.[350] In such patients, restoration of normal hemodynamics, the administration of mannitol to enhance urine flow and improve intrarenal blood distribution, and alkalinization of the urine to prevent

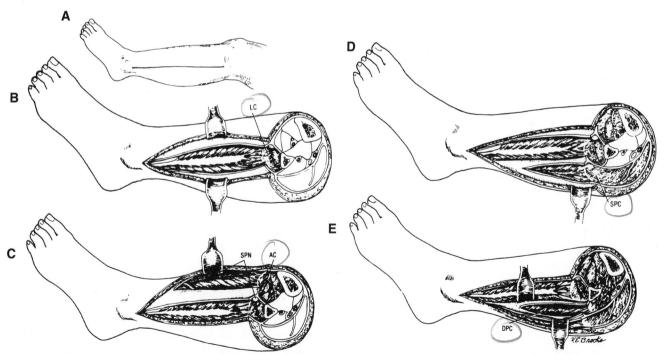

FIGURE 7–17 • Parafibular decompression of all four compartments of the leg. *A*, The skin incision runs the length of the fibula. *B*, The lateral compartment (LC) is opened directly beneath the skin incision. *C*, The anterior compartment (AC) is exposed by retracting the anterior skin flap and is opened over the entire length. Care is taken to preserve the superficial peroneal nerve (SPN). *D*, The superficial posterior compartment (SPC) is exposed by retracting the posterior skin flap and is opened over its entire length. *E*, The lateral compartment is retracted anteriorly, and the superficial posterior compartment is retracted posteriorly after the fibular origin of the soleus muscle is released (not shown). This exposes the deep posterior compartment (DPC), which is opened over its entire length. (From Matsen FA, Winquist RA, Krugmire RB: Diagnosis and management of compartmental syndromes. J Bone Joint Surg 62:286-291, 1980.)

precipitation of myoglobin within the renal tubules are specific therapeutic measures.[350] Prevention of the reperfusion syndrome has been shown in selected patients after the administration of hypertonic mannitol, presumably as a result of its free radical scavenging.[351] Deep muscle infections are uncommon but potentially life-threatening sequelae.

A rare but well-described form of compartment syndrome is exertional compartment syndrome seen in highly trained athletes.[352] As with other forms, the anterolateral compartments are most frequently affected. The diagnosis can be made by measuring compartment pressures at the point of exertional pain in affected individuals, with pressures in excess of 25 mm Hg consistent with the diagnosis. Turnipseed recently described his experience of 276 patients with documented exertional compartment syndrome undergoing surgical treatment with open fasciectomy.[353] Ninety-two percent of patients had complete relief of symptoms and return to normal activities.

Homocystinuria

Homocystinuria, an inborn error of metabolism in which homocysteine accumulates abnormally in plasma, tissues, and urine, is the second most treatable aminoacidopathy following phenylketonuria, with a reported incidence of 1 in 344,000.[354] First described in 1963, this disorder results in multiple abnormalities, including ectopia lentis, mental retardation, thromboembolic disorders, and rapidly progressive arteriosclerotic vascular disease.[355,356] Three specific enzyme deficiencies, each of which may be responsible for homocystinuria, have been identified: cystathionine β-synthetase (CβS) deficiency,[357] homocysteine methyltransferase (HMT) deficiency,[358] and methylene tetrahydrofolate reductase (MTHFR) deficiency.[359] These enzymes require cofactors, including folate, vitamin B_6 (pyridoxine), and vitamin B_{12} (cobalamin).[360-362] Regardless of the primary cause, all forms of homocystinuria in humans have been associated with premature atherosclerosis, frequently complicated by thrombosis.[356] The occurrence of the same clinical syndrome in patients with different enzyme deficiencies that all result in abnormal accumulation of homocysteine is strong evidence that homocysteine itself is toxic.

Homocysteine is an intermediary, nonstructural amino acid involved in the transulfuration pathway leading to the production of cysteine. In this pathway, a sulfur group is transferred from methionine to serine to produce cysteine. The enzymes CβS, HMT, and MTHFR, as well as the cofactors folate, vitamin B_6, and vitamin B_{12}, are all involved. Any deficiency in these enzymes or cofactors leads to the accumulation of homocysteine. Harker and colleagues showed that infusion of homocysteine into laboratory animals produces endothelial cell injury and rapid proliferation of atherosclerotic lesions.[363] Treatment of homocystinemic animals with vitamin B_6, folate, or both improved some of the laboratory and clinical manifestations of homocystinemia.[364]

Homocysteine exists in human plasma in at least three forms: as the mixed disulfide homocysteine-cysteine, as free homocysteine, and as the disulfide homocystine.[365] In nonhomocystinuric conditions, most homocysteine exists in the plasma bound to protein. Men have higher levels of plasma homocysteine than women, and premenopausal women have lower levels than postmenopausal women.[366] Accumulation of homocysteine leads the liver to produce homocysteine

thiolactone, which has been implicated as the toxic substance in homocystinemic atherogenesis. Homocysteine thiolactone alters surface charges and may predispose to cellular aggregation within the vascular lumen.[367] Interestingly, the metabolism of homocysteine thiolactone appears to be abnormal in patients with arteriosclerosis but without homocystinemia.

The detection of elevated plasma homocysteine has historically required the use of a cumbersome dietary methionine load. Kang and associates simplified these investigations when they demonstrated elevated levels of protein-bound homocysteine in patients with coronary artery disease, without any requirement for dietary methionine loading, through the use of high-performance liquid chromatography.[368] This enables accurate levels to be obtained without the need for fasting or for methionine loading and has become the standard clinical assay.[369]

The arteriosclerotic lesions occurring in homocystinuria, whether resulting from CβS deficiency, HMT deficiency, or MTHFR deficiency, are typical fibrous plaques.[370] Microscopic evaluation reveals medial hypertrophy, elaboration of extracellular matrix and collagen, and degeneration and destruction of the elastic laminae. Lipid deposition in the plaques is characteristically absent.[370]

The prevalence of mild homocystinemia in the general population is estimated to be 5% to 7%. If a genetic defect is necessary, homozygous thermolabile MTHFR and heterozygous CβS and MTHFR deficiency are the most probable factors.[371] These deficiencies cause an approximately 50% reduction in corresponding enzyme activities and are estimated to occur in 5% to 6% of the population. However, other factors, such as vitamin deficiency and environment, must be involved, as phenotypic expression is not complete.[372] Increasing evidence indicates that mildly elevated levels of plasma homocysteine may be associated with symptomatic atherosclerotic disease, although a causal relationship has not been established.[373]

Evaluation of our patients with peripheral vascular disease has confirmed elevated total plasma homocysteine levels in a significant number of patients compared with age- and sex-matched controls.[374] Stampfer and colleagues, in a retrospective review of prospectively obtained blood samples in the Physicians' Health Study, demonstrated an association between elevated plasma homocysteine levels and myocardial infarction.[375] Arnesen and coauthors showed that elevated homocysteine levels predicted myocardial infarction in a general population in Norway.[376] Both Perry and coauthors[377] and Verhoef and associates[378] found that elevated homocysteine levels were related to ischemic strokes.

Our data have established elevated homocysteine levels as an independent risk factor for death from cardiovascular disease in patients with lower extremity disease and cerebrovascular disease.[379] Norwegian investigators prospectively demonstrated a strong relationship between homocysteine levels and early mortality rates in patients with established coronary artery disease.[380]

Investigations have focused on lowering these supranormal plasma homocysteine levels through alteration of the homocysteine-methionine pathways using pharmacologic doses of the cofactors for these enzymatic pathways, specifically folic acid, vitamin B_6, and vitamin B_{12}.[381,382] Elevated levels of plasma homocysteine can reliably be reduced to normal by the administration of folate in most patients. Patients who are resistant to folate therapy often respond to vitamin B_6, vitamin B_{12}, choline, or betaine. These substances appear to be able to reduce homocysteine levels regardless of the underlying cause of the elevation.

Treatment of homocystinemia with various vitamins has the potential to be essentially nontoxic. At present, however, there are no convincing data that lowering the homocysteine level in patients with vascular disease will yield any true benefit. Although intuitively one would expect clinical improvement once the toxic homocysteine levels have declined, serial evaluation of the progression of peripheral vascular disease in groups randomized to treatment and nontreatment is necessary to determine clinical benefit.

KEY REFERENCES

Espinosa G, Font J, Tassies D, et al: Vascular involvement in Behçet's disease. Am J Med 112:37-43, 2002.

Gio HVL, Greene PS, Alejo DE, et al: Replacement of the aortic root in patients with Marfan's syndrome. N Engl J Med 340:1307-1313, 1999.

Miyata T, Sato O, Koyama H, et al: Long-term survival after surgical treatment of patients with Takayasu's arteritis. Circulation 108:1474-1480, 2003.

Olin JW: Current concepts: Thromboangiitis obliterans (Buerger's disease). N Engl J Med 343:864-869, 2000.

Salvarani C, Cantini F, Boiardi L, Hunder GG: Polymyalgia rheumatica and giant-cell arteritis. N Engl J Med 347:261-271, 2002.

Slovut DP, Olin JW: Current concepts: Fibromuscular dysplasia. N Engl J Med 350:1862-1871, 2004.

Turnipseed WD: Popliteal entrapment syndromes. J Vasc Surg 35:910-915, 2002.

Wigley F: Raynaud's phenomenon. N Engl J Med 347:1001-1008, 2002.

REFERENCES

1. Edwards JM: Raynaud's syndrome: Basic data. Ann Vasc Surg 8:509-513, 1994.
2. Fraenkel L, Zhang Y, Chaisson CE, et al: Different factors influencing the expression of Raynaud's phenomenon in men and women. Arthritis Rheum 42:306-310, 1999.
3. Planchon B, Pistorius MA, Beurrier P, De Faucal P: Primary Raynaud's phenomenon: Age of onset and pathogenesis in a prospective study of 424 patients. Angiology 45:677-686, 1994.
4. Freedman RR, Mayes MD: Familial aggregation of primary Raynaud's disease. Arthritis Rheum 39:1189-1191, 1996.
5. Lewis T: Experiments relating to the peripheral mechanism involved in spasmodic arrest of the circulation in the fingers, a variety of Raynaud's disease. Heart 15:7, 1929.
6. Kontos HA, Wasserman AJ: Effect of reserpine in Raynaud's phenomenon. Circulation 39:259-266, 1969.
7. Harker CT, Ousley PJ, Bowman CJ, Porter JM: Cooling augments alpha-2-adrenoceptor-mediated contractions in the rat tail artery. Am J Physiol 260:H1166-H1171, 1991.
8. Graafsma SJ, Wollersheim H, Droste HT, et al: Adrenoceptors on blood cells from patients with primary Raynaud's phenomenon. Clin Sci 80:325, 1991.
9. Keenan EJ, Porter JM: Alpha$_2$-adrenergic receptors in platelets from patients with Raynaud's syndrome. Surgery 94:204, 1983.
10. Edwards JM, Phinney ES, Taylor LM, et al: Alpha$_2$-adrenergic receptor levels in obstructive and spastic Raynaud's syndrome. J Vasc Surg 5:38, 1987.
11. Coffman JD, Cohen RA: Alpha$_2$-adrenergic and 5-HT$_2$ receptor hypersensitivity in Raynaud's phenomenon. J Vasc Med Biol 2:101-106, 1990.
12. Cooke JP, Creager SJ, Scales KM, et al: Role of digital artery adrenoceptors. Vasc Med 2:1-7, 1997.
13. Smith PJ, Ferro CJ, McQueen DS, Webb DJ: Impaired cholinergic dilator response of resistance arteries isolated from patients with Raynaud's disease. Br J Clin Pharmacol 47:507-513, 1999.
14. Zamora MR, O'Brien RF, Rutherford RB, et al: Serum endothelin-1 concentrations and cold provocation in primary Raynaud's phenomenon. Lancet 336:1144, 1990.
15. Leppert J, Ringquist A, Karlberg BE, Ringquist I: Whole-body cooling increases plasma endothelin-1 levels in women with primary Raynaud's phenomenon. Clin Physiol 18:420-425, 1998.
16. Shawket S, Dickerson C, Hazelman B, et al: Selective suprasensitivity to calcitonin gene-related peptide in the hands in Raynaud's phenomenon. Lancet 2:1354-1357, 1989.
17. Allen EV, Brown GE: Raynaud's disease: A critical review of minimal requisites for diagnosis. Am J Med Sci 83:187-200, 1932.
18. McLafferty RB, Edwards JM, Ferris BL, et al: Raynaud's syndrome in workers who use vibrating pneumatic air knives. J Vasc Surg 30:1-7, 1999.
19. Landry G, Edwards JM, McLafferty RM, et al: Long-term outcome of Raynaud's syndrome in a prospective analyzed cohort. J Vasc Surg 23:76-86, 1996.
20. Priollet P, Vayssairat M, Housset E: How to classify Raynaud's phenomenon: Long-term follow-up study of 73 cases. Am J Med 83:494-498, 1987.
21. Harper FE, Maricq HR, Turner RE, et al: A prospective study of Raynaud's phenomenon and early connective tissue disease: A five-year report. Am J Med 72:883-888, 1982.
22. Edwards JM, Porter JM: Associated diseases with Raynaud's syndrome. Vasc Med Rev 1:51-58, 1990.
23. Ziegler S, Brunner M, Eigenbauer E, Minar E: Long-term outcome of primary Raynaud's phenomenon and its conversion to connective tissue disease: A 12-year retrospective patient analysis. Scand J Rheum 32:343-347, 2003.
24. De Angelis R, Del Medico P, Blasetti P, Cervini C. Raynaud's phenomenon: Clinical spectrum of 118 patients. Clin Rheum 22:279-284, 2003.
25. Porter JM, Snider RL, Bardana EJ, et al: The diagnosis and treatment of Raynaud's phenomenon. Surgery 77:11, 1975.
26. Holmgren K, Baur GM, Porter JM: The role of digital photoplethysmography in the evaluation of Raynaud's syndrome. Bruit 5:5-9, 1981.
27. Sumner D, Strandness DE: An abnormal finger pulse associated with cold sensitivity. Ann Surg 175:294-298, 1972.
28. Wigley F: Raynaud's phenomenon. N Engl J Med 347:1001-1008, 2002.
29. Proud G, Burke F, Lawson IJ, et al: Cold provocation testing and hand-arm vibration syndrome—an audit of the results of the Department of Trade and Industry scheme for the evaluation of miners. Br J Surg 90:1076-1079, 2003.
30. Nielson SL, Lassen NA: Measurement of digital blood pressure after local cooling. J Appl Physiol 43:907-910, 1977.
31. Gates KH, Tyburczy JA, Zupan T, et al: The noninvasive quantification of digital vasospasm. Bruit 8:34-37, 1984.
32. Clark S, Campbell F, Moore T, et al: Laser Doppler imaging—a new technique for quantifying microcirculatory flow in patients with primary Raynaud's phenomenon and systemic sclerosis. Microvasc Res 57:284-291, 1999.
33. Kanetaka T, Komiyama T, Onozuka A, et al: Laser Doppler skin perfusion in the assessment of Raynaud's phenomenon. Eur J Vasc Endovasc Surg 27:414-416, 2004.
34. Brown KM, Middaugh SJ, Haythornthwaite JA, Bielory L: The effects of stress, anxiety, and outdoor temperature on the frequency and severity of Raynaud's attacks: The Raynaud's Treatment Study. J Behav Med 24:137-153, 2001.
35. Palesch YY, Valter I, Carpentier PH, Maricq HR: Association between cigarette and alcohol consumption and Raynaud's phenomenon. J Clin Epidemiol 52:321-328, 1999.
36. Mills JL, Friedman EI, Taylor LM Jr, et al: Upper extremity ischemia caused by small artery disease. Ann Surg 206:521, 1987.
37. Rodeheffer RJ, Rommer JA, Wigley F, et al: Controlled double-blind trial of nifedipine in the treatment of Raynaud's phenomenon. N Engl J Med 308:880-883, 1983.
38. Fisher M, Grotta J: New uses for calcium channel blockers. Drugs 46:961-975, 1993.
39. Sturgill MG, Seibold JR: Rational use of calcium-channel antagonists in Raynaud's phenomenon. Curr Opin Rheumatol 10:584-588, 1998.
40. Weber A, Bounameaux H: Effects of low-dose nifedipine on a cold provocation test in patients with Raynaud's disease. J Cardiovasc Pharmacol 15:853-855, 1990.
41. Wigley FM, Wise RA, Seibold JR, et al: Intravenous iloprost infusion in patients with Raynaud phenomenon secondary to systemic sclerosis. Ann Intern Med 120:199-206, 1994.
42. Wigley FM, Seibold JR, Wise RA, et al: Intravenous iloprost treatment of Raynaud's phenomenon and ischemic ulcers secondary to systemic sclerosis. J Rheumatol 19:1407-1414, 1992.
43. Kyle MV, Belcher G, Hazleman BL: Placebo-controlled study showing therapeutic benefit of iloprost in the treatment of Raynaud's phenomenon. J Rheumatol 19:1403-1406, 1992.

44. Black CM, Halkier-Sorensen L, Belch JJ, et al: Oral iloprost in Raynaud's phenomenon secondary to systemic sclerosis: A multicentre, placebo-controlled, dose-comparison study. Br J Rheumatol 37:952-960, 1998.

45. Vayssairat M: Controlled multicenter double blind trial of an oral analog of prostacyclin in the treatment of primary Raynaud's phenomenon. J Rheumatol 23:1917-1920, 1996.

46. Wigley FM, Korn JH, Csuka ME, et al: Oral iloprost treatment in patients with Raynaud's phenomenon secondary to systemic sclerosis: A multicenter, placebo-controlled, double-blind study. Arthritis Rheum 41:670-677, 1998.

47. Wise RA, Wigley F: Acute effects of misoprostol on digital circulation in patients with Raynaud's phenomenon. J Rheumatol 21:80-83, 1994.

48. Katoh K, Kawai T, Narita M: Use of prostaglandin E_1 (lipo-PGE_1) to treat Raynaud's phenomenon associated with connective tissue disease: Thermographic and subjective assessment. J Pharm Pharmacol 44:442-444, 1992.

49. Pancera P, Sansone S, Secchi S, et al: The effects of thromboxane A_2 inhibition (picotamide) and angiotensin II receptor blockade (losartan) in primary Raynaud's phenomenon. J Intern Med 242:373-376, 1997.

50. Dziadzio M, Denton CP, Smith R, et al: Losartan therapy for Raynaud's phenomenon and scleroderma: Clinical and biochemical findings in a fifteen-week, randomized, parallel-group, controlled trial. Arthritis Rheum 42:2646-2655, 1999.

51. Coleiro B, Marshall SE, Denton CP, et al: Treatment of Raynaud's phenomenon with the serotonin reuptake inhibitor fluoxetine. Rheumatology 40:1038-1043, 2001.

52. Pope J, Fenlon D, Thompson A, et al: Prazosin for Raynaud's phenomenon in progressive systemic sclerosis. Cochrane Database Syst Rev 2:CD000956, 2000.

53. Rajagopalan S, Pfenninger D, Somers E, et al: Effects of cilostazol in patients with Raynaud's syndrome. Am J Cardiol 92:1310-1315, 2003.

54. Freedman RR: Physiological mechanisms of temperature biofeedback. Biofeedback Self Regul 16:95-115, 1991.

55. Comparison of sustained-release nifedipine and temperature biofeedback for treatment of primary Raynaud's phenomenon: Results from a randomized clinical trial with 1-year follow up. Arch Intern Med 160:1101-1108, 2000.

56. Mulder P, Dompeling EC, van Slochteren-van der Boor JC, et al: Transcutaneous electrical nerve stimulation (TENS) in Raynaud's phenomenon. Angiology 42:414-417, 1991.

57. Appiah R, Hiller S, Caspary L, et al: Treatment of primary Raynaud's syndrome with traditional Chinese acupuncture. J Intern Med 241:119-124, 1997.

58. Lowell RC, Gloviczki P, Cherry KJ, et al: Cervicothoracic sympathectomy for Raynaud's syndrome. Int Angiol 12:168, 1993.

59. Matsumoto Y, Ueyama T, Endo M, et al: Endoscopic thoracic sympathectomy for Raynaud's phenomenon. J Vasc Surg 36:57-61, 2002.

60. Janoff KA, Phinney ES, Porter JM: Lumbar sympathectomy for lower extremity vasospasm. Am J Surg 150:147-151, 1985.

61. Watarida S, Shiraishi S, Fujimura M, et al: Laparoscopic lumbar sympathectomy for lower-limb disease. Surg Endosc 16:500-503, 2002.

62. Yee AM, Hotchkiss RN, Paget SA: Adventitial stripping: A digit saving procedure in refractory Raynaud's phenomenon. J Rheumatol 25:269-276, 1998.

63. McCall TE, Petersen DP, Wong LB: The use of digital artery sympathectomy as a salvage procedure for severe ischemia of Raynaud's disease and phenomenon. J Hand Surg [Am] 24:173-177, 1999.

64. Balogh B, Mayer W, Vesely M, et al: Adventitial stripping of the radial and ulnar arteries in Raynaud's disease. J Hand Surg [Am] 27:1073-1080, 2002.

65. Jones NF, Raynor SC, Medsger TA: Microsurgical revascularization of the hand in scleroderma. Br J Plast Surg 40:264-269, 1987.

66. Nehler MR, Dalman RL, Harris EJ, et al: Upper extremity arterial bypass distal to the wrist. J Vasc Surg 16:633-642, 1992.

67. King TA, Marks J, Berrettone BA: Arteriovenous reversal for limb salvage in unreconstructable upper extremity arterial occlusive disease. J Vasc Surg 17:924-933, 1993.

68. Spencer-Green G: Outcomes in primary Raynaud's phenomenon: A meta-analysis of the frequency, rates, and predictors of transition to secondary diseases. Arch Intern Med 158:595-600, 1998.

69. Lie JT: Vasculitis, 1815 to 1991: Classification and diagnostic specificity. J Rheumatol 19:83-89, 1992.

70. Jennette JC, Falk RJ, Andrassy K, et al: Nomenclature of systemic vasculitides: Proposal of an international consensus conference. Arthritis Rheum 37:187-192, 1994.

71. Sheperd RFJ, Rooke T: Uncommon arteriopathies: What the vascular surgeon needs to know. Semin Vasc Surg 16:240-251, 2003.

72. Savage COS: Pathogenesis of systemic vasculitis. In Churg A, Churg J (eds): Systemic Vasculitides. New York, Igaku-Shoin, 1991, pp 7-30.

73. Gauthier VJ, Mannik M: Immune complexes in the pathogenesis of vasculitis. In LeRoy EC (ed): Systemic Vasculitis: The Biological Basis. New York, Marcel Dekker, 1992, pp 401-420.

74. Sheps SG, McDuffie FC: Vasculitis. In Juergens JL, Spittell JA, Gairbaim JF (eds): Peripheral Vascular Disease. Philadelphia, WB Saunders, 1980, pp 493-553.

75. Jacobs MR, Allen NB: Giant cell arteritis. In Churg A, Churg J (eds): Systemic Vasculitides. New York, Igaku-Shoin, 1991, pp 143-158.

76. Joyce JW: Uncommon arteriopathies. In Rutherford RB (ed): Vascular Surgery. Philadelphia, WB Saunders, 1989, pp 276-286.

77. Michel BA, Arend WP, Hunder GG: Clinical differentiation between giant cell (temporal) arteritis and Takayasu's arteritis. J Rheumatol 23:106-111, 1996.

78. Salvarani C, Gabriel SE, O'Fallon WM, Hunder GG: The incidence of giant cell arteritis in Olmsted County, Minnesota: Apparent fluctuations in a cyclic pattern. Ann Intern Med 123:192-194, 1995.

79. Duhaut P, Bosshard S, Calvet A, et al: Giant cell arteritis, polymyalgia rheumatica, and viral hypotheses: A multicenter, prospective case-control study. J Rheumatol 26:361-369, 1999.

80. Pountain G, Hazleman B: Polymyalgia rheumatica and giant cell arteritis. BMJ 310:1057-1059, 1995.

81. Salvarani C, Cantini F, Boiardi L, Hunder GG: Polymyalgia rheumatica and giant-cell arteritis. N Engl J Med 347:261-271, 2002.

82. Mehler MF, Rabinowich L: The clinical neuro-ophthalmologic spectrum of temporal arteritis. Am J Med 85:839-844, 1988.

83. Gonzalez-Gay MA, Blanco R, Rodriguez-Valverde V, et al: Permanent visual loss and cerebrovascular accidents in giant cell arteritis: Predictors and response to treatment. Arthritis Rheum 41:1497-1504, 1998.

84. Evans JM, O'Fallon M, Hunder GG: Increased incidence of aortic aneurysm and dissection in giant cell (temporal) arteritis. Ann Intern Med 122:502-507, 1995.

85. Stanson AW: Imaging findings in extracranial (giant cell) temporal arteritis. Clin Exp Rheumatol 18(Suppl 20):S43-S48, 2001.

86. Klein RG, Hunder GG, Stanson AW, et al: Large artery involvement in giant cell temporal arteritis. Ann Intern Med 83:806-812, 1975.

87. Rivers SP, Baur GM, Inahara T, et al: Arm ischemia secondary to giant cell arteritis. Am J Surg 143:554-558, 1982.

88. Kay RH, Pale R, Herman MV: Unsuspected giant cell arteritis diagnosed at open heart surgery. Arch Intern Med 112:1378-1379, 1982.

89. Hunder GG, Bloch DA, Michel BA, et al: The American College of Rheumatology 1990 criteria for the classification of giant cell arteritis. Arthritis Rheum 33:1122-1128, 1990.

90. Salvarini C, Hunder GG: Giant cell arteritis with low erythrocyte sedimentation rate: Frequency of occurrence in a population-based study. Arthritis Rheum 45:140-145, 2001.

91. Cantini F, Salvarani C, Olivieri I, et al: Erythrocyte sedimentation rate and C-reactive protein in the evaluation of disease activity and severity in polymyalgia rheumatica: A prospective follow-up study. Semin Arthritis Rheum 30:17-24, 2000.

92. Achkar AA, Lie JT, Hunder GG, et al: How does previous corticosteroid treatment affect the biopsy findings in giant cell (temporal) arteritis? Ann Intern Med 120:987-992, 1994.

93. Boyer LR, Miller NR, Green WR: Efficacy of unilateral versus bilateral temporal artery biopsies for the diagnosis of giant cell arteritis. Am J Ophthalmol 128:211-215, 1999.

94. Schmidt WA, Kraft HE, Vorpahl K, et al: Color duplex ultrasonography in the diagnosis of temporal arteritis. N Engl J Med 337:1336-1342, 1997.

95. Jover JA, Hernandez-Garcia C, Morado IC, et al: Combined treatment of giant-cell arteritis with methotrexate and prednisone: A randomized, double blind, placebo-controlled trial. Ann Intern Med 134:106-114, 2001.

96. Cantini F, Niccoli L, Salvarani C, et al: Treatment of longstanding active giant cell arteritis with infliximab: Report of four cases. Arthritis Rheum 44:2933-2935, 2001.

97. Matteson EL, Gold KN, Bloch DA, Hunder GG: Long-term survival of patients with giant cell arteritis in the American College of Rheumatology giant cell arteritis classification criteria cohort. Am J Med 100:193-196, 1996.

98. Numano F, Okawara M, Inomata H, et al: Takayasu's arteritis. Lancet 356:1023-1025, 2000.

99. Sharma BK, Jain S: A possible role of sex in determining distribution of lesions in Takayasu arteritis. Int J Cardiol 66:S81-S84, 1998.

100. Lupi-Herrera E, Sanchez-Torres G, Marcustiamer J, et al: Takayasu's arteritis: Clinical study of 107 cases. Am Heart J 93:94-103, 1977.
101. Sharma S, Rajani M, Talwar KK: Angiographic morphology in non-specific aortoarteritis (Takayasu's arteritis): A study of 126 patients from north India. Cardiovasc Intervent Radiol 15:160-165, 1992.
102. Sun Y, Yip PK, Jeng JS, et al: Ultrasonographic study and long-term follow-up of Takayasu's arteritis. Stroke 27:2178-2182, 1996.
103. Taniguchi N, Itoh K, Honda M, et al: Comparative ultrasonographic and angiographic study of carotid arterial lesions in Takayasu's arteritis. Angiology 48:9-20, 1997.
104. Park JH, Chung JW, Lee KW, et al: CT angiography of Takayasu's arteritis: Comparison with conventional angiography. J Vasc Intervent Radiol 8:393-400, 1997.
105. Yamazaki M, Takano H, Miyauchi H, et al: Detection of Takayasu arteritis in early stage by computed tomography. Int J Cardiol 85:305-307, 2002.
106. Tso E, Flamm SD, White RD, et al: Takayasu arteritis: Utility and limitations of magnetic resonance imaging in diagnosis and treatment. Arthritis Rheum 46:1634-1642, 2002.
107. Kerr GS, Hallahan CW, Giordano J, et al: Takayasu arteritis. Ann Intern Med 120:919-929, 1994.
108. Joyce JW: The giant cell arteritides: Diagnosis and the role of surgery. J Vasc Surg 3:827-832, 1986.
109. Robbs JV, Abdool-Carrim ATO, Kadwa AM: Arterial reconstruction for non-specific arteritis (Takayasu's disease): Medium to long term results. Eur J Vasc Surg 8:401-407, 1994.
110. Miyata T, Sato O, Koyama H, et al: Long-term survival after surgical treatment of patients with Takayasu's arteritis. Circulation 108:1474-1480, 2003.
111. Tyagi S, Kaul UA, Nair M, et al: Balloon angioplasty of the aorta in Takayasu's arteritis: Initial and long-term results. Am Heart J 124:876-882, 1992.
112. Rao SA, Mandalam KR, Rao VR, et al: Takayasu arteritis: Initial and long-term follow-up in 16 patients after percutaneous transluminal angioplasty of the descending thoracic and abdominal aorta. Radiology 189:173-179, 1993.
113. Tyagi S, Verma PK, Gambhir DS, et al: Early and long-term results of subclavian angioplasty in aortoarteritis (Takayasu's disease): Comparison with atherosclerosis. Cardiovasc Intervent Radiol 21:219-224, 1998.
114. Madrazo AA, Keane WF: Radiation vasculitis. In Churg A, Churg J (eds): Systemic Vasculitides. New York, Igaku-Shoin, 1991, pp 343-349.
115. Sugihara T, Hattori Y, Yamamoto Y, et al: Preferential impairment of nitric oxide-mediated endothelium-dependent relaxation in human cervical arteries after radiation. Circulation 100:635-641, 1999.
116. Fonkalsrud EW, Sanchez M, Zervbavel R, et al: Serial changes in arterial structure following radiation therapy. Surg Gynecol Obstet 145:395-400, 1977.
117. McCready RA, Hyde GL, Bivins BA, et al: Radiation induced arterial injuries. Surgery 93:306-312, 1983.
118. August M, Wang J, Plante D, et al: Complications associated with therapeutic neck radiation. J Oral Maxillofac Surg 54:1409-1415, 1996.
119. Andros G, Schneider PA, Harris RW, et al: Management of arterial occlusive disease following radiation therapy. Cardiovasc Surg 9:135-142, 1996.
120. Phillips GR 3rd, Peer RM, Upson JE, Ricotta JJ: Late complications of revascularization for radiation-induced arterial disease. J Vasc Surg 16:921-924, 1992.
121. Roubin GS, New G, Iyer SS, et al: Immediate and late clinical outcomes of carotid artery stenting in patients with symptomatic and asymptomatic carotid artery stenosis: A five-year prospective analysis. Circulation 103:532-537, 2001.
122. Branchereau AP, Berthet JP, Marty-Ane MH: Carotid artery stenting for stenosis following revascularization or cervical irradiation. J Endovasc Ther 9:14-19, 2002.
123. Modrall JG, Sadjadi J: Early and late presentations of radiation arteritis. Semin Vasc Surg 16:209-214, 2003.
124. Arkin A: A clinical and pathological study of periarteritis nodosa. Am J Pathol 6:401-427, 1930.
125. Rosen S, Falk RJ, Jennette JC: Polyarteritis nodosa, including microscopic form and renal vasculitis. In Churg A, Churg J (eds): Systemic Vasculitides. New York, Igaku-Shoin, 1991, pp 57-77.
126. Staud R, Williams RC: Antineutrophilic cytoplasmic antibodies (ANCA) and vasculitis. Compr Ther 20:623-627, 1994.
127. Travers RL, Allison DJ, Brettle RP, et al: Polyarteritis nodosa: A clinical and angiographic analysis of 17 cases. Semin Arthritis Rheum 8:184-199, 1979.
128. Ewald EA, Griffin D, McCune WJ: Correlation of angiographic abnormalities with disease manifestations and disease severity in polyarteritis nodosa. J Rheumatol 14:952-956, 1987.
129. Selke FW, Williams GB, Donovan DL, et al: Management of intra-abdominal aneurysms associated with periarteritis nodosa. J Vasc Surg 4:294-299, 1986.
130. Fauci AS, Katz P, Haynes BF, et al: Cyclophosphamide therapy of severe systemic necrotizing vasculitis. N Engl J Med 301:325-328, 1979.
131. McCauley RL, Johnston MR, Fauci AS: Surgical aspects of systemic necrotizing vasculitis. Surgery 97:104-108, 1985.
132. Cohen RD, Conn DL, Ilstrup DM: Clinical features, prognosis, and response to treatment in polyarteritis. Mayo Clin Proc 55:140-144, 1980.
133. Allen NB, Bressler PB: Diagnosis and treatment of systemic and cutaneous necrotizing vasculitis syndromes. Med Clin North Am 8:243-259, 1997.
134. Guillevin L, Lhote F, Gayraud M, et al: Prognostic factors in polyarteritis nodosa and Churg-Strauss syndrome: A prospective study in 342 patients. Medicine (Baltimore) 75:17-28, 1996.
135. Kawasaki T: MCLS—clinical observations of 50 cases. Jpn J Allergy 16:178-182, 1967.
136. Kawasaki T, Kosaki F, Okawa S, et al: A new infantile acute febrile mucocutaneous lymph node syndrome (MLNS) prevailing in Japan. Pediatrics 54:271-276, 1974.
137. Feigen RD, Schleien CL: Kawasaki disease. Curr Clin Top Infect Dis 4:30, 1983.
138. Yanagawa H, Yashiro M, Nakamura Y, et al: Epidemiologic pictures of Kawasaki disease in Japan: From the nationwide incidence survey in 1991 and 1992. Pediatrics 95:475-479, 1995.
139. Barron KS, Shulman ST, Rowley A, et al: Report of the National Institutes of Health Workshop on Kawasaki disease. J Rheumatol 26:170-190, 1999.
140. Arav-Boger R, Assia A, Jurgenson U, Spirer Z: The immunology of Kawasaki disease. Adv Pediatr 41:359-367, 1994.
141. Nadh MC, Shah V, Dillon MJ: Soluble cell adhesion molecules and von Willebrand factor in children with Kawasaki disease. Clin Exp Immunol 101:13-17, 1995.
142. Landing BH, Larson EJ: Pathological features of Kawasaki disease (mucocutaneous lymph node syndrome). Am J Cardiovasc Pathol 1:215-229, 1987.
143. Laupland KB, Dele Davies H: Epidemiology, etiology, and management of Kawasaki disease: State of the art. Pediatr Cardiol 20:177-183, 1999.
144. Capannari TE, Daniels SR, Meyer RA, et al: Sensitivity, specificity, and predictive value of two-dimensional echocardiography in detecting coronary artery aneurysms in patients with Kawasaki disease. J Am Coll Cardiol 7:355-360, 1986.
145. Gribetz D, Landing BH, Larson EJ: Kawasaki disease: Mucocutaneous lymph node syndrome (MCLS). In Churg A, Churg J (eds): Systemic Vasculitides. New York, Igaku-Shoin, 1991, pp 257-272.
146. Kato H, Ichinose E, Yoshioka F, et al: Fate of coronary aneurysms in Kawasaki disease: Serial coronary angiography and long term follow-up study. Am J Cardiol 49:1758-1766, 1982.
147. Inoue O, Akagi T, Ichinose E, et al: Systemic artery involvement in Kawasaki disease. In Proceedings of the Third International Kawasaki Disease Symposium, Tokyo, November 29 to December 2, 1988. New York, Allan R Liss, 1988, p 53.
148. Koren G, Rose V, Lavi S, Rowe R: Probable efficacy of high dose salicylates in reducing coronary involvement in Kawasaki disease. JAMA 254:767-769, 1985.
149. Saalouke MG, Venglarcik JS III, Barker DR, et al: Rapid regression of coronary dilatation in Kawasaki disease with intravenous gamma-globulin. Am Heart J 12:905-909, 1991.
150. Freeman AF, Shulman ST: Refractory Kawasaki disease. Pediatr Infect Dis J 23:463-464, 2004.
151. Kitamura S, Kawashima Y, Fujita T, et al: Aortocoronary bypass grafting in a child with coronary obstruction due to a mucocutaneous lymph node syndrome. Circulation 53:1035-1040, 1976.
152. Myers JL, Gleason MM, Cyren SE, Baylen BG: Surgical management of coronary insufficiency in a child with Kawasaki's disease: Use of bilateral mammary arteries. Ann Thorac Surg 46:459-461, 1988.
153. Kitamura S: The role of coronary bypass operation on children with Kawasaki disease. Coron Artery Dis 13:437-447, 2002.
154. Takeuchi Y, Gomi A, Okamura Y, et al: Coronary revascularization in a child with Kawasaki disease: Use of a right gastroepiploic artery. Ann Thorac Surg 50:294-296, 1990.

155. Kitamura S, Kameda Y, Seki T, et al: Long-term outcome of myocardial revascularization in patients with Kawasaki coronary artery disease: A multicenter cooperative study. J Thorac Cardiovasc Surg 107:663-673, 1994.
156. Checchia PA, Pahl E, Shaddy RE, Shulman ST: Cardiac transplantation for Kawasaki disease. Pediatrics 100:695-699, 1997.
157. Sethi S, Ott DA, Nihill M: Surgical management of the cardiovascular complications of Kawasaki's disease. Tex Heart Inst J 10:343-348, 1983.
158. Mockel M, Kampf D, Lobeck H, et al: Severe panarteritis associated with drug abuse. Intensive Care Med 25:113-117, 1999.
159. Yu Y, Cooper DR, Wellenstein DE: Cerebral angiitis and intracerebral hemorrhage associated with methamphetamine abuse. J Neurosurg 58:109-111, 1983.
160. Fredericks RK, Lefkowitz DS, Challa VR, Troost BT: Cerebral vasculitis associated with cocaine abuse. Stroke 22:1437-1439, 1991.
161. Bingham C, Beaman M, Nicholls AJ, Anthony PP: Necrotizing renal vasculopathy resulting in chronic renal failure after ingestion of methamphetamine and 3,4-methylenedioxymethamphetamine ("ecstasy"). Nephrol Dial Transplant 13:2654-2655, 1998.
162. Ellertson DG, Lazarus AM, Averbach R: Patterns of acute vascular injury after intra-arterial barbiturate injection. Am J Surg 126:813-817, 1973.
163. Lindell TD, Porter JM, Langston C: Intraarterial injection of oral medications: A complication of drug addiction. N Engl J Med 287:1132-1133, 1972.
164. Woodburn KR, Murie JA: Vascular complications of injecting drug misuse. Br J Surg 83:1329-1334, 1996.
165. Behçet H: Über rezidivierende Aphthose durch ein Virus verursachte Geschwur am Mund, am Maule und an den Genitalien. Dermatol Wochenschr 105:1152-1157, 1937.
166. Espinosa G, Font J, Tassies D, et al: Vascular involvement in Behçet's disease. Am J Med 112:37-43, 2002.
167. Shimutzu T, Ehrlich GE, Inaba G, Hayashi K: Behçet's disease (Behçet's syndrome). Semin Arthritis Rheum 8:223-260, 1979.
168. Ehrlich GE: Vasculitis in Behçet's disease. Int Rev Immunol 14:81-88, 1997.
169. Hamzaoui K, Hamzaoui A, Hentati F, et al: Phenotype and functional profile of T cells expressing gamma-delta receptor from patients with active Behçet's disease. J Rheumatol 21:2301-2306, 1994.
170. Sakane T, Takeno M, Suzuki N, Inaba G: Behçet's disease. N Engl J Med 341:1284-1291, 1999.
171. Mizuki N, Inoko H, Ohno S: Pathogenic gene responsible for the predisposition to Behçet's disease. Int Rev Immunol 14:33-48, 1997.
172. Lehner T: The role of heat shock protein, microbial and autoimmune agents in the aetiology of Behçet's syndrome. Int Rev Immunol 14:21-32, 1997.
173. Schwartz P, Weisbrott M, Landau M, Antebi E: Peripheral false aneurysms in Behçet's disease. Br J Surg 74:67-68, 1987.
174. Tuzun H, Besirli K, Sayin A, et al: Management of aneurysms in Behçet's syndrome: An analysis of 24 patients. Surgery 121:150-156, 1997.
175. Vasseur MA, Haulon S, Beregi JP, et al: Endovascular treatment of abdominal aneurysmal aortitis in Behçet's disease. J Vasc Surg 27:974-976, 1998.
176. Kasirajan K, Marek JM, Langsfeld M: Behçet's disease: Endovascular management of a ruptured peripheral arterial aneurysm. J Vasc Surg 34:127-129, 2001.
177. Yurdakul S, Hamuryudan V, Yazici H: Behçet syndrome. Curr Opin Rheumatol 16:38-42, 2004.
178. Freyrie A, Paragona O, Cenacchi G, et al: True and false aneurysms in Behçet's disease: Case report with ultrastructural observations. J Vasc Surg 17:762-767, 1993.
179. St Clair EW, McCallum RW: Cogan's syndrome. Curr Opin Rheumatol 11:47-52, 1999.
180. Ho AC, Roat MI, Venbrux A, Hellmann DB: Cogan's syndrome with refractory abdominal aortitis and mesenteric vasculitis. J Rheumatol 26:1404-1407, 1999.
181. Tseng JF, Cambria RP, Aretz HT, Brewster DC: Thoracoabdominal aortic aneurysm in Cogan's syndrome. J Vasc Surg 30:565-568, 1999.
182. Covelli M, Lapadula G, Pipitone V: Cogan's syndrome: Unsuccessful outcome with early combination therapy. Clin Exp Rheumatol 17:479-483, 1999.
183. Fortin PR, Esdaile JM: Vasculitis and malignancy. In Churg A, Churg J (eds): Systemic Vasculitides. New York, Igaku-Shoin, 1991, pp 327-341.
184. Greer JM, Longley S, Edwards NL, et al: Vasculitis associated with malignancy. Medicine 67:220-230, 1988.
185. Fortin PR: Vasculitides associated with malignancy. Curr Opin Rheumatol 8:30-33, 1996.
186. Kurzrock R, Cohen PR, Markowitz A: Clinical manifestations of vasculitis in patients with solid tumors: A case report and review of the literature. Arch Intern Med 154:334-340, 1994.
187. Andrasch RH, Bardana EJ, Porter JM, et al: Digital ischemia and gangrene preceding renal neoplasm. Arch Intern Med 136:486-488, 1976.
188. Levo Y, Gorevic PD, Kassab HJ, et al: Association between hepatitis B virus and essential mixed cryoglobulinemia. N Engl J Med 296:1501-1504, 1977.
189. Taylor LM, Baur GM, Porter JM: Finger gangrene caused by small artery occlusive disease. Ann Surg 193:453, 1981.
190. Danning CL, Illei GG, Boumpas DT: Vasculitis associated with primary rheumatologic disease. Curr Opin Rheumatol 10:58-65, 1998.
191. Panush RS, Katz P, Longley S, et al: Rheumatoid vasculitis: Diagnostic and therapeutic decisions. Clin Rheumatol 2:321-330, 1983.
192. Braun MG, Csernok E, Schmitt WH, Gross WL: Incidence, target antigens, and clinical implications of antineutrophil cytoplasmic antibodies in rheumatoid arthritis. J Rheumatol 23:826-830, 1996.
193. Voskuyl AE, Zwinderman AH, Westedt ML, et al: Factors associated with the development of vasculitis in rheumatoid arthritis: A case-control study. Ann Rheum Dis 55:190-192, 1996.
194. D'Cruz D: Vasculitis in systemic lupus erythematosus. Lupus 7:270-274, 1998.
195. Witte T, Hartung K, Matthias T, et al: Association of IgA anti-dsDNA antibodies with vasculitis and disease activity in systemic lupus erythematosus. Rheumatol Int 18:63-69, 1998.
196. Navarro M, Cervera R, Font J, et al: Anti-endothelial cell antibodies in systemic autoimmune diseases: Prevalence and clinical significance. Lupus 6:521-526, 1997.
197. Roman MJ, Shanker BA, Davis A, et al: Prevalence and correlates of accelerated atherosclerosis in systemic lupus erythematosus. N Engl J Med 349:2399-2406, 2003.
198. Doria A, Shoenfeld Y, Wu R, et al: Risk factors for subclinical atherosclerosis in a prospective cohort of patients with systemic lupus erythematosus. Ann Rheum Dis 62:1071-1077, 2003.
199. Martin-Suarez I, D'Cruz D, Mansoor M, et al: Immunosuppressive treatment in severe connective tissue diseases: Effect of low dose intravenous cyclophosphamide. Ann Rheum Dis 56:481-487, 1997.
200. Buerger L: Thromboangiitis obliterans: A study of the vascular lesions leading to presenile spontaneous gangrene. Am J Med Sci 136:567-580, 1908.
201. Mills JL: Buerger's disease in the 21st century: Diagnosis, clinical features, and therapy. Semin Vasc Surg16:179-189, 2003.
202. Olin JW: Current concepts: Thromboangiitis obliterans (Buerger's disease). N Engl J Med 343:864-869, 2000.
203. Cutler DA, Runge MS: 86 years of Buerger's disease—what have we learned? Am J Med Sci 309:74-75, 1995.
204. Abu-Dalu J, Giler SH, Urca I: Thromboangiitis obliterans of the iliac artery. Angiology 24:359-364, 1973.
205. Lie JT: Visceral intestinal Buerger's disease. Int J Cardiol 66(Suppl 1): S249-S256, 1998.
206. Papa M, Bass A, Adar R, et al: Autoimmune mechanisms in thromboangiitis obliterans (Buerger's disease): The role of tobacco antigen and the major histocompatibility complex. Surgery 111:527-531, 1992.
207. Spittell JA: Thromboangiitis obliterans—an autoimmune disorder. N Engl J Med 308:1157-1158, 1983.
208. Simi CL, Pirnat L: Immunological aspects of smoking in patients with thromboangiitis obliterans. Vasa 14:349-352, 1985.
209. Adar R, Papa MZ, Halpern Z, et al: Cellular sensitivity to collagen in thromboangiitis obliterans. N Engl J Med 308:1113-1116, 1983.
210. Eichhorn J, Sima D, Lindschau C, et al: Antiendothelial cell antibodies in thromboangiitis obliterans. Am J Med Sci 315:17-23, 1998.
211. Kobayashi M, Ito M, Nakagawa A, et al: Immunohistochemical analysis of arterial wall cellular infiltration in Buerger's disease (endarteritis obliterans). J Vasc Surg 29:451-458, 1999.
212. Mills JL, Porter JM: Buerger's disease: A review and update. Semin Vasc Surg 6:14-23, 1993.
213. Shionoya S: Diagnostic criteria of Buerger's disease. Int J Cardiol 66(Suppl):S243-S245, 1998.
214. Matsushita M, Shionoya S, Matsumoto T: Urinary cotinine measurement in patients with Buerger's disease: Effects of active and passive smoking on the disease process. J Vasc Surg 14:53-58, 1992.

215. Mills JL, Friedman EI, Taylor LM Jr, Porter JM: Upper extremity ischemia caused by small artery disease. Ann Surg 206:521-528, 1987.
216. Borner C, Heidrich H: Long-term follow-up of thromboangiitis obliterans. Vasa 27:80-86, 1998.
217. Ohta T, Ishioashi H, Hosaka M, Sugimoto I: Clinical and social consequences of Buerger's disease. J Vasc Surg 39:176-180, 2004.
218. Swigris JJ, Olin JW, Mekhail NA: Implantable spinal cord stimulator to treat the ischemic manifestations of thromboangiitis obliterans (Buerger's disease). J Vasc Surg 29:928-935, 1999.
219. Largiader J, Schneider E, Bruner U, Bollinger A: Arterial reconstruction in Buerger's disease (thromboangiitis obliterans). Vasa 15:174-179, 1986.
220. Sasajima T, Kubo Y, Inaba M, et al: Role of infrainguinal bypass in Buerger's disease: An eighteen-year experience. Eur J Vasc Endovasc Surg 13:186-192, 1997.
221. Talwar S, Jain S, Porwal R, et al: Pedicled omental transfer for limb salvage in Buerger's disease. Int J Cardiol 72:127-132, 2000.
222. Verstraete M, European TAO Study Group: Oral iloprost in the treatment of thromboangiitis obliterans (Buerger's disease): A double-blind, randomized, placebo-controlled trial. Eur J Vasc Endovasc Surg 15:300-307, 1998.
223. Isner JM, Baumgartner I, Rauh G, et al: Treatment of thromboangiitis obliterans (Buerger's disease) by intramuscular gene transfer of vascular endothelial growth factor: Preliminary results. J Vasc Surg 28:964-973, 1998.
224. Hollister DW, Godfrey MP, Sakai LY, et al: Immunohistologic abnormalities of the microfibrillar-fiber system in the Marfan syndrome. N Engl J Med 323:152-159, 1990.
225. Kainulainen K, Pulkkinen L, Savolainen A, et al: Location on chromosome 15 of the gene defect causing Marfan syndrome. N Engl J Med 323:935-939, 1990.
226. Dietz HC, Cutting GR, Pyeritz RE, et al: Marfan syndrome caused by a recurrent de novo missense mutation in the fibrillin gene. Nature 353:337-339, 1991.
227. Nijbroek G, Sood S, McIntosh I, et al: Fifteen novel FBN1 mutations causing Marfan syndrome detected by heteroduplex analysis of genomic amplicons. Am J Hum Genet 57:8-21, 1995.
228. Auyama T, Francke U, Dietz MC, Furthmayr H: Quantitative differences in biosynthesis and extracellular deposition of fibrillin in cultured fibroblasts distinguish five groups of Marfan syndrome patients and suggest distinct pathogenetic mechanisms. J Clin Invest 94:130-137, 1994.
229. McKusick VA: The defect in Marfan syndrome. Nature 352:279-281, 1991.
230. Schaefer GB, Godfrey M: Quantitation of fibrillin immunofluorescence in fibroblast cultures in the Marfan syndrome. Clin Genet 47:144-149, 1995.
231. Wang M, Mata J, Price CE, et al: Prenatal and presymptomatic diagnosis of the Marfan syndrome using fluorescence PCR and an automated sequencer. Prenat Diagn 15:499-507, 1995.
232. Perejda AJ, Abraham PA, Carnes WH, et al: Marfan syndrome: Structural, biochemical, and mechanical studies of the aortic media. J Lab Clin Med 106:376-383, 1985.
233. Segura AM, Lyna RE, Horiba K, et al: Immunohistochemistry of matrix metallo proteinases and their inhibitors in thoracic aortic aneurysms and aortic valves in patients with Marfan's syndrome. Circulation 98(Suppl):II331-II337, 1998.
234. Hirata K, Triposkiadis F, Sparks E, et al: The Marfan syndrome: Abnormal elastic properties. J Am Coll Cardiol 18:57-63, 1991.
235. Kornbluth M, Schnittger I, Eyngorina I, et al: Clinical outcome in the Marfan syndrome with ascending aortic dilatation followed annually by echocardiography. Am J Cardiol 84:752-755, 1999.
236. Rios AS, Silber EN, Bavishi N, et al: Effect of long-term beta blockade on aortic root compliance in patients with Marfan syndrome. Am Heart J 137:1057-1061, 1999.
237. Shores J, Berger KR, Murphy EA, Pyeritz RE: Progression of aortic dilatation and the benefit of long-term β-adrenergic blockade in Marfan's syndrome. N Engl J Med 330:1335-1341, 1994.
238. Fleck TM, Hutschala D, Tschernich H, et al: Stent graft placement of the thoracoabdominal aorta in a patient with Marfan syndrome. J Thorac Cardiovasc Surg 125:1541-1543, 2003.
239. Finkbohner R, Johnston D, Crawford ES, et al: Marfan syndrome: Long-term survival and complications after aortic aneurysm repair. Circulation 91:728-733, 1995.
240. Gio HVL, Greene PS, Alejo DE, et al: Replacement of the aortic root in patients with Marfan's syndrome. N Engl J Med 340:1307-1313, 1999.
241. Van Meekeren JA: De dilatabilitate extraordinaria cutis. In Observations Medicochirugicae. Amsterdam, 1682.
242. Ehlers E: Cutis laxa Neigung zu Haemorrhagien in der Haut, Lockerung mehrere Artikulationen. Dermatol Z 8:173-174, 1901.
243. Danlos M: Un cas de cutis laxa avec tumeurs par contusion chronique des condes et des genoux (xanthome juvénile pseudodiabè-tique de M. M. Hallopeault Mace de Lepinay). Bull Soc F Dermatol Syphilis 19:70, 1908.
244. Tsipouras P, Byers PH, Schwartz RC, et al: Ehlers-Danlos syndrome type IV: Cosegregation of the phenotype to a COL3A1 allele of type III procollagen. Hum Genet 74:41-46, 1986.
245. Prockop DJ, Kivirikko KI: Heritable diseases of collagen. N Engl J Med 34:376, 1984.
246. Freeman RK, Swegle J, Sise MJ: The surgical complications of Ehlers-Danlos syndrome. Am Surg 62:869-873, 1996.
247. Pepin M: Clinical and genetic features of Ehlers-Danlos syndrome type IV, the vascular type. N Engl J Med 342:673-680, 2000.
248. Bellenot F, Boisgard S, Kantelip B, et al: Type IV Ehlers-Danlos syndrome with isolated arterial involvement. Ann Vasc Surg 4:15-19, 1990.
249. Serry C, Agomuoh OS, Goldin MD: Review of Ehlers-Danlos syndrome: Successful repair of rupture and dissection of abdominal aorta. J Cardiovasc Surg 29:530-534, 1988.
250. Mattar SG, Kumar AG, Lumsden AB: Vascular complications in Ehlers-Danlos syndrome. Am Surg 60:827-831, 1994.
251. Erdheim J: Medionecrosis aortae idiopathica cystica. Virchows Arch 276:187-229, 1930.
252. Maraslese DI, Moodie DS, Lytle B, et al: Cystic medial necrosis of the aorta in patients without Marfan's syndrome: Surgical outcome and long-term follow-up. J Am Coll Cardiol 16:68-73, 1990.
253. Roberts AJ, Jaffe RB, Michaels LL, et al: Cystic medial necrosis: A correctable cause of the superior vena cava syndrome. Arch Surg 109:84, 1974.
254. Tredal SM, Carter JB, Edwards JE: Cystic medial necrosis of the pulmonary artery. Arch Pathol 97:183, 1974.
255. Millar AJ, Gilbert RD, Brown RA, et al: Abdominal aortic aneurysms in children. J Pediatr Surg 31:1624-1628, 1996.
256. Read RC, Wolf P: Symptomatic disseminated cystic medial necrosis. N Engl J Med 271:816, 1964.
257. Struk B, Neldner KH, Rao VS, et al: Mapping of both autosomal recessive and dominant variants of pseudoxanthoma elasticum to chromosome 16p13.1. Hum Mol Genet 6:1823-1828, 1997.
258. Van Soest S, Swart J, Tijmes N, et al: A locus for autosomal recessive pseudoxanthoma elasticum, with penetrance of vascular symptoms in carriers, maps to chromosome 16p13.1.Genome Res 7:830-834, 1997.
259. Hu X, Plomp AS, van Soest S, et al: Pseudoxanthoma elasticum: A clinical, histopathological, and molecular update. Surv Ophthalmol 48:424-438, 2003.
260. Carter DJ, Vince FP, Woodword DAK: Arterial surgery in pseudoxanthoma elasticum. Postgrad Med J 52:291, 1976.
261. Slade AK, John RM, Swanton RH: Pseudoxanthoma elasticum presenting with myocardial infarction. Br Heart J 63:372-373, 1990.
262. Kevorkian JP, Masque C, Kural-Menasche S, et al: New report of severe coronary artery disease in an eighteen year old girl with pseudoxanthoma elasticum: Case report and review of the literature. Angiology 48:735-741, 1997.
263. Takaro TK, Coodley GO: Pentoxifylline for ischemic pain in pseudoxanthoma elasticum. West J Med 159:689-690, 1993.
264. Leriche R: Dolicho et méga-artère: Dolicho et méga-veine. Presse Med 51:554, 1943.
265. Randall PA, Omar MM, Rohner R, et al: Arteria magna revisited. Radiology 132:295, 1979.
266. Thomas ML: Arteriomegaly. Br J Surg 71:690, 1971.
267. Lawrence PF, Wallis C, Dobrin PB, et al: Peripheral aneurysms and arteriomegaly: Is there a familial pattern? J Vasc Surg 28:599-605, 1998.
268. Quain R: Partial coarctation of the abdominal aorta. Trans Pathol Soc Lond 1:244, 1847.
269. Glenn F, Keefer EB, Speer DS, et al: Coarctation of the lower thoracic and abdominal aorta immediately proximal to the celiac axis. Surg Gynecol Obstet 94:561, 1952.
270. Hallett JW, Brewster CD, Darling RC, et al: Coarctation of the abdominal aorta: Current options in surgical management. Ann Surg 191:430, 1980.
271. Meacham PW, Dean RH, Lawson JW, et al: Study of the renal pressor system in experimental coarctation of the abdominal aorta. Am Surg 43:771, 1977.

272. Paroni R, Astuni M, Baroni C, et al: Abdominal aortic coarctation inducing aortic occlusion and renovascular hypertension. J Cardiovasc Surg 32:770-773, 1991.

273. Stanley JC, Graham LM, Whitehouse WM: Developmental occlusive disease of the abdominal aorta and the splenic and renal arteries. Am J Surg 142:190, 1981.

274. Siassi B, Glyman G, Emmonouilides GC: Hypoplasia of the abdominal aorta associated with the rubella syndrome. Am J Dis Child 120:426, 1970.

275. Sen PK, Kinore SG, Engineer SD, et al: The middle aortic syndrome. Br Heart J 25:610, 1963.

276. Lande A: Takayasu's arteritis and congenital coarctation of the descending thoracic and abdominal aorta: A critical review. AJR Am J Roentgenol 127:277, 1976.

277. Messina ML, Goldstone J, Ferrell LD, et al: Middle aortic syndrome: Effectiveness and durability of complex arterial revascularization techniques. Ann Surg 204:331-339, 1986.

278. Lillehei CW, Shamberger RC: Staged reconstruction for middle aortic syndrome. J Pediatr Surg 36:1252-1254, 2001.

279. Mickley V, Fleiter T: Coarctations of descending and abdominal aorta: Long-term results of surgical therapy. J Vasc Surg 28:206-214, 1998.

280. Brzezinska-Rajszys G, Qureshi SA, Ksiazyk J, et al: Middle aortic syndrome treated by stent implantation. Heart 81:166-170, 1999.

281. Eliason JL, Passman MA, Guzman RJ, Naslund TC: Durability of percutaneous angioplasty and stent implantation for the treatment of abdominal aortic coarctation: A case report. Vasc Surg 35:397-401, 2001.

282. Suarez de Lezo J, Pan M, Romero M, et al: Immediate and follow-up findings after stent treatment for severe coarctation of aorta. Am J Cardiol 83:400-406, 1999.

283. Shortell CK, Illig KA, Ouriel K, Green RM: Fetal internal iliac artery: Case report and embryologic review. J Vasc Surg 28:1112-1114, 1998.

284. Greebe J: Congenital anomalies of the iliofemoral artery. J Cardiovasc Surg 18:317, 1977.

285. Steele G, Saunders RJ, Riley J, et al: Pulsatile buttock masses: Gluteal and persistent sciatic artery aneurysms. Surgery 82:201-204, 1977.

286. Gasecki AP, Ebers GC, Vellet AD, Buchan A: Sciatic neuropathy associated with persistent sciatic artery. Arch Neurol 49:967-968, 1992.

287. Shutze WP, Garrett WV, Smith BL: Persistent sciatic artery: Collective review and management. Ann Vasc Surg 7:303-310, 1993.

288. Wolf YG, Gibbs BF, Guzzetta VJ, Bernstein EF: Surgical treatment of aneurysm of the persistent sciatic artery. J Vasc Surg 17:218-221, 1993.

289. Maldini G, Teruya TH, Kamida C, Eklof B: Combined percutaneous endovascular and open surgical approach in the treatment of a persistent sciatic artery aneurysm presenting with acute limb-threatening ischemia: A case report and review of the literature. Vasc Endovasc Surg 36:403-409, 2002.

290. Stuart TP: A note on a variation in the course of the popliteal artery. J Anat Physiol 13:162, 1879.

291. Hamming JJ: Intermittent claudication at an early age, due to an anomalous course of the popliteal artery. Angiology 10:369-371, 1959.

292. Love JW, Whelan TJ: Popliteal artery entrapment syndrome. Am J Surg 109:620-624, 1965.

293. Murray A, Halliday M, Croft RJ: Popliteal artery entrapment syndrome. Br J Surg 78:1414-1419, 1991.

294. Rich NM, Collins GJ, McDonald PT, et al: Popliteal vascular entrapment: Its increasing interest. Arch Surg 114:1377-1384, 1979.

295. Levien LJ: Popliteal artery entrapment syndrome. Semin Vasc Surg 16:223-231, 2003.

296. Turnipseed WD: Popliteal entrapment syndromes. J Vasc Surg 35:910-915, 2002.

297. Gibson MH, Mills JG, Johnson GE, et al: Popliteal entrapment syndrome. Ann Surg 185:341-348, 1977.

298. Naylor SJ, Levien LJ, Kooper K: Histological features of the popliteal artery entrapment syndrome. Vasc Surg 34:665-672, 2000.

299. diMarzo L, Cavallaro A, Sciacca V, et al: Diagnosis of popliteal artery entrapment syndrome: The role of duplex scanning. J Vasc Surg 13:434-438, 1991.

300. Collins PS, McDonald PT, Lim RC: Popliteal artery entrapment: An evolving syndrome. J Vasc Surg 10:484-490, 1989.

301. Rizzo RJ, Flinn WR, Yao JST, et al: Computed tomography for evaluation of arterial disease in the popliteal fossa. J Vasc Surg 11:112-119, 1990.

302. Fermand M, Houlle D, Fiessinger JN, et al: Entrapment of the popliteal artery: MR findings. AJR Am J Roentgenol 154:425-426, 1990.

303. Levien LJ, Veller MG: Popliteal artery entrapment syndrome: More common than previously recognized. J Vasc Surg 30:587-598, 1999.

304. Lambert AW, Wilkins DC: Popliteal artery entrapment syndrome. Br J Surg 86:1365-1370, 1999.

305. Ohara N, Miyata T, Oshiro H, et al: Surgical treatment for popliteal artery entrapment syndrome. Cardiovasc Surg 9:141-144, 2001.

306. Luscher TF, Lie JT, Stanson AW, et al: Arterial fibromuscular dysplasia. Mayo Clin Proc 62:931-952, 1987.

307. Stanley JC, Gewertz BL, Bove EL, et al: Arterial fibrodysplasia: Histopathologic character and current etiologic concepts. Arch Surg 110:561-566, 1975.

308. Leadbetter WF, Burkland CE: Hypertension in unilateral renal disease. J Urol 39:611-626, 1938.

309. Descotes J, Pelissier PH, Chignier E: Dystrophy of the media with aneurysmal tendency in the abdominal aorta-iliac segments. J Cardiovasc Surg 17:413, 1976.

310. Harrington OB, Crosby VG, Nicholas L: Fibromuscular hyperplasia of the internal carotid artery. Ann Thorac Surg 9:516-524, 1970.

311. Pannier-Moreau I, Grimbert P, Fiquet-Kempf B, et al: Possible familial origin of multifocal renal artery fibromuscular dysplasia. J Hypertens 15:1797-1801, 1997.

312. Bofinger A, Hawley C, Fisher P, et al: Polymorphisms of the renin-angiotensin system in patients with multifocal renal arterial fibromuscular dysplasia. J Hum Hypertens 15:185-190, 2001.

313. Olin JW, Piedmonte M, Young JR, et al: Utility of duplex scanning of the renal arteries for diagnosing significant renal artery stenosis. Ann Intern Med 122:833-838, 1995.

314. Radermacher J, Chavan A, Bleck J, et al: Use of Doppler ultrasonography to predict the outcome of therapy for renal artery stenosis. N Engl J Med 344:410-417, 2001.

315. Slovut DP, Olin JW: Current concepts: Fibromuscular dysplasia. N Engl J Med 350:1862-1871, 2004.

316. Anderson CA, Hansen KJ, Benjamin ME, et al: Renal artery fibromuscular dysplasia: Results of current surgical therapy. J Vasc Surg 22:207-216, 1995.

317. Reiher L, Pfeiffer T, Sandmann W: Long-term results after surgical reconstruction for renal artery fibromuscular dysplasia. Eur J Vasc Endovasc Surg 20:556-559, 2000.

318. Marekovic Z, Mokos I, Krhen I, et al: Long-term outcome after surgical kidney revascularization for fibromuscular dysplasia and atherosclerotic renal artery stenosis. J Urol 171:1043-1045, 2004.

319. O'Neill JA Jr: Long-term outcome with surgical treatment of renovascular hypertension. J Pediatr Surg 33:106-111, 1998.

320. Birrer M, Do DD, Mahler F, et al: Treatment of renal artery fibromuscular dysplasia with balloon angioplasty: A prospective follow-up study. Eur J Vasc Endovasc Surg 23:146-152, 2002.

321. Surowiec SM, Sivamurthy N, Rhodes JM, et al: Percutaneous therapy for renal artery fibromuscular dysplasia. Ann Vasc Surg 17:650-655, 2003.

322. de Fraissinette B, Garcier JM, Dieu V, et al: Percutaneous transluminal angioplasty of dysplastic stenoses of the renal artery: Results on 70 adults. Cardiovasc Intervent Radiol 26:46-51, 2003.

323. Davidson RA, Barri Y, Wilcox CS: Predictors of cure of hypertension in fibromuscular renovascular disease. Am J Kidney Dis 28:334-338, 1996.

324. Mettinger KL, Ericson K: Fibromuscular dysplasia and the brain. I. Observations on angiographic, clinical and genetic characteristics. Stroke 13:46, 1982.

325. Chiche L, Bahnini A, Koskas F, Kieffer E: Occlusive fibromuscular disease of arteries supplying the brain: Results of surgical treatment. Am Vasc Surg 11:496-504, 1997.

326. Flanigan DP, Burnham SJ, Goodreau JJ, et al: Summary of cases of adventitial cystic disease of the popliteal artery. Ann Surg 189:165-175, 1979.

327. Ejrup B, Hiertonn T: Intermittent claudication: Three cases treated by free vein graft. Acta Chir Scand 108:217, 1954.

328. Galle C, Cavenaile JC, Hoang AD, et al: Adventitial cystic disease of the popliteal artery communicating with the knee joint. J Vasc Surg 28:738-741, 1998.

329. Levien LJ, Benn CA: Adventitial cystic disease: A unifying hypothesis. J Vasc Surg 28:193-205, 1998.

330. Miller A, Salenius JP, Sacks BA, et al: Noninvasive vascular imaging in the diagnosis and treatment of adventitial cystic disease of the popliteal artery. J Vasc Surg 26:715-720, 1997.

331. Do DD, Braunschweig M, Baumgartner I, et al: Adventitial cystic disease of the popliteal artery: Percutaneous US-guided aspiration. Radiology 203:743-746, 1997.

332. Macfarlane R, Livesey SA, Pollard S, Dunn DC: Cystic adventitial arterial disease. Br J Surg 74:89-90, 1987.

333. Pursell R, Torrie EPH, Gibson M, Galland RB: Spontaneous and permanent resolution of cystic adventitial disease of the popliteal artery. J R Soc Med 97:77-78, 2004.

334. Tsolakis IA, Walvatne CS, Caldwell MD: Cystic adventitial disease of the popliteal artery: Diagnosis and treatment. Eur J Vasc Endovasc Surg 15:188-194, 1998.

335. Koman M, Hardaker WT, Goldner JL: Wick catheter in evaluating and treating compartment syndromes. South Med J 73:303-309, 1981.

336. Eaton RG, Green WT: Volkmann's ischemia: A volar compartment syndrome of the forearm. Clin Orthop 117:58-64, 1975.

337. Jepson PS: Ischemic contracture: Experimental study. Ann Surg 84:785, 1926.

338. Matsen FA: Compartmental Syndrome: A Unified Concept. New York, Grune & Stratton, 1980.

339. DelMaestro RF: An approach to free radicals in medicine and biology. Acta Physiol Scand Suppl 492:153-168, 1980.

340. Perler BA, Tohmeh AG, Bulkley GB: Inhibition of the compartment syndrome by ablation of free radical-mediated reperfusion injury. Surgery 108:40-47, 1990.

341. Mileski WJ, Winn RK, Vetter NB, et al: Inhibition of CD18-dependent neutrophil adherence reduces organ injury after hemorrhagic shock in primates. Surgery 108:206, 1990.

342. Mubarak SJ, Hargens AR: Acute compartment syndromes. Surg Clin North Am 63:539-551, 1983.

343. Mills JL, Porter JM: Basic data related to clinical decision-making in acute limb ischemia. Ann Vasc Surg 5:96-98, 1991.

344. Rudoff J, Ebner S, Canepa C: Limb-compartmental syndrome with thrombolysis. Am Heart J 128:1267-1268, 1994.

345. Whitesides TE, Haney TC, Morimoto K, et al: Tissue pressure measurements as a determinant of the need of fasciotomy. Clin Orthop 113:43-49, 1975.

346. Mubarak SJ, Owen CA, Hargens AR: Acute compartment syndromes: Diagnosis and treatment with the aid of the Wick catheter. J Bone Joint Surg Am 60:1091-1095, 1978.

347. McDermott AGP, Marble AE, Yabsley RH: Monitoring acute compartment pressures with the STIC catheter. Clin Orthop 190:192-197, 1984.

348. Mars M, Hadley GP: Raised intracompartmental pressure and compartment syndromes. Injury 29:403-411, 1998.

349. Mabee JR: Compartment syndrome: A complication of acute extremity trauma. J Emerg Med 12:651-656, 1994.

350. Perry MO: Compartment syndromes and reperfusion injury. Surg Clin North Am 68:853-864, 1988.

351. McCord JM: Oxygen-derived free radicals in post-ischemic tissue injury. N Engl J Med 313:154-157, 1985.

352. Blackman PG: A review of chronic exertional compartment syndrome in the lower leg. Med Sci Sports Exerc 32(Suppl):S4-S10, 2000.

353. Turnipseed WD: Diagnosis and management of chronic compartment syndrome. J Vasc Surg 132:613-619, 2002.

354. Yap S: Classical homocystinuria: Vascular risk and its prevention. J Inherit Metab Dis 26:259-265, 2003.

355. Carson HAJ, Cusworth DC, Dent CE, et al: Homocystinuria: A new inborn error of metabolism associated with mental deficiency. Arch Dis Child 38:425, 1963.

356. McCully KS: Homocysteine theory of atherosclerosis: Development and current status. Atheroscler Rev 11:157-247, 1983.

357. Mudd SH, Finkelstein JD, Irrevere F, Laster L: Homocystinuria: An enzymatic defect. Science 143:1443-1445, 1964.

358. Mudd SH, Levy HL, Abeles RH: A derangement in the metabolism of vitamin B₁₂ leading to homocystinuria, cystathionuria, and methyl malonic aciduria. Biochem Biophys Res Commun 35:21-26, 1969.

359. Deloughery TG, Evans A, Sadeghi A, et al: Common mutation in methylenetetrahydrofolate reductase: Correlation with homocysteine metabolism and late-onset vascular disease. Circulation 94:3074-3078, 1996.

360. Smolin LA, Crenshaw TD, Kurtyca D, Benevenga NJ: Homocysteine accumulation in pigs fed diets deficient in vitamin B₆ (pyridoxine): Relationship to atherosclerosis. J Nutr 133:2022-2028, 1983.

361. Kang SS, Wong PWK, Norusis M: Homocysteine due to folate deficiency. Metabolism 36:458-465, 1987.

362. Brattstrom L, Israelsson B, Lindgarde X, et al: Higher total plasma homocysteine in vitamin B₁₂ deficiency than in heterozygosity for homocystinuria due to cystathionine beta-synthetase deficiency. Metabolism 37:175-182, 1988.

363. Harker LA, Ross R, Slichter SJ, Scott CR: Homocystinemia: Vascular injury and arterial thrombosis. N Engl J Med 291:537-543, 1974.

364. Hladovec J: Experimental homocystinemia, endothelial lesions and thrombosis. Blood Vessels 16:202-205, 1979.

365. Refsum H, Helland S, Ueland PM: Radioenzymatic determination of homocysteine in plasma and urine. Clin Chem 31:624-628, 1985.

366. Boers GHK, Smals AGH, Trijbels FJM: Unique efficiency of methionine metabolism in premenopausal women may protect against vascular disease in the reproductive years. J Clin Invest 72:1971-1975, 1983.

367. McCully KS, Carvalho ACA: Homocysteine thiolactone, N-homocysteine thiolactonyl retinamide, and platelet aggregation. Res Commun Chem Pathol Pharmacol 6:349-360, 1987.

368. Kang SS, Wong PWK, Cook HY, et al: Protein bound homocysteine: A possible risk factor for coronary artery disease. J Clin Invest 77:1482-1486, 1986.

369. Fortin LJ, Genest J: Measurement of homocyst(e)ine in the prediction of arteriosclerosis. Clin Biochem 28:155-162, 1995.

370. McCully KS: Vascular pathology of homocysteinemia: Implications for the pathogenesis of atherosclerosis. Am J Pathol 56:111-128, 1969.

371. Kang SS: Critical points for determining moderate hyperhomocyst(e)inemia. Eur J Clin Invest 25:806-808, 1995.

372. Boers GHK, Smals AGH, Trijbels FJM, et al: Heterozygosity for homocystinuria in premature peripheral and cerebral occlusive arterial diseases. N Engl J Med 313:709-714, 1985.

373. Nehler MR, Taylor LM Jr: Homocysteinemia as a risk factor for atherosclerosis: A review. Cardiovasc Surg 5:559-567, 1997.

374. Taylor LM, DeFrang RD, Harris EJ, Porter JM: The association of elevated plasma homocyst(e)ine with progression of symptomatic peripheral arterial disease. J Vasc Surg 13:128-136, 1991.

375. Stampfer MJ, Malinow MR, Willett WC, et al: A prospective study of plasma homocyst(e)ine and risk of myocardial infarction in US physicians. JAMA 268:877-881, 1992.

376. Arnesen E, Refsum H, Bonaa KM, et al: Serum total homocysteine and coronary heart disease. Int J Epidemiol 24:704-709, 1995.

377. Perry IJ, Refsum H, Morris RW, et al: Prospective study of serum homocysteine concentration and risk of stroke in middle aged men. Lancet 346:1395-1398, 1995.

378. Verhoef P, Hennekens CH, Malinow MR, et al: A prospective study of plasma homocyst(e)ine and risk of ischemic stroke. Stroke 25:1924-1930, 1994.

379. Taylor LM Jr, Moneta GL, Sexton GJ, et al: Prospective blinded study of the relationship between plasma homocysteine and progression of symptomatic peripheral arterial disease. J Vasc Surg 29:8-21, 1999.

380. Nygard O, Nordrehaug JE, Refsum H, et al: Plasma homocysteine levels and mortality in patients with coronary heart disease. N Engl J Med 337:230-236, 1997.

381. Brattstrom L: Vitamins as homocysteine-lowering agents. J Nutr 126:S1276-S1280, 1996.

382. Wilcken DEL, Wilcken B: The natural history of vascular disease in homocystinuria and effects of treatment. J Inherit Metab Dis 20:295-300, 1997.

Questions

1. **Which group with Raynaud's syndrome has the lowest risk of developing a connective tissue disease?**
   - (a) Vasospastic, negative serologies
   - (b) Vasospastic, positive serologies
   - (c) Obstructive, negative serologies
   - (d) Obstructive, positive serologies
   - (e) Obstructive, unknown serologies

2. **Vasculitis is a central feature in all of the following syndromes except**
   - (a) Kawasaki disease
   - (b) Cogan's syndrome
   - (c) Behçet's disease
   - (d) Takayasu's disease
   - (e) Gilbert's disease

3. The majority of patients with temporal arteritis are encompassed in which of the following groups?
   (a) 50 years, male, white
   (b) 50 years, female, nonwhite
   (c) 50 years, male, nonwhite
   (d) 50 years, male and female, nonwhite
   (e) 50 years, female, white

4. What is the optimal initial treatment for subacute upper extremity ischemia caused by temporal arteritis?
   (a) Steroids
   (b) Endarterectomy
   (c) Saphenous vein bypass
   (d) Thrombolytic therapy
   (e) Warfarin anticoagulation

5. Which of the following is of greatest benefit in the treatment of patients with Buerger's disease?
   (a) Sympathectomy
   (b) Oral vasodilators
   (c) Arterial reconstructive surgery
   (d) Warfarin anticoagulation
   (e) Cessation of tobacco use

6. Extensive vascular calcification in a young patient with normal parathyroid function suggests which of the following?
   (a) Hyperlipidemia
   (b) Hurler's syndrome
   (c) Pseudoxanthoma elasticum
   (d) Marfan's syndrome
   (e) Ehlers-Danlos syndrome

7. Abdominal coarctation is most frequently discovered during evaluation for which symptom?
   (a) Claudication
   (b) Blue toe syndrome
   (c) Weight loss
   (d) Hypertension
   (e) Abdominal pain

8. Calf claudication in a nonsmoker younger than 30 years is most commonly caused by which disorder?
   (a) Popliteal entrapment syndrome
   (b) Atherosclerosis
   (c) Polyarteritis nodosa
   (d) Takayasu's disease
   (e) Homocystinemia

9. The early objective diagnosis of anterior compartment syndrome is best made by which finding?
   (a) Absent dorsal pedal pulse
   (b) Footdrop
   (c) Tense swelling
   (d) Localized compartment pain
   (e) Compartment pressure measurement with Wick or the "solid-state transducer in catheter" monitor

10. All of the following are important in homocysteine metabolism except
   (a) Vitamin B_6
   (b) Folate
   (c) Cobalamin
   (d) Ornithine transcarbamoylase
   (e) Homocysteine methyltransferase

Answers

1. a	2. e	3. e	4. a	5. e
6. c	7. d	8. a	9. e	10. d

Influence of Diabetes Mellitus on Vascular Disease and Its Complications

Diabetes is described in the *Ebers Papyrus*, an Egyptian text dating to about 1552 BC. Nevertheless, despite being recognized for 4 millennia, the disease in many ways remains undefined. Diabetes mellitus is a heterogeneous collection of syndromes characterized by hyperglycemia. It is estimated to affect approximately 14 million inhabitants of the United States.[1] With new criteria for its diagnosis,[2] the prevalence of diabetes may be as high as 16 million. Owing to the high prevalence of diabetes mellitus in patients with peripheral arterial disease, screening for this disorder is now recommended for all patients on vascular wards who do not already carry the diagnosis.[3]

Insulin-dependent diabetes mellitus (IDDM), or type 1 diabetes, accounts for approximately 10% of diabetic patients; the majority have non-insulin-dependent diabetes mellitus (NIDDM), or type 2 diabetes. Other types of diabetes include gestational diabetes mellitus, which occurs de novo during pregnancy; a type that can occur from toxins or trauma to the insulin-secreting cells (β cells) of the pancreatic islets of Langerhans; or secondary diabetes mellitus due to another disease that impairs pancreatic function or induces insulin resistance, such as occurs in iron overload syndromes, acromegaly, or Cushing's disease.

IDDM, or the type characterized by low or undetectable insulin secretion and a need for insulin administration to sustain life, is generally accepted as primarily autoimmune in etiology.[4] The genetic vulnerabilities and the environmental insults that elicit IDDM are under intense study but remain uncharacterized. The complexity of these interactions is illustrated by the fact that less than 50% of monozygotic twins of a diabetic proband develop IDDM. NIDDM is a highly concordant genetic disease, with nearly 100% of monozygotic twins

of a diabetic proband acquiring the disease. The concordance for first- and second-degree relatives increases given the challenge of obesity. NIDDM subjects tend to have insulin levels in the normal to high range yet remain "insulin resistant," with an inadequate ability to secrete insulin in a manner sufficient to lower blood glucose into the normal range.[5]

Clinical practice guidelines are published yearly by the American Diabetes Association.[6] These guidelines define diabetes as a fasting glucose higher than 126 mg/dL and impaired glucose tolerance as a fasting glucose between 110 and 126 mg/dL.

Persons with either IDDM or NIDDM tend to be at double jeopardy for the development of vascular disease because they have both glucose toxicity as a result of elevated blood glucose levels, the hallmark of the disease, and insulin toxicity as a result of elevated insulin levels from peripheral insulin injection (IDDM and some NIDDM) or elevated endogenous insulin secretion (most NIDDM). The nature of these toxicities is described in some detail later. This chapter also emphasizes the importance of minimizing these two toxicities through therapeutic approaches that target normal glucose levels without unduly raising insulin levels or promoting hypoglycemia.[7]

The recognition of vascular disease as an obligatory concomitant of diabetes mellitus occurred during the 20th century. Osler noted in 1908 that "the thickening of the arteries in … diabetes … may be due to the action on the blood vessels of poisons retained within the system."[8] In the 1945 edition of his textbook, 20 years after the use of insulin had become common, Joslin noted that "arteriosclerosis in the form of gangrene of the lower extremities has decreased while at the same time it has increased in the heart as coronary disease and in the brain as apoplexy."[9]

It is now generally agreed that diabetes mellitus accelerates the initiation and propagation of vascular disease. At present, 84% of diabetic subjects who live longer than 20 years after diagnosis have some form of vascular disease, and 75% of persons with diabetes now die of vascular disease

This chapter was written by Charles M. Peterson in his private capacity. The views expressed in the chapter do not necessarily represent the views of the National Institutes of Health, the Department of Health and Human Services, or the United States.

or its complications, primarily myocardial infarction and stroke.[10] Thus, persons with diabetes, regardless of type, have an increased risk for disease of the large and small vessels. In addition, the distribution of large vessel disease is more diffuse.

Diabetes remains problematic for the vascular surgeon for several reasons. The diagnosis of vascular disease in a person with diabetes may be confounded by the presence of sensorimotor polyneuropathy, which may mask typical pain patterns. The outcome of surgical intervention tends to be less favorable in persons with diabetes because the hospital stay is generally longer, the risk for infection is greater, and the probability of an adverse outcome is higher than in persons without diabetes. In the 1960s, mortality rates in diabetic patients who had surgery were reported to be 3.6% to 13.2%.[11] In 1983, Hjortrup and colleagues studied morbidity in diabetic and nondiabetic patients who had major vascular surgery and found that there were no deaths in either group and comparable morbidity.[12] Although their theories were unproved, the authors hypothesized that the improvement in statistical outcome in the intervening 20 years was due to improvements in diabetes care.

There appears to be little doubt that diabetes care enhances the outcome of perioperative infection. From 1990 to 1995, Golden and coworkers at Johns Hopkins evaluated 411 adults with diabetes who underwent coronary artery surgery, conducting glucose surveillance six times a day.[13] After adjusting for age, sex, race, underlying comorbidity, acute severity of illness, and length of stay in the surgical intensive care unit, patients with higher mean glucose readings were at increased risk of developing infections. Thus, the investigators concluded that in patients with diabetes who undergo coronary artery surgery, postoperative hyperglycemia is an independent predictor of short-term infectious complications.

This chapter reviews the epidemiologic data as well as the mechanisms behind the factors that make individuals with diabetes vulnerable to the initiation and propagation of vascular disease, with an emphasis on the effects on the large vessels. The chapter also details protocols that have proved useful for the control of glucose in patients with IDDM and NIDDM. In view of the increasing evidence that both acute and chronic risk can be modified by intensive diabetes control protocols, these approaches should be part of the therapeutic armamentarium of surgeons as well as specialists in diabetes care. Control of blood pressure and blood lipids is also especially important in patients with diabetes, as explained later in this chapter.

Cerebrovascular, Cardiovascular, and Peripheral Vascular Disease and Diabetes

There are now several large studies across multiple cultures that attest to the adverse effect of elevated glucose levels on the various forms of large vessel disease. Elevated glucose not only accelerates the appearance of vascular disease but also predicts vascular events and prognosis once a vascular event has occurred. This section reviews the major large studies because they address the issues of stroke, cardiovascular disease (CVD), and peripheral vascular disease.

A number of studies documented that the glucose level at the time of hospital admission is a predictor of outcome and extent of neurologic deficit in persons with acute stroke.

For example, Toni and associates attempted to identify predictors and possible pathogenic mechanisms of early neurologic deterioration in patients with acute ischemic strokes and to evaluate their impact on clinical outcome.[14] They studied a continuous series of 152 patients with first-ever ischemic hemispheric strokes who were hospitalized within 5 hours of onset, evaluated according to the Canadian Neurological Scale, and assessed with a computed tomography (CT) scan. The initial subset of 80 patients also underwent angiography. A repeat CT scan or autopsy was performed within 5 to 9 days of a patient's stroke. Progressing neurologic deficit was defined as a decrease of 1 point or more in the global neurologic scale score during hospitalization compared with the score at entry. Those whose condition deteriorated had been hospitalized earlier and had higher serum glucose levels at admission.

The Oslo Study also found that diabetes and the level of nonfasting glucose predicted the outcome of stroke.[15] That study, started in 1972, included 16,209 men aged 40 to 49 years. Of these, 16,172 had no previous history of stroke and 151 were known to have diabetes. Five diabetic and 80 nondiabetic subjects died of stroke during the 18 years of follow-up, giving a rate ratio of 7.87 (95% confidence interval [CI], 2.48 to 19.14) for diabetic subjects. The rate of mortality for all causes in diabetic subjects was more than five times that of those who were nondiabetic. Nonfasting serum glucose was a predictor of fatal stroke in all participants (diabetic subjects included) without a history of stroke in age-adjusted univariate analysis. The relative risk (RR) was 1.13 (95% CI, 1.03 to 1.25) by an increase of 1 mmol/L (18 mg/dL) of serum glucose, according to results of proportional hazards regression analysis.

Similar observations were made in Scotland, where women were found to be more vulnerable to the effects of glucose than were men.[16] Sex-specific CVD, ischemic heart disease, and stroke mortality rates and relative risks for asymptomatic hyperglycemic subjects (top 5%) were compared with those of normoglycemic individuals (bottom 95%) during a mean follow-up of 11.6 years (range, 10 to 14 years) of 4696 men and 5714 women in western Scotland aged 45 to 64 years at entry. Univariate analysis showed that asymptomatic hyperglycemia was associated with increased risk of all causes of CVD, ischemic heart disease, and stroke mortality in both men and women. The degree of this association was greater in women than in men. Using multiple logistic regression analysis to take into account differences in age, systolic and diastolic blood pressure, serum cholesterol, body mass index (BMI), and cigarette smoking, a high causal blood glucose level was still a significant risk factor for CVD mortality in both men and women.

Within the diabetic population, the level of complications such as retinopathy, preexisting nephropathy, and coronary and peripheral vascular disease, in addition to age, is a predictor of outcome.[17] In a cohort of 2124 diabetic persons identified at multiphasic health checkups from 1979 through 1985, 56 suffered a nonembolic ischemic stroke during the follow-up period, which extended through 1991. For each case subject, one diabetic control subject, matched by sex and year of birth, was selected from the same cohort of diabetic subjects. The estimated relative risk of stroke in diabetic subjects with retinopathy was 2.8 (95% CI, 1.2 to 6.9). After adjustment for age, sex, smoking, use of insulin, average systolic blood pressure, and average random glucose level, the estimated relative risk was 4.0 (95% CI, 1.0 to 14.5). The relative risk of stroke in diabetic subjects with retinopathy remained elevated after the exclusion of those with complications other than retinopathy.

The Honolulu Heart Program also confirmed a poorer prognosis for vascular disease associated with hyperglycemia.[18] This study examined the association between a variety of baseline lifestyle and biologic factors in a middle-aged cohort of Japanese American men and the 20-year incidence rates of total atherosclerotic end points and each of the initial clinical manifestations of this disease, including fatal and nonfatal coronary heart disease, angina pectoris, thromboembolic stroke, and aortic aneurysm. Japanese American men ($N = 2710$) between the ages of 55 and 64 years at the time of the initial clinical examination (1965 through 1968) who had no evidence of coronary heart disease, cerebrovascular disease, cancer, or aortic aneurysm were studied. Among these men, 602 atherosclerotic events developed during the 23-year follow-up period (1965 through 1988). After adjustment for each of the baseline characteristics examined, significant positive associations between quartile cutoffs of BMI, systolic blood pressure, serum glucose levels, cholesterol, triglycerides, and uric acid, as well as cigarette smoking, and the occurrence of any atherosclerotic end point were noted.

Within the diabetic population, nonfatal or small infarction, especially with multiple occurrences, is a feature of cerebrovascular disease complicating diabetes mellitus and correlates with elevated blood glucose and blood pressure.[19] Asymptomatic cerebral infarction is not rare in diabetic subjects and can now be pathologically and clinically evaluated with accuracy using magnetic resonance imaging (MRI).

The Wisconsin Epidemiologic Study also confirmed the finding of elevated risk for vascular disease in the diabetic population.[20] The association of glycemia with cause-specific mortality in a diabetic population was studied in a cohort design based in a primary care setting. All participants ($N = 1210$) had diabetes, were taking insulin, and were diagnosed when they were younger than 30 years. They were compared with a random sample of diabetic persons diagnosed when they were 30 years or older ($n = 1780$). Thus, both IDDM and NIDDM were studied, although the National Diabetes Data Group criteria for diagnosis were not used.[21] Glycosylated hemoglobin levels were obtained at baseline examinations. Median follow-up was 10 years in patients with an earlier onset and 8.3 years in those with a later onset. The main outcome measure was cause-specific mortality determined from death certificates. In the early-onset group, after controlling for other risk factors in proportional hazards models and considering the underlying cause of death, the glycosylated hemoglobin level as an index of average glucose control was significantly associated with mortality from diabetes (hazard ratio [HR] for a 1% change in glycosylated hemoglobin, 1.25; 95% CI, 1.13 to 1.38) and ischemic heart disease (HR, 1.18; 95% CI, 1.00 to 1.40). In the later-onset group, glycosylated hemoglobin was significantly associated with mortality from diabetes (HR, 1.32; 95% CI, 1.21 to 1.43), ischemic heart disease (HR, 1.10; 95% CI, 1.04 to 1.17), and stroke (HR, 1.17; 95% CI, 1.05 to 1.30), but not cancer (HR, 0.99; 95% CI, 0.88 to 1.10). The authors concluded that "these results suggest ... benefit to the control of glycemia with respect to death due to vascular disease and diabetes."[21]

The Copenhagen Stroke Study also found that diabetes is a risk factor for stroke and that diabetes influences the nature of stroke.[22] The study evaluated stroke type, stroke severity, prognosis, and the relation between admission glucose levels and stroke severity and mortality. This community-based study included 1135 acute stroke patients, of whom 233 (20%) had diabetes. All patients were evaluated until the end of rehabilitation by weekly assessment of neurologic deficits (Scandinavian Stroke Scale) and functional disabilities (Barthel index). A CT scan was performed in 83% of stroke cases. The diabetic stroke patient was 3.2 years younger than the nondiabetic stroke patient ($P < 0.001$) and had hypertension more frequently (48% vs. 30%; $P < 0.0001$). Intracerebral hemorrhages were six times less frequent in diabetic patients ($P = 0.002$). Initial stroke severity, lesion size, and site were comparable between the two groups; mortality was higher in diabetic patients (24% vs. 17%; $P = 0.03$), and diabetes independently increased the relative death risk by 1.8 (95% CI, 1.04 to 3.19). Outcome was comparable in surviving patients with and without diabetes, but patients with diabetes recovered more slowly. Mortality increased with higher glucose levels on admission in nondiabetic patients, independent of stroke severity (odds ratio [OR], 1.2 per 1 mmol/L; 95% CI, 1.01 to 1.42; $P = 0.04$). Thus, diabetes influences stroke in terms of age, subtype, speed of recovery, and mortality. The authors concluded that "the effect of reducing high admission glucose levels in nondiabetic stroke patients should be examined in future trials."[22]

A Finnish study, although of short duration, confirmed the excess risk of elderly diabetic women for acute stroke.[23] The study examined whether NIDDM, its metabolic control and duration, and insulin level predict stroke. Cardiovascular risk factors, including glucose tolerance, plasma insulin, and glycosylated hemoglobin, were determined in a Finnish cohort of 1298 subjects aged 65 to 74 years, and the impact of these risk factors on the incidence of both fatal and nonfatal stroke was investigated during 3.5 years of follow-up. Of 1298 subjects participating in the baseline study, 1069 did not have diabetes and 229 had NIDDM. During the 3.5-year follow-up, 3.4% ($n = 36$) of nondiabetic subjects and 6.1% ($n = 14$) of NIDDM subjects had a nonfatal or fatal stroke. The incidence of stroke was significantly higher in diabetic women compared with nondiabetic women (OR, 2.25; 95% CI, 1.65 to 3.06). In multivariate logistic regression analyses including all study subjects, fasting and 2-hour glucose ($P < 0.01$ and $P < 0.05$, respectively), glycosylated hemoglobin (Hb) A_{1c} ($P < 0.01$), atrial fibrillation ($P < 0.05$), hypertension ($P < 0.05$), and previous stroke ($P < 0.01$) predicted stroke events. In diabetic subjects, fasting and 2-hour glucose ($P < 0.01$ and $P < 0.05$, respectively), glycosylated Hb A_{1c} ($P < 0.05$), duration of diabetes ($P < 0.05$), and atrial fibrillation ($P < 0.05$) were the baseline variables predicting stroke events. Finally, fasting insulin ($P < 0.05$), hypertension ($P < 0.05$), and previous stroke ($P < 0.01$) were associated with stroke incidence in nondiabetic subjects.

The longer-term Honolulu Heart Program confirmed that, for men, diabetes confers extra risk of thromboembolic stroke but not hemorrhagic stroke.[24] The goal of this study was to determine whether glucose intolerance and diabetes increase the risk of thromboembolic, hemorrhagic, and total stroke, independent of other risk factors. Among the 7549 Japanese American men aged 45 to 68 years and free of coronary heart disease and stroke from 1965 to 1968, a total of 374 thromboembolic, 128 hemorrhagic, and 36 type-unknown strokes occurred. The incidence of thromboembolic but not hemorrhagic stroke increased with the worsening glucose tolerance category. Compared with the low-normal (glucose < 151 mg/dL) group, subjects in the high-normal (151 to 224 mg/dL), asymptomatic high (≥ 225 mg/dL), and known diabetes groups all had significantly elevated age-adjusted relative risks of thromboembolic stroke. After adjustment for other risk factors, relative risks remained significantly elevated for the asymptomatic high and known diabetes groups (RR, 1.43 and 2.45; 95% CI, 1.00 to 2.04 and 1.73 to 3.47, respectively). Associations were the same in hypertensive and nonhypertensive subjects and similar but slightly stronger in younger (45 to 54 years) than in older (55 to 68 years) men.

The Northern Manhattan Stroke Study found that an admission blood glucose level greater than 140 mg/dL was an important predictor of mortality in stroke.[25] Ethanol abuse (RR, 2.5), hypertension requiring discharge medications (RR, 1.6), and elevated blood glucose within 48 hours of index ischemic stroke (RR, 1.2/50 mg/dL) were found to be independent predictors of recurrence.

The aforementioned review emphasizes that the relationship between glucose and vascular disease appears to hold across various cultures and genetic backgrounds. In a study in Taiwan of 479 NIDDM patients 40 years or older from four community primary care health centers, cholesterol, high-density lipoprotein cholesterol, plasma glucose, and Hb A_{1c} were studied.[26] The duration of diabetes was associated with the development of stroke, with a relative risk of 1.063 for every 1-year increment ($P = 0.07$). Significant risk factors were serum cholesterol and Hb A_{1c} levels. For every 1-mg/dL increase in mean total cholesterol level, the relative risk of developing vascular disease increased 1.016-fold ($P = 0.04$). For every 1% (approximately 35 mg/dL) increase in Hb A_{1c}, the relative risk of developing vascular disease increased 1.170-fold ($P = 0.01$). Female diabetic subjects had a higher relative risk than male subjects did. The risk of CVD is therefore two to three times higher in diabetic than nondiabetic subjects. There is a gender difference; the incidence is two times higher in diabetic men and three times higher in diabetic women.[27-30]

In the nondiabetic group in the Honolulu Heart Program, there was a dose-response relation between glucose intolerance at baseline and coronary heart disease incidence, coronary heart disease mortality, and total mortality. This risk was independent of other risk factors in this cohort of 8006 middle-aged and older Japanese American men.[31] Therefore, even in the normal range, glucose levels predict risk for vascular disease.

Persons with diabetes have shorter life spans. About 75% of increased mortality in men and 50% in women is caused by CVD. Kleinman and colleagues found that the relative risk of mortality from ischemic heart disease was 2.8 for men and 2.5 for women after controlling for other confounding variables of hypertension, obesity, age, serum cholesterol, and smoking.[27] In a Utah population, CVD accounted for 48% of all-cause mortality in diabetic subjects.[28] Not only do diabetic subjects have an increased mortality from acute myocardial infarction; they also have an increased rate of congestive heart failure, cardiogenic shock, and dysrhythmias, not necessarily correlated with the size of the infarct.[30,32] It is thought that the increased rate of congestive heart failure is secondary to hypocontractility, which may be due to microvascular disease, the metabolic effects of diabetes leading to cardiomyopathy, and autonomic dysfunction.[32]

Disease of the large vessels in one area of the vascular tree appears to predict disease in other areas. Associations of vascular disease are also found with perturbations in coagulation.[33] Heinrich and coworkers investigated the vessel status of coronary and peripheral arteries and those arteries supplying the brain in 929 consecutive male patients admitted to a coronary rehabilitation unit.[33] The severity of coronary atherosclerosis was scored using coronary angiography. Changes in extracranial brain vessels and manifest CVD were determined by B-mode ultrasound and Doppler examination. Peripheral arterial disease was diagnosed using baseline and stress oscillography. There was a significant increase in plasma fibrinogen, plasminogen, D-dimer, and C-reactive protein with increasing severity of coronary heart disease. Compared with men who had unaffected arteries, men with three diseased coronary arteries had 58% greater D-dimer concentrations. Patients with cerebrovascular disease and peripheral vascular disease also had significantly higher fibrinogen, D-dimer, and C-reactive protein concentrations.

Many of the vascular lesions may also be asymptomatic, emphasizing the potential role of prophylactic screening for vascular lesions in other parts of the vascular tree when an index lesion is identified in a diabetic subject.[34] In a prospective population-based study of Dutch white inhabitants between 50 and 75 years of age, 2484 subjects were screened with respect to glucose tolerance. A group of 173 people with diabetes and a representative age- and sex-stratified sample of 288 nondiabetic subjects were studied in the vascular laboratory. Carotid artery disease was investigated with duplex scanning, and arm and leg artery obstructions were evaluated with real-time frequency analysis of continuous-wave Doppler signals and indirect blood pressure measurements. Comparing diabetic with nondiabetic subjects, the authors found significantly more obstructions of the carotid arteries (8.7% vs. 2.8%), arm arteries (2.3% vs. 0%), and leg arteries (31.8% vs. 18.4%). This was also true if only crural artery obstructions were compared (23.7% vs. 16.0%). More than half the subjects with carotid artery obstructions also had leg artery obstructions.[34]

The same group investigated the cross-sectional association between peripheral arterial disease and glycemic level, age, sex, and glucose tolerance.[35] The prevalence rates of ankle-brachial index (ABI) less than 0.90 were 7.0%, 9.5%, 15.1%, and 20.9% in normal glucose-tolerant, impaired glucose-tolerant, NIDDM, and known diabetic subjects under treatment, respectively (chi-square test for linear trend, $P < 0.01$). Prevalence rates of any peripheral arterial disease (ABI < 0.90, at least one monophasic or absent Doppler flow curve, or vascular surgery) were 18.1%, 22.4%, 29.2%, and 41.8% in these categories (chi-square test for linear trend, $P < 0.0001$). Logistic regression analyses showed that any arterial disease was significantly associated with Hb A_{1c}, fasting, and 2-hour postload plasma glucose after correction for cardiovascular risk factors (OR, 1.35, 1.20, and 1.06, respectively; 95% CI, 1.10 to 1.65, 1.06 to 1.36, and 1.01 to 1.12, respectively). These authors did not find an association between insulin levels and vascular disease.

Diabetes-related peripheral vascular disease remains a huge public health problem.[36] Although rates of lower extremity amputation and arterial reconstruction declined from 1983 to 1992, by 1996, the rate of major amputation had increased 10.6% since 1979. The earlier 12-year decline was positively correlated with reductions in the prevalence of smoking, hypertension, and heart disease, but not diabetes.[37]

Diabetic subjects with peripheral vascular disease are more likely to have small vessel disease of the foot, as well as large vessel disease elsewhere.[38] These findings may contribute to the higher risk for the development of chronic foot ulcers in diabetic patients with peripheral vascular disease. Other independent predictors of amputation include sensory neuropathy and foot ulcers.[39]

Doppler studies using the ABI appear to be as useful in diabetic as in nondiabetic populations for identifying vascular disease, as documented by the Cardiovascular Health Study of 5084 participants.[40] Risk factors associated with an ABI of less than 1.0 in multivariate analysis included smoking (OR, 2.55), history of diabetes (OR, 3.84), increasing age (OR, 1.54), and nonwhite race (OR, 2.36). In the 3372 participants free of clinical coronary vascular disease, other noninvasive measures of subclinical CVD, including carotid stenosis by duplex scanning, segmental wall motion abnormalities by echocardiogram, and major electrocardiographic abnormalities, were inversely related to the ABI (all $P < 0.01$). Therefore, the lower the ABI, the greater the increase in CVD risk; however, even those with modest, asymptomatic reductions in the ABI (0.8 to 1.0) had an increased risk of coronary vascular disease.

The risk for amputation in diabetic subjects appears to parallel the risk for vascular disease in general.[41] A case-control study was carried out among 10,068 patients from a large health maintenance organization at a multiphasic health checkup between 1964 and 1984, with an average length of follow-up after baseline of 13.2 years. Case patients were 150 cohort members with a first nontraumatic lower extremity amputation after baseline. Control subjects were 278 cohort members who did not experience an amputation during follow-up, matched to patients by age, sex, and year of baseline. Level of glucose control ($P < 0.0001$), duration of diabetes ($P = 0.04$), and baseline systolic blood pressure

($P = 0.004$) were independent predictors of amputation, as were microvascular complications (retinopathy, neuropathy, and nephropathy). The observation that type of diabetes (or genetic background) did not predict amputation but that glycemia was predictive lends credence to the "glucose toxicity" hypothesis of vascular risk.

Clinical Studies of Intervention

As noted earlier, there seems to be a consensus that there is a relationship between glucose levels and cardiovascular events that shows a dose response within both normal and diabetic populations.[42] There have been several intervention studies that tested the glucose toxicity hypothesis, as well as studies of blood pressure control and lipid control in patients with diabetes mellitus. Table 8-1 summarizes the results of prospective glucose-lowering trials and CVD in people with diabetes mellitus. As can be seen, a significant risk reduction was demonstrated in seven of the eight published trials in type 1 and type 2 diabetes.

A Stockholm study provided convincing evidence that control of glycemia prevents microvascular complications in IDDM.[43] The Diabetes Control and Complications Trial (DCCT) clearly confirmed that tight control decreased the incidence of microvascular complications in IDDM.[44] The DCCT showed a trend of decreased incidence of CVD, but the result was not statistically significant. The DCCT was not designed primarily to test the hypothesis that blood glucose control would influence the risk for CVD. The patients were too young and it was too early in the course of their diabetes to expect significant cardiovascular event rates. Nevertheless, 17 initial major cardiovascular events were recorded: 14 in the conventional treatment group and 3 in the intensive treatment group.[45] Total major cardiovascular and peripheral vascular events numbered 40 in the conventional group, compared with 23 in the intensive group. Thus, with intensive treatment, the risk for cardiac events was reduced by 78%, and the risk for combined cardiac and peripheral vascular events was reduced by 42%. As noted earlier, these risk differences did not achieve the defined limits for statistical significance. In contrast, a meta-analysis published in 1999 clearly shows that intervention with intensive glucose control has a beneficial

TABLE 8–1	Glucose-Lowering Trials and Cardiovascular Disease in Diabetes Mellitus (DM)					
Study	Duration of Trial (yr)	Hb A$_{1c}$ Intense (%)	Hb A$_{1c}$ Control (%)	Treatment	Outcome	Relative Risk Reduction (%)
UKPDS[48]	10	7.0	7.9	Insulin and sulfonylurea	MI	16
UKPDS[49]	10.7	7.4	8.0	Metformin	MI	39
Kumamoto[49a]	6.0	7.1	9.4	Insulin	CV events	46
VACSDM[49b]	2.3	7.1	9.3	Insulin and sulfonylurea	CV events	−40
DIGAMI[47,49c]	1.0	7.1	7.9	Insulin	Mortality	29
Type 1 DM meta-analysis[46]	2-7	7.6	8.7	Insulin	Any event	45
Type 1 DM meta-analysis[46]	2-7	7.6	8.7	Insulin	First event	28

CV, cardiovascular; DIGAMI, Diabetes and Insulin Glucose Infusion in Acute Myocardial Infarction; Hb, hemoglobin; MI, myocardial infarction; UGDP, University Group Diabetes Program; UKPDS, United Kingdom Prospective Diabetes Study; VACSDM, Veterans Affairs Cooperative Study on Glycemic Control and Complications in NIDDM.

effect on the incidence of the first and any cardiovascular event in type 1 patients (see Table 8-1).[46]

As summarized in Table 8-1, the results in persons with type 2 diabetes are even more convincing. Of particular note is the Diabetes and Insulin Glucose Infusion in Acute Myocardial Infarction (DIGAMI) study, which documented that acute management with intense insulin treatment at the time of myocardial infarction with subsequent insulin therapy has a significant impact on mortality at 1 year.[47] The 1998 publication of the United Kingdom Prospective Diabetes Study reinforced the clinical goal of obtaining Hb A_{1c} values at or below 7% in these patients.[48,49]

My own studies of peripheral vascular risk in IDDM show that an intensive program of glucose control documented by glycosylated hemoglobin and multiple daily blood glucose self-monitoring measures can reverse lesions of the red blood cell, polymorphonuclear leukocyte, platelet, and fluid phase of coagulation associated with diabetes.[50-54] In addition, basement membrane thickening, nerve conduction, and the ABI were found to improve after a 9-month program of intensive glucose control and exercise. In view of the association between the ABI and the risk in diabetic subjects noted earlier, these studies still provide some of the most compelling evidence for programs of glucose control and exercise in persons with diabetes to avoid or even facilitate the reversal of large vessel disease. The goal is to aggressively treat elevated blood glucose and blood pressure and abnormal lipid profiles.

Table 8-2 summarizes the major lipid-lowering trials in patients with type 2 diabetes. There are three primary randomized trials for primary prevention and an equal number for secondary prevention of CVD. Meta-analysis of these trials shows an overall relative risk reduction of 55% for primary prevention and 29% for secondary prevention. The 4S study also documented the cost-effectiveness of lipid lowering.[55] In persons with coronary heart disease with normal fasting glucose levels, simvastatin reduced the average cost of CVD-related hospitalization by $3585, which offset 60% of the cost of drug. For those with impaired fasting glucose

levels, average CVD-related hospitalization costs were reduced by $4478, which offset 74% of the drug cost. For diabetic subjects, there was a net cost savings of $1801 per subject. Current American Diabetes Association guidelines recommend low-density lipoprotein cholesterol targets of less than 2.59 mmol/L (100 mg/dL) for diabetic subjects with one additional cardiovascular risk factor and an intervention level of 3.36 mmol/L (130 mg/dL), with a target of 2.59 mmol/L for all other subjects with diabetes.[56] As shown by the Long-Term Intervention with Pravastatin in Ischaemic Disease Study, patients appear to benefit from statin therapy over a wide range of initial lipid levels.[57]

Table 8-3 summarizes the trials of blood pressure lowering in persons with type 2 diabetes. As emphasized in a 1998 Cochrane Library review,[58] primary intervention trials indicate a treatment benefit for coronary vascular disease but not for total mortality in people with diabetes. For both short- and long-term secondary prevention, there is a benefit for total mortality in persons with diabetes. Most of the published data from randomized, controlled trials of antihypertensive therapy in diabetes for all-cause mortality and CVD outcomes are taken from hypertension trials that are not specific to diabetes.

It has been suggested that it is cost-effective to treat all patients with type 2 diabetes with angiotensin-converting enzyme inhibitors.[59] This approach is reinforced by the publication of the Heart Outcomes Prevention Evaluation, a placebo-controlled study of more than 9000 subjects that indicated that ramipril substantially lowers the risk of death, heart attack, stroke, coronary revascularization, heart failure, and complications related to diabetes mellitus in a high-risk group of patients with preexisting vascular disease. The results are remarkable both for the magnitude of the treatment effect (an overall reduction of 22% in the primary outcome of myocardial infarction, stroke, or death from cardiovascular causes) and for the rather small reduction (3.2 mm Hg) in blood pressure. The authors also noted a marked reduction in the incidence of complications related to diabetes and new cases of diabetes in those taking ramipril.[59]

TABLE 8–2	Lipid-Lowering Trials and Cardiovascular Disease in Type 2 Diabetes Mellitus					
Study	**No. of Patients**	**Follow-up (yr)**	**Decreased LDL (%)**	**First Treatment**	**Outcome**	**Relative Risk Reduction (%)**
Helsinki Heart[54a]	135	5.0	10	Gemfibrozil	CHD death, nonfatal MI	69
WOSCOPS[54b]	76	4.9	26	Pravastatin	CHD death, nonfatal MI	NA
AF/Tex CAPS[54c]	155	5.2	25	Lovastatin	CHD death, nonfatal MI, angina	37
Meta-analysis of primary prevention trials above						55
4S[55]	202	5.5	34	Simvastatin	CHD death, nonfatal MI	55
CARE[56]	586	4.9	27	Pravastatin	CHD death, nonfatal MI	13
LIPID[57]	782	6.1	25	Pravastatin	CHD death, nonfatal MI	19
Meta-analysis of secondary prevention studies above[58]						29

AF/Tex CAPS, Air Force/Texas Coronary Atherosclerosis Prevention Study; CARE, Cholesterol and Recurrent Events; CHD, coronary heart disease; 4S, Scandinavian Simvastatin Survival Study; LDL, low-density lipoprotein; LIPID, Long-Term Intervention with Pravastatin in Ischaemic Disease; MI, myocardial infarction; NA, not available; WOSCOPS, West of Scotland Primary Prevention Study.

TABLE 8–3	Blood Pressure (BP)–Lowering Trials and Cardiovascular Disease in Type 2 Diabetes Mellitus					
Study	**Duration of Trial (yr)**	**BP Intervention (mm Hg)**	**BP Control (mm Hg)**	**First Treatment**	**Outcome**	**Relative Risk Reduction (%)**
UKPDS[49]	9.0	144/82	154/87	Captopril/atenolol	CVD	29
					Stroke	20
					MI	42
SHEP[54c]	4.5	145/70	155/70	Chlorthalidone	CVD	45
					Stroke	26
Syst-Eur[54c]	2.0	153/78	162/82	Nitrendipine	CVD	62
					Stroke	69
HOT[54c]	3.8	140/81	144/85	Felodipine	CVD + stroke	51
ABCD[54c]	5.6	130/80	135/85	Nisoldipine/enalapril	MI	–12
Overall primary prevention[54c]						38
Cochrane primary prevention[54c]	5.0			Various	CVD mortality and morbidity	30
Cochrane secondary prevention[54c]	>1			Various	CVD mortality and morbidity	11

ABCD, Appropriate Blood Pressure Control in Diabetes; CVD, cardiovascular disease; HOT, Hypertension Optimal Treatment; MI, myocardial infarction; SHEP, Systolic Hypertension in the Elderly; Syst-Eur, Systolic Hypertension in Europe Trial; UKPDS, United Kingdom Prospective Diabetes Study.

There has been less enthusiasm for calcium channel blockers in persons with diabetes.[60] Nevertheless, there is evidence that they can be effective as well, as shown in Table 8-3.

Evidence for the Influence of Glucose on the Pathophysiology of Vascular Disease

Hyperglycemia is associated with vascular disease, as documented earlier. The reasons for this association remain speculative. Table 8-4 documents some of the hypothesized means by which glucose might influence pathologic vascular changes. These factors are discussed here in some detail.

GLYCATION AND ADVANCED GLYCATION END PRODUCTS, OR EARLY AND LATE MAILLARD REACTIONS

In 1976, it became clear that a minor hemoglobin component, Hb A_{1c}, resulted from a post-translational modification of hemoglobin A by glucose and that there was a clinical relationship between Hb A_{1c} and fasting plasma glucose, the peak on the glucose tolerance test, the area under the curve on the glucose tolerance test, and mean glucose levels over the preceding weeks.[61-64] It soon became apparent that an improvement in ambient blood glucose levels resulted in correction of Hb A_{1c} levels[50-54] and that these nonenzymatic glycosylation reactions might provide a hypothesis that could explain a number of the pathologic sequelae of diabetes mellitus via toxicity arising from glucose adduct formation with proteins or nucleic acids.[64]

As early as 1912, Maillard suggested that the chemical reactions that now bear his name might play a role in the pathologic changes associated with diabetes mellitus.[65]

The ability of reducing sugars to react with the amino groups of proteins is now widely recognized, as is the natural occurrence of many nonenzymatically glycosylated proteins. Important details about the nature of such reactions are still unclear, however.

The initial step (or early Maillard reaction) involves the condensation of an amino moiety with the aldehyde form of a particular sugar. Only a very small fraction of most common sugars is normally present in the aldehyde form.[66,67] A number of transformations are possible following the addition of an amine to a sugar carbonyl group. Considerable evidence now exists that supports the involvement of an Amadori-type rearrangement for the adduct of glucose with the N-terminal

TABLE 8–4	Glucose Toxicity Hypothesis: Hyperglycemia Initiates or Propagates Vascular Disease by Multiple Mechanisms

Glycation of proteins and genetic material leading to dysfunctional or toxic products

Interference with the fluid, vascular, and platelet phases of coagulation

Perturbations in oxidation-reduction pathways

Production of abnormal lipid metabolism

Vascular volume shifts associated with changes in glycemia, or intracellular osmotic shifts associated with alternative metabolic pathways invoked when glucose is elevated, are toxic to the vascular tree

Abnormal insulin or proinsulin levels in response to hyperglycemia contribute to vascular disease

Perturbations in the immune system, including lymphokine production and polymorphonuclear leukocyte function, contribute to vascular disease of the β chain of hemoglobin. The labile Schiff base aldimine adduct is transformed into a relatively stable ketoamine adduct via the Amadori rearrangement.

Because hemoglobin circulates in its red blood cell for approximately 120 days, there is little opportunity in this cell for late Maillard reactions, or nonenzymatic browning, to occur. In these late Maillard reactions, the Amadori product is degraded into deoxyglucosones that react again with free amino groups to form chromophores, fluorophores, and protein cross-links.[68,69] In tissues that are longer lived, these reactions may be important mediators of diabetic changes as well as the aging process. Although the structure of a large number of nonenzymatic browning products has been elucidated, few have been obtained under physiologic conditions, thus making detection in vivo difficult and their pathologic role uncertain.[70] Table 8-5 summarizes some of the observations and hypotheses whereby glycation might promote pathologic changes in persons with elevated blood glucose.

The Maillard reaction is ubiquitous in nature. The accumulation of advanced glycation end products (AGEs) in tissues in the human body has been implicated in the complications of diabetes, aging, and renal failure.[71] The links between these reactions and the pathogenesis of nephropathy, macro- and microangiopathy, and cataracts in diabetic subjects are increasingly strong.[72] AGEs accumulate in vivo on long-lived proteins in the vascular wall collagen and basement membranes as a function of age and levels of glycemia.[73] They are capable of producing cross-linking of proteins and have been shown to display diverse biologic activities, including increased endothelial cell permeability,[74] binding to receptors on macrophages and endothelial mesangial cells,[75-77] activation of macrophages with secretion of cytokines after AGE ligand-receptor interaction,[78] quenching of nitric oxide with the consequent inhibition of vascular dilatation,[79] enhancement of oxidative stress,[80] and oxidation of low-density lipoprotein.[81] Thus, there is a growing body of evidence supporting a connection between circulating and tissue-accumulated AGEs and diabetic complications.

COAGULATION FACTORS

The coagulation cascade has been implicated in diabetes-related complications through disorders of the platelet, fluid phase, and vascular components of clotting. The following sections briefly review the abnormalities in glucose metabolism and their relationship to these factors.

Platelet

The platelet, when obtained from patients with diabetes mellitus, has long been recognized as showing abnormal behavior in in vitro[50] and in vivo studies.[54] In general, the correction of hyperglycemia is associated with an improvement in platelet behavior and release. The potential role of the platelet in vascular disease in general is discussed elsewhere in this book. The lesion of the platelet associated with hyperglycemia appears to be related to a hypersensitivity to stimuli. Thus, platelet aggregation in vitro may occur spontaneously by stirring in plasma obtained from persons with Hb A_{1c} greater than 10%, with concomitant release of vasoactive substances including serotonin, adenosine diphosphate, prostaglandins, and so on. The increased functional properties of diabetic platelets result in part from the primary release of larger platelets with enhanced thromboxane formation capacity and increased numbers of the functional glycoprotein (GP) receptors GP Ib and GP IIb/IIIa, which are synthesized in megakaryocytes.[82] Insulin exerts an antiaggregating effect, but that effect is diminished in the obese and in subjects with NIDDM.[83] Increased platelet aggregation to arachidonic acid has also been linked to reduced antioxidant properties seen in persons with diabetes.[84]

Platelet-rich or fibrin clots are less amenable to lysis in patients with diabetes than in controls.[85] Further, the release of platelet plasminogen activator inhibitor-1 (PAI-1) in whole blood has been found to be increased in NIDDM subjects.[86] PAI-1 levels have been noted to decrease with the lowering of blood glucose in NIDDM.[87] Therefore, the platelet contributes not only to a prethrombotic state in persons with

TABLE 8–5	Hypotheses Regarding the Potential Role of Nonenzymatic Glycation and Browning in the Pathologic Changes Associated with Diabetes Mellitus

I. Structural proteins
  A. Collagen: decreased turnover, flexibility, solubility, strength; increased aggregating potential for platelets; binding of immunoglobulins; cross-linking; and immunogenicity
  B. Lens crystallina and membrane: opacification, increased vulnerability to oxidative stress
  C. Basement membrane: increased permeability, decreased turnover, increased thickness
  D. Extracellular matrix: changes in binding to other proteins
  E. Hemoglobin: change in oxygen binding
  F. Fibrin: decreased enzymatic degradation
  G. Red blood cell membrane: increased rigidity
  H. Tubulin: cell structure and transport
  I. Myelin: altered structure and immunologic recognition
II. Carrier proteins
  A. Lipoproteins: alternative degradative pathways and metabolism by macrophages and endothelial cells, increased immunogenicity
  B. Albumin: alteration in binding properties for drugs and in handling by the kidney
  C. IgG: altered binding
III. Enzyme systems
  A. Copper-zinc superoxide dismutase: altered redox defense
  B. Fibrinogen: altered coagulation
  C. Antithrombin III: hypercoagulable state
  D. Purine nucleoside phosphorylase: aging of erythrocytes
  E. Alcohol dehydrogenase: substrate metabolism
  F. Ribonuclease A: loss of activity
  G. Cathepsin B: loss of activity
  H. N-acetyl-D-glucosaminidase: loss of activity
  I. Calmodulin: decreased calcium binding
IV. Nucleic acids
  A. Age-related changes, congenital malformations
V. Potentiation of other diseases of postsynthetic protein modification
  A. Carbamoylation-associated disorders in uremia
  B. Steroid cataract formation
  C. Acetaldehyde-induced changes in alcoholism

diabetes but also to problems of clot lysis in hyperglycemic subjects.

The Evaluation of Platelet IIb/IIIa Inhibitor for Stenting Trial substudy is the most extensive evaluation of stenting and platelet IIb/IIIa blockade in persons with diabetes and provides additional evidence for the platelet's role in the morbidity and mortality of heart disease and the associated processes in diabetes.[88] The trial involved 491 diabetic patients who were divided into three groups: the first group received both a stent and abciximab, the second group underwent balloon angioplasty and also received the drug, and the third group had a stent implanted but received only a placebo. The reblockage rate was cut in half in the patients who received both the stent and the drug. Those patients had an 8.1% reblockage rate in the 6 months after the procedure, which was about half that of the other two groups. Ongoing trials of eptifibatide and tirofiban should help determine whether platelet IIb/IIIa receptor blockers should be used routinely to reduce restenosis after stenting in diabetic subjects, as well as the role of activated platelets and endothelium in pathologic conditions.[88] These agents will become more attractive, in part because of the report of thrombotic thrombocytopenic purpura associated with ticlopidine in the setting of coronary artery stents.[89]

Fluid Phase of Coagulation

Fibrinogen is increasingly recognized as a potential cardiovascular risk factor.[90-92] Fibrinogen levels generally have been found to be elevated in diabetes. Fibrinogen synthesis is increased in part because of increased turnover and feedback to the liver with fragment D and because insulin increases fibrinogen synthesis.[93]

Early studies of fibrinogen kinetics in diabetic subjects documented a reversible disorder associated with hyperglycemia that was corrected with normal glucose levels or heparin administration, consistent with a lesion of antithrombin III activity in hyperglycemic subjects.[94,95] These findings were confirmed by the PLAT Group study.[96]

Oxidative stress, which is accentuated in diabetic subjects, has been linked to thrombin activation, and a correlation between markers of oxidative stress and fibrinogen has been reported in diabetic subjects. Thus, oxidative stress, which is mediated by hyperglycemia and compounded by glycation, may represent an additional link between diabetes and hyperfibrinogenemia.[97-99] Glycated fibrin is also less susceptible to plasmin degradation.[100]

Endothelial Phase of Coagulation

Studies indicate that elevated glucose levels can be toxic to vascular endothelial cells through multiple mechanisms.[101] Having observed that glucose levels mimicking diabetic hyperglycemia induce in vitro endothelial cell overexpression of extracellular matrix molecules, decreased replication, and increased levels of transforming growth factor-β (TGF-β) messenger RNA (mRNA), Cagliero and colleagues examined whether the effects of high glucose are mediated by autocrine TGF-β.[101] Whereas the inhibitory effect of high glucose levels on endothelial cell replication was reversible, that of TGF-β was not. Both perturbations induced upregulation of fibronectin expression, but the effects were additive.

Thus, there are growth-inhibitory effects of high glucose levels that are independent of TGF-β, and high glucose levels and TGF-β exert their effects through distinct pathways and at different loci.

Pieper and coworkers attempted to evaluate the relative roles of hyperglycemia and insulin lack on endothelial cell dysfunction in diabetes.[102] Rats were continuously infused with glucose or saline for 72 hours to achieve peak plasma glucose concentrations of approximately 25 mM. Plasma insulin rose by 12-fold in glucose-infused rats. Blood pressure was not altered by this intervention. Aortic rings taken from control rats relaxed to the administration of the endothelium-dependent vasodilators acetylcholine and A-23187 and the endothelium-independent vasodilator nitroglycerin. Relaxation to acetylcholine but not to A-23187 or nitroglycerin was impaired in glucose-infused rat aortic rings. Incubation in vitro with either indomethacin or superoxide dismutase did not restore the impaired relaxation to acetylcholine in rings taken from glucose-infused rats. Thus, hyperglycemia with hyperinsulinemia selectively impairs receptor-dependent, endothelium-dependent relaxation. These studies are consistent with the idea that elevated glucose may be a common pathway leading to endothelial dysfunction in IDDM and NIDDM.

Baumgartner-Parzer and associates showed that adhesion molecule gene expression can be modulated by ambient glucose levels as well.[103] These authors found an increase in intercellular adhesion molecule-1 (ICAM-1) but not platelet endothelial cell adhesion molecule expression in response to a high glucose level in human umbilical vein endothelial cells. These findings are also consistent with the specific abnormalities in endothelial dysfunction occurring in diabetes.

In vivo–generated nitric oxide circulates in plasma mainly as an adduct of serum albumin. Compared with free nitric oxide, this nitric oxide adduct is relatively long-lived and exhibits vasodilating and platelet inhibitory properties. Farkas and Menzel documented that proteins lose their nitric oxide–stabilizing function after advanced glycosylation, thus providing another mechanism by which AGE-modified proteins can promote vascular disease.[104]

LIPIDS

Hyperlipidemia is a normal concomitant of hyperglycemia. Both triglyceride and cholesterol levels tend to improve with normalization of blood glucose levels, as documented by ambient glucose levels and glycated hemoglobin levels.[51] Further, glycation of low-density lipoproteins and modification by AGEs leads to a more atherogenic pattern of lipid metabolism.[81] The presence of renal failure accelerates the pathologic changes associated with the presence of AGEs.[105,106] Thus, improvement in glycemia corrects at least some of the perturbations of lipid metabolism unique to the individual with diabetes.

Oxidation-Reduction Pathways

Both the metabolism of excess glucose and the Amadori rearrangement product resulting from excess glycation can promote pro-oxidant activity.[107,108] Lipid peroxides are thought to be formed by free radicals and may play an important role in the development of atheromatous vascular disease.

Velazquez and colleagues investigated the relationship among lipids, lipoproteins, coagulation factors, and lipid peroxides (measured as thiobarbituric acid reacting species [TBARS]) in NIDDM patients with macrovascular disease.[109] Eighteen diabetic and 20 nondiabetic subjects with clinical evidence of ischemic heart disease or peripheral vascular disease were investigated, together with 28 healthy subjects without evidence of vascular disease. TBARS concentration, as a measure of oxidation status, did not differ significantly in nondiabetic (mean, 5.0 mmol/L [95% CI, 4.5 to 5.7]) and diabetic (5.6 [range, 5.1 to 6.0] mmol/L) groups with macrovascular disease, although values were higher in both groups of patients with vascular disease compared with control subjects (2.7 [range, 2.4 to 3.1] mmol/L; $P < 0.001$). Significant univariate correlations between TBARS concentration and measures of blood glucose control (fructosamine, blood glucose, and Hb A_{1c}) were found for all 66 subjects ($P < 0.001$ to 0.01). Thus, diabetes confers a pro-oxidant internal environment consistent with the promotion of vascular disease.

VASCULAR VOLUME SHIFTS

In studies of fibrinogen turnover, it became apparent that it was important to correct for vascular volume shifts induced by changes in glucose. When blood glucose was elevated from 100 mg/dL to 300 mg/dL, a rise in vascular volume of 8% was documented by double-labeling techniques.[95] The implications for these types of recurrent volume shifts and the resultant stresses on the vascular tree have not been studied.

INSULIN LEVELS

In NIDDM there is thought to be an increased atherogenic potential related to the presence of insulin resistance, hyperinsulinemia, central obesity, and dyslipidemia. This syndrome, now known as syndrome X,[110] was previously called CHAOS (coronary artery disease, hypertension, NIDDM, obesity, stroke) or the "deadly quartet" of upper body obesity, glucose intolerance, hypertriglyceridemia, and hypertension. All were associated with the early development of coronary artery disease. Because of these syndromes, insulin resistance with hyperinsulinemia has been studied as a risk factor for CVD. There have been several epidemiologic studies showing a correlation of hyperinsulinemia with CVD.[110-112] Angiographically documented coronary artery disease has been linked with impaired glucose and insulin metabolism.[110]

The proposed pathophysiology of hyperinsulinemia and atherosclerotic disease is complicated. Hyperinsulinemia is associated with increased triglycerides, increased very-low-density lipoproteins, decreased high-density lipoproteins, central obesity, vascular intimal hyperplasia, and possibly hypertension, each of which may accelerate the development of atheroma. However, some studies implicate proinsulin as the culprit, rather than insulin itself, and suggest that exogenous insulin does not increase the risk of CVD.[113,114] Intervention studies of the effect of glucose control on the initiation and progression of large vessel disease in persons with diabetes mellitus are sorely needed. These interactions have been modified to include a role for insulin and glucose in regulating central sympathetic activity.[115] Thus, the links among obesity, diet, insulin resistance, hyperinsulinemia,

sympathetic activity, and lipid disorders are becoming better defined.

IMMUNOLOGIC MECHANISMS

There are multiple potential interactions of the immune system in the genesis of vascular disease. A number of the cytokine-lymphokine perturbations induced by glycation were discussed earlier. Immune perturbations specific to diabetes and the development of vascular disease have not yet been identified. Because diabetes is heterogeneous and exhibits similar vascular changes despite the cause or the phenotype, it is unlikely that a particular genetic lesion of the immune system will be linked to the accelerated vascular disease seen in diabetes.

The one lesion in the immune system of importance to the surgeon is that of the polymorphonuclear leukocyte. The polymorphonuclear leukocyte functions abnormally in a person with hyperglycemia, with decreased adherence, migration, chemotaxis, and killing.[50,116] The lesion of the polymorphonuclear leukocyte reverses within a marrow transit time of 14 days.[50] Therefore, the optimal surgical candidate is one who has had normoglycemia for 2 weeks before surgery.

INFLAMMATORY PROCESSES

The Atherosclerosis Risk in Communities study found a role for inflammation and endothelial dysfunction in the pathogenesis of type 2 diabetes.[117] It also appears that circulating inflammatory factors such as tumor necrosis factor-α and interleukin-6 may cause insulin resistance and obesity.[118,119]

SMOKING

The Speedwell study emphasized the critical role of smoking in the genesis of vascular disease, especially in persons with diabetes.[120] Systolic blood pressure, fasting plasma glucose, triglycerides, and white blood cell count were all independently associated with the development of intermittent claudication, angina, and death, but the most striking association was with smoking.

Other Risk Factors for Diabetes- or Hyperglycemia-Associated Vascular Disease

IMPAIRED GLUCOSE TOLERANCE

Approximately 16% of American adults aged 40 to 74 years have impaired glucose tolerance (IGT), and approximately 6.6% have diabetes.[121] Because 1% to 5% of those with IGT and 5% to 10% of those at high risk for NIDDM become diabetic each year, IGT is an important risk factor for diabetes.[122-130] In addition, macrovascular disease is present, and mortality rates are higher in individuals with IGT.[123,127,130] It appears that individuals with IGT have diabetic risk factor values (defined later) that fall between the values for normoglycemic individuals and those for diabetic individuals. Harris suggested "that IGT and NIDDM may have similar natural histories and may reflect a continuum of declining glucose tolerance from IGT to overt diabetes."[128]

PHYSICAL INACTIVITY AND OBESITY

Over the last few decades, the importance of physical activity for disease prevention and health maintenance has been increasingly recognized. The benefits of exercise and increased physical activity include enhanced insulin sensitivity and glucose effectiveness, decreased risk for hypertension, improved plasma lipids and lipoproteins, decreased obesity and improved body fat distribution, enhanced immunologic function, decreased anxiety and depression, improved sleep, improved psychological characteristics in both normal and psychiatric patients, and disease prevention.[131]

Obesity and an unfavorable body fat distribution, with increased abdominal fat, are well-established risk factors for diabetes, confounded by ethnicity and family history.[132-134] For obese individuals, the rates of diabetes are higher in Hispanics than in African Americans, and the rates in African Americans are higher than those in whites. Up to 50% of obese Native Americans develop diabetes.[122] Data from the Second National Health and Nutrition Examination Survey revealed that 24.2% of men and 27.1% of women aged 20 to 74 years were overweight (BMI = 27.8 kg/m² for men and BMI = 27.3 kg/m² for women).[135] It is estimated that in the United States there are 34 million overweight adults, 12.5 million of whom are "severely overweight."[136]

In a study of 8715 men (mean age, 42 years) followed for an average of 8.2 years, the age-adjusted death rate increased with higher levels of fasting glucose, and fit men had a lower age-adjusted all-cause death rate compared with unfit men regardless of glycemic status.[137] Fit men with a fasting blood glucose (FBG) less than 6.4 mM had the lowest age-adjusted death rate (21.4 per 10,000 person-years). Within each class of glycemic status (FBG < 6.4 mM, FBG 6.4 to 7.8 mM, FBG ≥ 7.8 mM, or diagnosed NIDDM), those who were fit had lower mortality rates than those who were unfit. Men who were fit but in the highest glycemic status group had an age-adjusted all-cause mortality rate (45.9 per 10,000 person-years) similar to that of men who were unfit but in the lowest glycemic status group. The data suggest that the risk of death for fit men with an FBG of 7.8 mM or with NIDDM is similar to that of men who are unfit with a normal FBG. The authors suggested that because cardiorespiratory fitness can be improved by regular physical activity, using exercise to improve fitness could be a "cornerstone to the effective management of patients with abnormal blood glucose profiles or NIDDM."[137]

No primary prevention projects for NIDDM have used increased physical activity or exercise as the sole intervention for the prevention or deferment of disease.[137-139] Nevertheless, there is evidence of an association between exercise and diabetes from societies that have abandoned a traditional active lifestyle for a more sedentary "modern" lifestyle. There is a dramatic increase in NIDDM in people who become more sedentary.[140,141] Conversely, physically active societies have lower rates of NIDDM than do more sedentary societies.[142-147]

ETHNICITY

Ethnic minority populations in the United States have high rates of IGT and are at higher risk for NIDDM.[147] Minorities are especially afflicted with obesity, especially minority women. The age-adjusted percentages of overweight and severely overweight individuals are 24.6% and 9.6%, respectively, for white women, 45.1% and 19.7% for African American

women, and 41.5% and 16.7% for Mexican American women. It is acknowledged that although some races tend to be "heavier" than others, without adverse health effects, and that perhaps the norms and standards need to be adjusted for different races, maintaining a normal weight according to the overall population norm was associated with a 23% lower risk of mortality compared with being persistently overweight.

Results from the National Health and Nutrition Examination Survey Epidemiologic Follow-up Study suggest that the higher rate of lower extremity amputations in black compared with white Americans with diabetes is not attributable to biologic causes but rather to a combination of social and environmental factors, including obesity.[148] The findings included an analysis of more than 14,000 people who participated, 2240 of whom had diabetes at baseline or developed it during the study. The authors found that during 20 years of follow-up, the age-adjusted rate of all lower extremity amputations was 2.8 times higher in black than in white subjects. Diabetes and its duration were strong predictors of risk, as were hypertension, smoking, low educational level, and low socioeconomic status.[148]

POSITIVE FAMILY HISTORY

Mitchell and colleagues compared the prevalence of NIDDM and IGT in 4914 subjects of white, African American, and Hispanic origin.[149] Men with a parental history of diabetes (in one or both parents, regardless of which one) had a higher prevalence of diabetes and IGT than did men without a parental history. In women, only a maternal history of diabetes (or both maternal and paternal, but not paternal alone) was associated with a higher prevalence of NIDDM and IGT.

GESTATIONAL DIABETES

A history of gestational diabetes mellitus, defined as glucose intolerance of variable severity with an onset or first recognition during pregnancy,[150] represents an independent risk factor for the development of subsequent diabetes.[151-163] (Gestational diabetes is generally viewed by obstetricians as a potential risk factor for adverse pregnancy outcome.) The original criteria put forth by O'Sullivan and Mahan for the diagnosis of gestational diabetes were developed and validated for their predictive value for subsequent diabetes.[164]

Because of the different means used to diagnose diabetes during pregnancy and to define diabetes outside of pregnancy, the prevalence of subsequent diabetes after gestational diabetes has been reported to be 19% to 87% for combined glucose intolerance and diabetes and 6% to 62% for diabetes alone. When only the O'Sullivan and Mahan criteria were used for the diagnosis of gestational diabetes,[164] the prevalence of subsequent diabetes using the National Diabetes Data Group criteria[21] varied from 2.7% to 20.9%, depending on the length of follow-up.

Protocols to Improve Glucose Control Before, During, and After Surgery

The rationale for maintaining near-normal glucose levels was established earlier. Another consideration for a patient with diabetes who faces surgery is the possibility of hemodynamic instability during anesthesia due to dehydration and osmotic shifts. In addition, as noted earlier and in a 1999 review,[165] a diabetic patient is more prone to infection,[13,166] has slower wound healing,[167] and may have increased free fatty acids, the metabolism of which requires greater myocardial oxygen consumption.[121] This section provides guidelines for various situations encountered preoperatively, perioperatively, and postoperatively.

PREPARATION FOR ELECTIVE SURGERY

Ideally, all patients with diabetes should have attained good glucose control before elective surgery. *Good glucose control is* defined as the glycemic level that provides the optimal setting for elective surgery, minimizes the risk of infection, facilitates healing, and prevents thrombogenesis. The ideal targets for glucose control are 80 to 100 mg/dL before meals and no higher than 180 mg/dL 1 hour after meals. Maintenance of these glucose targets achieves an Hb A_{1c} level that is associated with the lowest risk of diabetic complications (<7%).

STANDING INSULIN ORDERS: IMPROVING GLUCOSE CONTROL IN THE HOSPITAL

When a patient with diabetes is admitted to the hospital, the usual outpatient dose of insulin is not appropriate. First, the patient is generally put to bed, with a resultant increase in insulin requirements of 10% to 20%, depending on his or her usual daily activity level. Second, there is an increased insulin requirement associated with the psychological and physical stress (infection, trauma, inflammation, surgery) of hospitalization. Therefore, the patient's usual dose of insulin generally needs to be adjusted. The only way to achieve a "perfect" dose of insulin is to measure the blood glucose frequently. Alternatively, the admitting orders could be written to start with a prescription that is near the estimated needs and allow the staff to automatically adjust each insulin dose based on the blood glucose response to that dose. To this end, we developed the standing orders described later. In the following discussion, NPH (neutral protamine Hagedorn) insulin and regular insulin are emphasized because of clinicians' long-term familiarity with them. Those interested in newer insulins may wish to consult a 1999 review.[168] Short-acting insulins such as insulin lispro may be substituted for regular insulin; their advantages include a rapid onset of action and peak effect, with less delayed hyperinsulinemia and hypoglycemia.

The protocol for standing insulin orders was designed to go hand in hand with a 40% carbohydrate diet consisting of three meals and three snacks. The diet is generally calculated based on body weight. A general guideline is 30 kcal/kg for malnourished adults, 25 kcal/kg for persons of ideal body weight, and 18 kcal/kg for obese patients.

Calculating the 24-Hour Insulin Requirement

The insulin requirements for increasingly stressful states are listed in Table 8-6. Standing orders (Fig. 8-1) start with a default calculation of 0.6 unit/kg per 24 hours in persons who are not NPO (nothing by mouth). This dose is safe and is generally an undercalculation. If, however, it is clear to the

TABLE 8–6	Increased Insulin Requirements for Stress

The 24-hour insulin requirement (BIG I) is calculated based on the degree of stress the patient is experiencing:

    I = 0.6 unit × the patient's weight in kilograms for a person who is healthy and physically active

    I = 0.7 unit × the patient's weight in kilograms for a person who is premenstrual or is placed on bed rest or who is mildly stressed (whether infectious, physical trauma, or psychological stress)

    I = 0.8-2.0 units × the patient's weight in kilograms for a person who is moderately to severely stressed. Note that stress doses of steroids may require 1-2 units/kg.

Patient's weight: _____ kg

Constant chosen for BIG I: _____

Thus, I = _____ units/24 hr

BIG I is then fractioned into

4/9 I = prebreakfast NPH = _____ units of NPH

2/9 I = prebreakfast reg = _____ units of reg

1/6 I = predinner reg = _____ units of reg

1/6 I = 11 PM NPH = _____ units of NPH

NPH, neutral protamine Hagedorn (insulin); reg, regular insulin.

admitting physician that 0.6 unit/day is too low, the standing orders state that all handwritten orders will be followed. Thus, one may override the standing orders by writing in a higher constant when calculating the 24-hour insulin requirement.

Frequency of Monitoring and Charting Glucose

To ensure that the peak response to insulin and the peak postprandial response to food are monitored, eight blood glucose tests are required each day: before and 1 hour after each meal, before bed, and at 3 AM. These blood glucose levels are charted on the insulin worksheet illustrated in Figure 8-2. The initial calculations of such insulin requirements are written on the worksheet, as are all subsequent insulin changes.

The standing orders allow the nurses to adjust each of the injections daily. The percentage change for the sliding scale is 3% of the total insulin requirement. The sliding scale is adjusted as a percentage of the total dose, because these orders apply to small children as well as obese adults. A 2-unit change to correct for the following day is included to make orders slightly easier to follow, but if a patient is very small or very large, one may override the orders and rewrite them, making smaller or larger changes for the subsequent dose.

Automatic Adjustments by Standing Orders

Each dose of insulin is changed as outlined in the established orders (see Fig. 8-1) by the nursing staff. The morning dose of NPH insulin is adjusted according to the predinner blood sugar. For example, if the predinner blood sugar is too low, the following morning NPH insulin dose will be decreased by 2 units.

The NPH insulin dose at bedtime requires three blood glucose checks before it can be safely adjusted. The NPH insulin dose before bed is designed to "fix the fasting" or conquer the wake-up blood glucose for the following morning.

☐ 1. Routine: NPH plus regular schedule.

Nursing will calculate and administer the starting dose of insulin as outlined below:

I = 0.6 × weight kg/24 hours divided so that 4/9 of dose is NPH given before breakfast and 1/6 of dose is NPH given before bedtime.

Regular insulin is given before breakfast as 2/9 of dose and before dinner as 1/6 of dose. The regular insulin is titrated on the blood glucose.

0730: NPH = 4/9 dose = _____.

    Check last predinner BS:

        If the predinner BS is <70, then decrease the AM NPH by 2 units.
        If the predinner BS is 71–120, then no change in the AM NPH.
        If the predinner BS is >120, then increase the AM NPH by 2 units.

    Regular = 2/9 dose = _____ to be adjusted according to the following scale:

        BS < 70 = _____ = (2/9 I dose) − 3% of the total insulin requirement.
        71–100 = _____ = 2/9 I dose.
        101–140 = _____ = (2/9 I dose) + 3% of I.
        >141 = _____ = (2/9 I dose) + 6% of I.

    If the BS 1 hour after the meal is <110, then decrease the corresponding next-day mealtime regular insulin by 2 units.
    If the BS 1 hour after the meal is 111–150, no change in the corresponding next-day mealtime regular insulin.
    If the BS 1 hour after the meal is >151, then increase the corresponding next-day mealtime regular insulin by 2 units.

1130 prelunch: Regular insulin is given based on the following scale:

        BS < 120 = 0 insulin.
        121–140 = 1/181 = _____.
        141–180 = 1/181 + 2 units = _____.
        >181 = 1/181 + 4 units = _____.

1700 predinner: Regular is 1/6 dose = _____ and based on the following scale:

        BS < 70 = _____ = (1/6 I dose) − 3% of I.
        71–100 = _____ = 1/6 I dose.
        101–140 = _____ = (1/6 I dose) + 3% of I.
        >141 = _____ = (1/6 I dose) + 6% of I.

    If the BS 1 hour after the meal is <110, then decrease the corresponding next-day mealtime regular insulin by 2 units.
    If the BS 1 hour after the meal is 111–150, no change in the corresponding next-day mealtime regular insulin.
    If the BS 1 hour after the meal is >151, then increase the corresponding next-day mealtime regular insulin by 2 units.

2330 bedtime NPH: Give 1/6 dose = _____.

    If the prebreakfast BS is <70, then decrease the bedtime NPH by 2 units.
    If the prebreakfast BS is 71–120, then no change in the bedtime NPH.
    If the prebreakfast BS is >121, then check the last HS and 3 AM BS:

    If the HS, 3 AM, and prebreakfast BS are >121, then increase the bedtime NPH by 2 units.
    If the 3 AM BS is <70 (regardless of the HS or prebreakfast BS), decrease the bedtime NPH by 2 units.
    If the HS and the 3 AM BS are 70–120, but the prebreakfast is >121, then increase the bedtime NPH by 2 units.

NOTE: ALL ORDERS CHECKED OR HANDWRITTEN WILL BE FOLLOWED

_____   _____   _____
Physician's signature   Date   Time

FIGURE 8–1 • Standing orders for insulin for hospitalized diabetic patients. BS, blood sugar; HS, hour of sleep; NPH, neutral protamine Hagedorn.

Other forces come into play, however, that may make the interpretation of a high fasting blood glucose difficult. There are six ways to end up with a high fasting blood glucose level:

1. One can go to bed with a high glucose level because of a persisting high dinner level and stay elevated all night long. The cause is either not enough regular insulin at dinner or too much food at dinner.
2. One can go to bed with a normal blood glucose level but have a bedtime snack, which then produces a high wake-up glucose level. This can be avoided by having a smaller bedtime snack.

	DATE										
	0300 Blood glucose										
B R E A K F A S T	AC Basal NPH insulin										
	AC Regular insulin										
	<70 =										
	71–100 =										
	101–140 =										
	>140 =										
	AC Blood glucose	AC	PC	AC	PC	AC	PC	AC	PC	AC	PC
L U N C H	AC Regular insulin										
	<120 =										
	121–140 =										
	141–180 =										
	>180 =										
	AC Blood glucose	AC	PC	AC	PC	AC	PC	AC	PC	AC	PC
D I N N E R	AC Regular insulin										
	<70 =										
	71–100 =										
	101–140 =										
	>140 =										
	AC Blood glucose	AC	PC	AC	PC	AC	PC	AC	PC	AC	PC
	2330 Blood glucose										
	2330 Basal NPH insulin										
	COMMENTS										
	INITIALS										

FIGURE 8–2 • Insulin worksheet for charting blood glucose levels. AC, before meal; PC, after meal; NPH, neutral protamine Hagedorn.

3. One can go to bed with a normal blood glucose level but "drift up" throughout the night because the NPH insulin dose at bedtime was inadequate.

4. One can go to bed with a normal blood glucose level, become hypoglycemic in the middle of the night, and wake up with a high level because of the counterregulatory hormonal response to the low blood glucose. The cause is too much bedtime NPH insulin or an inadequate bedtime snack.

5. One can go to bed with a high glucose level but still have a hypoglycemic reaction in the middle of the night, mount a counterregulatory response, and wake up with a high glucose level. In this case, the cause is not enough regular insulin at dinner (or too much food at dinner) and too much bedtime NPH insulin.

6. One can have a normal bedtime glucose level that stays normal until after 3 AM, when the blood glucose level rises with increasing insulin needs (the dawn phenomenon). More bedtime insulin is needed.

Thus, the adjustment of the bedtime dose of NPH requires all three readings: bedtime, 3 AM, and wake-up blood glucose levels.

If the wake-up blood glucose level is low (<70 mg/dL), decrease the bedtime NPH insulin dose by 2 units. If the wake-up level is high and if the previous night's bedtime and 3 AM levels were also high, the 11 PM NPH insulin dose should be increased by 2 units. If the 3 AM glucose reading is low, no matter what the bedtime or the wake-up blood glucose is, cut back on the bedtime dose of NPH insulin. Here, the physician would need to write separate orders to indicate whether the quantity of food at dinner or at the bedtime snack should be adjusted. The established orders (see Fig. 8-1) would also increase the NPH insulin dose before bedtime if the wake-up blood glucose level is high but the bedtime and 3 AM blood glucose levels are normal, because there is room for a little more bedtime NPH insulin to conquer the fasting.

The 3 AM "Touch-up" Insulin Dose

One additional order that can speed the normalization process is to prescribe regular insulin at 3 AM. If the blood glucose level is high at 3 AM, it will definitely be high at 7:30 AM due to the dawn-associated rise in counterregulatory hormones. Therefore, a convenient and worthwhile addition to these orders is a sliding scale for regular insulin at 3 AM, which is generally the same as the lunchtime "touch-up":

$$BS < 120 = 0$$

$$BS\ 121\ to\ 140 = 1/18\ I$$

$$BS\ 141\ to\ 180 = 1/18\ I + 2\ units$$

$$BS > 181 = 1/18\ I + 4\ units$$

where BS is blood sugar and I is total insulin dose per 24 hours.

It is worth noting that bedtime regular insulin is dangerous. Between the hours of 11 PM and 3 AM, patients are more sensitive to regular insulin because of low levels of counterregulatory hormones. It is generally preferable to leave a high bedtime glucose level untreated but wake the patient at 3 AM and give regular insulin at that time if the blood glucose is still elevated.

Hypoglycemia Prevention

Although the standing orders for insulin begin with 0.6 unit/kg per 24 hours, which is most likely an undercalculation, it is always best to pair this protocol with a protocol for hypoglycemia. Suggested hypoglycemia orders are given in Table 8-7.

Deriving the "Personal Lag Time" for Insulin Action

At times, the health care professional may actually create brittle diabetes. All that may be needed is an injection of regular insulin at the moment the meal is ingested. The simple sugars in foods peak as sugar in the bloodstream in 15 to 20 minutes. Complex carbohydrates peak as sugar in the bloodstream in 60 minutes.

Regular insulin injected under the skin requires about 45 minutes before an effect can be documented in terms of a decrement in blood glucose. The hypoglycemic action of the injected insulin does not peak for 2 to 3 hours. The result is that after an injection of insulin given at the same time as a meal with a fairly large percentage of calories as carbohydrate,

TABLE 8–7	Standing Orders for Hypoglycemia

Routine: nursing staff will carry out the protocol outlined below:

1. For BS < 60 mg/dL:
   Give 8 oz milk and recheck BS in 15 min.
2. For symptomatic BS < 60 mg/dL:
   Give 8 oz milk and recheck BS in 15 min.
   If BS is still <60 mg/dL, give another 8 oz milk and recheck BS in 15 min.
   If BS is still <60 mg/dL, give 8 oz orange juice and a slice of bread.
3. If the patient is unable to take fluids, lethargic, or argumentative:
   Give 0.15 mg glucagon SC and recheck BS in 10 min.
   If BS is still <60 mg/dL, give another 0.15 mg glucagon SC and recheck BS in 10 min.
   Once BS is >60 mg/dL but <120 mg/dL and patient is able to hear, give 8 oz milk.
4. When patient is unresponsive:
   Give 1.0 mg glucagon IM and call the physician.
   Check BS in 10 min.
   If patient is still unresponsive, start IV line of 1000 mL D_{10} to run wide open.
   Recheck BS in 10 min; turn down IV line to 100 mL/hr when BS is >80 mg/dL.

BS, blood sugar; D_{10}, 10% dextrose in water; IV, intravenous; SC, subcutaneous.

blood glucose peaks at about 1 hour after the start of the meal, and the patient is hypoglycemic at 3 hours, concomitant with the peak in insulin action. Such an occurrence might be referred to as iatrogenic reactive hypoglycemia. Counterregulatory hormones secreted (and extra food ingested) in response to the hypoglycemia lead to a marked rise in glucose (usually 250 to 350 mg/dL) approximately 3 hours later, which in turn prompts the need for additional insulin.

To convert this type of brittle diabetes into a smoother glycemic profile, one needs to change the timing of the injection of regular insulin in relationship to the meal. Increasing the lag time between the insulin injection and the ingestion of food can dampen glycemic excursions despite no change in meal plan or dose of insulin. The usual optimal lag time for abdominal injections is 30 to 40 minutes. The usual lag time for leg injections is 40 to 50 minutes.

Several approaches can shorten the lag time between insulin injection and action. First, insulin lispro has a rapid peak and rapid disposal compared with regular insulin. Thus, it can be given when food arrives or even after ingestion of a meal, with calculation of the ingested carbohydrate. Second, the warmer the skin temperature, the faster the insulin is absorbed. A hot washcloth placed over the injection site accelerates absorption. Third, muscle activity at the site of injection shortens lag time. Thus, exercise can speed insulin absorption.

Suggested Sliding Scale for Insulin

A simple way to think about insulin action is to assume that hypoglycemia increases insulin sensitivity and hyperglycemia increases insulin resistance. Therefore, a premeal sliding scale for regular insulin might include not only a scale of graded doses of insulin but also a scale of lag times for beginning the meal after the injection. In practice, it is often prudent on a busy inpatient ward to await the arrival of food before injecting insulin, to avoid hypoglycemia. As noted earlier, the use of insulin lispro obviates the problem.

Nothing by Mouth (NPO) Orders

Compliance with NPO orders might be simpler if all patients used an insulin infusion pump; then the patient merely skips the breakfast bolus and maintains the basal infusion of insulin. However, this advice presupposes that the patient is on a perfectly calculated basal infusion of insulin (the dose of insulin that keeps the patient normoglycemic during fasting). Unfortunately, the basal infusion rate is often adjusted higher than the basal need in order to provide extra insulin to cover extra calories or foods that convert slowly to glucose (e.g., protein and high-fiber carbohydrates). Thus, even "well-controlled" patients using a pump may need to be instructed to decrease the basal infusion rate by 20% for as long as they are NPO or to adjust the calculated basal infusion to 0.25 unit/kg per 24 hours, whichever is lower. A good starting point is 0.3 unit/kg per 24 hours as a basal constant infusion. The blood glucose is measured before bed, at 3 AM, at 7 AM, and every 2 hours thereafter. These frequent checks allow one to increase or decrease the basal rate or to "touch up" with insulin, intravenous (IV) glucose, or glucagon, as needed.

If a patient is on an NPH insulin system, the doses during the fasting period are calculated (0.1 × weight [kg]) to be given every 8 hours that the patient is NPO. The blood glucose should be measured at midnight, 3 AM, 8 AM, and then every 2 hours until the operation. If the blood glucose is elevated, touch-up doses of regular insulin, similar to the Ultralente insulin protocol, may be given.

If the patient is hospitalized and an IV line is started, hypoglycemia and hyperglycemia can be avoided with IV infusions at 2 mL/kg per hour based on blood glucose checks every hour (during the procedure and recovery) or every other hour. The guidelines for maintaining normoglycemia on IV infusion are outlined in Table 8-8.

These algorithms for the maintenance of normoglycemia during periods of fasting are essentially the same as those used to prescribe a true basal insulin dose or the dose of insulin that maintains normal blood glucose levels in a person with IDDM when he or she does not eat. During periods of increasing stress, such as surgery, extra insulin may be needed. Nevertheless, these guidelines and the surveillance system provide a relatively simple and safe approach to fasting for patients with IDDM or NIDDM.

ENTERAL AND PARENTERAL NUTRITION IN DIABETIC PATIENTS

Given a severely stressful situation, or after the administration of high-dose corticosteroids, the population estimated to be frankly hyperglycemic rises to over 25% (referred to as "stress-induced" diabetes). Further, when highly concentrated glucose solutions are given intravenously during stressful situations, the percentage of hyperglycemic individuals rises to over 50%.[169] It can be seen that a significant number of surgical patients require additional attention to enteral

TABLE 8–8	Guidelines for Intravenous Infusion Based on Blood Glucose Values
Blood Glucose (mg/dL)	**Infusion at 2 mL/kg/hr**
<70	D_{10}
70-120	D_5
>120	Normal saline
>150	Use touch-up IV insulin (0.02 unit) while normal saline is continued at 2 mL/kg/hr and adjust rate based on hourly readings

D_5, 5% dextrose in water; D_{10}, 10% dextrose in water.

and parenteral nutrition because of elevated blood glucose values if optimal glucose levels are to be maintained.

Enteral Route

There are multiple formulas for tube feeding. They differ by protein concentration and composition, density, fat, and carbohydrate percentage. These basic formulas contain 45% to 60% carbohydrates. The elemental formulas contain low residue and thus are completely absorbed from the jejunum. These elemental diets have more than 70% carbohydrates and sugars. Corn syrup is usually the carbohydrate used. There are two formulas with a low percentage of carbohydrates: one is for pulmonary patients to help lower the respiratory quotient (28% carbohydrates); the other is designed for diabetic patients, with 38% high-fiber carbohydrates. The carbohydrate content of the formula directly affects the blood glucose level achieved; the lower the carbohydrate content of a formula, the lower the resultant blood glucose level. If hyperglycemia is documented by blood glucose determinations every 4 hours, insulin may be given as a constant IV infusion or subcutaneously. One unit of regular insulin per 10 g of carbohydrate is given over 24 hours in the formula. Table 8-9 summarizes the protocol for blood glucose monitoring and initiating insulin in a nondiabetic patient.

TABLE 8–9	Enteral Nutrition: Normal Fasting for Patients with Normal Glucose Tolerance and for Patients with Non-Insulin-Dependent Diabetes Mellitus and Normal Fasting Glucose without Insulin

1. Monitor fingerstick blood glucose q6h for 2 days. If all glucose levels remain <180 mg/dL, the frequency of monitoring may be decreased to once a day.
2. If hyperglycemia occurs, continue to monitor blood glucose q6h and proceed to step 3.
3. Begin insulin as a continuous infusion while the enteral nutrition is being infused: 1 unit of regular insulin for every 10 g of carbohydrate in the feeding.
4. Based on the blood glucose level q6h, change the insulin dose for tomorrow as follows:
   ≤80: decrease ratio (0.5 unit/10 g carbohydrate)
   81-180: no change in ratio (1.0 unit/10 g carbohydrate)
   ≥181: increase ratio (1.5 units/10 g carbohydrate)

If a patient with known NIDDM has a normal fasting blood glucose level before the enteral infusion is started, the patient may be given insulin with the enteral infusion at a dose of 1 unit of regular insulin for every 10 g of carbohydrate given over 24 hours (Fig. 8-3). Most severely stressed NIDDM patients have fasting hyperglycemia even if their interim fasting glucose levels are normal. In the majority of cases, NIDDM patients require both a basal insulin infusion, calculated as 0.3 unit of regular insulin times the patient's weight in kilograms, and the "meal requirement," which is 1 unit of regular insulin for every 10 g of carbohydrate in the formula (Table 8-10).

IDDM patients who require enteral nutrition may also be given insulin for their basal and formula-related needs (see Table 8-10). If the patient is severely ill or is also taking glucocorticoids, the basal insulin dose may be calculated as 1 unit/kg body weight, and the formula-related insulin dose may start at 1 unit/10 g carbohydrate. The blood glucose should be checked every 4 to 6 hours, and if it is elevated, additional regular insulin may be given subcutaneously by the floor nursing staff, using the following scale:

$$BS < 180 = \text{no extra regular insulin}$$

$$BS\ 181\ to\ 240 = 6\ \text{units regular insulin}$$

$$BS\ 241\ to\ 300 = 8\ \text{units regular insulin}$$

$$BS \geq 301 = 10\ \text{units regular insulin}$$

ENTERAL NUTRITION ORDER

DATE AND TIME	**1. FEEDING TUBE:**		
	☐ Nasogastric ☐ Nasoduodenal ☐ Gastrostomy ☐ Jejunostomy		
	Feeding tube: Type _____ French Size _____		
	☐ Abdominal x-ray to confirm tube placement and termination point prior to		
	feeding initiation.		
	2. FORMULA:	**DESCRIPTION**	**INDICATIONS**
	ISOTONIC (1 kcal/mL)		
	☐ Jevity	Contains fiber	Normal bowel function
	☐ Glucerna	Low carbohydrate	Abnormal glucose tolerance
	☐ Osmolite HN	High nitrogen	Low intestinal residue
	HYPERTONIC (1.5 kcal/mL)		
	☐ Ensure Plus	High calorie	Increased caloric needs,
			volume restriction
	☐ Pulmocare	High fat/Low carbohydrate	Respiratory failure
	ELEMENTAL (1 kcal/mL)		
	☐ Vital HN	Hydrolyzed	Impaired GI function
	OTHER:		
	3. DELIVERY:		
	METHOD: ☐ Continuous Other:		
	STRENGTH: ☐ Full ☐ 3/4 ☐ 1/2 Other:		
	RATE/FEEDING SCHEDULE: ☐ 25 mL/hr ☐ 50 mL/hr Other: _____ mL/hr		
	Increase rate to _____ mL/hr after _____ hrs		
	Other feeding schedule:		
	ADDITIONAL WATER: Total additional water volume, including		
	flushes/medications, to be _____ mL/24 hr.		
	Briskly irrigate tubing with 30 mL water BEFORE and AFTER		
	medication administration or if feeding is interrupted for more		
	than 5 minutes.		
	4. MONITORING:		
	GASTRIC RESIDUALS: Check residuals every _____ hrs. If greater than _____ mL,		
	hold feeding for _____ hr(s). Recheck residual. Restart		
	feeding at _____ mL/hr, when residual less than _____ mL.		
	EXAMPLE: For 50 mL/hr, check residual q 4 hr and hold if 200 mL.		
	WEIGHT: ☐ Weigh patient on intiation of feeding and M/W/F.		
	5. LABORATORY: ☐ CHEM 20 AND TRANSFERRIN NOW AND WEEKLY		
	OTHER LABORATORY:		
	DATE **TIME** **SIGNATURE**		
	NOTE: ALL ORDERS CHECKED OR HANDWRITTEN WILL BE FOLLOWED		

FIGURE 8–3 • Enteral nutrition order form for diabetic patients.

TABLE 8–10	Enteral Nutrition for Patients with Known Non-Insulin-Dependent Diabetes and Elevated Fasting Glucose

1. Monitor blood glucose q6h.
2. Begin enteral nutrition and insulin infusion at the same time.
3. Insulin infusion is calculated as the sum of the basal and carbohydrate-related need.
   Basal need is dependent on stress level and weight:

Stress Level	*Units of Regular Insulin*
Mild	$0.3 \times$ weight (kg)
Moderate	$0.5 \times$ weight (kg)
Severe	$1.0 \times$ weight (kg)
Steroid therapy (maximum doses) regardless of degree of illness	$1.0 \times$ weight (kg)

   Carbohydrate-related need: 1 unit regular insulin for every 10 g carbohydrate in enteral nutrition.
4. Adjustment for tomorrow's dose: the insulin-carbohydrate ratio is changed based on today's blood glucose levels:
   ≤80: decrease ratio (0.5 unit/10 g carbohydrate)
   81-180: no change in ratio (1.0 unit/10 g carbohydrate)
   ≥181: increase ratio (1.5 units/10 g carbohydrate)

If the blood glucose level is between 80 and 180 mg/dL, no change in the carbohydrate ratio is necessary. If the blood glucose level is less than 80 mg/dL, the ratio may be decreased to 0.5 unit regular insulin per 10 g carbohydrate. If the blood glucose level is greater than 180 mg/dL, the insulin-carbohydrate ratio should be increased to 1.5 units/10 g carbohydrate (Table 8-11).

Intravenous Parenteral Nutrition

Most normal, healthy persons become hyperglycemic if they are given IV solutions with a concentration of 20% dextrose (D_{20}) or more. For a person with normal glucose tolerance,

TABLE 8–11	Intravenous Nutrition for Patients with Normal Glucose Tolerance and Patients with Non-Insulin-Dependent Diabetes Mellitus and Normal Fasting Blood Glucose

1. Monitor blood glucose q6h for 2 days and then twice a day as long as blood glucose remains normal.
2. If hyperglycemia occurs, continue to monitor q6h.
3. Regular insulin may be given SC q6h for the immediate treatment of hyperglycemia:
   ≤ 180: 0 units
   181-240: 6 units
   241-300: 8 units
   ≥ 301: 10 units
4. Begin with an IV solution containing 1 unit of regular insulin for every 10 g of dextrose in the bag.
5. Adjust tomorrow's insulin dose based on today's blood glucose levels, as follows:
   ≤ 80: decrease ratio (0.5 unit/10 g carbohydrate)
   81-180: no change in ratio (1.0 unit/10 g carbohydrate)
   ≥ 181: increase ratio (1.5 units/10 g carbohydrate)

IV, intravenous; SC, subcutaneous.

only the dextrose load needs to be covered with insulin, at a dose of 1 unit regular insulin per 10 g dextrose. For example, if 500 g of dextrose is infused over 24 hours (usually 2.5 L of a D_{20} solution), 50 units of regular insulin may be placed in the dextrose solution to be infused over 24 hours. The blood glucose should be checked every 4 to 6 hours and extra regular insulin given as detailed earlier. The dose of insulin for the following day may be adjusted based on blood glucose levels: if the blood glucose level is 80 to 180 mg/dL, no change in the ratio of 1 unit regular insulin per 10 g dextrose is necessary; if the blood glucose is less than 80 mg/dL, the ratio may be decreased to 0.5 unit/10 g dextrose; if the blood glucose level is greater than 180 mg/dL, the ratio may be increased to 1.5 units/10 g dextrose. If a patient remains hyperglycemic while receiving 500 g of dextrose over 24 hours despite 50 units of insulin, the insulin dose may be increased to 75 units of regular insulin for 500 g dextrose (1.5 units/10 g dextrose) (Fig. 8-4 and Table 8-12).

For the patient with fasting hyperglycemia before parenteral nutrition is started, a basal insulin need must be added to the dextrose-insulin–related need. The basal dose depends on body weight, severity of illness, and the administration of steroids. Tables 8-11 and 8-12 list the incremental increase in insulin response with increasing need in NIDDM. The dextrose-related need must be added to the basal need for all diabetic patients.

The parenteral solutions may have both the basal insulin need and the dextrose need placed in the bottles to be infused over 24 hours. The three-in-one bags contain an entire day's nutritional needs in one bag. In addition, the day's insulin requirement (basal plus dextrose-related needs) may all be put in one bag.

There is a new product available for peripheral nutrition that substitutes dextrose with glycerol. Because glycerol does not require insulin for metabolism, this product (ProcalAmine) does not raise the blood glucose level of diabetic patients.

In summary, prevention and treatment of hyperglycemia in up to 50% of all patients given parenteral or enteral nutrition is necessary to optimize care in the severely ill patient. The protocols outlined here are designed to monitor and avoid potentially dangerous iatrogenic hyperglycemia.

MATCHING INSULIN TO FOOD

The correlation of postprandial glucose to percentage carbohydrate in a fixed caloric meal is excellent for the dinner meal and quite good for breakfast and lunch. The amount of insulin required to cover carbohydrate in the evening meal is generally about 1.0 unit/10 g carbohydrate and for breakfast, about 1.5 units/10 g carbohydrate. The amount of insulin required to cover lunch usually falls between that required to cover breakfast and dinner. Nevertheless, the above ratios are approximations. An insulin-carbohydrate ratio for each meal is ideally established for each patient. The advantage in developing the skill of matching insulin and carbohydrate lies in the freedom to vary meal composition. It is useful not only for persons on an insulin pump but also for patients on a fixed meal plan if they choose to eat out or vary the meal plan. If an individual knows that an ingested meal is going to exceed the normal carbohydrate quota for a meal, an upward adjustment in the insulin dose may be made by calculating

TOTAL PARENTERAL NUTRITION ORDER FORM

ADMINISTER OVER 24 HOURS: ALL TPN SOLUTIONS WILL BEGIN AT 1800 HOURS DAILY.
ALL CHANGES, ADDITIONS, OR DELETIONS <u>MUST</u> BE RECEIVED BY 1400 HOURS.

1. Select One Only:
☐ **Custom** FORMULA AND RATE   **or**   ☐ **Standard** FORMULA (SET RATES DO NOT CHANGE)

CUSTOM:		PER DAY
Usual requirements:		
Total daily kcals:	25–35 kcal/kg/day	
Protein: 1–2 g/kg or	10–15% of total kcal	
Dextrose:	45–55% of total kcal	
Lipids:	25–35% of total kcal	
PROTEIN: (4 kcal/g)		g/day
DEXTROSE: (3.4 kcal/g)		kcal/day
LIPIDS: (10 kcal/g)		kcal/day
RATE: (for custom only)		_____mL/hr

Start at _____ mL/hr for 4 hours, then increase to rate above.

NOTE: TPN typically requires 2–3 liters.
Call pharmacy at ext. XXXX for LEAST POSSIBLE VOLUME, or assistance.

STANDARD:			PER DAY
☐ PERIPHERAL		2.4 L	1652 kcal
Protein 3.5%		84 g	336 kcal
Dextrose 10%		240 g	816 kcal
Lipids 20% 250 mL		50 g	500 kcal
Total Volume = 2400 mL		**Rate: 100 mL/hr**	
☐ CENTRAL		2 L	1564 kcal
Protein 3.5%		70 g	280 kcal
Dextrose 13%		260 g	884 kcal
Lipids 20% 200 mL		40 g	400 kcal
Total Volume = 2000 mL		**Rate: 83 mL/hr**	
*** for 50-kg patient (30 kcal/kg)			
☐ CENTRAL		2.4 L	2214 kcal
Protein 4.25%		102 g	408 kcal
Dextrose 16%		384 g	1306 kcal
Lipids 20% 250 mL		50 g	500 kcal
Total Volume = 2400 mL		**Rate: 100 mL/hr**	
*** for 70-kg patient (30 kcal/kg)			

☐ Delete lipids
☐ Start at 50 mL/hr for 4 hr

2. Select Additives FOR ALL TPN
(BOTH CUSTOM AND STANDARD)

ADDITIVES:				PER DAY
mark this box for standard additives ⟶			Custom and/or additional orders	
Item	Range	☐ ↵		
NaCl	60–150	20		mEq/day
Na Acetate		50		mEq/day
Na Phosphate	10–25 mM	12		mM/day
K Phosphate		✕		mM/day
K Acetate		✕		mEq/day
KCl	40–80	40		mEq/day
MgSO₄	15–30	10		mEq/day
Ca Gluconate	9–18	9		mEq/day
Vitamins [MVI–12]	10 mL	10		mL/day
Trace elements	3 mL	3		mL/day
Reg insulin 1 U/10 g or 3 U/100 kcal dextrose (if diabetic add 0.3 U/kg)		✕		U/day
Heparin 1000 U/L	2–3000 U	✕		U/day
Folic acid	1 mg			mg/day
Vit. K 10 mg Monday to MWF	1–3x wk	✕		mg/day every Monday

OTHER:_____
_____
_____

3. MONITORING:

☐ Glucose monitoring Q6H × 5D, then BID.
☐ Renal panel, phosphorus, and magnesium ordered daily × 3, then MWF.
☐ Serum transferrin, CHEM 20 ordered now and 1 week after start of TPN.
☐ Triglycerides now and 48 hrs after start of TPN.
☐ Daily weights.
☐ Other:_____

NOTE HOSPITAL POLICY:

• Dextrose 10% will replace TPN during interruptions at same rate.
• Nutrition Support Team (NST) will provide basic assessment and monitoring.
• For new orders received by pharmacy after 1800, Standard Peripheral TPN formula will be used until 1800 the following day per physician approval. Rate and additives will remain as ordered.

_____   _____
Physician signature   Date

FIGURE 8–4 • Intravenous parenteral nutrition order form for diabetic patients.

TABLE 8–12	Intravenous Nutrition for Patients with Insulin-Dependent Diabetes Mellitus and Patients with Non-Insulin-Dependent Diabetes Mellitus and Fasting Hyperglycemia

1. Monitor blood glucose q6h.
2. Begin IV solution and insulin together in the same bag.
3. Insulin dosage is calculated as the sum of the basal and the dextrose-related insulin needs.
   Basal need is dependent on stress level and weight:

Stress Level	*Units of Regular Insulin*
Mild	0.3 × weight (kg)
Moderate	0.5 × weight (kg)
Severe	1.0 × weight (kg)
Steroid therapy (maximum doses) regardless of degree of illness	1.0 × weight (kg)

   Dextrose-related need: 1 unit regular insulin for every 10 g dextrose in the infusion solution.
4. Adjustment for tomorrow's dose: the insulin-carbohydrate ratio is changed based on today's blood glucose levels:
   ≤80: decrease ratio (0.5 unit/10 g carbohydrate)
   81-180: no change in ratio (1.0 unit/10 g carbohydrate)
   ≥181: increase ratio (1.5 units/10 g carbohydrate)

the extra insulin needed from the number of grams of carbohydrate to be ingested above the established quota of the prescribed diet. The approach is equally useful when calories and carbohydrate are eliminated from a meal or diet as might occur in a weight-loss program.

Oral Hypoglycemic Agents and Suggested Protocols for NIDDM Patients Outside the Hospital

Outside the hospital, the goal is to achieve a target glycosylated hemoglobin of less than 7%. If a given treatment protocol is not achieving a fasting blood glucose level of 80 mg/dL and a 1-hour postprandial glucose level less than 180 mg/dL, the present medications may be discontinued and the following scheme followed:

1. Glipizide 10 mg three times a day (30 minutes before each meal, with an additional 10 mg given if there is a particularly problematic meal).[170]
2. If the fasting blood glucose and postprandial glucose levels are not in the target ranges after 2 weeks of this scheme, glipizide may be discontinued and a trial of glyburide 10 mg twice a day prescribed.[171]
3. If the fasting blood glucose and postprandial glucose levels are not in the target ranges after 2 weeks, metformin may be added, starting at a dose of 500 mg twice a day and titrated upward until target blood glucose levels are achieved or a maximum of 2500 mg/day is reached.[172-175] Contraindications to metformin include renal or hepatic disease or cardiac compromise.

If the target fasting blood glucose is not achieved despite the maximum doses of metformin and sulfonylurea agents, NPH insulin may be started at bedtime beginning at a dose of 0.1 unit/kg and increasing the dose by increments of 2 units/day until the fasting blood glucose is in the target range.[175-178]

Acarbose at a dosage up to 100 mg three times a day may be considered as adjunctive therapy. This agent is a disaccharidase inhibitor and therefore prevents the postprandial rise in glucose after complex carbohydrate ingestion. Also on the horizon are several new classes of drugs, including "insulin sensitizers" and drugs that increase the first phase of insulin secretion from the beta cells. These new agents may minimize the need for insulin therapy when sulfonylurea agents and metformin fail to improve glucose control.

The main class of insulin-sensitizing drugs includes the thiazolidinediones. Troglitazone, the first agent on the market, has been associated with poorly understood hepatic toxicity and hence should be avoided in patients with hepatic disease. Whether the newer approved agents rosiglitazone and pioglitazone have such toxicity remains to be seen.

Meglitinides stimulate insulin secretion and have been found to be useful in type 2 diabetes. These agents are taken 15 to 30 minutes before a meal. Repaglinide is the first drug of this class to become available. It appears to be effective, and the behavioral modification associated with premeal drug delivery may be an advantage.

Table 8-13 outlines an ongoing care protocol for persons with diabetes who are at risk for or have vascular disease. For the reasons detailed throughout the chapter, the emphasis is on control of blood glucose, lipids, and blood pressure. In addition, the issues of aspirin or platelet therapy, vaccination against influenza and pneumonia, smoking cessation, foot care, exercise, and nutrition should be considered as part of the management plan. Although these issues, with the exception of blood glucose control, do not differ qualitatively from those associated with vascular disease in the nondiabetic

TABLE 8–13	Diabetes Maintenance Therapy for Vascular Disease Prevention

I. Blood glucose control
   A. Target hemoglobin A$_{1c}$ ≤ 7%
   B. Monitor blood glucose and target premeal values of 80-120 mg/dL and bedtime values of 100-140 mg/dL
II. Blood pressure control
   A. Angiotensin-converting enzyme inhibitor for all adults with diabetes or if microalbuminuria is present
   B. Target level < 130/85 mm Hg
III. Blood lipid control
   A. Target low-density lipoprotein level < 100 mg/dL
   B. Target triglyceride level < 200 mg/dL
IV. Antiplatelet therapy
   A. Aspirin if age > 30 yr
   B. Clopidogrel
   C. Ticlopidine (associated with thrombotic thrombocytopenic purpura)
   D. Platelet IIb/IIIa inhibitor
IV. Miscellaneous treatment
   A. Vaccination for influenza and pneumonia
   B. Smoking cessation
   C. Foot care program
   D. Exercise plan
   E. Nutrition plan

population, a few points are noteworthy. Every patient with diabetes needs to be considered for angiotensin-converting enzyme inhibitor therapy. The findings of the Heart Outcomes Prevention Evaluation reinforce previously noted findings that ramipril substantially lowers the risk of death, heart attack, stroke, coronary revascularization, heart failure, and complications related to diabetes mellitus in a high-risk group of patients with preexisting vascular disease. The study was stopped early by the data and safety monitoring board because of the obvious benefit of ramipril.[179]

Another treatment that warrants some comment is aspirin. It is generally agreed that aspirin is underutilized by persons with diabetes for a number of reasons.[180] Aspirin has been found to have greater benefit in diabetic patients than in those without diabetes in improving survival in the presence of coronary artery disease.[181] Also of note is that in the Wisconsin Epidemiologic Study of Diabetic Retinopathy, daily aspirin use by persons with diabetes was inversely associated (OR, 0.11) with lower extremity amputation.[182] Thus, the American Diabetes Association recommends aspirin for all diabetic patients older than 30 years.[178]

KEY REFERENCES

American Diabetes Association: Clinical Practice Recommendations 2005. Diabetes Care 28(Suppl 1):S1-S76, 2005.

Diabetes Control and Complications Trial Research Group: The effect of intensive treatment of diabetes on the development and progression of long-term complications in insulin-dependent diabetes mellitus. N Engl J Med 329:977-986, 1993.

Diabetes Control and Complications Trial Research Group: The effect of intensive diabetes management on macrovascular events and risk factors in the Diabetes Control and Complications Trial. Am J Cardiol 75:894-903, 1995.

Herman WH, Alexander CM, Cook JR, et al: Effect of simvastatin treatment on cardiovascular resource utilization in impaired fasting glucose and diabetes: Findings from the Scandinavian Simvastatin Survival Study. Diabetes Care 22:1771-1778, 1999.

Malmberg K, Ryden L, Efendic S, et al: Randomized trial of insulin-glucose infusion followed by subcutaneous insulin treatment in diabetic patients with acute myocardial infarction (DIGAMI study): Effects on mortality at 1 year. J Am Coll Cardiol 26:57-65, 1995.

Moss SE, Klein R, Klein BE: The 14 year incidence of lower extremity amputations in a diabetic population. The Wisconsin Epidemiologic Study of Diabetic Retinopathy. Diabetes Care 22:951-959, 1999.

United Kingdom Prospective Diabetes Study Group: Relative efficacy of randomly allocated diet, sulphonylurea, insulin or metformin in patients with newly diagnosed non-insulin dependent diabetes followed for three years. BMJ 310:83-88, 1995.

UK Prospective Diabetes Study (UKPDS) Group: Intensive blood glucose control with sulphonylureas or insulin compared with the conventional treatment and risk of complications in patients with type 2 diabetes (UKPDS 33). Lancet 352:837-853, 1998.

REFERENCES

1. Garber AJ: Clinical perspectives on type 2 diabetes in North America. Diabetes Metab Rev 11(Suppl 1):S81-S86, 1995.
2. Schwartz LM, Woloshin S: Changing disease definitions: Implications for disease prevalence. Analysis of the Third National Health and Nutrition Examination Survey, 1988-1994. Effective Clin Pract 2:96-99, 1999.
3. Stuart WP, Wolf B, Macaulay EM, Cross KS: Screening for diabetes on a vascular ward: Lessons from an audit. J R Coll Surg Edinb 43:11-12, 1998.
4. Lernmark A: Insulin-dependent diabetes mellitus. In Davidson JK (ed): Clinical Diabetes Mellitus. New York, Georg Thieme, 1991, p 35.
5. Reaven GM, Laws A: Insulin resistance, compensatory hyperinsulinaemia, and coronary heart disease. Diabetologia 37:948-952, 1994.
6. American Diabetes Association: Clinical Practice Recommendations 2005. Diabetes Care 28(Suppl 1):S1-S76, 2005.
7. Clark CM, Adlin V (eds): Risks and benefits of intensive management in non-insulin dependent diabetes mellitus. Ann Intern Med 124(Suppl): 1-186, 1996.
8. Osler W, McCrae T: Diseases of the arteries. In Osler W (ed): Modern Medicine, Its Theory and Practice, 4th ed. Philadelphia, Lea & Febiger, 1908, pp 426-427.
9. Joslin EP: A Diabetic Manual. Philadelphia, Lea & Febiger, 1945, p 141.
10. Wellman KF, Volk BW: Historical review. In Volk BW, Wellman KF (eds): The Diabetic Pancreas. New York, Plenum Press, 1977, pp 1-14.
11. Galloway JA, Shuman CR: Diabetes and surgery: A study of 667 cases. Am J Med 34:177-192, 1963.
12. Hjortrup A, Rasmussen B, Kehlet H: Morbidity in diabetic and non-diabetic patients after major vascular surgery. BMJ 257:1107-1108, 1983.
13. Golden SH, Peart-Vigilance C, Kao WHL, Brancati FL: Perioperative glycemic control and the risk of infectious complications in a cohort of adults with diabetes. Diabetes Care 22:1408-1414, 1999.
14. Toni D, Fiorelli M, Gentile M, et al: Progressing neurological deficit secondary to acute ischemic stroke: A study on predictability, pathogenesis, and prognosis. Arch Neurol 52:670-675, 1995.
15. Haheim LL, Holme I, Hjermann I, Leren P: Nonfasting serum glucose and the risk of fatal stroke in diabetic and nondiabetic subjects: 18-year follow-up of the Oslo Study. Stroke 26:774-777, 1995.
16. Janghorbani M, Jones RB, Gilmour WH, et al: A prospective population based study of gender differential in mortality from cardiovascular disease and "all causes" in asymptomatic hyperglycaemics. J Clin Epidemiol 47:397-405, 1994.
17. Petitt DB, Bhatt H: Retinopathy as a risk factor for nonembolic stroke in diabetic subjects. Stroke 26:593-596, 1995.
18. Goldberg RJ, Burchfiel CM, Benfante R, et al: Lifestyle and biologic factors associated with atherosclerotic disease in middle-aged men: 20-year findings from the Honolulu Heart Program. Arch Intern Med 155:686-694, 1995.
19. Kameyama M, Fushimi H, Udaka F: Diabetes mellitus and cerebral vascular disease. Diabetes Res Clin Pract 24(Suppl):S205-S208, 1994.
20. Moss SE, Klein R, Klein BE, Meuer SM: The association of glycemia and cause-specific mortality in a diabetic population. Arch Intern Med 154:2473-2479, 1994.
21. National Diabetes Data Group: Classification and diagnosis of diabetes mellitus and other categories of glucose intolerance. Diabetes 28: 1039-1057, 1979.
22. Jorgensen H, Nakayama H, Raaschou HO, Olsen TS: Stroke in patients with diabetes. The Copenhagen Stroke Study. Stroke 25:1977-1984, 1994.
23. Kuusisto J, Mykkanen L, Pyorala K, Laakso M: Non-insulin-dependent diabetes and its metabolic control are important predictors of stroke in elderly subjects. Stroke 125:1157-1164, 1994.
24. Burchfiel CM, Curb JD, Rodriguez BL, et al: Glucose intolerance and 22-year stroke incidence. The Honolulu Heart Program. Stroke 25:951-957, 1994.
25. Sacco RL, Shi T, Zamanillo MC, Kargman DE: Predictors of mortality and recurrence after hospitalized cerebral infarction in an urban community. The Northern Manhattan Stroke Study. Neurology 44:626-634, 1994.
26. Fu CC, Chang CJ, Tseng CH, et al: Development of macrovascular diseases in NIDDM patients in northern Taiwan: A 4-year follow-up study. Diabetes Care 16:137-143, 1993.
27. Kleinman JC, Donahue RP, Harris MI, et al: Mortality among diabetics in a national sample. Am J Epidemiol 128:389-401, 1988.
28. Cardiovascular disease risk factors and related preventive health practices among adults with and without diabetes—Utah, 1988-1993. MMWR Morb Mortal Wkly Rep 44:804-809, 1995.
29. Nathan DM: The pathophysiology of diabetic complications: How much does the glucose hypothesis explain? Ann Intern Med 124:86-89, 1996.
30. Kannel WB, McGee DL: Diabetes and glucose tolerance as risk factors for cardiovascular disease. The Framingham Study. Diabetes Care 2:120-126, 1979.
31. Rodriquez BL, Lau N, Burchfiel CM, et al: Glucose intolerance and 23-year risk of coronary heart disease and total mortality. The Honolulu Heart Program. Diabetes Care 22:1262-1265, 1999.
32. Fava S, Azzopardi J, Muscat HA, Fenech FF: Factors that influence outcome in diabetic subjects with myocardial infarction. Diabetes Care 16:1615-1618, 1993.
33. Heinrich J, Schulte H, Schonfeld R, et al: Association of variables of coagulation, fibrinolysis and acute-phase with atherosclerosis in coronary and peripheral arteries and those arteries supplying the brain. Thromb Haemost 73:374-379, 1995.

34. Mackay AJ, Beks PJ, Dur AH, et al: The distribution of peripheral vascular disease in a Dutch Caucasian population: Comparison of type II diabetic and non-diabetic subjects. Eur J Vasc Endovasc Surg 9:170-175, 1995.

35. Beks PJ, Mackaay AJ, de Neeling JN, et al: Peripheral arterial disease in relation to glycaemic level in an elderly Caucasian population: The Hoorn study. Diabetologia 38:86-96, 1995.

36. Akbari CM, LoGerfo FW: Diabetes and peripheral vascular disease. J Vasc Surg 30:373-384, 1999.

37. Feinglass J, Brown JL, LoSasso A, et al: Rates of lower-extremity amputation and arterial reconstruction in the United States, 1979-1996. Am J Public Health 89:1222-1227, 1999.

38. Adler AI, Boyko EJ, Ahroni JH, Smith DG: Lower-extremity amputation in diabetes: The independent effects of peripheral vascular disease, sensory neuropathy, and foot ulcers. Diabetes Care 22:1029-1035, 1999.

39. Jorneskog G, Brismar K, Fagrell B: Skin capillary circulation is more impaired in the toes of diabetic than non-diabetic patients with peripheral vascular disease. Diabet Med 12:36-41, 1995.

40. Newman AB, Siscovick DS, Manolio TA, et al: Ankle-arm index as a marker of atherosclerosis in the Cardiovascular Health Study. Cardiovascular Heart Study (CHS) Collaborative Research Group. Circulation 88:837-845, 1993.

41. Selby JV, Zhang D: Risk factors for lower extremity amputation in persons with diabetes. Diabetes Care 18:509-516, 1995.

42. Coutinho M, Gerstein HC, Wang Y, Yusuf S: The relationship between glucose and incident cardiovascular events: A metaregression analysis of published data from 20 studies of 95,783 individuals followed for 12.4 years. Diabetes Care 22:233-240, 1999.

43. Reichard P, Nilsson BY, Rosenqvist U: The effect of long term intensified insulin treatment on the development of microvascular complications of diabetes mellitus. N Engl J Med 329:304-309, 1993.

44. Diabetes Control and Complications Trial Research Group: The effect of intensive treatment of diabetes on the development and progression of long-term complications in insulin-dependent diabetes mellitus. N Engl J Med 329:977-986, 1993.

45. Diabetes Control and Complications Trial Research Group: The effect of intensive diabetes management on macrovascular events and risk factors in the Diabetes Control and Complications Trial. Am J Cardiol 75:894-903, 1995.

46. Lawson M, Gerstein HC, Tsui E, Zinman B: Effect of intensive therapy on early macrovascular disease in young individuals with type 1 diabetes: A systematic review and meta-analysis. Diabetes Care 22(Suppl 2):B35-B39, 1999.

47. Malmberg K, Ryden L, Efendic S, et al: Randomized trial of insulin-glucose infusion followed by subcutaneous insulin treatment in diabetic patients with acute myocardial infarction (DIGAMI study): Effects on mortality at 1 year. J Am Coll Cardiol 26:57-65, 1995.

48. UK Prospective Diabetes Study (UKPDS) Group: Intensive blood glucose control with sulphonylureas or insulin compared with the conventional treatment and risk of complications in patients with type 2 diabetes (UKPDS 33). Lancet 352:837-853, 1998.

49. UK Prospective Diabetes Study (UKPDS) Group: Effect of intensive blood glucose control with metformin on complications in overweight patients with type 2 diabetes (UKPDS 34). Lancet 352:954-965, 1998.

49a. Ohkubo Y, Kishikawa H, Araki E, et al: Intensive insulin therapy prevents the progression of diabetic microvascular complications in Japanese patients with non-insulin-dependent diabetes mellitus: a randomized prospective 6-year study. Diabetes Res Clin Pract 28:103-117, 1995.

49b. Colwell JA: The feasibility of intensive insulin management in non-insulin-dependent diabetes mellitus. Implications of the Veterans Affairs Cooperative Study on Glycemic Control and Complications in NIDDM. Ann Intern Med 124(1 Pt 2):131-135, 1996.

49c. Malmberg K: Prospective randomised study of intensive insulin treatment on long term survival after acute myocardial infarction in patients with diabetes mellitus. DIGAMI (Diabetes Mellitus, Insulin Glucose Infusion in Acute Myocardial Infarction) Study Group. BMJ 314:1512-1515, 1997.

50. Peterson CM, Jones RL, Koenig RJ, et al: Reversible hematologic sequelae of diabetes mellitus. Ann Intern Med 86:425-429, 1977.

51. Peterson CM, Koenig RJ, Jones RL, et al: Correlation of serum triglyceride levels and hemoglobin A_{1c} concentrations in diabetes mellitus. Diabetes 26:507-509, 1977.

52. Peterson CM, Jones RL, Dupuis A, et al: Feasibility of improved glucose control in patients with insulin dependent diabetes mellitus. Diabetes Care 2:329-335, 1979.

53. Peterson CM, Jones RL, Esterly JA, et al: Changes in basement membrane thickening and pulse volume concomitant with improved glucose control and exercise in patients with insulin dependent diabetes mellitus. Diabetes Care 3:586-589, 1980.

54. Jones RL, Paradise C, Peterson CM: Platelet survival in diabetes mellitus. Diabetes 30:486-489, 1981.

54a. Brown WV: Clinical trials including an update on the Helsinki Heart Study. Am J Cardiol 66:11A-15A, 1990.

54b. Streja L, Packard CJ, Shepherd J, Cobbe S, Ford I; WOSCOPS Group: Factors affecting low-density lipoprotein and high-density lipoprotein cholesterol response to pravastatin in the West Of Scotland Coronary Prevention Study (WOSCOPS). Am J Cardiol 90:731-736, 2002.

54c. Reviewed in Laakso M: Cardiovascular disease in type 2 diabetes: challenge for treatment and prevention. J Intern Med 249:225-235, 2001.

55. Herman WH, Alexander CM, Cook JR, et al: Effect of simvastatin treatment on cardiovascular resource utilization in impaired fasting glucose and diabetes: Findings from the Scandinavian Simvastatin Survival Study. Diabetes Care 22:1771-1778, 1999.

56. Goldberg RB: The benefits of lowering cholesterol in subjects with mild hyperglycemia. Arch Intern Med 159:2627-2628, 1999.

57. Long-Term Intervention with Pravastatin in Ischaemic Disease (LIPID) Study Group: Prevention of cardiovascular events and death with pravastatin in patients with coronary heart disease and a broad range of initial cholesterol levels. N Engl J Med 339:1349-1357, 1998.

58. Fuller J, Stevens LK, Chaturvedi N, Holloway JF: Antihypertensive therapy in diabetes mellitus. In The Cochrane Library, issue 4. Oxford, Update Software, 1998.

59. Golan L, Birkmeyer JD, Welch HG: The cost-effectiveness of treating all patients with type 2 diabetes with angiotensin-converting enzyme inhibitors. Ann Intern Med 131:660-667, 1999.

60. Tuomilehto J, Rastenyte D, Birkenhager WH, et al: Effects of calcium-channel blockade in older patients with diabetes and systolic hypertension. Systolic Hypertension in Europe Trial Investigators. N Engl J Med 340:677-684, 1999.

61. Bunn HF, Haney DN, Kamin S, et al: The biosynthesis of human hemoglobin A_{1c}. J Clin Invest 57:1652-1659, 1976.

62. Koenig RJ, Peterson CM, Kilo C, et al: Hemoglobin A_{1c} as an indicator of the degree of glucose intolerance in diabetes. Diabetes 25:230-232, 1976.

63. Koenig RJ, Peterson CM, Jones RL, et al: Correlation of glucose regulation and hemoglobin A_{1c} in diabetes mellitus. N Engl J Med 295:417-420, 1976.

64. Peterson CM, Jones RL: Minor hemoglobins, diabetic "control" and diseases of postsynthetic protein modification. Ann Intern Med 87:489-491, 1977.

65. Maillard L-C: Réaction générale des acides amines sur les sucres; conséquences biologiques. CR Acad Sci III 154:66-68, 1912.

66. Angyal SJ: The composition of reducing sugars in solution. In Harmon RE (ed): Asymmetry in Carbohydrates. New York, Marcel Dekker, 1979, pp 15-30.

67. Benkovic SJ: Anomeric specificity of carbohydrate utilizing enzymes. Methods Enzymol 63:370-379, 1979.

68. Hayase F, Nagaraj RH, Miyata S, et al: Aging of proteins: Immunological detection of a glucose-derived pyrrole formed during Maillard reaction in vivo. J Biol Chem 263:37858-37864, 1989.

69. Peterson CM (ed): Proceedings of a conference on nonenzymatic glycosylation and browning reactions: Their relevance to diabetes mellitus. Diabetes 31(Suppl 3):1-82, 1982.

70. Horiuchi S, Shiga M, Araki N, et al: Evidence against in vivo presence of 2-(2-furoyl)-4(5)-(2-furanyl)-1H-imidazole, a major fluorescent advanced end product generated by nonenzymatic glycosylation. J Biol Chem 263:18821-18826, 1988.

71. Vlassara H, Bucala R, Striker L: Pathogenic effects of advanced glycosylation: Biochemical, biological, and clinical implications for diabetes and aging. J Lab Invest 70:138-151, 1994.

72. Brownlee M: Glycation and diabetic complication. Diabetes 43:836-841, 1994.

73. Bucala R, Cerami A: Advanced glycosylation: Chemistry, biology and implications for diabetes and aging. Adv Pharmacol 23:1-19, 1992.

74. Schmidt AM, Mora R, Cao K, et al: The endothelial cell binding site for advanced glycation end products consists of a complex: An integral membrane protein and a lactoferrin-like polypeptide. J Biol Chem 269:9882-9888, 1994.

75. Doi T, Vlassara H, Kirstein M, et al: Receptor specific increase in extracellular matrix production in mouse mesangial cells by advanced glycation end products is mediated via platelet derived growth factor. Proc Natl Acad Sci U S A 89:2873-2877, 1992.

76. Neper M, Schmidt AM, Brett J, et al: Cloning and expression of RAGE: A cell surface receptor for advanced glycation end products of proteins. J Biol Chem 267:14998-15004, 1992.

77. Vlassara H, Moldawer L, Chan B: Macrophage/monocyte receptor for nonenzymatically glycosylated proteins is up-regulated by cachectin/tumor necrosis factor. J Clin Invest 84:1813-1820, 1989.

78. Vlassara H, Brownlee M, Cerami A: Novel macrophage receptor for glucose-modified protein is distinct from previously described scavenger receptors. J Exp Med 164:1301-1309, 1988.

79. Bucala R, Tracey KJ, Cerami A: Advanced glycosylation products quench nitric oxide and mediate defective endothelium-dependent vasodilation in experimental diabetes. J Clin Invest 87:432-438, 1991.

80. Yan DS, Schmidt AM, Anderson GM, et al: Enhanced cellular oxidant stress by the interaction of advanced glycation end products with their receptors/binding proteins. J Biol Chem 269:9889-9897, 1994.

81. Bucala R, Makita Z, Vega G, et al: Modification of low density lipoprotein by advanced glycation end products contributes to the dyslipidemia of diabetes and renal insufficiency. Proc Natl Acad Sci U S A 91:7742-7746, 1994.

82. Tschoeppe D: The activated megakaryocyte-platelet-system in vascular disease: Focus on diabetes. Semin Thromb Hemost 21:152-160, 1995.

83. Trovati M, Mularoni EM, Burzacca S, et al: Impaired insulin-induced platelet antiaggregating effect in obesity and in obese NIDDM patients. Diabetes 44:1318-1322, 1995.

84. Di Simpliciao P, de Giorgio LA, Cardaioli E, et al: Glutathione, glutathione utilizing enzymes and thioltransferase in platelets of insulin-dependent diabetic patients: Relation with platelet aggregation and with microangiopathic complications. Eur J Clin Invest 25:665-669, 1995.

85. Udvardy M, Posan E, Harsfalvi J: Altered lysis resistance of platelet-rich clots in patients with insulin-dependent diabetes mellitus. Thromb Res 79:57-63, 1995.

86. Jokl R, Klein RL, Lopes-Virella MF, Colwell JA: Release of platelet plasminogen activator inhibitor 1 in whole blood is increased in patients with type II diabetes. Diabetes Care 18:1150-1155, 1995.

87. Bahru Y, Kesteven P, Alberti KGMM, Walker M: Decreased plasminogen activator inhibitor-1 activity in newly diagnosed type 2 diabetic patients following dietary modification. Diabet Med 10:802-806, 1993.

88. Marso SP, Lincoff AM, Ellis SG, et al: Optimizing the percutaneous interventional outcomes for patients with diabetes mellitus: Results of the EPISTENT (Evaluation of Platelet IIb/IIIa Inhibitor for Stenting Trial) Diabetic Substudy. Circulation 100:2477-2484, 1999.

89. Bennet CL, Davidson CJ, Raisch DW, et al: Thrombotic thrombocytopenia purpura associated with ticlopidine in the setting of coronary artery stents and stroke prevention. Arch Intern Med 159:2524-2528, 1999.

90. Dormandy J, Ernst E, Matrai A, Flute PT: Hemorrheological changes following acute myocardial infarction. Am Heart J 104:1364-1367, 1982.

91. Handa K, Kono S, Saku K, et al: Plasma fibrinogen levels as an independent indicator of severity of coronary atherosclerosis. Atherosclerosis 77:209-213, 1989.

92. ECAT Angina Pectoris Study Group: ECAT Angina Pectoris Study: Baseline associations of haemostatic factors with extent of coronary arteriosclerosis and other coronary risk factors in 3000 patients with angina pectoris undergoing coronary angiography. Eur Heart J 14:8-17, 1993.

93. Ceriello A, Taboga C, Giacomello R, et al: Fibrinogen plasma levels as a marker of thrombin activation in diabetes. Diabetes 43:430-432, 1994.

94. Jones RL, Peterson CM: Reduced fibrinogen survival in diabetes mellitus: A reversible phenomenon. J Clin Invest 63:485-493, 1979.

95. Jones RL, Jovanovic L, Forman S, Peterson CM: The time course of reversibility of accelerated fibrinogen disappearance in diabetes mellitus: Association with intravascular volume shifts. Blood 63:22-30, 1984.

96. Cortellaro M, Cofrancesco E, Boschetti C, et al: Association of increased fibrin turnover and defective fibrinolytic capacity with leg atherosclerosis. The PLAT Group. Thromb Haemost 72:292-296, 1994.

97. Collier A, Rumley AG, Paterson JR, et al: Free radical activity and hemostatic factors in NIDDM patients with and without microalbuminuria. Diabetes 41:909-913, 1992.

98. Knobl P, Schernthaner G, Schack C, et al: Thrombogenic factors are related to urinary albumin excretion rate in type 1 (insulin-dependent) and type 2 (non-insulin-dependent) diabetic patients. Diabetologia 36:1045-1050, 1993.

99. Ceriello A, Giugliani D, Quatraro A, et al: Metabolic control may influence the increased superoxide anion generation in diabetic serum. Diabet Med 8:540-542, 1991.

100. Brownlee M, Vlassara H, Cerami A: Nonenzymatic glycosylation reduces the susceptibility of fibrin to degradation by plasmin. Diabetes 32:680-684, 1983.

101. Cagliero E, Roth T, Taylor AW, Lorenzi M: The effects of high glucose on human endothelial cell growth and gene expression are not mediated by transforming growth factor-beta. Lab Invest 73:667-673, 1995.

102. Pieper GM, Meier DA, Hager SR: Endothelial dysfunction in a model of hyperglycemia and hyperinsulinemia. Am J Physiol 269:H845-H850, 1995.

103. Baumgartner-Parzer SM, Wagner L, Pettermann M, et al: Modulation by high glucose of adhesion molecule expression in cultured endothelial cells. Diabetologia 38:1367-1370, 1996.

104. Farkas J, Menzel EJ: Proteins lose their nitric oxide stabilizing function after advanced glycosylation. Biochim Biophys Acta 1245:305-310, 1995.

105. Gugliucci A, Bendaya M: Renal fate of circulating advanced glycated end products (AGE): Evidence for reabsorption and catabolism of AGE-peptides by renal proximal tubular cells. Diabetologia 39: 149-160, 1996.

106. Friedlander MA, Wu YC, Elgawish A, Monnier VM: Early and advanced glycosylation end products. J Clin Invest 97:728-735, 1996.

107. Smith MA, Sayre LM, Vitek MP, et al: Early AGEing and Alzheimer's. Nature 374:316, 1995.

108. Kobayashi K, Watanabe J, Umeda F, et al: Metabolism of oxidized glycated low-density lipoprotein in cultured bovine aortic endothelial cells. Horm Metab Res 27:356-362, 1995.

109. Velazquez E, Winocour PH, Kesteven P, et al: Relation of lipid peroxides to macrovascular disease in type 2 diabetes. Diabet Med 8:752-758, 1991.

110. Reaven GM: Banting Lecture 1998: Role of insulin resistance in human disease. Diabetes 37:1595-1607, 1988.

111. Shinozaki K, Suzuki M, Ikebuchi M, et al: Demonstration of insulin resistance in coronary artery disease documented with angiography. Diabetes Care 19:1-7, 1996.

112. Stout RW: Insulin and atheroma: 20-year perspective. Diabetes Care 13:631-654, 1990.

113. Wingard DL, Barrett-Connor EL, Ferrara A: Is insulin really a heart disease risk factor? Diabetes Care 18:1299-1304, 1995.

114. Genuth S: Exogenous insulin administration and cardiovascular risk in non-insulin-dependent diabetes mellitus. Ann Intern Med 124: 104-109, 1996.

115. Reaven GM, Lithell H, Landsberg L: Hypertension and associated metabolic abnormalities: The role of insulin resistance and the sympathoadrenal system. N Engl J Med 334:374-381, 1995.

116. Bagdade JD: Phagocytic and microbiological function in diabetes mellitus. Acta Endocrinol (Copenh) 83:27-31, 1976.

117. Duncan BB, Schmidt MI, Offenbacher S, et al: Factor VIII and other hemostasis variables are related to incident diabetes in adults. Diabetes Care 22:767-772, 1999.

118. Pickup JC, Mattock MB, Chusney GD, et al: NIDDM as a disease of the innate immune system: Association of acute-phase reactants and interleukin-6 with metabolic syndrome X. Diabetologia 40:1286-1292, 1997.

119. Tracy RP: The relationship between inflammation, coagulation and CVD. Paper presented at the 59th Annual Scientific Sessions of the American Diabetes Association, 1999, San Diego.

120. Bainton D, Sweetnam P, Baker I, Elwood P: Peripheral vascular disease: Consequence for survival and association with risk factors in the Speedwell prospective heart disease study. Br Heart J 72:128-132, 1994.

121. Wahlquist MI, Kayser L, Lassers BW: Fatty acids as a determinant of myocardial substrate and oxygen metabolism in man at rest and during prolonged exercise. Acta Med Scand 193:83-96, 1973.

122. Saad MF, Knowler WC, Pettitt DJ, et al: The natural history of impaired glucose tolerance in Pima Indians. N Engl J Med 319: 1500-1506, 1988.

123. Sartor G, Schersten B, Carlstrom S, et al: Ten-year follow-up of subjects with impaired glucose intolerance. Diabetes 29:41-49, 1980.

124. Jarrett RJ, Keen H, McCartney P: The Whitehall study: Ten-year follow-up on men with impaired glucose tolerance with reference to worsening to diabetes and predictors of death. Diabet Med 1:279-283, 1984.

125. Jarrett RJ, Keen H, Fuller JH, McCartney M: Worsening to diabetes in men with impaired glucose tolerance ("borderline diabetes"). Diabetologia 16:25-30, 1979.

126. Kadowaki T, Miyake Y, Hagura R, et al: Risk factors for worsening to diabetes in subjects with impaired glucose tolerance. Diabetologia 26:44-49, 1984.

127. King H, Zimmet P, Raper LR, Balkau B: The natural history of impaired glucose tolerance in the Micronesian population of Nauru: A six-year follow-up study. Diabetologia 26:39-43, 1984.

128. Harris MI: Impaired glucose tolerance in the US population. Diabetes Care 12:464-474, 1989.

129. Keen H, Rose G, Pyke DA, et al: Blood-sugar and arterial disease. Lancet 2:505-508, 1965.

130. Fuller JH, Shipley MJ, Rose G, et al: Coronary heart disease risk and impaired glucose tolerance. Lancet 1:1373-1376, 1980.

131. Blair SN, Kohl HW, Gordon NF, Paffenbarger RS Jr: How much physical activity is good for health? Annu Rev Public Health 13:99-126, 1992.

132. Bjorntorp P: Regional patterns of fat distribution. Ann Intern Med 103:994-995, 1985.

133. Flegel KG, Ezzati TM, Harris MI, et al: Prevalence of diabetes in Mexican Americans, Cubans, and Puerto Ricans from the Hispanic Health and Nutrition Examination Survey, 1982-84. Diabetes Care 14:628-638, 1991.

134. National Center for Health Statistics: Plan and Operation of the Hispanic Health and Nutrition Examination Survey 1982-1984 (DHHS Publication No. 85-1321). Washington, DC, Government Printing Office, 1985.

135. National Center for Health Statistics: Plan and Operation of the Second National Health and Nutrition Examination Survey, United States—1976-1980. Vital and Health Statistics, Series 1, No. 15 (DHEW Publication No. PHS 81-1317). Washington, DC, Government Printing Office, 1981.

136. Kuczmarski RJ: Prevalence of overweight and weight gain in the United States. Am J Clin Nutr 55:495S-502S, 1992.

137. Kohl HW, Gordon NF, Villegas JA, Blair SN: Cardiorespiratory fitness, glycemic status, and mortality risk in men. Diabetes Care 15:184-192, 1992.

138. Stern MP: Kelly West Lecture: Primary prevention of type II diabetes mellitus. Diabetes Care 14:399-410, 1991.

139. King H, Kriska AM: Prevention of type II diabetes by physical training. Diabetes Care 15(Suppl 4):1794-1799, 1992.

140. Kriska AM, LaPorte RE, Pettitt DJ, et al: The association of physical activity with obesity, fat distribution and glucose intolerance in Pima Indians. Diabetologia 36:863-869, 1993.

141. Kawate R, Yamakido M, Nishimoto Y, et al: Diabetes and its vascular complications in Japanese migrants on the island of Hawaii. Diabetes Care 2:161-170, 1979.

142. West KM: Epidemiology of Diabetes and Its Vascular Lesions. New York, Elsevier, 1978.

143. Eaton SB, Konner M, Shostak M: Stone Agers in the fast lane: Chronic degenerative disease in evolutionary perspective. Am J Med 84:739-749, 1988.

144. Lindgarde F, Saltin B: Daily physical activity, work capacity and glucose tolerance in lean and obese normoglycemic middle-aged men. Diabetologia 20:134-138, 1981.

145. Cederholm J, Wibell L: Glucose tolerance and physical activity in a health survey of middle-aged subjects. Acta Med Scand 217:373-378, 1985.

146. Eriksson K-F, Lindgarde F: Impaired glucose tolerance in a middle-aged male urban population: A new approach for identifying high-risk cases. Diabetologia 33:526-531, 1990.

147. Harris MI: Epidemiological correlates of NIDDM in Hispanics, whites, and blacks in the US population. Diabetes Care 14(Suppl 3):639-648, 1991.

148. Resnick HE, Vlsania P, Phillips CL: Diabetes mellitus and nontraumatic lower extremity amputation in black and white Americans. The National Health and Nutrition Examination Survey Epidemiologic Follow-up Study, 1971-1992. Arch Intern Med 159:2470-2475, 1999.

149. Mitchell BD, Valdez R, Hazuda HP, et al: Differences in the prevalence of diabetes and impaired glucose tolerance according to maternal or paternal history of diabetes. Diabetes Care 16:1262-1267, 1993.

150. Metzger BE: Summary and recommendations of the Third International Diabetes Workshop-Conference on Gestational Diabetes. Diabetes 40(Suppl 2):197-201, 1991.

151. Kjos SL, Buchanan TA, Greenspoon JS, et al: Gestational diabetes mellitus: The prevalence of glucose intolerance and diabetes mellitus in the first two months post partum. Am J Obstet Gynecol 163:93-98, 1990.

152. O'Sullivan JB: Diabetes mellitus after GDM. Diabetes 40(Suppl 2): 131-135, 1991.

153. Lam KSL, Li DF, Lauder IJ, et al: Prediction of persistent carbohydrate intolerance in patients with gestational diabetes. Diabetes Res Clin Pract 12:181-186, 1991.

154. Catalano PM, Vargo KM, Bernstein IM, Amini SB: Incidence and risk factors associated with abnormal post partum glucose tolerance in women with gestational diabetes. Am J Obstet Gynecol 165:914-919, 1991.

155. Damm P, Kuhl C, Bertelsen A, Molsted-Pedersen L: Predictive factors for the development of diabetes in women with previous gestational diabetes mellitus. Am J Obstet Gynecol 167:607-661, 1992.

156. Stangenberg M, Agarwal N, Rahman F, et al: Frequency of HLA genes and islet cell antibodies and result of post partum oral glucose tolerance tests (OGTT) in Saudi Arabian women with abnormal OGTT during pregnancy. Diabetes Res Clin Pract 14:9-13, 1990.

157. Larsson G, Spjuth J, Ranstam J, et al: Prognostic significance of birth of large infant for subsequent development of maternal non-insulin dependent diabetes: A prospective study over 20-27 years. Diabetes Care 9:359-364, 1986.

158. O'Sullivan JB: Gestational diabetes: Factors influencing the rates of subsequent diabetes. In Sutherland HW, Stowers JM (eds): Carbohydrate Metabolism in Pregnancy and the Newborn. New York, Springer-Verlag, 1978, pp 425-435.

159. Coustan DR, Carpenter MW, O'Sullivan PS, Carr SR: Gestational diabetes: Predictors of subsequent disordered glucose metabolism. Am J Obstet Gynecol 168:1139-1145, 1993.

160. Dornhorst A, Bailey PC, Anyaoku V, et al: Abnormalities of glucose intolerance following gestational diabetes. Q J Med 77:1219-1228, 1990.

161. Mestman JH, Anderson GV, Guadalupe V: Follow-up study of 360 subjects with abnormal glucose metabolism during pregnancy. Obstet Gynecol 39:421-425, 1972.

162. Persson B, Hanson U, Hartling SG, Binder C: Follow-up of women with previous gestational diabetes: Insulin, C-peptide, and proinsulin response to oral glucose load. Diabetes 40(Suppl 2):136-141, 1991.

163. Benjamin E, Winters D, Mayfield J, Gohdes D: Diabetes in pregnancy in Zuni Indian women. Diabetes Care 16:1231-1235, 1993.

164. O'Sullivan JB, Mahan CM: Criteria for the oral glucose tolerance test in pregnancy. Diabetes 13:278-285, 1964.

165. Jacober SJ, Soweres JR: An update on perioperative management of diabetes. Arch Intern Med 159:2405-2411, 1999.

166. Cruse PJ, Foord R: A 5-year prospective study of 23,649 surgical wounds. Arch Surg 107:206-210, 1973.

167. Goodson WH, Hunt TK: Studies of wound healing in experimental diabetes mellitus. J Surg Res 22:221-227, 1977.

168. Bolli GB, Di Marchi RD, Park GD, et al: Insulin analogues and their potential in the management of diabetes mellitus. Diabetologia 42:1151-1167, 1999.

169. Harris M: Diabetes in America. Alexandria, Va, American Diabetes Association, 1995.

170. Peterson CM, Sims RV, Jones RL, Rieders F: Bioavailability of glipizide and its effect on blood glucose and insulin levels in patients with non-insulin dependent diabetes. Diabetes Care 5:497-450, 1982.

171. United Kingdom Prospective Diabetes Study Group: Relative efficacy of randomly allocated diet, sulphonylurea, insulin or metformin in patients with newly diagnosed non-insulin dependent diabetes followed for three years. BMJ 310:83-88, 1995.

172. Jackson RA, Hawa MI, Jaspan JB, et al: Mechanism of metformin action in non-insulin-dependent diabetes. Diabetes 36:632-640, 1987.

173. Hermann LS, Schersten B, Bizen PO, et al: Therapeutic comparison of metformin and sulfonylurea, alone and in various combinations: A double-blind controlled study. Diabetes Care 17:1100-1109, 1994.

174. Defronzo RA, Goodman AM, Multicenter Metformin Study Group: Efficacy of metformin in patients with non-insulin dependent diabetes mellitus. N Engl J Med 333:541-549, 1995.

175. United Kingdom Prospective Diabetes Study Group: Study design, progress, and performance. Diabetologia 34:877-890, 1991.

176. Stolar MW, Endocrine Fellows Foundation Study Group: Clinical management of the NIDDM patient: Impact of the American Diabetes Association practice guidelines, 1985-1993. Diabetes Care 18:701-707, 1995.

177. Bloomgarden ZT: The American Diabetes Association annual meeting, 1994: Treatment issues for NIDDM. Diabetes Care 17:1078-1084, 1994.

178. Colwell JA: Aspirin therapy in diabetes. Diabetes Care 20:1767-1771, 1997.

179. Yusuf S, Sleight P, Pogue J, et al: Effects of an angiotensin-converting-enzyme inhibitor, ramipril, on cardiovascular events in high-risk patients. The Heart Outcomes Prevention Evaluation Study Investigators. N Engl J Med 342:145-153, 2000.

180. Wood DM, Plehwe WE, Colman PB: Aspirin usage in a large teaching hospital diabetes clinic setting. Diabet Med 16:605-608, 1999.
181. Hepaz D, Gottlieb S, Graff E, et al: Effects of aspirin treatment on survival in non-insulin-dependent diabetic patients with coronary artery disease. Israeli Bezafibrate Infarction Prevention Study Group. Am J Med 105:494-499, 1998.
182. Moss SE, Klein R, Klein BE: The 14 year incidence of lower extremity amputations in a diabetic population. The Wisconsin Epidemiologic Study of Diabetic Retinopathy. Diabetes Care 22:951-959, 1999.

Questions

1. **Which of the following statements most accurately reflects the course of diabetic patients following the discovery of insulin?**
   (a) Life expectancy is longer
   (b) Mortality from coma and sepsis is decreased
   (c) Mortality from vascular disease is increased
   (d) Control of glucose prevents microvascular disease of the eye and kidney as well as neuropathy
   (e) All of the above

2. **Abnormal glucose tolerance or diabetes is found more frequently in which of the following?**
   (a) Relatives of a person with diabetes
   (b) Hispanic and black minorities
   (c) Women with a history of gestational diabetes
   (d) The obese and unfit
   (e) All of the above

3. **Which statement is most accurate?**
   (a) Diabetes is a single known genetic disease
   (b) Diabetes is characterized by low insulin levels
   (c) A person with diabetes may be at excess risk for vascular disease because of both increased insulin levels and increased glucose levels
   (d) Diabetes in pregnancy does not increase the risk of eye disease

4. **Which of the following statements is not true?**
   (a) Diabetic patients tend to have a higher prevalence of stroke, myocardial infarction, and peripheral vascular disease
   (b) Diabetic patients tend to have more diffuse large vessel disease
   (c) The most likely cause of death in a person with diabetes is vascular disease
   (d) Most cardiovascular deaths in persons with diabetes are the result of microvascular disease

5. **Which of the following statements regarding stroke is not true?**
   (a) Nonfasting serum glucose predicts outcome, including speed of recovery and mortality
   (b) Women are less vulnerable to the increased vascular risk associated with hyperglycemia than men
   (c) Systolic and diastolic blood pressures predict risk in diabetic patients
   (d) Cholesterol and body mass index are risk factors for stroke
   (e) Glycosylated hemoglobin predicts risk
   (f) Persons with diabetes are at increased risk for thrombotic but not hemorrhagic stroke

6. **Which statement is not true?**
   (a) The risk of cardiovascular disease is two to three times higher in persons with diabetes than in nondiabetic subjects
   (b) The risk of vascular disease associated with diabetes is secondary to obesity, lipid disorders, and increased blood pressure, but not diabetes per se
   (c) The increased prevalence of congestive heart failure in diabetic patients with coronary artery disease has been attributed to microvascular disease and autonomic dysfunction
   (d) Large vessel disease in one area of the vascular tree predicts disease in other areas as well
   (e) Many vascular lesions in persons with diabetes are asymptomatic

7. **Which of the following statements is not true?**
   (a) The ABI is not a good screening tool for persons with diabetes
   (b) Intervention studies in persons with diabetes have shown improvement in the ABI after 9 months of normoglycemia and exercise
   (c) The prevalence of foot ulcers in diabetic patients with peripheral vascular disease is increased in part by problems with the microcirculation and neuropathy
   (d) Glucose control, blood pressure, and duration of diabetes are all independent predictors of amputation

8. **Which of the following probably contributes to vascular disease in hyperglycemic subjects?**
   (a) Glycation and advanced glycation end products
   (b) Perturbations in the fluid phase of coagulation
   (c) Increased reactivity of the platelet
   (d) Endothelial cell dysfunction
   (e) Increased oxidative stress
   (f) Vascular volume shifts
   (g) All of the above

9. **Which of the following statements is most accurate regarding the indications for vascular reconstruction in a diabetic patient?**
   (a) It should be performed primarily for limb salvage rather than claudication
   (b) It should be avoided in subjects with severe neuropathy
   (c) It should be performed less frequently because of poorer outcome statistics
   (d) It should be performed for the same indications in diabetic and nondiabetic patients

10. **Physiologic blood glucose control with careful glucose monitoring before, during, and after surgery is important for which of the following reasons?**
    (a) To minimize the risk of infection
    (b) To increase wound healing and strength
    (c) To avoid hypoglycemia
    (d) To minimize the risk of a prothrombotic state
    (e) All of the above

Answers

1. e	2. e	3. c	4. d	5. b
6. b	7. a	8. g	9. d	10. e

9

Todd D. Reil

Pharmacology of Drugs Used in the Management of Vascular Disease

Anticoagulants

HEPARIN

STRUCTURE AND MECHANISM OF ACTION. Heparin is an anticoagulant composed of a heterogeneous group of straight-chain glycosaminoglycans with molecular weights ranging from 5 to 30 kD (mean, 15 kD).[1] It is strongly acidic secondary to its high content of sulfate and carboxyl groups. Heparin is a naturally occurring substance excreted by mast cells and basophils in the process of clot formation. Standard, unfractionated heparin is derived commercially from porcine gut mucosa or bovine lung tissue. Heparin acts at multiple points within the coagulation system. Its major anticoagulant effect is via interaction with antithrombin III, leading to the inactivation of factor Xa and subsequent inhibition of the conversion of prothrombin to thrombin.[2,3] Heparin further inhibits coagulation by inactivating thrombin, preventing the conversion of fibrinogen to fibrin.[4] Heparin also prevents stable fibrin clot formation through the inhibition of fibrin stabilization factor. Heparin has no fibrinolytic activity and therefore does not lyse existing clots.

Heparin's onset of action is immediate with intravenous injection. It can also be administered subcutaneously. Response to heparin is monitored by measuring the activated partial thromboplastin time (aPTT) and activated clotting time (ACT). An aPTT 1.5 to 2.5 times normal has been shown to prevent recurrent thromboembolism.[5] Weight-adjusted nomograms have been shown to be useful in dosing.[6]

The anticoagulant activity of heparin varies greatly among patients. The heterogeneous clinical response is primarily due to nonspecific binding of heparin to variable concentrations of plasma and cellular proteins, limiting heparin's bioavailability. This leads to marked variability of the anticoagulant response.[2] There also appear to be natural inhibitors of heparin that can be released by sites of active thrombus.[7] Further, the biophysical limitations of the large heparin–antithrombin III complex can block receptors on thrombin to heparin cofactor 2, limiting heparin's effectiveness.[7]

CLINICAL USE. Heparin is indicated for intraoperative anticoagulation in vascular and cardiac surgery, for the prophylaxis and treatment of deep venous thrombosis, for the prevention of pulmonary embolism in surgical patients, and in patients with atrial fibrillation and embolization.[2]

ADVERSE REACTIONS. Heparin therapy is associated with increased risk of bleeding. It also can cause skin lesions, including papules, plaques, and necrosis.[8] Heparin therapy can lead to hypoaldosteronism,[9] priapism,[10] and osteoporosis.[11] Thrombocytopenia is a known complication of heparin administration. Heparin-induced thrombocytopenia (HIT) can lead to thromboembolic complications, including skin necrosis, extremity gangrene, myocardial infarction, pulmonary embolism, and stroke.[2]

Heparin-Induced Thrombocytopenia. Two major forms of HIT are recognized. Type I HIT is an early-onset, benign, reversible thrombocytopenia with no associated platelet antibodies. It is non–immune mediated and is usually self-limited without complications.[12] Type II HIT is a more serious immune-modulated thrombocytopenia.[13] It is caused by platelet IgG antibodies that target platelet factor 4, a heparin binding protein, leading to platelet activation.[14,15] Activation of platelets and endothelium and neutralization of heparin all contribute to a highly thrombogenic state.[2] Patients with type II HIT have a high risk of developing thrombotic complications.[2] Fortunately, most patients who develop HIT antibodies do not develop thrombocytopenia or thrombosis. Further, almost all patients who develop mild to moderate thrombocytopenia during the first 4 days of heparin treatment do not have antibodies. Type II HIT should be considered a clinicopathologic syndrome with a combination of thrombocytopenia and associated clinical events, including thrombosis and confirmation of platelet antibodies.[2] The management of HIT is aimed at preventing thromboembolic complications. All heparin should be discontinued and an alternative anticoagulant initiated.

PROTAMINE

STRUCTURE AND MECHANISM OF ACTION. Protamine is made up of a heterogeneous group of low-molecular-weight proteins. These proteins are rich in arginine and are strongly basic. They occur naturally in the sperm of salmon and certain other fish species. The mechanism of action for heparin reversal is through electrostatic bonding. Heparin is highly acidic and forms a strong bond with the highly basic protamine molecules, forming an inactive complex.[16]

CLINICAL USE. Protamine is used clinically as a heparin antidote. When administered alone, protamine has an anticoagulant effect similar to that of heparin. However, in the presence of heparin, it forms a stable salt, and the anticoagulant activity of both is lost. Protamine has a rapid onset of action; within 5 minutes of administration, it begins to neutralize heparin.

ADVERSE REACTIONS. Too rapid administration can have serious side effects, including hypotension and anaphylaxis.[17] Decreased blood pressure, pulmonary hypertension, shortness of breath, flushing, and urticaria have all been associated with rapid administration.[18] Protamine should be administered slowly over 10 minutes, with a goal of 1 mg of protamine to neutralize every 90 units of heparin. Further dosing should be guided by coagulation studies.[16] Patients with allergies to fish products may be allergic to protamine.[19]

LOW-MOLECULAR-WEIGHT HEPARINS

STRUCTURE AND MECHANISM OF ACTION. Low-molecular-weight heparins (LMWHs) are collections of heparin molecules that have significantly lower molecular weights than standard, unfractionated heparin.[20] LMWHs are derived from unfractionated heparin via chemical or enzymatic depolymerization. This produces fragments one third the size of heparin, with mean molecular weights of 4 to 5 kD (range, 1 to 10 kD). Similar to unfractionated heparin, LMWHs are heterogeneous in terms of both molecular size and anticoagulant activity.[21] The LMWHs have distinct differences from standard heparin. LMWHs have reduced ability to catalyze the inactivation of thrombin, because the smaller fragments cannot bind to thrombin. However, LMWHs retain the ability to inactivate factor Xa. There is a reduction in nonspecific protein binding and subsequent improved predictability in dose-response relationships.[21] LMWHs have an increased half-life compared with standard heparin. This is thought to be secondary to reduced macrophage binding. Similarly, there is reduced binding to platelets and a decrease in the incidence of HIT.[21] LMWHs also have been associated with a reduction in bone loss compared with standard heparin.

CLINICAL USE. The LMWHs have been examined extensively in the prevention of deep venous thrombosis in patients undergoing major abdominal surgery or knee and hip replacement surgery and in patients with restricted mobility.[20] LMWHs have also been investigated for the treatment of acute deep venous thrombosis and pulmonary embolism.[20] LMWHs are used in patients with acute coronary syndromes

and unstable angina.[22] The advantages of LMWHs over standard heparin are longer plasma half-life and a more predictable anticoagulant response, allowing for simple dosing and decreasing the need for laboratory monitoring.[21]

ADVERSE REACTIONS. Adverse reactions to LMWHs are similar to those associated with standard heparin. Bleeding, ecchymosis, and thrombocytopenia can all occur with LMWH administration. The incidence of HIT is decreased compared with standard heparin, but LMWHs can cause HIT, and patients should be monitored for this complication.[23]

WARFARIN

STRUCTURE AND MECHANISM OF ACTION. Warfarin is a coumarin derivative that produces an anticoagulant effect through the inhibition of vitamin K–dependent coagulation factors (II, VII, IX, X) and the anticoagulant proteins C and S. Warfarin interferes with the conversion of vitamin K to 2,3-epoxide.[24] Vitamin K is an essential cofactor for postribosomal synthesis of clotting factors, acting through the carboxylation of glutamine residues in the protein.[25] Carboxylation promotes binding of vitamin K–dependent coagulation factors to phospholipid surfaces.[24] Coumarins specifically block vitamin K epoxide reductase, preventing the carboxylation of the factors rendering them inactive.[26] The vitamin K antagonists also inhibit carboxylation of the regulatory anticoagulant proteins C and S.[26]

Warfarin is a racemic mixture of two optically active isomers.[24] Absorption from the gastrointestinal tract is rapid, reaching maximal plasma levels within 90 minutes. Warfarin has a half-life of 36 to 42 hours. Response is variable owing to certain genetic factors, drug interactions, various disease states, and diet. The anticoagulant effect can be overcome by low doses of vitamin K_1, as vitamin K_1 bypasses vitamin K epoxide reductase.[24] Warfarin anticoagulation is monitored via measurement of the prothrombin time (PT). The PT reflects the depression of the vitamin K–dependent factors. PT measurement is laboratory dependent, and physicians should be aware of the specific method used to measure it at their institutions.

CLINICAL USE. Warfarin is indicated for the prophylaxis or treatment of venous thrombosis and thromboembolism. It is also indicated for the prophylaxis or treatment of the thromboembolic complications associated with atrial fibrillation and cardiac valve replacement. Warfarin has been shown to reduce the risk of death, recurrent myocardial infarction, and thromboembolic events such as stroke or systemic embolization after myocardial infarction.[24]

Warfarin has been studied in terms of its usefulness in promoting the patency of infrainguinal bypass grafts.[27-30] A recent publication on antithrombotic and thrombolytic therapy provided guidelines based on a review of the clinical data available.[31] Although some studies suggest improved patency of infrainguinal bypass grafts with warfarin or a combination of warfarin and aspirin, the data are not strong enough to warrant its routine use, except in patients at high risk of bypass occlusion and limb loss.[31] These conclusions are based on small improvements in patency in the face of relatively high rates of bleeding complications.

ADVERSE REACTIONS. Warfarin therapy is associated with an increased risk of hemorrhagic complications. It also can cause necrosis and gangrene of skin or other tissues. It should be used with caution in patients with HIT, because it can lead to increased thrombotic complications early in the treatment of HIT.[32]

DIRECT THROMBIN INHIBITORS

The direct thrombin inhibitors are small molecules that act directly at the active site of thrombin, without the use of an intermediate such as antithrombin III with heparin. There are five direct thrombin inhibitors currently available for clinical use: lepirudin, desirudin, bivalirudin, argatroban, and melagatran/ximelagatran.

Thrombin is the central enzyme in hemostasis. It is a serine protease that catalyzes the conversion of fibrinogen to fibrin. In addition, thrombin serves many other roles, including the activation of various coagulation factors, platelets, smooth muscle cells, fibroblasts, and endothelium.[33] Thrombin is chemotactic, stimulates secretion of vasoactive proteins from platelets and inflammatory cells, and plays a role in angiogenesis and restenosis.[33]

Antithrombin III, the major regulator of thrombin, forms an irreversible complex with thrombin to block its active site.[21] For years, this has been the main target for thrombin inhibition and anticoagulation via heparin. However, the use of heparin is limited by several major factors: (1) the development of HIT; (2) heparin's inability to penetrate clot, leading to the release of active thrombin from clots; and (3) the variable anticoagulant response, owing to heparin's propensity to bind to plasma proteins.[34] The rationale for the development of direct thrombin inhibitors was to create a small molecule with site-specific thrombin inhibition.[34] With an increased understanding of the detailed molecular structure of thrombin, site-specific agents have been developed with a high specificity for thrombin.[35]

HIRUDIN. Hirudin, the first direct thrombin inhibitor, was originally isolated from the salivary gland of the medicinal leech *Hirudo medicinalis* after it was noted that leech saliva had anticoagulant properties.[35] It is now produced via recombinant technology as lepirudin and desirudin. It is a 65– to 66–amino acid polypeptide. The amino terminus forms a tight bond with thrombin's active site, and the carboxy terminus binds to the thrombin exosite-1 (fibrinogen binding site).[36] Peak plasma levels are reached after parenteral administration in 20 to 30 minutes. Hirudin is rapidly cleared by the kidneys, having a half-life of 1 to 3 hours. Some hepatic excretion also occurs but is not clinically significant. Hirudin should not be used in patients with renal failure, as no specific antidote exists should overdosage occur.

BIVALIRUDIN. Bivalirudin is a recombinant protein based on hirudin. It is a 20–amino acid peptide that interacts with the active site of thrombin.[33] It has a short half-life of 25 minutes. In contrast to hirudin, renal excretion is not the major route of excretion.[35]

ARGATROBAN. Argatroban is a synthetic, small-molecule arginine derivative that interacts only with the active site of thrombin.[33,35] It is metabolized by the liver, with a half-life of 45 minutes. Dose reduction may be necessary in patients with liver dysfunction. The anticoagulant effect can be monitored with the aPTT or ACT.

MELAGATRAN/XIMELAGATRAN. There is great interest in the development of oral direct thrombin inhibitors. Ximelagatran is a prodrug of melagatran, a synthetic active-site direct inhibitor of thrombin. Melagatran is poorly absorbed from gastrointestinal tract, but ximelagatran is rapidly absorbed. Once it is absorbed, it is converted to melagatran via two intermediate metabolites. The half-life is about 3 hours, and the drug is excreted primarily by the kidneys.[33,37]

CLINICAL USE. Direct thrombin inhibitors have been studied in the treatment of HIT with thrombosis, the treatment of acute coronary events, and the prevention and treatment of deep venous thrombosis, pulmonary embolism, and stroke.[33,35]

FACTOR X INHIBITORS

FONDAPARINUX. Fondaparinux is a pentasaccharide that activates antithrombin III in a manner similar to heparin, leading to inactivation of factor X.[38] It differs in one major respect from heparin, in that the pentasaccharide is unable to mediate the inactivation of thrombin by antithrombin III.[38] It is administered subcutaneously and does not require laboratory monitoring. It is renally excreted and is contraindicated in patients with renal failure. Fondaparinux has been evaluated in multiple trials for preventing deep venous thrombosis in patients undergoing major hip fracture and knee replacement surgery.[39-42] It also has been evaluated in the treatment of deep venous thrombosis[43] and acute coronary syndromes.[44]

Antiplatelet Agents
ASPIRIN

STRUCTURE AND MECHANISM OF ACTION. Aspirin inhibits platelet aggregation by irreversibly acetylating prostaglandin synthase, inhibiting its cyclooxygenase activity. This blocks prostaglandin metabolism and, most importantly, the synthesis of thromboxane A_2, a potent stimulator of platelet aggregation.[45,46] There are two isoforms of the cyclooxygenase enzyme: COX-1 and COX-2.[47] COX-1 is constitutively expressed in many cell types, including platelets, whereas COX-2 is present only in inflammatory cells. Aspirin is 50- to 100-fold more potent in inhibiting COX-1 than COX-2; thus, lower doses are required to obtain antiplatelet compared with anti-inflammatory effects.[47] Several other mechanisms for platelet inhibition have been proposed, including inhibiting neutrophil activation of platelets[48] and interfering with prostacyclin synthesis by endothelium.[49] There are also data suggesting an antioxidant role for aspirin[50,51] and the improvement of endothelial cell function by aspirin.[52] It is primarily the antiplatelet and antithrombotic effects of aspirin that result in cardiovascular benefits. Aspirin is rapidly absorbed by the upper gastrointestinal tract, with measurable platelet effects within 1 hour.[47] Enteric coating significantly impairs its absorption, taking up to 4 hours to reach peak plasma levels. Although the plasma half-life is only 20 minutes, the effect on COX-1 and the platelet is permanent, as the anucleate platelet cannot synthesize new enzyme. The life span of a platelet is approximately 10 days. After a single dose of aspirin and with normal platelet turnover of approximately 10% per day, it may take 10 days for renewal of the platelet population. However, data suggest that as little as 20% of platelets with normal COX enzyme activity is required for normal hemostasis.[47,53]

CLINICAL USE. The benefit of aspirin therapy is determined largely by the patient's absolute risk of vascular events. Those at high risk and those with unstable angina or prior myocardial infarction or stroke derive the most benefit.[54]

Primary Prevention. Aspirin for primary disease prevention has been carefully evaluated in multiple clinical trials.[55-59] The combined data demonstrated a significant reduction in myocardial infarction with aspirin but did not demonstrate a decrease in overall mortality. There was a slightly increased risk of bleeding complications with aspirin, so the benefits and risks must be balanced. Generally, the greater the thrombotic risk, the greater the benefits of aspirin for primary prevention.[54]

Secondary Prevention. The benefits of aspirin in preventing cardiovascular disease complications have been clearly demonstrated in several large clinical trials.[60] The Antiplatelet Trialists Committee published a meta-analysis that included 287 trials with more than 300,000 patients.[57,61] In high-risk patients—those with a history of myocardial infarction, angina, or stroke—long-term therapy with aspirin significantly decreased the risk of nonfatal myocardial infarction, nonfatal ischemic stroke, and vascular death.[57]

Aspirin is also recommended in patients undergoing prosthetic inguinal bypass grafting or carotid endarterectomy and those with asymptomatic and recurrent carotid stenosis.[31] Aspirin has been demonstrated to improve long-term vessel patency in patients undergoing lower extremity angioplasty with or without stenting.[31]

ADVERSE REACTIONS. The most significant adverse reactions associated with aspirin therapy include bleeding and gastrointestinal irritation. These side effects appear to be dose related. Aspirin dosing varied widely in the Antiplatelet Trialists Committee overview, and there was no significant benefit associated with higher doses.[61] Daily dosing of 75 to 150 mg of aspirin appears to be as effective as higher doses for long-term treatment.[57] Because of the increased side effects with higher doses and the lack of any conclusive data favoring higher doses, the concept of lower dosing is supported.[62]

THIENOPYRIDINES (CLOPIDOGREL AND TICLOPIDINE)

STRUCTURE AND MECHANISM OF ACTION. Adenosine diphosphate (ADP) plays a central role in platelet aggregation and activation. ADP released from activated platelets induces further platelet activation and adhesion through binding to the ADP receptor on the platelet surface. The ADP receptor is a membrane-bound, G-protein–coupled receptor.[63,64] There are two main types of ADP receptors, $P2Y_1$ and $P2Y_{12}$.[63] The overall effect of platelet ADP receptor binding is increased platelet activation and aggregation.[63]

Ticlopidine and clopidogrel are selective antiplatelet agents that inhibit the $P2Y_{12}$ receptor. Their chemical structures are similar, with clopidogrel having an extra carboxymethyl side group. Both parent compounds are quickly metabolized in the liver to active metabolites that covalently bind to the ADP receptor. Clopidogrel is six times more potent than ticlopidine. The effect is permanent over the life

span of the platelet, and overall platelet function generally recovers within 7 to 10 days after stopping the drug.[63]

CLINICAL USE. Ticlopidine has been evaluated in several clinical trials in patients with peripheral arterial disease and has been associated with a reduction in the risk of myocardial infarction, stroke, and vascular death.[65,66] However, ticlopidine's clinical usefulness is limited by the potential for severe hematologic side effects, particularly neutropenia.[67-69]

Clopidogrel, which has fewer side effects than ticlopidine, has been approved for use in patients with recent myocardial infarction, stroke, or established peripheral vascular disease for the reduction of thrombotic events. The Food and Drug Administration (FDA) has also approved it for use in patients with non-ST elevation acute coronary syndromes and percutaneous coronary interventions. A landmark study of clopidogrel was the Clopidogrel versus Aspirin in Patients at Risk of Ischemic Events (CAPRIE) trial.[70] This randomized, prospective, double-blinded trial compared the efficacy of aspirin and clopidogrel in reducing the risk of ischemic stroke, myocardial infarction, or vascular death. The study of nearly 20,000 patients with atherosclerotic disease (those with recent stroke, myocardial infarction, or established peripheral arterial disease) found that clopidogrel resulted in an 8.7% relative risk reduction in vascular death, ischemic stroke, or myocardial infarction compared with aspirin. Remarkably, this was not a placebo comparison but a comparison with a known effective antiplatelet agent already proved to confer a 25% risk reduction.[57,71] Subset analyses of CAPRIE showed an even greater benefit in high-risk patients, diabetics, and those with previous vascular interventions.[72]

Thienopyridines have been used in vascular surgery practice as antithrombotic therapy for lower extremity balloon angioplasty and stenting. This has not yet been examined in randomized clinical trials, so there are insufficient data to recommend thienopyridine use in this setting.[31] Ticlopidine (Ticlid) has been demonstrated to improve the patency of infrainguinal bypass grafts, but its clinical use has been superseded by clopidogrel's significantly fewer adverse effects.[31,73] Currently, there are no controlled trials looking specifically at clopidogrel and infrainguinal graft patency, so it cannot be recommended at this time.

ADVERSE REACTIONS. Side effects of clopidogrel include gastrointestinal complaints and skin rash. Bleeding complications are similar to those associated with aspirin. Neutropenia is a rare complication with clopidogrel but is much more frequent with ticlopidine.[69,74] Neutropenia can be severe and has resulted in fatalities. It generally occurs within 3 months after instituting therapy, and strict hematologic monitoring is recommended.[63] Diarrhea and skin rashes are also common with ticlopidine.[72] Thrombotic thrombocytopenic purpura is a recognized complication of thienopyridine treatment, with an incidence between 1:1600 and 1:5000 patients.[75]

GLYCOPROTEIN IIb/IIIa RECEPTOR INHIBITORS

STRUCTURE AND MECHANISM OF ACTION. The glycoprotein (GP) receptor is an integrin found in high concentrations on the platelet membrane. The GP receptor (GP IIb/IIIa) represents a final common pathway to platelet aggregation and subsequent thrombus formation.[76] Once activated, the receptor undergoes a conformational change that permits the binding of fibrinogen. This allows cross-linking of platelets and aggregation, with the formation of the hemostatic platelet plug.[77] Selective inhibition of the GP IIb/IIIa receptor is a logical target for more specific antiplatelet therapy. There are three main inhibitors approved for clinical use: abciximab (ReoPro), eptifibatide (Integrilin), and tirofiban (Aggrastat).

Abciximab. Abciximab was the first GP IIb/IIIa receptor inhibitor developed. It is a macromolecule composed of the Fab fragment of the chimeric human murine monoclonal antibody c7E3.[78] It has a high binding affinity for the GP IIb/IIIa receptor, which accounts for its prolonged antiplatelet effect after cessation of infusion, with up to 10 days of low-level receptor blockade.[78] Platelet aggregation is almost completely inhibited by 2 hours after infusion, with recovery evident 48 hours after discontinuing the drug. However, platelet-bound drug can still be detected for up to 10 days.[79]

Tirofiban. Tirofiban is a small, nonpeptide antagonist of the GP IIb/IIIa receptor.[79] It is a tyrosine derivative with a molecular weight of 495 kD. At standard doses, platelet function is inhibited as early as 5 minutes after infusion, with bleeding time and platelet aggregation normalizing within 3 to 8 hours after discontinuation.[79]

Eptifibatide. Eptifibatide is a nonimmunogenic, cyclic heptapeptide that inhibits the GP IIb/IIIa receptor. It is derived from the structure of barbourin from the venom of a species of rattlesnake.[80] It has a short plasma half-life of 15 minutes, with peak platelet effects within 15 minutes of infusion; platelet function returns to 50% of baseline by 4 hours after terminating the infusion.[81]

CLINICAL USE. The GP IIb/IIIa receptor antagonists have been shown to reduce cardiac event rates in patients with acute coronary syndromes treated by medicine alone or in combination with percutaneous coronary intervention.[82] Evidence supporting their use in percutaneous coronary interventions is good. It confers significant long-term mortality benefits and decreases ischemic events.[76,77,83-85] There are currently no large, randomized clinical trials of GP IIb/IIIa inhibitors specifically in vascular surgery patients.

ADVERSE REACTIONS. Bleeding is the principal adverse effect of all the GP inhibitors. Nearly all trials demonstrate an increase in serious bleeding rates. Fatal bleeding is rare, less than 0.1%, which is similar to the rate with combined heparin and aspirin therapy.[79] Thrombocytopenia is also associated with GP inhibition. Abciximab causes severe thrombocytopenia (<20,000/µL) in 0.7% of patients, and eptifibatide and tirofiban in 0.2% of patients.[79]

The optimal patients to receive GP inhibitors are those with acute coronary syndrome who undergo percutaneous coronary intervention and are at high risk for early failure. The value of GP inhibition in other vascular interventions is not yet established.[79]

Medical Treatment of Claudication

PENTOXIFYLLINE

STRUCTURE AND MECHANISM OF ACTION. Pentoxifylline is an antithrombotic agent whose exact mechanism of action is unknown. It is thought to improve blood flow by increasing red cell deformity, decreasing platelet adhesiveness, and decreasing blood viscosity, leading to increased flow in the microcirculation.[86-88]

CLINICAL USE. Multiple clinical trials of pentoxifylline have demonstrated conflicting results in the treatment of claudication. Some suggested improved walking distance with pentoxifylline,[89-94] while others showed little benefit compared with placebo.[95-98] Based on such conflicting data, it is currently not recommended for use in claudication.

CILOSTAZOL

STRUCTURE AND MECHANISM OF ACTION. Cilostazol is a type III phosphodiesterase inhibitor that increases cellular cyclic adenosine monophosphate and acts to inhibit platelet aggregation and thrombus formation. It is also a direct vasodilator.[31] Cilostazol has been shown to improve claudication symptoms, but the exact mechanism is unknown. It is absorbed after oral administration and extensively metabolized by hepatic cytochrome P-450 enzymes, with two main active metabolites being produced.[11] Excretion is predominantly urinary.

CLINICAL USE. Cilostazol was approved in 1999 by the FDA for the treatment of intermittent claudication, based on randomized clinical trials that demonstrated increased walking distance and quality of life.[99-101] Compared with those given placebo, patients taking cilostazol experienced significant increases in walking distance. The effect was apparent as early as 2 to 4 weeks after initiating therapy. Cilostazol is more effective than pentoxifylline in improving claudication.[11] Current recommendations are that cilostazol should be used only by those with disabling claudication who are not revascularization candidates.[31] Cilostazol has weak antiplatelet effects, but there are no clinical data to support its use as an antiplatelet agent.[31]

ADVERSE REACTIONS. Because cilostazol is a phosphodiesterase inhibitor, it should not be used in patients with congestive heart failure. The only adverse effect in study patients leading to discontinuation of the drug was headache, likely secondary to its vasodilatory effects. Other more common side effects include palpitations and diarrhea.

Agents to Prevent Contrast-Induced Nephropathy

Contrast nephropathy (CN) is the third leading cause of acute renal failure in hospitalized patients.[102,103] Most cases of CN are reversible and nonoliguric; however, up to 25% to 30% of patients who develop CN have a permanent decline in renal function.[104] In addition, patients who develop acute renal failure have increased morbidity and mortality.[105] The main risk factors for developing CN are underlying renal insufficiency and diabetes.[106] The exact mechanism behind the development of CN remains unknown but is likely a combination of direct renal tubule epithelial cell toxicity and renal medullary ischemia.[106,107]

The use of low volumes of low-osmolar and iso-osmolar contrast agents appears to reduce the risk of CN when compared with the use of high-osmolar contrast agents.[108-110] Multiple trials have demonstrated that saline hydration is also beneficial in preventing CN.[111,112]

N-ACETYLCYSTEINE

STRUCTURE AND MECHANISM OF ACTION. N-acetylcysteine (NAC) is the acetylated form of the amino acid L-cysteine. NAC has been in clinical use for more than 30 years, mostly as a mucolytic.[113] NAC is an antioxidant and a free radical scavenger. It can stimulate glutathione synthesis and has vasodilatory properties through its effects on nitric oxide.[114]

CLINICAL USE. Clinical data on the value of NAC in preventing CN are mixed. NAC initially demonstrated a significant reduction in CN in patients with preexisting renal insufficiency.[115] The frequency of CN in patients receiving hydration plus NAC was 2%, compared with 22% in those receiving hydration alone. This was followed by other studies demonstrating similar protective effects of NAC.[116,117] However, subsequent trials have not demonstrated a clear benefit in the prevention of CN.[118,119] Proponents of NAC argue that its ease of administration, relatively low cost, and limited side effects make this an appealing agent in high-risk patients. However, inconsistent clinical data currently preclude recommending its routine use.

FENOLDOPAM

STRUCTURE AND MECHANISM OF ACTION. Fenoldopam is a selective dopamine-1 agonist that increases both cortical and medullary renal blood flow. Unlike dopamine, fenoldopam does not stimulate the α- and β-adrenergic receptors or the dopamine-2 receptors, which can produce vasoconstriction.[120,121] Fenoldopam has been shown to increase the glomerular filtration rate and induce diuresis.[120]

CLINICAL USE. Early retrospective studies suggested that fenoldopam reduced the incidence of CN.[121-123] However, more recent prospective, randomized trials have not shown that it offers any protection against CN.[124,125] Therefore, fenoldopam cannot be recommended for the prevention of CN.

THEOPHYLLINE

STRUCTURE AND MECHANISM OF ACTION. Theophylline blocks adenosine receptors in the kidney. Adenosine is an important intrarenal mediator that can cause a decrease in glomerular filtration rate through vasoconstriction of afferent arterioles and vasodilatation of efferent arterioles and mesangial cell contraction.[126] It also induces cortical vasoconstriction and increases free radical generation in the tubular cells.[126] Animal studies suggest a benefit of adenosine receptor blockade in the renal vascular response to contrast media.[126]

CLINICAL USE. Initial clinical trials suggested a benefit of theophylline in the prevention of CN.[127,128] Another study demonstrated that theophylline offered no addition protection compared with hydration alone.[129] Thus, with no convincing clinical data, theophylline cannot currently be recommended for the prevention of CN.

OTHER AGENTS

PROSTAGLANDIN E₁. Prostaglandin E_1 has vasodilatory effects that may be beneficial in preventing CN.[106] One randomized trial suggested protection in patients receiving prostaglandin E_1, but this was not statistically significant.[130] Further trials are needed.

ENDOTHELIN ANTAGONISTS. Endothelin-1 is an endogenous vasoconstrictor. It has been examined as a possible cause of CN.[102] Blockade of the endothelin-1 receptor with endothelin-α antagonists has been shown in animal models to reduce the incidence of nephropathy.[131] However, a clinical trial actually demonstrated decreased renal function after radiocontrast with endothelin receptor antagonism.[132] There are currently no data to support endothelin receptor blockade in the prevention of CN.

CALCIUM CHANNEL BLOCKERS. Calcium channel blockers prevent the influx of calcium into smooth muscle cells, causing a vasodilatory effect in all vascular beds, including the kidney. They also offer some cytoprotective effects.[133] Animal studies have shown that calcium channel blockade confers protection against CN,[133] but there is no consensus among clinical trials.[134-138] Large-scale clinical trials of calcium channel blockers are required.

DOPAMINE. Dopamine has variable effects, depending on dose. Low-dose dopamine activates DA-1 and DA-2 receptors. Medium doses activate β-adrenergic receptors, and high doses activate α receptors.[139] The DA-1 receptor causes renal vasodilatation, and low-dose dopamine has been investigated with regard to preventing CN.[102] There are conflicting data regarding dopamine and protection against CN, however[139-142]; therefore, dopamine is not currently recommended for the prevention of CN.

DIURETICS. Furosemide and mannitol have had disappointing results when examined for the prevention of CN. The majority of the evidence is against their use, as they may exacerbate renal dysfunction.[111,143]

Statins

Statin therapy has been demonstrated to reduce cardiovascular morbidity and mortality in multiple patient populations.[117,144-148] Although the primary mechanism of action is to reduce cholesterol levels, the benefits of statin therapy appear to extend beyond that effect.[149]

STRUCTURE AND MECHANISM OF ACTION. Statins decrease cholesterol levels through inhibition of the HMG-CoA reductase enzyme, the rate-limiting step through which cells synthesize cholesterol. Inhibition of cholesterol synthesis leads to increased hepatocyte expression of low-density lipoprotein (LDL) receptors, with increased cellular uptake of LDL and a reduction in plasma LDL and cholesterol levels.[149] Statins also reduce the rate at which apolipoprotein B particles are secreted by the liver.[149]

CLINICAL USE. There are considerable data to support the use of statins in patients with cardiovascular disease. The Scandinavian Simvastatin Survival Study (4S) clearly established that lipid-lowering therapy was safe, and it reduced morbidity and mortality in patients with ischemic heart disease who had elevated cholesterol levels.[145] Statin treatment reduced major coronary events, coronary mortality, and overall mortality. Multiple subsequent studies of patients with elevated cholesterol demonstrated a significant reduction in cardiovascular events and overall mortality with statin therapy.[146,150,151]

Statins are also beneficial in patients with cardiovascular disease who have normal lipid levels.[144,148,151,152] In addition, statin therapy is associated with a reduction in the risk of stroke in patients with cardiovascular disease.[153,154]

Besides lowering cholesterol, statins are thought to have significant so-called pleiotropic effects.[149] Statins can improve endothelial cell function[155,156] and reduce inflammation and thrombosis, leading to plaque stabilization.[149,152,157,158]

The majority of studies support the aggressive use of statins in patients at high risk for coronary or cerebrovascular events, particularly in those with established disease, irrespective of their baseline cholesterol levels.

Specific studies focusing on vascular surgery patients are few. Subgroup analysis of patients with peripheral vascular disease in the major statin trials demonstrated a significant decrease in myocardial infarction and cardiovascular events.[159] The 4S trial found that the incidence of new-onset or worsening intermittent claudication was reduced 38% with statin therapy.[145] Statin treatment in patients undergoing noncardiac vascular surgery has been shown to reduce cardiac morbidity and mortality.[160-162] Statins also improve vein graft patency.[163]

ADVERSE REACTIONS. High-dose statin therapy leads to hepatic necrosis in animal models.[164] In clinical trials, statins have not been demonstrated to cause significant liver enzyme elevations compared with controls.[165] Current recommendations are to monitor hepatic enzymes for 4 to 6 weeks after initiating treatment. In high-risk patients or those taking certain medications, closer monitoring may be warranted.

The most serious risks associated with statin therapy are myositis and rhabdomyolysis.[164,166] Cerivastatin was withdrawn from the market owing to deaths from such complications.[167] Risks for rhabdomyolysis are increased with small body size, advanced age, renal or hepatic dysfunction, diabetes, and hypothyroidism.[167] Patients on statins should be monitored closely for symptoms of myopathy.

KEY REFERENCES

Antithrombotic Trialists' Collaboration: Collaborative meta-analysis of randomised trials of antiplatelet therapy for prevention of death, myocardial infarction, and stroke in high risk patients. BMJ 324:71-86, 2002.

Becker RC, Fintel DJ, Green D (eds): Antithrombotic Therapy, 2nd ed. West Islip, New York, Professional Communications, 2002, pp 63-76.

Clagett GP, Sobel M, Jackson MR, et al: Antithrombotic therapy in peripheral arterial occlusive disease: The Seventh ACCP Conference on Antithrombotic and Thrombolytic Therapy. Chest 126(3 Suppl): 609S-626S, 2004.

Collaborative overview of randomised trials of antiplatelet therapy. I. Prevention of death, myocardial infarction, and stroke by prolonged antiplatelet therapy in various categories of patients. Antiplatelet Trialists' Collaboration. BMJ 308:81-106, 1994.

Cox CD, Tsikouris JP: Preventing contrast nephropathy: What is the best strategy? A review of the literature. J Clin Pharmacol 44:327-337, 2004.

Dawson DL, Cutler BS, Hiatt WR, et al: A comparison of cilostazol and pentoxifylline for treating intermittent claudication. Am J Med 109: 523-530, 2000.

Frangos SG, Chen AH, Sumpio B: Vascular drugs in the new millennium. J Am Coll Surg 191:76-92, 2000.

Hiatt WR: Pharmacologic therapy for peripheral arterial disease and claudication. J Vasc Surg 36:1283-1291, 2002.

Hirsh J, Raschke R: Heparin and low-molecular-weight heparin: The Seventh ACCP Conference on Antithrombotic and Thrombolytic Therapy. Chest 126(3 Suppl):188S-203S, 2004.

Kam PC, Nethery CM: The thienopyridine derivatives (platelet adenosine diphosphate receptor antagonists), pharmacology and clinical developments. Anaesthesia 58:28-35, 2003.

Kaplan KL: Direct thrombin inhibitors. Expert Opin Pharmacother 4:653-666, 2003.

Patrono C, Coller B, FitzGerald GA, et al: Platelet-active drugs: The relationships among dose, effectiveness, and side effects: The Seventh ACCP Conference on Antithrombotic and Thrombolytic Therapy. Chest 126(3 Suppl):234S-264S, 2004.

Poldermans D, Bax JJ, Kertai MD, et al: Statins are associated with a reduced incidence of perioperative mortality in patients undergoing major noncardiac vascular surgery. Circulation 107:1848-1851, 2003.

Randomised trial of cholesterol lowering in 4444 patients with coronary heart disease: The Scandinavian Simvastatin Survival Study (4S). Lancet 344:1383-1389, 1994.

REFERENCES

1. Johnson EA, Mulloy B: The molecular-weight range of mucosal-heparin preparations. Carbohydr Res 51:119-127, 1976.
2. Hirsh J, Raschke R: Heparin and low-molecular-weight heparin: The Seventh ACCP Conference on Antithrombotic and Thrombolytic Therapy. Chest 126(3 Suppl):188S-203S, 2004.
3. Lindahl U, Backstrom G, Hook M, et al: Structure of the antithrombin-binding site in heparin. Proc Natl Acad Sci U S A 76:3198-3202, 1979.
4. Tollefsen DM, Majerus DW, Blank MK: Heparin cofactor II: Purification and properties of a heparin-dependent inhibitor of thrombin in human plasma. J Biol Chem 257:2162-2169, 1982.
5. Basu D, Gallus A, Hirsch J, Cade J: A prospective study of the value of monitoring heparin treatment with the activated partial thromboplastin time. N Engl J Med 287:324-327, 1972.
6. Raschke RA, Gollihare B, Peirce JC: The effectiveness of implementing the weight-based heparin nomogram as a practice guideline. Arch Intern Med 156:1645-1649, 1996.
7. Haas S: The present and future of heparin, low molecular weight heparins, pentasaccharide, and hirudin for venous thromboembolism and acute coronary syndromes. Semin Vasc Med 3:139-146, 2003.
8. Warkentin TE: Heparin-induced skin lesions. Br J Haematol 92:494-497, 1996.
9. Laidlaw JC, Abbott EC, Sutherland DJ, Stiefel M: The influence of a heparin-like compound on hypertension, electrolytes and aldosterone in man. Trans Am Clin Climatol Assoc 77:111-124, 1965.
10. Klein LA, Hall RL, Smith RB: Surgical treatment of priapism: With a note on heparin-induced priapism. J Urol 108:104-106, 1972.
11. Dawson DL, Cutler BS, Hiatt WR, et al: A comparison of cilostazol and pentoxifylline for treating intermittent claudication. Am J Med 109:523-530, 2000.
12. Comunale ME, Van Cott EM: Heparin-induced thrombocytopenia. Int Anesthesiol Clin 42:27-43, 2004.
13. Warkentin TE: Clinical presentation of heparin-induced thrombocytopenia. Semin Hematol 35(4 Suppl 5):9-16, discussion 35-36, 1998.
14. Kelton JG, Sheridan D, Brian H, et al: Clinical usefulness of testing for a heparin-dependent platelet-aggregating factor in patients with suspected heparin-associated thrombocytopenia. J Lab Clin Med 103:606-612, 1984.
15. Arepally GM, Mayer IM: Antibodies from patients with heparin-induced thrombocytopenia stimulate monocytic cells to express tissue factor and secrete interleukin-8. Blood 98:1252-1254, 2001.
16. Park KW: Protamine and protamine reactions. Int Anesthesiol Clin 42:135-145, 2004.
17. Horrow JC: Protamine: A review of its toxicity. Anesth Analg 64:348-361, 1985.
18. Horrow JC: Adverse reactions to protamine. Int Anesthesiol Clin 23:133-144, 1985.
19. Knape JT, Schuller JL, de Haan P, et al: An anaphylactic reaction to protamine in a patient allergic to fish. Anesthesiology 55:324-325, 1981.
20. White RH, Ginsberg JS: Low-molecular-weight heparins: Are they all the same? Br J Haematol 121:12-20, 2003.
21. Hirsh J, Warkentin TE, Raschke R, et al: Heparin and low-molecular-weight heparin: Mechanisms of action, pharmacokinetics, dosing considerations, monitoring, efficacy, and safety. Chest 114(5 Suppl):489S-510S, 1998.
22. Kaul S, Shah PK: Low molecular weight heparin in acute coronary syndrome: Evidence for superior or equivalent efficacy compared with unfractionated heparin? J Am Coll Cardiol 35:1699-1712, 2000.
23. Warkentin TE, Greinacher A: Heparin-induced thrombocytopenia: Recognition, treatment, and prevention. The Seventh ACCP Conference on Antithrombotic and Thrombolytic Therapy. Chest 126(3 Suppl): 311S-337S, 2004.

24. Hirsh J, Fuster V, Ansell J, et al: American Heart Association/American College of Cardiology Foundation guide to warfarin therapy. J Am Coll Cardiol 41:1633-1652, 2003.

25. Nelsestuen GL, Suttie JW: The mode of action of vitamin K: Isolation of a peptide containing the vitamin K-dependent portion of prothrombin. Proc Natl Acad Sci U S A 70:3366-3370, 1973.

26. Whitlon DS, Sadowski JA, Suttie JW: Mechanism of coumarin action: Significance of vitamin K epoxide reductase inhibition. Biochemistry 17:1371-1377, 1978.

27. Kretschmer G, Herbst F, Prager M, et al: A decade of oral anticoagulant treatment to maintain autologous vein grafts for femoropopliteal atherosclerosis. Arch Surg 127:1112-1115, 1992.

28. Holm J, Arfvidsson B, Jivegard L, et al: Chronic lower limb ischaemia: A prospective randomised controlled study comparing the 1-year results of vascular surgery and percutaneous transluminal angioplasty (PTA). Eur J Vasc Surg 5:517-522, 1991.

29. Sarac TP, Huber TS, Back MR, et al: Warfarin improves the outcome of infrainguinal vein bypass grafting at high risk for failure. J Vasc Surg 28:446-457, 1998.

30. Johnson WC, Williford WO: Benefits, morbidity, and mortality associated with long-term administration of oral anticoagulant therapy to patients with peripheral arterial bypass procedures: A prospective randomized study. J Vasc Surg 35:413-421, 2002.

31. Clagett GP, Sobel M, Jackson MR, et al: Antithrombotic therapy in peripheral arterial occlusive disease: The Seventh ACCP Conference on Antithrombotic and Thrombolytic Therapy. Chest 126(3 Suppl): 609S-626S, 2004.

32. Warkentin TE, Elavathil LJ, Hayward CP, et al: The pathogenesis of venous limb gangrene associated with heparin-induced thrombocytopenia. Ann Intern Med 127:804-812, 1997.

33. Kaplan KL: Direct thrombin inhibitors. Expert Opin Pharmacother 4:653-666, 2003.

34. Bauer KA: Selective inhibition of coagulation factors: Advances in antithrombotic therapy. Semin Thromb Hemost 28(Suppl 2):15-24, 2002.

35. Weitz JI, Crowther M: Direct thrombin inhibitors. Thromb Res 106:V275-V284, 2002.

36. Stone SR, Hofsteenge J: Kinetics of the inhibition of thrombin by hirudin. Biochemistry 25:4622-4628, 1986.

37. Weitz J: Orally active direct thrombin inhibitors. Semin Vasc Med 3:131-138, 2003.

38. Bauer KA: Fondaparinux: A new synthetic and selective inhibitor of factor Xa. Best Pract Res Clin Haematol 17:89-104, 2004.

39. Eriksson BI, Lassen MR: Duration of prophylaxis against venous thromboembolism with fondaparinux after hip fracture surgery: A multicenter, randomized, placebo-controlled, double-blind study. Arch Intern Med 163:1337-1342, 2003.

40. Eriksson BI, Dahl OE: Prevention of venous thromboembolism following orthopaedic surgery: Clinical potential of direct thrombin inhibitors. Drugs 64:577-595, 2004.

41. Bauer KA, Eriksson BI, Lassen MR, et al: Fondaparinux compared with enoxaparin for the prevention of venous thromboembolism after elective major knee surgery. N Engl J Med 345:1305-1310, 2001.

42. Turpie AG, Eriksson BI, Lassen MR, Bauer KA: A meta-analysis of fondaparinux versus enoxaparin in the prevention of venous thromboembolism after major orthopaedic surgery. J South Orthop Assoc 11:182-188, 2002.

43. Treatment of proximal deep vein thrombosis with a novel synthetic compound (SR90107A/ORG31540) with pure anti-factor Xa activity: A phase II evaluation. The Rembrandt Investigators. Circulation 102: 2726-2731, 2000.

44. Coussement PK, Bassand JP, Convens C, et al: A synthetic factor-Xa inhibitor (ORG31540/SR9017A) as an adjunct to fibrinolysis in acute myocardial infarction. The PENTALYSE study. Eur Heart J 22:1716-1724, 2001.

45. Burch JW, Majerus PW: The role of prostaglandins in platelet function. Semin Hematol 16:196-207, 1979.

46. Burch JW, Stanford N, Majerus PW: Inhibition of platelet prostaglandin synthetase by oral aspirin. J Clin Invest 61:314-319, 1978.

47. Patrono C, Coller B, FitzGerald GA, et al: Platelet-active drugs: The relationships among dose, effectiveness, and side effects: The Seventh ACCP Conference on Antithrombotic and Thrombolytic Therapy. Chest 126(3 Suppl):234S-264S, 2004.

48. Lopez-Farre A, Caramelo C, Esteban A, et al: Effects of aspirin on platelet-neutrophil interactions: Role of nitric oxide and endothelin-1. Circulation 91:2080-2088, 1995.

49. Bolz SS, Pohl U: Indomethacin enhances endothelial NO release— evidence for a role of PGI$_2$ in the autocrine control of calcium-dependent autacoid production. Cardiovasc Res 36:437-444, 1997.

50. Farivar RS, Chobanian AV, Brecher P: Salicylate or aspirin inhibits the induction of the inducible nitric oxide synthase in rat cardiac fibroblasts. Circ Res 78:759-768, 1996.

51. Steer KA, Wallace TM, Bolton CH, Hartog M: Aspirin protects low density lipoprotein from oxidative modification. Heart 77:333-337, 1997.

52. Husain S, Andrews NP, Mulcahy D, et al: Aspirin improves endothelial dysfunction in atherosclerosis. Circulation 97:716-720, 1998.

53. Bradlow BA, Chetty N: Dosage frequency for suppression of platelet function by low dose aspirin therapy. Thromb Res 27:99-110, 1982.

54. Becker RC, Fintel DJ, Green D (eds): Antithrombotic Therapy, 2nd ed. West Islip, NY, Professional Communications, 2002, pp 63-76.

55. Physician's health study: Aspirin and primary prevention of coronary heart disease. N Engl J Med 321:1825-1828, 1989.

56. Peto R, Gray R, Collins R, et al: Randomised trial of prophylactic daily aspirin in British male doctors. BMJ (Clin Res Ed) 296:313-316, 1988.

57. Collaborative overview of randomised trials of antiplatelet therapy. I. Prevention of death, myocardial infarction, and stroke by prolonged antiplatelet therapy in various categories of patients. Antiplatelet Trialists' Collaboration. BMJ 308:81-106, 1994.

58. Hansson L, Zanchetti A, Carruthers SG, et al: Effects of intensive blood-pressure lowering and low-dose aspirin in patients with hypertension: Principal results of the Hypertension Optimal Treatment (HOT) randomised trial. HOT Study Group. Lancet 351:1755-1762, 1998.

59. Thrombosis Prevention Trial: Randomised trial of low-intensity oral anticoagulation with warfarin and low-dose aspirin in the primary prevention of ischaemic heart disease in men at increased risk. The Medical Research Council's General Practice Research Framework. Lancet 351:233-241, 1998.

60. Tendera M, Wojakowski W: Role of antiplatelet drugs in the prevention of cardiovascular events. Thromb Res 110:355-359, 2003.

61. Antithrombotic Trialists' Collaboration: Collaborative meta-analysis of randomised trials of antiplatelet therapy for prevention of death, myocardial infarction, and stroke in high risk patients. BMJ 324:71-86, 2002.

62. Elwood P: Gastric safety and enteric-coated aspirin. Lancet 349:432, 1997.

63. Kam PC, Nethery CM: The thienopyridine derivatives (platelet adenosine diphosphate receptor antagonists), pharmacology and clinical developments. Anaesthesia 58:28-35, 2003.

64. Jacobson AK: Platelet ADP receptor antagonists: Ticlopidine and clopidogrel. Best Pract Res Clin Haematol 17:55-64, 2004.

65. Janzon L: The STIMS trial: The ticlopidine experience and its clinical applications. Swedish Ticlopidine Multicenter Study. Vasc Med 1:141-143, 1996.

66. Hiatt WR: Pharmacologic therapy for peripheral arterial disease and claudication. J Vasc Surg 36:1283-1291, 2002.

67. Bennett CL, Weinberg PD, Rozenberg-Ben-Dror K, et al: Thrombotic thrombocytopenic purpura associated with ticlopidine: A review of 60 cases. Ann Intern Med 128:541-544, 1998.

68. Hankey GJ, Sudlow CL, Dunbabin DW: Thienopyridine derivatives (ticlopidine, clopidogrel) versus aspirin for preventing stroke and other serious vascular events in high vascular risk patients. Cochrane Database Syst Rev 2000(2):CD001246, 2000.

69. Hass WK, Easton JD, Adams HP Jr, et al: A randomized trial comparing ticlopidine hydrochloride with aspirin for the prevention of stroke in high-risk patients. Ticlopidine Aspirin Stroke Study Group. N Engl J Med 321:501-507, 1989.

70. A randomised, blinded, trial of clopidogrel versus aspirin in patients at risk of ischaemic events (CAPRIE). CAPRIE Steering Committee. Lancet 348:1329-1339, 1996.

71. Frangos SG, Chen AH, Sumpio B: Vascular drugs in the new millennium. J Am Coll Surg 191:76-92, 2000.

72. Barer D: CAPRIE trial. Lancet 349:355-356, 1997.

73. Becquemin JP: Effect of ticlopidine on the long-term patency of saphenous-vein bypass grafts in the legs. Etude de la Ticlopidine apres Pontage Femoro-Poplite and the Association Universitaire de Recherche en Chirurgie. N Engl J Med 337:1726-1731, 1997.

74. Hankey GJ: Current oral antiplatelet agents to prevent atherothrombosis. Cerebrovasc Dis 11(Suppl 2):11-17, 2001.

75. Bennett CL, Connors JM, Carwile JM, et al: Thrombotic thrombocytopenic purpura associated with clopidogrel. N Engl J Med 342: 1773-1777, 2000.

76. Bhatt DL, Topol EJ: Current role of platelet glycoprotein IIb/IIIa inhibitors in acute coronary syndromes. JAMA 284:1549-1558, 2000.

77. Chun R, Orser BA, Madan M: Platelet glycoprotein IIb/IIIa inhibitors: Overview and implications for the anesthesiologist. Anesth Analg 95:879-888, 2002.

78. Madan M, Kereiakes DJ, Hermiller JB, et al: Efficacy of abciximab readministration in coronary intervention. Am J Cardiol 85:435-440, 2000.

79. Rosove MH: Platelet glycoprotein IIb/IIIa inhibitors. Best Pract Res Clin Haematol 17:65-76, 2004.

80. Phillips DR, Scarborough RM: Clinical pharmacology of eptifibatide. Am J Cardiol 80:11B-20B, 1997.

81. Harrington RA, Kleiman NS, Kottke-Marchant K, et al: Immediate and reversible platelet inhibition after intravenous administration of a peptide glycoprotein IIb/IIIa inhibitor during percutaneous coronary intervention. Am J Cardiol 76:1222-1227, 1995.

82. Becker RC: The scientific basis for combined platelet and thrombin-directed pharmacotherapy in acute coronary syndromes. J Invasive Cardiol 12(Suppl E):E19-E24, discussion E25-E28, 2000.

83. Tcheng JE: Glycoprotein IIb/IIIa receptor inhibitors: Putting the EPIC, IMPACT II, RESTORE, and EPILOG trials into perspective. Am J Cardiol 78:35-40, 1996.

84. Topol EJ: Novel antithrombotic approaches to coronary artery disease. Am J Cardiol 75:27B-33B, 1995.

85. Harrington RA, Becker RC, Ezekowitz M, et al: Antithrombotic therapy for coronary artery disease: The Seventh ACCP Conference on Antithrombotic and Thrombolytic Therapy. Chest 126(Suppl 3): 513S-548S, 2004.

86. Angelkort B, Boateng K, Maurin N: Blood fluidity and coagulation phenomena in chronic arterial occlusive disease. J Int Med Res 8:242-246, 1980.

87. Angelkort B, Maurin N, Boateng K: Influence of pentoxifylline on erythrocyte deformability in peripheral occlusive arterial disease. Curr Med Res Opin 6:255-258, 1979.

88. Johnson WC, Sentissi JM, Baldwin D, et al: Treatment of claudication with pentoxifylline: Are benefits related to improvement in viscosity? J Vasc Surg 6:211-216, 1987.

89. Hood SC, Moher D, Barber GG: Management of intermittent claudication with pentoxifylline: Meta-analysis of randomized controlled trials. CMAJ 155:1053-1059, 1996.

90. Di Perri T, Guerrini M: Placebo controlled double blind study with pentoxifylline of walking performance in patients with intermittent claudication. Angiology 34:40-45, 1983.

91. Roekaerts F, Deleers L: Trental 400 in the treatment of intermittent claudication: Results of long-term, placebo-controlled administration. Angiology 35:396-406, 1984.

92. Strano A, Davi G, Avellone G, et al: Double-blind, crossover study of the clinical efficacy and the hemorheological effects of pentoxifylline in patients with occlusive arterial disease of the lower limbs. Angiology 35:459-466, 1984.

93. Lindgarde F, Jelnes R, Bjorkman H, et al: Conservative drug treatment in patients with moderately severe chronic occlusive peripheral arterial disease. Scandinavian Study Group. Circulation 80:1549-1556, 1989.

94. Porter JM, Cutler BS, Lee BY, et al: Pentoxifylline efficacy in the treatment of intermittent claudication: Multicenter controlled double-blind trial with objective assessment of chronic occlusive arterial disease patients. Am Heart J 104:66-72, 1982.

95. Gallus AS, Gleadow F, Dupont P, et al: Intermittent claudication: A double-blind crossover trial of pentoxifylline. Aust N Z J Med 15: 402-409, 1985.

96. Perhoniemi V, Salmenkivi K, Sundberg J, et al: Effects of flunarizine and pentoxifylline on walking distance and blood rheology in claudication. Angiology 35:366-372, 1984.

97. Reilly DT, Quinton DN, Barrie WW: A controlled trial of pentoxifylline (Trental 400) in intermittent claudication: Clinical, haemostatic and rheological effects. N Z Med J 100:445-447, 1987.

98. Tonak J, Knecht H, Groitl H: [Treatment of circulation disorders with pentoxifylline: A double-blind study with Trental.] Med Monatsschr 31:467-472, 1977.

99. Dawson DL, Cutler BS, Meissner MH, et al: Cilostazol has beneficial effects in treatment of intermittent claudication: Results from a multicenter, randomized, prospective, double-blind trial. Circulation 98:678-686, 1998.

100. Beebe HG, Dawson DL, Cutler BS, et al: A new pharmacological treatment for intermittent claudication: Results of a randomized, multicenter trial. Arch Intern Med 159:2041-2050, 1999.

101. Money SR, Herd JA, Isaacsohn JL, et al: Effect of cilostazol on walking distances in patients with intermittent claudication caused by peripheral vascular disease. J Vasc Surg 27:267-274; discussion 274-275, 1998.

102. Waybill MM, Waybill PN: Contrast media-induced nephrotoxicity: Identification of patients at risk and algorithms for prevention. J Vasc Interv Radiol 12:3-9, 2001.

103. Agrawal M, Stouffer GA: Cardiology grand rounds from the University of North Carolina at Chapel Hill: Contrast induced nephropathy after angiography. Am J Med Sci 323:252-258, 2002.

104. Madyoon H, Croushore L, Weaver D, Mathur V: Use of fenoldopam to prevent radiocontrast nephropathy in high-risk patients. Catheter Cardiovasc Interv 53:341-345, 2001.

105. Murphy SW, Barrett BJ, Parfrey PS: Contrast nephropathy. J Am Soc Nephrol 11:177-182, 2000.

106. Cox CD, Tsikouris JP: Preventing contrast nephropathy: What is the best strategy? A review of the literature. J Clin Pharmacol 44:327-337, 2004.

107. Brezis M, Rosen S: Hypoxia of the renal medulla—its implications for disease. N Engl J Med 332:647-655, 1995.

108. Rudnick MR, Goldfarb S, Wexler L, et al: Nephrotoxicity of ionic and nonionic contrast media in 1196 patients: A randomized trial. The Iohexol Cooperative Study. Kidney Int 47:254-261, 1995.

109. Barrett BJ, Carlisle EJ: Metaanalysis of the relative nephrotoxicity of high- and low-osmolality iodinated contrast media. Radiology 188:171-178, 1993.

110. Chalmers N, Jackson RW: Comparison of iodixanol and iohexol in renal impairment. Br J Radiol 72:701-703, 1999.

111. Solomon R, Werner C, Mann D, et al: Effects of saline, mannitol, and furosemide to prevent acute decreases in renal function induced by radiocontrast agents. N Engl J Med 331:1416-1420, 1994.

112. Trivedi HS, Moore H, Nasr S, et al: A randomized prospective trial to assess the role of saline hydration on the development of contrast nephrotoxicity. Nephron Clin Pract 93:C29-C34, 2003.

113. Ide JM, Lancelot E, Pines E, Corot C: Prophylaxis of iodinated contrast media-induced nephropathy: A pharmacological point of view. Invest Radiol 39:155-170, 2004.

114. Morcos SK: Prevention of contrast media nephrotoxicity—the story so far. Clin Radiol 59:381-389, 2004.

115. Tepel M, van der Giet M, Schwarzfeld C, et al: Prevention of radiographic-contrast-agent-induced reductions in renal function by acetylcysteine. N Engl J Med 343:180-184, 2000.

116. Kay J, Chow WH, Chan TM, et al: Acetylcysteine for prevention of acute deterioration of renal function following elective coronary angiography and intervention: A randomized controlled trial. JAMA 289:553-558, 2003.

117. Diaz-Sandoval LJ, Kosowsky BD, Losordo DW: Acetylcysteine to prevent angiography-related renal tissue injury (the APART trial). Am J Cardiol 89:356-358, 2002.

118. Durham JD, Caputo C, Dokko J, et al: A randomized controlled trial of N-acetylcysteine to prevent contrast nephropathy in cardiac angiography. Kidney Int 62:2202-2207, 2002.

119. Hoffmann U, Fischereder M, Kruger B, et al: The value of N-acetylcysteine in the prevention of radiocontrast agent-induced nephropathy seems questionable. J Am Soc Nephrol 15:407-410, 2004.

120. Kini AS, Mitre CA, Kim M, et al: A protocol for prevention of radiographic contrast nephropathy during percutaneous coronary intervention: Effect of selective dopamine receptor agonist fenoldopam. Catheter Cardiovasc Interv 55:169-173, 2002.

121. Chamsuddin AA, Kowalik KJ, Bjarnason H, et al: Using a dopamine type 1A receptor agonist in high-risk patients to ameliorate contrast-associated nephropathy. AJR Am J Roentgenol 179:591-596, 2002.

122. Kini AA, Sharma SK: Managing the high-risk patient: Experience with fenoldopam, a selective dopamine receptor agonist, in prevention of radiocontrast nephropathy during percutaneous coronary intervention. Rev Cardiovasc Med 2(Suppl 1):S19-S25, 2001.

123. Madyoon H: Clinical experience with the use of fenoldopam for prevention of radiocontrast nephropathy in high-risk patients. Rev Cardiovasc Med 2(Suppl 1):S26-S30, 2001.

124. Allaqaband S, Tumuluri R, Malik AM, et al: Prospective randomized study of N-acetylcysteine, fenoldopam, and saline for prevention of radiocontrast-induced nephropathy. Catheter Cardiovasc Interv 57:279-283, 2002.

125. Stone GW, McCullough PA, Tumlin JA, et al: Fenoldopam mesylate for the prevention of contrast-induced nephropathy: A randomized controlled trial. JAMA 290:2284-2291, 2003.

126. Oldroyd SD, Fang L, Haylor JL, et al: Effects of adenosine receptor antagonists on the responses to contrast media in the isolated rat kidney. Clin Sci (Lond) 98:303-311, 2000.

127. Arakawa K, Suzuki H, Naitoh M, et al: Role of adenosine in the renal responses to contrast medium. Kidney Int 49:1199-1206, 1996.

128. Katholi RE, Taylor GJ, McCann WP, et al: Nephrotoxicity from contrast media: Attenuation with theophylline. Radiology 195:17-22, 1995.

129. Erley CM, Duda SH, Rehfuss D, et al: Prevention of radiocontrast-media-induced nephropathy in patients with pre-existing renal insufficiency by hydration in combination with the adenosine antagonist theophylline. Nephrol Dial Transplant 14:1146-1149, 1999.

130. Koch JA, Plum J, Grabensee B, Modder U: Prostaglandin E_1: A new agent for the prevention of renal dysfunction in high risk patients caused by radiocontrast media? PGE_1 Study Group. Nephrol Dial Transplant 15:43-49, 2000.

131. Hermann M, Schulz E, Ruschitzka F, Muller GA: Preventive strategies in endothelin-induced renal failure. Kidney Int Suppl 67:S202-S204, 1998.

132. Wang A, Holcslaw T, Bashore TM, et al: Exacerbation of radiocontrast nephrotoxicity by endothelin receptor antagonism. Kidney Int 57:1675-1680, 2000.

133. Wang YX, Jia YF, Chen KM, Morcos SK: Radiographic contrast media induced nephropathy: Experimental observations and the protective effect of calcium channel blockers. Br J Radiol 74:1103-1108, 2001.

134. Neumayer HH, Junge W, Kufner A, Wenning A: Prevention of radiocontrast-media-induced nephrotoxicity by the calcium channel blocker nitrendipine: A prospective randomised clinical trial. Nephrol Dial Transplant 4:1030-1036, 1989.

135. Carraro M, Mancini W, Artero M, et al: Dose effect of nitrendipine on urinary enzymes and microproteins following non-ionic radiocontrast administration. Nephrol Dial Transplant 11:444-448, 1996.

136. Rodicio JL, Morales JM, Alcazar JM, Ruilope LM: Calcium antagonists and renal protection. J Hypertens Suppl 11:S49-S53, 1993.

137. Spangberg-Viklund B, Berglund J, Nikonoff T, et al: Does prophylactic treatment with felodipine, a calcium antagonist, prevent low-osmolar contrast-induced renal dysfunction in hydrated diabetic and nondiabetic patients with normal or moderately reduced renal function? Scand J Urol Nephrol 30:63-68, 1996.

138. Esnault VL: Radiocontrast media-induced nephrotoxicity in patients with renal failure: Rationale for a new double-blind, prospective, randomized trial testing calcium channel antagonists. Nephrol Dial Transplant 17:1362-1364, 2002.

139. Hans SS, Hans BA, Dhillon R, et al: Effect of dopamine on renal function after arteriography in patients with pre-existing renal insufficiency. Am Surg 64:432-436, 1998.

140. Kapoor A, Sinha N, Sharma RK, et al: Use of dopamine in prevention of contrast induced acute renal failure—a randomised study. Int J Cardiol 53:233-236, 1996.

141. Gare M, Haviv YS, Ben-Yehuda A, et al: The renal effect of low-dose dopamine in high-risk patients undergoing coronary angiography. J Am Coll Cardiol 34:1682-1688, 1999.

142. Abizaid AS, Clark CE, Mintz GS, et al: Effects of dopamine and aminophylline on contrast-induced acute renal failure after coronary angioplasty in patients with preexisting renal insufficiency. Am J Cardiol 83:260-263, A5, 1999.

143. Weisberg LS, Kurnik PB, Kurnik BR: Risk of radiocontrast nephropathy in patients with and without diabetes mellitus. Kidney Int 45:259-265, 1994.

144. Downs JR, Clearfield M, Weis S, et al: Primary prevention of acute coronary events with lovastatin in men and women with average cholesterol levels: Results of AFCAPS/TexCAPS. Air Force/Texas Coronary Atherosclerosis Prevention Study. JAMA 279:1615-1622, 1998.

145. Randomised trial of cholesterol lowering in 4444 patients with coronary heart disease: The Scandinavian Simvastatin Survival Study (4S). Lancet 344:1383-1389, 1994.

146. West of Scotland Coronary Prevention Study: Identification of high-risk groups and comparison with other cardiovascular intervention trials. Lancet 348:1339-1342, 1996.

147. Prevention of cardiovascular events and death with pravastatin in patients with coronary heart disease and a broad range of initial cholesterol levels. The Long-Term Intervention with Pravastatin in Ischaemic Disease (LIPID) Study Group. N Engl J Med 339:1349-1357, 1998.

148. Sacks FM, Pfeffer MA, Moye, LA, et al: The effect of pravastatin on coronary events after myocardial infarction in patients with average cholesterol levels. Cholesterol and Recurrent Events Trial investigators. N Engl J Med 335:1001-1009, 1996.

149. Mason JC: Statins and their role in vascular protection. Clin Sci (Lond) 105:251-266, 2003.

150. Shepherd J, Cobbe SM, Ford I, et al: Prevention of coronary heart disease with pravastatin in men with hypercholesterolemia. West of Scotland Coronary Prevention Study Group. N Engl J Med 333:1301-1307, 1995.

151. LaRosa JC, He J, Vupputuri S: Effect of statins on risk of coronary disease: A meta-analysis of randomized controlled trials. JAMA 282:2340-2346, 1999.

152. Ong HT: Protecting the heart: A practical review of the statin studies. Med Gen Med 4:1, 2002.

153. White HD, Simes RJ, Anderson NE, et al: Pravastatin therapy and the risk of stroke. N Engl J Med 343:317-326, 2000.

154. Collins R, et al: Effects of cholesterol-lowering with simvastatin on stroke and other major vascular events in 20,536 people with cerebrovascular disease or other high-risk conditions. Lancet 363:757-767, 2004.

155. O'Driscoll G, Green D, Taylor RR: Simvastatin, an HMG-coenzyme A reductase inhibitor, improves endothelial function within 1 month. Circulation 95:1126-1131, 1997.

156. Tsunekawa T, Hayashi T, Kano H, et al: Cerivastatin, a hydroxymethylglutaryl coenzyme A reductase inhibitor, improves endothelial function in elderly diabetic patients within 3 days. Circulation 104:376-379, 2001.

157. Liao JK: Beyond lipid lowering: The role of statins in vascular protection. Int J Cardiol 86:5-18, 2002.

158. Rosenson RS, Tangney CC: Antiatherothrombotic properties of statins: Implications for cardiovascular event reduction. JAMA 279:1643-1650, 1998.

159. Farmer JA, Gotto AM Jr: The Heart Protection Study: Expanding the boundaries for high-risk coronary disease prevention. Am J Cardiol 92:3i-9i, 2003.

160. Durazzo AE, Machado FS, Ikeoka DT, et al: Reduction in cardiovascular events after vascular surgery with atorvastatin: A randomized trial. J Vasc Surg 39:967-975, discussion 975-976, 2004.

161. Schillinger M, Exner M, Mlekusch W, et al: Statin therapy improves cardiovascular outcome of patients with peripheral artery disease. Eur Heart J 25:742-748, 2004.

162. Poldermans D, Bax JJ, Kertai MD, et al: Statins are associated with a reduced incidence of perioperative mortality in patients undergoing major noncardiac vascular surgery. Circulation 107:1848-1851, 2003.

163. Abbruzzese TA, Havens J, Belkin M, et al: Statin therapy is associated with improved patency of autogenous infrainguinal bypass grafts. J Vasc Surg 39:1178-1185, 2004.

164. Federman DG, Hussain F, Walters AB: Fatal rhabdomyolysis caused by lipid-lowering therapy. South Med J 94:1023-1026, 2001.

165. de Denus S, Spinler SA, Miller K, Peterson AM: Statins and liver toxicity: A meta-analysis. Pharmacotherapy 24:584-591, 2004.

166. Omar MA, Wilson JP, Cox TS: Rhabdomyolysis and HMG-CoA reductase inhibitors. Ann Pharmacother 35:1096-1107, 2001.

167. Thompson PD, Clarkson P, Karas RH: Statin-associated myopathy. JAMA 289:1681-1690, 2003.

Questions

1. What is the most common serious side effect associated with statin therapy?
   - (a) Rhabdomyolysis
   - (b) Liver failure
   - (c) Renal failure
   - (d) Stroke

2. Which of these therapies has clearly been shown to prevent contrast-induced nephropathy?
   - (a) High-osmolar contrast agents
   - (b) Intravenous hydration
   - (c) Fenoldopam
   - (d) Theophylline
   - (e) Lasix

3. Which agent has been associated with severe neutropenia?
   - (a) Clopidogrel
   - (b) Ticlopidine
   - (c) Tirofiban
   - (d) Hirudin

4. True or false: Higher-dose aspirin therapy (325 mg or more) has been shown to be more effective than low-dose therapy (81 mg) in providing cardiovascular protection.

5. Which of the following is not a documented side effect of heparin therapy?
   - (a) Hypothyroidism
   - (b) Osteoporosis
   - (c) Priapism
   - (d) Skin lesions
   - (e) Cushing's syndrome

6. Which antigen is thought to be associated with the development of heparin-induced thrombocytopenia?
   - (a) Platelet factor 4
   - (b) Von Willebrand's factor
   - (c) Factor X
   - (d) Platelet ADP receptor

7. Patients with a history of fish allergy may have an increased risk of reaction to which of the following?
   - (a) Protamine
   - (b) Heparin
   - (c) Argatroban
   - (d) Tirofiban
   - (e) Clopidogrel

8. True or false: Argatroban, being renally excreted, needs to be dosed carefully in patients with renal failure.

9. Which of the following has clear indications for use in the treatment of intermittent claudication?
   - (a) Ticlopidine
   - (b) Clopidogrel
   - (c) Cilostazol
   - (d) Pentoxifylline
   - (e) Tirofiban

10. Aspirin exerts its anti-inflammatory effects via which of the following?
    - (a) Cyclooxygenase-1
    - (b) Cyclooxygenase-2
    - (c) Platelet factor 4
    - (d) Adenosine diphosphate

Answers

1. a	2. b	3. b	4. false	5. e
6. a	7. a	8. false	9. c	10. a

Hugh A. Gelabert

Primary Arterial Infections and Antibiotic Prophylaxis

Primary Arterial Infections

In general terms, a primary arterial infection is a condition in which an infectious agent invades and destroys the wall of an artery, resulting in disruption and pseudoaneurysm formation. Such infections may be difficult to recognize and manage. The essential feature is the destruction of a major artery by an infectious process; the secondary manifestations are aneurysm formation, embolization, and hemorrhage in the face of systemic septic illness. The presentation varies from indolent to cataclysmic. Successful management requires familiarity with the processes involved and the ability to make prompt decisions at the time of surgery. The goal of this chapter is to review primary arterial infections in terms of their pathophysiology, diagnosis, and treatment.

HISTORICAL PERSPECTIVE

One of the earliest reports of arterial infection was offered by Paré in the 16th century. He described suture ligation and excision of vessels that had become infected after battle injuries. This early treatment became a mainstay of therapy and, in combination with the modern techniques of vessel substitution, remains so today. Rokitansky and others recognized, in the 19th century, an association between arterial infection and aneurysm formation.[1,2] Osler, in 1885, presented the first comprehensive description of this relationship.[3] In addressing the Royal College of Physicians, he described a 30-year-old man who had died from fever, chills, and pneumonia. At autopsy, the patient was found to have endocarditis involving the aortic valve, as well as multiple aneurysms of the thoracic aorta. Based on carefully described pathologic findings, Osler proposed a causal relationship between infection of the aortic wall and subsequent aneurysm formation. Because of a similarity between the beaded appearance of these aneurysms and fungal vegetations, he introduced the term *mycotic aneurysm* and thus the concept of primary arterial infection.

DEFINITIONS

There is no universally accepted definition of primary arterial infection. Moreover, there continues to be confusion regarding the general classification of native arterial infections. Although the term *mycotic aneurysm* initially signified an infected aneurysm found in association with bacterial endocarditis, it has come to denote an infected aneurysm of any type. Additionally, the majority of the published literature has focused on specific subtypes of arterial infections—namely, aneurysmal dilatation associated with arterial infection and illnesses resulting from infection of traumatic pseudoaneurysms. Another problem is that there is considerable disparity among the several definitions that have been proposed. Finally, it should be recognized that, with the exception of a secondarily infected arterial aneurysm, most of these lesions are actually infected pseudoaneurysms. Most arise by means of the local destruction of the arterial wall and the fibrous encapsulation of an expanding hematoma; thus, these lesions do not have the histologic components of an arterial wall.

In this chapter, *primary arterial infection* is defined as follows: the direct invasion or extension of a specific pathogen into the intima, media, or adventitia of a native artery, irrespective of the preexisting state of the underlying artery or source of the pathogen. The term *mycotic aneurysm* is used to denote both true aneurysms and false aneurysms.

PATHOGENESIS

Five basic mechanisms have been implicated in the development of primary arterial infections. They may broadly be grouped as (1) mycotic aneurysms, (2) microbial arteritis with aneurysm formation, (3) infected aneurysms, (4) mechanical injury with contamination, and (5) arteritis from contiguous spread.

Mycotic Aneurysms

Osler, in coining the term *mycotic aneurysm*, both named the condition and described what would be the most prevalent cause of primary arterial infection in the preantibiotic era. As he described it, the true mycotic aneurysm is limited to the unique clinical condition characterized by bacterial endocarditis with septic embolization from valvular vegetations. These septic emboli lodge within the arterial wall, where a suppurative infection develops. The arterial wall is destroyed by the infection, and the resultant pseudoaneurysm is recognized as a mycotic aneurysm.

Considerable confusion has arisen because the term *mycotic aneurysm* has been applied to various types of infected aneurysms. Crane attempted to classify mycotic aneurysms as primary and secondary types.[4] He introduced the term *primary mycotic aneurysm* to refer to infected aortic aneurysms not associated with endocarditis or an infectious focus; *secondary* types were those that formed as a result of preceding endocarditis. Ponfick[5] and Eppinger[6] were among the first to characterize the anatomic features of these aneurysms pathologically. Ponfick proposed that the initial insult to the arterial wall was a mechanical injury inflicted by the embolization of septic material.[5] Eppinger in 1887 provided further support for the theory of septic emboli by culturing the same strain of bacteria from both vegetative lesions and the wall of an aneurysm in a patient with endocarditis. He applied the term *embolomycotic* to describe the combination of infectious and embolic components that led to the formation of mycotic aneurysms.[6]

Microbial Arteritis with Aneurysm Formation

The second mechanism of arterial infection involves the microbial "seeding" of arteries during an episode of bacteremia. Microbial arteritis with aneurysm formation occurs when a normal or atherosclerotic artery becomes infected and the weakened artery becomes aneurysmal.

In 1906, the German pathologist Weisel described distinctive pathologic changes in arterial walls that occurred during the course of an infectious disease but were not of embolic origin.[7] Lewis and Schrager[8] and Cathcart[9] presented case reports of infected peripheral aneurysms that developed in normal arteries of patients with osteomyelitis and typhoid fever, respectively. Despite these reports, nearly 30 years passed before consideration was given to the mechanism by which bacteremia led to arterial infection. Crane, in 1937, described an infected aneurysm in a patient with hypoplasia of the aorta but no associated bacterial endocarditis or other identifiable source of infection.[4] He proposed that the combination of the "force of the blood stream" and abnormal development of the aorta allowed bacteria to invade that portion of the aorta. This resulted in an arterial infection, disruption of the aortic wall, and an infected pseudoaneurysm. Revell extended the concept of aortic bacterial seeding one step further and proposed that the route of infection was through the aortic vasa vasorum.[10] Hawkins and Yeager, acknowledging the resistance of arterial intima to infection, suggested that

an intimal defect such as that produced by arteriosclerosis allowed bacterial localization and infection.[11]

Infected Aneurysms

The term *infected aneurysm* refers to an infection of a preexisting aneurysm, most often by hematogenous microbiologic seeding of the aneurysm. The original aneurysm is most commonly atherosclerotic; however, it may also be the result of trauma or arteritis. The diseased artery becomes host to bacterial pathogens when these lodge within the intramural thrombus and arteriosclerotic intima. Although some of these infected aneurysms may proceed to rapid expansion and rupture, many appear to remain quiescent. These are often discovered in the course of incidental microbiologic investigation of aneurysm contents.

Mechanical Injury with Contamination

Another cause of arterial infections is mechanical arterial injury by contaminated instruments. This type of infection can occur after an inadvertent arterial puncture with a contaminated needle in a drug abuser, as an accidental contamination during radiologic procedures, during placement of hemodynamic monitoring catheters, or as a result of traumatic injury. The combination of mechanical disruption of the intima and seeding of the arterial lesion with pathogenic bacteria leads to the formation of suppurative arteritis and destroys a portion of the arterial wall. This subsequently becomes an infected arterial pseudoaneurysm.

Arteritis from Contiguous Spread

Arterial infections can also develop through the spread of infection from a contiguous focus. Contiguous infections that have been recognized as potential sources of bacteria include lesions such as osteomyelitis, infected lymph nodes, tuberculous lymph nodes, and abscesses from narcotic injection.[12] Bacteria and, less commonly, mycobacteria or fungi invade the artery either by direct extension or via lymphatics. They subsequently produce a necrotizing invasive infection of the arterial wall, with eventual destruction of the wall. This process, depending on the rate of progression, leads to either pseudoaneurysm formation or free arterial rupture.

Other Forms of Arterial Infection

There are three other, less common forms of infected aneurysms: syphilitic aortitis, true fungal aneurysms, and primary (spontaneous) aortoenteric fistulas. Because of significant differences in the pathogens and pathogenesis of these lesions, they merit separate discussion.

Syphilitic aneurysms are a rarely encountered complication of advanced syphilis. These lesions occur in approximately 10% of patients with the tertiary form of the disease.[13] These aneurysms commonly arise in the ascending aorta, frequently involve the aortic valve, and are secondary to treponemal invasion of the vasa vasorum. The reasons why *Treponema* prefers this portion of the aorta remain unclear. After spirochete penetration, an infiltrate develops within the vessel wall consisting of plasma cells, epidermal cells, and giant cells. This infiltrate results in destruction of the elastic and muscular components of the tunica media, replacement of the normal wall with fibrous tissue, and dilatation and subsequent formation of saccular aneurysms.

Fungal arterial infections are also extremely rare and occur most often in patients who are immunosuppressed. Common risk factors include diabetes, immunosuppressive medications, and chronic hematologic disorders such as leukemia or lymphoma. The species most often implicated are *Histoplasma capsulatum*, *Aspergillus fumigatus*, *Candida albicans*, and *Penicillium* species. These lesions most commonly result from either colonization of a preexisting aneurysm or infection of a damaged artery.

Spontaneous or "primary" aortoenteric fistulas (AEFs) arise as a consequence of progressive aneurysmal enlargement, with gradual erosion into the adjacent gastrointestinal tract. The erosion is thought to be facilitated by the indurated, atherosclerotic artery pressing against a tethered portion of bowel. The most common location for this erosion is the third portion of the duodenum. In their 1951 review of a series of 16,633 autopsies, Hirst and Affeldt reported the incidence of this type of fistula to be 0.05%.[14] Because the majority of patients diagnosed with aortic aneurysms now undergo elective operation, the incidence of these lesions is thought to be considerably lower today. Patients with spontaneous AEFs may have an initial or "herald" bleed, which represents the initial hemorrhage of blood into the duodenum. It may stop for a while and then resume in a more prolonged and dramatic manner. Clot within the AEF is responsible for the intermittent nature of the bleeding episodes. This condition is considerably different from that associated with aortic graft infection, or secondary AEF. Secondary AEF is more common, more dangerous, and more difficult to manage.

Graft excision and remote reconstruction are the standard management of secondary AEF. In contrast, significant evidence exists that primary AEF can be managed by closure of the duodenal rent, débridement of the aorta, and in situ reconstruction with a Dacron prosthesis. The prerequisites of this approach are the absence of purulence at the fistula site, a small defect in the duodenum, and a relatively healthy patient. It should be noted that the management of primary aortic infections (mycotic aneurysms) is similar to that of primary AEF, in that the absence of gross infection along with adequate débridement may allow in situ graft reconstruction of the aorta.[15]

CAUSATIVE ORGANISMS

The organism most commonly associated with microbial aortitis is *Salmonella*. This is followed, in order of frequency, by *Streptococcus*, *Bacteroides*, *Arizona hinshawii*, *Escherichia coli*, and *Staphylococcus aureus*.[15] Studies that focus on subpopulations such as intravenous (IV) drug abusers or those with femoral mycotic aneurysms tend to identify a predominance of gram-positive bacteria such as staphylococci and streptococci, along with gram-negative organisms such as *E. coli* and *Pseudomonas* species.

The bacteriology of primary arterial infections has undergone considerable transformation since its original description in the mid-1800s (Fig. 10-1). Brown and colleagues and others suggested that the reason for this change is antibiotic selective pressure leading to bacterial adaptation.[16] Also, there has been a change in the relative incidence of pathogenic mechanisms with the more common use of invasive diagnostic modalities, as well as the increased illicit use of IV drugs. The majority of arterial infections during the preantibiotic era were true mycotic aneurysms; that is, they were related to bacterial endocarditis. The bacteriology of arterial infections during this period, therefore, was that of endocarditis. Stengal and Wolferth[17] in the 1920s and Revell[10] in the 1940s reported that the predominant organisms were nonhemolytic streptococci, staphylococci, and pneumococci. Magilligan and Quinn, in a 1986 review, subdivided 91 patients with bacterial endocarditis into two groups: those known to be IV drug abusers (36 patients) and those who were not (55 patients).[18] Of the first group, the most common organisms were *S. aureus* (36%), *Pseudomonas* species (16%), polymicrobial organisms (15%), *Streptococcus faecalis* (13%), and *Streptococcus viridans* (11%). Organisms in the second group (non-IV drug abusers) were *S. viridans* (22%), *S. aureus* (20%), *S. faecalis* (14%), and *Staphylococcus epidermidis* (11%). The declining incidence of rheumatic fever and the adoption of early, appropriate antibiotic treatment have resulted in a significant decrease in bacterial endocarditis. This in turn has resulted in a decline in the incidence of Oslerian mycotic aneurysms in recent decades.

Concurrent with the declining incidence of mycotic aneurysms has been an increase in various other types of primary arterial infections. Principal among these are microbial arteritis and infected aneurysms. This may be due, in part,

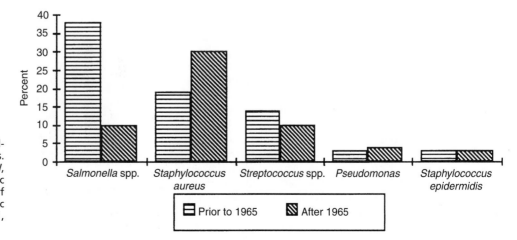

FIGURE 10–1 • Organisms cultured from mycotic aneurysms. (From Brown SL, Busuttil RW, Baker JD, et al: Bacteriologic and surgical determinants of survival in patients with mycotic aneurysms. J Vasc Surg 1:541, 1984.)

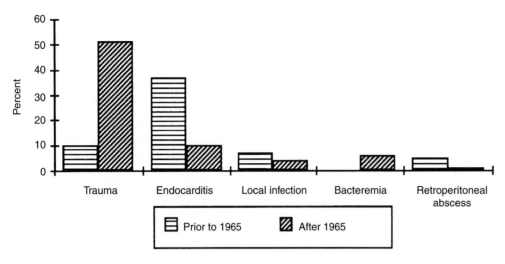

FIGURE 10–2 • Causes of mycotic aneurysms. (From Brown SL, Busuttil RW, Baker JD, et al: Bacteriologic and surgical determinants of survival in patients with mycotic aneurysms. J Vasc Surg 1:541, 1984.)

to the increasing age of the population and the simultaneous increase in the prevalence of atherosclerosis. The bacteriology of these arterial infections is different from that of mycotic aneurysms. The microorganisms most commonly associated with microbial arteritis are *Salmonella* species, *Staphylococcus* species, and *E. coli*. *Salmonella* species, in particular, have a striking propensity for invading diseased (atherosclerotic) aortas. In selected series, the involvement of *Salmonella* species has been reported to be as high as 50%. The most virulent species, *Salmonella choleraesuis* and *Salmonella typhimurium*, account for more than 60% of the reported cases of *Salmonella* arteritis.[19] Less commonly reported organisms associated with microbial arteritis include fungi and anaerobic organisms. Among the latter, *Bacteroides fragilis* has been reported in association with supraceliac aortic aneurysms.

The bacteriology of infected aneurysms is similar to that of both mycotic aneurysms and microbial arteritis. Despite this, some variation exists among reported series. Although Bennett and Cherry reported a 66% incidence of *Salmonella* infections,[20] Jarrett and associates described a predominance of gram-positive cocci (59%), with *S. aureus* representing 41%.[21] In two prospective studies of patients undergoing aneurysmectomy, cultures obtained from both the aneurysm wall and the bowel bag revealed a predominance of gram-positive organisms.[21,22] Both of these series are thought to represent cases of bacterial colonization. Despite the relative infrequency of gram-negative organisms observed in Jarrett's series, the distinction between gram-negative and gram-positive cultures proved clinically important. Patients with gram-negative bacteria demonstrated a greater likelihood of aortic rupture than did those with gram-positive organisms. Specifically, the rupture rate associated with gram-negative bacterial isolates was 84%, whereas that associated with gram-positive bacterial cultures was 10%.

According to Brown and associates, the most common infected aneurysms since 1965 are those that occur as a result of mechanical arterial injury with contamination of the vessel wall.[16] The organism most frequently implicated in this type of arterial infection is *S. aureus*, which Brown's group cultured in as many as 30% of cases. Reddy and associates, in a series of infected femoral false aneurysms, reported a 65% incidence of *S. aureus* and a 33% rate of polymicrobial infection.[23] Although arterial infections secondary to

contiguous spread are most commonly bacterial, mycobacterial and fungal infections also occur in these lesions. As with microbial arteritis, *Salmonella* organisms are the predominant pathogen, and *Staphylococcus* organisms are second in frequency (Fig. 10-2).

ANATOMIC DISTRIBUTION

The anatomic distribution of primary arterial infections varies somewhat, depending on the pathologic type. True mycotic aneurysms, owing to their embolic etiology, may occur in any artery larger than capillaries. They most often involve the larger muscular and elastic arteries. Both Lewis and Schrager[8] and Brown and colleagues,[16] in retrospective reviews, found the most common sites of infection to be the abdominal aorta and the femoral and superior mesenteric arteries (Fig. 10-3). The predisposition for aortic involvement is thought to be related to the higher incidence of underlying atherosclerotic aneurysms in this location compared with other anatomic sites.

Microbial arteritis with aneurysm formation occurs when a pathogen localizes at the site of an arterial lesion such as an atherosclerotic plaque. As one would anticipate, the arteries most commonly involved are the ones that demonstrate

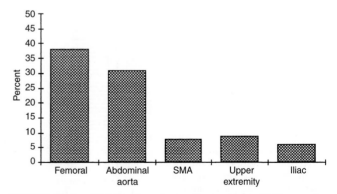

FIGURE 10–3 • Distribution of mycotic aneurysms. SMA, superior mesenteric artery. (From Brown SL, Busuttil RW, Baker JD, et al: Bacteriologic and surgical determinants of survival in patients with mycotic aneurysms. J Vasc Surg 1:541, 1984.)

advanced atherosclerotic changes—namely, the distal aorta and the femoral, iliac, and popliteal vessels. Infected aneurysms may, in theory, occur at any site within the arterial tree where there is a preexisting aneurysm. It is curious that all series in the literature demonstrate a strong propensity for involvement of the abdominal aorta. Involvement of this artery has been reported in up to 79% of cases. Whether this represents a tendency of the bacteria to infect aortic aneurysms or a study bias toward aortic aneurysms is not clear. Certainly, aortic aneurysms have been subjected to closer scrutiny than have other peripheral arterial aneurysms. This may account, in part, for this reported predilection.

Arterial infections due to mechanical injury with contamination most commonly involve arteries that have minimal soft tissue coverage. There are three main causes: accidental drug injection, vascular access, and trauma. Because these causes are related to the accessibility of the arteries and their superficial locations, these infections most commonly involve the femoral or brachial arteries. These locations also have an important impact on the presentation of these lesions, because femoral and brachial artery aneurysms are usually identified by the prominence, erythema, and tenderness of the aneurysm itself rather than by symptoms of arterial sepsis.

CLINICAL PRESENTATION

The most common clinical presentation in patients with primary arterial infection is fever, leukocytosis, and tenderness over the affected artery. Patients may have a wide range of signs and symptoms, depending on the pathophysiology, bacteriology, and location of the infected artery or arteries. Most components of the clinical presentation can be assigned to one of two general groups: signs and symptoms resulting from infection or bacteremia, and signs and symptoms occurring secondary to local arterial involvement or aneurysm formation. Night sweats, general malaise, arthralgias, and increased fatigability in conjunction with fever and leukocytosis occur as a consequence of the recurrent bacteremias associated with primary arterial infections. These are the signs of sepsis caused by the arterial infection. In certain patients, these signs may also be attributed to the primary source of bacteremia. In patients with true mycotic aneurysms, the clinical signs and symptoms of bacterial endocarditis may be difficult to distinguish from those associated with the arterial infection. Similarly, symptoms in patients with arterial lesions that developed by spread from a contiguous suppurative source may derive from either infectious focus.

The second group of signs and symptoms occurs as a result of inflammation and aneurysmal dilatation of the infected artery. Localized tenderness is the most readily recognized symptom related to the inflammatory destruction of the arterial wall. Characteristics such as abdominal or peripheral bruits, neurologic defects from nerve compression, or pulsatile masses may be included in this group.

Thrombosis and thromboembolization are common sequelae of such arterial aneurysms. When they appear, they elicit a host of associated symptoms, such as ischemic digital or limb pain. Initially, these embolic presentations may be indistinguishable from similar events in uninfected aneurysms. If the embolic material is infected and causes a secondary arterial infection, the mycotic nature of the lesion may be revealed.

Other findings of arterial infection include petechial skin lesions and septic arthritis.

Arterial rupture is not uncommon in cases of infected arterial aneurysms. This presentation is identical to that of any arterial rupture. If the damaged artery is contained and supported by a capsule of fibrous connective tissue, it may progress to form a pseudoaneurysm, and the principal symptom would be pain. If the rupture is uncontrolled, the presentation is that of hypotensive shock. If the rupture is in a superficial artery that erodes through the skin, the presentation is that of evident life-threatening hemorrhage.

Periarterial gas formation signals the presence of a gas-producing organism and should be a clear signal that urgent treatment is needed. Although this is not a common presentation, it should be considered in any patient who has unexplained periaortic gas and symptoms suggestive of sepsis.

DIAGNOSTIC TESTING

The diagnosis of a primary arterial infection is based on elements of the clinical presentation, along with appropriate testing modalities. The primary factor in making such a diagnosis is a high clinical suspicion, followed by a search for evidence to support the diagnosis of a primary arterial infection. The choice and use of diagnostic tests are of singular importance in identifying and substantiating the presence of an arterial infection. Because of the potentially fulminant course of these infections and the fatal outcome of improperly managed cases, diagnostic speed and accuracy are crucial. The basic elements of diagnostic testing include bacteriologic and radiologic techniques.

Blood Cultures

The demonstration of bacterial organisms in association with an arterial lesion is central to the diagnosis of an arterial infection. The bacteria may be detected by either blood cultures or cultures of the arterial wall itself. Blood cultures, by virtue of their availability, are frequently one of the first tests done in patients suspected of having a significant infection. If the patient is floridly bacteremic, the blood culture may detect the circulating bacteria. However, several problems limit the usefulness of blood cultures. The incidence of negative blood cultures testifies to the fact that they are helpful in only a fraction of symptomatic patients; many patients with arterial infections never have positive blood cultures. In the review of Brown and associates, only 60% of patients had positive preoperative blood cultures.[16] In addition, blood cultures may not detect the infectious organism until several days or weeks have elapsed, limiting the test's impact on clinical management.

The presence of bacteria in the blood may be an important early clue to an arterial infection, but the information from such tests must be evaluated in the proper clinical context. Most bacteremic patients have an evident source of bacteremia that should be identified and treated. Patients with positive blood cultures and no clinical evidence of a concurrent infection should be examined for possible arterial lesions. The significance of a positive blood culture in an otherwise asymptomatic patient is difficult to determine without considering the patient's underlying problems and risk factors. It should also be noted that patients who are relatively asymptomatic (no systemic manifestations of sepsis) tend to have fewer positive blood cultures. Thus, in Wakefield and coworkers' study of patients undergoing clean arterial procedures, only 2% of blood cultures were positive, whereas 12% of arteries and 14% of periarterial adipose tissues harbored bacteria.[24] Obvious clues, such as a recently noted aneurysm or a history of drug abuse, may promote further investigation.

The type of organism identified in blood cultures may suggest a source of the infection. Certain pathogens are related to certain types of infections. The association between gram-negative bacteria and urinary tract infections is one example. Similarly, if a blood culture reveals *Salmonella* species in a patient with an aneurysm, an arterial infection should be seriously considered. Although *Staphylococcus* organisms are a common pathogen in arterial infections, their ubiquitous presence on skin often confuses the diagnosis and calls into question the results of the blood culture.

The importance of the preoperative blood culture is difficult to understate. It represents the earliest reliable clue to the presence of an arterial infection. Even in the event of a delayed result, such as when several days are required before the blood culture can identify the bacteria, the information provided may be invaluable in managing the patient.

Arterial Cultures

Arterial wall cultures may also secure the diagnosis of an arterial infection. The principal drawback to arterial wall cultures is the time required before any information about the infection is available. Patient management must therefore depend on other factors, such as the clinical setting, the index of suspicion, the presence of prior blood culture data, and the results of angiographic studies. The patient's presentation may be important, because Wakefield and coworkers discovered that tissue cultures in asymptomatic patients had a significantly higher sensitivity than did blood cultures.[24] This stands in contrast to symptomatic patients, in whom blood cultures tend to have a higher sensitivity than do arterial cultures.

Because clinical decisions cannot always be based on arterial culture results, other techniques are often considered, such as intraoperative Gram staining and frozen section of the arterial tissue. Unfortunately, these methods may not provide significant improvement in the detection of bacteria. In the study of Brown and associates, although 60% of patients had positive preoperative blood cultures, only 20% of intraoperative Gram stains were positive.[16] Arterial wall frozen sections have not seen widespread use, but they may prove helpful. Histologic findings of inflammation and bacterial invasion are strong evidence supporting the diagnosis of arterial infection.

When obtaining blood or arterial wall cultures, it should be kept in mind that the type of organism may affect the yield of the tests. Brown and associates noted that 60% of arterial wall cultures were negative.[16] About 25% of their cultures failed to detect any organism at all. Presumably, these were difficult organisms to collect and culture. *S. epidermidis* may be difficult to culture without sonicating the specimen. *Treponema pallidum* may require darkfield examination for identification. *Mycobacterium tuberculosis* is a fastidious organism that is difficult to grow. These considerations should prompt the special attention of the pathology laboratory, as well as the collection of adequate specimens.

Nuclear Imaging: Tagged White Blood Cell Scans

Nuclear imaging has become an important tool in the identification of arterial graft infections, but it has not played as important a role in identifying primary arterial infections. The technique is based on the ability of various radioisotope markers to become involved in an inflammatory process. The advantages of these tests are their relatively low risk to the patient and the facility of their application. The principal drawback is that the tests may detect many inflammatory lesions, not just those that are the result of an arterial infection. Interpreting the results of a nuclear scan must take into account the clinical condition of the patient. Although the usefulness of these tests has been debated, in the absence of recent trauma or infection, the use of radiolabeled indium or gallium as markers may allow localization of an arterial infection.

Perhaps the most significant problem with the isotopic detection of arterial infections is that these techniques have not been widely applied to this situation, and their role is not well established. As a consequence, in cases in which the diagnosis of arterial infection is apparent, the tests are forsaken. When the diagnosis of an arterial infection has not been established, other testing modalities are often used first. Lesions that are not clearly apparent, such as intra-abdominal aneurysms, are often better visualized by other forms of imaging, such as angiography, computed tomography (CT), or magnetic resonance imaging (MRI). Finally, the specificity and selectivity of the nuclear imaging tests are not well established in these lesions.

Computed Tomography and Magnetic Resonance Imaging

The success of techniques such as CT and MRI in identifying primary arterial infections depends largely on their ability to resolve the characteristic anatomic features of the lesions. Because of the detailed anatomic data these scans present, they have become very popular in the evaluation of intra-abdominal vascular lesions. There are some significant limitations, however, with regard to their ability to secure the diagnosis of an arterial infection.

The essential diagnostic characteristics of arterial infections include the presence of a focal defect in the wall of the aorta, the saccular shape of the aneurysm, and the tissue edema that accompanies the inflammatory reaction. Routine reconstruction of CT images does not readily allow recognition of the diagnostic features of mycotic aneurysms; three-dimensional reconstruction does allow their recognition, but such reconstruction is not routinely performed and must be specifically requested.

MRI represents an improvement over CT scanning because current computer analysis allows a more flexible assemblage of the data and facilitates the recognition of essential diagnostic characteristics. Additionally, the resolution of MRI may be better than that of CT. MRI does not require intravascular contrast agents, which are frequently needed with CT. Finally, MRI is able to detect tissue differences with regard to certain molecular constituents. Another advantage of MRI is its ability to detect the accumulation of water in tissues; this

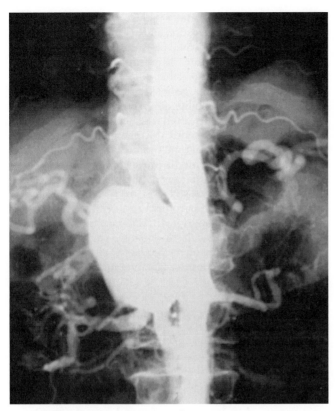

FIGURE 10-4 • Angiogram of mycotic aortic aneurysm.

tissue edema is frequently the hallmark of an inflammatory process and may identify an arterial infection.

Angiography

Angiography is the most widely used technique for the investigation and definition of arterial infections (Fig. 10-4). It can image both central (abdominal and thoracic) and peripheral arterial lesions. Historically, it was the first method by which the characteristics of primary arterial infections, specifically infectious aortic aneurysms, were identified. Thus, angiography not only identified but also defined the characteristics of these lesions. Not surprisingly, angiography surpasses computed imaging in identifying the characteristic signs of arterial infections. Additionally, angiography is clearly superior in areas such as the intestinal mesentery and the visceral vessels, where the size of the arterial lesion may be below the resolution of computed techniques. In the case of aortic mycotic aneurysms, the angiogram usually provides excellent definition of the defect in the aortic wall, the saccular pseudoaneurysm, and the contiguous arterial anatomy. Finally, the arteriogram offers the best definition of the relationship between the visceral vessels and the arterial defect—an essential step in planning patient management. The strength of angiography, then, is its ability to detect arterial lesions and define the arterial anatomy. These two elements are essential in planning an arterial reconstruction.

The role of arteriography in the management of a peripheral arterial infection has been questioned. Because some peripheral arterial infections are managed with ligation and débridement without reconstruction, an angiogram may not be necessary; however, it is important to assess the native circulation before attempting arterial ligation. Should the limb require urgent revascularization after arterial ligation, an angiogram obtained before the ligation would be very helpful in planning the revascularization. It should be noted that an arteriogram obtained after ligation and resection of the vessel is often less than satisfactory. For this reason, an arteriogram of the involved vessels is required in all but emergent cases.

TIMING OF DIAGNOSIS

The diagnosis of a primary arterial infection may be made preoperatively, intraoperatively, or postoperatively. Should the diagnosis be suspected before surgery, preoperative antibiotics may be commenced, and the patient can be better informed about potential problems. Plans can also be drawn for contingencies that might require alternative reconstructions.

The diagnosis may be established or confirmed by the findings at surgery. The presence of gross purulence, engorged lymph nodes, and inflamed tissues helps establish the diagnosis conclusively. Adjunctive tests such as the Gram stain and bacterial cultures may be performed. The intraoperative findings help determine the mode of arterial reconstruction; gross infection and pus should be taken as indications for débridement and remote reconstruction, whereas minimal evidence of infection may suggest reasonably good results from in situ reconstruction.

If the diagnosis is confirmed in the postoperative period by positive bacterial cultures, a prolonged course of antibiotics and graft surveillance is advisable.

NATURAL HISTORY

Given the pathogenesis of a primary arterial infection—bacterial invasion, colonization, and destruction of an artery—the sequence of events after this initial insult is predictable and inexorable. Destruction of the arterial wall leads to either the development of an arterial pseudoaneurysm or a life-threatening hemorrhage. Which of these two events occurs is probably related to the rate of progression of the infection, its location, and the subsequent development of an inflammatory response. If the destruction of the arterial wall is gradual and accompanied by a vigorous inflammatory response, the arterial infection may produce a pseudoaneurysm. If the process of arterial infection leads to a rapid loss of arterial integrity, the arterial infection may result in hemorrhage.

Complications of arterial infections include those common to all aneurysms: embolization, thrombosis, and rupture. The incidence of rupture is thought to be increased when the arterial wall is invaded by infectious pathogens. The high rupture rate is reflected in both the virulent course (rapid expansion and progression to rupture) and the high mortality of these lesions. For these reasons, mycotic aneurysms are urgent cases that should be repaired as soon as possible. One final complication, which is significantly increased in cases of primary arterial infection, is the rate of infection of the vascular reconstruction. Although the anticipated incidence of graft infection in "clean" cases is less than 1% or 2%, the incidence of graft infection after remote (extra-anatomic) reconstruction in cases of primary arterial infection may be as high as 15%. In older series, when in situ reconstruction was performed in the face of a purulent infection and without concurrent antibiotics, the reinfection rate approached 100%.

PRINCIPLES OF MANAGEMENT

Once the diagnosis has been established, early definitive intervention must be initiated. Two elemental principles form the basis of therapy in primary arterial infections: (1) control of sepsis and (2) establishment of arterial continuity.

Control of Sepsis

Antibiotic therapy and surgical débridement represent the primary treatment modalities for the control of sepsis in arterial infections. All infected arterial tissue must be débrided. It is important that the arterial resection encompass all inflamed tissues and continue to the point where the arterial tissue is normal and healthy. This helps prevent recurrence of the infection and disruption of the arterial suture line.

Soft tissues adjacent to the infected artery that appear to be involved are also débrided. Major structures such as the vena cava and ureters are left intact. Retroperitoneal tissues that appear to be involved are resected as well. Once all infected tissues have been removed, the wound is thoroughly irrigated with an antibiotic solution—ideally, one that contains antibiotic directed toward the suspected pathogens (as detected by preoperative blood cultures). Surgical drains are useful when there is clear evidence of purulence. In the absence of an abscess or fluid collection, drains may not be required. When collateral circulation allows, the excision may be accompanied by proximal and distal ligation and no effort to reconstruct the artery, as first described by Paré.

The use of antibiotics is mandatory in these situations. Broad-spectrum antibiotics must be initiated as soon as a strong clinical suspicion of arterial infection has been established. Blood cultures should be obtained before the initiation of antibiotics. When positive, these cultures are then used to select an antibiotic regimen with the highest therapeutic value and the fewest side effects. Negative cultures should not preclude the institution of broad-spectrum antibiotics when arterial infection is suspected. The use of high-dose preoperative antibiotics is directed toward sterilizing the aneurysm and adjacent tissues to minimize bacteremia and local contamination during surgical manipulation of infected tissues. Antibiotics must be continued until the source of the bacteremia has been corrected either surgically or medically. Similarly, the primary source of bacteremia or local bacterial invasion must be controlled as a mainstay of therapy in all types of primary arterial infections. In patients with true mycotic aneurysms, specific consideration must be given to sterilization of cardiac valvular vegetations.

The duration of antibiotic treatment is somewhat controversial, and several competing regimens have been proposed. Several authors suggest that IV antibiotics be initiated before surgery and extended for no less than 6 weeks postoperatively.[25-27] Additionally, these authors recommend that patients with prosthetic reconstructions, especially in situ prosthetic reconstructions, be placed on lifelong oral regimens of suppressive antibiotics. Typically, oral trimethoprim-sulfamethoxazole (Bactrim), a sulfa drug, or a first-generation cephalosporin or penicillin is the agent of choice.

Important technical points include the use of monofilament suture material in ligation and oversewing of the arteries. This recommendation is based on the superiority of monofilaments over braided suture in resisting recurrent infection. Additionally, whenever possible, the resected arterial stump should be covered with a pedicle of healthy, viable tissue to further reduce the possibility of a recurrent infection and to accelerate healing of the arterial segment. In the abdomen, this tissue pedicle is frequently the omentum. A flap of fascia from the prevertebral fascia and ligaments can be used to reinforce the aortic suture line. In the periphery, muscle transposition is the preferred means of obtaining tissue coverage. In the femoral region, this is most readily accomplished by rotating the head of the sartorius.

Nonoperative therapy for arterial infections in specific subsets of patients has been proposed by Kaufman and coworkers.[28] This treatment modality, although effective anecdotally, remains controversial, and further investigation is necessary.

Reestablishment of Arterial Continuity

Lack of adequate arterial collateralization results in end-organ ischemia when infected arteries are ligated and resected. Accordingly, in these situations, some form of arterial reconstruction must be performed to avoid tissue ischemia. This situation is most common with infections involving the visceral arteries, the aorta, and the femoral artery bifurcation.

Blakemore, in 1947, was among the first to employ a graft to replace an infected artery when he implanted a Vitallium tube. Since then, a wide range of bypass materials has been used, with varying success rates. These include autologous tissues such as saphenous vein and arterial homografts, as well as various synthetic materials such as polytetrafluoroethylene (PTFE) and Dacron.

Prosthetic grafts are the first choice for routine arterial reconstruction, but their use in cases of mycotic aneurysm is limited by their vulnerability to infection. Accordingly, most prosthetic graft reconstructions are found in extra-anatomic bypasses. In rare instances, they are used for in situ reconstruction of the paravisceral aorta, along with long-term antibiotics.

Vein grafts are superior to prosthetic material in resisting recurrent infection. Also, they are durable and familiar to most vascular surgeons. Their use is limited by the need to procure these grafts and the size and length constraints imposed by the individual patient's anatomy.

Arterial homografts have recently been the subject of considerable interest—in particular, their application to arterial reconstruction in the face of infection. Although they are not immune to infection, the risk of recurrent infection is dramatically reduced with these grafts. However, these grafts are subject to late aneurysmal degeneration with resultant thrombosis, occlusion, and embolization.

Successful management of arterial infections depends largely on the location and size of the affected artery. General principles indicate that when bypass procedures must be performed, autologous materials, such as the patient's own arteries or veins harvested from clean sites, should be the graft of first choice. When prosthetic grafts must be used, every attempt should be made to place them through clean planes, including extra-anatomic bypass when necessary.

Infrarenal Aortic Infections

Traditional management of primary arterial infections of the infrarenal aorta invariably requires excision and graft reconstruction. The standard therapy that has evolved for infections in this location combines excision and débridement of the aneurysm and adjacent tissues with extra-anatomic (e.g., axillofemoral) bypass. In a review of spontaneous abdominal aortic infections, Ewart and associates demonstrated a 23% to 63% reoperation rate for graft infection after immediate in situ reconstruction and a 7% recurrent infection rate when patients were initially treated with arterial débridement and remote reconstruction.[29]

Brown and associates, in their review of 51 cases of mycotic aneurysms, noted that the mortality of local graft reconstruction was 32%, whereas extra-anatomic reconstruction was associated with a 13% mortality rate.[16] Still, the authors advocated in situ reconstruction in selected cases; they proposed that if no gross purulence was encountered intraoperatively, and if the result was gram-negative, in situ reconstruction using prosthetic material (Dacron) could be safely performed. This approach is predicated on the recommendation that postoperative antibiotics be continued for a minimum of 6 to 8 weeks. Brown and associates demonstrated 63% survival and 19% reinfection rates for aneurysms treated with this approach. In comparison, the rate of infection of extra-anatomic bypasses following repair of mycotic aortic aneurysms was as high as 13%.[16]

Experience with in situ reconstruction for primary aortoduodenal fistulas has encouraged some authors to proceed with in situ graft reconstruction of the aorta when there is minimal contamination, no pus, and little extent of the infectious process.[15] Approximately 70% of aneurysms associated with primary aortoduodenal fistulas are not due to arterial infection; the majority of the remaining aneurysms are thought to be infectious in origin.[30] In the case of a primary mycotic aortoduodenal fistula, extensive débridement and extra-anatomic bypass graft are recommended for significant infection and obvious involvement of the arterial bed. In situ graft replacement has been performed successfully in cases in which the level of contamination was mild. When the aneurysm is not of infectious origin, in situ reconstruction has been advised by a number of authors.[30,31]

The benefit of this approach is that it may reduce the length of surgery, improve graft patency, and simplify technical management of the case. The risk associated with this reconstruction is that the new arterial prosthesis may become infected.

A fundamental technical issue involves the material used for aortic reconstruction. Alternatives include antibiotic-impregnated prosthetic grafts and human tissue, such as autogenous veins or cadaveric allografts.

Antibiotic-Impregnated Grafts

Experimental and clinical evidence suggests that in situ reconstruction with antibiotic-impregnated prosthetic grafts is feasible. Bandyk and colleagues reported 27 patients operated on with rifampin-impregnated grafts as treatment for a variety of arterial infections.[32] At least four recurrent infections were reported, including two that resulted in death. They concluded that in situ replacement using a rifampin-bonded prosthetic graft was most effective for low-grade staphylococcal arterial infection. An added caveat was that in the presence of virulent and antibiotic-resistant bacterial strains, this therapy usually failed.[32] A more recent experience of 27 patients with both graft infections and mycotic aneurysms managed with silver-coated polyester grafts was published by Batt and associates.[33] There were 7 perioperative deaths and 20 long-term survivors. Of the long-term (actuarial period, 24 months) survivors, one developed a recurrent infection.

Autogenous Reconstruction

VEINS. Aortoilac reconstruction with autogenous veins has been performed with both saphenous and femoral veins. An initial experience using femoral veins for aortic and iliac reconstruction was reported by Schulman and associates in 1986.[34] The use of superficial femoral and popliteal veins has been advocated by Clagett and associates for a number of infectious indications, including primary aortoiliac arterial infections.[35] In their series of 38 patients with aortofemoral infections who underwent successful reconstruction with autogenous superficial femoral vein, the long-term primary patency was 85% at 5 years.

HUMAN ALLOGRAFTS. In situ reconstruction with human allografts for infected aneurysms in the aortoiliac region has been reported with good results—low mortality and good durability. Reinfection rates after prolonged administration of culture-directed antibiotics are generally very low. The most common problem associated with allograft reconstruction is the eventual degradation of the allograft, which is subject to aneurysmal degeneration.

Kieffer and associates reported their experience with 43 patients with infected infrarenal aortic prosthetic grafts who underwent in situ replacement using preserved allografts obtained from cadavers.[36] In the early postoperative period, there were five septic complications, including two pseudoaneurysm ruptures; two cases of septic shock; and one instance of peritonitis from colon perforation. In follow-up, one late death may have been related to persistent infection. A report focusing on mycotic aortic aneurysms was published by Leseche and associates.[37] They reported a series of 28 patients operated on for a variety of vascular infections, including five mycotic aneurysms. There were five perioperative deaths, two from sepsis and two from multisystem organ failure. The long-term outcomes were good. There were no recurrent infections and only three instances of aneurysmal degeneration of the allograft.

Endovascular Repair

Endovascular techniques have been used in the management of infected aortic aneurysms. One concern about such an intervention is that it places a graft in direct proximity to the infection and does not afford the opportunity to débride the infected tissue. This leads to the possibility of a significant rate of recurrent infections and septic complications. The principal advantage is that because many patients with arterial infections are debilitated, the less invasive approach may be better tolerated.

The few reports of endovascular treatment to date indicate that, in combination with prolonged antibiotic administration and the use of drainage, some patients may achieve resolution of the arterial infection, with no infection of the endoprosthesis.[38,39] In 2002, Berchtold and colleagues reported a case of *Salmonella*-associated mycotic infrarenal aortic aneurysm managed with an endovascular graft and prolonged antibiotics.[38] After a 4-year follow-up period, repeat CT scans demonstrated resolution of the aneurysm and no sign of residual infection. More recently, Koeppel and associates reported successful endovascular repair of a mycotic aneurysm of the infrarenal aorta associated with a retroperitoneal abscess.[39] The aneurysm was treated with an endoprosthesis, and the abscess was drained percutaneously. Antibiotics were continued for 6 months. A CT scan done 1 year after implantation revealed no sign of retroperitoneal inflammation. These investigators noted that endovascular repair was particularly attractive in critically ill patients who might not be able to tolerate an open surgical repair.

Suprarenal Aneurysms

Because of their unique anatomic characteristics, arterial infections of the paravisceral and suprarenal aorta almost always require immediate in situ arterial reconstruction. It is nearly impossible to bypass the visceral vessels without traversing the bed of the infected paravisceral aorta. Experience gained from the repair of suprarenal mycotic aneurysms has given credence to the concept of in situ repair with adjunctive lifelong antibiotic therapy.

When combined with débridement of grossly infected tissue and appropriate use of antibiotics, most series reporting this type of reconstruction have demonstrated acceptable morbidity and mortality rates. Chan and associates reported a series of 22 patients with mycotic aneurysms of the thoracic and abdominal aorta.[25] Of these, 13 had involvement of the paravisceral aorta, all of which required in situ reconstruction. Twelve of the 13 patients survived surgery and were placed on lifelong suppressive antibiotics. None had clinical recurrence of the infection. In the overall series, three patients died; two of the deaths were attributed to multisystem organ failure and one to aspiration pneumonia. The authors concluded that in situ reconstruction, along with surgical débridement and lifelong antibiotics, offers the best chance of survival in these difficult-to-treat patients. It should be noted that although this form of therapy (in situ reconstruction) is inescapable in the reconstruction of infected paravisceral aneurysms, its application to arterial infections at other sites (e.g., infrarenal aorta or femoral artery) is less well established and should be approached with caution.

Femoral, Iliac, and Mesenteric Arterial Infections

Other anatomic locations where primary arterial infections are considered relatively common include the femoral, superior mesenteric, and celiac arteries. Attempts at ligation and excision of these vessels for the treatment of primary arterial infections may be associated with a high rate of irreversible ischemia. Currently, the patients who are at greatest risk of developing these infections are IV drug abusers. Because of these patients' recidivistic tendencies, they are at risk of reinfecting their arterial reconstructions. This has generated debate regarding the best treatment for these patients. The simplest approach is to ligate, resect, and then observe the ligated

vascular bed for signs of severe ischemia. Revascularization is performed only if severe ischemia develops. The second choice is to proceed with an autogenous reconstruction at the time of resection of the infected lesion.

Infected Femoral Pseudoaneurysms

Infections of the vessels of the femoral region are the most common type of arterial infection. In the review by Brown and colleagues, these lesions accounted for 38% of all arterial infections.[16] The most common manifestation is an inflamed, tender, pulsatile inguinal mass. The more common complications include erosion through the skin with hemorrhage, embolization, compression of adjacent structures (femoral vein and nerve), and thrombosis. Of these, erosion and hemorrhage are the most feared complications.

The debate regarding reconstruction is of particular interest in the subset of patients with infected pseudoaneurysms of the femoral bifurcation that are the result of IV drug abuse. Because of the addict's tendency to reuse femoral sites for drug administration, the arterial reconstruction may be in jeopardy of recurrent infection. If the reconstruction required prosthetic material, the resultant reinfection would be all the more complicated and dangerous. Finally, the incidence of graft infection after immediate reconstruction is sufficient by itself to warrant hesitation in such reconstructions. Because of these concerns, some authors have advocated simple arterial ligation and resection of the infected tissues. The problem is that simple ligation of the femoral arteries at the level of the arterial bifurcation may result in a subsequent amputation rate approaching 33%.[23,40]

An alternative school of thought holds that the limbs should be reconstructed, and if they subsequently become infected, the infection should be dealt with as necessary. In the course of these reconstructions, the infected arteries and adjacent tissues should be débrided and the reconstruction coursed through uninfected tissues.[41] Finally, the reconstruction should be performed with autogenous tissue if possible.

The third option is to combine both approaches so that the arterial lesion is resected and the adjacent tissues are débrided. The artery is ligated, but no reconstructions are performed in the initial setting. The limb is observed for signs of severe ischemia. If the limb appears viable with collateral perfusion alone, no effort is made to reconstruct. If the limb appears severely ischemic, revascularization is attempted. Femoral artery reconstruction should be carried out either with in situ saphenous vein interposition grafting or through an extra-anatomic approach, such as a transobturator bypass.

Infection and pseudoaneurysm of the common femoral, superficial femoral, and deep femoral arteries do not appear to suffer a similar fate. These vessels stand a far better chance of tolerating simple ligation without requiring reconstruction. Wright and Shepard reported a very low incidence of amputation following ligation and resection in this circumstance.[42] In a series of 39 patients with such infections, they noted an amputation rate of 5%; these amputations occurred in two patients who had impaired collateral circulation from prior (contralateral) common femoral artery ligation. In the absence of these two cases, the amputation rate in this group of patients was 0%.[42]

Mesenteric Artery Infections

Mesenteric artery infections tend to appear as pseudo-aneurysms within the mesentery of the intestine. These lesions may be asymptomatic, but the more common presentation is abdominal pain. These lesions may develop as a consequence of IV drug abuse. Pathophysiologically, they are considered to be the result of mycotic embolization. Because of this, it is necessary to consider the source of the emboli as well as the possibility of other embolic targets. In practical terms, this means that these patients should be screened for both cardiac vegetations and other arterial lesions. Preoperative angiography is recommended if possible. Postoperative angiography should be considered if a preoperative study was not obtained.

Mesenteric artery infections tend to develop rapid expansion and intramesenteric hemorrhage. Alternatively, these aneurysms may result in thrombosis and infarction of the intestine. Management of these vessels is related to the location of the lesion, the available collateral circulation, and the presence and extent of intestinal infarction. Lesions of the proximal mesenteric arteries frequently require reconstruction with autogenous tissues. More distally located pseudoaneurysms can often be managed by simple excision. If a small area of intestinal ischemia develops, a limited bowel resection may also be necessary. In instances of extensive intestinal ischemia, a second-look celiotomy may be advisable after restoration of intestinal perfusion.

Arterial Infections of the Upper Extremity

Infections of the arteries of the upper extremities are fairly rare. Collectively, they represented about 10% of arterial infections in the review by Brown and colleagues.[16] Frequently, these lesions are associated with trauma. Like other infections of peripheral vessels, these lesions may present in a number of ways, with the most common presentation being an inflamed, tender, pulsatile mass. In the upper extremities, careful inspection should detect evidence of digital embolization—splinter hemorrhages and ischemic lesions.

Because of the extensive collateral blood supply to the upper extremities, arterial infections there can often be treated with simple ligation and excision. This is particularly true when the involved segment is between the thyrocervical trunk and the subscapular artery or distal to the deep brachial artery. Reconstruction, when required, should be accomplished with a saphenous vein graft or similar autogenous tissues. As with all mycotic aneurysms, pre- and postoperative antibiotics should be given for a prolonged period.

CONCLUSIONS

Primary arterial infections are relatively rare, but they are frequently lethal. They often follow a rapidly progressive course toward expansion and rupture. Only an astute diagnosis and correct management can improve a patient's chance of survival. The diagnosis is established by a high index of suspicion, along with identification of risk factors and appropriate testing. Once an arterial infection is identified, management must be tailored to the organism involved and the site and severity of the infection, as well as the condition of the patient. Surgical excision is almost always necessary in the course of management. Long-term (6 weeks) IV antibiotics are almost always required, and the use of lifelong oral antibiotic suppression is strongly recommended for these patients. Optimal care may reduce the mortality of these lesions from nearly 100% to less than 10% to 15%.

Prophylactic Antibiotic Therapy

Although infections of implanted vascular prostheses are relatively uncommon, when they do occur, they are associated with significant morbidity and mortality. Complications of graft infection include pseudoaneurysm, anastomotic disruption, hemorrhage, fistula formation, and sepsis. Infection of a vascular graft almost always requires partial or complete graft removal, which is associated with a high incidence of amputation. Vascular graft infection leads to the patient's death in one fourth to one half of cases in contemporary series. These dire consequences have prompted laboratory and clinical investigation into the role of antibiotics in the prevention of vascular graft infection. The widespread use of prophylactic antibiotics in vascular surgery has significantly altered the microbiology and clinical presentation of graft infections. New insights have been gained into the pathogenesis of this process, and alternative methods of antibiotic delivery have been developed in animal models. This section presents the bacteriology and current understanding of the pathogenesis of graft infection, a historical overview of the development of antibiotic prophylaxis in vascular surgery, current recommendations for prophylaxis, and new directions in antibiotic delivery.

CLINICAL SIGNIFICANCE OF GRAFT INFECTION

The reported incidence of infection after the placement of vascular prostheses ranges from 1% to 6%. This relatively low rate of infection has remained stable over time, despite improvements in technique and the introduction of routine preoperative antibiotic prophylaxis. Two early series, from Hoffert and colleagues[43] in 1965 and Fry and Lindenauer[44] in 1967, reported graft infection rates of 6.0% (12 of 201) and 1.34% (12 of 890), respectively. In 1972, Szilagyi and colleagues reported a large series of 3397 cases in which the graft infection rate was 1.9%.[45] Later reports detailed similar findings. The series of Lorentzen and coauthors from 1985 described graft infections in 62 of 2411 patients, a rate of 2.6%.[46] Although the overall incidence of infection has not changed significantly, the use of antibiotic prophylaxis has clearly changed the clinical presentation of most vascular graft infections. Suppurative infections appearing in the first few weeks after graft implantation have given way to more insidious, low-grade, chronic infections.[47,48]

Infection in prosthetic grafts remains a critical issue in vascular surgery. Reported mortality rates from graft infection range from 25% to 75% (Table 10-1).[43,44,47,49-52] Mortality is greatest for proximal grafts, with almost uniform lethality reported in aortic stump sepsis.[44,45,49,53] Despite attempts to reduce mortality in aortic graft infection, it remains relatively high at 24% to 43%.[54-58] Peripheral graft infections are generally associated with lower mortality rates (as low as 6%).[59] Amputation rates are similar for survivors of aortic and peripheral graft infections, ranging from 22.5% to 43%.[45,50,60]

TABLE 10–1		Influence of Graft Site on Incidence and Outcome of Graft Infection					
Author	Year	Type of Graft	No. of Patients	Graft Infection Rate (%)*	Amputation Rate (%)†	Mortality Rate (%)
Hoffert et al[43]	1965	Aortoiliac	84	0	NA	NA
		Aortofemoral	30	0	NA	NA
		Iliofemoropopliteal	83	13.0	75	25
Szilagyi et al[45]	1972	Aortoiliac	418	0.7	0	66
		Aortofemoral	1244	1.6	21	53
		Iliofemoropopliteal	270	3.0	40	7
Bouhoutsos et al[69]	1974	Aortoiliac/aortofemoral	412	1.5	0	50
		Iliofemoropopliteal	108	7.4	25	0
Liekweg and Greenfield[50]	1977	Aortoiliac	NR	NR	3	58
		Aortofemoral	NR	NR	11	47
		Iliofemoropopliteal	NR	NR	30	13
Yashar et al[52]	1978	Aortoiliac	300	1.0	0	33
		Aortofemoral	210	2.9	33	50
		Iliofemoropopliteal	65	4.6	67	0
Casali et al[115]	1980	Aortoiliac	NR	NR	0	50
		Aortofemoral	NR	NR	25	67
		Iliofemoropopliteal	NR	NR	33	33
Lorentzen et al[46]	1985	Aortoiliac	515	0.0	NA	NA
		Aortofemoral	1497	3.0	22	29
		Iliofemoropopliteal	489	3.5	53	18
Edwards et al[63]	1987	Aortic/aortoiliac	769	0.0	NA	NA
		Aortofemoral	1060	0.47	20	40
		Iliofemoropopliteal	583	2.9	12	18

*Primary graft infections only; excludes aortoenteric fistulas.
†Amputation rate among survivors.
NA, not applicable; NR, not reported.

In more recent series, reported amputation rates range from 24% to 27%.[57-59]

PRINCIPLES OF ANTIBIOTIC PROPHYLAXIS

The goal of prophylactic antibiotic therapy is to prevent infection after surgery. The most important indication for antibiotic prophylaxis in vascular reconstructive surgery is the use of prosthetic materials. Synthetic materials provide a protective substrate for bacterial colonization and proliferation. Experimental studies have demonstrated that the presence of a foreign body increases the infectivity of S. aureus 10,000-fold.[61] In light of the potentially catastrophic consequences of vascular graft infection, prophylactic antibiotics are recommended in patients undergoing procedures in which prosthetic materials are employed.

The ideal prophylactic antibiotic should be bactericidal for the most common pathogens causing postoperative infection and adequately concentrated in serum and at the site of surgery. It should be present in adequate concentrations throughout the surgical procedure and nontoxic to the patient. In addition, its cost should be reasonable enough to justify its routine use.

Most vascular graft infections are caused by a few specific bacteria. Therefore, broad-spectrum antibiotic prophylaxis is unnecessary. Selecting an antibiotic with the narrowest spectrum of activity that includes the most common pathogens involved in graft infection will limit the emergence of resistant organisms. Antibiotics that are the principal line of therapy in difficult infections (such as vancomycin in the treatment of S. epidermidis infections) should be reserved for that indication and not used in prophylaxis.

BACTERIOLOGY OF GRAFT INFECTION

Gram-positive cocci, the predominant flora of the skin and dermal appendages, are most often responsible for vascular graft infections. Although the bacteriology of graft infection varies somewhat by anatomic site, when all sites are considered together, approximately 60% to 65% of reported cases are currently due to gram-positive organisms. The remaining 35% to 40% are largely due to gram-negative rods, which account for approximately half of all infections in intra-abdominal (aortic, aortoiliac) grafts. Although S. aureus has historically been the most frequently cultured pathogen, the introduction of routine antibiotic prophylaxis and improved culture techniques have led to the emergence of S. epidermidis and other coagulase-negative staphylococci as the most frequent cause of vascular graft infection (Table 10-2). The most commonly cultured gram-negative rod is E. coli, followed by Proteus species, Pseudomonas species, and Klebsiella species.

In early reports from the 1960s and 1970s, S. aureus was identified as the predominant pathogen in vascular graft infections. In 1965, Hoffert and colleagues reported that S. aureus was cultured in 67% (8 of 12) of aortic, femoral, and popliteal reconstructions.[43] Likewise, in a series of 890 aortic grafts

| TABLE 10–2 | Effect of Antibiotic Prophylaxis on the Microbiology of Graft Infection |

Author	Year	Type of Graft	Prophylactic Antibiotics	Cultured Organisms (%)*				Culture Negative (%)
				S. aureus	S. epidermidis	E. coli	Other GNRs	
Hoffert et al[43]	1965	Aortic and distal	No	67	17	8	25	17
Fry and Lindenauer[44]	1967	Aortic	No	67	0	25	8	8
Goldstone and Moore[47]	1974	Aortic and distal	In some cases†	41	26	15	11	7
Liekweg and Greenfield[50]	1977	Aortic and distal	No	50	4	13	18	NR
Bandyk et al[48]	1984	Aortofemoral	Yes	10	60	13	23	10
Yeager et al[58]	1985	Aortic	Yes	0	50	0	0	33
		Distal	Yes	14	14	0	29	43
Quiñones-Baldrich et al[64]	1991	Aortic	Yes	13	21	18	45	21

*Expressed as the percentage of cases from which each organism was cultured.
†Prophylaxis administered in 10 of 27 cases of graft infection.
GNR, gram-negative rod; NR, not reported.

from Fry and Lindenauer in 1967, S. aureus was cultured in 67% (8 of 12) of cases.[44] In 1967, Smith and colleagues reported on nine cases of femoropopliteal graft infection, eight of which were due to S. aureus.[62] In a review of 108 published cases of vascular graft infection reported between 1959 and 1974, Liekweg and Greenfield noted that S. aureus was responsible for 50% of cases.[50] The next most common pathogens were gram-negative rods (30.5%) and streptococci (8.5%); only 3.6% of cases were due to S. epidermidis.

Goldstone and Moore were among the first to note the impact of antibiotic prophylaxis on the presentation and bacteriology of graft infection.[47] They retrospectively reviewed the incidence of graft infection before and after the initiation of routine antibiotic prophylaxis. During the preantibiotic prophylaxis period (1959 to 1966), the vascular graft infection rate was 4.1% (9 of 222). From 1966 to 1973, when prophylactic antibiotic use became routine, the graft infection rate dropped to 1.5% (5 of 344). Of all staphylococcal infections treated at my institution between 1959 and 1973, 14 of 18 (78%) occurred before the routine use of prophylactic antibiotics.

Reviews of graft infection since the advent of routine antibiotic prophylaxis demonstrate an increasing incidence of late infections due to fastidious organisms such as S. epidermidis and other coagulase-negative staphylococci. Bandyk and colleagues presented a report of 30 patients treated for aortofemoral graft infections from 1972 to 1982; 60% of these infections were due to S. epidermidis.[48] The time of presentation influenced the microbiology of graft infection. Four of five early (<4 months) infections were due to gram-negative rods. Late infections (>4 months) were much more common, totaling 25; of these, 15 (60%) were due to S. epidermidis.

In 1985, Yeager and associates reported a 9-year experience in which they managed 14 aortic and 11 peripheral graft infections.[58] Whereas peripheral graft infections appeared, on average, 8 months after surgery, aortic graft infections appeared, on average, 5 years postoperatively. Of five primarily infected aortic grafts (not graft-enteric fistulas or erosions) with positive cultures, four were due to S. epidermidis. A wide range of organisms was cultured from peripheral grafts, including coagulase-positive and -negative staphylococci, gram-negative rods, anaerobic streptococci, and diphtheroids.

Edwards and associates reported on 24 infections from a series of 2614 aortofemoropopliteal grafts over a 10-year period from 1975 to 1986; the majority (29%) were due to S. aureus.[63] The authors noted, however, that in only 7 of 24 cases were prophylactic antibiotics administered according to the departmental protocol; thus, this series may be more representative of the preantibiotic era. This observation is supported by the fact that 63% of these infections appeared within 3 months of implantation. Additionally, cultures were negative in 21% of patients, suggesting that the presence of fastidious organisms such as S. epidermidis may have been underestimated. In 1991, Quiñones-Baldrich and colleagues reported an 18-year experience (1970 to 1988) with 45 aortic graft infections.[64] Culture results were available for 38 of 45 patients. Gram-negative organisms, most commonly Pseudomonas species (21%) and E. coli (18%), were cultured from 24 patients (63%). Gram-positive cocci, most frequently S. epidermidis (21%), were cultured from 21 patients (55%). Of note is the fact that cultures grew multiple organisms in 39% of cases, and there were eight (21%) negative cultures, again suggesting that the incidence of infection due to fastidious organisms may have been underestimated.

PATHOGENESIS OF GRAFT INFECTION

Although there is no definitive explanation of how graft infection occurs, the two principal routes of infection are thought to be direct contamination (bacteria present in the surgical wound) and hematogenous or lymphatogenous seeding. It is generally thought that most graft infections are caused by direct intraoperative contamination of the prosthesis. Potential sources of infecting organisms include the patient's skin, breaks in aseptic technique, adjacent active infections, transudation of bowel flora into the peritoneal space, and the diseased arterial tree itself, which may become colonized with pathogenic bacteria.

Skin Flora

The normal skin flora is the most important source of bacteria. Accordingly, preoperative skin preparation influences subsequent infection rates. Kaiser and coworkers noted a higher rate of infection with a hexachlorophene-ethanol preparation compared with povidone-iodine.[65] Close and colleagues reported that hexachlorophene is more effective alone than when used in combination with ethanol.[66] In a prospective study, Cruse demonstrated that preoperative hexachlorophene showering can be effective in reducing wound infection rates, and overzealous shaving may actually increase the risk of infection.[67] Wooster and colleagues demonstrated that vascular grafts routinely become contaminated with skin organisms intraoperatively and suggested that careful attention to aseptic technique can significantly reduce this occurrence.[68]

Groin incisions appear to have special significance in the development of vascular graft infections. Grafts involving an inguinal wound have a higher incidence of infection than do those that avoid this region.[45,47,69] Jamieson and colleagues reported that the presence of a groin incision increased the risk of graft infection 3.5 times; the presence of a groin complication such as a seroma or hematoma increased the risk of infection ninefold over patients without groin complications.[49] Up to 33% of groin incisions with hematomas may develop infections.[52] Lorentzen and associates reported that the highest incidence of infection was in patients who underwent aortobifemoral grafting for abdominal aortic aneurysms (5.9%), whereas there were no infections in 425 patients who underwent aortoiliac bypass for aneurysms (213) and occlusive atherosclerosis (212).[46]

Gastrointestinal Flora

The gastrointestinal tract is a potential source of contamination during aortic reconstruction. Cultures of intestinal bag fluid have been reported by some investigators to yield enteric bacteria[50] and skin organisms such as coagulase-negative staphylococci.[22] In a report of 109 bowel bag cultures from abdominal aortic reconstructions, Scobie and colleagues found positive cultures in 14% of patients.[70] S. epidermidis was the single most common organism isolated (n = 11), whereas enteric flora were cultured in 12.

The impact of concomitant gastrointestinal surgery in the development of vascular graft infection is unclear. In separate series, DeBakey and coauthors,[71] Stoll,[72] and Hardy and coworkers[73] reported a total of 670 patients who underwent aortic graft placement and simultaneous gastrointestinal procedures, with no episodes of graft infection. These authors concluded that such coincident procedures can be undertaken safely. Other investigators, however, described the development of graft infection in patients undergoing simultaneous appendectomy,[47] cholecystectomy and gastrostomy,[74] and anterior resection.[69]

Arterial Colonization

The native arterial tree may harbor bacteria. The presence of pathogenic bacteria, particularly coagulase-negative staphylococci, in vascular tissues not previously operated on has been widely documented (Table 10-3). Lalka and colleagues postulated that transient bacteremias resulting from breaks in the skin or mucous membranes may lead to arterial colonization.[75] Bacterial contamination of vascular prostheses may therefore be inevitable in some cases. It is not yet clear, however, to what extent the presence of positive arterial wall cultures influences the likelihood of subsequent graft infection.

The 1977 report of Ernst and associates of abdominal aortic aneurysmal wall cultures was one of the first to highlight the presence of pathogenic organisms in the native aorta.[22] The overall incidence of positive cultures was 15%, and cultures were more likely to be positive when atherosclerotic disease was more advanced. Asymptomatic aneurysms were less likely to be culture positive (9%) than were symptomatic (13%) or ruptured aneurysms (35%). S. epidermidis was the most frequently isolated organism. The late graft sepsis rate was 10% in the culture-positive group versus 2% in the culture-negative group. In a similar report, Buckels and coauthors described

TABLE 10–3	Positive Arterial Wall Cultures: Incidence and Significance				
Author	**Year**	**Culture Source**	**Positive Cultures (%)**	**Associated with Subsequent Infection?**	**Frequency of S. epidermidis among Positive Cultures (%)**
Ernst et al[22]	1977	Aortic aneurysms	15	Yes	53
Scobie et al[70]	1979	Aortic aneurysms	23	No	71
Macbeth et al[77]	1984	Femoropopliteal specimens	43	Yes	71
McAuley et al[116]	1984	Aortic thrombus	14	No	NR
Buckels et al[76]	1985	Aortic aneurysms	8	Yes	30
Durham et al[78]	1987	Aortofemoropopliteal specimens	44	Yes	56
Schwartz et al[117]	1987	Aortic aneurysms	10	No	54
Ilgenfritz and Jordan[118]	1988	Aortic aneurysms and atrial septal defects	20	No	55
Brandimarte et al[119]	1989	Aortic aneurysms	31	No	NR
Wakefield et al[24]	1990	Aortofemoropopliteal specimens	12	No	60

NR, not reported.

an 8% (22 of 275) incidence of positive cultures from aortic aneurysm contents.[76] The incidence of graft sepsis was 32% (7 of 22) in patients with positive cultures, compared with 2.4% (6 of 253) in the culture-negative group.

Similar data suggest that lower extremity arteries can also become infected. In 1984, Macbeth and colleagues reported on cultures of arterial wall specimens from 88 clean, elective lower extremity revascularization procedures.[77] Control cultures were taken from adjacent adipose or lymphatic tissue. Although all control cultures were negative, arterial wall cultures were positive in 43% of cases (38 of 88). Of these, 71% (27 of 38) grew *S. epidermidis*. The authors described three graft infections in 335 cases (0.9% infection rate), all of which had positive arterial wall cultures. Also included in this report was a retrospective review of 22 cases of graft infection for which arterial and graft culture data were available. Of the patients with positive arterial cultures, 57% (8 of 14) had suture line disruption, whereas there were no disruptions in the culture-negative group.[77] Durham and colleagues reported a series of 102 patients undergoing vascular reconstruction with a 74% (75 of 102) incidence of positive arterial wall cultures.[78] *S. epidermidis* accounted for 56% of the cultured organisms. Six infections (3.5%) occurred over 18 months; all these patients had prior positive arterial cultures. No patients with negative arterial cultures developed graft infection. The greatest risk for graft infection appeared to be in patients with positive arterial wall cultures undergoing reoperation.

Hematogenous and Lymphatogenous Seeding

Hematogenous seeding of vascular prostheses is another potential source of graft infection. Anecdotal reports implicate urinary tract infection,[46,47] abdominal sepsis,[47,52,70] and other infections[45] in the development of vascular graft infections. Laboratory models demonstrate that bacteremia reliably produces prosthetic graft infections.[79-81]

Other Local and Systemic Factors

Open wounds on the distal lower extremities may be a source of contaminating bacteria. Hoffert and colleagues noted that 75% of patients with graft infections (9 of 12) had open, infected lesions on the distal lower extremity at the time of graft implantation.[43] Liekweg and Greenfield reported that 33% of inguinal infections (20 of 60) occurred proximal to open foot infections.[50] Bunt and Mohr described the presence of bacteria cultured from a distally infected extremity in the inguinal lymph nodes of two patients undergoing lower extremity revascularization; both patients developed graft infection.[82]

Prior vascular surgery has been implicated as a risk factor for vascular graft infection. Dense scar tissue, increased bleeding, and lymphatic leak may all contribute to this phenomenon. Goldstone and Moore noted that 45% of patients (12 of 27) with graft infections had undergone one or more revisions of the original graft before developing an infection in the same region.[47] In 8 of the 12 patients, the infection was in the groin. In the series of Edwards and coworkers, 9 of 18 patients (50%) had undergone a previous vascular surgery at the site of the graft infection.[63] Similarly, a report from Reilly and colleagues described a history of multiple previous vascular procedures at the site of graft infection in 40% of cases.[56]

Johnson and associates found that prior vascular procedures were not a significant risk factor for graft infection; however, only 12 of 135 patients in this series had prior operations at the site of infection.[83]

The immunologic status of patients with vascular disease may also have an impact on the development of graft infection. Systemic disease, malnutrition, and medical debility may suppress the host response to invading microorganisms. Kwaan and colleagues reported on 12 patients with advanced, fulminating graft infections, all of whom had critical deficiencies in immune status as determined by serum albumin, hemoglobin, immunoglobulin, and lymphocyte assays and by response to standard skin test antigens.[84] Eight of 12 patients who received total parenteral nutrition had significant enhancement of immune response and accelerated recovery from the graft infection. Of the four patients who did not receive nutritional support, two had a prolonged convalescence, and two subsequently died from complications of graft infection.

EXPERIMENTAL INVESTIGATIONS

The suggestion that prophylactic antibiotic therapy may be effective in the prevention of surgical infections was first made 50 years ago.[85-89] In the early 1960s, Alexander and colleagues demonstrated the efficacy of penicillin prophylaxis in experimental wound infections.[90,91]

Lindenauer and associates reported an experimental demonstration of the importance of antibiotics in preventing graft infection.[51] Three groups of dogs underwent femoral arteriotomy with primary, Teflon patch, or vein patch closure. A fourth group received sham operation alone. Wounds were contaminated with 10,000 to 100,000 S. *aureus* organisms. All subjects, except controls, received intramuscular (IM) procaine penicillin. Among control animals, the infection rate was 94% (8 of 9 shams, 3 of 3 arteriotomies, 3 of 3 Teflon patches, 3 of 3 vein patches). In animals treated with penicillin, the infection rate was 0% (15 shams, 5 arteriotomies, 5 Teflon patches, 5 vein patches). Thus, antibiotic therapy may sterilize a contaminated wound even in the presence of a prosthetic arterial patch.

Moore and colleagues tested the utility of antibiotic prophylaxis in a canine model of hematogenous aortic graft contamination.[92] Thirty minutes before laparotomy, dogs were infused intravenously with 10 million S. *aureus* organisms and then underwent placement of a Dacron infrarenal aortic graft. The experimental group received an IV dose of cephalothin (25 mg/kg), which was started just before the skin incision and continued for 30 minutes after the procedure. Experimental animals then received IM cephalothin three times a day for 5 days; control animals received no antibiotics. Control animals experienced a significantly increased rate of positive cultures (72%) compared with animals that received perioperative cephalothin (24%).

CLINICAL INVESTIGATIONS

Early Experience

Up until the mid-1970s, the use of antibiotics in vascular reconstruction with synthetic materials was largely based on personal preference. It is notable that in the series of Szilagyi and colleagues from 1972, the graft infection rate among

2145 cases in which prophylactic antibiotics were not administered was 1.5%.[45] Fry and Lindenauer reported an incidence of 1.34% in 890 cases in which no antibiotics were used.[44] These infection rates were comparable with, and often lower than, those reported in series in which prophylactic antibiotics were used.[49] Noting the preponderance of *S. aureus* in vascular graft infections, particularly in cases involving an inguinal incision, Szilagyi and colleagues suggested a clinical trial of an antibiotic directed at this organism in reconstructions that required an inguinal anastomosis.[45]

In 1974, Goldstone and Moore published a review of the San Francisco Veterans Administration Hospital experience with vascular prosthetic infection.[47] This series of 566 aortofemoropopliteal reconstructions was divided into two time periods: 1959 to 1965, when antibiotics were administered only postoperatively; and 1966 to 1973, when prophylaxis included pre-, intra-, and postoperative antibiotics. The incidence of graft infection in the former group was 4.1% (9 of 222), compared with 1.5% (5 of 344) in the latter. Although the investigators conceded that greater experience and skill may have contributed to the lower incidence of infection, they maintained that the major factor responsible was the more appropriate use of antibiotics in the second group of patients. The following year, Perdue published a similar retrospective review that suggested that the institution of routine antibiotic prophylaxis reduced the incidence of wound infections and other nosocomial infections in patients undergoing major arterial reconstructive procedures.[93]

Prospective Trials

The first large, prospective, randomized, blinded clinical study of antibiotic prophylaxis in vascular reconstructive surgery was published by Kaiser and colleagues in 1978.[65] In that series, 462 patients undergoing aortofemoropopliteal reconstruction were randomized to receive either 1 g of cefazolin or a saline placebo. There were no graft infections among 225 patients who received cefazolin, compared with 4 of 237 placebo recipients (1.7%). When superficial skin infections and subcutaneous skin infections were considered in the analysis (Szilagyi classes I and II), the overall infection rates were 0.9% in the cefazolin group and 6.8% in the placebo group. Given no adverse drug reactions and no noted cefazolin resistance, the authors strongly recommended a short course of cefazolin prophylaxis in patients undergoing arterial reconstructive surgery.

In 1980, Pitt and colleagues reported the results of a controlled study of cephradine prophylaxis in vascular procedures involving groin incisions in which topical, systemic, and topical plus systemic administration were compared.[94] Of 205 patients, 52 had prosthetic grafts placed, whereas the remainder received vein grafts. Infection rates were equivalent in these two groups. Wound infection rates were 0% for those receiving topical administration alone and systemic administration alone, 5.9% for patients receiving both, and 24.5% for controls. No distinction was made between graft (Szilagyi class III) and isolated wound (Szilagyi classes I and II) infections. Minimum follow-up was 4 weeks, but the mean length of follow-up was not indicated. Patients in whom synthetic graft material was used did not experience a higher incidence of wound infection. The authors concluded that topical and systemic prophylaxis were equally efficacious and

that combined prophylaxis was unnecessary. The follow-up interval in this study, however, was not long enough to make conclusive statements.

The benefit of a short course of systemic cephalosporin prophylaxis in vascular reconstructive surgery was subsequently confirmed in a number of other prospective, randomized trials. In 1983, Salzmann reported a trial of cefuroxime (a second-generation agent) and later cefotaxime (a third-generation agent) versus placebo in 300 patients undergoing aortofemoropopliteal reconstruction.[95] The prophylaxis regimen was changed from cefuroxime to cefotaxime midway through the study because the latter was found to be more effective in vitro against the most common graft infection pathogens at the author's institution. Graft infection rates were 2.4% for the placebo group and 0.8% for the prophylaxis group. The incidence of wound infection was 15.1% in the placebo group and 3.0% in the prophylaxis group. No differences in infection rate were noted between the two antibiotics, and the author concluded that either agent could be used effectively in the prophylaxis of postoperative infection.

Addressing the question of duration of treatment for antibiotic prophylaxis, Hasselgren and colleagues compared 1- and 3-day courses of cefuroxime versus placebo in lower extremity arterial reconstruction.[96] There was only one graft infection in this small cohort of 110 patients, and this occurred in the placebo group. The wound infection rate was 16.7% for patients receiving placebo, compared with 3.8% in the 1-day and 4.3% in the 3-day prophylaxis groups. The investigators recommended that prophylactic antibiotic therapy be limited to a short-term course.

Bennion and colleagues examined the utility of antibiotic prophylaxis in patients with chronic renal insufficiency undergoing placement of a prosthetic arteriovenous shunt for hemodialysis.[97] Patients were randomized to receive cefamandole or placebo just before placement of a PTFE graft, followed by two subsequent doses. The wound infection rate for the cefamandole group was 10.5% (2 of 19), with one graft (Szilagyi class III) infection. The wound infection rate in the placebo group was 42.1% (8 of 19), with three graft infections.[97] This high rate of infection is not uncommon in renal failure patients, and the study emphasized the importance of perioperative antibiotic prophylaxis.

Robbs and associates reported a trial of cloxacillin plus gentamicin versus cefotaxime in infrainguinal arterial reconstruction.[98] This group had adopted a 48-hour course of cloxacillin plus gentamicin as their routine prophylaxis owing to the predominance of *S. aureus* and gram-negative infections at their institution. Length of follow-up ranged from 6 to 20 months. The wound infection and graft infection rates for patients receiving cloxacillin plus gentamicin were 5.4% (7 of 129 wounds) and 1.5% (1 of 63 grafts), respectively. The rates for patients receiving cefotaxime were 6.3% (8 of 127 wounds) and 3.3% (2 of 61 grafts). The differences were not statistically significant. The authors concluded that the multiagent 2-day regimen conferred no advantage over the shorter, single-agent regimen.

Comparisons of Antibiotic Regimens

Because it has become evident that a short course of a cephalosporin antibiotic is the ideal prophylaxis for vascular reconstructive procedures, several studies have focused on whether the most widely used cephalosporin, cefazolin, is the best choice. A large number of graft infections, particularly in abdominal grafts, are due to gram-negative rods. A theoretical disadvantage of first-generation cephalosporins such as cefazolin is that they are more vulnerable to gram-negative beta-lactamase than are second- and third-generation agents. Gram-negative activity is thus limited to E. coli, Proteus species, and Klebsiella species, and many hospital-acquired strains of these organisms are cefazolin resistant. It has also been demonstrated that other cephalosporins, such as the second-generation agent cefamandole, have greater in vitro activity against coagulase-negative staphylococci, which have been found to colonize the native arterial wall in a large number of patients. It is clear from previous studies by Salzmann[95] and by Hasselgren[96] and Robbs[98] and their coworkers that second- and third-generation cephalosporins can be used effectively in vascular surgery prophylaxis.

In 1989, Lalka and colleagues examined this issue in a prospective study of arterial wall microbiology and antibiotic penetration.[75] Forty-seven patients undergoing aortofemoropopliteal reconstruction were randomized to receive perioperative cefazolin or cefamandole, 1 g every 6 hours for nine doses. Serial samples of serum, subcutaneous fat, thrombus, atheroma, and arterial wall were obtained for culture and assay of drug levels by high-performance liquid chromatography. Serum and tissue levels of cefazolin were significantly higher than those of cefamandole at almost all time points. Positive arterial wall cultures were obtained in 41.4% of patients, and 68.8% of bacterial isolates were coagulase-negative staphylococci (half of these were slime producers). At times, the arterial wall concentration of both antibiotics fell below the geometric mean minimal inhibitory concentration for all organisms combined, but this occurred significantly more often with cefamandole. The investigators concluded that both antibiotics needed to be administered in larger doses (cefazolin, 1.5 g every 4 hours; cefamandole, 2 g every 3 hours) and that the antibiotics were essentially equal in efficacy if administered appropriately. This study corroborated the findings of Mutch and colleagues,[99] who noted that serum antibiotic levels did not correlate well with aortic tissue concentrations of bioactive antibiotic, and it suggested that arterial tissue levels rather than serum levels should be the standard for comparison of antibiotic efficacy.

Edwards and colleagues reported, in 1992, a prospective trial of cefazolin versus the more beta-lactamase–stable second-generation cephalosporin cefuroxime in patients undergoing aortic and peripheral vascular reconstruction.[100] Prior studies had suggested that some failures of cefazolin prophylaxis were due to this agent's susceptibility to staphylococcal beta-lactamase and that other cephalosporins might provide better protection in cardiac surgery.[65,101,102] Antibiotics were administered just before surgery, redosed intraoperatively, and continued every 6 hours postoperatively for 24 hours. Dosage and administration schedules were based on a prior pharmacokinetic study. The infection rate in the cefazolin group was 1% (3 of 287), versus 2.6% (7 of 272) in the cefuroxime group. This difference was not statistically significant. Cefuroxime exhibited lower trough concentrations than did cefazolin, and the length of the operative procedure was found to be a risk factor for infection only in the cefuroxime group. The investigators concluded that despite its lower resistance to beta-lactamase, cefazolin provides better perioperative prophylaxis because of its greater antistaphylococcal potency and superior pharmacokinetic profile.[100] Data from this and other studies[65] suggest that intraoperative redosing of cefazolin should be more frequent in prolonged procedures than in routine therapeutic administration—that is, every 4 hours rather than every 6 hours.

CURRENT STATUS OF ANTIBIOTIC PROPHYLAXIS

Antibiotic Selection

Cefazolin is currently the antibiotic of choice for routine vascular surgery prophylaxis. It is relatively inexpensive, has negligible toxicity and a low incidence of severe allergic reactions, and is active against many of the bacteria commonly implicated in graft infection (Tables 10-4 and 10-5). Its pharmacokinetic profile is ideal for this indication, with reliably high peak serum concentrations and a long half-life of elimination compared with other cephalosporins.[100,103] It penetrates arterial tissue well, with drug concentrations exceeding the minimal inhibitory concentration of common graft infection pathogens in most instances.[75] Cefazolin is active against S. aureus (including penicillinase-producing strains), some strains of S. epidermidis, and the more commonly encountered gram-negative rods E. coli, Proteus species, and Klebsiella species. Most other gram-negative rods are resistant, including indole-positive Proteus vulgaris. Cephalothin, the other first-generation agent in common clinical use, is somewhat more resistant to staphylococcal beta-lactamase, but it is less active against gram-negative organisms. More important, it is cleared from plasma four to five times as rapidly as cefazolin.[103]

Later-generation cephalosporins have greater gram-negative activity and the potential benefit of increased resistance to staphylococcal beta-lactamase; however, in vitro and in vivo activity against gram-positive cocci is reduced. Many investigators have tailored their choice of antibiotic to the

Prophylaxis	No. of Infections	No. of Patients	Infected (%)	Class I Infections (%)	Class II Infections (%)	Class III Infections (%)
Cefazolin	2	225	0.9*	0	2	0
Placebo	16	237	6.8*	4	8	4
Total	18	462	3.9	4	10	4

TABLE 10–4 Wound Infections among Patients Receiving Cefazolin or Placebo Prophylaxis

*Difference is significant at P < 0.001. Brachiocephalic procedures are not included.
From Kaiser AB, Clayson KR, Mulherin JL, et al: Antibiotic prophylaxis in vascular surgery. Ann Surg 188:283, 1978.

TABLE 10–5	Antibacterial Spectrum of Selected Antibiotics				
	Antibacterial Activity (MIC-90 in µg/mL)*				
Antibiotic	*S. aureus*	*S. epidermidis*	*E. coli*	*Klebsiella* spp.	*Pseudomonas* spp.
Cefazolin	1.0	0.8	5.0	6.0	R
Cephalothin	1.0	0.5	5.0	32.0	R
Cefamandole	1.0	2.0	4.0	8.0	R
Cefuroxime	2.0	1.0	4.0	R	R
Cefotaxime	2.0	8.0	0.25	0.25	>32.0
Vancomycin	1.0	3.0	R	R	R
Penicillin V	ALP+: >25.0	0.02[†]	R	R	R
	ALP–: 0.03				
Oxacillin	0.25	0.2[†]	R	R	R
Gentamicin	0.6	2.0[†]	4.0	1.0	2.0
Ciprofloxacin	0.5	0.25	0.03	0.125	0.5
Rifampin	0.015	0.015	16.0	32.0	64.0

*MIC-90 is the minimal inhibitory concentration for 90% of strains. MIC > 64 µg/mL is considered resistant. Values are approximate and may vary among institutions.
[†]Many strains are resistant.
ALP, alkaline phosphatase; R, resistant.
Data from Mandell RGD (ed): Principles and Practice of Infectious Diseases, 3rd ed. New York, Churchill Livingstone, 1989.

predominant organisms responsible for graft infection at their particular institutions. Cefamandole,[75] cefuroxime,[104] and cefotaxime[98] have all been used effectively as prophylactic agents in prospective trials. However, cefamandole has fallen out of favor for routine use owing to an association with hypoprothrombinemia and bleeding, particularly in elderly patients and those with renal insufficiency. Cefuroxime has been shown to have antistaphylococcal potency and pharmacokinetic properties inferior to those of cefazolin.[100] The third-generation agents such as cefotaxime have broad anti–gram-negative activity but are generally less active against staphylococci. Moreover, the later-generation cephalosporins are, in most instances, significantly more expensive than the first-generation agents. Cefazolin, therefore, remains the antibiotic of choice, except in specific instances when in vitro testing has revealed that another agent more adequately covers the principal pathogens of graft infection.

A potential disadvantage of cefazolin prophylaxis is the inconsistent activity of this agent against the organism that is currently responsible for the greatest number of graft infections, *S. epidermidis*. It has been shown that during hospitalization, patients acquire multiply resistant strains of this bacterium.[105,106] Up to 75% of *S. epidermidis* isolates at some institutions are now cefazolin resistant. Vancomycin is highly active against both *S. epidermidis* and *S. aureus*; resistance in these organisms is rarely encountered. Vancomycin, however, provides no gram-negative coverage. It is the drug of choice for prophylaxis in patients with a history of anaphylaxis to beta-lactam antibiotics, often in combination with an aminoglycoside in procedures in which there is significant risk of gram-negative infection, such as aortic reconstruction. Vancomycin is also considered the antibiotic of choice for the prophylaxis of prosthetic hemodialysis access grafts and for patients known to be colonized with methicillin-resistant *S. aureus*. It is excreted primarily by glomerular filtration and therefore persists in high serum concentrations in patients with end-stage renal disease.

The broad antibacterial spectrum, excellent tissue penetration, and low toxicity of the fluoroquinolones make them potentially ideal agents for the prophylaxis of surgical infections. Limited data are available concerning the use of fluoroquinolones for this indication, but there are reports of efficacy equal or superior to that of cephalosporin antibiotics in the prophylaxis of colorectal,[107,108] biliary,[107,109] and urologic surgery.[110-112] Auger and coauthors reported a randomized study of pefloxacin, a nalidixic acid analog, and cefazolin in patients undergoing cardiac surgery.[113] Of 111 patients, 14 receiving pefloxacin developed bacterial colonization at culture sites, compared with 11 in the cefazolin group. One patient who received cefazolin developed mediastinitis from a cefazolin-resistant strain of *S. epidermidis*. As yet, there are no published clinical trials of a fluoroquinolone versus a cephalosporin in the prophylaxis of peripheral vascular surgery procedures.

Antibiotic Administration

Prophylactic antibiotics are administered just before surgery and redosed intraoperatively during long procedures. Pharmacokinetic studies suggest that prophylactic antibiotics should be administered more frequently and in higher doses during surgery than is recommended for routine therapeutic indications (e.g., cefazolin 1.5 g every 4 hours).[65,100,114] Prophylaxis is usually continued postoperatively for up to 24 hours and possibly longer when there is a theoretical risk of postoperative bacteremia from indwelling venous catheters, arterial lines, bladder catheters, and endotracheal tubes. The advantage of continuing coverage beyond the operating room, however, has not been clearly demonstrated. In the absence of these risk factors, there is clearly no advantage in extending antibiotic prophylaxis for longer than 24 hours.

Regimens of prophylaxis should be tailored to the type of vascular reconstruction undertaken. Cefazolin prophylaxis is recommended in all procedures involving the placement of prosthetic materials. It is probably not necessary in "clean" vascular procedures of the neck and upper extremities that do not involve the use of synthetic grafts. In contrast, the marked colonization and favorable bacterial environment of the lower abdomen and groin necessitate the use of antibiotic prophylaxis in all aortofemoropopliteal vascular procedures. The risk of gram-negative infection in aortic reconstruction may necessitate the addition of an aminoglycoside, particularly in institutions with a high degree of cefazolin resistance among gram-negative isolates. Alternatively, a second- or third-generation cephalosporin with broader anti–gram-negative activity may be substituted, as this obviates the risk of aminoglycoside-associated nephrotoxicity.

Cephalosporins should be avoided in patients with a history of anaphylaxis to beta-lactam antibiotics. Patients with a history of minor allergic reactions to penicillin antibiotics may be given a cephalosporin test dose to determine whether cross-reactivity is present. Reduced dosing of cefazolin and most other cephalosporins is recommended in renal insufficiency, based on the calculated creatinine clearance.

There is evidence that remote bacteremia may be implicated in vascular graft infection. Accordingly, oral prophylaxis for procedures that are highly associated with bacteremia, such as tooth extraction, cystoscopy, and colonoscopy, is recommended. Wooster and colleagues demonstrated in 200 vascular surgery patients undergoing cystoscopy that the incidence of bacteremia was 64% among inpatients and 8% among outpatients.[68] For procedures such as tooth extraction and colonoscopy, prophylaxis must be tailored to the most common normal flora of the traumatized site. Penicillins are appropriate choices for major dental procedures, whereas broader gram-negative and anaerobic coverage may be warranted in colonoscopy. It should be emphasized, however, that the true risk of graft infection after procedures associated with bacteremia is unclear, and there is currently no consensus on the role of antibiotic prophylaxis in this setting.

REFERENCES

1. Rokitansky K: Handbuch der pathologischen Anatomie, 2nd ed. 1844, p 55.
2. Koch L: Über Aneurysma der Arteriae mesenterichae superioris [dissertation]. Erlangen, Germany, 1851.
3. Osler W: The Gulstonian lectures on malignant endocarditis. BMJ 1:467, 1885.
4. Crane A: Primary multilocular mycotic aneurysm of the aorta. Arch Pathol 24:634, 1937.
5. Ponfick E: Über embolische Aneurysmen, nebst Bemerkungen über das acute Herzaneurysma (Herzgeschwur). Virchows Arch 58:528, 1873.
6. Eppinger H: Pathogenese (Histogeneses und Aetiologie) der Aneurysmen einschliesslich des Aneurysma equiverminosum. Arch Klin Chir 35:404, 1887.
7. Weisel J: Die Erkrankungen arterieller Gefässe im Verlaufe akuter Infektionen. Z Heilkd 27:269, 1916.
8. Lewis D, Schrager V: Embolomycotic aneurysms. JAMA 53:1808, 1909.
9. Cathcart R: False aneurysms of the femoral artery following typhoid fever. South Med J 2:593, 1909.
10. Revell S: Primary mycotic aneurysms. Ann Intern Med 22:431, 1943.
11. Hawkins J, Yeager G: Primary mycotic aneurysm. Surgery 40:747, 1956.
12. Yellin A: Ruptured mycotic aneurysm, a complication of parenteral drug abuse. Arch Surg 112:981, 1977.
13. Lande A, Beckman Y: Aortitis—pathologic, clinical and arteriographic review. Radiol Clin North Am 14:219, 1976.
14. Hirst AJ, Affeldt J: Abdominal aortic aneurysm with rupture into the duodenum: A report of eight cases. Gastroenterology 10:504, 1951.
15. Reddy DJ, Ernst CB: Infected aneurysms: Recognition and management. Semin Vasc Surg 1:541, 1984.
16. Brown SL, Busuttil RW, Baker JD, et al: Bacteriologic and surgical determinants of survival in patients with mycotic aneurysms. J Vasc Surg 1:541, 1984.
17. Stengal A, Wolferth C: Mycotic (bacterial) aneurysms of intravascular origin. Arch Intern Med 31:527, 1923.
18. Magilligan D, Quinn E: Active infective endocarditis. In Magilligan DJ, Quinn E (eds): Endocarditis: Medical and Surgical Management. New York, Marcel Dekker, 1986, p 207.
19. Wilson S, Van Wagenen P, Passaro EJ: Arterial infection. Curr Probl Surg 15:5, 1978.
20. Bennett D, Cherry J: Bacterial infection of aortic aneurysms: A clinicopathological study. Am J Surg 113:321, 1967.
21. Jarrett F, Darling R, Mundth E, et al: Experience with infected aneurysms of the abdominal aorta. Arch Surg 10:1281, 1975.
22. Ernst C, Campbell H, Daugherty M, et al: Incidence and significance of intra-operative bacterial cultures during abdominal aortic aneurysmectomy. Ann Surg 185:626, 1977.
23. Reddy D, Smith R, Elliot JJ, et al: Infected femoral artery false aneurysms in drug addicts: Evolution of selective vascular reconstruction. J Vasc Surg 3:718, 1986.
24. Wakefield T, Pierson C, Schoberg D, et al: Artery, periarterial adipose tissue, and blood microbiology during vascular reconstructive surgery: Perioperative and postoperative observations. J Vasc Surg 11:624, 1990.
25. Chan F, Crawford E, Coselli J, et al: In situ prosthetic graft replacement for mycotic aneurysm of the aorta. Ann Thorac Surg 47:193, 1989.
26. Crawford E, Crawford J: Diseases of the Aorta Including an Atlas of Angiographic Pathology and Surgical Techniques. Baltimore, Williams & Wilkins, 1984.
27. Mundth E, Darling R, Alvarado RH, et al: Surgical management of mycotic aneurysms and the complications of infections in vascular reconstructive surgery. Am J Surg 110:460, 1969.
28. Kaufman J, Smith R, Capel G, et al: Antibiotic therapy for arterial infection: Lessons from the successful treatment of a mycotic femoral artery aneurysm without surgical reconstruction. Ann Vasc Surg 4:592, 1990.
29. Ewart J, Burke M, Bunt T: Spontaneous abdominal aortic infections: Essentials of diagnosis and management. Am Surg 49:37, 1983.
30. Lemos D, Raffetto J, Moore T, Menzoian J: Primary aortoduodenal fistula: A case report and review of the literature. J Vasc Surg 37:686, 2003.
31. Daugherty M, Shearer GR, Ernst CB: Primary aortoduodenal fistula: Extra-anatomic vascular reconstruction not required for successful management. Surgery 86:399, 1979.
32. Bandyk DF, Novotney ML, Johnson BL, et al: Use of rifampin-soaked gelatin-sealed polyester grafts for in situ treatment of primary aortic and vascular prosthetic infections. J Surg Res 95:44, 2001.
33. Batt M, Magne J, Alric P, et al: In situ revascularization with silver-coated polyester grafts to treat aortic infection: Early and midterm results. J Vasc Surg 38:983, 2003.
34. Schulman ML, Badhey MR, Yatco R, Pillari G: An 11-year experience with deep leg veins as femoropopliteal bypass grafts. Arch Surg 121:1010, 1986.
35. Clagett GP, Valentine RJ, Hagino RT: Autogenous aortoiliac/femoral reconstruction from superficial femoral-popliteal veins: Feasibility and durability. J Vasc Surg 25:255, 1997.
36. Kieffer E, Bahnini A, Koskas F, et al: In situ allograft replacement of infected infrarenal aortic prosthetic grafts: Results in forty-three patients. J Vasc Surg 17:349, 1993.
37. Leseche G, Castier Y, Petit MD, et al: Long-term results of cryopreserved arterial allograft reconstruction in infected prosthetic grafts and mycotic aneurysms of the abdominal aorta. J Vasc Surg 34:616, 2001.
38. Berchtold C, Eibl C, Seelig MH, et al: Endovascular treatment and complete regression of an infected abdominal aortic aneurysm. J Endovasc Ther 9:543, 2002.
39. Koeppel TA, Gahlen J, Diehl S, et al: Mycotic aneurysm of the abdominal aorta with retroperitoneal abscess: Successful endovascular repair. J Vasc Surg 40:164, 2004.
40. Johnson J, Ledgerwood A, Lucas C: Mycotic aneurysms: New concepts in therapy. Arch Surg 118:577, 1983.
41. Patel K, Semel L, Clauss R: Routine revascularization with resection of infected femoral pseudoaneurysm from substance abuse. J Vasc Surg 8:322, 1988.
42. Wright D, Shepard A: Infected femoral artery aneurysm associated with drug abuse. In Stanley J, Ernst C (eds): Current Therapy in Vascular Surgery. Philadelphia, BC Decker, 1990, p 350.
43. Hoffert P, Gensler S, Haimovichi H: Infection complicating arterial grafts. Arch Surg 90:427, 1965.
44. Fry WJ, Lindenauer SM: Infection complicating the use of plastic arterial implants. Arch Surg 94:600, 1967.

45. Szilagyi DE, Smith RF, Elliott JP, Vrandecic MP: Infection in arterial reconstruction with synthetic grafts. Ann Surg 106:321, 1972.
46. Lorentzen JE, Nielsen OM, Arendrup H: Vascular graft infection: An analysis of sixty-two graft infections in 2411 consecutively implanted synthetic vascular grafts. Surgery 98:81, 1985.
47. Goldstone J, Moore WS: Infection in vascular prostheses: Clinical manifestations and surgical management. Am J Surg 128:225, 1974.
48. Bandyk D, Berni G, Thiele B, Towne J: Aortofemoral graft infection due to *Staphylococcus epidermidis*. Arch Surg 119:102, 1984.
49. Jamieson G, DeWeese J, Rob C: Infected arterial grafts. Ann Surg 181:850, 1975.
50. Liekweg WG, Greenfield LJ: Vascular prosthetic infections: Collected experience and results of treatment. Surgery 81:335, 1977.
51. Lindenauer S, Fry W, Schaub G, Wild D: The use of antibiotics in the prevention of vascular graft infections. Surgery 62:487, 1967.
52. Yashar J, Weyman A, Burnard R, Yashar J: Survival and limb salvage in patients with infected arterial prostheses. Am J Surg 135:499, 1978.
53. Buchbinder D, Pasch AR, Rollins DL, et al: Results of arterial reconstruction of the foot. Arch Surg 121:673, 1986.
54. Edwards MJ, Richardson D, Klamer TW: Management of aortic prosthetic infections. Am J Surg 155:327, 1988.
55. O'Hara PJ, Hertzer NR, Beven EG, Krajewski LP: Surgical management of infected abdominal aortic grafts: Review of a 25-year experience. J Vasc Surg 3:725, 1986.
56. Reilly L, Stoney R, Goldstone J, Ehrenfeld W: Improved management of aortic graft infection: The influence of operation sequence and staging. J Vasc Surg 5:421, 1987.
57. Reilly LM, Altman H, Lusby RJ, et al: Late results following surgical management of vascular graft infection. J Vasc Surg 1:36, 1984.
58. Yeager R, McConnell D, Sasaki T, Vetto R: Aortic and peripheral prosthetic graft infection: Differential management and causes of mortality. Am J Surg 150:36, 1985.
59. Samson RH, Veith FJ, Janko GS, et al: A modified classification and approach to the management of infections involving peripheral arterial prosthetic grafts. J Vasc Surg 8:147, 1988.
60. Conn J, Hardy J, Chavez C, et al: Infected arterial grafts. Ann Surg 101:704, 1970.
61. Elek S, Conen P: The virulence of *Staphylococcus pyogenes* for man: A study of the problems of wound infection. Br J Exp Pathol 38:573, 1957.
62. Smith R, Lowry K, Perdue G: Management of the infected arterial prosthesis in the lower extremity. Am Surg 33:711, 1967.
63. Edwards W, Martin R, Jenkins J, et al: Primary graft infections. J Vasc Surg 6:235, 1987.
64. Quiñones-Baldrich WJ, Hernandez JJ, Moore WS: Long-term results following surgical management of aortic graft infection. Arch Surg 126:507, 1991.
65. Kaiser A, Clayson K, Mulherin J: Antibiotic prophylaxis in vascular surgery. Ann Surg 188:283, 1978.
66. Close A, Stengel B, Love H: Preoperative skin preparation with povidone-iodine. Am J Surg 108:398, 1964.
67. Cruse P: A five-year prospective study of 23,649 surgical wounds. Arch Surg 107:206, 1973.
68. Wooster D, Louch R, Kradjen S: Intraoperative bacterial contamination of vascular grafts: A prospective study. Can J Surg 28:407, 1985.
69. Bouhoutsos J, Chavatsas D, Martin P, Morris T: Infected synthetic arterial grafts. Br J Surg 61:108, 1974.
70. Scobie K, McPhail N, Barber G, Elder R: Bacteriologic monitoring in abdominal aortic surgery. Can J Surg 22:368, 1979.
71. DeBakey M, Ochsner J, Cooley D: Associated intraabdominal lesions encountered during resection of aortic aneurysms: Surgical considerations. Dis Colon Rectum 3:485, 1960.
72. Stoll W: Surgery for intraabdominal lesions associated with resection of aortic aneurysms. WMJ 65:89, 1966.
73. Hardy J, Tompkins W, Chavez C, Conn J: Combining intra-abdominal arterial grafting with gastrointestinal or biliary tract procedure. Am J Surg 126:598, 1973.
74. Becker R, Blundell P: Infected aortic bifurcation grafts: Experience with 14 patients. Surgery 80:544, 1976.
75. Lalka S, Malone J, Fisher D, et al: Efficacy of prophylactic antibiotics in vascular surgery: An arterial wall microbiologic and pharmacokinetic perspective. J Vasc Surg 10:501, 1989.
76. Buckels J, Fielding J, Black J, et al: Significance of positive bacterial cultures from aortic aneurysm contents. Br J Surg 72:440, 1985.
77. Macbeth G, Rubin J, McIntyre KJG, Malone J: The relevance of arterial wall microbiology to the treatment of prosthetic graft infections: Graft infection vs arterial infection. J Vasc Surg 1:750, 1984.
78. Durham J, Malone J, Bernhard V: The impact of multiple operations on the importance of arterial wall cultures. J Vasc Surg 5:160, 1987.
79. Moore WS, Chvapil M, Sieffert G, Keown K: Development of an infection resistant vascular prosthesis. Arch Surg 116:1403, 1981.
80. White J, Benvenisty A, Reemtsma K, et al: Simple methods for direct antibiotic protection of synthetic vascular grafts. J Vasc Surg 1:372, 1984.
81. Chervu A, Moore WS, Gelabert HA, et al: Prevention of graft infection by use of prostheses bonded with a rifampin/collagen release system. J Vasc Surg 14:521, 1991.
82. Bunt TJ, Mohr J: Incidence of positive inguinal lymph node cultures during peripheral revascularization. Am J Surg 50:522, 1984.
83. Johnson JA, Cogbill TH, Strutt PJ, Gundersen AL: Wound complications after infrainguinal bypass: Classification, predisposing factors, and management. Arch Surg 123:859, 1988.
84. Kwaan J, Dahl R, Connolly J: Immunocompetence in patients with prosthetic graft infection. J Vasc Surg 1:45, 1984.
85. Pulaski E, Schaeffer J: The background of antibiotic therapy in surgical infections. Surg Gynecol Obstet 93:1, 1951.
86. Pulaski E: Discriminate antibiotic prophylaxis in elective surgery. Surg Gynecol Obstet 108:385, 1959.
87. Linton R: The appropriate use of antibiotics in clean surgery. Surg Gynecol Obstet 112:218, 1961.
88. Altemeier W, Culbertson W, Vetto M: Prophylactic antibiotic therapy. Arch Surg 71:2, 1955.
89. Altemeier W, Culbertson W, Sherman R, et al: Critical re-evaluation of antibiotic therapy in surgery. JAMA 157:305, 1955.
90. Alexander J, McGloin J, Altemeier W: Penicillin prophylaxis in experimental wound infections. Surg Forum 11:299, 1960.
91. Alexander J, Altemeier W: Penicillin prophylaxis of experimental staphylococcal wound infection. Surg Gynecol Obstet 120:243, 1965.
92. Moore W, Rosson C, Hall A: Effect of prophylactic antibiotics in preventing bacteremic infection in vascular prostheses. Surgery 69:825, 1971.
93. Perdue G: Antibiotics as an aid in the prevention of infections after peripheral arterial surgery. Am Surg 41:296, 1975.
94. Pitt H, Postier R, MacGowan W, et al: Prophylactic antibiotics in vascular surgery. Ann Surg 192:356, 1980.
95. Salzmann G: Perioperative infection prophylaxis in vascular surgery: A randomized prospective study. Thorac Cardiovasc Surg 31:239, 1983.
96. Hasselgren P, Ivarsson L, Risberg B, Seeman T: Effects of prophylactic antibiotics in vascular surgery. Ann Surg 200:86, 1984.
97. Bennion R, Hiatt J, Williams R, et al: A randomized prospective study of perioperative microbial prophylaxis for vascular surgery. J Cardiovasc Surg 26:270, 1985.
98. Robbs J, Reddy E, Ray R: Antibiotic prophylaxis in aortic and peripheral arterial surgery in the presence of infected extremity lesions. Drugs 35(Suppl 2):141, 1988.
99. Mutch D, Richards G, Brown R, et al: Bioactive antibiotic levels in the human aorta. Surgery 92:1068, 1982.
100. Edwards W, Kaiser A, Kernodle D, et al: Cefuroxime versus cefazolin as prophylaxis in vascular surgery. J Vasc Surg 15:35, 1992.
101. Kernodle D, Classen D, Burke J, et al: Failure of cephalosporins to prevent surgical wound infections. JAMA 263:961, 1990.
102. Slama T, Sklar S, Misinski J, et al: Randomized comparison of cefamandole, cefazolin, and cefuroxime in open-heart surgery. Antimicrob Agents Chemother 29:744, 1986.
103. Mandell G, Sande M: Penicillins, cephalosporins and other beta-lactam antibiotics. In Gilman A, Rall T, Nies A, Taylor P (eds): Goodman and Gilman's The Pharmacologic Basis of Therapeutics, 8th ed. Elmsford, NY, Pergamon Press, 1990, p 1065.
104. Herbst A, Kamme C, Norgren L, et al: Infections and antibiotic prophylaxis in reconstructive vascular surgery. Br J Vasc Surg 3:303, 1989.
105. Levy M, Schmitt D, Edmiston C, et al: Sequential analysis of staphylococcal colonization of body surfaces of patients undergoing vascular surgery. J Clin Microbiol 28:664, 1990.
106. Archer G, Tenenbaum M: Antibiotic-resistant *Staphylococcus epidermidis* in patients undergoing cardiac surgery. Antimicrob Agents Chemother 10:269, 1980.
107. Cooreman F, Ghyselen J, Penninckx F: Pefloxacin vs cefuroxime for prophylaxis of infections after elective colorectal surgery. Rev Infect Dis 11(Suppl 5):S1301, 1989.
108. Offer C, Weuta H, Bodner E: Efficacy of perioperative prophylaxis with ciprofloxacin or cefazolin in colorectal surgery. Infection 16(Suppl 1):S46, 1988.
109. Kujath P: Brief report: Antibiotic prophylaxis in biliary tract surgery: Ciprofloxacin vs ceftriaxone. Am J Med 87(Suppl 5A):255S, 1989.

110. Gombert M, DuBouchet L, Aulicino T, et al: Brief report: Intravenous ciprofloxacin versus cefotaxime prophylaxis during transurethral surgery. Am J Med 87(Suppl 5A):250S, 1989.

111. Cox C: Comparison of intravenous ciprofloxacin and intravenous cefotaxime for antimicrobial prophylaxis in transurethral surgery. Am J Med 87(Suppl 5A):252S, 1989.

112. Christensen M, Nielsen K, Knes J, et al: Brief report: Single-dose preoperative prophylaxis in transurethral surgery: Ciprofloxacin versus cefotaxime. Am J Med 87(Suppl 5A):258S, 1989.

113. Auger P, Leclerc Y, Pelletier L, et al: Efficacy and safety of pefloxacin vs cefazolin as prophylaxis in elective cardiovascular surgery. Rev Infect Dis 11(Suppl 5):S1302, 1989.

114. Guglielmo B, Salazar T, Rodondi L, et al: Altered pharmacokinetics of antibiotics during vascular surgery. Am J Surg 157:410, 1989.

115. Casali R, Tucker W, Thompson B, Read R: Infected prosthetic grafts. Arch Surg 115:577, 1980.

116. McAuley C, Steed D, Webster M: Bacterial presence in aortic thrombus at elective aneurysm resection: Is it clinically significant? Am J Surg 147:322, 1984.

117. Schwartz J, Powell T, Burnham S, Johnson G Jr: Culture of abdominal aortic aneurysm contents, an additional series. Arch Surg 122:777, 1987.

118. Ilgenfritz F, Jordan F: Microbiological monitoring of aortic aneurysm wall and contents during aneurysmectomy. Arch Surg 123:506, 1988.

119. Brandimarte C, Santini C, Venditti M, et al: Clinical significance of intraoperative cultures of aneurysm walls and contents in elective abdominal aortic aneurysmectomy. Eur J Epidemiol 5:521, 1989.

Questions

1. True or false: Arterial trauma is involved in the pathogenesis of most primary arterial infections.

2. When should prosthetic grafts be used to replace excised mycotic aneurysms?
   (a) If the surgical field is laved with antibiotics
   (b) In the upper extremities
   (c) Only in carefully selected instances
   (d) In fungal arterial infections
   (e) Never

3. Since 1965, what organism is most commonly associated with microbial aortitis?
   (a) *Salmonella* species
   (b) Fungi
   (c) Mycobacteria
   (d) *Pseudomonas* species
   (e) *Staphylococcus aureus*

4. In the management of a mycotic mesenteric aneurysm located in the distal arterial arcade (adjacent to the intestine), what is the recommended management?
   (a) Reconstruction with a Dacron graft
   (b) Reconstruction with a PTFE graft
   (c) Reconstruction with an umbilical vein graft
   (d) Reconstruction with a vein graft
   (e) Ligation and excision without reconstruction

5. True or false: The recommended management of an infrarenal mycotic aneurysm involves the use of antibiotics, débridement of infected tissues, and reconstruction through a remote (extra-anatomic) uninfected field.

6. What is the average reported incidence of prosthetic graft infection?
   (a) 1% to 6%
   (b) 6% to 10%
   (c) 10% to 15%
   (d) Greater than 15%
   (e) 0% to 1%

7. True or false: The study by Pitt and colleagues revealed that intravenous antibiotics were much more effective than antibiotic irrigation.

8. Risk factors for prosthetic graft infection include which of the following?
   (a) Multiple reoperations
   (b) Inguinal incisions
   (c) Open, infected wounds on the extremities
   (d) Prior graft infections
   (e) Positive arterial wall cultures
   (f) All of the above

9. Avenues of infection include which of the following?
   (a) Skin
   (b) Arterial wall
   (c) Open wounds on the distal limb
   (d) Intestinal transudate accumulated during aortic bypass
   (e) Foley catheter
   (f) All of the above

10. What are the most common organisms found in prosthetic graft infections?
    (a) *Proteus* species
    (b) *Escherichia coli*
    (c) *Staphylococcus aureus*
    (d) *Streptococcus viridans*
    (e) *Staphylococcus epidermidis*

Answers

1. true	2. c	3. a	4. e	5. true
6. a	7. false	8. f	9. f	10. e

11

Peter Gloviczki

Vascular Malformations

Vascular malformations (VMs) are developmental abnormalities of the vascular system. They should be differentiated from vascular tumors or hemangiomas, because they have different causes, growth patterns, treatments, and outcomes. Malformations may involve any segment of the vascular tree: arteries, capillaries, veins, or lymphatics. High-flow arteriovenous malformations are associated with shunting of large amounts of arterial blood into the venous system; these lesions can have alarming hemodynamic manifestations, such as venous engorgement, distal limb ischemia, and high-output cardiac failure. Predominantly venous malformations are the most common type seen at vascular clinics; most have a benign clinical course and require no special treatment. In one series, the ratio of venous to arteriovenous malformations was 4:1.[1] Most VMs are mixed, and some complex malformations such as Klippel-Trénaunay syndrome or Parkes Weber syndrome are associated with developmental abnormalities of other tissues, including bone and soft tissue overgrowth or digital abnormalities.[2-4]

Historical Notes

Birthmarks and congenital deformities have been described by historians and depicted by painters for centuries. One of the first detailed medical descriptions of an arteriovenous malformation with pulsating varices of the head, caused by a so-called cirsoid aneurysm, dates back to the 16th century.[5] Slowing of the heart rate after compression of a high-shunt congenital arteriovenous malformation was first described by Nicoladoni in 1875.[6] This so-called bradycardia sign of arteriovenous fistulas was observed later by Branham in a patient with acquired arteriovenous fistula.[7] Excellent early descriptions of arteriovenous malformations can be found in the works of Reid,[8] Holman,[9] de Takats,[10] and Coursley and associates.[11] Malan and Puglionisi presented a detailed classification of vascular malformations (angiodysplasia),[12] although the first practical guidelines for clinical classification and treatment were given by Szilagyi and coworkers.[13,14] In excellent reviews, Rutherford and colleagues[15] and Rosen and Riles[16] summarized the state of the art of VMs. Of the multiple classifications published, the Hamburg classification is the one used most frequently today.[1,17,18] Although surgical excision may be

recommended for local lesions, selective catheterization, embolotherapy, and percutaneous sclerotherapy (usually with absolute alcohol) have changed the management of VMs in the last 2 decades.[19-22]

Definitions

Vascular malformations are localized errors of angiogenic development, whereas hemangiomas are vascular tumors. Mulliken and colleagues defined the endothelial characteristics and cell biology of VMs and vascular tumors.[23-25] The term *hemangioma* should be reserved for vascular tumors alone. During the proliferative phase they undergo growth, and then they resolve. The proliferative phase occurs during the first year, and spontaneous involution of hemangiomas is observed in 95% of cases by age 7 years. The female-male ratio is 5:1. Thirty percent of hemangiomas are present at birth, and the rest develop within the first 3 months of life. Endothelial hyperplasia is evident on biopsies obtained from hemangiomas; these cells grow in tissue culture, and in the proliferative phase they incorporate ^{3}H-thymidine and have an increased mast cell count.[25] Most patients with hemangiomas require no treatment at all.

In contrast, VMs are developmental, congenital abnormalities. There is increasing evidence that aberrant signaling at the molecular level results in dysfunction of normal proliferation, differentiation, maturation, and apoptosis of the vascular cells.[26] Localized, superficial, mostly venous or capillary VMs—"birthmarks" of the skin and mucosa—are most common, but VMs also occur in the skeletal muscles, the pelvis or chest, visceral organs such as the lungs, the gastrointestinal system, and the brain.[15,16,26] The abnormal vascular channels are lined by a continuous endothelium and surrounded by an abnormal complement of mural cells. Ninety percent of them are present at birth, and the male-female ratio is 1:1. VMs show no endothelial proliferation, and no cell growth is observed in tissue culture; the cells do not incorporate ^{3}H-thymidine, and no mast cells have been observed in biopsy specimen.[23-25] Clinically, no proliferation or spontaneous involution has been observed in VMs. The growth of the malformation is usually commensurate with the growth of the child, although hemodynamic factors (arteriovenous shunting, venous stasis) can accelerate growth and morbidity. Most low-flow VMs have a benign course, although complications such as bleeding, thrombophlebitis, skin changes, or infection may need treatment. High-flow arteriovenous malformations usually have a more ominous course and a worse prognosis. Treatment of these lesions is frequently needed.

Development of the Vascular System

Because the classification, clinical presentation, and prognosis of VMs depend to a great extent on the point at which there is an arrest or abnormality in the development of the vascular system, it is worthwhile to review briefly the normal development of the vascular tree of the limbs. Primitive vascular channels first appear in the third week of gestation. During its development, the vascular system undergoes differentiation through multiple stages, first described by Woollard in 1922.[27] Stage 1 is the *undifferentiated* stage, with only a capillary network being present. Stage 2 is the *retiform* stage, when large plexiform structures can be seen. In stage 3, by the third week of gestation, the *maturation* stage includes the development of large channels, arteries, and veins.

Vascular endothelial growth factor (VEGF), secreted by keratinocytes, has been found to be responsible for inducing the penetration of capillary vessels into the avascular epidermis.[28,29] This invasion and the subsequent arterial differentiation are also guided by VEGF originating from sensory nerves.[30] A defective migratory response of endothelial cells to VEGF is the consequence of abnormal signaling of VEGF receptors. Malformations develop if the differentiation is abnormal and there is an arrest in the development of normal vascular tissue. It is the persistence of the normal embryonic vascular system and any additional abnormal development that result in VMs.

Classification

Because of the complex presentation and frequently mixed nature of VMs, classification has been difficult. Malan and Puglionisi attempted to separate them based on anatomic appearance and the presence or absence of arteriovenous shunting.[12] The classification of Szilagyi and colleagues[13,14] was based primarily on Woollard's stages of embryologic development. Capillary malformations develop when there is an arrest in stage 1 (Fig. 11-1). Although Szilagyi named these malformations *hemangiomas*, they are not tumors but capillary or cavernous VMs. Microfistulous or macrofistulous arteriovenous malformations develop if there is an arrest in stage 2 (see Fig. 11-1). Persistence of large embryonic veins that develop in stage 3 is seen in patients with persistent sciatic vein (Fig. 11-2) or in those with large lateral veins of the leg (Fig. 11-3). There are many mixed VMs owing to involvement of several segments of the vascular system (capillaries, veins, lymphatics).

Forbes and associates distinguished VMs based on hemodynamics and contrast angiographic appearance.[20] Depending on the amount of blood supplying the malformation, high-flow and low-flow lesions are distinguished. These are called *high-shunt* and *low-shunt* lesions; the size of the shunt is determined by the volume of blood that enters the feeding vessels. High-shunt lesions correspond with macrofistulous arteriovenous malformations, whereas microfistulous arteriovenous

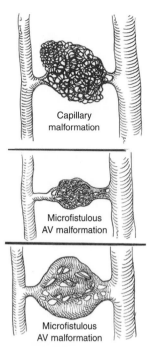

FIGURE 11–1 • Capillary malformation, microfistulous arteriovenous (AV) malformation, and macrofistulous arteriovenous malformation.

malformations are low-shunt lesions. Between these two extremes, a whole spectrum of malformations exists.

The most recent and now widely used classification is the 1988 Hamburg classification, with modifications by Rutherford and Lee (Table 11-1).[1,17,18] A malformation is first

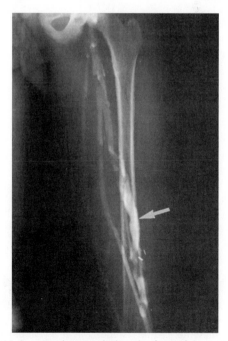

FIGURE 11–2 • Persistent sciatic vein *(arrow)* in a 12-year-old girl. Surgical resection of the painful vein through a posterior approach resulted in an excellent clinical result at 7 years' follow-up. The dilated vein contained no valves. (From Cherry KJ, Gloviczki P, Stanson AW: Persistent sciatic vein: Diagnosis and treatment of a rare condition J Vasc Surg 23:490-497, 1996.)

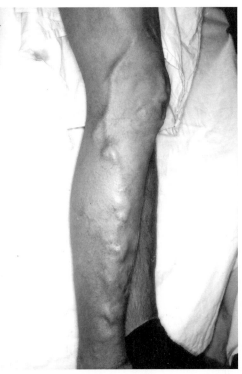

FIGURE 11–3 • Persistent lateral embryonic veins in a 19-year-old man with Klippel-Trénaunay syndrome. (From Noel AA, Gloviczki P, Cherry KJ Jr, et al: Surgical treatment of venous malformations in Klippel-Trenaunay syndrome. J Vasc Surg 32:840-847, 2000.)

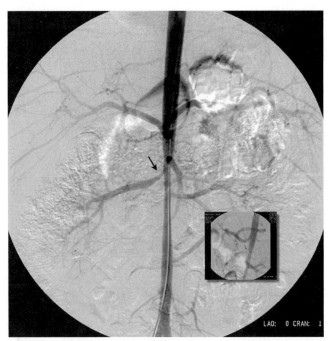

FIGURE 11–4 • Abdominal aortic coarctation associated with renal and mesenteric artery stenosis in a 9-year-old boy with renovascular hypertension. The *arrow* indicates right renal artery stenosis; the *arrow* in the inset shows superior mesenteric artery stenosis. (From West CA, Delis KT, Service G, et al: Middle aortic syndrome: Surgical treatment in a child with neurofibromatosis, renovascular hypertension, superior mesenteric artery stenosis and intermittent claudication. J Vasc Surg [in press].)

TABLE 11–1	The Hamburg Classification of Vascular Malformations (Revised)
Affected Segment of the Vascular System	**Anatomic Forms**

Arterial malformations	Truncular forms
	  Aplasia or obstruction
	  Dilatation
	Extratruncular forms
	  Infiltrating
	  Limited

Venous malformations	Truncular forms
	  Aplasia or obstruction
	  Dilatation
	Extratruncular forms
	  Infiltrating
	  Limited

Arteriovenous (AV) malformations (with shunting)	Truncular forms
	  Deep AV fistula
	  Superficial AV fistula
	Extratruncular forms
	  Infiltrating
	  Limited

Lymphatic malformations	Truncular forms
	  Aplasia or obstruction
	  Dilatation
	Extratruncular forms
	  Infiltrating
	  Limited

Combined vascular malformations	Truncular forms
	  Arterial and venous
	  Hemolymphatic
	Extratruncular forms
	  Infiltrating hemolymphatic
	  Limited hemolymphatic

classified by the predominant vascular defect (arterial, venous, arteriovenous, lymphatic, or combined); it is further classified into truncular or extratruncular form, depending on the involvement of major axial vessels or branches of major arteries or veins.

The truncular forms of predominantly *arterial* VMs include aplasia or obstruction, stenosis, coarctation, dilatation, and aneurysm. These include malformations such as the persistent sciatic artery or an aberrant left subclavian artery that runs behind the esophagus and causes the typical syndrome of dysphagia lusoria.[31] Thoracic or abdominal aortic coarctation (Fig. 11-4),[32] anomalies of the aortic arch, and persistence of embryonic mesenteric vessels are other examples of these malformations. The extratruncular forms can be diffuse or localized.

Predominantly *venous* malformations may also be truncular; these include aplasia or obstruction, stenosis or hypoplasia, dilatation, and aneurysm. Many patients with Klippel-Trénaunay syndrome have persistence of large embryonic veins or hypoplasia, dilatation, or aneurysmal dilatation of the deep veins of the limb (Fig. 11-5).[33-36] The estimated prevalence of deep venous anomalies in patients with predominantly venous malformations was 47% in one study.[35] Phlebectasia was the most common (36%), followed by

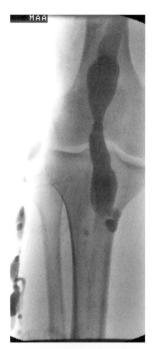

FIGURE 11–5 • Aneurysmal dilatation of the popliteal vein with bandlike narrowing associated with atypical lateral varicosity in a 19-year-old man with Klippel-Trénaunay syndrome. (From Noel AA, Gloviczki P, Cherry KJ Jr, et al: Surgical treatment of venous malformations in Klippel-Trenaunay syndrome. J Vasc Surg 32:840-847, 2000.)

aplasia or hypoplasia of the deep venous trunks (8%) and venous aneurysms (8%).

Extratruncular venous VMs are the most frequent malformations, and they can be diffuse (Fig. 11-6; see color plate) or localized. Most venous malformations are localized defects of vascular morphogenesis that present as single or multiple bluish purple lesions, mainly in the skin and the mucosa.[26] Specimens obtained at biopsy show enlarged, endothelial-lined veinlike channels with abnormal smooth muscle cells.

Predominantly *arteriovenous* malformations are divided into truncular and extratruncular lesions; both can be either localized or diffuse. Lesions with clinical or angiographic evidence of arteriovenous communication in the limbs (Parkes Weber–type malformations) or pelvis are the type most frequently seen by vascular surgeons. Low-shunt (Fig. 11-7) and high-shunt (Fig. 11-8) malformations are distinguished. The hereditary arteriovenous VMs in the lung and sometimes in the brain and gut are part of hereditary hemorrhagic telangiectasia syndrome.[37] Arteriovenous malformations are perhaps most frequent in the central nervous system, and vascular surgeons performing carotid arteriography and stenting should recognize and be familiar with arteriovenous VMs and high-flow arteriovenous fistulas of the brain.

Capillary malformations, or port-wine stains, are frequent. These cutaneous lesions appear as a red macular stain that darkens over years (Fig. 11-9). Capillary malformations are typical in patients with Sturge-Weber syndrome, Klippel-Trénaunay syndrome, and Parkes Weber syndrome.[38,39]

Lymphatic malformations are also frequent findings in some series. Truncular forms include obstruction or hypoplasia causing congenital lymphedema[40-43] or dilatation leading to valvular incompetence and rupture of lymphatics, causing chylous effusions or chylocutaneous fistulas due to reflux of chyle.[44] Most lymphatic cysts and "lymphangiomas" are lymphatic malformations, and many venous malformations contain lymphatic tissue.

More than 70% of VMs are mixed, and these complex abnormalities may include arterial, capillary, venous, or lymphatic elements as well. Although the Hamburg classification discourages the use of eponyms, some of them were named after the physicians who first described the conditions, and these names have become widely accepted and used. The list of clinical syndromes of VM includes Parkes Weber, Klippel-Trénaunay, Servelle-Martorell (Fig. 11-10; see color plate), Sturge-Weber, Rendu-Osler-Weber, von Hippel-Lindau, Kasabach-Merritt, Proteus (Fig. 11-11; see color plate), and Mafucci's syndromes, among others (Table 11-2).[15,16,38,39,45-47]

Genetics

Genetic information on VMs has greatly increased in recent years. Most VMs are sporadic, but autosomal dominant inheritance has also been described. Genetic studies of families have resulted in the identification of mutated genes,[26,39,48-54] which play an important role in angiogenesis. These mutated genes in some patients encode tyrosine kinase receptors and intracellular signaling molecules.[26] Vikkula and coworkers identified the endothelial-specific angiopoietin receptor TIE2/TEK, located on chromosome 9p21, as the cause of familial mucocutaneous VMs.[26,52] Glomuvenous malformations (venous malformations with glomus cells, or glomangiomas) are similar to VMs; most of these lesions are inherited, and Boon and colleagues identified the gene glomulin, a novel locus on the short arm of chromosome 1.[53]

Port-wine stains have also been observed in families, and a genetic susceptibility for capillary malformations was suggested. Eerola and associates identified a large locus, CMC1, on chromosome 5q.[39] These authors used genetic fine mapping to identify a positional candidate gene, RASA1; heterozygous inactivating RASA1 mutations were detected in families manifesting capillary malformations. Of interest, arteriovenous malformation, arteriovenous fistula, or Parkes Weber syndrome was also documented in all the families with this mutation.

Arteriovenous malformations in the lungs, brain, or gut may be part of hereditary hemorrhagic telangiectasia (HHT).[37] Two genes encoding proteins associated with transforming growth factor-β receptor have been identified, causing HHT1 and HHT2, respectively.

Primary congenital lymphedema can be hereditary (Milroy disease), and late-onset primary lymphedema has been observed in multiple members of the same families (Meige disease).[40-43] Congenital lymphedema has been linked to chromosome 5q35.3, where the VEGFR3 gene is located. It is likely that congenital lymphedema is caused by lack of sufficient signaling via the VEGFR3 receptor.[26]

Incidence

Vascular malformations occur in 1.5% of the population.[35] Published series of VMs seen at referral centers suggest that predominantly venous malformations are the most common

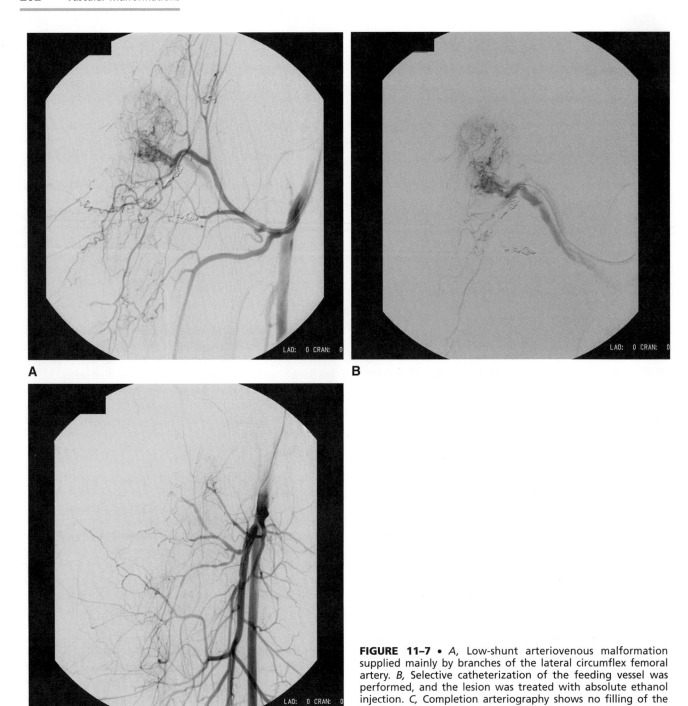

FIGURE 11–7 • *A*, Low-shunt arteriovenous malformation supplied mainly by branches of the lateral circumflex femoral artery. *B*, Selective catheterization of the feeding vessel was performed, and the lesion was treated with absolute ethanol injection. *C*, Completion arteriography shows no filling of the lesion. (Courtesy of Michael A. McKusick, MD, Mayo Foundation.)

vascular anomalies.[35] They are estimated to occur in 1 in 5000 to 10,000 childbirths.[26] Venous malformations are certainly the most frequent type that requires medical attention. Still, it is likely that capillary malformations or port-wine stains of the skin and mucosa are the most frequent VMs, occurring in 0.3% of childbirths.[39] Among 797 patients with VMs reported by Lee and colleagues, 40% had predominantly lymphatic malformations.[1] Arteriovenous shunts occurred in 9.5% of the cases in their series.

Clinical Presentation

Patients with VMs are frequently asymptomatic, and a birthmark of the skin or mucosa is often only a cosmetic deformity. However, those patients who seek consultation with a vascular surgeon may have a complex presentation, and the limbs or pelvis may be extensively involved. Clinical presentations include varicose veins (see Fig. 11-3), limb edema or overgrowth (Fig. 11-12; see color plate), port-wine stain, and

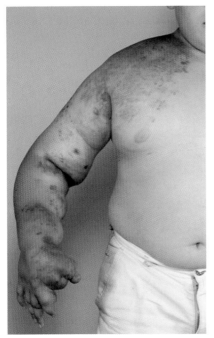

FIGURE 11–6 • Diffuse extratruncular venous malformation involving the right arm. (Courtesy of David J. Driscoll, MD, Mayo Foundation)

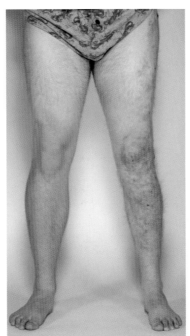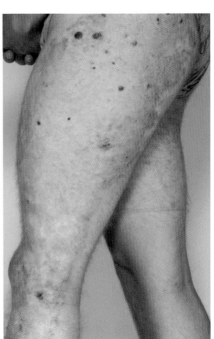

A   **B**

FIGURE 11–10 • In Servelle-Martorell syndrome, the typical venous malformation is extratruncular and diffuse. The affected extremity is shorter, there are phleboliths present on plain radiographs, and there is no arteriovenous shunting. Spontaneous bone fracture and osteopenia are frequent. Usually there are no port-wine stains. (Courtesy of David J. Driscoll, MD, Mayo Foundation.)

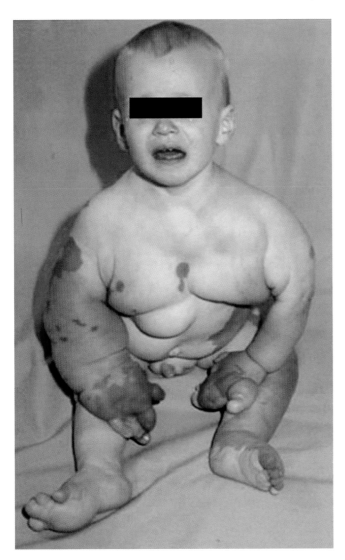

FIGURE 11–11 • Patient with Proteus syndrome consisting of disproportionate overgrowth of multiple tissues, vascular malformations, and connective tissue or linear epidermal nevi. The patient had multiple lipomas and hyperostosis. (Courtesy of David J. Driscoll, MD, Mayo Foundation.)

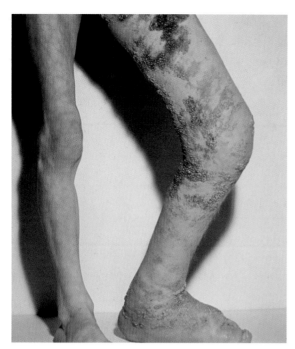

FIGURE 11–12 • Klippel-Trénaunay syndrome with overgrowth of the left lower extremity by 12 cm.

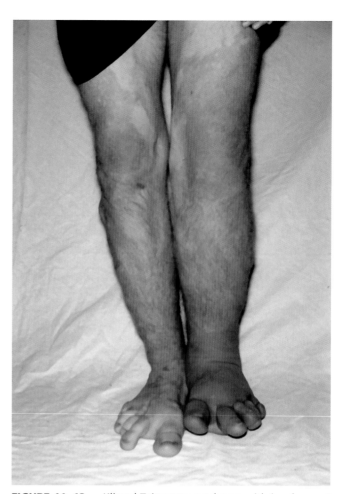

FIGURE 11–13 • Klippel-Trénaunay syndrome with involvement of both lower extremities. Note the port-wine stains and digital anomalies.

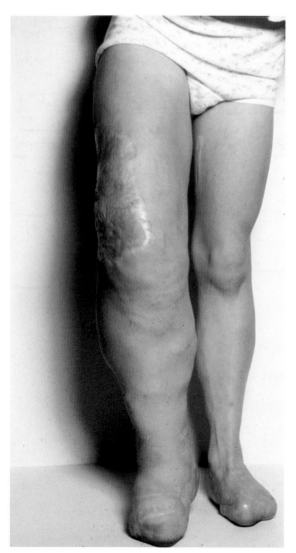

FIGURE 11–14 • Bilateral leg involvement in Klippel-Trénaunay syndrome. Bilateral transmetatarsal amputations were needed because of digital anomalies.

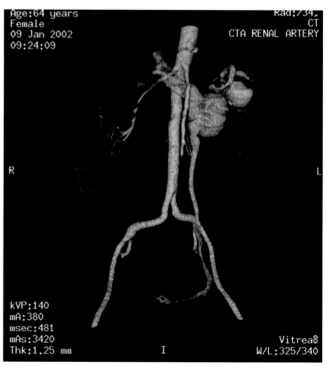

FIGURE 11–18 • Three-dimensional CT reconstruction of a venous malformation involving the left renal vein and the hilum of the left kidney. (Courtesy of Terri J. Vrtiska, MD, Mayo Foundation.)

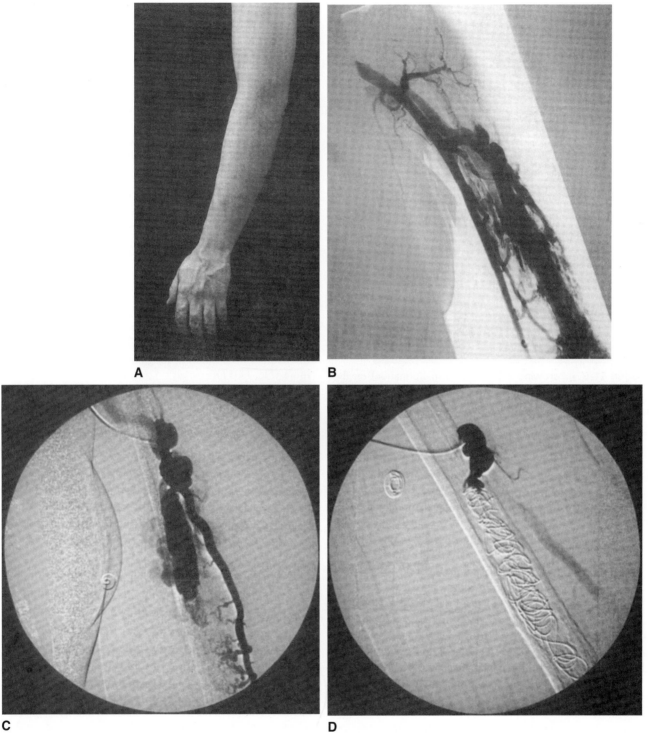

FIGURE 11–8 • *A*, High-shunt, high-flow arteriovenous malformation involving the left arm and hand of a 26-year-old woman. *B*, Left arm arteriogram reveals an extensive arteriovenous malformation with involvement of the bone and soft tissue. *C*, Selective injection of the deep brachial artery reveals involvement of the interosseous branches of the humerus as well. *D*, The large arteriovenous fistula in the medullary cavity of the humerus was embolized using numerous coils and three strands of No. 2-0 silk sutures. Almost complete occlusion of the arteriovenous fistula in the humerus was noted. (Courtesy of A. W. Stanson, MD, Mayo Foundation.)

digital anomalies (Figs. 11-13 and 11-14; see color plate). The affected limb or pelvis may harbor a mass that is pulsatile; there may be a systolic-diastolic bruit and a palpable thrill. The varicose veins are usually atypical, lateral or suprapubic, although varicosity occasionally involves the great saphenous vein and its tributaries. Bleeding or leakage of lymph fluid from VMs is not infrequent. Thrombophlebitis, cellulitis and lymphangitis, skin lesions, induration, pigmentation, and ulcerations can be signs of chronic venous insufficiency. Many patients with mixed lesions have associated lymphedema.

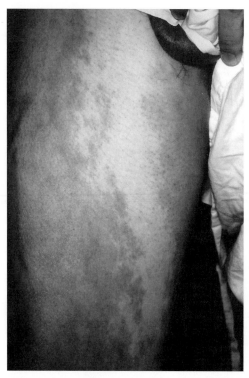

FIGURE 11–9 • Port-wine stain (capillary malformation) on the affected extremity of a patient with Klippel-Trénaunay syndrome. Note also the large lateral embryonic vein of the thigh. (From Noel AA, Gloviczki P, Cherry KJ Jr, et al: Surgical treatment of venous malformations in Klippel-Trenaunay syndrome. J Vasc Surg 32:840-847, 2000.)

Patients with pelvic involvement may present with hematuria and rectal bleeding. Any patient with varicose veins or port-wine stains with a longer or shorter limb must be suspected of having an underlying VM. Patients with primary or secondary lymphedema have limbs of identical length.

In a Mayo Clinic study of 185 patients with arteriovenous malformations of the extremities and pelvis, the most frequent clinical sign was skin discoloration (43%), and the most frequent symptom was pain (37%).[55] Thirty-five percent had a palpable mass, and 34% had limb hypertrophy. A bruit was present in 26%, and 20% of patients had some skin necrosis or ulceration. Increased skin temperature at the level of the lesion, decreased distal pulses, pulsatile veins, and edema of the extremity were additional clues to the diagnosis.

Evaluation

Diagnostic tests should focus on evaluating the type and extent of the malformation; the presence or absence of any arteriovenous shunting must also be established. Physical examination of limb and pelvic lesions should be complemented by segmental systolic limb pressure measurement and establishment of the ankle-brachial index. Pulse volume recording is helpful in patients with arteriovenous shunting (Fig. 11-15). Placement of a tourniquet on a limb with a high-flow, high-shunt arteriovenous malformation and occlusion of the fistula will increase systolic blood pressure, followed by a slowing of the heart rate due to a vagal response in the baroreceptors in the aorta and carotid arteries (bradycardia sign). Duplex scans can confirm other hemodynamic

consequences of an arteriovenous shunt (Fig. 11-16), such as a low-resistance waveform in the arteries and pulsatile flow in the veins. Duplex scans can also establish the patency of the superficial and deep veins, as well as other abnormalities such as aneurysm or dilatation, hypoplasia, or valvular incompetence.

To document arteriovenous shunting, labeled microspheres are useful. Technetium 99m–labeled human albumin microspheres are injected into the artery proximal to an arteriovenous shunt. Less than 3% of the microspheres should pass through a normal capillary bed. The percentage of the shunted material is calculated based on radioactivity in the lungs, measured after a separate injection of the colloid in a vein of the body.[15]

Contrast echocardiography is also useful to establish arteriovenous shunting. It can detect the appearance of indocyanine green on the venous side, after intra-arterial injection; the test was used by Pritchard and coworkers to determine residual shunts after surgical excision.[56,57]

Imaging Studies

Scanograms are performed to document any length discrepancy between the limbs. Scanograms are long bone radiographic films that provide the most accurate measurement of the length of the different long bones of the upper and lower limbs (Fig. 11-17).

Computed tomography (CT) scans and three-dimensional CT-angiography have progressed rapidly in recent years, and they provide excellent pictures of the malformations; high-quality angiography is also possible with the advent of new CT technology (Fig. 11-18; see color plate). CT can show the extent of involvement, but arteriovenous malformations may not always be distinguishable from venous malformations. Because intravenous contrast is required, appropriate timing of the imaging is necessary, depending on the amount of blood shunted in the VM.

Magnetic resonance imaging and magnetic resonance angiography have multiple advantages. They can differentiate muscle, bone, fat, and vascular tissue without the need for radiation or intravenous contrast, which may be harmful to the kidneys. Axial, coronal, and sagittal images can be generated (Fig. 11-19), and gadolinium enhancement provides high-quality angiography. High-flow and low-flow fistulas can be distinguished.

Contrast arteriography is reserved for patients who are potential candidates for arterial embolization (Figs. 11-20 and 11-21). Arteriovenous shunting is confirmed by contrast arteriography, which also delineates the feeding arteries and excludes the presence of any vascular tumor (see Fig. 11-8). The size of the feeding arteries can be measured, and the size of the arteriovenous shunts (2 mm in large shunts, 100 to 200 μm in small shunts) can be estimated based on the appearance of contrast in the vein. The flow volume is determined by the size and rate of opacification of the feeding arteries, whereas the shunt volume can be estimated with acceptable accuracy by the time and appearance of contrast medium in the veins.

Contrast venography is reserved for patients who are potential candidates for venous intervention (see Fig. 11-5). Contrast venography is frequently done through multiple injections in the limb, with the use of a tourniquet or Esmarch bandage to visualize the deep system, and with direct injection into the malformation before or after ethanol sclerotherapy.

TABLE 11–2	Clinical Syndromes Associated with Vascular Malformations					
Syndrome	**Inheritance**	**Type**	**Location**	**Characteristic Features**	**Treatment**	**Prognosis**
Parkes Weber	Somatic mutations	AVM (intraosseous or close to epiphyseal plate) Port-wine stain	Extremities Pelvis	Soft tissue and bone hypertrophy Varicosity (atypical) Capillary and high-flow, high-shunt AVM	Observation Elastic support Embolization ± excision (localized lesions only)	Deep, diffuse lesions have poor prognosis
Klippel-Trénaunay	Somatic mutations	No- or low-shunt AVM Venous or lymphatic Port-wine stains	Extremities Pelvis Trunk	Soft tissue and bone hypertrophy Varicosities (lateral lumbar to foot pattern) Capillary or venous vascular malformation, lymphatic malformation	Elastic support Seldom: epiphyseal stapling or selective excision or ablation of varicose veins	Usually good
Rendu-Osler-Weber (hereditary hemorrhagic telangiectasia)	Autosomal dominant	Punctate angioma Telangiectasia GI tract AVM	Skin Mucous membranes Liver Lungs Kidneys Brain Spinal cord	Epistaxis Hematemesis, melena Hematuria Hepatomegaly Neurologic symptoms	Transfusions Embolization vs. laser treatment ± excision	Good if bleeding can be controlled and no CNS manifestations
Sturge-Weber (encephalo-trigeminal angiomatosis)	No	Port-wine stains	Trigeminal area Leptomeninges Choroid Oral mucosa	Convulsions Hemiplegia Ocular deformities Mental retardation Glaucoma Intracerebral calcification	Anticonvulsants Neurosurgical procedure	Guarded Depends on intracranial lesion
von Hippel-Lindau (oculocerebellar hemangioblastomatosis)	Autosomal dominant	Hemangioma	Retina Cerebellum	Cysts in cerebellum, pancreas, liver, adrenals, kidneys	Excision of cysts	Depends on intracranial lesion
Blue rubber bleb nevus	Autosomal dominant	Cavernous venous malformation	Skin GI tract Spleen Liver CNS	Bluish, compressible rubbery lesions GI bleeding, anemia	Transfusions Electrocoagulation Excision	Depends on CNS and GI involvement
Kasabach-Merritt	Autosomal dominant	Large cavernous venous malformation	Trunk Extremities	Thrombocytopenia Hemorrhage Anemia Ecchymosis Purpura	Compression Transfusion of blood, platelets	Death from hemorrhage or infection
Maffucci's (dyschondroplasia with vascular hamartoma)	Probably autosomal dominant	AVM Cavernous lymphangioma	Fingers Toes Extremities Viscera	Enchondromas Spontaneous fractures Deformed, shorter extremity Vitiligo	Orthopedic management	Chance of malignancy 20%

AVM, arteriovenous malformation; CNS, central nervous system; GI, gastrointestinal.
Adapted from Gloviczki AA, Noel AA, Hollier LH: Arteriovenous fistulas and vascular malformations. In Ascher E (ed): Haimovici's Vascular Surgery, 5th ed. Malden, Mass, Blackwell, 2004, pp 991-1014.

Treatment

INDICATIONS

There are absolute and relative indications for the treatment of VMs. The absolute indications include hemorrhage, ischemia, refractory ulcers, and congestive heart failure. Bleeding from malformations may occur through defects in the skin or mucosa, or the patient may have intramuscular or retroperitoneal hematoma, hematuria, rectal bleeding, hematemesis, hemoptysis, or intracerebral or intraspinal bleeding. Relative indications for treatment include pain, claudication, functional impairment, limb asymmetry, and cosmetic reasons. A multidisciplinary approach in the evaluation and treatment of VMs provides the best result for

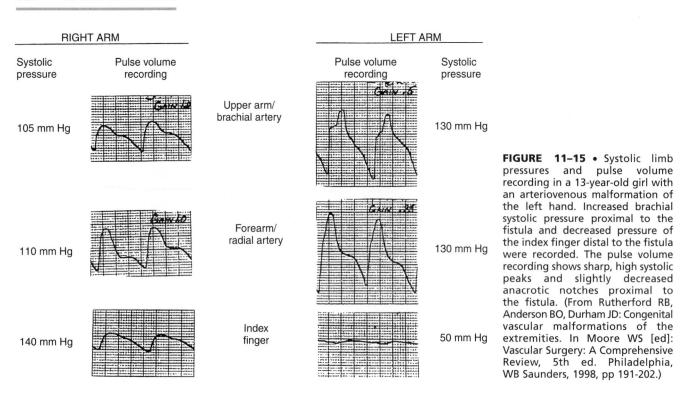

FIGURE 11–15 • Systolic limb pressures and pulse volume recording in a 13-year-old girl with an arteriovenous malformation of the left hand. Increased brachial systolic pressure proximal to the fistula and decreased pressure of the index finger distal to the fistula were recorded. The pulse volume recording shows sharp, high systolic peaks and slightly decreased anacrotic notches proximal to the fistula. (From Rutherford RB, Anderson BO, Durham JD: Congenital vascular malformations of the extremities. In Moore WS [ed]: Vascular Surgery: A Comprehensive Review, 5th ed. Philadelphia, WB Saunders, 1998, pp 191-202.)

the patient. The team may include a pediatrician; pediatric, orthopedic, plastic, and vascular surgeons; an interventional radiologist; a cardiologist or vascular internist; and a physical therapy physician. Conservative treatment is used for most patients. Laser therapy has been used effectively for capillary malformations (port-wine stains). Effective minimally invasive percutaneous techniques include transcatheter embolization and percutaneous or transcatheter sclerotherapy. Surgical excision is reserved for the minority of patients with localized superficial lesions or for those who have symptomatic juvenile varicose veins or localized venous malformations.

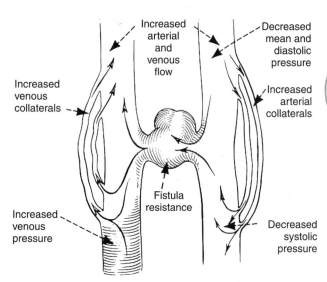

FIGURE 11–16 • Hemodynamic consequences of an arteriovenous fistula. (Courtesy of the Mayo Foundation.)

CONSERVATIVE TREATMENT

Treatment of VMs is usually conservative. An elastic garment or bandage, local wound care, compression dressings, special orthopedic footwear, and lifestyle modification may be required to manage daily life and improve limb function. Lymphedema is frequently managed using elastic garments, intermittent compression treatment, or lymphatic massage treatment by a physical therapist. The psychological problems caused by a visible deformity should not be underestimated. Long-term antibiotic therapy may be needed for recurrent cellulitis, and patients with recurrent deep vein thrombosis are treated with lifelong anticoagulants.

EMBOLIZATION

Embolization with selective catheterization has emerged as the primary therapy of arteriovenous malformations. Materials for embolization include polyvinyl alcohol particles (100 to 500 μm in size), absolute ethanol, stainless steel coils (usually with tufted Dacron), absorbable gelatin pledgets, powder coils, and cyanoacrylate adhesives. Each of these agents acts at different levels in the arterial system. Coils are equivalent to surgical ligation, although the tufted Dacron and the addition of thrombin generate more extensive arterial thrombosis than that achieved with ligation alone. Coils occlude medium to small arteries; liquid agents and the smaller-diameter particles occlude at the arteriolar level or the capillary bed.[56]

Forbes and associates reported on 31 therapeutic embolizations of 23 patients with extra-axial VMs of the head.[20] Of the nine patients with arteriovenous malformations, embolization produced excellent results in seven; the degree of obstruction was 80% or more. Two patients with high-shunt flow needed combined radiological-surgical treatment.

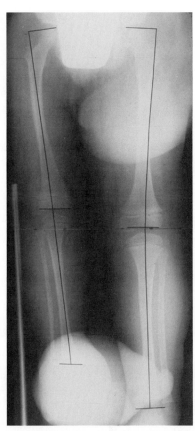

FIGURE 11–17 • Long bone film (scanogram) confirms leg length discrepancy in bilateral Klippel-Trénaunay syndrome.

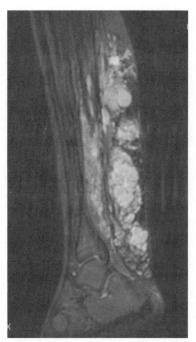

FIGURE 11–20 • Magnetic resonance image of a predominantly venous malformation involving the superficial and deep compartments of the distal calf.

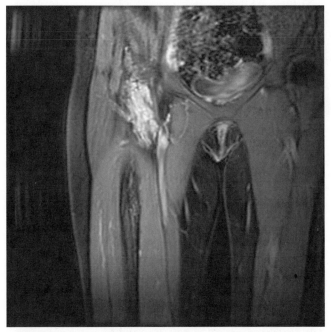

FIGURE 11–19 • Sagittal magnetic resonance image of an arteriovenous malformation involving the head of the right femur.

Rosen and Riles reported that 25% of 215 patients were cured 3 years after treatment of arteriovenous malformations with embolization.[16] Overall, improvement was noted in 76%. Four percent of the patients were worse, with complications including temporary hemiparesis or massive hematuria. High-flow, high-shunt arteriovenous malformations are difficult to treat, and major complications, including tissue necrosis, pulmonary embolization, and limb amputations, have also been reported by others.[15,16,55]

Jacobowitz and colleagues reported on transcatheter embolization of pelvic arteriovenous malformations in 35 patients.[58] A mean of 2.4 embolization procedures (range, 1 to 11 procedures) were needed over a mean period of 23.3 months (range, 1 to 144 months), using rapidly polymerizing acrylic adhesives most frequently. More than one procedure was performed in 53% of the patients. Adjunctive surgical excision was done in only five patients (15%). Eighty-three percent of patients were asymptomatic or significantly improved at a mean follow-up of 84 months (range, 1 to 204 months).

SCLEROTHERAPY

Absolute ethanol induces denaturation of tissue protein, precipitating protoplasm, and destroys the endothelial cells. It is delivered through selective arterial catheterization for arteriovenous malformations and through direct percutaneous injections into the lesions for predominantly venous malformations (see Figs. 11-7 and 11-21). Unfortunately, alcohol sclerotherapy causes significant pain; therefore, general anesthesia and pain control are required. Absolute ethanol can also cause significant side effects; treatment should be performed selectively, and it must be done by a physician with

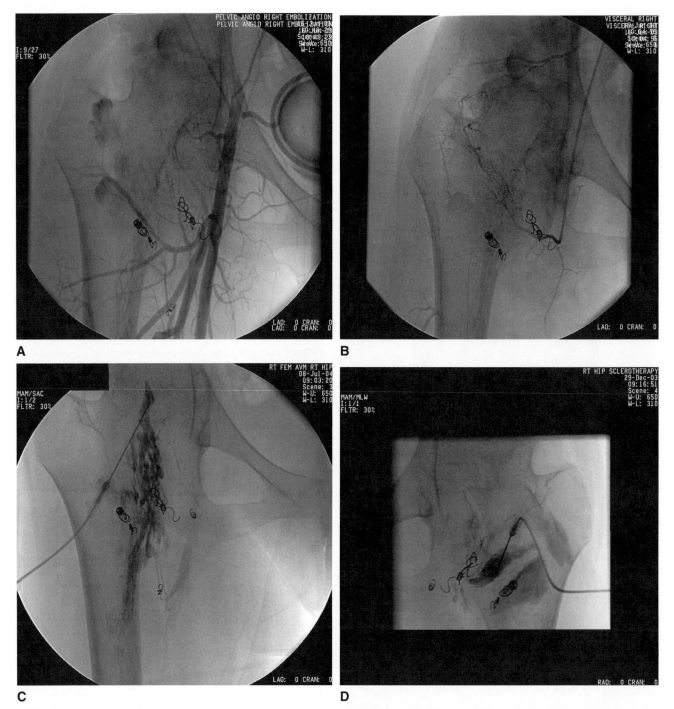

FIGURE 11–21 • *A,* Large arteriovenous malformation surrounding the right hip, with partial destruction of the hip joint. Previous embolization of the feeding vessels with coils was performed. *B,* Repeat embolization with Ivalon particles and with absolute alcohol was performed through selective catheterization of the lateral circumflex femoral artery. *C* and *D,* Additional ethanol sclerotherapy with direct percutaneous injections of absolute alcohol into the lesion. (Courtesy of Michael A. McKusick, MD, Mayo Foundation.)

expertise and knowledge of the dose and toxicity-related complications.

For large arteriovenous malformations, pulmonary artery catheter and arterial pressure line monitoring is suggested by Coldwell[59] and Yakes[60] and their respective coauthors, who also recommend giving dexamethasone sodium phosphate, 3 to 10 mg, intravenously before the procedure. The maximum dose should not exceed 1.0 mL/kg body weight.

Pulmonary hypertension should be monitored when large doses are given, and nitroglycerin can be used to treat pulmonary vasospasm. Yakes reported a complication rate that ranged from 10% to 30%, depending on the physician's years of experience.[60] Tissue necrosis, sloughing of the skin, and pulmonary hypertension are the most frequent side effects, followed by deep vein thrombosis and motor and sensory nerve injury.

One of the largest experiences using ethanol sclerotherapy for venous malformations was compiled by Lee and coworkers and reported in multiple publications.[1,21,22] In 87 patients who underwent 399 sessions of sclerotherapy for the treatment of VMs, Lee reported an initial success rate of 95%. The mean follow-up was 24 months, and 71 of the 87 patients (82%) showed no recurrence of the treated lesion. Minor to major complications, mostly skin damage, developed after 47 sessions (12%) in 24 patients (28%). There was one permanent facial nerve palsy and one peroneal nerve palsy. The authors concluded that absolute ethanol sclerotherapy can deliver excellent results to patients with diffuse venous malformation, with a 25% rate of early complications and a 3% rate of permanent complications. The low complication rate in this series was remarkable; most authors report complication rates between 10% and 30%. Complication rates in predominantly venous malformations are significantly less than in those patients who have arteriovenous shunting. The benefits and potential major complications of absolute alcohol sclerotherapy were emphasized in an editorial by Villavicencio.[61]

Other materials that have been used for sclerotherapy include sotradecol and polidocanol foam.[61-67] The advantage of foam detergent solutions is that smaller amounts can be used to achieve thrombosis. Polidocanol is less allergenic and produces less pain and inflammatory response than do other sclerosing solutions. Tessari uses 1% polidocanol for duplex-guided foam sclerotherapy: two syringes are attached by a three-way stopcock—one is filled with polidocanol, the other with air—and the foam is obtained by mixing the contents of the two syringes.[62,63] Five to 10 mL of the foam is injected under duplex and venographic guidance into the venous malformation. Foam has been used with increasing frequency and with good results for both occlusion of varicose veins and venous malformations.[61-67] Although longer follow-up is required, early complication rates are lower than those associated with ethanol sclerotherapy, and foam may have great promise in the treatment of venous malformations.

LASER TREATMENT

Cutaneous capillary malformations (port-wine stains) were initially treated with argon lasers, with good results in many patients; however, scarring occurred in 5% to 24% of patients.[68] The best results were obtained in adults with purple, well-vascularized lesions. Scarring has become less frequent with the introduction of the yellow light lasers.[69,70] The best results today are achieved with the flashlamp-pumped pulsed dye laser. The 585-nm wavelength achieves deep tissue penetration while maintaining vascular specificity.[70] Both pale and dark skins can be treated with minimal intraoperative discomfort and a low chance of postoperative epidermal damage or pigmentary change. As stated by Tanzi and coworkers, the pulsed dye laser has revolutionized the treatment of superficial vascular lesions, especially port-wine stains and facial telangiectasias.[70]

SURGICAL EXCISION

Surgical excision of arteriovenous malformation is rarely curative. In the classic series of Szilagyi,[13,14] 18 of 82 patients underwent surgical treatment, and improvement was documented

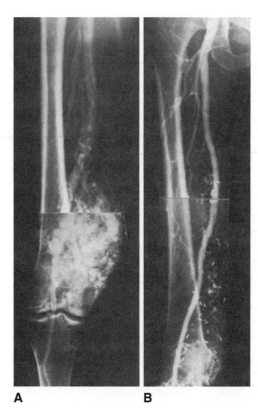

FIGURE 11–22 • *A,* Large macrofistulous arteriovenous malformation of the right thigh. *B,* Arteriogram 5 months after surgical resection, which was preceded by multiple embolizations of the lesion. (From Gloviczki AA, Noel AA, Hollier LH: Arteriovenous fistulas and vascular malformations. In Ascher E [ed]: Haimovici's Vascular Surgery, 5th ed. Malden, Mass, Blackwell, 2004, pp 991-1014.)

in only 10 patients. Surgical attempts at excision can result in significant blood loss, and ligation of major feeding vessels is not a good option. It prevents the later use of selective catheterization and embolotherapy. Excision of venous malformations, if they are localized, can be done with a higher rate of success. Exsanguination of the limb with an elastic (Esmarch) bandage and the use of a proximal tourniquet greatly decrease blood loss and make the operation technically easier.[71] If excision is decided on, preoperative sclerotherapy or embolization should be considered to minimize bleeding (Fig. 11-22). Use of the rapid cell saver is mandatory. In high-flow, high-shunt lesions, the only operation that can be performed in some patients is amputation. Trout and colleagues attempted surgical treatment of large lower extremity arteriovenous malformations, but two of the four patients required amputation.[72] Schwartz and associates reported on 82 patients treated at the Mayo Clinic for arteriovenous malformations; 18 patients required amputation at various levels of the extremity.[55] Still, for many patients, amputation means cure, and a prosthesis offers the possibility of functional recovery.

Complex Malformations

For vascular surgeons, the management of two complex clinical syndromes involving VMs deserves a separate discussion. These are Parkes Weber syndrome and Klippel-Trénaunay syndrome.

PARKES WEBER SYNDROME

Congenital arteriovenous malformation of a limb associated with soft tissue and bony hypertrophy was described as "hemangiectatic hypertrophy" in 1907 and again in 1918.[73,74] Parkes Weber syndrome should be differentiated from Klippel-Tréaunay syndrome, which is done by establishing the presence of arteriovenous shunting. Patients with Parkes Weber syndrome have clinically significant microfistulous or macrofistulous arteriovenous shunts, affecting usually one extremity. There is associated soft tissue and skeletal hypertrophy of the affected limb, and there are port-wine stains, usually on the lateral aspect of the limb. The patient has dilated, frequently pulsatile varicose veins and other visible signs of arteriovenous shunting. There is a palpable mass, the temperature of the skin is frequently elevated, and there is a cutaneous blush.[75] The abnormality is sporadic; it is likely a somatic mutation. There is frequent intraosseous involvement. These patients may develop cardiac failure due to the long-standing arteriovenous shunting; progression of the disease, because of hemodynamic involvement, is much more frequent in Parkes Weber syndrome than in Klippel-Tréaunay syndrome.

Management is initially conservative, using elastic compression. In limbs with high-flow lesions, repeated embolization may be required to treat the malformation, decrease pain, and diminish the hemodynamic effects of the high-shunt fistula. Occasionally, amputation of the limb is the only alternative.

KLIPPEL-TRÉNAUNAY SYNDROME

The clinical triad of Klippel-Tréaunay syndrome is capillary malformations (port-wine stains); soft tissue and bone hypertrophy; and atypical, usually lateral varicosity and venous and lymphatic malformations (see Figs. 11-3, 11-5, 11-12, and 11-13). This mixed malformation was described at the turn of the 20th century by the French physicians it is named for.[76] The deep veins are frequently affected; the most common deep venous anomalies include ectasia or aneurysm, external compression, hypoplasia, aplasia, and persistent sciatic veins.[2,3] Klippel-Tréaunay syndrome is clearly a mixed VM that includes predominantly venous, lymphatic, and capillary elements but no arteriovenous shunting. Many patients have lymphedema, and some have cavernous lymphatic malformations.

In 1998, Jacob and colleagues from the Mayo Clinic reported a retrospective review of 252 patients with Klippel-Tréaunay syndrome.[3] Of these, 246 (98%) had capillary malformations, 236 (94%) had soft tissue or bone hypertrophy, and 182 (72%) had varicosities or venous malformations. The lower extremities were involved in 70%, and the malformation was bilateral in 19%. The upper extremity was involved in 74 of 252 patients (29%). In this review, symptoms of Klippel-Tréaunay syndrome included swelling (70%), pain (7%), and bleeding (17%). Thirty-nine patients (15%) had a history of superficial phlebitis, 4% had a history of deep vein thrombosis, and 4% had pulmonary embolism, which was fatal in one patient. Lateral varicose veins were frequent (56%). One percent had suprapubic varicosities due to iliac vein agenesis or aplasia, and 19% of the patients had medial varicosities.

Management of Klippel-Tréaunay syndrome is largely conservative. Most patients who undergo surgical treatment do so because of overgrowth of one limb; these patients are managed with epiphysiodesis, with good results.[3,33,34] Vascular interventions must be preceded by careful evaluation of the patency of the deep venous system.[2,34,77-80] Noel and colleagues from the Mayo Clinic reported on 20 patients who underwent surgical treatment.[2] All had varicosities with a lateral distribution, although 65% had medial varicosities as well. Stripping and avulsion were performed in all patients; avulsion of varicose veins and excision of superficial venous malformations were usually accomplished with the help of a thigh tourniquet. Additional concomitant or staged procedures included release of the constricted popliteal veins, deep vein reconstruction, perforator ligation, and excision of an incompetence, persistent sciatic vein. Mean follow-up was 64 months. The results were excellent or good in 18 patients; only 2 patients showed no improvement. Twelve percent developed hematomas that required drainage, but no deep vein thrombosis, pulmonary embolism, or nerve injury was observed in this group of patients. The improvement was excellent in patients with varicosities, although some recurrence was noted in half of the patients. The clinical severity score significantly decreased in the entire group—from 4.3 to 3.1—documenting significant clinical benefits. In patients with a history of deep vein thrombosis, preoperative placement of a vena cava filter should be considered.

Because of the rarity of this disorder and the presence of a mixed malformation, a multidisciplinary management approach is clearly warranted.

Conclusion

Vascular malformations are caused by developmental abnormalities of the vascular system. They should be classified based on the predominant vascular structure and the presence or absence of arteriovenous shunting. Careful evaluation by a multidisciplinary team is required. Duplex scanning, CT-angiography, or magnetic resonance imaging can reveal the type and extent of the lesion. Arteriovenous shunting, if detected, can be treated using transcatheter embolotherapy. Symptomatic, predominantly venous malformations can be managed by percutaneous sclerotherapy, whereas localized capillary malformations of the skin respond well to laser therapy. High-flow, high-shunt malformations may develop severe complications, in spite of combined radiological-surgical management, and amputation may be the only option for optimal treatment. In patients with Klippel-Tréaunay syndrome, conservative management is favored, but vascular interventions can be beneficial, with ablation of the symptomatic incompetent superficial veins if the deep venous system is patent. As molecular genetic information about VMs is rapidly gained, traditional treatment strategies of destroying the intravascular spaces with sclerotherapy and lasers or excising the lesions with surgery may be replaced, at least in part, by gene therapy to prevent or treat angiogenic disorders.

KEY REFERENCES

Lee BB, Do YS, Yakes W, et al: Management of arteriovenous malformations: A multidisciplinary approach. J Vasc Surg 39:590-600, 2004.

Lee BB, Kim I, Huh S, et al: New experiences with absolute ethanol sclerotherapy in the management of a complex form of congenital venous malformation. J Vasc Surg 33:764-772, 2002.

Mulliken JB, Young AE: Vascular Birthmarks: Hemangiomas and Malformations. Philadelphia, WB Saunders, 1988.

Noel AA, Gloviczki P, Cherry KJ Jr, et al: Surgical treatment of venous malformations in Klippel-Trenaunay syndrome. J Vasc Surg 32:840-847, 2000.

Rutherford RB: Classification of peripheral congenital vascular malformations. In Ernst C, Stanley J (eds): Current Therapy in Vascular Surgery. St. Louis, Mosby, 1995, pp 834-838.

Vikkula M, Boon LM, Mullikan JB: Molecular genetics of vascular malformations. Matrix Biol 20:327-335, 2001.

REFERENCES

1. Lee BB, Do YS, Yakes W, et al: Management of arteriovenous malformations: A multidisciplinary approach. J Vasc Surg 39:590-600, 2004.
2. Noel AA, Gloviczki P, Cherry KJ Jr, et al: Surgical treatment of venous malformations in Klippel-Trenaunay syndrome. J Vasc Surg 32:840-847, 2000.
3. Jacob AG, Driscoll DJ, Shaughnessy WJ, et al: Klippel-Trenaunay syndrome: Spectrum and management. Mayo Clin Proc 73:28-36, 1998.
4. McGrory BJ, Amadio PC: Klippel-Trenaunay syndrome: Orthopaedic considerations. Orthop Rev 22:41-50, 1993.
5. Virchow R: Pathologie des tumeurs: cours professé à l'Université de Berlin, vol 4. Paris, Germer-Bailliére, 1876, p 169.
6. Nicoladoni C: Phlebarteriectasie der rechten oberen Extremität. Arch Kim Chir 18:252, 1875.
7. Branham HH: Aneurismal varix of the femoral artery and vein following a gunshot wound. Int J Surg 3:250, 1890.
8. Reid MR: Studies on abnormal arteriovenous communicanons, acquired and congenital. I. Report of a series of cases. Arch Surg 10:601, 1925.
9. Holman E: Arteriovenous Aneurysm: Abnormal Communications between the Arterial and Venous Circulations. New York, Macmillan, 1937.
10. de Takats G: Vascular anomalies of the extremities: Report of five cases. Surg Gynecol Obstet 55:227, 1932.
11. Coursley G, Ivins JC, Barker NW: Congenital arteriovenous fistulas in the extremities: An analysis of sixty-nine cases. Angiology 7:201, 1956.
12. Malan E, Puglionisi A: Congenital angiodysplasias of the extremities: Generalities and classifications: Venous dysplasias. J Cardiovasc Surg 5:87-130, 1964.
13. Szilagyi DE, Elliott JP, et al: Peripheral congenital arteriovenous fistulas. Surgery 57:61, 1965.
14. Szilagyi DE, Smith RF, et al: Congenital arteriovenous anomalies of the limbs. Arch Surg 111:423-429, 1976.
15. Rutherford RB, Anderson BO, Durham JD: Congenital vascular malformations of the extremities. In Moore WS (ed): Vascular Surgery: A Comprehensive Review, 5th ed. Philadelphia, WB Saunders, 1998, pp 191-202.
16. Rosen RJ, Riles TS: Congenital vascular malformations. In Rutherford RB (ed): Vascular Surgery, 5th ed. Philadelphia, WB Saunders, 2000, pp 1451-1465.
17. Belov ST: Anatomopathological classification of congenital vascular defects. Semin Vasc Surg 6:219-224, 1993.
18. Rutherford RB: Classification of peripheral congenital vascular malformations. In Ernst C, Stanley J (eds): Current Therapy in Vascular Surgery. St. Louis, Mosby, 1995, pp 834-838.
19. Natali J, Merland JJ: Superselective arteriography and therapeutic embolisation for vascular malformations (angiodysplasias). J Cardiovasc Surg (Torino) 17:465, 1976.
20. Forbes G, Earnest FIV, et al: Therapeutic embolization angiography for extra-axial lesions in the head. Mayo Clin Proc 61:427, 1986.
21. Lee BB: Critical issues in management of congenital vascular malformation. Ann Vasc Surg 18:380-392, 2004.
22. Lee BB, Kim I, Huh S, et al: New experiences with absolute ethanol sclerotherapy in the management of a complex form of congenital venous malformation. J Vasc Surg 33:764-772, 2002.
23. Mulliken JB, Zetter BR, Folkman J: In vitro characteristics of endothelium from hemangiomas and vascular malformations. Surgery 92:348, 1982.
24. Glowacki J, Mulliken JB: Mast cells in hemangiomas and vascular malformations. Pediatrics 70:48, 1982.
25. Mulliken JB, Glowacki J: Hemangiomas and vascular malformations in infants and children: A classification based on endothelial characteristics. Plast Reconstr Surg 69:412-420, 1982.
26. Vikkula M, Boon LM, Mullikan JB: Molecular genetics of vascular malformations. Matrix Biol 20:327-335, 2001.
27. Woollard RH: The development of the principal arterial stems in the forelimb of the pig. Contrib Embryol 14:139-154, 1922.
28. Ballaun C, Weninger W, Uthman A, et al: Human keratinocytes express the three major splice forms of vascular endothelial growth factor. J Invest Dermatol 104:710, 1995.
29. Brown LF, Yeo KT, Berse B, et al: Expression of vascular permeability factor (vascular endothelial growth factor) by epidermal keratinocytes during wound healing. J Exp Med 176:1375-1379, 1992.
30. Mukouyama YS, Shin D, Britsch S, et al: Sensory nerves determine the pattern of arterial differentiation and blood vessel branching in the skin. Cell 109:693-705, 2002.
31. Nicholson CP, Gloviczki P: Embryology and development of the vascular system. In White RA, Hollier LH (eds): Vascular Surgery: Basic Science and Clinical Correlations. Philadelphia, JB Lippincott, 1994. pp 3-20.
32. West CA, Delis KT, Service G, et al: Middle aortic syndrome: Surgical treatment in a child with neurofibromatosis, renovascular hypertension, superior mesenteric artery stenosis and intermittent claudication. J Vasc Surg (in press).
33. Gloviczki P, Hollier LR, et al: Surgical implications of Klippel-Trenaunay syndrome. Ann Surg 197:353, 1983.
34. Gloviczki P, Stanson AW, et al: Klippel-Trenaunay syndrome: The risks and benefits of vascular interventions. Surgery 110:469-479, 1991.
35. Eifert S, Villavicencio L, Kao TG, et al: Prevalence of deep venous anomalies in congenital vascular malformations of venous predominance. J Vasc Surg 31:462-471, 2000.
36. Servelle M: Klippel Trenaunay syndrome: 768 operated cases. Ann Surg 201:365-373, 1985.
37. Guttmacher AE, Marchuk DA, White RI: Hereditary hemorrhagic telangiectasia. N Engl J Med 33:918-924, 1995.
38. Gloviczki AA, Noel AA, Hollier LH: Arteriovenous fistulas and vascular malformations. In Ascher E (ed): Haimovici's Vascular Surgery, 5th ed. Malden, Mass, Blackwell, 2004, pp 991-1014.
39. Eerola I, Boon LM, Mulliken JB, et al: Capillary malformation-arteriovenous malformation, a new clinical and genetic disorder caused by RASA1 mutations. Am J Hum Genet 73:1240-1249, 2003.
40. Milroy WF: An undescribed variety of hereditary edema. N Y Med J 56:505, 1892.
41. Milroy WF: Chronic hereditary edema: Milroy's disease. JAMA 91:1172, 1928.
42. Meige H: Dystrophie oedemateuse hereditaire. Presse Med 2:341, 1898.
43. Gloviczki P, Wahner HW: Clinical diagnosis and evaluation of lymphedema. In Rutherford RB (ed): Vascular Surgery, 5th ed. Philadelphia, WB Saunders, 2000, pp 2123- 2142.
44. Noel A, Gloviczki P, Bender CE, et al: Treatment of symptomatic primary chylous disorders. J Vasc Surg 34:785-791, 2001.
45. Collins PS, Han W, Williams LR, et al: Maffucci's syndrome (hemangiomatosis osteolytica): A report of four cases J Vasc Surg 16:364-371, 1992.
46. Lublin M, Schwartzentruber DJ, Lukish J, et al: Principles for the surgical management of patients with Proteus syndrome and patients with overgrowth not meeting Proteus criteria. J Pediatr Surg 37:1013-1020, 2002.
47. Tasnadi G: Epidemiology and etiology of congenital vascular malformations. Semin Vasc Surg 6:200-203, 1993.
48. Boon LM, Mulliken JB, Vikkula M, et al: Assignment of a locus for dominantly inherited venous malformations to chromosome 9p. Hum Mol Genet 3:1583-1587, 1994.
49. Vikkula M, Boon LM, Mulliken JB, Olsen BR: Molecular basis of vascular anomalies. Trends Cardiovasc Med 8:281-292, 1998.
50. Timur AA, Sadgephour A, Graf M, et al: Identification and molecular characterization of a de novo supernumerary ring chromosome 18 in a patient with Klippel-Trenaunay syndrome. Ann Hum Genet 68:353-361, 2004.
51. Tian XL, Kadaba R, You SA, et al: Identification of an angiogenic factor that when mutated causes susceptibility to Klippel-Trenaunay syndrome. Nature 427:640-645, 2004.
52. Vikkula M, Boon LM, Carraway KLI, et al: Vascular dysmorphogenesis caused by an activating mutation in the receptor tyrosine kinase TIE2. Cell 87:1181-1190, 1996.
53. Boon LM, Brouillard P, Irrthum A, et al: A gene for inherited cutaneous venous anomalies ("glomangiomas") localizes to chromosome 1p21-22. Am J Hum Genet 65:125-133, 1999.
54. Boon LM, Mulliken JB, Enjolras O, Vikkula M: Glomuvenous malformation (glomangioma) and venous malformation: Distinct clinico-pathologic and genetic entities. Arch Dermatol 140:971-976, 2004.

55. Schwartz RS, Osmundson PJ, Rollier LH: Treatment and prognosis in congenital arteriovenous malformation of the extremity. Phlebology 1:171, 1986.

56. Pritchard DA, Maloney JD, et al: Surgical treatment of congenital pelvic arteriovenous malformation. Mayo Clin Proc 53:607, 1978.

57. Pritchard DA, Maloney JD, et al: Peripheral arteriovenous fistula: Detection by contrast echocardiography. Mayo Clin Proc 52:186, 1977.

58. Jacobowitz GR, Rosen RJ, Rockman CB, et al: Transcatheter embolization of complex pelvic vascular malformations: Results and long-term follow-up. J Vasc Surg 33:51-55, 2001.

59. Coldwell DM, Stokes KR, Yakes WF: Embolotherapy: Agents, clinical applications, and techniques. Radiographics 14:623-643, 1994.

60. Yakes WF, Rossi P, Odink H: How I do it: Arteriovenous malformation management. Cardiovasc Intervent Radiol 19:65-71, 1996.

61. Villavicencio JL: Primum non nocere: Is it always true? The use of absolute ethanol in the management of congenital vascular malformations J Vasc Surg 33:904-906, 2001.

62. Yamaki T, Nozaki M, Fujiwara O, Yoshida E: Duplex-guided foam sclerotherapy for the treatment of the symptomatic venous malformations of the face. Dermatol Surg 28:619-622, 2002.

63. Tessari L: Nouvelle technique d'obtention de la sclero-mousee. Phlebologie 53:129, 2000.

64. Tessari L, Cavezzi A, Frullini A: Preliminary experience with a new sclerosing foam in the treatment of varicose Monfreux A. Traitement sclérosant des troncs saphènies et leurs collatérals de gros caliber par le method MUS. Phlebologie 50:3513, 1997.

65. Henriet JP: Un an de pratique quotidienne de la sclérothérapie (veines reticulaires et télangiectasies) par mousse de polidocanol faisabilité, resultants, complications. Phlebologie 50:355-360, 1997.

66. Cavezzi A, Frullini A: The role of sclerosing foam in ultrasound guided sclerotherapy of the saphenous veins and of recurrent varicose veins: our personal experience. Aust N Z J Phlebol 3:4950, 1999.

67. Cabrera Garrido JR, Cabrera Garcia-Olmedo JR, Garcia-Olmedo Dominguez MA: Elargissement des limites de la sclérothérapie: Nouveaux produits sclérosants. Phlebologie 50:1818, 1997.

68. Noe JM, Barsky SH, et al: Port wine stains and the response to argon laser therapy: Successful treatment and the predictive role of color, age, and biopsy. Plast Reconstr Surg 65:130, 1980.

69. Goldman MP, Fitzpatrick RE, Ruiz-Esparza J: Treatment of port-wine stains (capillary malformation) with the flashlamp-pumped pulsed dye laser. J Pediatr 122:71-77, 1993.

70. Tanzi EL, Lupton JR, Alster TS: Lasers in dermatology: Four decades of progress. J Am Acad Dermatol 49:1-31, 2003.

71. Villavicencio JL, Gillespie DL, Kreishman P: Controlled ischemia for complex venous surgery: The technique of choice. J Vasc Surg 34:947-951, 2001.

72. Trout RH III, McAllister RA Jr, et al: Vascular malformations. Surgery 97:36, 1985.

73. Weber FP: Angioma-formation in connection with hypertrophy of limbs and hemi-hypertrophy. Br J Dermatol 19:231, 1907.

74. Weber FP: Haemangiectatic hypertrophy of limbs: Congenital phlebarteriectasis and so-called congenital varicose veins. Br J Child Dis 15:13, 1918.

75. Mulliken JB, Young AE: Vascular Birthmarks: Hemangiomas and Malformations. Philadelphia, WB Saunders, 1988.

76. Klippel M, Trénaunay P: Du naevus variquex osteohypertrophique. Arch Gen Med (Paris) 3:641-672, 1900.

77. Baskerville PA, Ackroyd JS, Lea TM, Browse NL: The Klippel-Trenaunay syndrome: Clinical, radiological and haemodynamic features and management. Br J Surg 72:232-236, 1985.

78. Lindenauer SM: The Klippel-Trenaunay syndrome: Varicosity, hypertrophy and hemangioma with no arteriovenous fistula. Ann Surg 162:303-313, 1965.

79. Villavicencio JL: Congenital vascular malformations of venous predominance: Klippel-Trenaunay syndrome. In Raju S, Villavicencio JL (eds): Surgical Management of Venous Disease. Baltimore, Williams & Wilkins, 1997, pp 445-461.

80. Baskerville PA, Ackroyd JS, Browse NL: The etiology of the Klippel-Trenaunay syndrome. Ann Surg 202:624-627, 1985.

Questions

1. **Which predominant type of vascular malformation is seen most often in vascular clinics?**
   (a) Venous
   (b) Arterial
   (c) Arteriovenous
   (d) Lymphatic

2. **Temporary occlusion of flow to a vascular malformation with a high-flow arteriovenous fistula will result in which of the following?**
   (a) Tachycardia
   (b) Venous hypertension proximal to the fistula
   (c) Arrhythmia
   (d) Bradycardia
   (e) Decrease of mean arterial pressure

3. **Microfistulous arteriovenous malformations are caused by an inborn error at which stage of limb bud development?**
   (a) Undifferentiated
   (b) Retiform
   (c) Syncytial
   (d) Maturational

4. **Which of the following statements regarding hemangiomas encountered during infancy is not true?**
   (a) They have a high endothelial turnover
   (b) They may exhibit high-flow characteristics
   (c) The female-male ratio is 5:1
   (d) Their growth is commensurate with the child's growth

5. **Which of the following presentations is not typical of Klippel-Trénaunay syndrome?**
   (a) Increased limb size
   (b) Increased pulsatility with a palpable thrill
   (c) Varicose veins
   (d) Capillary malformation (port-wine stain)
   (e) Malformation of the deep veins

6. **Which noninvasive test finding is not characteristic of a high-flow arteriovenous malformation (fistula) of the thigh?**
   (a) Increased systolic pressure proximal to the lesion
   (b) High end-diastolic velocity in the proximal artery
   (c) Elevated pulse volume recording (plethysmographic tracing) distally in the foot
   (d) Decreased ankle-brachial index
   (e) Elevated venous pressure distal to the malformation

7. **In young patients with symptomatic lateral varicose veins, preoperative evaluation must establish which of the following findings?**
   (a) Patency of the deep veins
   (b) Presence of port-wine stains
   (c) Limb length discrepancy
   (d) Positive family history of varicosity
   (e) History of hematuria or rectal bleeding

8. **Which of the following malformations is not considered hereditary?**
   (a) Milroy disease
   (b) Meige disease
   (c) Glomuvenous malformation
   (d) Klippel-Trénaunay syndrome
   (e) HHT1

9. **Which of the following is not true about catheter-directed injections of absolute alcohol into the nidus of a vascular malformation?**
   (a) They require multiple sessions
   (b) They must be done under general anesthesia
   (c) They selectively destroy endothelium and cause thrombosis without resulting in surrounding tissue necrosis
   (d) They can cause permanent nerve injury in as many as 10% of cases
   (e) They can permanently control some vascular malformations

10. **Neither excision of a localized malformation nor embolotherapy is justified for which of the following indications in patients with vascular malformations?**
    (a) Recurrent hemorrhage from skin lesions
    (b) Uneven limb growth
    (c) Ischemic ulcer
    (d) Symptomatic arterial steal

Answers

1. a	2. d	3. b	4. d	5. b
6. c	7. a	8. d	9. c	10. b

12

Ralph G. DePalma

Vasculogenic Erectile Dysfunction

Impotence, or male erectile dysfunction (ED), is defined as "the persistent or repeated inability to attain and/or maintain an erection sufficient for satisfactory performance in the absence of an ejaculatory disorder."[1] ED is now better understood and more effectively treated than in the past. Comprehension of the physiology of erection and the central role of cavernous sinus smooth muscle relaxation[2] resulted in the development of medical therapy for men with ED.[3] Vascular surgeons require information about the prevention of ED and other sexual dysfunctions, including ejaculatory and orgasmic disorders, particularly as these conditions relate to aortoiliac interventions. They also need to be able to assess the contribution of macrovascular disease to vasculogenic ED and to treat occlusive or aneurysmal disease that contributes to ED. Aortoiliac reconstruction itself can cause ED by failing to perfuse the internal iliac arteries or by damaging autonomic genital nerves.[4] Techniques of particular importance to vascular surgeons are those that minimize or completely avoid damage to the pelvic nerves while restoring or maintaining flow into the internal iliac arteries. These techniques may prevent sexual dysfunction and, in selected cases, restore potency after aortoiliac interventions.[5,6]

This chapter describes surgical approaches for the prevention of postoperative ED during aortoiliac interventions. Vasculogenic ED due to small vessel disease, cavernous smooth muscle dysfunction, and primary ED are complex disorders; some of the pertinent approaches to treatment are summarized here, and readers with a specific interest in the subject are referred to the comprehensive volume *Male Sexual Function*.[7] Microvascular procedures for vasculogenic ED, which are now performed infrequently, are briefly described. Vascular surgeons should also be aware of female sexual dysfunction (FSD), which may occur after aortoiliac surgery[8] and radical hysterectomy.[9] Nerve-sparing and revised operative techniques may prevent or minimize these effects in gynecologic surgery.[10,11]

Physiology of Erection

Penile erection requires adequate arterial inflow and closure of cavernosal outflow, mediated by a complex interplay between neural and local factors.[12,13] Erection results primarily through relaxation of the smooth muscle of the corporal bodies.

These endothelium-mediated relaxation responses are stimulated by neural mechanisms.[14] The roles of nitric oxide (NO) as the chemical mediator,[15] as well as the importance of blood flow and oxygenation of the cavernous smooth muscle,[16] are fundamental to an understanding of erectile physiology. With increased intracavernosal flow, a greater amount of oxygen stimulates NO synthesis by cavernosal nerves and endothelium. Cavernosal oxygenation promotes penile erection, whereas hypoxemia is inhibitory. Testosterone, in addition to its central effects, has been shown in animals to stimulate NO synthase activity in corporal tissues,[17] thus enhancing sensitivity to cavernosal nerve stimulation. NO, in turn, activates conversion of guanosine triphosphate to cyclic guanosine monophosphate (GMP). The latter provides the message leading to relaxation of the smooth muscle within the corpora cavernosa.[18] Agents that inhibit hydrolysis of cyclic GMP increase messenger cyclic GMP and facilitate smooth muscle relaxation to promote penile erection.[19] Cyclic nucleotide phosphodiesterase (PDE) isoenzymes increase hydrolysis of cyclic GMP; among these, PDE-5 and PDE-6 are specific for the substrate in human cavernosal tissue.[20] Specific PDE-5 inhibitors constitute an important new class of oral agents, including sildenafil, vardenafil, and tadalafil. PDE-5 inhibitors are currently available and widely used for the treatment of ED. As corporal arterial pressure increases, draining emissary veins are compressed against the tunica albuginea, causing venous outflow occlusion. During full erection, cavernosal artery flow virtually ceases. During flaccidity, a constant venous leak balances baseline penile inflow and outflow. With insufficient arterial inflow, the corpora do not pressurize adequately, and secondary venous leakage occurs. Intracavernous pressure increases from 10 to 15 mm Hg to levels ranging from 80 to 90 mm Hg in the erect state. Intracavernous pressures higher than systemic pressure, generated by perineal muscle contraction,[13] contribute to penile rigidity.

Approaches to the Investigation of Erectile Dysfunction

Table 12-1 summarizes general factors contributing to erectile dysfunction. In modern practice, more cases are now recognized as being organic in origin than were previously appreciated;

TABLE 12–1	General Causative Factors in Erectile Dysfunction

Vasculogenic
Neurogenic
Endocrine
Drug induced
Psychogenic

however, men with organic impotence may exhibit psychogenic problems as well. Of 1023 impotent men screened for diagnosis and treatment, 461 demonstrated some type of arterial inflow problem, based on noninvasive criteria using the penile brachial index and pulse volume recordings.[21,22] However, many men exhibited other contributing factors, including diabetes, neuropathy (about 20%), antihypertensive medication, and other types of cavernous dysfunction, including Peyronie's disease. Older men with multiple factors contributing to ED are generally not candidates for vascular surgical intervention for this complaint alone. About 6% to 7% of the men who were investigated ultimately became candidates for vascular intervention. In my experience, only 15.6% of men with decreased arterial perfusion exhibited large vessel disease. Thus, imposing a selective screening sequence for surgical case selection yields a sharp funnel effect that minimizes candidacy for vascular intervention for ED.[22] However, for young men with small vessel disease or men of any age with macrovascular disease, vascular intervention is a logical first step for those who fail aggressive medical therapy and for those who do not desire prosthetic implantation.[23]

Table 12-2 offers an updated classification of vasculogenic ED. Some type of small vessel, cavernosal, or arteriolar cause appears to be present in 43.3% of men exhibiting abnormal penile perfusion. An additional 41.1% of men with the primary complaint of impotence exhibit a combination of large and small vessel involvement, as ascertained by noninvasive and physical criteria. Most men with the primary complaint of ED are more likely to have small vessel or cavernosal disorders than macrovascular disease. Importantly, the complaint

TABLE 12–2	Classification of Vasculogenic Erectile Dysfunction

Arterial

Large vessel	Aorta and branches to internal iliac artery
Small vessel	Anterior division of internal iliac artery and penile arteries
Combined	Atheroembolism from aortoiliac segment

Cavernosal

Fibrosis	Postpriapic, drug injection, idiopathic with aging
Peyronie's disease	Deformity; venous leakage
Refractory states	Hormonal, diabetic, blood pressure medication

Venous

Acquired	Various patterns; dorsal vein, crural, spongiotic
Congenital	Cavernous spongiosis leak

of impotence has also been associated with occult aortoiliac occlusive or aneurysmal disease.

In men with Leriche syndrome,[24,25] impotence as a sentinel complaint sometimes precedes the onset of claudication. Men younger than 55 years are often potent before reconstruction for aneurysm or occlusive disease, and an accurate history of their sexual activity must be obtained. Despite the best surgical techniques to preserve sexual function, ED and other sexual disabilities continue to occur after reconstructions for aneurysms and occlusive disease. Therefore, before intervention, the surgeon must make careful inquiries into the patient's sexual function and, when necessary, assess preoperative penile artery perfusion. A detailed history and noninvasive testing are particularly important when postoperative sexual function is an expressed concern of the patient.

History and Physical Examination

A history of gradual erectile failure, in the absence of traumatic life events and correlated with symptoms such as claudication, suggests large vessel arteriogenic ED. In these men, both the intensity and the duration of atherosclerotic risk factors, mainly cigarette smoking, hypertension, diabetes, and hypercholesterolemia, contribute to atherosclerosis. This pattern signals patients who have involvement of the aorta or the iliac system. Abdominal aneurysms or ulcerated aortoiliac disease can cause penile vessel emboli.[21] In such instances, the onset of ED is characteristically sudden. Perineal injury predisposes to thrombosis of the pudendal arteries. The immediate onset of erectile failure after urologic, vascular, or rectal operations is an important diagnostic clue suggesting neurovascular damage. Although either neural or vascular interruption can cause ED, periaortic, sympathetic, or hypogastric neural interruption can cause ejaculatory disorders. Alcohol and drug abuse contributes to progressive erectile failure, along with drugs used to treat hypertension because of their neuropathic and metabolic effects. Other hormonal disorders, such as hypogonadism, rarely seem to cause ED. Our group detected two prolactinomas during the screening of approximately 1400 men; these men exhibited dramatic responses to medical therapy.

The major findings of aortoiliac disease on physical examination are decreased femoral pulses, bruits, or palpation of an abdominal aortic aneurysm in those whose waists measure less than 38 to 40 inches. Sensory testing of the extremities, perineum, or glans occasionally reveals neuropathies associated with diabetic impotence. However, these abnormalities are most reliably quantified by neurovascular testing, using pudendal evoked potentials and measurement of bulbocavernosus reflex times.[26,27] Currently, neurologic screening is not routinely performed initially, because medical treatment with vasoactive agents is often effective, even in cases of neuropathy. In cases of postoperative or post-traumatic dysfunction, neurologic testing is an important factor in decision making, particularly in recommending prosthetic implantation as an option. Considerable overlap exists between vascular and neurologic ED.

The prostate must be examined, and nodular abnormalities investigated. Prostate-specific antigen determinations should routinely be obtained before the prostate examination. Methodical palpation of the corpora cavernosa for Peyronie's plaques and estimation of testicular size complete the examination. In most men presenting with primary ED, the physical examination is completely normal.

At this point, the erectile mechanism can be tested in the clinic by intracavernous injection of 10 to 20 μg of Prostin E1.[28] Rigid erection sufficient for intercourse demonstrates adequate arterial inflow and veno-occlusive mechanisms. Provided that aneurysmal disease has been ruled out (e.g., by sonography), treatment with oral, injectable, or intra-arterial vasoactive agents is the first step. Such treatment may succeed in up to 70% to 80% of cases.

Multiple factors contribute to ED, which is a symptom, not a single disease. These factors, summarized in Table 12-1, help guide approaches to the diagnosis and treatment of sexual dysfunction and, in some respects, are relevant to both sexes. An important area, hitherto neglected, has been the study of female sexual dysfunction (FSD), which appears in women with diabetes[29,30] or cardiovascular disease[31] and in postmenopausal women as disordered sexual arousal,[32] failure to achieve orgasm, and dyspareunia with failure to lubricate. Feminine arousal and vaginal lubrication are difficult to assess, whereas penile erection can be seen and quantified. Progress in understanding the cause, physiology, and treatment of FSD continues.[33] Treatment modalities similar to those suggested in men have been proposed, and treatment trials have included oral PDE-5 inhibitors[34,35] (which are probably not as effective as in men) and topical alprostadil.[36] From the standpoint of aortic reconstruction, vascular surgeons should now recognize the potential benefits of nerve-sparing dissections with preserved internal iliac flow for women as well as for men.

No universally accepted approach to managing ED exists; as mentioned, ED is a symptom, not a single disease. The initial approach is directed by the patient's goals and depends on the response to simple therapy.[37] When oral medication fails, more elaborate investigations might be considered.[38] Should the intracavernous administration of vasoactive agents fail and vacuum constrictor devices prove ineffective, and if vascular intervention is an option, evaluation may progress to more elaborate invasive tests that delineate abnormal physiology.

Neurovascular Testing

Neurovascular testing was initially used for all patients by our group[22] to screen candidates for reconstructive procedures[23] and to help determine the initial dosage for intracavernous injection of vasoactive agents; patients with neurologic deficits are often exquisitely sensitive to such agents, and their dosage must be reduced to avoid priapism. With the advent of giving a trial of oral medication as the first step in treatment, such testing is needed less frequently. Testing may be useful for the investigation of postoperative onset or traumatic ED or when legal issues exist.

The penile brachial index (PBI) is the ratio between systolic pressure detected by a Doppler probe placed distal to the penile cuff and systemic or brachial arm pressure.[39] A cuff of 2.5 cm is used for an average-size penis. The cuff is inflated, then deflated, and the reappearance of Doppler signals in the dorsal artery branch proximal to the corona signals reflow. Normally, this pressure approaches systemic pressure. A PBI above 0.75 suggests no major obstacle between the aorta and the distal measurement point. Generally, PBIs less than 0.6

relate to major vascular obstructions in the aortoiliac bed, whereas PBIs between 0.6 and 0.75 are considered abnormal.

Flow can be further characterized by penile pulse volume recording, which uses a pneumoplethysmographic cuff (Buffington) with a contained transducer. This test is performed with the penis in the flaccid state. The variables recorded are the same as those used for the lower extremity. These include crest time, waveform, and the presence or absence of a dicrotic notch. This technique measures the total pulsation of all penile arteries as the cuff compresses the cavernous tissues. The measurements are taken with the cuff inflated to mean arterial pressure and are calculated as diastolic pressure plus one third of systemic pulse pressure. Waveforms on a polygraph with a chart speed of 25 mm/sec and a sensitivity setting of 1 demonstrate in normal patients that the upstroke of the waveform is completed by 0.2 second, whereas normal waveform amplitudes vary from 5 or 6 to 30 mm in height. Waveforms might be distinctly abnormal with small vessel disease or cavernosal disorders, whereas PBI is normal.

These noninvasive tests are not completely sensitive and specific. I found that the combination of PBI and pulse volume recording predicts an abnormal arteriogram with a sensitivity of 85% and a specificity of 70%. In suspected cases of venogenic impotence (i.e., normal arterial noninvasive tests), 23% of men examined with normal noninvasive studies had associated arterial lesions demonstrated angiographically.[40] Therefore, before small vessel interventions, which are done only for those failing medical therapy,[18] both pudendal arteriography and dynamic infusion cavernosography are required for proper case selection.

PBI detects inadequate arterial inflow from large arteries. Vasculogenic impotence caused by venous leak, Peyronie's disease, or cavernosal fibrosis is not detected. In these instances, color-flow duplex scanning after an intracavernous injection to produce erection or tumescence has been used extensively by urologists, sometimes in combination with visual erotic stimulation, to measure deep cavernosal and dorsal blood flow velocity at intervals after the injection of a vasodilator.[41] Based on these studies, ED can be classified as arterial, venous, or mixed vascular. Studies of local blood flow dynamics yield little information about proximal macrovascular inflow. Radionuclide phallography and pelvic magnetic resonance imaging are currently research applications.

Nocturnal penile tumescence and rigidity monitoring, using noninvasive strain gauge techniques, are ideally performed in a sleep laboratory over several nights. Home monitoring devices are available. A normal rigid erection during sleep rules out organic impotence.[42]

Cavernosometry and Cavernosal Artery Occlusion Pressure

Invasive studies provide quantitative information about arterial inflow and veno-occlusive mechanisms.[43] A calibrated pump provides a flow of warm, heparinized saline via 20-gauge needles inserted into the corpora. During maximal erection, intracavernous pressure at some point equilibrates with arterial inflow pressure, and flow in the deep cavernosal artery stops. This value is called cavernosal artery occlusion pressure, and it is measured by using Doppler insonation at the point of full erection. Normal is considered greater than 90 mm Hg. A pressure gradient from brachial levels greater than 30 mm Hg suggests arterial inflow occlusion. Dynamic infusion cavernosography measures the flow required to maintain erection. This value is normally 40 mL or less after intracavernous injection of a standard papaverine-phentolamine mixture. Nonionic dilute contrast is injected to visualize venous leaks. Spot filming in various obliquities identifies specific abnormal or leaking veins when cavernosography is positive. As mentioned previously, failure of erection is associated with an excess of venous leakage over inflow. Venous leakage can be due to arterial insufficiency, so before contemplated venous ablation, I recommend highly selective pudendal arteriography.

Aortoiliac Reconstruction Principles

Given the standard indications for large vessel aortoiliac reconstruction (i.e., aneurysm or occlusive disease), the procedure, whether endovascular[44,45] or open,[46,47] should be planned to provide perfusion of both internal iliac arteries whenever possible. Flushing of debris into the internal iliacs should be avoided, and endovascular repair should attempt to maintain internal iliac flow—at least to one internal iliac artery.[17] The dissection in open cases must spare the neural fibers about the aorta and the iliac arteries (which are especially rich on the left side) and about the inferior mesenteric artery. In all these cases, a specific history of preoperative sexual activity must be sought. If an elderly person manifests no interest in this activity, complicated preoperative testing is unnecessary. However, when interest exists, preoperative PBI and pulse volume recordings are helpful for comparison with postoperative findings. In addition, positive findings of abnormal pudendal and somatosensory evoked potentials are helpful to demonstrate neuropathy.

Operative Techniques

Operative techniques have been described previously,[46] and illustrations have been reproduced from prior reviews.[47] Exposure for aortoiliac reconstruction is best accomplished by dissecting the aortoiliac segment from the right and sparing the nerves and inferior mesenteric artery. In cases of aortoiliac aneurysm, perfusion of the internal iliac is ensured by an inlay technique, illustrated in Figure 12-1. Again, the aneurysmal sac is incised well to the right, avoiding interruption of a dominant left periaortic nerve plexus. The inferior mesenteric artery is sutured from within the aneurysmal sac. Figures 12-2 and 12-3 show the techniques for occlusive disease. In men with buttock claudication and impotence related to local disease in the arterial distribution of the internal iliac artery, an extraperitoneal approach with endarterectomy or bypass is not a difficult procedure, although endovascular interventions have been also used. This open approach uses a longitudinal incision along the edge of the rectus muscle, with reflection of the peritoneum medially (Fig. 12-4). In renal transplant patients, end-to-side renal artery anastomosis to the external iliac artery avoids division of an internal iliac artery.

Fredberg and Mouritzen described sexual dysfunction resulting from conventional aortoiliac operations.[48] In their series,

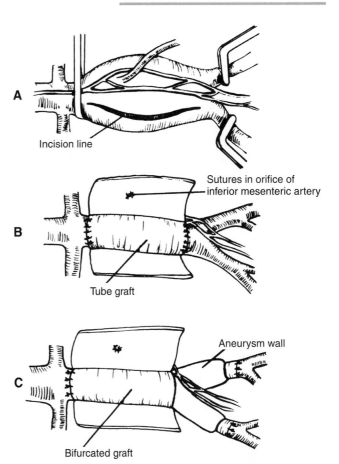

FIGURE 12–1 • Inlay nerve-sparing techniques for aneurysm repair. Note the incision on the right side of the aneurysm. (From DePalma RG: Prevention of sexual dysfunction in aortoiliac surgery. In Jamieson CW [ed]: Current Operative Surgery. Eastborne, East Sussex, England, Bailliere-Tindall, 1985, pp 781-788.)

55% of men (11 of 20) with aneurysms were preoperatively impotent, whereas 95% (19 of 20) were postoperatively impotent. Among those with occlusive disease, 31% (15 of 48) were preoperatively impotent, and 60% (29 of 48) were postoperatively impotent. Miles and colleagues found that about 22% of 76 patients receiving conventional aortoiliac operations reported preoperative sexual dysfunction; an additional 30% of those operated on for aneurysm or occlusive disease were rendered impotent.[49] Impotence was twice as common in men reporting unspecified preoperative "minor dysfunction." It seems unlikely that prospective trials comparing conventional aortic reconstructions with nerve-sparing, internal iliac revascularization techniques will surface, given that attention to the details of these procedures imposes little additional surgical burden or risk.

Rich interconnections of the vegetative nervous system about the aortoiliac vessels and the inferior mesenteric artery include both sympathetic and parasympathetic fibers that promote normal ejaculatory function. Damage to these fibers also causes other types of sexual dysfunction: retrograde ejaculation with or without erection and orgasm, anejaculation, failure of emission, and, rarely, normal erection with failure to achieve either ejaculation or orgasm. Ejaculatory disorders are reportedly the most prevalent sexual dysfunction, occurring in nearly 40% of men.[50] This condition is more likely to be encountered in urologic[51] or fertility practices and has not

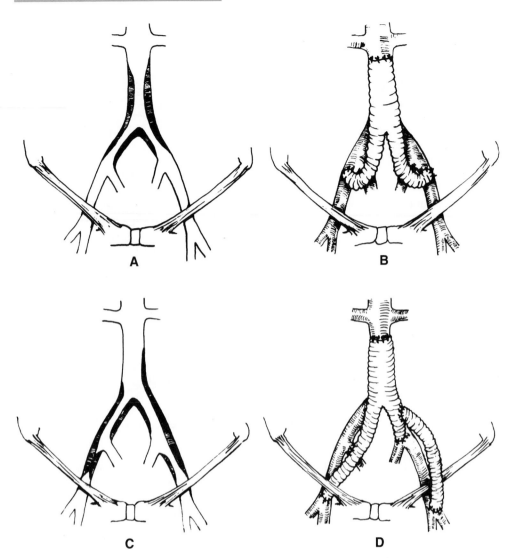

FIGURE 12–2 • Techniques for aortoiliac or aortofemoral bypass: *A* and *B*, End-to-end aortic anastomosis with suprainguinal end-to-side bypass in which the external iliac and common femoral arteries are spared. *C* and *D*, End-to-end aortic anastomosis with side-to-side reconstruction of the right internal iliac artery and two limbs on the left side. (From DePalma RG: Prevention of sexual dysfunction in aortoiliac surgery. In Jamieson CW [ed]: Current Operative Surgery. Eastborne, East Sussex, England, Bailliere-Tindall, 1985, pp 781-788.)

been a prominent complaint in vascular practice. Ejaculatory disorders should be differentiated from ED, although the psychological consequences of ejaculatory disorders can interfere with erection.

Women were once thought to be less susceptible to sexual dysfunction after aortoiliac surgery.[52] In my experience, three women regained arousal, lubrication, and orgasm after aortoiliac surgery using nerve-sparing aortoiliac reconstructions that provided internal iliac flow. In this anecdotal experience, the operations were performed using the same technique as in men. The approach was chosen out of habit, with no intention of influencing sexual function; these women reported favorable effects later. Scanty data exist; few women in their sexually active years require aortoiliac reconstruction, and objective measurement of female arousal is difficult to perform. Hultgren and coworkers described sexual dysfunction, based on questionnaires, in women before and after aortoiliac operation.[8] They stressed the possibility of iatrogenic nerve damage as a cause of postoperative sexual dysfunction.

Several reports indicated that up to 25% of men regained erectile function after aortoiliac reconstructions using open repairs in patients of varying ages for obstructive disease or aneurysms.[53-61] The prevalence and exact cause of preoperative

ED in various series are difficult to assess with accuracy. Erectile function depends on age; comorbid factors, including the use of drugs; and methods of subjective or objective documentation available to clinicians. Flanigan and coworkers stated that, with planning to avoid the diversion of pelvic blood flow, nerve-sparing aortoiliac dissections, and selective use of indirect methods, iatrogenic impotence can be minimized, and a significant proportion of patients can regain normal sexual function postoperatively.[54] In their series of 110 patients using direct and indirect aortoiliac revascularization, 45% of patients with preoperative vasculogenic impotence regained normal sexual function postoperatively, no patients with normal preoperative sexual function were rendered impotent, and two men developed retrograde ejaculation.

A series of men I operated on using techniques previously described were followed for at least 3 years (up to 1990) using direct interrogation and penile plethysmography. Of 126 men who underwent operation for aortoiliac disease, 4 became impotent as a result of emergency operations or the presence of internal iliac aneurysms. In all the instances of ED, penile plethysmography showed flat-line recordings, and PBIs were well below 0.5. Fifty-three men, average age 64.6 years, were impotent both preoperatively and postoperatively; 30 men,

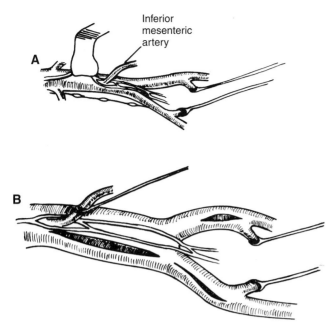

Inferior
mesenteric
artery

A

B

FIGURE 12–3 • Dissection of infrarenal aorta for endarterectomy. *A*, Aorta exposed without mobilization, and inferior mesenteric artery spared along with neural fibers. *B*, Internal iliacs controlled, and common or external iliacs clamped with minimal mobilization. (From DePalma RG: Prevention of sexual dysfunction in aortoiliac surgery. In Jamieson CW [ed]: Current Operative Surgery. Eastborne, East Sussex, England, Bailliere-Tindall, 1985, pp 781-788.)

average age 57 years (range, 39 to 71), were potent both preoperatively and postoperatively; 39 men, average age 58.0 years (range, 38 to 69), were impotent preoperatively and regained function postoperatively. Thus, among 126 men undergoing aortoiliac surgery, about 3% were rendered impotent, commonly in emergency settings. Overall, function was restored or maintained in 54% of men requiring aortoiliac surgery. The data from these series are necessarily retrospective and nonconcurrent.

A recent randomized trial compared immediate elective repair to imaging surveillance of abdominal aortic aneurysms measuring 4.0 to 5.5 cm in men aged 50 to 79 years.[62] Quality of life, impotence, and activity level were later assessed using the SF-36 health status instrument in men followed from 3.5 to 8 years (mean, 4.9 years). For most measures and times, there was no difference between the randomized groups, but overall, significantly more men became impotent after immediate repair than after surveillance ($P < 0.03$). There was a higher prevalence of impotence in the surgical group more than 1 year after randomization, paradoxically associated with an improved perception of health during the first 2 years. The data suggest that open intervention for small abdominal aortic aneurysms carries a finite risk of sexual dysfunction, and decreasing potency with age does not appear to be related to patient perception of health status. Possibly, the loss of erectile function was not considered important by some of these older men. Schiavi showed that age-related changes in frequency, duration, and degree of nocturnal penile tumescence correlated with desire, arousal, and coital frequency.[63] Thus, the age of a patient preoperatively and normal postoperative aging contribute to diminished sexual function. This decrement in function with age does not appear to be linearly related to arterial inflow compromise.

A retrospective questionnaire study of 90 men showed that sexual orgasmic and erectile function deteriorated after open aneurysm repair compared with endovascular repair.[64] In my experience, the focus of endovascular interventions for ED has been directed toward the common or external iliac arteries.[45] Others have described selective dilatation of the internal iliac arteries, with modest success.[65,66] Procedures attempting endovascular intervention below this level—that is, in the pudendal arteries—have failed.[67] Recently, Lin and associates reported severe pelvic ischemia and erectile dysfunction due to internal iliac embolization associated with endovascular repair.[68] The severity of ischemia was related to both bilateral embolization and the presence of disease in the deep femoral arteries. Endovascular repair may require occlusion of the orifice of one or both internal iliac arteries to achieve safe and adequate landing sites. Bilateral internal iliac occlusion is associated with a finite risk of pelvic ischemia; adequate hypogastric flow, through at least one of these vessels, relates to normal sexual function. The risk of internal iliac occlusion is not absolute; femoral collaterals sometimes compensate for internal iliac occlusion, and femoral artery branches have been shown to provide significant collateral circulation to the penis in the face of hypogastric artery occlusion.[69] Internal iliac collateral flow in the presence of acute hypogastric artery ligation is more dependent on the ipsilateral external iliac artery than it is on the contralateral internal iliac artery, even though abundant collateralization between the left and right internal iliac arteries is common in chronic ischemia.[70,71] The variability of responses to internal iliac embolization before endovascular repair has been emphasized.[72] Buttock or thigh claudication and late ischemic complications, seen in 3 of 10 patients after 6 months, led the investigators to suggest limiting bilateral internal iliac embolization before endovascular repair to only those patients considered unfit for open aortic repair. Clearly, more work is needed to make pelvic perfusion a regular facet of endovascular repair.

Femorofemoral bypass combined with intraluminal dilatation of donor external or common iliac arteries is an excellent choice for certain candidates with occlusive disease (Fig. 12-5). The procedure completely avoids aortoiliac dissection, and patency remains quite durable. Objective information from pulse volume recordings before and after femorofemoral bypass correlates with improved patterns of penile plethysmography and pressures after reconstruction.[73] Common iliac artery transluminal dilatation is both practical and useful. Transluminal dilatation of the external iliac arteries can also improve penile perfusion by relieving steal via the internal iliac and gluteal arteries. Although transluminal dilatation of the common iliac arteries is effective, the internal iliac arteries can be difficult to dilate. A report in the Italian literature describes three successful cases among 25 men treated with endovascular interventions for ED.[66] Transluminal dilatation of the pudendal and penile arteries was plagued by restenosis.[74]

Microvascular Procedures

Small vessel reconstructions initially used direct arterialization of the corpus cavernosum, but this approach was soon abandoned. These procedures induced priapism or thrombosis due to fibrosis at the anastomosis between the artery and the corpus cavernosum. Although interest in small vessel

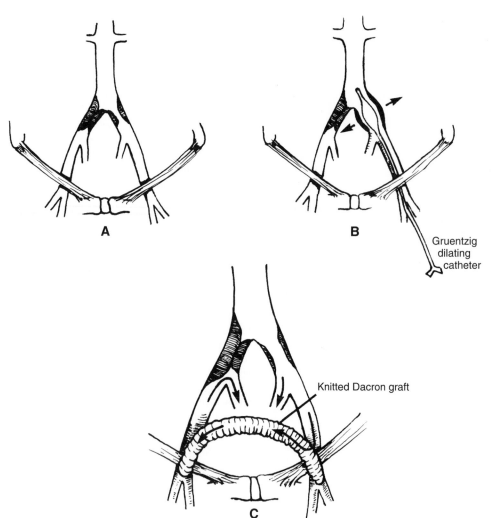

FIGURE 12–4 • Femorofemoral bypass with transluminal angioplasty. *A,* Initial lesion. *B,* Left iliac angioplasty. *C,* Femorofemoral bypass using dilated left iliac donor limb. (From DePalma RG: Prevention of sexual dysfunction in aortoiliac surgery. In Jamieson CW [ed]: Current Operative Surgery. Eastborne, East Sussex, England, Bailliere-Tindall, 1985, pp 781-788.)

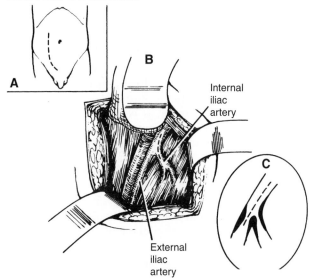

FIGURE 12–5 • Isolated iliac artery endarterectomy. *A,* Incision for retroperitoneal exposure. *B,* Incision for isolated plaque of internal iliac artery. *C,* Linear incision when the external iliac artery is also involved. (From DePalma RG: Prevention of sexual dysfunction in aortoiliac surgery. In Jamieson CW [ed]: Current Operative Surgery. Eastborne, East Sussex, England, Bailliere-Tindall, 1985, pp 781-788.)

reconstruction persists,[75] a 1996 meta-analysis by a urology guidelines panel stated that the chances of success with venous or arterial surgery did not justify its routine use.[76] These procedures are applicable to men who fail to respond to medical therapy and who do not wish to have prostheses. With the availability of effective vasoactive drugs, these procedures are rarely performed. Two types of microvascular bypasses have been used: bypass into the dorsal artery, and arterialization of the deep dorsal vein. The inferior epigastric artery is a readily available inflow source, behaving much like the internal mammary artery. Some use a vein graft originating from the femoral artery. I recommend using the inferior epigastric artery and direct arterial reconstruction rather than deep dorsal vein arterialization.

Patient and Procedure Selection

Candidates for microvascular correction of ED must be rigorously screened. They must have failed to respond to lifestyle alterations, maximal oral PDE-5 inhibitors, and other measures such as cavernosal or intraurethral injection therapy and vacuum erection devices. The options, risks, and benefits of prosthetic insertion should be explored with these patients. Candidates for microvascular surgery are young men with a history of trauma or localized disease.[21,23] Some exhibit diffuse distal penile lesions of unknown origin. Candidates should be free of neural, hormonal, and medication-induced causes of impotence. All patients require selective pudendal arteriography. Communication between the dorsal penile artery and the cavernosal artery requires detailed visualization of individual penile vessels after intracavernous injection of a vasoactive agent to produce tumescence. As mentioned previously, a full erection masks inflow into the cavernosal artery and is not appropriate for evaluation of the penile microvasculature. The inferior epigastric artery, dissected in continuity, is turned down for microvascular anastomosis to the appropriate dorsal artery, anatomy permitting.

DEEP DORSAL VEIN ARTERIALIZATION

Candidates for deep dorsal vein arterialization are younger men with small vessel disease whose dorsal arteries are not suitable for direct bypass. The rationale of this operation was postulated to be reverse flow via emissary veins into the corpus cavernosum. However, my own arteriographic observations and those of others indicate that flow is largely by the circumflex veins into the spongiosum. Follow-up data at 12 to 84 months (average, 34.5 months) showed that 33% of these men attained spontaneous erections, 47% responded to intracavernous injections, and 21% remained impotent.[21] A microvascular anastomosis is done between the inferior epigastric artery and the deep dorsal vein. Glans hyperperfusion is a serious, specific complication of venous arterialization. Venous hypertension, often preceded by urinary spraying due to edema, ultimately causes glans ulceration and necrosis. To minimize this complication, the anastomosis should be performed proximally under the arch of the pubis, and the dorsal vein is ligated proximally and distally, sparing the circumflex veins, which provide outflow. This complication, which can occur late, urgently requires further distal penile vein ligation or ligation of the inflow source.

VENOUS INTERRUPTION

Reported success rates for venous ligation vary considerably, and opinions about this procedure range from advocacy to qualified reservation to condemnation. This variability

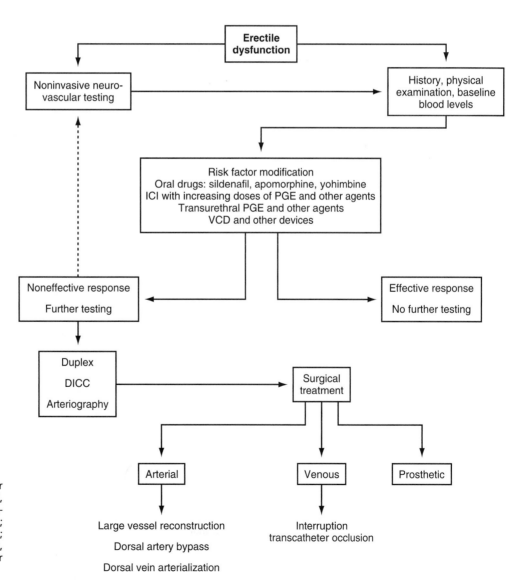

FIGURE 12–6 • Algorithm for erectile dysfunction. DICC, Dynamic Infusion Cavernosometry and Cavernosography; ICI, intracavernous injection; PGE, prostaglandin E_1; VCD, vacuum erection constrictor device.

probably relates to patient selection and failure to evaluate all factors, including arterial supply or prior penile trauma that can cause venous leakage. At follow-up ranging from 12 to 100 months (average, 48 months), 33% of men functioned spontaneously, 44% used intracavernous injection, and the remainder were impotent.[21,23] Venous ligation requires direct ligation and excision of the veins in cases selected by dynamic infusion cavernosography. I confine these procedures to excision of the dorsal vein and do not approach the crural veins directly.[77] Other draining veins can be occluded using coils inserted by an invasive radiologist. At times, an introducing catheter inserted via the deep dorsal vein is useful. Yu and associates recommend routine dynamic cavernosography and cavernosometry at 3 months in all cases of venous ligation to rule out sham effect.[78] At this time, embolization for recurrent leaks can be done; with these procedures, about 70% of men can regain erectile function and are able to function with supplemental intracavernous injection.

Medical Treatment

Once aneurysms, large vessel disease, and uncontrolled diabetes have been ruled out, the branched logic sequence shown in Figure 12-6 can be used. Treatment begins with control of risk factors such as cigarette smoking, hyperlipidemia, and obesity. It is possible to minimize the necessity for antihypertensive treatment by weight control or exercise or to minimize the sexual effects of such treatment by changing drugs (e.g., to an angiotensin-converting enzyme inhibitor). Some men improve after one or two intracavernous injections have produced artificial erection, and they then resume spontaneous function.

Specific medical therapy and risk factor modification are done synchronously with initial oral therapy using selected PDE-5 inhibitors widely available in oral form. With dosage titration, sildenafil was effective in 59% of individuals, compared with 20% in the placebo group.[79] Administration of nitrates, antihypertensive agents, or alpha blockers is a specific contraindication to PDE-5 therapy. Other oral agents include apomorphine, recently formulated for sublingual administration; approval of phentolamine mesylate for ED has been delayed because of toxicologic concerns.[80] Men with ED who fail oral agents can progress to intraurethral or cavernosal injections. Vacuum devices can also be prescribed.

Conclusion

Vascular surgeons must recognize the basic requirements for open and endovascular aortoiliac interventions that prevent or relieve ED associated with large vessel disease. They need to collaborate with urologists and other experts in treating men with primary ED. After screening and medical treatment, few individuals are candidates for vascular surgical intervention for the sole purpose of treating a sexual disability. Those with macrovascular disease, occult aneurysms, and poorly controlled diabetes, however, need attention. Treating men and, more rarely, women with sexual disabilities requires a unique sensitivity to individual needs. Outcomes of medical treatment and surgical interventions continue to improve in concert with more accurate diagnosis, advances in technique, and meticulous patient selection.

KEY REFERENCES

DePalma RG, Levine SB, Feldman S: Preservation of erectile function after aortoiliac reconstruction. Arch Surg 113:958, 1978.

DeTejada IS, Goldstein I, Azadzoi K, et al: Impaired neurogenic and endothelium-mediated relaxation of penile smooth muscle from diabetic men with impotence. N Engl J Med 32:1025, 1989.

Flanigan DP, Schuler JJ, Keifer T, et al: Elimination of iatrogenic impotence and improvement of sexual dysfunction after aortoiliac revascularization. Arch Surg 117:544, 1982.

Goldstein I, Lue TF, Padma-Nathan H, et al: Oral sildenafil in the treatment of erectile dysfunction. N Engl J Med 338:1397, 1998.

Harris JD, Jepson RP: Aorto-iliac stenosis: A comparison of two procedures. Aust J Surg 34:211, 1965.

Leriche R, Morel A: The syndrome of thrombotic obliteration of the aortic bifurcation. Ann Surg 127:193, 1948.

Merchant RF Jr, DePalma RG: Effects of femorofemoral grafts on postoperative sexual function: Correlation with penile pulse volume recordings. Surgery 90:962, 1981.

Rajfer J, Aronson WJ, Bush PA, et al: Nitric oxide as a mediator of the corpus cavernosum in response to nonadrenergic noncholinergic neurotransmission. N Engl J Med 326:90, 1992.

REFERENCES

1. Process of Care Consensus Panel, position paper: The process of care model for evaluation and treatment of erectile dysfunction. Int J Impot Res 11:59, 1999.
2. DePalma RG: New developments in the diagnosis and treatment of impotence. West J Med 164:54, 1996.
3. DePalma RG: The best treatment for impotence. Vasc Surg 32:519, 1998.
4. May AG, DeWeese JA, Rob CG: Changes in sexual function following operations on the abdominal aorta Surgery 65:41, 1969.
5. DePalma RG, Levine SB, Feldman S: Preservation of erectile function after aortoiliac reconstruction. Arch Surg 113:958, 1978.
6. DePalma RG, Kedia K, Persky L: Surgical options in the correction of vasculogenic impotence. Vasc Surg 14:92, 1980.
7. Mulcahy JJ (ed): Male Sexual Function: A Guide to Clinical Management. Totowa, NJ, Humana Press, 2001.
8. Hultgren R, Sjogren B, Soderberg M, et al: Sexual function in women suffering from aortoiliac occlusive disease. Eur J Vasc Endovasc Surg 17:306, 1999.
9. Saini J, Kuczynski E, Gretz HF 3rd, Sills ES: Supracervical hysterectomy versus total abdominal hysterectomy: perceived effects on sexual function. BMC Women's Health 2:1, 2002.
10. Graesslin O, Martin-Morille C, Leguillier-Armour MC, et al: Local investigation concerning psychic and sexual functioning a short time after hysterectomy. Gynecol Obstet Fertil 6:474, 2002.
11. Trimbos JB, Maas CP, Deruiter MC, et al: A nerve sparing radical hysterectomy: Guidelines and feasibility in Western patients. Int J Gynecol Cancer 11:180, 2001.
12. Andersson KE, Wagner G: Physiology of penile erection. Physiol Rev 75:191, 1995.
13. DePalma RG: Anatomy and physiology of normal erections: Pathogenesis of impotence. In Sidawy AN, Sumpio BE, DePalma RG (eds): Basic Science of Vascular Disease. Armonk, NY, Futura, 1996, pp 761-773.
14. DeTejada IS, Goldstein I, Azadzoi K, et al: Impaired neurogenic and endothelium-mediated relaxation of penile smooth muscle from diabetic men with impotence. N Engl J Med 32:1025, 1989.
15. Rajfer J, Aronson WJ, Bush PA, et al: Nitric oxide as a mediator of the corpus cavernosum in response to nonadrenergic noncholinergic neurotransmission. N Engl J Med 326:90, 1992.
16. Azadzoi KM, Nehra A, Siroky MB: Effects of cavernosal hypoxia and oxygenation on penile erection [abstract]. Int J Impot Res 6(Suppl I): A26, 1994.
17. Brock GB, Zvara P, Sioufi R, et al: Nitric oxide synthase is testosterone dependent [abstract]. Int J Impot Res 6(Suppl I):D42, 1994.
18. Burnett AL: Role of nitric oxide in the physiology of erection. Biol Report 52:485, 1995.
19. Beavo JA: Cyclic nucleotide phosphodiesterases: Functional implication of multiple isoforms. Physiol Rev 75:725, 1995.
20. Gingell C, Ballard SA, Tang K, et al: Cyclic nucleotide phosphodiestrase and erectile function. Int J Impot Res 9(Suppl I):510, 1997.

21. DePalma RG, Olding M, Yu GW, et al: Vascular interventions for impotence: Lessons learned. J Vasc Surg 21:576, 1995.
22. DePalma RG, Emsellem HA, Edwards CM, et al: A screening sequence for vasculogenic impotence. J Vasc Surg 5:228, 1987.
23. DePalma RG: Vascular surgery for impotence: A review. Int J Impot Res 9:61, 1997.
24. Leriche R, Morel A: The syndrome of thrombotic obliteration of the aortic bifurcation. Ann Surg 127:193, 1948.
25. Leriche R: Des oblitérations artériele hautes (oblitération de la términation de l'aorte) comme cause de insuffances circulatoires des membres inférieurs [abstract]. Bull Mem Soc Chir 49:1404, 1923.
26. Fabra M, Porst H: Bulbocavernosus-reflex latencies and pudendal nerve SSEP compared to penile vascular testing in 669 patients with erectile failure and other sexual dysfunction. Int J Impot Res 11:167, 1999.
27. Emsellem HA, Bergsrud DW, DePalma RG, et al: Pudendal evoked potentials in the evaluation of impotence [abstract]. J Clin Neurophysiol 359:5, 1988.
28. Stackl W, Hasun R, Marberger M: Intracavernous injection of prostaglandin E_1 in impotent men. J Urol 140:66, 1988.
29. Guay AT: Sexual dysfunction in the diabetic patient. Int J Impot Res 13(Suppl 5):S47, 2001.
30. Enzlin P, Mathieu C, Van den Bruel A, et al: Sexual dysfuntion in women with type 1 diabetes: A controlled study. Diabetes Care 25:672, 2002.
31. DeBusk R, Drory Y, Goldstein I, et al: Management of sexual dysfunction in patients with cardiovascular disease: Recommendations of the Princeton Consensus Panel. Am J Cardiol 86:62F, 2000.
32. Meston CM, Worcel M: The effects of yohimbine plus L-arginine glutamate on sexual arousal in postmenopausal women with sexual arousal disorder. Arch Sex Behav 31:323, 2002.
33. Berman JR, Berman LA, Lin H, Goldstein I: Female sexual dysfunction: Epidemiology, physiology and treatment. In Mulcahy JJ (ed): Male Sexual Function: A Guide to Clinical Management. Totowa, NJ, Humana Press, 2001, pp 123-140.
34. Caruso S, Intelisano G, Lupo L, Agnello C: Premenopausal women affected by sexual disorder treated with sildenafil: A double blind, crossover, placebo-controlled study. BJOG 108:623, 2001.
35. Laan E, van Lunsen RH, Everaerd W, et al: The enhancement of vaginal vasocongestion by sildenafil in healthy premenstrual women. J Womens Health Gend Based Med 11:357, 2002.
36. Islam A, Mitchell J, Rosen R, et al: Topical alprostadil in the treatment of female sexual arousal disorder: A pilot study. J Sex Marital Ther 27:531, 2001.
37. Lue TF: Impotence: A patient's goal-directed approach to treatment. World J Urol 8:67, 1990.
38. DePalma RG: What constitutes an adequate impotence workup? World J Urol 10:157, 1992.
39. DePalma RG, Michal V: Point of view: Déjà vu-again: Advantages and limitations of methods for assessing penile arterial flow. Urology 36:199, 1990.
40. DePalma RG, Dalton CM, Gomez CA, et al: Predictive value of a screening sequence for venogenic impotence. Int J Impot Res 4:143, 1992.
41. Sanchez-Ortiz RF, Broderick GA: Vascular evaluation of erectile dysfunction. In Mulcahy JJ (ed): Male Sexual Function: A Guide to Clinical Management. Totowa, NJ, Humana Press, 2001, pp 167-202.
42. Levine LA, Elterman L: Nocturnal penile tumescence and rigidity testing. In Mulcahy JJ (ed): Male Sexual Function: A Guide to Clinical Management. Totowa, NJ, Humana Press, 2001, pp 151-166.
43. DePalma RG: New developments in the diagnosis and treatment of impotence. West J Med 164:54, 1996.
44. Reis JM, Alves CR, Garro MA, et al: Endovascular surgery for erectile dysfunction. Int J Impot Res 10(Suppl 3):398, 1998.
45. DePalma RG: Iliac artery occlusive disease: Impotence and colon ischemia. In Moore WS, Ahn SS (eds): Endovascular Surgery. Philadelphia, WB Saunders, 2001, pp 335-360.
46. DePalma RG, Edwards CM, Schwab FJ, Steinberg DL: Modern management of impotence associated with aortic surgery. In Bergen JJ, Yao JST (eds): Arterial Surgery: New Diagnostic and Operative Techniques. Orlando, Fla, Grune & Stratton, 1988, pp 337-348.
47. DePalma RG: Prevention of sexual dysfunction in aortoiliac surgery. In Jamieson CW (ed): Current Operative Surgery: Vascular Surgery. London, Bailliere-Tindall, 1988, pp 80-84.
48. Fredberg U, Mouritzen C: Sexual dysfunction as a symptom of arteriosclerosis and as a complication to reconstruction of the aortoiliac segment. J Cardiovasc Surg 29:149, 1988.
49. Miles JR, Miles DG, Johnson G Jr: Aortoiliac operations and sexual dysfunction. Arch Surg 117:1177, 1982.
50. Laumann EO, Paik A, Rosen RC: The epidemiology of erectile dysfunction: Results from the National Health and Social Life Survey. Int J Impot Res 11:S60, 1999.
51. McCullough AR Jr: Ejaculatory disorders. In Mulcahy JJ (ed): Male Sexual Function: A Guide to Clinical Management. Totowa, NJ, Humana Press, 2001, pp 351-370.
52. Queral LA, Flinn WR, Bergan JJ, et al: Pelvic hemodynamics after aortoiliac reconstruction. Surgery 86:799, 1979.
53. DePalma RG, Levine SB, Feldman S: Preservation of erectile function after aortoiliac reconstruction. Arch Surg 113:958, 1978.
54. Flanigan DP, Schuler JJ, Keifer T, et al: Elimination of iatrogenic impotence and improvement of sexual dysfunction after aortoiliac revascularization. Arch Surg 117:544, 1982.
55. Hallbrook T, Holmquist B: Sexual disturbances following dissection of the aorta and the common iliac arteries. J Cardiovasc Surg 11:255, 1970.
56. Harris JD, Jepson RP: Aorto-iliac stenosis: A comparison of two procedures. Aust J Surg 34:211, 1965.
57. Castaneda-Zuniga WR, Smith A, Kaye K, et al: Transluminal angioplasty for treatment of vasculogenic impotence. AJR Am J Roentgenol 139:371, 1982.
58. Sabri S, Cotton LT: Sexual function following aortoiliac reconstruction. Lancet 2:1218, 1971.
59. Spiro M, Cotton LT: Aorto-iliac thrombo-endarterectomy. Br J Surg 57:161, 1979.
60. Weinstein MH, Machleder HI: Sexual function after aortoiliac surgery. Ann Surg 181:787, 1975.
61. DePalma RG: Impotence as a complication in aortoiliac reconstruction. In Bernhard VM, Towne JB (eds): Complications in Vascular Surgery. New York, Grune & Stratton, 1980, pp 427-442.
62. Lederle FA, Johnson GR, Wilson SE, et al: Quality of life, impotence, and activity level in a randomized trial of immediate repair versus surveillance of small abdominal aortic aneurysm. J Vasc Surg 38:745, 2003.
63. Schiavi RC, Schreiner-Engel P, Mandeli J, et al: Healthy aging and male sexual function. Am J Psychiatry 147:766, 1990.
64. Xenos ES, Stevens SL, Freeman MB, et al: Erectile function after open or endovascular abdominal aortic aneurysm repair. Ann Vasc Surg 17:530, 2003.
65. Lee CW, Kaufman JA, Fan CM, et al: Clinical outcome of internal iliac occlusions during endovascular treatment of aortoiliac aneurysmal disease. J Vasc Interv Radiol 11:567, 2000.
66. Urigo F, Pischedda A, Maiore M, et al: The role of arteriography and percutaneous transluminal angioplasty in the treatment of arteriogenic impotence [Italian]. Radiol Med (Torino) 88:80, 1994.
67. Valji K, Bookstein JJ: Transluminal angioplasty in the treatment of arteriogenic impotence. Cardiovasc Intervent Radiol 11:245, 1988.
68. Lin PH, Bush RL, Chen C, et al: A prospective evaluation of hypogastric artery embolization in endovascular aortoiliac aneurysm repair. J Vasc Surg 36:500, 2002.
69. Kawai M: Pelvic hemodynamics before and after aortoiliac vascular reconstruction: The significance of penile blood pressure. Jpn J Surg 18:514, 1988.
70. Iliopoulos JI, Horwanitz PE, Pierce GE, et al: The critical hypogastric circulation. Am J Surg 154:671, 1987.
71. Iliopoulos JI, Hermreck AS, Thomas JH, et al: Hemodynamics of the hypogastric arterial circulation. J Vasc Surg 9:637, 1989.
72. Engelke C, Elford J, Morgan RA, Belli AM: Internal iliac artery embolization with bilateral occlusion before endovascular aortoiliac aneurysm repair: Clinical outcome of simultaneous and sequential intervention. J Vasc Interv Radiol 13:667, 2002.
73. Merchant RF Jr, DePalma RG: Effects of femorofemoral grafts on postoperative sexual function: Correlation with penile pulse volume recordings. Surgery 90:962, 1981.
74. Bookstein JJ, Valji K: The arteriolar component in impotence: A possible paradigm shift. AJR Am J Roentgenol 157:932, 1991.
75. Jarrow JP: Vascular surgery for erectile dysfunction. In Mulcahy JJ (ed): Male Sexual Function: A Guide to Clinical Management. Totowa, NJ, Humana Press, 2001, pp 293-306.
76. Montague DK, Barada JH, Belker AM, et al: Clinical Guidelines Panel on Erectile Dysfunction: Summary report on the treatment of organic erectile dysfunction. American Urological Association. J Urol 156:2007, 1996.

77. DePalma RG, Schwab F, Druy EM, et al: Experience in diagnosis and treatment of impotence caused by cavernosal leak syndrome. J Vasc Surg 10:117, 1989.
78. Yu GW, Schwab FJ, Melograna FS, et al: Preoperative and postoperative dynamic cavernosography and cavernosometry: Objective assessment of venous ligation for impotence. J Urol 147:618, 1992.
79. Goldstein I, Lue TF, Padma-Nathan H, et al: Oral sildenafil in the treatment of erectile dysfunction. N Engl J Med 338:1397, 1998.
80. Padma-Nathan H, Guiliano F: Oral pharmocotherapy. In Mulcahy JJ (ed): Male Sexual Function: A Guide to Clinical Management. Totowa, NJ, Humana Press, 2001, pp 203-224.

Questions

1. **Which of the following occurs during full penile erection?**
   (a) Deep cavernosal artery flow increases
   (b) Venous valves close
   (c) Cavernosal oxygen tension falls
   (d) Cavernosal smooth muscle relaxes
   (e) Arterial pressure in the dorsal arteries falls

2. **Men with erectile dysfunction most often exhibit which of the following?**
   (a) Decreased dorsal arterial flow
   (b) Failure to respond to PDE-5 inhibition
   (c) Occult aneurysms
   (d) Neurologic abnormalities
   (e) Normal physical examination

3. **Which of the following statements about endovascular aortoiliac procedures is true?**
   (a) They require bilateral internal iliac artery occlusion
   (b) They may result in buttock ischemia
   (c) They may result in more ED postoperatively
   (d) They spare periaortic nerves
   (e) They may increase the bulbocavernosus reflex time

4. **When does the penile brachial index (PBI) indicate aortoiliac occlusive disease?**
   (a) PBI between 0.6 and 0.75
   (b) PBI 0.6 or less
   (c) PBI 0.8 or less
   (d) PBI 0.8, accompanied by flat pulse volume waves
   (e) PBI 0.75, accompanied by abnormally shaped pulse waves

5. **Women with female sexual dysfunction may have which of the following?**
   (a) Failure to lubricate
   (b) Dyspareunia
   (c) Aortoiliac occlusive disease
   (d) Arousal failure
   (e) All of the above

6. **When a sexually active man expresses concern about possible erectile dysfunction before aneurysm repair, what should the physician do?**
   (a) Reassure the patient and spouse that this is preventable
   (b) Refer the patient to a psychiatrist
   (c) Measure baseline levels of testosterone and prolactin
   (d) Obtain preoperative penile brachial index and pulse volume recordings
   (e) Perform preoperative selective pudendal arteriography

7. **Useful techniques in preventing sexual dysfunction after aortic surgery include which of the following?**
   (a) Restoration of flow to internal iliac arteries
   (b) Suture of inferior mesenteric artery within the aortic sac
   (c) Avoidance of the aortic bifurcation
   (d) Retrograde flushing of internal iliacs
   (e) All of the above

8. **Age most likely affects potency by what means?**
   (a) Decreasing arterial inflow
   (b) Causing nerve deterioration
   (c) Causing smooth muscle dysfunction
   (d) Causing progressive venous fibrosis
   (e) Decreasing cardiovascular function

9. **Artificial erection is most safely obtained by which of the following?**
   (a) Intracavernous papaverine injection
   (b) Intracavernous prostaglandin E_1 injection
   (c) Intracavernous phentolamine injection
   (d) Roller pump cavernosal infusion of 40 mL normal saline per minute
   (e) All of the above

10. **Screening and medical treatment for erectile dysfunction most often require which of the following?**
    (a) PDE-5 inhibitors
    (b) Cavernosometry
    (c) Arteriography
    (d) Psychotherapy
    (e) Psychological counseling along with medical therapy

Answers

1. d	2. e	3. d	4. b	5. e
6. d	7. e	8. c	9. b	10. a

13

R. Eugene Zierler • D. Eugene Strandness, Jr.*

Hemodynamics for the Vascular Surgeon

Blood flow in human arteries and veins can be described in terms of strict hemodynamic principles. Although the elements of hemodynamics are derived from engineering, mathematics, and physiology, these principles also form the theoretical foundation for the surgical treatment of vascular disease.

The major mechanisms of arterial disease are obstruction of the lumen and disruption of the vessel wall. Arterial obstruction or narrowing may result from atherosclerosis, emboli, thrombi, fibromuscular dysplasia, trauma, or external compression. The clinical significance of an obstructive lesion depends on its location, severity, and duration, as well as on the ability of the circulation to compensate by increasing cardiac output and developing collateral pathways. Surgical treatment requires the identification and correction of arterial lesions associated with significant hemodynamic disturbances. Disruption of the arterial wall is caused by ruptured aneurysm or trauma. The tendency of aneurysms to rupture is determined by arterial wall characteristics, intraluminal pressure, and size. In this situation, the role of surgery is to prevent rupture or to reestablish arterial continuity after rupture occurs.

On the venous side of the circulation, the major hemodynamic mechanisms of disease are obstruction and valvular incompetence. These are generally the sequelae of thrombosis in the deep venous system, and they produce venous hypertension in the circulation distal to the involved venous segment. The clinical consequences of venous hypertension are the signs and symptoms of the post-thrombotic syndrome: pain, edema, subcutaneous fibrosis, pigmentation, stasis dermatitis, and ulceration. Treatment of this condition involves elevation, external compression, venous interruption, and, rarely, direct venous reconstruction.

This chapter begins with a discussion of the hemodynamic principles and wall properties that govern arterial flow. The hemodynamic alterations produced by arterial stenoses and their effect on flow patterns in human limbs are considered next. These principles are then related to the treatment of arterial obstruction. Finally, the hemodynamics of the venous system are briefly reviewed and related to the pathophysiology and treatment of venous disease.

*Deceased

Basic Principles of Arterial Hemodynamics

FLUID PRESSURE

The pressure in a fluid system is defined as force per unit area (given in dynes per square centimeter). Intravascular arterial pressure (P) has three components: (1) the dynamic pressure produced by contraction of the heart, (2) the hydrostatic pressure, and (3) the static filling pressure. Hydrostatic pressure is determined by the specific gravity of blood and the height of the point of measurement above a specific reference level. The reference level in the human body is considered to be the right atrium. The hydrostatic pressure is given by the following equation:

$$P \text{ (hydrostatic)} = -\rho g h \qquad [1]$$

where ρ is the specific gravity of blood (approximately 1.056 g/cm^3), g is the acceleration due to gravity (980 cm/sec^2), and h is the distance in centimeters above or below the right atrium. The magnitude of hydrostatic pressure may be quite large. In a man 5 feet 8 inches tall, this pressure at ankle level is approximately 89 mm Hg.[1]

The static filling pressure represents the residual pressure that exists in the absence of arterial flow. This pressure is determined by the volume of blood and the elastic properties of the vessel wall, and it is usually in the range of 5 to 10 mm Hg.

FLUID ENERGY

Blood flows through the arterial system in response to differences in total fluid energy. Although pressure gradients are the most obvious forces involved, other forms of energy drive the circulation.[2] Total fluid energy (E) can be divided into potential energy (E_p) and kinetic energy (E_k). The components of potential energy are intravascular pressure (P) and gravitational potential energy.

The factors contributing to intravascular pressure have already been discussed. Gravitational potential energy represents the ability of a volume of blood to do work because of its height above a specific reference level. The formula for gravitational potential energy is the same as that for hydrostatic pressure (see Equation 1) but with an opposite sign: $+\rho gh$. Because the gravitational potential energy and hydrostatic pressure usually cancel each other out and the static filling pressure is relatively low, the predominant component of potential energy is the dynamic pressure produced by cardiac contraction. Potential energy can be expressed as follows:

$$E_p = P + (\rho gh) \qquad [2]$$

Kinetic energy represents the ability of blood to do work on the basis of its motion. It is proportional to the specific gravity of blood and the square of blood velocity (v), in centimeters per second:

$$E_k = \tfrac{1}{2}\rho v^2 \qquad [3]$$

By combining Equations 2 and 3, an expression for the total fluid energy per unit volume of blood (in ergs per cubic centimeter) can be obtained:

$$E = P + \rho gh + \tfrac{1}{2}\rho v^2 \qquad [4]$$

FLUID ENERGY LOSSES

Bernoulli's Principle

$E_p + E_k = Ct_{\mp}$

When fluid flows from one point to another, its total energy (E) along any given streamline is constant, provided that flow is steady and there are no frictional energy losses. This is in accordance with the law of conservation of energy and constitutes Bernoulli's principle:

$$P_1 + \rho gh_1 + \tfrac{1}{2}\rho v_1^2 = P_2 + \rho gh_2 + \tfrac{1}{2}\rho v_2^2 \qquad [5]$$

This equation expresses the relationship among pressure, gravitational potential energy, and kinetic energy in an idealized fluid system. In the horizontal diverging tube shown in Figure 13-1, steady flow between point 1 and point 2 is accompanied by an increase in cross-sectional area and a decrease in flow velocity. Although the fluid moves against a pressure gradient of 2.5 mm Hg and therefore gains potential energy, the total fluid energy remains constant because of the lower velocity and a proportional loss of kinetic energy. In other words, the widening of the tube results in the conversion of kinetic energy to potential energy in the form of pressure. In a converging tube, the opposite would occur; a pressure drop and increase in velocity would result in potential energy being converted to kinetic energy.

The situation depicted in the preceding example is not observed in human arteries because the ideal flow conditions specified in the Bernoulli relationship are not present. The fluid energy lost in moving blood through the arterial circulation is dissipated mainly in the form of heat. When this source of energy loss is accounted for, Equation 5 becomes the following:

$$P_1 + \rho gh_1 + \tfrac{1}{2}\rho v_1^2 = P_2 + \rho gh_2 + \tfrac{1}{2}\rho v_2^2 + heat \qquad [6]$$

Viscous Energy Losses and Poiseuille's Law

Energy losses in flowing blood occur either as viscous losses resulting from friction or as inertial losses related to changes in the velocity or direction of flow. The term *viscosity* describes

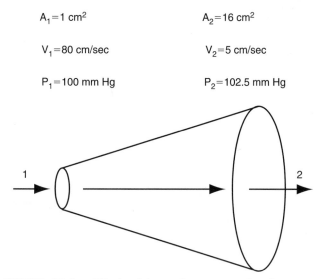

$A_1 = 1\ cm^2$ $A_2 = 16\ cm^2$

$V_1 = 80\ cm/sec$ $V_2 = 5\ cm/sec$

$P_1 = 100\ mm\ Hg$ $P_2 = 102.5\ mm\ Hg$

FIGURE 13–1 • Effect of increasing cross-sectional area on pressure in a frictionless fluid system. While pressure increases, total fluid energy remains constant as a result of a decrease in velocity. (Redrawn from Sumner DS: The hemodynamics and pathophysiology of arterial disease. In Rutherford RB [ed]: Vascular Surgery. Philadelphia, WB Saunders, 1977.)

the resistance to flow that arises because of the intermolecular attractions between fluid layers. The coefficient of viscosity (η) is defined as the ratio of shear stress (τ) to shear rate (D):

$$\eta = \frac{\tau}{D} \qquad [7]$$

Shear stress is proportional to the energy loss due to friction between adjacent fluid layers, whereas shear rate refers to the relative velocity of adjacent fluid layers. Fluids with particularly strong intermolecular attractions offer a high resistance to flow and have high coefficients of viscosity. For example, motor oil has a higher coefficient of viscosity than water.[3] The unit of viscosity is the poise, which equals 1 dyne-sec/cm². Because it is difficult to measure viscosity directly, relative viscosity is often used to relate the viscosity of a fluid to that of water. The relative viscosity of plasma is approximately 1.8, whereas for whole blood, the relative viscosity is in the range of 3 to 4.

Because viscosity increases exponentially with increases in hematocrit, the concentration of red blood cells is the most important factor affecting the viscosity of whole blood. The viscosity of plasma is determined largely by the concentration of plasma proteins. These constituents of blood are also responsible for its non-Newtonian character. In a Newtonian fluid, viscosity is independent of shear rate or flow velocity. Because blood is a suspension of cells and large protein molecules, its viscosity can vary greatly with shear rate (Fig. 13-2). Blood viscosity increases rapidly at low shear rates but approaches a constant value at higher shear rates. In most of the arterial circulation, the prevailing shear rates place the blood viscosity on the asymptotic portion of the curve. Thus, for arteries with diameters greater than about 1 mm, human blood resembles a constant-viscosity, or Newtonian, fluid.

Poiseuille's law describes the viscous energy losses that occur in an idealized flow model. This law states that the pressure gradient along a tube ($P_1 - P_2$, in dynes per square centimeter) is directly proportional to the mean flow velocity

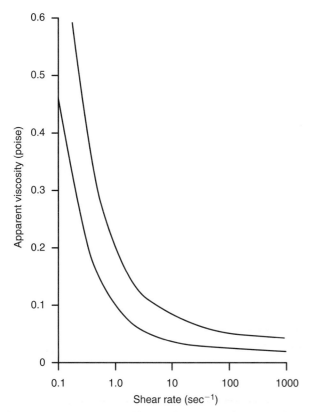

FIGURE 13–2 • Viscosity of human blood as a function of shear rate. Values range between the two lines. (From Strandness DE, Sumner DS: Hemodynamics for Surgeons. New York, Grune & Stratton, 1975.)

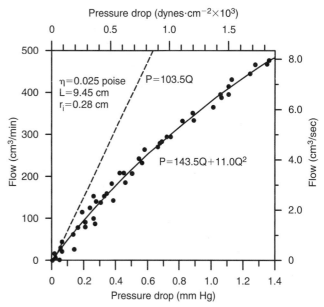

FIGURE 13–3 • Pressure drop across a 9.45-cm length of canine femoral artery at varying flow rates. The experimental data line *(solid)* has both linear and squared terms, corresponding to viscous and inertial energy losses. The pressure-flow curve predicted by Poiseuille's law *(dashed line)* depicts much lower energy losses than those actually observed. (From Sumner DS: The hemodynamics and pathophysiology of arterial disease. In Rutherford RB [ed]: Vascular Surgery. Philadelphia, WB Saunders, 1977.)

($\overline{V}$, in centimeters per second) or volume flow ($\overline{Q}$, in cubic centimeters per second), the tube length (L, in centimeters), and the fluid viscosity (η, in poises), and is inversely proportional to either the second or fourth power of the radius (r, in centimeters):

$$P_1 - P_2 = \overline{V}\frac{8L\eta}{r^2} = \overline{Q}\frac{8L\eta}{\pi r^4} \qquad [8]$$

When this equation is simplified to pressure = flow × resistance, it is analogous to Ohm's law of electrical circuits.

The strict application of Poiseuille's law requires the steady, laminar flow of a Newtonian fluid in a straight, rigid, cylindrical tube. Because these conditions seldom exist in the arterial circulation, Poiseuille's law can only estimate the minimum pressure gradient or viscous energy losses that may be expected in arterial flow. Energy losses due to inertial effects often exceed viscous energy losses, particularly in the presence of arterial disease.

Inertial Energy Losses

Energy losses related to inertia (ΔE) are proportional to a constant (K), the specific gravity of blood, and the square of blood velocity:

$$\Delta E = K\tfrac{1}{2}\rho v^2 \qquad [9]$$

Because velocity is the only independent variable in this equation, inertial energy losses result from the acceleration and deceleration of pulsatile flow, variations in lumen diameter, and changes in the direction of flow at points of curvature and branching.

The combined effects of viscous and inertial energy losses are illustrated in Figure 13-3. When the pressure drop across an arterial segment is measured at varying flow rates, the experimental data fit a line with both linear (viscous) and squared (inertial) terms. The viscous energy losses predicted by Poiseuille's law are considerably less than the total energy loss actually observed.

Vascular Resistance

Hemodynamic resistance (R) can be defined as the ratio of the energy drop between two points along an artery ($E_1 - E_2$) to the mean blood flow (Q):

$$R = \frac{E_1 - E_2}{Q} \cong \frac{P_1 - P_2}{Q} \qquad [10]$$

If the kinetic energy term ($\tfrac{1}{2}\rho v^2$) is considered to be a small component of the total energy, and the artery is assumed to be horizontal so that the gravitational potential energy terms (ρgh) cancel, Equation 4 can be used to express resistance as the simple ratio of pressure drop ($P_1 - P_2$) to flow. Thus, Equation 10 becomes a rearranged version of Poiseuille's law (Equation 8), and the minimum resistance or viscous energy losses are given by the resistance term:

$$R = \frac{8L\eta}{\pi r^4} \qquad [11]$$

The hemodynamic resistance of an arterial segment increases as the flow velocity increases, provided that the lumen size

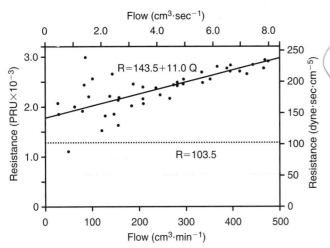

FIGURE 13–4 • Resistance derived from the pressure-flow curve in Figure 13-3. The resistance increases with increasing flow. Constant resistance predicted by Poiseuille's law is shown by the *dotted line*. PRU, peripheral resistance unit. (From Sumner DS: The hemodynamics and pathophysiology of arterial disease. In Rutherford RB [ed]: Vascular Surgery. Philadelphia, WB Saunders, 1977.)

remains constant (Fig. 13-4). These additional energy losses are related to inertial effects and are proportional to $\frac{1}{2}P + \rho v^2$.

According to Equation 11, the predominant factor influencing hemodynamic resistance is the fourth power of the radius. The relationship between radius and pressure drop for various flow rates along a 10-cm vessel segment is shown in Figure 13-5. For a wide range of flow rates, the pressure drop

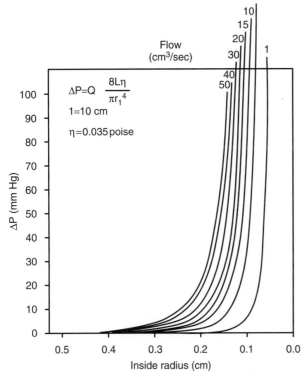

FIGURE 13–5 • Relationship of pressure drop to inside radius of a cylindrical tube 10 cm in length at various rates of steady laminar flow. Flow rates are comparable to those in the human iliac artery. (From Strandness DE, Sumner DS: Hemodynamics for Surgeons. New York, Grune & Stratton, 1975.)

is negligible until the radius is reduced to about 0.3 cm; for radii less than 0.2 cm, the pressure drop increases rapidly. These observations may explain the frequent failure of femoropopliteal autogenous vein bypass grafts less than 4 mm in diameter.[4]

The calculation of total resistance (R_t) depends on whether the component resistances ($R_1 \dots R_n$) are arranged in series or in parallel. This is also analogous to electrical circuits.

$$R_t \text{ (series)} = R_1 + R_2 + \dots R_n \qquad [12]$$

$$\frac{1}{R_t \text{ (parallel)}} = \frac{1}{R_1} + \frac{1}{R_2} + \dots + \frac{1}{R_n} \qquad [13]$$

The standard physical units of hemodynamic resistance are dyne-seconds per centimeter to the fifth power. A more convenient way of expressing resistance is the peripheral resistance unit (PRU), which has the dimensions of millimeters of mercury per cubic centimeter per minute. One PRU is approximately 8×10^4 dyne-sec/cm^5.

In the human circulation, approximately 90% of the total vascular resistance results from flow through the arteries and capillaries, whereas the remaining 10% results from venous flow. The arterioles and capillaries are responsible for more than 60% of the total resistance, whereas the large and medium-size arteries account for only about 15%.[2] Thus, the arteries that are most commonly affected by atherosclerotic occlusive disease are normally vessels with very low resistance.

BLOOD FLOW PATTERNS

Laminar Flow

In the steady-state conditions specified by Poiseuille's law, the flow pattern is laminar. All motion is parallel to the walls of the tube, and the fluid is arranged in a series of concentric layers, or laminae, like those shown in Figure 13-6. While the velocity within each lamina remains constant, the velocity is lowest adjacent to the tube wall and increases toward the center of the tube. This results in a velocity profile that is parabolic in shape (Fig. 13-7). As previously discussed, the

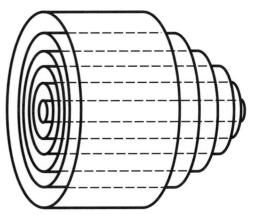

FIGURE 13–6 • Concentric laminae of fluid in a cylindrical tube. Flow is from left to right. The center laminae move more rapidly than those near the periphery, and the flow profile is parabolic. (From Strandness DE, Sumner DS: Hemodynamics for Surgeons. New York, Grune & Stratton, 1975.)

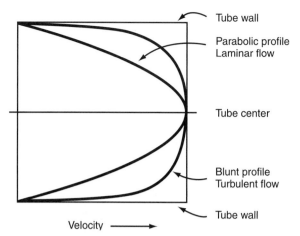

FIGURE 13–7 • Velocity profiles of steady laminar and turbulent flow. Velocity is lowest adjacent to the tube wall and maximal in the center. (From Sumner DS: The hemodynamics and pathophysiology of arterial disease. In Rutherford RB [ed]: Vascular Surgery. Philadelphia, WB Saunders, 1977.)

energy expended in moving one lamina of fluid over another is proportional to viscosity.

Turbulent Flow

In contrast to the linear streamlines of laminar flow, turbulence is an irregular flow state in which velocity varies rapidly with respect to space and time. These random velocity changes result in the dissipation of fluid energy as heat. The point of transition between laminar and turbulent flow depends on the tube diameter (d, in centimeters), the mean velocity, the specific gravity of the fluid, and the fluid viscosity. These factors can be expressed as a dimensionless quantity called the Reynolds number (Re), which is the ratio of inertial forces to viscous forces acting on the fluid:

$$Re = \frac{d\overline{V}\rho}{\eta} \qquad [14]$$

In flowing blood at Reynolds numbers greater than 2000, inertial forces may disrupt laminar flow and produce fully developed turbulence. With values less than 2000, localized flow disturbances are damped out by viscous forces. In the normal arterial circulation, Reynolds numbers are usually less than 2000, and true turbulence is unlikely to occur; however, Reynolds numbers greater than 2000 can be found in the ascending aorta, where small areas of turbulence develop.[3] Although turbulent flow is uncommon in normal arteries, the arterial flow pattern is often disturbed.[5] The condition of disturbed flow is an intermediate state between stable laminar flow and fully developed turbulence. It is a transient perturbation in the laminar streamlines that disappears as the flow proceeds downstream. Arterial flow may become disturbed at points of branching and curvature.

When turbulence is the result of a stenotic arterial lesion, it generally occurs immediately downstream from the stenosis and may be present only over the systolic portion of the cardiac cycle when the critical value of the Reynolds number is exceeded. Under conditions of turbulent flow, the velocity profile changes from the parabolic shape of laminar flow to a rectangular or blunt shape (see Fig. 13-7). Because of the

random velocity changes, energy losses are greater for a turbulent or disturbed flow state than for a laminar flow state. Consequently, the linear relationship between pressure and flow expressed by Poiseuille's law cannot be applied. This deviation from Poiseuille's law in arterial flow is shown in Figure 13-3.

Boundary Layer Separation

In fluid flowing through a tube, the portion of fluid adjacent to the tube wall is referred to as the boundary layer. This layer is subject to both frictional interactions with the tube wall and viscous forces generated by the more rapidly moving fluid toward the center of the tube. When the tube geometry changes suddenly, such as at points of curvature, branching, or alteration in lumen diameter, small pressure gradients are created that cause the boundary layer to stop or reverse direction. This results in a complex, localized flow pattern known as an area of flow separation or separation zone.[6]

Areas of boundary layer separation have been observed in models of arterial anastomoses and bifurcations.[7,8] In the carotid artery bifurcation shown in Figure 13-8, the central rapid flow stream of the common carotid artery is compressed along the inner wall of the carotid bulb, producing a region of high shear stress. An area of flow separation has formed along the outer wall of the carotid bulb that includes helical flow patterns and flow reversal. The region of the carotid bulb adjacent to the separation zone is subject to relatively low shear stresses. Distal to the bulb, in the internal carotid artery, flow reattachment occurs, and a more laminar flow pattern is present.

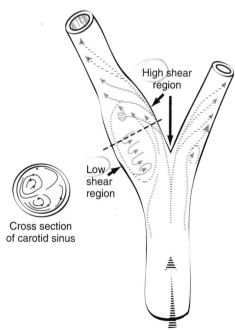

FIGURE 13–8 • Carotid artery bifurcation showing an area of flow separation adjacent to the outer wall of the bulb. Rapid flow is associated with high shear stress, whereas the slower flow of the separation zone produces a region of low shear. (From Zarins CK, Giddens DP, Glagov S: Atherosclerotic plaque distribution and flow velocity profiles in the carotid bifurcation. In Bergan JJ, Yao JST [eds]: Cerebrovascular Insufficiency. New York, Grune & Stratton, 1983.)

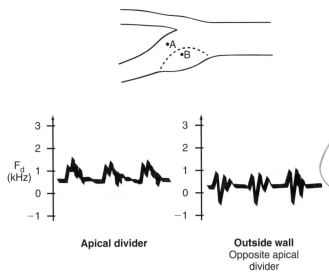

F_d (kHz)

Apical divider

Outside wall
Opposite apical divider

FIGURE 13–9 • Flow separation in the normal carotid bulb shown by pulsed Doppler spectral analysis. The flow pattern near the apical divider (A) is forward throughout the cardiac cycle, but near the outside wall (B) the spectrum contains both forward (positive) and reverse (negative) flow components. The latter pattern indicates an area of flow separation. F_d, Doppler shift frequency, in kHz. (Courtesy of J. F. Primozich, BS, and D. J. Phillips, PhD.)

The complex flow patterns described in models of the carotid bifurcation have also been documented in human subjects by pulsed Doppler studies.[9,10] As shown in Figure 13-9, the Doppler spectral waveform obtained near the inner wall of the carotid bulb is typical of the forward, quasi-steady flow pattern found in the internal carotid artery. However, sampling of flow along the outer wall of the bulb demonstrates lower velocities with periods of both forward and reverse flow. These spectral characteristics are consistent with the presence of flow separation and are considered to be a normal finding, particularly in young individuals.[10] Alterations in arterial distensibility with increasing age make flow separation less prominent in older individuals.[11]

The clinical importance of boundary layer separation is that these localized flow disturbances may contribute to the formation of atherosclerotic plaques.[12] Examination of human carotid bifurcations, both at autopsy and during surgery, indicates that intimal thickening and atherosclerosis tend to occur along the outer wall of the carotid bulb, whereas the inner wall is relatively spared.[8] These findings suggest that atherosclerotic lesions form near areas of flow separation and low shear stress. Whether flow separation represents a true causative factor or simply promotes the development of previously existing lesions is not known.

Pulsatile Flow

In a pulsatile system, pressure and flow vary continuously with time, and the velocity profile changes throughout the cardiac cycle. The hemodynamic principles already discussed are based on steady flow, and they are not adequate for a precise description of pulsatile flow in the arterial circulation; however, as previously stated, they can be used to determine the minimal energy losses occurring in a specific flow system.

The complex interactions of cardiac contraction, arterial wall characteristics, and blood flow are extremely difficult to

define rigorously. For example, estimation of the inertial energy losses in pulsatile flow requires a value for the velocity term (Equation 9); however, in pulsatile flow, velocity varies with both time and position across the flow profile. Further, skewing of the velocity profile may occur as a result of curvature or branching. The resistance term of Poiseuille's law (Equation 11) estimates viscous energy losses in steady flow, but it does not account for the inertial effects, arterial wall elasticity, and wave reflections that influence pulsatile flow. The term *vascular impedance* is used to describe the resistance or opposition offered by a peripheral vascular bed to pulsatile blood flow.[3]

Pulsatile flow appears to be important for optimal organ function. For example, when a kidney is perfused by steady flow instead of pulsatile flow, a reduction in urine volume and sodium excretion occurs.[13] The critical effect of pulsatile flow is probably exerted on the microcirculation. Although the exact mechanism is unknown, transcapillary exchange, arteriolar tone, and lymphatic flow are all influenced by the pulsatile nature of blood flow.

Bifurcations and Branches

The branches of the arterial system produce sudden changes in the flow pattern that are potential sources of energy loss. However, the effect of branching on the total pressure drop in normal arterial flow is relatively small. Arterial branches commonly take the form of bifurcations. Flow patterns in a bifurcation are determined mainly by the area ratio and the branch angle. The *area ratio* is defined as the combined area of the secondary branches divided by the area of the primary artery.

Bifurcation flow can be analyzed in terms of pressure gradient, velocity, and transmission of pulsatile energy. According to Poiseuille's law, an area ratio of 1.41 would allow the pressure gradient to remain constant along a bifurcation. If the combined area of the branches equals the area of the primary artery, the area ratio is 1.0, and there is no change in the velocity of flow.[14] For efficient transmission of pulsatile energy across a bifurcation, the vascular impedance of the primary artery should equal that of the branches, a situation that occurs with an area ratio of 1.15 for larger arteries and 1.35 for smaller arteries.[15] Human infants have a favorable area ratio of 1.11 at the aortic bifurcation, but there is a gradual decrease in the ratio with age. In the teenage years, the average area ratio is less than 1.0; in the 20s, it is less than 0.9; and by the 40s, it drops below 0.8.[16] This decline in the area ratio of the aortic bifurcation leads to an increase in both the velocity of flow in the secondary branches and the amount of reflected pulsatile energy. For example, with an area ratio of 0.8, approximately 22% of the incident pulsatile energy is reflected in the infrarenal aorta. This mechanism may play a role in the localization of atherosclerosis and aneurysms in this arterial segment.[17]

The curvature and angulation of an arterial bifurcation can also contribute to the development of flow disturbances. As blood flows around a curve, the high-velocity portion of the stream is subjected to the greatest centrifugal force; rapidly moving fluid in the center of the vessel tends to flow outward and be replaced by the slower fluid originally located near the arterial wall. This can result in complex helical flow patterns, such as those observed in the carotid bifurcation.[9]

As the angle between the secondary branches of a bifurcation is increased, the tendency to develop turbulent or disturbed flow also increases. The average angle between the human iliac arteries is 54 degrees; however, with diseased or tortuous iliac arteries, this angle can approach 180 degrees.[3] In the latter situation, flow disturbances are particularly likely to develop.

PHYSICAL PROPERTIES OF THE ARTERIAL WALL

Composition

Blood vessels are viscoelastic tubes. In this context, viscosity refers to the resistance of a material to shear, and elasticity describes the tendency of a material to return to its original shape after being subjected to a deforming force. As blood proceeds from the large arteries of the thorax and abdomen to the medium-size arteries of the extremities, the relative amount of elastic tissue in the vessel wall decreases as the amount of collagen and smooth muscle increases. At the level of the arteriole, the wall consists almost entirely of smooth muscle. Thus, the viscoelastic properties of an artery depend primarily on the elastin-collagen ratio. Elastin is the predominant component of the thoracic aorta that allows energy to be stored during cardiac systole and returned to the system in diastole. Because collagen is much less extensible than elastin, the more distal arteries, such as the brachial and femoral, do not store much of the pulsatile energy but serve mainly as conduits for blood. The function of the muscular arterioles is to control blood pressure and flow by actively altering the lumen diameter.

As the structure of the arterial wall changes, each successive branching also increases the total cross-sectional area of the arterial tree. The cross-sectional area at the arteriolar level is approximately 125 times that of the aorta; at the capillary level, it has increased approximately 800 times.[3] The reduced elastin-collagen ratio and increased stiffness of the peripheral arteries result in a more rapid pulse wave velocity and a high vascular impedance. Although the impedance of the thoracic aorta must be low to minimize cardiac work, the impedance of peripheral arteries should match the high arteriolar impedance to decrease the reflected components of the pulse wave.

Tangential Stress and Tension

The tangential stress (τ) within the wall of a fluid-filled cylindrical tube can be expressed as follows:

$$\tau = P\frac{r}{\delta} \qquad [15]$$

where P is the pressure exerted by the fluid (in dynes per square centimeter), r is the internal radius (in centimeters), and δ is the thickness of the tube wall (in centimeters). Stress (τ) has the dimensions of force per unit area of tube wall (dynes per square centimeter). Thus, tangential stress is directly proportional to pressure and radius but inversely proportional to wall thickness.

Equation 15 is similar to Laplace's law, which defines tangential tension (T) as the product of pressure and radius:

$$T = Pr \qquad [16]$$

Tension is given in units of force per tube length (dynes per centimeter). The terms *stress* and *tension* have different

dimensions and describe the forces acting on the tube wall in different ways. Laplace's law can be used to characterize thin-walled structures such as soap bubbles; however, it is not suitable for describing the stresses in arterial walls.

Arterial Wall Properties in Specific Conditions

AGING AND ATHEROSCLEROSIS. Arterial walls become less distensible with age. This increase in stiffness cannot be explained on the basis of atherosclerosis alone.[3] Alterations in the elastin fibers and elastic lamellae, together with an increase in wall thickness, probably account for this increase in arterial stiffness. Changes associated with aging include fragmentation of elastic lamellae and deposition of collagen between the elastin layers. This tends to maintain the elastin fibers in the extended state. Calcium is also deposited near the elastin fibers and contributes to the increased thickness of the arterial wall.

The effects of atherosclerosis on the mechanical properties of the arterial wall are complex and difficult to distinguish from those due to aging. In the early stages, arterial distensibility may actually increase as elastin fibers are disrupted; however, as the disease progresses, fibrosis and calcification tend to make the arterial wall less distensible.

ENDARTERECTOMY. During an endarterectomy the atherosclerotic plaque is removed, along with the intima and a portion of the media, leaving behind a tube consisting of the outer media and adventitia. This reduces the wall thickness to approximately one third of its original value and should result in an increase in tangential stress, according to Equation 15. As would be expected, endarterectomy decreases the stiffness of an artery to circumferential expansion.[18] Still, the endarterectomized artery remains stiffer and less distensible than a normal artery. This indicates that the components responsible for strength and stiffness are concentrated in the outer layers of the arterial wall. It is because of this anatomic arrangement that endarterectomy is possible.

ANEURYSMS. When the structural components of the arterial wall are weakened, aneurysms may form. Rupture occurs when the tangential stress within the arterial wall becomes greater than the tensile strength. Figure 13-10 shows a tube with an outside diameter of 2.0 cm and a wall thickness of 0.2 cm, dimensions similar to those of atherosclerotic aortas.[1] If the internal pressure is 150 mm Hg, the tangential wall stress is 8.0×10^5 dynes/cm^2. Expansion of the tube to form an aneurysm with a diameter of 6.0 cm results in a decrease in wall thickness to 0.06 cm. The increased radius and decreased wall thickness increase the wall stress to 98.0×10^5 dynes/cm^2, assuming that the pressure remains constant. In this example, the diameter has been enlarged by a factor of 3, and the wall stress has increased by a factor of 12.

Although the tensile strength of collagen is extremely high, it constitutes only about 15% of the aneurysm wall.[19] Further, the collagen fibers in an aneurysm are sparsely distributed and subject to fragmentation. The tendency of larger aneurysms to rupture is readily explained by the effect of increased radius on tangential stress (Equation 15) and the degenerative changes in the arterial wall. The relationship between tangential stress and blood pressure accounts for the contribution of hypertension to the risk of rupture.

The diverging and converging geometry of aneurysms can result in complex flow patterns that include areas of

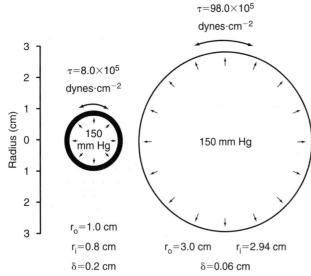

FIGURE 13–10 • End-on view of a cylinder, 2 cm in diameter, that is expanded to 6 cm in diameter while the wall area remains constant. δ, wall thickness, r_i, inside radius, r_o, outside radius; t, wall stress. (From Sumner DS: The hemodynamics and pathophysiology of arterial disease. In Rutherford RB [ed]: Vascular Surgery. Philadelphia, WB Saunders, 1977.)

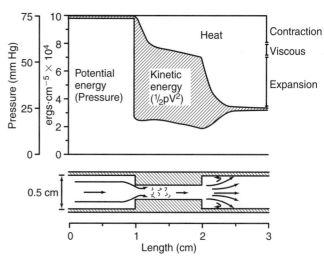

FIGURE 13–11 • Energy losses resulting when blood flows steadily through a 1-cm-long stenosis. Inertial losses (contraction and expansion) are more significant than viscous losses. (From Sumner DS: The hemodynamics and pathophysiology of arterial disease. In Rutherford RB [ed]: Vascular Surgery. Philadelphia, WB Saunders, 1977.)

boundary layer separation and flow reversal.[20] These patterns explain the frequent accumulation of clot in aneurysms, which confines the flow stream to an area not much larger than the native artery. Because this clot increases the effective thickness of the vessel wall, it may reduce tangential stress and provide some protection against rupture. However, the tensile strength of clot and arterial wall is not the same, and the contribution of clot to the integrity of an aneurysm is impossible to predict.[3] Further, the clot within an aneurysm is often not circumferential. In this situation, Equation 15 can be applied to the wall segment without clot, and the tangential stress at that site depends on the maximum internal radius.

Another factor to consider is that in about 55% of ruptured abdominal aortic aneurysms, the site of rupture is in the posterolateral aspect of the aneurysm wall.[21] The posterior wall of the aorta is relatively fixed against the spine, and repeated flexion of the wall in that area could result in structural fatigue. This would produce a localized area of weakness that might predispose to rupture.

Hemodynamics of Arterial Stenosis

ENERGY LOSSES

According to Poiseuille's law (Equation 8), the radius of a stenotic segment has a much greater effect on viscous energy losses than does its length. Inertial energy losses, which occur at the entrance (contraction effects) and exit (expansion effects) of a stenosis, are proportional to the square of blood velocity (Equation 9). Energy losses are also influenced by the geometry of a stenosis; a gradual tapering results in less energy loss than an irregular or abrupt change in lumen size. A converging vessel geometry tends to stabilize laminar flow and flatten the velocity profile, whereas a diverging vessel produces an elongated velocity profile and a less stable flow pattern. The energy lost at the exit of a stenosis may be

quite significant because of the sudden expansion of the flow stream and dissipation of kinetic energy in a zone of turbulence.

The energy lost in expansion (ΔP) can be expressed in terms of the flow velocity distal to the stenosis (v) and the radii of the stenotic lumen (r_s) and the normal distal lumen (r):

$$\Delta P = k \frac{\rho}{2} \vartheta^2 \left[\left(\frac{r}{r_s} \right)^2 - 1 \right]^2 \qquad [17]$$

Figure 13-11 illustrates the energy losses related to a 1-cm-long stenosis. The viscous losses are relatively small and occur within the stenotic segment. Inertial losses due to contraction and expansion are much greater. Because most of the energy loss in this example results from inertial effects, the length of the stenosis is relatively unimportant.[1]

BRUITS AND POSTSTENOTIC DILATATION

The presence of an audible sound or bruit over an artery is usually regarded as a clinical sign of arterial disease. Stenoses or irregularities of the vessel lumen produce turbulent flow patterns that set up vibrations in the arterial wall. These vibrations generate displacement waves that radiate through the surrounding tissues and can be detected as audible sounds. Such vibrations are probably the main source of sound in the arterial system.[3]

Generally, a soft, midsystolic bruit is associated with a relatively minor lesion that does not significantly reduce flow or pressure. A bruit with a loud diastolic component suggests a stenosis severe enough to reduce flow and produce a pressure drop. Thus, the intensity and duration of a bruit serve as a rough guide to the severity of an arterial stenosis. A bruit may be absent when an artery is nearly occluded or when the flow rate is extremely low.

A dilated area distal to a stenosis is a common clinical finding. Poststenotic dilatation has been observed in the thoracic aorta below coarctations, distal to arterial stenoses at the thoracic outlet, and distal to atherosclerotic lesions. The most likely explanation for this phenomenon is that arterial wall vibrations result in structural fatigue of elastin fibers. In a series of animal model studies, poststenotic dilatations did not develop unless a bruit was present distal to the stenosis.[22] It appears that vibrations in the audible range may weaken elastin fibers and break down links between collagen fibers. When this occurs, the arterial wall distal to the stenosis becomes more distensible and subject to localized dilatation.

CRITICAL ARTERIAL STENOSIS

The degree of arterial narrowing required to produce a significant reduction in blood pressure or flow is called a *critical stenosis*. Because the energy losses associated with a stenosis are inversely proportional to the fourth power of the radius at that site (Equations 8 and 17), there is an exponential relationship between energy loss (pressure drop) and reduction in lumen size. When this relationship is illustrated graphically, the curves have a single sharp bend (Fig. 13-12; also see Fig. 13-5). These observations provide theoretical support for the concept of critical stenosis.[23,24]

As previously noted, blood flow velocity is a major determinant of fluid energy losses (Equations 8, 9, and 17). Thus, the pressure drop across a stenosis varies with the flow rate. Because flow velocity depends on the distal hemodynamic resistance, the critical stenosis value also varies with the resistance of the runoff bed. In Figure 13-12, a system with a high flow velocity (low resistance) shows a reduction in pressure with less narrowing than a system with low flow velocity (high resistance). The higher flow velocities produce curves that are less sharply bent, making the point of critical stenosis less distinct.

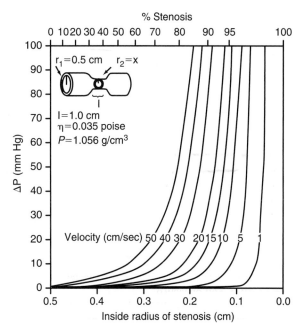

FIGURE 13–12 • Relationship of pressure drop across a stenosis to the radius of the stenotic segment and the flow velocity. (From Strandness DE, Sumner DS: Hemodynamics for Surgeons. New York, Grune & Stratton, 1975.)

Another observation related to critical stenosis is that the decrease in flow is linearly related to the increase in pressure gradient, as long as the peripheral resistance remains constant[24] (Fig. 13-13). In this situation, the curves for pressure drop and flow reduction are mirror images of each other,

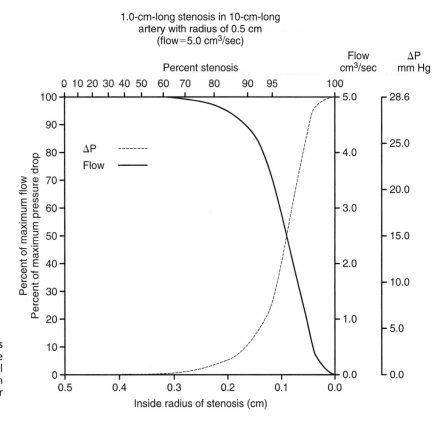

FIGURE 13–13 • Effect of increasing stenosis on blood flow and pressure drop across the stenotic segment. Collateral and peripheral resistances are considered to be fixed. (From Strandness DE, Sumner DS: Hemodynamics for Surgeons. New York, Grune & Stratton, 1975.)

and the critical stenosis value is the same for both. Many vascular beds are able to maintain a constant level of blood flow over a wide range of perfusion pressures by the mechanism of autoregulation. This is achieved by constriction of resistance vessels in response to an increase in blood pressure and dilatation of resistance vessels when blood pressure decreases. For example, autoregulation permits the brain to maintain normal flow rates down to perfusion pressures in the range of 50 to 60 mm Hg.[25]

Significant changes in pressure and flow begin to occur when the arterial lumen has been reduced by about 50% of its diameter or 75% of its cross-sectional area; however, the concept of critical stenosis is strictly valid only when the flow conditions are specified. Consequently, a stenosis that is not significant at resting flow rates may become critical when flow rates are increased by reactive hyperemia or exercise. For example, iliac stenoses that do not appear severe by arteriography may be associated with significant pressure gradients during exercise.[26] Because of the complex geometry of atherosclerotic lesions and the wide variation in arterial flow rates, it is often difficult to predict the hemodynamic significance of a lesion based on the apparent reduction in lumen size. Therefore, physiologic testing by blood pressure measurement must be used to document the clinical severity of arterial lesions.[27,28]

EFFECT OF STENOSIS LENGTH AND MULTIPLE STENOSES

Poiseuille's law predicts that the radius of a stenosis will have a much greater effect on viscous energy losses than will its length (Equation 8). If the length of a stenosis is doubled, the viscous energy losses are also doubled; however, reducing the radius by one half increases energy losses by a factor of 16. Further, inertial energy losses are independent of stenosis length and are especially prominent at the exit of a stenosis (see Fig. 13-11 and Equation 17). Because energy losses are primarily due to entrance and exit effects, separate short stenoses tend to be more significant than a single longer stenosis. It has been shown experimentally that when stenoses that are not significant individually are arranged in series, large reductions in pressure and flow can occur.[29] Thus, multiple subcritical stenoses may have the same effect as a single critical stenosis.

Based on the preceding discussion, several points can be made about stenoses in series. When two stenoses are of similar diameter, removal of one provides only a modest increase in blood flow. If the stenoses have different diameters, removal of the least severe has little effect, whereas removal of the most severe improves blood flow significantly.

These principles apply only to unbranched arterial segments such as the internal carotid. In the presence of a severe stenosis in the carotid siphon, removal of a less severe lesion at the carotid bifurcation is not likely to result in significant hemodynamic improvement. In contrast, when the proximal lesion involves an artery that supplies a collateral bed that parallels a distal lesion, removal of the proximal lesion can be beneficial. For example, when there is an iliac stenosis and superficial femoral occlusion, removal of the iliac lesion usually improves perfusion of the lower leg by increasing flow through the profunda-geniculate collateral system.

Arterial Flow Patterns in Human Limbs

COLLATERAL CIRCULATION

When arterial obstruction occurs, blood must pass through a network of collateral vessels to bypass the diseased segment. The functional capacity of the collateral circulation varies according to the level and extent of occlusive lesions. As mentioned in the preceding example, the profunda-geniculate system can compensate to a large degree for an isolated superficial femoral artery occlusion; however, the addition of an iliac lesion severely limits collateral flow.

A typical hemodynamic circuit includes the diseased major artery, a parallel system of collateral vessels, and the peripheral runoff bed (Fig. 13-14). The collateral system consists of stem arteries, which are large distributing branches; a midzone of smaller intramuscular channels; and reentry vessels that join the major artery distal to the point of obstruction.[30] These vessels are preexisting pathways that enlarge when flow through the parallel major artery is reduced. The main stimuli for collateral development are an abnormal pressure gradient across the collateral system and increased velocity of flow through the midzone vessels.[31] This mechanism is consistent with the gradual improvement in collateral circulation that results from a regular exercise program in patients with lower extremity arterial occlusive disease.[32]

Collateral vessels are smaller, longer, and more numerous than the major arteries they replace. Although considerable enlargement may occur in the midzone vessels, collateral

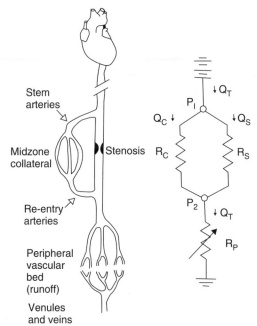

FIGURE 13–14 • Major components of a hemodynamic circuit containing a stenotic artery. The analogous electrical circuit is shown on the right, with the heart represented as a battery and the central veins as a ground. Flows are represented by Q_T (total), Q_C (collateral), and Q_S (stenosis). Resistances are represented by R_C (collateral), R_S (stenosis), and R_P (peripheral runoff); R_C and R_S are fixed, and R_P is variable. (From Sumner DS: The hemodynamics and pathophysiology of arterial disease. In Rutherford RB [ed]: Vascular Surgery. Philadelphia, WB Saunders, 1977.)

resistance is always greater than that of the original unobstructed artery. In addition, the acute changes in collateral resistance during exercise are minimal.[33] Therefore, the resistance of a collateral system is, for practical purposes, fixed.

DISTRIBUTION OF VASCULAR RESISTANCE AND BLOOD FLOW

Unlike collateral resistance, the resistance of a peripheral runoff bed is quite variable. The muscular arterioles are primarily responsible for regulating peripheral resistance and controlling the distribution of blood flow to various capillary beds. Arteriolar tone is mainly determined by the sympathetic nervous system, but it is also subject to the influence of locally produced metabolites.

When discussing blood flow in the lower limb, it is useful to separate vascular resistance into segmental and peripheral components. Segmental resistance consists of the relatively fixed parallel resistances of the major normal or diseased artery and the bypassing collateral vessels, such as the superficial femoral artery and the profunda-geniculate system. Peripheral resistance includes the highly variable resistances of the distal calf muscle arterioles and cutaneous circulation. The total vascular resistance of the limb can be estimated by adding the segmental and peripheral resistances (Equations 12 and 13).

Normally, the resting segmental resistance is very low and the peripheral resistance is relatively high; therefore, the pressure drop across the femoropopliteal segment is minimal. With exercise, the peripheral resistance falls, and flow through the segmental arteries increases by a factor of up to 10, with little or no pressure drop.

With moderate arterial disease, such as an isolated superficial femoral artery occlusion, the segmental resistance is increased as a result of collateral flow, and an abnormal pressure drop is present across the thigh. Because of a compensatory decrease in peripheral resistance, the total resistance of the limb and the resting blood flow often remain in the normal range.[34] During exercise, the segmental resistance remains high and fixed, whereas the peripheral resistance decreases further. However, the capacity of the peripheral circulation to compensate for a high segmental resistance is limited, and exercise flow is less than normal. In this situation, exercise is associated with a still larger pressure drop across the diseased arterial segment. The clinical result is calf muscle ischemia or claudication.

When arterial disease becomes severe, as in combined iliofemoral and tibioperoneal occlusive disease, the compensatory decrease in peripheral resistance may be unable to provide normal blood flow at rest. In this case, there is a marked pressure drop across the involved arterial segments and little or no increase in blood flow with exercise. Claudication is severe, and ischemic rest pain or ulceration may develop.

These changes in the distribution of vascular resistance in the lower limb explain the alterations in blood pressure and flow observed in patients with arterial occlusive disease.

ARTERIAL PULSES AND WAVEFORMS

The heart generates a complex pressure pulse that is modified by arterial wall properties and changes in vascular resistance as it progresses distally. Normally, the peak systolic pressure is amplified as it passes down the lower limb.[3] This is due to

a progressive decrease in arterial compliance and reflections originating from the relatively high peripheral resistance. Consequently, the systolic pressure at the ankle is higher than that in the upper arm, and the ankle-arm pressure ratio is greater than 1. However, the diastolic and mean pressures gradually decrease as the blood moves distally.

When blood flows through an arterial stenosis or a high-resistance collateral bed, the distal pulse pressure is reduced to a greater extent than the mean pressure.[35] This indicates that the systolic pressure beyond a lesion is a more sensitive indicator of hemodynamic significance than is the mean pressure. It is well known that palpable pedal pulses in patients with superficial femoral artery stenosis can disappear after leg exercise. This occurs when increased flow through high-resistance vessels causes a reduction in pulse pressure. The contour of the pressure pulse also reflects the presence of proximal arterial disease. These changes can be demonstrated plethysmographically and include a delayed upslope, rounded peak, and bowing of the downslope away from the baseline.[36]

Changes in the flow pulse are also useful to characterize the state of the arterial system. As the peak pressure increases, the peak of the flow pulse decreases as the periphery is approached.[3] The flow pattern in the major arteries of the leg is normally triphasic (Fig. 13-15). An initial large forward-velocity phase resulting from cardiac systole is followed by a brief phase of flow reversal in early diastole and a third smaller phase of forward flow in late diastole. This triphasic pattern is modified by a variety of factors, including proximal arterial disease and changes in peripheral resistance. For example, body heating, which causes vasodilatation and decreased resistance, abolishes the second phase of flow reversal; on exposure to cold, resistance increases and the reverse-flow phase becomes more prominent. Because a stenotic lesion is

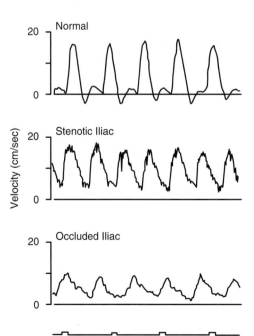

FIGURE 13–15 • Velocity flow waveforms obtained with a directional Doppler velocity detector from the femoral artery of a normal subject, a patient with external iliac stenosis, and a patient with common iliac occlusion. (From Strandness DE, Sumner DS: Hemodynamics for Surgeons. New York, Grune & Stratton, 1975.)

accompanied by a compensatory decrease in peripheral resistance, one of the earliest changes noted distal to a stenosis is the disappearance of the reverse-flow phase (see Fig. 13-15). As a stenosis becomes more severe, the distal flow pattern becomes monophasic, with a slow rise, a rounded peak, and a gradual decline toward the baseline in diastole. The character of the flow pulse proximal to an arterial obstruction is variable and depends on the capacity of the collateral circulation. These flow patterns can be studied noninvasively using a Doppler velocity detector and strip-chart recorder.

PRESSURE AND FLOW IN NORMAL LIMBS

As the pressure pulse moves distally, the systolic pressure rises, the diastolic pressure falls, and the pulse pressure becomes wider. The fall in mean arterial pressure between the heart and ankle is normally less than 10 mm Hg. In normal individuals at rest, the ratio of ankle systolic pressure to brachial systolic pressure (ankle-brachial index) has a mean value of 1.11 ± 0.10.[37] Moderate exercise in normal extremities produces little or no drop in ankle systolic pressure. Strenuous effort may be associated with a drop of several millimeters of mercury; however, pressures return rapidly to resting levels after cessation of exercise.

The average blood flow in the normal human leg is in the range of 300 to 500 mL/minute under resting conditions.[3] Blood flow to the muscles of the lower leg is approximately 2.0 mL/100 g per minute. With moderate exercise, total leg blood flow increases by a factor of 5 to 10, and muscle blood flow rises to around 30 mL/100 g per minute. During strenuous exercise, muscle blood flow may reach 70 mL/100 g per minute. After cessation of exercise, blood flow decreases rapidly and returns to resting values within 1 to 5 minutes.

PRESSURE AND FLOW IN LIMBS WITH ARTERIAL OBSTRUCTION

If an arterial lesion is hemodynamically significant at rest, there is a measurable reduction in distal blood pressure. Generally, limbs with a lesion at one anatomic level have an ankle-brachial index between 0.9 and 0.5, whereas limbs with occlusions at multiple anatomic levels have an index less than 0.5.[28] The ankle-brachial index also correlates with the clinical severity of disease: in limbs with intermittent claudication, the index has a mean value of 0.59 ± 0.15; in limbs with ischemic rest pain, 0.26 ± 0.13; and in limbs with impending gangrene, 0.05 ± 0.08.[37]

Because of the increased segmental vascular resistance in limbs with arterial occlusive disease, the ankle systolic blood pressure falls dramatically during leg exercise. As indicated in Figures 13-16 to 13-18, the extent and duration of the pressure drop are proportional to the severity of the arterial lesions. Recovery of pressure to resting levels may require up to 30 minutes.[28]

Resting leg or calf blood flow in patients with intermittent claudication is not significantly different from values obtained in normal individuals. However, the capacity to increase limb blood flow during exercise is quite limited, and pain occurs in the muscles that have been rendered ischemic. The pain of claudication is presumably due to the accumulation of metabolic products that are removed under normal flow conditions. As the occlusive process becomes more severe,

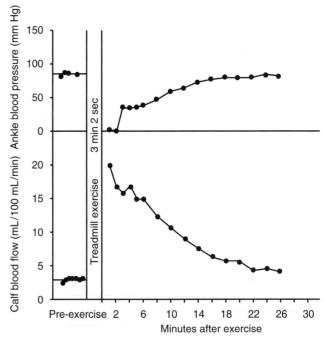

FIGURE 13–16 • Pre-exercise and postexercise ankle blood pressure and calf blood flow in a patient with severe stenosis of the superficial femoral artery. (From Sumner DS, Strandness DE: The relationship between calf blood flow and ankle blood pressure in patients with intermittent claudication. Surgery 65:763-771, 1969.)

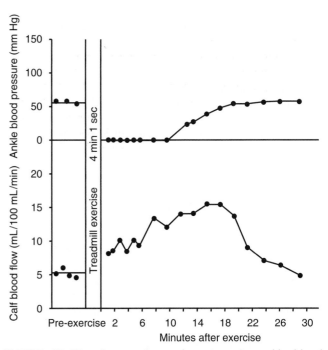

FIGURE 13–17 • Pre-exercise and postexercise ankle blood pressure and calf blood flow in a patient with iliac stenosis and superficial femoral artery occlusion. (From Sumner DS, Strandness DE: The relationship between calf blood flow and ankle blood pressure in patients with intermittent claudication. Surgery 65:763-771, 1969.)

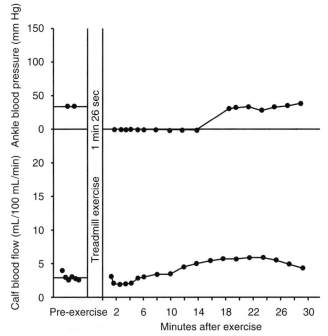

FIGURE 13–18 • Pre-exercise and postexercise ankle blood pressure and calf blood flow in a patient with occlusion of the iliac, common femoral, and superficial femoral arteries. This patient had moderate rest pain and severe claudication. (From Sumner DS, Strandness DE: The relationship between calf blood flow and ankle blood pressure in patients with intermittent claudication. Surgery 65:763-771, 1969.)

the decrease in peripheral vascular resistance can no longer compensate, and resting flow may be less than normal. When this occurs, ischemic rest pain or ulceration may appear. As shown in Figures 13-16 to 13-18, the capacity to increase calf blood flow with exercise depends on the severity of arterial disease. With increasing degrees of disease, the hyperemia that follows exercise becomes more prolonged, and the peak calf blood flow is both decreased and delayed. In some cases, flow may fall below resting levels.[28] The ankle blood pressure returns to normal after peak flows have started to decline.

The changes in blood pressure and flow in lower limbs with arterial occlusive disease provide the basis for noninvasive diagnostic tests. By monitoring the ankle systolic pressure before and after treadmill exercise or reactive hyperemia, two components of the physiologic response can be evaluated: (1) the magnitude of the immediate pressure drop, and (2) the time for recovery to resting pressure. The changes in both of these parameters are proportional to the severity of arterial disease.[38]

VASCULAR STEAL

Hemodynamic arrangements in which one vascular bed draws blood away or "steals" from another can occur in a variety of situations. A vascular steal may arise when two runoff beds with different resistances must be supplied by a limited source of inflow.

Multiple-Level Occlusive Disease

One example of the steal phenomenon involves a limb with lesions in both the iliac and superficial femoral arteries.[1]

Between the fixed resistances of these two arterial lesions is the profunda orifice, which supplies the variable resistance of the thigh. The resistance of the distal calf runoff bed is also variable. Under resting conditions, normal leg blood flow can be maintained by a nearly maximal decrease in calf resistance and a moderate decrease in thigh resistance. This is apparent clinically as an abnormally low ankle systolic pressure. With the increased metabolic demands of exercise, the thigh resistance can decrease further, but the calf resistance has already reached its lower limit. This results in a further pressure drop across the proximal iliac lesion, which reduces the pressure perfusing the calf. Blood flow to the calf is decreased until the thigh resistance rises and thigh blood flow begins to fall. In this situation, the effect of exercise is to increase thigh blood flow, decrease calf blood flow, and decrease distal blood pressure. The thigh steals blood from the calf because the proximal iliac lesion restricts inflow to both runoff beds.

Subclavian Steal Syndrome

In the subclavian steal syndrome, reversal of flow in the vertebral artery is associated with subclavian artery occlusion and symptoms of brainstem ischemia.[39] When occlusion is present in the proximal subclavian artery on the left or the innominate artery on the right, the pressure at the origin of the ipsilateral vertebral artery is reduced. This can result in reversal of flow in the vertebral artery, which then serves as a source of collateral circulation to the arm. The increased demands of arm exercise tend to augment the reversed flow, and the patient may experience ischemia of the brainstem. The hemodynamic effect is more severe with innominate artery occlusion than with isolated subclavian occlusion. With innominate occlusion, the origin of the right common carotid is also subject to reduced pressure, and the patterns of collateral circulation to the arm and brain become quite complicated. Blood passing down the vertebral artery on the side of the occlusion may be recovered, in part, by the right common carotid artery; however, during arm exercise, flow in the right common carotid may be reduced.

It is important to distinguish between symptomatic and asymptomatic subclavian steal. The presence of reversed vertebral artery flow, as demonstrated by arteriography, may be a normal variant without clinical significance.[40] In true subclavian steal syndrome, there is often a definite relationship between arm exercise and symptoms of brainstem ischemia. There will also be objective evidence of decreased blood flow to the involved arm, such as a diminished radial pulse and lowered brachial blood pressure relative to the contralateral arm.[41]

Extra-anatomic Bypass Grafts

When an extra-anatomic bypass is performed, a single donor artery must supply several vascular beds. In the case of a femorofemoral crossover graft, one iliac is the donor artery, the leg ipsilateral to the donor artery is the donor limb, and the contralateral leg is the recipient limb. Studies of crossover grafts in animal models have shown that the immediate effect of the graft is to double the flow in the donor artery.[42,43] When an arteriovenous fistula is created in the recipient limb, graft flows may increase by a factor of 10 without any evidence of a steal from the donor limb.

These experimental observations are consistent with hemodynamic data from patients with femorofemoral grafts.[44] Improvement in the ankle-brachial index on the recipient side can be achieved, even in the presence of significant occlusive disease in both the donor and recipient limbs. Although the ankle-brachial index may decrease slightly on the donor side, a symptomatic steal is extremely uncommon. The most important factor contributing to vascular steal with a femorofemoral graft is stenosis of the donor iliac artery. With iliac stenosis, a steal is most likely to occur during exercise, when flow rates are increased. A mildly stenotic iliac can be used as a donor artery when high flow rates are not needed, such as in the treatment of ischemic rest pain. However, when increased flow rates are required to improve the walking distance of a patient with claudication, stenosis of the donor iliac may result in a steal from the donor limb. Occlusive disease in the arteries of the donor limb distal to the origin of the graft does not result in a steal, provided that the donor iliac artery is normal.

These principles also apply to other types of extra-anatomic bypass grafts, including axillary-axillary, carotid-subclavian, and axillofemoral grafts.[42,45]

Hemodynamic Principles and the Treatment of Arterial Disease

It should be apparent from the preceding discussion that the high fixed segmental resistance of the diseased major arteries and collaterals is responsible for decreased peripheral blood flow. Therefore, to be most effective in improving peripheral blood flow and relieving ischemic symptoms, therapy must be directed toward lowering this abnormally high segmental resistance. Because the peripheral resistance has already been lowered to compensate for the increased segmental resistance, attempts to further reduce the peripheral resistance are seldom beneficial.[46]

Although exercise therapy has been shown to improve collateral function, the degree of clinical improvement is usually modest.[32] In general, exercise therapy is best suited for patients with mild, stable claudication who are not candidates for direct intervention. Another method for improving peripheral blood flow in limbs with arterial disease is medically induced hypertension.[46] The administration of mineralocorticoid and sodium chloride raises systemic blood pressure and increases the head of pressure perfusing the diseased arterial segment. Although this technique has not been widely applied, it has been used successfully in patients with severe distal ischemia and ulceration.

DIRECT ARTERIAL INTERVENTION

The most satisfactory approach to reducing the fixed segmental resistance is direct intervention by surgical or radiological techniques. Depending on the nature of the lesions, endarterectomy, embolectomy, replacement grafting, or bypass grafting may be indicated. Percutaneous transluminal angioplasty may also be appropriate in selected cases.[47] In patients with occlusive disease involving a single anatomic level, a successful procedure should return all hemodynamic parameters to normal or near normal. This should be evident as an increase in the ankle-brachial index and an improvement

in the ankle pressure response to leg exercise.[48] However, because it is seldom possible to perform a perfect arterial reconstruction, it is common to detect a minor degree of residual hemodynamic impairment. When occlusions involve multiple levels, the treatment of one level should result in significant improvement, and the persisting hemodynamic abnormality should then reflect the remaining untreated disease. In such cases, the improvement is usually sufficient to increase claudication distance or relieve ischemic rest pain. The relative severity of lesions at different levels is often difficult to determine clinically; however, the basic principle is to initially treat the most proximal level of hemodynamically significant occlusive disease.

The factors required for optimal function of arterial bypass grafts can be analyzed in terms of basic hemodynamic principles. As previously noted, vessel diameter is the main determinant of hemodynamic resistance, so the diameter of a graft is considerably more important than its length. All prosthetic grafts develop a pseudointimal layer of variable thickness that further reduces the effective diameter.[3] Therefore, whenever the situation permits, a graft with a relatively large diameter should be used. Graft diameter is often limited by arterial size. To minimize energy losses associated with entrance and exit effects, the diameter of a graft should approximate that of the adjacent artery. When arteries of unequal size must be joined, a gradual transition is preferable. Thus, the graft should be slightly smaller than the proximal artery and slightly larger than the distal artery.

Theoretically, end-to-end anastomoses are preferable to those done end to side, because the end-to-end configuration eliminates energy losses due to curvature and angulation. However, these losses appear to be minimal under physiologic conditions, and in most clinical situations the anastomotic angle is determined by technical factors. For example, reversed angulation has been used successfully in the construction of aortorenal and femorofemoral bypass grafts. Nevertheless, as a general rule, the smallest anastomotic angle that is technically feasible should be used. The width of an end-to-side anastomosis should be approximately equal to the diameter of the graft; the length of an anastomosis is less important but does serve as the main determinant of anastomotic angle. A carefully everted suture line also helps minimize energy losses at anastomoses.

Bifurcation grafts, such as those used for aortofemoral bypass, are subject to the same general hemodynamic considerations as arterial bifurcations and branches. Most commercially available grafts have secondary limbs with diameters that are one half that of the primary tube, resulting in an area ratio of 0.5. In this configuration, each of the secondary limbs has 16 times the resistance of the primary tube, and in parallel they offer 8 times the primary tube resistance. The flow velocity in the secondary limbs is doubled, and almost 50% of the incident pulsatile energy is reflected at the graft bifurcation.[3] As previously discussed, the area ratio determines the hemodynamic characteristics of a bifurcation with respect to pressure gradient, flow velocity, and transmission of pulsatile energy. However, the optimal area ratio for grafts has not been established, and the geometry of bifurcation grafts has received relatively little attention. Instead, the development of prosthetic grafts has emphasized features such as graft material, porosity, and surface characteristics. Despite their theoretical disadvantages, commercially available grafts have functioned extremely well in a variety of clinical applications.

VASODILATORS

The rationale for the use of vasodilators is that they lower peripheral vascular resistance and improve limb blood flow. Although this may occur in normal limbs, it is unlikely to be beneficial in limbs in which peripheral resistance is already decreased as a result of arterial disease. There is even a theoretical possibility that dilating vessels in relatively normal areas could divert blood away from the areas of ischemia. Most clinical studies of vasodilator therapy have failed to show a significant effect.[49,50] There is no conclusive evidence that vasodilators can increase flow in either collateral vessels or severely ischemic tissues. Consequently, there is no theoretical or clinical support for vasodilator therapy.

SYMPATHECTOMY

Because the purpose of sympathectomy is to reduce peripheral resistance by release of vasomotor tone, it is subject to the same general criticisms as vasodilator therapy. Because sympathectomy has little, if any, influence on collateral resistance, there is no rational basis for its use in the treatment of intermittent claudication.[51] Further, exercise-induced muscle ischemia alone is a potent stimulus for peripheral vasodilatation.

The use of sympathectomy for cutaneous ischemia has some physiologic basis, because the predominant effect is dilatation of cutaneous arterioles. However, clinical improvement can occur only if the ischemic tissues are capable of further vasodilatation, as demonstrated by reactive hyperemia testing.[36] Beneficial results have been obtained in patients with mild rest pain and superficial ischemic ulcers; patients with severe rest pain and extensive tissue loss are not likely to respond.[51] Although sympathectomy has been recommended as an adjunct to arterial operations, there is little objective evidence that it improves either the early or the late results of arterial reconstructive surgery.[52]

RHEOLOGIC AGENTS

According to Poiseuille's law, hemodynamic resistance is directly proportional to blood viscosity (Equations 8 and 11). If the pressure remains constant and viscosity is reduced, flow increases in proportion to the fall in viscosity. Procedures for lowering blood viscosity are most often used in the immediate postoperative period to increase flow through a reconstructed arterial segment.

Low-molecular-weight dextran (molecular weight 40,000) is the most commonly used agent for reducing blood viscosity. The increased peripheral blood flow observed after intravenous administration of low-molecular-weight dextran is the result of both peripheral vasodilatation secondary to blood volume expansion and changes in viscosity due to hemodilution.[3] Dextran solutions also influence red blood cell aggregation and platelet function.[53]

An orally administered rheologic agent, pentoxifylline, has been evaluated in a multicenter clinical trial for the treatment of patients with intermittent claudication.[54] Pentoxifylline reduces blood viscosity by improving the membrane flexibility of red blood cells. The drug also has an inhibitory effect on platelet aggregation. During the clinical trial, the distance walked before the onset of claudication increased in both the pentoxifylline and the placebo groups; however, the degree of improvement was significantly greater in those receiving pentoxifylline. It was concluded that pentoxifylline is a safe and effective drug for use in patients with intermittent claudication. Although this agent may provide a modest degree of functional improvement in some patients, its effect on the progression of arterial disease is unknown.

Hemodynamics of the Venous System

The structure of the vein wall is considerably different from that of the companion arteries. Some of these major differences are as follows: (1) the vein wall is much thinner, being anywhere from one third to one tenth as thick as that of the systemic arteries; (2) there is very little elastic tissue in the wall of the vein; (3) the venous media is almost exclusively a muscular layer; (4) venules have no media and no smooth muscle; and (5) a major part of the walls of the larger veins is composed of adventitia. An important characteristic of the veins is the presence of valves, which are essential for proper function. The distribution and number of valves correspond quite well to those regions in which the effects of gravity are greatest. They have a bicuspid structure with a fine connective tissue skeleton covered by endothelium on both surfaces. Their major function is to ensure antegrade flow and prevent reflux from the deep to the superficial veins.

From a clinical standpoint, the area of greatest interest is below the knee. This is the most common site for the development of venous thrombosis, and it is also the region of the leg where the complications of post-thrombotic syndrome are evident. The veins of the soleus muscle are often termed the "soleal sinuses" because of their capacious size and lack of venous valves. These sinuses are the most common site for the development of venous thrombosis.

The perforating veins that normally carry blood from the superficial to the deep veins are key elements in venous function. These short channels have the following features: they penetrate the deep fascia; they contain valves; they are found predominantly below the knee; the majority are small and inconstant in location; and they vary in number from 90 to 200.[55] Although not commonly thought of as such, the greater and lesser saphenous veins have all the characteristics of perforating veins. One relatively constant large perforator can be found on the medial aspect of the distal thigh, and this is one of the few that establishes a direct communication between the greater saphenous vein and the deep venous system. A common misconception is that the perforating veins along the medial aspect of the lower leg communicate directly with the greater saphenous vein. In fact, they communicate most commonly with its major tributary, the posterior arch vein. Normally, there are four relatively constant perforators that join the posterior arch vein, and when these are diseased, they contribute to the pathogenesis of post-thrombotic syndrome. The region in the vicinity of the lowest two perforating veins is often referred to as the gaiter area.[55]

As discussed later in this chapter, the function of the venous wall and its associated valves becomes evident when the effects of gravity and the calf muscle pump are considered.

NORMAL PRESSURE AND FLOW RELATIONSHIPS

A major factor in venous physiology that explains the capacitance function of these vessels is that they can undergo large changes in volume with very little change in transmural pressure. This is due not to the elastic properties of the walls but rather to the fact that they tend to collapse under the influence of a low transmural pressure. Veins are actually stiffer than arteries when compared at the same distending pressure. This results from the paucity of elastic tissue and the very prominent adventitia, which consists largely of collagen.

One of the remarkable features of the venous system is the wide range of flow rates that can be found—from high flows to nearly complete stasis. Flow rates depend on a host of complex interactive factors such as body position, level of activity, vascular fluid volume, and ambient temperature. Because it is virtually impossible to measure instantaneous venous flow in either the superficial or the deep veins, it is necessary to look at measurements of venous pressure and relate these to specific conditions or disease states.

Resting Venous Pressure

The pressures that exist in the absence of pulsatile flow are shown in Figure 13-19, which is the hydrostatic model of a 6-foot-tall "dead man." If the case of an open rigid tube is considered, pressure at the top would be zero (atmospheric). In the body, the arteries and veins can be represented as a series of parallel tubes, with the veins being collapsible and the arteries rigid. When the system is filled with fluid, but not enough to entirely distend the collapsible tube (venous), the pressure in the collapsed portion of the tube is atmospheric. Pressures in the rigid tube (arterial) must be equal to those in the collapsible tube up to the zero point. Above the zero pressure point, the pressures in the rigid tube are negative, because the collapsed tube representing the veins prevents free communication between the two segments.

When we examine the pressure relationships in a living man, supine and erect, some important facts can be noted[56] (Fig. 13-20). There is a point just below the diaphragm where the pressures in the arteries and veins remain constant regardless of position. This has been termed the *hydrostatic indifferent point* (HIP). This point changes only when the subject is placed head down, and then it is located at the level of the

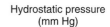

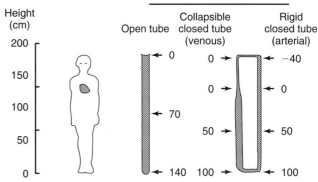

FIGURE 13–19 • Hydrostatic pressures measured in the upright "dead man." The pressures in the open tube are those expected in a rigid tube of equal height. The pressures in the closed tubes are those expected in a system of closed, connected parallel tubes. (From Strandness DE, Sumner DS: Hemodynamics for Surgeons. New York, Grune & Stratton, 1975.)

right atrium. The zero pressure level is in the region of the right atrium, usually at the level of the fourth intercostal space. The effect of gravity is the same throughout the vascular system in a supine subject. Raising an arm above the head in the erect position produces some dramatic changes. The arteriovenous pressure gradient in the foot remains the same (83 mm Hg), but in the hand it falls to a level of 31 mm Hg.[57]

Although there is no difference in the pressure gradient across the capillaries in the feet between the supine and the standing positions, some important changes do occur. On assuming the standing position, there is a translocation of blood into the veins of the legs, about 500 mL.[58] There is also a marked increase in the transmural venous pressure at the foot as a result of the effect of gravity. With this increase in pressure, fluid is forced out of the capillaries into the tissues. Although some of this fluid may be picked up by the lymphatics, other factors must come into play if edema is to be prevented. The single most important element in preventing the continued accumulation of interstitial fluid is the calf muscle pump. This can dramatically lower the pressure in the veins and capillaries, thus promoting the return of interstitial fluid to the circulation.

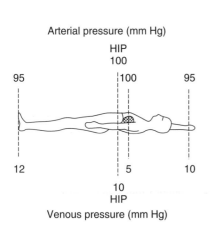

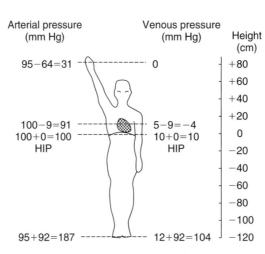

FIGURE 13–20 • Intravascular pressures present in the normal supine and erect human. The hydrostatic indifferent point (HIP) is located just below the diaphragm. (From Strandness DE, Sumner DS: Hemodynamics for Surgeons. New York, Grune & Stratton, 1975.)

Pressure Changes during Exercise

Features that distinguish normal subjects from patients with venous disease are best understood by examining the pressure changes that occur with leg exercise. Although patients with chronic arterial disease can usually be distinguished from normal subjects under resting conditions by measurement of distal arterial blood pressure, this is not the case with venous disease. For patients with venous problems, it is only when the muscle pump is activated that the abnormality is apparent. The calf muscle pump produces important changes in venous volume, flow rate, and flow direction. The muscle pump fulfills three useful functions: it lowers the venous pressure in the dependent limb; it reduces venous volume in the exercising limb; and it increases venous return.

With quiet standing, the venous pressure at the level of the foot remains constant, but this is dramatically altered with even a single step (Fig. 13-21). As noted in Figure 13-21, at the completion of a single step, the venous pressure is very low and requires several seconds to return to the prestep level.[59] When a normal subject walks, the venous pressure remains at a low and steady level throughout the period of exercise. Calf volume initially falls but gradually increases during exercise as the arterial inflow rises (Fig. 13-22). It is essential to understand that the observed pressure changes at the level of the foot are entirely dependent on intact and functioning venous valves in the distal limb. The calf muscle pump essentially empties the local venous system during contraction. With relaxation, the veins are nearly empty, and the venous pressure is very low. These changes are vital to maintaining normal venous return and protecting the limb. As shown later in the chapter, destruction of the valves dramatically alters these changes.

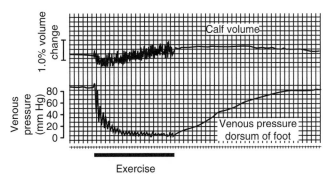

FIGURE 13–22 • Normal calf volume and venous pressure response to calf muscle exercise. Pressure changes were measured in a dorsal foot vein. Venous pressure falls rapidly, remains low throughout the period of exercise, and returns slowly to the baseline after calf muscle contraction ceases. (From Strandness DE, Sumner DS: Hemodynamics for Surgeons. New York, Grune & Stratton, 1975.)

Venous Flow Patterns

Flow on the venous side of the circulation is influenced by a variety of factors, including respiration, the filling pressure of the right heart, body position, the activity of the calf muscle pump, and the amount of arterial inflow. The patterns of blood flow in the femoral artery and vein are shown in Figure 13-23. Flow velocity in the normal femoral vein is lowest at peak inspiration, when the intra-abdominal pressure resulting from descent of the diaphragm is at its maximum. In theory, the changes in velocity of venous flow in the subclavian vein should be opposite to those in the femoral vein—that is, highest at peak inspiration, when intrathoracic pressure is at its minimum.

As noted earlier, the presence of competent valves prevents reflux of blood and an increase in venous pressure. This can be shown when the pressure is suddenly increased above a competent iliofemoral valve (Fig. 13-24). A cough and a Valsalva maneuver result in a sharp increase in pressure above the valve but not below it. There is no reflux of blood flow through the valve during either of these maneuvers.

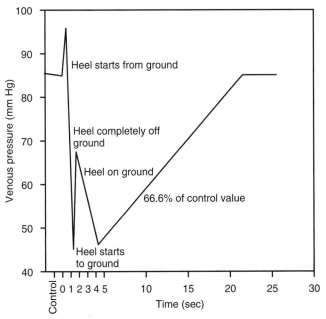

FIGURE 13–21 • Changes in the mean saphenous vein pressure measured at the level of the ankle that occur with a single step. (Redrawn from Pollack AA, Wood EH: Human venous pressure in the saphenous vein at the ankle in during exercise and changes in posture. J Appl Physiol 1:649-662, 1949.)

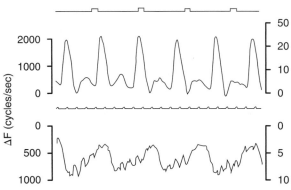

FIGURE 13–23 • Comparison of the flow velocity patterns in the common femoral artery (top) and vein (bottom) in the supine position with normal respiration. The venous velocity patterns are dominated by the pressure changes that occur with respiration. F, Doppler shift frequency, which is proportional to velocity. (From Strandness DE, Sumner DS: Hemodynamics for Surgeons. New York, Grune & Stratton, 1975.)

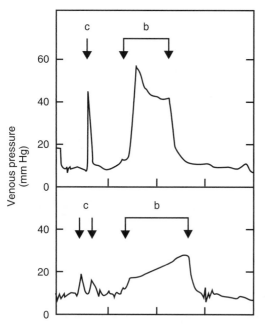

FIGURE 13–24 • Effect of a cough (c) and a Valsalva maneuver (b) on the venous pressure in a patient with a competent valve at the iliofemoral level. *Upper panel,* Pressure changes above the valve. *Lower panel,* Pressure changes below the valve. (From Ludbrook J, Beale G: Femoral venous valves in relation to varicose veins. Lancet 1:79-81, 1962.)

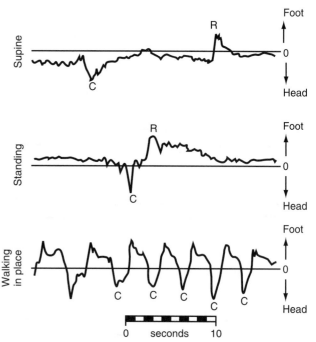

FIGURE 13–25 • Venous velocity changes recorded from an incompetent greater saphenous vein in a patient with primary varicose veins. The effects of muscular contraction (C) and relaxation (R) are indicated for the supine and standing positions. The bidirectional flow that occurs with walking is also shown. (From Strandness DE, Sumner DS: Hemodynamics for Surgeons. New York, Grune & Stratton, 1975.)

ABNORMAL PRESSURE AND FLOW RELATIONSHIPS

The most common manifestations of abnormal venous function are primary varicose veins and the post-thrombotic syndrome. Current evidence suggests that primary varicose veins are often familial. The initial abnormality in this condition appears to be incompetence of the terminal valves of the greater and lesser saphenous veins, which permits reflux of blood. With the passage of time, progressive incompetence of the other valves occurs. Dodd and Cockett also include patients with idiopathic perforator vein incompetence in the primary varicose vein group.[60] Although this may be valid, it is likely that many of these incompetent perforators occur secondary to episodes of calf vein thrombosis that result in destruction of the valves.

The flow abnormality produced by loss of valvular competence at any level of the venous system is easily demonstrated with a Doppler ultrasonic velocity detector. The flow patterns shown in Figure 13-25 are from the greater saphenous vein of a patient with primary varicose veins. In the supine position, flow with calf contraction is antegrade, with a slight and transient period of reflux during relaxation; however, with standing, the opposite is noted, with flow being toward the foot. Walking in place clearly illustrates the rapid changes in direction that occur with each step as a result of loss of valvular competence. When the pressure in the veins on the dorsum of the foot is measured during exercise in a patient with primary varicose veins, the deviations from normal are evident (Fig. 13-26). The pressure does not fall to normally low levels, and it returns to the pre-exercise level much faster when walking is stopped. If a tourniquet is placed around the upper calf, this

pattern is normalized as long as the valves in the deep system are competent.

With the development of acute deep vein thrombosis, two major factors determine the long-term outcome: the location and extent of the residual venous obstruction, and the condition of the valves below the knee in the area of the calf

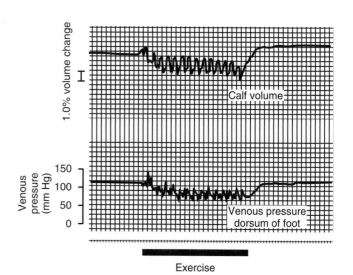

FIGURE 13–26 • Calf volume and venous pressure changes recorded from a dorsal foot vein of a patient with primary varicose veins. The pressure does not fall to the low levels seen in normal subjects, and it returns to the baseline much faster. (From Strandness DE, Sumner DS: Hemodynamics for Surgeons. New York, Grune & Stratton, 1975.)

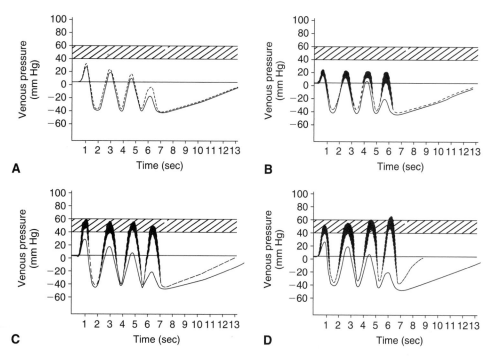

FIGURE 13–27 • Pressure changes in the greater saphenous vein at the ankle during four steps. In each panel, the normal response is noted by the solid line. *A,* Primary varicose veins and no leg ulcers. *B,* Varicose veins, incompetent ankle perforators, normal deep veins, no leg ulcers. *C,* Varicose veins, incompetent ankle perforators, normal deep veins, leg ulcers present. *D,* Varicose veins, incompetent ankle perforators, abnormal deep veins, leg ulcers present. (From Arnoldi CC, Linderholm H: On the pathogenesis of the venous leg ulcer. Acta Chir Scand 134:427-440, 1968.)

muscle pump.[61-64] Because these vary greatly from one patient to another, it is not surprising that the pressure responses also show a wide variation. Four examples of the types of patterns that can be observed are shown in Figure 13-27. It is clear that even with primary varicose veins, the pressure changes at the level of the foot are abnormal with exercise (see Figs. 13-26 and 13-27). However, patients with this very common condition generally complain of minimal edema and rarely develop ulceration. The factors that appear to be responsible for the development of post-thrombotic syndrome relate primarily to the status of the deep veins below the knee and the perforating veins. The most abnormal venous pressures and flows occur in the area where ulceration develops and are due to valvular incompetence in both the distal deep veins and their connections with the superficial venous system. With this combination, the very high pressures that can be generated by activation of the calf muscle pump result in ambulatory venous hypertension in the lower leg.

Browse and Burnand, in 1978, offered a reassessment of the factors responsible for the development of post-thrombotic syndrome.[65] They recognized that the clinical condition could occur only with damage to the deep venous system and postulated that the abnormally high venous pressures would lead to the development of multiple new capillaries in the dermis, with large pores in the venular side. As a result, there would be extravasation of large molecules such as fibrinogen and coagulation factors. These, in conjunction with tissue factors, would lead to the conversion of fibrinogen to fibrin. If this were combined with inadequate fibrinolysis, fibrin would accumulate in the tissues and produce a barrier to the diffusion of both oxygen and nutrients. The end result would be tissue anoxia and death of the skin in the affected region.

Hemodynamic Principles and the Treatment of Venous Disease

In contrast to the arterial side of the circulation, there are very few direct therapeutic approaches that can correct the underlying hemodynamic abnormalities of venous disease. Although obstruction of inflow to a limb is the most commonly treated arterial abnormality, mechanical interference with venous outflow is a rare cause of chronic venous insufficiency.

One exception to this observation is the patient with venous claudication. This entity is uncommon and may not be recognized. It occurs in the specific clinical setting of chronic iliofemoral venous occlusion. In most cases, the major deep veins distal to the groin are patent and competent. With vigorous exercise, the patient is unable to adequately decompress the deep venous system, and the thigh becomes tense and very painful. After the patient stops exercising, it often requires 15 to 30 minutes for the pain and tightness to disappear. It is important to recognize that this syndrome rarely occurs with ordinary exercise and thus tends to be seen in relatively young patients who indulge in vigorous activities such as jogging, skiing, or tennis. The underlying mechanism of venous claudication involves the collateral veins that bypass the obstructed segment and have a relatively high, fixed resistance.[66] This high outflow resistance results in a marked increase in venous volume during exercise. In some circumstances, it may be feasible to provide therapeutic relief with a crossover saphenous vein graft using the proximal saphenous vein from the opposite limb. This is rarely done, however, because the symptoms in most patients produce only minimal disability.

Other surgical procedures designed to treat chronic venous insufficiency do so by either removing the offending vein or interrupting it at some point in its course. This is done to eliminate sites of reflux and restore the pressure-flow relationship to normal. The value of this particular approach is limited because the most common site of the disease responsible for chronic venous insufficiency is the distal deep veins, an area that is not amenable to direct surgical intervention.

There has been a good deal of interest in promoting valvular competence in the proximal superficial femoral vein. This has been done by a direct surgical approach through a longitudinal venotomy or by transposition of a competent venous valve.[67,68] The validity of these techniques is questionable, however, because there is no evidence to support the concept of the so-called critical valve; the alterations of pressure and flow are nearly always secondary to deep venous abnormalities in the distal limb, and proof of the effectiveness of such an approach is currently lacking.

The most common form of therapy for chronic venous insufficiency is the use of support stockings that provide external compression and thus minimize the amount of edema that occurs during ambulation.[69] The exact mechanism of compression therapy remains poorly understood.[70] In theory, the stocking should reduce the transmural venous pressure gradient in a graduated fashion, with the highest compression pressures in the ankle area and diminishing pressures proximally up the limb. The amount of pressure exerted by a stocking depends on the elastic tension in the garment and the radius of the limb. Compression pressure should be in the range of 80 to 90 mm Hg while standing, 50 to 60 mm Hg while sitting, and 0 mm Hg in the recumbent position. This is obviously not possible with any single stocking, so a compromise must be accepted.

Elevation of the legs above the level of the heart is also a standard method for relieving the symptoms of chronic venous insufficiency. The physiologic basis for the use of elevation depends on three major effects: it reduces venous pressure by decreasing the hydrostatic component related to gravity; it promotes the reabsorption of edema fluid; and it prevents ambulatory venous hypertension. Periodic elevation and external compression therapy are essential for the treatment of chronic venous insufficiency. When strictly adhered to, a regimen of elevation and compression minimizes edema, improves skin nutrition, and avoids ulceration in the majority of patients.

Conclusion

The fundamental principles of hemodynamics often seem remote from the everyday clinical problems faced by vascular surgeons. The purpose of this chapter has been to show how these mathematical and physical concepts provide the basis for a rational approach to the pathophysiology, diagnosis, and treatment of vascular disease. These principles are also important for understanding the noninvasive diagnostic techniques that are discussed elsewhere in this book. The use of objective hemodynamic data is an essential step in the clinical evaluation of patients. This increased reliance on physiologic testing should encourage vascular surgeons to consider patients with vascular disease in terms of basic hemodynamic principles.

KEY REFERENCES

Berguer R, Hwang NHC: Critical arterial stenosis—a theoretical and experimental solution. Ann Surg 180:39-50, 1974.

Carter SA: Response of ankle systolic pressure to leg exercise in mild or questionable arterial disease. N Engl J Med 287:578-582, 1972.

Flanigan DP, Tullis JP, Streeter VL, et al: Multiple subcritical arterial stenosis: Effect on poststenotic pressure and flow. Ann Surg 186:663-668, 1977.

Johnson BF, Manzo RA, Bergelin RO, et al: Relationship between changes in the deep venous system and the development of the postthrombotic syndrome after an acute episode of lower limb deep vein thrombosis: A one-to six-year follow-up. J Vasc Surg 21:307-313, 1995.

Killewich LA, Martin R, Cramer M, et al: Pathophysiology of venous claudication. J Vasc Surg 1:507-511, 1984.

Ku DN, Giddens DP, Phillips DJ, et al: Hemodynamics of the normal human carotid bifurcation—in vitro and in vivo studies. Ultrasound Med Biol 1:13-26, 1985.

May AG, Van de Berg L, DeWeese JA, Rob CG: Critical arterial stenosis. Surgery 54:250-259, 1963.

Phillips DJ, Greene FM Jr, Langlois Y, et al: Flow velocity patterns in the carotid bifurcations of young, presumed normal subjects. Ultrasound Med Biol 1:39-49, 1983.

Sumner DS, Strandness DE Jr: The hemodynamics of the femorofemoral shunt. Surg Gynecol Obstet 134:629-636, 1972.

Sumner DS, Strandness DE Jr: The relationship between calf blood flow and ankle blood pressure in patients with intermittent claudication. Surgery 65:763-771, 1969.

REFERENCES

1. Sumner DS: The hemodynamics and pathophysiology of arterial disease. In Rutherford RB (ed): Vascular Surgery. Philadelphia, WB Saunders, 1977, pp 25-46.
2. Burton AC: Physiology and Biophysics of the Circulation, 2nd ed. St. Louis, Mosby-Year Book, 1972, pp 86-94.
3. Strandness DE Jr, Sumner DS: Hemodynamics for Surgeons. New York, Grune & Stratton, 1975.
4. Barnes RW: Hemodynamics for the vascular surgeon. Arch Surg 115:216-223, 1980.
5. Attinger EO: Flow patterns in vascular geometry. In Attinger EO (ed): Pulsatile Blood Flow. New York, McGraw-Hill, 1964, pp 179-200.
6. Gutstein WH, Schneck DJ, Marks JO: In vitro studies of local blood flow disturbance in a region of separation. J Atheroscler Res 8:381-388, 1968.
7. Logerfo FW, Soncrant T, Teel T, Dewey F: Boundary layer separation in models of side-to-end arterial anastomoses. Arch Surg 114:1364-1373, 1979.
8. Zarins CK, Giddens DP, Glagov S: Atherosclerotic plaque distribution and flow velocity profiles in the carotid bifurcation. In Bergan JJ, Yao JST (eds): Cerebrovascular Insufficiency. New York, Grune & Stratton, 1983, pp 19-30.
9. Ku DN, Giddens DP, Phillips DJ, et al: Hemodynamics of the normal human carotid bifurcation—in vitro and in vivo studies. Ultrasound Med Biol 1:13-26, 1985.
10. Phillips DJ, Greene FM Jr, Langlois Y, et al: Flow velocity patterns in the carotid bifurcations of young, presumed normal subjects. Ultrasound Med Biol 1:39-49, 1983.
11. Reneman RS, van Merode T, Hick P, et al: Flow velocity patterns in and distensibility of the carotid artery bulb in subjects of various ages. Circulation 71:500-509, 1985.
12. Fox JA, Hugh AE: Localization of atheroma: A theory based on boundary layer separation. Br Heart J 28:388-394, 1966.
13. Milnor WR: Pulsatile blood flow. N Engl J Med 287:27-34, 1972.
14. Malan E, Noseda G, Longo T: Approach to fluid dynamic problems in reconstructive vascular surgery. Surgery 66:994-1003, 1969.
15. McDonald DA: Blood Flow in Arteries, 2nd ed. London, Edward Arnold, 1974.
16. Goaling RG, Newman DL, Bowden NLR, et al: The area ratio of normal aortic junctions—aortic configuration and pulse wave reflection. Br J Radiol 44:850-853, 1971.
17. Lalleman RC, Gosling RG, Newman DL: Role of the bifurcation in atheromatosis of the abdominal aorta. Surg Gynecol Obstet 137:987-990, 1973.
18. Sumner DS, Hokanson DE, Strandness DE Jr: Arterial walls before and after endarterectomy, stress-strain characteristics and collagen-elastin content. Arch Surg 99:606-611, 1969.

19. Sumner DS, Hokanson DE, Strandness DE Jr: Stress-strain characteristics and collagen-elastin content of abdominal aortic aneurysms. Surg Gynecol Obstet 130:459-466, 1970.
20. Scherer PW: Flow in axisymmetrical glass model aneurysms. J Biomech 6:695-700, 1973.
21. Darling RC: Ruptured arteriosclerotic abdominal aortic aneurysms—a pathologic and clinical study. Am J Surg 119:397-401, 1970.
22. Roach MR: Changes in arterial distensibility as a cause of poststenotic dilatation. Am J Cardiol 12:802-815, 1963.
23. Berguer R, Hwang NHC: Critical arterial stenosis—a theoretical and experimental solution. Ann Surg 180:39-50, 1974.
24. May AG, Van de Berg L, DeWeese JA, Rob CG: Critical arterial stenosis. Surgery 54:250-259, 1963.
25. James IM, Millar RA, Purves MY: Observations on the intrinsic neural control of cerebral blood flow in the baboon. Circ Res 25:77-93, 1969.
26. Moore WS, Hall AD: Unrecognized aortoiliac stenosis—a physiologic approach to the diagnosis. Arch Surg 103:633-638, 1971.
27. Carter SA: Response of ankle systolic pressure to leg exercise in mild or questionable arterial disease. N Engl J Med 287:578-582, 1972.
28. Sumner DS, Strandness DE Jr: The relationship between calf blood flow and ankle blood pressure in patients with intermittent claudication. Surgery 65:763-771, 1969.
29. Flanigan DP, Tullis JP, Streeter VL, et al: Multiple subcritical arterial stenosis: Effect on poststenotic pressure and flow. Ann Surg 186:663-668, 1977.
30. Longland CJ: The collateral circulation of the limb. Ann R Coll Surg Engl 13:161-176, 1953.
31. John HT, Warren R: The stimulus to collateral circulation. Surgery 49:14-25, 1961.
32. Skinner JS, Strandness DE Jr: Exercise and intermittent claudication. II. Effect of physical training. Circulation 36:23-29, 1967.
33. Ludbrook J: Collateral artery resistance in the human lower limb. J Surg Res 6:423-434, 1966.
34. Sumner DS, Strandness DE Jr: The effect of exercise on resistance to blood flow in limbs with an occluded superficial femoral artery. Vasc Surg 4:229-237, 1970.
35. Keitzer WF, Fry WT, Kraft RO, et al: Hemodynamic mechanism for pulse changes seen in occlusive vascular disease. Surgery 57:163-174, 1965.
36. Strandness DE Jr, Bell JW: Peripheral vascular disease: Diagnosis and objective evaluation using a mercury strain gauge. Ann Surg 161(Suppl):1-35, 1965.
37. Yao JST: Hemodynamic studies in peripheral arterial disease. Br J Surg 57:761-766, 1970.
38. Zierler RE, Strandness DE Jr: Doppler techniques of lower extremity arterial diagnosis. In Zwiebel WJ (ed): Introduction to Vascular Ultrasonography, 2nd ed. New York, Grune & Stratton, 1986, pp 305-331.
39. Reivich MH, Holling HE, Roberts B, Toole JF: Reversal of blood flow through the vertebral artery and its effect on the cerebral circulation. N Engl J Med 265:878-885, 1961.
40. Gonzales L, Weintraub RA, Wiot JF, Lewis C: Retrograde vertebral artery blood flow: A normal phenomenon. Radiology 82:211-216, 1964.
41. Kelly WA, Strandness DE Jr: The subclavian steal syndrome. In Strandness DE Jr (ed): Collateral Circulation in Clinical Surgery. Philadelphia, WB Saunders, 1969, pp 570-582.
42. Ehrenfeld WK, Harris JD, Wylie EJ: Vascular "steal" phenomenon—an experimental study. Am J Surg 116:192-197, 1968.
43. Shin CS, Chaudhry AG: The hemodynamics of extraanatomic bypass grafts. Surg Gynecol Obstet 148:567-570, 1979.
44. Sumner DS, Strandness DE Jr: The hemodynamics of the femorofemoral shunt. Surg Gynecol Obstet 134:629-636, 1972.
45. Mozersky DJ, Sumner DS, Barnes RW, et al: The hemodynamics of the axillary-axillary bypass. Surg Gynecol Obstet 135:925-929, 1972.
46. Larsen DA, Lassen NA: Medical treatment of occlusive arterial disease of the legs—walking exercise and medically induced hypertension. Angiologica 6:288-301, 1969.
47. Freiman DB, Ring EJ, Oleaga JA: Transluminal angioplasty of the iliac, femoral, and popliteal arteries. Radiology 132:285-288, 1979.
48. Strandness DE Jr, Bell JW: Ankle pressure responses after reconstructive arterial surgery. Surgery 59:514-516, 1966.
49. Coffman JD, Mannick JA: Failure of vasodilator drugs in arteriosclerosis obliterans. Ann Intern Med 76:35-39, 1972.
50. Strandness DE Jr: Ineffectiveness of isoxsuprine on intermittent claudication. JAMA 213:86-88, 1970.
51. Strandness DE Jr: Role of sympathectomy in the treatment of arteriosclerosis obliterans and thromboangiitis obliterans. In Strandness DE Jr (ed): Collateral Circulation in Clinical Surgery. Philadelphia, WB Saunders, 1969, pp 450-459.
52. Barnes RW, Baker WH, Shanik G: Value of concomitant sympathectomy in aortoiliac reconstruction. Arch Surg 112:1325-1330, 1977.
53. Gruber UF: Dextran and the prevention of postoperative thromboembolic complications. Surg Clin North Am 55:679-696, 1975.
54. Porter JM, Cutler BS, Lee BY, et al: Pentoxifylline efficacy in the treatment of intermittent claudication: Multicenter controlled double-blind trial with objective assessment of chronic occlusive disease patients. Am Heart J 104:66-72, 1982.
55. Strandness DE Jr, Thiele BL: Anatomy of the venous system of the lower limb. In Selected Topics in Venous Disorders. New York, Futura, 1981, pp 1-26.
56. Gauer OH, Thron HL: Postural changes in the circulation. In Hamilton WF, Dow P (eds): Handbook of Physiology. Section 2: Circulation, vol 3. Washington, DC, American Physiological Society, 1965, pp 2409-2439.
57. Holling HE, Verel D: Circulation of the elevated forearm. Clin Sci 16:197-213, 1957.
58. Henry JP, Slaughter OL, Greiner T: A medical massage suit for continuous wear. Angiology 6:482-494, 1955.
59. Pollack AA, Wood EH: Venous pressure in the saphenous vein at the ankle in man during exercise and changes in posture. J Appl Physiol 1:649-662, 1949.
60. Dodd H, Cockett FB: The Pathology and Surgery of the Veins of the Lower Limbs. Edinburgh, Churchill Livingstone, 1976.
61. Strandness DE Jr, Langlois YE, Cramer M, et al: Long-term sequelae of acute venous thrombosis. JAMA 250:1289-1292, 1983.
62. van Bemmelen PS, Bedford G, Beach K, et al: Status of the valves in the superficial and deep venous system in chronic venous disease. Surgery 109:730-734, 1990.
63. Markel A, Manzo RA, Bergelin RO, et al: Valvular reflux after deep vein thrombosis: Incidence and time of occurrence. J Vasc Surg 15:377-384, 1992.
64. Johnson BF, Manzo RA, Bergelin RO, et al: Relationship between changes in the deep venous system and the development of the postthrombotic syndrome after an acute episode of lower limb deep vein thrombosis: A one- to six-year follow-up. J Vasc Surg 21:307-313, 1995.
65. Browse NL, Burnand KG: The postphlebitic syndrome—a new look. In Bergan JJ, Yao JST (eds): Venous Problems. St Louis, Mosby-Year Book, 1978, pp 395-404.
66. Killewich LA, Martin R, Cramer M, et al: Pathophysiology of venous claudication. J Vasc Surg 1:507-511, 1984.
67. Kistner RL: Transvenous repair of the incompetent femoral vein valve. In Bergan JJ, Yao JST (eds): Venous Problems. St Louis, Mosby-Year Book, 1975, pp 493-509.
68. Queral LA, Whitehouse WM, Flinn WR, et al: Surgical correction of chronic deep venous insufficiency by valvular transposition. Surgery 87:688-695, 1980.
69. Husni EA, Ximenes JOC, Goyette EM: Elastic support of the lower limbs in hospital patients—a critical study. JAMA 214:1456-1462, 1970.
70. Mayberry JC, Moneta GL, DeFrang RD, et al: The influence of elastic compression stockings on deep venous hemodynamics. J Vasc Surg 13:91-100, 1991.

Questions

1. **Viscous energy losses in flowing blood result from which of the following?**
   (a) Changes in the velocity and direction of flow
   (b) Friction between adjacent layers of moving blood
   (c) Turbulent flow in areas of stenosis
   (d) Disturbed flow at points of branching
   (e) Areas of boundary layer separation

2. **Poiseuille's law states that pressure gradients in an idealized flow model are inversely proportional to which of the following?**
   (a) Mean flow velocity
   (b) Tube or stenosis length
   (c) Blood viscosity
   (d) Tube or stenosis radius
   (e) Volume flow rate

3. Inertial energy losses in blood flow are related primarily to which of the following?
   (a) Changes in the velocity and direction of flow
   (b) Blood viscosity
   (c) Specific gravity of blood
   (d) Friction between adjacent layers of moving blood
   (e) Mean blood pressure

4. The critical stenosis value for a particular artery depends on which of the following?
   (a) Length of the arterial segment
   (b) Tangential wall stress
   (c) Blood viscosity
   (d) Compliance of the arterial wall
   (e) Flow rate and peripheral vascular resistance

5. Which of the following statements about the collateral circulation is false?
   (a) Collateral vessels are preexisting pathways that enlarge when the parallel major artery is occluded
   (b) The vascular resistance of the collateral bed is relatively fixed
   (c) Collateral artery resistance is usually less than that of the original unobstructed parallel artery
   (d) An abnormal pressure gradient across the collateral bed may stimulate the further development of collateral pathways
   (e) The midzone of the collateral bed consists of small, intramuscular vessels

6. Which of the following is not related to tangential stress and rupture of arterial aneurysms?
   (a) Volume flow rate through the aneurysm
   (b) Arterial blood pressure
   (c) Internal radius of the aneurysm
   (d) Tensile strength of collagen
   (e) Thickness of the aneurysm wall

7. With an extra-anatomic bypass, such as a femoro-femoral crossover graft, a vascular steal from the "donor" limb is most likely to occur in which of the following circumstances?
   (a) There is occlusive disease in both the donor and the recipient limbs
   (b) There is an occlusive lesion in the donor artery
   (c) Severe occlusive disease is present in the donor limb
   (d) The recipient limb has only mild occlusive disease
   (e) The donor limb is hemodynamically normal

8. Venous claudication is characterized by all of the following except
   (a) Chronic iliofemoral venous occlusion
   (b) Thigh pain with vigorous exercise
   (c) High-resistance venous collaterals
   (d) Minimal disability with ordinary activities
   (e) Valvular incompetence in the tibial veins

9. Which of the following is not a function of the calf muscle pump?
   (a) It lowers venous pressure in the dependent limb
   (b) It reduces venous volume in the exercising limb
   (c) It improves arterial blood flow to the exercising muscle
   (d) It increases venous return to the right heart
   (e) It minimizes the accumulation of interstitial fluid in the distal limb

10. All of the following contribute to the pathogenesis of the post-thrombotic syndrome except
   (a) Deep vein thrombosis with chronic obstruction of the deep veins
   (b) Extravasation of blood components into the subcutaneous tissues
   (c) Incompetence of the venous valves in the deep veins below the knee
   (d) The presence of primary varicose veins
   (e) Ambulatory venous hypertension

Answers

1. b	2. d	3. a	4. e	5. c
6. a	7. b	8. e	9. c	10. d

14

J. Dennis Baker

The Noninvasive Vascular Laboratory

In the early days of vascular surgery, patient assessment was based on a careful history and physical examination. Although a few clinicians used the Collins oscillometer to estimate the pulse pressure in an extremity, there was little help available in terms of quantitative assessment of arterial or venous disease. Angiography provided the only objective determination of pathologic changes. Early experience with arteriography and phlebography highlighted some of the limitations of these techniques, especially the problem of underestimating the severity of stenotic lesions on single-plane studies. In addition, the cost, patient discomfort, and risk of complications associated with contrast studies precluded their routine use for screening evaluations and follow-up.

The growing interest in more accurate differential diagnosis, localization of disease, determination of its severity, and documentation of progression stimulated the development of objective measurement techniques. In the 1960s, investigators started working with different plethysmographic techniques to quantitate arterial occlusive disease in the leg. Modification of ultrasound equipment to measure blood flow by the Doppler shift principle represented an important step forward in instrumentation and led to the rapid development of noninvasive studies. Additional techniques were designed to evaluate carotid artery disease as well as deep venous occlusion and insufficiency. This chapter describes the main diagnostic techniques used in the noninvasive laboratory and discusses their clinical application for patients with vascular disease. With an understanding of the merits and limitations of each method, clinicians can make the best use of these tests.

Instrumentation

DOPPLER VELOCITY MEASUREMENT TECHNIQUES

High-frequency sound waves (2 to 10 MHz) penetrate soft tissues and are reflected by the different interfaces encountered. Reflection from a moving interface results in the reflected frequency being increased if the motion is toward the point of observation and decreased if the motion is away

from it. The magnitude of the shift is determined by the following equation:

$$f_s = \frac{2Vf_0 \cos\phi}{C}$$

where f_s is the frequency shift, V the velocity, f_0 the transmitted frequency, ϕ the angle between the ultrasound beam and the velocity vector, and C the speed of sound in tissue (1540 m/sec). For a given velocity, a greater frequency shift is obtained with a higher transmitting frequency. In contrast, tissue penetration varies inversely with probe frequency, so the selection of a frequency for a given application is a balance between depth and velocity requirements.

Continuous-wave detectors are the simplest systems. The probe has two separate crystals, one transmitting and one receiving continuously. This system detects all velocities within the intersecting paths of the sound beams. If this zone includes more than one vessel (e.g., an artery and a vein), the resulting signal represents a combination of both velocities. Pulsed Doppler systems use a single crystal that repeatedly transmits a short burst of sound followed by a waiting period, during which the crystal functions in a receiving mode. By selecting the time and duration of the listening phase, one can define a sample volume, or the portion of the vessel from which velocity is to be measured. Modern duplex scanners use complex scan probes made up of many elements in an array, but the principle of selective sampling is the same.

The shifted frequency obtained from a vessel is within the audible range, so the data can be presented to the examiner as an audio signal. Although qualitative interpretation is helpful in some patient examinations, quantitative measurements provide more objective testing. Spectral analyzers are used to determine the main frequency components obtained from a given vessel. This information is usually displayed on a sonogram, which shows the frequency content in time (Fig. 14-1).

In some applications, it is more useful to have a measure of velocity rather than the raw frequency data. If the probe angle can be measured, the velocity is estimated using the Doppler equation. The accuracy of the estimate depends greatly on the accuracy of the angle measurement. Errors are greatest when the probe is at a right angle to flow and

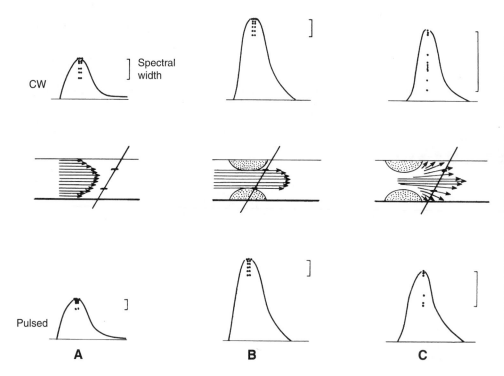

FIGURE 14–1 • Comparison of sonograms from continuous-wave (CW) and pulsed Doppler systems. Sonograms display the different frequency contents detected at each point in time. The CW system detects all velocities across the vessel, whereas the pulsed system detects only those velocity vectors within the sample volume, indicated by the marks on the ultrasound beam. *A*, Normal arterial signals. CW has more low-frequency content, because it detects flow near the walls as well as in the center stream. *B*, Within stenosis, there is increased peak frequency, and the frequency distributions of both types of Doppler systems are similar, because the sample volume encompasses the entire flow stream. *C*, Beyond stenosis, peak frequency is elevated, with increased frequency distribution resulting from turbulent flow. Spectral width is greater with CW systems.

least when it is at a low angle. Whenever possible, velocities should be measured with an angle less than 60 degrees.

DUPLEX SCAN

During the 1960s, B-mode ultrasound imaging was used for visualization of soft tissue structures. Although early devices had only crude resolution, equipment has improved to the point that clear, detailed images of vessels can be produced in real time (Fig. 14-2). In general, experience shows that when high-quality imaging is obtained, the diagnostic accuracy is very high; however, in patients with advanced atherosclerosis, it is difficult to obtain optimal studies, and diagnostic accuracy is lower. A common problem is incomplete imaging of the vessel wall as a result of calcification, which is present in varying degrees in up to half of patients studied. The extent of interference may be limited, but in some vessels there is no visualization of substantial portions of the artery. Although calcified plaques stand out sharply in the ultrasound image, some atheromas are visualized poorly or not at all. A major source of error is that recent thrombus may have the same echo density as flowing blood, so that an occluded vessel may look normal on the ultrasound image.

To overcome the limitations of ultrasound imaging, the research team at the University of Washington developed the duplex scanner, combining a real-time B-mode ultrasound image system with a pulsed Doppler detector.[1] The ultrasound image shows not only the vessel under study but also the location of the sample volume of the Doppler beam so that the examiner can position it to study velocity patterns at specific locations in the vessel. The device can study calcified vessels by analyzing the Doppler velocity signal distal to the areas of calcification. The evaluation of the Doppler signal from the common carotid artery and its branches is carried out using spectral analysis (Fig. 14-3). Based on the peak systolic velocity, end-diastolic velocity, velocity ratios, and

degree of spectral broadening, a category of stenosis is assigned to the vessel segment.

In the past 20 years, there has been extensive improvement of duplex scanners in terms of both image resolution and Doppler signal processing. The early devices were limited to the study of superficial vessels; however, the availability of low-frequency probes (2.0 to 3.5 MHz) permits the evaluation of abdominal vessels, including the aorta, vena cava, and main visceral branches. Study of intracranial artery branches is also possible.

The most recent development is the color-coded Doppler system. A linear array transducer composed of many separate elements is used to produce a grid of sample volumes encompassing the area covered by the B-mode image (Fig. 14-4). A portion of the grid is selected for color coding of velocity information. Each of the sample volumes within the area is examined. If the returning ultrasound signal has no change in phase or frequency, the amplitude information is used to create the gray-scale image at that point in the matrix. If there is a change in phase or frequency, the information is analyzed in terms of velocity. A color is assigned to represent the mean velocity occurring at that point in the field. Red and blue show flow toward and away from the transducer, respectively. The magnitude of the velocity is represented by the hue of the color: a dark shade indicates slow flow, and a lighter shade or white indicates high flow. The aggregate of the color representation from the sample volumes detecting motion produces a real-time representation of the flow patterns within the vessels superimposed on the gray-scale image of the stationary tissue. Figure 14-5 (see color plate) illustrates examples of the advantages of color duplex scans. A more recent development is color coding of the Doppler power (as opposed to velocity) detected. Power is proportional to the square of the velocity, so this measurement provides more sensitive detection of very slow flow or flow in small vessels. A good example of the benefit of power imaging is the detection of

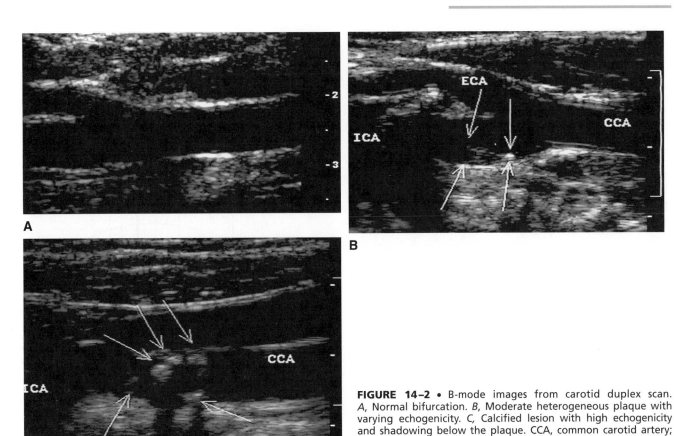

FIGURE 14–2 • B-mode images from carotid duplex scan. *A*, Normal bifurcation. *B*, Moderate heterogeneous plaque with varying echogenicity. *C*, Calcified lesion with high echogenicity and shadowing below the plaque. CCA, common carotid artery; ECA, external carotid artery; ICA, internal carotid artery.

an internal carotid string sign. Squaring the velocity eliminates the positive or negative value, so that power values have no directional representation. Power is represented in a single color, usually orange.

Carotid Artery Studies

The internal carotid artery (ICA) poses a unique challenge to physical examination, because it is impossible to palpate a distal pulse. It is not uncommon to find a patient whose carotid pulse in the neck is normal to palpation but who has occlusion of the internal carotid branch. This limitation stimulated the development of physiologic tests to assess the status of the ICA. Most of the early tests provided indirect measurement by detecting distal changes in blood flow characteristics produced by advanced stenosis. Common features of the indirect methods are that they detect only lesions that are sufficiently advanced to reduce mean blood flow, and they cannot separate a tight stenosis from an occlusion because the physiologic changes in the distal bed may be indistinguishable. These methods achieved a variable degree of clinical use in the 1970s and 1980s but were ultimately replaced by duplex scanning.

DUPLEX SCAN

The routine examination covers as much of the common carotid artery (CCA) and its branches as can be visualized with the configuration of the transducer used. In some patients,

the origins of the CCAs can be visualized. Figures 14-2A and 14-5A (see color plate) show normal carotid bifurcations. The color image demonstrates the reverse velocity detected in the carotid bulb as a result of the complex flow pattern at the bifurcation. Many older patients have tortuosity that precludes the CCA, the bulb, and the branches from being visualized in a single plane; in such cases, careful scanning is required to obtain satisfactory imaging. Figure 14-5B (see color plate) shows an example of tortuosity in an elderly patient. Although such arteries can be studied with a conventional scanner, the color-coded unit simplifies the examination. The scan usually identifies the pathologic regions, but with advanced atherosclerosis, it is often difficult to get an adequate image to accurately estimate the degree of stenosis. Much of the classification of stenosis is based on interpretation of the Doppler signal. The two branches are distinguished by the image and the velocity signals. The ICA has a low peripheral resistance at all times, resulting in forward flow throughout diastole, whereas the high resistance in the external carotid artery results in a diastolic flow of zero. Stenoses produce an increased velocity at the site of the lesion and turbulence beyond it (see Fig. 14-1). The turbulence is identified as spectral broadening on the sonogram (see Fig. 14-3). Mild stenoses may not produce a significant increase in peak systolic velocity but are identified by a moderate degree of spectral broadening.

Based on the peak systolic velocity and the degree of spectral broadening, the ICA is placed into one of six diagnostic categories. There are two sets of criteria that have been

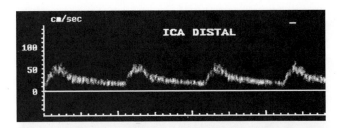

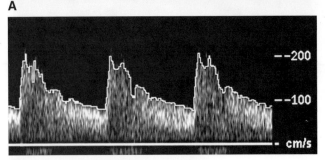

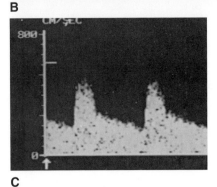

FIGURE 14–3 • Doppler sonograms from carotid duplex scans. *A*, Normal study with normal spectral width. *B*, Moderate stenosis with spectral broadening but no increase in peak frequency. (Note that frequency scales are different in the three records.) *C*, Severe stenosis with high peak velocity and extensive spectral broadening.

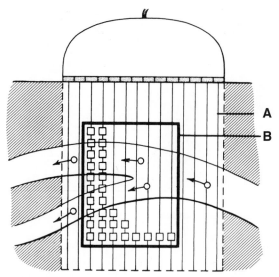

FIGURE 14–4 • Color-coded duplex system. A linear array transducer is used to create a matrix of sample volumes. A gray-scale image is created within area A. Most examinations are carried out with color coding of velocities limited to a portion of the image (area B). Within this portion of the matrix, ultrasound signals from sample volumes with a change in phase or frequency are interpreted as velocity data. Otherwise, the data are coded as part of the gray-scale image.

used for many years, and although some laboratories have made modifications or adjustments, the basic principles continue to be applied. The criteria developed at the University of Washington use primarily ICA velocity parameters (Table 14-1).[2] Further improvements in accuracy may be obtained using ratios of ICA velocities to CCA velocities in normal portions of the artery (Table 14-2).[3] The diagnosis of ICA occlusion must be based on image as well as Doppler information, because the very low flow found with some

"string signs" is below the velocity detection threshold of many scanners. Newer color duplex devices have improved our ability to find small residual flow channels, especially using power flow mapping. Both the stippled appearance of chronic thrombus and a small diameter of the ICA point to occlusion. Overall, low-grade stenoses are best assessed with the image, whereas advanced lesions are best evaluated with the Doppler information.

There has been a rapid growth in the use of duplex scanning for carotid diagnosis. Different investigators have demonstrated that the technique can be highly accurate. Studies have shown rates of 92% to 96% accuracy in the identification of severe stenosis.[4-6] When these studies are analyzed in terms of correct category of stenosis, exact agreement is found in 77% to 87%, with poor agreement in only 1% to 2%. Of particular importance is the fact that experienced laboratories make very few errors in separating severe stenosis from occlusion. Mansour and coauthors reported a 98% positive predictive value and 99% negative predictive value in the correct determination of ICA occlusion.[7]

TABLE 14–1	Categories of Internal Carotid Artery (ICA) Stenosis: University of Washington Criteria	
ICA Stenosis	**ICA Velocity**	**Spectrum**
Normal vessel	Peak systolic velocity < 125 cm/sec	No broadening
1-19%	Peak systolic velocity < 125 cm/sec	Limited broadening in late systole
20-59%	Peak systolic velocity < 125 cm/sec	Broadening throughout systole
60-79%	Peak systolic velocity < 125 cm/sec; end-diastolic velocity < 125 cm/sec	Broadening throughout systole
80-99%	End-diastolic velocity < 125 cm/sec (severe stenosis may have very low velocity)	Broadening throughout systole
Occlusion	No ICA Doppler signal; flow to zero in common carotid artery	

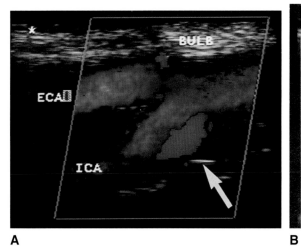

A

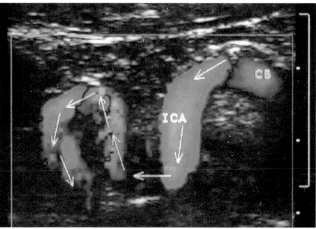

B

ECA▯

BULB

ICA

ICA

CB

IMAGING COMPATIBLE
WITH PLAQUE ULCERATION

ICA   CB   CCA

C

FIGURE 14–5 • Advantages of using color duplex scanning, *A,* Normal carotid bifurcation, illustrating the reverse flow occurring in the bulb during peak systole *(arrow). B,* Marked tortuosity of internal carotid artery (ICA) is easily demonstrated with color scan. *C,* Conventional gray-scale image does not provide clear identification of a large ulcer.

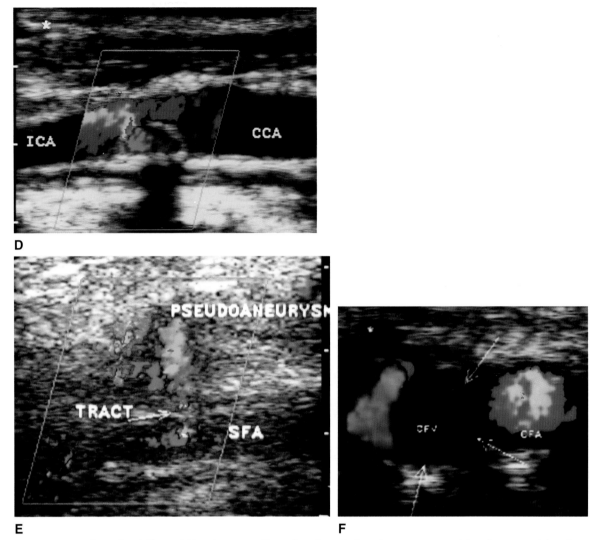

FIGURE 14–5 • Cont'd *D,* Blood flow within plaque confirms the ulcer. *E,* Pseudoaneurysm resulting from arterial catheterization. *F,* Blood flow around partial occluding venous thrombus. CCA, common carotid artery; CB, carotid bifurcation; CFA, common femoral artery; CFV, common femoral vein; ECA, external carotid artery.

TABLE 14–2	Categories of Internal Carotid Artery (ICA) Stenosis: Bluth Criteria		
ICA Stenosis	**Peak Systolic Velocity**	**Diastolic Velocity**	**ICA/CCA Velocity**
Normal vessel	<110 cm/sec	<40 cm/sec	<1.8
1-39%	<115 cm/sec	<40 cm/sec	<1.8
40-59%	<130 cm/sec	>40 cm/sec	<1.8
60-79%	>130 cm/sec	>40 cm/sec	>1.8
80-99%	>250 cm/sec (severe stenosis may have very low velocity)	>100 cm/sec	>3.7
Occlusion	No ICA Doppler signal	No ICA Doppler signal	No ICA Doppler signal

CCA, common carotid artery.

In addition to estimating the severity of a stenosis, scanners are now being used to study the plaque itself. Most investigators merely distinguish between homogeneous- and heterogeneous-appearing plaques and describe the surface as either smooth or irregular. More elaborate approaches to the description of morphology are being evaluated, but no single approach has been widely adopted.

Although the majority of attention has been focused on the carotid circulation, laboratories routinely investigate the status of the vertebral arteries as well. The examination seeks two types of problems: stenosis in the vertebral artery itself, and the abnormal flow produced by subclavian steal. In the majority of cases of significant vertebral stenosis, the lesion is located at the origin of the vessel. In some cases of severe occlusive disease, there is sufficient asymmetry in the waveforms of the two vertebral arteries to point to the problem side. However, a more complete assessment is obtained by examining the origins. Because of its deeper location, the left vertebral artery is more difficult to study than the right. Ackerstaff and associates found that the status of the ostium could be studied satisfactorily in about 80% of patients.[8] When adequate evaluation of the prevertebral portion was possible, a sensitivity of 80% and a specificity of 97% were achieved in the detection of reductions greater than 50% in diameter. Most clinical cases of subclavian steal are demonstrated by a reverse flow in the vertebral artery on the affected side. Von Reutern and Pourcelot demonstrated that in some cases of subclavian stenosis there is distortion of the waveform rather than complete reversal of flow.[9] The abnormal waveforms may have attenuation of the systolic component or an alternating pattern with reverse flow in systole and forward flow in diastole (Fig. 14-6). Such cases can be more fully assessed by recording the Doppler signal after arm exercise or the induction of reactive hyperemia. In the presence of advanced subclavian stenosis, this stress test produces full reversal of flow.

APPLICATIONS

Symptomatic Patients

A large number of transient ischemic attacks and strokes are caused by thromboembolization from arterial plaques in the carotid bifurcation. In most situations, a duplex scan is the initial workup, identifying the location and severity of lesions in the carotid system. Many centers use the ultrasound study as the definitive test on which to base the decision to operate. Having an experienced vascular laboratory with a validated

record of high accuracy in carotid scanning is the critical element in using duplex scanning as the definitive test. In other settings, additional confirmation is obtained with magnetic resonance or computed tomography angiography.

Asymptomatic Carotid Stenosis

Increasing numbers of asymptomatic patients are being referred to vascular laboratories for the evaluation of cervical bruits. Although some of these patients have bruits radiating from the heart or the great vessels, in a considerable number of them the sound originates from the carotid bifurcation. Duplex scanning can provide accurate separation according to category of stenosis (see Tables 14-1 and 14-2). Patients with severe stenosis are considered at increased risk of stroke and are evaluated for prophylactic carotid endarterectomy. Lesions that fall in the moderate category should have follow-up testing to detect those that progress into the high-risk group. Most people with normal vessels or early disease do not require routine follow-up.

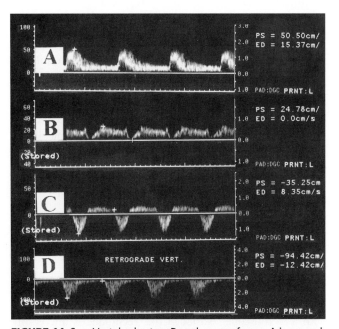

FIGURE 14–6 • Vertebral artery Doppler waveforms. A is normal. B to D are signals recorded on the side of severe subclavian stenosis. B shows attenuated systolic flow; C illustrates reversed flow in systole, with forward flow in diastole; and D shows complete flow reversal.

Another indication is the screening of patients with advanced atherosclerotic disease in the coronary or peripheral vessels. Owing to the diffuse nature of atherosclerosis, some of these patients have occult carotid bifurcation lesions, with a resulting increased risk of stroke. Screening is carried out most often in patients who are being considered for cardiac or major peripheral arterial operations to detect carotid lesions that may substantially increase the risk of perioperative stroke. Although screening may be appropriate for patients with multiple risk factors or severe occlusive disease in other arteries, routine testing of large populations results in a low yield of stenoses in the 80% to 99% category and is not cost-effective, especially if duplex scanning is used.

Intraoperative Assessment

Over the years, there has been increasing use of completion studies to evaluate the status of the operated artery before closing. Contrast angiography is the most common technique used, usually with a single injection into the CCA below the level of the endarterectomy. Another approach is to examine the repair using a simple continuous-wave Doppler unit with subjective evaluation of the signals. This method detects severe residual stenoses but is not sensitive to less severe problems. Increasingly, completion duplex scanning is now being used to detect residual defects requiring correction, and studies have shown satisfactory results.[10-12] Bandyk and colleagues used a peak systolic velocity greater than 180 cm/second or a velocity ratio greater than 2.4 as the criterion to carry out a confirmatory angiogram or to proceed directly to repair.[13]

Postoperative Follow-up

Recurrent stenosis after carotid endarterectomy remains a clinical problem. Early studies reported as much as 5% symptomatic restenosis and 8% asymptomatic restenosis (as identified by noninvasive testing).[14,15] More recent studies applying life-table analysis have found restenosis rates of 20% to 32% with greater than 50% diameter reduction.[16,17] It has been shown that a substantial proportion of restenoses occurs early in the postoperative period. A common practice is to obtain an early postoperative study that can be used as a baseline. Follow-up evaluations are done 6 and 12 months after surgery. If the study remains normal, noninvasive studies are repeated yearly. More recent studies show that in the presence of a normal completion angiogram or duplex scan, follow-up need not be performed until 1 year after operation.[18,19]

Lower Extremity Arterial Studies

SEGMENTAL EXTREMITY PRESSURE MEASUREMENT

Indirect measurement of extremity pressures has been performed since the beginning of the 20th century using a sphygmomanometer and auscultation of the Korotkoff sounds with a stethoscope. Although this technique is universally used to measure pressures in the brachial artery, its application in the lower extremity is less practical because of the difficulty of listening for Korotkoff sounds in the popliteal space. The technique is certainly not applicable in the distal portions of the extremity because of the small size of the vessels involved. Investigators have overcome this limitation by using a variety of plethysmographic devices. In 1959, Winsor first described the clinical measurement of arterial gradients using a plethysmograph.[20] Systolic pressures in the lower extremity were normally higher than those in the upper extremity. He described the blood pressure index (blood pressure of arm/blood pressure of leg), which in normal persons is less than 1.0. A value greater than 1.0 indicates clinically significant occlusive disease proximal to the point of measurement. (Note that the ratio described is the inverse of the currently used ankle-brachial index.) Likewise, a gradient between two sampling sites localizes the occlusive disease in the intervening segment. The main limitation of this method is that it detects only occlusive lesions that are sufficiently advanced to reduce the systolic pressure, so that it is not possible to detect early disease. Introduction of the Doppler velocity detector greatly simplified the indirect measurement of extremity pressures. For this application, the Doppler device is used merely to detect the presence or absence of the movement of blood in the artery. Measurements made by this method are reproducible but do not provide diastolic pressure. Plethysmographic techniques are cumbersome and are not used routinely.

In clinical practice, simple screening can be carried out by measuring the pressure at the brachial arteries and at the dorsal pedal and posterior tibial arteries on each side. The ankle-brachial index (ABI) is determined by dividing the ankle pressure on each side by the higher of the two brachial pressures. The resulting value reflects the severity of the occlusive disease for the entire extremity. Normally, the ABI should be greater than 1.0, and values less than 0.95 are abnormal. Figure 14-7 summarizes the general relation between ABI values and clinical status. It must be emphasized that this is only a rough correlation and that patients with similar values may have substantial differences in exercise tolerance. Likewise, the index at which rest pain appears varies considerably from patient to patient, ranging from 0.30 to 0.50.

An important limitation of the indirect measurement of extremity pressure is seen in patients with abnormal stiffening of the vessel wall, most often due to heavy calcification. Such conditions occur with diabetes mellitus but can also be found with other disorders. In these cases, the systolic pressure measured reflects the cuff pressure required to collapse the vessel wall in addition to the pressure required to overcome the intraluminal pressure. In a few patients, it is not possible to stop the flow of blood at all. Error due to wall stiffness should be suspected whenever the ABI is greater than 1.3 or its value is out of proportion to the patient's clinical status. In general, a leg with a normal ABI should have an easily palpable ankle pulse. In some patients with stiff arteries, it may be possible to obtain an accurate evaluation by measuring the toe pressure. In the normal person, there is a gradient of 20 to 30 mm Hg between the ankle and the toe, so a correction must be made when toe pressures are being used.

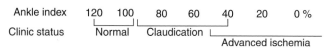

FIGURE 14-7 • Relation of ankle-brachial index to patient symptoms.

Additional information on the localization of occlusive disease can be obtained by measuring the pressures at different levels of the leg. Segmental pressure measurements are usually performed by applying cuffs at the thigh, the upper calf, and immediately above the ankle. A standard adult-sized cuff (12 cm wide) is satisfactory for calf and ankle determinations, but a thigh cuff (18 cm) should be used above the knee. (Using a narrower cuff above the knee results in artificially high pressure measurements as a result of the size discrepancy between the cuff and the diameter of the thigh. Thigh measurements with an arm cuff usually result in determinations that are 20 to 30 mm Hg higher than those obtained with the wider cuff.) A thigh pressure lower than the brachial pressure indicates obstruction proximal to the location of the thigh cuff. Gradients of more than 20 mm Hg between measuring sites are diagnostic of occlusive disease in the intervening segment, and higher gradients are usually associated with more severe lesions.

An important limitation of the use of the wide cuff for thigh measurement is that it is possible to make only a single thigh measurement. As a result, it is not possible to distinguish occlusive disease above the ligament from that in the proximal portion of the superficial femoral artery, because both conditions may result in the same thigh pressure measurement. To overcome this problem, some investigators have recommended using 12-cm-wide cuffs to obtain two separate thigh measurements. When this is done, it is necessary to take into account the 20- to 30-mm Hg artifact that results. In a study comparing the wide-cuff with the two narrow-cuff techniques in the same group of patients, Heintz and coworkers reported an increased accuracy in the localization of disease using the two-cuff technique.[21] Both methods of thigh pressure measurement are still being used, so it is important to know which method is being reported when reviewing the results of patient studies. Although segmental pressures have been used extensively to detect proximal disease, diagnostic errors may occur in 25% of patients. Other techniques should be used when an accurate assessment of the segmental localization is needed.

STRESS TESTING

Most patients with advanced arterial insufficiency are adequately evaluated by measurements at rest; however, less severe lesions may not produce a sufficient disturbance at resting flow rates to be detected by the usual methods. An example of this problem is a patient with typical symptoms of claudication who has normal or borderline leg pressures. A more complete evaluation can be obtained by increasing the flow to accentuate the hemodynamic effect of the stenosis. The simplest and most normal way to increase blood flow is to have the patient walk. Exercise produces a decrease in vascular resistance in the leg, with a resulting increase in flow to the leg. With moderate levels of exercise, there is no change in distal pressures in a normal extremity, but increasing the flow through a moderate stenosis causes an increased resistance at the lesion. The resulting energy loss can be detected by noninvasive tests such as a pressure gradient or the attenuation of the pulse waveform.

The stress test is performed by having the patient walk on a treadmill for 5 minutes or until symptoms force the patient to stop. Most protocols use a low level of exercise

(2 miles/hour with a 10% to 12% grade). This level of stress is sufficient to yield an abnormal result in most claudication patients, without undue cardiac stress. Baseline arm and ankle pressures are measured with the Doppler detector. As soon as walking is completed, the patient lies down on the examining table for repeat pressure measurements, made at 30-second intervals during the first 2 minutes and at 60-second intervals for the remainder of the examination, usually 5 to 10 minutes. The examiner always asks the patient why he or she stopped walking, because in some cases, the limiting factor is angina or shortness of breath rather than claudication. Identification of these limitations is an important benefit of the stress test, because it may uncover or emphasize the significance of these other conditions.

One objective measurement of the severity of occlusive disease is exercise tolerance (i.e., the time the patient walks at the standardized rate). Further assessment is based on the changes in extremity pressures. Figure 14-8 shows the time-pressure relations seen in control subjects and in different categories of occlusive disease. Normal people have no significant change in ankle pressures with the modest level of exercise used for the stress test. In contrast, patients with flow-limiting stenoses have a drop in distal pressures as a result of vasodilatation in the muscles. The amounts of the drop in both ABI and recovery time are increased with more severe occlusive disease. Multiple lesions produce more marked depression of the recovery curve than do single lesions.

There are some situations in which treadmill exercise is not practical or does not offer the best evaluation. In such cases, reactive hyperemia can be used to increase blood flow in the extremities. A thigh cuff inflated above systolic pressure produces local circulatory arrest, resulting in hypoxia and local vasodilatation. When the cuff is released, there is a transient increase in flow, the duration of which is related to the period of ischemia and to the total blood flow to the leg. The magnitude of the pressure drop is comparable to that seen after walking, but the recovery is always more rapid with reactive hyperemia. In contrast to exercise, reactive hyperemia does produce a transient pressure drop (with a rapid

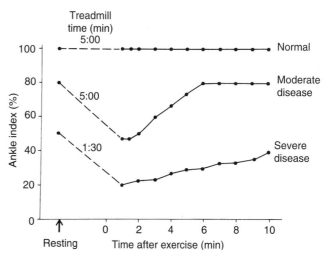

FIGURE 14-8 • Changes in ankle-brachial index with exercise. The severity of the arterial stenosis is related to the exercise tolerance and the magnitude of the drop in ankle pressure and recovery time.

recovery) in normal subjects. Criteria for a normal result are (1) lowest ABI greater than 0.80 and (2) return of the index to 90% of the baseline value within 1 minute.[22] The technique provides a useful test method for patients who cannot walk on the treadmill because of disabilities or those who are unwilling to perform adequately on the treadmill, and for the full evaluation of the less-involved limb in patients with marked asymmetry of their occlusive disease.

In general, stress testing is not routinely needed in a large proportion of patients seen in the vascular laboratory. Patients with significant abnormalities at rest always have abnormal responses to exercise. This additional evaluation can be reserved for patients with typical symptoms of arterial insufficiency but normal or near-normal resting studies and those with confusing symptoms in whom one wants to exclude arterial insufficiency as a cause. The stress examination is also useful for research studies in which more sensitivity for the detection of improvement or deterioration is needed.

DOPPLER WAVEFORM EVALUATION

Most commercial Doppler detectors provide an analog signal that is proportional to the velocity of the blood in the vessel studied. This signal can be displayed on a screen or recorded. The overall shape of the waveform reflects the status of the vessel proximal to the point studied (Fig. 14-9). In the lower extremity, the normal velocity wave is triphasic, with reverse flow in early diastole. Proximal stenosis first eliminates the reverse flow; with more severe lesions, there is blunting of the systolic upstroke and increasing flow during diastole. The simplest analysis of Doppler waveforms is a qualitative interpretation of the curves, allowing the identification of broad categories of disease. One specific application has been the assessment of the aortoiliac segment. However, the method suffers from a high false-positive rate resulting from the fact that an attenuated wave can be caused by proximal disease, distal disease, or a combination of the two.

A variety of techniques for quantitative analysis of the Doppler waveform have been described over the years. These include the pulsatility index, Gosling damping factor, LaPlace transform analysis, and principal component analysis. These investigations have largely focused on separating significant inflow occlusive disease from that below the inguinal ligament. Although each of these methods offers some additional diagnostic benefit, none has achieved wide application. Burnham and colleagues proposed the measurement of common femoral artery acceleration time (onset of systole to peak systole) to identify significant aortoiliac disease. An acceleration time greater than 133 msec is found with proximal stenosis.[23]

SEGMENTAL PLETHYSMOGRAPHY

During systole, the blood entering a limb normally causes an increase in the total volume of the extremity, with a return to resting volume during diastole. This phenomenon is responsible for the pulse pressure oscillations seen with the sphygmomanometer while taking blood pressure. The total volume change is small and can be detected only with the aid of sensitive devices. A variety of plethysmographic recorders have been devised using a mercury strain gauge, water displacement, capacitance, and impedance systems, but the majority of these systems have proved to be impractical for routine clinical application. In the early 1970s, the pulse-volume recorder was designed specifically for peripheral arterial diagnosis. The system uses a calibrated recording air plethysmograph with standard blood pressure cuffs applied at the thigh, calf, and ankle levels. The cuffs are inflated to 65 mm Hg to ensure optimal contact of the cuff around the extremity. A sensitive transducer detects the small increase in pressure within the cuff resulting from the volume increase of the extremity during systole. The recorder provides a hard-copy tracing of the pulse wave, which has been demonstrated to be quite similar to arterial pressure waves measured directly.

The primary diagnosis is based on a qualitative evaluation of the pulse-volume waveform.[24] The tracing from each level is categorized as normal, mildly abnormal, moderately abnormal, or severely abnormal. The normal tracing has a brisk, sharp rise to the systolic peak and usually displays a prominent dicrotic notch (Fig. 14-10). Early disease is characterized by the absence of a dicrotic notch and a more gradual, prolonged downslope. Moderate disease is characterized by a rounded systolic peak. Severe occlusive disease produces a flattened wave with a slow upstroke and downstroke. The absolute amplitude measurements are of limited value from patient to patient, because substantial changes result from variations in cardiac output and vasomotor tone. Comparison of amplitudes from each side in the same patient can be of value in assessing unilateral disease. In the presence of bilateral disease, it can be helpful to standardize the amplitude measurements in the lower extremities by comparing them with arm tracings, because most patients do not have major upper extremity occlusive disease. Serial pulse-volume measurements have been shown to be reproducible in patients with stable disease, so that amplitude changes indicate progression of disease.

The pulse-volume recorder has received extensive application in the past 20 years. In most situations, the plethysmographic studies are used in combination with segmental Doppler pressure measurements. Vascular laboratories using the device report that it is a useful adjunct to routine pressure measurements. One particular advantage is the ability to

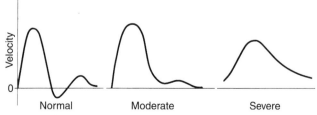

FIGURE 14–9 • Doppler velocity tracings in the leg. Increasing stenosis results in elimination of reverse flow, decrease in systolic peak, and increase in flow during diastole.

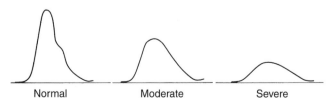

FIGURE 14–10 • Pulse-volume recorder tracings in the leg. Increasing stenosis results in loss of the dicrotic notch and flattening of the curve.

accurately assess the presence or absence of occlusive disease in patients with rigid arteries. In addition, the pulse-volume recorder has improved the detection of aortoiliac stenosis. Kempczinski reported the correct identification of advanced inflow disease in 95% of extremities.[25]

DUPLEX SCAN

In recent years, the duplex scan has been used more frequently to evaluate peripheral arteries. With appropriate scan heads, Doppler signals can be obtained from the aorta down to the tibial branches. Screening for occlusive disease can be done by comparing signals from the distal aorta and more distal sites. A more complete assessment is obtained by examining the full length of the segment in question, looking for the increased velocity and spectral broadening produced by a stenosis. The color-coded Doppler scan makes tracking of the vessels and localizing of significant stenoses considerably easier than with conventional scanners. The most common practice is to use the ratio of the peak systolic velocity recorded at the tightest part of the stenosis to the peak systolic velocity recorded in a normal portion of the same artery. A ratio greater than 2.0 defines a greater than 50% diameter reduction of the lumen.[26,27] Some groups have established additional criteria to distinguish stenosis greater than 75%. Cossman and colleagues consider the stenosis to be greater than 75% if the velocity ratio is greater than 4.0 or the peak velocity in the lesion is greater than 400 cm/second.[28] Gonsalves and Bandyk identify a severe lesion by a velocity ratio greater than 4.0, a peak velocity greater than 300 cm/second, or an end-diastolic velocity greater than 100 cm/second.[29]

Scanning is also used for visceral vessels, including the arteries of normal and transplanted kidneys. The anterior approach to visceral branches can be difficult owing to the presence of bowel gas. Flank approaches and examination of a fasting patient increase the rate of successful studies. Most renal artery stenoses occur at the origins, so it is necessary to obtain recordings from the proximal part of the vessel. As with peripheral lesions, the focus has been on identifying hemodynamically significant stenoses. A peak systolic velocity greater than 180 cm/second identifies an abnormal vessel, and a ratio of the peak velocity in the stenosis to the peak velocity in the aorta at the level of the renal arteries greater than 3.5 predicts a stenosis with a greater than 60% lumen diameter reduction.[30-32] Another approach has been to use the waveform recorded in the renal hilum.[33] Although recording hilar signals is usually easier than examining the main renal arteries, this approach does not seem to be as accurate in the diagnosis of significant stenoses.[32] An important limitation of the duplex scan in the evaluation of renal disease is that accessory branches are rarely found.

Duplex scanning has also been used to study the mesenteric branches. The celiac trunk and the proximal superior mesenteric artery can be easily located. In contrast, the inferior mesenteric artery is often not found unless it provides significant collateral flow because of occlusions in other branches. Unlike the situation with the kidneys, the perfusion to the gut is quite variable, depending on physiologic responses to feeding. Therefore, it is important to obtain baseline studies of patients in a fasting state. There has not been as much investigation of quantitative criteria to define severe mesenteric disease as there has been of other duplex scan applications. Severe stenosis is identified by a significant focal increase in velocity combined with poststenotic turbulence and reduced velocity beyond the stenosis.[34]

APPLICATIONS

Severity and Location of Arterial Lesions

The primary use of noninvasive tests in patients with lower extremity problems is to obtain objective determinations to supplement the physical examination. Such measurements permit reproducibility between different examiners as well as from one time to another. In addition, the tests are valuable in measuring the progression of arterial disease and assessing arterial reconstructions. Extremity pressures and pulse plethysmographic recordings are valuable to assess disease severity; however, duplex scanning must be used for an accurate determination of the level and extent of lesions. Kohler and associates found a sensitivity of 89% and a specificity of 90% in the identification of iliac stenosis greater than 50%.[26] Legemate and coworkers used a velocity increase of 150% and found a sensitivity of 92% and specificity of 98%.[35] It is possible to estimate common femoral artery blood flow with duplex scan measurements, but the high variability in repeat measurements in individual patients limits the clinical usefulness of this approach.[36] Although further refinement of quantitative criteria is required, it is clear that duplex scanning can play an increasing role in the evaluation of peripheral arterial insufficiency.

Following the lead of those performing carotid endarterectomy without preoperative angiography, investigators have reported the feasibility of planning arterial operations with only the ultrasound scan.[28,37-40] Wain and coauthors reported that duplex mapping is quite accurate down to the popliteal level, but in their experience, the technique is not as good at defining an appropriate target vessel at the crural level.[40] More recent studies have shown improved results with mapping of the entire lower leg in order to plan the appropriate bypass operation, including selection of the site of distal anastomosis.[41,42] Adequate visualization of the peroneal artery in the lower calf remains one of the challenges for the examiner.

Intraoperative Assessment

As with carotid surgery, duplex scanning provides an excellent tool for completion assessment after certain other arterial operations. In many operating rooms, scanning can be done more quickly and provide a more complete examination than can a conventional contrast angiogram. Often, short focal defects such as a retained valve are easily seen on a scan but may not be well demonstrated angiographically, especially with a single film study. Bandyk and associates reported on scanning after infrainguinal bypass grafts.[43] The examination involves scanning the full length of the graft, including both anastomoses. A peak systolic velocity greater than 180 cm/second or a velocity ratio greater than 2.4 indicates problem areas for which revision must be considered. Bandyk and associates reported intraoperative revision rates of 14% to 16%. Fifty-two percent of the legs with significant duplex findings that were not repaired at the time of the original operation underwent subsequent revision.

Intraoperative duplex scanning has also been advocated for renal artery repairs to reduce the risk of early occlusion and possible loss of the kidney. Studies from both Bowman Gray and the Mayo Clinic reported an 11% incidence of the detection of defects requiring repair at the time of the original procedure.[44,45] A focal high-velocity jet with a peak systolic velocity greater than 200 cm/second combined with distal turbulence identifies a tight stenosis, whereas lack of flow in the vessel indicates acute thrombosis.[44] Both these findings mandate immediate revision.

Graft Surveillance

Because of the poor secondary patency of vein grafts that thrombose, careful attention has been given to follow-up. As early as 1972, some surgeons advocated noninvasive testing to identify hemodynamic changes. For many years, graft status was monitored with pressure measurements; however, this technique is limited for patients with stiff arteries or with small-caliber distal bypasses. In 1985, Bandyk and associates reported good results with graft surveillance using the duplex scanner to measure the peak systolic velocity.[46] In this study, a peak velocity of less than 40 cm/second was associated with early graft thrombosis. In later years, the surveillance protocol was expanded to include not just a sampling of the graft velocity but also a scan of the entire graft.[47,48] Such mapping permits the identification of the specific site of stenosis. A peak systolic velocity of 180 to 200 cm/second indicates a problem. Bandyk and Johnson recommended intervention for any lesion with a peak systolic velocity greater than 300 cm/second or a velocity ratio greater than 3.5.[48] A large proportion of stenoses are found within the first postoperative year, so a program of close surveillance is advocated by many authors.[49-51] The fact that significant problems can appear later is a reason to continue surveillance beyond the first year, albeit at a reduced frequency.

Venous Disease

The correct diagnosis of venous disease can be challenging. In contrast to arterial occlusive disease, venous disease may be difficult to distinguish from other problems on the basis of the physical examination. In the past, diagnosis depended on phlebography, which, in addition to being painful, can precipitate thrombosis in a normal venous system. In the 1960s, Strandness and coworkers[52] and Sigel and colleagues[53] used the simple continuous-wave Doppler velocity detector to identify normal and abnormal flow patterns in the veins of the leg. With the subsequent development of noninvasive techniques for the arterial system, there was a parallel growth in the methods of venous diagnosis. The 1970s and 1980s saw extensive use of physiologic methods such as impedance phlebography, but these tests have been replaced by duplex scanning.

DOPPLER VENOUS EXAMINATION

The flow in the extremity veins can be evaluated qualitatively with a continuous-wave Doppler detector. The patient is examined in the supine position with the head slightly elevated. The deep veins are found adjacent to the accompanying arteries. A normal vein has spontaneous flow with a phasic variation with respiration. Breath-holding or a Valsalva maneuver decreases or abolishes flow; with release, there is a transient augmentation of the signal. A quick compression of the extremity distal to the probe produces a brisk augmentation, often followed by a transient decrease on release. Proximal compression decreases or abolishes the flow signal, with augmentation coming on release. Examination of a thrombosed segment of vein shows no flow, and adjacent collateral veins have a high-pitched signal. The patent portion of the vein distal to an obstruction has a continuous flow with no respiratory variation, and the Valsalva maneuver produces no change. Limb compression may produce limited augmentation, but clearly less than that in the normal vein. The vein segment proximal to an occlusion may have phasic flow similar to normal, but the compression produces little change. The Doppler examination is sensitive to alterations in venous flow patterns, and different forms of extrinsic compression can produce similar changes. Abnormal studies can result from large hematomas, massive edema, or ruptured popliteal cysts. A false-positive test can also occur with advanced pregnancy, ascites, morbid obesity, or abdominal masses compressing the inferior vena cava.

The Doppler venous examination can also detect venous valvular insufficiency. Normally, there should be no flow produced by compression proximal to the probe, because the valves prevent flow toward the probe. With incompetent valves, proximal compression (or a Valsalva maneuver) produces augmentation as a result of the retrograde flow. Demonstration of significant reverse flow is clear evidence of post-thrombotic syndrome.

The Doppler venous examination was once an important test for acute deep venous thrombosis (DVT) in the leg, but it has been supplanted by quantitative and imaging techniques. Because of the simplicity of the Doppler examination, it is still used, primarily as an extension of the physical examination. An abnormal flow pattern in a patient with borderline physical findings can trigger more complete evaluation by the vascular laboratory. Simple Doppler examination is also helpful in detecting deep venous reflux in a patient with varicose veins.

DUPLEX SCAN

The high resolution available with duplex scanners makes it possible to visualize venous thrombosis. In this application, the emphasis is on imaging. Thrombus is seen within the vein lumen with varying degrees of echogenicity (Fig. 14-11). On occasion, fresh thrombus may look no different from flowing blood; in these instances, additional assessment is obtained by compressing the vein with the probe. Normally, gentle pressure flattens the vein completely (Fig. 14-12). A partially or totally occluding thrombus prevents collapse in response to external pressure. Compression is performed in the transverse mode to ensure accurate evaluation with the maneuver. When examining in the longitudinal orientation, it is possible to move the ultrasound beam off the center of the vein so that the vein appears to collapse when it does not.

Occluded segments can also be identified by the lack of flow on Doppler examination, and examination of flow characteristics should be part of every study. Abnormalities in Doppler velocity signals either at rest or in response to augmentation maneuvers point to lesions that may not be evident with imaging. Color-coded Doppler is especially helpful

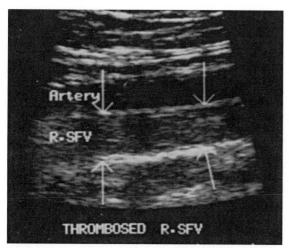

FIGURE 14–11 • B-mode scan of venous thrombus. Note the appearance of the vein lumen compared with the normal flow in the adjacent artery. R-SFV, right superficial femoral vein.

in detecting partial occluding thrombi (Fig. 14-5F; see color plate). The color scanner has also improved the examination of the tibial veins.

Most centers using duplex scanning carry out a detailed examination from the inguinal ligament to the distal end of the popliteal vein. The common and superficial femoral veins are examined in the supine position with moderate leg dependency. (The deep femoral vein is usually not followed beyond its origin.) The popliteal vein is best imaged with the patient in the lateral or prone position. In addition to the deep system, superficial veins can be imaged. The greatest difficulty in many examinations is following the vein through the adductor canal. Many studies do not trace all the infra-popliteal branches; however, these should be examined whenever the patient has focal calf symptoms. The other problem area is detecting thrombus in the common or external iliac veins. It is difficult to image these veins; therefore, one must often rely on indirect evidence given by the flow signal from the common femoral vein. Proximal occlusion causes a loss of phasic variation with respiration and limited or no change with the Valsalva maneuver. Vogel and coworkers described using the change in common femoral vein diameter during

the Valsalva maneuver: an increase of less than 10% indicates iliofemoral thrombosis.[54]

Duplex scanning of the deep leg veins for thrombus is technically difficult and requires considerable experience for an accurate diagnosis. Experienced investigators have reported sensitivities and specificities of about 95% for the diagnosis of thrombus.[54-57] Although most studies have focused on acute thrombosis, Rollins and associates demonstrated the same high accuracy in the identification of chronic disease.[56] In addition, they reported 89% accuracy in the evaluation of calf veins, compared with 93% for the proximal veins.

The duplex scan is also used to evaluate reflux in specific venous segments. Many laboratories perform this evaluation in a casual fashion, examining patients in the recumbent position and using manual compression to cause valve closure. Van Bemmelen and associates emphasized the need to examine the patient in the standing position to re-create the maximum stimulus for reflux.[58] In addition, they recommended using a pneumatic cuff with rapid decompression to provide the necessary reverse flow. A reverse velocity of 30 cm/second is necessary for consistent valvular closure.[59] Manual compression produces a variable amount of reverse flow and often results in incomplete closure. In such a case, slow reverse flow may occur through a normal valve, leading to the interpretation of an abnormal segment.

VENOUS REFLUX PHOTOPLETHYSMOGRAPHY

The venous reflux resulting from valvular insufficiency has long been recognized as the primary cause of the symptoms and complications of post-thrombotic syndrome. The first method used to study venous hypertension was direct measurement achieved by inserting a needle into a superficial foot vein and determining pressures before, during, and after walking. The response to this test is defined by the magnitude of the pressure drop during walking and the time required for the pressure to return to baseline. The main drawback of ambulatory venous pressure measurement is the need to place the needle into a foot vein, a procedure that can be difficult or impossible in some patients with advanced post-thrombotic syndrome.

Photoplethysmography (PPG) has been used to study reflux. A light in the probe shines into the superficial layers of the skin, and a photoelectric detector measures the reflected light.

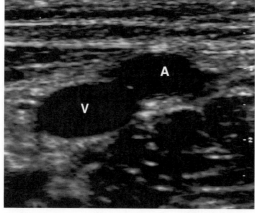
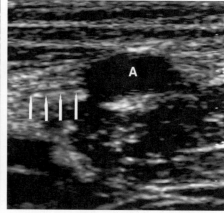

FIGURE 14–12 • Transverse duplex scans. *A*, Normal appearance of vein. *B*, Complete collapse of vein in response to external compression with the probe. V, vein; A, artery.

A   **B**

The intensity of light reflected varies with the amount of blood in the underlying microcirculation, and the device produces a pulse-wave trace, which is displayed on a strip-chart recorder. The technique is sensitive enough to record the arterial pulsation in the skin. The PPG tracing varies with the venous congestion of the skin, which varies with the venous pressure in the limb. Studies of simultaneous recordings of venous pressure and PPG signals have demonstrated similar tracing configurations by these two methods.[60,61]

The test is usually performed with the patient in the sitting position. The sensor is attached with double-sided clear tape over the medial malleolus, but it should not be directly over a superficial vein. After a short baseline tracing is obtained, the patient is instructed to contract the calf five times in quick succession and then relax the leg. The recording is continued until the tracing has fully returned to the baseline level. The recovery time is measured from the end of the calf exercise to the point at which the curve returns to baseline (Fig. 14-13). A normal recovery is more than 20 seconds, with many subjects having times of 30 to 60 seconds. Times less than 20 seconds indicate venous reflux, with the severity of the condition being inversely proportional to the recovery time. If an abnormal tracing is obtained, the examination is repeated with a Penrose drain tourniquet (or a narrow cuff inflated to 50 mm Hg) placed above or below the knee to exclude the effect of reflux down a superficial system insufficiency in the face of a normal deep system. Commonly, the tracing improves without being completely normal, indicating combined deep and superficial disease. In some cases of severe reflux combined with persisting iliofemoral occlusion, there may be either no change or a rise in the tracing. These findings indicate very severe disease.

PPG provides a simple, objective method for quantifying venous reflux. The test is easy to perform and interpret. Unlike the Doppler venous examination, which identifies the presence or absence of flow reversal at given levels, the PPG reflects the overall effect of the venous insufficiency in the leg. A limitation of the test is the possibility of having reflux in the deep system with competent valves in the perforating veins. In this situation, the abnormal congestion of the deep system would not be transmitted to the skin, and the PPG tracing would be normal.[62]

APPLICATIONS

Acute Deep Venous Thrombosis

Clinicians are aware of the fallibility of physical findings in the diagnosis of acute DVT of the leg, so most of the effort toward the noninvasive diagnosis of venous disease has focused on acute occlusion. In the past 15 years, duplex scanning has become the primary modality used to diagnose acute DVT. Many institutions perform contrast phlebography only in patients with nondiagnostic scans or when the scan cannot be obtained. This practice has been justified by the high accuracy achieved by different investigators.[54-57] A major advantage of scanning over impedance phlebography is the ability to identify the specific location of disease, especially when there are thrombi at multiple levels. Another important advantage is the detection of partially occluding thrombi, a key limitation of the physiologic techniques used in the past. In addition to confirming the initial diagnosis, scanning can be used to document change during therapy.

Recurrent Deep Venous Thrombosis

The diagnosis of recurrent DVT in patients with postthrombotic syndrome presents a great challenge to clinicians. Exacerbation of symptoms may mimic the symptoms of the original thrombosis, and in many cases, patients are readmitted for heparin therapy without objective evidence of recurrence. Noninvasive testing may be used to obtain an objective diagnosis. Duplex scanning can identify residual chronic thrombus by its high echogenicity. Other characteristics include thickened vein walls, fibrosed segments of occluded veins, and valvular insufficiency with reverse flow on Doppler examination. These features allow the examiner to use a duplex scan to distinguish recent from chronic clot. This contrasts with the phlebogram, which shows all lesions as filling defects.

Venous Insufficiency

The complications of chronic stasis are usually obvious, but it may be difficult to assess the relative contributions of outflow obstruction and reflux. Although the initial conservative management is similar, further surgical treatment must be directed to the specific cause. Doppler examination or PPG can determine the presence of venous reflux and whether it involves the deep or the superficial system. More recently, duplex scanning has been used to evaluate specific segments, especially in the deep system. Measurement of reverse blood velocities or flows provides a quantitative assessment that is not available with the simpler tests.[58,63] This information can help in the selection of procedures such as long saphenous stripping, interruption of communicating veins, and, possibly, the newer methods of venous valve transfer or transposition.

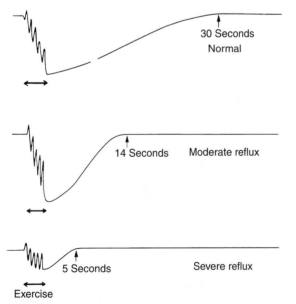

30 Seconds
Normal

14 Seconds   Moderate reflux

5 Seconds   Severe reflux

Exercise

FIGURE 14–13 • Photoplethysmography in the evaluation of venous reflux. Incompetent valves result in a recovery time less than 20 seconds. Severe insufficiency causes incomplete emptying of the calf during exercise, seen as a limited downward deflection of the tracing.

Preoperative Vein Mapping

With the growing use of the greater saphenous vein for in situ bypass grafts, knowledge of the patient's specific anatomy has become more important. Using contrast phlebograms, Shah and associates demonstrated that only 65% of thighs and 45% of calves had a single saphenous trunk.[64] The rest had variants of double systems and cross-connections. Because many surgeons are concerned about the possibility of contrast phlebography's inducing acute thrombosis, there has been increasing use of preoperative duplex scanning to map the superficial veins in both the arms and the legs.[65,66] The high resolution of the images available on contemporary machines permits a satisfactory demonstration of size, course, double segments, and varicosities in most patients. These findings correlate closely with anatomy demonstrated at operation.

Screening Asymptomatic High-Risk Patients

Patients with obesity or previous venous thrombosis and those undergoing major hip, pelvic, or intracranial operations are all at high risk of developing DVT during or shortly after surgery. Some physicians use prophylaxis against thrombosis, whereas others prefer to treat only if thrombosis occurs. Studies of asymptomatic, high-risk patients have compared scanning and contrast venography. Although specificity ranges from 94% to 100%, sensitivity is only 63% to 79%.[67-69] The results indicate that a negative study may miss asymptomatic thrombi in a significant proportion of patients, particularly with thrombi that do not occlude the lumen. The screening role for scanning requires further evaluation to determine the appropriate patient populations and the timing of examinations.

Conclusions

The rapid development of noninvasive vascular laboratory techniques has increased the amount of objective data that can be accumulated about a patient. As is the case with other diagnostic modalities, it is critical to remember that the different tests should always supplement, not replace, the information gained from a careful history and physical examination. It is increasingly common to find medical students or young house staff presenting patients in terms of the results of vascular laboratory tests rather than describing presenting symptoms and physical findings. Another area of concern is the common practice of sending patients to the noninvasive laboratory for "diagnosis of vascular condition" without their having been examined. This practice results in too many inappropriate tests (with the corresponding unnecessary costs to patients).

Optimal use of noninvasive test results requires an understanding of the limitations and errors of the specific examinations. The choice of tests must be based on the questions to be answered. There are some questions that cannot be answered by any of these techniques; for example, they cannot detect small ulcers in the carotid arteries. In addition, it must be remembered that errors, both false-positives and false-negatives, occur with all diagnostic methods, so it is important to be aware of the accuracy of the tests being used. Published studies often represent the best that can be expected, and newly established laboratories often do not achieve optimal results. Therefore, to apply noninvasive results appropriately,

it is important to know the accuracy obtained by the laboratory performing the test.

ACKNOWLEDGMENTS

I thank Vicki Carter, RN, RVT, and Christina M. Watts, ARRT, RDMS, RVT, for providing the images used in this chapter.

KEY REFERENCES

AbuRhama A, Bergan J (eds): Noninvasive Vascular Diagnosis. New York, Springer-Verlag, 2000.

Mansour MA, Labropoulos N (eds): Vascular Diagnosis. Philadelphia, Elsevier, 2004.

Polak J: Peripheral Vascular Sonography, 2nd ed. Philadelphia, Lippincott, Williams & Wilkins, 2004.

Strandness DE: Duplex Scanning in Vascular Disorders, 3rd ed. Philadelphia, Lippincott, Williams & Wilkins, 2002.

Zwiebel WJ (ed): Introduction to Vascular Ultrasonography, 5th ed. Philadelphia, Elsevier, 2004.

REFERENCES

1. Blackshear WM, Phillips DJ, Thiele BL, et al: Detection of carotid occlusive disease by ultrasonic imaging and pulsed Doppler spectrum analysis. Surgery 86:698-706, 1979.
2. Strandness DE: Extracranial arterial disease. In Strandness DE (ed): Duplex Scanning in Vascular Disorders, 3rd ed. Philadelphia, Lippincott Williams & Wilkins, 2002, pp 84-117.
3. Bluth EI, Stavros AT, Marich KW, et al: Carotid duplex sonography: A multicenter recommendation for standardized imaging and Doppler criteria. Radiographics 8:487-506, 1988.
4. Bendick PJ, Jackson VP, Becker GJ: Comparison of ultrasound scanning/Doppler with digital subtraction angiography in evaluation of carotid arterial disease. Med Instrum 17:220-222, 1983.
5. Langlois Y, Roederer GO, Chan A, et al: Evaluating carotid artery disease—the concordance between pulsed Doppler/spectrum analysis and angiography. Ultrasound Med Biol 9:51-63, 1983.
6. Londrey GL, Spadona DP, Hodgson KJ, et al: Does color-flow imaging improve the accuracy of duplex carotid evaluation? J Vasc Surg 13:659-662, 1991.
7. Mansour MA, Mattos MA, Hood DB, et al: Detection of total occlusion, string sign and preocclusive stenosis in the internal carotid artery by color-flow duplex scanning. Am J Surg 170:154-158, 1995.
8. Ackerstaff RGA, Grosvelt WJHM, Eikelbloom BC, Ludwig JW: Ultrasonic duplex scan of the prevertebral segment of the vertebral artery in patients with cerebral atherosclerosis. Eur J Vasc Surg 2:387-393, 1988.
9. von Reutern GM, Pourcelot L: Cardiac cycle-dependent alternating flow in vertebral arteries with subclavian stenosis. Stroke 9:229-236, 1978.
10. Kinney EV, Seabrook GR, Linney LY, et al: The importance of intraoperative detection of residual flow abnormalities after carotid artery endarterectomy. J Vasc Surg 17:912-923, 1993.
11. Lipski DA, Bergamini TM, Garrison RN, Fulton RL: Intraoperative duplex scanning reduces the incidence of residual stenosis after carotid endarterectomy. J Surg Res 60:3117-3120, 1966.
12. Papanicolaou G, Toms C, Yellin AE, et al: Relationship between intraoperative color-flow duplex findings and early restenosis after carotid endarterectomy: A preliminary report. J Vasc Surg 24:588-596, 1996.
13. Bandyk DF, Mills JL, Gahtan V, Esses G: Intraoperative duplex scanning of arterial reconstructions: Fate of repaired and unrepaired defects. J Vasc Surg 20:426-433, 1994.
14. Kremen JE, Gee W, Kaupp HA, McDonald KM: Restenosis or occlusion after carotid endarterectomy. Arch Surg 114:608-610, 1979.
15. Salvian A, Baker JD, Machleder HI, et al: Etiology and noninvasive detection of restenosis following carotid endarterectomy. Am J Surg 146:29-34, 1983.
16. DeGroote RD, Lynch TG, Jamil Z, Hobson RW: Carotid restenosis: Long-term noninvasive follow-up after carotid endarterectomy. Stroke 18:1031-1036, 1987.
17. Healy DA, Zierler RE, Nichols SC, et al: Long-term follow-up and clinical outcome of carotid restenosis. J Vasc Surg 10:662-669, 1989.
18. Roth SM, Back MR, Bandyk DF et al: A rational algorithm for duplex scan surveillance after carotid endarterectomy. J Vasc Surg 30:453-460, 1999.

19. Pross C, Shortsleeve CM, Baker JD, et al: Carotid endarterectomy with normal findings from completion study: Is there need for early duplex scan? J Vasc Surg 33:963-967, 2001.

20. Winsor T: Influence of arterial disease on the systolic blood pressure gradients of the extremity. Am J Med Sci 220:117-126, 1959.

21. Heintz SE, Bone GE, Slaymaker EE, et al: Value of arterial pressure measurements in the proximal and distal part of the thigh in arterial occlusive disease. Surg Gynecol Obstet 146:337-343, 1978.

22. Baker JD: Poststress Doppler ankle pressures. Arch Surg 113:1171, 1978.

23. Burnham SJ, Jaques P, Burnham CB: Noninvasive detection of iliac artery stenosis in the presence of superficial femoral artery obstruction. J Vasc Surg 16:445-453, 1992.

24. Raines JK: Pulse volume recording in the diagnosis of peripheral vascular disease. In AbuRhama A, Bergan J (eds): Noninvasive Vascular Diagnosis. New York, Springer-Verlag, 2000, pp 231-239.

25. Kempczinski RK: Segmental volume plethysmography in the diagnosis of lower extremity arterial occlusive disease. J Cardiovasc Surg 23: 125-129, 1982.

26. Kohler TR, Nance DR, Cramer MM, et al: Duplex scanning for diagnosis of aortoiliac and femoropopliteal disease: A prospective study. Circulation 76:1074-1080, 1987.

27. Leng G, Whyman MR, Donnan PT, et al: Accuracy and reproducibility of duplex ultrasonography in grading femoropopliteal stenoses. J Vasc Surg 17:510-517, 1993.

28. Cossman DV, Ellison JE, Wagner WH, et al: Comparison of contrast angiography to arterial mapping with color-flow duplex imaging in the lower extremities. J Vasc Surg 10:522-529, 1989.

29. Gonsalves A, Bandyk DF: Duplex scanning for lower extremity arterial disease. In AbuRhama A, Bergan J (eds): Noninvasive Vascular Diagnosis. New York, Springer-Verlag, 2000, pp 241-252.

30. Hoffman U, Edwards JM, Carter S, et al: Role of duplex scanning for the detection of atherosclerotic renal artery disease. Kidney Int 39:1232-1239, 1991.

31. Hansen KJ, Tribble RW, Reavis SW, et al: Renal duplex sonography: Evaluation of clinical utilities. J Vasc Surg 12:227-236, 1990.

32. Neumyer MM: Duplex evaluation of the renal arteries. In AbuRhama A, Bergan J (eds): Noninvasive Vascular Diagnosis. New York, Springer-Verlag, 2000, pp 379-390.

33. Stavros TA, Parker SH, Yakes YF, et al: Segmental stenosis of the renal artery: Pattern recognition of the tardus and parvus abnormalities with duplex sonography. Radiology 184:487-492, 1992.

34. Flinn WR, Sandager G: Duplex ultrasonography of the mesenteric circulation. In AbuRhama A, Bergan J (eds): Noninvasive Vascular Diagnosis. New York, Springer-Verlag, 2000, pp 391-399.

35. Legemate DA, Teeuwen C, Hoeneveld H, et al: The potential of duplex scanning to replace aorto-iliac and femoro-popliteal angiography. Eur J Vasc Surg 3:49-54, 1989.

36. Lewis P, Psaila JV, Davies WT, et al: Measurement of volume flow in the human common femoral artery using a duplex ultrasound system. Ultrasound Med Biol 12:777-784, 1986.

37. Kohler TR, Andros G, Porter JM, et al: Can duplex scanning replace arteriography for lower extremity arterial disease? Ann Vasc Surg 4:280-287, 1990.

38. Bodily K, Buttorff J, Nordesgaard A, et al: Aorto-iliac reconstruction without arteriography. Am J Surg 171:505-507, 1996.

39. Pemberton M, Nydahl S, Hartshorne T, et al: Can lower extremity reconstruction be based on colour duplex imaging alone? Eur J Vasc Endovasc Surg 12:452-454, 1996.

40. Wain RA, Berdejo GL, Delvalle WN, et al: Can duplex scan arterial mapping replace contrast arteriography as the test of choice before infrainguinal revascularization? J Vasc Surg 29:100-109, 1999.

41. Ascher E, Hingorani A, Markevich N, et al: Acute lower limb ischemia: The value of duplex ultrasound arterial mapping (DUAM) as the sole preoperative imaging technique. Ann Vasc Surg 17:284-289, 2003.

42. Grassbaugh JA, Nelson PR, Rzucidio EM, et al.: Blinded comparison of preoperative duplex ultrasound scanning and contrast arteriography for planning revascularization at the level of the tibia. J Vasc Surg 37:1186-1190, 2003.

43. Bandyk DF, Johnson BL, Gupta AK, Esses GE: Nature and management of duplex abnormalities encountered during infrainguinal bypass grafting. J Vasc Surg 24:430-438, 1996.

44. Hansen KJ, O'Niel EA, Reavis SW, et al: Intraoperative duplex sonography during renal artery reconstruction. J Vasc Surg 14:364-374, 1991.

45. Dougherty MJ, Hallett JW, Naessens JM, et al: Optimizing technical success of renal revascularization: The impact of intraoperative color-flow duplex ultrasonography. J Vasc Surg 17:849-857, 1993.

46. Bandyk DF, Cato RF, Towne JB: A low flow velocity predicts failure of femoropopliteal and femorotibial bypass grafts. Surgery 98:799-809, 1985.

47. Bandyk DF, Schmitt DD, Seabrook GR, et al: Monitoring functional patency of in situ saphenous vein bypasses: The impact of a surveillance protocol and elective revision. J Vasc Surg 9:286-296, 1989.

48. Bandyk DF, Johnson BL: Duplex surveillance of infrainguinal bypass grafts. In AbuRhama A, Bergan J (eds): Noninvasive Vascular Diagnosis. New York, Springer-Verlag, 2000, pp 253-267.

49. Bandyk DF, Seabrook GR, Moldenhauer P, et al: Hemodynamics of vein graft stenosis. J Vasc Surg 8:688-695, 1988.

50. Buth J, Disselhoff B, Sommeling C, et al: Color-flow duplex criteria for grading stenoses in infrainguinal vein grafts. J Vasc Surg 14:716-728, 1991.

51. Mattos MA, van Bemmelen PS, Hodgson KJ, et al: Does correction of stenoses identified by color duplex scanning improve infrainguinal graft patency? J Vasc Surg 17:54-66, 1993.

52. Strandness DE, Schultz RD, Summer DS, Rushmer RF: Ultrasonic flow detection—a useful technique in the evaluation of peripheral vascular disease. Am J Surg 113:311-320, 1967.

53. Sigel B, Popky GL, Wagner DK, et al: A Doppler ultrasound method for diagnosing lower extremity venous disease. Surg Gynecol Obstet 127:339-350, 1968.

54. Vogel P, Laing FC, Jeffrey RB, Wing VW: Deep venous thrombosis of the lower extremity: US evaluation. Radiology 163:747-751, 1987.

55. Cronan JJ, Dorfman GS, Scola FH, et al: Deep venous thrombosis: US assessment using venous compression. Radiology 162:191-194, 1987.

56. Rollins DL, Semrow CM, Friedell ML, et al: Progress in the diagnosis of deep venous thrombosis: The efficacy of real-time B-mode ultrasonic imaging. J Vasc Surg 7:638-641, 1988.

57. Sullivan ED, Peter DJ, Cranley JJ: Real-time B-mode venous ultrasound. J Vasc Surg 1:465-471, 1984.

58. van Bemmelen PS, Bedord G, Beach K, Strandness DE: Quantitative segmental evaluation of venous valvular reflux with duplex ultrasound scanning. J Vasc Surg 10:425-431, 1989.

59. van Bemmelen PS, Bedford G, Beach K, Strandness DE: The mechanism of venous valve closure. Arch Surg 125:617-619, 1990.

60. Abramowitz HB, Queral LA, Flinn WR, et al: The use of photoplethysmography in the assessment of venous insufficiency: A comparison to venous pressure measurements. Surgery 86:434-441, 1979.

61. Nicolaides AN, Miles C: Photoplethysmography in the assessment of venous insufficiency. J Vasc Surg 5:405-412, 1987.

62. Barnes RW, Yao JST: Photoplethysmography in chronic venous insufficiency. In Bernstein EF (ed): Noninvasive Diagnostic Techniques in Vascular Disease, 2nd ed. St Louis, Mosby-Year Book, 1982, pp 514-521.

63. Vasdekis SN, Clarke GH, Nicolaides AN: Quantification of venous reflux by means of duplex scanning. J Vasc Surg 10:670-677, 1989.

64. Shah DM, Chang BB, Leopold PW, et al: The anatomy of the greater saphenous venous system. J Vasc Surg 3:273-283, 1986.

65. Ruoff BA, Cranley JJ, Haannan LA, et al: Real-time duplex ultrasound mapping of the greater saphenous vein before in situ infrainguinal revascularization. J Vasc Surg 6:107-113, 1987.

66. Salles-Cunha SX, Andros G, Harris RW, et al: Preoperative noninvasive assessment of arm veins to be used as bypass grafts in the lower extremities. J Vasc Surg 3:813-816, 1986.

67. Borris LC, Christiansen HM, Lassen MR, et al: Real-time ultrasonography in the diagnosis of deep vein thrombosis in non-symptomatic high-risk patients. Eur J Vasc Surg 4:473-475, 1990.

68. Woolson ST, McCrory DW, Walter JF, et al: B-mode ultrasound scanning in the detection of proximal venous thrombosis after total hip replacement. J Bone Joint Surg Am 72:983-987, 1990.

69. Mattos MA, Londrey GL, Leutz DW, et al: Color-flow duplex scanning for the surveillance and diagnosis of acute deep venous thrombosis. J Vasc Surg 15:366-376, 1992.

Questions

1. Measuring thigh pressure with a regular arm blood pressure cuff affects the determination in what way?
   - (a) It is higher than the actual pressure
   - (b) It is equal to the actual pressure
   - (c) It is lower than the actual pressure

2. The right ankle index is calculated by dividing the higher ankle pressure by which of the following?
   - (a) Right brachial pressure
   - (b) Left brachial pressure
   - (c) Higher brachial pressure
   - (d) Lower brachial pressure

3. An ankle-brachial index of 1.60 indicates which of the following?
   - (a) Normal arterial system
   - (b) Significant arterial insufficiency
   - (c) Pathologic vessel wall stiffness
   - (d) Arteriovenous fistula in the extremity
   - (e) None of the above

4. When evaluating a patient with an exercise stress test, the severity of occlusive disease is evaluated by what means?
   - (a) Walking time
   - (b) Magnitude of drop in ankle-brachial index
   - (c) Recovery time
   - (d) All of the above
   - (e) None of the above

5. Noninvasive cerebrovascular techniques are accurate for all of the following except
   - (a) Detecting advanced stenosis of the internal carotid artery
   - (b) Detecting internal carotid occlusion
   - (c) Detecting arterial ulceration
   - (d) Detecting abnormal turbulence in the internal carotid artery

6. For a given arterial velocity, the magnitude of the Doppler frequency shift is related to which of the following?
   - (a) Distance from the probe
   - (b) Frequency of the probe
   - (c) Type of system (pulse or continuous wave)
   - (d) All of the above
   - (e) None of the above

7. Which of the following statements is true about spectral broadening of a Doppler signal?
   - (a) It is greatest proximal to a stenosis
   - (b) It is greatest in the stenosis
   - (c) It is greatest just beyond a stenosis
   - (d) It is the same at all the above sites

8. Asymptomatic deep venous thrombosis of the leg is best detected by which of the following means?
   - (a) Impedance plethysmography
   - (b) Duplex scan
   - (c) Both
   - (d) Neither

9. A venous reflux photoplethysmographic examination of a patient with postphlebitic syndrome will show which of the following?
   - (a) Increased recovery time
   - (b) Unchanged recovery time
   - (c) Decreased recovery time

10. Suitability of a superficial femoral artery for treatment with balloon dilatation can be determined by which of the following?
    - (a) Segmental pressures
    - (b) Volume plethysmography
    - (c) Duplex scan
    - (d) All of the above
    - (e) None of the above

Answers

1. a	2. c	3. c	4. d	5. c
6. b	7. c	8. b	9. c	10. c

15

Gregory L. Moneta • Erica L. Mitchell • Gregory J. Landry

Natural History and Nonoperative Treatment of Chronic Lower Extremity Ischemia

Despite the focus on operative and endovascular interventions in vascular surgery, most patients with peripheral chronic lower extremity ischemia do not require intervention. Nonoperative therapy and risk factor modification are the primary elements of treatment for the majority of patients.

Although only 1% to 2% of people younger than 50 years suffer from symptoms of intermittent claudication, this figure rises to 5% in those aged 50 to 70 years and to 10% in those older than 70.[1-3] It is estimated that 8 million to 12 million people in the United States,[4] and 27 million people in North America and Europe,[5] suffer from peripheral arterial disease (PAD), and this number is expected to rise as the population ages.

Stratification and Epidemiology

Chronic lower extremity ischemia represents a clinical spectrum. Clinical severity ranges from asymptomatic disease to intermittent claudication with ambulation to critical limb ischemia with impending tissue loss. Claudication history is typically reported as the number of blocks a patient can walk on level ground at a normal speed without having to stop; however, patients are frequently poor judges of objective walking distance. Pharmaceutical trials have stratified patients based on walking distances (initial or absolute claudication distances) or claudication times during either fixed or graded load treadmill testing. Recently, tools such as the Walking Impairment Questionnaire have assisted in the stratification of claudication history.[6] Combining the objective measurements of ischemia (ankle-brachial pressure index, toe pressure, pulse-volume recordings) with the clinical situation helps define the natural history of various patient groups with chronic lower extremity ischemia.

Lower extremity PAD is an independent risk factor for cardiovascular morbidity and mortality. Atherosclerotic cardiovascular disease is a systemic process affecting multiple arterial beds, including the coronary, cerebrovascular, upper and lower extremities, and visceral arteries. There may be significant disease overlap in the various arterial segments.[7,8] A number of large population-based epidemiologic studies have reported on the incidence and prevalence of PAD, which are dependent on the definition of PAD used.

ASYMPTOMATIC ARTERIAL INSUFFICIENCY

Asymptomatic PAD is defined as a decreased ankle-brachial index (ABI) without lower extremity symptoms. Most studies use an ABI of less than 0.9 as a reference standard for PAD.[5] The presence of asymptomatic lower extremity occlusive disease varies, but available data indicate that for every patient with intermittent claudication, there are probably three others with similar disease who do not complain of symptoms.[9] Ratios of symptomatic to asymptomatic patients range from 1:1.8 to 1:5.3.[1,2,10,11]

The prevalence of asymptomatic PAD was 25.5% among 1537 participants in the Systolic Hypertension in the Elderly Program.[12] Data from a recent nationwide cross-sectional study, based on more than 350 primary care practices, demonstrated that 13% of 6979 patients older than 50 years had abnormal ABIs, with or without symptoms of intermittent claudication.[7] Only 24% of patients with chronic lower extremity ischemia had previously been diagnosed with PAD. Asymptomatic patients accounted for 48% of newly diagnosed patients with PAD.

INCIDENCE OF SYMPTOMATIC PERIPHERAL ARTERIAL DISEASE

The majority of epidemiologic studies of PAD have focused on patients with intermittent claudication, defined as leg pain (most often calf pain, but it may involve the thighs and buttocks as well) induced by exercise and relieved by rest. The reported incidence of PAD varies between 2.2% of a population aged 33 to 82 years and 17% of a population aged 55 to 70 years.[1,2] In the Framingham Heart Study, the incidence of PAD was based on symptoms of intermittent claudication in subjects 29 to 62 years old. The annual incidence of intermittent claudication per 10,000 subjects at risk rose from 6 in men and 3 in women aged 30 to 44 years to 61 in men and 54 in women aged 65 to 74.[13] The average rate of development of intermittent claudication over a 2-year period in subjects older than age 50 was 0.7% in men and 0.4% in women.[13]

In the Edinburgh Artery Study of almost 1600 subjects older than 55 years, the 5-year cumulative incidence of PAD was 9%.[14] Bowlin and coworkers followed 8343 Israeli men over a 21-year period and found a cumulative incidence of 43.1 per 1000 population.[15] In the Quebec Cardiovascular Study of 4570 men followed over 12 years, an incidence of 41 per 10,000 population per year was noted.[16] In the large prospective Physicians' Health Study, 433 incident cases of PAD were reported among 22,071 relatively healthy men.[17]

PREVALENCE OF SYMPTOMATIC PERIPHERAL ARTERIAL DISEASE

Epidemiologic studies have employed both questionnaires and noninvasive vascular laboratory screening to estimate the prevalence of PAD in the elderly adult population. Before the development of reliable noninvasive testing, the diagnosis of PAD was based on standardized patient questionnaires. Among questionnaires, the WHO/Rose Questionnaire and the Edinburgh Classification Questionnaire (ECQ) have been the most extensively studied. The ECQ appears to be more robust, with a sensitivity of 91% and a specificity of 99% for the diagnosis of intermittent claudication.[18] Using the ECQ, the prevalence of lower extremity arterial disease was estimated to be 4.6% in the Edinburgh Artery Study in men and women between the ages of 55 and 74 years.[2] Other studies have found the prevalence of intermittent claudication in adults older than age 45 to be approximately 1% to 5% (Table 15-1).

When the ABI is used as a reference standard, the detected prevalence of lower extremity arterial occlusive disease is even greater, likely due to the inclusion of patients who are asymptomatic. The overall age-adjusted prevalence of PAD diagnosed on the basis of the ABI is approximately 12%; for intermittent claudication, it is 1% to 2% up to age 50 and 5% to 7% from the seventh decade onward.[19] In the Cardiovascular Health Study, the prevalence of a decreased ABI (<0.9) was 12.4% in adults aged 65 or older in four U.S. communities.[12] Using the same criteria, investigators in the Rotterdam Study reported a PAD prevalence of 19% in subjects older than 55.[10] In the Edinburgh Artery Study, the prevalence of lower extremity arterial occlusive disease diagnosed using ABI was 17% in subjects between the ages of 55 and 74 years.[2] In a Danish study, the prevalence of lower extremity arterial occlusive disease in 60-year-old subjects was 16% for men and 13% for women (Table 15-2).[20] Thus, objective standards of measurement identify a greater number of patients with PAD than does reliance on patients' description of symptoms.

Several factors may explain the lack of sensitivity of questionnaires and the increased prevalence of PAD with noninvasive testing.[2,21] First, symptoms may not occur until the disease is advanced. This is particularly relevant in elderly patients who may rarely walk more than one or two blocks at a time in the performance of their activities of daily living, or who may assume that leg pain while walking is a natural part of the aging process. Second, patients with PAD may have other comorbidities, such as arthritis, cardiac disease, or pulmonary disease, which affect their walking ability to a greater degree than PAD.

TABLE 15–1 Prevalence of Intermittent Claudication by History or Questionnaire in Large Population Studies

Study	No. of Patients	Age (Yr)	Intermittent Claudication Prevalence (%)
Schroll and Munck (1981)[11]	360 men	60	5.8
	306 women	60	1.3
Reunanen et al (1982)[247]	5738 men	30-59	2.1
	5224 women	30-59	1.8
Fowkes et al (1991)[2]	1592 men and women	55-74	4.5
Stoffers et al (1991)[248]	3654 men and women	45-54	0.6
		55-64	2.5
		65-74	8.8
Smith et al (1990)[110]	18,388 men	40-64	0.8
Skau and Jonsson (1993)[249]	7254 men and women	50-89	4.1
Newman et al (1993)[12]	5084 men and women	65-85	2.0
Stoffers et al (1996)[19]	1719 men	55-75	1.5
	1935 women	55-75	2.8
Zheng et al (1997)[250]	15,106 men and women	45-64	1.0
Meijer et al (1998)[10]	3052 men	70	2.2
	4663 women	70	1.2

TABLE 15–2	Prevalence of Peripheral Arterial Disease Based on Ankle-Brachial Index Abnormalities in Large Population Studies		
Study	**No. of Patients**	**Age (Yr)**	**Intermittent Claudication Prevalence (%)**
Schroll and Munck (1981)[11]	360 men	60	16.0
	306 women	60	13.0
Criqui et al (1985)[1]	613 men and women	38-82	11.7
Hiatt et al (1990)[251]	950 men and women	44-68	11.9
Newman et al (1991)[252]	1592 men and women	55-74	24.6
Coni et al (1992)[21]	265 men and women	>65	9.1
Newman et al (1993)[12]	2214 men	>65	13.9
	2870 women	>65	11.4
Stoffers et al (1991)[248]	1719 men	55-75	11.0
	1935 women	55-75	8.6
Meijer et al (1998)[10]	2589 men	>55	16.9
	3861 women	>55	20.5

Risk Factors

SMOKING

The specific mechanisms by which tobacco exerts its adverse effects on arteries remain poorly understood; however, a direct relationship between tobacco smoking and peripheral vascular disease has been well established.[22] All epidemiologic studies of lower extremity arterial disease have confirmed cigarette smoking as a strong risk factor for the development of such disease, with relative risk ratios ranging from 1.7 to 7.5.[1,10,12,23-27] A case-control study revealed a sevenfold higher risk of developing PAD in ex-smokers compared with those who had never smoked, and the risk increased to 16-fold in current smokers compared with those who had never smoked.[28] The diagnosis of lower extremity arterial disease is made up to a decade earlier in smokers compared with nonsmokers. More than 90% of all patients referred to vascular clinics for PAD have a history of smoking.[29]

In addition to the chronic effects of smoking on the development of atherosclerosis, smoking has acute effects on lower extremity function. Smoking two cigarettes within a 10-minute period resulted in an acute lowering of the ABI in chronic smokers from 0.64 ± 0.14 to 0.55 ± 0.11 ($P = 0.008$).[30] In addition to having adverse influences on atherosclerosis, the carbon monoxide in tobacco smoke may directly contribute to claudication. Smoking is associated with acute drops in treadmill walking distances, presumably owing to carbon monoxide.[31] An immediate and significant decrease in the time or distance that patients can walk on the treadmill before they get claudication symptoms has been demonstrated when air containing carbon monoxide is breathed.[31,32] Smokers have an increased risk of peripheral vascular disease progression,[33] myocardial infarction, stroke, and death.[34] Smokers also have an increased risk of major amputation.[35,36]

DIABETES MELLITUS

A strong association exists between diabetes mellitus and PAD. Two types of vascular disease are seen in patients with diabetes: microcirculatory dysfunction involving the capillaries and arterioles of the kidneys, retina, and peripheral nerves,

and a macroangiopathy involving the peripheral and coronary arterial circulation.[37] The Framingham Study was one of the first major epidemiologic studies to demonstrate the association between diabetes and PAD. Diabetes increased the risk of claudication by a factor of 3.5 in men and 8.6 in women.[38] Numerous subsequent studies have associated impaired glucose tolerance with a two- to fourfold increase in the risk of developing intermittent claudication.[39-44] In an elderly white population, 20.9% of patients with diabetes mellitus and 15.1% of patients with an abnormal glucose tolerance test had an ABI less than 0.9.[45] In a Swedish study, 21% of patients with diabetes had signs of PAD.[46] The duration and severity of diabetes mellitus correlate strongly with the incidence and severity of PAD.

Patients with diabetes mellitus often develop symptomatic forms of PAD and have poorer lower extremity function than do those with PAD alone.[47] The prevalence of diabetes in patients undergoing lower extremity revascularization ranges from 25% to 50%, compared with a prevalence of 6% in the general population.[48] The rate of lower extremity amputation is 7- to 10-fold higher in diabetic patients than in those without diabetes,[23,49-51] and in fact, diabetes leads to most nontraumatic lower extremity amputations in the United States. In addition to diabetes, insulin resistance and hyperinsulinemia are risk factors for PAD.[26,52]

GENDER

Early epidemiologic studies focused on the prevalence of PAD in men. The popular notion based on the Framingham Study was that symptomatic PAD in women lagged behind men by 10 years[53] and that women were generally not affected by PAD until after menopause. However, more recent epidemiologic studies indicate that PAD prevalence and incidence in men and women are similar. Several studies have demonstrated that the age-adjusted incidence of intermittent claudication is equal in both genders,[20,54] with the frequency of PAD among diabetic women markedly higher than that among diabetic men.[20] Among subjects with a low ABI, coronary artery disease was less prevalent among women. Women also had a lower frequency of cerebrovascular disease.[54] In another study, the prevalence of PAD was almost identical in men and women; however, other cardiovascular disease was twice as prevalent in men.[7] Progression of PAD in men and women is the same, with correction for other risk factors.[55]

Epidemiologic studies have shown that women may be more susceptible to aortoiliac arterial occlusive disease than men are.[56] Autopsy findings also provide important information about gender differences in the occurrence of atherosclerotic changes in various arterial beds. Compared with men, women have a greater extent of fatty streaks in the abdominal aorta, but not in the coronary arteries.[57]

It is possible that PAD is underdiagnosed in women to a greater degree than in men. Studies have shown that women are less likely than men to be diagnosed with PAD on the basis of symptoms, even if clinically significant PAD is present on noninvasive examinations.[58,59] Also, it has been shown that infrainguinal arterial reconstructions performed on women tend to be for more advanced disease compared with men, and the women tend to be older.[60,61] The reasons for the more advanced presentation in women are unclear. It has been speculated that because women more frequently assume a caretaker role, they are more likely to ignore their own medical care; or perhaps women are more likely to ignore mild to moderate pain, attributing it to a consequence of "old age."[62] It is clear that the previous dictum of PAD being primarily a disease of men is changing as more data about its effect on women emerge.

RACE

Few studies have assessed differences in PAD prevalence among different ethnic groups. One early study indicated that African American patients with PAD typically had a higher occurrence of infrapopliteal atherosclerosis, which was associated with a greater incidence of limb loss.[63] More recent studies indicate that PAD may be underreported in the African American population. In the Atherosclerosis Risk in Communities Study, more than 4000 African Americans were screened for PAD. Despite a greater prevalence of hypertension and diabetes, the prevalence of PAD measured by questionnaire was lower among African American men than among white men. However, 3.3% of African Americans had an ABI less than 0.9, compared with only 2.3% of whites.[54] In the Cardiovascular Health Study, the nonwhite population tested had a 3.5-fold increased frequency of an ABI less than 0.8.[12]

HYPERLIPIDEMIA

It is estimated that up to 50% of patients with lower extremity arterial disease have hyperlipidemia. In the Framingham Study, a fasting cholesterol level over 270 mg/dL was associated with a doubling of the incidence of intermittent claudication.[53] Population studies have demonstrated that the relative risk of PAD is 2.05 in patients with hypercholesterolemia,[64] 1.7 in patients with hypertriglyceridemia,[24] and 2.0 in patients with elevated levels of lipoprotein (a).[65] Other studies have shown that triglyceride levels are not an independent risk factor for PAD when corrected for other serum lipid variables.[24,66]

Ridker and colleagues evaluated multiple plasma lipid constituents, including total cholesterol, high-density lipoprotein (HDL) and low-density lipoprotein (LDL) cholesterol,

lipoprotein (a), and apolipoproteins A-I and B-100, and the risk of developing PAD.[67] Of the lipid markers tested, the ratio of total cholesterol to HDL cholesterol was the strongest predictor of PAD development, and the addition of screening for other lipid abnormalities did not improve predictive values. The addition of screening for two nonlipid variables—C-reactive protein and fibrinogen—did, however, improve the prediction of PAD risk.

HYPERHOMOCYSTEINEMIA

A number of prospective and retrospective studies have suggested an association between elevated levels of plasma homocysteine and premature vascular disease in the coronary, cerebrovascular, and peripheral circulation.[68-71] Early studies suggesting this association, however, were based on small numbers of patients. Darius and colleagues evaluated plasma homocysteine levels as an independent risk factor for PAD in 6880 primary care patients older than 65 years.[72] Although PAD (defined as an ABI <0.9) was more frequently diagnosed in patients in the highest quintile of homocysteine levels (24.3%) than in the lowest quintile (13.0%; crude odds ratio 2.1), the association was less strong after adjusting for other atherosclerotic risk factors (odds ratio 1.4). Thus, the association between hyperhomocysteinemia and atherosclerosis is likely mild.

SERUM MARKERS

Fibrinogen and C-reactive protein have been implicated in the pathogenesis of PAD in numerous studies.[34,73-78] The role of these factors in the pathogenesis of atherosclerosis is unclear; however, they are thought to be potential markers of endothelial dysfunction.[79] Elevated fibrinogen levels were independent risk factors for the development of PAD in both the Edinburgh and Rotterdam studies.[10,80]

C-reactive protein is an acute phase reactant that is elevated in acute inflammatory conditions. Persistent elevations are observed in chronic inflammatory disorders. The elevation of this factor in patients with atherosclerosis has led to the theory that inflammation contributes to the development of atherosclerosis. Whether C-reactive protein itself causes atherosclerosis is unknown. Other atherogenic risk factors such as age,[81,82] smoking,[83] diabetes,[84] and hyperlipidemia[85] are associated with elevated levels of C-reactive protein in the absence of PAD. Therefore, elevated C-reactive protein may be an epiphenomenon associated with, but not causative of, an atherogenic state.

McDermott and colleagues evaluated the association of elevated inflammatory biomarkers and physical performance in patients with PAD.[86] Both elevated C-reactive protein and D-dimer, a marker of ongoing fibrin formation and degradation, were associated with poorer physical functioning in PAD patients. Measurements of walking distance, walking speed, and balance were significantly worse in patients with elevated C-reactive protein and D-dimer.

INFECTION

Although controversial, there is some evidence that atherosclerosis may be associated with an inflammatory process caused by chronic infection with *Chlamydia pneumoniae*.[87,88]

Most existing studies have explored the role of *Chlamydia* infection in coronary artery disease.[89-91] A recent meta-analysis was performed in which the pooled data from 38 studies were examined.[92] The overall odds ratio was 1.6, suggesting only a mild causative role at best. Skeptics argue that *C. pneumoniae* is an innocent bystander in the atherosclerotic process rather than a cause. In support of this, the association between atherosclerosis and *C. pneumoniae* appears to be higher in retrospective cross-sectional and case-control studies than in prospective case-control studies, and the association is inversely proportional to length of follow-up.[92]

ALCOHOL CONSUMPTION

There is growing evidence that mild to moderate alcohol consumption is associated with a reduced risk of cardiovascular disease and reduced cardiac mortality.[93-96] Several epidemiologic studies have also suggested an inverse relationship between alcohol consumption and PAD.[17,97-100] In nonsmoking men, researchers from the Rotterdam Study found an odds ratio for PAD of 0.68 with consumption of more than 20 g of alcohol per day, with an odds ratio of 0.41 in a comparable group of women. The beneficial effects of alcohol are thought to be due to its influence on hemostasis,[80] lipid profile,[101] or the generation of oxygen free radicals.[102]

Natural History

Once the diagnosis has been made, patients and physicians fear both disease progression and limb loss, in addition to the functional limitations caused by intermittent claudication. Multiple longitudinal studies of large groups of claudicants with objective criteria for enrollment provide an accurate database.[103-106]

VASCULAR OVERLAP

Because atherosclerosis is a systemic process, significant overlap exists between PAD and other forms of cardiovascular disease—namely, coronary artery disease and cerebrovascular disease. Hertzer and colleagues clearly demonstrated a high incidence of coronary artery disease in vascular surgery patients.[107] Their conclusions were based on a series of 1000 patients undergoing major vascular surgery in whom they performed preoperative coronary angiography, regardless of the history of coronary artery disease or symptoms. More than 90% of patients had clinically significant coronary artery disease, much of which was asymptomatic. The authors also found an increased frequency of severe coronary artery disease with age, from 22% among patients younger than 50 years to 41% among patients 70 years or older. Table 15-3 summarizes the data from this important study.

In the Cardiovascular Health Study, 60% of patients with PAD had a history of other symptomatic cardiovascular disease, such as myocardial infarction, angina, or stroke.[12] Conversely, 40% of patients with coronary artery or significant cerebrovascular disease also had PAD. Similar findings were reported in the large epidemiologic study of Aronow and Ahn, in which 1886 patients older than 62 years were screened for cardiovascular disease.[8] Seventy percent of patients with PAD had associated coronary artery or cerebrovascular disease (34% cerebrovascular, 58% coronary artery). The well-recognized

TABLE 15–3	Incidence of Coronary Artery Disease (CAD) in 1000 Consecutive Patients with Peripheral Vascular Disease Screened by Angiography			
	Unsuspected		**Suspected**	
Extent of Disease	*No. of Patients*	*(%)*	*No. of Patients*	*(%)*
Normal coronary arteries	64	14	21	4
Mild to moderate CAD	218	49	99	18
Advanced compensated CAD	97	22	192	34
Severe correctable CAD	63	14	188	34
Severe incorrectable CAD	4	1	54	10

Data from Hertzer NR, Beven EG, Young JR, et al: Coronary artery disease in peripheral vascular patients: A classification of 1000 coronary angiograms and results of surgical management. Ann Surg 199: 223-233, 1984.
Table from Taylor LM Jr, Porter JM: Natural history and nonoperative treatment in chronic lower extremity ischemia. In Moore WS (ed): Vascular Surgery: A Comprehensive Review. Philadelphia, WB Saunders, 1993.

overlap between PAD and other types of cardiovascular disease has been confirmed in numerous large epidemiologic studies and clinical trials (Table 15-4).

PROGRESSION OF SYMPTOMS

Knowledge of the natural history of PAD is essential when planning therapeutic strategies. When patients with intermittent claudication are followed for 5 years, approximately 50% to 75% have either no change in symptoms or experience improvement. Approximately 25% experience symptom progression, with 5% to 25% requiring therapeutic intervention and only 2% to 4% requiring major amputation.[19,108] Both continued tobacco use[33] and diabetes mellitus[108] are correlated with progressive deterioration. However, the most important consistent predictor is the severity of objectively determined arterial occlusive disease at the first patient encounter.[51]

TABLE 15–4	Concomitant Cerebrovascular and Coronary Artery Disease in Patients with Peripheral Arterial Disease	
Study	**Cerebrovascular Disease (%)**	**Coronary Artery Disease (%)**
Ogren et al (1993)[253]	33	51
Szilagyi et al (1986)[254]	19	47
Mendelson et al (1998)[255]	35	62
Aronow and Ahn (1994)[8]	34	58
CAPRIE (1996)[122]	19	40
Meijer et al (1998)[10]		
Men	9	39
Women	8	14

LIFE EXPECTANCY

In contrast to the relatively benign lower extremity prognosis in patients with PAD, the prognosis for morbidity and mortality from other manifestations of cardiovascular disease is worse. Life expectancy is clearly reduced in patients with PAD, attributable primarily to an increase in cardiovascular disease (Table 15-5).[1,2,12,14,20,109-114] The relative risk of a claudicant having a fatal or nonfatal myocardial infarction or stroke is two to three times that of a nonclaudicant. All-cause mortality is also two to four times higher, with 60% of deaths from myocardial infarction and 15% from stroke.[109,111] According to the TransAtlantic Inter-Society Consensus document, the 5-year mortality of the average claudicant is 30%, with the majority of deaths due to manifestations of cardiovascular disease.[20] Another 5% to 10% will experience a nonfatal cardiovascular event.[19] The prevalence of asymptomatic carotid artery disease in patients with chronic lower extremity disease has also been examined. Screening carotid duplex scans before infrainguinal revascularization showed a 30% incidence of asymptomatic internal carotid artery stenosis greater than 50%.[115,116] Given the demonstrated prevalence of concomitant coronary and carotid vascular disease, reduced long-term survival in patients with chronic lower extremity ischemia is not surprising.

Multiple risk factors have been defined as important contributors to the increased long-term cardiovascular mortality of patients with lower extremity arterial occlusive disease. These include advanced age, continued tobacco use,[34] diabetes,[117] and dialysis dependence.[118-120] Of these, end-stage renal disease is the most pronounced, predicting 2-year survival rates of 50% to 65%.

Survival is inversely related to the degree of objectively determined chronic lower extremity ischemia at presentation.[121] McDermott and coworkers showed that patients with an ABI less than 0.3 had significantly higher mortality than those with an ABI of 0.3 to 0.9 (relative risk 1.8).[121] In a group of patients followed for 10 years, Criqui and associates demonstrated progressively decreasing survival with increasing PAD disease severity.[109] Among patients with a normal ABI, asymptomatic PAD, symptomatic PAD, and severe symptomatic PAD, 10-year survival rates were approximately

85%, 55%, 40%, and 25%, respectively. In another study, Vogt and coworkers found that patients with multilevel PAD had a relative mortality risk of 7.2 compared with controls.[113] In contrast, patients with PAD confined to the aortoiliac arterial segment had a relative mortality risk of 2.0 compared with controls. Multiple randomized trials in large coronary populations indicate that aggressive risk factor modification reliably reduces near-term cardiac mortality.[122-128]

CRITICAL LIMB ISCHEMIA

At the far end of the spectrum of clinical severity are those patients with critical limb ischemia (CLI). CLI is defined as arterial blood flow that is inadequate to accommodate the metabolic needs of resting tissue. Clinically, it describes a group of patients with limb-threatening ischemia and includes patients with rest pain, ischemic ulcerations, and gangrene. Objective circulatory measurement of CLI populations provides the best stratification of prognosis. The likelihood of near-term limb loss is related to the severity of ischemia at the time of patient presentation.

Data on the incidence and prevalence of CLI are less definitive than those for intermittent claudication. Using multiple different extrapolation methods, it is estimated that between 500,000 and 1 million new cases occur each year.[129,130] Roughly speaking, this means that one new patient per year develops CLI for every 100 patients with intermittent claudication in the population. Most of these patients are elderly. Only a few epidemiologic studies of CLI exist, compared with the myriad studies addressing the epidemiology of intermittent claudication. In a 7-year prospective study from the Lombardy region of northern Italy, CLI was estimated by three methods: conversion of intermittent claudication to CLI in prospectively followed patients, hospital admissions for CLI over a 3-month period, and rates of major limb amputations.[129] Surprisingly similar results were obtained with each method, with the incidence of CLI ranging from 450 to 650 cases per million per year. A national survey of the Vascular Surgical Society of Great Britain and Ireland found a similar incidence of 400 patients per million population per year.[130]

Patients with CLI and those with intermittent claudication share similar risk factors. Major risk factors for advanced limb ischemia include age, smoking, and diabetes. The incidence of major amputation rises markedly with age. A Danish national discharge survey reported that the incidence of major lower extremity amputations increased from 0.3 per 100,000 per year for patients younger than 40 years to 226 per 100,000 per year for those older than 80 years.[131] Smoking is an independent risk factor for the development and progression of PAD, a correlation stronger than that between tobacco use and coronary artery disease.

Diabetes is also a major risk factor PAD. Although diabetes affects only 2% to 5% of Western populations, 40% to 45% of all major amputees have diabetes. Major amputation is more than 10 times more frequent in diabetic patients with peripheral vascular disease than in nondiabetic patients with peripheral vascular disease.[132] The correlation is independent of age and smoking, but diabetic smokers require amputation earlier in life than do nondiabetic smokers.[130]

Not all patients with CLI initially experience claudication. Clearly, patients with progressive gangrenous changes and constant ischemic pain have an unstable clinical situation

TABLE 15–5	Relative Risk of Mortality in Patients with Peripheral Arterial Disease Compared with Those Without		
Study	**No. of Patients**	**Follow-up (Yr)**	**Relative Risk**
Reunanen et al (1982)[247]	5738 men	5	3.0
McKenna et al (1991)[112]	744 men and women	5	2.4
Criqui et al (1992)[109]	565 men and women	10	3.1
Ogren et al (1993)[253]	477 men	10	2.5
Vogt et al (1993)[113]	1492 women	4	4.0
Kornitzer et al (1995)[114]	1592 men	10	3.3
Leng et al (1996)[14]	1592 men and women	5	1.6

TABLE 15–6	Chronic Lower Extremity Ischemia in Younger Patients					
Study	No. of Patients	Follow-up (Yr)	Stable/Improved (%)	Worse (%)	Dead (%)	Amputated (%)
McCready et al (1984)[143]	21	4-6	38	52	10	—
Pairolero et al (1984)[142]	50	13.5	64	36	10	30
Evans et al (1987)[141]	153	5.5	—	—	17	16
Valentine et al (1990)[138]	22	2.2	76	24	4.5	0
Levy et al (1994)[256]	109	2.3	—	—	—	27

requiring prompt therapy. However, abundant clinical experience indicates that patients who have CLI with intermittent rest pain may experience noticeable improvement at times, presumably secondary to improved cardiac hemodynamics. Small ulcerations may heal with protective dressings alone. Several randomized pharmacologic trials have documented ulcer healing in up to 40% of CLI patients randomized to placebo,[133,134] although in most of these trials, less than half the control patients were alive without a major amputation after 6 months.[135,136]

CHRONIC LOWER EXTREMITY ISCHEMIA IN YOUNGER PATIENTS

Lower extremity ischemia in patients younger than 40 years is infrequent. Peripheral vascular disease in young patients has several unique features that must be considered (Table 15-6).[137-143] These patients are almost universally heavy smokers. One prospective study performed detailed evaluations for hypercoagulable states in younger patients with chronic lower extremity ischemia and demonstrated that 90% had laboratory abnormalities (deficiencies in natural anticoagulants, defective fibrinolytic activity, or antiphospholipid antibodies).[140] Another study demonstrated significant abnormalities in LDL cholesterol oxidation in younger patients with PAD compared with older PAD patients.[137]

Younger patients who manifest limb-threatening symptoms frequently progress rapidly to limb loss, despite attempts at revascularization, because of the limited survival of reconstructions and the need for more frequent operative revisions required in these patients.[137,144] Although survival is reduced in younger patients with peripheral vascular disease compared with age-matched controls, on balance, their coronary atherosclerosis does not appear to be as aggressive as that affecting their lower extremities.[145,146] Nonoperative management with aggressive risk factor modification (cessation of tobacco use, lipid control) is the initial therapy of choice in younger patients with claudication. However, the greater functional expectations and frequent limitations on gainful employment experienced by younger patients with claudication complicate their ability to tolerate a prolonged course of nonoperative therapy. Despite this, revascularization attempts should be made judiciously, with an understanding of the diminished longevity of these procedures in this age group and the higher amputation rate after failure.

AMPUTATION

It is worthwhile to review the natural history of patients undergoing lower extremity amputation. The incidence of major lower extremity amputation appears to have reached a plateau or decreased in the last decade, possibly owing to improved methods of revascularization and limb salvage.[147-149] Patients who undergo major amputation often do not experience a steady disease progression from claudication to rest pain to tissue necrosis to amputation, with or without revascularization attempts. In a review of 713 patients who were undergoing below-knee amputations for ischemia, more than half had experienced no ischemic symptoms as recently as 6 months before the amputation.[150]

Overall, the ratio of below-knee amputations to above-knee amputations is equal and has not significantly changed in several decades.[145,151-153] However, the introduction of aggressive limb salvage teams has increased the rate of below-knee amputations at selected centers.[154] Primary healing of below-knee amputations ranges from 30% to 90%.[154,155] Revision to attempt below-knee salvage varies from 4% to 30%.[156-158] Half of all below-knee amputees who fail to achieve primary healing ultimately require above-knee amputation.[159-161]

More below-knee than above-knee amputees achieve ambulation.[152,162,163] Overall, however, only a small number of major amputees for ischemic disease achieve meaningful independent ambulation. Initial rehabilitation can take 9 months or longer. After 2 years, 30% of amputees who had been walking no longer use their prostheses.[152] Advanced age and female gender bode poorly for ambulation.[164] Fifteen percent of amputees require contralateral amputation, and another 20% to 30% die within 2 years.[152,154,165]

Nonoperative Treatment

The nonoperative treatment of chronic lower extremity ischemia includes risk factor modification, exercise, and pharmacologic therapy.

MANAGEMENT OF RISK FACTORS

The first step in the management of PAD patients is the treatment of recognized risk factors. Multiple randomized trials in large coronary populations indicate that aggressive risk factor modification (lipid reduction, antiplatelet therapy, diabetes management, and blood pressure control) reliably reduces near-term cardiac mortality.[122,123,125-128] Table 15-7 describes basic guidelines for risk factor modification based on these trials. Evidence is accumulating that multiple pharmacologic interventions in these high-risk patients can improve long-term survival.

Smoking Cessation

Smoking cessation is by far the most important treatment for patients with PAD. Their symptoms are unlikely to progress

TABLE 15–7	Recommendations for Risk Factor Reduction in Patients with Chronic Lower Extremity Ischemia	
Parameter	**Target Goal**	**Therapy**
LDL cholesterol	<100 mg/dL	Diet, statins
HDL cholesterol	Men, ≥35 mg/dL Women, ≥45 mg/dL	Diet, exercise, niacin, fibrates
Triglycerides	<150 mg/dL	Diet, exercise, gemfibrozil, niacin
Blood pressure	Systolic < 130 Diastolic < 85	Beta blockers, ACE inhibitors
Antiplatelet therapy	All patients on some form	Aspirin, clopidogrel
Diabetes	Hb A_{1c} < 7%	Insulin, ↑ insulin sensitivity
Tobacco cessation	Complete abstinence	Nicotine replacement, antidepressant

ACE, angiotensin-converting enzyme; Hb A_{1c}, glycosylated hemoglobin; HDL, high-density lipoprotein; LDL, low-density lipoprotein.

and may even improve once smoking is stopped completely.[166] In patients with intermittent claudication, improvement in walking distance up to 40% has been reported.[166,167] Improved patency of arterial repairs in nonsmokers has been demonstrated for both aortofemoral and femoropopliteal reconstructions,[168-171] and degree of tobacco use (measured by carboxyhemoglobin levels) bears directly on the incidence of graft occlusion.[172]

Patients with PAD are often unaware of the strong association between smoking and lower extremity disease. In one study, only 37% of smokers with PAD recognized smoking as a risk factor.[173] The initial effort, therefore, on the part of all physicians must be to educate patients about the relationship between tobacco use and PAD and to inform patients unequivocally that smoking is the most important factor responsible for their leg condition. Studies have shown that strong and repeated advice by physicians to quit smoking results in abstinence in more than one third of smokers.[174]

In addition, physicians must be prepared to provide a plan to help the patient achieve the goal of smoking cessation. Reassuring the patient is extremely important, because multiple attempts at quitting are common. For most people who eventually quit, 2 to 5 years and an average of six abstinence-relapse cycles are required.[175] Although half of all smokers make an attempt to discontinue tobacco use each year, as few as 3% to 5% remain abstinent at 1 year.[176]

Pharmacologic adjuncts for the treatment of smoking addiction may be helpful in facilitating cessation. Current adjuncts include nicotine replacement therapy and antidepressant therapy. Most nicotine replacement agents provide up to 30% of a smoker's regular daily nicotine intake and thus reduce or prevent withdrawal symptoms. Nicotine gum is the oldest form of nicotine replacement and is currently available without prescription. Drawbacks include the requirement of specific chewing techniques to maximize nicotine release and drug inactivation with pH changes if beverages are consumed during use. Nicotine transdermal patches (dose ranging from 7 to 21 mg/24 hours) are easier to use. Reported success

with this technique has been modest. Reviews of randomized, double-blinded nicotine replacement trials for smoking cessation therapy in younger patients (30 to 40 years old) document biochemically confirmed 6-month abstinence rates of 20% to 45% in the treatment groups, compared with 5% to 25% in the control groups, depending on the setting (with treatment initiation in a smoking cessation clinic superior to that in a primary care office).[177,178] No benefit was derived from treatment longer than 8 weeks or from the tapering of nicotine. Intermediate-dose (14 mg/24 hour) nicotine patches have been used cautiously in patients with symptomatic coronary artery disease.[179] Older patients with cardiovascular disease have only half the abstinence rates compared with controlled trials in a younger population.[180] These patients must be warned about the danger of continued smoking while wearing the patch, owing to the potential risk of myocardial infarction. Finally, nicotine and citrate inhalers have been used in several small, randomized trials with or without nicotine patches.[181,182] These devices maintain reinforcement of the ritual, sensory phenomena of smoking. Although short-term abstinence with these devices has been achieved in 20% to 30% of cases, long-term success has been disappointing.

Smoking cessation programs now focus on depression as an important component of the smoker profile and as a major factor in withdrawal symptoms.[183] The antidepressant agents buproprion and fluoxetine have been used in randomized trials, with 12-week biochemically confirmed cessation rates of 30% to 40%.[184] In addition to diminishing withdrawal symptoms (which share many characteristics with chronic depression), these agents appear to attenuate some of the weight gain observed with smoking cessation. These agents have also been used in combination with nicotine replacement (patch or inhaler), with improved results compared with either agent alone.[185]

Finally, research on smoking cessation has centered on the effects of nicotine and neurotransmitters in the brain. Smoking one to two cigarettes increases plasma endorphin levels up to 200% and correlates with nicotine levels.[186] However, a 12-week randomized trial of naltrexone, an opioid antagonist, in 100 smokers did not demonstrate efficacy.[187]

Treatment of Diabetes

Although diabetes is clearly recognized as a risk factor for PAD, it is not clear how optimizing glycemic control affects the progression of PAD. There is evidence that glycemic control prevents the microvascular complications of diabetes; however, its effect on macrovascular complications is less clear.[188] In the Diabetes Control and Complications Trial, 1440 patients with type 1 diabetes were randomized to intensive versus conventional insulin therapy. Although patients receiving intensive insulin had fewer cardiovascular events, there was no effect on the progression of PAD.[189] Similarly, in the United Kingdom Prospective Diabetes Study, in which 3867 patients with type 2 diabetes were randomized to drug treatment with sulfonylureas or insulin versus dietary control, intensive treatment resulted in fewer deaths from myocardial infarction but no difference in amputations or death from PAD.[190] Thus, recommendations for optimal glycemic control (hemoglobin A_{1C} < 7%) are based primarily on its beneficial effect on cardiac rather than on peripheral arterial end points.

Treatment of Hyperlipidemia

Hyperlipidemia is a risk factor for all manifestations of atherosclerotic arterial occlusive disease, including PAD. A number of studies have evaluated the effects of treatment of hyperlipidemia on the progression of PAD. In general, lipid-lowering therapies are associated with stabilization or regression of PAD, as measured by angiography and severity of symptoms.[188,191] In the Cholesterol Lowering Atherosclerosis Study, 188 men with PAD and coronary artery disease were randomized to treatment with colestipol and niacin versus placebo. Lipid-lowering therapy was associated with stabilization of femoral atherosclerosis.[192] In the Program on Surgical Control of the Hyperlipidemias study, 838 patients with a history of myocardial infarction and hyperlipidemia were randomized to ileal bypass surgery versus placebo and followed for 10 years. A significant reduction in PAD progression was noted in the surgical group, with a 44% risk reduction for the development of an abnormal ABI (<0.95) and a 30% risk reduction for the development of symptomatic intermittent claudication.[193] Similar results were found in the Scandinavian Simvastatin Survival Study, in which cholesterol reduction was associated with a 38% reduction in the risk of new or worsening symptoms of intermittent claudication.[194] By consensus agreement, the goals of lipid-lowering therapy are an LDL level less than 100 mg/dL and a triglyceride level less than 150 mg/dL.[195] Initial recommended therapy is a 3-hydroxy-3-methylglutaryl-coenzyme A (HMG-CoA) reductase inhibitor ("statin"); however, niacin is an important adjunct in increasing HDL levels and decreasing triglyceride levels.[196]

Treatment of Hypertension

Although hypertension is a risk factor for PAD, there is little evidence that management of hypertension alters disease progression. Therefore, the goal of hypertension management in patients with PAD is to reduce the risk of myocardial infarction and stroke. There was some concern that the use of beta blockers might result in a worsening of PAD symptoms, based on early reports of reduced blood flow to the lower extremities.[197] However, meta-analyses found no evidence that beta blockers adversely affect mild to moderate claudication.[198]

In the Heart Outcomes Prevention Evaluation Study, the angiotensin-converting enzyme inhibitor ramipril was shown to significantly decrease rates of myocardial infarction, stroke, and cardiovascular death in patients at high risk for these events, 44% of whom had a history of PAD.[123] These results could not be explained solely on the basis of blood pressure lowering, because most patients did not have hypertension at the time of study entry, and the mean reduction in systolic blood pressure was only 3 mm Hg.

Treatment of Hyperhomocysteinemia

Hyperhomocysteinemia is a recognized risk factor for PAD and other manifestations of cardiovascular disease. Elevated plasma homocysteine levels can be lowered with vitamin B and folate supplements. There is, however, no evidence that treatment of hyperhomocysteinemia alters the course of PAD; therefore, specific recommendations cannot be made.

ANTIPLATELET THERAPY

Although there is no clear evidence of improvement in PAD symptoms with antiplatelet therapy, there is growing evidence that patients with PAD benefit from antiplatelet therapy to reduce the risk of cardiovascular morbidity and mortality. The most frequently used antiplatelet medications include aspirin and the glycoprotein IIa/IIIb inhibitors (clopidogrel, ticlopidine).

Aspirin

The Antiplatelet Trialists' Collaboration reviewed 189 controlled studies involving the prevention of cardiovascular events in more than 100,000 patients with clinical evidence of cardiovascular disease. Overall, there was a 25% reduction in fatal and nonfatal myocardial infarction, stroke, and cardiovascular death.[199] However, in a subgroup analysis of 3295 claudicants, the risk reduction in these end points after a mean follow-up of 27 months was not significantly different. The small number of patients in the subgroup analysis may have accounted for this lack of statistical difference. The benefit persisted for 3 years and was similar for aspirin doses ranging from 75 to 350 mg/day. Similar benefits of aspirin therapy were noted in the Physicians' Health Study, in which 22,071 male physicians were enrolled; aspirin at a dose of 325 mg every other day resulted in a 54% risk reduction in the subsequent need for peripheral arterial surgery compared with placebo.[200] Based on these findings, aspirin has been recommended as antiplatelet therapy in patients with PAD by groups such as the American College of Chest Physicians[201] and the TransAtlantic Inter-Society Consensus.[20]

Glycoprotein IIb/IIIa Inhibitors

The glycoprotein IIb/IIIa inhibitors inhibit platelet activation by blocking adenosine diphosphate receptors. Drugs in this class include ticlopidine and clopidogrel.

Ticlopidine

Ticlopidine has been shown to significantly lower the risk of ischemic events, including stroke and fatal and nonfatal myocardial infarction,[202] and to decrease the need for lower extremity revascularization procedures compared with placebo in patients with PAD.[203] Despite this success, ticlopidine has fallen into disfavor because of rare but severe hematologic side effects, including thrombotic thrombocytopenic purpura, thrombocytopenia, and neutropenia, for which extensive hematologic monitoring is required.[204]

Clopidogrel

The most recently and extensively studied antiplatelet medication is clopidogrel. In the Clopidogrel versus Aspirin in Patients at Risk of Ischemic Events (CAPRIE) trial, 19,185 patients with recent stroke, myocardial infarction, or stable PAD were randomized to receive clopidogrel 75 mg daily or aspirin 325 mg daily.[122] The study showed a significant relative risk reduction of 8.7% ($P = 0.04$) for subsequent cardiovascular events (myocardial infarction, ischemic stroke, or vascular death) among all participants. In the subgroup of more than 6000 patients with PAD, the relative risk reduction was even greater, at 24%.

The safety profiles of aspirin and clopidogrel were comparable in the CAPRIE study. Although their antiplatelet effects are comparable, clopidogrel has a distinct advantage over ticlopidine, being associated with fewer side effects. The risk of thrombotic thrombocytopenic purpura in patients taking clopidogrel is estimated at 4 per million; therefore, routine hematologic monitoring is not necessary.[205]

EXERCISE THERAPY

Patients with intermittent claudication typically reduce their walking in response to the discomfort. Severely affected individuals may become nearly housebound. Most patients believe that the pain from claudication indicates injury and avoid walking to prevent any further adverse consequences. Exercise therapy in the management of claudication has been studied for more than 30 years. It is the best documented therapy and is an essential component of the nonoperative treatment of intermittent claudication. Regular walking exercise results in a measurable improvement in walking distance, quality of life, and community-based functional capacity in most patients with claudication.[206-209] The major limitation of exercise therapy is the presence of associated medical conditions that limit the ability to exercise. Initial evaluation includes functional assessment followed by exercise testing to maximal claudication pain. Success is defined as improvement in initial and maximal claudication distances on the treadmill, improvement in scores on the questionnaire, or both.

The improvement produced by exercise programs ranges from an 80% to a 234% increase in walking distance.[206,207] Although better results have been achieved with supervised exercise programs, some benefit has consistently been measured in simple physician-recommended programs as well. A meta-analysis of supervised programs found a mean increase of 179% in patients' initial claudication distance (the point at which pain with walking first develops) and a mean increase of 122% in maximal walking distance.[208]

The optimal frequency and duration of exercise are unclear; however, in a recent Cochrane analysis, significant benefits in claudication symptoms were detectable with 30 minutes of exercise 3 days a week.[210] In randomized trials that compared exercise to other treatment modalities, exercise therapy was superior to angioplasty at 6 months. Surgery may be more effective than exercise, but the attendant morbidities and potential mortality must be considered.[210]

The mechanism by which walking exercise improves symptoms of claudication is not completely understood. Neither ankle blood pressure nor calf muscle blood flow is objectively improved in claudicants with improved walking tolerance after an exercise program,[207,211-213] although elevated levels of proangiogenic vascular endothelial growth factor have been detected in exercised muscle.[214] The current belief is that adaptation of the muscle cells, likely by enzyme induction, to the relatively decreased oxygen delivery in an ischemic limb is largely responsible for the improved muscle performance seen with exercise training. Other possible mechanisms include improved hemorheologic blood cell characteristics, changes in gait with more efficient use of muscle groups, better fatty acid metabolism, and an increased ratio of muscle fibers to capillaries after regular exercise.[211,212,215]

PHARMACOLOGIC THERAPY

Intermittent Claudication

The initial focus of treatment for patients with intermittent claudication is risk factor modification. Pharmacologic therapy should also be considered and is occasionally useful in improving symptoms. A number of drug classes, including vasodilators, hemorheologic agents, prostaglandins, antiplatelet agents, and anticoagulants, have been studied in recent years for the treatment of claudication symptoms. Currently two drugs, pentoxifylline and cilostazol, have been approved by the U.S. Food and Drug Administration for the treatment of patients with intermittent claudication.

Pentoxifylline

Patients with chronic lower extremity ischemia have abnormal hemorheology. Blood from patients with claudication demonstrates reduced flow rates through filters with uniform pore size.[216] Multiple studies have demonstrated decreased erythrocyte and leukocyte deformability, increased platelet aggregation, increased leukocyte and platelet adhesion, and increased blood viscosity in patients with chronic lower extremity ischemia.[217,218] Pentoxifylline is a hemorheologic agent that decreases blood viscosity and platelet aggregation and improves red blood cell flexibility. A modest improvement in claudication symptoms can be anticipated in some patients treated with pentoxifylline.[219,220] Less than 10% of patients demonstrate greater than 100% improved walking distances. Patients with ABIs less than 0.80 and symptoms of less than 1 year's duration appear to experience the most benefit.

The results of a 1982 randomized, placebo-controlled, multicenter trial showed an improvement in both initial and absolute claudication distances in patients treated with 1200 mg/day pentoxifylline compared with placebo.[220] The most common side effect is gastrointestinal distress. A meta-analysis was performed that examined the results of randomized, placebo-controlled clinical trials from 1976 to 1994 in which pentoxifylline was compared with placebo in patients with intermittent claudication.[219] In a total of 612 patients (308 in treatment groups and 304 in placebo groups), there was an absolute increase in initial claudication distance of 29.4 m in the treatment group, and an increase in absolute claudication distance of 48.4 m compared with the placebo group.

Cilostazol

Cilostazol is a phosphodiesterase inhibitor that has a multifactorial mechanism of action, including vasodilatation, inhibition of platelet aggregation and smooth muscle proliferation, and improvement of lipid profile. Randomized, multicenter, placebo-controlled trials have demonstrated the superiority of cilostazol over placebo in improving initial and absolute claudication distances in patients with intermittent claudication.[221-224] These trials demonstrated an improvement in initial claudication distance of 35% to 59%, and an improvement in absolute claudication distance of 41% to 51%, after 12 to 24 weeks of treatment with cilostazol versus placebo. Effects seem to disappear after discontinuation of the drug.[225] The usual dose of cilostazol is 100 mg orally twice a day.

One randomized, prospective trial comparing pentoxifylline to cilostazol has been published, showing significantly greater improvement in walking distance in patients receiving cilostazol compared with pentoxifylline or placebo.[226] In 54 centers, 698 patients were randomized to receive pentoxifylline (n = 232), cilostazol (n = 227), or placebo (n = 239). After 24 weeks of treatment, mean maximal walking distance in patients receiving cilostazol had increased by 107 m, compared with 64 m in patients receiving pentoxifylline and 65 m in those receiving placebo. Quality-of-life assessments using Medical Outcome Study SF-36 questionnaires also demonstrated cilostazol's efficacy. Side effects include headache, diarrhea, and dizziness.

Other Pharmacologic Agents

A number of additional pharmacologic agents have been investigated in the treatment of intermittent claudication. Although each has exhibited some benefit in limited, small trials, none has proved efficacious in large randomized trials.

NAFTIDROFURYL. Naftidrofuryl is a vasoactive drug frequently used for intermittent claudication in Europe. It is not available in the United States. Naftidrofuryl is a serotonin antagonist that improves aerobic metabolism in oxygen-depleted tissues (via stimulation of carbohydrate and fat entry into the tricarboxylic acid cycle). It may also reduce both erythrocyte and platelet aggregation.[227] Systematic reviews of randomized, controlled trials comparing naftidrofuryl with placebo revealed modest but statistically significant increases in both pain-free walking distance and total walking distance. Treatment with naftidrofuryl does not change ABI.[228]

CARNITINE. Intermittent claudication is the result of not only blood flow abnormalities to the lower extremities but also metabolic abnormalities in skeletal muscle. Carnitine metabolism has been shown to be abnormal in patients with intermittent claudication; they have an accumulation of acylcarnitines (intermediates of oxidative metabolism) in skeletal muscle, inhibiting transport of free fatty acids into the mitochondria.[229] The amount of acylcarnitine in muscle corresponds to the degree of walking impairment. This has led to the hypothesis that carnitine supplementation can improve muscle performance. The mechanism of action includes promoting pyruvate entry into the citric acid cycle and facilitating transport of free fatty acids into the mitochondria. These actions have been demonstrated in several small phase II trials. In three randomized, multicenter trials, treatment of patients with intermittent claudication with carnitine analogs (L-carnitine or propionyl L-carnitine) resulted in significant improvements in treadmill walking and quality of life compared with placebo.[230-232] Carnitine is not approved for use in the United States.

PROSTAGLANDIN ANALOGS. Prostaglandin analogs (synthetic prostaglandin E_1 and prostaglandin I_2, or prostacyclin) are potent vasodilators that inhibit platelet aggregation.[233] Prostaglandins have been evaluated primarily for the treatment of critical limb ischemia, with fewer trials performed in patients with claudication. Intravenous prostaglandin E_1 was evaluated in two randomized, controlled trials, demonstrating significant improvements in maximal walking distance (371% increase in absolute claudication distance) and quality of life compared with placebo.[234,235] Side effects include frequent vasoactive flushing and headache.

Because intravenous preparations are not practical for widespread use in patients with intermittent claudication, oral prostaglandin analogs have been developed. Beraprost sodium is an oral prostacyclin analog with vasodilatory and antiplatelet effects. A multicenter, randomized European trial suggested that beraprost increased walking distance in claudicants.[236] However, a recent large, multicenter, randomized, placebo-controlled trial in the United States failed to show any statistical benefit.[237]

VASODILATORS. Vasodilator drugs were the first class of drugs used to treat intermittent claudication. Examples include alpha blockers, calcium channel blockers, and direct-acting vasodilators such as papaverine. Several controlled trials have shown that vasodilators have no efficacy in treating intermittent claudication.[238] In theory, the reason for this is that ischemic muscle beds are already maximally vasodilated during exercise. Vasodilators therefore do not augment arterial flow in muscle beds distal to stenoses, but they may cause vasodilatation of nonischemic muscle beds, thereby creating a "steal" phenomenon, taking blood away from ischemic tissue.

ANTICOAGULANTS. Anticoagulants (heparin, low-molecular-weight heparin, oral anticoagulants) result in no significant improvement in either pain-free or maximal walking distances. An increased risk of bleeding has been noted with these agents. Anticoagulants are not indicated for the treatment of intermittent claudication.[239]

BUFLOMEDIL. Buflomedil, a vasoactive, hemorheologic agent, has been used for the treatment of intermittent claudication in Europe for many years. Blufomedil reduces vasoconstriction through both α_1 and α_2 adrenolysis. The use of this medication is based on scant clinical evidence. A recent meta-analysis examining clinical trials of buflomedil found only two small trials that conformed to accepted reporting standards. Although modest improvements in walking distance have been reported, the data are not strong enough to support the recommendation of this medication. It is not available in the United States.[240]

L-ARGININE. L-Arginine is an amino acid demonstrated to enhance nitric oxide formation and endothelium-dependent vasodilatation in patients with atherosclerosis. Two small trials demonstrated improvements in initial and absolute claudication distances, but larger trials are needed to define L-arginine's role in claudication therapy.[241,242]

CRITICAL LIMB ISCHEMIA

The mainstay of treatment for chronic CLI is either surgical or endovascular revascularization; however, this is not always required when the only manifestations are intermittent rest pain or shallow ulcers. The natural history of intermittent rest pain is not necessarily one of inevitable progression to gangrene and limb loss. This was clearly shown in randomized, controlled trials of prostaglandin treatment in patients with CLI, in which approximately 50% of patients with rest pain or ulcer improved on placebo.[133,243] In situations in which patients refuse surgery or are not surgical candidates owing to severe comorbidities or lack of target vessels, small ulcers or rest pain does improve on occasion without revascularization. Gene-induced angiogenesis using recombinant angiogenic growth factors is an area of emerging interest in patients with PAD. Tissue perfusion may be enhanced through the growth and proliferation of blood vessels in response to the delivery of angiogenic growth factors using protein or gene transfer approaches and viral or plasmid vectors. Vascular endothelial growth factor is a mitogenic agent designed to develop collateral channels in arterial occlusive disease. Increased collateral vessel development and capillary density have been documented in rabbit skeletal muscle.[244] Early clinical trials have suggested a beneficial effect of vascular endothelial growth factor in achieving therapeutic angiogenesis in patients with chronic CLI.[245] A recent clinical trial showed no benefit in treating patients with unilateral intermittent claudication with vascular endothelial growth factor, however.[246]

Conclusion

Appropriate management of patients with chronic lower extremity ischemia is complex. Despite advances in revascularization, much can be done regarding education, risk factor modification, and nonoperative therapy for these patients.

REFERENCES

1. Criqui MH, Fronek A, Barrett-Connor E, et al: The prevalence of peripheral arterial disease in a defined population. Circulation 71:510-515, 1985.
2. Fowkes FG, Housley E, Cawood EH, et al: Edinburgh Artery Study: Prevalence of asymptomatic and symptomatic peripheral arterial disease in the general population. Int J Epidemiol 20:384-392, 1991.
3. Novo S, Avellone G, Di Garbo V, et al: Prevalence of risk factors in patients with peripheral arterial disease: A clinical and epidemiological evaluation. Int Angiol 11:218-229, 1992.
4. Criqui MH, Denenberg JO, Langer RD, et al: The epidemiology of peripheral arterial disease: Importance of identifying the population at risk. Vasc Med 2:221-226, 1997.
5. Weitz JI, Byrne J, Clagett GP, et al: Diagnosis and treatment of chronic arterial insufficiency of the lower extremities: A critical review. Circulation 94:3026-3049, 1996.
6. Coyne KS, Margolis MK, Gilchrist KA, et al: Evaluating effects of method of administration on Walking Impairment Questionnaire. J Vasc Surg 38:296-304, 2003.
7. Hirsch AT, Criqui MH, Treat-Jacobson D, et al: Peripheral arterial disease detection, awareness, and treatment in primary care. JAMA 286:1317-1324, 2001.
8. Aronow WS, Ahn C: Prevalence of coexistence of coronary artery disease, peripheral arterial disease, and atherothrombotic brain infarction in men and women ≥62 years of age. Am J Cardiol 74:64-65, 1994.
9. Hiatt WR, Hoag S, Hamman RF: Effect of diagnostic criteria on the prevalence of peripheral arterial disease: The San Luis Valley Diabetes Study. Circulation 91:1472-1479, 1995.
10. Meijer XT, Hoes AW, Rutgers D, et al: Peripheral arterial disease in the elderly: The Rotterdam Study. Arterioscler Thromb Vasc Biol 18:185-192, 1998.
11. Schroll M, Munck O: Estimation of peripheral arteriosclerotic disease by ankle blood pressure measurements in a population study of 60-year-old men and women. J Chronic Dis 34:261-269, 1981.
12. Newman AB, Siscovick DS, Manolio TA, et al: Ankle-arm index as a marker of atherosclerosis in the Cardiovascular Health Study. Cardiovascular Heart Study (CHS) Collaborative Research Group. Circulation 88:837-845, 1993.
13. Kannel WB, McGee DL: Update on some epidemiologic features of intermittent claudication: The Framingham Study. J Am Geriatr Soc 33:13-18, 1985.
14. Leng GC, Lee AJ, Fowkes FG, et al: Incidence, natural history and cardiovascular events in symptomatic and asymptomatic peripheral arterial disease in the general population. Int J Epidemiol 25:1172-1181, 1996.
15. Bowlin SJ, Medalie JH, Flocke SA, et al: Intermittent claudication in 8343 men and 21-year specific mortality follow-up. Ann Epidemiol 7:180-187, 1997.
16. Dagenais GR, Maurice S, Robitaille NM, et al: Intermittent claudication in Quebec men from 1974-1986: The Quebec Cardiovascular Study. Clin Invest Med 14:93-100, 1991.
17. Camargo CA Jr, Stampfer MJ, Glynn RJ, et al: Prospective study of moderate alcohol consumption and risk of peripheral arterial disease in US male physicians. Circulation 95:577-580, 1997.
18. Leng GC, Fowkes FG: The Edinburgh Claudication Questionnaire: An improved version of the WHO/Rose Questionnaire for use in epidemiological surveys. J Clin Epidemiol 45:1101-1109, 1992.
19. Stoffers HE, Rinkens PE, Kester AD, et al: The prevalence of asymptomatic and unrecognized peripheral arterial occlusive disease. Int J Epidemiol 25:282-290, 1996.
20. Management of peripheral arterial disease (PAD): TransAtlantic Inter-Society Consensus (TASC). Eur J Vasc Endovasc Surg 19(Suppl A): S5-S44, 2000.
21. Coni N, Tennison B, Troup M: Prevalence of lower extremity arterial disease among elderly people in the community. Br J Gen Pract 42: 149-152, 1992.
22. Lord JW Jr: Cigarette smoking and peripheral atherosclerotic occlusive disease. JAMA 191:249-251, 1965.
23. Hughson WG, Mann JI, Garrod A: Intermittent claudication: Prevalence and risk factors. BMJ 1:1379-1381, 1978.
24. Fowkes FG, Housley E, Riemersma RA, et al: Smoking, lipids, glucose intolerance, and blood pressure as risk factors for peripheral atherosclerosis compared with ischemic heart disease in the Edinburgh Artery Study. Am J Epidemiol 135:331-340, 1992.
25. Gofin R, Kark JD, Friedlander Y, et al: Peripheral vascular disease in a middle-aged population sample: The Jerusalem Lipid Research Clinic Prevalence Study. Isr J Med Sci 23:157-167, 1987.
26. Criqui MH, Browner D, Fronek A, et al: Peripheral arterial disease in large vessels is epidemiologically distinct from small vessel disease: An analysis of risk factors. Am J Epidemiol 129:1110-1119, 1989.
27. Meijer WT, Grobbee DE, Hunink MG, et al: Determinants of peripheral arterial disease in the elderly: The Rotterdam study. Arch Intern Med 160:2934-2938, 2000.
28. Cole CW, Hill GB, Farzad E, et al: Cigarette smoking and peripheral arterial occlusive disease. Surgery 114:753-756, discussion 756-757, 1993.
29. Fowkes FG: Epidemiological research on peripheral vascular disease. J Clin Epidemiol 54:863-868, 2001.
30. Yataco AR, Gardner AW: Acute reduction in ankle/brachial index following smoking in chronic smokers with peripheral arterial occlusive disease. Angiology 50:355-360, 1999.
31. Aronow WS, Stemmer EA, Isbell MW: Effect of carbon monoxide exposure on intermittent claudication. Circulation 49:415-417, 1974.
32. Celermajer DS, Sorensen KE, Georgakopoulos D, et al: Cigarette smoking is associated with dose-related and potentially reversible impairment of endothelium-dependent dilation in healthy young adults. Circulation 88:2149-2155, 1993.
33. Cronenwett JL, Warner KG, Zelenock GB, et al: Intermittent claudication: Current results of nonoperative management. Arch Surg 119:430-436, 1984.
34. Violi F, Criqui M, Longoni A, et al: Relation between risk factors and cardiovascular complications in patients with peripheral vascular disease: Results from the ADEP study. Atherosclerosis 120:25-35, 1996.
35. Juergens JL, Barker NW, Hines EA Jr: Arteriosclerosis obliterans: Review of 520 cases with special reference to pathogenic and prognostic factors. Circulation 21:188-195, 1960.
36. McGrath MA, Graham AR, Hill DA, et al: The natural history of chronic leg ischemia. World J Surg 7:314-318, 1983.
37. Akbari CM, LoGerfo FW: Diabetes and peripheral vascular disease. J Vasc Surg 30:373-384, 1999.
38. Kannel WB, McGee DL: Diabetes and cardiovascular disease: The Framingham study. JAMA 241:2035-2038, 1979.
39. Laakso M, Ronnemaa T, Pyorala K, et al: Atherosclerotic vascular disease and its risk factors in non-insulin-dependent diabetic and nondiabetic subjects in Finland. Diabetes Care 11:449-463, 1988.
40. Ohlson LO, Bjuro T, Larsson B, et al: A cross-sectional analysis of glucose tolerance and cardiovascular disease in 67-year-old men. Diabet Med 6:112-120, 1989.
41. Wingard DL, Barrett-Connor EL, Scheidt-Nave C, et al: Prevalence of cardiovascular and renal complications in older adults with normal or impaired glucose tolerance or NIDDM: A population-based study. Diabetes Care 16:1022-1025, 1993.
42. Newman AB, Sutton-Tyrrell K, Vogt MT, et al: Morbidity and mortality in hypertensive adults with a low ankle/arm blood pressure index. JAMA 270:487-489, 1993.

43. Beckman JA, Creager MA, Libby P: Diabetes and atherosclerosis: Epidemiology, pathophysiology, and management. JAMA 287:2570-2581, 2002.

44. Murabito JM, D'Agostino RB, Silbershatz H, et al: Intermittent claudication: A risk profile from the Framingham Heart Study. Circulation 96:44-49, 1997.

45. Beks PJ, Mackaay AJ, de Neeling JN, et al: Peripheral arterial disease in relation to glycaemic level in an elderly Caucasian population: The Hoorn Study. Diabetologia 38:86-96, 1995.

46. Lundman B, Engstrom L: Diabetes and its complications in a Swedish county. Diabetes Res Clin Pract 39:157-164, 1998.

47. Dolan NC, Liu K, Criqui MH, et al: Peripheral artery disease, diabetes, and reduced lower extremity functioning. Diabetes Care 25:113-120, 2002.

48. Farkouh ME, Rihal CS, Gersh BJ, et al: Influence of coronary heart disease on morbidity and mortality after lower extremity revascularization surgery: A population-based study in Olmsted County, Minnesota (1970-1987). J Am Coll Cardiol 24:1290-1296, 1994.

49. Jonason T, Ringqvist I: Factors of prognostic importance for subsequent rest pain in patients with intermittent claudication. Acta Med Scand 218:27-33, 1985.

50. Jude EB, Oyibo SO, Chalmers N, et al: Peripheral arterial disease in diabetic and nondiabetic patients: A comparison of severity and outcome. Diabetes Care 24:1433-1437, 2001.

51. Dormandy J, Heeck L, Vig S: Predicting which patients will develop chronic critical leg ischemia. Semin Vasc Surg 12:138-141, 1999.

52. Price JF, Lee AJ, Fowkes FG: Hyperinsulinaemia: A risk factor for peripheral arterial disease in the non-diabetic general population. J Cardiovasc Risk 3:501-505, 1996.

53. Kannel WB, Skinner JJ Jr, Schwartz MJ, et al: Intermittent claudication: Incidence in the Framingham Study. Circulation 41:875-883, 1970.

54. Mittelmark MB, Psaty BM, Rautaharju PM, et al: Prevalence of cardiovascular diseases among older adults: The Cardiovascular Health Study. Am J Epidemiol 137:311-317, 1993.

55. van der Meer IM, Iglesias del Sol A, Hak AE, et al: Risk factors for progression of atherosclerosis measured at multiple sites in the arterial tree: The Rotterdam Study. Stroke 34:2374-2379, 2003.

56. Smith FB, Lee AJ, Fowkes FG, et al: Variation in cardiovascular risk factors by angiographic site of lower limb atherosclerosis. Eur J Vasc Endovasc Surg 11:340-346, 1996.

57. McGill HC Jr, McMahan CA, Malcom GT, et al: Effects of serum lipoproteins and smoking on atherosclerosis in young men and women: The Pathobiological Determinants of Atherosclerosis in Youth (PDAY) Research Group. Arterioscler Thromb Vasc Biol 17:95-106, 1997.

58. Gardner AW: Sex differences in claudication pain in subjects with peripheral arterial disease. Med Sci Sports Exerc 34:1695-1698, 2002.

59. Higgins JP, Higgins JA: Epidemiology of peripheral arterial disease in women. J Epidemiol 13:1-14, 2003.

60. Eugster T, Gurke L, Obeid T, et al: Infrainguinal arterial reconstruction: Female gender as risk factor for outcome. Eur J Vasc Endovasc Surg 24:245-248, 2002.

61. Roddy SP, Darling RC 3rd, Maharaj D, et al: Gender-related differences in outcome: An analysis of 5880 infrainguinal arterial reconstructions. J Vasc Surg 37:399-402, 2003.

62. Cheanvechai V, Harthun NL, Graham LM, et al: Incidence of peripheral vascular disease in women: Is it different from that in men? J Thorac Cardiovasc Surg 127:314-317, 2004.

63. Gordon WC Jr, Freeman JM, Roberts MH: A new look at peripheral vascular disease in blacks: A two-year update. J Natl Med Assoc 72:1177-1183, 1980.

64. Bowlin SJ, Medalie JH, Flocke SA, et al: Epidemiology of intermittent claudication in middle-aged men. Am J Epidemiol 140:418-430, 1994.

65. Cheng SW, Ting AC, Wong J: Lipoprotein (a) and its relationship to risk factors and severity of atherosclerotic peripheral vascular disease. Eur J Vasc Endovasc Surg 14:17-23, 1997.

66. Pomrehn P, Duncan B, Weissfeld L, et al: The association of dyslipoproteinemia with symptoms and signs of peripheral arterial disease: The Lipid Research Clinics Program Prevalence Study. Circulation 73:I100-I107, 1986.

67. Ridker PM, Stampfer MJ, Rifai N: Novel risk factors for systemic atherosclerosis: A comparison of C-reactive protein, fibrinogen, homocysteine, lipoprotein(a), and standard cholesterol screening as predictors of peripheral arterial disease. JAMA 285:2481-2485, 2001.

68. Homocysteine and risk of ischemic heart disease and stroke: A meta-analysis. JAMA 288:2015-2022, 2002.

69. Wald DS, Law M, Morris JK: Homocysteine and cardiovascular disease: Evidence on causality from a meta-analysis. BMJ 325:1202, 2002.

70. Boushey CJ, Beresford SA, Omenn GS, et al: A quantitative assessment of plasma homocysteine as a risk factor for vascular disease: Probable benefits of increasing folic acid intakes. JAMA 274:1049-1057, 1995.

71. Graham IM, Daly LE, Refsum HM, et al: Plasma homocysteine as a risk factor for vascular disease: The European Concerted Action Project. JAMA 277:1775-1781, 1997.

72. Darius H, Pittrow D, Haberl R, et al: Are elevated homocysteine plasma levels related to peripheral arterial disease? Results from a cross-sectional study of 6880 primary care patients. Eur J Clin Invest 33: 751-757, 2003.

73. Rossi E, Biasucci LM, Citterio F, et al: Risk of myocardial infarction and angina in patients with severe peripheral vascular disease: Predictive role of C-reactive protein. Circulation 105:800-803, 2002.

74. Ridker PM, Cushman M, Stampfer MJ, et al: Plasma concentration of C-reactive protein and risk of developing peripheral vascular disease. Circulation 97:425-428, 1998.

75. Libby P, Ridker PM, Maseri A: Inflammation and atherosclerosis. Circulation 105:1135-1143, 2002.

76. Mosca L: C-reactive protein—to screen or not to screen? N Engl J Med 347:1615-1617, 2002.

77. Ridker PM: Clinical application of C-reactive protein for cardiovascular disease detection and prevention. Circulation 107:363-369, 2003.

78. Yeh ET, Willerson JT: Coming of age of C-reactive protein: Using inflammation markers in cardiology. Circulation 107:370-371, 2003.

79. Brevetti G, Silvestro A, Di Giacomo S, et al: Endothelial dysfunction in peripheral arterial disease is related to increase in plasma markers of inflammation and severity of peripheral circulatory impairment but not to classic risk factors and atherosclerotic burden. J Vasc Surg 38:374-379, 2003.

80. Lowe GD, Fowkes FG, Dawes J, et al: Blood viscosity, fibrinogen, and activation of coagulation and leukocytes in peripheral arterial disease and the normal population in the Edinburgh Artery Study. Circulation 87:1915-1920, 1993.

81. Strandberg TE, Tilvis RS: C-reactive protein, cardiovascular risk factors, and mortality in a prospective study in the elderly. Arterioscler Thromb Vasc Biol 20:1057-1060, 2000.

82. Pirro M, Bergeron J, Dagenais GR, et al: Age and duration of follow-up as modulators of the risk for ischemic heart disease associated with high plasma C-reactive protein levels in men. Arch Intern Med 161: 2474-2480, 2001.

83. Tracy RP, Psaty BM, Macy E, et al: Lifetime smoking exposure affects the association of C-reactive protein with cardiovascular disease risk factors and subclinical disease in healthy elderly subjects. Arterioscler Thromb Vasc Biol 17:2167-2176, 1997.

84. Ford ES: Body mass index, diabetes, and C-reactive protein among US adults. Diabetes Care 22:1971-1977, 1999.

85. Frohlich M, Imhof A, Berg G, et al: Association between C-reactive protein and features of the metabolic syndrome: A population-based study. Diabetes Care 23:1835-1839, 2000.

86. McDermott MM, Greenland P, Green D, et al: D-dimer, inflammatory markers, and lower extremity functioning in patients with and without peripheral arterial disease. Circulation 107:3191-3198, 2003.

87. Lindholt JS, Vammen S, Lind I, et al: The progression of lower limb atherosclerosis is associated with IgA antibodies against *Chlamydia pneumoniae*. Eur J Vasc Endovasc Surg 18:527-529, 1999.

88. Siscovick DS, Schwartz SM, Caps M, et al: *Chlamydia pneumoniae* and atherosclerotic risk in populations: The role of seroepidemiology. J Infect Dis 181(Suppl 3):S417-S420, 2000.

89. Danesh J, Collins R, Peto R: Chronic infections and coronary heart disease: Is there a link? Lancet 350:430-436, 1997.

90. Danesh J, Whincup P, Walker M, et al: *Chlamydia pneumoniae* IgG titres and coronary heart disease: Prospective study and meta-analysis. BMJ 321:208-213, 2000.

91. Siscovick DS, Schwartz SM, Corey L, et al: *Chlamydia pneumoniae*, herpes simplex virus type 1, and cytomegalovirus and incident myocardial infarction and coronary heart disease death in older adults: The Cardiovascular Health Study. Circulation 102:2335-2340, 2000.

92. Bloemenkamp DG, Mali WP, Visseren FL, et al: Meta-analysis of seroepidemiologic studies of the relation between *Chlamydia pneumoniae* and atherosclerosis: Does study design influence results? Am Heart J 145:409-417, 2003.

93. Goldberg RJ, Burchfiel CM, Reed DM, et al: A prospective study of the health effects of alcohol consumption in middle-aged and elderly men: The Honolulu Heart Program. Circulation 89:651-659, 1994.

94. Hein HO, Suadicani P, Gyntelberg F: Alcohol consumption, serum low density lipoprotein cholesterol concentration, and risk of ischaemic heart disease: Six year follow up in the Copenhagen male study. BMJ 312:736-741, 1996.

95. Gaziano JM, Gaziano TA, Glynn RJ, et al: Light-to-moderate alcohol consumption and mortality in the Physicians' Health Study enrollment cohort. J Am Coll Cardiol 35:96-105, 2000.

96. Rehm JT, Bondy SJ, Sempos CT, et al: Alcohol consumption and coronary heart disease morbidity and mortality. Am J Epidemiol 146:495-501, 1997.

97. Jepson RG, Fowkes FG, Donnan PT, et al: Alcohol intake as a risk factor for peripheral arterial disease in the general population in the Edinburgh Artery Study. Eur J Epidemiol 11:9-14, 1995.

98. Fabsitz RR, Sidawy AN, Go O, et al: Prevalence of peripheral arterial disease and associated risk factors in American Indians: The Strong Heart Study. Am J Epidemiol 149:330-338, 1999.

99. Djousse L, Levy D, Murabito JM, et al: Alcohol consumption and risk of intermittent claudication in the Framingham Heart Study. Circulation 102:3092-3097, 2000.

100. Vliegenthart R, Geleijnse JM, Hofman A, et al: Alcohol consumption and risk of peripheral arterial disease: The Rotterdam study. Am J Epidemiol 155:332-338, 2002.

101. Rimm EB, Williams P, Fosher K, et al: Moderate alcohol intake and lower risk of coronary heart disease: Meta-analysis of effects on lipids and haemostatic factors. BMJ 319:1523-1528, 1999.

102. Stein JH, Keevil JG, Wiebe DA, et al: Purple grape juice improves endothelial function and reduces the susceptibility of LDL cholesterol to oxidation in patients with coronary artery disease. Circulation 100:1050-1055, 1999.

103. Dormandy JA, Murray GD: The fate of the claudicant—a prospective study of 1969 claudicants. Eur J Vasc Surg 5:131-133, 1991.

104. O'Riordain DS, O'Donnell JA: Realistic expectations for the patient with intermittent claudication. Br J Surg 78:861-863, 1996.

105. Cox GS, Hertzer NR, Young JR, et al: Nonoperative treatment of superficial femoral artery disease: Long-term follow-up. J Vasc Surg 17:172-181, discussion 181-182, 1993.

106. Fowl RJ, Gewirtz RJ, Love MC, et al: Natural history of claudicants with critical hemodynamic indices. Ann Vasc Surg 6:31-33, 1992.

107. Hertzer NR, Beven EG, Young JR, et al: Coronary artery disease in peripheral vascular patients: A classification of 1000 coronary angiograms and results of surgical management. Ann Surg 199:223-233, 1984.

108. McDaniel MD, Cronenwett JL: Basic data related to the natural history of intermittent claudication. Ann Vasc Surg 3:273-277, 1989.

109. Criqui MH, Langer RD, Fronek A, et al: Mortality over a period of 10 years in patients with peripheral arterial disease. N Engl J Med 326:381-386, 1992.

110. Smith GD, Shipley MJ, Rose G: Intermittent claudication, heart disease risk factors, and mortality: The Whitehall Study. Circulation 82:1925-1931, 1990.

111. Fowkes FG: Epidemiology of atherosclerotic arterial disease in the lower limbs. Eur J Vasc Surg 2:283-291, 1988.

112. McKenna M, Wolfson S, Kuller L: The ratio of ankle and arm arterial pressure as an independent predictor of mortality. Atherosclerosis 87:119-128, 1991.

113. Vogt MT, Cauley JA, Newman AB, et al: Decreased ankle/arm blood pressure index and mortality in elderly women. JAMA 270:465-469, 1993.

114. Kornitzer M, Dramaix M, Sobolski J, et al: Ankle/arm pressure index in asymptomatic middle-aged males: An independent predictor of ten-year coronary heart disease mortality. Angiology 46:211-219, 1995.

115. Gentile AT, Taylor LM Jr, Moneta GL, et al: Prevalence of asymptomatic carotid stenosis in patients undergoing infrainguinal bypass surgery. Arch Surg 130:900-904, 1995.

116. Marek J, Mills JL, Harvich J, et al: Utility of routine carotid duplex screening in patients who have claudication. J Vasc Surg 24:572-577, discussion 577-579, 1996.

117. Hertzer NR, Lees CD: Fatal myocardial infarction following carotid endarterectomy: Three hundred thirty-five patients followed 6-11 years after operation. Ann Surg 194:212-218, 1981.

118. Johnson BL, Glickman MH, Bandyk DF, et al: Failure of foot salvage in patients with end-stage renal disease after surgical revascularization. J Vasc Surg 22:280-285, discussion 285-286, 1995.

119. Sanchez LA, Goldsmith J, Rivers SP, et al: Limb salvage surgery in end stage renal disease: Is it worthwhile? J Cardiovasc Surg (Torino) 33:344-348, 1992.

120. Edwards JM, Taylor LM Jr, Porter JM: Limb salvage in end-stage renal disease (ESRD): Comparison of modern results in patients with and without ESRD. Arch Surg 123:1164-1168, 1988.

121. McDermott MM, Feinglass J, Slavensky R, et al: The ankle-brachial index as a predictor of survival in patients with peripheral vascular disease. J Gen Intern Med 9:445-449, 1994.

122. A randomised, blinded, trial of clopidogrel versus aspirin in patients at risk of ischaemic events (CAPRIE): CAPRIE Steering Committee. Lancet 348:1329-1339, 1996.

123. Yusuf S, Sleight P, Pogue J, et al: Effects of an angiotensin-converting-enzyme inhibitor, ramipril, on cardiovascular events in high-risk patients: The Heart Outcomes Prevention Evaluation Study Investigators. N Engl J Med 342:145-153, 2000.

124. Summary of the second report of the National Cholesterol Education Program (NCEP) Expert Panel on Detection, Evaluation, and Treatment of High Blood Cholesterol in Adults (Adult Treatment Panel II). JAMA 269:3015-3023, 1993.

125. Gould AL, Rossouw JE, Santanello NC, et al: Cholesterol reduction yields clinical benefit: Impact of statin trials. Circulation 97:946-952, 1998.

126. Grundy SM: Statin trials and goals of cholesterol-lowering therapy. Circulation 97:1436-1439, 1998.

127. MacGregor AS, Price JF, Hau CM, et al: Role of systolic blood pressure and plasma triglycerides in diabetic peripheral arterial disease: The Edinburgh Artery Study. Diabetes Care 22:453-458, 1999.

128. Miettinen TA, Pyorala K, Olsson AG, et al: Cholesterol-lowering therapy in women and elderly patients with myocardial infarction or angina pectoris: Findings from the Scandinavian Simvastatin Survival Study (4S). Circulation 96:4211-4218, 1997.

129. Catalano M: Epidemiology of critical limb ischaemia: North Italian data. Eur J Med 2:11-14, 1993.

130. Critical limb ischaemia: Management and outcome. Report of a national survey. The Vascular Surgical Society of Great Britain and Ireland. Eur J Vasc Endovasc Surg 10:108-113, 1995.

131. Eickhoff JH, Hansen HJ, Lorentzen JE: The effect of arterial reconstruction on lower limb amputation rate: An epidemiological survey based on reports from Danish hospitals. Acta Chir Scand Suppl 502:181-187, 1980.

132. Da Silva A, Widmer LK, Ziegler HW, et al: The Basle longitudinal study: Report on the relation of initial glucose level to baseline ECG abnormalities, peripheral artery disease, and subsequent mortality. J Chronic Dis 32:797-803, 1979.

133. Schuler JJ, Flanigan DP, Holcroft JW, et al: Efficacy of prostaglandin E_1 in the treatment of lower extremity ischemic ulcers secondary to peripheral vascular occlusive disease: Results of a prospective randomized, double-blind, multicenter clinical trial. J Vasc Surg 1:160-170, 1984.

134. Cronenwett JL, Zelenock GB, Whitehouse WM Jr, et al: Prostacyclin treatment of ischemic ulcers and rest pain in unreconstructible peripheral arterial occlusive disease. Surgery 100:369-375, 1986.

135. Belch JJ, McKay A, McArdle B, et al: Epoprostenol (prostacyclin) and severe arterial disease: A double-blind trial. Lancet 1:315-317, 1983.

136. Norgren L, Alwmark A, Angqvist KA, et al: A stable prostacyclin analogue (iloprost) in the treatment of ischaemic ulcers of the lower limb: A Scandinavian-Polish placebo controlled, randomised multicenter study. Eur J Vasc Surg 4:463-467, 1990.

137. Levy PJ, Gonzalez MF, Hornung CA, et al: A prospective evaluation of atherosclerotic risk factors and hypercoagulability in young adults with premature lower extremity atherosclerosis. J Vasc Surg 23:36-43, discussion 43-45, 1996.

138. Valentine RJ, MacGillivray DC, DeNobile JW, et al: Intermittent claudication caused by atherosclerosis in patients aged forty years and younger. Surgery 107:560-565, 1990.

139. Valentine RJ, Grayburn PA, Vega GL, et al: Lp(a) lipoprotein is an independent, discriminating risk factor for premature peripheral atherosclerosis among white men. Arch Intern Med 154:801-806, 1994.

140. Valentine RJ, Kaplan HS, Green R, et al: Lipoprotein (a), homocysteine, and hypercoagulable states in young men with premature peripheral atherosclerosis: A prospective, controlled analysis. J Vasc Surg 23:53-61, discussion 61-63, 1996.

141. Evans WE, Hayes JP, Vermillion BD: Atherosclerosis in the younger patient: Results of surgical management. Am J Surg 154:225-229, 1987.

142. Pairolero PC, Joyce JW, Skinner CR, et al: Lower limb ischemia in young adults: Prognostic implications. J Vasc Surg 1:459-464, 1984.

143. McCready RA, Vincent AE, Schwartz RW, et al: Atherosclerosis in the young: A virulent disease. Surgery 96:863-869, 1984.

144. Harris LM, Peer R, Curl GR, et al: Long-term follow-up of patients with early atherosclerosis. J Vasc Surg 23:576-580, discussion 581, 1996.

145. Valentine RJ, Myers SI, Inman MH, et al: Late outcome of amputees with premature atherosclerosis. Surgery 119:487-493, 1996.

146. Valentine RJ, Myers SI, Hagino RT, et al: Late outcome of patients with premature carotid atherosclerosis after carotid endarterectomy. Stroke 27:1502-1506, 1996.

147. Karlstrom L, Bergqvist D: Effects of vascular surgery on amputation rates and mortality. Eur J Vasc Endovasc Surg 14:273-283, 1997.

148. Mattes E, Norman PE, Jamrozik K: Falling incidence of amputations for peripheral occlusive arterial disease in western Australia between 1980 and 1992. Eur J Vasc Endovasc Surg 13:14-22, 1997.

149. Tunis SR, Bass EB, Steinberg EP: The use of angioplasty, bypass surgery, and amputation in the management of peripheral vascular disease. N Engl J Med 325:556-562, 1991.

150. Dormandy J, Belcher G, Broos P, et al: Prospective study of 713 below-knee amputations for ischaemia and the effect of a prostacyclin analogue on healing: Hawaii Study Group. Br J Surg 81:33-37, 1994.

151. Dowd GS: Predicting stump healing following amputation for peripheral vascular disease using the transcutaneous oxygen monitor. Ann R Coll Surg Engl 69:31-35, 1987.

152. Kihn RB, Warren R, Beebe GW: The "geriatric" amputee. Ann Surg 176:305-314, 1972.

153. Ratliff DA, Clyne CA, Chant AD, et al: Prediction of amputation wound healing: The role of transcutaneous pO_2 assessment. Br J Surg 71:219-222, 1984.

154. Rush DS, Huston CC, Bivins BA, et al: Operative and late mortality rates of above-knee and below-knee amputations. Am Surg 47:36-39, 1981.

155. Mooney V, Wagner W Jr, Waddell J, et al: The below-the-knee amputation for vascular disease. J Bone Joint Surg Am 58:365-368, 1976.

156. Yamanaka M, Kwong PK: The side-to-side flap technique in below-the-knee amputation with long stump. Clin Orthop 1985:75-79, 1985.

157. Robinson KP: Long posterior flap amputation in geriatric patients with ischaemic disease. Ann R Coll Surg Engl 58:440-451, 1976.

158. Silverman DG, Roberts A, Reilly CA, et al: Fluorometric quantification of low-dose fluorescein delivery to predict amputation site healing. Surgery 101:335-341, 1987.

159. Tripses D, Pollak EW: Risk factors in healing of below-knee amputation: Appraisal of 64 amputations in patients with vascular disease. Am J Surg 141:718-720, 1981.

160. Finch DR, Macdougal M, Tibbs DJ, et al: Amputation for vascular disease: The experience of a peripheral vascular unit. Br J Surg 67:233-237, 1980.

161. Burgess EM, Matsen FA 3rd, Wyss CR, et al: Segmental transcutaneous measurements of PO_2 in patients requiring below-the-knee amputation for peripheral vascular insufficiency. J Bone Joint Surg Am 64:378-382, 1982.

162. Pollock SB Jr, Ernst CB: Use of Doppler pressure measurements in predicting success in amputation of the leg. Am J Surg 139:303-306, 1980.

163. Gregg RO: Bypass or amputation? Concomitant review of bypass arterial grafting and major amputations. Am J Surg 149:397-402, 1985.

164. Cameron HC, Lennard-Jones JE, Robinson MP: Amputations in the diabetic outcome and survival. Lancet 18:605-607, 1964.

165. Whitehouse FW, Jurgensen C, Block MA: The later life of the diabetic amputee: Another look at fate of the second leg. Diabetes 17:520-521, 1968.

166. Lepantalo M, Lassila R: Smoking and occlusive peripheral arterial disease: Clinical review. Eur J Surg 157:83-87, 1991.

167. Quick CR, Cotton LT: The measured effect of stopping smoking on intermittent claudication. Br J Surg 69(Suppl):S24-S26, 1982.

168. Robicsek F, Daugherty HK, Mullen DC, et al: The effect of continued cigarette smoking on the patency of synthetic vascular grafts in Leriche syndrome. J Thorac Cardiovasc Surg 70:107-113, 1975.

169. Provan JL, Sojka SG, Murnaghan JJ, et al: The effect of cigarette smoking on the long term success rates of aortofemoral and femoropopliteal reconstructions. Surg Gynecol Obstet 165:49-52, 1987.

170. Myers KA, King RB, Scott DF, et al: The effect of smoking on the late patency of arterial reconstructions in the legs. Br J Surg 65:267-271, 1978.

171. Ameli FM, Stein M, Prosser RJ, et al: Effects of cigarette smoking on outcome of femoral popliteal bypass for limb salvage. J Cardiovasc Surg (Torino) 30:591-596, 1989.

172. Wiseman S, Kenchington G, Dain R, et al: Influence of smoking and plasma factors on patency of femoropopliteal vein grafts. BMJ 299:643-646, 1989.

173. Clyne CA, Arch PJ, Carpenter D, et al: Smoking, ignorance, and peripheral vascular disease. Arch Surg 117:1062-1065, 1982.

174. Kirk CJ, Lund VJ, Woolcock NE, et al: The effect of advice to stop smoking on arterial disease patients, assessed by serum thiocyanate levels. J Cardiovasc Surg (Torino) 21:568-569, 1980.

175. Stachnik T, Stoffelmayr B: Worksite smoking cessation programs: A potential for national impact. Am J Public Health 73:1395-1396, 1983.

176. Hughes JR, Gulliver SB, Fenwick JW, et al: Smoking cessation among self-quitters. Health Psychol 11:331-334, 1992.

177. Fiore MC, Smith SS, Jorenby DE, et al: The effectiveness of the nicotine patch for smoking cessation: A meta-analysis. JAMA 271:1940-1947, 1994.

178. Silagy CA, Neil HA: A meta-analysis of the effect of garlic on blood pressure. J Hypertens 12:463-468, 1994.

179. Daughton DM, Fortmann SP, Glover ED, et al: The smoking cessation efficacy of varying doses of nicotine patch delivery systems 4 to 5 years post-quit day. Prev Med 28:113-118, 1999.

180. Joseph AM, Norman SM, Ferry LH, et al: The safety of transdermal nicotine as an aid to smoking cessation in patients with cardiac disease. N Engl J Med 335:1792-1798, 1996.

181. Schneider NG, Olmstead R, Nilsson F, et al: Efficacy of a nicotine inhaler in smoking cessation: A double-blind, placebo-controlled trial. Addiction 91:1293-1306, 1996.

182. Westman EC, Behm FM, Rose JE: Airway sensory replacement combined with nicotine replacement for smoking cessation: A randomized, placebo-controlled trial using a citric acid inhaler. Chest 107:1358-1364, 1995.

183. Glassman AH, Helzer JE, Covey LS, et al: Smoking, smoking cessation, and major depression. JAMA 264:1546-1549, 1990.

184. Jorenby DE, Leischow SJ, Nides MA, et al: A controlled trial of sustained-release bupropion, a nicotine patch, or both for smoking cessation. N Engl J Med 340:685-691, 1999.

185. Blondal T, Gudmundsson LJ, Tomasson K, et al: The effects of fluoxetine combined with nicotine inhalers in smoking cessation—a randomized trial. Addiction 94:1007-1015, 1999.

186. Pomerleau OF, Fertig JB, Seyler LE, et al: Neuroendocrine reactivity to nicotine in smokers. Psychopharmacology (Berl) 81:61-67, 1983.

187. Wong GY, Wolter TD, Croghan GA, et al: A randomized trial of naltrexone for smoking cessation. Addiction 94:1227-1237, 1999.

188. Hiatt WR: Medical treatment of peripheral arterial disease and claudication. N Engl J Med 344:1608-1621, 2001.

189. Effect of intensive diabetes management on macrovascular events and risk factors in the Diabetes Control and Complications Trial. Am J Cardiol 75:894-903, 1995.

190. Intensive blood-glucose control with sulphonylureas or insulin compared with conventional treatment and risk of complications in patients with type 2 diabetes (UKPDS 33): UK Prospective Diabetes Study (UKPDS) Group. Lancet 352:837-853, 1998.

191. Regensteiner JG, Hiatt WR: Treatment of peripheral arterial disease. Clin Cornerstone 4:26-40, 2002.

192. Blankenhorn DH, Azen SP, Crawford DW, et al: Effects of colestipol-niacin therapy on human femoral atherosclerosis. Circulation 83:438-447, 1991.

193. Buchwald H, Bourdages HR, Campos CT, et al: Impact of cholesterol reduction on peripheral arterial disease in the Program on the Surgical Control of the Hyperlipidemias (POSCH). Surgery 120:672-679, 1996.

194. Pedersen TR, Kjekshus J, Pyorala K, et al: Effect of simvastatin on ischemic signs and symptoms in the Scandinavian Simvastatin Survival Study (4S). Am J Cardiol 81:333-335, 1998.

195. Ansell BJ, Watson KE, Fogelman AM: An evidence-based assessment of the NCEP Adult Treatment Panel II guidelines: National Cholesterol Education Program. JAMA 282:2051-2057, 1999.

196. Elam MB, Hunninghake DB, Davis KB, et al: Effect of niacin on lipid and lipoprotein levels and glycemic control in patients with diabetes and peripheral arterial disease: The ADMIT study: A randomized trial. Arterial Disease Multiple Intervention Trial. JAMA 284:1263-1270, 2000.

197. Solomon SA, Ramsay LE, Yeo WW, et al: Beta blockade and intermittent claudication: Placebo controlled trial of atenolol and nifedipine and their combination. BMJ 303:1100-1104, 1991.

198. Radack K, Deck C: Beta-adrenergic blocker therapy does not worsen intermittent claudication in subjects with peripheral arterial disease: A meta-analysis of randomized controlled trials. Arch Intern Med 151:1769-1776, 1991.

199. Collaborative overview of randomised trials of antiplatelet therapy. I. Prevention of death, myocardial infarction, and stroke by prolonged antiplatelet therapy in various categories of patients. Antiplatelet Trialists' Collaboration. BMJ 308:81-106, 1994.

200. Goldhaber SZ, Manson JE, Stampfer MJ, et al: Low-dose aspirin and subsequent peripheral arterial surgery in the Physicians' Health Study. Lancet 340:143-145, 1992.

201. Sachdev GP, Ohlrogge KD, Johnson CL: Review of the Fifth American College of Chest Physicians Consensus Conference on Antithrombotic Therapy: Outpatient management for adults. Am J Health Syst Pharm 56:1505-1514, 1999.

202. Blanchard J, Carreras LO, Kindermans M: Results of EMATAP: A double-blind placebo-controlled multicentre trial of ticlopidine in patients with peripheral arterial disease. Nouv Rev Fr Hematol 35:523-528, 1994.

203. Bergqvist D, Almgren B, Dickinson JP: Reduction of requirement for leg vascular surgery during long-term treatment of claudicant patients with ticlopidine: Results from the Swedish Ticlopidine Multicentre Study (STIMS). Eur J Vasc Endovasc Surg 10:69-76, 1995.

204. Bennett CL, Weinberg PD, Rozenberg-Ben-Dror K, et al: Thrombotic thrombocytopenic purpura associated with ticlopidine: A review of 60 cases. Ann Intern Med 128:541-544, 1998.

205. Bennett CL, Connors JM, Carwile JM, et al: Thrombotic thrombocytopenic purpura associated with clopidogrel. N Engl J Med 342:1773-1777, 2000.

206. Clifford PC, Davies PW, Hayne JA, et al: Intermittent claudication: Is a supervised exercise class worthwhile? BMJ 280:1503-1505, 1980.

207. Ekroth R, Dahllof AG, Gundevall B, et al: Physical training of patients with intermittent claudication: Indications, methods, and results. Surgery 84:640-643, 1978.

208. Gardner AW, Poehlman ET: Exercise rehabilitation programs for the treatment of claudication pain: A meta-analysis. JAMA 274:975-980, 1995.

209. Nehler MR, Hiatt WR: Exercise therapy for claudication. Ann Vasc Surg 13:109-114, 1999.

210. Leng GC, Fowler B, Ernst E (eds): Exercise for Intermittent Claudication. Oxford, Cochrane Review, 2002.

211. Stewart KJ, Hiatt WR, Regensteiner JG, et al: Exercise training for claudication. N Engl J Med 347:1941-1951, 2002.

212. Dahllof AG, Holm J, Schersten T, et al: Peripheral arterial insufficiency, effect of physical training on walking tolerance, calf blood flow, and blood flow resistance. Scand J Rehabil Med 8, 1976.

213. Johnson EC, Voyles WF, Atterbom HA, et al: Effects of exercise training on common femoral artery blood flow in patients with intermittent claudication. Circulation 80:III59-III72, 1989.

214. Gustafsson T, Puntschart A, Kaijser L, et al: Exercise-induced expression of angiogenesis-related transcription and growth factors in human skeletal muscle. Am J Physiol 276:H679-H685, 1999.

215. Hiatt WR, Regensteiner JG, Wolfel EE, et al: Effect of exercise training on skeletal muscle histology and metabolism in peripheral arterial disease. J Appl Physiol 81:780-788, 1996.

216. Reid HL, Dormandy JA, Barnes AJ, et al: Impaired red cell deformability in peripheral vascular disease. Lancet 1:666-668, 1976.

217. Ernst EE, Matrai A: Intermittent claudication, exercise, and blood rheology. Circulation 76:1110-1114, 1987.

218. Johnson G Jr, Keagy BA, Ross DW, et al: Viscous factors in peripheral tissue perfusion. J Vasc Surg 2:530-535, 1985.

219. Hood SC, Moher D, Barber GG: Management of intermittent claudication with pentoxifylline: Meta-analysis of randomized controlled trials. CMAJ 155:1053-1059, 1996.

220. Porter JM, Cutler BS, Lee BY, et al: Pentoxifylline efficacy in the treatment of intermittent claudication: Multicenter controlled double-blind trial with objective assessment of chronic occlusive arterial disease patients. Am Heart J 104:66-72, 1982.

221. Beebe HG, Dawson DL, Cutler BS, et al: A new pharmacological treatment for intermittent claudication: Results of a randomized, multicenter trial. Arch Intern Med 159:2041-2050, 1999.

222. Dawson DL, Cutler BS, Meissner MH, et al: Cilostazol has beneficial effects in treatment of intermittent claudication: Results from a multicenter, randomized, prospective, double-blind trial. Circulation 98:678-686, 1998.

223. Elam MB, Heckman J, Crouse JR, et al: Effect of the novel antiplatelet agent cilostazol on plasma lipoproteins in patients with intermittent claudication. Arterioscler Thromb Vasc Biol 18:1942-1947, 1998.

224. Money SR, Herd JA, Isaacsohn JL, et al: Effect of cilostazol on walking distances in patients with intermittent claudication caused by peripheral vascular disease. J Vasc Surg 27:267-274, discussion 274-275, 1998.

225. Dawson DL, DeMaioribus CA, Hagino RT, et al: The effect of withdrawal of drugs treating intermittent claudication. Am J Surg 178:141-146, 1999.

226. Dawson DL, Cutler BS, Hiatt WR, et al: A comparison of cilostazol and pentoxifylline for treating intermittent claudication. Am J Med 109:523-530, 2000.

227. Waters KJ, Craxford AD, Chamberlain J: The effect of naftidrofuryl (Praxilene) on intermittent claudication. Br J Surg 67:349-351, 1980.

228. Girolami B, Bernardi E, Prins MH, et al: Treatment of intermittent claudication with physical training, smoking cessation, pentoxifylline, or nafronyl: A meta-analysis. Arch Intern Med 159:337-345, 1999.

229. Hiatt WR, Koziol BJ, Shapiro JI, et al: Carnitine metabolism during exercise in patients on chronic hemodialysis. Kidney Int 41:1613-1619, 1992.

230. Brevetti G, Perna S, Sabba C, et al: Superiority of L-propionylcarnitine vs L-carnitine in improving walking capacity in patients with peripheral vascular disease: An acute, intravenous, double-blind, cross-over study. Eur Heart J 13:251-255, 1992.

231. Brevetti G, Chiariello M, Ferulano G, et al: Increases in walking distance in patients with peripheral vascular disease treated with L-carnitine: A double-blind, cross-over study. Circulation 77:767-773, 1998.

232. Hiatt WR, Regensteiner JG, Creager MA, et al: Propionyl-L-carnitine improves exercise performance and functional status in patients with claudication. Am J Med 110:616-622, 2001.

233. Weeks JR, Sekhar NC, Ducharme DW: Relative activity of prostaglandins E_1, A_1, E_2 and A_2 on lipolysis, platelet aggregation, smooth muscle and the cardiovascular system. J Pharm Pharmacol 21:103-108, 1969.

234. Belch JJ, Bell PR, Creissen D, et al: Randomized, double-blind, placebo-controlled study evaluating the efficacy and safety of AS-013, a prostaglandin E_1 prodrug, in patients with intermittent claudication. Circulation 95:2298-2302, 1997.

235. Diehm C, Balzer K, Bisler H, et al: Efficacy of a new prostaglandin E_1 regimen in outpatients with severe intermittent claudication: Results of a multicenter placebo-controlled double-blind trial. J Vasc Surg 25:537-544, 1997.

236. Lievre M, Morand S, Besse B, et al: Oral beraprost sodium, a prostaglandin I_2 analogue, for intermittent claudication: A double-blind, randomized, multicenter controlled trial. Beraprost et Claudication Intermittente (BERCI) Research Group. Circulation 102:426-431, 2000.

237. Melian EB, Goa KL: Beraprost: A review of its pharmacology and therapeutic efficacy in the treatment of peripheral arterial disease and pulmonary arterial hypertension. Drugs 62:107-133, 2002.

238. Coffman JD: Vasodilator drugs for peripheral vascular disease. N Engl J Med 301:159-160, 1979.

239. Cosmi B, Conti E, Coccheri S: Anticoagulants (Heparin, Low Molecular Weight Heparin and Oral Anticoagulants) for Intermittent Claudication. Oxford, Cochrane Review, 2002.

240. De Backer TLM, Vander Stichele RH, Bogaert MG: Buflomedil for Intermittent Claudication. Oxford, Cochrane Review, 2002.

241. Boger RH, Bode-Boger SM, Thiele W, et al: Restoring vascular nitric oxide formation by L-arginine improves the symptoms of intermittent claudication in patients with peripheral arterial occlusive disease. J Am Coll Cardiol 32:1336-1344, 1998.

242. Maxwell AJ, Anderson BE, Cooke JP: Nutritional therapy for peripheral arterial disease: A double-blind, placebo-controlled, randomized trial of HeartBar. Vasc Med 5:11-19, 2000.

243. Eklund AE, Eriksson G, Olsson AG: A controlled study showing significant short term effect of prostaglandin E_1 in healing of ischaemic ulcers of the lower limb in man. Prostaglandins Leukot Med 8:265-271, 1982.

244. Tsurumi Y, Takeshita S, Chen D, et al: Direct intramuscular gene transfer of naked DNA encoding vascular endothelial growth factor augments collateral development and tissue perfusion. Circulation 94:3281-3290, 1996.

245. Manninen HI, Makinen K: Gene therapy techniques for peripheral arterial disease. Cardiovasc Intervent Radiol 25:98-108, 2002.

246. Rajagopalan S, Mohler ER 3rd, Lederman RJ, et al: Regional angiogenesis with vascular endothelial growth factor in peripheral arterial disease: A phase II randomized, double-blind, controlled study of adenoviral delivery of vascular endothelial growth factor 121 in patients with disabling intermittent claudication. Circulation 108:1933-1938, 2003.

247. Reunanen A, Takkunen H, Aromaa A: Prevalence of intermittent claudication and its effect on mortality. Acta Med Scand 211:249-256, 1982.

248. Stoffers HEJH, Kaiser V, Knottnerus JA: Prevalence in general practice. In Epidemiology of Peripheral Vascular Disease. London, Springer-Verlag, 1991, pp 109-115.

249. Skau T, Jonsson B: Prevalence of symptomatic leg ischaemia in a Swedish community—an epidemiological study. Eur J Vasc Surg 7:432-437, 1993.

250. Zheng ZJ, Sharrett AR, Chambless LE, et al: Associations of ankle-brachial index with clinical coronary heart disease, stroke and preclinical carotid and popliteal atherosclerosis: The Atherosclerosis Risk in Communities (ARIC) Study. Atherosclerosis 131:115-125, 1997.

251. Hiatt WR, Marshall JA, Baxter J, et al: Diagnostic methods for peripheral arterial disease in the San Luis Valley Diabetes Study. J Clin Epidemiol 43:597-606, 1990.

252. Newman AB, Sutton-Tyrrell K, Rutan GH, et al: Lower extremity arterial disease in elderly subjects with systolic hypertension. J Clin Epidemiol 44:15-20, 1991.

253. Ogren M, Hedblad B, Isacsson SO, et al: Non-invasively detected carotid stenosis and ischaemic heart disease in men with leg arteriosclerosis. Lancet 342:1138-1141, 1993.

254. Szilagyi DE, Elliott JP Jr, Smith RF, et al: A thirty-year survey of the reconstructive surgical treatment of aortoiliac occlusive disease. J Vasc Surg 3:421-436, 1986.

255. Mendelson G, Aronow WS, Ahn C: Prevalence of coronary artery disease, atherothrombotic brain infarction, and peripheral arterial disease: Associated risk factors in older Hispanics in an academic hospital-based geriatrics practice. J Am Geriatr Soc 46:481-483, 1998.

256. Levy PJ, Hornung CA, Haynes JL, et al: Lower extremity ischemia in adults younger than forty years of age: A community-wide survey of premature atherosclerotic arterial disease. J Vasc Surg 19:873-881, 1994.

Questions

1. **An abnormal ankle-brachial index (ABI) is present in approximately what percentage of patients older than 50 years?**
   (a) 1%
   (b) 2%
   (c) 15%
   (d) 25%
   (e) 35%

2. **What is the increased risk of developing peripheral arterial disease in current smokers versus those who have never smoked?**
   (a) 2 times
   (b) 4 times
   (c) 8 times
   (d) 16 times
   (e) 32 times

3. **What disease process leads to the most nontraumatic amputations in the United States?**
   (a) Diabetes
   (b) Buerger's disease
   (c) Tobacco abuse
   (d) Obesity
   (e) Connective tissue disorders

4. **What is the prevalence of peripheral arterial disease in women versus that in men?**
   (a) 10% that in men
   (b) 50% that in men
   (c) 75% that in men
   (d) Equal to that in men
   (e) 150% that in men

5. **The relative risk of a patient with intermittent claudication having a myocardial infarction or stroke compared with a nonclaudicant is increased by what factor?**
   (a) One to two times
   (b) Two to three times
   (c) Four to five times
   (d) Six to eight times
   (e) Ten times

6. **What proportion of patients undergoing amputation for ischemia experienced ischemic symptoms 6 months before the amputation?**
   (a) Less than 50%
   (b) 60% to 70%
   (c) 70% to 80%
   (d) 80% to 90%
   (e) 100%

7. **The relative risk reduction for myocardial infarction, ischemic stroke, or vascular death in patients with peripheral arterial disease managed with clopidogrel versus aspirin is approximately which of the following?**
   (a) 5%
   (b) 10%
   (c) 15%
   (d) 20%
   (e) 25%

8. **The most likely mechanism by which exercise therapy improves walking distance in patients with intermittent claudication is which of the following?**
   (a) Increase in ankle-brachial index
   (b) Muscle cell adaptation to decreased oxygen delivery
   (c) Increased collateral formation
   (d) Improved cardiac output
   (e) Improved blood hemorheology

9. **Which of the following is currently the most effective drug available in the United States for improving walking distance in patients with peripheral arterial disease and intermittent claudication?**
   (a) Cilostazol
   (b) Pentoxifylline
   (c) Warfarin
   (d) Aspirin
   (e) Carnitine

10. **Which of the following is a contraindication to the use of cilostazol for the treatment of intermittent claudication?**
    (a) Congestive heart failure
    (b) Walking distance less than 100 feet
    (c) CYP 3A inhibitors
    (d) Warfarin therapy
    (e) Use of beta blocker drugs

Answers

1. d	2. d	3. a	4. d	5. b
6. a	7. e	8. b	9. a	10. a

16

Antoinette S. Gomes

Principles of Imaging in Vascular Disease

Two new imaging techniques are now available for performing angiography: magnetic resonance angiography (MRA) and multislice computed tomography-angiography (CTA). These techniques, although representing distinctly different technologies, provide images of the vascular system that are competitive with those obtained from conventional catheter-based angiography. Although the image resolution of these two techniques is less than that of conventional angiography, the image quality is such that these methods have the potential to supplant, and in many instances already do supplant, conventional diagnostic angiography.

The benefits of conventional angiography are high resolution; the ability to repeat injections of contrast; and, with the use of digital subtraction techniques, the ability to visualize small vessels. Endovascular treatments can be performed at the same time as arteriography.

Limitations of conventional angiography are its invasive nature, with the requirement for catheter placement; the need for conscious sedation; the length of the study; and radiation exposure. The need for patient monitoring both before and after the procedure and the need for patient recovery time add significantly to the cost of the procedure.

Magnetic Resonance Angiography

Magnetic resonance imaging (MRI) uses radiofrequency waves and magnetic field gradients to generate images. It is characterized by high contrast between soft tissue and flowing blood. The different pulse sequences used during MRI permit the enhancement or reduction of signal from different tissues based on their hydrogen density and their response to varying magnetic field gradients. MRI can be used to obtain static images of the body and images of the vascular system.

A variety of pulse sequences have been used to perform MRA. These include two-dimensional time-of-flight, phase-contrast, and, more recently, three-dimensional time-of-flight gadolinium-enhanced MRA.

TIME-OF-FLIGHT ANGIOGRAPHY

Time-of-flight angiography is performed using a flow-compensated gradient refocused sequence. Data are typically acquired as a stack of two-dimensional slices or as a single three-dimensional volume. In this technique, stationary tissues in the slice or volume of interest are saturated from repeated radiofrequency pulses and have low signal intensity.[1-3] Blood flowing into the imaging has not been subjected to these radiofrequency pulses and is therefore fully magnetized (unsaturated). When it flows into the volume, it is bright compared with the stationary background tissues. This inflow technique works well in relatively normal arteries and veins, such as carotid arteries, the cerebral vasculature, vessels of the feet, the inferior vena cava, and iliac veins. Selective saturation pulses can be applied, allowing selective saturation of blood entering the imaging volume, such that either the arterial or the venous signal can be suppressed. With this technique, separate images of the arterial and venous system can be acquired.

A limitation of this technique is in-plane saturation, which results in signal dropout when the long axis of the vessel coincides with the scan plane or in the presence of slowly flowing blood in tortuous arteries. Another limitation is turbulence-induced signal loss in and distal to a stenosis.[4,5] Additionally, the relatively long echo times required for gradient moment nulling make time-of-flight imaging sensitive to susceptibility artifacts from bowel gas, implanted metallic objects (e.g., clips), or other air-tissue interfaces. These artifacts are a primary reason for the inaccuracy of time-of-flight MRA. In addition, imaging times are lengthy because vessels need to be imaged perpendicular to the long axis of the vessel and a stack of slices must be acquired. Long acquisition times can lead to artifacts due to slice misregistration or patient motion.

PHASE-CONTRAST ANGIOGRAPHY

Phase-contrast angiography uses velocity-induced phase shifts, which occur as blood flows through a magnetic field in the presence of flow-encoding gradients.[1,6,7] Two images created with opposite bipolar flow-encoding gradients are subtracted from each other; in the phase difference image, the residual phase is proportional to velocity. Stationary tissues do not undergo a velocity-induced phase shift in either image; they are suppressed and therefore subtract completely. The flow-encoding gradients can be in any direction or in multiple directions, depending on the selected flow sensitivity. Phase-contrast angiography can be performed as a two- or three-dimensional gradient refocused sequence and is improved after contrast administration.[8] It has been employed in the evaluation of the renal arteries, carotid arteries, and portal veins. It is also used to measure flow velocity. When used with cardiac gating, a time-resolved velocity profile can be generated, providing quantitative measurement of the flow rate.

There are limitations to the technique. The amplitude of the preselected bipolar gradient (VENC) determines the degree of velocity encoding. Phase-contrast sequences encode only a specified range of velocities.[9] In occlusive disease, turbulence causes a wide spectrum of rapidly changing velocities, which produce intravoxel phase dispersion and signal loss. Artifactual signal loss at sites of vessel stenosis is common. The sequence is also susceptible to measurement degradation from cardiac, respiratory, and translational motion. Background subtraction can be problematic.

THREE-DIMENSIONAL CONTRAST-ENHANCED MAGNETIC RESONANCE ANGIOGRAPHY

Three-dimensional time-of-flight gadolinium-enhanced MRA is the most widely employed and useful of the MRA techniques. It does not rely on motion of blood to create flow signal. A contrast agent, typically gadolinium chelate, is given to shorten the T1 (spin-lattice) relaxation time of blood so that it is significantly shorter than that of surrounding tissues. Blood is imaged directly using a T1-weighted sequence. This technique reduces the sensitivity to turbulence, and in-plane saturation effects are eliminated.[4,5] With this technique, a limited number of slices are oriented in the plane of the target vessels, permitting rapid imaging of a large field of view covering a large region of the vascular system. Contrast-enhanced MRA is fast and affords high-quality breath-hold and non–breath-hold angiograms. Dynamic contrast-enhanced MRA exploits the transient shortening in blood T1 after the intravenous administration of a contrast agent using a fast three-dimensional spoiled gradient echo sequence. This is a first-pass technique, because the contrast agents currently used are extracellular agents and the gadolinium chelate rapidly leaks into the extravascular space. Typical repetition times (TR) for contrast-enhanced MRA are less than 5 to 6 msec, with echo times (TE) of 1 to 2 msec and total scan times of 10 to 30 seconds. The sequences that use T1-weighted gradient echo (SPGR), T1 fast field echo (FFE), or fast low-angle shot (FLASH) have high spatial resolution and a high signal-to-noise ratio. The images can be acquired in a breath-hold fashion and reformatted in any plane.[10-14] Because intravascular signal is dependent on T1 relaxation rather than inflow or phase accumulation, in-plane saturation and signal loss due to turbulence are not significant.[4]

Blood is bright relative to background tissues during the arterial phase of three-dimensional contrast-enhanced MRA, because contrast transiently reduces the arterial blood T1 to less than that of the brightest background tissue (fat). During the first-pass arterial phase, imaging is done before vascular contrast equilibration. Utilizing a first-pass technique, steady-state background signal is nearly eliminated. Once the contrast is injected and dynamic imaging is done, however, a second bolus injection of contrast material must be given in order to repeat the process. When the second dose is given, residual soft tissue enhancement can obscure vascular detail.[15] Subtraction techniques, using a precontrast mask, are typically used to remove background tissues. When the second or third dose of contrast is used, subtraction is mandatory. Timing is important in contrast-enhanced MRA. Unlike CT, MRA does not map spatial data linearly over time.[16] With three-dimensional MRI, all the three-dimensional Fourier or K-space data (the information from which the image is constructed) are collected before individual slices are reconstructed. K-space maps spatial frequencies rather than spatial data. Consequently, K-space data do not correspond to image space directly. Different portions of K-space determine the features of the image. The center of K-space, which records low spatial frequencies, affects contrast, whereas the periphery of K-space records high spatial frequencies, which contribute to the fine details, such as edges.[16,17]

Intravascular T1 signal intensity is determined by the gadolinium concentration at the time the center of K-space is collected.[17] The timing is synchronized so the midportion of the bolus arrives at the desired site as the center of K-space is being collected. Perfect timing produces maximal arterial signal with minimal venous signal. If central K-space data are acquired too early, while arterial gadolinium is increasing rapidly, ringing or banding artifacts may be generated. Acquiring central K-space data too late leads to reduced arterial signal intensity and enhancement of venous structures. Several methods have been used to obtain proper bolus timing, including simple estimates of the travel time of the bolus from the site of injection to the region of interest. For example, in a normal patient, the travel time from the antecubital vein to the aorta is approximately 15 seconds; in a patient with cardiac disease or an aneurysm, it is 25 to 35 seconds. To estimate contrast travel time more precisely, a test bolus can be used. In this technique, 1 to 2 mL of contrast followed by a 10- to 15-mL saline flush is injected at the same rate as the planned injection. Multiple single-slice fast gradient echo images of the appropriate vascular regions are then obtained as rapidly as possible—typically, every 1 to 2 seconds for a given period—and the time to peak enhancement (contrast travel time) is determined in the region of interest. A limitation of this technique is the setup time; also, the redistribution of the test bolus to the interstitial space may add to background signal.

Other techniques used include MR fluoroscopy.[18] In this technique, two two-dimensional sagittal gradient refocused images are obtained rapidly (<1 second per image) throughout the region of interest. Images are generated in near–real time and updated at a rate greater than one image every second; the bolus time is watched, and when it arrives, the operator switches over to the three-dimensional MRA sequence. This technique may be helpful in cases of asymmetrical flow due to asymmetrical stenoses.

Another technique is a temporally resolved method in which multiple three-dimensional data sets are rapidly acquired (over 2 to 8 seconds) without any predetermined timing; injection and scanning are begun simultaneously.[19-23] The operator then selects the desired image set. Other techniques used to facilitate MRA involve simply scanning faster using parallel imaging techniques and using alternative K-space acquisition techniques.

Respiratory motion causes image blurring, ghosting, and signal loss. In three-dimensional imaging, blurring occurs in the direction of motion, whereas ghosting is more pronounced in the phase-encoding direction.[24] Before the availability of fast imaging systems, MRA techniques were too long to permit breath-holding. Breath-holding results in improved images in abdominal and thoracic MRA and facilitates the visualization of small vessels, such as the renal arteries.[25] It does not appear to be as critical in the evaluation of the carotids. Most ambulatory patients can hold their breath 20 to 30 seconds, and imaging is usually done on inspiration.

Patient Preparation

Patient cooperation is required for optimal contrast-enhanced MRA, because motion and improper breath-holding can render the MRA study nondiagnostic. Valuable scanner time is often squandered during attempts to image an uncooperative patient. Patients should be relaxed, and the procedure should be explained to them beforehand. For patients who are particularly anxious, premedication with a sedative such as diazepam or fentanyl may be helpful. The intravenous (IV) line should be placed before the imaging is started and before the patient is in the magnet. A 22-gauge or larger IV line is placed in the antecubital fossa or below if the arms are to be extended above the head.

Gadolinium-Based Contrast Agents

Currently, almost all contrast-enhanced MRA studies are performed using gadolinium-based contrast agents. Gadolinium is a paramagnetic metal ion. Paramagnetic atoms or molecules possess unpaired electrons that, when placed in a magnetic field, undergo magnetization (attain magnetic susceptibility). The electrons set up circulating currents in response to the externally applied field. These induce an internal magnetization that augments or opposes the external field. When the direction of internal magnetization is the same as that of the external field, the effective field within the object is enhanced. This magnetic field enhancement is known as paramagnetism.

Gadolinium decreases both spin-lattice (T1) and spin-spin (T2) relaxation times. Gadolinium is chelated with ligands, such as gadopentetate dimeglumine, gadoteridol, or gadodiamide, to form MR contrast agents.[26] These are extracellular agents that pass from the intravascular compartment into the interstitial space in a matter of minutes.[4,5] Unlike iodinated contrast agents, these agents have a very low rate of adverse effects and essentially no nephrotoxicity, which makes them advantageous for evaluating patients with impaired renal function.

Measurements of T1 shortening at different cardiac outputs have shown that injection rates greater than approximately 2 mL/second do not increase T1 shortening. Signal intensity increases asymptotically as the injection rate increases, with negligible increases seen beyond a rate of 4 to 5 mL/second.[27,28]

Most contrast-enhanced MR studies are performed with 0.1 mmol/kg of gadolinium or a double dose of 0.2 mmol/kg, or with a set volume of 20 or 30 mL with an injection rate of 1.5 to 2.5 mL/second. Contrast can be injected manually or, preferably, with a power injector. Either technique is followed rapidly by a 15- to 20-mL saline flush.

With contrast-enhanced MRA, once arterial data are collected, the sequence is repeated to capture the venous and equilibrium phases. With longer scanning times, the patient may take a short breath before repeating the sequences.

Postprocessing Techniques

Three-dimensional contrast-enhanced MRA produces a contiguous volume of data. In most body MRA studies, the volume is asymmetrical (e.g., $400 \times 300 \times 64$). The slice is typically viewed interactively using a computer workstation. Thin multiplanar reformatting (MPR) can be done,[1,28] and 1- to 2-mm slices can be viewed in multiple planes (axial, sagittal, and oblique).[29,30]

Because the thin sections do not display the entire vessel, the maximum-intensity projection (MIP) processing technique is often used.[31,32] With this algorithm, the user first selects the volume or portion of the volume to be evaluated. The algorithm then generates rays perpendicular to the viewing plane, records the maximum intensity of any voxel encountered along that ray, and assigns that maximum value to the corresponding pixel in the output image. This results in images similar in appearance to conventional angiograms.

The MIP algorithm has some limitations. A major problem occurs when stationary tissue or structures within stationary tissue have a higher signal intensity than the vessels of interest. This can occur in the presence of crossing vessels, hemorrhage, fat, metallic susceptibility artifacts, or motion artifacts. This results in mapping of these extra signals into the projection image, producing a discontinuity in vessel signal that mimics vessel stenosis.[1] Reducing the thickness of the MIP subvolume to exclude as much extraneous tissue as possible can mitigate this limitation. Underestimation of vessel diameter is another limitation of the technique.

Subtraction techniques are also employed to improve vessel visibility. This is performed by a complex subtraction of precontrast and postcontrast raw data sets[33,34] and is routinely used in contrast-enhanced MRA of the extremities.

Three-dimensional volume rendering is another postprocessing technique that allows separation of overlapping structures. In many instances, this is preferred over standard MIP images.

CLINICAL APPLICATIONS

Extracranial Carotid Arteries

The carotid arteries can be well seen with contrast-enhanced MRA (Fig. 16-1). The short circulation time of the carotid circulation (4 to 6 seconds) makes timing critical; otherwise, venous overlap of the images results. Both long and short imaging times have been used to overcome this problem.

High-resolution imaging with short TE is recommended. A major problem that impedes accurate stenosis assessment is the occurrence of high-speed turbulent jets at the site of stenosis. Specialized coils are recommended. The origins of the vessels from the aorta should be included in the imaging plane. Numerous studies have shown a high degree of correlation between stenosis measurement with contrast-enhanced MRA and digital subtraction angiography.[35-40]

Thoracic Aorta

Contrast-enhanced MRA is now routinely used to evaluate the thoracic aorta. It is the standard of practice for following

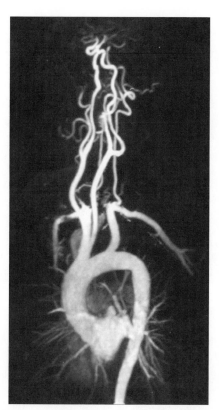

FIGURE 16–1 • Contrast-enhanced MRA of normal carotid arteries. Sagittal oblique MIP of the thoracic aorta shows normal carotid arteries.

the status of dissections and monitoring aneurysm enlargement (Fig. 16-2). Imaging is usually performed in the oblique sagittal plane or coronal plane. In dissections, the origins of the brachiocephalic vessels should be included. A phased array body coil is recommended when the aneurysm is confined to the thoracic aorta. Both the ascending and descending aortas are evaluated. A full evaluation of the aorta should include multiplanar cardiac-gated black blood imaging of the aortic wall to detect intramural hematoma.

Abdominal Aorta and Pelvic Vessels

Contrast-enhanced MRA is most often performed in this region to evaluate for aortic dissection or abdominal aortic aneurysm or as part of an evaluation for peripheral artery disease. The images are acquired in the coronal plane using a phased array body coil. A localizer image is obtained first in the sagittal plane, preferably with breath-holding, to determine that the entire volume of the aneurysm will be in the field of view. It is important to note that vessel calcifications are typically not seen with MRA (see Fig. 16-2A).

Renal Arteries

Renal contrast-enhanced MRA is performed similarly to an abdominal aortic study, although a thinner coronal slab may be used, allowing decreased slice thickness or acquisition time. High-resolution imaging is preferred. A true slice thickness of less than 2.4 mm is recommended, and breath-holding is critical. Otherwise, distal renal artery branches and accessory renal arteries may be difficult to visualize. Typically, renal arteries

can be seen out to the interlobar branches. Review of the raw data is critical for full assessment (Fig. 16-3).

Small intrarenal branches are not well seen with current techniques. If resolution is not adequate or if motion occurs, fibromuscular dysplasia may not be detected. Examination of the source images can provide information regarding renal size and cortical thickness. A transit time can be calculated for each kidney. Renal transplant arteries can also be seen with contrast-enhanced MRA. Newer techniques that shorten acquisition time and reduce motion artifacts should result in improved visualization of the renal arteries. Although there are multiple studies describing the value of renal artery MRA, it is used largely as a screening tool. In hypertensive patients, if the renal arteries are normal, conventional arteriography is usually deferred. If an abnormality is detected, conventional arteriography is usually performed, at which time angioplasty or stent placement can be done (Fig. 16-4). Using conventional angiography as a reference standard, the reported sensitivity and specificity of contrast-enhanced MRA for diagnosing renal artery stenosis are 88% to 100% and 70% to 100%, respectively.[41]

Mesenteric Vessels

The proximal portions of the mesenteric arteries are usually well seen on renal or abdominal MRA. Contrast-enhanced MRA is used often to evaluate for mesenteric ischemia due to proximal vessel stenosis or occlusion. Evaluation of the source images and MPR are useful.[42-45] Distal small vessels are usually not visualized well enough to exclude distal small vessel disease. Thin slices are recommended.

Portal Venous System

Contrast-enhanced MRA provides high-quality images of the portal system and hepatic veins. Following arterial phase images, delayed acquisitions are obtained that routinely show the portal and hepatic veins.[45,46] Portal vein thrombosis and collaterals are also seen (Fig. 16-5). Again, a review of the source data and three-dimensional volume rendering are necessary.

Peripheral Vessels

Initially, contrast-enhanced MRA of the runoff vessels of the lower extremities was limited by the restricted field of view of MR scanners.[47] The field of view of most scanners, typically 400 to 500 mm, required repeat injections to cover the entire lower extremity. This was typically performed by first imaging the smaller vessels of the calf, followed by repeat injections while positioning over the knee and thigh. A complete abdominal aorta and peripheral runoff study could not be performed in one setting owing to soft tissue enhancement from extracellular gadolinium contrast agent. Newer scanners are equipped with a moving table, which allows image acquisition similar to that of conventional arteriography, whereby a single bolus of contrast can be followed and imaged multiple times as it travels from the aorta to the feet (Figs. 16-6 to 16-8). Newer scanners also permit whole-body MRA (Fig. 16-9).

It is important to note that optimal visualization of peripheral vessels requires that they be imaged before venous enhancement occurs and obscures arterial vessels. In addition,

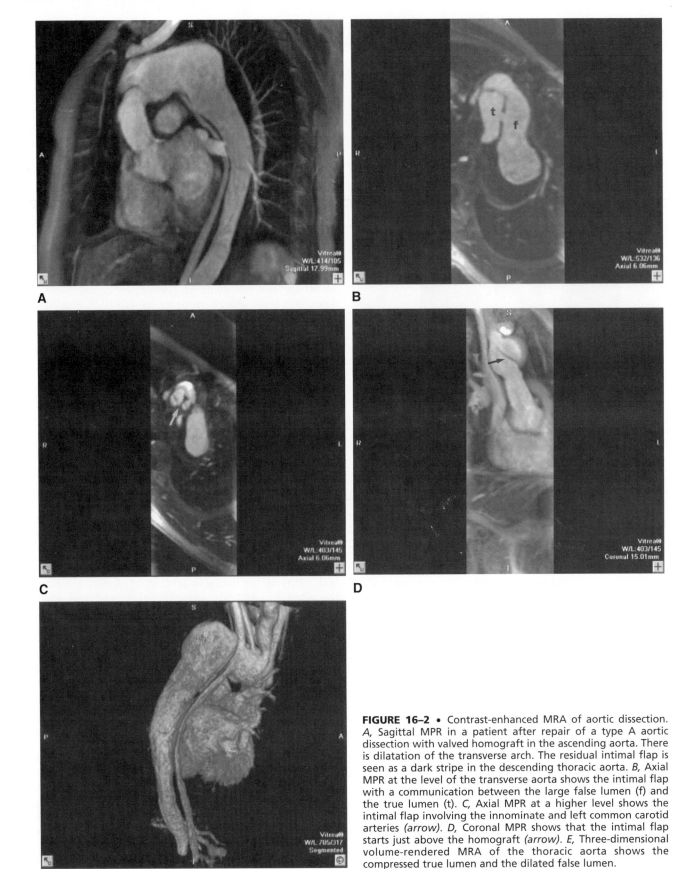

FIGURE 16–2 • Contrast-enhanced MRA of aortic dissection. *A*, Sagittal MPR in a patient after repair of a type A aortic dissection with valved homograft in the ascending aorta. There is dilatation of the transverse arch. The residual intimal flap is seen as a dark stripe in the descending thoracic aorta. *B*, Axial MPR at the level of the transverse aorta shows the intimal flap with a communication between the large false lumen (f) and the true lumen (t). *C*, Axial MPR at a higher level shows the intimal flap involving the innominate and left common carotid arteries *(arrow)*. *D*, Coronal MPR shows that the intimal flap starts just above the homograft *(arrow)*. *E*, Three-dimensional volume-rendered MRA of the thoracic aorta shows the compressed true lumen and the dilated false lumen.

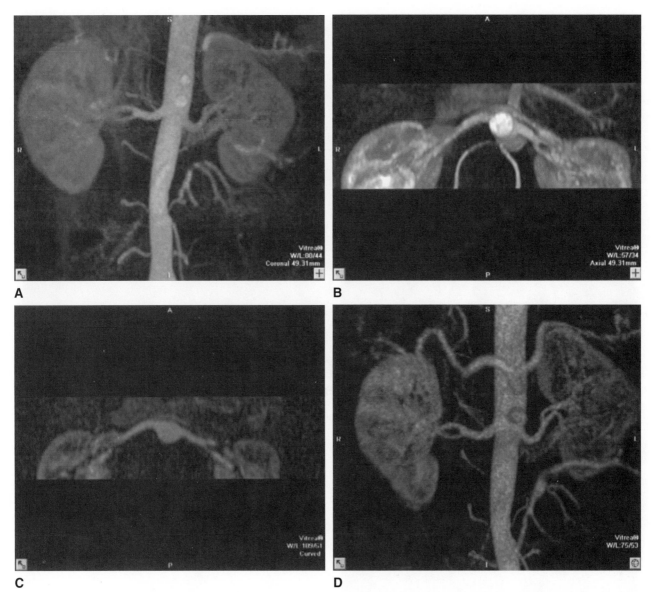

FIGURE 16–3 • Contrast-enhanced MRA of normal renal arteries. *A,* MIP of renal arteries shows normal right and left renal arteries. A plaque is seen in the descending aorta. *B,* Thick-slab MIP in the axial plane shows the origins of the right and left renal arteries. *C,* Curved MPR allows visualization of the interlobar arteries. *D,* Three-dimensional volume-rendered image affords visualization of the right and left renal arteries and the proximal interlobar branches.

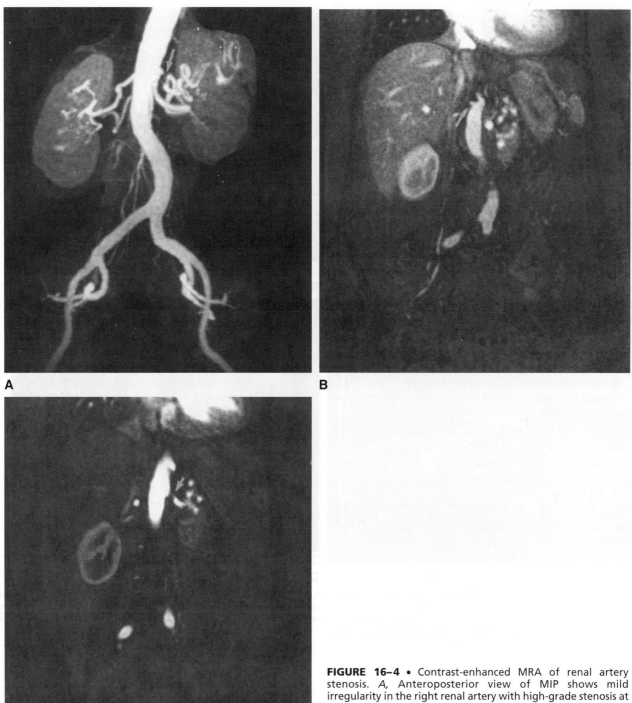

FIGURE 16–4 • Contrast-enhanced MRA of renal artery stenosis. *A,* Anteroposterior view of MIP shows mild irregularity in the right renal artery with high-grade stenosis at the origin of the left renal artery. *B,* Review of raw data shows the origin of the right renal artery *(arrow). C,* Adjacent slice of raw data shows high-grade stenosis at the origin of the left renal artery *(arrow).* Inspection of raw data slices from the slab volume is often necessary for accurate diagnosis.

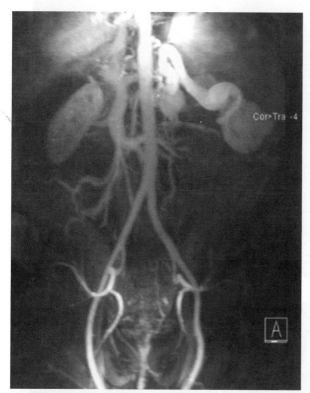

FIGURE 16–5 • Venous phase of abdominal contrast-enhanced MRA. The superior mesenteric vein and portal vein are seen. Large dilated varices are seen in the splenic bed draining into the left renal vein, producing a spontaneous splenorenal shunt.

because they are smaller than pelvic vessels, calf vessels must be imaged with parameters that afford higher resolution. Typically, with bolus-chase techniques, MRI is performed faster and with lower resolution in the pelvis and thigh, and the infusion rate is low to ensure a long bolus. Injection rates of 0.3 to 2.0 mL/second for 30 to 60 seconds may be used. Subtraction improves image quality. The issue of venous enhancement is related not only to imaging delay and contrast injection but also to the underlying disease process. In general, patients with claudication usually do not exhibit venous enhancement until very late, whereas patients with inflammatory processes, such as cellulitis or venous ulcers, tend to have early venous enhancement. The examination must therefore be tailored to the patient. This has prompted some imagers to perform two injections; the first injection targets the lower station, and the second injection evaluates the upper and middle stations. This technique has proved to be advantageous.[48]

Magnetic Resonance Venography

MR venography of the pelvis and extremities can also be obtained during the late phase of a contrast-enhanced MR angiogram. Axial two-dimensional time-of-flight imaging has been used to evaluate venous structures in the upper extremities and venous thrombus in the lower extremities. However, with these studies, vessels parallel to the imaging plane undergo "in-plane saturation," resulting in signal dropout; this can be problematic when evaluating the great veins of the chest because the subclavian and axillary veins are in-plane during an axial acquisition performed to evaluate the superior vena cava. Two-dimensional time-of-flight imaging may also be degraded by patient motion, magnetic field inhomogeneity, and susceptibility artifacts. Nonetheless, it is useful in evaluating the pelvic veins and inferior vena cava.[49,50]

Contrast-enhanced MRA overcomes many of the limitations of two-dimensional time-of-flight imaging and is particularly useful for evaluating the veins of the upper extremity, superior vena cava, jugular veins, inferior vena cava, and renal veins. These structures can be imaged by obtaining delayed acquisition images on a standard contrast-enhanced MRA study (Figs. 16-10 and 16-11). The initial acquisition is timed for the first pass through the arterial system, and multiple acquisitions are obtained following the arterial phase. These late images usually have both arterial and venous enhancement. A selective venous study can be obtained by subtracting the arterial phase study from a mixed venous-arterial phase study.[51,52] Direct venography of upper extremity veins can also be performed by direct injection of a diluted or full-strength gadolinium contrast agent.[53,54]

Newer techniques, such as true FISP, a steady-state gradient echo sequence, have also been used with some success to evaluate the arterial and venous systems. A rapidly acquired stack of true FISP images provides thin-section viewing of arteries and veins, which are seen as bright blood.

Source data and postprocessing techniques are important in the assessment of venous thrombus, because low-signal-intensity thrombus may not be seen with MIP. The differentiation of acute and chronic thrombus may be difficult with two-dimensional time-of-flight images. With acute thrombus, contrast-enhanced images may show dense periadventitial enhancement.[55] This enhancement is usually not seen with chronic clots and vessel size reductions. At our center, venous mapping using contrast-enhanced MRA is routine. It is also useful for quantifying clot burden and determining the presence and size of collaterals. This information is helpful in assessing alternative access sites in patients with venous obstruction from long-term central venous catheters. Contrast-enhanced MRA can also differentiate bland from tumor thrombus in patients with neoplasms that extend into the venous system. Tumor thrombus enhancement distinguishes it from bland thrombus that does not enhance. At our institution, MR venography is routinely used to evaluate the patency of upper extremity veins, jugular veins, and the superior vena cava.

FUTURE DIRECTIONS—NEW CONTRAST AGENTS

New gadolinium chelate agents formulated at 1.0 M (e.g., gadobutrol), rather than the current 0.5 M, and agents with higher relaxivity owing to weak protein interactions (e.g., gadobenate dimeglumine) demonstrate greater intravascular signal than do conventional agents.[56-58] These agents provide better visualization of both large and small vessels. Intravascular blood pool agents are under development, and two main types are currently being evaluated. One type (e.g., MS-325) has a strong affinity for serum albumin,[59-61] and the other type (e.g., gadomer-17) is a macromolecular agent whose size precludes rapid extravasation.[62] Full exploitation of these intravascular agents will necessitate sophisticated subtraction techniques to separate the arteries from the veins.

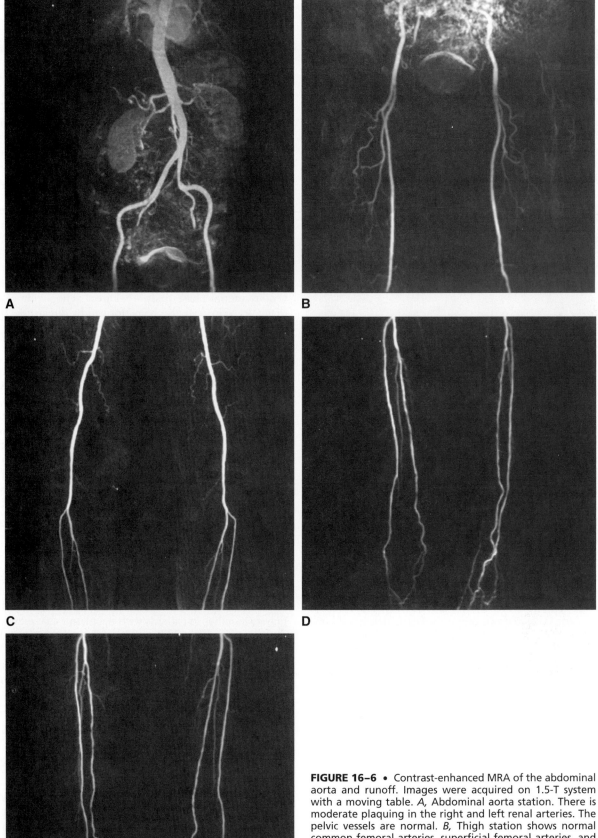

FIGURE 16–6 • Contrast-enhanced MRA of the abdominal aorta and runoff. Images were acquired on 1.5-T system with a moving table. *A,* Abdominal aorta station. There is moderate plaquing in the right and left renal arteries. The pelvic vessels are normal. *B,* Thigh station shows normal common femoral arteries, superficial femoral arteries, and deep femoral arteries. *C,* Knee station shows normal popliteal arteries, anterior tibial arteries, and tibioperoneal trunk. The proximal posterior tibial arteries and peroneal arteries are seen. *D,* Calf station. Anteroposterior projection shows three-vessel runoff bilaterally, including views of the plantar arch. *E,* Calf station oblique view allows separation of the runoff vessels.

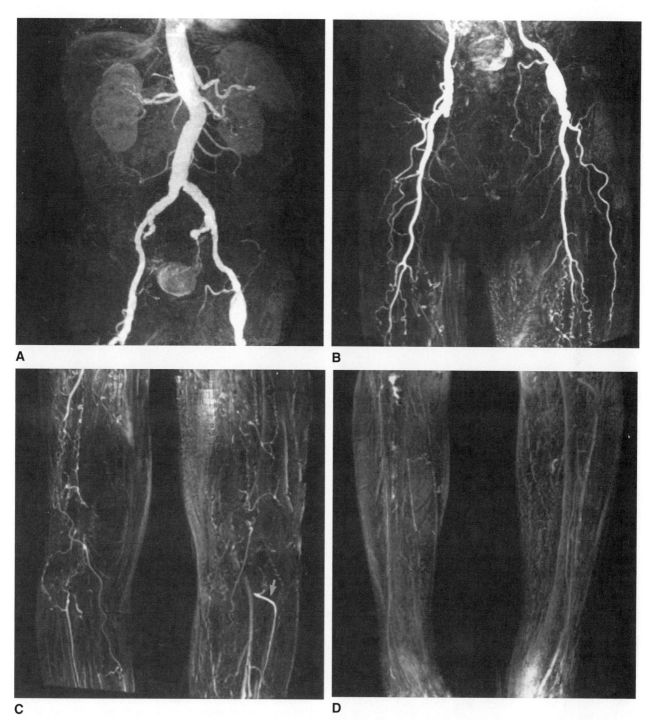

FIGURE 16–7 • Contrast-enhanced MRA abdominal aortogram and runoff in a patient with severe peripheral vascular disease. *A,* Abdominal station shows atherosclerotic changes in the common iliac vessels. An aneurysm is seen in the left common iliac artery. *B,* Thigh station shows occlusion of the right and left superficial femoral arteries, with bilateral enlarged deep femoral collaterals. *C,* Knee station shows severe occlusive disease. There is no filling of either popliteal artery. On the right, collaterals reconstitute a segment of the anterior tibial artery *(arrow)* and a segment of the posterior tibial artery. On the left, a segment of the proximal anterior tibial artery is reconstituted by collaterals. *D,* Calf station. On the right, a diffusely diseased anterior tibial artery is faintly seen. An isolated segment of the posterior tibial artery is identified. On the left, a portion of the anterior tibial artery is faintly seen, and a small portion of the peroneal artery is identified *(arrow)*.

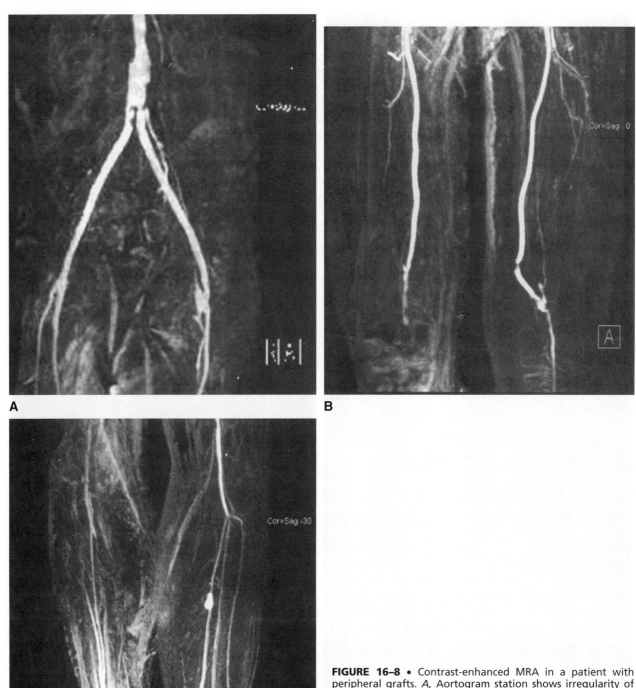

FIGURE 16–8 • Contrast-enhanced MRA in a patient with peripheral grafts. *A,* Aortogram station shows irregularity of the distal abdominal aorta and a patent aortobifemoral graft. A filling defect is seen at the origin of the right limb of the graft. *B,* Thigh station shows bilateral superficial femoral artery grafts. The left graft has a tight stenosis proximal to the distal anastomosis. The right graft is occluded distally. *C,* Calf station on the right shows poor filling of a portion of the anterior tibial artery. On the left, the popliteal artery is patent, with three-vessel runoff. A small aneurysm is seen in the posterior tibial artery.

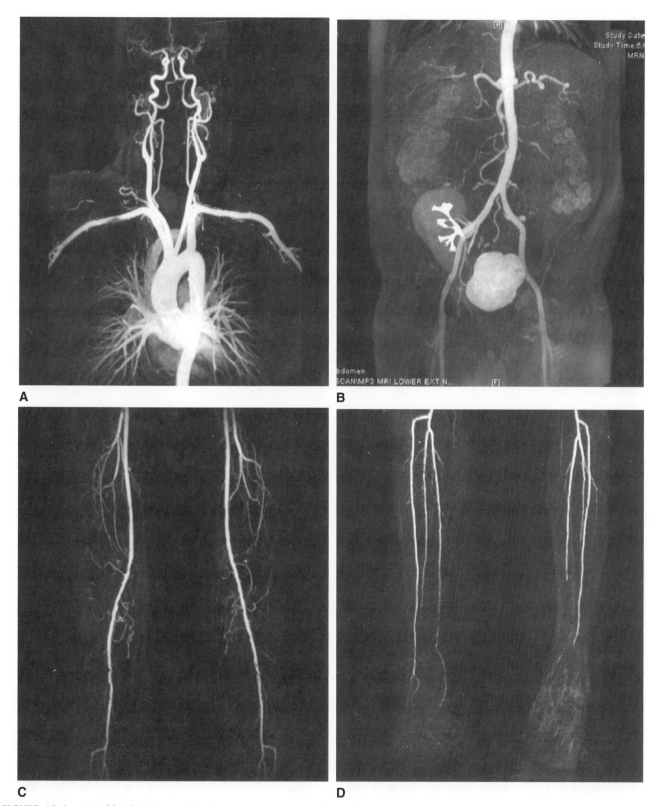

FIGURE 16–9 • Total-body MRA. *A,* The thoracic aorta is normal. *B,* Abdominal aorta and pelvis station show right renal transplant. *C,* Thigh and knee station show mild atherosclerotic plaquing in the superficial femoral arteries. *D,* Calf station. Timing is too early on the left, with poor filling of the left calf vessels.

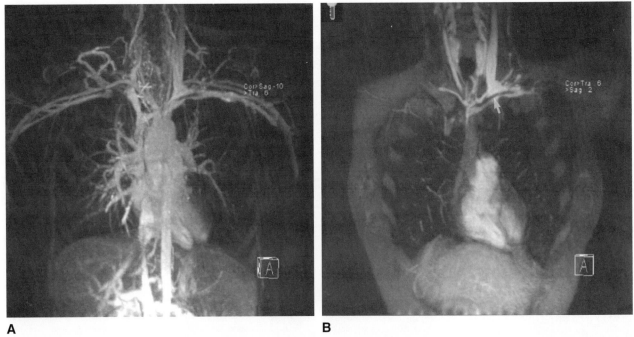

A   **B**

FIGURE 16–10 • Contrast-enhanced MRA venogram of the upper extremities. *A,* Venouse phase MIP shows occlusion of the right internal jugular vein with multiple collaterals. There is localized occlusion of the right subclavian vein. A dark linear structure is seen in the left subclavian vein and superior vena cava. This represents a catheter. *B,* Thin MIP shows the catheter to better advantage *(arrow)*.

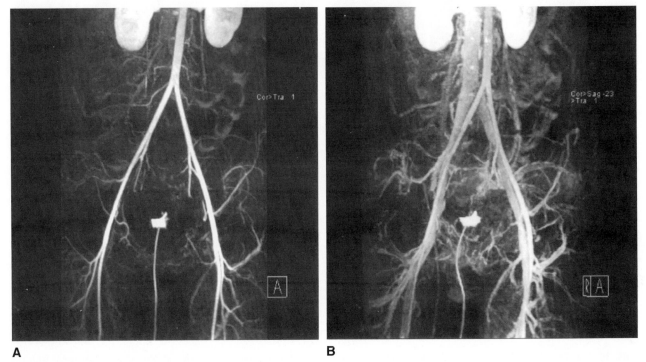

A   **B**

FIGURE 16–11 • Contrast-enhanced MRA pelvic venogram. *A,* Arterial phase shows normal arterial vessels. *B,* Delayed phase shows good filling of pelvic veins and inferior vena cava.

Multidetector Row Computed Tomography Angiography (MDCT CTA)

The widespread use of CT for imaging the vascular system has been made possible by the development of multidetector row computed tomography (MDCT) scanners. This outgrowth of spiral (helical) CT permits the rapid acquisition of data and increased data collection with each rotation. Initial spiral scanners were single-slice scanners, but the development of multidetector row arrays, faster gantry rotation times, stronger x-ray tubes, and improved reconstruction algorithms has resulted in shorter image acquisition times and improved volume coverage. The three fundamental improvements—speed, volume coverage, and section thickness—are important for CTA, making it an excellent noninvasive imaging technique. The speed of acquisition is such that the contrast bolus can be imaged as it traverses the arterial system. The evolution of 4-, 8-, 16-, 32-, and now 64-slice MDCT scanners has resulted in incremental increases in volume coverage and spatial and temporal resolution and reductions in scan time. Scanners with an even greater number of detector rows are currently under development. With a 4-row scanner, the entire thoracoabdomial aorta and iliac arteries can be imaged in 15 to 30 seconds using a 2.5-mm section thickness throughout the entire scan volume. With a 16-row CT scanner, the same anatomic territory can be imaged in 8 to 10 seconds using a 1.25-mm section thickness. CTA is used to image not only large vessels, such as the thoracic and abdominal aortas, but also the major visceral branches of the abdominal aorta, the carotids, and the pulmonary arteries. With faster scans, MDCT now permits the entire abdominal aorta and lower extremity runoff to be imaged in a single, high-spatial-resolution scan. Using a 1.25-mm collimation and a table speed of 27.5 seconds (1.6-mm effective section thickness), a distance of 1300 mm can be covered in less than 30 seconds. Sixteen-slice MDCT permits 100 cm to be covered in 21.4 seconds, and with the 64-slice scanner, 153 cm can be covered in approximately 15.6 seconds. Most scanners used in vascular work have 4, 8, 16, or 64 row detectors. Although not every case requires the use of a 16-row scanner to achieve diagnostic images, it is generally accepted that 16-row scanners result in more scans being diagnostic, particularly when large anatomic coverage or small vessel detail is required. Experience with 64-slice scanners is still limited.

The speed of multislice CT shortens breath-hold examination times and reduces the amount of contrast medium needed to achieve consistent high-quality vascular enhancement.[63-66] The speed of MDCT allows large-volume coverage in a short time. This image acquisition speed can also be used to increase spatial resolution with the acquisition of thinner slices in order to increase the flexibility of a data set. High-resolution imaging requires that thin-slice collimation data be reconstructed to produce a near-isotropic data set of thin, overlapping, transverse images. The 16-row scanner permits the acquisition of 0.625- to 0.75-mm nominal slice thicknesses with nearly isotropic voxels with almost equal in-plane and through-plane resolution. Acquisition of extensive volumes with submillimeter resolution generates nearly isotropic data that can be arranged in arbitrary imaging planes with the same high spatial resolution as the original axial section. The acquisition of high-resolution data enhances the image quality of two-dimensional displays and three-dimensional volume rendering.[67-72]

The rapid acquisition time of MDCT scans allows image acquisition during a breath-hold. Image noise is an important consideration, particularly when images are to be reviewed with three-dimensional volume rendering. The visibility of a structure in the body is dependent on the ratio of that structure and its immediate background to the noise (contrast-to-noise ratio). During CTA, this ratio is affected by the amount of arterial opacification and the noise in the scan. As section thickness is halved, image noise increases by approximately 40%. The goal of decreasing section thickness in order to visualize small blood vessels and to obtain better detail in large vessels must be balanced with the goal of reducing image noise. Fortunately, image noise is influenced by other factors that do not affect spatial resolution. These include x-ray current and potential and the reconstruction algorithm or kernel used. Depending on the scanner, the pitch can influence scan noise indirectly. According to International Electrotechnical Commission (IEC) specifications, pitch (p) equals the table feed per rotation divided by the total width of the collimated beam. It shows whether data acquisition occurs with gaps (p > 1) or with overlap in the transverse direction (p < 1). Greater tube current is required to compensate for reconstruction strategies that avoid an increase in the effective section thickness as the pitch is increased. For many acquisitions, an increase in pitch will not affect noise. If the maximum tube current is selected for a scan with a given pitch value, and the pitch value is increased, no more current can be supplied to compensate, and the noise will increase.

With MDCT, slice thickness is a reconstruction parameter rather than an acquisition parameter. The narrowest section thickness that can be reconstructed is dependent on the width of the detector groups. Images can be reconstructed at thicker intervals. When images are acquired with thin sections, as long as the raw data are saved, thicker sections can be reconstructed, and the data set that provides the best diagnostic information can be used.

As noted earlier, images with 0.625- to 0.75-mm nominal thickness can be acquired with the 16-row scanner With the 64-slice MDCT, pitch-independent visualization of 0.4-mm isotropic voxels is possible. Although slice thickness of this degree is not necessary for all CT studies, it enhances visualization of small vessels in the central nervous system, coronary and mesenteric vessels, and vessels of the calf.

CONTRAST MEDIUM ADMINISTRATION

Iodinated contrast material is used for CTA. This is the same contrast material used for conventional arteriography and therefore presents the same risks of idiosyncratic allergic reaction and nephrotoxicity. Optimized vessel opacification is an important aspect of CTA because with each new scanner generation, acquisition time decreases and correct synchronization of CT acquisition relative to arterial enhancement becomes more critical.[73] Image acquisition techniques are modified depending on the number of detector rows in the scanner. With 16-slice MDCT, the entire chest, abdomen, and pelvis can be imaged in less than 15 seconds. With the 16-slice scanner, care must be taken not to outrun the contrast bolus when imaging the peripheral vessels. With MDCT, the scanning delay following an injection of contrast needs to be timed relative to the patient's contrast transit time (from intravenous injection site to the arterial region of interest). This transit time can be obtained with the injection of a small test bolus. Many scanners have this capability built into the system. When contrast is injected, a series of low-dose scans is acquired while the attenuation in the region of interest is monitored. The transit time equals the time when a predetermined enhancement threshold is reached (e.g., 100 Hounsfield units). The minimum trigger delay to start the CT acquisition after the threshold is reached depends on the scanner (range, 2 to 8 seconds) and on the longitudinal distance between the monitoring series and the starting position of the CT series.[74] Automatic triggering is used, coupled with a dual-head contrast injector that permits a saline flush. The saline flush reduces the total contrast used by eliminating contrast left in the tubing; it also reduces perivenous streak artifacts by removing dense contrast material from the brachiocephalic veins and superior vena cava in thoracic and cardiac CT scans. In routine clinical practice, the injection duration should match the acquisition time. With 4-row scanners, injection duration is usually equal to the image acquisition time. With 8- and 16-slice scanners, the injection duration may be longer. Faster acquisitions require less contrast material volume. Long acquisition times benefit from biphasic injections, with an initially high injection rate followed by a lower one, because they lead to a more uniform enhancement plateau. To ensure adequate vessel opacification with fast MDCT acquisitions, the iodine administration needs to be increased. This is done by increasing the injection flow rate or using contrast material with a higher iodine concentration.

RADIATION DOSE

A variety of measurements have been used to measure or describe CTA dose. Studies using 4-slice CTA have shown increased effective collective doses compared with multislice CT. There are few data on 16-row scanners using dose-optimized protocols. In dose-optimized protocols using tube current modulation, the dose is delivered according to the attenuation of the tissues scanned, and the dose is reduced over thinner areas. Depending on scan volume, the dose may be reduced by 10% to 30%.[75] At least two studies have shown an average reduction in dose using the 16-row scanner as compared with 4-row multislice CT.[75] Nonetheless, the radiation dose of CTA is lower than that of conventional angiography.

IMAGE RECONSTRUCTION

The large data sets obtained with 4-, 8-, and 16-row multislice CT require three-dimensional workstation viewing. Typically, comprehensive image analysis is performed, consisting of rapidly scrolling all axial images on a dedicated workstation and performing three-dimensional reconstructions using a variety of algorithms. Postprocessing techniques consist of MPR, MIP, volume rendering, and shaded surface displays. In vascular imaging, heavy calcifications and intravascular stents may impede luminal visualization, but review of the axial transverse images and longitudinal or curved MPR usually permits the evaluation of the vessel lumen.

APPLICATIONS

MDCT angiography (CTA) is used for imaging most major vessels and even some smaller vessels in the body.

Carotid Arteries

CTA provides high-quality images of the carotid arteries and permits visualization of carotid plaque. CTA with MPR provides views of the plaque and vessel lumen, making it a useful technique for assessing carotid artery stenosis.[76-78] Quantification of plaque is feasible. The combined use of noncontrast cranial CT with CT perfusion imaging and CTA of the cerebral vessels is safe and feasible,[79] and such a protocol can facilitate the triage of patients with suspected carotid disease.

Pulmonary Arteries

CTA is now routinely used as the first-line imaging technique to assess for pulmonary artery embolism. It has largely replaced conventional invasive arteriography for diagnosis. A main advantage of the technique is that in addition to having a high positive and negative predictive value, it reliably demonstrates alternative or additional disease causing the patient's symptoms. In the past, the major limitation of CTA was inadequate visualization of the peripheral lung bed.[80] Newer MDCT scanners, such as the 16-row scanner, cover the entire thorax with submillimeter slices in one short breath-hold (10 seconds), with near-isotropic voxels allowing visualization of the proximal and distal vessels.[75] Scans can be acquired with high resolution (thin 0.5- and 1-mm collimation), or in severely dyspneic patients, a faster protocol with wider collimation (2.5 and 1.5 mm) can be acquired. The optimal protocol depends on the equipment used.[75,80-82]

MDCT CTA has been used for the combined study of the pulmonary arteries and the deep veins of the legs using the same injected bolus of contrast.[83] Because of the high positive and negative predictive value of CTA of the pulmonary arteries and the added radiation dose required to study the legs, the current recommendation is that if pulmonary embolism is present, the deep venous system should be evaluated with ultrasonography, except in carefully selected patients such as those with suspected involvement of the inferior vena cava.[84,85]

CTA is useful for assessing the presence of other vascular anomalies of the pulmonary arteries, such as pulmonary artery arteriovenous malformations. It is also used for mapping and evaluating abnormalities of the pulmonary veins.

Thoracic Aorta

CT has long been used to evaluate the thoracic aorta. With current 8- and 16-slice scanners, the entire thoracic and abdominal aorta can be imaged with near-isotropic resolution (Fig. 16-12). The traditional helical CT indications for imaging the thoracic aorta have been re-emphasized and strengthened with the introduction of MDCT.[86] The availability, speed, and ease of modern MDCT make it the imaging technique of choice for the diagnosis of acute aortic pathology such as aortic trauma, dissection, intramural hematoma, and aneurysm (Fig. 16-13; see color plate).[87]

MDCT CTA is faster, more readily available, and less operator dependent than echocardiography, and it provides more

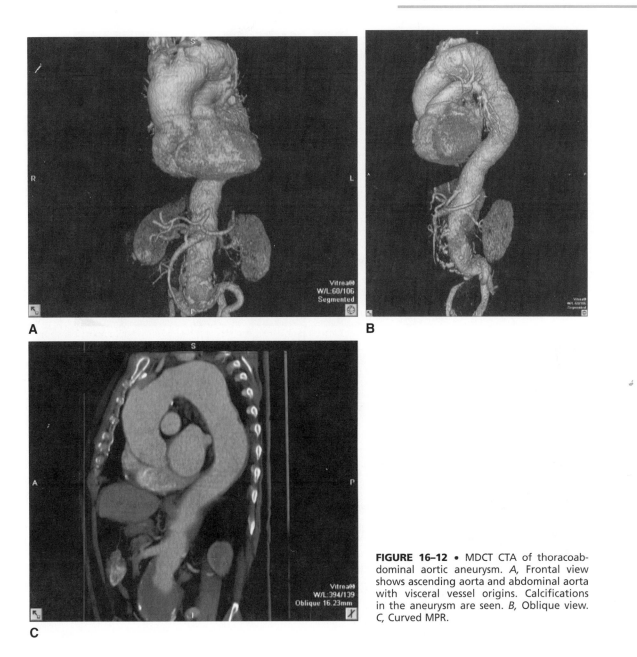

FIGURE 16–12 • MDCT CTA of thoracoab-dominal aortic aneurysm. *A,* Frontal view shows ascending aorta and abdominal aorta with visceral vessel origins. Calcifications in the aneurysm are seen. *B,* Oblique view. *C,* Curved MPR.

complete organ visualization. It is faster than both MRA and conventional arteriography. It is more suitable than MRA for unstable patients, and it is less invasive than conventional arteriography. The ability to perform multiplanar reformatting and the ability to see both the lumen of the aorta and the wall are distinct advantages over conventional arteriography. Imaging of the thoracic aorta typically is done with noncontrast images of the thorax to identify regions of hyperdensity within the aortic wall suggesting intramural hematoma. This may be performed with wider collimation and slice thicknesses of 5 to 7 mm. Narrow-slice collimation is necessary for CTA and requires thin slices of 1 to 2.5 mm to provide adequate spatial resolution and image quality for postprocessing.[75] In cases of aortic root pathology, electrocardiographic synchronization of the scan acquisition using either prospective or, more commonly, retrospective electrocardiographic gating removes cardiac motion artifact, allowing evaluation of this region.

Abdominal Aorta and Iliac Arteries

The volume coverage capabilities of MDCT have had a major impact on imaging of the abdominal aorta. With 8- and 16-row scanners, the entire abdominal aorta and iliac vessels can be covered with near-isotropic resolution (Fig. 16-14; see color plate for Fig. 16-14C). The high scan speed allows the use of less contrast material.[88]

In the abdomen, traditional indications for CTA include diagnosis and surveillance of aneurysms, preoperative evaluation of endograft placement and postplacement monitoring, and tumor diagnosis and staging (Fig. 16-15). Other routine uses include evaluation of abnormalities of the mesenteric vessels,[89-91] renal artery stenosis, and portal venous system abnormalities. MDCT CTA is now routinely used in the evaluation of potential renal donors[92] and liver donors[93-95] (Fig. 16-16). It is also used in the assessment of patients

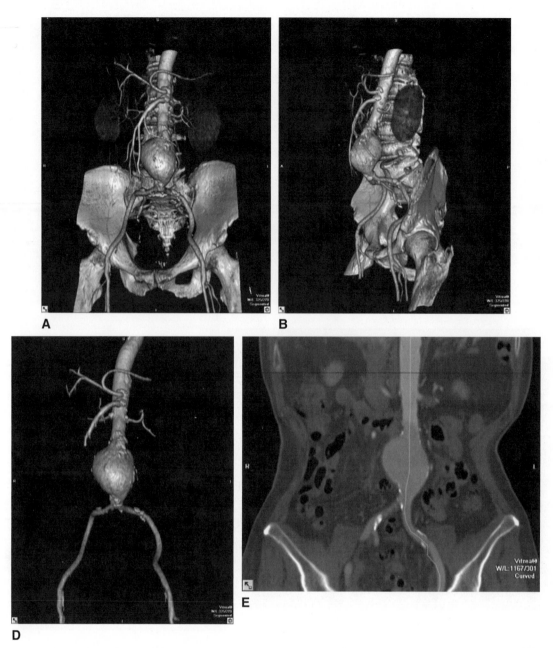

FIGURE 16–14 • MDCT CTA of infrarenal abdominal aortic aneurysm. *A,* Three-dimensional volume-rendered image of the abdominal aorta and branch vessels. The celiac artery and superior mesenteric arteries are seen. The infrarenal saccular aneurysm extends to just above the aortic bifurcation. *B,* Oblique view of the aorta. *C,* Partial removal of bone shows the renal arteries and superior mesenteric artery branches. See color plate. *D,* Images with full bone and soft tissue removal show the aneurysm. Note that vessel calcifications are well seen on the CTA images. *E,* Curved MPR allows measurement of vessel diameter.

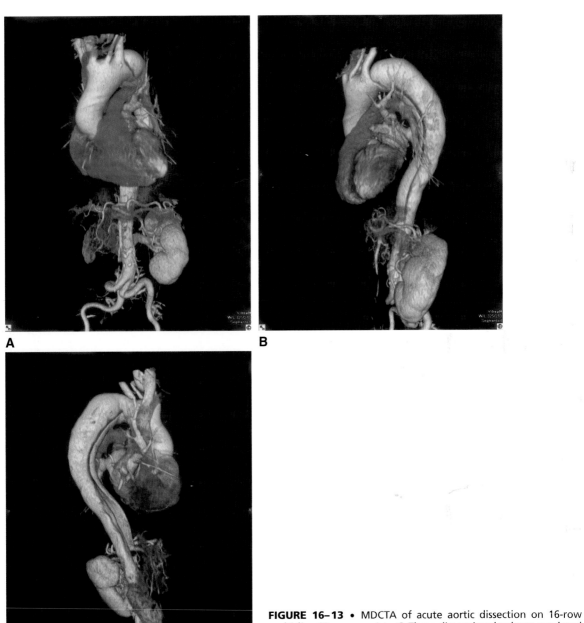

A

B

C

FIGURE 16–13 • MDCTA of acute aortic dissection on 16-row multislice CT scanner. *A* to *C*, Three-dimensional volume-rendered images of type B aortic dissection showing the intimal flap and the true and false lumens. Note the clear delineation of the origins of the major branch vessels.

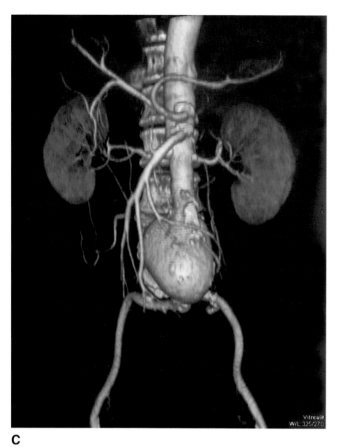

C

FIGURE 16–14 • *C,* Partial removal of bone shows the renal arteries and superior mesenteric artery branches.

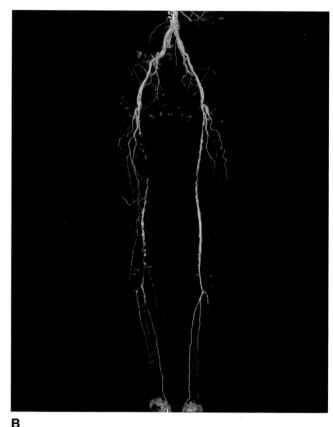

B

FIGURE 16–18 • *B,* Three-dimensional volume rendering may also be performed.

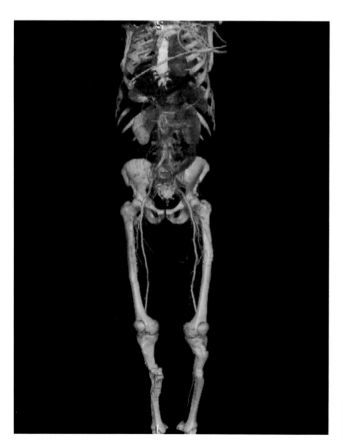

FIGURE 16–19 • Total-body MRA. Imaging of the entire body is possible using a 16- or 64-row MDCT scanners. Extensive postprocessing is required to remove bone and soft tissue.

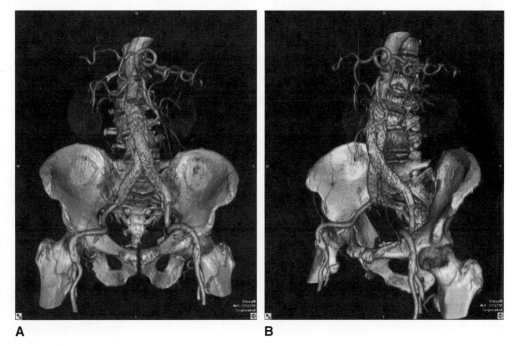

FIGURE 16–15 • MDCT CTA of aortic endograft. *A,* Abdominal study shows a bifurcated endograft in the aorta. *B,* Oblique view shows that the limbs of the endograft are crossed; no obstruction is seen.

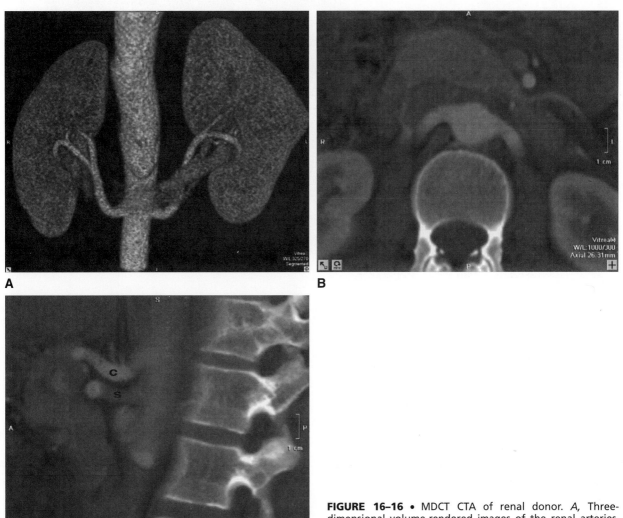

FIGURE 16–16 • MDCT CTA of renal donor. *A,* Three-dimensional volume-rendered images of the renal arteries. *B,* MPR of the origin of the renal arteries. *C,* Note that the origins of the celiac (c) and superior mesenteric (s) arteries are well seen on sagittal MPR.

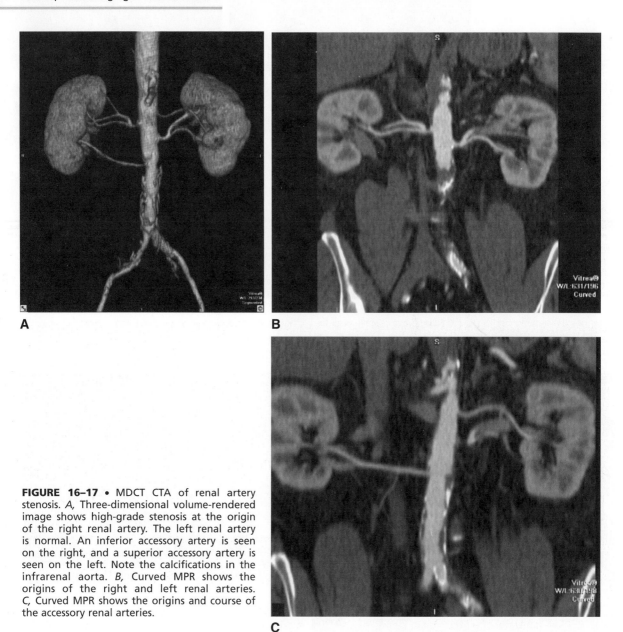

FIGURE 16–17 • MDCT CTA of renal artery stenosis. *A,* Three-dimensional volume-rendered image shows high-grade stenosis at the origin of the right renal artery. The left renal artery is normal. An inferior accessory artery is seen on the right, and a superior accessory artery is seen on the left. Note the calcifications in the infrarenal aorta. *B,* Curved MPR shows the origins of the right and left renal arteries. *C,* Curved MPR shows the origins and course of the accessory renal arteries.

undergoing liver lesion embolization. The use of thin collimation reduces volume averaging that impedes small vessel visualization; the improved z-axis resolution allows clear assessment of small mesenteric vessels and the degree of renal artery stenosis. Using a 0.5-second MDCT scanner, Willmann and colleagues obtained excellent-quality CT angiograms with 92% sensitivity and 99% specificity for the detection of aortoiliac and renal artery stenosis[89] (Fig. 16-17). The decision to use MRA or CTA to evaluate the abdominal aorta is determined largely by the patient's ability to cooperate, the status of the patient's renal function, and the degree of resolution required for diagnosis.

Peripheral Arteries

Imaging of the peripheral arteries is one of the new and exciting applications of CTA. With multislice CTA, noninvasive imaging of the entire abdominal aorta and runoff vessels can be accomplished with high resolution, providing angiogram-like images of the runoff vessels (Fig. 16-18; see color plate for Fig. 16-18B). Using 4-slice MDCT, high correlation has been found between MDCT results and digital subtraction angiography in the evaluation of lower extremity athereosclerotic vascular disease.[96,97] The ability to see the relationship of vessel calcifications and the ability to perform multiplanar reformatting are advantages that are not available with conventional arteriography. Although disadvantages such as the use of ionizing radiation, the need for iodinated contrast material, and the demanding postprocessing requirements need to be considered, there are circumstances when MDCT CTA is preferred. Calcifications can be seen and provide useful pretreatment information about whether to use angioplasty alone or stents. Patients who have had prior stent placement are better evaluated with CTA, which allows the vessel lumen to be visualized. In some situations, such as preoperative endograft planning, CTA is sufficient and angiography is unnecessary. Careful bolus timing is required. With 4-row scanners, imaging delay may result in venous opacification,

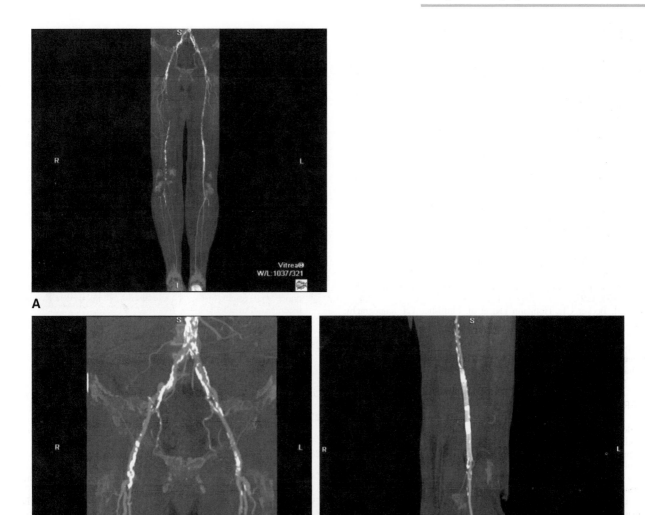

FIGURE 16–18 • MDCT CTA of peripheral runoff. *A,* MIP of peripheral runoff study done on a 16-row scanner. Note full coverage of extremities. *B,* Three-dimensional volume rendering may also be performed. See color plate. *C,* Zoomed images of pelvis station show the dense calcifications in the aorta and pelvic vessels. Occlusion of the right superficial femoral artery (SFA) is seen. *D,* Zoomed MIP images of the left distal SFA show the vascular stents.

obscuring the arteries of the feet. With 16-row scanners, care must be taken not to outstrip the bolus and acquire images too early, before vessels are filled. Sixty-four-slice scanners are available, and 256-row scanners are under development. The rapid rate of CT development has outstripped our ability to perform studies to assess the accuracy of CTA techniques, and formal investigations are awaited.

Magnetic Resonance Angiography versus Computed Tomography Angiography

The determination to use CTA versus MRA is dependent on the nature of the vascular bed to be studied, the information to be obtained, and the status of the patient. MDCT CTA is faster, requires less patient cooperation, and affords higher resolution than MRA, but it involves exposure to ionizing radiation and the use of potentially nephrotoxic iodinated contrast material. MRA has lower resolution, takes longer, and requires more patient cooperation, but it does not involve the use of ionizing radiation, and the gadolinium-containing contrast material is not nephrotoxic. Patients with metallic stents and implants are better evaluated with MDCT CTA because of artifacts that occur with MRA. Patients with pacemakers are not routinely studied with MRA.

Both techniques permit the acquisition of volume data, which can be manipulated with postprocessing techniques. Both techniques provide large data sets, which require workstation viewing. Subtraction techniques currently available with MRA make postprocessing faster than with CTA, which requires time-consuming background and bone removal (Fig. 16-19; see color plate). Both these techniques, however, are noninvasive and are likely to supplant conventional angiography in the diagnosis of vascular disease. As technology improves, other applications of CTA and MRA are anticipated. Improved small vessel visualization is expected, and accurate imaging of other vascular beds such as the coronary arteries is anticipated.

KEY REFERENCES

Binkert C, Baker P, Petersen B, et al: Peripheral vascular disease: Blinded study of dedicated calf MR angiography versus standard bolus-chase MR angiography and film hard-copy angiography. Radiology 232:860-866, 2004.

Fleischmann D: High concentration contrast media in MDCT angiography: Principles and rationale. Eur Radiol 13(Suppl 3):N39-N43, 2003.

Foley WD, Karcaaltincaba M: Computed tomography angiography: Principles and clinical applications. J Comput Assist Tomogr 27(Suppl 1):S23-S30, 2003.

Gotway MB, Dawn SK: Thoracic aorta imaging with multislice CT. Radiol Clin North Am 41:521-543, 2003.

Napoli V, Fleischmann D, Chan FP, et al: Computed tomography angiography: State-of-the-art imaging using multidetector-row technology. J Comput Assist Tomogr 28(Suppl 1):S32-S45, 2004.

Phillips CD, Bubash LA: CT angiography and MR angiography in the evaluation of extracranial carotid vascular disease. Radiol Clin North Am 420:783-798, 2002.

Prince M: Body MR angiography with gadolinium contrast agents. Magn Reson Imaging Clin N Am 4:11-24, 1996.

Prokop M, Shin HO, Schanz A, Schaefer-Prokop CM: Use of maximum intensity projection in CT angiography: A basic review. Radiographics 17:433-451, 1997.

Shoepf UJ, Becker CR, Hofmann LK, et al: Multislice CT angiography. Eur Radiol 13:629-636, 2003.

Willmann JK, Wildermuth S, Pfammatter T, et al: Aortoiliac and renal arteries: Prospective intraindividual comparison of contrast-enhanced three-dimensional MR angiography and multi-detector row CT angiography. Radiology 226:798-811, 2003.

REFERENCES

1. Saloner D: MRA: Principles and display. In Higgins C, Hricak H, Helms C (eds): Magnetic Resonance Imaging of the Body. Philadelphia, Lippincott-Raven, 1997, pp 1345-1368.
2. Gullberg G, Wherli F, Shimakawa A, Simmons M: MR vascular imaging with a fast gradient refocusing pulse sequence and reformatted images from transaxial sections. Radiology 165:241-246, 1997.
3. Doumolin C, Cline H, Souza S, et al: Three-dimensional time-of-flight magnetic resonance angiography using spin saturation. Magn Reson Imaging 11:35-46, 1989.
4. Prince M: Gadolinium-enhanced MR aortography. Radiology 191:155-164, 1994.
5. Prince M: Body MR angiography with gadolinium contrast agents. Magn Reson Imaging Clin N Am 4:11-24, 1996.
6. Bryant D, Payne J, Firmin D, Longmore D: Measurement of flow with NMR imaging using a gradient pulse and phase difference technique. Comput Assist Tomogr 8:588-593, 1984.
7. Gedroye W: Magnetic resonance angiography of renal arteries. Urol Clin North Am 21:201-214, 1994.
8. Bass J, Prince M, Londy F, Chenevert T: Effect of gadolinium on phase-contrast MR angiography of the renal arteries. AJR Am J Roentgenol 168:261-266, 1997.
9. Turski P, Korosec F: Technical features and emerging clinical applications of phase-contrast magnetic resonance angiography. Neuroimaging Clin N Am 2:785, 1992.
10. Moseley M, Sawyer A: Imaging techniques: Pulse sequences. In Higgins C, Hricak H, Helms C (eds): Magnetic Resonance Imaging of the Body. Philadelphia, Lippincott-Raven, 1997, pp 43-69.
11. Wehrli F: Principles of magnetic resonance. In Stark D, Bradley W (eds): Magnetic Resonance Imaging. St. Louis, Mosby-Year Book, 1992, pp 3-20.
12. Prince M, Marashimham D, Stanley J, et al: Breath-hold gadolinium-enhanced MR angiography of the abdominal aorta and its major branches. Radiology 197:785-792, 1995.
13. Snidow J, Johnson S, Harris V, et al: Three-dimensional gadolinium-enhanced MR angiography of the aortoiliac inflow assessment plus renal artery screening in a single breath hold. Radiology 198:725-732, 1996.
14. Leung D, McKinnon G, Davis C, et al: Breath-hold contrast-enhanced, three-dimensional MR angiography. Radiology 201:569-571, 1996.
15. Weinman H, Laniado M, Mutzel W: Pharmacokinetics of Gd-DTPA/dimeglumine after intravenous injection into healthy volunteers. Physiol Chem Phys Med NMR 16:167-172, 1984.
16. Barnes G, Lakshminarayann A: Conventional and spiral computed tomography. In Lee J, Sagel S, Stanely R, Heiken J (eds): Computed Body Tomography with MRI Correlation. Philadelphia, Lippincott-Raven, 1998, pp 1-20.
17. Maki J, Prince M, Londy F, Chenevert T: The effects of time varying intravascular signal intensity on three-dimensional MR angiography image quality. J Magn Reson Imaging 6:642-651, 1996.
18. Reiderer S, Tasciyan T, Farzaneh F: MR fluoroscopy: Technical feasibility. Magn Reson Med 8:1-15, 1988.
19. Levy R, Maki J: Three-dimensional contrast-enhanced MR angiography of the extracranial carotid arteries: Two techniques. AJNR Am J Neuroradiolol 19:688-690, 1998.
20. Korosec F, Grist T, Frayne R, Mistretta C: Time-resolved contrast-enhanced 3D MR angiography. Magn Reson Med 36:345-351, 1996.
21. Mistretta C, Grist T, Korosec F, Frayne R: 3D time-resolved contrast-enhanced MR DSA: Advantages and tradeoffs. Magn Reson Med 40:571-581, 1998.
22. Schoenberg S, Bock M, Floemer F, et al: High-resolution pulmonary arterio- and venography using multiple-bolus multiphase 3D-Gd-MRA. J Magn Reson Imaging 10:339-346, 1999.
23. Schoenberg S, Essig M, Hallscheidt P, et al: Multiphase magnetic resonance angiography of the abdominal and pelvic arteries: Results of a bicenter multireader analysis. Invest Radiol 37:20-28, 2002.
24. Wood M, Runge V, Henkelman R: Overcoming motion in abdominal MR imaging AJR Am J Roentgenol 150:513-522, 1988.
25. Holland G, Dougherty L, Carpenter J, et al: Breath-hold ultrafast three-dimensional gadolinium-enhanced MR angiography of the aorta and the renal and other visceral abdominal arteries. AJR Am J Roentgenol 166:971-981, 1996.
26. Schima W, Mukerjee A, Saini S: Contrast-enhanced MR imaging. Clin Radiol 51:235-244, 1996.
27. Haney T, Schmidt M, Hilfiker P, et al: Optimization of contrast dosage for gadolinium-enhanced 3D MRA of the pulmonary and renal arteries. Magn Reson Imaging 16:901-906, 1998.
28. Shetty A, Bis K, Kirsch M, et al: Contrast-enhanced breath-hold three dimensional magnetic resonance angiography in the evaluation of renal arteries: Optimization of techniques and pitfalls. J Magn Reson Imaging 12:912-923, 2000.
29. Prince M, Grist T, Debatin J: 3D Contrast MR Angiography. Berlin, Springer-Verlag, 1997.
30. De Marco J, Nesbit G, Wesbey G, Richardson D: Prospective evaluation of extracranial carotid stenosis: MR angiography with maximum-intensity projections and multiplanar reformation compared with conventional angiography. AJR Am J Roentgenol 163:1205-1212, 1994.
31. Laub G: Displays for MR angiography. Magn Reson Med 14:222-229, 1990.
32. Rossnick S, Laub G, Braeckle R: Three-dimensional display of blood vessels in MRI. In Proceedings of the IEEE: Computers in Cardiology. New York, IEEE, 1986, pp 193-195.
33. Douck P, Revel U, Chazel S, et al: Fast MR angiography of the aortoiliac arteries and arteries of the lower extremity: Value of bolus enhanced, whole-volume subtraction technique. AJR Am J Roentgenol 165:431-437, 1995.
34. Wang Y, Johnston DL, Breen JF, et al: Dynamic MR digital subtraction angiography using contrast enhancement, fast data acquisition, and complex subtraction. Magn Reson Med 36:551-556, 1996.
35. Sardanelli F, et al: MR angiography of internal carotid arteries: Breath-hold Gd-enhanced 3D fast imaging with steady-state precession versus unenhanced 2D and 3D time-of-flight techniques. J Comput Assist Tomogr 23:208-215, 1999.
36. Hartnell GG: Imaging of aortic aneurysm and dissection: CT and MRI. J Thorac Imaging 16:35-46, 2001.
37. Remonda L, et al: Contrast-enhanced 3D MR angiography of the carotid artery: Comparison with conventional digital subtraction angiography. AJNR Am J Neuroradiol 23:213-219, 2002.
38. Lenhart M, et al: Time-resolved contrast-enhanced magnetic resonance angiography of the carotid arteries: Diagnostic accuracy and inter-observer variability compared with selective catheter angiography. Invest Radiol 37:535-541, 2002.
39. Khan IA, Nair CK: Clinical, diagnostic, and management perspective of aortic dissection. Chest 122:311-328, 2002.
40. Nederkoorn PJ, et al: Cartoid artery stenosis: Accuracy of contrast-enhanced MR angiography for diagnosis. Radiology 228:677-682, 2002.

41. Zhang H, Schoenberg S, Prince MR: MR angiography of the renal arteries. In Schneider G, Prince MR, Meaney JFM, Ho VB(eds): Magnetic Resonance Angiography: Techniques, Indications and Practical Applications. New York, Springer, 2005, pp 209–229.

42. Meaney JFM, Prince MR, Nostrand TT, et al: Gadolinium-enhanced magnetic resonance angiography in patients with suspected chronic mesenteric ischemia. J Magn Reson Imaging 7:171-176, 1997.

43. Baden J, Racy D, Grist T: Contrast-enhanced three-dimensional magnetic resonance angiography of the mesenteric vasculature. J Magn Reson Imaging 10:369-375, 1999.

44. Carlos RC, Stanley JC, Stafford-Johnson D, et al: Interobserver variability in the evaluation of chronic mesenteric ischemia with gadolinium-enhanced MR angiography. Acad Radiol 8:879-887, 2001.

45. Laissy J, Trillaud H, Douek P: MR angiography: Non-invasive vascular imaging of the abdomen. Abdom Imaging 27:488-506, 2002.

46. Kreft B, Strunk H, Flacke S, et al: Detection of thrombosis in the portal venous system: Comparison of contrast-enhanced MR angiography with intraarterial digital subtraction angiography. Radiology 216:86-92, 2000.

47. Maki JH, Knopp MV, Prince M: Contrast-enhanced MR angiography. Appl Radiol 32:182-210, 2003.

48. Binkert C, Baker P, Petersen B, et al: Peripheral vascular disease: Blinded study of dedicated calf MR angiography versus standard bolus-chase MR angiography and film hard-copy angiography. Radiology 232:860-866, 2004.

49. Laissy JP, Cinqualbre A, Loshkajian A, et al: Assessment of deep venous thrombosis in the lower limbs and pelvis: MR venography versus duplex Doppler sonography. AJR Am J Roentgenol 167:971-975, 1996.

50. Fraser DG, Moody AR, Morgan PS, et al: Diagnosis of lower-limb deep venous thrombosis: A prospective blinded study of magnetic resonance direct thrombosis imaging. Ann Intern Med 136:89-98, 2002.

51. Lebowitz JA, Rofsky NM, Krinsky GA, Weinreb JC: Gadolinium-enhanced body MR venography with subtraction technique. AJR Am J Roentgenol 169:755-758, 1997.

52. Fraser DG, Moody AR, Davidson R, et al: Deep venous thrombosis: Diagnosis by using venous enhanced subtracted peak arterial MR venography versus conventional venography. Radiology 226:812-820, 2003.

53. Li W, David V, Kaplan A, Edelman AR: Three-dimensional low dose gadolinium-enhanced peripheral MR venography. J Magn Reson Imaging 8:630-633, 1998.

54. Ruehm SG, Wiesner W, Debatin JF: Pelvic and lower extremity veins: Contrast-enhanced three-dimensional MR venography with a dedicated vascular coil—initial experience. Radiology 215:421-427, 2000.

55. Froehlich JB, Prince MR, Greenfield U, et al: "Bull's-eye" sign on gadolinium-enhanced magnetic resonance venography determines thrombus presence and age: A preliminary study. J Vasc Surg 26:809-816, 1997.

56. Goyen M, Lauenstein T, Herborn C, et al: 0.5 M Gd chelate (Magnevist) versus 1.0 M Gd chelate (Gadovist): Dose-independent effect in image quality of pelvic three-dimensional MR angiography. J Magn Reson Imaging 14:602-607, 2001.

57. Knopp M, Schoenberg S, Rehnl C, et al: Assessment of gadobenate dimeglumine (GdBOPTA) for MR angiography phase I studies. Invest Radiol 37:706-715, 2002.

58. Herborn C, Lauenstein T, Ruehrn S, et al: Intraindividual comparison of gadopentetate dimeglumine, gadobenate dimeglumine and gadobutrol for pelvic 3D magnetic resonance angiography. Invest Radiol 38:27-33, 2003.

59. Grist T, Korosec F, Peters D, et al: Steady-state and dynamic MR angiography with MS-325: Initial experience in humans. Radiology 207:539-544, 1998.

60. Lauffer R, Parmelee D, Dunham S, et al: MS-325: Albumin-targeted contrast agent for MR angiography. Radiology 207:529-538, 1998.

61. Bluemke D, Stillman A, Bis K, et al: Carotid MR angiography: Phase II study of safety and efficacy of MS-325. Radiology 219:114-122, 2001.

62. Dong Q, Hurst D, Weinmann H, et al: Magnetic resonance angiography with gadomer-17: An animal study original investigation. Invest Radiol 33:699-708, 1998.

63. Bae K, Heinken JP, Brink JA: Aortic and hepatic peak enhancement at CT: Effect of contrast medium injection rate—pharmacokinetic analysis and experimental porcine model. Radiology 206:455-464, 1998.

64. Fleischmann D, Hittmair K: Mathematical analysis of arterial enhancement and optimization of bolus geometry for CT angiography using the discrete Fourier transform. J Comput Assist Tomogr 23:474-484, 1999.

65. Fleischmann D, Rubin GD, Bankier AA, Hittmair K: Improved uniformity of aortic enhancement with customized contrast medium injection protocols at CT angiography. Radiology 214:363-371, 2000.

66. Bae KT, Tran HQ, Heiken JP: Multiphasic injection method for uniform prolonged vascular enhancement at CT angiography: Pharmacokinetic analysis and experimental porcine model. Radiology 216:872-880, 2000.

67. Van Hoe L, Vandermeulen D, Gryspeerdt S, et al: Assessment of accuracy of renal artery stenosis grading in helical CT angiography using maximum intensity projections. Eur Radiol 6:658-664, 1996.

68. Becker C, Soppa C, Fink U, et al: Spiral CT angiography and 3D reconstruction in patients with aortic coarctation. Eur Radiol 7:1473-1477, 1997.

69. Prokop M, Shin HO, Schanz A, Schaefer-Prokop CM: Use of maximum intensity projection in CT angiography: A basic review. Radiographics 17:433-451, 1997.

70. Remy J, Remy-Jardin M, Artaud D, Fribourg M: Multiplanar and three-dimensional reconstruction techniques in CT: Impact on chest diseases. Eur Radiol 8:335-351, 1998.

71. Johnson PT, Halpern EJ, Kuszyk BS, et al: Renal artery stenosis: CT angiography comparison of real-time volume-rendering and maximum intensity projection algorithms. Radiology 211:337-343, 1999.

72. Marcus CD, Ladam-Marcus VJ, Bigot JL, et al: Carotid arterial stenosis: Evaluation at CT angiography with the volume-rendering technique. Radiology 211:775-780, 1999.

73. Fleischmann D: High concentration contrast media in MDCT angiography: Principles and rationale. Eur Radiol 13(Suppl 3):N39-N43, 2003.

74. Napoli V, Fleischmann D, Chan FP, et al: Computed tomography angiography: State-of-the-art imaging using multidetector-row technology. J Comput Assist Tomogr 28(Suppl 1):S32-S45, 2004.

75. Shoepf UJ, Becker CR, Hofmann LK, et al: Multislice CT angiography. Eur Radiol 13:629-636, 2003.

76. Phillips CD, Bubash LA: CT angiography and MR angiography in the evaluation of extracranial carotid vascular disease. Radiol Clin North Am 420:783-798, 2002.

77. Alvarez-Linera J, Benito-Leon J, Escribano J, et al: Prospective evaluation of carotid artery stenosis: Elliptic centric contrast-enhanced MR angiography and spiral CT angiography compared with digital subtraction angiography. AJNR Am J Neuroradiol 24:1012-1019, 2003.

78. Foley WD, Karcaaltincaba M: Computed tomography angiography: Principles and clinical applications. J Comput Assist Tomogr 27(Suppl 1): S23-S30, 2003.

79. Na DG, Ryoo JW, Lee KH, et al: Multiphasic perfusion computed tomography in hyperacute ischemic stroke: Comparison with diffusion and perfusion magnetic resonance imaging. J Comput Assist Tomogr 27:194-206, 2003.

80. Goodman L, Curtin JJ, Mewissen MW, et al: Detection of pulmonary embolism in patients with unresolved clinical and scintigraphic diagnosis: Helical CT versus angiography. AJR Am J Roentgenol 164:1369-1374, 1995.

81. Marcus CD, Ladam-Marcus VJ, Bigot JL, et al: Carotid arterial stenosis: Evaluation at CT angiography with the volume-rendering technique. Radiology 211:775-780, 1999.

82. Becker CR, Ohnesorge BM, Schoepf UJ, Reiser MF: Current development of cardiac imaging with multidetector-row CT. Eur J Radiol 36:97-103, 2000.

83. Schoepf UJ, Kessler MA, Rieger CT, et al: Multislice CT imaging of pulmonary embolism. Eur Radiol 11:2278-2286, 2001.

84. Katz DS, Loud PA, Bruce D, et al: Combined CT venography and pulmonary angiography: A comprehensive review. Radiographics 22:S3-S19, 2002.

85. Krestan CR, Klein N, Fleischmann D, et al: Value of negative spiral CT angiography in patients with suspected acute PE: Analysis of PE occurrence and outcome. Eur Radiol 14:93-98, 2004.

86. Gotway MB, Dawn SK: Thoracic aorta imaging with multislice CT. Radiol Clin North Am 41:521-543, 2003.

87. Rubin GD: MDCT imaging of the aorta and peripheral vessels. Eur J Radiol 45(Suppl 1):S42-S49, 2003.

88. Rubin GD, Shiau MC, Leung AN, et al: Aorta and iliac arteries: Single versus multiple detector-row helical CT angiography. Radiology 215:670-676, 2000.

89. Willmann JK, Wildermuth S, Pfammatter T, et al: Aortoiliac and renal arteries: Prospective intraindividual comparison of contrast-enhanced three-dimensional MR angiography and multi-detector row CT angiography. Radiology 226:798-811, 2003.

90. Laghi A, Iannaccone R, Catalano C, et al: Multislice spiral computed tomography angiography of mesenteric arteries. Lancet 358:638-639, 2001.
91. Lawler LP, Fishman EK: Celiomesenteric anomaly demonstration by multidetector CT and volume rendering. J Comput Assist Tomogr 25:802-804, 2001.
92. Kim JK, Park SY, Kim HJ, et al: Living donor kidneys: Usefulness of multi-detector row CT for comprehensive evaluation. Radiology 229:869-876, 2003.
93. Erbay N, Raptopoulos V, Pomfret EA, et al: Living donor liver transplantation in adults: Vascular variants important in surgical planning for donor and recipients. AJR Am J Roentgenol 181:109-114, 2003.
94. Byun JH, Kim TK, Lee SS, et al: Evaluation of the hepatic artery in potential donors for living donor liver transplantation by computed tomography angiography using multidetector-row computed tomography: Comparison of volume rendering and maximum intensity projection techniques. J Comput Assist Tomogr 27:125-131, 2003.
95. Lee SS, Kim TK, Byun JH, et al: Hepatic arteries in potential donors for living related liver transplantation: Evaluation with multi-detector row CT angiography. Radiology 227:391-399, 2003.
96. Rubin GD, Schmidt AJ, Logan LJ, Sofilos MC: Multi-detector row CT angiography of lower extremity arterial inflow and runoff: Initial experience. Radiology 221:146-158, 2001.
97. Martin ML, Tay KH, Flak B, et al: Multidetector CT angiography of the aortoiliac system and lower extremities: A prospective comparison with digital subtraction angiography. AJR Am J Roentgenol 180:1085-1091, 2003.

Questions

1. **True or false: MRA and CTA provide similar images because they are based on the same technology and use ionizing radiation.**

2. **Which of the following statements regarding MRA is correct?**
   (a) Two-dimensional time-of-flight techniques are best for visualizing tortuous vessels with slow flow
   (b) Contrast-enhanced MRA techniques use conventional iodinated contrast material
   (c) Gadolinium-containing contrast material is more nephrotoxic than conventional iodinated contrast material
   (d) Subtraction techniques are used to remove background tissue in both digital subtraction angiography and MRA

3. **Which of the following techniques have been used for MRA?**
   (a) Two-dimensional time of flight
   (b) Three-dimensional time-of-flight contrast-enhanced MRA
   (c) Phase-contrast techniques
   (d) All of the above

4. **Contrast-enhanced MRA is useful for evaluating which of the following vascular beds?**
   (a) Arch vessels
   (b) Abdominal aorta
   (c) Runoff vessels
   (d) Deep veins of the upper and lower extremities
   (e) Tertiary branches of the mesenteric artery

5. **Which of the following statements regarding MDCT CTA is true?**
   (a) It has lower resolution than contrast-enhanced MRA
   (b) Image acquisition time is shorter than for contrast-enhanced MRA
   (c) Postprocessing of images to remove bone and soft tissue is easier with MDCT CTA

6. **Which of the following statements regarding MDCT CTA are true?**
   (a) It is frequently used for the diagnosis of acute aortic dissection
   (b) It is preferred over contrast-enhanced MRA for follow-up studies in patients with chronic aortic dissection
   (c) It is better than contrast-enhanced MRA in patients with limited ability to cooperate

7. **True or false: Accuracy of stenosis assessment is equal with MDCT CTA and contrast-enhanced MRA.**

8. **True or false: Peripheral runoff studies can be performed with both MDCT CTA and contrast-enhanced MRA.**

9. **Which of the following statements regarding MDCT CTA is correct?**
   (a) Scanners with 4 detector rows have larger volume coverage than scanners with 16 detector rows
   (b) Slice thickness is a reconstruction parameter with MDCT
   (c) MDCT has higher accuracy than contrast-enhanced MRA for evaluating accessory renal arteries in renal donors
   (d) All of the above

10. **Postprocessing techniques used for MDCT CTA and contrast-enhanced MRA include which of the following?**
    (a) MIP
    (b) Three-dimensional volume rendering
    (c) MPR
    (d) All of the above

Answers

1. false   2. d   3. d   4. a, b, c, d   5. b
6. a, c   7. false   8. true   9. d   10. d

17

George Andros • Michael B. Silva, Jr. • Paul B. Haser •
Sheila M. Coogan • Peter A. Schneider

Arterial Access; Guidewires, Catheters, and Sheaths; and Balloon Angioplasty Catheters*

Arterial Access

Endovascular intervention begins with vascular access. The fundamentals are technical skill and familiarity with the use and organization of essential tools (e.g., needles, guidewires, catheters, and sheaths) and the sequence of how they fit together. The interventionist then learns angiography, both primary and selective, and progresses to more advanced procedures: angioplasty, stenting, and thrombolysis. As the surgeon's experience expands, new procedures with alternative methods and devices are added. The road to proficiency begins with mastery of percutaneous vascular access, the subject of this chapter. Access by way of a surgically exposed artery is essentially identical to percutaneous access, and for the experienced vascular surgeon, little elaboration is necessary.

SELECTING THE ACCESS SITE

Selection of the access site is a two-part process. First, an artery with a secure, direct, and uninterrupted pathway to the target lesion or the arterial territory of interest is selected (Fig. 17-1). Then the artery is cannulated based on specific local landmarks (Figs. 17-2 and 17-3).

Although there are pros and cons to the use of each of the access sites (Table 17-1), the femoral approach (preferably from the right) is the first choice for angiography and most interventions. By using retrograde femoral puncture, access

*This material was adapted from a previously published book: Moore WS, Ahn SS (eds): Endovascular Surgery, 3rd ed. Philadelphia, WB Saunders, 2001, Chapters 5-7, pp 37-63.

to the entire thoracoabdominal aorta (and its ramifications) is standard; catheterization of the contralateral iliofemoral tree and runoff is readily performed. With antegrade femoral puncture, the interventionist can selectively catheterize vessels as distal as the infrapopliteal arteries and beyond.

Arterial puncture in the upper extremity (usually the left) also provides access to both the thoracic and the abdominal aortas and their runoffs. Every interventionist should acquire experience in gaining upper extremity access at one or more of the available sites. Generally, however, the use of upper extremity access is limited to instances in which the common femoral arteries are occluded or otherwise unavailable (e.g., a recently implanted aortofemoral bypass graft).

Cannulation of the artery at the selected site is a standardized procedure, irrespective of the artery selected. It begins with arterial puncture, and there are two methods of achieving intra-arterial access (Fig. 17-4A):

1. Through-and-through puncture completely across both walls of the artery. The needle is then withdrawn *backward* into the lumen.
2. Single-wall entry, in which only the anterior wall is punctured by gentle pressure as the arterial pulsation is "palpated" through the slowly advancing needle. Pulsatile flow signals entry into the arterial lumen.

For each method of entry, there are appropriate types of needles. For single-wall entry, a simple disposable needle, preferably with a stabilizing flange, is used. We believe that this is the safest method of accessing arteries and veins. The bevel is placed anteriorly. Through-and-through puncture, or double-wall entry, can also be performed with a single-wall entry needle; alternatively, a multipart needle, of which there are many types, can be used. The multipart needle, with its inner core, is used to puncture both walls of the artery.

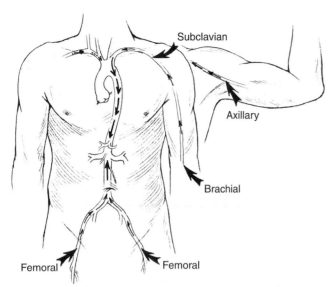

FIGURE 17–1 • Sites for arterial access. (From Moore WS, Ahn SS [eds]: Endovascular Surgery, 3rd ed. Philadelphia, WB Saunders, 2001, p 37.)

The inner needle is then removed, and the outer needle is withdrawn backward into the arterial lumen. The original Seldinger needle comprised four parts, including an obturator.

Puncture of small arteries, such as the brachial artery at the antecubital fossa, is facilitated by the use of a multipart "micropuncture kit," available from several manufacturers. A small-caliber needle is inserted first, followed by a 0.018-inch guidewire. Next, the needle is exchanged for paired coaxial catheters. The smaller inner catheter accommodates the guidewire and permits the larger outer catheter to dilate the subcutaneous track. After both catheters are securely advanced into the artery, the guidewire and the small inner catheter are removed; the remaining larger catheter then accepts a 0.035-inch guidewire, which is capable of supporting larger devices.

THE SELDINGER TECHNIQUE

The Seldinger method, first described in 1953, is the fundamental technique of vascular access (Fig. 17-5). So widespread

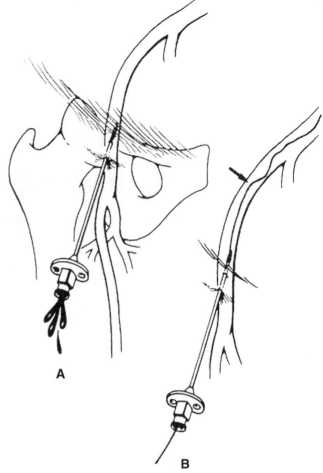

FIGURE 17–2 • Common femoral artery puncture. *A,* Entry into the common femoral artery. *B,* Guidewire passed with the floppy portion well advanced. (From Moore WS, Ahn SS [eds]: Endovascular Surgery, 3rd ed. Philadelphia, WB Saunders, 2001, p 38.)

is its application for the insertion of catheters that virtually every medical student has some personal hands-on experience with its elegant simplicity. The steps include the following:

1. Localization of the entry point by palpation of the appropriate arterial pulse.

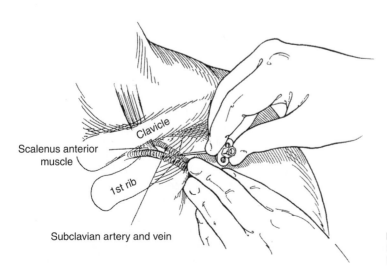

FIGURE 17–3 • Left subclavian artery puncture. (From Moore WS, Ahn SS [eds]: Endovascular Surgery, 3rd ed. Philadelphia, WB Saunders, 2001, p 39.)

TABLE 17–1	Comparison of Sites for Arterial Access		
Site	**Advantages**	**Disadvantages**	**Comments**
Femoral	Easily accessed Large vessel SPR set up for right-handed access Most devices designed for femoral access Right or left artery available Permits brachiocephalic and aortic runoff access Easily compressed Puncture complication easily managed	Possible tortuosity Long pathway for catheter manipulations to remote targets May be compromised by ASO	First choice among sites Obesity may complicate puncture Left side accessed from the patient's right Predictable complications
Brachial	Usually patent and disease free Either side accessible Most target lesions are accessible	Prone to thrombosis Patient comfort compromised by arm board Long, tortuous route for catheter manipulations	Second-choice site "Micropuncture" set is a useful adjunctive device Brachial site best for angiography and some simple interventions
Axillary	Large vessel Short working distance to the aorta Access from the left avoids crossing the cerebrovascular orifices	Major complication, "short hematoma" Brachial plexopathy Uncomfortable patient position	Small catheters are best used by experienced operators Use is best limited to angiography
Subclavian	Large vessel Very short working distance to the aorta Accessible bilaterally; left side preferred Access to arch, thoracic aorta, and entire runoff Each leg may be accessed antegradely	Potential for pneumothorax Prolonged bimanual compression Increased risk of hematoma with larger catheters	Useful for angiography, PTA and stenting, thrombolysis Angle of approach desirable for renal angioplasty Sheath removed when PTT returns to normal Most difficult access; requires experience
Radial	Ease of access and compression for early patient discharge Radial artery may be expandable	Very long working distance Radial artery may thrombose; later unusable for bypass graft Hand ischemia potential Nerve damage potential	A novelty

ASO, arteriosclerosis obliterans; PTA, percutaneous transluminal angioplasty; PTT, partial thromboplastin time; SPR, special procedures room.
From Moore WS, Ahn SS (eds): Endovascular Surgery, 3rd ed. Philadelphia, WB Saunders, 2001, p 39.

2. Angulated entry into the vessel lumen (Fig. 17-4B.) As previously noted, anterior single-wall entry with the bevel pointed anteriorly is preferred.
3. Verification of the intraluminal position by pulsatile flow from the arterial hub. When in doubt, a puff of contrast material is administered under fluoroscopic guidance. A guidewire is passed into the arterial lumen and advanced so that the stiff portion is securely inside the lumen. If the tissues surrounding the punctured artery are fibrotic, as they might be in the case of previous arterial catheterization, or if the artery is calcified and rigid, the needle is exchanged for a dilator or a series of graduated dilators to enlarge the track.
4. Finally, the needle or the dilating catheter is exchanged for the intended catheter or the appropriate sheath. The guidewire can then be safely removed or exchanged.

GUIDEWIRES AND SHEATHS

Several features distinguish guidewires. Variations in the tip of the catheter include J-shaped tips of various sizes with or without a movable core. Tips can also be flexible or "floppy," such as the Bentson wire; steerable, such as the Wholey wire; platinum tipped for visibility in negotiating tortuous arteries; and so forth. Guidewires are of various lengths and stiffnesses to permit exchanges over the reinforced portion of the wire and to allow devices to be exchanged and deployed. Appropriate guidewire coatings, such as the hydrophilic coating of the Terumo Glidewire (Boston Scientific, Quincy, Mass.) facilitate wire advancement through tortuous and irregular channels.

Introducing sheaths are composed of a catheter portion, with a hydrostatic valve with a side arm for fluid injection, and an inner dilator. The diameter, length, and construction of the sheath are dictated by its purpose, which may include:

1. Securing access for one or more catheter or guidewire exchanges.
2. Securing access through fibrotic subcutaneous tissue (such as groin) that has undergone previous intervention, either surgically or with catheter techniques.
3. Securing smooth access through calcified or sclerotic arteries.
4. Straightening of tortuous arteries.
5. Passage and guidance of interventional devices such as balloon angioplasty catheters, stents, selective

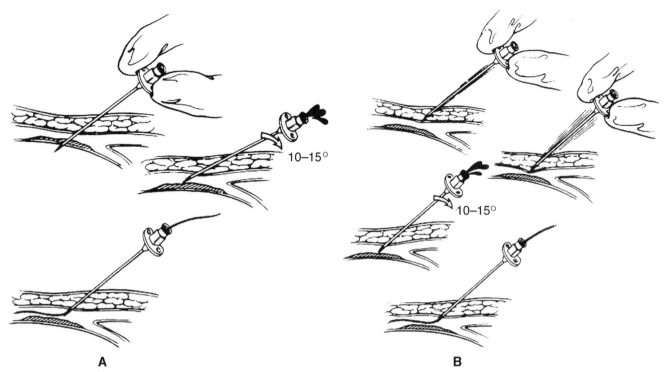

FIGURE 17–4 • *A*, Through-and-through (double-wall) puncture. *B*, Single (anterior wall) puncture. (From Moore WS, Ahn SS [eds]: Endovascular Surgery, 3rd ed. Philadelphia, WB Saunders, 2001, p 40.)

angiography catheters, thrombolysis and thrombectomy catheters, and other catheters (e.g., guiding catheters).

6. Facilitating intraprocedural angiography to assess the status of an intervention (e.g., angioplasty and stent placement).

FOUR ESSENTIAL TECHNIQUES

After the fundamentals have been learned, there are four essential access techniques that every interventionist must master (and perhaps a fifth, if one includes learning to obtain access by way of an upper extremity artery).

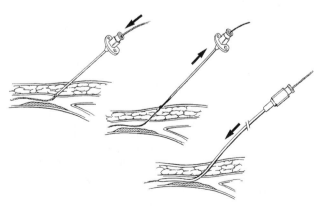

FIGURE 17–5 • The Seldinger technique. (From Moore WS, Ahn SS [eds]: Endovascular Surgery, 3rd ed. Philadelphia, WB Saunders, 2001, p 40.)

Retrograde Femoral Puncture

Puncture of the femoral artery is simplified by knowledge of its position referable to osseous anatomic landmarks. In the majority of cases, there is approximately 3 cm of common femoral artery between the inguinal ligament and the femoral bifurcation suitable for the introduction of a needle, guidewire, and catheter; it lies over the junction of the medial third and middle third of the femoral head. Importantly, this relationship varies little with the patient's body habitus, age, and so forth (Fig. 17-6). This point is commonly designated as lying two fingerbreadths lateral to the pubic symphysis on a line joining the symphysis with the anterior iliac spine. Because increasing numbers of patients undergoing arterial catheterization are obese, it may be difficult to orient the common femoral artery to the standard landmarks. Hence, it is useful to lay the entry needle directly on the patient and to identify its relationship to the femoral head using fluoroscopy.

Attempts to enter the femoral artery may result in a puncture that is too distal into either the deep or the superficial femoral artery, especially in an obese patient. Catheterization of either of these vessels carries an increased risk of postprocedural hematoma or pseudoaneurysm development. By establishing the relationship between the skin puncture wound and the femoral head, it is easier to puncture the common femoral artery. If there is any concern regarding the intraluminal passage of the guidewire once the needle tip has entered the femoral artery, the guidewire should be advanced under fluoroscopic guidance. Alternatively, a "puff" of contrast material, together with road-mapping, assists in negotiating passage of a guidewire. Using the standard Bentson guidewire, at least 20 cm of guidewire is advanced through

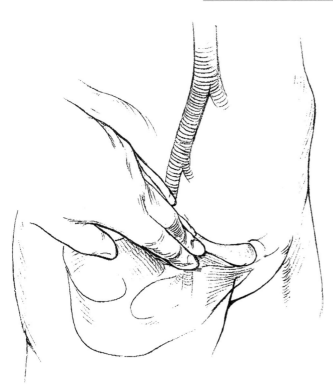

FIGURE 17–6 • Retrograde femoral puncture orientation. (From Moore WS, Ahn SS [eds]: Endovascular Surgery, 3rd ed. Philadelphia, WB Saunders, 2001, p 41.)

the needle so that exchanges can be done safely. It is usually safe to let the Bentson guidewire tip buckle so that the stiffer portion is safely within the artery. After the 18 French thin-walled needle has punctured the artery and the 0.035-inch guidewire has passed into the artery, a 4 French dilator is exchanged for the needle to permit passage of a No. 5 catheter or sheath. If, however, the groin is densely scarred and fibrotic, it may be desirable to pass a No. 6 dilator in anticipation of introducing a 5 French sheath. With access established and the sheath in place, the next step, crossing the iliac arteries, can be taken.

Antegrade Femoral Puncture

Antegrade femoral puncture is a simple technique of achieving direct access to the common femoral artery and its superficial femoral and popliteal artery runoff (Fig. 17-7). It is an optimal technique for selective distal angiography or ipsilateral intervention. The most common error, again often a result of patient obesity, is puncture of the superficial or deep femoral artery. Less commonly, the external iliac artery is punctured; entry into this artery may result in either difficult passage of the guidewire at the beginning of the procedure or a retroperitoneal hematoma at the end (Fig. 17-8). A three-dimensional sense of the location of the common femoral artery is invaluable; when in doubt, revert to the "needle on the skin under fluoroscopy" technique.

After preliminary skin infiltration with lidocaine and the establishment of cutaneous access, the needle is inserted in an antegrade direction just distal to the anterior iliac spine and passes through the inguinal ligament to engage the common femoral artery. If the patient is very obese, it is often

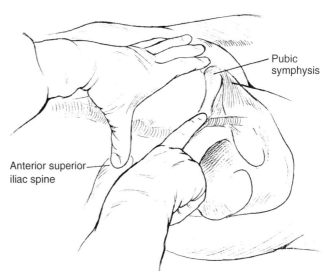

FIGURE 17–7 • Antegrade femoral puncture orientation. (From Moore WS, Ahn SS [eds]: Endovascular Surgery, 3rd ed. Philadelphia, WB Saunders, 2001, p 42.)

necessary for an assistant to retract the abdominal panniculus in a cephalad direction to allow an appropriate angle of entry. As in the case of retrograde femoral puncture, it is sometimes useful to pass the guidewire under fluoroscopic control, supplemented by contrast agent administration with or without road-mapping. If the guidewire enters the deep femoral artery, the needle tip may be moved either medially or laterally to redirect it into the superficial femoral artery. This may not be possible if the needle has entered the artery too close to the femoral bifurcation. This circumstance should be ascertained by angling the image intensifier into an anterior oblique position and injecting contrast material to localize the entry point of the needle. This will also help in redirecting the guidewire into the superficial femoral artery. In those instances when the guidewire enters the deep femoral artery, it is possible to "bounce" the guidewire tip off the lateral

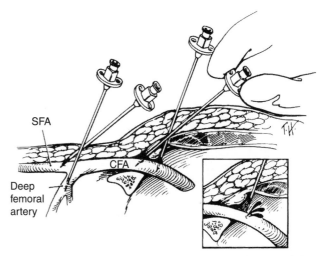

FIGURE 17–8 • Antegrade femoral puncture with external iliac puncture and extraperitoneal hemorrhage *(inset)*. CFA, common femoral artery; SFA, superior femoral artery. (From Moore WS, Ahn SS [eds]: Endovascular Surgery, 3rd ed. Philadelphia, WB Saunders, 2001, p 43.)

aspect of the femoral artery to redirect it to the more medially placed orifice of the superficial femoral artery; alternatively, the guidewire tip can be steered with a Wholey wire.

Our preferred technique of redirecting the guidewire down the superficial femoral artery is to exchange the needle for a 30-cm-long cobra catheter. This is securely positioned in the deep femoral artery and is slowly withdrawn under fluoroscopic guidance as contrast material is injected with the image intensifier in a right anterior oblique angle, which opens a space between the deep and the superficial femoral arteries. The catheter tip is directed anteromedially as it is withdrawn and will "pop" into the superficial femoral artery orifice. The guidewire is then reinserted, and it advances almost invariably into the superficial femoral artery; the catheter follows (Fig. 17-9).

Puncturing the Pulseless Femoral Artery

If no femoral pulse can be palpated to enable retrograde femoral puncture and arterial access, there are eight techniques that can be used to overcome this challenge (Fig. 17-10):

1. Even if the iliac artery is completely occluded, the femoral artery usually has a "soft," compliant spot, as is often noted in patients with complete aortic occlusions who undergo aortofemoral bypass. Similarly, when a patient is sedated on the angiographic table, the pulse that was previously nonpalpable in the office may be detected. The artery believed to be pulseless may, in fact, have a sufficient pulse to guide needle placement.
2. The arterial fibrosis and calcification associated with arteriosclerosis render the common femoral artery itself palpable. The surgically exposed artery feels like a thickened cord, and it can be palpated transcutaneously as well.

A needle can be effectively directed into this thickened, calcified vessel.

3. Under magnified fluoroscopy, careful examination of the region of the femoral head can reveal arterial calcification to help localize the common femoral artery.
4. When the contralateral iliofemoral system is patent, lumbar aortography is usually performed before intervention. This angiogram visualizes the common femoral artery distal to the iliac occlusive lesion. Using the angiogram and bony references, the needle can be directed to the site of the femoral artery, as visualized on the preintervention lumbar aortogram; a complementary technique is to perform lumbar aortography and road-mapping. By using the road map and direct fluoroscopy, the needle can be directed while watching the live image on the screen. Of course, when working with fluoroscopy, lead gloves should be used.
5. Ultrasound techniques have been used to localize the common femoral artery. An ultrasound probe or a duplex machine can be brought to the special procedures room and used to determine the position of the common femoral artery. The position is then marked on the skin to facilitate puncture.
6. A second ultrasound technique employs the so-called smart needle, which has an ultrasound probe at its tip. As the needle approaches the artery, the needle emits an ultrasound signal, which identifies proximity to the pulseless vessel.
7. Occasionally, attempts to enter the common femoral artery result in puncture of the common femoral vein and the appearance of dark, nonpulsatile venous blood. If the needle is in the common femoral vein, it can be withdrawn and reinserted 1 to 2 cm laterally, the normal

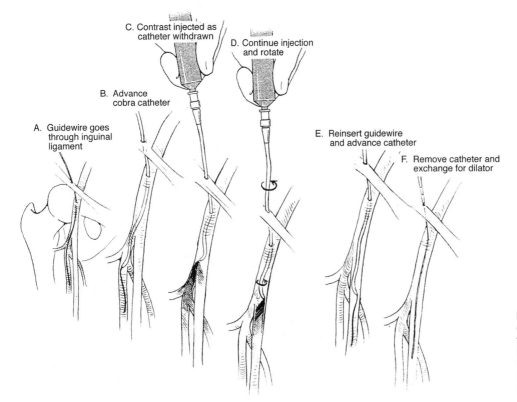

FIGURE 17–9 • Redirecting the catheter from the deep to the superficial femoral artery. (From Moore WS, Ahn SS [eds]: Endovascular Surgery, 3rd ed. Philadelphia, WB Saunders, 2001, p 44.)

C. Contrast injected as catheter withdrawn

D. Continue injection and rotate

B. Advance cobra catheter

A. Guidewire goes through inguinal ligament

E. Reinsert guidewire and advance catheter

F. Remove catheter and exchange for dilator

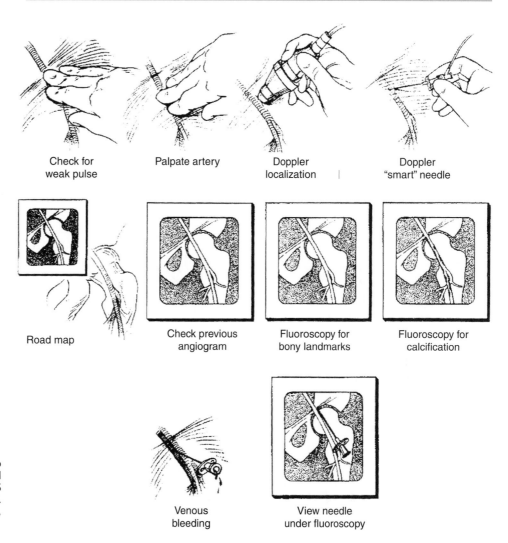

FIGURE 17–10 • Adjuncts to puncture of the pulseless femoral artery. (From Moore WS, Ahn SS [eds]: Endovascular Surgery, 3rd ed. Philadelphia, WB Saunders, 2001, p 45.)

distance between the artery and the vein. Bear in mind, however, that the pulseless femoral artery often has low pressure and low pulse pressure, so that the arterial blood may be dark and may resemble venous blood; what appears to be a venous puncture may, in fact, be an arterial puncture. If the origin of the dark, minimally pulsatile blood flow is in doubt, the needle should not be withdrawn. A puff of dye is injected to identify the location of the needle.

8. The junction of the middle third and the medial third of the femoral head is the normal location of the common femoral artery, as visualized fluoroscopically. A needle aimed at this point, especially if it encounters a firm, "crunchy" sclerotic structure, often engages the nonpulsatile artery.

With one of these techniques, percutaneous access can be obtained in virtually every instance. Once access to the lumen has been attained, the Seldinger technique is employed.

Crossing over the Top

Gaining access to the iliofemoropopliteal system from the contralateral femoral artery over the aortic bifurcation is an indispensable technique. Moreover, it can be learned with

surprising ease. Several maneuvers and devices facilitate the procedure (Fig. 17-11).

The aortic bifurcation can be localized not only by its usual position in relation to L-4 but also by its relation to the iliac crests. If there is aortic calcification, this also helps with localization and orientation. It is sometimes helpful to angle the image intensifier obliquely to view the iliac artery orifice. This widens the apparent angle of entry into the iliac artery and facilitates passage of the guidewire down the external iliac artery rather than the internal iliac artery. A preliminary lumbar aortogram, with or without road-mapping, also helps establish landmarks.

The choice of catheter to cannulate the contralateral iliac artery is decisive. We generally use a Tennis Racquet catheter to perform lumbar aortograms. If the aorta is of normal width, the same catheter can be withdrawn under fluoroscopic guidance to the aortic bifurcation; the tip tends to uncoil and usually "hooks" the iliac artery orifice. At least 6 to 8 inches of a soft guidewire, such as a Bentson or Wholey wire, can then be directed into the iliac system; guidewire buckling is permissible. The catheter is then passed over the wire to secure access before catheter and guidewire exchanges are effected.

For narrower aortas, particularly in women, we find the Sos catheter useful. It is advanced into the distal lumbar aorta

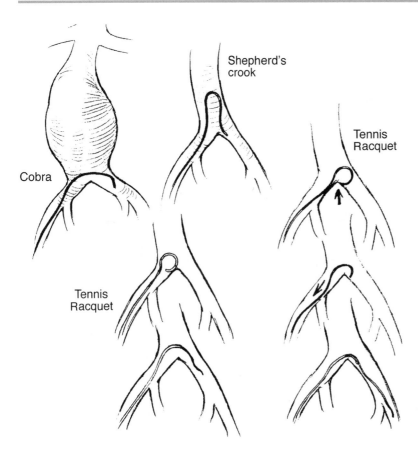

FIGURE 17–11 • Directing a catheter and a guidewire over the aortic bifurcation ("over the top"). (From Moore WS, Ahn SS [eds]: Endovascular Surgery, 3rd ed. Philadelphia, WB Saunders, 2001, p 45.)

and reconfigured so that the tip points distally. With about 1 cm of guidewire exposed, the catheter tip is then dragged retrogradely into the orifice of the common iliac artery. The guidewire is advanced until it is securely positioned in the iliofemoral system before exchanges are attempted.

It is worth noting that when guided over the aortic bifurcation, in almost all cases the guidewire tends to pass from the external iliac artery through the common femoral artery directly into the superficial femoral artery rather than down the deep femoral artery.

In the case of a wide aortic bifurcation, such as in the presence of an aneurysm, a cobra catheter is effective in directing the guidewire over the aortic bifurcation. Some interventionists recommend the use of a Balken guiding sheath for this purpose; this device has the advantage of permitting antegrade angiography to monitor the course of interventions.

Calcification with stenosis and tortuosity often make crossing the aortic bifurcation difficult. The need to traverse extensive iliofemoral occlusive disease is a relative contraindication to gaining access to the contralateral femoropopliteal segment, because this may cause damage to the inflow of an outflow artery intended for treatment. In this instance, an alternative approach should be used. Tortuosity is often a problem in torquing and directing catheters and guidewires, particularly when traversing the aortic bifurcation. The effect of tortuosity can be reduced by employing a 15- or 20-cm introducing sheath, which helps straighten the artery.

There are many opportunities to gain skill in the over-the-top technique. We often use it to perform selective femoral, popliteal, and tibial angiography after lumbar aortography

to visualize the distal runoff of the contralateral limb. This selective catheterization technique produces angiograms of startlingly improved quality and permits acquisition of femoral angiograms with multiple projections. By incorporating these techniques into routine angiographic practice, experience can be gained not only in these so-called diagnostic procedures but also in subsequent and concomitant interventions.

COMPLICATIONS OF ARTERIAL ACCESS

Complications of catheter-based interventions, like all conditions, are better managed with prevention rather than treatment. Damage to the arteries at the puncture site and at remote locations of secondary catheterization is lessened by puncturing the proper artery. Hematomas, pseudoaneurysms, and arteriovenous fistulas in the groin usually result from failure to puncture the common femoral artery or from selecting a very diseased artery to gain access. Technique in handling catheters and guidewires is important. They should be manipulated and advanced in small increments, gently and without force, to avoid dissections. The liberal use of sheaths of the smallest appropriate size helps forestall damage to the entry artery. Dye-induced nephropathy, particularly in diabetic patients, can be virtually eliminated with the use of mannitol and diuretics (to establish diuresis, by either single injection or infusion) and with dopamine infusion (to enhance renal flow). Direct injection of contrast material into the renal arteries should be avoided, and the minimal amount of contrast material, diluted if possible, should always be employed, whatever the status of renal function. Carbon dioxide angiography should be considered.

COMMENTS

The performance of angiograms provides the best opportunity to gain skill in the use of needles, guidewires, sheaths, and catheters. We believe that vascular surgeons should obtain their own angiograms in the special procedures room. Vascular surgeons are the ones who know, in intimate detail, the information needed for vascular reconstruction, as well as which lesions are best treated with endovascular techniques and which with open surgery. After gaining expertise in the primary skills of angiography, more advanced techniques, such as antegrade femoral puncture and other techniques mentioned in this chapter, can be attempted. There are, however, hindrances to gaining this skill. Among the roadblocks to gaining endovascular skills is interspecialty rivalry with interventional radiologists and, increasingly, invasive cardiologists.

Vascular surgeons who master endovascular techniques and perform them in the special procedures room will seldom find it necessary to combine inflow angioplasty with femorodistal or femorofemoral bypass. Angiography and endoluminal intervention can be performed as a single procedure, with bypass grafting done at a later date. Surgeons who attain skill in percutaneous techniques will soon realize that minimally invasive procedures using a cutdown are seldom necessary. Likewise, scheduling of percutaneous procedures in the operating room would become rare. Those cases that require multiple sites of access—such as bilateral femoral puncture for kissing balloon techniques, the seldom-performed popliteal puncture, and the manipulation of multiple guidewires—can be undertaken far more easily in the special procedures room than in the operating room with a mobile C-arm and a radiolucent table.

Gaining percutaneous arterial access for diagnostic and therapeutic procedures is akin to making an incision in open surgery. Just as the position, size, and orientation of the incision can optimize visualization of the organs to be examined and treated, properly selected and performed arterial access allows remote interrogation and treatment of arterial lesions. Knowledge of when to use forceps, needle holders, and retractors is analogous to expertise in the selection and use of needles, guidewires, sheaths, and endoluminal devices. No surgeon can progress without skill and experience in the use of the former, and no endovascular surgeon can gain technical mastery without training and experience in the latter.

Guidewires, Catheters, and Sheaths

Most interventionists acquire their knowledge of guidewires, catheters, and sheaths through actual handling of the devices, with little thought given to the complex scientific and engineering processes that led to their development. Suppliers of these products are eager to offer a variety of devices that are tailored to specific needs and may have subtly different handling characteristics, making the task of selecting and stocking an inventory difficult for the practitioner.

The maturation of an endovascular practice goes through predictable phases in the buildup and use of this fundamental inventory. Initially, only a few variants are available, and the interventionist makes do with what is on hand. With growing experience, more difficult anatomic challenges, and a wider offering of therapeutic endovascular alternatives, the perceived need for additional wire, catheter, and sheath options increases substantially. In this second phase, a number of competing products are tested, and inventory increases markedly. Ultimately, the interventionist becomes facile with a wider selection of devices and is able to adapt their different shapes and handling characteristics to a greater number of anatomic conditions. In this mature phase, inventory stabilizes, with new products being introduced as new technologies are developed or significant improvements are made.

This chapter does not promote any particular brand or list of products necessary for the successful conduct of an endovascular practice; rather, it offers background and definitions that may be useful in assisting the practitioner in sorting through the myriad options presented for consideration. The number and variety of products needed are directly related to the number and variety of procedures performed and the previously mentioned phase of maturation of the particular endovascular practice.

GUIDEWIRES

Design Characteristics

Guidewires are designed to have the characteristics of "pushability" and flexibility. Most guidewires have a single steel core, called a mandrel, surrounded by a coiled wire and coated with a substance to make the guidewire slippery. The tip of the guidewire, always more flexible than the rigid body, is frequently made of a smaller wire that is bonded to the distal tip of the mandrel. These design characteristics— slipperiness and maximal flexibility—allow the tip of the guidewire to be manipulated past tortuous lesions or tight stenoses while limiting the risk of dissection or perforation. (This is why turning the wire around and using the rigid back end is not recommended.)

Guidewire tips are available in three shapes: straight, angled, or J-shaped. The type of tip chosen imparts variable degrees of steerability under fluoroscopic guidance. Steerability refers to the ability to direct the intravascular tip of the guidewire through manipulation of the extra-anatomic portion by twisting, pulling, and pushing.

Guidewires are sized by their maximal transverse diameter (in hundredths of inches) and by their length (in centimeters). The guidewires most commonly used in peripheral vascular procedures come in three diameters: 0.035, 0.018, and 0.014 inch. For most angiographic procedures and most aortoiliac interventions, a 0.035-inch guidewire is used. Trackability of a wire refers to the ability of a catheter or an endovascular device such as a balloon catheter or stent to pass over the wire through tortuous anatomic configurations. Generally, a larger-diameter wire that is stiffer provides better trackability than one that is smaller and more flexible.

For infrageniculate lesions or tight renal and carotid stenoses, a 0.014- or 0.018-inch wire can be used. These smaller wires allow the operator to advance a lower-profile balloon across a tight lesion in a smaller artery. A balloon with a lower profile has a smaller transverse diameter in its folded or uninflated state, which allows it to traverse a tighter stenosis than one with a higher profile.

Occasionally, a 0.038-inch wire is needed for passage of a large-diameter sheath or delivery of an endograft through a tortuous iliac artery. Passage of these large devices may be facilitated by the additional trackability of a stiffer wire with a greater diameter.

Guidewires come in a variety of lengths. The most commonly used lengths for general-purpose guidewires are 145 and 150 cm. Exchange wires, which allow the exchange of catheters or interventional devices without losing access across a remote lesion, are usually 180 or 260 cm long. Longer wires are more difficult to handle and increase the chance of contamination. When performing any intervention, one should try to maintain the wire across the lesion until the completion angiogram has been obtained and is satisfactory. This allows additional interventional procedures, such as stent placement, to be performed after suboptimal intermediate interventions through a constant channel. A good formula for selecting wire length is as follows:

$$\text{Total length of wire needed} = \text{length of wire from insertion site to lesion} + \text{length of catheter or interventional device} + 10 \text{ cm}$$

With a shorter wire, it may not be possible to remove the catheter while maintaining fixation of the wire across the lesion. Docking devices are available in some wire systems that allow extension of the length of the wire in place by adding a second wire to the end of the first via an attachable dock. These docking systems are of sufficiently low profile that they allow for subsequent passage of catheters and interventional devices over the added wire, over the docking system, and onto the initial wire.

Guidewire tip shapes and coatings facilitate function. Non–hydrophilic-coated J-tip catheters are useful for initial catheter introduction via the Seldinger technique. Although dissection can occur with any type of wire, these wires have characteristics that may reduce the frequency of this complication compared with hydrophilic wires with angled or straight tips. J-tip wires are also useful for passage of a wire through a stent when use of an angled or straight wire may lead to inadvertent passage through a fenestration in the stent. Angled- or shapeable-tip guidewires are steerable and are therefore useful in manipulating the catheter across a tight stenosis or into a specific branch vessel. We limit the use of straight wires to catheter exchanges.

Most guidewires have a hydrophilic coating of either polytetrafluoroethylene or silicone, which decreases the coefficient of friction during catheter exchange or while traversing a stenosis. The interventionist should be aware of the tactile differences noted with different wires as they are advanced into an artery. For example, the passage of a very hydrophilic wire or a reduced-diameter wire in the subintimal plane may offer so little resistance that the technician is unaware that dissection has occurred. In contrast, attempted passage of a standard J-tip wire through an introducer needle and into an artery in an extraluminal plane may offer enough resistance that the operator feels the need to confirm the location with a hand-held injection of contrast agent. For the beginning interventionist, this is our recommended starting wire. A good practice is to wipe the guidewire with a sponge soaked in heparin and saline solution frequently and routinely between each catheter manipulation. This minimizes the amount of thrombotic debris that accumulates on the wire and decreases friction during subsequent catheter or wire exchanges. Care must be taken when wiping a wire not to inadvertently remove any length of the wire from its intended position. The practice of wiping toward the body reduces this possibility.

Selection

As one gains experience with catheter-based therapy, the number of guidewires and catheters needed to complete an intervention successfully may become fewer. Our recommendations should serve as a reference for the reader but are by no means comprehensive (Table 17-2). For initial entry into the artery, we recommend a J-tip wire, which is associated with the lowest risk of dissection. J-tip wires come in a wide variety; some have a movable core that can convert the distal end of the wire from a flexible state to a rigid one. For initial introduction, a nonhydrophilic guidewire with medium rigidity should be chosen. The Bentson wire has a floppy tip, is of medium to firm rigidity and, although straight in its packaged state, forms a large, functional J-tip when being advanced through an artery or vein.

Glidewires (Boston Scientific, Quincy, Mass.) can be either straight or angled and are hydrophilic. Angled Glidewires are steerable and may be manipulated with torque at the skin level, with or without an external torquing device. We do not recommend the use of straight Glidewires during initial access because they are associated with the greatest chance of dissection. If dissection is suspected but not confirmed, a few simple tests can be performed. If a J-tip wire is used, one can attempt to spin the wire under fluoroscopy. The curved J-tip will not move freely in a subintimal plane. One can also perform hand-held contrast agent injection.

Smaller-diameter wires include 0.018- and 0.014-inch wires. These may be useful in renal, carotid, or infrageniculate manipulations. Use of these wires requires use of appropriately sized catheters, balloon angioplasty catheters, and stents. This may necessitate an expanded inventory and some redundancy, however (e.g., one may use 4-mm balloon angioplasty catheters with a 0.018-inch system and different 4-mm balloon catheters with a 0.035-inch system). We have found small wires preferable in many instances when introduction of the lowest-profile balloon catheters is needed. Recent advances in the design of 0.014-inch wires have made their bodies more rigid, allowing for improved trackability. The 0.014-inch system is currently our preferred system for angioplasty and stenting of renal arteries.

Infusion wires have been designed for use during thrombolytic infusion therapy. These wires have a proximal infusion port and a lumen that allows infusion through the distal aspect of the wire. Typically, these wires are passed through a multiside hole infusion catheter, such as a Mewissen Infusion Catheter (Boston Scientific, Quincy, Mass.). Using a coaxial system and a Tuohy-Borst adapter (Cook, Bloomington, Ind.), thrombolytic agents can be infused directly into the clot through the infusion catheter while simultaneously infusing either additional thrombolytic agent or heparin into the distal circulation via the infusion wire.

TABLE 17–2	Types of Guidewires and Catheters			
Guidewire	**Diameter (0.001 × in)**	**Length (cm)**	**Features**	**Function**
General				
J-tip (Cook, Bloomington, Ind.)	18, 21, 25, 28, 32, 35, 38	80, 100, 125, 145	Variable tip curve 1.5, 3, 7.5, 15 TFE coated	Catheter introduction Passage through stents or tortuous vessels
Bentson (Cook, Bloomington, Ind.)	18, 21, 25, 28, 32, 35, 38	145, 180	15-cm flexible tip with distal 5 cm soft	Atraumatic negotiation of tortuous or strictured vessel
Glidewire (Boston Scientific, Quincy, Mass.)	18, 25, 32, 35	120, 150, 180, 260	Hydrophilic; angled or shapeable tip	Crossing difficult lesions
Exchange				
Amplatz Super Stiff (Cook, Bloomington, Ind.)	35, 38	80, 145, 180, 260	Stiff mandrel with flexible tip	Catheter exchange, good trackability Straightens acute aortoiliac bifurcation
Rosen (Boston Scientific, Quincy, Mass.)	35	150, 180, 260	1.5-mm J-tip	Good trackability Supports advancing catheter
Wholey (Mallinckrodt, St. Louis, Mo.)	35	145, 190, 300	17-cm floppy tip	Steerable tip, stiff core catheterization
Lunderquist-Ring (Cook, Bloomington, Ind.)	38	125	Very stiff	Used through a catheter, flossing, straightening tortuous iliac arteries for endograft delivery
Renal				
TAD (Mallinckrodt, St. Louis, Mo.)	35 tapers to 18 tip	145, 200	36-cm tapered tip Guidewire extension available	Good for crossing a stenosis with little trauma Good trackability with little trauma
TAD II Spartacore (Guidant, Santa Clara, Calif.)	Same as TAD 14	145, 180	20-cm tapered tip Atraumatic tip, 1:1 torquing	Short renal arteries Rigid support Low-profile 14 system

TFE, tetrafluoroethyl.
From Moore WS, Ahn SS (eds): Endovascular Surgery, 3rd ed. Philadelphia, WB Saunders, 2001, p 50.

CATHETERS

Design

Catheters are made from polyurethane, polyethylene, polypropylene, Teflon, or nylon, with polyurethane catheters having the highest coefficient of friction and Teflon having the lowest. Catheters are sized according to their outer diameter (in French) and their length (in centimeters). Although catheters that have smaller internal diameters are available, most catheters used in angiography will accommodate a 0.035-inch guidewire. We stock and use mostly 5 French catheters, but 4 and 6 French catheters are occasionally used. These are matched with appropriately sized sheaths. The most commonly used catheter lengths are 65 and 100 cm.

Functionally, catheters can be either selective or nonselective. Nonselective or flush catheters, which have multiple side and end holes that allow a large cloud of contrast agent to be infused over a short period, are used for large-vessel opacification and in high-flow systems. These nonselective catheters may be straight, or they may have shaped ends (e.g., Tennis Racquet or pigtail catheters). There are numerous variations of the curled pigtail shape, with subtle modifications of the tightness of the curls. We have found them to be interchangeable.

Selective catheters have only a single hole at the tip and are used to intubate vascular families (branches off the aorta) before advancement of the wire. With angiography that includes selective catheterization, one uses smaller amounts of contrast material at lower injection rates to obtain adequate arterial opacification. When using selective catheters, care must be taken to avoid intimal injury or dissection of the artery from either direct catheter tip advancement or the forceful injection of contrast material. Additionally, a "jet effect" can occur when forceful injection of contrast material pushes the catheter out of the vessel of interest and back into the aorta. Lengthening the "rise of rate" of injection on the power injector control panel can limit these negative effects.

Catheter information, such as maximal flow rate, bursting pressure, inner diameter, outer diameter, and length, is detailed on the package label. We routinely review the catheter package before opening it. This allows us to reaffirm the catheter's compatibility with the wire and the introducer sheath while visually assessing the shape of the tip relative to the anatomic angles we are attempting to navigate.

Flow rate (Q) through a catheter varies with its internal radius and is inversely proportional to catheter length.

TABLE 17–3	Catheter Maximal Flow Rate	
Size (French)	Length (cm)	Rate of Contrast Agent (mL/sec)
5	65	15
5	100	11
6	65	21
6	100	17

From Moore WS, Ahn SS (eds): Endovascular Surgery, 3rd ed. Philadelphia, WB Saunders, 2001, p 51.

Poiseuille's equation can be used to describe the factors associated with flow through a catheter:

$$Q = \frac{P\pi R^4}{8\eta L}$$

where Q is flow (cc/min), P is the pressure drop (mm Hg) over the length of the catheter, R is the internal radius (mm), η is the viscosity of the fluid, and L is the length of the catheter (mm). Table 17-3 shows the effect of altering radius and length on flow rates for several commonly used catheters.

Selection

Prevention of thrombus formation is desired in any vascular cannulation. There is an increasing likelihood of thrombus formation as catheter size increases with respect to the internal diameter of the vessel lumen. This risk can be minimized by selecting the smallest catheter that will achieve the intended purpose and by removing the catheter as early as possible. Thrombus may also form within a catheter while it is in the lumen of the vessel. We recommend regular aspiration of blood from catheters before planned injection and flushing with heparinized saline solution once the catheter is found to be free of clot.

The head shape of a catheter determines its function. All catheters, regardless of shape, should be advanced over a wire to limit the potential for intimal injury during advancement and positioning. Nonselective catheters, such as the pigtail catheter, are designed to be used in larger-diameter vessels, such as the aorta. Once the wire has been withdrawn and the curl of the pigtail has been formed in the aorta, the leading edge of the catheter curl offers a relatively blunt profile. As such, these catheters can be carefully advanced or repositioned distally without reinserting the wire. We recommend, however, that a wire be reinserted before removing any shaped catheter through the iliac or brachial artery into which it is introduced. This practice limits the potential for the catheter tip to score and injure the intima as it is removed.

To cannulate the contralateral iliac artery for selective iliac injection, the nonselective flush catheter used for the initial aortogram can often be used. The wire is reinserted and advanced to the tip of the catheter orifice to open the angle of the curl. The catheter is withdrawn to the bifurcation so that the tip engages the orifice of the contralateral iliac artery. The wire is then advanced distally, and the catheter is advanced over the wire. To minimize arterial injury, care should be taken not to advance or withdraw the unfurled pigtail catheter without reintroducing the wire.

For selective cannulation of branches of the aorta, one should choose a catheter with a head shape that corresponds to the anatomic angle of the branch to be entered. In selective catheterization, the catheter tip itself is manipulated into the orifice of the branch vessel. Injections at lower pressures may be performed after this step; however, for higher-pressure injections, the catheter must be advanced farther into the branch to prevent losing access as a result of catheter whip and recoil. This is accomplished by passing the wire more distally and advancing the catheter over it and into the target vessel.

For arch vessels, we recommend starting with a vertebral catheter. This catheter has perhaps the most minimally selective design, with a 1-cm tip angled at approximately 30 degrees to the straight access. With practice, however, it is possible to use this catheter for each of the thoracic arch vessels. Alternatively, a number of elaborately designed catheters have been developed to facilitate cannulation of arch vessels. The headhunter or the Simmons may be appropriate for this task; if these are unsuccessful, one may try the Mani, the Vitek, or the HN4.

Most of the more elaborately shaped selective catheters are designed to be re-formed in the aortic arch or the abdominal aorta proximal to the vessel that one is attempting to intubate. Once the catheter is re-formed into its planned shape, the operator withdraws and rotates the catheter under fluoroscopic guidance until it engages the orifice of the desired branch vessel.

For renal and visceral arteries, we recommend a cobra catheter or a Shepherd hook. The catheter should be advanced above the intended artery and rotated as it is gently pulled inferiorly. This manipulation will result in intubation of the renal or the visceral orifice; its position can be confirmed with a puff of contrast material. Once the orifice of the intended artery has been intubated, a guidewire with a floppy tip is advanced into it distally so that the catheter can then be advanced over the stiffer portion of the wire.

In arteries of the lower extremity, we use a simple selective straight catheter over a guidewire for selective arteriography. Occasionally, when a guidewire cannot be manipulated across a tight stenosis, the catheter can be advanced to the area of stenosis to support the wire as an additional attempt to cross the lesion is made.

A number of catheters have been designed for specific functions or unusual situations. Catheters with a hydrophilic coating, called Glidecaths (Boston Scientific, Quincy, Mass.) or Slip-Caths (Cook, Bloomington, Ind.), may be helpful in crossing tight stenoses. For thrombolytic therapy, the Mewissen Infusion Catheter is used in conjunction with Cragg or Katzen wires (Boston Scientific, Quincy, Mass.). When assessing a patient with an aneurysm for the potential use of an aortic endograft, aortography is performed with a 6 French pigtail catheter that is marked with radiopaque markers at 1-cm increments. This allows for the measurement of aortic and iliac segments and aids in the selection of appropriately tailored limbs for the endoprosthesis. Additionally, a catheter with radiopaque markings spaced 2.8 cm apart is available. This catheter is useful in obtaining an inferior venacavogram before vena cava filter placement. The 2.8-cm measurement can then be used to determine the transverse diameter of the vena cava and identify those vessels that are too large for standard filter placement.

With the proliferation of accurate noninvasive imaging techniques and the growing acceptance of the appropriateness of endovascular intervention for the treatment of atherosclerotic disease, purely diagnostic angiography is performed infrequently in our practice. More commonly, our patients undergoing catheterization are candidates for potential intervention in addition to angiographic inspection. As such, we routinely perform catheterizations through introducer sheaths with hemostatic valves. This facilitates the introduction of various endovascular devices while minimizing blood loss and trauma to the artery at the insertion site.

SHEATHS

Introducer Sheaths

Once percutaneous access has been obtained and wire access to the blood vessel has been established, we prefer to dilate the track gradually with progressively enlarging dilators. Dilators, like catheters, are sized according to their outer diameter (in French). Sheaths, in contradistinction, are sized according to their inner diameter (also in French). Consequently, if we are planning to use a 5 French sheath, we sequentially pass 4, 5, and 6 French dilators. The final size of the hole in the artery is determined by the outer size of the 5 French sheath, which is just over 6 French. Progressive dilatation causes less trauma to the common femoral artery and, we believe, reduces the potential for iatrogenic injury.

Introducer sheaths all have hemostatic valves and side infusion ports. The side port may be used to monitor pressure or, in some cases, to inject contrast agent and eliminate the need for a catheter. Sheaths come in multiple lengths (measured in centimeters). Most commonly, we use 15- or 25-cm lengths. A shorter 6-cm sheath is ideally suited for working on arteriovenous grafts or fistulas. These shorter sheaths are adapted for high-volume infusion and may be left in the graft for dialysis after the procedure if the patient requires same-day dialysis. Occasionally, we use a long 5 French sheath to assist with passage of a catheter through a tortuous iliac artery. When one is planning to perform angioplasty or stenting, the initial 5 French sheath placed for diagnostic angiography is exchanged for a larger-diameter sheath, usually 7 French, through which the interventional devices can be passed. We use the smallest size sheath required for the planned intervention.

Guiding Catheters and Guiding Sheaths

Both guiding catheters and guiding sheaths are used to facilitate passage of a smaller catheter or an endovascular device through a tortuous area to a desired treatment location. The larger size of the guiding catheter or the guiding sheath may allow contrast agent injection around the smaller endovascular treatment device while it is in place. For visceral, renal, and carotid artery angioplasty and stenting, use of a guiding catheter or a guiding sheath is preferred. In addition to facilitating passage of the endovascular device, they promote precise positioning by allowing contrast agent injections around the device, with concomitant maintenance of wire access across the lesion.

Although the terms *guiding catheter* and *guiding sheath* are sometimes used interchangeably, there are differences between them. Guiding catheters are designed with a stronger external reinforcement material, which aids in supporting balloon or catheter passage through long distances in the aorta to branch vessels. Unlike guiding sheaths, guiding catheters have no hemostatic valve and require the use of a Tuohy-Borst side-arm adapter. Another important distinction between sheaths and catheters is that guiding sheaths are sized according to their internal diameter, whereas guiding catheters are sized according to their outer diameter (both in French).

Sheaths are packaged with a tapered internal obturator for introduction and advancement into an artery. Not all guiding catheters come with internal obturators. The size discrepancy between the internal diameter of the guiding catheter and the wire is usually significant. Advancement of a guiding catheter that is much larger than its wire can be associated with injury to the intima of the artery and an unintentional endarterectomy. To reduce the size mismatch, one can advance a selective catheter over the wire to just beyond the tip of the guiding catheter and then advance both as a unit. We prefer, however, to use only guiding sheaths and guiding catheters supplied with internal obturators. Both sheaths and catheters are available with radiopaque tips. These are preferred because they allow for accurate identification of the end of the guide in relation to the endovascular device and the lesion being treated.

Guides are available with preformed distal shapes for use in many anatomic scenarios. Use of a hockey stick–shaped catheter that forms a 90-degree angle is useful in the deployment of a renal artery stent. When using a guide to facilitate delivery of a balloon-expandable stent, we attempt to advance the guide past the lesion to be stented. If successful, this allows delivery of the stent through a protected sleeve, limiting the potential for dislodging the stent from its delivery balloon as it traverses the atherosclerotic lesion. The guide is then withdrawn to the orifice of the involved artery, and contrast material is injected for accurate positioning just before deployment.

We have used an externally supported long-shuttle catheter with a straight but malleable tip for angioplasty and stenting of the brachiocephalic vessels. Newer guide sheaths with a variety of tips shaped specifically for accessing the arch vessels and those with hemostatic valves, radiopaque tips, and obturators are currently being developed, which will make carotid angioplasty and stenting less complex.

Guiding sheaths are particularly useful when performing interventions in the contralateral iliac system. In addition to facilitating passage of stents up and over the bifurcation, they protect the ipsilateral iliac artery from the repetitive passage of balloon catheters, diagnostic catheters, and stents. Most important, they allow for intermediate assessment of the results of preliminary angioplasty with pericatheter puff angiography while maintaining wire access across the lesion. If angioplasty of a contralateral iliac artery is performed without a guide sheath, assessment of the results requires removing the balloon catheter and advancing a diagnostic catheter over the wire. The wire must then be removed, and the catheter must be pulled back above the lesion undergoing angioplasty to perform angiography. If it is determined that a stent is required owing to suboptimal angioplasty results, it becomes necessary to recross the freshly treated lesion. If the wire does not pass through the center of the lumen but rather tracks through a portion of the fractured plaque, subsequent stenting may prove catastrophic. We recommend use of a guiding sheath for contralateral iliac endovascular interventions.

When using guiding catheters or guiding sheaths, the operator should note that their diameters are much larger than those of devices used in simple angiographic procedures. The larger the diameter of the introducer, the higher the rate of complications in the iliac and femoral systems. In a smaller patient, the catheter may be of sufficient size to occlude the artery or significantly diminish flow distal to the insertion site, subjecting the ipsilateral extremity to some degree of ischemia and predisposing to thrombosis. We anticoagulate the patient once these large-diameter devices are in place. Use of these catheters should be limited, and their removal from a vessel should be prompt. With devices of 8 French or larger, percutaneous closure devices may be of benefit.

SUMMARY

In our endovascular training program, we teach three rules of endovascular surgery:
  1. The inviolate rule: once across a lesion with a wire, do not remove it until the case is finished. Unfortunately, wires still get pulled out inadvertently.
  2. Read the package. As we have described in this chapter, sizing methodology for wires, catheters, and sheaths was clearly an afterthought. Wire diameters are in hundredths of an inch, and their lengths are in centimeters; dilators and catheters are described in French by their outer diameters; and sheaths are described in French by their inner diameters with their lengths in centimeters. For guiding sheaths, the inner diameter is in French; for guiding catheters, the outer diameter is in French. Balloon catheters and stents are described by their outer diameter in French in the undeployed state and in millimeters once they are inflated or deployed. The challenge is putting together pieces that fit. Mercifully, all the information needed is on the front of the package for each of these devices. The corollary to this rule is that the package will be found in the trashcan.
  3. Everything falls on the floor. This is both self-explanatory and prophetic. We recommend having at least two of everything.

Balloon Angioplasty Catheters

ROLE OF BALLOON ANGIOPLASTY IN ENDOVASCULAR INTERVENTION

Endoluminal blood vessel manipulation by means of balloon angioplasty has become a cornerstone of contemporary vascular therapy. The usefulness of balloon angioplasty has increased steadily since 1980, and at present, balloon angioplasty contributes significantly to the management of occlusive disease in most vascular beds. Improvements in technology and catheter-based techniques have broadened the spectrum of lesions that are amenable to percutaneous transluminal angioplasty (PTA). The development of vascular stents has further increased the number of applications for balloon angioplasty.

PTA (with stent placement, as needed) is an essential option in the management of aortoiliac, femoropopliteal, and renovascular occlusive disease.[1-6] Subclavian, common carotid, and innominate lesions, although less common, have been managed with PTA, with reasonable initial results.[7,8] The results of PTA of the carotid bifurcation, the intracranial vasculature, and the tibial and pedal vessels are less clear, but there is substantial interest in pursuing these applications.[9-12]

Balloon angioplasty may be used to treat some lesions within bypass grafts and dialysis grafts. PTA shows promise in the central venous system and represents a potentially significant advance in venous reconstruction.

This section presents the concepts, equipment, and techniques that make balloon angioplasty an integral part of contemporary vascular practice.

STRUCTURE OF BALLOON ANGIOPLASTY CATHETERS

Balloon angioplasty is performed using a disposable coaxial catheter selected from among many sizes and types to meet the demands of the particular lesion being treated. The function of a balloon angioplasty catheter is to exert a dilating force on the endoluminal surface of a blood vessel at a desired location. Although a balloon angioplasty catheter is a relatively simple tool, there are multiple variables that must be considered when choosing a catheter for a given situation. These features include balloon diameter and length, catheter size and length, balloon type, and catheter profile (Fig. 17-12).

The angioplasty catheter has two lumens: one that permits the catheter to pass over a guidewire during placement, and one to inflate the balloon once it is appropriately placed. Balloon diameters range from 1.5 to 24 mm and are selected with the intent to slightly overdilate the artery being treated (Table 17-4). Balloon lengths range from 1.5 to 10 cm and should be sufficient to dilate the lesion, with a slight overhang into the adjacent artery. Radiopaque markers on the catheter at each end of the balloon permit the operator to place the catheter precisely. The shoulder is the tapered balloon end that extends beyond the radiopaque marker. Because the body of the balloon is always cylindrical, the taper of the shoulder helps define the balloon's overall shape when it is fully inflated. A short shoulder is desirable when angioplasty is performed adjacent to an area where dilatation is contraindicated, such as a smaller-diameter branch vessel or an ulcerated or aneurysmal segment. The tip of the catheter, which is the segment that extends beyond the end of the balloon, also varies in length.

The shaft length varies from 40 to 150 cm. The shaft must be long enough to reach from the remote access site to the lesion. In general, the shortest catheter that is able to reach the target site is desirable, because it is less cumbersome and more responsive to manipulation, requires shorter guidewires, and makes exchanges simpler. Angioplasty catheters that pass over a 0.035-inch guidewire are available over a broad range of balloon sizes (3 to 18 mm). Catheter shaft sizes range from 3 to 7 French and are determined by the balloon type and diameter. Standard angioplasty in its most common working range (diameters from 3 to 8 mm) can be performed using 5 French catheters. Larger-diameter balloons or heavy-duty (high-pressure) balloons require larger catheter shafts (5.8 to 7 French). Smaller-diameter balloons (2 to 4 mm) are available on 3.8 French shafts, which pass over 0.018-inch guidewires.

FUNCTION OF BALLOON ANGIOPLASTY CATHETERS

The type of balloon is determined by its material. Standard balloons are constructed of polyethylene, polyethylene terephthalate, or other low-compliance plastic polymers.

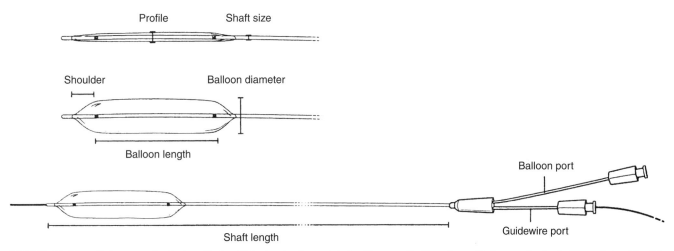

FIGURE 17–12 • Balloon angioplasty catheter. This simple disposable tool has applications in multiple vascular beds. (From Schneider PA: Endovascular Skills. St. Louis, Quality Medical Publishing, 1998; and Moore WS, Ahn SS [eds]: Endovascular Surgery, 3rd ed. Philadelphia, WB Saunders, 2001, p 55.)

Burst pressures range from 8 to 12 atmospheres. At higher pressures, low-compliance balloons will exert force without an increase in diameter or the risk of vessel rupture. Thinner-walled balloons are available, which permit a lower profile (discussed later). These are more easily passed through a preocclusive or tortuous lesion, but they are less puncture resistant and are not useful for heavily calcified lesions or stent placement. Reinforced high-pressure polymer balloons, such as the Blue Max (Boston Scientific, Quincy, Mass.), have burst pressures that exceed 17 atmospheres and may be pressurized to more than 20 atmospheres. These have larger shafts (usually by approximately 1 French) than standard balloons. These thick-walled balloons are useful for treating heavily calcified or sharp lesions and recalcitrant lesions, such as those caused by intimal hyperplasia.

The performance of the catheter can be enhanced by a hydrophilic coating applied by the manufacturer to the balloon surface to permit the balloon to track and cross easily. There are multiple potential applications of this concept of modifying the balloon surface (e.g., antithrombotic therapy and brachytherapy).

The profile of the catheter is the overall diameter of the catheter shaft with the balloon wrapped around it. After a balloon has been inflated, its profile increases in size because the balloon no longer wraps as neatly around the catheter. The used balloon material forms wings, which may be manually rewrapped around the catheter if necessary. The profile of the balloon affects its ability to pass through a lesion. In general, preinflation of the balloon is not performed because this may make it more difficult to pass it across the lesion. Catheter profile is the main factor limiting the size of the percutaneous access site and is an important consideration in every angioplasty.

MECHANISM OF REVASCULARIZATION WITH BALLOON ANGIOPLASTY

Balloon angioplasty causes desquamation of endothelial cells and histologic damage proportional to the diameter of the balloon and the duration of inflation. Longitudinal fracture of the atherosclerotic plaque and stretching of the media and adventitia increase the cross-sectional area of the

TABLE 17–4	Structure and Function of Balloon Angioplasty Catheters
Structure	**Function**
Balloon diameter	Exert dilating pressure to appropriate diameter on endoluminal surface of blood vessel
Balloon length	Dilate entire length of lesion with slight overhang of balloon onto adjacent artery
Catheter size	Deliver appropriate balloon to lesion on smallest possible catheter
Catheter length	Reach lesion through chosen access site without excessive catheter length
Balloon type	Promote use for high-pressure inflation, low-profile catheter passage, stent placement, or scratch resistance based on various materials
Catheter profile	Determine size of access sheath required
Shoulder	Taper balloon to the catheter shaft and determine inflated shape of balloon
Balloon port	Provide lumen along catheter shaft and into balloon used for inflation
Guidewire port	Provide guidewire lumen for delivery of catheter to its intended site
Radiopaque markers	Mark end of balloon for correct placement

From Moore WS, Ahn SS (eds): Endovascular Surgery, 3rd ed. Philadelphia, WB Saunders, 2001, p 56.

diseased vessel.[13,14] Plaque compression does not appreciably add to the newly restored luminal diameter.[15] Postangioplasty arteriography almost always reveals areas of dissection and plaque separation caused by PTA. Areas of dissection are seen more frequently with dilatation of calcified lesions. The plaque may become partially separated from the artery wall at the angioplasty site and may remain attached to the proximal and distal arterial walls. Medial dissection occurs at plaque edges or at plaque rupture sites and tends to be somewhat unpredictable.[13,15] The media opposite the plaque becomes thinner. Because most fractures in the plaque are oriented in the direction of flow, there is a relatively low incidence of acute occlusion at the angioplasty site (due to dissection) or distally (due to atheroembolization).[13-16]

Platelets and fibrin cover the damaged surface, and some endothelialization and surface remodeling soon follow. Follow-up angiography shows that most dissection planes have healed within 1 month.[17]

MECHANISM OF BALLOON DILATATION

The dilating force generated by the balloon is proportional to the balloon diameter, the balloon pressure, and the surface over which the balloon material is applied.[18,19] The dilating force is a result of the hydrostatic pressure within the balloon, the wall tension generated by balloon expansion, and the force vector that results from deformation of the balloon by the lesion.

Hydrostatic pressure is proportional to both the inflation pressure and the endoluminal surface area of the lesion that is dilated by the balloon. At any established level of hydrostatic pressure, wall tension is dependent on Laplace's law and is therefore proportional to the radius of the balloon. This explains why larger balloons are more likely to rupture at a given pressure: the larger radius results in increased wall tension.

Most atherosclerotic lesions require 8 atmospheres of pressure or less for dilatation. When the balloon is inflated, the proximal and distal ends fill first, and the middle section or the body of the balloon, which is usually located at the segment of most severe stenosis, forms a waist (Fig. 17-13). This waist-like shape also contributes to the dilating force of the balloon. As the balloon waist is expanded by increasing wall tension, a radial vector force is generated, which is greatest when the waist is tightest. Once the balloon is fully inflated, further inflation to treat a small area of residual stenosis will not contribute to the dilating force but will increase the likelihood of balloon rupture. For a given stenosis for which there is a choice of possible balloon diameters, a larger balloon will generate a much higher dilating force. The larger diameter increases the wall tension, and the larger balloon size results in a tighter waist at the point of maximal stenosis and a higher radial force vector.

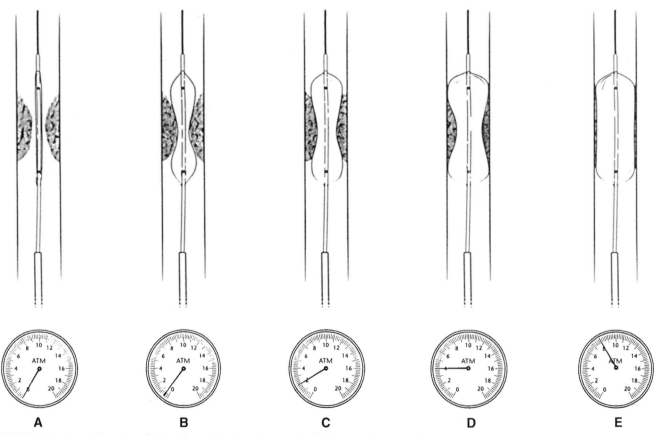

FIGURE 17–13 • Dilatation of the atherosclerotic waist. *A*, The balloon catheter is advanced through the lesion. *B*, The proximal and distal ends of the balloon begin to fill at very low pressure. *C*, At 2 atmospheres of pressure, a waist develops where the stenosis caused by the plaque is most severe. *D*, Stenosis remains at 4 atmospheres of pressure as the waist persists. *E*, The waist has been fully dilated. (From Schneider PA: Endovascular Skills. St. Louis, Quality Medical Publishing, 1998; and Moore WS, Ahn SS [eds]: Endovascular Surgery, 3rd ed. Philadelphia, WB Saunders, 2001, p 57.)

THE PERFECT ANGIOPLASTY CATHETER

Balloon angioplasty catheters, like all other catheters, must be pushable and trackable. The balloon material must be durable and resistant to rupture and must permit very high pressures (20 atmospheres or more). The compliance of the balloon should be low; once the balloon has reached its intended diameter, further increases in pressure should not be followed by an increase in diameter. The balloon must be scratch resistant, puncture resistant, and reusable and must collapse to the lowest possible profile. The lumen filling the balloon must be large enough to inflate and deflate the balloon in a short time. The catheter must be small enough in caliber to be used safely via standard percutaneous approaches.[18,20]

Present technology does not permit the optimization of all these factors in a single catheter; however, most balloon angioplasty catheters are designed to feature one or more of these strengths. Basic categories of balloons are as follows:

1. A wide variety of lesions that require pressures of 2 to 10 atmospheres and intended diameters of 4 to 10 mm may be treated using standard polyethylene balloons through 5 or 6 French sheaths placed over 0.035-inch guidewires.
2. Small-caliber balloons (1.5 to 4 mm in diameter) are available that can be placed through 4 French sheaths over 0.018-inch guidewires. These catheters confer advantages in specific situations that require small-caliber balloons. Trackability and pushability are poor, however, especially from a very remote puncture site.
3. High-pressure balloons are made of more durable polymer material and may be inflated to pressures in excess of 20 atmospheres. The shaft size is larger (5.8 French or more), and the profile of the thicker balloon material is higher because the wings of the previously expanded balloon material are not completely collapsible. This requires use of a 7 French or larger sheath.
4. Larger-diameter balloons (>10 mm) are available for aortic or central venous angioplasty. Balloons up to 18 mm in diameter are available on 5.8 French shafts; however, the profile of these balloons is high, they require more time to inflate and deflate, and they are often more compliant than is desired.
5. Scratch-resistant balloons have been designed and are being marketed for stent placement. Sharp stent edges may cause balloon rupture. When this occurs during stent placement, it can cause stent embolization or migration.

CURRENT PRACTICE OF BALLOON ANGIOPLASTY

Indications for balloon angioplasty vary significantly from one vascular bed to another.[21,22] Balloon angioplasty plays a role, however, in the management of most vascular occlusive problems. In general, the best candidates for balloon angioplasty are those with less extensive disease or those with medical comorbidities that contraindicate open surgery.[21,22] The lesions that are most amenable to balloon angioplasty are focal stenoses located in large vessels with good runoff.[2,21] Stents have had a significant influence on the feasibility of balloon angioplasty, making it possible to treat more extensive lesions.[23,24]

The advantage of balloon angioplasty is that it permits mechanical intervention with less morbidity than that associated with most open surgical options; however, its use is limited by several factors. Many patients present with disease that is too extensive to be treated with angioplasty. Balloon angioplasty offers limited long-term success in many settings; the patency and durability are less than with surgery. Applications of angioplasty and short- and long-term success are limited in smaller-diameter arteries, especially those less than 5 mm in diameter. The required administration of iodinated contrast agents cannot be tolerated by many patients with renal insufficiency.

TECHNIQUE OF BALLOON ANGIOPLASTY

Equipment

A wide selection of balloon angioplasty catheters should be readily available to the operator. A facility with trained support staff, an inventory of other endovascular supplies, and satisfactory radiographic imaging capabilities are essential. Supplies that should be opened and placed on the sterile field are listed in Table 17-5.[25-27]

Approach to the Lesion

Before balloon angioplasty, the approach must be planned, based on the location of the lesion, its suitability for angioplasty, and the timing of PTA performance. If the lesion's location and appearance are known as a result of a prior imaging study (e.g., duplex mapping, magnetic resonance angiography, standard arteriography) and it is deemed suitable for angioplasty, the puncture site for remote access may be chosen accordingly. When arteriography is performed initially and PTA is added to the same procedure, the access site chosen for arteriography may be converted to use for the

TABLE 17–5	Supplies for Balloon Angioplasty

Endovascular Inventory
Balloon angioplasty catheters
Stents
Access sheaths
Guidewires
Angiographic catheters

Supplies for Sterile Field
4- × 4-inch gauze
Entry needle
No. 11 scalpel
Mosquito clamp
Iodinated contrast agent
Lidocaine (local anesthetic agent)
10-mL syringe
20-mL syringe or larger
25-gauge needle
Inflation device
Gown
Gloves, drapes

From Moore WS, Ahn SS (eds): Endovascular Surgery, 3rd ed. Philadelphia, WB Saunders, 2001, p 58.

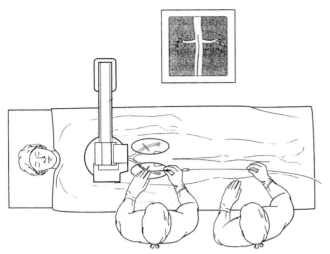

FIGURE 17–14 • Working forehand. In this case, the right-handed operator works forehand to manipulate catheters and guidewires. The assistant stands to the side. The fluoroscopic image is observed on the monitor placed on the opposite side of the table. (From Schneider PA: Endovascular Skills. St. Louis, Quality Medical Publishing, 1998; and Moore WS, Ahn SS [eds]: Endovascular Surgery, 3rd ed. Philadelphia, WB Saunders, 2001, p 59.)

therapeutic procedure, or a new access site may be selected. The shortest distance that provides adequate working room is usually best. The operator should work forehand for best catheter control (Fig. 17-14).

After the lesion has been identified, it is marked with external markers placed on the field by the observation of bony landmarks or by road-mapping. Heparin is administered if required. When stent placement is also anticipated, antibiotics are administered.

The lesion should be crossed with an appropriate guidewire before placing a sheath or opening angioplasty catheters. If the guidewire does not pass easily, the operator may decide on a different approach. If the lesion is preocclusive, the guidewire

alone may inhibit flow and induce thrombus formation. In that situation, the patient should be adequately heparinized, and the operator should proceed directly with PTA.

Arteriography does not usually require a hemostatic access sheath. When an arteriographic procedure is converted to an angioplasty procedure, a sheath is usually placed to minimize injury to the access vessel. The smallest sheath adequate for the intended balloon catheter is best, because complications increase with increasing French size. Midprocedure sheath changes are cumbersome and inconvenient; therefore, the operator should attempt to place the correct sheath when the decision is made to proceed with PTA. Guidelines for sheath sizing are presented in Table 17-6. The required sheath is selected based on the desired type and diameter of the balloon, the size of the catheter, and the need for a stent.

Balloon Catheter Selection

A slight overdilatation at the angioplasty site is generally recommended. The ranges of balloon sizes available for specific PTA sites are listed in Table 17-7. The diameter of the normal vessel just distal to the lesion is measured to help assess the required balloon diameter (Fig. 17-15). Cut film provides a 10% to 20% magnification of the artery, and the diameter of the artery may be taken directly from the radiographic film measurement. Digital subtraction filming requires the use of software measuring packages or the use of catheters with graduated measurement markers for size comparisons. In general, if there is uncertainty about the final desired diameter, it is best to begin with a smaller-diameter balloon and to upsize as needed to avoid overdilatation.

The balloon should be long enough so that there is a short overhang into the adjacent artery. If the lesion is lengthy or is juxtaposed to an area where dilatation is contraindicated, it is best to choose a shorter balloon and to dilate the lesion with several sequential balloon inflations. The length of the catheter shaft must be adequate to cover the distance from the access site to the lesion.

TABLE 17–6	Sheath Sizing Guidelines for Balloon Angioplasty		
Sheath (French)	**Balloon Diameter (mm)**	**Balloon Shaft (French)**	**Anticipated Procedure**
4	2-4	3.8	Small-vessel PTA (0.018-inch guidewire)
5	3-6	5	Infrainguinal, renal, or dialysis graft PTA without stent (0.035-inch guidewire)
6	Up to 8	5	Standard PTA—aortoiliac, infrainguinal, renal, or subclavian
	Up to 7	5	Placement of medium Palmaz stent with low-profile balloon
	Up to 6	5.8	PTA with high-pressure balloon
7	Up to 12	5.8	Aortic PTA
	Up to 8	5.8	PTA with high-pressure balloon
	Up to 9	5	Placement of medium Palmaz stent (4-9 mm)
			Placement of Wallstent (≤10 mm)
9	Up to 18	5.8	Aortic PTA
	6-8	5	Placement of 8 French guiding catheter for renal, subclavian, or carotid PTA-stent
	8-12	5.8	Placement of large Palmaz stent (up to 12 mm)
			Placement of large Wallstent (≥12 mm)

PTA, percutaneous transluminal angioplasty.
From Moore WS, Ahn SS (eds): Endovascular Surgery, 3rd ed. Philadelphia, WB Saunders, 2001, p 59.

TABLE 17–7	Selection of Balloon Angioplasty Catheters				
			Shaft Length (cm)		
Lesion Site	**Balloon Diameter (mm)**	**Balloon Length (cm)**	*Femoral Access*	*Axillary Access*	
Common carotid artery	6-8	2 or 4	120	—	
Subclavian artery	6-8	2 or 4	120	75	
Axillary artery	5-7	2 or 4	120	30	
Renal artery	5-7	2 or 4	75	75	
Aorta	8-18	4	75	—	
Common iliac artery	6-10	2, 4, or 6	75*	120	
External iliac artery	6-8	2, 4, or 6	75*	120	
Superficial femoral artery	4-7	2, 4, 6, or 10	75†	120	
Popliteal artery	3-6	2, 4, or 6	75†	120‡	
Infrageniculate artery	2-4	2 or 4	75†	120‡	

*Approaching these lesions via a contralateral femoral access site usually requires a 75-cm catheter.
†Approaching these lesions via a contralateral femoral access site usually requires a 120-cm catheter and occasionally may require a 150-cm catheter.
‡May occasionally require a 150-cm catheter.
From Moore WS, Ahn SS (eds): Endovascular Surgery, 3rd ed. Philadelphia, WB Saunders, 2001, p 60.

Balloon Catheter Placement

The selected balloon catheter is wiped and flushed with heparinized saline solution but is not preinflated. After placement of the correctly sized sheath, the angioplasty catheter is passed over the guidewire, through the sheath, and into the lesion. The catheter should pass easily through the sheath because the balloon has not yet been inflated. The balloon catheter should track along the guidewire and advance across the lesion using predetermined markers of the lesion's location. The balloon is centered so that its body dilates the portion of the lesion with the most critical stenosis. This is where the force vector will contribute substantially to the dilating force.

The balloon material may break by snagging on a protruding calcific lesion or a previously placed stent. If this is a concern, a longer sheath may be used to deliver the balloon to the lesion. If the balloon catheter will not track along the guidewire, this may be due to distance, lack of shaft strength, tortuosity, or even subintimal guidewire positioning. If this occurs, consider a stiffer guidewire or a longer sheath.

Occasionally, the lesion itself may be so tight that the balloon catheter cannot be advanced across it. If the balloon will cross the lesion only partially, do not start angioplasty. Withdraw the PTA catheter, and confirm guidewire positioning. Consider (1) adequate anticoagulation, (2) "Dottering" the lesion by advancing a van Andel graduated-tip catheter or a straight 5 French angiographic catheter across the lesion, (3) predilatation with a smaller-diameter (lower-profile) balloon, or (4) a balloon with a hydrophilic coating.

Balloon Inflation

After catheter placement, the balloon is inflated without delay to avoid thrombus formation. The balloon is inflated using a 50% contrast agent solution so that the outline of the balloon is visible under fluoroscopy. This permits the operator to observe the location and severity of the atherosclerotic waist as it is being dilated. Solution is forced into the balloon using an inflation device, which also measures the pressure required to dilate the lesion.

The balloon is usually inflated for 30 to 60 seconds, deflated, and then reinflated for another 30 to 60 seconds. A spot film of the inflated balloon is often obtained to document its full expansion. After complete deflation of the balloon, but before moving the catheter, fluoroscopy is used to visualize the balloon and ensure that it is fully deflated. Partially flared balloon wings may disrupt fractured atherosclerotic plaque or may damage the tip of the access sheath on withdrawal. During removal of the balloon catheter, the guidewire must be maintained in place across the lesion.

Completion Arteriography

After the balloon catheter is removed, completion arteriography is performed to evaluate the results of PTA. This is usually done through the same access site used for balloon angioplasty. The guidewire may be exchanged for an angiographic catheter, which is placed upstream from the lesion. If the tip of the sheath is in proximity to the lesion, contrast material may be injected through the side arm of the sheath to obtain an arteriogram. Occasionally, it is necessary to perform a second puncture to obtain access for completion arteriography.

When completion arteriography shows a widely patent PTA site without residual stenosis or significant dissection, the procedure is complete. When residual stenosis or dissection is present, its significance may be evaluated using adjunctive means of assessment (Table 17-8). Inadequate angioplasty results may be treated with stent placement.[23,24]

COMPLICATIONS OF BALLOON ANGIOPLASTY

The balloon angioplasty procedure is less likely to result in complications when the catheters are handled with excellent technique. Advice about the use of balloon catheters is presented in Table 17-9.

The tremendous advantage of PTA is that the incidence and severity of complications are generally low. Because the durability is not as good as with surgical reconstruction,

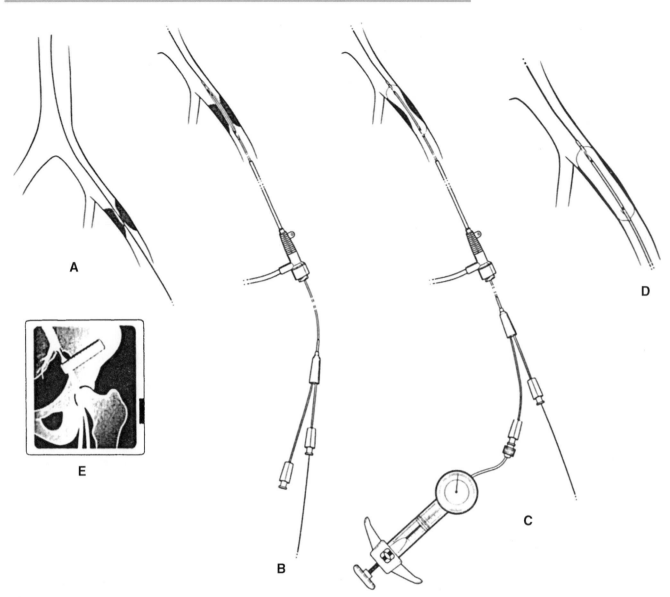

FIGURE 17–15 • Balloon angioplasty. *A*, Stenosis of the left external iliac artery is treated. A guidewire is placed across the lesion. *B*, The balloon diameter is selected, based on the diameter of the adjacent uninvolved artery. This is determined either by measuring cut-film images directly or, if using digital subtraction imaging, by comparing the artery with a known standard such as a catheter with graduated markers. *C*, The angioplasty catheter is passed over the guidewire, through the access sheath, and across the stenosis. *D*, The balloon is inflated using the inflation device. *E*, The fully dilated shape of the balloon is confirmed using fluoroscopy. (From Schneider PA: Endovascular Skills. St. Louis, Quality Medical Publishing, 1998; and Moore WS, Ahn SS [eds]: Endovascular Surgery, 3rd ed. Philadelphia, WB Saunders, 2001, p 61.)

TABLE 17–8	Assessing the Results of Balloon Angioplasty
Method	**Comments**
Completion arteriography	Only method required in most cases; usually performed in projection used for PTA (anteroposterior)
Oblique views	Useful in assessing posterior wall residual stenosis or postangioplasty dissection
Magnified views	Evaluation for dissection flaps or contrast trapping in arterial wall
Pressure measurement	Only quantitative hemodynamic assessment available; time-consuming; results variable; catheter placement across lesion may affect pressure in small-diameter artery
Vasodilator use	Adjunct to pressure measurement when there is no gradient despite the appearance of substantial lesion
Intravascular ultrasonography	Expensive; particularly effective in finding and measuring diameter of residual stenosis

PTA, percutaneous transluminal angioplasty.
From Moore WS, Ahn SS (eds): Endovascular Surgery, 3rd ed. Philadelphia, WB Saunders, 2001, p 61.

TABLE 17–9	Handling Balloon Catheters

Pick catheters before the case to save time and ensure that you have what you need

Flush and wipe catheter with heparinized saline solution to decrease thrombogenicity

Keep profile of catheter low by avoiding preinflation

Check catheter size before placement to avoid unintended overdilatation

When correct catheter shaft length is unclear, measure outside the body with angiographic catheter of known length for a quick estimation

When best arterial diameter is unclear, underestimate to avoid overdilatation

Be sure guidewire is intraluminal before advancing and inflating balloon catheter

Push catheter from the tip when entering the hub of the access sheath to avoid kinking the guidewire and catheter

Have some options when the catheter will not advance along the guidewire (see text discussion)

Be ready to inflate as soon as the balloon crosses the lesion

Magnify field of view at the PTA site if necessary to ensure correct balloon position

Know what to do next when catheter will not advance through lesion (see text discussion)

Deflate balloon by aspirating with a large syringe before withdrawal of catheter

Rotate catheter to fold its wings before pulling it into the sheath

Employ fluoroscopy during inflation to confirm the location and severity of the lesion

Take a spot film of expanded balloon after complete inflation for documentation and size comparisons

Maintain guidewire across the lesion until completion study is satisfactory

If balloon bursts, inflate rapidly until it will no longer hold pressure, then exchange it for a new balloon

If there is evidence of arterial rupture, reinflate balloon at same location to tamponade

PTA, percutaneous transluminal angioplasty.
From Moore WS, Ahn SS (eds): Endovascular Surgery, 3rd ed. Philadelphia, WB Saunders, 2001, p 62.

PTA is useful only when complication rates are acceptable. Patients with extensive disease (category 3 or 4 lesions) are poor candidates for endovascular intervention and have a high chance of experiencing complications if it is attempted.[21]

Complications may occur at the access site, at the PTA site, in the runoff, or systemically. Systemic complications and

TABLE 17–10	Complications of Balloon Angioplasty		
Systemic	**Puncture Site**	**PTA Site**	**Runoff**
Renal failure	Hemorrhage	Dissection	Embolization
Fluid overload	AV fistula	Residual stenosis	Thrombosis
Contrast agent allergy	Hematoma	Thrombosis	Spasm
	Ecchymosis	Rupture	
	Pseudoaneurysm		
	Thrombosis		

AV, arteriovenous; PTA, percutaneous transluminal angioplasty.
From Moore WS, Ahn SS (eds): Endovascular Surgery, 3rd ed. Philadelphia, WB Saunders, 2001, p 62.

some access site complications may occur with arteriography alone. The total complication rate should be less than 10%, and the rate of serious complications (or those requiring operative intervention) should be less than 5% (Table 17-10).[2,21,22]

KEY REFERENCES

Abele JE: Balloon catheters and transluminal dilatation: Technical considerations. AJR Am J Roentgenol 135:901, 1980.

Becker GJ: Intravascular stents: General principles and status of lower extremity arterial applications. Circulation 83(Suppl):I122, 1991.

Block PC, Baughman KL, Pasternak RC, et al: Transluminal angioplasty: Correlation of morphologic and angiographic findings in an experimental model. Circulation 61:778, 1980.

Johnston KW: Iliac arteries: Reanalysis of results of balloon angioplasty. Radiology 186:207, 1993.

Pentecost MJ, Criqui MH, Dorros G, et al: Guidelines for peripheral percutaneous transluminal angioplasty of the abdominal aorta and lower extremity arteries. Circulation 89:511, 1994.

Roubin GS, Yadav S, Iyer SS, et al: Carotid stent-supported angioplasty: A neurovascular intervention to prevent stroke. Am J Cardiol 78:8, 1996.

Sapoval MR, Chatellier G, Long AR, et al: Self-expandable stents for the treatment of iliac artery obstructive lesions: Long-term success and prognostic factors. AJR Am J Roentgenol 166:1173, 1996.

Schneider PA, Rutherford RB: Endovascular interventions in the management of chronic lower extremity ischemia. In Rutherford RB (ed): Vascular Surgery, 5th ed. Philadelphia, WB Saunders, 2000, p 1035.

Zarins CK, Lu CT, Gewertz BL, et al: Arterial disruption and remodeling following balloon dilatation. Surgery 92:1086, 1982.

REFERENCES

1. Becker GJ, Katzen BT, Dake MD: Noncoronary angioplasty. Radiology 170:921, 1989.
2. Johnston KW: Iliac arteries: Reanalysis of results of balloon angioplasty. Radiology 186:207, 1993.
3. O'Donovan RM, Gutierrez OH, Izzo JL: Preservation of renal function by percutaneous renal angioplasty in high-risk elderly patients: Short-term outcome. Nephron 60:187, 1992.
4. Englund R, Brown MA: Renal angioplasty for renovascular disease: A reappraisal. J Cardiovasc Surg 32:76, 1991.
5. Krepel VM, van Andel GJ, van Erp WFM, et al: Percutaneous transluminal angioplasty of the femoropopliteal artery: Initial and long-term results. Radiology 156:325, 1985.
6. Becker GJ: Intravascular stents: General principles and status of lower extremity arterial applications. Circulation 83(Suppl):I122, 1991.
7. Selby JB, Matsumoto AH, Tegtmeyer CJ, et al: Balloon angioplasty above the aortic arch: Immediate and long-term results. AJR Am J Roentgenol 160:631, 1993.
8. Motarjeme A, Keifer JW, Zuska AJ, et al: Percutaneous transluminal angioplasty for treatment of subclavian steal. Radiology 155:611, 1985.
9. Saab MH, Smith DC, Aka PK, et al: Percutaneous transluminal angioplasty of the tibial arteries for limb salvage. Cardiovasc Intervent Radiol 15:211, 1992.
10. Brown KT, Moore ED, Getrajdman GI, et al: Infrapopliteal angioplasty: Long-term follow up. J Vasc Interv Radiol 4:139, 1993.
11. Dietrich EB, Ndiaye M, Reid DB: Stenting in the carotid artery: Initial experience in 110 patients. J Endovasc Surg 3:42, 1996.
12. Roubin GS, Yadav S, Iyer SS, et al: Carotid stent-supported angioplasty: A neurovascular intervention to prevent stroke. Am J Cardiol 78:8, 1996.
13. Castaneda-Zuniga WR, Formanek A, Tadavarthy M, et al: The mechanism of balloon angioplasty. Radiology 135:565, 1980.
14. Block PC, Baughman KL, Pasternak RC, et al: Transluminal angioplasty: Correlation of morphologic and angiographic findings in an experimental model. Circulation 61:778, 1980.
15. Szlavy L, Taveras JM: Pathomechanism of percutaneous transluminal angioplasty. In Szlavy L, Taveras JM (eds): Noncoronary Angioplasty and Interventional Radiologic Treatment of Vascular Malformations. Baltimore, Williams & Wilkins, 1995, p 21.
16. Jain A, Demer LL: In vivo assessment of vascular dilatation during percutaneous transluminal coronary angioplasty. Am J Cardiol 60:988, 1987.

17. Zarins CK, Lu CT, Gewertz BL, et al: Arterial disruption and remodeling following balloon dilatation. Surgery 92:1086, 1982.
18. Abele JE: Balloon catheters and transluminal dilatation: Technical considerations. AJR Am J Roentgenol 135:901, 1980.
19. Orron DE, Kim D: Percutaneous transluminal angioplasty. In Orron DE, Kim D: Peripheral Vascular Imaging and Intervention. St. Louis, Mosby-Year Book, 1992, p 380.
20. Gerlock AJ, Regen DM, Shaff MI: An examination of the physical characteristics leading to angioplasty balloon rupture. Radiology 144:421, 1982.
21. Pentecost MJ, Criqui MH, Dorros G, et al: Guidelines for peripheral percutaneous transluminal angioplasty of the abdominal aorta and lower extremity arteries. Circulation 89:511, 1994.
22. Schneider PA, Rutherford RB: Endovascular interventions in the management of chronic lower extremity ischemia. In Rutherford RB (ed): Vascular Surgery, 5th ed. Philadelphia, WB Saunders, 2000, p 1035.
23. Katzen BT, Becker GJ: Intravascular stents: Status and development of clinical applications. Surg Clin North Am 72:941, 1992.
24. Sapoval MR, Chatellier G, Long AR, et al: Self-expandable stents for the treatment of iliac artery obstructive lesions: Long-term success and prognostic factors. AJR Am J Roentgenol 166:1173, 1996.
25. Hinink MGM, Kandarpa K: Extremity balloon angioplasty. In Kandarpa K, Aruny JE (eds): Handbook of Interventional Radiologic Procedures. Boston, Little, Brown, 1996, p 69.
26. Schneider PA: Balloon angioplasty: Minimally invasive autologous revascularization. In Schneider PA: Endovascular Skills. St. Louis, Quality Medical Publishing, 1998, p 107.
27. Ahn SS, Obrand DI: Percutaneous transluminal angioplasty. In Handbook of Endovascular Surgery. Georgetown, Tex, KargerLandes, 1997, p 59.

Questions

1. **Which of the following statements is most appropriate with regard to selecting an access site for endovascular procedures?**
   (a) Use the brachial artery, because thrombosis is well tolerated
   (b) Use an artery closest to the target lesion
   (c) Use an artery that provides antegrade access
   (d) Use an artery that provides secure and direct access to the target lesion

2. **Which size guidewire is most commonly used?**
   (a) 0.014 inch
   (b) 0.035 inch
   (c) 0.028 inch
   (d) 0.018 inch

3. **What should one do to avoid arterial thrombosis?**
   (a) Use the smallest catheter-to-arterial diameter ratio
   (b) Remove the catheter as soon as possible
   (c) Flush the catheter frequently with heparinized saline
   (d) All of the above

4. **Which is the most frequently used catheter for renal artery imaging?**
   (a) HM 4
   (b) Pigtail
   (c) Cobra
   (d) Tennis Racquet

5. **Which of the following statements is correct?**
   (a) For guiding sheaths, the inner diameter is measured in French; for guiding catheters, the outer diameter is measured in French
   (b) Balloon catheters and stents are described by their outer undeployed diameter in French and their outer deployed diameter in millimeters
   (c) The outer diameter of guiding sheaths and the inner diameter of guiding catheters are measured in French
   (d) Balloon catheters and stents are measured in millimeters for both the deployed and undeployed states

Answers

1. d   2. b   3. d   4. c   5. a

18

Ruth L. Bush • Peter H. Lin • Alan B. Lumsden

Angioplasty and Stenting for Aortoiliac Disease: Technique and Results

History of Endoluminal Treatment

The concept of endovascular therapy of atherosclerotic occlusive disease was introduced 4 decades ago when Dotter performed the first transluminal angioplasty in a patient with ischemic extremities.[1] His novel technique, however, could not reliably maintain luminal patency and did not receive wide acceptance as a treatment of vascular occlusive lesions. Subsequent device modifications led to the development of an angioplasty balloon composed of latex material. The clinical success of this new construct was limited, due in part to its improved compliance, which could not fully dilate a calcified lesion. The introduction of an angioplasty balloon made of polyvinyl chloride in 1976 by Gruntzig, followed by rigid balloons composed of polyethylene and polyetheylene terephthalate, marked a significant advance in endovascular therapy. The latter angioplasty balloons displayed a low compliance and high radial force in a fully inflated condition.[2] As the technology and techniques of endovascular therapy continued to improve over the past 2 decades, transluminal balloon angioplasty evolved to become an important modality in the treatment of peripheral vascular disease.

Despite numerous studies that demonstrate the short-term clinical success of transluminal angioplasty, it has several limitations, due in part to the architectural variation of atherosclerotic lesions. Early restenosis or occlusion following angioplasty may occur because of either elastic recoil of the arterial wall or intimal dissection.[3,4] Vessels that are heavily calcified or completely occluded or that contain ulcerated plaques may not be amenable to balloon angioplasty. Moreover, residual luminal irregularities following angioplasty occasionally trigger mural thrombus formation, leading to thrombotic occlusion.[5,6] Late restenosis following angioplasty may occur as a result of intimal hyperplasia or atherosclerotic progression.[7-9]

In an effort to deal with these limitations of transluminal angioplasty, researchers proposed the concept of intravascular stents as a means of maintaining vessel patency against the restenotic process, as well as improving the clinical outcome of balloon angioplasty. Since Dotter first reported his successful deployment of intravascular stents in canine femoral and popliteal arteries in 1969,[10] a variety of stent devices composed of various materials have been introduced.[11-14] Intravascular stenting is recognized as a potentially effective modality in overcoming elastic recoil of the arterial wall, stabilizing intimal dissection at the site of angioplasty, and maintaining the luminal patency of arteries with calcified and eccentric atherosclerotic plaques.

General Principles of Endoluminal Stents

Given that stenting provides a mechanical scaffold within a stenotic vessel to maintain luminal patency, certain characteristics are desirable in an intravascular stent. The stent should be flexible and durable, with a simple deployment mechanism. It should have a relatively small profile before deployment, along with the capacity to expand to a larger profile when it is fully deployed. Moreover, the stent should have noticeable radiographic opacity to facilitate visualization. The structural material used in stent construction should have a low thrombogenic nature and a high radial force upon expansion. Finally, the ideal stent would be biocompatible, to promote endothelialization without causing intimal hyperplasia.

Intravascular stents can be separated into two distinct types, based on design concepts: self-expanding stents and balloon-expandable stents. Within each of these categories, there are numerous stents with different structural materials, deployment devices, and biocompatible characteristics.[11,12,15-18] Many of these stents are currently under clinical trials; only the Wallstent (Schneider Inc., Minneapolis, Minn.) and the Palmaz stent (Cordis Corp, Warren, N.J.) have been

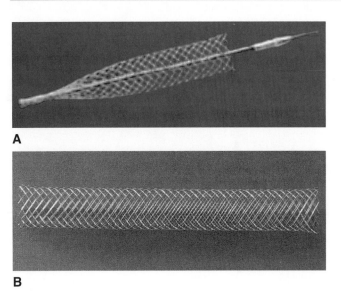

FIGURE 18–1 • *A,* Deployment of the Wallstent is achieved by withdrawing the constraining sheath. *B,* The fully deployed Wallstent.

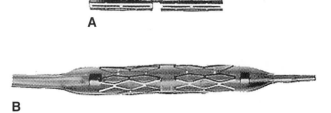

FIGURE 18–2 • *A,* The Palmaz stent is crushed to a small caliber and mounted on an angioplasty balloon. Sizes most commonly used for iliac interventions are already premounted by the manufacturer. *B,* The Palmaz stent is deployed by inflating the angioplasty balloon.

approved by the U.S. Food and Drug Administration (FDA) for iliac artery placement. These two representative stents are described and discussed in this chapter.

SELF-EXPANDING STENTS

Self-expanding stents are generally manufactured so that the stents are constrained within a delivery sheath. The prosthesis is placed intravascularly through an introducer sheath that is advanced over a guidewire for deployment. Deployment is achieved by withdrawing the constraining sheath while keeping the stent in position, thus permitting the stent to self-expand and anchor to the vessel lumen (Fig. 18-1). Stents in this category are generally noted for their ease of deployment and high degree of flexibility. Compared with balloon-expandable stents, however, they may have lower hoop strength or radial force, which is the resistance to radial compression. Most delivery systems of self-expanding stents have a smaller diameter compared with those of balloon-expandable stents. Besides the Wallstent, the Gianturco-Z stent (Cook, Inc., Bloomington, Ind.) is available.

Another type of self-expanding stent is the nitinol stent, which was first introduced by Dotter and colleagues in 1983.[19] Nitinol is a nickel-titanium alloy that has a unique temperature-associated memory property. The nitinol wires can be shaped into a coil spring configuration to serve as a stent when heated to 500°C. As it cools down to 0°C, the nitinol coil straightens into a linear alignment that can be constrained into a delivery catheter for stent deployment. The exposure to warm body temperature after deployment causes the nitinol stent to resume its original coil spring shape. Several clinical studies have evaluated the application of these stents in vascular occlusive lesions.[19-22] Common examples of nitinol stents include the Symphony stent (Boston Scientific Vascular, Watertown, Mass.), Cragg stent (Mintech, France), Smart stent (Cordis Corp, Miami, Fla.), and Memotherm stent (Bard/Angiomed, Karlsruhe, Germany).

BALLOON-EXPANDABLE STENTS

The balloon-expandable stent is first mounted and compressed onto an angioplasty balloon. The original stents were all operator mounted; newer stents are premounted by the manufacturer. Once the stent is positioned intraluminally, it is deployed by inflating the balloon to expand the stent (Fig. 18-2). Unlike a self-expanding stent, the balloon-expandable stent can be expanded further by a larger angioplasty balloon catheter beyond its predetermined diameter. Most balloon-expandable stents are characterized by excellent hoop strength owing to intrinsic stent rigidity once deployed, which can be advantageous in treating stenotic vessels containing calcified plaques. The rigid property of such a stent, however, may create a technical dilemma when treating lesions in tortuous vessels. Moreover, it makes a contralateral approach for iliac artery stenting a challenge, although newer stents are more trackable and flexible. Common examples of balloon-expandable stents include the Palmaz stent (Johnson & Johnson Interventional Systems, Warren, N.J.), Strecker stent (Boston Scientific Vascular, Watertown, Mass.), Gianturco-Roubin stent (Cook, Bloomington, Ind.), AVE stent (Arterial Vascular Engineering, Santa Rosa, Calif.), Absolute Stent (Medtronic, San Diego, Calif.), and IntraStent (IntraTheapeutic, Minneapolis, Minn.).

Indications for Stent Placement

Indications approved by the FDA for iliac stent placement include (1) stenotic or occlusive atherosclerotic lesions or (2) failed or inadequate balloon angioplasty in the iliac artery. The latter condition can be assessed by either angiographic or hemodynamic means. Angiographic detection of residual stenosis of 30% or greater, unstable intimal flaps, and dissection along the subintimal or medial layers are all considered inadequate angioplasty results that warrant intraluminal stent placement. Further, a trans-stenotic pressure gradient of 5 to 10 mm Hg or greater following angioplasty is considered an indication for iliac stent placement. Provocative testing using pharmacologic agents that stimulate vasodilatation may be necessary to identify a hemodynamically significant lesion. Up to 75% of patients without a translesion pressure gradient will have a significant gradient following injection of a vasodilator. Either 100 to 200 μg/mL of nitroglycerin or 30 to 60 mg of papaverine can be injected directly into the vessel in question. Immediate arterial dilatation is induced, thus mimicking exercise. A 10 mm Hg or more pressure drop is considered indicative of a hemodynamically significant stenosis.

In addition to the FDA-approved indications for iliac artery stenting, certain other conditions may be considered for stent placement. In the case of early restenosis following balloon angioplasty, stent placement is appropriate rather than repeat angioplasty alone. The 2-year patency rate of the iliac artery following angioplasty is between 65% and 81% and is affected by numerous factors, such as the degree of stenosis, the length of narrowing, and the distal vessel patency.[3,23,24] Restenosis of the iliac artery frequently occurs at the original angioplasty site,[7,9,11,25] which can be caused by neointimal hyperplasia or rapid atherosclerotic progression. Iliac artery stenting in such a condition may delay the restenotic process. The combination of autologous or prosthetic graft and stents has been used in the treatment of iliac aneurysms, occlusive lesions, and traumatic arteriovenous fistulas.[26-28] Although the use of these stent-graft devices in these conditions is not FDA approved, several reports have indicated technical feasibility and early success. The application of stent-grafts is discussed elsewhere in this book.

Primary stent placement, as opposed to stenting following inadequate angioplasty, has been used more frequently in the treatment of difficult iliac lesions. Nearly or totally occluded iliac arteries may be appropriate for primary stenting because angioplasty alone in these situations generally yields poor long-term patency rates.[14,29-33] Stenotic iliac vessels with ulcerative plaques may cause distal embolization when treated with balloon angioplasty.[6,34] It is appropriate to perform primary stent placement in such a condition to prevent plaque dislodgment. Moreover, primary stenting may be used as an adjunctive procedure to improve iliac inflow when combined with a planned infrainguinal bypass operation.[35-37] Although primary stent placement has been advocated by several interventionalists for the treatment of all iliac lesions,[14,32] prospective, randomized trials are needed to define the long-term benefit of primary stenting in the treatment of iliac artery lesions.

Contraindications to Stent Placement

Table 18-1 summarizes the contraindications to intravascular stent placement. Arterial perforation as a result of balloon angioplasty, as evidenced by contrast extravasation, is considered a contraindication to intra-arterial stent placement. Stent placement in such a condition may lead to severe hemorrhagic complications or pseudoaneurysm formation. In these challenging situations, placement of a covered stent may be more appropriate.[38,39] Stent placement should also be avoided in aneurysmal arteries, because persistent blood flow around the stent may lead to further aneurysm expansion unless a covered stent is used. Because balloon-expandable stents, such as the Palmaz stent, are relatively rigid, they are less than ideal in tortuous vessels. Self-expanding stents, such as the Wallstent, have greater flexibility and are more appropriate in vessels with marked tortuosity. Severely calcified arteries often are not amenable to balloon angioplasty; similarly, stent placement should not be expected to restore the normal vessel lumen because stent deployment requires the same basic techniques as balloon angioplasty. Long-standing arterial occlusion is considered a relative contraindication to stent placement. In this setting, the risk of plaque embolization resulting from stent expansion may outweigh the potential benefit of arterial recanalization. Finally, stent deployment should be avoided in arteries that might serve as either the proximal or distal site of a bypass grafting procedure. In a stented artery, application of vascular clamps may not only cause significant damage to the arterial wall but also crush the stent so that re-expansion may be impossible. If vascular control is needed in a stented artery, intraluminal occlusion balloon catheter should be used rather than vascular clamps.

Aortic Disease

In the infrarenal aorta, short segment stenoses may occur that are unrelated to the bifurcation. Atherosclerotic occlusive disease is the culprit in the vast majority of cases. Primary stent implantation for the endovascular treatment of such focal atherosclerotic stenoses has been demonstrated in small series to be technically feasible and relatively easy to perform, with satisfactory midterm results (Fig. 18-3).[40-42] These patients usually present with disabling claudication and are between 30 and 70 years of age. The disease may be a focal infrarenal stenosis or, more commonly, involve the origins of the common iliac arteries. The spectrum of symptoms is referred to as the Leriche syndrome, a combination of diminished or absent femoral pulses, thigh and buttock claudication, and erectile dysfunction in men. Women may present with these types of lesions owing to the intrinsically small caliber of their vessels. Female patients tend to be younger, be heavy smokers, and have elevated lipid levels. Alternatively, distal embolization presenting as blue toe syndrome may be the first manifestation of disease.

In patients deemed appropriate for intervention, noninvasive studies to determine the physiologic nature of the obstruction and angiography (conventional, magnetic resonance angiography, or computed tomography-angiography) are valuable in analyzing the extent of the lesion and planning appropriate treatment. The type of lesion, patient characteristics, concomitant comorbidities, and acuteness of symptoms are all factors to consider in choosing percutaneous therapy versus surgical modalities. Percutaneous techniques are a viable alternative to major surgical reconstruction, with lower costs, morbidity, and mortality.

TABLE 18–1	Contraindications to Intravascular Stent Placement

Arterial perforation with contrast extravasation in the target vessel
Severely calcified vessels
Marked vessel tortuosity (not a contraindication for Wallstent placement)
Target lesions cross areas of flexion, such as the inguinal ligament, knee, or shoulder
Coexistent aneurysmal disease requiring surgical intervention
Successful balloon angioplasty
Presence of hypercoagulable disorder
Long-standing arterial occlusion
Target vessels that may serve as the proximal or distal site of a bypass grafting procedure

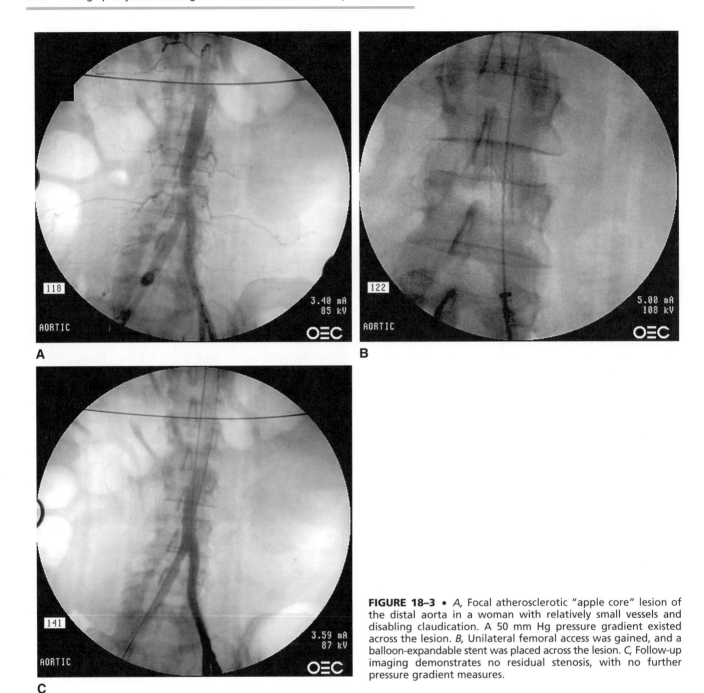

FIGURE 18–3 • *A,* Focal atherosclerotic "apple core" lesion of the distal aorta in a woman with relatively small vessels and disabling claudication. A 50 mm Hg pressure gradient existed across the lesion. *B,* Unilateral femoral access was gained, and a balloon-expandable stent was placed across the lesion. *C,* Follow-up imaging demonstrates no residual stenosis, with no further pressure gradient measures.

Aortic Stenosis

Techniques used for angioplasty, with or without stenting, of the aorta and iliac segments are similar. Although percutaneous transluminal angioplasty (PTA) has demonstrated excellent results in focal stenoses of the abdominal aorta and iliacs, primary stenting may reduce the degree of restenosis with PTA alone and decrease distal embolization.[29,32,40,42-45]

Focal aortic stenoses are treated by mounting a balloon-expandable stent on a larger-caliber angioplasty balloon or using a large self-expanding stent. The role of covered stents, such as cuffs made for endoluminal abdominal aortic aneurysm repair, has not been rigorously studied. The aortic diameter should be sized with a calibrated catheter or by preintervention computed tomography scanning to avoid undersizing. Balloon size usually ranges from 12 to 18 mm. A single stent is generally required in most cases with no special technical requirements; large Palmaz-type stents (Palmaz XXL) have been used successfully and may be inflated up to 25 mm in diameter. Concentric aortic stenosis may encroach on the inferior mesenteric artery, and coverage of this vessel may be unavoidable. Further, only midabdominal aortic lesions should be treated in this fashion. Different techniques (described later) are employed when the lesion involves the aortic bifurcation. For focal aortic stenoses, technical success, safety, and adequate patency rates have been reported with primary stent placement.[32,41,42,46,47] Durability seems satisfactory in properly selected patients.

Iliac Stenosis or Occlusion

Patients with iliac lesions present with a wide spectrum of symptoms, depending on the amount of involvement of the iliac arteries, whether the lesions are focal or multisegmental, and the degree of infrainguinal disease. Indications for intervention are severe disabling claudication, rest pain, tissue loss, or blue toe syndrome. Individual risk factors and possible adverse outcomes associated with each procedure must also be taken into consideration when deciding on the best treatment option. Initially, iliac artery angioplasty with subsequent stent placement was used for only focal lesions; with technologic advances, however, more complex multisegmental lesions are now approached endoluminally. In 2000, the TransAtlantic Inter-Society Consensus (TASC) working group published recommendations for treatment approaches to peripheral arterial disease.[48] This multidisciplinary endeavor sought to classify iliac lesions according to complexity and anatomic specificity (types A through D). Table 18-2 presents the classification system and the recommended treatments for each lesion category.

Results of Iliac Angioplasty and Stenting

Multiple studies have documented excellent results following both focal and complex iliac artery stenting procedures, with most reporting superior results over angioplasty alone (Figs. 18-4 and 18-5).[13,14,21,23,29,36,49-57] In a large, representative systematic review by Bosch and Hunink, technical success with angioplasty alone was 91%; with stent placement, it was 96%.[57] This report of more than 2100 patients compared the PTA cohort ($n = 1300$) with the stent cohort ($n = 816$) and demonstrated similar complication rates between the two groups; however, the stented patients had improved long-term patency rates. When performed for claudication, 4-year primary patency rates were 65% for stenosis and 54% for occlusion after angioplasty, versus 77% for stenosis and 61%

for occlusion after stenting. The rate differential was similar, although the overall percentages were lower, when procedures were performed for critical limb ischemia. Statistical analysis showed a 39% reduction in long-term failure after stent placement compared with PTA.

As seen in Table 18-2, there is currently no consensus about the best treatment for moderately severe iliac artery lesions (TASC type B and C lesions). In a review of their experience with percutaneous and surgical treatment of these complex iliac lesions, Timaran and associates evaluated the primary outcome of patency and also analyzed potential variables that may preclude successful revascularization.[23] At all time points (1, 3, and 5 years), surgically reconstructed patients ($n = 52$) had higher patency rates than stented patients ($n = 136$). Poor runoff was the only independent predictor of primary failure in either cohort. Further, in patients with poor runoff, iliac stenting was associated with inferior outcomes compared with surgical reconstruction. This finding has been supported by other studies of either surgical or endovascular interventions.[51,58,59] In a review of the treatment of TASC type D lesions, the most severe type, Ballard and colleagues found that ipsilateral superficial femoral artery obstruction was also an independent predictor of both stent and bypass graft failure.[59]

In most gender-based comparisons, women have inferior results following iliac stent placement compared with their male counterparts.[59-61] Conversely, in a retrospective study of 44 women having iliac angioplasty compared with men matched for comorbidities, female gender was not a negative predictor of outcome. Although women in this series had smaller vessels and a higher incidence of pretreatment total occlusion, no statistically significant difference existed in 2-year primary patency, percutaneous primary-assisted patency, or limb salvage rates. However, stent placement was not performed in these patients. Perhaps the use of stents in smaller vessels in women should be limited. Full critical evaluation awaits future prospective trials or larger retrospective series.

Complications of Intraluminal Stent Placement

The complication profile is similar for either aortic or iliac interventions (Table 18-3). Because the deployment of a

TABLE 18–2	TransAtlantic Inter-Society Consensus: Morphologic Stratification of Iliac Lesions	
Type	**Definition**	**Treatment Choice**
A	Single stenosis < 3 cm long (unilateral or bilateral) of CIA or EIA	Percutaneous endovascular procedure
B	Single stenosis 3-10 cm long, not extending into CFA	Unresolved
	Two stenoses totaling < 5 cm long, not extending into CFA	
	Unilateral CIA occlusion	
C	Bilateral stenosis of CIA, EIA, or both, 5-10 cm long, not extending into CFA	Unresolved
	Unilateral EIA occlusion not extending into CFA	
	Unilateral EIA stenosis extending into CFA	
	Bilateral CIA occlusion	
D	Diffuse stenosis of CIA, EIA, and CFA > 10 cm long	Open surgery
	Unilateral occlusion of CIA and EIA	
	Bilateral EIA occlusion	
	Iliac stenosis in conjunction with AAA or other lesion requiring operative intervention	

AAA, abdominal aortic aneurysm; CFA, common femoral artery; CIA, common iliac artery; EIA, external iliac artery.

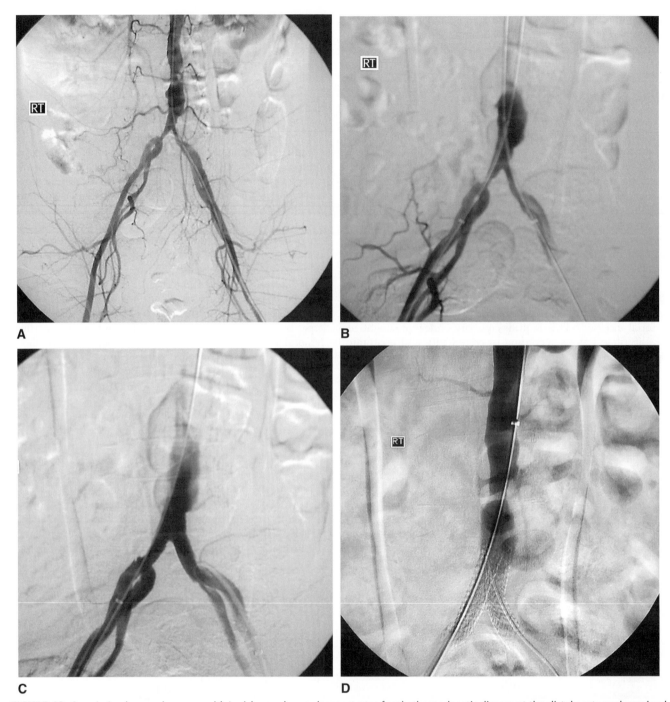

FIGURE 18–4 • *A,* Angiogram in a man with Leriche syndrome demonstrates focal atherosclerotic disease at the distal aorta and proximal common iliac arteries. *B,* Bilateral percutaneous femoral access was obtained with placement of 6 French sheaths. *C,* Initial improved result after angioplasty of the common iliac arteries. *D,* Completion angiogram after deployment of bilateral "kissing" balloon-expandable stents.

balloon-expandable stent requires the physical mounting of the stent on a balloon catheter, accidental dislodgment of the stent from the catheter delivery system may occur. Similar complications occur that are nonspecific for percutaneous procedures, including those related to puncture sites, arterial dissection, and vessel rupture. Unlike with self-expanding stents, which constantly exert an outward radial force, external compression on balloon-expandable stents due to vascular clamping injury can result in permanent stent deformity. Although short-term failure is mainly due to thrombosis in

the stented vessel, long-term patency can be adversely affected by restenosis induced by intimal hyperplasia. Factors associated with stented artery thrombosis are iliac artery occlusion, multiple stent deployment, and hypercoagulable disorders. Stent placement in an occluded iliac artery is particularly prone to restenosis, due in part to the lack of an endothelial lining in the occluded vessel. Stent deployment may further denude the intimal lining, thereby reducing the protective antithrombotic function of endothelium. Additionally, the incidence of distal embolization following the stent placement

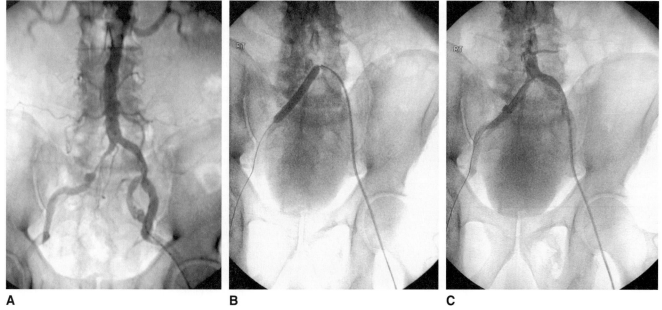

A   **B**   **C**

FIGURE 18–5 • *A*, High-grade lesion of the right common iliac artery. *B*, Access from the contralateral femoral artery was used for initial angioplasty. *C*, Results after balloon angioplasty, with no apparent residual stenosis. The patient went on to have a self-expanding stent placed across the lesion (not shown).

is 2.4% to 7.8%.[34] As with all radiographic interventions, transient contrast-induced nephropathy may occur following an interventional procedure.

Conclusions

Intravascular stent placement has proved to be an invaluable tool in both the primary treatment of aortoiliac occlusive disease and the management of complications of balloon angioplasty. Clinical application of iliac stents has also extended to the treatment of patients with total iliac occlusion and restenosis. Although balloon angioplasty has met with limited success in treating totally occluded iliac arteries, the use of intravascular stents has improved the success rate to approximately 80% at 3 years, with a late occlusion rate

similar to that of stenotic lesions. The benefit of primary stenting of the iliac artery has been demonstrated in several series, with a favorable 5-year patency rate of greater than 90%, which is comparable to conventional surgical reconstruction. The Achilles heel of intravascular stenting is the induction of intimal hyperplasia leading to restenosis. The incidence of restenosis within 1 year of stent placement has been shown to be greater than 20%. There are many areas for future research to focus on in an attempt to solve this dilemma. Promising techniques, including the use of drug-eluting stents, vascular brachytherapy, cutting balloons, and aggressive antiplatelet regimens, are being tested to improve clinical outcomes.[62-68]

KEY REFERENCES

Ballard JL, Bergan JJ, Singh P, et al: Aortoiliac stent deployment versus surgical reconstruction: Analysis of outcome and cost. J Vasc Surg 28:94-101, 1998.

Brewster DC: Current controversies in the management of aortoiliac occlusive disease. J Vasc Surg 25:365-379, 1997.

Dormandy JA, Rutherford RB: Management of peripheral arterial disease (PAD). TASC Working Group. TransAtlantic Inter-Society Consensus (TASC). J Vasc Surg 31:S1-S296, 2000.

Dotter CT, Judkins MP: Transluminal treatment of arteriosclerotic obstruction: Description of a new technic and a preliminary report of its application. Circulation 30:654-670, 1964.

Greiner A, Dessl A, Klein-Weigel P, et al: Kissing stents for treatment of complex aortoiliac disease. Eur J Vasc Endovasc Surg 26:161-165, 2003.

Harnek J, Zoucas E, Stenram U, et al: Insertion of self-expandable nitinol stents without previous balloon angioplasty reduces restenosis compared with PTA prior to stenting. Cardiovasc Intervent Radiol 25:430-436, 2002.

Martin D, Katz SG: Axillofemoral bypass for aortoiliac occlusive disease. Am J Surg 180:100-103, 2000.

Mohamed F, Sarkar B, Timmons G, et al: Outcome of "kissing stents" for aortoiliac atherosclerotic disease, including the effect on the non-diseased contralateral iliac limb. Cardiovasc Intervent Radiol 25:472-475, 2002.

Murphy TP, Ariaratnam NS, Carney WI Jr, et al: Aortoiliac insufficiency: Long-term experience with stent placement for treatment. Radiology 231:243-249, 2004.

TABLE 18–3	Complications Associated with Intravascular Stent Placement

Local complications
    Hematoma
    Pseudoaneurysm
    Arteriovenous fistula
    Plaque distal embolization
Stent dislodgment in delivery system
Stent migration and embolization
Stent misplacement
Contrast allergic reaction
Vessel perforation
Side branch occlusion
Accelerated intimal hyperplasia
Extrinsic compression of stent
Stent infection

Schneider JR, Besso SR, Walsh DB, et al: Femorofemoral versus aorto-bifemoral bypass: Outcome and hemodynamic results. J Vasc Surg 19:43-55, 1994.

Stoeckelhuber BM, Meissner O, Stoeckelhuber M, et al: Primary endovascular stent placement for focal infrarenal aortic stenosis: Initial and midterm results. J Vasc Interv Radiol 14:1443-1447, 2003.

Timaran CH, Prault TL, Stevens SL, et al: Iliac artery stenting versus surgical reconstruction for TASC (TransAtlantic Inter-Society Consensus) type B and type C iliac lesions. J Vasc Surg 38:272-278, 2003.

Timaran CH, Stevens SL, Freeman MB, et al: Infrainguinal arterial reconstructions in patients with aortoiliac occlusive disease: The influence of iliac stenting. J Vasc Surg 34:971-978, 2001.

Treiman GS, Schneider PA, Lawrence PF, et al: Does stent placement improve the results of ineffective or complicated iliac artery angioplasty? J Vasc Surg 28:104-112, 1998.

Waksman R: Vascular brachytherapy vs drug-eluting stents for the treatment of in-stent restenosis: The jury's still out. Catheter Cardiovasc Interv 62:290-291, 2004.

REFERENCES

1. Dotter CT, Judkins MP: Transluminal treatment of arteriosclerotic obstruction: Description of a new technic and a preliminary report of its application. Circulation 30:654-670, 1964.
2. Gruntzig A, Hopff H: [Percutaneous recanalization after chronic arterial occlusion with a new dilator-catheter (modification of the Dotter technique).] Dtsch Med Wochenschr 99:2502-2510, 2511, 1974.
3. Becker GJ, Katzen BT, Dake MD: Noncoronary angioplasty. Radiology 170:921-940, 1989.
4. Wilson SE, Wolf GL, Cross AP: Percutaneous transluminal angioplasty versus operation for peripheral arteriosclerosis: Report of a prospective randomized trial in a selected group of patients. J Vasc Surg 9:1-9, 1989.
5. Becker GJ, Palmaz JC, Rees CR, et al: Angioplasty-induced dissections in human iliac arteries: Management with Palmaz balloon-expandable intraluminal stents. Radiology 176:31-38, 1990.
6. Gardiner GA Jr, Meyerovitz MF, Stokes KR, et al: Complications of transluminal angioplasty. Radiology 159:201-208, 1986.
7. Richter GM, Palmaz JC, Noeldge G, et al: Relationship between blood flow, thrombus, and neointima in stents. J Vasc Interv Radiol 10:598-604, 1999.
8. Richter GM, Palmaz JC, Noeldge G, et al: Blood flow and thrombus formation determine the development of stent neointima. J Long Term Eff Med Implants 10:69-77, 2000.
9. Salam TA, Taylor B, Suggs WD, et al: Reaction to injury following balloon angioplasty and intravascular stent placement in the canine femoral artery. Am Surg 60:353-357, 1994.
10. Dotter CT: Transluminally-placed coilspring endarterial tube grafts: Long-term patency in canine popliteal artery. Invest Radiol 4:329-332, 1969.
11. Sigwart U, Puel J, Mirkovitch V, et al: Intravascular stents to prevent occlusion and restenosis after transluminal angioplasty. N Engl J Med 316:701-706, 1987.
12. Chronos NA, Sigwart U: New technologies in interventional cardiology. Curr Opin Cardiol 7:634-641, 1992.
13. Hausegger KA, Lammer J, Hagen B, et al: Iliac artery stenting—clinical experience with the Palmaz stent, Wallstent, and Strecker stent. Acta Radiol 33:292-296, 1992.
14. Onal B, Ilgit ET, Yucel C, et al: Primary stenting for complex atherosclerotic plaques in aortic and iliac stenoses. Cardiovasc Intervent Radiol 21:386-392, 1998.
15. Diethrich EB: Endovascular treatment of abdominal aortic occlusive disease: The impact of stents and intravascular ultrasound imaging. Eur J Vasc Surg 7:228-236, 1993.
16. Palmaz JC: Intravascular stents: Tissue-stent interactions and design considerations. AJR Am J Roentgenol 160:613-618, 1993.
17. Palmaz JC, Richter GM, Noeldge G, et al: Intraluminal stents in atherosclerotic iliac artery stenosis: Preliminary report of a multicenter study. Radiology 168:727-731, 1988.
18. Henry M, Klonaris C, Amor M, et al: State of the art: Which stent for which lesion in peripheral interventions? Tex Heart Inst J 27:119-126, 2000.
19. Henry M, Amor M, Beyar R, et al: Clinical experience with a new nitinol self-expanding stent in peripheral arteries. J Endovasc Surg 3:369-379, 1996.
20. Harnek J, Zoucas E, Stenram U, et al: Insertion of self-expandable nitinol stents without previous balloon angioplasty reduces restenosis compared with PTA prior to stenting. Cardiovasc Intervent Radiol 25:430-436, 2002.
21. Hausegger KA, Cragg AH, Lammer J, et al: Iliac artery stent placement: Clinical experience with a nitinol stent. Radiology 190:199-202, 1994.
22. Kinoshita Y, Suzuki T, Hosokawa H, et al: Usefulness of the Symphony nitinol stent for arteriosclerosis obliterans. Circ J 66:1000-1002, 2002.
23. Timaran CH, Prault TL, Stevens SL, et al: Iliac artery stenting versus surgical reconstruction for TASC (TransAtlantic Inter-Society Consensus) type B and type C iliac lesions. J Vasc Surg 38:272-278, 2003.
24. Murphy TP, Ariaratnam NS, Carney WI Jr, et al: Aortoiliac insufficiency: Long-term experience with stent placement for treatment. Radiology 231:243-249, 2004.
25. Glover JL, Bendick PJ, Dilley RS, et al: Efficacy of balloon catheter dilatation for lower extremity atherosclerosis. Surgery 91:560-565, 1982.
26. Gravereaux EC, Marin ML: Endovascular repair of diffuse atherosclerotic occlusive disease using stented grafts. Mt Sinai J Med 70:410-417, 2003.
27. Rzucidlo EM, Powell RJ, Zwolak RM, et al: Early results of stent-grafting to treat diffuse aortoiliac occlusive disease. J Vasc Surg 37:1175-1180, 2003.
28. Krajcer Z, Sioco G, Reynolds T: Comparison of Wallgraft and Wallstent for treatment of complex iliac artery stenosis and occlusion: Preliminary results of a prospective randomized study. Tex Heart Inst J 24:193-199, 1997.
29. Treiman GS, Schneider PA, Lawrence PF, et al: Does stent placement improve the results of ineffective or complicated iliac artery angioplasty? J Vasc Surg 28:104-112, 1998.
30. Cambria RP, Faust G, Gusberg R, et al: Percutaneous angioplasty for peripheral arterial occlusive disease: Correlates of clinical success. Arch Surg 122:283-287, 1987.
31. Colapinto RF, Stronell RD, Johnston WK: Transluminal angioplasty of complete iliac obstructions. AJR Am J Roentgenol 146:859-862, 1986.
32. Nyman U, Uher P, Lindh M, et al: Primary stenting in infrarenal aortic occlusive disease. Cardiovasc Intervent Radiol 23:97-108, 2000.
33. Raillat C, Rousseau H, Joffre F, et al: Treatment of iliac artery stenoses with the Wallstent endoprosthesis. AJR Am J Roentgenol 154:613-616, 1990.
34. Lin PH, Bush RL, Conklin BS, et al: Late complication of aortoiliac stent placement—atheroembolization of the lower extremities. J Surg Res 103:153-159, 2002.
35. Sinci V, Kalaycioglu S, Halit V, et al: Long-term effects of combined iliac dilatation and distal arterial surgery. Int Surg 85:13-17, 2000.
36. Timaran CH, Ohki T, Gargiulo NJ 3rd, et al: Iliac artery stenting in patients with poor distal runoff: Influence of concomitant infrainguinal arterial reconstruction. J Vasc Surg 38:479-484, 2003.
37. Timaran CH, Stevens SL, Freeman MB, et al: Infrainguinal arterial reconstructions in patients with aortoiliac occlusive disease: The influence of iliac stenting. J Vasc Surg 34:971-978, 2001.
38. Murthy R, Arbabzadeh M, Richard H 3rd, et al: Axillary artery traumatic pseudoaneurysm managed with a Wallgraft endoprothesis. J Vasc Interv Radiol 14:117-118, 2003.
39. Parodi JC, Schonholz C, Ferreira LM, et al: Endovascular stent-graft treatment of traumatic arterial lesions. Ann Vasc Surg 13:121-129, 1999.
40. Yilmaz S, Sindel T, Yegin A, et al: Primary stenting of focal atherosclerotic infrarenal aortic stenoses: Long-term results in 13 patients and a literature review. Cardiovasc Intervent Radiol 27:121-128, 2004.
41. Stoeckelhuber BM, Meissner O, Stoeckelhuber M, et al: Primary endovascular stent placement for focal infrarenal aortic stenosis: Initial and midterm results. J Vasc Interv Radiol 14:1443-1447, 2003.
42. Eftekhar K, Young N, Fletcher J, et al: Clinical efficacy of metal stents for the treatment of focal abdominal aortic stenosis. Australas Radiol 48:17-20, 2004.
43. Hallisey MJ, Meranze SG, Parker BC, et al: Percutaneous transluminal angioplasty of the abdominal aorta. J Vasc Interv Radiol 5:679-687, 1994.
44. Hedeman Joosten PP, Ho GH, Breuking FA Jr, et al: Percutaneous transluminal angioplasty of the infrarenal aorta: Initial outcome and long-term clinical and angiographic results. Eur J Vasc Endovasc Surg 12:201-206, 1996.
45. Saha S, Gibson M, Torrie EP, et al: Stenting for localised arterial stenoses in the aorto-iliac segment. Eur J Vasc Endovasc Surg 22:37-40, 2001.
46. Lim MC, Choo M, Tan HC: Stenting of stenosis of the abdominal aorta. Singapore Med J 36:562-565, 1995.
47. McPherson SJ, Laing AD, Thomson KR, et al: Treatment of infrarenal aortic stenosis by stent placement: A 6-year experience. Australas Radiol 43:185-191, 1999.
48. Dormandy JA, Rutherford RB: Management of peripheral arterial disease (PAD). TASC Working Group. TransAtlantic Inter-Society Consensus (TASC). J Vasc Surg 31:S1-S296, 2000.
49. Hassen-Khodja R, Sala F, Declemy S, et al: Value of stent placement during percutaneous transluminal angioplasty of the iliac arteries. J Cardiovasc Surg (Torino) 42:369-374, 2001.

50. Henry M, Amor M, Ethevenot G, et al: Percutaneous endoluminal treatment of iliac occlusions: Long-term follow-up in 105 patients. J Endovasc Surg 5(3):228-235, 1998.
51. Hood DB, Hodgson KJ: Percutaneous transluminal angioplasty and stenting for iliac artery occlusive disease. Surg Clin North Am 79:575-596, 1999.
52. Mendelsohn FO, Santos RM, Crowley JJ, et al: Kissing stents in the aortic bifurcation. Am Heart J 136:600-605, 1998.
53. Mohamed F, Sarkar B, Timmons G, et al: Outcome of "kissing stents" for aortoiliac atherosclerotic disease, including the effect on the non-diseased contralateral iliac limb. Cardiovasc Intervent Radiol 25:472-475, 2002.
54. Schurmann K, Mahnken A, Meyer J, et al: Long-term results 10 years after iliac arterial stent placement. Radiology 224:731-738, 2002.
55. Toogood GJ, Torrie EP, Magee TR, et al: Early experience with stenting for iliac occlusive disease. Eur J Vasc Endovasc Surg 15:165-168, 1998.
56. Powell RJ, Fillinger M, Bettmann M, et al: The durability of endovascular treatment of multisegment iliac occlusive disease. J Vasc Surg 31:1178-1184, 2000.
57. Bosch JL, Hunink MG: Meta-analysis of the results of percutaneous transluminal angioplasty and stent placement for aortoiliac occlusive disease. Radiology 204:87-96, 1997.
58. Brewster DC: Current controversies in the management of aortoiliac occlusive disease. J Vasc Surg 25:365-379, 1997.
59. Ballard JL, Bergan JJ, Singh P, et al: Aortoiliac stent deployment versus surgical reconstruction: Analysis of outcome and cost. J Vasc Surg 28:94-101, 1998.
60. Timaran CH, Stevens SL, Grandas OH, et al: Influence of hormone replacement therapy on the outcome of iliac angioplasty and stenting. J Vasc Surg 33(2 Suppl):S85-S92, 2001.
61. Timaran CH, Stevens SL, Freeman MB, et al: External iliac and common iliac artery angioplasty and stenting in men and women. J Vasc Surg 34:440-446, 2001.
62. Duda SH, Poerner TC, Wiesinger B, et al: Drug-eluting stents: Potential applications for peripheral arterial occlusive disease. J Vasc Interv Radiol 14:291-301, 2003.
63. Ellozy SH, Carroccio A: Drug-eluting stents in peripheral vascular disease: Eliminating restenosis. Mt Sinai J Med 70:417-419, 2003.
64. Rastogi S, Stavropoulos SW: Infrapopliteal angioplasty. Tech Vasc Interv Radiol 7:33-39, 2004.
65. Waksman R: Vascular brachytherapy vs drug-eluting stents for the treatment of in-stent restenosis: The jury's still out. Catheter Cardiovasc Interv 62:290-291, 2004.
66. Engelke C, Morgan RA, Belli AM: Cutting balloon percutaneous transluminal angioplasty for salvage of lower limb arterial bypass grafts: Feasibility. Radiology 223:106-114, 2002.
67. Munneke GJ, Engelke C, Morgan RA, et al: Cutting balloon angioplasty for resistant renal artery in-stent restenosis. J Vasc Interv Radiol 13:327-331, 2002.
68. Bradberry JC: Peripheral arterial disease: Pathophysiology, risk factors, and role of antithrombotic therapy. J Am Pharm Assoc (Wash) 44(2 Suppl 1):S37-S44, 2004.

Questions

1. All of the following are indications for stent placement except
   (a) Intimal dissection
   (b) Residual stenosis greater than 15%
   (c) Recurrent stenosis following angioplasty alone
   (d) Symptomatic atherosclerotic iliac lesions

2. Which of the following statements about pharmacologic agents in angiography are true?
   (a) They may induce peripheral vasodilatation that unmasks significant stenosis
   (b) Either papaverine or nitroglycerin may be used
   (c) They are injected directly into the intra-arterial catheter or sheath in the vessel under investigation
   (d) They cause significant vasospasm

3. Covered stents may be used in the iliac arteries in all of the following conditions except
   (a) Arteriovenous fistulas
   (b) Vessel ruptures
   (c) Aneurysms
   (d) Mycotic aneurysms
   (e) Atherosclerotic occlusive lesions

4. Complications of iliac stent placement include which of the following?
   (a) Distal embolization
   (b) Thrombosis
   (c) Stent malposition
   (d) Vessel rupture
   (e) All of the above

5. The classic definition of Leriche syndrome consists of all of the following except
   (a) Decreased femoral pulses
   (b) Blue toe syndrome
   (c) Buttock claudication
   (d) Impotence

6. Iliac stenting has been recommended as the primary treatment for which of the following lesions?
   (a) TASC type A
   (b) TASC type B
   (c) TASC type C
   (d) TASC type D

7. The outcome after stenting of which vessel most closely approximates surgical results?
   (a) Common iliac artery
   (b) External iliac artery
   (c) Common femoral artery

8. Long-term patency of intravascular stents is limited by which of the following?
   (a) Vessel size
   (b) Neointimal hyperplasia
   (c) Progression of atherosclerosis
   (d) Stent durability

9. Complications common to percutaneous procedures include which of the following?
   (a) Contrast-induced nephropathy
   (b) Puncture site hematoma
   (c) Vascular injury
   (d) Nerve damage

10. All of the following are (relative) contraindications for intravascular stent placement except
    (a) Target area across from an area of flexion, such as the knee joint
    (b) Arterial perforation with contrast extravasation
    (c) Residual stenosis of 40% following balloon angioplasty
    (d) Multisegmental iliac disease

Answers

1. b	2. a, b, c	3. d	4. e	5. b
6. a	7. a	8. b, c	9. a, b, c	10. c

19

Douglas B. Hood • Kim J. Hodgson

Endovascular Treatment of Renovascular Disease

Although surgical revascularization of renal artery occlusive disease has long been known to benefit patients with renovascular hypertension, as well as selected patients with renal insufficiency, the associated morbidity and mortality of these procedures discouraged their use in all but the most severe cases. Endovascular renal revascularization offers the opportunity to gain the therapeutic benefits of surgery with reduced periprocedural risk and recovery time, albeit with potentially less durability. This has led to an explosion in renal artery interventions, often with little preprocedural evaluation and frequently for the perceived benefit of "renal salvage," although data to support this indication, as reviewed later, are not compelling. Nonetheless, all endovascular surgeons should know the indications for and the technique of percutaneous renal revascularization, because a significant number of patients seen in the average vascular surgery practice will benefit from this procedure.

Renal artery stenosis (RAS) is the most common cause of secondary hypertension, with an estimated incidence of 5% in the hypertensive population. Congenital anomalies, arteritis, trauma, arterial dissection, fibromuscular dysplasia, and atherosclerosis are recognized causes of RAS. Among these, atherosclerosis is by far the most common, accounting for 60% to 80% of all cases of clinically significant renal artery disease. This chapter summarizes the current status of endovascular management of atherosclerotic RAS, with a focus on recently reported technical and clinical results.

Natural History

Atherosclerosis affecting the renal arteries is a progressive disease that most often results from encroachment of aortic plaque into or across the renal artery orifice. Because of this characteristic pattern, most clinically relevant atherosclerotic renal artery lesions are ostial in location, occurring within the most proximal 5 mm of the vessel. Once RAS becomes hemodynamically significant (>60%), progression to renal artery occlusion is a real possibility. Using sequential angiograms, Tollefson and Ernst found that RAS progressed at approximately 5% per year, irrespective of the level of stenosis, and that occlusion was associated with greater degrees of stenosis.[1] Caps and associates reported in 1998 that 49% of patients with RAS greater than 60% measured by duplex ultrasonography showed disease progression over a 3-year period.[2] Zierler and colleagues reported that in renal arteries with a stenosis greater than 60%, the cumulative progression to occlusion was 5% at 1 year and 11% at 2 years.[3] Renal artery occlusion is associated with atrophy of the kidney parenchyma, with a mean decrease in kidney length of 1.8 cm in Zierler's report. Renal atrophy can also occur in association with stenotic but nonoccluded renal arteries.[2]

Diagnosis

Patients with atherosclerotic RAS are more often male and older than 60 years, and they have the typical atherosclerotic risk factors of diabetes, hyperlipidemia, tobacco use, and hypertension. The diagnosis of renovascular hypertension is suggested by unstable or accelerated hypertension in isolation or in combination with a progressive deterioration of renal function (ischemic nephropathy). Development of malignant hypertension in a patient with a prior history of easily controlled essential hypertension is particularly suggestive of RAS. A less common clinical scenario is rapidly progressive renal insufficiency associated with mild hypertension. Flash pulmonary edema in the setting of accelerated hypertension may also indicate the existence of significant RAS. The physical finding of an abdominal or flank bruit supports the diagnosis but is present in only 25% of patients. Laboratory findings consistent with RAS include refractory hypokalemia and an elevated peripheral renin assay, but each is found in only an occasional patient. Any of these clinical findings, alone or in combination, raises the index of suspicion and should prompt diagnostic imaging of the renal arteries.

Imaging Studies

In the past, renal artery imaging required invasive angiographic procedures. The need for angiography and its associated morbidity dissuaded many practitioners from aggressively pursuing the diagnosis of RAS in patients who were medically compromised. The development of less invasive imaging techniques that provide a thorough investigation of renal artery anatomy has increased the recognition of RAS.

Renal duplex ultrasonography has emerged as an excellent test to screen patients for RAS. Although it requires significant technical expertise, it is a safe and relatively inexpensive modality that provides information concerning kidney size, cortical thickness, renal artery hemodynamics, and velocity profiles, as well as nonvascular anatomic renal abnormalities such as cysts. Several authors have documented the accuracy of using renal artery peak systolic velocities to detect RAS. A peak systolic velocity greater than 180 to 220 cm/second has a reported sensitivity and specificity of 84% to 91% and 85% to 99%, respectively. In our experience, a peak systolic velocity greater than 220 cm/second identified RAS with a sensitivity and specificity of 91% and 85%, respectively.[4] Importantly, the negative predictive value of 95% of this threshold value in our laboratories essentially eliminated the possibility of RAS, making duplex ultrasonography a highly useful screening test.

Magnetic resonance angiography (MRA) using gadolinium is also a useful tool for evaluating renal artery anatomy. It has a sensitivity of 90% to 100% and a specificity of 76% to 94% when compared with conventional arteriography.[6,7] As a screening modality, MRA is more expensive and less patient-friendly than duplex scanning, but it has become a valuable diagnostic tool and is the first-line screening test in institutions without reliable results with duplex scanning.

Advances in computed tomography (CT) imaging, including multislice CT–angiography, have provided very accurate reconstructions of abdominal vascular anatomy and pathology. Images can be computer reconstructed into three-dimensional models for viewing from a variety of angles. The major limitations to widespread use of this modality for RAS screening are the need for iodinated contrast and the significant cost, both of which also limit the use of this modality for surveillance of known subcritical stenoses.

Using any of these modalities, the diagnosis of RAS can be reliably excluded, but conventional angiography is required for confirmation of positive results and to guide endovascular interventions. In the presence of renal insufficiency, carbon dioxide or gadolinium can be used instead of iodinated contrast agents.[8-10] Although both carbon dioxide and gadolinium have limitations, and the image quality is inferior to that obtained using conventional iodinated contrast agents, renal artery imaging is possible and reproducible. These alternative agents are particularly valuable for patients with ischemic nephropathy, in whom even small amounts of iodinated contrast may be injurious.

When considering intervention for RAS, the clinician must recognize that the mere presence of anatomic RAS does not necessarily establish it as the pathophysiologic cause of hypertension or renal dysfunction. Consequently, the decision to intervene is ultimately a clinical judgment and can never be made with absolute certainty of benefit. In our opinion, physiologic tests such as peripheral or renal vein renin sampling and nuclear scanning are not sufficiently reliable to be of value in selecting patients for treatment. At our institution, intervention is considered when unilateral or bilateral RAS of greater than 60% is documented and any of the following clinical parameters is present: poorly controlled blood pressure despite aggressive medical management, hypertension complicated by congestive heart failure or flash pulmonary edema, or progressive renal insufficiency.

Endovascular Management

Following is a description of the techniques that we have used successfully for the endovascular management of renal artery lesions. It should be noted, however, that there are many variations of this technique, and an operator may find different combinations of sheaths, guidewires, and other instruments equally efficacious.

Groin access via the femoral artery is used most commonly, although a brachial artery approach should be considered for renal arteries with significant caudal angulation or in patients with significant aortoiliac occlusive disease (Fig. 19-1). For unilateral RAS, we prefer to access the contralateral femoral artery, which usually provides a straighter path to the target lesion. Following percutaneous arterial access and placement of a 5 French sheath, a multi-side-hole catheter is placed in the abdominal aorta and positioned at approximately the level of the L-1–L-2 vertebral interspace for flush aortography. Complete visualization of the renal artery origins usually requires anteroposterior and oblique views. For moderate angiographic stenoses (40% to 60%), catheterization of one or both renal arteries may be required for better renal angiographic detail. Translesion pressure measurements may be performed for lesions of questionable hemodynamic significance, although we seldom find this necessary. Documentation of significant RAS is followed by upsizing to a longer 6 or 7 French sheath. Several sheaths with preformed curves at their tips are available for this purpose, or the operator may prefer to use a standard 12- to 25-cm-long femoral sheath in combination with a shaped guiding catheter to minimize trauma to the arterial puncture site from repeated catheter manipulations or exchanges.

If the operator has chosen to use a long, straight sheath rather than a shaped sheath or guiding catheter, the sheath is manipulated into position in the juxtarenal aorta, and after systemic heparinization, the renal ostium is engaged with a curved (Cobra 2, Simmons 1, or Sos) catheter. Catheter selection is individualized, depending on renal artery anatomy and angulation. For most patients, a Cobra 2 catheter is sufficient. The renal artery lesion is then traversed with a guidewire. We usually use either an angled, hydrophilic 0.035-inch wire (Glidewire, Boston Scientific, Natick, Mass.) or a flexible-tipped 0.018-inch wire (Thruway, Boston Scientific). The wire tip is placed into a proximal segmental renal branch. Caution must be exercised with the passage of any wire, because renal artery or parenchymal perforation is possible, particularly with the hydrophilic wires. The catheter is advanced over the wire, with its tip placed well into the renal artery; it is then used as a guide to advance the long sheath up to the renal orifice. Use of a shaped sheath or guiding catheter obviates the need for the Cobra-type catheter and 0.035-inch guidewire, as well as the need to cross the lesion with the catheter; the shaped tip of the sheath or guiding catheter serves the directional function of the Cobra catheter and provides "external" support for the subsequent passage of guidewires, balloons, and stent delivery systems.

Placement of the sheath or guiding catheter at the renal orifice allows small amounts of contrast to be injected through

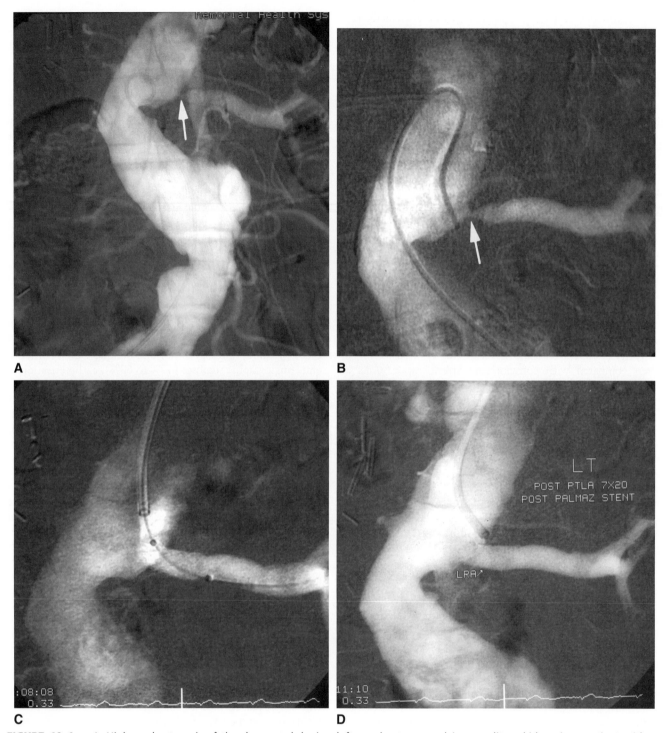

FIGURE 19-1 • *A,* High-grade stenosis of the downward-sloping left renal artery supplying a solitary kidney in a patient with an abdominal aortic aneurysm and aortoiliac tortuosity. *B,* Difficult selective catheterization from the femoral approach. *C,* Simplified access from the left brachial approach. *D,* Completion arteriogram after angioplasty and stenting.

the sheath's side arm to guide the precise placement of angioplasty balloons and stents (Fig. 19-2). In addition, with the "external" support provided by the sheath or guiding catheter positioned at the orifice, the chance of the wire "kicking" out of the renal artery and into the aorta when the various devices are advanced is lessened. This arrangement also allows completion imaging without the loss of the guidewire crossing the lesion.

Atherosclerotic lesions in the midportion of the main renal artery may be well treated with balloon angioplasty alone, but the more common ostial lesions generally require stent placement. We prefer premounted, balloon-expandable stents, especially the new 0.014-inch monorail (rapid-exchange) delivery systems, several of which are available commercially. These systems are much more flexible and have lower crossing profiles than the 0.035-inch systems of

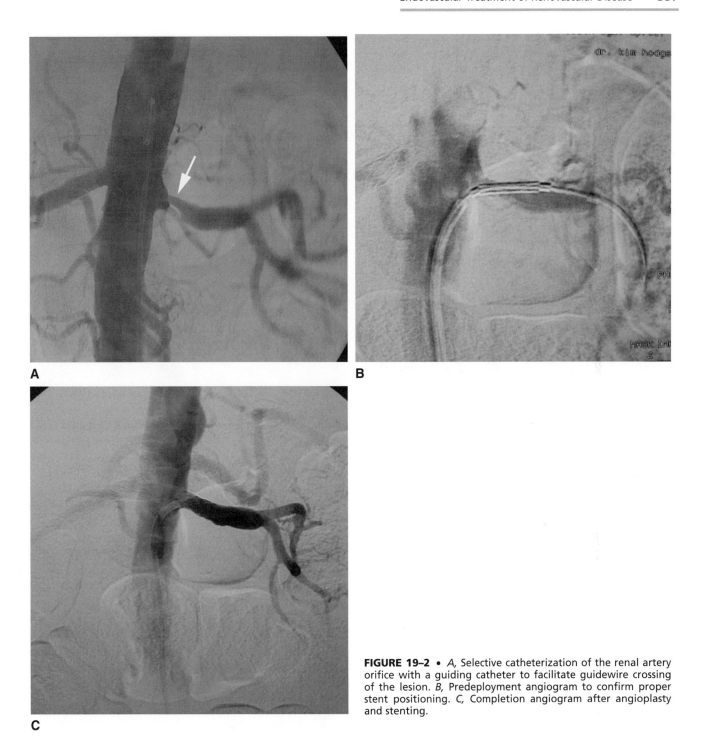

FIGURE 19–2 • *A,* Selective catheterization of the renal artery orifice with a guiding catheter to facilitate guidewire crossing of the lesion. *B,* Predeployment angiogram to confirm proper stent positioning. *C,* Completion angiogram after angioplasty and stenting.

the past. Predilatation is generally not required and may be associated with microembolization of plaque fragments to the renal parenchyma. Most cases require a stent 20 mm long or less mounted on a 5- or 6-mm balloon. The stent is positioned across the lesion, with 2 to 3 mm of stent projecting into the aorta for ostial lesions. Once the stent is deployed, the balloon is deflated and withdrawn, being careful to maintain wire access across the lesion.

Completion angiography is performed with contrast injected through the side arm of the sheath or guiding catheter. The completion study should be critically assessed for technical success (<30% residual stenosis) and for the complications of renal artery dissection, thrombosis, emboli, or perforation of the renal parenchyma. Having confirmed a satisfactory result, we generally use a closure device to seal the femoral puncture site after the sheath is removed.

Results

Prospective trials comparing endovascular intervention with medical management or open surgical repair of RAS are few, but a substantial body of nonrandomized descriptive literature is available. In general, published reports describe the results of endovascular treatment according to technical success, blood pressure response, renal function, and survival criteria.

INITIAL TECHNICAL SUCCESS AND PROCEDURAL COMPLICATIONS

A number of series have analyzed the initial technical results of endovascular intervention. Interpretation of technical results in the various studies is sometimes challenging because of the varying definitions of success and the inconsistent use of postprocedural imaging and pre- and postangioplasty pressure measurements. Technical success is most commonly defined as a residual stenosis of less than 30%, with no evidence of flow-limiting dissection (Fig. 19-3), perforation, or branch vessel compromise. Inability to traverse the lesion with a guidewire is the most common cause of technical failure and occurs in 2% to 5% of cases.[11]

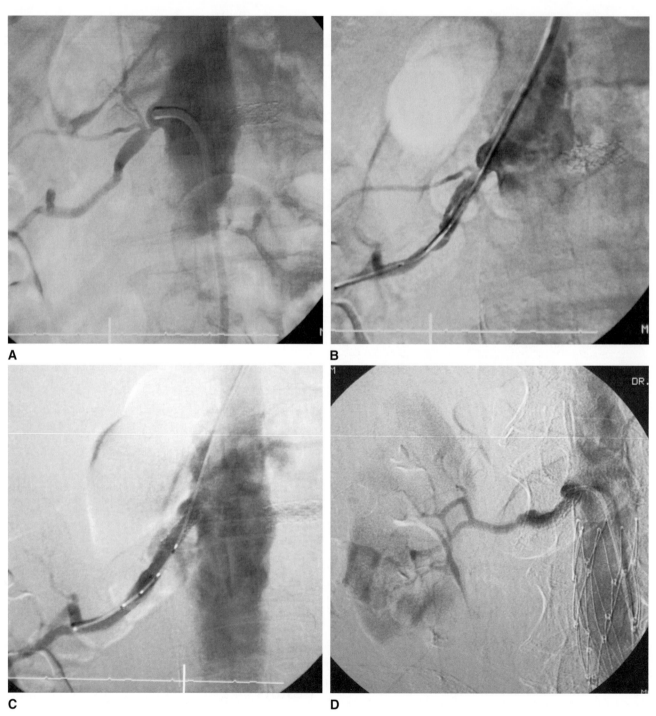

A

B

C

D

FIGURE 19–3 • *A,* Scout angiogram of the right renal artery demonstrating a high-grade stenosis with a caudally angulated renal artery. *B,* Guidewire-induced dissection of the right renal artery approached from a femoral access site, now crossed with a guidewire from the brachial approach. *C,* Successful stenting of the dissection. *D,* Follow-up angiogram 6 months later.

The use of stents has resulted in increased technical success and patency rates when compared with balloon angioplasty alone. In series published during the 1990s, technical success rates varied between 24% and 91% using primary angioplasty alone, with stenting reserved only for rescue indications.[11] In an effort to clarify the role of primary stenting in the treatment of atherosclerotic ostial stenosis, van de Ven and coworkers performed a randomized, prospective study that included 84 hypertensive patients.[12] Ostial stenosis was defined as a 50% or greater reduction in luminal diameter within the first 10 mm of the aortic lumen. Immediate technical success was significantly better in the stent group than in the angioplasty group (88% vs. 57%), with equivalent complication rates. Analyzed on an intent-to-treat basis, the rate of primary patency (free of restenosis) at 6 months was only 29% in the angioplasty group and 75% in the stent group. Secondary patency (including treatment of restenosis) at 6 months was 51% and 80%, respectively (Fig. 19-4). Clinical results at

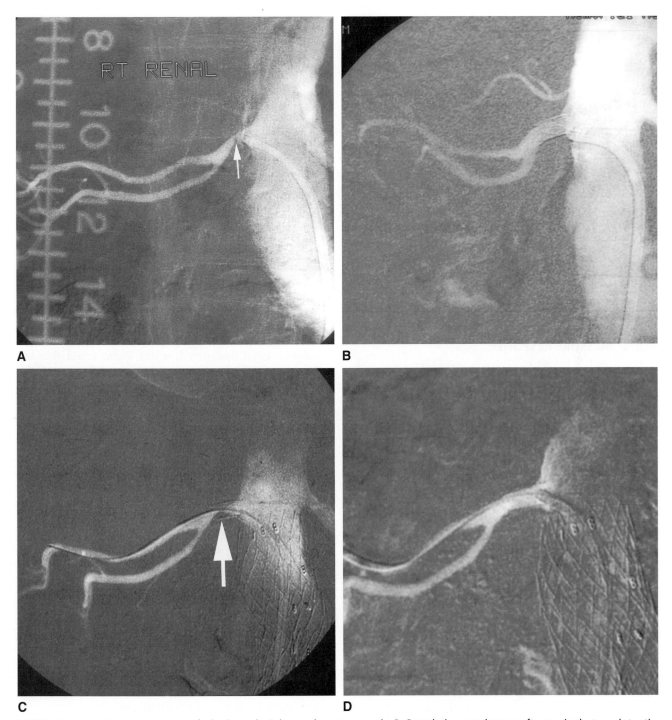

FIGURE 19–4 • *A,* Scout angiogram of a high-grade right renal artery stenosis. *B,* Completion arteriogram after angioplasty and stenting. *C,* In-stent recurrent stenosis at 6 months. *D,* Result after simple repeat balloon angioplasty of in-stent restenosis.

6 months showed no difference between the groups in terms of blood pressure or serum creatinine levels. In all, 12 patients in the angioplasty group received stents during follow-up, either for an unsuccessful initial result (5) or for recurrent stenosis (7). These authors concluded that by following a policy of selective stenting, with stent placement used only for technical failures and recurrent stenoses, stents could be avoided in about 40% of patients. However, because of the need for repeat interventions in those patients treated initially with angioplasty alone, primary stenting is probably more efficacious for patients with atherosclerotic ostial RAS. A meta-analysis of primary renal artery stenting by Isles and associates documented a technical success of 96% to 100%.[13] Restenosis rates following primary stenting were 9% and 39% at 6 and 12 months, respectively. A more recent publication by Sivamurthy and colleagues reported primary patency of 82% and primary assisted patency of 100% at 5 years.[14]

The rate of procedural complications has also been evaluated. Alhadad and coworkers found a 30-day mortality rate of 2% for renal artery interventions.[15] Beutler and coauthors reported initial technical success in 61 of 63 patients (97%), with a 6% renovascular complication rate.[16] More importantly, in Beutler's series, 8% of patients showed clinical signs of cholesterol emboli, and at least 20% of patients experienced a decrease in renal function. Martin and associates reviewed complication rates from two large series and two meta-analyses to determine weighted complication rates.[17] Periprocedural complication rates ranged from 12% to 36%. The most common complications were groin hematoma and puncture site trauma, both occurring in approximately 5% of patients. The incidence of renal artery embolization varied from 1% to 8%, with renal artery occlusion rates between 0.8% and 2.5%.

BLOOD PRESSURE RESPONSE

Three randomized trials have compared the blood pressure response to endovascular intervention and pharmacologic therapy. Webster and coworkers published the first randomized trial of angioplasty versus medical therapy in 1998, including 55 patients with hypertension and RAS in excess of 50%.[18] Both medical and angioplasty groups demonstrated a significant reduction in blood pressure, with no significant difference between groups. Subgroup analysis, however, showed that patients with bilateral RAS had an improved blood pressure response with angioplasty. Plouin and associates randomized 49 patients to either angioplasty alone or medical therapy.[19] There was no significant difference in mean blood pressure between the two groups at 6 months, but significantly more patients were rendered free of pharmacologic treatment in the endovascular group. Van Jaarsveld and colleagues also prospectively compared the results of medical therapy versus angioplasty and failed to show a compelling difference in blood pressure control between groups.[20] Nevertheless, the number of antihypertensive medications prescribed was significantly lower in the angioplasty group. Of note, 44% of patients in the medical arm ultimately underwent angioplasty after 3 months owing to poor blood pressure control.

These prospective, randomized trials compared renal artery angioplasty with or without selective stent placement to medical therapy. The benefit of routine primary stenting

(stenting without attempting angioplasty alone) compared with medical therapy has not been evaluated. However, given the improved technical outcome with primary stenting compared with selective stenting, it would be reasonable to conclude that primary stenting may provide better blood pressure benefit than was demonstrated in these early series. A more recent retrospective study of 100 patients with RAS by Pizzolo and associates supports this assumption.[21] In this study, primary stenting was performed in the majority of patients (67%) undergoing endovascular therapy. A significant improvement in blood pressure control was observed when compared with patients treated medically. Almost twice as many patients manifested an improvement in blood pressure control with endovascular intervention (57% vs. 29%). No patient in either group was cured.

A summary analysis of these cited studies suggests that the endovascular management of RAS results in a better blood pressure response than that achieved with medical therapy, requiring fewer antihypertensive agents for control. Further, it appears that this response can be enhanced by the use of stents.

RENAL FUNCTION

The results of endovascular intervention for ischemic nephropathy have been less compelling. The randomized trials already cited also examined the renal response to intervention, and all failed to show consistent improvement in renal function compared with preintervention status. In the reports by Plouin and van Jaarsveld, mean serum creatinine levels and creatinine clearance at 6 and 12 months were unchanged from pretreatment values.[19,20] Webster's study documented no change in serum creatinine levels; creatinine clearance was not evaluated.[18]

However, in a retrospective study of patients with rapidly declining renal function, Beutler's group found that stent placement resulted in stabilization of renal function in 87% of patients.[16] No effect on renal function was evident when patients with stable renal function were treated. Consistent with Beutler's findings is a report by Ramos and coworkers, in which patients with lower glomerular filtration rates (GFRs) had larger improvements in GFR following endovascular intervention than did patients with higher preprocedure GFRs.[22] In addition, when considering all patients as a group, a significant increase in renal function was evident. Burket and colleagues reported that 43% of patients with baseline renal insufficiency showed significant improvement in renal function after intervention.[23] A recent retrospective review by Hodgson and colleagues of 79 patients who had undergone renal artery stenting revealed that 25% experienced an increase in their serum creatinine of 20% or more over the average follow-up period of 24 months, despite maintenance of anatomic patency (<50 restenosis) in 88%.[24] Of note, dialysis was ultimately required in 44% of patients with baseline pre-PTA (percutaneous transluminal angioplasty) creatinine levels of ≥2.0 mg% but in only 3.4% of patients with pre-PTRA (percutaneous transluminal renal angioplasty) creatinine levels of <2.0 mg%, suggesting that early angioplasty, prior to the development of renal excretory dysfunction, may be important for overall preservation of renal function.

Surgical revascularization remains the one other option available for the treatment of ischemic nephropathy due to RAS. Randomized comparisons between surgical and endovascular therapy for ischemic nephropathy are not available. Reports by Marone, Hansen, and Hallett and their respective coauthors all documented that surgical revascularization provides a substantial improvement in renal function, particularly if the RAS is bilateral or affects a solitary kidney.[25-28] Further, the proportion of patients achieving a benefit after surgical revascularization is generally greater than that observed following endovascular therapy. Additionally, the more severe the renal insufficiency, the greater the benefit seen.

There are two primary explanations of why endovascular intervention has had a less beneficial effect on renal function than expected, despite excellent technical results. First, iodinated contrast agents may cause injury from which the compromised kidney cannot recover. The use of less nephrotoxic contrast agents, such as carbon dioxide, in patients with compromised renal function (serum creatinine > 1.8 mg/dL) may lessen the impact of this toxin. Satisfactory renal artery imaging using carbon dioxide with digital imaging can guide endovascular revascularization. At the very least, the use of carbon dioxide drastically reduces the amount of iodinated contrast required for renal interventions and thereby limits contrast-induced parenchymal injury. The second explanation for the less than expected response is cholesterol embolization. This has led to the recent use of distal protection devices originally designed for coronary and carotid interventions. Holden and Hill described their results using a distal protection device in 37 patients, 14 of whom exhibited improved renal function at 1-year follow-up.[29] In contrast, in 20 patients who underwent stenting without the use of a protection device, none had an improvement in renal function at 1 year. Further prospective studies are needed to confirm this observation. If these results can be duplicated, the use of protection devices will certainly expand the indications for endovascular intervention in patients with renal dysfunction.

SURVIVAL

The expectation that improvement in blood pressure control and renal function following endovascular intervention will result in enhanced survival has yet to be conclusively documented. Only two studies have addressed this issue. Pillay and coworkers found an overall mortality of 30% at 2 years in patients with either unilateral or bilateral RAS.[30] No significant difference in survival was evident between patients who underwent endovascular treatment versus patients receiving optimal medical management.[9] However, patients in the endovascular group had a significantly higher baseline serum creatinine level. In contrast, Pizzolo's group found that 87% of patients treated with stent placement were alive at a median follow-up of 28 months, compared with 67% of patients treated medically.[21] Subsequent regression analysis, used in an effort to explain the observed benefit, found endovascular treatment to be the sole independent predictor of improved survival.

Summary

The technical success of primary stenting, along with the low incidence of morbidity and mortality, has made endovascular management the primary therapy for atherosclerotic RAS in many institutions. Surgical revascularization of atherosclerotic RAS is now limited to patients with renal artery

occlusions, multiple renal arteries, hilar or segmental renal artery lesions, or dissections or those who fail endovascular management.

The recent advances in stent technology and renal endovascular management have provided a technically reproducible method of percutaneously treating atherosclerotic RAS. In many centers, this has resulted in endovascular management being the primary therapy for atherosclerotic RAS. Although still controversial, it appears that endovascular management of RAS by primary stent deployment provides better blood pressure control than that afforded by best medical management. The impact on renal function is less than that found for hypertension, but there is evidence that the use of protection devices and primary stenting may enhance renal function. Whether the ultimate benefit of enhanced survival will follow remains an important question and should be the subject of future prospective studies.

REFERENCES

1. Tollefson DFJ, Ernst CB: Natural history of atherosclerotic renal artery stenosis associated with aortic disease. J Vasc Surg 14:327-331, 1991.
2. Caps MT, Perissinotto C, Zierler RE, et al: Prospective study of atherosclerotic disease progression in the renal artery. Circulation 98:2866-2872, 1998.
3. Zierler R, Bergelin RO, Isaacson JA, Strandness DE Jr: Natural history of atherosclerotic renal artery stenosis: A prospective study with duplex ultrasonography. J Vasc Surg 19:250-258, 1998.
4. Hua HT, Hood DB, Jensen CC, et al: The use of colorflow duplex scanning to detect significant renal artery stenosis. Ann Vasc Surg 14:118-124, 2000.
5. Radermacher J, Mengel M, Ellis S, et al: The renal arterial resistance index and renal allograft survival. N Engl J Med 349:115-124, 2003.
6. Kent KC, Edelman RR, Kim D, et al: Magnetic resonance imaging: A reliable test for the evaluation of proximal atherosclerotic renal arterial stenosis. J Vasc Surg 13:311-318, 1991.
7. Schoenberg SO, Rieger J, Johannson LO, et al: Diagnosis of renal artery stenosis with magnetic resonance angiography: Update 2003. Nephrol Dial Transplant 18:1252-1256, 2003.
8. Spinosa DJ, Matsumoto AH, Angle JF, et al: Gadolinium-based contrast and carbon dioxide angiography to evaluate renal transplants for vascular causes of renal insufficiency and accelerated hypertension. J Vasc Interv Radiol 9:909-916, 2003.
9. Sam AD II, Morasch MD, Collins J, et al: Safety of gadolinium contrast angiography in patients with chronic renal insufficiency. J Vasc Surg 38:313-318, 2003.
10. Schreier D, Weaver FA, Frankhouse J, et al: A prospective study of carbon dioxide-digital subtraction vs standard contrast arteriography in the evaluation of the renal arteries. Arch Surg 131:503-508, 1996.
11. Leertouwer TC, Gussenhoven EJ, Bosch JL, et al: Stent placement for renal arterial stenosis: Where do we stand? A meta-analysis. Radiology 216:78-85, 2000.
12. van de Ven PJG, Kaatee R, Beutler JJ, et al: Arterial stenting and balloon angioplasty in ostial atherosclerotic renovascular disease: A randomized trial. Lancet 353:282-286, 1999.
13. Isles CG, Robertson S, Hill D: Management of renovascular disease: A review of renal artery stenting in ten studies. Q J Med 92:159-167, 1999.
14. Sivamurthy N, Surowiec SM, Culakova E, et al: Divergent outcomes after percutaneous therapy for symptomatic renal artery stenosis. J Vasc Surg 39:565-574, 2004.
15. Alhadad A, Ahle M, Ivancev K, et al: Percutaneous transluminal renal angioplasty (PTRA) and surgical revascularization in renovascular disease: A retrospective comparison of results, compilations, and mortality. Eur J Vasc Endovasc Surg 27:151-156, 2004.
16. Beutler JJ, Van Ampting JMA, van de Ven PJG, et al: Long-term effects of arterial stenting on kidney function for patients with ostial atherosclerotic renal artery stenosis and renal insufficiency. J Am Soc Nephrol 12:1475-1481, 2001.
17. Martin LG, Rundback JH, Sacks D, et al: Quality improvement guidelines for angiography, angioplasty, and stent placement in the diagnosis and treatment of renal artery stenosis in adults. J Vasc Interv Radiol 14:S297-S310, 2003.

18. Webster J, Marshall F, Abdalla M, et al: Randomised comparison of percutaneous angioplasty vs continued medical therapy for hypertensive patients with atheromatous renal artery stenosis: Scottish and Newcastle Renal Artery Stenosis Collaborative Group. J Hum Hypertens 12:329-335, 1998.

19. Plouin P-F, Chatellier G, Darne B, Raynaud A: Blood pressure outcome of angioplasty in atherosclerotic renal artery stenosis: A randomized trial. Hypertension 31:823-829, 1998.

20. van Jaarsveld BC, Krijnen P, Pieterman H, et al: The effect of balloon angioplasty on hypertension in atherosclerotic renal artery stenosis. N Engl J Med 342:1007-1014, 2000.

21. Pizzolo F, Mansueto G, Minniti S, et al: Renovascular disease: Effect of ACE gene deletion polymorphism and endovascular revascularization. J Vasc Surg 39:140-147, 2004.

22. Ramos F, Kotliar C, Alvarez D, et al: Renal function and outcome of PTRA and stenting for atherosclerotic renal artery stenosis. Kidney Int 63:276-282, 2003.

23. Burket MW, Cooper CJ, Kennedy DJ, et al: Renal artery angioplasty and stent placement: Predictors of a favorable outcome. Am Heart J 139:64-71, 2000.

24. Gruneiro LA, McLafferty RB, Ayerdi J, et al: Renal preservation following renal artery angioplasty. Paper presented at the Society for Clinical Vascular Surgery Meeting, March 8, 2003, Miami.

25. Marone LK, Clouse WD, Dorer DJ, et al: Preservation of renal function with surgical revascularization in patients with atherosclerotic renovascular disease. J Vasc Surg 39:322-329, 2004.

26. Hansen KJ, Starr SM, Sands RE, et al: Contemporary surgical management of renovascular disease. J Vasc Surg 16:319-331, 1992.

27. Hallett JW Jr, Fowl R, O'Brien PC, et al: Renovascular operations in patients with chronic renal insufficiency: Do the benefits justify the risks? J Vasc Surg 5:622-627, 1987.

28. Hallett JW, Textor SC, Kos PB, et al: Advanced renovascular hypertension and renal insufficiency: Trends in medical comorbidity and surgical approach from 1970 to 1993. J Vasc Surg 21:750-760, 1995.

29. Holden A, Hill A: Renal angioplasty and stenting with distal protection of the main renal artery in ischemic nephropathy: Early experience. J Vasc Surg 38:962-968, 2003.

30. Pillay WR, Kan YM, Crinnion JN, Wolfe JHN: Prospective multicentre study of the natural history of atherosclerotic renal artery stenosis in patients with peripheral vascular disease. Br J Surg 89:737-740, 2002.

Questions

1. **What is the most common cause of secondary hypertension?**
   (a) Pheochromocytoma
   (b) Renal artery stenosis
   (c) Hyperthyroidism
   (d) Coarctation of the aorta

2. **What is the most likely cause of renal artery occlusive disease?**
   (a) Takayasu's arteritis
   (b) Fibromuscular dysplasia
   (c) Post-traumatic dissection
   (d) Atherosclerosis

3. **In patients with hemodynamically significant renal artery stenosis, progression to vessel occlusion occurs in what percentage at 1 year?**
   (a) 1%
   (b) 5%
   (c) 25%
   (d) 40%

4. **Abdominal or flank bruits are audible in up to what percentage of patients with renal artery stenosis?**
   (a) 5%
   (b) 15%
   (c) 25%
   (d) 50%

5. **Noninvasive methods of renal artery imaging include all of the following except**
   (a) Duplex scanning
   (b) Magnetic resonance angiography
   (c) Computed tomography–angiography
   (d) Renal scintigraphy

6. **Alternatives to iodinated contrast agents that may be used for angiography in patients with renal insufficiency include which of the following?**
   (a) Iopamidol
   (b) Carbon dioxide
   (c) Oxygen
   (d) Gadolinium

7. **What is the most common cause of technical failure of renal artery interventions?**
   (a) Inability to traverse the lesion with a guidewire
   (b) Residual stenosis greater than 30%
   (c) Vessel perforation
   (d) Branch vessel compromise

8. **True of false: In the treatment of renal artery ostial stenosis due to atherosclerosis, primary stenting produces an inferior result compared with angioplasty alone.**

9. **True or false: Compared with medical therapy, endovascular management of renal artery stenosis provides at least an equivalent blood pressure response, with fewer antihypertensive agents required.**

10. **Endovascular intervention may have little beneficial effect on renal function, despite adequate technical results, owing to which of the following?**
    (a) Intrinsic renal parenchymal disease
    (b) Use of nephrotoxic contrast agents
    (c) Intraprocedural microembolization
    (d) All of the above

Answers

1. b	2. d	3. b	4. c	5. d
6. b, d	7. a	8. false	9. true	10. d

20

Michael T. Caps • Peter A. Schneider

Angioplasty and Stenting for Infrainguinal Disease: Technique and Results

This chapter reviews our current technique and the results of balloon angioplasty and stent placement for infrainguinal arterial occlusive disease. Management of this disease is continuing to move away from open surgery and toward percutaneous procedures, and the number of percutaneous options is growing rapidly. We focus on the standard techniques for dealing with arterial stenoses and short-segment occlusions in the femoropopliteal arterial segment, but we also touch on evolving techniques for treating long-segment occlusions, bypass graft lesions, and tibial artery occlusive disease.

Technique

PATIENT SELECTION

Infrainguinal occlusive disease can usually be diagnosed by history and physical examination. Confirmatory studies are usually performed—either duplex mapping or magnetic resonance angiography (MRA)—in order to plan the therapeutic approach and limit the amount of contrast required for arteriography. Diagnostic arteriography does not exist in many practices today. Most of our patients do not undergo arterial access unless there is an intention to treat. Occasionally, what initially appeared to be a lesion appropriate for angioplasty based on duplex scanning or MRA turns out to be more complex, and only an arteriogram is obtained. This is most likely to occur with tibial lesions.

Infrainguinal occlusive disease can be classified by its morphology, which assists in determining which patients are best managed with endovascular intervention and which require surgery. The TransAtlantic Inter-Society Consensus (TASC) classification (Table 20-1) and others have defined disease morphology in an effort to clarify the issue of lesion severity.[1] The general concept is that endovascular techniques are preferred in patients with less severe forms of disease and among those with shorter life expectancies or greater periprocedural risk factors. Conversely, open surgical approaches have a better risk-benefit profile in patients with fewer

medical comorbidities or more severe forms of disease, such as long-segment occlusions, in which endovascular procedures are less durable. The recommendation from the TASC group is that type A lesions be treated with endovascular intervention, type D lesions be treated with surgery, and types B and C lesions be treated with either, at the operator's discretion, pending further evaluation.

Over the past 5 years, our practice has seen a steady movement toward the use of endovascular techniques for infrainguinal arterial occlusive disease. Currently, we treat all TASC type A lesions and the majority of types B and C lesions with

---

TABLE 20–1	TransAtlantic Inter-Society Consensus Classification of Femoropopliteal Lesions

Type A Lesions
Single stenosis < 3 cm

Type B Lesions
Single stenosis 3-10 cm long, not involving the distal popliteal artery
Heavily calcified stenosis up to 3 cm
Multiple lesions, each < 3 cm (stenosis or occlusion)
Single or multiple lesions in the absence of tibial runoff to improve inflow for distal surgical bypass

Type C Lesions
Single stenosis or occlusion > 5 cm long
Multiple stenoses or occlusions, each 3-5 cm

Type D Lesions
Occlusion of the common femoral artery, popliteal artery, proximal trifurcation arteries
Occlusion of the superficial femoral artery > 10 cm long

From Schneider PA, Nelken N, Caps MT: Angioplasty and stenting for infrainguinal lesions. In Yao JST, Pearse WH, Matsumura JS (eds): Trends in Vascular Surgery. Chicago, Parmentier Publishing, 2003, p 292.

angioplasty, with or without stenting. We continue to treat all common femoral and popliteal artery occlusions and most long superficial femoral artery (SFA) occlusions surgically. In our practice, approximately 60% of patients requiring treatment for femoropopliteal disease and 15% of patients with tibial disease are treated with endovascular surgery. It is likely that these proportions will continue to increase as additional technologic improvements become clinically available in the coming years.

APPROACHES

Balloon angioplasty and stent placement in the infrainguinal arteries are usually performed through the contralateral femoral artery using an up-and-over approach or through the ipsilateral femoral artery using an antegrade approach (Table 20-2). Infrainguinal interventions can also be performed through the brachial artery, but this approach is rarely required and may be more challenging owing to the longer distances involved. The primary advantages of the up-and-over approach, which is most commonly used, are the following: an aortogram with runoff can be easily converted to endovascular therapy; it permits evaluation of the inflow aortoiliac arteries before treatment of infrainguinal lesions; only a simple retrograde femoral puncture is required; and it facilitates selective catheterization of the SFA orifice and treatment of proximal SFA lesions, which can be difficult via the ipsilateral antegrade approach. Further, puncture site management is contralateral to the intervention site rather than proximal to it. The antegrade approach may be used for better guidewire and catheter control in infrapopliteal intervention and also in patients who have contraindications to the up-and-over approach. The likely approach is determined before the procedure to facilitate room setup and the availability of supplies, but both groins are always prepared in case an alternative approach is required during the procedure.

PLATFORMS

Most balloon angioplasty and stent placement in the infrainguinal arteries can be performed using the standard 0.035-inch platform. The standard platform includes 0.035-inch-diameter guidewires, 4 and 5 French flush and selective catheters, 5 French balloon angioplasty catheters, and 6 French self-expanding stent delivery catheters. The standard platform has several advantages: the guidewires and catheters are easy to handle, the inventory is usually readily available, the fluoroscopic visualization of these larger-caliber devices is simpler, long balloons are available (up to 10 cm) to treat longer SFA lesions, and the larger guidewires and catheters are useful if an occlusion must be crossed or subintimal angioplasty is required. However, there are also some significant disadvantages of 0.035-inch systems: the larger-caliber guidewires and catheters may not easily cross critically diseased segments and may be more prone to cause arterial damage; at longer distances, these catheters lose their "pushability" owing to high friction; and in small arteries such as tibial vessels, the standard platform devices may be too big. In addition to their smaller crossing profiles, the smaller 0.018- and 0.014-inch platforms tend to be more trackable in small, tortuous vessels at distant locations from the access site, especially when using monorail (rapid-exchange) systems with longer guiding sheaths or catheters. Another significant advantage of the smaller platforms is that contrast agent is more easily injected through standard-sized guide sheaths or catheters with the balloon or stent delivery catheter in place, thus permitting more precise angioplasty and stent deployment. Most of the coronary devices are on a 0.014-inch platform, so the array of available balloon catheters and stents is much broader with this system. The balloon catheters are 3 French and can be placed through a 4 French sheath. Monorail balloon catheters permit better "pushability" because the friction of the guidewire on the balloon catheter lumen occurs over a much shorter distance than with coaxial balloon catheters. Monorail systems have the additional advantages of greater ease of use (especially with a single operator), shorter required guidewire lengths, and less guidewire movement during catheter exchanges.

SHEATHS

The access sheath is usually 5 French for balloon angioplasty and 6 French for stent placement. If stent placement is unlikely, we usually place a 5 French sheath, although angioplasty can

TABLE 20–2	Comparison of Approaches to Infrainguinal Interventions: Up-and-Over versus Antegrade	
	Up-and-Over Approach	**Antegrade Approach**
Puncture	Simple retrograde femoral	More challenging, less working room
Catheterization	Challenging with tortuous arteries, narrow or diseased aortic bifurcation; easier to catheterize SFA when going up and over	Entering SFA from antegrade approach requires proximal femoral puncture and selective catheter
Guidewire and catheter control	Fair	Excellent
Catheter inventory	More supplies needed	Minimal, shorter catheters
Specialty items	Up-and-over sheath, long balloon catheters	None
Indications	Proximal SFA disease, CFA disease ipsilateral to infrainguinal lesion, obesity	Infrapopliteal disease, patients with contraindication to up-and-over approach

CFA, common femoral artery; SFA, superior femoral artery.
From Schneider PA: The infrainguinal arteries—advice about balloon angioplasty and stent placement. In Endovascular Skills, 2nd ed. New York, Marcel Dekker, 2003, p 316.

be performed entirely through a 4 French sheath with the use of 0.014- or 0.018-inch platforms. If there is a reasonable likelihood of stent placement, we usually place a 6 French sheath. When using monorail systems, it is helpful to use longer guide sheaths to minimize the amount of unattached delivery catheter extruding outside the sheath; this maintains maximum trackability and reduces the chance of arterial injury. Self-expanding stents are now available that have monorail delivery and can be placed through a 5 French sheath up to 8 mm in diameter. Balloon-expandable coronary stents can be placed in the tibial arteries through a 5 French sheath. In addition, if a 0.014-inch guidewire is used, devices that accommodate a 0.018-inch guidewire will be compatible. It is important to note that with the advent of better percutaneous closure devices, sheath size has become a less important consideration because the larger puncture holes can be safely and easily closed percutaneously in most patients without the need to hold pressure.

UP-AND-OVER APPROACH

Supplies required for an up-and-over approach are listed in Table 20-3. This approach requires longer guidewires, catheters, and sheaths than the antegrade approach. A standard retrograde common femoral artery puncture is performed contralateral to the symptomatic side. A floppy-tipped guidewire is passed into the aorta. A hook-shaped, multi-side-hole flush catheter, such as a 65-cm, 4 French Omni-flush catheter (AngioDynamics, Inc., Queensbury, N.Y.), is passed into the aorta, and an aortoiliac arteriogram is obtained. If bilateral runoff is required, it may be performed at that time with the catheter head placed in the infrarenal aorta. When only unilateral runoff on the symptomatic side is indicated, the catheter is passed over the aortic bifurcation, and lower extremity arteriography is performed. After evaluating the infrainguinal

lesions, determining that the aortic bifurcation can accommodate an access sheath, and deciding that the up-and-over approach is best, an up-and-over sheath is placed (Fig. 20-1).

The aortic flush catheter is withdrawn to the aortic bifurcation, and its tip is rotated toward the contralateral side to direct the guidewire into the contralateral iliac artery. The advancing guidewire, usually a steerable, angled-tip Glidewire (Medi-Tech, Westwood, Mass.), must be steered into the external iliac artery and then into the infrainguinal arteries. From this approach, the guidewire usually tends to select the contralateral internal iliac artery if there is tortuosity of the iliac system. It also tends to select the SFA rather than the deep femoral artery. Either of these destinations for the guidewire is satisfactory from the standpoint of sheath placement, as long as the guidewire is well anchored distal to the groin. The catheter is advanced over the bifurcation, and an exchange guidewire is placed. The tip of the exchange guidewire should be distal to the groin as far as it will easily travel. If there is a proximal SFA lesion that is planned for treatment, the guidewire is usually directed into the deep femoral artery. A 180-cm-long, 0.035-inch Rosen guidewire is usually adequate for sheath placement. If there is a lot of tortuosity in the iliac system, an Amplatz superstiff guidewire may be required.

Dilators are used to enlarge the arteriotomy. Because dilators are sized by their outside diameter and sheaths are sized by their inside diameter, if a 6 French sheath is planned for placement, the tract should be dilated using a 7 French dilator. The guide sheath is placed on the guidewire; when a curved sheath is used, it is oriented such that its curved end is pointing toward the contralateral side and the side arm of the sheath is on the side of the operator. The sheath is advanced over the guidewire using fluoroscopy. Passage over a narrow or diseased aortic bifurcation is performed with care and patience. The sheath is advanced to its hub, if possible. Remember that the tip of the dilator extends beyond the

TABLE 20–3	Supplies for Up-and-Over Approach to Infrainguinal Intervention				
Category	**Type**	**Function**	**Diameter**	**Length**	**Other Features**
Guidewires	Bentson	Starting	0.035 inch	145 cm	
	Glidewire	Selective, therapy	0.035, 0.018 inch	150, 260 cm	Steerable
	Rosen	Exchange	0.035 inch	180 cm	Sheath placement
	Amplatz	Exchange	0.035 inch	180 cm	Sheath placement
	Ironman	Therapy	0.014 inch	190, 300 cm	
Catheters	Omni-flush	Flush, selective	4 French	65 cm	
	Straight	Flush, exchange	5 French	90 cm	Multi–side hole
	Glidecath	Selective, exchange	4, 5 French	100 cm	Angled tip
Sheaths	Destination	Guide sheath	5, 6 French	45 cm	Straight
	Rabbe	Guide sheath	6 French	45, 70 cm	Straight
Balloons	Multiple	PTA infrainguinal	0.035, 0.018, 0.014 inch	75, 90, 110 cm OTW Rapid exchange	Balloon diameters, 2-6 mm Balloon lengths, 2, 4, 6, 10 cm
Stents	SMART	Stent SFA, popliteal Self-expanding	0.035 inch	80, 120 cm OTW	Stent diameters, 7-8 mm Stent lengths, 4, 6, 10 cm
	Precise	Stent SFA, popliteal Self-expanding	0.018 inch	120 cm OTW Rapid exchange	Stent diameters, 7-8 mm Stent length, 4 cm
	Multiple	Stent tibials Balloon-expandable	0.014 inch	150 cm Rapid exchange	Stent diameters, 2.5-4 mm Stent length, 2 cm

OTW, over the wire; PTA, percutaneous transluminal angioplasty; SFA, superficial femoral artery.

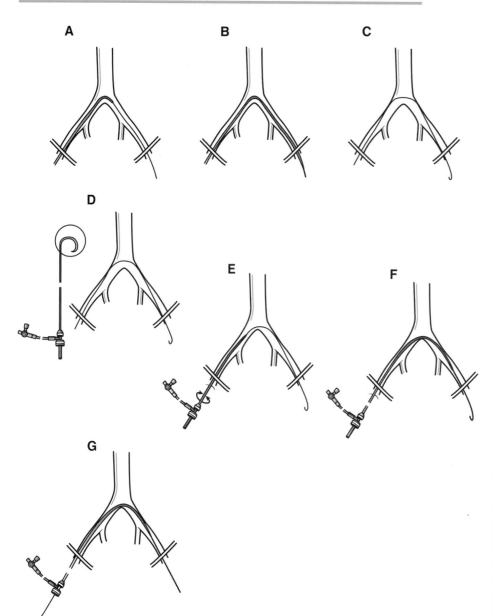

FIGURE 20–1 • Placement of an up-and-over sheath. *A,* A guidewire and catheter are passed over the aortic bifurcation. *B,* The catheter is advanced to the contralateral femoral artery. *C,* An exchange guidewire is placed, and the catheter is removed. *D,* The sheath is oriented with its tip pointing toward the contralateral side. *E,* The sheath is advanced over the guidewire. This is visualized using fluoroscopy. *F,* The sheath is advanced to its hub. There must be enough guidewire ahead of the sheath tip to permit a smooth advance. *G,* The dilator is removed, and the sheath is ready to use. (From Schneider PA: The infrainguinal arteries—advice about balloon angioplasty and stent placement. In Endovascular Skills, 2nd ed. New York, Marcel Dekker, 2003, p 195.)

radiopaque marker on the end of the sheath tip for a short distance. The tip of the sheath will end up somewhere between the mid external iliac artery and the very proximal SFA, depending on the height of the patient. Heparin is usually administered (50 to 75 U/kg) as the sheath is placed.

Figure 20-2 demonstrates the steps required for infrainguinal balloon angioplasty using an up-and-over approach. The exchange guidewire is replaced with a steerable Glidewire, usually 260 cm long. Through the side arm of the sheath, the diseased infrainguinal segment is road-mapped, and the Glidewire is used to cross the lesion to be treated. If treatment of tibial lesions is planned, a 4 or 5 French, 100-cm-long catheter is advanced into the distal popliteal artery, and road-mapping is performed through this catheter; a low-profile guidewire, usually 0.014-inch, is used to cross the tibial lesions. An angled Glidecath (Medi-Tech) may be used to direct the guidewire across the lesion. Interval arteriography may be

performed through the side arm of the sheath or through the selective catheter using a Tuohy-Borst adapter.

The balloon catheter is selected to treat the lesion. Most superficial femoral and popliteal artery lesions are treated with a 5- or 6-mm balloon. Occasionally, a 4- or 7-mm balloon is required. Tibial arteries range from 1 to 4 mm in diameter, but most are between 2 and 3.5 mm. Standard platform balloons are most commonly delivered in 4-cm lengths, but 2-, 6-, 8-, or 10-cm lengths may also be used. Longer lesions can be treated faster by using longer balloons to minimize the number of inflations. Small platform balloons are usually 2 cm long, but 4-cm balloons are available. Small platform balloons may be either noncompliant, like the larger platform balloons, or compliant. An example of a compliant balloon would be a 4-mm balloon with a nominal pressure of 8 atmospheres. At 4 atmospheres, the balloon diameter might be 3.6 mm, but at 14 atmospheres, it might be 4.3 mm. Catheter length must be

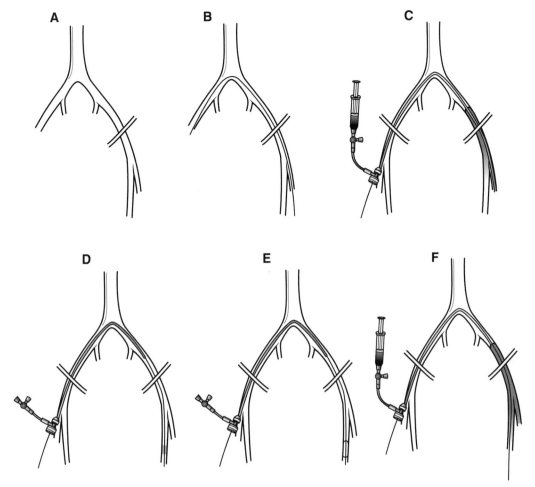

FIGURE 20–2 • Balloon angioplasty of the femoral and popliteal arteries through an up-and-over approach. *A*, A superficial femoral artery lesion is identified. *B*, A guidewire is introduced through the contralateral femoral artery and passed over the aortic bifurcation. *C*, An up-and-over sheath is placed, and arteriography is performed. *D*, The guidewire crosses the lesion. *E*, Balloon angioplasty is performed. *F*, Completion arteriography is performed through the sheath. (From Schneider PA: The infrainguinal arteries—advice about balloon angioplasty and stent placement. In Endovascular Skills, 2nd ed. New York, Marcel Dekker, 2003, p 323.)

anticipated before selecting the balloon. Most of the standard platform balloons are on shafts that are either 75 to 80 cm long or 120 to 130 cm long, depending on the manufacturer. A 75-cm balloon catheter shaft passed up and over will reach anywhere from the common femoral artery to the distal SFA, depending on the patient's height. An estimation of the distance to the lesion can be obtained by using a 75-cm-long straight exchange catheter for guidewire exchanges. The up-and-over sheath also provides clues because its length is known.

The balloon angioplasty catheter is passed over the guidewire and into the lesion. The location of the lesion may be marked using road-mapping or an external marker. Balloon angioplasty is performed by inflating the balloon until the waist on the balloon profile is resolved. The duration of balloon inflation is anywhere from a few seconds to several minutes. Inflation pressure may be as low as 3 or 4 atmospheres to open the waist or as high as 15 to 20 atmospheres. The completion arteriogram is obtained through the side arm of the sheath. Balloon angioplasty of the superficial femoral and popliteal arteries almost always produces some evidence of dissection on completion arteriography. In this setting, deciding which patients require a stent may be challenging. In the

pre-stent era, most dissections that occurred after percutaneous transluminal angioplasty (PTA) healed. Because primary stent placement has not proved to be of value in enhancing durability, stents should be placed selectively. This issue is discussed in greater detail in the section about stents.

The completion arteriogram is assessed. If it shows a satisfactory result, the sheath is withdrawn so that its tip is pulled back over the aortic bifurcation. The guidewire is removed, a dressing is placed, and the patient is moved to another area where the sheath is removed. Alternatively, in patients with favorable anatomy, the puncture site can be closed with a percutaneous closure device.

ANTEGRADE APPROACH

Supplies required for an antegrade approach are listed in Table 20-4. An antegrade common femoral artery puncture is performed ipsilateral to the symptomatic side. This approach is well suited to patients who have normal aortoiliac inflow, especially if tibial angioplasty is required or if there is a need to limit the use of contrast material. The puncture should be performed as proximally along the common femoral artery as

TABLE 20–4	Supplies for Antegrade Approach to Infrainguinal Intervention				
Category	**Type**	**Function**	**Diameter**	**Length**	**Other Features**
Guidewires	Wholey	Starting, selective	0.035 inch	145 cm	Steerable
	Glidewire	Selective, therapy	0.035 inch	150, 180 cm	Steerable
	Rosen	Exchange	0.035 inch	180 cm	Sheath placement
	Ironman	Therapy	0.014 inch	190 cm	
Catheters	Kumpe	Selective, exchange	5 French	40 cm	Short, angled tip
	Glidecath	Selective, exchange	4, 5 French	70 cm	Angled tip
	Straight	Flush, exchange	5 French	70 cm	Multi–side hole
Sheaths	Standard	Access, guide	5, 6 French	12-20 cm	Straight
Balloons	Multiple	PTA infrainguinal	0.035, 0.018, 0.014 inch	75, 90 cm	Balloon diameters, 2-6 mm Balloon lengths, 2, 4, 6 cm
Stents	SMART	Stent SFA, popliteal Self-expanding	0.035 inch	80 cm OTW	Stent diameters, 7-8 mm Stent lengths, 4, 6, 10 cm
	Precise	Stent SFA, popliteal Self-expanding	0.018 inch	80 cm OTW Rapid exchange	Stent diameters, 7-8 mm Stent length, 4 cm
	Multiple	Stent tibials Balloon-expandable	0.014 inch	100 cm Rapid exchange	Stent diameters, 2.5-4 mm Stent length, 2 cm

OTW, over the wire; PTA, percutaneous transluminal angioplasty; SFA, superficial femoral artery.

possible to leave some working room between the puncture and the origin of the SFA. A steerable guidewire, such as the Wholey guidewire (Mallinckrodt, Inc., Hazelwood, Md.), is used; the shaft of this guidewire is more supportive for catheter and sheath passage than a Glidewire. The Wholey guidewire can often be steered anteromedially into the SFA. If not, the guidewire is advanced into the deep femoral artery, and an angled-tip catheter is placed over it (Fig. 20-3). The image intensifier is placed in the ipsilateral anterior oblique position to open the femoral bifurcation, and the catheter is withdrawn enough to perform road-mapping by refluxing contrast material into the SFA. The catheter is used to steer the guidewire into the SFA.

If the lesion is in the proximal to mid-SFA, the artery is road-mapped using the catheter, and the guidewire is advanced across the lesion (Fig. 20-4). The same guidewire can be used for sheath placement. If the lesion is more distal in the artery, the guidewire is advanced without crossing the lesion, and the sheath is placed. The sheath required may be 4, 5, or 6 French, depending on the platform used and whether balloon angioplasty will be followed by stent placement. An appropriately sized dilator is used to enlarge the arteriotomy before sheath placement.

After the sheath is placed, femoral arteriography is performed through its side arm. Heparin is administered. Standard-length 150-cm, 0.035-inch guidewires may be used for lesions above the knee. Longer guidewires, 180 or 260 cm, are used for infrageniculate balloon angioplasty, especially in tall patients. A 75- or 80-cm-long balloon angioplasty catheter may be used to the midtibial level. Longer catheters are required for more distal lesions. The lesion is evaluated angiographically. A steerable Glidewire is used to cross the lesion. Arteriography is repeated after the guidewire is across the lesion to be certain that the guidewire is in the distal artery and not in a perigenicular collateral. The balloon catheter is selected and passed over the guidewire, and balloon angioplasty

is performed. Completion arteriography is done through the sheath while maintaining guidewire control until the results are assessed.

STENTS

Stents may be used to manage poor immediate postangioplasty results without resorting to emergent surgery. Stents are placed for postangioplasty residual stenosis or flow-limiting dissection. Some residual stenosis at the angioplasty site is acceptable, but when residual stenosis exceeds 30%, a stent should be strongly considered. Dissection can be identified after almost every balloon angioplasty in the femoral and popliteal arteries. Mild dissections do not require treatment. However, if there is substantial residual stenosis from the dissection or flow limitation, or if there is contrast trapping in the wall of the artery, a stent should be placed. Primary stent placement should be performed in most cases when recanalizing an occlusion or performing a subintimal balloon angioplasty.

Most of the stents placed in the femoral and popliteal arteries are self-expanding stents (Fig. 20-5). These stents are flexible and must be oversized—1 to 3 mm larger than the intended artery segment. The newer nitinol stents foreshorten only minimally and can be obtained with markers on the ends for better visualization. Stent delivery catheters are either 80 or 120 cm long, based on the length of the balloon catheter required. Self-expanding stents deploy by unfurling from the tip end of the catheter, back toward the hub end. Most stents are deployed with the same mechanism: the pushing rod is held steady while the stent delivery catheter hub is pulled back. This withdraws the membrane covering the stent, and it deploys. The stent is visualized with fluoroscopy. The constrained stent is passed slightly beyond the lesion and pulled back slightly with a fine-tuning adjustment as its tip end begins to open. After the stent is deployed, repeat balloon angioplasty is performed.

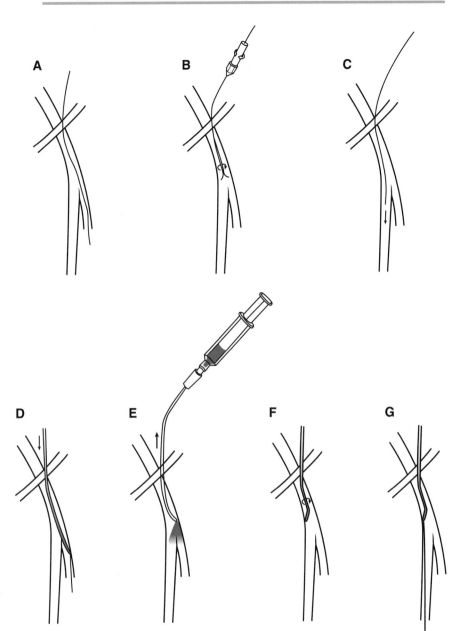

FIGURE 20–3 • Catheterization of the superficial femoral artery (SFA) through an ipsilateral antegrade approach. *A,* After antegrade femoral puncture, the guidewire tends to advance into the profunda (deep) femoral artery (PFA). *B,* A Wholey guidewire may be used with a torque device to direct the guidewire into the SFA. *C,* The guidewire tip is rotated anteriorly and medially to enter the SFA. *D,* Another option is to pass an angled-tip catheter into the PFA. *E,* The guidewire is removed, and the catheter is slowly withdrawn while puffing contrast material to demonstrate the femoral bifurcation. *F,* The catheter tip is rotated toward the SFA. *G,* The guidewire is advanced through the catheter into the SFA. (From Schneider PA: The infrainguinal arteries—advice about balloon angioplasty and stent placement. In Endovascular Skills, 2nd ed. New York, Marcel Dekker, 2003, p 109.)

Results

FEMOROPOPLITEAL BALLOON ANGIOPLASTY

Data accumulated over 20 years provide an understanding of femoropopliteal balloon angioplasty. In a summary of studies covering 1241 patients, the results (weighted averages) for femoropopliteal balloon angioplasty were as follows: 90% technical success rate, 4.3% complication rate, 1-year patency of 61%, and 5-year patency of 48%.[1] In a review of several large studies published in the early to mid-1990s, before the broad availability and use of stents, patency rates ranged from 47% to 63% at 1 year and 26% to 48% at 5 years.[2] Multiple factors affect the results of femoropopliteal PTA, including lesion length, clinical stage (claudication vs. limb salvage), runoff, lesion type (stenosis vs. occlusion), proximal location, and lack of residual stenosis after PTA (Tables 20-5 and 20-6).[3-5]

Meta-analyses have demonstrated the impact of lesion type and clinical stage (see Table 20-5).[6,7] Lesion length is not addressed in as many studies, and length classifications have not been standardized; however, it appears that length also has a significant impact on results (see Table 20-6).[8-11]

The patency of PTA of a short femoropopliteal lesion under favorable circumstances is 70% to 80% at 1 year and 50% to 60% at 5 years. This type of lesion is ideally suited to PTA. Endovascular intervention is cost-effective in comparison to surgery in this setting and is the treatment of choice.[12] Unfortunately, most situations in which femoropopliteal balloon angioplasty is considered are more complex and factors are not as favorable. In addition, balloon angioplasty is no longer a stand-alone procedure since stent placement has become more common in endovascular surgery of the infrainguinal arteries.

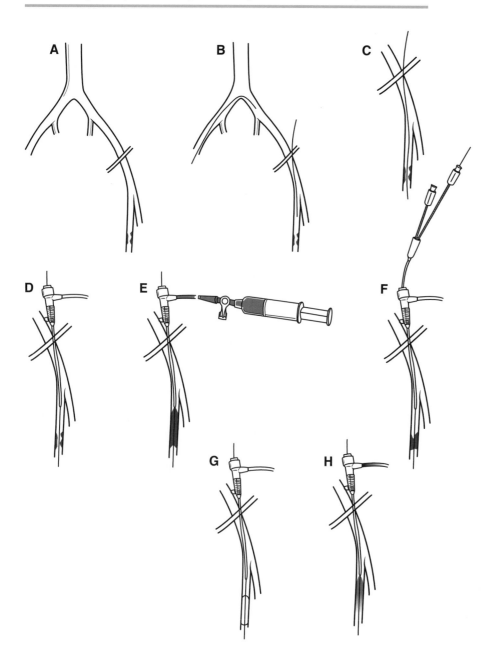

FIGURE 20–4 • Balloon angioplasty of the superficial femoral artery (SFA) and popliteal artery through an antegrade approach. *A*, Stenosis of the SFA is suitable for balloon angioplasty. *B*, The lesion may be approached from either the contralateral or the ipsilateral femoral artery. *C*, The guidewire is placed across the stenosis through an antegrade approach. *D*, An access sheath is placed into the proximal SFA. *E*, Arteriography is performed through the side arm of the sheath to evaluate the lesion and confirm guidewire position. *F*, The balloon angioplasty catheter is passed over the guidewire and advanced into the lesion. *G*, Balloon angioplasty is performed. *H*, Completion arteriography is performed. Guidewire position is maintained until the results are assessed. (From Schneider PA: The infrainguinal arteries—advice about balloon angioplasty and stent placement. In Endovascular Skills, 2nd ed. New York, Marcel Dekker, 2003, p 318.)

TABLE 20–5	Meta-analyses of Femoropopliteal Balloon Angioplasty: Effect of Lesion Type and Clinical Stage				

				Primary Patency (%)		
Author	No. of Limbs	Lesion Type	Clinical Stage	1 Year	3 Years	5 Years
Hunink et al[6]	4800	Stenosis	Claudication	79	74	68
		Stenosis	Limb threat	62	54	47
		Occlusion	Claudication	52	43	35
		Occlusion	Limb threat	26	18	12
Muradin et al[7]	923	Stenosis	Claudication		61	
		Stenosis	Limb threat		43	
		Occlusion	Claudication		48	
		Occlusion	Limb threat		30	

From Schneider PA, Nelken N, Caps MT: Angioplasty and stenting for infrainguinal lesions. In Yao JST, Pearse WH, Matsumura JS (eds): Trends in Vascular Surgery. Chicago, Parmentier Publishing, 2003, p 293.

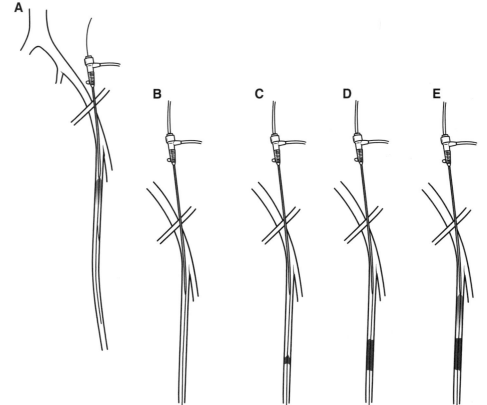

FIGURE 20–5 • Stent placement in the superficial femoral artery. *A*, Dissection is present after balloon angioplasty. *B*, A self-expanding stent delivery catheter is placed over the guidewire and advanced into the segment of dissection. *C*, The stent is deployed from the tip end to the hub end of the catheter. *D*, Post-stent balloon angioplasty is performed to bring the stent to its appropriate profile. *E*, Completion arteriography is performed. (From Schneider PA: The infrainguinal arteries—advice about balloon angioplasty and stent placement. In Endovascular Skills, 2nd ed. New York, Marcel Dekker, 2003, p 321.)

FEMOROPOPLITEAL STENT PLACEMENT

Over the past 5 years, stent placement has become integrated into infrainguinal intervention. This evolution has been prompted by the development of a variety of simple, low-profile, user-friendly, self-expanding stents that can be easily placed when needed or when the immediate results of PTA are not satisfactory.

There is no evidence that routine or primary stent placement improves long-term results. Several randomized trials have shown no significant difference in patency 1 to 4 years after intervention in comparisons of primary and selective stent placement (Table 20-7).[13-16] Because stent technology is a rapidly developing field, it must be acknowledged that the results of these studies, which evaluated primarily balloon-expandable stents, may not be applicable to the current generation of self-expanding stents. Recent data suggest that self-expanding nitinol stents may significantly improve results (70% to 80% primary patency at 3 years).[17-19] Stents that deliver medications or are covered with graft material to prevent intimal hyperplasia are also likely to become clinically

TABLE 20–6	Effect of Lesion Length on Results of Femoropopliteal Balloon Angioplasty		
Author	**Lesion Length (cm)**	**Patency (%)**	**Follow-up**
Murray et al[8]	<7	81	6 mo
	>7	23	6 mo
Currie et al[9]	<5	59	6 mo
	>5	4	6 mo
Jeans et al[10]	<1	76	5 yr
	>1	50	5 yr
Krepel et al[11]	<2	77	5 yr
	>2	54	5 yr

From Schneider PA, Nelken N, Caps MT: Angioplasty and stenting for infrainguinal lesions. In Yao JST, Pearse WH, Matsumura JS (eds): Trends in Vascular Surgery. Chicago, Parmentier Publishing, 2003, p 293.

TABLE 20–7	Results of Randomized Trials Comparing Primary versus Selective Stent Placement for Femoropopliteal Occlusive Disease			
Author	**Year**	**Primary**	**Selective**	**Follow-up (Yr)**
Vroegindeweij et al[13]	1997	74	85	1
Cejna et al[14]	2001	65	65	2
Grimm et al[15]	2001	62	68	3
Becquemin et al[16]	2003	44	57	4

From Schneider PA, Nelken N, Caps MT: Angioplasty and stenting for infrainguinal lesions. In Yao JST, Pearse WH, Matsumura JS (eds): Trends in Vascular Surgery. Chicago, Parmentier Publishing, 2003, p 293.

useful in the near future.[20-22] Spiral-shaped stents that have high radial strength and flexibility; the ability to accommodate bending, shortening, and elongation; and the capability to preserve potentially important collaterals may also play an important role in endovascular infrainguinal revascularization.[23]

Although primary stent placement is not warranted, selective stent placement plays an important role. The immediate success of intervention is higher with the availability of stents. About 15% of patients undergoing PTA alone require selective stent placement or experience immediate failure.[14,16] The least favorable results of PTA come from the treatment of long lesions, occlusions, residual stenoses, and limb-threatening ischemia. Stents are an essential tool if endovascular intervention is to be an option in treating these complex lesions and unfavorable clinical situations. The day-to-day reality is that PTA is being performed on a broad array of infrainguinal lesions, partially because the availability of stents makes endovascular intervention a more reasonable option and less likely to cause an ischemic emergency. A meta-analysis of 423 stent implantations for femoropopliteal occlusive disease demonstrated 66% patency at 3 years, which was not dependent on clinical indication or lesion type.[7] Stents have also yielded promising results with long, chronic occlusions.[24]

SUBINTIMAL ANGIOPLASTY AND STENTING FOR FEMOROPOPLITEAL OCCLUSIONS

The technique of subintimal angioplasty with or without stenting for long-segment occlusions of the femoropopliteal arteries was first described in the late 1980s.[25,26] The technique involves the intentional creation of and entry into a subintimal dissection plane created just proximal to the occlusion using an angled Glidewire and supporting angled catheter. The wire typically forms a loop that is advanced through the subintimal plane until the occlusion is passed; the true lumen is then reentered, followed by angioplasty and adjunctive stenting as indicated. Technical success rates range from approximately 70% to 90%.[27-29] The major obstacle to technical success is the difficulty in reentering the true lumen distal to the occlusion. Preliminary results using two commercially available systems designed for true lumen reentry are promising and may improve technical success rates.[30,31] In the largest study with long-term follow-up, patency rates following technically successful procedures were 71% and 58% at 1 and 3 years, respectively.[28]

INFRAINGUINAL BYPASS GRAFT STENOSIS

The results of balloon angioplasty for failing infrainguinal bypass grafts have been mixed.[32,33] This is due in part to the nature of lesions caused by myointimal hyperplasia. These lesions are smooth and fibrous and are often not sufficiently remodeled by standard balloon angioplasty; there is a relatively high probability of elastic recoil. Preliminary studies on the use of cutting balloons for infrainguinal bypass graft stenoses have demonstrated promising results.[34,35] Cutting balloons are available on a 0.014-inch platform and contain three or four longitudinally placed atherotomes designed to create a controlled series of incisions in the lesion, thereby promoting more effective remodeling. Currently, the largest available cutting balloon diameter is 4 mm. Cutting balloon angioplasty is frequently followed by larger standard balloon angioplasty to improve luminal diameter.

INFRAPOPLITEAL LESIONS

The patency of infrapopliteal balloon angioplasty is not as well established as that for more proximal lesions. Most of these patients have limb-threatening ischemia, multilevel disease, and multiple or diffuse tibial lesions that require treatment. Results have been assessed most often by evaluating limb salvage rather than patency. A meta-analysis of 1282 treated limbs demonstrated a technical success rate of 93% and a 2-year limb salvage rate of 74%.[36] Stent placement is technically feasible using low-profile, balloon-expandable coronary stents on a 0.014-inch platform. Although this approach may help salvage an unsuccessful tibial balloon angioplasty, there are insufficient data to determine whether stents are of any significant value in the infrapopliteal arteries.

Other Evolving Technologies

Other evolving technologies for treating infrainguinal arterial occlusive disease include cryoplasty and atherectomy. Both technologies are expensive, and data regarding their efficacy are relatively sparse.[37,38] Cryoplasty is performed using nitrous oxide as the balloon inflation medium, thereby causing freezing and cellular apoptosis of the smooth muscle layer with a theoretical reduction in myointimal hyperplasia and restenosis. Cryoplasty has the additional advantage of causing less extensive dissection at the treatment site and a reduction in the need for adjunctive stenting. Currently, one system is commercially available, employing a 0.014-inch platform for smaller balloons (≤4 mm) and a 0.035-inch platform for larger balloons (4 to 8 mm). Access sheath requirements range from 5 to 8 French, depending on balloon size and platform.

Directional atherectomy has been used in the coronary circulation with mixed results for many years. The newest-generation device has shown promising results in the treatment of infrainguinal arterial stenoses and occlusions, with low rates of recurrent stenosis and distal embolization.[38] The device contains a battery-operated rotating atherectomy blade that removes a core of atheroma with each pass; multiple passes are typically required in order to achieve adequate vessel remodeling. Adjunctive stenting is usually not required. The device is available on a 0.014-inch platform with multiple tip lengths.

Conclusions

Although the results of endovascular intervention for occlusive disease of the iliac arteries are excellent, whether this success can be extrapolated to the infrainguinal arteries remains controversial. The lower periprocedural morbidity and rapid recovery associated with endovascular approaches make them attractive to physicians as well as patients. A full-service vascular practice must include a broad variety of both endovascular and surgical options for treating infrainguinal arterial occlusive disease. Infrainguinal endovascular intervention and its growing cadre of associated options have a high likelihood of improving the care of vascular patients in the years to come.

REFERENCES

1. TransAtlantic Inter-Society Consensus: Management of peripheral vascular disease: Femoropopliteal PTA. J Vasc Surg 31:S103-S107, 2000.
2. Schneider PA: Endovascular interventions in the management of chronic lower extremity ischemia. In Rutherford RB (ed): Vascular Surgery, 5th ed. Philadelphia, WB Saunders, 2000, pp 1055-1058.
3. Capek P, McLean GK, Berkowitz HD: Femoropopliteal angioplasty: Factors influencing long-term success. Circulation 83(2 Suppl):I70-I80, 1991.
4. Hunink MG, Donaldson MC, Meyerovitz MF, et al: Risks and benefits of femoropopliteal percutaneous balloon angioplasty. J Vasc Surg 17:183-192, 1993.
5. Johnston KW: Femoral and popliteal arteries: Reanalysis of results of balloon angioplasty. Radiology 183:767-771, 1992.
6. Hunink MG, Wong JB, Donaldson MC, et al: Patency results of percutaneous and surgical revascularization for femoropopliteal arterial disease. Med Decis Making 14:71-81, 1994.
7. Muradin GS, Bosch JL, Stijnen T, Hunink MG: Balloon dilation and stent implantation for treatment of femoropopliteal arterial disease: Meta-analysis. Radiology 221:137-145, 2001.
8. Murray JG, Apthorp LA, Wilkins RA: Long-segment (≥10 cm) femoropopliteal angioplasty: Improved technical success and long-term patency. Radiology 195:158-162, 1995.
9. Currie IC, Wakeley CJ, Cole SE, et al: Femoropopliteal angioplasty for severe limb ischaemia. Br J Surg 81:191-193, 1994.
10. Jeans WD, Armstrong S, Cole SE, et al: Fate of patients undergoing transluminal angioplasty for lower-limb ischemia. Radiology 177:559-564, 1990.
11. Krepel VM, van Andel GJ, van Erp WF, Breslau PJ: Percutaneous transluminal angioplasty of the femoropopliteal artery: Initial and long-term results. Radiology 156:325-328, 1985.
12. Hunink MG, Wong JB, Donaldson MC, et al: Revascularization for femoropopliteal disease: A decision and cost-effectiveness analysis. JAMA 274:165-171, 1995.
13. Vroegindeweij D, Vos LD, Tielbeek AV, et al: Balloon angioplasty combined with primary stenting versus balloon angioplasty alone in femoropopliteal obstructions: A comparative randomized study. Cardiovasc Intervent Radiol 20:420-425, 1997.
14. Cejna M, Thurnher S, Illiasch H, et al: PTA versus Palmaz stent placement in femoropopliteal artery obstructions: A multicenter prospective randomized study. J Vasc Interv Radiol 12:23-31, 2001.
15. Grimm J, Muller-Hulsbeck S, Jahnke T, et al: Randomized study to compare PTA alone versus PTA with Palmaz stent placement for femoropopliteal lesions. J Vasc Interv Radiol 12:935-942, 2001.
16. Becquemin JP, Favre JP, Marzelle J, et al: Systematic versus selective stent placement after superficial femoral artery balloon angioplasty: A multicenter prospective randomized study. J Vasc Surg 37:487-494, 2003.
17. Cho L, Roffi M, Mukherjee D, et al: Superficial femoral artery occlusion: Nitinol stents achieve better flow and reduce the need for medications than balloon angioplasty alone. J Invasive Cardiol 15:198-200, 2003.
18. Lugmayr HF, Holzer H, Kastner M, et al: Treatment of complex arteriosclerotic lesions with nitinol stents in the superficial femoral and popliteal arteries: A midterm follow-up. Radiology 222:37-43, 2002.
19. Mewissen MW: Self-expanding nitinol stents in the femoropopliteal segment: Technique and mid-term results. Tech Vasc Interv Radiol 7:2-5, 2004.
20. Duda SH, Pusich B, Richter G, et al: Sirolimus-eluting stents for the treatment of obstructive superficial femoral artery disease: Six-month results. Circulation 106:1505-1509, 2002.
21. Jahnke T, Andresen R, Muller-Hulsbeck S, et al: Hemobahn stent-grafts for treatment of femoropopliteal arterial obstructions: Midterm results of a prospective trial. J Vasc Interv Radiol 14:41-51, 2003.
22. Saxon RR, Coffman JM, Gooding JM, et al: Long-term results of EPTFE stent-graft versus angioplasty in the femoropopliteal artery: Single center experience from a prospective, randomized trial. J Vasc Interv Radiol 14:303-311, 2003.
23. Rosenthal D, Martin JD, Schubart PJ, et al: Remote superficial femoral artery endarterectomy and distal aSpire stenting: Multicenter medium-term results. J Vasc Surg 40:67-72, 2004.
24. Conroy RM, Gordon IL, Tobis JM, et al: Angioplasty and stent placement in chronic occlusion of the superficial femoral artery: Technique and results. J Vasc Interv Radiol 11:1009-1020, 2000.
25. Bolia A, Miles KA, Brennan J, Bell PR: Percutaneous transluminal angioplasty of occlusions of the femoral and popliteal arteries by subintimal dissection. Cardiovasc Intervent Radiol 13:357-363, 1990.
26. Bolia A, Brennan J, Bell PR: Recanalisation of femoro-popliteal occlusions: Improving success rate by subintimal recanalisation. Clin Radiol 40:325, 1989.
27. Lipsitz EC, Ohki T, Veith FJ, et al: Does subintimal angioplasty have a role in the treatment of severe lower extremity ischemia? J Vasc Surg 37:386-391, 2003.
28. London NJ, Srinivasan R, Naylor AR, et al: Subintimal angioplasty of femoropopliteal artery occlusions: The long-term results. Eur J Vasc Surg 8:148-155, 1994.
29. McCarthy RJ, Neary W, Roobottom C, et al: Short-term results of femoropopliteal subintimal angioplasty. Br J Surg 87:1361-1365, 2000.
30. Hausegger KA, Georgieva B, Portugaller H, et al: The Outback catheter: A new device for true lumen re-entry after dissection during recanalization of arterial occlusions. Cardiovasc Intervent Radiol 27:26-30, 2004.
31. Saketkhoo RR, Razavi MK, Padidar A, et al: Percutaneous bypass: Subintimal recanalization of peripheral occlusive disease with IVUS guided luminal re-entry. Tech Vasc Interv Radiol 7:23-27, 2004.
32. Alexander JQ, Katz SG: The efficacy of percutaneous transluminal angioplasty in the treatment of infrainguinal vein bypass graft stenosis. Arch Surg 138:510-513, 2003.
33. Avino AJ, Bandyk DF, Gonsalves AJ, et al: Surgical and endovascular intervention for infrainguinal vein graft stenosis. J Vasc Surg 29:60-70, 1999.
34. Engelke C, Morgan RA, Belli AM: Cutting balloon percutaneous transluminal angioplasty for salvage of lower limb arterial bypass grafts: Feasibility. Radiology 223:106-114, 2002.
35. Kasirajan K, Schneider PA: Early outcome of "cutting" balloon angioplasty for infrainguinal vein graft stenosis. J Vasc Surg 39:702-708, 2004.
36. Kandarpa K, Becker GJ, Hunink MG, et al: Transcatheter interventions for the treatment of peripheral atherosclerotic lesions: Part I. J Vasc Interv Radiol 12:683-695, 2001.
37. Fava M, Loyola S, Polydorou A, et al: Cryoplasty for femoropopliteal arterial disease: Late angiographic results of initial human experience. J Vasc Interv Radiol 15:1239-1243, 2004.
38. Zeller T, Rastan A, Schwarzwalder U, et al: Percutaneous peripheral atherectomy of femoropopliteal stenoses using a new-generation device: Six-month results from a single-center experience. J Endovasc Ther 11:676-685, 2004.

Questions

1. **Which of the following is an advantage of endovascular intervention over open surgery for infrainguinal arterial occlusive disease?**
   (a) Less morbidity
   (b) Improved patency
   (c) Superior durability
   (d) All of the above

2. **The ipsilateral antegrade femoral approach for infrainguinal intervention is preferred over the contralateral up-and-over approach in which of the following circumstances?**
   (a) Preprocedural imaging demonstrates absence of iliac inflow disease
   (b) Chronic renal insufficiency
   (c) Planned infrapopliteal intervention
   (d) All of the above

3. **Which of the following is an advantage of the smaller (0.014- or 0.018-inch) platforms over standard (0.035-inch) systems in infrainguinal endovascular intervention?**
   (a) Smaller crossing profiles
   (b) Better fluoroscopic visualization
   (c) Improved ability to cross chronic occlusions
   (d) All of the above

4. **When using smaller platforms, why are monorail (rapid-exchange) catheters preferred over coaxial catheters?**
   (a) Less friction and improved trackability
   (b) Reduced guidewire movement during catheter exchanges
   (c) Shorter required guidewire lengths
   (d) All of the above

5. **Which of the following statements regarding sheath selection for infrainguinal endovascular intervention is true?**
   (a) Balloon angioplasty requires a sheath sized 6 French or larger
   (b) Stent placement requires a sheath sized 6 French or smaller
   (c) Sheaths are sized according to their outer diameter
   (d) All of the above

6. **Which of the following factors is associated with improved outcome in patients undergoing femoropopliteal balloon angioplasty?**
   (a) Long lesions
   (b) Absence of residual stenosis after angioplasty
   (c) Poor outflow
   (d) All of the above

7. **Which of the following statements regarding the use of stents for femoropopliteal disease is true?**
   (a) All stenotic lesions should be stented primarily
   (b) Balloon-expandable stents are more effective than self-expanding stents
   (c) Postangioplasty dissection with contrast trapping should be stented
   (d) All of the above

8. **Major obstacles to technical success with infrainguinal subintimal angioplasty include which of the following?**
   (a) Entering the subintimal plane from the true lumen above the occlusion
   (b) Reentering the true lumen below the occlusion
   (c) Perforation
   (d) All of the above

9. **Endovascular intervention for infrainguinal bypass graft stenoses differs from de novo atherosclerotic lesions in which of the following respects?**
   (a) Increased incidence of elastic recoil
   (b) Increased incidence of dissection
   (c) Increased need for stents
   (d) All of the above

10. **Which of the following statements regarding infrapopliteal balloon angioplasty is true?**
    (a) Patency rates are well established
    (b) Unsuccessful PTA can be salvaged with balloon-expandable coronary stents
    (c) Contralateral up-and-over approach is preferred over ipsilateral antegrade approach
    (d) All of the above

Answers

1. a	2. d	3. a	4. d	5. b
6. b	7. c	8. b	9. a	10. b

21

Takao Ohki • Carlos H. Timaran • Jay Yadav

Technique of Carotid Angioplasty and Stenting

The efficacy of carotid endarterectomy (CEA) in preventing stroke in a select group of patients with significant internal carotid stenosis has been proved by multiple randomized trials. Therefore, CEA remains the gold standard of treatment for the majority of patients. However, CEA is not a panacea, nor is it perfect. Cumulative complication rates between 17% and 23% have been reported in these randomized trials.[1,2] Moreover, a well-defined group of patients for whom CEA presents a high risk has been identified. These patients include those with severe medical comorbidities, recurrent stenosis, a hostile neck, and unusually low or high lesions.[3] Carotid angioplasty and stenting (CAS) has emerged as an alternative to CEA in patients with such risk factors. During the last decade, CAS has evolved rapidly and has become a safe and effective procedure. For example, the Stenting and Angioplasty with Protection in Patients at High Risk for Endarterectomy (SAPPHIRE) trial proved that CAS was not inferior to CEA in a high-risk patient cohort.[4] This chapter describes the techniques of CAS as well as the early results of observational studies and registries and the current status of randomized clinical trials assessing CAS for the treatment of carotid disease.

Results of Observational Studies and Clinical Trials

With the advent of new endovascular techniques, CAS has become a safe and effective procedure.[5-12] The introduction of nitinol stents, smaller stent delivery systems, and cerebral protection devices (CPDs) will certainly result in the improvement and refinement of CAS techniques, which will probably translate into better outcomes. These technologic advances, however, create challenges for the performance of randomized clinical trials comparing CAS and CEA, because surgical procedures and techniques may be outdated before the completion of such trials.

The role of CEA in the treatment of symptomatic and asymptomatic carotid occlusive disease has been well defined by major randomized clinical trials.[1,2] Conversely, although many single- and multicenter studies of CAS have been reported, only two randomized, prospective multicenter trials have been published to date.[4,13] The results of other clinical trials of CAS have been partially reported, and peer-reviewed publications are expected in the near future. Although most of the evidence available on CAS originates primarily from observational studies, such information is pivotal in recommending this procedure, as well as in designing future clinical trials.

Single-center studies performed from 1990 to 1999 reported significantly higher rates of stroke or death for CAS than for CEA, as elucidated by a systematic review of the 30-day outcome of both procedures for symptomatic carotid lesions.[14] In that report, which covered 33 studies (13 CAS and 20 CEA), the risk of any stroke or death was 7.8% for CAS and 4% for CEA, whereas the risk of major stroke or death was 3.9% after CAS and 2.2% after CEA. Although the authors of the review concluded that CAS should not be recommended for the treatment of symptomatic carotid lesions, that recommendation was based on CAS procedures with several technical limitations. For instance, carotid stents were deployed in only 44% of patients undergoing carotid angioplasty, and only two case series (82 of 714 CAS procedures) included patients who underwent CAS with the use of CPDs.

Initial attempts to perform randomized clinical trials comparing CAS and CEA were unsuccessful, and the trials were stopped prematurely because of the poor results from CAS. The Leicester trial, which randomized patients with severe symptomatic carotid stenosis to CEA or CAS, was terminated after the enrollment of 17 patients.[15] Of note, this trial had no exclusion criteria, and all patients with symptomatic carotid stenosis were enrolled. Five of seven patients undergoing unprotected CAS had periprocedural stroke, whereas none of the 10 patients treated with CEA had neurologic complications. Although the adverse outcome of CAS was probably related to a lack of adequate patient selection, dedicated devices, and operator experience, this study underscores the risk of embolization during CAS. The Wallstent trial was another industry-supported randomized, prospective trial comparing CEA and CAS that was terminated after the enrollment of 219 symptomatic patients.[16] CAS procedures were performed without CPDs and with antiplatelet therapy that would not be considered adequate according to current standards. The 30-day rate of any stroke or death was 4.5% for CEA and 12.1% for unprotected CAS. The authors appropriately concluded that CAS without embolic protection was not equivalent to CEA with respect to safety.

One of the two completed randomized clinical trials of CAS, the Carotid and Vertebral Artery Transluminal Angioplasty Study (CAVATAS), demonstrated similar outcomes of unprotected CAS and CEA in 504 patients with symptomatic internal carotid artery (ICA) stenoses.[13] The technical success rate of CAS was 89%. The 30-day rate of any stroke or mortality was approximately 10% in both the CAS and the CEA groups, and the rate of major stroke was 6% in both groups. The applicability of the clinical information derived from this study is questionable, however, because of several technical limitations. Most carotid endovascular procedures in CAVATAS were treated with angioplasty alone, whereas only 26% of cases underwent carotid stenting. CPDs were not used in this trial. Although similar results for unprotected CAS and CEA were reported in this study, there is strong clinical and experimental evidence supporting the use of CPDs in all patients undergoing CAS.[17,18]

The recognition that embolization of plaque debris to the brain is the most significant complication of CAS has prompted intense investigation of CPDs.[19] Although Theron performed the first CAS procedure with cerebral protection in 1993,[8] the use of CPDs did not become widespread for many years. However, there is considerable evidence, both clinical and experimental, that embolization takes place during all CAS procedures. In addition, the development of more sophisticated protection devices and their availability have made the concept of cerebral protection more acceptable, and there is now a consensus among specialists that protection devices should be used in all CAS procedures.[3] As a matter of fact, several observational studies have shown improved outcomes of CAS when CPDs are used. Our initial experience with CPDs revealed that CAS under cerebral protection can be performed safely with a high technical success rate (97%).[12] Although most patients who underwent treatment with CAS were at high risk, the neurologic complication rate was low, with a combined 30-day stroke and death rate close to 3%. During a mean follow-up period of 17 months, one subacute occlusion of a stent occurred but did not result in a stroke. Three other patients had duplex scan–proven in-stent restenosis, and two underwent treatment with repeat percutaneous transluminal angioplasty, with good results. No patient had a stroke during the follow-up period. In a recent systematic review of studies published between 1990 and 2002, early outcome of CAS with and without CPDs was assessed.[18] Of 3433 CAS procedures included in this study, 2537 were performed without CPDs, and 896 were performed under cerebral protection. The combined 30-day stroke and death rate was 1.8% in patients treated with CPDs, compared with 5.5% in patients treated without cerebral protection. These results were attributed primarily to a decreased occurrence of all strokes in CAS procedures with CPDs, because death rates were almost identical (0.8%).

The SAPPHIRE trial was the first completed randomized clinical trial that showed the benefit of CAS using CPDs.[4] Moreover, this trial proved that the outcome of protected CAS was not inferior to that of CEA and in fact could be superior in selected high-risk patients (Table 21-1). In this trial, 307 patients were randomized to CEA or CAS with CPDs. The 30-day stroke and death rates were 7.3% for CEA and 4.4% for CAS (Table 21-2). The total major adverse event rate (any stroke, myocardial infarction, or death) was 12.6% for CEA and 5.8% for CAS. One-year results were similar, and major adverse event (death or ipsilateral stroke at 31 to 360 days) rates were 19.9% for CEA and 11.9% for CAS. At 1 year, there were thus no statistical differences in the rates of death or myocardial infarction, but there were significant reductions in major ipsilateral stroke or any myocardial infarction after CAS (Fig. 21-1). The 2-year results were recently reported, with the same trend shown in the 30-day and 1-year results. The major adverse event rate for CEA was 25.2%, whereas for CAS it was 18.4%. Of note, the outcomes of asymptomatic patients in this trial have been criticized because the stroke and death rates (6.1% for CEA and 5.8% for CAS) were significantly worse than those associated with medical therapy alone in the Asymptomatic Carotid Atherosclerosis Study (ACAS) and higher than those recommended by the American Heart Association guidelines.[20,21] These results should be interpreted with caution, however, because the SAPPHIRE trial had broader end points and included a different patient population from the major clinical trials assessing CEA for the treatment of carotid occlusive disease. Also, unlike the ACAS trial, which included asymptomatic stenosis greater than 60%, the SAPPHIRE trial included only those with greater than 80% stenosis.

Several "high-risk" registries further support the safety and efficacy of CAS in patients considered to be at high risk when undergoing CEA (Table 21-3). Although direct comparison between CAS and CEA is not performed, information relative to the feasibility of CAS in high-risk patients is provided by these registries, which generally use historical CEA outcomes in high-risk cohorts for comparisons. The AccuLink for Revascularization of Carotids in High-Risk Patients (ARCHeR) trial was a prospective, nonrandomized, multicenter, single-arm study that treated 513 patients at 41 sites in North and South America using the investigational AccuLink Carotid Stent System (Guidant, Menlo Park, Calif.).[22] ARCHeR results revealed that CAS is safe and effective in

TABLE 21–1	Definition of High-Risk Patients*

Congestive heart failure (CCS class III or IV) or known severe left ventricular dysfunction (ejection fraction < 30%)
Open heart surgery needed within 6 wk
Recent myocardial infarction (> 24 hr and < 4 wk)
Unstable angina (CCS class III or IV)
Severe pulmonary disease
Contralateral carotid occlusion
Contralateral laryngeal nerve palsy
Radiation therapy to neck
Previous CEA with recurrent stenosis
High cervical ICA lesions or CCA lesions below the clavicle
Severe tandem lesions
Age older than 80 yr

*Based on the SAPPHIRE trial. At least one factor is required.
CCA, common carotid artery; CCS, Canadian Cardiac Society; CEA, carotid endarterectomy; ICA, internal carotid artery.

TABLE 21–2	Cumulative Incidence of Adverse Events at 30 Days					
	Intention-to-Treat Analysis: No. of Patients (%)			Actual Treatment Analysis: No. of Patients (%)		
Event	*Stent* (n = 167)	*Endarterectomy* (n = 167)	*P Value*	*Stent* (n = 159)	*Endarterectomy* (n = 151)	*P Value*
Death	2 (1.2)	4 (2.5)	0.39	1 (0.6)	3 (2.0)	0.29
Stroke	6 (3.6)	5 (3.1)	0.77	5 (3.1)	5 (3.3)	0.94
Major ipsilateral	1 (0.6)	2 (1.2)	0.55	0	2 (1.3)	0.15
Major nonipsilateral	1 (0.6)	1 (0.6)	1.00	1 (0.6)	1 (0.7)	0.97
Minor ipsilateral	4 (2.4)	1 (0.6)	0.18	4 (2.5)	1 (0.7)	0.20
Minor nonipsilateral	1 (0.6)	1 (0.6)	1.00	1 (0.6)	1 (0.7)	0.97
Myocardial infarction	4 (2.4)	10 (6.1)	0.10	3 (1.9)	10 (6.6)	0.04
Q wave	0	2 (1.2)	0.15	0	2 (1.3)	0.15
Non-Q wave	4 (2.4)	8 (4.9)	0.23	3 (1.9)	8 (5.3)	0.11
Death, stroke, or myocardial infarction	8 (4.8)	16 (9.8)	0.09	7 (4.4)	15 (9.9)	0.06
Major vascular complications	2 (1.2)	1 (0.6)	0.57	2 (1.3)	1 (0.7)	0.60

From Yadav JS, Wholey MH, Kuntz RE, et al: Protected carotid-artery stenting versus endarterectomy in high-risk patients. N Engl J Med 351: 1493-1501, 2004.

high-risk patients. This trial was performed in stages as the CAS technique evolved and was refined. ARCHeR 1 used just the stent, ARCHeR 2 included the stent under embolic protection, and ARCHeR 3 used rapid-exchange systems for delivering the stent and the CPD. The major stroke or death rate in the first 30 days was low in all trials: 3.8%, 2.5%, and 2.8% for ARCHeR 1, 2, and 3, respectively (Fig. 21-2). At 1 year, the major adverse event rate was 8.3% and 10.2% for ARCHeR 1 and 2, respectively. Another high-risk registry, the Study to Evaluate the NeuroShield Bare Wire Cerebral Protection System and Xact Stent in Patients at High Risk for Carotid Endarterectomy (SECURITY), enrolled 305 patients and assessed the outcome of CAS with the MedNova NeuroShield bare wire filter and the Xact self-expanding carotid stent system (Abbott Laboratories, Abbott Park, Ill.).[23] The composite rate of death, any stroke, and myocardial infarction at 30 days was 7.2%, whereas the expected rate in these patients (based on historical controls of CEA) would be 11% to 15%. The Boston Scientific/EPI: A Carotid Stenting Trial for High Risk Surgical Patients (BEACH) is another single-arm, prospective, nonrandomized trial that completed the enrollment of 480 patients in the pivotal phase of the trial. Early results were presented but have not been published yet.[24] Figure 21-2 summarizes the reported outcomes of various trials.

Because the majority of patients with carotid stenosis are either asymptomatic or not considered high risk for CEA, efforts have focused on defining the role of CAS in "real-world" patients with carotid disease. The multicenter, prospective, nonrandomized Carotid Revascularization Using Endarterectomy or Stenting Systems (CARESS) clinical trial was designed as an equivalence cohort study to determine whether the stroke and death rates following CAS with CPD were comparable to those for CEA in treating all patients with symptomatic (≥50%) and asymptomatic (≥75%) carotid stenosis.[25] At 14 centers, 397 patients with carotid disease were treated—254 with CEA, and 143 with CAS. Both the 30-day and 1-year results of this phase I trial have been reported, with equivalent stroke and death rates following CAS with cerebral protection and CEA in a broad risk population of patients with carotid stenosis. The 30-day combined all-cause mortality and stroke rate for CEA and CAS was the same (2%), whereas the 30-day all-cause mortality, stroke, and myocardial infarction rates were 2% for CAS and 3% for CEA. The 1-year combined all-cause mortality and stroke rate was 13.6% for CEA and 10.0% for CAS, whereas the 1-year combined all-cause mortality, stroke, and acute myocardial infarction rate was 14.3% for CEA and 10.9% for CAS.

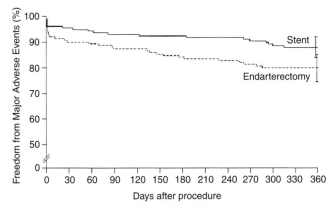

FIGURE 21–1 • Freedom from major adverse events at 1 year. The rate of event-free survival at 1 year was 88.0% among patients who received a stent, compared with 79.9% among those who underwent endarterectomy (*P* = 0.048). I-bars represent 1.5 times the standard error. (From Yadav JS, Wholey MH, Kuntz RE, et al: Protected carotid-artery stenting versus endarterectomy in high-risk patients. N Engl J Med 351: 1493-1501, 2004.).

TABLE 21–3	Carotid Stenting Trials				
Trial Name	**Type**	**Patient Population**	**Sponsor**	**Stent**	**CPD**
SAPPHIRE	Randomized and registry	High risk	Cordis, JNJ	Precise	AngioGuard
CREST	Randomized	Low risk	NINDS, Guidant	AccuLink	AccuNet
ARCHeR	Registry	High risk	Guidant	AccuLink	AccuNet
SECURITY	Registry	High risk	MedNova, Abbott	Xact	NeuroShield
MAVERIC	Registry	High risk	Medtronic	Exponent	GuardWire
BEACH	Registry	High risk	BSC	Wallstent	EPI FilterWire
CABERNET	Registry	High risk	BSC	Nexstent	EPI FilterWire
ArteriA	Registry	High and low risk	ArteriA	Wallstent	PAEC
CARESS	Registry	High and low risk	ISES	Wallstent	GuardWire

BSC, Boston Scientific Corporation; CPD, cerebral protection device; ISES, International Society for Endovascular Specialists; JNJ, Johnson and Johnson; NINDS, National Institute for Neurological Disorders; PAEC, Parodi Anti-Embolization Catheter.

The Carotid Revascularization Endarterectomy versus Stent Trial (CREST) is the first randomized, multicenter clinical trial funded by the National Institutes of Health to assess the safety and efficacy of CAS in symptomatic patients eligible for CEA (see Table 21-3). In fact, the inclusion and exclusion criteria of CREST are very similar to those of the North American Symptomatic Carotid Endarterectomy Trial (NASCET); therefore, CREST will enroll only patients with standard surgical risks for CEA. To compare CAS and CEA, approximately 2500 patients with symptomatic severe carotid stenosis (i.e., those with ≥70% stenosis by duplex criteria or ≥50% by NASCET angiographic criteria) will be enrolled. A preliminary result was recently presented, showing that CAS was associated with a 13% stroke and death rate in patients older than 80 years.[26] This was statistically higher than the rate in patients younger than 80 years. As a result, the trial has stopped enrolling octogenarians. Until the results of this clinical trial are available, CAS should be reserved for patients for whom CEA would be considered a high-risk procedure.

Patient Selection for Carotid Angioplasty and Stenting

As mentioned earlier, CEA remains the gold standard therapy for carotid stenosis. Although ongoing trials comparing the efficacy and safety of CEA and CAS may prove that CAS is also indicated for good-risk patients, CAS is currently indicated only in select high-risk cases.

Patients considered high-risk surgical candidates for CEA can be grouped into two main categories according to anatomic and physiologic conditions.[3,4] Anatomic characteristics associated with a high risk for CEA include (1) restenosis after previous CEA, particularly because of the risk of cranial nerve injury; (2) high or low lesions, defined as those above C-2 or below the clavicle, respectively; (3) "hostile" neck, related primarily to previous radical neck dissection, radiation therapy, presence of a permanent tracheostomy, or a frozen neck; or (4) other carotid lesions, including tandem lesions within the same carotid artery or contralateral ICA occlusion. Physiologic characteristics are associated with the presence of significant comorbid conditions, which include (1) class III or IV angina or congestive heart failure; (2) severe chronic obstructive pulmonary disease (forced expiratory volume ≤ 1 or the need for home oxygen); or (3) cardiac disease necessitating open heart surgery within 4 weeks. Although CAS has also been performed in patients not considered at high risk for CEA as part of several clinical trials, definite results and clinical evidence from these trials are not available; therefore, CAS should be reserved for high-risk surgical patients (see Table 21-1). In addition, because the Center for Medicare and Medicaid Services' national noncoverage

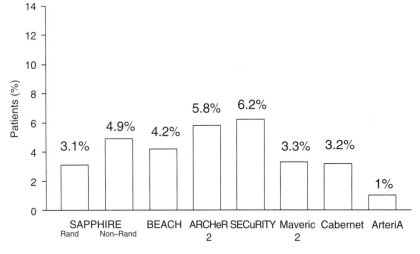

FIGURE 21–2 • Thirty-day risk of stroke in high-risk carotid stenting registries.

policy will still be in effect for good-risk patients after CAS is approved for high-risk patients, there will be no reimbursement if CAS is performed on the former.

Because the learning curve for CAS is prolonged, patient selection is critical when experience with the procedure is limited.[10,11] Medical and anatomic risk factors may affect the safety of both CEA and CAS, but anatomic factors may influence CAS to a greater extent.[5,27] Details of factors that make CAS difficult and dangerous are discussed in the angiography section.

Antiplatelet and Anticoagulant Therapy

Patients should receive aspirin 325 mg and clopidogrel 75 mg daily for at least 3 days before the procedure.[28] Patients not treated preoperatively with clopidogrel should be loaded with 300 mg at least 4 hours before the procedure; if this is not possible, the procedure should be rescheduled. The improved results of modern CAS series owe a lot to the use of dual antiplatelet treatment. For example, the Schneider Wallstent trial was terminated prematurely owing to a high complication rate following CAS, which is thought to be due in part to the fact that clopidogrel was not used.[16] Dual antiplatelet therapy should be continued for at least 30 days after the procedure. In certain situations, particularly if there is a need for major surgery, antiplatelet therapy can be stopped after 2 weeks, but it should be restarted immediately postoperatively. Heparin should be administered to maintain the activated clotting time (ACT) at longer than 250 seconds. If one is using a CPD, especially a filter type, it is advisable to maintain the ACT at longer than 275 seconds, because these devices carry the risk of thrombosis and thrombus formation if the patient is inadequately anticoagulated. Because there is significant patient variability in the response to heparin, it is important to monitor ACT intraprocedurally in all patients. Recently, direct thrombin inhibitors such as bivalirudin (Angiomax) have been shown to reduce complications associated with heparin, such as groin hematomas, but there is a lack of firm data relative to the use of these agents for CAS.

Some investigators have used glycoprotein (GP) IIb/IIIa inhibitors during CAS to reduce the microcirculatory impact of distal embolization.[29] However, because CPDs are now widely available and higher rates of major bleeding complications have been reported with these agents, the use of GP IIb/IIIa inhibitors has largely been abandoned during uncomplicated CAS. GP IIb/IIIa inhibitors may be beneficial for treating embolic complications.

As is the case with CEA, postprocedure blood pressure control is also important to avoid hyperperfusion syndrome and intracranial hemorrhage.

Diagnostic Aortic Arch, Cervical Carotid, and Cerebral Angiography

There are four purposes in obtaining a carotid and cerebral angiogram: stratifying risk, confirming the degree of stenosis, understanding the intracranial collateral circulation, and obtaining a baseline cerebral angiogram that can be compared with the postprocedure angiogram. Diagnostic angiography is usually performed at the time of CAS, but during the learning phase, it may be advisable to perform it beforehand so that one can carefully assess the difficulty of the case and select the appropriate techniques and tools. Either way, it is essential to have a good-quality, complete diagnostic cerebral angiogram before performing CAS. Digital subtraction capabilities are critical in performing intracranial angiography. Although it may be desirable to perform CAS in an angiography suite with a fixed C-arm, it can be done equally well with a high-quality portable C-arm with high resolution, such as the GE/OEC 9800 series (OEC, Salt Lake City, Utah). The recent development of a motorized, portable C-arm has narrowed the gap between fixed and portable even further.

It is also important to perform the procedure using only local anesthesia without sedation, so as not to impair the intraprocedural neurologic evaluation.

AORTIC ARCH ANGIOGRAPHY

The ability to safely deliver the stent to the lesion is probably the most difficult part of the procedure, and the level of difficulty can be assessed with the diagnostic aortic arch and carotid angiogram. The aortic arch angiogram is probably the most important diagnostic image because it helps determine the difficulty of CAS. It should be obtained in a 20- to 45-degree left anterior oblique orientation to open up the aortic arch adequately. A 5 French pigtail catheter with markers is inserted through a 5 French femoral sheath. Contrast material injected at a rate of 20 mL over 1.5 seconds is generally sufficient for good opacification, particularly when using digital subtraction techniques. A nonionic contrast medium is preferred. The field of view should be large enough to visualize the origin of the great vessels, as well as the carotid bifurcations. Arch anatomy has been categorized into three types, based on the relationship between the origins of the great vessels and a transverse line drawn at the level of the apex of the aortic arch (Fig. 21-3).[30] In type I aortic arches, all the great vessels originate at the same level, and carotid cannulation is easy. If the origins of the innominate or the left common carotid artery (CCA) are progressively lower than this line, the arch is classified as type II (two fingerbreadths) or type III (more than three fingerbreadths). Aortic arch angiograms are also helpful in demonstrating any anatomic anomalies such as the bovine origin of the left CCA.

Delivering a stent to the target site is difficult and challenging in patients with type III arches and in those with anomalies such as a bovine takeoff of the left CCA. With type II or III arches, catheters advanced from the descending aorta tend to prolapse into the ascending aorta when cannulation of the inferiorly located great vessels is attempted. Although experience and advanced technical skills can overcome these difficult situations, one should reassess the risks and benefits of CAS, CEA, and medical treatment before proceeding. When faced with difficult anatomy, it is perfectly reasonable to abort CAS and perform CEA later or treat the patient with medical therapy. Patient selection and sound judgment are the keys in achieving a good outcome.

SELECTIVE CATHETERIZATION AND CERVICAL CAROTID ANGIOGRAPHY

The type of aortic arch helps determine which diagnostic catheter is preferable. Although a variety of diagnostic catheters

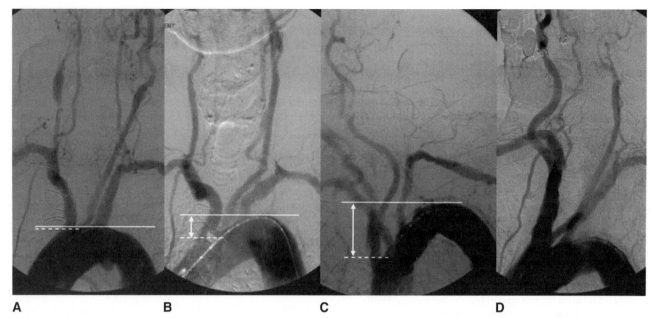

FIGURE 21–3 • Classification of aortic arch. *A,* Type I aortic arch. All the great vessels originate at the same level as the apex of the aortic arch. *B,* Type II aortic arch. The innominate artery orifice is one fingerbreadth below the apex of the arch. *C,* Type III aortic arch. *D,* Bovine origin of the left common carotid artery.

are available for cerebral angiography, one does not need to be familiar with every type. For example, we perform 95% of our angiograms with a Vitek catheter, a Headhunter, or an angled vertebral catheter (Cook, Inc., Indianapolis, Ind.) (Fig. 21-4). In types I and II arches, the Headhunter or the vertebral catheter can be used to rapidly access all the great vessels. For a type III arch or a bovine takeoff of the left CCA, a Vitek or Simmons catheter is more appropriate (see Figs. 21-3 and 21-4). The Simmons 1.5 catheter is usually reserved for type III arches because it requires a certain amount of manipulation within the arch to re-form its shape and is thus associated with an increased risk of embolization. One should choose three or four catheters and become familiar with their use, indications, strengths, and weaknesses (Table 21-4; Figs. 21-5 and 21-6).

With the exception of the left CCA angiogram, which can be obtained as soon as the catheter engages the vessel, a guidewire must be used to advance the catheter selectively into the right CCA or the vertebral artery. For the right common carotid angiogram, the catheter first must be placed in the innominate artery. Then an angiogram can be obtained to visualize the takeoff of the right CCA and the carotid bifurcation. Alternatively, the initial aortic arch angiogram may suffice for this purpose. Using these images as a road map, a 0.038- or 0.035-inch stiff Glidewire (Terumo Inc., Somerset, N.J.) is advanced into the right CCA. Care is taken not to advance the Glidewire into the lesion, because this can cause embolization. Because the guidewire purchase is limited, use of a stiff Glidewire is critical; it enables passage of the catheter with less purchase compared with a standard Glidewire (Fig. 21-7). It is especially important to choose stiff Glidewires when using a reversed curve catheter such as the Vitek or Simmons catheter. The same principle applies when one is obtaining a selective vertebral angiogram.

After selective catheterization, anteroposterior and lateral angiograms are taken. In addition, a magnified "worst-view" angiogram of the lesion is taken; this view varies from patient to patient and may not be either the anteroposterior or the lateral. Angiographic assessment of the degree of stenosis is done using the NASCET criterion of comparing the smallest diameter at the lesion with a reference diameter of the distal ICA in a segment with parallel walls.[1] Care is taken to avoid air embolization by confirming return of blood into the syringe before injecting contrast material.

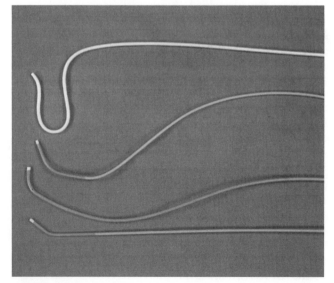

FIGURE 21–4 • Commonly used selective catheters for carotid angioplasty and stenting. From top: vertebral, AL 4, Headhunter, Vitek.

The target carotid artery angiogram should be obtained after obtaining the contralateral carotid and vertebral angiograms. By doing so, one can proceed directly to CAS

TABLE 21–4   Characteristics of Various Selective Catheters

	JR, Vertebral	Headhunter	Vitek	Simmons
Indication	Type I arch	Type I, II arch	Type I, II, III arch	Type III arch
Use in anomalous left CCA	No	No	Yes	Yes
Ease of use	Easy	Easy	Moderate	Difficult
Ease of advancement	Easy	Easy	Moderate	Difficult
Risk of emboli	Minimal	Minimal	Minimal	Moderate

CCA, common carotid artery.

after obtaining the angiogram and minimize the number of selective catheterizations.

Lesions that may make CAS difficult include very tight stenoses with the string sign, acute occlusions, lesions with intraluminal thrombus, those with dense calcification, tandem lesions, and severe stenosis or tortuosity within the CCA (Table 21-5; Fig. 21-8). Tight stenosis makes passage of the CPD difficult and may require predilatation. Intraluminal thrombus increases the chance of embolization during passage of the CPD, balloon, and stent (see Fig. 21-8). Dense calcification may result in acute recoil refractory to repeat balloon dilatation, and it may cause difficulty in passing the stent. In addition, although the likelihood is very remote, the risk of vessel rupture is increased with dense calcification. Tortuous

vessels make passage of the CPD and stent challenging. The tortuosity is exaggerated distal to the stent after stent implantation because current stents tend to straighten out the vessel, extending the tortuosity distally. Tandem lesions in the CCA in addition to the ICA pose a challenge. An occluded external carotid artery (ECA) makes safe cannulation of the CCA difficult. As discussed earlier in the aortic arch section, these lesions should be avoided if alternative treatment options are feasible. Although simultaneous treatment of bilateral carotid artery stenosis is possible, it should generally be staged at least 30 days apart, as it is with CEA. The major risks of a simultaneous bilateral approach are severe bradycardia and hypotension due to overstimulation of both carotid sinuses, as well as cerebral hyperperfusion syndrome.

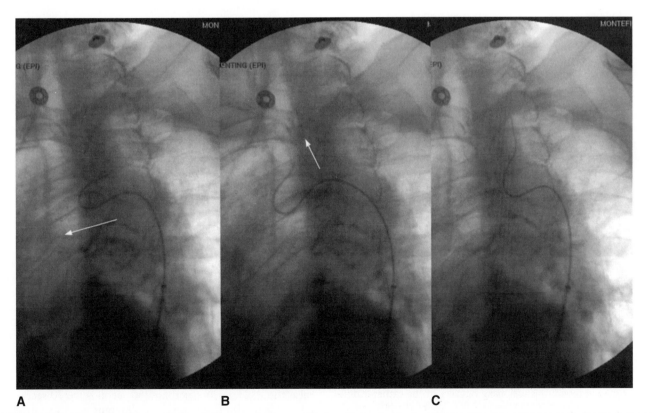

A   **B**   **C**

FIGURE 21–5 • Use of the Vitek catheter. *A,* The reversed curve Vitek catheter is a push catheter. After the catheter re-forms its shape in the descending thoracic aorta, it is slowly pushed proximally *(arrow). B,* Once it engages the great vessel, the tip of the Vitek catheter flips cranially *(arrow). C,* Then the catheter should be pulled back. This maneuver puts the catheter farther into the target vessel. A Glidewire is used to selectively cannulate the right common carotid or the vertebral artery.

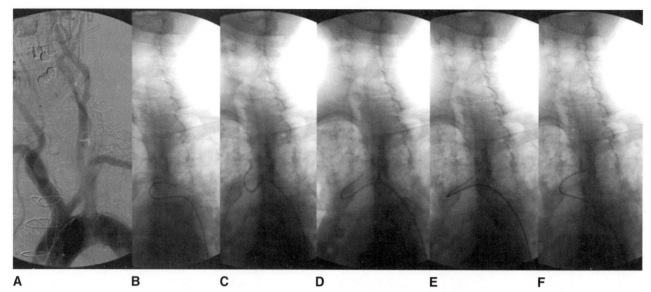

A   B   C   D   E   F

FIGURE 21–6 • Technique to cannulate a bovine left common carotid artery (CCA). *A,* Arch angiogram shows bovine origin of the left CCA. *B,* The Vitek catheter is re-formed in the distal arch and then slowly pushed forward. *C,* As it engages the innominate artery, the tip of the catheter "flicks" cranially. *D,* The catheter is pushed farther proximally. Counterclockwise rotation of the catheter may be helpful. *E,* A Glidewire is used to probe the left CCA. *F,* Once the left CCA is cannulated with the Glidewire, the Glidewire and the catheter should be pulled back as a unit to enter the CCA. If counterclockwise rotation were applied earlier, clockwise rotation should be applied as one pulls the catheter-Glidewire complex back.

CEREBRAL ANGIOGRAPHY

A complete cerebral angiogram requires defining the intracranial anatomy of both carotid arteries as well as one vertebral artery, preferably the dominant one. Anteroposterior and lateral views are obtained for each injection of 7 to 10 mL of

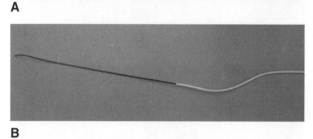

A

B

FIGURE 21–7 • The difference between 0.035- and 0.038-inch Glidewire. *A,* A 0.035-inch regular-stiffness Glidewire is placed inside the Vitek catheter. Note that the catheter has not completely straightened; this will make delivery of the catheter difficult because it will prolapse in the arch. *B,* A 0.038-inch Glidewire has been placed inside the Vitek catheter. Note that with the same amount of purchase as in *A,* the catheter has straightened significantly, allowing the catheter to be introduced into the target vessel.

contrast agent over 1 second. Digital subtraction angiography is very useful. A parenchyma-gram, which can be obtained by increasing the gain of the late-phase image, is useful in understanding the perfusion of the brain parenchyma (Fig. 21-9). This baseline image can be compared with the postprocedure image to quickly identify the presence or absence of emboli. In the presence of cerebral emboli, there would be an area that does not stain in either the anteroposterior or the lateral projection.

It is crucial to define the collateral circulation to the brain hemisphere of interest. These collaterals include the anterior and posterior communicating arteries. The use of CPDs of the balloon occlusion type mandates a good understanding of the collateral circulation to the hemisphere to be treated. In the absence of good collateral circulation, the patient may not tolerate the procedure with the use of occlusive CPDs, which could necessitate a rapid or even aborted procedure.

Introducing the Sheath into the Common Carotid Artery

Although direct cervical carotid percutaneous and open approaches, as well as a brachial approach, have been used for CAS, the transfemoral route is preferred. After the diagnostic angiogram has been obtained and the decision to proceed with CAS has been made, a sheath or a guiding catheter must be placed into the CCA so that one can safely introduce the stent and perform angiography during percutaneous transluminal angioplasty and stent deployment. Before introducing the sheath, 70 to 100 IU/kg of heparin is administered to raise the ACT to longer than 250 seconds (>270 seconds if a CPD is used). There are three different ways to introduce the sheath or guiding catheter: the sequential over-the-wire technique, the telescoping technique, and the direct coronary technique. Each has advantages and disadvantages that

TABLE 21–5	Causes of Difficult Access		
Iliac Artery	**Aortic Arch**	**Great Vessels**	**Carotid Artery**
Tortuosity	Type III arch	Ostial stenotic lesion	Occluded ECA
Stenosis or occlusion	Bovine arch	Anomalous origin	Tortuous ICA at and distal to lesion
	Diseased arch	Tortuous CCA	Heavy calcification

CCA, common carotid artery; ECA, external carotid artery; ICA, internal carotid artery.

are discussed in the following sections. The operator needs to be familiar with each technique, because the approach used is generally related to the nature of the aortic arch.

In addition to choosing the access technique, one needs to decide whether to use a sheath or a guiding catheter. The pros and cons of each are described in Table 21-6. Because the current stent delivery systems are mostly 6 French and smaller, a long 6 French sheath or an 8 French guiding catheter is sufficient in most cases. We prefer to use a 90-cm 6 French Shuttle sheath (Cook, Inc., Indianapolis, Ind.) in the majority of the cases; it has a smooth transition and a flexible tip, allowing safe introduction. Guiding catheters may be helpful in placing both CPDs and the capturing sheaths needed to retrieve CPDs. In addition, guiding catheters may be repositioned when they slide out of the CCA, which is generally not possible when a sheath prolapses out of the CCA during CPD or stent delivery (Fig. 21-10). Another advantage of guiding catheters in cases of severe tortuosity and elongation of the left CCA is the possibility of using an angulated stiff

guidewire to cannulate the CCA; this allows CAS to be performed without having to advance the sheath into the carotid artery itself, thereby avoiding exaggerated kinking of the vessel.

SEQUENTIAL OVER-THE-WIRE TECHNIQUE

This approach is probably the safest and is definitely most useful when there is severe arch tortuosity (types II, III; see Fig. 21-3). It is, however, the most time-consuming approach, requiring more steps than the others. This approach is most appropriate if one has not decided to perform CAS at the time of the diagnostic angiogram (Table 21-7). The selective catheter that was used to engage the CCA is used to obtain an angiogram that adequately separates the ECA and ICA. The image intensifier should be positioned such that one can view the ECA-ICA bifurcation as well as the aortic arch (Fig. 21-11). By doing so, one can keep an eye on the tip of the guidewire as well as monitor the behavior of the sheath

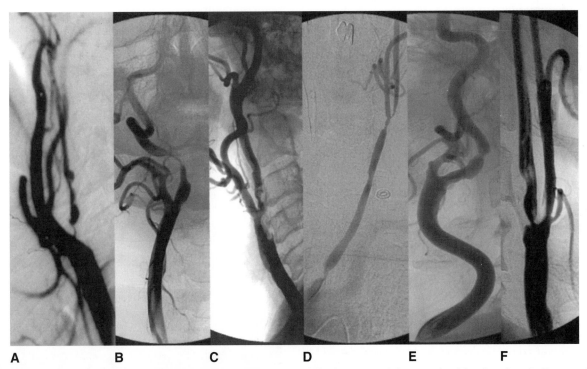

FIGURE 21–8 • Anatomies that make carotid angioplasty and stenting difficult. *A,* Very tight stenosis with string sign. *B,* Tortuous internal carotid artery (ICA). *C,* Dense calcification. *D,* Tandem lesion in the common carotid artery (CCA) orifice and ICA. *E,* Tortuosity within the CCA. *F,* Lesion with mural thrombus.

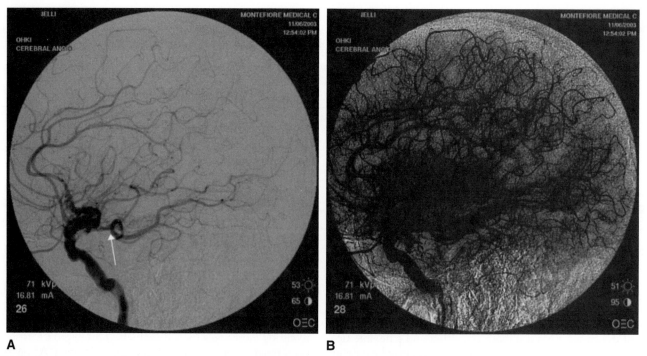

A　　　　　　　　　　　　　　　　　**B**

FIGURE 21–9 • Intracranial angiogram. *A,* Lateral view shows normal anterior and middle cerebral arteries. Note the presence of a fetal posterior communicating artery *(arrow). B,* Parenchyma-gram of the angiogram shown in *A.*

within the aortic arch as it is introduced. Posteroanterior or left anterior oblique views are usually adequate for this purpose. Use of road-mapping may be helpful in selectively cannulating the ECA. Right anterior oblique views are often better for opening up the right carotid bifurcation, but visualization of the aortic arch may be suboptimal. A stiff or a 0.038-inch angled Glidewire is advanced deep into the ECA, and the diagnostic catheter is advanced over the wire into the ECA. The Glidewire is then exchanged for a Meier (Meditech) or Amplatz superstiff guidewire (Meditech), and the diagnostic catheter is removed, along with the 5 French sheath that was initially placed in the femoral artery (Fig. 21-12). It is important to use a 260-cm-long guidewire so that one can maintain guidewire position during catheter removal. Manual pressure is applied to the femoral artery as the 5 French sheath is removed to prevent groin hematoma. The 6 or 7 French Shuttle sheath is then advanced over the stiff wire. With a type II or III aortic arch, the sheath may not track the guidewire and may prolapse into the ascending aorta. This is one of the critical steps in CAS. A useful maneuver is to perform the "push-and-pull" technique, whereby the guidewire is gently

TABLE 21–6	Sheath versus Guiding Catheter
Sheath	**Guiding Catheter**
Smaller hole in femoral artery (6-7 French)	Less likely to kink
Tracks better in difficult arch (type II, III)	Better torque control (beneficial in guiding CPD, retrieval catheters in tortuous anatomy)
Smooth dilator permits atraumatic insertion into CCA	Allows direct access to CCA without cannulating ECA

CCA, common carotid artery; CPD, cerebral protection device; ECA, external carotid artery.

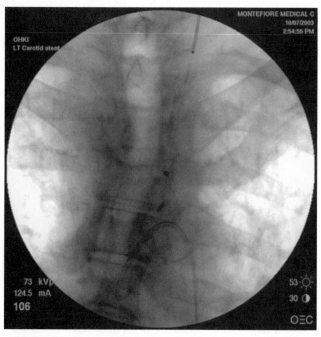

FIGURE 21–10 • Prolapse of the sheath during stent delivery.

TABLE 21–7	Sequential Over-the-Wire Technique

Introduce 5 French groin sheath

Perform arch angiography and other diagnostic studies

Make the decision whether to stent

Engage target CCA with diagnostic catheter

Road-map in low-magnification anteroposterior or left anterior oblique projection; visualize arch and ECA-ICA

Advance 0.038-inch Glidewire into ECA

Advance catheter into ECA; exchange for superstiff wire, Meier or Amplatz

Remove selective catheter and 5 French sheath while maintaining superstiff wire access

Insert 6 French shuttle sheath over superstiff wire

Advance sheath into mid-CCA over stiff wire into ECA

CCA, common carotid artery; ECA, external carotid artery; ICA, internal carotid artery.

retracted as the sheath is introduced around the aortic arch (see Fig. 21-12). Because there is little guidewire purchase, the tip of the guidewire must be monitored to avoid pulling it out of the ECA. The radiopaque tip of the Meier wire, as well as its stiffness, ensures the safety of this step, making it the preferred wire. Also, it is important to advance the sheath very slowly during this step. Deep inspiration or exhalation may change the angle of the CCA and the aortic arch and may assist in the delivery of the sheath. The sheath should be introduced deep enough into the CCA so that it will not prolapse during the CPD or stent delivery phase.

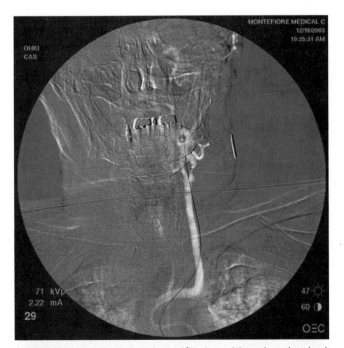

FIGURE 21–11 • The image intensifier is positioned so that both the arch and the carotid bifurcation can be visualized. Using the road-mapping function, one can selectively cannulate the external carotid artery with a Glidewire.

Conversely, the sheath should not be introduced too deep into the CCA, because this can exaggerate the preexisting tortuosity of the vessel (Fig. 21-13). Also, a deeply placed sheath can interfere with stent deployment. It is important to position the sheath appropriately at this time and avoid moving it later during the procedure.

This technique may not be possible if the target lesion is located in the CCA or if the ECA is occluded. In these cases, a loop can be created in the stiff wire that generally prevents the wire from advancing through the lesion (Fig. 21-14). Alternatively, the coronary technique (described later) for vascular access should be used.

TELESCOPING TECHNIQUE

A 6 or 7 French Shuttle sheath or a guiding catheter is introduced into the descending thoracic aorta. A 125-cm Vitek, JR4, or Multi-purpose catheter (Cordis, Johnson and Johnson, Warren, N.J.) is inserted through the Shuttle sheath or the 8 French H1 guiding catheter (Cordis). Guidewires, diagnostic catheters, CPDs, and stents are passed through a Tuohy-Borst valve. With the telescoping technique, it is important to use a 120- to 125-cm catheter because the long sheath or guiding catheter is at least 90 cm long. Selective cannulation of the CCA is performed with the angiographic catheter. As described in the section on the sequential technique, an angiogram is obtained that distinguishes the ECA and ICA. The image intensifier should be positioned so that one can view the ECA as well as the aortic arch. Then, a stiff or 0.038-inch angled Glidewire is passed through the diagnostic catheter and into the ECA; the diagnostic catheter is advanced into the mid-CCA over the Glidewire. The Glidewire and the diagnostic catheter are then used as a rail to advance the sheath or guiding catheter into the mid-CCA. Small rotational movements of the sheath may be necessary to advance it into position. Again, the "push-and-pull" technique may be useful. The diagnostic catheter and Glidewire are now ready to be withdrawn; this requires the application of some countertraction to the guiding catheter or sheath, which tends to jump forward as the diagnostic catheter and Glidewire are removed. Back-bleeding from the guiding catheter or sheath must be allowed to wash out any debris that may have accumulated during positioning of the catheter or sheath.

The telescoping approach is contraindicated when the CCA ostium is diseased. Sliding the sheath over the diagnostic catheter may cause plaque disruption and embolization because there is a gap between the diagnostic catheter and the larger sheath. In these cases, the sequential over-the-wire technique should be used to minimize trauma and embolization.

CORONARY TECHNIQUE

The CCA can also be cannulated directly with an H1 guiding catheter using an approach similar to that used with the coronary arteries. This coronary approach may be safe and fast, but it requires greater experience and a favorable arch configuration (i.e., type I or II). In the presence of a bovine arch, where the left CCA originates from the innominate artery, it is more convenient to use an AL 1 guide to cannulate the ostium and proximal left CCA. When a bovine takeoff is combined with severe CCA disease or occlusion of the ECA, which makes it almost impossible to advance a 0.038-inch

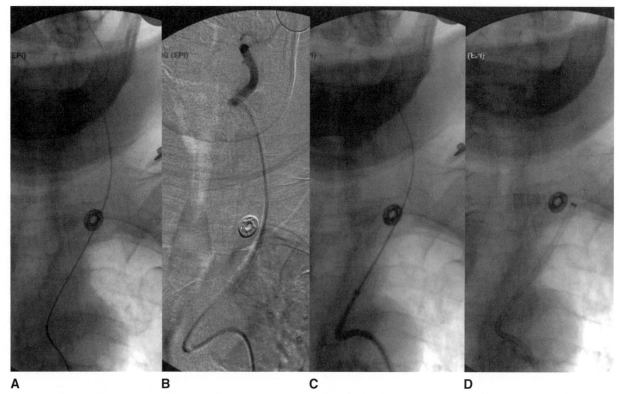

A   **B**   **C**   **D**

FIGURE 21–12 • Use of the external carotid artery (ECA) as the anchoring vessel for sheath insertion. *A,* The Glidewire is introduced into the ECA. *B,* The Vitek catheter is introduced into the ECA over the Glidewire. The angiogram confirms correct positioning of the catheter. A superstiff wire is then introduced deep into the ECA, and the catheter and the 5 French sheath in the groin are removed. *C,* As the Shuttle sheath is introduced into the common carotid artery (CCA), a gentle "push-pull" technique may be useful. It is important to position the image intensifier so that both the tip of the guidewire and the aortic arch can be visualized. *D,* Once the sheath is in a good position, the dilator and the superstiff wire are removed in preparation for carotid angioplasty and stenting.

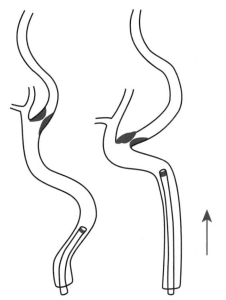

FIGURE 21–13 • Exaggeration of the tortuosity of the common carotid artery caused by introduction of the sheath.

wire into the left CCA, the use of an AL 1 guide may be particularly helpful. In this situation, in addition to the stent delivery wire (CPD wire), a stiff 0.018-inch wire may need to be placed in the CCA or ECA to maintain guide stability because, unlike with a sheath, sufficient purchase of the CCA is lacking.

OTHER APPROACHES

A brachial approach may be necessary in rare cases.[31] The right CCA should be accessed via the left brachial artery and the left CCA via the right brachial artery (Fig. 21-15). A helpful approach in these situations involves the use of a 6 French Ansel sheath (Cordis, Warren, N.J.) and a Simmons 1, 1.5, or 2 catheter placed into the ipsilateral CCA. A stiff wire is then advanced into the ECA. At this point, the Simmons catheter can be replaced by the introducer of the Ansel sheath, which allows the sheath to be advanced into the CCA.

Percutaneous or open carotid access through a cervical approach has been described, but because of the lower profile and increased trackability of current stents, this approach is seldom necessary. Complications related to a cervical carotid puncture include carotid dissection, carotid thrombosis while achieving hemostasis after sheath removal, and airway compromise from hematomas. The cervical approach may, however, be the last resort in patients with severe tortuosity of the CCA and an unfavorable arch anatomy (Fig. 21-16).

If there is severe occlusive disease at the ostium of the innominate or left CCA, this lesion needs to be treated before introducing the sheath, because the sheath may cause complete cessation of blood flow. Percutaneous transluminal angioplasty of the ostial lesion is performed to achieve an adequate lumen so that flow will be maintained after sheath insertion. The sheath can then be introduced into the CCA, CAS is performed, and a stent is placed in the ostial lesion (Fig. 21-17). Stenting of the ostial lesion before CAS should be avoided because the stent may be dislodged as the sheath is advanced into the CCA; also, the stent may damage the sheath. These cases are technically demanding and should be avoided during the leaning phase.

Cerebral Protection during Carotid Angioplasty and Stenting

There is considerable evidence that embolization takes place during all carotid stenting procedures, with most emboli being released at the time of balloon deflation, as detected by transcranial Doppler monitoring and confirmed in ex vivo experiments (Fig. 21-18).[17,32] Moreover, with the development and availability of lower profile and more sophisticated CPDs, the concept of cerebral protection has become widely accepted, and there is a consensus among specialists that protection devices should be used routinely (Table 21-8; Fig. 21-19).[3] The results of the SAPPHIRE trial and others have furnished the evidence for routine use of protection devices (see Fig. 21-2).[4]

The use of CPDs, however, is not without complications and may in fact add risks to the procedure. Intrinsic problems associated with the use of protection devices relate to the difficulty

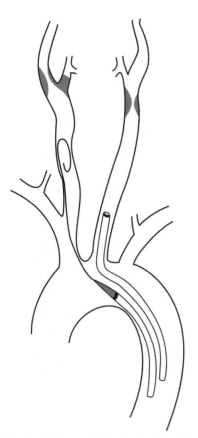

FIGURE 21–14 • Technique of introducing the sheath into the common carotid artery (CCA) when the external carotid artery (ECA) is occluded or when there is a lesion in the CCA. A pigtail shape is created at the tip of the stiff wire, providing sufficient support without excessive purchase. A direct introduction can be performed using an appropriately shaped guiding catheter (coronary technique).

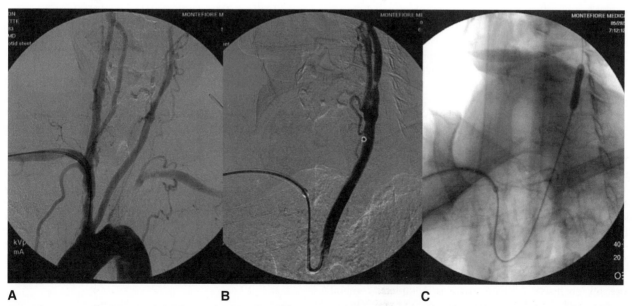

A   B   C

FIGURE 21–15 • Brachial access in a patient with aortoiliac occlusion. This patient had aortic occlusion, precluding femoral access. *A,* Arch angiogram shows bovine origin of the left common carotid artery (CCA) and occlusion of the left subclavian artery. *B,* Selective catheterization of the left CCA is performed with a Sos-Omni catheter. The angiogram shows severe recurrent stenosis in the left internal carotid artery (ICA). *C,* Carotid angioplasty and stenting are performed.

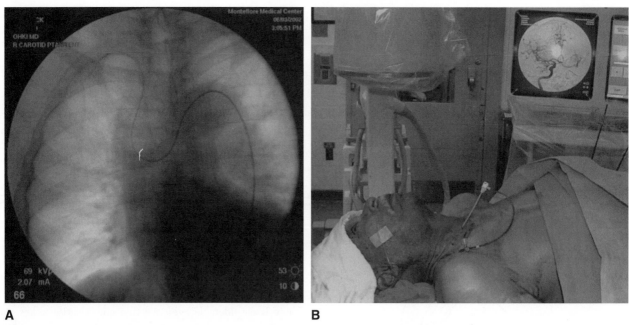

A

B

FIGURE 21–16 • Direct common carotid artery (CCA) access in a patient with a type III arch. *A,* This patient's type III arch made introduction of the sheath difficult and risky. *B,* The patient was not a surgical candidate owing to a hostile neck and severe congestive heart failure. Therefore, a direct CCA puncture was performed to gain access.

of introducing and deploying the device, the effectiveness of emboli capture, CPD-induced vessel injury, and the difficulty in recapturing and withdrawing the device.[33] A number of papers have been published demonstrating the safety and efficacy of cerebral protection during CAS, however.[34-40]

CPDs are basically of two types: occlusive and nonocclusive. Occlusive devices work through proximal or distal occlusion relative to the carotid lesion. Nonocclusive devices are either filters with supportive nitinol endoskeletons or unsupported devices that resemble a windsock. These devices have intrinsic advantages and disadvantages and specific technical features. Familiarity with several devices is helpful, allowing the most appropriate device to be selected for a particular lesion and anatomy.

Once the sheath is in place, an appropriate working view must be selected. This view should allow clear visualization of the carotid lesion with maximum separation of the external and internal carotid arteries. Before we used CPDs, the lateral view was used most frequently; however, in this view, the guiding catheter or sheath in the CCA is generally not visible. When CPDs are used, visualization of the sheath should be maintained at all times, because prolapse of the sheath into the aortic arch could result in withdrawal of the deployed CPD through the lesion. An anteroposterior or ipsilateral oblique view is preferred now that CPDs are used routinely (Fig. 21-20). This view allows visualization of the entire field, including the CPD and the distal portion of the sheath.[41]

GUARDWIRE

Before an occlusive CPD is used, a complete cerebral angiogram, including the collateral circulation to both hemispheres, must be obtained because incomplete collateral circulation to the affected hemisphere may contraindicate the use of this device. The GuardWire (PercuSurge, Medtronic,

Sunnyvale, Calif.) consists of a 0.014-inch guidewire with a central lumen connected to a compliant distal occlusion balloon (Table 21-9). Nominal balloon diameters are 5 to 6 mm. After testing for integrity, the balloon is fully deflated and introduced into the Shuttle sheath. To minimize occlusion time, it is best to have the predilatation balloon loaded on the GuardWire before occluding the ICA. The predilatation angioplasty balloon (4-mm by 4-cm Aviator, Cordis, Warren, N.J.; or Soft SV, Boston Scientific Corp., Natick, Mass.) is loaded onto the GuardWire and kept just below the lesion. Then the GuardWire is advanced across the lesion, and the GuardWire balloon is inflated until vessel size is reached (Fig. 21-21). If there is severe tortuosity in the lesion or within the distal ICA that precludes insertion of the GuardWire, a separate "buddy wire" (0.014-inch Reflex or Stabilizer, Cordis) may be placed across the lesion to straighten the vessel and facilitate insertion of the GuardWire. This technique is seldom needed because the second-generation GuardWire Plus is very flexible. An angiogram is obtained to verify complete occlusion of the ICA. The predilatation balloon within the Shuttle sheath is then advanced across the lesion, and angioplasty is performed. Following stent deployment and dilatation, the PercuSurge export aspiration catheter is introduced to aspirate the blood column as well as the embolic particles. Finally, the GuardWire occlusion balloon is deflated and removed. Once the GuardWire balloon is inflated, it is not possible to obtain an angiogram in the ICA; therefore, it is important to obtain a good angiogram beforehand, with bony landmarks that can be used as a reference during predilatation and stent deployment.

DISTAL FILTER PROTECTION DEVICE

A filter with a diameter matching the distal cervical ICA is advanced through the lesion (Table 21-10). It is advisable to

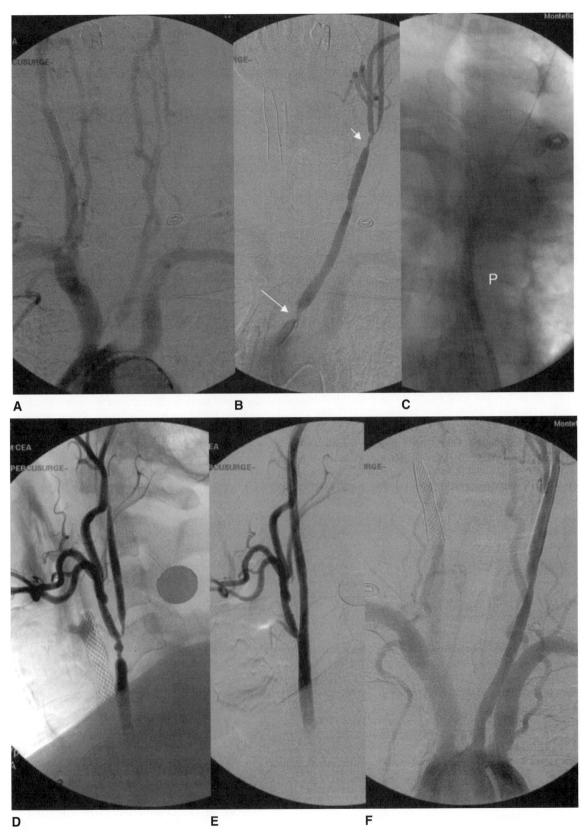

FIGURE 21–17 • Management of tandem lesions. *A* and *B,* Arch angiograms show severe stenosis at the takeoff of the left common carotid artery (CCA) *(long arrow),* distal CCA, and internal carotid artery (ICA) *(short arrow). C,* Percutaneous transluminal angioplasty (P) is performed at the orificial lesion to maintain flow after insertion of the sheath. *D,* Flow is maintained with the sheath inserted into the CCA. *E,* Carotid angioplasty and stenting are performed in the standard manner. *F,* A stent is placed at the orifice of the previously angio-plastied site. Stenting is not performed until the end, because introduction of the sheath may dislodge the stent.

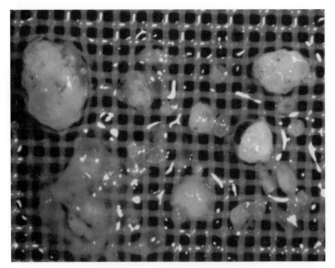

FIGURE 21–18 • Embolic particles released during percutaneous transluminal angioplasty and stenting. (From Ohki T, Marin ML, Lyon RT, et al: Ex vivo human carotid artery bifurcation stenting: Correlation of lesion characteristics with embolic potential. J Vasc Surg 27:463-471, 1998.)

place the filter device at the level of the distal ICA immediately before the petrous portion unless prohibitive tortuosity is present. The floppy distal tip of the wire should be kept in the petrous portion (Figs. 21-22 and 21-23). The CPD can then be stabilized in this position, decreasing forward displacement. Then the outer sheath of the filter is retrieved, and the filter deployed. It is important to obtain an angiogram to confirm good flow and circumferential opposition of the filter to the vessel wall, preferably using at least two perpendicular views (Fig. 21-24). In cases in which the stenosis is extremely tight, a 2-mm coronary balloon may be used to dilate the lesion before filter insertion. In tortuous lesions, a buddy wire is often needed to straighten the vessel; filter devices are generally stiffer than the GuardWire and may not be able to negotiate tortuous vessels. An angiogram is obtained to confirm correct positioning of the filter, as well as preservation of prograde ICA flow.

TABLE 21–8	Cerebral Protection Devices	
Type	**Product**	**Manufacturer**
Distal occlusion	GuardWire	PercuSurge, Medtronic
	Kensy Nash	Tri-Activ
Distal filter	AccuNet	Guidant
	AngioGuard	Cordis
	FilterWire	EPI/Boston Scientific Corp.
	Interceptor	Medtronic
	NeuroShield	MedNova/Abbott
	Spider	EV3
	Rubicon filter	Rubicon
Proximal occlusion	PAES	ArteriA
	MOMA	InvaTec

An angiogram must always be obtained to assess flow before collapse and removal of the filter. Large amounts of emboli may have been released, and the filter surface may be saturated; this would be suggested angiographically by reduced or absent flow through the ICA. Because of the large amount of embolic debris captured by the filter, there is a stagnant column of blood in the ICA with suspended particles, which could be carried distally into the brain once the filter is collapsed. Filters full of emboli may be difficult to withdraw because of the resistance to full capture of the device. In these instances, the filter should be only partially captured, because forcefully pulling the filter completely into the capture sheath may squeeze and release emboli. Generally, the filter can be removed safely after only the proximal part has been captured. This phenomenon may occur in approximately 5% of cases when filter devices are used. Therefore, it is essential to aspirate the proximal ICA before collapsing the filter. The PercuSurge export catheter or a 125-cm-long, 5 French multipurpose catheter can be used for this purpose. Occasionally, it may be difficult to remove a CPD because the capture sheath hits the edge of the stent, hindering its advancement. Further dilatation of the proximal end of the stent or angling the guiding catheter to change the orientation of the capture sheath may be necessary. Alternatively, placing a small balloon on a buddy wire next to the catheter sheath may displace the CPD wire, allowing the capture sheath to enter the stent. When the CPD is withdrawn from the sheath or guiding catheter, the Tuohy-Borst valve should be completely opened, and some back-bleeding should be allowed in case particles have been released into the sheath or guiding catheter during CPD withdrawal.

ARTERIA PARODI ANTI-EMBOLIZATION SYSTEM

When using the ArteriA device (ArteriA, San Francisco) instead of the Shuttle sheath, the Parodi Anti-Embolization Catheter (PAEC) is introduced into the CCA over a super-stiff wire placed into the ECA (Table 21-11; see Fig. 21-19). The Parodi External Carotid Balloon (PEB) is introduced through the main lumen of the PAEC into the ECA (Fig. 21-25). Finally, a 5 French sheath is inserted percutaneously into the contralateral femoral vein and connected to the Parodi Blood Recovery System (PBRS), which has a filter to capture the emboli. After completing these steps, a 0.014-inch standard guidewire and a predilatation balloon are inserted through the PAEC and kept just below the lesion. Both the occlusion balloon attached at the distal end of the PAEC and the PEB are inflated to occlude prograde flow of the CCA and retrograde flow from the ECA. Finally, the proximal end of the PAEC is connected to the femoral vein through the PBRS. Contrast material is injected into the ICA to confirm reversal of flow. The guidewire positioned inside the PAEC is then used to traverse the lesion, and angioplasty and stenting are performed. Both the PEB and the PAEC balloon are deflated at the completion of the stenting procedure. Proximal occlusive CPDs are particularly helpful in lesions associated with mural thrombus, which may result in distal embolization during wire passage. Also, lesions with severe stenosis or severe tortuosity, both of which make the use of distal CPDs difficult, are ideally treated with the ArteriA device because it allows the use of any guidewire (see Fig. 21-25). Moreover, this approach probably has the highest efficiency

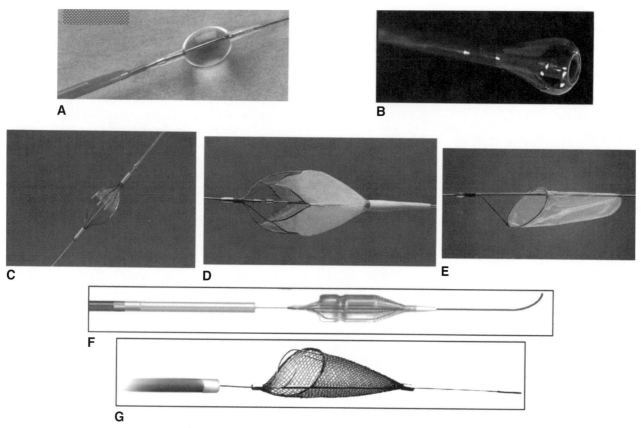

FIGURE 21–19 • Cerebral protection devices. *A,* Medtronic/PercuSurge GuardWire Plus; *B,* ArteriA Parodi Anti-Embolization Catheter; *C,* Cordis AngioGuard; *D,* Guidant AccuLink; *E,* Boston Scientific FilterWire EZ; *F,* Abbott/MedNova NeuroShield; *G,* EV3 Spider.

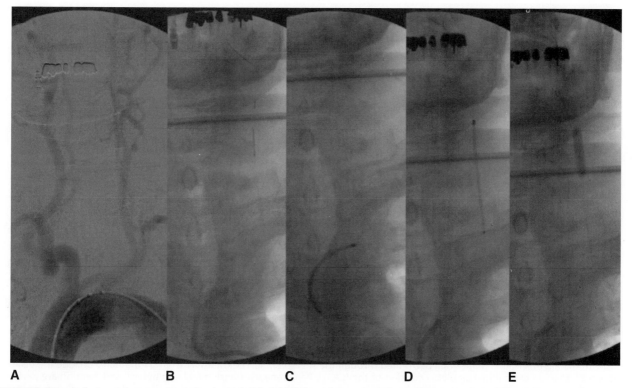

FIGURE 21–20 • *A,* Arch angiogram shows bovine origin of the left common carotid artery (CCA) and a severe stenosis in the left internal carotid artery (ICA). *B* to *E,* Subsequent procedures are performed in the anteroposterior–left anterior oblique view in order to visualize the cerebral protection device, the lesion, and the distal end of the sheath (guiding catheter). *B,* Filter passage. *C* and *D,* Delivery of the stent. *E,* Postdilatation.

TABLE 21–9	Strengths and Weaknesses of Distal Occlusion Balloon

Strengths

Better chance of crossing tight, tortuous lesion compared with filters
    Lower crossing profile
    More flexible

Weaknesses

Somewhat cumbersome
Prolonged procedure time
Inability to perform angiography during protection
Some patients (~10%) may not tolerate occlusion
Unprotected
    During passage
    Suction shadow
    Potential for ECA embolization

ECA, external carotid artery.

in terms of capturing emboli because protection can be initiated before touching the lesion, and emboli of any size are effectively recovered with the reversal of flow. These devices are also available in larger profiles and require occlusion of the ECA to create adequate proximal occlusion and flow reversal through the ICA.

Carotid Stents and Deployment

A number of stents are available for CAS or are being evaluated for this purpose. Carotid Wallstents and nitinol stents such as the Precise (Cordis, Warren, N.J.) or the AccuLink (Guidant, Melno Park, Calif.) are used most frequently (Fig. 21-26). They differ primarily in the way they are sized.[42] Wallstents are always substantially oversized because of significant foreshortening and reduced radial force; a 10- by 20-mm size works well for most bifurcation lesions (Figs. 21-27 and 21-28). When using the Wallstent, it is advisable to place it with sufficient proximal and distal lesion coverage because the stent can foreshorten proximally or distally later (Fig. 21-29; see also Fig. 21-28). Conversely, nitinol stents have minimal foreshortening and higher radial force; therefore, the nitinol stent diameter should be 1 to 2 mm greater than the artery diameter, and the stent should be 5 to 10 mm longer than the lesion (Fig. 21-30; see also Fig. 21-28). Additional advantages of nitinol stents include accurate deployment, good lesion coverage, and lesion conformability. Disadvantages include low radiopacity and the presence of stent struts protruding inside the vessel. An 8- by 30-mm Precise nitinol stent is appropriate for most lesions, whereas a 7- by 20-mm Precise stent is preferred for more focal lesions in the mid-ICA (see Fig. 21-28). It should be noted that either stent should be sized to the CCA if the stent is to be deployed across the bifurcation; therefore, there will be considerable oversizing within the ICA. For this reason, a tapered stent is being developed (see Fig. 21-26).

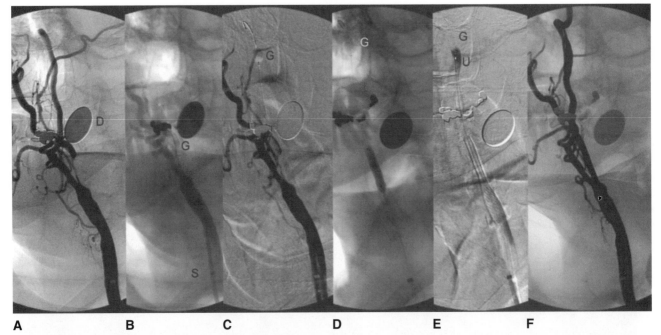

A   **B**   **C**   **D**   **E**   **F**

FIGURE 21–21 • Procedural steps for stenting with distal occlusion protection. *A,* Preprocedure angiogram shows severe stenosis in the left internal carotid artery (ICA). A dime (D) is placed on the ipsilateral neck for calibration. *B,* The GuardWire (G) is passed through the stenosis with the aid of a "puff" angiogram performed through the sheath (S). *C,* The GuardWire (G) is inflated to occlude the distal ICA. Angiogram is obtained to confirm complete occlusion of the ICA. *D,* Percutaneous transluminal angioplasty and stenting are performed under protection. *E,* Aspiration catheter is introduced to aspirate the embolic particles trapped by the protection device. Angiogram is performed to evaluate the completeness of the aspiration. Suction shadow (U) can be seen adjacent to the GuardWire (G). *F,* Completion angiogram is obtained after deflation of the GuardWire.

TABLE 21–10	Strengths and Weaknesses of Distal Filters

Strengths

Intuitive

Easier to use than distal balloon in straightforward cases

Preserves ICA flow

Weaknesses

Larger profile, less flexible, less torque; may need to predilate or use buddy wire

Unprotected

    During passage

    Small particles (<100 μm)

    Flow around filter

    During filter retrieval

Need sufficient landing zone in distal ICA

May thrombose; may plug up

Need to keep filter stable; may cause spasm or dissection in distal ICA

Difficult to introduce retrieval catheter through stent

Filter may get stuck in stent during recovery

Somewhat cumbersome procedure

Prolonged procedure time

ICA, internal carotid artery.

Although primary stenting (stent deployment without predilatation) of carotid lesions is performed by some operators, predilatation is generally required and recommended for most carotid lesions, which are usually quite stenotic and often associated with heavy calcification or fibrosis from previous endarterectomy. Without predilatation, there may be an increased risk of inability to cross the lesion with the stent delivery system, inability to withdraw the stent delivery system after deployment through the constricted portion of the stent, and inability to recross the stent for postdilatation. Primary stenting is a valid option only if the carotid lesion is severely ulcerated and not very stenotic. Another reason to perform predilatation is that the predilatation balloon can be used as a reference to confirm the diameter and length of the stent. We prefer 0.014-inch-based rapid-exchange balloons that are 4 mm in diameter and 30 to 40 mm long. Shorter balloons should be avoided because they can move cranially or caudally during inflation, a phenomenon called "watermelon seeding." Longer balloons prevent this because the proximal and distal portion of the balloon inflates to make a "doggy bone" shape, securing the balloon in position. Carotid lesion predilatation may also suggest the patient's hemodynamic response to carotid sinus stimulation.

If the sheath or the guiding catheter is appropriately positioned in the CCA, and if predilatation has been performed, introduction of the stent into the lesion should be easy and

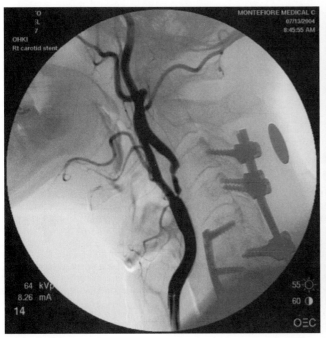

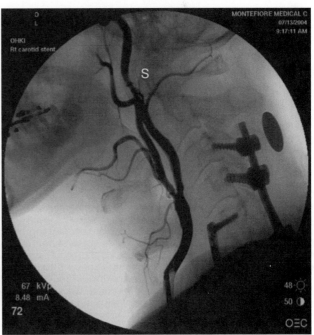

A **B**

FIGURE 21–22 • Procedural steps for stenting with distal filter protection. *A,* Preprocedure angiogram shows high-grade stenosis at the orifice of the internal carotid artery (ICA). Note that this patient has a fixation device in his cervical spine, making surgical exposure difficult. *B,* Completion angiogram shows minimal residual stenosis (5%). Also, mild spasm (S) is noted at the site of filter deployment.

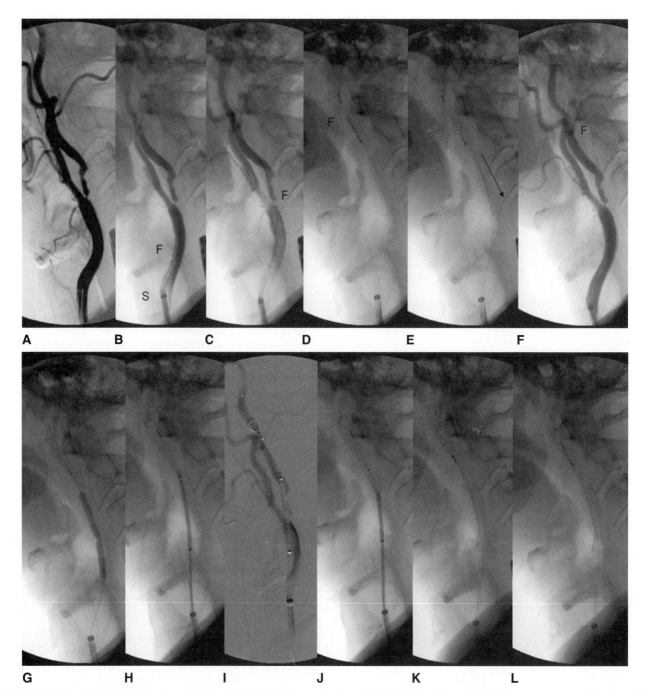

FIGURE 21–23 • Procedural steps for stenting with distal filter protection. *A,* Selective angiography shows severe stenosis in the right internal carotid artery (ICA). *B* and *C,* "Puff" angiogram is obtained through the sheath (S) to guide the filter (F) through the lesion. *D* and *E,* The filter is deployed by retracting the outer sheath *(arrow).* The filter should be kept in a straight segment so that it circumferentially apposes the vessel. *F,* Angiogram is obtained to confirm complete apposition of the filter and maintenance of flow. This should be obtained in two different directions. Note the presence of ICA spasm just distal to the filter. *G,* Predilatation is performed with a 4-mm by 4-cm balloon. Balloons 3 to 4 cm long should be used to avoid "watermelon seeding" of the balloon. *H* and *I,* The stent is delivered to the target lesion, and an angiogram is obtained to confirm positioning of the stent. *J* and *K,* Stenting is performed from the ICA to common carotid artery (CCA) to achieve full coverage of the lesion. Note accurate deployment and minimal foreshortening of the Presice stent. *L,* After postdilatation is performed with a 5-mm by 2-cm balloon, and after a completion angiogram is obtained, the filter is collapsed with the dedicated retrieval sheath and removed from the body.

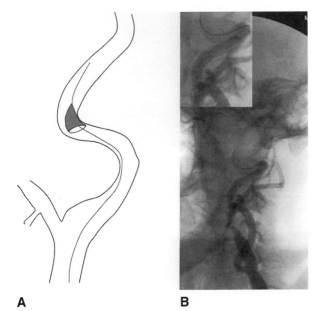

A   **B**

FIGURE 21–24 • Malapposition of a filter in a tortuous vessels. *A,* Schematic drawing of a filter placed in a tortuous vessel. *B,* Angiogram shows filter with incomplete apposition. *Inset,* Magnified view of the filter.

smooth in most cases. However, in type II or III aortic arches, those with severe tortuosity in the CCA or ICA, or lesions with severe recoil following predilatation, introduction of the stent may be difficult. As mentioned in the section on CPD deployment, the image intensifier should be positioned so that the tip of the CPD and the distal end of the sheath can be visualized simultaneously (see Fig. 21-20). If the CPD is pulled down or the sheath is pushed down during stent introduction, it should not be forced; this could lead to complete prolapse of the sheath into the aortic arch, or the CPD could be pulled down through the lesion (see Fig. 21-10). In such a case, repeat predilatation may be needed. Also, having the patient tilt the neck back and turn the head to the contralateral side may help reduce the resistance during stent delivery.

TABLE 21–11	Strengths and Weaknesses of Proximal Occlusion System

Strengths
Ability to obtain complete protection before manipulating lesion
Captures particles of all sizes
Ability to treat tight or tortuous lesions; can use guidewire of choice

Weaknesses
Counterintuitive
Interruption of flow during protection (although can perform angiography)
Potential to cause dissection or spasm in ECA or CCA
Requires larger puncture site hole in groin (9 French)

CCA, common carotid artery; ECA, external carotid artery.

Nitinol stents usually tend to jump forward during the initial phase of stent deployment. The longitudinal compression of the inner core of the delivery system during advancement of the stent through the lesion and the release of stored energy upon withdrawal of the sheath may cause this tendency. Advancing the delivery system to a point slightly cranial to where the stent should be deployed and then withdrawing it back may minimize stent jumping. Moreover, the initial sheath's pullback should be done gently so that only the first hoop of the stent is released, and the stent should be repositioned at this time. The carotid Wallstent has the ability to be recaptured and repositioned, although this maneuver is rarely needed (see Fig. 21-27). Stent length should be sufficient to adequately cover the lesion, because mild disease in the ICA can be quite extensive and impossible to exclude.

Stent placement does not reduce distal tortuosity or kinking and may in fact worsen it by reducing the arterial compliance as the kink is displaced upward to the skull base, where it is even more difficult to treat (see Fig. 21-25). Minimizing the stent length and using stents that conform to the artery may cause less straightening and less distal kinking. For this reason, patients with severe tortuosity or elongation of the CCA and ICA are better treated by surgical shortening of the artery with eversion endarterectomy.

Postdilatation is performed using 0.014-inch-based monorail balloons. Balloons up to 5.5 mm in diameter are usually adequate for most internal carotids. We typically use a 5- or 5.5-mm balloon for postdilatation. Extremely aggressive postdilatation to eliminate any degree of residual stenosis is not advised because most nitinol stents tend to keep expanding, and the large volume of emboli may overwhelm the CPD. Further, aggressive balloon dilatation may lead to severe and refractory hypotension and bradycardia. Residual stenosis of 10% to 20% is acceptable after CAS. Because postdilatation of the stent is the most emboligenic part of the procedure, extreme care should be taken to make sure that the CPD is in a good position and well opposed to the vessel wall. One should note that with CAS, "perfect is the enemy of good."

Hemodynamic Changes

The carotid sinus reflex pathways consist of two distinct components: a chronotropic mechanism affecting the sinus and atrioventricular nodes leading to bradycardia, and a vasodilatory component leading to hypotension. Maximum stimulation of the carotid sinus baroreceptors generally occurs during postdilatation of the stent. Because of anatomic considerations, carotid sinus stimulation is usually more pronounced when the carotid lesion is located in the proximal ICA or in the carotid bifurcation. A previous endarterectomy may reduce the carotid sinus response, although this is not always predictable.

Bradycardia is typically short-lived, whereas the vasodilatory response may be more persistent. Bradycardia usually responds to anticholinergic drugs such as atropine. A temporary pacemaker is rarely needed. Patients with severe baseline bradycardia secondary to beta blockers should not be given beta blockers on the day of the procedure. The vasodilatory response is best treated with volume expansion, which should be done before dilatation of the stent. Vasoconstrictors such as pseudoephedrine, norepinephrine, and dopamine are indicated only for refractory cases. Oral pseudoephedrine may be

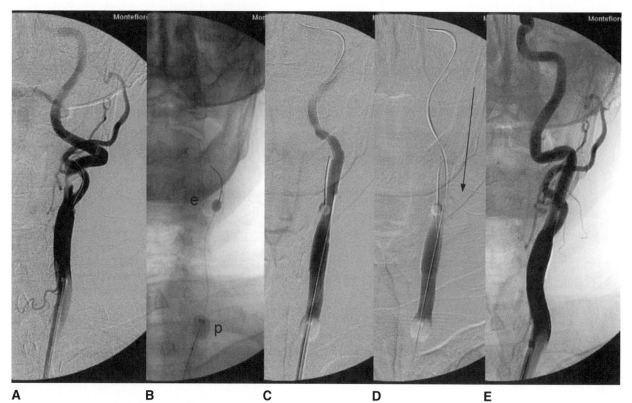

FIGURE 21–25 • ArteriA Parodi Anti-Embolization System. *A,* Preprocedure angiogram shows high-grade stenosis and severe tortuosity in the internal carotid artery (ICA) that will make the use of distal protection difficult. *B,* The proximal balloon (p) attached on the outside of the sheath is inflated to occlude the inflow. The external carotid artery is occluded by the external balloon (e). *C* and *D,* The proximal end of the sheath is connected to a femoral venous sheath, thereby creating a temporary arteriovenous fistula. Injected contrast agent initially travels toward the brain but quickly flows back toward the sheath, owing to the reversal of flow *(arrow)* created by the arteriovenous fistula. *E,* Completion angiogram is taken after carotid angioplasty and stenting and after the occlusion balloons are deflated. Note the exaggerated kink in the distal ICA. This is caused by the relatively stiff stent.

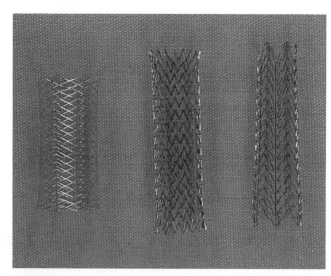

FIGURE 21–26 • Carotid stents. *From left,* Wallstent, Precise stent, AccuLink (tapered).

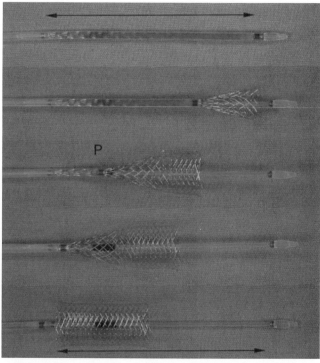

FIGURE 21–27 • Deployment of the Wallstent. The Wallstent is deployed by retracting the outer sheath. Note the significant fore-shortening. *Arrow* denotes the length of the stent before deployment. The Wallstent can be recaptured if the deployment has not exceeded the point of no return (P).

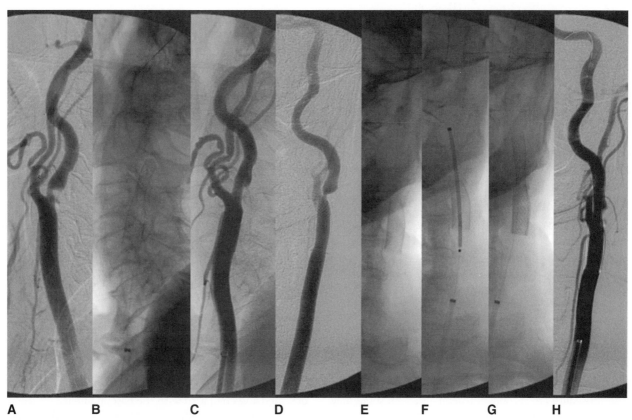

A   B   C   D   E   F   G   H

FIGURE 21–28 • Proximal migration of a Wallstent. *A,* Preprocedure angiogram (lateral view). *B,* The Wallstent is deployed. Note that it is slightly low. *C,* Completion angiogram shows satisfactory result. *D,* Follow-up duplex study obtained 3 months after stenting suggests recurrent stenosis. This angiogram (anteroposterior view) shows recurrent stenosis as well as proximal migration of the Wallstent. *E,* Note significant foreshortening of the stent. *F,* An additional stent was deployed within the previous stent. *G* and *H,* Satisfactory outcome.

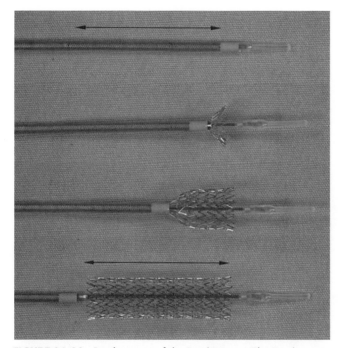

FIGURE 21–29 • Deployment of the Precise stent. The Precise stent is deployed by retracting the outer sheath. Note the minimal fore-shortening and accurate deployment. *Arrow* denotes the length of the stent before deployment.

given because it provides enough vasoconstriction to stabilize the blood pressure yet avoids the necessity of an intensive care unit stay. We do not believe that atropine should be used routinely because it has significant side effects, particularly in elderly patients, including urinary retention, severe dry mouth, and mental status changes. Occasionally, patients may develop significant tachycardia after atropine administration that may lead to myocardial ischemia in the presence of significant coronary artery disease. Patients with severe congestive heart failure may need to be managed with a pulmonary artery catheter for more precise management of their volume status. A pulmonary artery catheter and a pacemaker may also be necessary for patients with left main disease or severe aortic stenosis because of their risk of developing severe bradycardia or hypotension.

Neurologic Complications

The use of cerebral protection during CAS appears to have reduced the risk of intraprocedural stroke. Neurologic examinations should, however, be performed throughout a CAS procedure. Patients should be asked to speak and move the contralateral upper and lower extremities, which is sufficient evidence of adequate cerebral perfusion. Such brief examinations are particularly important during and after placement of the sheath or guiding catheter, initial crossing of the lesion with the CPD, predilatation, stent placement, postdilatation,

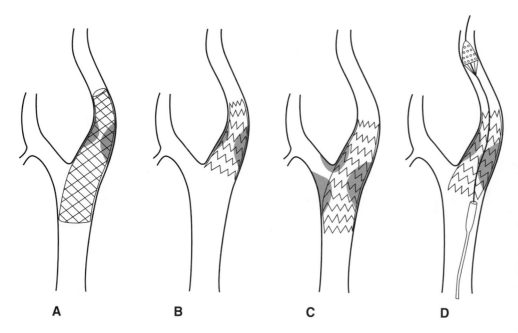

FIGURE 21–30 • Sizing and location of stent placement, depending on type of stent and lesion location. *A,* Deployment of a Wallstent. Owing to significant foreshortening, the Wallstent should always be deployed across the bifurcation. *B,* Deployment of a nitinol stent. If the lesion is isolated within the internal carotid artery (ICA) and does not involve the bifurcation, a nitinol stent can be deployed in just the ICA. In this case (as in most cases), a 7-mm by 2-cm stent is appropriate. *C,* Deployment of a nitinol stent. If the lesion involves the bifurcation, an 8-mm by 3-cm stent is commonly used. *D,* Avoid leaving the stent partially deployed in the bifurcation, because this makes it difficult to introduce balloons and the filter retrieval sheath.

and guiding catheter removal. Not all neurologic deficits during the procedure are secondary to embolization; some may be related to hemodynamic instability and cerebral ischemia from flow obstruction by the CPD. In these instances, the procedure should be completed swiftly, and particular attention should be given to anticoagulation, maintaining the ACT at longer than 300 seconds, and maintaining hemodynamic stability. The patient should be reassessed as soon as the procedure is completed and the CPD is removed. Careful posteroanterior and lateral cerebral angiography should be

performed at this point. A parenchyma-gram should be obtained and compared with the baseline image. In the presence of cerebral emboli, one would see an area that does not stain in either the anteroposterior or the lateral projection (Fig. 21-31). If there is no evidence of occlusion of the middle or anterior cerebral artery or one of their major branches, the patient will probably make a full recovery within a few hours. Attention to volume status and maintenance of adequate blood pressure are mandatory. Embolization with involvement of the M1 or M2 segments of the middle cerebral artery

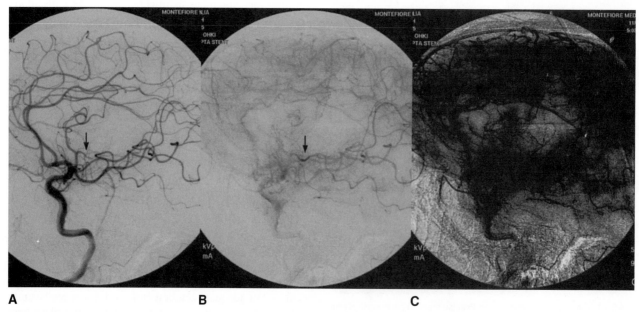

FIGURE 21–31 • Embolic complication shown on completion intracranial angiogram. *A,* A cutoff of the M3 segment of the middle cerebral artery is seen *(arrow). B,* Later phase shows stagnation of contrast material *(arrow). C,* The region of infarct becomes more obvious with parenchyma-gram. Note the lack of stain in the middle cerebral area.

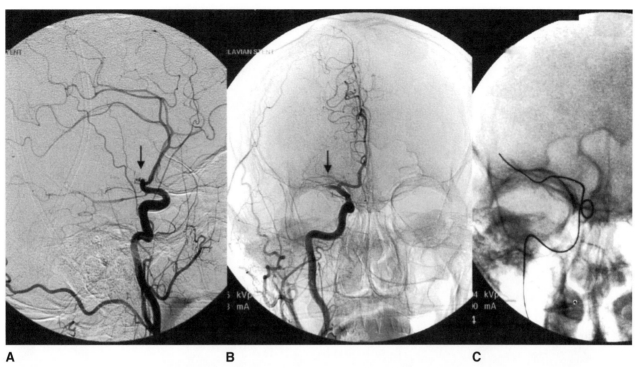

A   B   C

FIGURE 21–32 • Embolic complication. *A* and *B*, Completion angiogram shows abrupt cutoff of the right middle cerebral artery due to a major embolus. *C*, A microcatheter was introduced into the target vessel, and thrombolysis was initiated.

or A1 or A2 segment of the anterior cerebral artery requires intervention, because these patients have a low chance of complete spontaneous recovery. Intubation to secure the airway and provide maximum oxygenation may be beneficial. A microcatheter should be advanced into the lesion, and intra-arterial thrombolysis with urokinase or tissue plasminogen activator should be initiated (Figs. 21-32 and 21-33). Adjuvant therapy with systemic infusion of GP IIb/IIIa antagonists may be helpful, although this increases the risk of intracranial hemorrhage, especially in those with severe hypertension and a high ACT (>300 seconds). Conversely, a mechanical approach can be used. A small 1.5-mm coronary balloon is advanced to the occlusion, and gentle dilatation often dislodges the plaque fragment. Soft hydrophilic wires may also be used to cross the blockage, which may be enough to restore flow. In refractory cases, a small snare such as the NeuroNet (Guidant, Indianapolis, Ind.) may be used to remove the embolus.

Postoperative Management

Closure devices may be used with caution, particularly when diseased or calcified femoral arteries are used for access. In these instances, local compression is preferable. The patient is kept overnight in a telemetry unit and usually discharged the next day. Careful neurologic monitoring throughout the recovery period is essential because of the rare occurrence of embolization within a few hours after CAS. This probably occurs owing to plaque fragments that protrude through the stent struts. Continuous blood pressure monitoring is mandatory, and systolic pressure should be maintained between

100 and 140 mm Hg. Severe hypertension should be aggressively managed because it can lead to cerebral hyperperfusion syndrome and intracranial hemorrhage. A combination of intravenous beta blockers and nitroglycerin is the initial therapy to control severe hypertension. Cerebral hyperperfusion usually occurs in patients with chronic cerebral hypoperfusion who have maximal dilatation of intracranial arterioles after CAS and abnormal cerebral autoregulation, which may not be restored for several days.[43] Patients with severe stenosis (>90%), contralateral occlusions, and severe hypertension are at increased risk, similar to patients undergoing CEA. In these instances, patients usually complain of a headache ipsilateral to the CAS, which may progress to a focal neurologic deficit, confusion, stupor, and death. Cerebral hyperperfusion may occur in 0.9% of patients after CAS. Beta blockers and diuretics are the mainstays of treatment. Vasodilators should be used cautiously, because dilatation of the intracranial arteries may worsen the syndrome. Because CAS typically lowers the blood pressure for a few days postoperatively, antihypertensive medications are often reduced or stopped in the hospital. Continuous blood pressure monitoring after discharge is important, and patients should restart their antihypertensive medications as their blood pressure returns to baseline. Failure to do so may result in intracranial hemorrhage when hypertension returns.

Patients should be seen at 1 and 6 months after CAS and yearly thereafter. Carotid duplex scanning is performed before discharge and repeated at 1 month, 6 months, and then annually. Duplex scanning is the standard modality for postoperative surveillance. However, a pitfall of duplex surveillance is that flow velocities may be increased in the

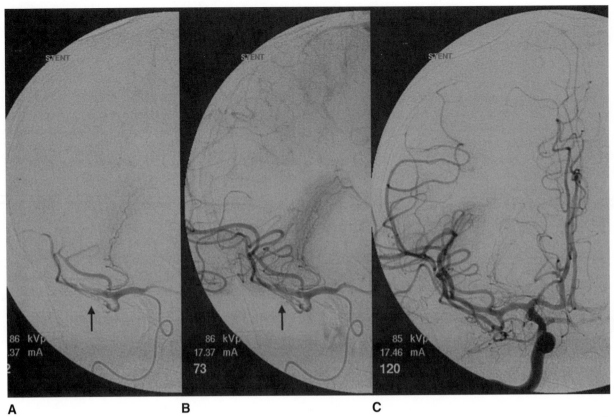

FIGURE 21–33 • Embolic complication. *A* and *B,* Thrombolysis of the embolus *(arrow)* with tissue plasminogen activator was performed through a microcatheter. Note the gradual resolution of the embolus. *C,* Completion angiogram shows complete lysis of the embolus, with good filling of the middle cerebral artery. Full neurologic recovery was achieved.

absence of hemodynamically significant lesions. This phenomenon is thought to be due to changes in arterial wall compliance associated with stent placement that produce alterations in flow velocities.[44] Specific criteria for in-stent restenosis should therefore be validated at each vascular laboratory, as these may vary and may overestimate the degree or residual and recurrent stenosis.[45]

KEY REFERENCES

Abou-Chebl A, Yadav JS, Reginelli JP, et al: Intracranial hemorrhage and hyperperfusion syndrome following carotid artery stenting: Risk factors, prevention, and treatment. J Am Coll Cardiol 43:1596-1601, 2004.

Alberts MJ, McCann R, Smith TP, et al: A randomized trial of carotid stenting vs endarterectomy in patients with symptomatic carotid stenosis: Study design. J Neurovasc Dis 2:228-234, 1997.

Endovascular versus surgical treatment in patients with carotid stenosis in the Carotid and Vertebral Artery Transluminal Angioplasty Study (CAVATAS): A randomised trial. Lancet 357:1729-1737, 2001.

Naylor AR, Bolia A, Abbott RJ, et al: Randomized study of carotid angioplasty and stenting versus carotid endarterectomy: A stopped trial. J Vasc Surg 28:326-334, 1998.

Ohki T, Veith FJ: Critical analysis of distal protection devices. Semin Vasc Surg 16:317-325, 2003.

Ouriel K, Hertzer NR, Beven EG, et al: Preprocedural risk stratification: Identifying an appropriate population for carotid stenting. J Vasc Surg 33:728-732, 2001.

Yadav JS, Wholey MH, Kuntz RE, et al: Protected carotid-artery stenting versus endarterectomy in high-risk patients. N Engl J Med 351:1493-1501, 2004.

REFERENCES

1. Beneficial effect of carotid endarterectomy in symptomatic patients with high-grade carotid stenosis. North American Symptomatic Carotid Endarterectomy Trial Collaborators. N Engl J Med 325:445-453, 1991.

2. MRC European Carotid Surgery Trial: Interim results for symptomatic patients with severe (70-99%) or with mild (0-29%) carotid stenosis. European Carotid Surgery Trialists' Collaborative Group. Lancet 337:1235-1243, 1991.

3. Veith FJ, Amor M, Ohki T, et al: Current status of carotid bifurcation angioplasty and stenting based on a consensus of opinion leaders. J Vasc Surg 33(2 Suppl):S111-S116, 2001.

4. Yadav JS, Wholey MH, Kuntz RE, et al: Protected carotid-artery stenting versus endarterectomy in high-risk patients. N Engl J Med 351:1493-1501, 2004.

5. Yadav JS, Roubin GS, King P, et al: Angioplasty and stenting for restenosis after carotid endarterectomy: Initial experience. Stroke 27:2075-2079, 1996.

6. Yadav JS, Roubin GS, Iyer S, et al: Elective stenting of the extracranial carotid arteries. Circulation 95:376-381, 1997.

7. Diethrich EB, Ndiaye M, Reid DB: Stenting in the carotid artery: Initial experience in 110 patients. J Endovasc Surg 3:42-62, 1996.

8. Theron JG, Payelle GG, Coskun O, et al: Carotid artery stenosis: Treatment with protected balloon angioplasty and stent placement. Radiology 201:627-636, 1996.

9. Mathias K, Jager H, Sahl H, et al: [Interventional treatment of arteriosclerotic carotid stenosis.] Radiologe 39:125-134, 1999.

10. Wholey MH, Wholey M, Mathias K, et al: Global experience in cervical carotid artery stent placement. Catheter Cardiovasc Interv 50:160-167, 2000.

11. Roubin GS, New G, Iyer SS, et al: Immediate and late clinical outcomes of carotid artery stenting in patients with symptomatic and asymptomatic

carotid artery stenosis: A 5-year prospective analysis. Circulation 103: 532-537, 2001.

12. Ohki T, Veith FJ, Grenell S, et al: Initial experience with cerebral protection devices to prevent embolization during carotid artery stenting. J Vasc Surg 36:1175-1185, 2002.

13. Endovascular versus surgical treatment in patients with carotid stenosis in the Carotid and Vertebral Artery Transluminal Angioplasty Study (CAVATAS): A randomised trial. Lancet 357:1729-1737, 2001.

14. Golledge J, Mitchell A, Greenhalgh RM, et al: Systematic comparison of the early outcome of angioplasty and endarterectomy for symptomatic carotid artery disease. Stroke 31:1439-1443, 2000.

15. Naylor AR, Bolia A, Abbott RJ, et al: Randomized study of carotid angioplasty and stenting versus carotid endarterectomy: A stopped trial. J Vasc Surg 28:326-334, 1998.

16. Alberts MJ, McCann R, Smith TP, et al: A randomized trial of carotid stenting vs endarterectomy in patients with symptomatic carotid stenosis: Study design. J Neurovasc Dis 2:228-234, 1997.

17. Ohki T, Marin ML, Lyon RT, et al: Ex vivo human carotid artery bifurcation stenting: Correlation of lesion characteristics with embolic potential. J Vasc Surg 27:463-471, 1998.

18. Kastrup A, Groschel K, Krapf H, et al: Early outcome of carotid angioplasty and stenting with and without cerebral protection devices: A systematic review of the literature. Stroke 34:813-819, 2003.

19. Ohki T, Veith FJ: Carotid artery stenting: Utility of cerebral protection devices. J Invasive Cardiol 13:47-55, 2001.

20. Endarterectomy for asymptomatic carotid artery stenosis: Executive Committee for the Asymptomatic Carotid Atherosclerosis Study. JAMA 273:1421-1428, 1995.

21. Biller J, Feinberg WM, Castaldo JE, et al: Guidelines for carotid endarterectomy: A statement for healthcare professionals from a Special Writing Group of the Stroke Council, American Heart Association. Circulation 97:501-509, 1998.

22. Wholey M: The ARCHeR trial: Prospective clinical trial for carotid stenting in high surgical risk patients—preliminary 30-day results. Paper presented at the American College of Cardiology Annual Meeting, March 6-9, 2003, Chicago.

23. Whitlow P: A registry study to evaluate the MedNova EmboShield bare-wire filter and MedNova Xact self-expanding carotid stent system in patients at high-risk for carotid endarterectomy (SECuRITY trial). Paper presented at TransCatheter Cardiovascular Therapeutics (TCT) Meeting, September 15-19, 2003, Washington, DC.

24. Iyer SS: Boston Scientific/EPI: A carotid stenting trial for high risk surgical patients (BEACH). Paper presented at the TransCatheter Cardiovascular Therapeutics (TCT) Meeting, September 27-October 1, 2004, Washington, DC.

25. The CARESS Steering Committee: Carotid Revascularization Using Endarterectomy or Stenting Systems (CARESS): Phase I clinical trial. J Endovasc Ther 6:1021-1030, 2003.

26. Hobson RW II, et al: Carotid artery stenting is associated with increased complications in octogenarians: 30-day stroke and death rates in the CREST lead-in phase. Paper presented at the Vascular 2004 Annual Meeting, June 3-6, 2004, Anaheim, Calif.

27. Ouriel K, Hertzer NR, Beven EG, et al: Preprocedural risk stratification: Identifying an appropriate population for carotid stenting. J Vasc Surg 33:728-732, 2001.

28. Bhatt DL, Kapadia SR, Bajzer CT, et al: Dual antiplatelet therapy with clopidogrel and aspirin after carotid artery stenting. J Invasive Cardiol 13:767-771, 2001.

29. Kapadia SR, Bajzer CT, Ziada KM, et al: Initial experience of platelet glycoprotein IIb/IIIa inhibition with abciximab during carotid stenting: A safe and effective adjunctive therapy. Stroke 32:2328-2332, 2001.

30. Myla S: Carotid access techniques: An algorithmic approach. Carotid Interv 3:2-12, 2001.

31. Criado E, Doblas M, Fontcuberta J, et al: Transcervical carotid artery angioplasty and stenting with carotid flow reversal: Surgical technique. Ann Vasc Surg 18:257-261, 2004.

32. Rapp JH, Pan XM, Sharp FR, et al: Atheroemboli to the brain: Size threshold for causing acute neuronal cell death. J Vasc Surg 32:68-76, 2000.

33. Ohki T, Veith FJ: Critical analysis of distal protection devices. Semin Vasc Surg 16:317-325, 2003.

34. Grube E, Gerckens U, Yeung AC, et al: Prevention of distal embolization during coronary angioplasty in saphenous vein grafts and native vessels using porous filter protection. Circulation 104:2436-2441, 2001.

35. Dietz A, Berkefeld J, Theron JG, et al: Endovascular treatment of symptomatic carotid stenosis using stent placement: Long-term follow-up of patients with a balanced surgical risk/benefit ratio. Stroke 32:1855-1859, 2001.

36. Al Mubarak N, Roubin GS, Vitek JJ, et al: Effect of the distal-balloon protection system on microembolization during carotid stenting. Circulation 104:1999-2002, 2001.

37. Tubler T, Schluter M, Dirsch O, et al: Balloon-protected carotid artery stenting: Relationship of periprocedural neurological complications with the size of particulate debris. Circulation 104:2791-2796, 2001.

38. Reimers B, Corvaja N, Moshiri S, et al: Cerebral protection with filter devices during carotid artery stenting. Circulation 104:12-15, 2001.

39. Angelini A, Reimers B, Della BM, et al: Cerebral protection during carotid artery stenting: Collection and histopathologic analysis of embolized debris. Stroke 33:456-461, 2002.

40. Al Mubarak N, Colombo A, Gaines PA, et al: Multicenter evaluation of carotid artery stenting with a filter protection system. J Am Coll Cardiol 39:841-846, 2002.

41. Topol EJ, Yadav JS: Recognition of the importance of embolization in atherosclerotic vascular disease. Circulation 101:570-580, 2000.

42. Mukherjee D, Kalahasti V, Roffi M, et al: Self-expanding stents for carotid interventions: Comparison of nitinol versus stainless-steel stents. J Invasive Cardiol 13:732-735, 2001.

43. Abou-Chebl A, Yadav JS, Reginelli JP, et al: Intracranial hemorrhage and hyperperfusion syndrome following carotid artery stenting: Risk factors, prevention, and treatment. J Am Coll Cardiol 43:1596-1601, 2004.

44. Timaran CH, Ohki T, Chen T, et al: Accuracy of duplex ultrasonography in evaluating in-stent restenosis after carotid angioplasty and stenting. Ann Vasc Surg (in press 2005).

45. Lal BK, Hobson RW, Goldstein J, et al: Carotid artery stenting: Is there a need to revise ultrasound velocity criteria? J Vasc Surg 39:58-66, 2004.

Questions

1. **What were the 30-day stroke and death rates for CEA and CAS in the SAPPHIRE trial?**
   (a) 7.3% versus 4.4%
   (b) 5.8% versus 0.3%
   (c) 4.4% versus 7.3%
   (d) 10% versus 10%
   (e) 0.3% versus 5.8%

2. **Which of the following characteristics is not considered as a high risk for CEA?**
   (a) Age older than 70 years
   (b) Recurrent stenosis following CEA
   (c) Unstable angina
   (d) Uncontrolled congestive heart failure
   (e) Contralateral ICA occlusion

3. **Which trial is not a high-risk registry?**
   (a) BEACH
   (b) CARESS
   (c) ARCHeR
   (d) SECURITY
   (e) CABERNET

4. **Which of the following is not a rationale for performing cerebral angiogram before CAS?**
   (a) Risk stratification for CAS
   (b) Rule out brain tumor
   (c) Confirmation of degree of stenosis
   (d) Understanding of intracranial collateral circulation
   (e) Obtaining a baseline cerebral angiogram

5. Which catheter is not commonly used for CAS?
   (a) Vitek
   (b) Vertebral
   (c) Headhunter
   (d) Simmons
   (e) Cobra

6. Which lesion is ideally treated with CAS?
   (a) Very tight stenosis with string sign
   (b) Acute occlusion
   (c) Dense calcification
   (d) Severe stenosis or tortuosity within the carotid artery
   (e) None of the above

7. Which of the following is a disadvantage of a sheath compared with a guiding catheter?
   (a) Larger puncture site hole
   (b) Lack of torque
   (c) Usability in type II or III arch
   (d) More traumatic introduction into the common carotid artery
   (e) Less trackable

8. Which of the following is an advantage of a filter-type protection device compared with balloon-based protection?
   (a) Does not require a straight landing zone
   (b) Can negotiate severe stenosis
   (c) Can obtain angiogram during stenting
   (d) Captures microemboli
   (e) Ideal for tortuous lesions

9. Which of the following is not an advantage of nitinol stents?
   (a) Accurate deployment
   (b) Strong radial force
   (c) Radiopacity
   (d) Good lesion coverage
   (e) Lesion conformability

10. Which of the following medications or techniques is commonly used for carotid sinus reflex?
    (a) Pseudoephedrine
    (b) Fluid resuscitation
    (c) Atropine
    (d) Transvenous pacing
    (e) Norepinephrine

Answers

1. a	2. a	3. b	4. b	5. e
6. e	7. b	8. c	9. c	10. d

Endovascular Repair of Abdominal Aortic Aneurysms: Technique and Results

History and General Design

The first endovascular aneurysm repair for an abdominal aortic aneurysm (AAA) was reported in 1986 by Volodos and colleagues.[1] However, it was not until Parodi's report in 1991 that interest in the endovascular treatment of AAA began to blossom.[2] The early grafts were physician-made devices consisting of a graft material placed over balloon-expandable or self-expanding stents. Many of the early grafts were single-unit, tubular designs. Later, the Malmo, Leicester, and Montefiore groups developed grafts that had a distal landing site in the common femoral artery.[3,4] The opposite iliac artery was occluded, and a femorofemoral bypass graft was constructed to provide arterial inflow for the contralateral extremity. During this same period, the Sydney group introduced the concept of modular components, making these grafts adaptable for use with the many dimensions an aneurysm can take.[5] Currently, most grafts use a modular system to account for the variability in the anatomy, length, and diameter of the patient's aorta (Figs. 22-1 and 22-2).

The graft material is either polyester (Dacron) or polytetrafluoroethylene (PTFE)—the same materials used in open repairs of AAAs. These materials are believed to be resistant to late deterioration, strong enough to prevent damage from the metallic stents, and thin enough to allow compression into small delivery catheters. Currently, other polymers are under investigation but are not yet approved by the U.S. Food and Drug Administration (FDA).

The method of fixation has generated considerable interest. The current systems use columnar stiffness; radial force to provide friction; hooks, anchors, or barbs for positive fixation by embedding into the aortic wall; or a combination of these. Suprarenal fixation is another option; bare metal stents with hooks provide fixation in the suprarenal aortic neck, which may be more resistant to late neck dilatation.

Preoperative Imaging

When evaluating a patient with an AAA who needs treatment with an aortic endograft, an imaging study is necessary to visualize aneurysm length and diameter, characteristics of the proximal and distal necks, characteristics of the access vessels, and amount of thrombus and calcification present within the vessels. An abdominal and pelvic computed tomography (CT) scan with 1- to 1.5-mm cuts and intravenous contrast enhancement provides this information. Using digital reconstruction or CT-angiography, the necessary preoperative measurements can usually be obtained (Table 22-1). This study also allows assessment of the major branch vessels of the aorta, as well as any aberrant vessels. Certain situations involving tortuosity and kinking or a questionable luminal diameter may require an arteriogram with a calibrating catheter. This catheter has radiopaque markers at 1-cm intervals to allow precise measurement of the vessels.[6]

Patient Selection

Certain anatomic criteria should be met, with slight variations based on the particular type of endograft (Fig. 22-3; Table 22-2). The most important area of interest is the proximal aortic neck.[7-9] A cylindrical neck distal to the renal arteries with a minimum length of 1.5 cm and a diameter of 2.8 cm or less is preferred. The neck should be relatively free of thrombus, allowing adequate room for proximal fixation. A conical neck flaring more than 4 mm from its proximal to distal end is less suitable for device placement. Neck angulation—the angle between the proximal neck and suprarenal aorta—of 60 degrees or greater is challenging for endovascular repair.

The second area of interest is the distal landing zone within the iliac arteries.[10,11] Patients with severe circumferential calcification of the iliac arteries, greater than 90-degree angles, or a maximal distal seal zone diameter that is less than 2 mm

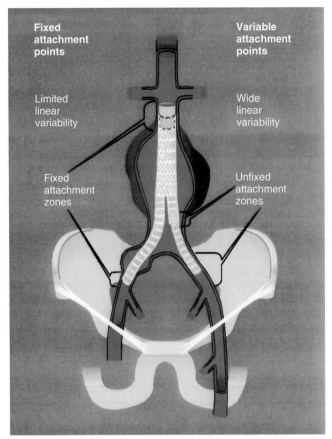

FIGURE 22–1 • Stent-graft design incorporating both limited and adjustable dimensional variability for maximum versatility. The fixed attachment points on the left have limited linear variability, whereas the adjustable fixation points on the right result in increased adaptability (From Allen RC, White RA, Zarins CK, et al: What are the characteristics of the ideal endovascular graft for abdominal aortic aneurysm exclusion? J Endovasc Surg 4:195-202, 1997.)

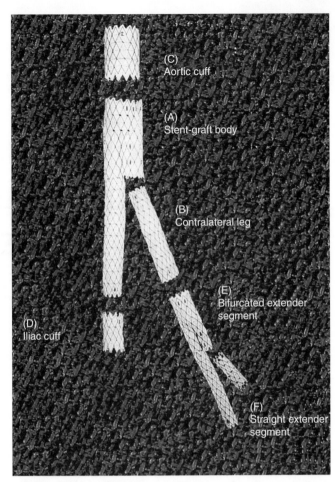

FIGURE 22–2 • Modular endovascular bifurcation prosthesis including main bifurcation segment (A), contralateral leg (B), proximal aortic cuff (C), iliac cuff (D), and bifurcated (E) or straight (F) extenders. (From Allen RC, White RA, Zarins CK, et al: What are the characteristics of the ideal endovascular graft for abdominal aortic aneurysm exclusion? J Endovasc Surg 4:195-202, 1997.)

smaller than the largest limb graft size available are suboptimal candidates. If the common iliac artery is short or the external iliac artery must be used as the landing vessel, the internal iliac artery may require embolization either before or during the procedure.[11,12] Usually, one hypogastric artery can be sacrificed without causing pelvic or spinal ischemia, provided the other hypogastric artery is normal. In the presence of iliac artery ectasia, aortic or flared cuffs can be used to allow part of the enlarged iliac artery to function as a seal zone for the endograft.[13] This is referred to as the bell-bottom technique. Tortuous or heavily calcified vessels cause graft kinking and prevent adequate graft-to-artery apposition.[14,15]

The third issue is the quality of the access vessels.[16] The femoral and iliac vessel lumen diameters must allow access of the introducer sheath, or a surgical conduit may be necessary. The outer diameter and trackability of the delivery sheaths vary, depending on the device. The degree of vessel tortuosity should be carefully evaluated. Tortuosity can usually be straightened using stiff guidewires and an introducer system or a brachial-femoral wire.[17] Most difficulties arise in situations of tortuosity combined with small-diameter vessels, calcification, and focal stenosis. In some situations, vessel recoil may occur as the vessel tries to resume its

TABLE 22–1	Required Anatomic Measurements
Computed Tomographic Measurements	**Angiographic Measurements (CTA or DSA)**
Proximal aortic neck diameter	Length from lowest renal artery to contralateral and ipsilateral distal fixation sites
Iliac artery diameter at ipsilateral distal fixation site	
Iliac artery diameter at contralateral distal fixation site	Length from lowest renal artery to aortic bifurcation
External iliac artery or common femoral artery diameter	Degree of lateral deviation and tortuosity of aorta and iliac vessels
Maximum aortic aneurysm diameter	Presence of aberrant or stenotic aortic branches
Length of aortic neck	

CTA, computed tomography-angiography; DSA, digital subtraction angiography.

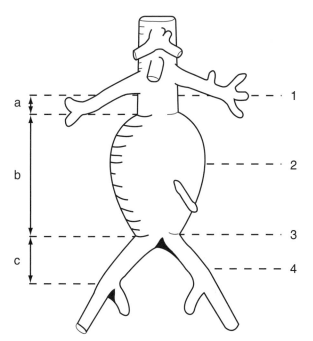

FIGURE 22–3 • Abdominal aortic aneurysm parameters measured with computed tomography-angiography (CTA) and digital subtraction angiography (DSA). For CTA, the maximal diameters shown are infrarenal (1), aneurysm (2), bifurcation (3), and common iliac arteries (4). Maximal lengths shown are for the proximal neck (a), aneurysm (b), and distal cuff (c). DSA shows arterial occlusive disease (visceral, renal, and iliac arteries), vascular anomalies (aberrant renal arteries), and tortuosity greater than 75 degrees in proximal iliac arteries.

smaller than original shape, causing kinking, malpositioning, or limb dislocation.

The patient should not have essential branch vessels that would be occluded by a stent-graft. For example, the intestinal circulation should not be dependent on the inferior mesenteric artery owing to superior mesenteric and celiac artery occlusion.

Finally, any patient being considered for an aortic endograft should be able and willing to comply with the follow-up protocol. Surveillance and reintervention are commonly needed to optimize long-term clinical outcomes.

TABLE 22–2	Patient Selection Criteria for Endovascular Repair of Abdominal Aortic Aneurysm

Fusiform AAA ≥ 5.5 cm in diameter
Saccular AAA
Suggested aortic morphology
   Proximal neck length ≥ 1.5 cm
   Neck diameter ≤ 2.8 cm
   Preservation of critical side branches
   Iliofemoral arteries of sufficient diameter for sheath access
   No severe iliac artery or aortic tortuosity
No hereditary connective tissue disorder
Anesthesia clearance for possible conversion to open repair if necessary

AAA, abdominal aortic aneurysm.

Setup

Endovascular AAA repair can be performed in a variety of environments. It is used both for elective repair and for emergent repair of ruptured aneurysms.[18] The procedure can be done in the operating room, radiology suite, or catheterization laboratory with general, regional, or local anesthesia.

The operating room environment is advantageous if rapid conversion to a major open procedure is necessary. Also, the operating room standards of sterility are maintained while the prosthetic device is being implanted into the body. When needed, open procedures can be performed simultaneously, such as a femorofemoral bypass or a distal peripheral vascular procedure.

Adequate imaging is provided by a portable C-arm unit with wide-field image intensifier, digital subtraction, road-mapping capabilities, and frame-by-frame replay. Ideally, a fixed unit system can be used because it provides many important features, including a larger field of view, better resolution, more heat capacity, and tableside controls and postprocessing.

In the operating room, the patient is prepped and draped the same way as for an open aneurysm repair. The primary endovascular specialist and assistant are positioned on opposite sides of the patient. A scrub nurse is positioned at the patient's feet, and an anesthesiologist or nurse should be present to monitor conscious sedation. It is helpful to have two monitors positioned, allowing the surgeon and the assistant an unobstructed view.

Graft Placement

Access to the common femoral arteries is obtained either through a surgical cutdown or percutaneously if a large vessel closure device is used. Angiography is performed, identifying the levels of the renal arteries, aortic bifurcation, and iliac bifurcations. Multiple magnified views with careful selection of imaging angles help optimize placement of the endograft. The main body of the graft is inserted and positioned so that the graft material is just inferior to the lowest renal artery. A second angiogram can be performed here to confirm the position of the lowest renal artery. When positioning a modular graft, it is important to orient it so that the contralateral limb gate can be easily accessed. Deployment of the main body occurs next, with some grafts allowing for minor placement alterations at points of partial deployment.

With modular systems, a directional catheter and guidewire are advanced through the contralateral femoral artery, and the contralateral gate is selectively catheterized. Anteroposterior and oblique fluoroscopic views or free rotation of a curved catheter in the proximal neck can assist in verification of device cannulation. Once the short-limb cannulation is ensured, an angiogram is obtained through the side port of the sheath to ascertain the position of the hypogastric artery. The contralateral limb size is selected to extend down to the planned distal landing zone and overlap the contralateral gate. When necessary, balloons can be used to mold the graft at the proximal and distal fixation sites.

A completion arteriogram is obtained to check side branch patency; assess limbs for kinking, which may affect patency; rule out types I and III endoleaks; and monitor for access-related arterial injury. Each graft varies slightly in terms of its introduction and deployment. The specifics of each graft are covered in individual training courses and product manuals.

Perioperative Complications

Several complications can occur in the immediate perioperative period. The most common are groin and wound complications. In this category are immediate postoperative bleeding, hematoma, or pseudoaneurysm formation. These are technical issues that are best avoided with diligence when initially accessing the femoral vessels and when subsequently repairing or closing the arteriotomy sites after removal of the endovascular devices. Liberal use of femoral completion arteriography and patch closure may minimize thromboembolic complications.

Injuries to the access vessels, particularly diseased or tortuous vessels, can occur when passing large-bore catheters and sheaths. In situations of difficult anatomy, access through the brachial artery, with passage of a wire through the thoracic aorta and subsequent capturing of that wire with a snare catheter, allows tension to be applied at both the femoral and brachial ends. This tension can result in straightening of the iliac artery (body floss technique).[17] The use of iliac conduits through a limited retroperitoneal approach also allows the operator to bypass unsuitable iliac anatomy.[16] In many situations, predilatation with a dilator or balloon allows the device to pass. If arterial dissection, avulsion, or rupture occurs, stents, stent-grafts, or conversion to open repair may be necessary.

Coverage of the internal iliac artery is commonly required during the endoluminal repair of extensive AAAs and internal iliac artery aneurysms. Studies have shown that the internal iliac artery can be embolized with minimal adverse consequences.[12] When bilateral iliac artery occlusion is necessary, a staged approach may be helpful, in the hope of developing collateral vessel formation. Alternatively, one of the internal iliac arteries may be revascularized.[11]

Distal embolization can result from manipulation of the endovascular devices within either the aneurysm sac or the access vessels.[19] Endovascular device manipulation within the aneurysm sac can also result in microembolization to the kidneys. Care should be taken to reduce manipulations in the aneurysm and at the renal and suprarenal levels, particularly if there is mural thrombus at this level. If distal embolization occurs, the same principles hold for endovascular repair as for open repair. Embolectomy catheters can be used to remove large pieces of distal debris, or a femoral or distal bypass can be performed to restore blood flow to the extremity, if necessary.

Postimplant syndrome is characterized by fever, malaise, and sometimes back pain.[20] Cultures for infection are often negative, but these symptoms can last up to 10 days. The cause may be related to cytokine release due to thrombosis within the aneurysm sac. The majority of practitioners consider this syndrome a benign event.

Late Complications

One of the principle reasons for failure of endovascular aneurysm repair is the presence of endoleak.[21-23] Endoleak is defined as persistent blood flow outside the graft and within the aneurysm sac. There are four general types of endoleak. Type I is persistent perigraft blood flow at the proximal or distal attachment site (or both) or blood flow around an iliac

occluder plug caused by an inadequate seal. Type II leaks occur due to retrograde flow from the inferior mesenteric artery, patent lumbar vessels, or other collateral vessels. Type III leaks are caused by disconnection of the modular graft components or by fabric tear, disruption, or disintegration. Type IV endoleaks occur when there is flow through porous graft fabric that is otherwise intact. Type IV endoleaks are observed only within the first 30 days after graft placement (Fig. 22-4; Table 22-3).

Endoleaks are managed by observation, a second endovascular procedure, an endoscopic procedure, or conversion to an open repair. Observation is used by those who believe that many endoleaks will seal spontaneously. This is the strategy employed with many type II endoleaks noticed on initial implantation of an aortic graft. There is no set time limit for observation; however, if the aneurysm sac is stable or shrinking, most physicians continue observation indefinitely. Type IV endoleaks are also observed, because the porosity of the graft should subside if it becomes incorporated and the graft interstices thrombose.

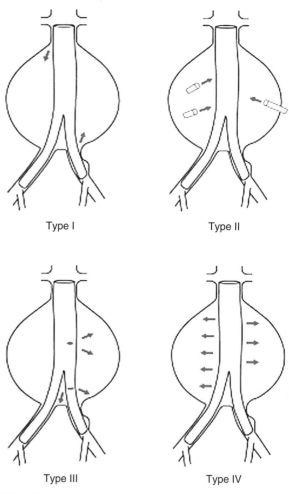

Type I   Type II

Type III   Type IV

FIGURE 22–4 • Type I endoleak (periprosthetic) occurs at the proximal or distal attachment zones, or both. Type II endoleak is caused by retrograde flow from patent lumbar or inferior mesenteric arteries. Type III endoleak arises from a defect in the graft fabric, inadequate intercomponent seal, or disconnection of modular graft components. Type IV endoleak is due to graft fabric porosity, often resulting in a generalized mild blush of contrast within the aneurysm sac.

TABLE 22–3	Types of Endoleaks	
Classification	**Causes of Perigraft Flow**	**Therapeutic Options**
Type I	Inadequate seal of proximal or distal end of endograft	Proximal or distal extension or cuff
	Inadequate seal of iliac occluder plug	Overstenting
		Embolization or glue
		Conversion
Type II	Flow from patent lumbar, middle sacral, or inferior mesenteric artery; hypogastric, accessory renal, or other visceral vessel	Observation
		Coil embolization or glue
		Laparoscopic ligation
		Conversion
Type III	Fabric disruption or tear	Secondary endograft or cuff
	Module disconnection	Conversion
Type IV	Flow from fabric porosity, suture holes (<30 days after graft placement)	Observation
Endoleak of undefined origin	Flow visualized from unidentified source	Observation
		Angiographic investigation

Most physicians prefer to treat types I and III endoleaks before leaving the procedure room. These are often treated with a secondary endoluminal procedure. Balloon dilatation to compress the device against the vessel wall or to increase graft-to-graft interposition is the first step. If balloon dilatation is unsuccessful, placement of a secondary stent or aortic cuff is the next step. In situations of perigraft blood flow at the iliac seal zone caused by the large diameter of the native vessel, using aortic or flared cuffs (bell-bottom technique) or occluding the iliac artery and extending the stent-graft to the external iliac artery can be effective. Occasionally, the primary procedure is long, and staged retreatment is another option.

Persistent type II endoleaks can be dealt with in a variety of ways. The vessels of interest can be coil embolized or treated with N-butyl cyanoacrylate glue or other thrombo-occlusive materials. Access to the vessel causing the leak can be through a translumbar, transperitoneal, or supraselective catheterization via the superior mesenteric or superior gluteal artery. Retroperitoneal endoscopic ligation of the lumbar arteries or inferior mesenteric artery is also practiced. Open conversion remains the ultimate treatment option.[24]

Migration is often defined as movement of a device more than 10 mm or any endograft displacement associated with the need for a secondary procedure.[25,26] Migration accounts for the majority of late type I endoleaks and is a significant risk factor for late rupture. Migration can occur when there is a fracture of the hooks or barbs or if there is initial failure of the attachment system to engage or penetrate the aortic wall. Another scenario occurs when there is aortic neck remodeling and dilatation, which alters the seal zone of the device.[20,27] Comparisons of devices are limited by the different definitions used and by whether only caudal migration of the proximal main trunk is assessed, but migration seems to be lowest with devices that have positive aortic fixation.[28] Also, longer seal zones help protect from catastrophic failure caused by migration.

Obstruction of a limb occurs at varying rates in most devices owing to thrombosis or kinking.[15,29] Early generations of grafts did not have enough external support structure to prevent kinking. Even in the newer grafts, morphologic changes within the AAA can lead to kinking of previously straight limbs, and late secondary procedures are occasionally needed to reopen and expand the graft limb.[24]

Morphologic changes occur in both the aneurysm sac and the aortic neck following endograft placement. Aneurysm sac size has been considered important in evaluating the success of the procedure. Shrinkage of the sac is often regarded as indicative of a successful repair, whereas growth is a cause for concern. However, the rates of sac shrinkage or enlargement vary with the type of graft placed, and as the grafts evolve (new graft materials), these rates will continue to change.[30-32] The clinical implications of sac enlargement may also vary among devices. Sac shrinkage causes a reduction in the length and transverse diameter of the AAA, which can lead to kinking or obstruction of the limbs of the graft. Aortic neck dilatation, most notably at a seal zone or fixation point, can lead to loss of the seal and subsequent migration or type I endoleak.[27] The cause of late increases in neck diameter may be a continuation of the original aneurysmal process or a result of device oversizing, with the continued outward force impacting the structural morphology of the aortic neck.

The infection rate associated with aortic stent-grafts is believed to be lower than that seen with open repair of AAAs. Anecdotal reports of stent-graft infection have implicated septicemic seeding of the endoluminal grafts. There have been few reports looking at primary endograft infection, and this is widely believed to be a rare event.[33]

Endotension is a state of elevated pressure within the aneurysm sac.[22,23] It is generally believed that for endotension to exist, an endoleak must also exist, or there must have been a recently sealed or clotted endoleak. In certain circumstances, pressure could theoretically be transmitted through the graft into the sac, or infection could result in endotension without an endoleak. Currently, the only means of detecting endotension is by noting sac enlargement on a CT scan. This is a crude, indirect method; however, work is currently being done to design micromachine pressure sensors to monitor aneurysm sac pressures.[34]

Sac hygroma is a translucent, highly viscous, gelatinous fluid found in the aneurysm sac after endovascular repair.[35] It results in a state of continued pressurization, even when no endoleak is present. The exact cause and incidence of this entity remain unknown. Originally, fibrinolysis and hyperosmolarity were hypothesized, but in some grafts, it is clear that the fluid is an ultrafiltrate through the graft material. Treatment recommendations vary and include observation, coaxial relining with a second endograft, aspiration, sac fenestration, sac excision, and open conversion.

Device failure usually occurs later in the follow-up period.[33] It can include fabric tears or disintegration, stent fractures, barb or hook fractures, spine fractures, and suture breaks causing separation and dislocation of the structural segments. Many of the newer designs have corrected the early causes of failure. However, the durability of these modified prostheses remains unknown. The full consequences may not become apparent until adequate follow-up is achieved.

Postoperative Surveillance

Surveillance is a key component of endovascular aneurysm therapy, and the compliance of the patient should be considered.[36,37] The postoperative surveillance program allows the identification of endoleaks, sac growth, migration, kinks and bends, and structural graft failure.[38] Through these detection methods, reinterventions can sometimes be performed before catastrophic failure.

Baseline abdominal radiographs are often obtained in multiple views. Abdominal radiographs allow visualization of tortuous areas, bends, and kinks, as well as structural abnormalities involving the attachment system and supporting structures. A baseline CT scan can be obtained within 30 days

of graft implantation. If there is no perigraft flow or endoleak detected, abdominal radiographs and CT scans may be obtained at 6- to 12-month intervals indefinitely. If there is perigraft flow other than a type I or III endoleak, suspicion of an endoleak, or failure of aneurysm sac shrinkage, CT scanning may be done more frequently. In patients with type I or III endoleaks or aneurysm sac enlargement greater than 5 mm, further evaluation and reintervention should be considered (Fig. 22-5). With newer devices and more data on long-term outcomes, it is likely that surveillance intervals will lengthen.

FDA-Approved Devices

ANCURE

The Guidant Ancure bifurcated endograft system is a unibody design (Fig. 22-6), unsupported except at the aortic and iliac attachment sites. The graft was approved on the basis of the comparison of 111 open controls and 573 patients with a 1-year follow-up and 319 patients selected for 5-year follow-up.[39]

Successful implantation was achieved in 531 of the 573 patients (92.7%). Reviewing the 30-day morbidity and mortality rates reveals several benefits in the endograft group. Only 29% of the Ancure group spent time in the intensive care unit, versus 94% of the control group. The operative time was slightly higher (184 vs. 167 minutes), but median blood loss was significantly lower (400 vs. 800 mL). There was no

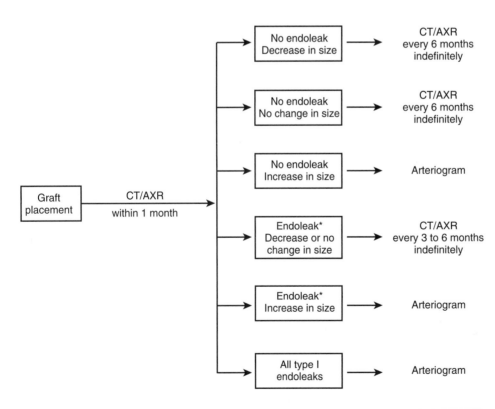

Significant size changes are an area of continuing controversy; however, a 3- to 5-mm diameter change relative to any prior comparable radiologic study may serve as a common theshold.
*Any perigraft flow other than a type I endoleak.

FIGURE 22–5 • Surveillance following endovascular repair of abdominal aortic aneurysm. AXR, abdominal x-ray; CT, computed tomography. (From Eskandari MK, Yao JST, Pearce WH, et al: Surveillance after endoluminal repair of abdominal aortic aneurysms. Cardiovasc Surg 9:469-471, 2001.)

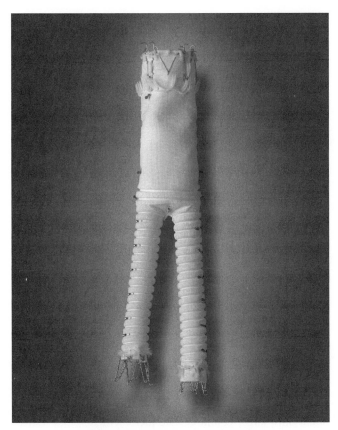

FIGURE 22–6 • Ancure endograft.

statistical difference in mortality at 30 days; however, the trend favored endograft placement (1.7% vs. 2.7%). The largest difference between the endograft and open groups was in the major complication rate, as defined by the investigational device exemption composite risk index. Major events occurred in 28.8% of the endograft group and 44.1% of the control group (P = 0.002), with the open control group experiencing significantly more bleeding, bowel, cardiac, and respiratory complications (P = 0.002), as well as a higher incidence of impotence (P = 0.026).

At 1 year there were no incidents of AAA rupture. Freedom from graft thrombosis (Kaplan-Meier method) was 94.6%, freedom from graft migration was 99.8%, and freedom from postoperative conversion was 99.4%. Unlike with other devices, approximately 30% of patients had intraoperative adjunctive stenting, and 9.8% required a postoperative intervention to treat compromised limb flow.

Five-year outcomes for the 319 endovascular patients and 111 standard open repair patients demonstrate a statistically insignificant trend in survival (68.1% endograft vs. 77.2% open repair) (Fig. 22-7). The causes of death in these two groups were similar. Neither group experienced aneurysm rupture. Nine of the 319 endograft patients (2.8%) underwent late conversion to open repair for endoleak, migration, prosthetic infection, limb occlusion, or aneurysm sac enlargement. Evaluation of aneurysm sac diameter in 42 patients having corelab follow-up demonstrated that 79% of patients had sac shrinkage, 19% had no change, and 2.4% experienced sac enlargement following endograft placement.[40] This rate of sac shrinkage is similar to that achieved with the Zenith graft and higher than that for the original AneuRx and Excluder grafts, both of which modified their graft material in 2004.

Overall, the Ancure graft demonstrates faster procedural recovery with a reduction in short-term morbidity. When the graft is successfully implanted, there are rare late problems requiring open conversion. Long-term mortality is comparable to that of open repair. Unfortunately, the manufacturer has withdrawn this device from the market despite these long-term results.

ANEURX

The AneuRx graft is a modular, bifurcated, woven polyester graft supported with a nitinol exoskeleton (Fig. 22-8). The graft was approved based on a comparison of 66 control patients and 1193 endograft patients. The AneuRx graft was associated with a significant reduction in operative blood loss, decreased transfusion requirements, decreased days in the intensive care unit, earlier return of gastrointestinal function, and earlier time to discharge. There were two intraoperative ruptures (0.17%), and three patients (0.25%) suffered from postoperative aneurysm rupture (<30 days). Major complications were reduced in the stent-graft group compared with the open group when deaths were excluded. The rate

FIGURE 22–7 • Kaplan-Meier graphic representation of freedom from mortality over 60 months. Data for the long-term experimental cohort, excluding patients who underwent immediate conversion to open repair, and for the control group were compared with log rank testing, with 95% confidence intervals noted *(vertical bars).* There are no statistically significant differences between the two groups.

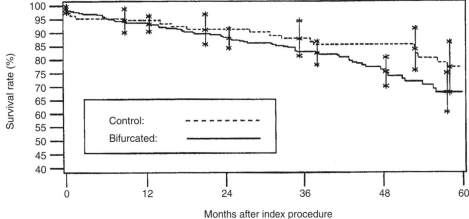

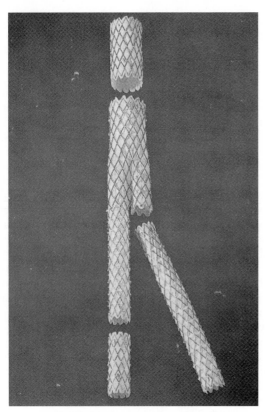

FIGURE 22–8 • AneuRx endograft.

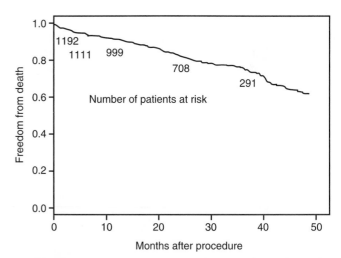

FIGURE 22–9 • Kaplan-Meier analysis of survival after endovascular aneurysm repair. (From Zarins CK, White RA, Moll FL, et al: The AneuRx stent graft: Four-year results and worldwide experience 2000. J Vasc Surg 33:S135-S145, 2001.)

EXCLUDER

The Excluder is a modular endoprosthesis composed of PTFE bonded to a nitinol exoskeleton (Fig. 22-10). This device was evaluated in a multicenter trial of 235 endovascular patients and 99 controls. Of note, the control group had larger aneurysms; larger common iliac measurements; and shorter, wider, more angulated proximal aneurysm necks.[44] There are 4-year controlled data available on this system.

All patients underwent successful aneurysm repair, either open or endograft, based on their assigned group. In the endograft group, 40% of the patients underwent repair with a local or regional anesthetic. Analysis of periprocedural outcomes

of surgical complications (reoperation, secondary procedures in the operating room, secondary endovascular procedures) was 12% with an open procedure and 9% with an endovascular procedure (P = not significant). The rate of medical complications (myocardial infarction, stroke, arrhythmia, renal failure) was 12% in the open group and 3% in the endovascular group ($P < 0.009$). The overall major complication rate was 23% for standard open repair and 12% for endograft repair ($P < 0.03$).[41]

Kaplan-Meier analysis of the endograft group revealed a freedom from AAA rupture of 99.5% at 1 year, 98.5% at 2 years, 98.4% at 3 years, and 98.4% at 4 years. Freedom from surgical conversion was 98.5% at 1 year, 96.9% at 2 years, 94.2% at 3 years, and 90.4% at 4 years.[41,42] The overall 4-year survival rate of the endovascular group was low, at 62.4% (Fig. 22-9). However, it should be noted that this group included high-risk patients. Comparison with the control group beyond 1 year was not done in the AneuRx clinical trial because controls were terminated after 1 year.

The AneuRx trial demonstrated an improved short-term reduction in morbidity and hospital stay when compared with open repair. Based on an analysis of the midterm data, the AneuRx graft is considered a safe, effective option for patients with infrarenal AAAs. The FDA released a notice in December 2003 noting that late AAA-related mortality might exceed that associated with open surgery. It estimated the AAA-related death rates to be 1.9% at 1 year after implantation, 2.2% at 2 years, and 2.7% at 3 years. The notice suggested that the graft be used in patients meeting the appropriate risk-benefit profile who can be treated in accordance with the manufacturer's instructions.[43]

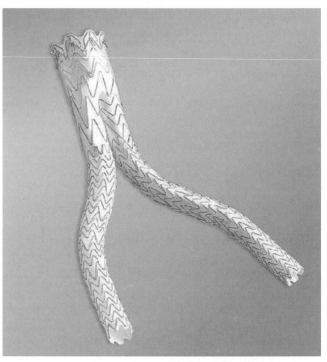

FIGURE 22–10 • Excluder endograft.

demonstrates shorter anesthesia and procedural times (196 vs. 144 minutes; $P < 0.0001$) in the endograft group. The endovascular group had less blood loss (1590 vs. 310 mL; $P < 0.0001$), shorter hospital stay (9.8 vs. 2 days; $P < 0.0001$), and a shorter complete recovery time, defined as time to return of normal activity (42 vs. 92 days; $P < 0.002$).

The endograft group had markedly decreased rates of major adverse events (57% vs. 14%; $P < 0.0001$). There were significant differences in the 30-day major bleeding, pulmonary, cardiac, bowel, and vascular complication rates, all favoring endograft repair. The rates of freedom from minor complications were 66% in endovascular patients and 33% in the control group at 30 days. Including early and late events, freedom from major adverse events favored the endovascular group at 1-year (36% control vs. 67% test group; $P < 0.0001$) and at 4-year follow-up (26% control vs. 34% test group; $P < 0.0001$). Kaplan-Meier survival estimates were 95% in the control group versus 94% in the test group at 1 year; no significant differences were seen using either univariable ($P = 0.13$) or multivariable analysis ($P = 0.388$).[45] At 4 years, survival was 82.4% (95% confidence interval 72.9 to 91.9) in the control group versus 75.8% (95% confidence interval 69.7 to 81.9) in the test group (Fig. 22-11); the trend is not statistically significant by log rank analysis.

Reintervention for endoleak or aneurysm enlargement was performed at rates of 6.4% during the first year, 5.4% during the second year, 3.6% during the third year, and 4.5% during the fourth year. Most reinterventions during the first 4 years were endovascular procedures, but five were open conversions. No aneurysm ruptures occurred over this period.[45] The Excluder has significantly lower rates of aneurysm sac shrinkage than does the Zenith or Ancure graft. At 4 years, 32% of aneurysms enlarged by 5 mm or more compared with baseline.[32]

The Excluder endograft demonstrates a marked reduction in recovery time and complication rates. The adverse event rates continue to favor the endograft group 4 years after repair, even when including reinterventions as adverse events. Survival is similar for open repair at 4 years. Continued follow-up is necessary to assess the durability of this device compared with the standard open repair. The high rate of sac enlargement has prompted a change in the graft material to a less porous composite.

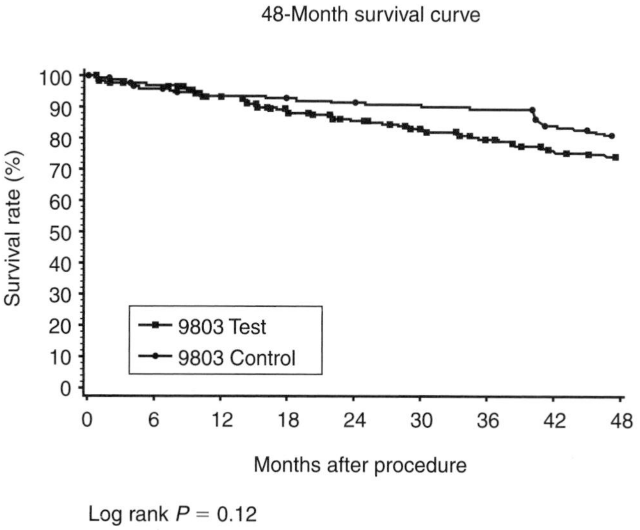

ZENITH

The Zenith endograft is a bifurcated, modular, three-component system (Fig. 22-12). It is made of woven Dacron sutured to stainless steel Z-stents, with a suprarenal stent component with positive fixation at the aortic attachment site. The pivotal trial was a comparison among four groups of patients: a surgical control group ($n = 80$), a roll-in training group ($n = 52$), a standard-risk (SR) group ($n = 200$), and a high-risk (HR) group ($n = 100$).[46]

Of the 352 patients, 351 (99.7%) underwent successful implantation of the endograft. A significantly decreased morbidity at 30 days was noted in cardiac ($P = 0.02$), pulmonary ($P < 0.001$), renal ($P = 0.01$), and vascular ($P < 0.001$) systems in the endograft group. Further, endovascular patients had fewer transfusion requirements, diminished blood loss, shorter hospital stay, shorter intensive care unit stay, and quicker return to daily activities.

Mortality within 30 days ranged from 0.5% to 2% in the stent groups (SR, roll-in, and HR) and was 2.5% in the open surgical control group. All-cause mortality at 12 months was 3.5% in the SR group, 9% in the HR group, 11% in the roll-in group, and 3.8% in the control group. Kaplan-Meier analysis demonstrated no difference in all-cause mortality

48-Month survival curve

Log rank $P = 0.12$

FIGURE 22–11 • Kaplan-Meier curves show subject survival by group. The control group *(circles)* consisted of 99 patients, and the test group *(squares)* consisted of 235 patients ($P = 0.12$).

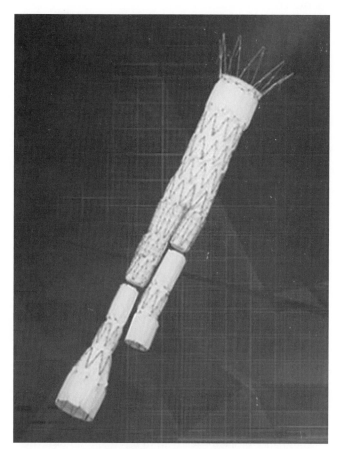

FIGURE 22–12 • Zenith endograft.

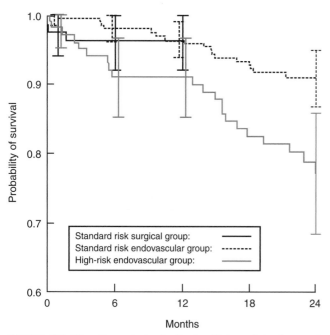

FIGURE 22–13 • Expanded-axis Kaplan-Meier plot of overall survival through 24 months in the standard-risk surgical group *(black line)*, standard-risk endovascular group *(dotted line)*, and high-risk endovascular group *(gray line)*. There was no statistical difference among the groups at 12 months.

and aneurysm-related death between the SR group and the control group (Fig. 22-13).

No acute conversions occurred in the study. Three late conversions were performed: one for endoleak, one for a rapidly expanding supraceliac pseudoaneurysm, and one for rupture at 222 days post procedure. In the last case, there was repressurization of the aneurysm sac following late migration of the iliac limb into the aneurysm. Eleven percent of the SR endograft group required secondary interventions, compared with 2.5% of the control group at 12 months. A decrease of 5 mm or greater was noted in 68% of patients at 12 months, with the rest of the aneurysms remaining stable in size.[46,47] This shrinkage rate is higher than with other endografts. There has been no evidence of renal function deterioration in follow-up as measured by serum creatinine level. Renal infarcts were observed in three patients in the SR group; these were attributed to coverage of accessory renal arteries.

In summary, the Zenith trial demonstrates a similar reduction in morbidity rates and improvement in recovery times. There is a high rate of aneurysm shrinkage at 1 year, and 1-year mortality is similar to that of open repair.

POWERLINK

The PowerLink endograft was approved by the FDA in November 2004. It is a one-piece design incorporating PTFE graft material with a cobalt-chromium stent. The pivotal clinical trial involved an endovascular group with a mean aneurysm sac size of 5.1 cm.[48] Because aneurysm-related death rates correlate with AAA size—6.1% for large aneurysms (>5.5 cm) versus 1.5% for small ones (<5.5 cm)—the vast predominance of small aneurysms in this trial is noteworthy.[49] Publication of the controlled study results is pending.

Endovascular versus Open Repair

In 2001, the lead article in the *British Journal of Surgery* declared the endovascular treatment of abdominal aortic aneurysms a failed experiment.[50] The authors noted poor reporting by individuals placing the grafts, high reintervention rates, prohibitive costs, and the fact that the best candidates for endovascular repair are also the best candidates for open repair.[51] Despite these comments and other reports documenting device structural failure,[52] endoleak,[21] migration,[25] rupture,[53] secondary interventions,[24] and the need for lifelong follow-up,[36,37] patients continue to request the procedure, and physicians continue to perform endovascular aneurysm repair. Various investigators have compared open and endovascular repair of AAAs using single-center experience and multicenter, statewide, and national databases. These databases include FDA-approved endografts, homemade endografts, and devices that never achieved FDA approval. These studies typically review immediate operative and postoperative results and quality-of-life issues.

Early reports from the mid- to late 1990s were underpowered but had similar perioperative mortality rates between the open and endovascular groups, and Kaplan-Meier survival curves did not demonstrate a statistically significant difference.[54,55] Benefits of endovascular repair were most striking in terms of less operative blood loss, shorter hospital stay, and fewer postoperative complications. As the learning curve for endovascular devices improved, centers also noted an overall decrease in operative times, while continuing to confirm the previously noted benefits.[54,56]

Single-institution studies examining the comorbidities of the patients selected for endovascular and open aortic repair demonstrated either that there were minimal differences in their preoperative medical conditions or that the endovascular repair patients suffered from higher rates of pulmonary, cardiac, and renal disease.[44,57] Endovascular AAA repair has also been shown experimentally to decrease the postoperative stress response, with significant differences in epinephrine, cortisol, insulin, and retinol-binding protein levels between the two groups.[58] In early endograft studies, endoluminally treated patients demonstrated better physical and function scores at 1 week after discharge, with an earlier return to baseline function. However, quality-of-life measures were similar after 6 months.[59,60]

Outcome research studies have shown that endovascular repair has good results in the community compared with university centers, where the devices were first tested.[61] In New York State, endovascular repair was associated with improved inpatient mortality rates from 2000 to 2002, decreasing from 3.05% to 0.8%.[55] This rate was statistically different from the open repair mortality rate, which remained at approximately 4.0% during all the measured years. There was also a statistically significant difference favoring endovascular repair in the three most commonly coded morbidities in the New York State hospital discharge database: cardiac complications, pulmonary insufficiency, and posthemorrhagic anemia. The average length of stay was markedly in the favor of endovascular repair (3.6 vs. 10.6 days). The benefits were seen despite the fact that patients undergoing endovascular repair were older and had higher rates of hypertension, coronary artery disease, diabetes mellitus, and hyperlipidemia. In reviewing the 2001 National Inpatient

Sample database, the overall in-hospital mortality rate was significantly less for endovascular repair (1.3%) than for open repair (3.8%).[56] Overall complication rates (open 28.7% vs. endovascular 17.8%) and cardiac complication rates (open 6.9% vs. endovascular 0.3%) were also significantly different. The average length of stay for endovascular repair was 5 days shorter than for open repair, with only 6% of endograft patients needing to go to a care facility other than home, compared with 14% of the open repair group.

The common trends of higher mortality in endograft cohorts compared with open controls in most industry-sponsored controlled studies has raised concerns that a significant difference in late mortality may be missed by smaller studies. Conversely, endovascular cohorts tend to be older, with more comorbidities, and may have better outcomes than expected. The issue requires adequately powered randomized trials, which are now under way.

The Endovascular Aneurysm Repair Trial 1 enrolled and randomized 1082 patients with an average age of 74 years and a mean aneurysm size of 6.5 cm. The early results of this trial demonstrated a short-term survival benefit with endovascular repair, with a 30-day mortality rate of 1.7% versus 4.7% in the open repair group.[62] In-hospital mortality was 2.1% for endovascular repair and 6.2% for open repair. These investigators concluded that the later results of the trial need to be assessed before changing the treatment paradigm of aneurysm repair.

The smaller Dutch Randomized Endovascular Aneurysm Management (DREAM) trial enrolled 345 patients with aneurysms 5 cm or larger. Although not statistically significant, similar point estimates were seen, with a 30-day operative mortality rate of 1.2% in the endovascular group and 4.6% in the open repair group. The combined rate of operative mortality and severe complications in the endovascular group was roughly half that of the open group (4.7% vs. 9.8%).[63] Similar randomized trials in France and the United States are ongoing.

Conclusions

Innovation has characterized endovascular aneurysm repair since its inception and will be necessary for continued improvements in this alternative therapy. Clinical research has clearly identified short-term benefits with endovascular repair, but late problems and specific device failure modes have also been recognized. Optimally, continued study and further engineering of devices will lead to durable endovascular repair, just as 5 decades of research and improvements have led to effective open AAA repair techniques.

KEY REFERENCES

Blum U, Voshage G, Lammer J, et al: Endoluminal stent-grafts for infrarenal abdominal aortic aneurysms. N Engl J Med 336:13-20, 1997.

Carpenter JP (for the Endologix investigators): Multicenter trial of the PowerLink bifurcated system for endovascular aortic aneurysm repair. J Vasc Surg 36:1129-1137, 2002.

Dattilo JB, Brewster DC, Fan CM, et al: Clinical failures of endovascular abdominal aortic aneurysm repair: Incidence, causes, and management. J Vasc Surg 35:1137-1144, 2002.

Eskandari MK, Yao JST, Pearce WH, et al: Surveillance after endoluminal repair of abdominal aortic aneurysms. Cardiovasc Surg 9:469-471, 2001.

EVAR trial participants: Comparison of endovascular aneurysm repair with open repair in patients with abdominal aortic aneurysm (EVAR trial 1), 30-day operative mortality results: Randomised controlled trial. Lancet 364:843-848, 2004.

Greenberg R (on behalf of the Zenith investigators): The Zenith AAA endovascular graft for abdominal aortic aneurysms: Clinical update. Semin Vasc Surg 16:151-157, 2003.

Kibbe MR, Matsumura JS (for the Excluder investigators): The Gore Excluder US multi-center trial: Analysis of adverse events at 2 years. Semin Vasc Surg 16:144-150, 2003.

Moore WS, Matsumura JS, Makaroun MS, et al: Five-year interim comparison of the Guidant bifurcated endograft with open repair of abdominal aortic aneurysm. J Vasc Surg 38:46-55, 2003.

Parodi JC, Palmaz JC, Barone HD: Transfemoral intraluminal graft implantation for abdominal aortic aneurysms. Ann Vasc Surg 5:491-499, 1991.

Prinssen M, Verhoeven ELG, Buth J et al: A randomized trial comparing conventional and endovascular repair of abdominal aortic aneurysms. N Engl J Med 351:1607-1618, 2004.

Veith FJ, Baum RA, Ohki T, et al: Nature and significance of endoleaks and endotension: Summary of opinions at an international conference. J Vasc Surg 35:1029-1035, 2002.

Zarins CK (for the AneuRx clinical investigators): The US AneuRx clinical trial: 6-year clinical update 2002. J Vasc Surg 37:904-908, 2003.

REFERENCES

1. Volodos NL, Shekhanin VE, Karpovich IP, et al: Self-fixing synthetic prosthesis for endoprosthetics of the vessels. Vestn Khir (Russia) 137:123-125, 1986.
2. Parodi JC, Palmaz JC, Barone HD: Transfemoral intraluminal graft implantation for abdominal aortic aneurysms. Ann Vasc Surg 5:491-499, 1991.
3. Ivancev K, Malina M, Lindblad B, et al: Abdominal aortic aneurysms: Experience with the Ivancev-Malmo endovascular system for aorto-monoiliac stent-grafts. J Endovasc Ther 4:242-251, 1997.
4. Ohki T, Veith FJ, Sanchez LA, et al: Varying strategies and devices for endovascular repair of abdominal aortic aneurysms. Semin Vasc Surg 10:242-256, 1997.
5. May J, White GH, Yu W, et al: Concurrent comparison of endoluminal versus open repair in the treatment of abdominal aortic aneurysms: Analysis of 303 patients by the life table method. J Vasc Surg 27:213-221, 1998.
6. Broeders IAMJ, Balm R, Blankensteijn JD, et al: Preoperative sizing of grafts for transfemoral endovascular management: A prospective comparative study of spiral CT angiography, arterial angiography and conventional CT imaging. J Endovasc Surg 4:252-261, 1997.
7. Sternbergh WC, Carter G, York JW, et al: Aortic neck angulation predicts adverse outcome with endovascular abdominal aortic aneurysm repair. J Vasc Surg 35:482-486, 2002.
8. Stanley BM, Semmens JB, Mai Q, et al: Evaluation of patient selection guidelines for endoluminal AAA repair with the Zenith stent-graft: The Australasian experience. J Endovasc Ther 8:457-464, 2001.
9. Albertini J, Kalliafas S, Travis S, et al: Anatomical risk factors for proximal perigraft endoleak and graft migration following endovascular repair of abdominal aortic aneurysms. Eur J Vasc Endovasc Surg 19:308-312, 2000.
10. Schumacher H, Eckstein HH, Kallinowski F, et al: Morphometry and classification in abdominal aortic aneurysms: Patient selection for endovascular and open surgery. J Endovasc Surg 4:39-44, 1997.
11. Rhee RY, Muluk SC, Tzeng E, et al: Can the internal iliac artery be safely covered during endovascular repair of abdominal aortic and iliac artery aneurysms? Ann Vasc Surg 16:29-36, 2002.
12. Schoder M, Zaunbauer L, Holzenbein T, et al: Internal iliac artery embolization before endovascular repair of abdominal aortic aneurysms: Frequency, efficacy, and clinical results. AJR Am J Roentgenol 177:599-605, 2001.
13. Kritpracha B, Pigott JP, Russel TE, et al: Bell-bottom aortoiliac endografts: An alternative that preserves pelvic blood flow. J Vasc Surg 35:874-881, 2002.
14. Carrocio A, Faries PL, Morrissey NJ, et al: Predicting iliac limb occlusions after bifurcated aortic stent grafting: Anatomic and device related causes. J Vasc Surg 36:679-684, 2002.
15. Dawson DL, Hellinger JC, Terramani TT, et al: Iliac artery kinking with endovascular therapies: Technical considerations. J Vasc Interv Radiol 13:729-733, 2002.
16. Abu-Ghaida AM, Clair DG, Greenberg RK, et al: Broadening the applicability of endovascular aneurysm repair: The use of iliac conduits. J Vasc Surg 36:111-117, 2002.

17. Criado FJ, Wilson EP, Abul-Khoudoud O, et al: Brachial artery catheterization to facilitate endovascular grafting of abdominal aortic aneurysm: Safety and rationale. J Vasc Surg 32:1137-1141, 2000.

18. Lachat ML, Pfammatter TH, Witzke HJ, et al: Endovascular repair with bifurcated stent-grafts under local anaesthesia to improve outcome of ruptured aortoiliac aneurysms. Eur J Vasc Endovasc Surg 23:528-536, 2002.

19. Hovsepian DM, Hein AN, Pilgram TK, et al: Endovascular abdominal aortic aneurysm repair in 144 patients: Correlation of aneurysm size, proximal aortic neck length, and procedure related complications. J Vasc Interv Radiol 12:1373-1382, 2001.

20. Blum U, Voshage G, Lammer J, et al: Endoluminal stent-grafts for infrarenal abdominal aortic aneurysms. N Engl J Med 336:13-20, 1997.

21. White GH, May J, Waugh RC, et al: Type II and type IV endoleak: Toward a complete definition of blood flow in the sac after endoluminal AAA repair. J Endovasc Surg 5:305-309, 1998.

22. Veith FJ, Baum RA, Ohki T, et al: Nature and significance of endoleaks and endotension: Summary of opinions at an international conference. J Vasc Surg 35:1029-1035, 2002.

23. Mehta M, Veith FJ, Ohki T, et al: Significance of endotension, endoleak, and aneurysm pulsatility after endovascular repair. J Vasc Surg 37:842-846, 2003.

24. Conner MS, Sternbergh WC, Carter G, et al: Secondary procedures after endovascular aortic aneurysm repair. J Vasc Surg 36:992-996, 2002.

25. Ebaugh JL, Eskandari MK, Finkelstein A, et al: Caudal migration of endoprostheses after treatment of abdominal aortic aneurysm. J Surg Res 107:14-17, 2002.

26. Zarins CK, Bloch DA, Crabtree T, et al: Stent graft migration after endovascular aneurysm repair: Importance of proximal fixation. J Vasc Surg 38:1264-1272, 2003.

27. Sternbergh WC, Money SR, Greenberg RK, et al: Influence of endograft oversizing on device migration, endoleak, aneurysm shrinkage, and aortic neck dilation: Results from the Zenith multicenter trial. J Vasc Surg 39:20-26, 2004.

28. Lee JT, Lee J, Aziz I, et al: Stent-graft migration following endovascular repair of aneurysms with large proximal necks: Anatomical risk factors and long-term sequelae. J Endovasc Ther 9:652-664, 2002.

29. Fransen GAJ, Desgranges P, Laheij RJF, et al: Frequency, predictive factors, and consequences of stent-graft kink following endovascular AAA repair. J Endovasc Ther 10:913-918, 2002.

30. Rhee RY, Garvey L, Missig-Carroll N, Makaroun MS: Does endograft support alter the rate of aneurysm sac shrinkage after endovascular repair? J Endovasc Ther 10:411-417, 2003.

31. Prinssen M, Blankensteijn JD: The sac shrinkage process after EAR does not start immediately in most patients. Eur J Endovasc Surg 23:426-430, 2002.

32. Cho J, Dillavou ED, Rhee RY, et al: Late abdominal aortic aneurysm enlargement after endovascular repair with the Excluder device. J Vasc Surg 39:1236-1242, 2004.

33. Dattilo JB, Brewster DC, Fan CM, et al: Clinical failures of endovascular abdominal aortic aneurysm repair: Incidence, causes, and management. J Vasc Surg 35:1137-1144, 2002.

34. Sonesson B, Dias N, Malina M, et al: Intra-aneurysm pressure measurements in successfully excluded abdominal aortic aneurysm after endovascular repair. J Vasc Surg 33:733-738, 2003.

35. Risberg B, Delle M, Lonn L, et al: Management of aneurysm sac hygroma. J Endovasc Ther 11:191-195, 2004.

36. Eskandari MK, Yao JST, Pearce WH, et al: Surveillance after endoluminal repair of abdominal aortic aneurysms. Cardiovasc Surg 9:469-471, 2001.

37. Fillinger MF: Postoperative imaging after endovascular AAA repair. Semin Vasc Surg 12:327-338, 1999.

38. Thurnher S, Cejna M: Imaging of aortic stent-grafts and endoleaks. Radiol Clin North Am 40:799-833, 2002.

39. Moore WS: The Guidant Ancure bifurcation endograft: Five-year follow-up. Semin Vasc Surg 16:138-143, 2003.

40. Moore WS, Matsumura JS, Makaroun MS, et al: Five-year interim comparison of the Guidant bifurcated endograft with open repair of abdominal aortic aneurysm. J Vasc Surg 38:46-55, 2003.

41. Zarins CK; AneuRx Clinical Investigators: The US AneuRx Clinical Trial: 6-year clinical update 2002. J Vasc Surg 37:904-908, 2003.

42. Zarins CK, White RA, Moll FL, et al: The AneuRx stent graft: Four-year results and worldwide experience 2000. J Vasc Surg 33:S135-S145, 2001.

43. FDA Public Health Notification: Updated data on mortality associated with Medtronic AVE AneuRx stent graft system. Dec 17, 2003.

44. Matsumura JS, Brewster DC, Makaroun MS, Naftel DC: A multicenter controlled clinical trial of open versus endovascular treatment of abdominal aortic aneurysm. J Vasc Surg 37:262-271, 2003.

45. Kibbe MR, Matsumura JS (for the Excluder investigators): The Gore Excluder US multi-center trial: Analysis of adverse events at 2 years. Semin Vasc Surg 16:144-150, 2003.

46. Greenberg R; Zenith Investigators: The Zenith AAA endovascular graft for abdominal aortic aneurysms: Clinical update. Semin Vasc Surg 16:151-157, 2003.

47. Abraham C, Chuter TAM, Reilly LM, et al: Abdominal aortic aneurysm repair with the Zenith stent graft: Short to midterm results. J Vasc Surg 36:217-225, 2002.

48. Carpenter JP; Endologix Investigators: Multicenter trial of the PowerLink bifurcated system for endovascular aortic aneurysm repair. J Vasc Surg 36:1129-1137, 2002.

49. Ouriel K, Srivastava SD, Sarac TP, et al: Disparate outcomes after endovascular treatment of small versus large abdominal aortic aneurysms. J Vasc Surg 37:1206-1212, 2003.

50. Collin J, Murie JA: Endovascular treatment of abdominal aortic aneurysms: A failed experiment. Br J Surg 88:1281-1282, 2001.

51. Hill BB, Wolf YG, Lee WA, et al: Open versus endovascular AAA repair in patients who are morphological candidates for endovascular treatment. J Endovasc Ther 9:255-261, 2002.

52. Rutherford RB, Krupski WC: Current status of open versus endovascular stent-graft repair of abdominal aortic aneurysm. J Vasc Surg 39:1129-1139, 2004.

53. Bernhard VM, Mitchell RS, Matsumura JS, et al: Ruptured abdominal aortic aneurysm after endovascular repair. J Vasc Surg 35:1155-1162, 2002.

54. Zarins CK, White RA, Schwarten D, et al: AneuRx stent graft versus open surgical repair of abdominal aortic aneurysms: Multicenter prospective clinical trial. J Vasc Surg 29:292-308, 1999.

55. Anderson PL, Arons RR, Moskowitz AJ, et al: A statewide experience with endovascular abdominal aortic aneurysm repair: Rapid diffusion with excellent early results. J Vasc Surg 39:10-19, 2004.

56. Lee WA, Carter JW, Upchurch G, et al: Perioperative outcomes after open and endovascular repair of intact abdominal aortic aneurysms in the United States during 2001. J Vasc Surg 39:491-496, 2004.

57. Ligush J, Pearce JD, Edwards MS, et al: Analysis of medical risk factors and outcomes in patients undergoing open versus endovascular abdominal aortic aneurysm repair. J Vasc Surg 36:492-499, 2002.

58. Salartash K, Sternbergh C, York JW, et al: Comparison of open transabdominal AAA repair with endovascular AAA repair in reduction of postoperative stress response. Ann Vasc Surg 15:53-59, 2001.

59. Schermerhorn ML, Finlayson SRG, Fillinger MF, et al: Life expectancy after endovascular versus open abdominal aortic aneurysm repair: Results of a decision analysis model on the basis of data from EUROSTAR. J Vasc Surg 36:1112-1120, 2002.

60. Aquino RV, Jones MA, Zullo TG, et al: Quality of life assessment in patients undergoing endovascular or conventional AAA repair. J Endovasc Ther 8:521-528, 2001.

61. Zarins CK, Shaver DM, Arko FR, et al: Introduction of endovascular aneurysm repair into community practice: Initial results with a new Food and Drug Administration-approved device. J Vasc Surg 36: 226-232, 2002.

62. EVAR trial participants: Comparison of endovascular aneurysm repair with open repair in patients with abdominal aortic aneurysm (EVAR trial 1), 30-day operative mortality results: Randomised controlled trial. Lancet 364:843-848, 2004.

63. Prinssen M, Verhoeven ELG, Buth J, et al: A randomized trial comparing conventional and endovascular repair of abdominal aortic aneurysms. N Engl J Med 351:1607-1618, 2004.

Questions

1. **What is the most important area when evaluating a patient for endovascular aortic aneurysm repair?**
   (a) Iliac vessels
   (b) Aneurysm size
   (c) Proximal aortic neck
   (d) Hypogastric arteries

2. **What is the cause of a type II endoleak?**
   (a) Tear in the graft fabric
   (b) Perigraft flow at the aortic neck
   (c) Porosity of the graft fabric
   (d) Retrograde flow from a patent branch vessel

3. **Which of the following can prevent graft migration?**
   (a) Radial force
   (b) Hooks or barbs
   (c) Proximal aortic seal zone 15 mm or greater
   (d) All of the above

4. **Which type of endoleak is often managed without intervention but with continued monitoring?**
   (a) Type I endoleak
   (b) Type II endoleak with stable aneurysm sac size
   (c) Type II endoleak with enlarging aneurysm sac
   (d) Type III endoleak

5. **Which of the following statements about baseline abdominal radiographs after endograft placement is true?**
   (a) They are unnecessary
   (b) They are used to rule out visceral perforation after endograft repair by looking for free air
   (c) They allow visualization of tortuous areas, bends, kinks, and structural failure or fractures
   (d) They can identify endoleaks

6. **True or false: All endografts cause aneurysm sac shrinkage at equal rates.**

7. **All of the following endografts use a modular system except**
   (a) AneuRx
   (b) PowerLink
   (c) Excluder
   (d) Zenith

8. **Which of the following statements about randomized trials comparing aortic endografts to open aneurysm repair is true?**
   (a) They demonstrate a decreased 30-day mortality
   (b) Patients in the endovascular group have lower rates of heart disease, diabetes mellitus, and hypertension
   (c) They lack randomization and proper controls
   (d) They demonstrate higher short-term morbidity in the endovascular group

9. **Match the technique (a-d) with the anatomic structure(1-4):**
   (a) Highly stenotic iliac arteries   (1) Stiff guidewire
   (b) Common iliac artery ectasia   (2) Internal iliac embolization
   (c) Tortuous iliac arteries   (3) Iliac conduit
   (d) Internal iliac artery aneurysm   (4) Bell-bottom technique

10. **Postoperative endograft surveillance involves which of the following?**
    (a) Lifelong CT scans at 6- to 12-month intervals
    (b) Physical examination alone
    (c) Baseline abdominal radiographs and CT scans at 3-month intervals for 1 year
    (d) Annual CT scans for 2 years

Answers

1. c	2. d	3. d	4. b	5. c
6. false	7. b	8. a	9. a-3, b-4, c-1, d-2	10. a

23

Carlos R. Gracia

Laparoscopic Aortic Surgery for Aneurysms and Occlusive Disease: Technique and Results

Minimally invasive surgical techniques and technologies have been evolving since the introduction of laparoscopic chole-cystectomy in 1989. Laparoscopic surgery has been recognized as beneficial in the performance of a growing number of surgical procedures. The advantages for patients include less postoperative pain, shorter hospital stay, and earlier return to work. Improved postoperative physiologic functions have also been documented.[1,2]

Endoaneurysmorrhaphy with intraluminal graft placement, described by Creech,[3] is the gold standard for abdominal aortic aneurysm (AAA) repair. The mortality rate is less than 5%, but systemic morbidity remains substantial.[4] For most patients with diffuse aortoiliac occlusive disease (AIOD), aorto-bifemoral (ABF) grafts are still the most durable and function-ally effective means of revascularization and should continue to be regarded as the gold standard with which other options are compared.[5] Overall, standard open procedures for AAA repair and AIOD are reliable, with durable results.[6,7] Operative mortality rates of less than 3% are reported, and primary patency rates are greater than 75% at 10 years.[8,9] In spite of this decreasing mortality and overall durability, conventional open procedures are associated with morbidity rates ranging from 10% to 35% owing to the long incision in the midline or flank required for exposure of the abdominal aorta.[10] Incisional hernias develop in more than 10% of midline laparotomies, and postoperative flank bulge is noted in up to 20% of retroperitoneal incisions extended into the intercostal space.[11] In addition, patients experience large fluid shifts, prolonged postoperative ileus, and significant postoperative pain.[12]

Minimally invasive approaches to aortic disease have been developed over the last 10 to 15 years to improve the treat-ment results for both AAA and AIOD. Improvements can be expected to reduce the mortality, morbidity, hospitalization, and costs associated with primary interventions. Improvements should also enhance long-term results, decreasing the need for secondary interventions and their associated morbidity and costs.

Endovascular prostheses were introduced to reduce the perioperative morbidity of AAA repair.[13] Although the early results were dramatically successful,[14-19] there are concerns regarding the midterm and long-term durability of these grafts, and their effectiveness in preventing rupture remains questionable.[20-23] The number of complications continues to increase with longer follow-up, leading to a significant rate of endovascular or surgical revision.[4,23] The reported exclusion rate for endovascular AAA repair is between 40% and 70%, owing to an unsuitable infrarenal neck or iliac artery access with endovascular stent-graft devices.[14,24-26] Until recently, patients not eligible for endovascular prostheses had no other option than to undergo conventional open repair.

Laparoscopic techniques have increasingly been used to overcome these drawbacks of standard open procedures. The objective of laparoscopic aortic surgery is to perform the conventional open repair for AAA and AIOD and achieve the same patency and durability without the associated morbidity. For AAA, the goal is to perform the endoaneurys-morrhaphy described by Creech with minimally invasive techniques and reduced surgical trauma. For AIOD, it must be possible to do both end-to-end and end-to-side aortic anastomoses. However, laparoscopic infrarenal aortic surgery is technically demanding; it requires the development of new skills to work in the two-dimensional, remote world of laparoscopy. Also, one must acquire knowledge of many new instruments and technologies, as well as the physiology encountered during laparoscopy.

Since the introduction of laparoscopic cholecystectomy in 1989, there has been a rapid proliferation of procedures on hollow viscous and solid organs. Although the first reports of laparoscopic aortic surgery were published in 1993, it was not until 2000 that significant numbers of procedures began to be performed. The slowness to adopt minimally invasive surgical techniques for the treatment of aortoiliac disease is due in part to three factors. First is the fact that laparoscopy has grown predominantly within nonvascular fields, limiting the current laparoscopic experience of vascular surgeons. Second, the technically challenging aspects of vascular surgery (exposure, vascular control, vascular occlusion, anastomosis of vessels and grafts, and hemostasis) could not be readily accomplished laparoscopically until 2000, when increasing numbers of laparoscopic vascular instruments began to appear. Third, the major investments (by both industry and surgeons) for technologic developments in minimally invasive vascular therapies have focused on endoluminal therapies. Also, for the last 10 years, industry investment has concentrated on minimally invasive cardiac surgery, not peripheral vascular reconstruction.

History and Development

AORTOILIAC OCCLUSIVE DISEASE

In 1991 and 1992, Dion and colleagues evaluated the possible access to and exposure of the aorta in a porcine model using an abdominal wall lifting device (Laborie Surgical, Ltd., Quebec, Canada). Gasless laparoscopy using an abdominal wall lift was chosen to avoid collapse of the working space if aggressive suction was necessary. It eliminated the risk of venous air embolism in the major venous structures of the retroperitoneum under insufflation. The valveless ports also allowed the insertion of conventional vascular instrumentation (particularly occlusive clamps and needle drivers), given that there were no laparoscopic vascular instruments at the time.

The result of this developmental work was the first application of laparoscopy to aortic reconstructive surgery (ABF bypass) for AIOD in 1993 by Dion and colleagues.[27] Clinical work by Berens and Herde followed.[28] Both groups used a transperitoneal route to the aorta; for dissection, Dion used insufflation, whereas Berens used an abdominal wall lift. Both performed a mini-laparotomy for clamping and a continuous sutured vascular anastomosis—an extremely tedious task. Patients demonstrated improved and shorter postoperative courses as a result of the minimally invasive surgery. Although time-consuming and lengthy, these early laparoscopy-assisted procedures reproduced the standard operative approach for aortoiliac arteriosclerotic occlusive disease. Procedural challenges centered on exposure of the abdominal aorta, which was hampered by the small intestine, which blinds the operative field, and laparoscopic suturing to complete the required anastomoses.

Limitations of the laparoscopy-assisted approach were noted. The variable thickness of the abdominal wall in patients of different sizes was problematic. With greater abdominal wall thickness, the incisions must be larger to maintain exposure. Thus, the advantages of minimizing access trauma were lessened. A completely laparoscopic approach might be more reproducible and overcome the limitations imposed by small incisions, but clamping and suturing are technically demanding, requiring improved instrumentation and laparoscopic suturing skills. The latter were perceived as much too difficult to acquire, although skill acquisition has been consistently demonstrated with appropriate training.[29]

As a result of our own laboratory experience[30-33] and the evaluation of a retroperitoneal approach for a completely laparoscopic ABF bypass in human cadavers, we began our clinical experience in March 1995. The first totally laparoscopic ABF bypass for AIOD using a retroperitoneal approach proved extremely difficult to complete, largely because of the problem of working in a gasless environment. In the second patient, use of insufflation to maintain the retroperitoneal space was a major improvement. Lack of suitable vascular instrumentation was also a significant problem. However, if exposure could be consistently achieved and maintained, and if basic vascular instrumentation for laparoscopy were available, vascular anastomoses could be safely completed in a totally laparoscopic environment without a mini-laparotomy.

These experiences were taken back to the laboratory to try to solve the problems related to exposure. The solution lay in working with the vulnerable area of the anterior peritoneum rather than avoiding it in order not to puncture it. By incising this area anteriorly under the left rectus sheath, a peritoneal "apron" could be constructed.[34] Suspending this apron with transabdominal sutures toward the right of the abdomen served several purposes. Containment of the abdominal viscera was consistent. Cutting the peritoneum in this fashion eliminated the consequences of competitive insufflation of the peritoneal cavity and retroperitoneum. With insufflation of the entire volume of the peritoneal cavity with 5 to 6 L of carbon dioxide, depending on the size of the patient, the working space would not collapse from aggressive suctioning using modern 20- to 30-L/minute insufflators. Finally, because this provided a left anteroloateral approach, as in a direct retroperitoneal approach, excellent visibility of the lumbar arteries was noted. This would later prove beneficial in clipping them during AAA repair, before opening the sac and after cross-clamping.

The apron technique was continually used for ABF bypass for AIOD through 1998. From March 1996 to May 1998, a total of 14 patients (11 men and 3 women) aged 42 to 76 years (mean age, 58 years) were operated on with the apron technique. The first three cases using this technique were reported,[34] followed by an additional seven cases, all completed with end-to-end anastomoses.[35] Indications for surgery in all cases were incapacitating claudication (ankle-brachial index < 0.60) with AIOD. All 14 patients had completed laparoscopic ABF bypass with 10 end-to-end anastomoses and 4 end-to-side anastomoses. Improvement in overall surgical times continued, with a range of 245 to 510 minutes (average, 367 minutes). Mean aortic cross-clamp time was 111 minutes (range, 65 to 189 minutes). Cross-clamp times also varied depending on whether additional reconstruction was required at the femoral or deep femoral vessels. Aortic anastomotic times ranged from 22 to 155 minutes (mean, 65 minutes). All anastomoses were completed with intracorporeal laparoscopic suturing using continuous running monofilament suture. The average amount of fluid administered was 6482 mL (range, 4000 to 8500 minutes).

AORTIC ANEURYSM

The successful application of minimally invasive surgical techniques to aneurysms is challenging. The earliest work on laparoscopic aortic aneurysm repair was reported by Chen and associates.[36] Endoluminal grafts were inserted by aortotomy and secured extraluminally by umbilical tapes. There were 15 successful graft insertions in 21 pigs undergoing transabdominal dissection of the aorta. Six were unsuccessful because of technical, anatomic, or bleeding difficulties. A retroperitoneal approach was attempted in two cases, but only one was successful; the other failed owing to a tear in the peritoneum. Operative time decreased from 6 to less than 2 hours, with a concomitant decrease in estimated blood loss from 1000 to less than 150 mL with experience.

Following these experiments, Chen and colleagues successfully completed laparoscopy-assisted repair of infrarenal AAA in humans.[36] The first case was performed with 10 trocars and a 10-cm mini-laparotomy. The approach was transabdominal, and bowel retraction was facilitated by a modified "fish" retractor for the special task. Decreased operative fluid requirements and early mobilization of fluids were observed, along with a more rapid return of bowel function and an earlier discharge. Kline and coworkers have since simplified the approach, further reducing the number of trocars and the operative time.[37] These experiments and the work of others have contributed to the feasibility of performing laparoscopic aortic surgery, whether totally laparoscopic or laparoscopy-assisted. Other studies confirm that laparoscopic AAA repair is possible.[38,39]

The endoaneurysmorrhaphy technique of suturing a graft in place with an intact back wall was completed totally laparoscopically in the laboratory.[40] Lumbar vessels were controlled intraluminally as well as extraluminally. In these attempts to develop minimally invasive surgical techniques to approach an aneurysm, one must recognize the limitations of animal models, such as the lack of an aneurysmal mass or calcification in the wall. Without this mass, the dissection is simpler, and without the calcification, there is no risk of distal embolization.

In April 1999, a 67-year-old woman with a 4.6-cm infrarenal AAA and rest pain from atherosclerotic iliac occlusive disease underwent the first reported totally laparoscopic aortic aneurysm resection with an ABF bypass.[41] Surgery lasted 230 minutes, with an aortic cross-clamp time of 76 minutes; the aortic anastomosis required 22 minutes to complete. Intraoperatively, the patient received a total of 4500 mL of crystalloid. No intraoperative transfusion was required, with a blood loss of 450 mL. Postoperatively, the patient recovered with no complications and was discharged home on the seventh postoperative day.

Percutaneous placement of endoluminal stent-grafts is directed at avoiding the morbidity and mortality associated with major abdominal surgery. Despite the technical success achieved in the majority of cases, endovascular grafts require a high degree of skill for implantation and are subject to complications. In a phase I trial, May reported a vascular complication rate of 10% for a tube graft, which rose to 43% for a bifurcated endovascular graft.[41a] In another phase I trial with 46 patients, Moore reported contrast enhancement outside the graft but within the aneurysmal sac in 17 grafts (44%), of which 9 (51%) resolved spontaneously.[41b] Hospital stay varied between 1 and 14 days. Uncontrolled lumbar vessels and endoleaks have raised concern over continued aneurysmal growth and risk of rupture.

Technologic improvements and additional clinical experience with endoluminal graft placement have improved the results achieved with endoluminal stent-grafts. Recent U.S. Food and Drug Administration approval of endoluminal devices in the United States has also changed the environment for minimally invasive aortic aneurysm repair. The numbers of patients undergoing repair with endoprostheses will steadily rise, providing more data for follow-up. An interesting approach to the treatment of AAA may be to combine laparoscopic and endovascular techniques. This may help solve many of the challenging problems encountered in the performance of each of these techniques alone.

Approaches to the Aorta

RETROPERITONEAL APPROACH

Gasless laparoscopy with an abdominal wall lift is not being used by the leading centers performing laparoscopic aortic surgery. In that technique, a mechanical retraction system creates a tent-shaped suspension with limited intra-abdominal working space.[42] This cannot compete with insufflation for exposure of the operative field. Insufflation, whether intraperitoneal or retroperitoneal, provides a dome-shaped exposure with a wider instrumental range of motion. Nearly all major centers and reports are using standard carbon dioxide insufflation to establish and maintain a working space, whether the procedure is totally laparoscopic or laparoscopy-assisted.

Approaching the aorta by the retroperitoneal approach would appear to be an ideal way to contain the abdominal viscera, as in the open retroperitoneal approach. Some authors indicate that extraperitoneal insufflation results in less cardiovascular impairment than does intraperitoneal insufflation.[43,44] However, the retroperitoneal approach involves several challenges. The first is creation of the retroperitoneal space. This dissection can be accomplished by a small 1- to 1.5-cm incision just lateral and superior to the left anterior superior iliac crest. The extraperitoneal space is identified, and with gentle, blunt dissection, a bladeless 10-mm trocar is inserted. With carbon dioxide insufflation of 10 to 12 mm Hg, a large retroperitoneal space can be created by continuous blunt dissection with a 0-degree, 10-mm laparoscope under direct vision while insufflating.[34] This establishes a pneumoretroperitoneum. A similar space can be dissected by the insertion and inflation of balloon dissectors.[45,46]

The retroperitoneal approach can expose a space extending proximally to the left renal vein and distally to the inguinal ligament on the left and the iliac bifurcation on the right. This would appear to be an ideal approach, with the small bowel fully compartmentalized within the peritoneal cavity. However, there are several problems. The first is that the retroperitoneal space is rather small, requiring 2 to 2.5 L of carbon dioxide to insufflate. When using a suction cannula, it does not take much suction to collapse the space. This can be a major problem in the event of bleeding; collapse of the space will seriously diminish exposure when it is most needed. Similarly, the smaller space and gas volume are more sensitive to leaks at trocar sites in the skin or when inserting or removing instruments and sutures, with the same result as suctioning.

There is also the problem of competitive insufflation between the retroperitoneal space and the peritoneal cavity. A tear in the peritoneum will leak air and may not be visible. If the tear is large, it may not be repairable, and the retroperitoneal space will collapse from the increasing intraperitoneal pressure. A large hole will also permit the small bowel to enter the retroperitoneal space, eliminating the advantage of keeping the small bowel away from the operative field. A small hole may be controlled with a simple, preformed, laparoscopic loop. This requires that another trocar already be safely in place to insert the loop. Finding the small hole and controlling it while the space is collapsing from increasing intraperitoneal insufflation are difficult tasks. Finally, even if the peritoneum is not violated, the anterior portions of the peritoneum under the rectus border are very thin. Over time, the carbon dioxide will diffuse across the peritoneum and fill the peritoneal cavity, and the retroperitoneal space will begin to collapse from the rising intraperitoneal pressure. A Veress needle can be placed in the peritoneal cavity to vent the intraperitoneal gas. This works with varying degrees of success.

The retroperitoneal approach provides limited working space internally without the dome-shaped cavity of the pneumoperitoneum, or externally for the placement of trocars.[46,47] Despite this, the retroperitoneal approach can provide very good exposure of the aorta. It is best reserved for limited work around the aorta, such as the clipping of lumbar arteries responsible for endoleaks, as described by Wisselink and coworkers.[48]

TRANSPERITONEAL APPROACH

The transperitoneal approach is a straightforward approach via the anterior abdominal wall directly into the peritoneal space. The problem with this approach is the difficulty in bowel retraction. Both Dion and colleagues[27] and Berens and Herde[28] noted in their first reports the major difficulties in maintaining retraction of the small bowel. Although the small bowel occupies less space as a result of the three-dimensional compressing effect of carbon dioxide under normal working pressures (12 to 15 mm Hg), it is still very difficult to keep it out of the operative field.[49]

During intraperitoneal laparoscopy, there are several options to provide retraction of the small bowel. The most useful is gravity with the Trendelenburg or reverse Trendelenburg position or lateral rotation left or right, depending on the direction one wishes to direct the small bowel. However, unlike in pelvic surgery or foregut surgery, where the extreme Trendelenburg or reverse Trendelenburg position is very effective in removing the small bowel from the operative field, this is not the case as one moves up the proximal infrarenal aorta. Another technique is to insert additional trocars as needed to place additional graspers to gently hold the bowel or to insert specific retracting devices.[37,50,51]

With a transperitoneal approach, it is usually necessary to use 30 degrees or more of the Trendelenburg position.[46,51,52] Prolonged increased intra-abdominal pressure by the pneumoperitoneum may have adverse effects on cardiopulmonary, intestinal, and hepatorenal function,[53,54] Although these effects are reportedly lessened by Trendelenburg positioning,[44] it appears that this is not well tolerated by patients undergoing laparoscopic aortic surgery by either the transperitoneal[49] or retroperitoneal[46] approach. It is not necessary to use as much Trendelenburg with a transperitoneal approach if an intraperitoneal retractor is used to contain the small bowel.[55]

OTHER APPROACHES

The modified retroperitoneal approach is to approach the retroperitoneum by a transabdominal route. This evolved out of efforts to overcome the problems with both the transperitoneal and the retroperitoneal approaches. There are three basic options in proceeding with a modified retroperitoneal approach. The first is the apron technique as originally described by Dion and Gracia.[34] The other is a transabdominal paracolic approach described by Said.[46] The final is a modification of the transabdominal paracolic approach—the transabdominal retrorenal approach described by Coggia.[56]

The apron technique was developed to provide stable retraction of the small bowel to expose and operate on the infrarenal aorta. The work that led to this technique was done with a transperitoneal mini-laparotomy-assisted approach. Both the transperitoneal approach and the mini-laparotomy made it difficult to perform ABF procedures, for the reasons previously described. The retroperitoneal approach had its own challenges, also described previously. Incision of the anterior peritoneum connected the transperitoneal and retroperitoneal spaces. If the peritoneum is incised very anteriorly, under the left rectus border, it can be pulled across the peritoneal cavity, with sutures placed through the anterior abdominal wall to suspend this "apron." This creates a natural sling that compartmentalizes the abdomen and contains the abdominal viscera.

There are several advantages to the apron technique. At the beginning of the procedure, transperitoneal access allows diagnostic laparoscopy. A larger retroperitoneal cavity is made with the apron technique than by a direct retroperitoneal approach, providing more working room. A larger volume of carbon dioxide insufflation is possible, thus insufflating the entire abdomen and making the space more resistant to collapse with suction. In fact, during suctioning or any other cause of decreasing insufflation pressure, the apron will seal itself against the anterior abdominal wall more securely as the anterior wall falls owing to the diminished pressure. This avoids the small bowel overcoming the retraction and falling into the operative field at the worst possible moment. The abdominal viscera are easier to retract with simple fan retractors because the peritoneum has no slits or fingers that the bowel can push through. The other advantages are at the end of the procedure, when it is possible to observe the left colon and check its viability after aortic surgery. Finally, with cessation of insufflation, the abdominal pressure returns to normal, as does the abdominal girth. The peritoneum of the apron lays back against the retroperitoneum and abdominal wall, providing coverage of the entire prosthetic vascular graft.

Positioning of the patient is less extreme with the apron technique, requiring only a 10-degree Trendelenburg position,[34] with the table tilted slightly to the right. In my early experience,[34] no adverse hemodynamic effects or elevation of blood carbon dioxide levels was observed. Intraoperative monitoring with transesophageal echocardiography was used in some patients. There were no changes in cardiac performance noted during the procedure, and only minimal hemodynamic alterations were observed after unclamping the aortic. Patients undergoing ABF bypass by a totally laparoscopic technique with the apron were also observed to require less intraoperative crystalloid infusion compared with open surgery.

The transabdominal paracolic approach does not require the sectioned left paracolic peritoneum to be sutured to the abdominal wall to keep the contents of the abdominal cavity off the aorta. Instead, it relies largely on gravity to displace intra-abdominal organs from the operative field by using a steep tilting of the patient to the right side.

The transabdominal retrorenal approach is indicated when a transabdominal left paracolic approach is not possible, as in the case of very thin patients or those with previous left colon or kidney surgery, where dissection along Toldt's membrane is difficult or impossible. The transabdominal retrorenal approach allows a larger working space, both externally for the placement of trocars and internally with the dome-shaped cavity of the pneumoperitoneum. Dissection can be continued above the renal arteries with the use of a complete right medial visceral rotation. It is useful when suprarenal clamping is needed. Totally laparoscopic superior mesenteric artery bypass has been done with this approach.[57]

Techniques

There are two basic techniques of performing laparoscopic aortic surgery: totally laparoscopic and laparoscopy-assisted. Laparoscopy-assisted techniques can be subdivided into mini-laparotomy and hand-assisted laparoscopy. Descriptions of the different laparoscopic techniques are not standardized, which generates confusion when reviewing results from different centers. Table 23-1 offers a standard nomenclature for the different laparoscopic techniques and identifies their components. These techniques can be combined with one of three different anatomic approaches to the aorta: transperitoneal, retroperitoneal, or modified retroperitoneal.

TOTALLY LAPAROSCOPIC APPROACH

Apron Technique

The patient is placed in a supine position. A padded gel roll is placed under the patient's left flank to elevate it and provide adequate access to the lateral abdominal wall. The right arm is preferentially tucked at the side, and the left arm is placed out at 90 degrees. The patient is then prepped and draped in the usual standard fashion to expose the entire abdomen and groins (Fig. 23-1).

A carbon dioxide pneumoperitoneum is instituted via an umbilical site to an intraperitoneal pressure of 14 mm Hg, followed by placement of a 10-mm trocar (trocar 1; Fig. 23-2). Trocars 2 and 3 (see Fig. 23-2) are then inserted under direct vision after first examining the peritoneal cavity. The retroperitoneal dissection is started at the site of trocar 4 (see Fig. 23-2), located 1.5 cm both medial and superior to the anterior superior iliac crest. Using S-retractors, a muscle-splitting 1.5-cm opening is made through the various layers of the lateral abdominal wall to identify the preperitoneal space. With gentle, blunt finger dissection, a small retroperitoneal space is created; the left iliac artery is commonly palpated, providing a useful landmark.

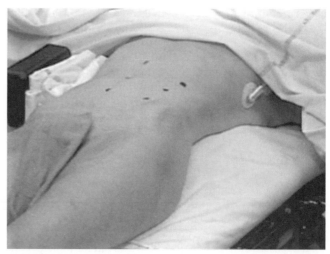

FIGURE 23–1 • The patient is positioned supine on the operating table, allowing simultaneous access to the abdomen and groins. A padded gel roll is placed under the patient's left flank to elevate it and provide adequate access to the lateral abdominal wall.

A 12-mm trocar is bluntly inserted into this retroperitoneal space and insufflated after releasing the prior intraperitoneal insufflation. With 12 mm Hg pressure, blunt dissection is performed with a 0-degree laparoscope to gently dissect the now crepitant retroperitoneal areolar tissue and create a large hemostatic retroperitoneal space. The best landmark is the left external iliac artery; this is followed to the common iliac artery and ureter, which is left posteriorly on the psoas muscle to avoid injury. The aorta is commonly seen pulsating as one dissects medially and superiorly. Dissection is carried cephalad and laterally under the lateral aspect of Gerota's fascia to mobilize the kidney (Fig. 23-3).

Intraperitoneal insufflation is now restored, and the peritoneum is cut to form the apron. Using the midline ports (numbered 1 to 3; see Fig. 23-2), the peritoneum is cut anteriorly under the lateral border of the rectus abdominis muscle from the point where the inferior epigastric vessels cross under the lateral border of the rectus abdominis to the costal margin. After it is cut, the peritoneum is mobilized laterally, connecting the intraperitoneal cavity with the previous retroperitoneal dissection. Dissection in the correct plane between the peritoneum and the posterior fascia proceeds quickly and hemostatically. The trocars numbered 5 and 6 (see Fig. 23-2) are inserted. It is also important to mobilize the peritoneum cephalad to above the costal margin in order to place trocar 7 in the best location for application of the aortic cross-clamp.

The peritoneal apron is now suspended to function as a retractor. It is sutured at its incised upper edge to the three

TABLE 23–1	Laparoscopic Techniques and Their Components					
Technique	**Dissection**	**Control**	**Clamping**	**Anastomosis**	**Instruments**	**Visualization**
Laparoscopy-assisted	Lap	Lap	Incision	Incision	Open	Direct
Laparoscopy-guided	Lap	Lap	Lap	Incision	Mixed	Scope
Hand-assisted laparoscopic	Lap	Lap	Lap	Lap	Lap	Scope
Totally laparoscopic	Lap	Lap	Lap	Lap	Lap	Scope

Lap, laparoscopic.

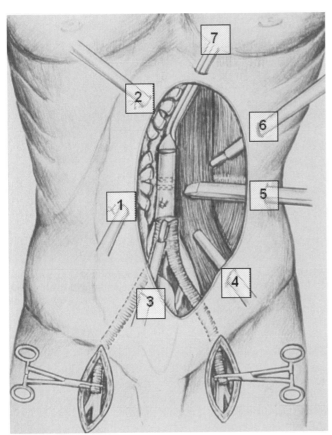

FIGURE 23–2 • Trocar sites and their order of insertion. Retraction is provided by fans behind the "apron" in trocars 1 and 2 (both 10 mm). The assistant uses port 3 (5 mm), and the surgeon uses ports 4, 5, and 6 (all 12 mm). The advantage of having all lateral 12-mm trocars is that endomechanicals or sutures can be inserted via any of these ports, depending on what is required. A vascular graft can also be readily inserted through a 12-mm trocar. The cross-clamp is placed through port 7, which is transrectus and as close to the midline as possible, providing an excellent angle for application in an anteroposterior direction. The DeBakey-style clamp can be advanced directly onto the spine, which is readily palpated as in open surgery, to ensure complete clamping across the aorta.

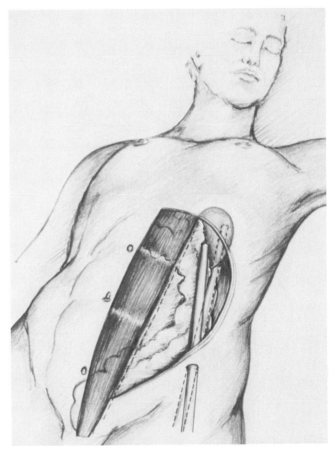

FIGURE 23–3 • Blunt scope dissection into the retroperitoneum. Dissection is continued cephalad and posterior to the left kidney. The correct landmark in this dissection is the left iliac artery; it is identified and followed up to the ureter, leaving it on the psoas muscle. The dissection is then continued medially and cephalad, as pictured here.

midline trocars. Using the lateral trocars, 0-nylon suture in a straight needle is placed through-and-through the abdominal wall behind each of the midline trocars. This needle is grasped and sutured through the upper cut edge of the peritoneum before being passed back through the abdominal wall. This creates a suspension suture that holds the peritoneal apron behind each midline trocar (Fig. 23-4). The midline trocars are now directed and remain behind the apron in the retroperitoneal space.

Two fan retractors are inserted through trocars 1 and 2 and behind the apron. The weight of the abdominal viscera contained behind the apron requires some retraction. It does not require forceful retraction, however, and only 100 degrees of Trendelenburg is required. The retractors are then fixed to an external fixation device secured to the rails of the operating table (Omni-Tract, Minnesota Scientific, Minneapolis, Minn.).

In this technique, the surgeon works from the patient's left while the assistant works from the right. This left anterolateral approach provides excellent visualization of the posterior aorta. Lumbar arteries can be clipped or divided as necessary

to mobilize the aorta for the site of anastomosis (Fig. 23-5). The seventh and final trocar, which is for the aortic cross-clamp, is inserted in a transrectus position (see Fig. 23-2). The trocar through which the laparoscopic aortic clamp is inserted stabilizes it into position (Fig. 23-6).

Upon completion of the procedure, the transabdominal apron sutures are removed, and the peritoneum is allowed to fall back into place. As the pneumoperitoneum is released, the peritoneum comes back to lie in its normal position and completely covers the prosthetic graft material. Trocar sites of 10 mm or greater should be closed to avoid bleeding or trocar site hernias.

Retrocolic Technique

Because this is a transabdominal approach to the retroperitoneum, there are a few similarities with the apron technique. This is a frontal approach, with the surgeon on the right side of the patient and the assistant on the left. This allows easier access for dissection of the right side of the aorta in the interaorticocaval space.

The patient is placed in a right lateral and rotated decubitus position, with the abdomen rotated at 45 degrees; an additional 20 degrees is provided by tilting the operating room table, for maximum lateral rotation of 65 degrees (Fig. 23-7).

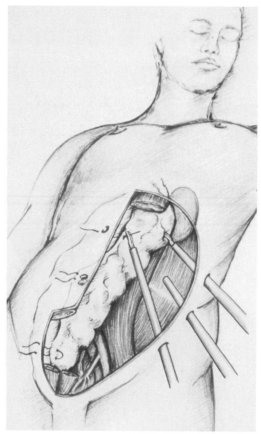

FIGURE 23–4 • Suspension of the peritoneal apron. A suture of 0 nylon on a straight needle is placed through-and-through the abdominal wall behind each of the midline trocars. This needle is grasped and sutured through the upper cut edge of the peritoneum before being passed back through the abdominal wall. This creates a suspension suture that suspends the peritoneal apron behind each midline trocar.

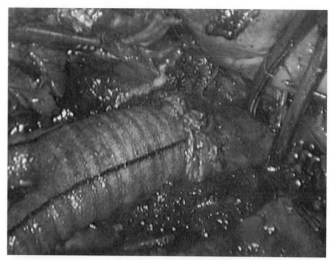

FIGURE 23–6 • Intraoperative photograph of a completed end-to-end anastomosis of a bifurcated Hemashield graft to the infrarenal aorta. The aortic cross-clamp has just been opened following conventional flushing techniques.

The surgeon is facing the patient's abdomen. The camera trocar is positioned through a 10-mm trocar introduced on the anterior axillary line 3 cm below the costal margin.

Figure 23-8 shows the position of the other trocars. A left retrocolic dissection is conducted along Toldt's fascia until the left renal vein is seen. The extreme right lateral decubitus position allows the small bowel and left mesocolon to fall to the right side of the abdomen (see Fig. 23-7). Exposure and dissection of the infrarenal aorta, on both its right and left sides, are now possible, extending down to the right and left common iliac arteries.

If exposure to the groins is required after dissection of the aorta and iliac arteries, the operating table is rotated to the left. This provides a conventional approach to the femoral arteries. When the vascular prosthesis is ready to be introduced into the abdomen and preparations are being made for cross-clamping the aorta, the operating table is placed in

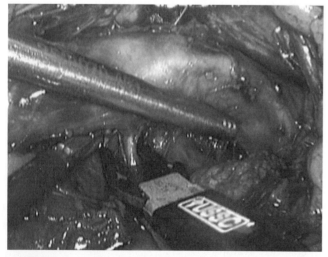

FIGURE 23–5 • The left anterolateral approach provides excellent visualization of the posterior aorta. Lumbar arteries can be clipped or divided as necessary to mobilize the aorta for the site of anastomosis. Generally, no more than one or two pairs require clipping or division.

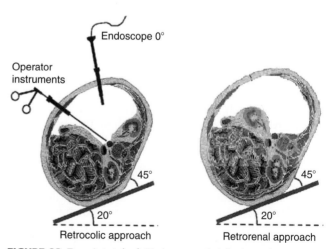

FIGURE 23–7 • A total of 65 degrees of right lateral rotation is provided for both the retrocolic and the retrorenal approaches to the aorta. The small bowel, left mesocolon, and spleen (retrorenal) drop into the right part of the abdomen, providing a stable exposure of the infrarenal and suprarenal (retrorenal) aorta.

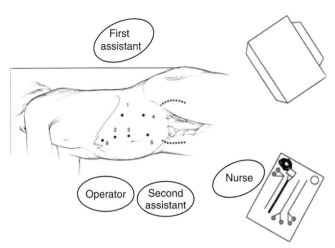

FIGURE 23–8 • Patient positioning for totally laparoscopic transabdominal retrocolic approach. The surgeon stands on the patient's right and the first assistant on the left. Trocar locations are identified as follows: 1, 10-mm trocar for laparoscope; 2 and 3, 10-mm trocars for operator instruments; 4, 5-mm trocar for suction and irrigation; 5 and 6, 10-mm trocars for proximal and distal coelioscopic aortic clamps.

maximal right rotation. As with any totally laparoscopic approach, the vascular prosthesis is delivered through one of the larger trocars.

This approach does not require retraction techniques to keep the viscera from falling into the operative field.[34,50] Instead, gravity is used as a retractor, providing a stable aortic exposure for dissection, control, and performance of the laparoscopic aortoprosthetic anastomosis. However, the extreme lateral rotation of the patient can cause difficulties, because movement of the left kidney toward the median line with lateral rotation may hamper the exposure. Construction of the anatomic tunnel for the right prosthetic limb may also be difficult, especially in obese patients.

Retrorenal Technique

A transperitoneal left retrorenal approach may be used when the left retrocolic approach is not possible. This may be the case in very thin patients or when prior surgery of the colon or kidney makes it difficult or impossible to dissect along Toldt's fascia. The patient positioning and trocar locations

are the same as for the retrocolic approach. Left retrorenal dissection is performed cranially and medially from the psoas muscle after incision of the retrorenal fascia. A complete right medial visceral rotation is performed, if necessary, so that dissection can be continued above the renal arteries. The small bowel, left mesocolon, left kidney, and spleen drop into the right part of the abdomen owing to the extreme lateral rotation (see Fig. 23-7). Maintenance of exposure can be aided with a retractor introduced through the subxiphoid port. The venous renal-azygos-lumbar trunk is divided to provide complete retraction of the kidney and permit dissection of the juxtarenal aorta. This is useful when suprarenal clamping is needed.

HAND-ASSISTED LAPAROSCOPY

Hand-assisted laparoscopy facilitates and accelerates complex laparoscopic operations, reduces the conversion rate to open surgery when total laparoscopic procedures are performed, and is superior to any mini-incision surgery in which a midline laparotomy is required.[58,59] The HandPort (Smith & Nephew Surgical, Andover, Mass.) enables the surgeon to use his or her hand while maintaining the pneumoperitoneum (Fig. 23-9). The protector-retractor device has an open-ended cylinder with a flexible ring at each end. One ring is inserted through the incision into the peritoneal cavity, and the other remains outside the incision. The retractor holds the incision open. The surgeon can introduce his or her nondominant hand through the HandPort mini-incision into the abdominal cavity to help in the dissection and exposure and for palpation and retraction.

Hand-assisted laparoscopy for aortic surgery is done via transperitoneal access and a midline mini-incision of 6 to 7 cm. Kolvenbach and coauthors reported using both the HandPort device and the Omniport (Advanced Surgical Concepts, Dublin).[58,60] The pneumoperitoneum is created, and a 10-mm trocar is inserted at the umbilicus. The incision for the HandPort is made after tracing the size of the incision on the abdominal wall with the abdomen insufflated. This provides an incision of minimal size, an airtight fit, and optimal planning in the placement of the ports.

The aorta is exposed using laparoscopic instruments and the surgeon's hand (see Fig. 23-9). Exposure is facilitated by placing the patient in a 60-degree Trendelenburg position and tilting the table to the right. Hand-assisted laparoscopy

FIGURE 23–9 • *A,* Illustration of hand inserted via a hand-assist device to palpate the aorta and retract the bowel in order to guide the dissection. The nondominant hand is inserted so that the dominant hand can manipulate the handle of the laparoscopic instrument. *B,* Insertion of a hand via a hand-assist device in an actual clinical case.

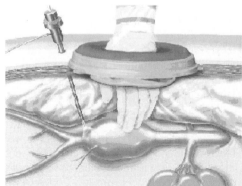

A

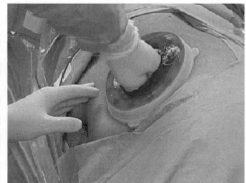

B

permits digital exploration of the aorta to determine the optimal sites for placing the clamp and for performing the proximal anastomosis.[61] Upon completion of the aortoiliac dissection, the protector-retractor device is removed, and two narrow, 2.5-cm blades of a conventional retractor can be inserted to retract the mini-incision. A conventional aortic cross-clamp is introduced through a 1-cm stab incision in the epigastrium. The anastomosis can be sutured using conventional instruments with access through the mini-incision.

In the presence of iliac artery aneurysms, the distal iliac anastomosis can also be performed through the mini-incision. If this cannot be accomplished under direct vision via the mini-incision, Kolvenbach and colleagues described a video-guided approach with conventional instruments and a gasless technique.[60] Conventional needle holders can be passed through the mini-incision, guided by the laparoscopic image on the monitor. Alternatively, two oblique incisions can be made above the inguinal ligament, and an anastomosis with the external iliac artery can be completed after stapler occlusion of both common iliac arteries, as described by Edoga and associates.[62]

The mini-incision for the hand-assist device must be placed strategically to minimize wound-related problems. It is widely recognized in open surgery that upper abdominal incisions can compromise ventilatory function and cause significant pain. There is a reported 30% incidence of ventral hernias in aneurysm patients undergoing open surgery, and ventral hernias developed in 18.7% of laparoscopic patients at the site where the hand-assist device was inserted. Although the incidence of ventral hernia is lower than that for open surgery, the benefit of minimally invasive access is lost if the patient requires reoperation for abdominal wall problems.

Kolvenbach and Ferrari noted that this 18.7% incidence of wound problems may have been exacerbated by the use of self-retaining retractors and the resulting transient tissue and muscle ischemia.[63] For this reason, the procedure is now performed completely laparoscopically under the pneumoperitoneum rather than working through the mini-incision with abdominal wall lift or retractors. It is recommended that a low transverse Pfannenstiel incision or a mini-incision be made in the left lower flank region (Fig. 23-10). By doing so, an overall reduction in wound-related problems to less than 2% can be achieved.[63] If a surgeon still chooses to perform the aortic anastomosis by direct suture through the mini-incision, a low transverse position for the hand-assist device does not compromise the ability to suture directly.

Hand-assisted laparoscopic aortic surgery is a safe and expeditious technique that can be performed almost as rapidly as open surgery.[58] The surgeon's hand is used to palpate, dissect, and retract while taking full advantage of the three-dimensional expansion of carbon dioxide insufflation. The new generation of hand-assist devices permits a laparoscopic aortic anastomosis to be performed expeditiously, with a faster learning curve than that associated with a total laparoscopic procedure. Rather than working with laparoscopic needle holders, a conventional and familiar needle holder introduced through the port can facilitate this part of the operation. The Omniport is an example of a new surgical device that can assist in performing advanced laparoscopic procedures such as aortoiliac reconstructions. It allows hand-assist techniques in a completely laparoscopic environment, preserving the surgeon's tactile feedback.

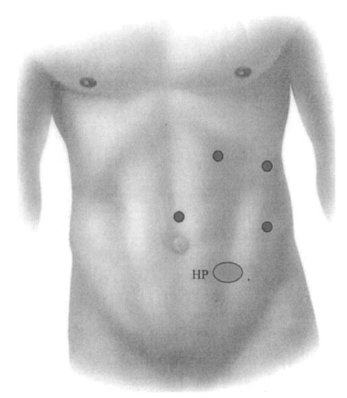

FIGURE 23–10 • Position of hand-assist device (HP) in the left lower abdomen for laparoscopic abdominal aortic aneurysm repair.

LAPAROSCOPY-ASSISTED TECHNIQUES

Laparoscopy-assisted techniques use laparoscopy to explore the abdominal cavity, accurately dissect the aorta, and place occlusive clamps. Alimi and coworkers found a mini-laparotomy to be beneficial when performing a laparoscopic aortoaortic or aortofemoral bypass for the treatment of AIOD and AAA, resulting in the performance of a faster aortoprosthetic anastomosis and decreased cross-clamp time compared with a totally laparoscopic technique.[64] The 5- to 8-cm mini-laparotomy is performed before cross-clamping so that suturing can be done under direct vision. Performing the aortic anastomosis through this mini-laparotomy enables the use of conventional instruments and retains the surgeon's normal tactile sense. This technique allows patients with conditions previously considered contraindications to mini-laparotomy (obesity; a short, angulated, or calcified proximal aortic neck; need for suprarenal aortic clamping; or AAA extension into the common iliac arteries) to be treated by a laparoscopy-assisted approach.[64]

Laparoscopy-assisted techniques have been used with both the transperitoneal and retroperitoneal approaches. The technique used by Alimi and colleagues for both AAA and AIOD is a transperitoneal approach.[64,65] The transperitoneal approach appears to be the most direct method, providing more exposure of the right aortic wall, the right lumbar and renal arteries, and the right iliac axis. However, it leads to problems with viscera retraction,[37,51,66] typically requiring 25 to 30 degrees or more of Trendelenburg to keep the small bowel from invading the operative field.[46,51,52,64] The use of a laparoscopic intestinal retractor (Fig. 23-11) enables a decrease in the Trendelenburg angle, requiring only 5 to 10 degrees to keep

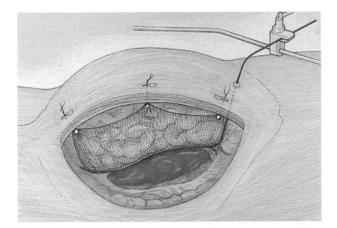

A

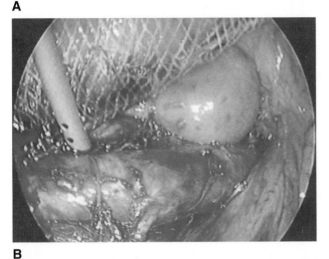

B

FIGURE 23–11 • Intraperitoneal bowel retractor provides the same exposure for the transperitoneal approach as the apron technique does for left anterolateral retroperitoneal approach. *A*, Overview diagram of the retractor in place with the mesh sutured through the anterior abdominal wall with retraction of the small intestine. *B*, Close-up of the intrarenal aorta with the retractor in place.

the bowel away from the operative site during laparoscopic dissection of the aorta and aortoprosthetic anastomoses through a mini-laparotomy.[65]

A laparoscopy-assisted retroperitoneal approach has been reported by Castronuovo and colleagues.[39] Patients are placed in a modified right lateral decubitus position (Fig. 23-12). Initial retroperitoneal access is gained through a 1.5-cm muscle-splitting incision in the left flank, just posterior to the anterior axillary line, midway between the costal margin and the iliac crest. A retroperitoneal approach is started with balloon dissectors, followed by insufflation and insertion of the remaining trocars. After aortoiliac dissection, the aortic cross-clamp is introduced via a puncture wound in the 10th intercostal space in the posterior axillary line. The iliac arteries are stapled with the Endo TA stapling device before placement of the aortic cross-clamp, to minimize the risk of distal embolization.

In Edoga and colleagues' early experience, the aortic anastomosis was performed with interrupted mattress sutures placed laparoscopically under insufflation of the retroperitoneum (pneumoretroperitoneum).[62] Owing to the lengthy nature of this technique, the anastomotic technique was changed to a running suture performed under laparoscopic visualization with standard instruments through a small incision (3 to 4 cm) connecting the laparoscopic and kidney retraction ports. This phase of the procedure is converted to gasless by deflating the retroperitoneum. The laparoscope remains in the trocar to provide visualization of the operative field during performance of the proximal anastomosis.

Results

LAPAROSCOPY-ASSISTED TECHNIQUES

Mini-laparotomy has been used in various laparoscopic procedures,[67] especially in more complex procedures such as colon and hepatic resection. In laparoscopy-assisted colon surgery, the mini-laparotomy is used to both extract the specimen and facilitate the anastomosis by insertion of endomechanical staple components. Laparoscopic hepatic resection is in its infancy and is undeniably complex; the exposure,

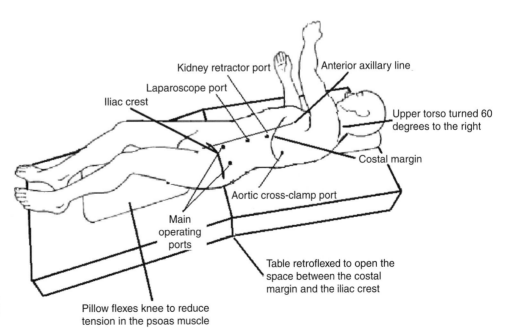

FIGURE 23–12 • Positioning for laparoscopy-assisted abdominal aortic aneurysm repair by Edoga.

TABLE 23–2	Results of Laparoscopy-Assisted Aortic Surgery with Mini-Laparotomy							
	No. of Patients	Type of Procedure (n)	Approach	Surgery Time (Mean)	Cross-clamp Time (Mean)	Conversion	Morbidity	Mortality
AIOD								
Alimi et al (2001)[55]	19	ABF (14) AF (2) Tube (3)	TP	273.3 min	78.03 min	0	5 (26.3%)	1 (5.3%)
	7*	ABF (5) AF (2)	TL/apron	350.7 min	127.9 min	1 (14.2%)	2 (28.5%)	0
Alimi et al (2004)[65]	First 29	ABF (25) AF (4)	TP	285 ± 67 min	76.4 ± 52 min	1 (3.4%)	3 (10.3%)	1 (3.4%)
	Next 29	ABF (27) Ao TEA (1) Tube (1)	TP	192 ± 30 min	31.8 ± 15 min	0	2 (6.9%)	1 (3.4%)
AAA								
Castronuovo et al (2000)[39]	LA 60	ABF (25) AF (4)	TP	7.7 (1.5-11.5) hr	112 (43-286) min	3 (5.0%)	8 (13.3%)	3 (5.0%)
	Open 100†	Tube (1) ABF (27) Ao TEA (1)	TP	5.0 (2.6-9.7) hr	90 (38-235) min	0	28 (28%)	4 (4.0%)
Alimi et al (2003)[64]	First 10	Tube (12) ABF (3) A-I (3)	TP	275 ± 50 min	101 ± 37 min	1 (10.0%)	3 (30.0%)	0
	Next 14			195 ± 26 min	52 ± 12 min	2 (14.3%)	1 (7.1%)	1 (7.1%)

*The first seven patients were operated on totally laparoscopically with the apron technique.
†Comparison of the 60 reported laparoscopy-assisted cases with a contemporary series of 100 consecutive AAA repairs performed by the same surgeons.
AAA, abdominal aortic aneurysm; AF, aortofemoral; ABF, aortobifemoral; A-I, aortoiliac; AIOD, aortoiliac occlusive disease; Ao, aorta; LA, laparoscopy-assisted; TEA, thromboendarterectomy; TL, totally laparoscopic; TP, transperitoneal.

hemostasis, and technology have not been completed converted from open liver applications to laparoscopic ones. Hepatic surgeons are facing these challenges with the same limited laparoscopic experience as vascular surgeons. The mini-laparotomy has been used by hepatic surgeons for exposure, insertion of open instruments, and specimen retrieval.[68]

The largest reported series of laparoscopy-assisted techniques for AIOD and AAA repair are summarized in Table 23-2. Alimi and coworkers reported experience with laparoscopy-assisted aortic reconstruction for AIOD in 2001 and and 2004.[55,65] In the earlier experience, 27 patients (23 men and 4 women) with a mean age of 58.2 years (range, 42 to 76 years) underwent aortoaortic (3), aortounifemoral (4), or aortobifemoral (20) bypass graft for AIOD (20), emboligenic aortitis (1), or AAA (6). A totally laparoscopic procedure was possible in seven patients, with a mean operative time of 350.7 minutes and a mean clamping time of 127.9 minutes.

For the next seven patients, a mini-laparotomy was made owing to technical difficulties caused by calcific aortic plaque and for construction of the proximal anastomosis. The mean operative and clamping times for these seven patients decreased to 316.4 minutes and 107.1 minutes, respectively. The next six patients underwent repair of AAAs, and a mini-laparotomy was done to control lumbar arteries and perform the proximal anastomosis. Mean operative and clamping times decreased again in this group to 269 minutes and 99 minutes, respectively. In the final six patients reported, all with AIOD, mini-laparotomy became a planned component of the technique. Mean operative surnd clamping times decreased again to 234.5 minutes and 28 minutes, respectively, and

were significantly lower both globally ($P = 0.021$) and individually ($P \leq 0.016$) when compared with those of the other three groups.

Alimi's group concluded that the significant decrease in operative and clamping times were the result of using the mini-laparotomy to deal with any technical problems.[55] In the case of AAA, mini-laparotomy facilitated thrombus removal and made it easier to deal with any bleeding lumbar arteries. The mini-laparotomy did not contribute to longer postoperative hospital stays when compared with totally laparoscopic procedures. However, the learning curve also affects the results of new procedures and techniques. An overall improvement in procedural times and fewer complications would be anticipated when comparing the first seven patients with the last seven, owing to greater experience and laparoscopic skills. Alimi and coworkers' experience with laparoscopy-assisted AAA repair further supports the learning curve effect.[64] Although they reported an early repeat intervention rate of 20.8%, comparison of the first 10 patients and last 14 patients demonstrated a significant decrease in mean operative and clamping times ($P < 0.0001$), as well as halving the percentage of early repeat interventions ($P = 0.61$).

In the experience of Castronuovo and associates, the operative and cross-clamp times for laparoscopy-assisted aneurysmectomy were longer than for open aneurysm repair.[39] However, the physiologic stress does not appear to increase mortality or morbidity rates in good- or moderate-risk patients (ASA class III or lower). Major complications attributable to technical errors included bleeding from the aortic anastomosis requiring reoperation, graft limb thrombosis, and ureteral injury. The authors stated that experience with this procedure should decrease the risk for such complications. In fact, the aortic cross-clamp time decreased from a mean of 146 minutes (range, 60 to 286 minutes) in the first 20 patients to a mean of 95 minutes (range, 43 to 165 minutes) in the last 24 patients as experience was gained with this procedure.

HAND-ASSISTED TECHNIQUE

The long operating times and the steep learning curve required for laparoscopic aortic surgery have discouraged some surgeons from performing these procedures. Hand-assisted laparoscopy is a novel technique that allows surgeons to use their hands along with laparoscopic instruments in the operative field while maintaining the advantages of the pneumoperitoneum. Hand-assisted laparoscopic surgery (HALS) is a safe and efficient method that makes it possible to combine the established convenience and safety of open surgery with the advantages of minimally invasive surgery.[69] Some authors report a reduced learning curve for HALS in comparison to advanced laparoscopy for donor nephrectomy and colon resection.[70-72] The main role of HALS is to simplify difficult intraoperative situations, reducing the need for conversion to an open procedure.[73] It is also useful in the training of unskilled surgeons. It is not meant to be an alternative to pure laparoscopic surgery.

Kolvenbach and colleagues reported the largest experiences with HALS for aortic surgery (Table 23-3). In one series of patients, HALS was applied to both AIOD and AAA.[61] The operative and cross-clamp times were significantly longer in patients with laparoscopic AAA repair compared with those with AIOD ($P < 0.001$). However, HALS can be performed in a wide variety of patients, rather than only in highly selected ones. Heavily calcified aortas were not excluded. Even suprarenal aorta cross-clamping was accomplished when necessary (two patients with AAA and one with AIOD). Dissection of the retroperitoneum using hand-assisted

laparoscopy and a pneumoperitoneum can be accomplished as rapidly as in conventional surgery.

HALS may offer advantages in controlling bleeding complications during laparoscopy that can lead to conversion to a standard laparotomy. These complication include loss of visibility by submersion of the operative field, suction collapsing the space, and increasing amounts of blood in the field that absorb light and reduce visibility further. Hemostasis can be quickly obtained with digital compression, preserving visibility and allowing time to place packing, stitches, or ligatures. In addition, the surgeon's tactile sensation is preserved with one hand in the operative field during laparoscopy.[74]

Kolvenbach and colleagues reported a second series of AAAs repaired by HALS.[60] In most cases, operative time ranged from 2.5 to 3 hours, and the mean aortic cross-clamp time was 1 hour or less. The data for a contemporary consecutive series of 24 AAA patients operated on conventionally are shown in Table 23-3. HALS for AAA resection increased the mean total operative time (198.2 minutes vs. 135.7 minutes) and cross-clamping time (59.2 minutes vs. 34.3 minutes) when compared with conventional surgery. However, postoperative recovery time and hospital stay were significantly shorter after the laparoscopic operation.

The size of the aneurysm was not a deterrent to laparoscopically dissecting the neck of the AAA. Suprarenal cross-clamping was necessary in seven patients in Kolvenbach's series, with mean renal ischemia of 23 minutes (range, 15 to 34 minutes). Obesity was not a contraindication for a laparoscopic operation. Procedures in obese patients required more time and were technically more demanding, however.

TOTALLY LAPAROSCOPIC TECHNIQUE

Clinical series of totally laparoscopic aortic surgery are summarized in Table 23-4. Two technical problems of total laparoscopic infrarenal aortic surgery are exposure of the aorta and performance of aortoprosthetic anastomoses. The apron

---

TABLE 23-3	Results of Hand-Assisted Laparoscopic Aortic Surgery							
	No. of Patients	Type of Procedure (n)	Approach	Surgery Time (Mean)	Cross-clamp Time (Mean)	Conversion	Morbidity	Mortality
AIOD and AAA*								
Kolvenbach et al (2000)[61]	AIOD 29	n/r	TP	148.5 ± 35.2 min	36.4 ± 7.9 min	3 (7.3%)	5 (12.1%)	1 (2.4%)
	AAA 12	n/r	TP	198.3 ± 19.5 min	43.0 ± 12.2 min			
	Open 20	n/r	TP	120.3 ± 43.8 min	30.7 ± 10.6 min	n/a	2 (10.0%)	0
AAA†								
Kolvenbach et al (2001)[60]	24	Tube (13) ABF (3) A-I (8)	TP	198 (95-395) min	59.2 (29-120) min	1 (4.1%)	4 (16.6%)	1
	EVAR 13	Vanguard (4) Stentor (1) Talent (8)	n/a	149 (85-245) min	15.7 min	0	4 (30.7%)	0
	Open 24	n/r	n/r	135.7 min	34.3 min	n/a	n/r	n/r

*Operative and cross-clamp times were significantly longer in patients with laparoscopic AAA repair than in those with AIOD ($P < 0.001$).
†Laparoscopic AAA repair by HALS was offered to 24 of 37 patients referred for EVAR who were not candidates for EVAR. The data are included for comparison of operative and cross-clamp times between HALS and conventional open AAA repair.
AAA, abdominal aortic aneurysm; ABF, aortobifemoral; A-I, aortoiliac; AIOD, aortoiliac occlusive disease; EVAR, endovascular aneurysm repair; HALS, hand-assisted laparoscopic surgery; n/a, not applicable; n/r, not reported; TP, transperitoneal.

TABLE 23–4		Results of Totally Laparoscopic Aortic Surgery						
	No. of Patients	Type of Procedure (n)	Approach	Surgery Time (Mean)	Cross-clamp Time (Mean)	Conversion	Morbidity	Mortality
AIOD								
Gracia and Dion (1999)[75]	21	ABF	Apron	326 min	100 min	3 (14.2%)	2 (9.5%)	1 (4.7%)
Coggia et al (2004)[76]	93	ABF (68) AF (25)	TAPA (78) TARA (8) RP (7)	240 (150-450) min	67.5 (30-135) min	2 (2.1%)	12 (13.5%)	4 (4.0%)
AAA								
Coggia et al (2004)[77]	30	Tube (11) ABF (4) A-I (15)	TAPA (27) TARA (2) RP (1)	290 (160-420) min	78 (35-230) min	4 (13.3%)	10 (33.3%)	2 (6.6%)
Kolvenbach et al (2004)[78]	47	Tube (8) Bifurcated (39)	TAPA/apron	227.8 ± 34.0 min 242.5 ± 40.5 min*	81.4 ± 31.0 min 95.9 ± 21.6 min*	8 to HALS (17.0%)	8 (14.8%)	0

*Separate times reported for 10 consecutive cases in which the aortoprosthetic anastomosis was completed with robotic assistance.
AAA, abdominal aortic aneurysm; ABF, aortobifemoral; AF, aortofemoral; A-I, aortoiliac; AIOD, aortoiliac occlusive disease; HALS, hand-assisted laparoscopic surgery; RP, retroperitoneal; TAPA, transabdominal paracolic approach; TARA, transabdominal retrorenal approach.

technique described by Dion and coworkers was the first stable aortic exposure.[41] The patient could be placed supine, with simultaneous access to the groins. Insufflation with carbon dioxide maintained the domelike, three-dimensional expansion effect of the pneumoperitoneum. The exposure remained stable, despite periods of aggressive and extended suction. This approach was consistently successful for exposure in AIOD, with overall decreasing operative and cross-clamp times. Exposure of an AAA is challenging with any laparoscopic approach. However, the rapidity and stability of the apron in exposing the aorta allowed it to be used in 1999 for the first reported totally laparoscopic AAA repair.[41]

Laparoscopic suture skills for an intracorporeal totally laparoscopic anastomosis were not a problem because of the large amount of training and development in the laboratory.[30-32,40] The challenge to aortoprosthetic anastomosis as reported by Gracia and Dion was calcified aortic plaque.[75] The three conversions noted in this experience all involved severe calcified plaque in the proximal aorta. In open surgery, the proximal aortic plaque can be fractured or removed by endarterectomy in order to drive a needle through the aortic wall. An endarterectomy was attempted and completed in one of the three patients laparoscopically. He was converted only for safety, to visually inspect the endarterectomized anastomosis, which required no manipulation. All three conversions were performed by mini-laparotomy in the midline, with insertion of curved, narrow retractors behind the apron to readily expose the infrarenal aorta.

Coggia and associates reported an impressive series of 93 patients with AIOD.[76] Extensive aortic calcifications have been considered contraindications to laparoscopy, owing to the previously noted difficulties. There was one conversion because of a heavily calcified distal aorta. However, infrarenal or juxtarenal circumferential calcifications were not contraindications to total laparoscopic AIOD repair when suprarenal clamping was possible. Associated occlusive lesions of the visceral arteries would be relative contraindications, based on the experience of the surgeons. Total occlusion of the superior

mesenteric artery was repaired in three patients during the laparoscopic bypass for AIOD reconstruction, and one laparoscopic reimplantation of the inferior mesenteric artery was performed because vascular flow to the left colon was compromised after aortic unclamping.[77]

Coggia and coworkers have reported increasing numbers of AAA cases.[77] Median blood loss for the laparoscopic surgery was comparable to that for conventional aortic surgery. Back-bleeding from the lumbar arteries was the main difficulty described during laparoscopic AAA repair. The aggressive suction required to control them can collapse the abdominal cavity. Calcified aortas were also problematic, resulting in the most extreme blood loss. In this series, the mortality rate was 6.6%.[77] However, there were no late deaths after the surgeons had surmounted the learning curve. They strongly emphasize the importance of training in laparoscopic suture skills to obtain the required level of expertise for laparoscopic anastomoses. Prior experience with laparoscopic AIOD reconstruction is essential before performing total laparoscopic AAA repair. These surgeons observed changes in laparoscopic surgical skills after 15 laparoscopic AAA repairs and discovered that approximately 50 procedures were necessary to achieve an appropriate level of expertise. Proper patient selection for laparoscopic AAA repair is mandatory. Inflammatory and ruptured AAAs are contraindications to total laparoscopic repair. An inferior mesenteric artery has also been laparoscoipcally reimplanted after laparoscopic AAA resection.[57]

Kolvenbach and colleagues reported their experience with totally laparoscopic aortic surgery[78] after extensive laparoscopic vascular experience with HALS.[59-61] Calcification of the iliac arteries was the main reason for technical problems and prolonged cross-clamping times. In one patient, transfemoral balloon occlusion of the common iliac artery and C-arm fluoroscopy were used when iliac artery clamping failed. Combining endovascular techniques with laparoscopic procedures can be an effective way to overcome these obstacles.[59,79,80]

Although conversion to HALS was required in 17% of cases because of technical difficulties, a total laparoscopic approach was used in the majority of patients.[78] HALS was used in these cases to avoid conversion to open surgery. Because the surgeon may be unaware of the time elapsed while performing totally laparoscopic procedures, strict time limits were set to avoid problems with ischemia and blood loss. Adherence to these limits in the interest of patient safety was another reason for the relatively high conversion rate of 17%. The most significant difference between total laparoscopy and HALS with a 7-cm mini-incision was the postoperative period required for full mobilization and the postoperative requirement for intravenous pain medication.

Robotics in Laparoscopic Aortic Surgery

Minimally invasive surgery is difficult to perform and perhaps even more difficult to teach. The surgeon must perform tasks remotely in a three-dimensional field while watching a two-dimensional image, which can lead to problems involving depth perception and orientation. The trocar creates a fixed fulcrum, making experience in correct trocar placement critical. Incorrectly placed ports may cause the surgeon to struggle to perform fine motor tasks because of the poor ergonomics and limited range of motion caused by the poor geometry. The "fulcrum effect" created by the trocar requires reversed motion; for example, to move the instrument tip to the left, the surgeon moves the hand to the right. Finally, the surgeon's motions become variably amplified; for instance, if an instrument is advanced deeply into the trocar, a small hand motion is translated into a large tip motion, and vice versa.

Additional limitations to laparoscopic surgery involve the need to adjust to differences from traditional laparoscopic instruments. The traditional digital tactile feedback that surgeons are familiar with is lacking; there is not a total loss of tactile sensation, but rather a change in the tactile experience that the surgeon must learn to interpret. The sum of these problems leads to a perceived lack of dexterity until the surgeon develops the minimally invasive surgery skill set. This perceived lack of dexterity translates to a loss of confidence, leading to a situation in which the surgeon no longer believes that he or she is in complete control of the operation.

The current impression of robot-assisted operations is of feasibility at the expense of longer operating time. The feasibility of performing complex laparoscopic gastrointestinal procedures with robotic instruments has been established.[81,82] Laparoscopic urologic surgery is also in development, along similar timelines as laparoscopic vascular surgery. Advances in surgical techniques have allowed surgeons to use robotic assistance in developing new approaches in extirpative and reconstructive urologic surgery, with improved outcomes.[83] Others report that the clinical outcome and results of robot-assisted laparoscopic surgery are no better than those of conventional or manual laparoscopic surgery.[84,85] The overall value of a robotic system for laparoscopic general surgery has yet to be defined. However, in laparoscopic vascular surgery for aortoiliac disease, use of a robotic system may facilitate laparoscopic suturing and knot tying, as reported for microvascular anastomoses in cardiac surgery.[86,87]

An experimental series evaluating the safety and efficacy of a robot-assisted totally laparoscopic aortic replacement compared with a human-performed laparoscopic procedure was reported by Ruurda and associates.[88] The da Vinci Robotic Surgical System (Intuitive Surgical, Sunnyvale, Calif.) was used, providing a true three-dimensional view based on a double optical system. Results demonstrate that the procedure can be performed more safely and efficiently with the da Vinci robot system. Overall procedure, suturing, and clamping times were significantly shorter in the robot group, and blood loss was less (Table 23-5).

The quality of the robotic anastomoses was judged superior to those of the human group as a result of decreased blood loss after unclamping and an increased number of sutures per anastomosis. There was no distance greater than 3 mm between sutures and no knot failures in the robot cases. Participating surgeons were capable of suturing an anastomosis with robotic assistance in approximately 20 minutes after as few as three cases. The time loss during the human laparoscopic procedures occurred while suturing the anastomosis, leading to a significantly longer clamping time. All 20 grafts were patent, with no anastomotic narrowing encountered.

The first report on robot-assisted laparoscopic ABF bypass was by Wisselink and colleagues.[89] Totally laparoscopic ABF

TABLE 23–5	Robotic versus Human Laparoscopic Aortic Surgery in Porcine Model		
Measured Parameter	**Laparoscopic Robotic (range)**	**Laparoscopic Human (range)**	**P Value**
Total no. of cases	10	10	n/a
Total operating time (min)	164 (116-225)	205 (162-244)	0.008
Aortic exposure time (min)	30 (20-55)	38 (20-50)	NS
Dissection time (min)	38 (31-78)	32 (20-78)	NS
Clamping time (min)	63 (37-95)	106 (79-151)	0.0003
Proximal anastomosis time (min)	22 (15-37)	40 (31-75)	0.0003
Stitches, proximal	15 (11-17)	13 (11-14)	NS
Time per stitch, proximal (min)	93 (53-149)	180 (143-409)	0.001
Total blood loss (mL)	55 (0-300)	280 (105-1700)	0.004
Blood loss after clamp removal (mL)	28 (0-200)	200 (50-1500)	0.01

All cases were performed totally laparoscopically using a retroperitoneal route with insufflation (pneumoretroperitoneum). The da Vinci Robotic Surgical System (Intuitive Surgical, Sunnyvale, Calif.) was used.

n/a, not applicable; NS, not significant.

From Ruurda JP, Broeders IA, Pulles B, et al: Manual robot assisted endoscopic suturing: Time-action analysis in an experimental model. Surg Endosc 18:1249-1252, 2004.

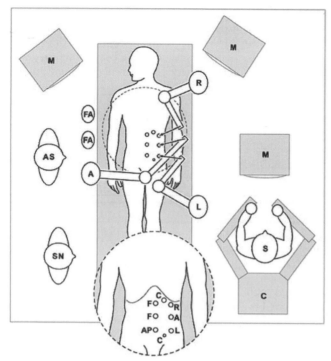

FIGURE 23–13 • Operating room setup for robot-assisted laparoscopic aortobifemoral bypass. A, surgical endoscope positioner (Aesop); AS, assistant surgeon; C, surgeon control console; FA, connection site for fan arm retraction holders; L, left robotic arm; M, monitor; R, right robotic arm; S, surgeon; SN, scrub nurse. *Inset,* Trocar positions in abdominal wall. AP, assistant port; C, aortic clamp; F, fan retractor.

bypass with the apron approach was performed in two patients with disabling intermittent claudication from severe AIOD. Proximal end-to-side anastomoses were constructed with robotic arms (ZEUS Surgical Robotic System, Computer Motion, Goleta, Calif.) mounted on the operating table and controlled from a separate console (Fig. 23-13). Operating times were 290 and 260 minutes, and aortic anastomosis times were 48 and 37 minutes (Table 23-6). No complications occurred, and blood loss was less than 200 mL in both cases.

A normal diet was resumed on the second postoperative day, with the patients discharged home on postoperative days 4 and 6.

Kolvenbach and associates also used the ZEUS robotic system in their first reported totally laparoscopic experience.[78] In 10 consecutive patients, the anastomosis was sutured robotically. Although the time required to suture the aortic anastomosis was significantly shorter in the robotic group (see Table 23-6), total operating time and aortic cross-clamping time were longer because of the setup time and mechanical problems with the robot ($P < 0.03$). In two cases, the surgeon had to complete the anastomosis laparoscopically.

Conclusions

The initial application of laparoscopic approaches and techniques to aortic disease were performed for AIOD[27,28] and AAA,[36,37,39] with the assistance of a mini-laparotomy by a transperitoneal route. The mini-laparotomy was used because of limitations in instrumentation and difficulties related to laparoscopic suturing of the anastomosis, which could be completed with conventional instruments under direct visualization. The procedures were long and difficult, with retraction of the bowel posing a major problem.

Totally laparoscopic approaches to the aorta for both AIOD[34,35,46,49,56] and AAA[38,41,90] have been performed and reported. These early experiences were also long and difficult procedures. As in all pioneering efforts, despite training with animal and cadaveric models, a learning curve exists and contributed to the length of these procedures. Lack of laparoscopic vascular instruments also contributed greatly to the inefficiency and length of procedures. However, these experiences provided knowledge about the advantages and disadvantages of different approaches to the aorta, and they encouraged the surgical industry to participate in meeting the technical needs identified. Development of appropriate instrumentation (primarily cross-clamps, needle holders, and dissection tools) has contributed greatly to improved efficiency, shorter procedural times, and enhanced safety.

Laparoscopic aortoiliac reconstructions are performed in only a few surgical centers and are not considered simple and

TABLE 23–6	Results of Robotic-Assisted Laparoscopic Aortic Surgery							
	No. of Patients	Approach	Surgery Time	Cross-clamp Time	Anastomotic Time	Conversion	Morbidity	Mortality
AIOD								
Wisselink et al (2002)[89]	2 (ABF)	Apron	290-260 min	n/r	48-37 min	0	0	0
AAA								
Kolvenbach et al (2004)[78]	10	TAPA/apron	242.5 ± 40.5 min (mean)	95.9 ± 21.6 min (mean)	40.8 ± 4.1 min	2 to HALS	8 (14.8%)†	0
	37		227.8 ± 34.0 min (mean)*	81.4 ± 31.0 min (mean)*	52.7 ± 9.0 min*	6 to HALS		0

The ZEUS Robotic Surgical System (Computer Motion, Goleta, Calif.) was used in both studies.
*Comparison times reported for 37 cases in the same series in which the aortoprosthetic anastomosis was completed laparoscopically by the surgeon.
†Morbidity for the overall experience, both robotic and nonrobotic.
AAA, abdominal aortic aneurysm; ABF, aortobifemoral; AIOD, aortoiliac occlusive disease; HALS, hand-assisted laparoscopic surgery; n/r, not reported, TAPA, transabdominal paracolic approach.

reproducible in the hands of the average surgeon. The operating time required for a total laparoscopic bypass graft can exceed 6 hours, combined with cross-clamp times of almost 2 hours, making this procedure relatively unattractive to the majority of surgeons. The learning curve to acquire the dexterity and skills needed for laparoscopic aortoiliac surgery is long and steep. In contrast to traditional open repairs, the overall technique is not standardized.[91] Long-term results are not yet known.

To safely advance into totally laparoscopic aortoiliac surgery, surgeons should consider undertaking laparoscopy-assisted repair with a small mini-laparotomy for suturing under direct vision as an intermediate step. However, HALS is the only technique that has been demonstrated to be a safe and effective modality for minimally invasive aortoiliac surgery and is the only proven technique that has allowed surgeons to advance to totally laparoscopic aortoiliac surgery.

The hand is one of the best-known intestinal retractors, and the ability to use the hand for retraction in laparoscopic AAA surgery greatly facilitates these operations. With HALS, palpation of the aorta is possible, and cross-clamping of a nondiseased or calcified segment can be performed with much greater confidence than in total laparoscopic aortic operations.[60] However, these procedures can be performed using a purely laparoscopic approach with near-equivalent safety and speed and without the higher incidence of wound-related complications associated with HALS.[63,70] It is important to remember that conversion with a short laparotomy is always possible when technical difficulties arise during the procedure, especially substantial bleeding or prolonged aortic clamping time.

Experience has been gained in the advantages and disadvantages of different approaches to the aorta. Specially designed laparoscopic vascular instrumentation is now available, and new technologies such as robotics are developing rapidly. New approaches to anastomotic devices, both intraluminal and extraluminal, are under development. Vascular surgeons entering specialized vascular training have gained experience in basic laparoscopy during general surgery residency. Laparoscopy has a growing number of applications in aortoiliac surgery. The main advantage of laparoscopy compared with endovascular procedures for AAA is the performance of a standard endoaneurysmorrhaphy that will provide the same excellent long-term results as conventional AAA repair. Laparoscopy is here to stay and has a growing role in the field of minimally invasive techniques for AIOD and AAA repair. Future studies, refinement of instrumentation, and consistent training to develop new skills are all necessary to continue to safely apply laparoscopic aortoiliac surgery in patients.

REFERENCES

1. Peters JH, Ortega A, Lehnerd SL, et al: The physiology of laparoscopic surgery: Pulmonary function after laparoscopic cholecystectomy. Surg Laparosc Endosc 3:370-374, 1993.
2. Poulin EC, Mamazza J, Breton G, et al: Evaluation of pulmonary function in laparoscopic cholecystectomy. Surg Laparosc Endosc 2:292-296, 1993.
3. Creech O: Endo-aneurysmorrhaphy and treatment of aortic aneurysm. Ann Surg 164:935-946, 1966.
4. Brewster DC, Cronenwett JL, Hallett JW Jr, et al: Guidelines for the treatment of abdominal aortic aneurysms: Report of a subcommittee of the Joint Council of the American Association for Vascular Surgery and Society for Vascular Surgery. J Vasc Surg 37:1106-1117, 2003.
5. Brewster DC: Current controversies in the management of aortoiliac occlusive disease. J Vasc Surg 25:365-379, 1997.
6. Vries SO, Hunink MG: Results of aortic bifurcation grafts for aortoiliac occlusive disease: A meta-analysis. J Vasc Surg 26:558-569, 1997.
7. Hertzer NR, Mascha EJ, Karafa MT, et al: Open infrarenal abdominal aortic aneurysm repair: The Cleveland Clinic experience from 1989 to 1998. J Vasc Surg 35:1145-1154, 2002.
8. McDaniel MD, Macdonald PD, Haver RA, Littenberg B: Published results of surgery for aortoiliac occlusive disease. Ann Vasc Surg 11:425-441, 1997.
9. Zarins CK, Harris EJ: Operative repair for aortic aneurysms: The gold standard. J Endovasc Surg 4:232-241, 1997.
10. Ernst CB: Abdominal aortic aneurysm. N Engl J Med 328:1167-1172, 1993.
11. Adye B, Luna G: Incidence of abdominal wall hernia in aortic surgery. Am J Surg 175:400-402, 1998.
12. Cambria RP, Brewster DC, Abbott WM, et al: Transperitoneal versus retroperitoneal approach for aortic reconstruction: A randomized prospective study. J Vasc Surg 11:314-325, 1990.
13. Parodi JC, Pamaz JC, Barone HD: Transfemoral intraluminal graft implantation for abdominal aortic aneurysms. Ann Vasc Surg 5:491-499, 1991.
14. Blum U, Voshage G, Lammer J, et al: Endoluminal stent-grafts for infrarenal abdominal aortic aneurysms. N Engl J Med 336:13-20, 1997.
15. Cuypers P, Buth J, Harris P, et al: Realistic expectations for patients with stent-graft treatment of abdominal aortic aneurysms: Results of a European multicentre registry. Eur J Vasc Endovasc Surg 17:507-516, 1999.
16. Brewster DC, Geller SC, Kaufman JA, et al: Initial experience with endovascular aneurysm repair: Comparison of early results with outcome of conventional open repair. J Vasc Surg 27:992-1003, 1998.
17. Zarins CK, White RA, Schwarten D, et al: AneuRx stent graft versus open surgical repair of abdominal aortic aneurysms: Multicenter prospective clinical trial. J Vasc Surg 29:292-308, 1999.
18. Moore WS, Kashyap VS, Vescera CL, Quinones-Baldrich J: Abdominal aortic aneurysm: A 6-year comparison of endovascular versus transabdominal repair. Ann Surg 230:20-30, 1999.
19. Moore WS, Brewster DC, Bernhard VM: Aorto-uni-iliac endograft for complex aorto-iliac aneurysms compared with tube/bifurcation endografts: Results of the EVT/Guidant trials. J Vasc Surg 33:511-520, 2001.
20. Zarins CK, White RA, Fogarty TJ: Aneurysm rupture after endovascular repair using the AneuRx stent graft. J Vasc Surg 31:960-970, 2000.
21. Holzbein TJ, Kretschmer G, Thurnher S, et al: Midterm durability of abdominal aortic aneurysm endograft repair: A word of caution. J Vasc Surg 33(2 Pt 2):46-54, 2001.
22. Harris PL, Vallabhaneni SR, Desgranges P, et al: Incidence and risk factors of late rupture, conversion, and death after endovascular repair of infrarenal aortic aneurysms: The EUROSTAR experience. European collaborators on stent/graft techniques for aortic aneurysm repair. J Vasc Surg 32:739-749, 2000.
23. Ohki T, Veith FJ, Shaw P, et al: Increasing incidence of mid and long-term complications after endovascular graft repair of AAAs: A note of caution based on a 9-year experience. Ann Surg 234:323-334, 2001.
24. Mortiz JD, Rotermund S, Keating DP, Oestmann JW: Infrarenal abdominal aortic aneurysms: Implications of CT evaluation of size and configuration for placement of endovascular aortic grafts. Radiology 198:463-466, 1996.
25. Schumacher H, Eckstein HH, Kallinowski F, Allenberg JR: Morphometry and classification in abdominal aortic aneurysms: Patient selection for endovascular and open surgery. J Endovasc Surg 4:39-44, 1997.
26. Wolf YG, Fogarty TJ, Olcott C IV, et al: Endovascular repair of abdominal aortic aneurysms: Eligibility rate and impact on the rate of open repair. J Vasc Surg 32:519-523, 2000.
27. Dion YM, Katkhouda N, Rouleau C, Aucoin A: Laparoscopy-assisted aortobifemoral bypass. Surg Laparosc Endosc 3:425-429, 1993.
28. Berens E, Herde JR: Laparoscopic vascular surgery: Four case reports. J Vasc Surg 22:73-79, 1995.
29. Rosser JC Jr, Rosser LE, Savalgi RS: Objective evaluation of a laparoscopic skill program for residents and senior surgeons. Arch Surg 133:657-661, 1998.
30. Dion YM, Gracia CR: Experimental laparoscopic aortic aneurysm resection and aortobifemoral bypass. Surg Laparosc Endosc 6:184-190, 1996.

31. Dion YM, Gaillard F, Demalsy JC, Gracia CR: Experimental laparoscopic aortobifemoral bypass for occlusive aortoiliac disease. Can J Surg 39:451-455, 1996.

32. Dion YM, Gracia CR: A reproducible animal model for laparoscopic retroperitoneal aortobifemoral bypass in aortoiliac occlusive disease. Surg Endosc 10:270, 1996.

33. Dion YM, Gracia CR, Demalsy JC, Estakhri M: Laparoscopic and laparoscopy-assisted aortoiliac surgery: Animal and clinical evaluation. J Endovasc Surg 3:114, 1996.

34. Dion YM, Gracia CR: A new technique for laparoscopic aortobifemoral grafting in occlusive aortoiliac disease. J Vasc Surg 26:685-692, 1997.

35. Dion YM, Gracia CR, Estakhri ME, et al: Totally laparoscopic aortobifemoral bypass: A review of 10 patients. Surg Laparosc Endosc 8:165-170, 1998.

36. Chen HM, Murphy EA, Levison J, Cohen JR: Laparoscopic aortic replacement in the porcine model: A feasibility study in preparation for laparoscopically assisted abdominal aortic aneurysm repair in humans. J Am Coll Surg 183:126-132, 1996.

37. Kline RG, D'Angelo AJ, Chen MH, et al: Laparoscopically assisted abdominal aortic aneurysm repair: First 20 cases. J Vasc Surg 27:81-87, 1998.

38. Edoga JK, James KV, Resnikoff M, et al: Laparoscopic aortic aneurysm resection. J Endovasc Surg 5:335-344, 1998.

39. Castronuovo JJ, James KV, Resnikoff M, et al: Laparoscopic-assisted aortic aneurysmectomy J Vasc Surg 32:224-233, 2000.

40. Dion YM, Cardon A, Gracia CR, Doillon C: A model for laparoscopic aortic aneurysm resection. Surg Endosc 13:654-657, 1999.

41. Dion YM, Gracia CR, El Kadi HB: Totally laparoscopic abdominal aortic aneurysm repair: A case report. J Vasc Surg 33:181-185, 2001.

41a. May J, White GH, Yu W, et al: Surgical management of complications following endoluminal grafting of abdominal aortic aneurysms. Eur J Vasc Endovasc Surg 10:51-59, 1995.

41b. Moore WS, Rutherford RB: Transfemoral endovascular repair of abdominal aortic aneurysm: Results of the North American EVT phase 1 trial. J Vasc Surg 23:543-553, 1996.

42. Gutt CN, Daume J, Schaeff B, Paolucci V: Systems and instruments for laparoscopic surgery without pneumoperitoneum. Surg Endosc 11:868-874, 1997.

43. Giebler RM, Kabatnik M, Stegen BH, et al: Retroperitoneal and intraperitoneal CO_2 insufflation have markedly different cardiovascular effects. J Surg Res 68:153-160, 1997.

44. Bannenberg JJG, Rademaker BMP, Froeling FM, Meijer D: Hemodynamics during laparoscopic extra and intraperitoneal insufflation. Surg Endosc 11:911, 1997.

45. Dion YM, Chin AK, Thompson TA: Experimental laparoscopic aortobifemoral bypass. Surg Endosc 9:894-897, 1995.

46. Said S, Mall J, Peter F, Muller JM: Laparoscopic aortofemoral bypass grafting: Human cadaveric and initial clinical experiences J Vasc Surg 29:639-648, 1999.

47. Alimi YS, Hartung O, Orsoni P, Juhan C: Abdominal aortic laparoscopic surgery: Retroperitoneal or transperitoneal approach? Eur J Vasc Endovasc Surg 19:21-26, 2000.

48. Wisselink W, Cuesta MA, Berends FJ, et al: Retroperitoneal endoscopic ligation of lumbar and inferior mesenteric arteries as a treatment of persistent endoleak after endoluminal aortic aneurysm repair. J Vasc Surg 31:1240-1244, 2000.

49. Barbera L, Mumme A, Metin S, et al: Operative results and outcome of twenty-four totally laparoscopic vascular procedures for aortoiliac occlusive disease. J Vasc Surg 28:136-142, 1998.

50. Alimi YS, Hartung O, Juhan C: Intestinal retractor for transperitoneal laparoscopic aortoiliac reconstruction: Experimental study on human cadavers and initial clinical experience. Surg Endosc 14:915-917, 2000.

51. Barbera L, Ludemann R, Grosefeld M, et al: Newly designed retraction devices for intestine control during laparoscopic aortic surgery: A comparative study in an animal model. Surg Endosc 14:63-66, 2000.

52. Ahn SS, Hiyama DT, Rudkin GH, et al: Laparoscopic aortobifemoral bypass. J Vasc Surg 26:128-132, 1997.

53. Taura P, Lopez A, Lacy AM, et al: Prolonged pneumoperitoneum at 15 mm Hg causes lactic acidosis. Surg Endosc 12:198-201, 1998.

54. Hashikura Y, Kawasaki S, Munakata Y, et al: Effects of peritoneal insufflation on hepatic and renal blood flow. Surg Endosc 8:759-761, 1994.

55. Alimi YS, Hartung O, Valerio N, Juhan C: Laparoscopic aortoiliac surgery for aneurysm and occlusive disease: When should a minilaparotomy be performed? J Vasc Surg 33:469-475, 2001.

56. Coggia M, Di Centa I, Javerliat I, et al: Total laparoscopic aortic surgery: Transperitoneal left retrorenal approach. Eur J Vasc Endovasc Surg 28:619-622, 2004.

57. Javerliat I, Coggia M, Bourriez A, et al: Total laparoscopic aortomesenteric bypass. Vascular 12:126-129, 2004.

58. Da Silva L, Kolvenbach R, Pinter L: The feasibility of hand-assisted laparoscopic bypass using a low transverse incision. Surg Endosc 16:173-176, 2002.

59. Kolvenbach R: Hand-assisted laparoscopic abdominal aortic aneurysm repair. Semin Laparosc Surg 8:168-177, 2001.

60. Kolvenbach R, Ceshire N, Pinter L, et al: Laparoscopy-assisted aneurysm resection as a minimally invasive alternative in patients unsuitable for endovascular surgery. J Vasc Surg 34:216-221, 2001.

61. Kolvenbach R, Da Silva L, Deling L, Schwierz E: Video-assisted aortic surgery. J Am Coll Surg 190:451-457, 2000.

62. Edoga JK, Asgarian K, Singh D, et al: Laparoscopic surgery for abdominal aortic aneurysm: Technical elements of the procedure and a preliminary report of the first 22 patients. Surg Endosc 12:1064-1072, 1998.

63. Kolvenbach R, Ferrari M: Hand-assisted advanced laparoscopic procedures—placement of the hand assist device is essential. Surg Endosc 17:1862-1863, 2003.

64. Alimi YS, Di Molfetta L, Hartung O, et al: Laparoscopy-assisted abdominal aortic aneurysm endoaneurysmorrhaphy: Early and mid-term results. J Vasc Surg 37:744-749, 2003.

65. Alimi YS, De Caridi G, Hartung O, et al: Laparoscopy-assisted reconstruction to treat severe aortoiliac occlusive disease: Early and midterm results. J Vasc Surg 39:777-783, 2004.

66. Fabiani JN, Mercier F, Carpentier A, et al: Video-assisted aortofemoral bypass: Results in seven cases. Ann Vasc Surg 11:273-277, 1997.

67. Fulton GJ, Gorey TF: Laparoscopic-assisted and hand-access laparoscopic surgery. Surg Technol Int 8:79-82, 2000.

68. Miyazawa M, Oishi T, Isobe Y, et al: Laparoscopic-assisted hepatectomy (LAH) for the treatment of hepatocellular carcinoma. Surg Laparosc Endosc Percutan Tech 10:404-408, 2000.

69. Meijer DW, Bannenberg JJ, Jakimowicz JJ: Hand-assisted laparoscopic surgery: An overview. Surg Endosc 14:891-895, 2000.

70. Maartense S, Bemelman WA, Gerritsen van der Hoop A, et al: Hand-assisted laparoscopic surgery (HALS): A report of 150 procedures. Surg Endosc 18:397-401, 2004.

71. Bemelman WA, van Doorn RC, de Wit LT, et al: Hand-assisted laparoscopic donor nephrectomy: Ascending the learning curve. Surg Endosc 15:442-444, 2001.

72. Mooney MJ, Elliott PL, Galapon DB, et al: Hand-assisted laparoscopic sigmoidectomy for diverticulitis. Dis Colon Rectum 41:630-635, 1998.

73. Targarona EM, Gracia E, Garriga J, et al: Prospective randomized trial comparing conventional laparoscopic colectomy with hand-assisted laparoscopic colectomy: Applicability, immediate clinical outcome, inflammatory response, and cost. Surg Endosc 16:234-239, 2002.

74. Memon M, Fitzgibbons R: Hand-assisted laparoscopic surgery (HALS): A useful technique for complex laparoscopic abdominal procedures. J Laparoendosc Adv Surg Tech A 8:143-150, 1998.

75. Gracia CR, Dion YM: Technological advances in laparoscopic aorto-occlusive surgery. Semin Laparosc Surg 6:164-174, 1999.

76. Coggia M, Javerliat I, Di Centa I, et al: Total laparoscopic bypass for aortoiliac occlusive lesions: 93-case experience. J Vasc Surg 40:899-906, 2004.

77. Coggia M, Javerliat I, Di Centa I, et al: Total laparoscopic infrarenal aortic aneurysm repair: Preliminary results. J Vasc Surg 40:448-454, 2004.

78. Kolvenbach R, Schwierz E, Wasilljew S, et al: Total laparoscopically and robotically assisted aortic aneurysm surgery: A critical evaluation. J Vasc Surg 39:771-776, 2004.

79. Kolvenbach R, Schwierz E: Combined endovascular/laparoscopic approach to aortic pseudoaneuyrsm repair. J Endovasc Surg 5:191-193, 1998.

80. Kolvenbach R, Pinter L, Raghunandan M, et al: Laparoscopic remodeling of abdominal aortic aneurysms after endovascular exclusion: A technical description. J Vasc Surg 36:1267-1270, 2002.

81. Cadiere GB, Himpens J, Germay O, et al: Feasibility of robotic laparoscopic surgery: 146 cases. World J Surg 25:1467-1477, 2001.

82. Ruurda JP, Broeders IA, Simmermacher RP, et al: Feasibility of robot-assisted laparoscopic surgery: An evaluation of 35 robot-assisted laparoscopic cholecystectomies. Surg Laparosc Endosc Percutan Tech 12:41-45, 2002.

83. Hemal AK, Menon M: Robotics in urology. Curr Opin Urol 14:89-93, 2004.

84. Cadiere GB, Himpens J, Vertruyen M, et al: Evaluation of telesurgical (robotic) Nissen fundoplication. Surg Endosc 15:918-923, 2001.
85. Marescaux J, Smith MK, Folscher D, et al: Telerobotic laparoscopic cholecystectomy: Initial clinical experience with 25 patients. Ann Surg 234:1-7, 2001.
86. Damiano RJ, Tabaie HA, Mack MJ, et al: Initial prospective multicenter clinical trial of robotically-assisted coronary artery bypass grafting. Ann Thorac Surg 72:1263-1268, 2001.
87. Boyd WD, Desai ND, Kiaii B, et al: A comparison of robot-assisted versus manually constructed endoscopic coronary anastomosis. Ann Thorac Surg 70:839-843, 2000.
88. Ruurda JP, Broeders IA, Pulles B, et al: Manual robot assisted endoscopic suturing: Time-action analysis in an experimental model. Surg Endosc 18:1249-1252, 2004.
89. Wisselink W, Cuesta MA, Gracia C, Rauwerda JA: Robot-assisted laparoscopic aortobifemoral bypass for aortoiliac occlusive disease: A report of two cases. J Vasc Surg 36:1079-1082, 2002.
90. Jobe BA, Duncan W, Swanstrom LL: Totally laparoscopic abdominal aortic aneurysm repair. Surg Endosc 13:77-79, 1999.
91. Kolvenbach R: The role of video-assisted vascular surgery. Eur J Vasc Endovasc Surg 15:377-379, 1998.

24

Niren Angle • William J. Quiñones-Baldrich

Thrombolytic Therapy for Vascular Disease

Thrombolytic therapy is an important modality in the treatment of patients with peripheral vascular disease. Randomized clinical trials have compared thrombolytic therapy with traditional surgical options, thus providing guidelines for patient selection. As a therapeutic intervention, lytic therapy may be the best alternative in certain clinical situations. In many other cases, it is just one aspect of the overall care of patients with thrombotic complications of peripheral vascular disease.

This chapter provides an overview of the fibrinolytic system and available agents. This information can be translated into guidelines to help clinicians select patients who may benefit from thrombolytic therapy. Methods, dosages, complications, and promising new areas are also discussed.

History

The fluidity of blood post mortem is an observation that dates to the Hippocratic school in the 4th century BC.[1] Almost 2000 years later, it was rediscovered by the Italian anatomist Malpighi.[2] In 1761, Morgagni noted that blood does not retain its liquid state after death but frequently forms clots.[3] This is followed by partial or complete reliquefaction.

In 1906, Morawitz observed that postmortem blood destroys fibrinogen and fibrin in normal blood.[4] Thus, the presence of an active fibrinolysin was postulated. The term *fibrinolysis* had been coined by Dastre in 1893 to describe the disappearance of fibrin in unclottable blood obtained from dogs subjected to repeated hemorrhage.[5] From the latter part of the 19th century until the present, intense investigation has been undertaken to elucidate the complex and vital functions of the fibrinolytic system. Its physiology, components, activators, and inhibitors are only partially understood; however, the role of the fibrinolytic system from a homeostatic point of view is fully appreciated. Its therapeutic potential has emerged in the last few decades, and results from prospective clinical trials are now available, providing guidelines to patient selection and therapy. Clearly, precise control of this system to resolve a thrombotic process is on the frontier of clinical medicine. For the vascular specialist, this represents one of the most promising therapeutic modalities. Unfortunately, currently available agents lack the precise control necessary to avoid the complications of an overactive

fibrinolytic system. Even so, thrombolytic therapy can be used successfully, and in some instances it is the preferred treatment.

The Fibrinolytic System

The complex and intricate relationships among all components of the fibrinolytic system are not fully understood. Much progress has been made, however, mostly owing to recognition of the importance of the fibrinolytic system as both a homeostatic system and a therapeutic alternative. The concept of dynamic equilibrium was proposed by Astrup in 1958.[6] In a delicate balance, fibrinolysis breaks down fibrin, which is continuously being deposited throughout the cardiovascular system. This is the result of limited activation of the coagulation system. This baseline fibrinolytic activity is probably under local and central control mechanisms. The feedback loop that prevents systemic fibrinolysis involves both inhibitors at the activator level and specific inhibitors of the proteolytic enzyme plasmin.

The final common pathway in the fibrinolytic system is the conversion of the proenzyme plasminogen to the active enzyme plasmin. Plasminogen is a glycoprotein produced by the liver. Full-sized plasminogen can be divided into a heavy N-terminal region that consists of five homologous but distinct triple-disulfide–bonded domains (kringles) fused to a lighter catalytic C-terminal domain. At least four forms occur in plasma, based on variations in the N-terminal and the degree of glycosylation. The two main forms are Glu-plasminogen and Lys-plasminogen.[7] Glu-plasminogen contains glutamic acid and exists in high concentrations in plasma. Lys-plasminogen, containing mostly lysin in the N-terminal, results from limited proteolysis of the Glu form; it has a shorter half-life and is found in higher concentrations in thrombus, most likely secondary to its higher affinity for fibrin.[8] A schematic view of the fibrinolytic system is presented in Figure 24-1.

The kringle portion of plasminogen is a nonprotease, or heavy chain, consisting of five homologous domains. These domains exhibit a high degree of sequence homology with one another and with domains found in prothrombin, tissue plasminogen activator (t-PA), urinary plasminogen activator, and factor XII. Kringle-4 shares homology with

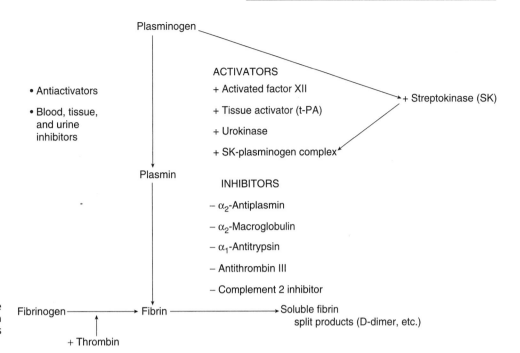

FIGURE 24–1 • Simplified scheme of the fibrinolytic system with endogenous and exogenous activators.

apolipoprotein A. The function of these kringles is thought to be of paramount importance in the binding of plasminogen and plasmin to fibrin, α_2-antiplasmin, and other macromolecules.[9,10] In addition, the kringle portion of plasminogen has been implicated in mediating neutrophil adherence to endothelial cells.[11] On binding, conformational changes occur that transform a closed structure into an open structure. ∈-Aminocaproic acid and tranexamic acid induce this change from the closed structure to the open structure. Because of this change, plasminogen is far more readily cleaved to the active enzyme plasmin by plasminogen activators. The open conformation also binds more readily to exposed lysine residues on fibrin's surface. Concentrations of lysine analogs, such as tranexamic acid and aminocaproic acid, that actually promote the more active, open conformation of Glu-plasminogen also prevent its binding to fibrin and therefore exhibit an antifibrinolytic effect.[12]

The primary substrates for the proteolytic activity of plasmin in circulation are fibrinogen and fibrin. Circulating fibrinogen is composed of three polypeptide chains known as the α, β, and γ chains. These chains are bonded together by disulfide bonds, which are also linked to a second identical chain, thus making fibrinogen a dimer of trimers. Thrombin, the common pathway of the coagulation cascade, removes several amino acid peptides from the end terminal of the α chain, the β chain (fibrinopeptide B), to form fibrin. As new sites are exposed, staggered polymerization is initiated.[7] Through catalysis by factor XIIIa, the domains are brought together and chemically cross-linked. Plasmin catalyzes the hydrolysis of these bonds, producing peptides that can be assayed in circulation. Specifically, those produced after the cleavage of fibrinogen consist of truncated polypeptides collectively known as X fragments. X fragments can be incorporated into both newly forming and existing thrombi, causing them to be more fragile. This has been proposed as an explanation of why fibrin-specific fibrinolytic agents such as t-PA do not result in fewer bleeding complications compared

with nonspecific agents. Because t-PA is such a potent fibrinolytic activator, the accumulation of these X fragments may make existing thrombi more susceptible to its fibrinolytic action. Several fragments are specifically produced by the action of plasmin on fibrin, as opposed to fibrinogen. Unique fragments such as D-dimers can be assayed, documenting fibrinolysis as opposed to fibrinogenolysis.[13]

Plasmin is a relatively nonspecific protease and thus can hydrolyze many proteins found in plasma and extracellular spaces. Known targets of plasmin are factors V and VIII and von Willebrand's factor.[1] Prothrombotic activity can be shown with the initial administration of fibrinolytic agents (specifically, t-PA and streptokinase, which may relate to the release of fibrinopeptide A). Plasminogen can also cause the release of kinin from high-molecular-weight kininogen. In addition, it can directly and indirectly activate prekallikrein, again inducing kinin formation.[14,15] Plasmin can also attack protein components of the basement membrane, as well as other active proteases within the matrix, including fibronectin, collagen, and laminin.[7]

Activation of factor XII by various stimuli results in initiation of the coagulation cascade, conversion of prekallikrein to kallikrein and kinin (inflammatory response), and formation of plasmin from plasminogen. This intrinsic mechanism of activation is complemented by a second intrinsic pathway that is not dependent on factor XII. The main pathway for plasminogen activation is known as the extrinsic system. Two activators are recognized in humans: urokinase-type plasminogen activator (u-PA) and t-PA. Their physiologic activity is controlled by inhibitors, mostly plasminogen activator inhibitor (PAI) type 1 (PAI-1) and type PAI-3. These inhibitors control the activity of the activators in plasma and possibly at the cellular level. PAI-1 is synthesized in the liver and vascular endothelial cells and is normally present in trace amounts in plasma. When pharmacologic doses of these agents are administered, the inhibitor activity is suppressed. It is estimated that one third to one half of the initial pharmacologic dose of urokinase, for example, becomes inactivated shortly after administration.[11] Once plasminogen has been converted to plasmin, inhibitors of plasmin come into play. The main physiologic inhibitor of plasmin is α_2-antiplasmin. This protease inhibitor is a single-chain glycoprotein that inhibits plasminogen in two steps: a fast reversible binding step, followed by the formation of a covalent complex involving the active site of plasmin.[7] The half-life of this complex is approximately 12 hours.[16] Other inhibitors of plasmin include α_2-macroglobulin, protease nexin, and aprotinin. Protease nexin is a broad-spectrum inhibitor of serine proteinases and inhibits, among others, trypsin, thrombin, urokinase, plasmin, and one- or two-chain t-PA. Once bound, these proteases are internalized via nexin receptors on the cell surface and rapidly degraded.[17] Aprotinin, also known as basic pancreatic trypsin inhibitor, has been isolated and purified and is sold under the name Trasylol (Bayer, West Haven, Conn.). It is also a potent inhibitor of trypsin and kallikrein, in addition to plasmin. The use of bovine aprotinin to reduce postoperative bleeding after major surgery has been reported.[18,19] In animal models, it has been shown to serve as an antidote to bleeding induced by the administration of recombinant t-PA (rt-PA).[20] Because aprotinin inhibits plasmin and not the activator, it should work with other plasminogen activators.

This complex system is capable of maintaining a balanced equilibrium between clotting and lysis, so that blood fluidity is ensured. It is important to recognize that although plasmin is highly selective for fibrin, it also digests fibrinogen and other plasma proteins. Circulating plasmin inhibitors prevent this otherwise disordered lytic action and preclude free circulating plasmin under normal conditions. Other important biologic functions of the plasminogen-plasmin system have now been recognized. The actions of plasminogen activators are facilitated by the presence of receptors of plasminogen, u-PA, and t-PA on cell surfaces, as well as in circulation. Expressions of these components have been observed in tissue cultures and in tissues. They are believed to be actively involved in biologic functions at the cellular level, such as embryogenesis, ovulation, neuron growth, muscle regeneration, wound healing, and angiogenesis, and in tumor growth and invasion.[21] It is now postulated that tumor cell invasion (as well as cell migration) and other important biologic processes are dependent on the plasminogen-plasmin system. Endothelial cells and smooth muscle cells that take an active role in thrombosis and atherogenesis may involve the plasminogen-plasmin system and cellular receptors in the reparative process following vascular injury. The expression seems to be modulated by a variety of cytokines, including interleukin and tumor necrosis factor; hormones such as steroid; gonadotropins; and growth factors, including platelet-derived growth factor.[21] Focal proteolysis, accomplished by the binding of these cellular receptors as part of the plasminogen-plasmin system, allows the migrating cell to penetrate its surrounding extracellular matrix. Further, u-PA has been found to be a growth stimulant and mitogenic for some tumor cells.[22-24] These findings suggest that proliferation of endothelial and smooth muscle cells during vascular repair and atherogenesis induces increased expression of u-PA in these cells. Both PAI-1 and PAI-2 are present on cell surfaces. Differences in distribution between u-PA and its inhibitor would allow proteolysis to occur at focal points

where the activator is located. The inhibitor would allow a foothold for the cell, aiding in its movement.

The synthesis and release of PAI-1 by the endothelial and hepatic cells may be under the control of plasma insulin. It has been suggested that insulin stimulates the synthesis and release of PAI-1 from hepatocytes; t-PA and PAI-1 are released simultaneously from endothelial cells because of an acute-phase response to chronic vascular disease and are then rapidly inactivated by complex formation.[25] A link between lipoprotein metabolism and fibrinolytic function has been suggested by the demonstration of significant homology between the amino acid sequence of apolipoprotein A and the structure of plasminogen. Thus, a prothrombotic function by virtue of interference with the numerous physiologic functions of plasminogen has been suggested in patients with increased levels of apolipoprotein A. Apolipoprotein A has also been found to competitively inhibit the binding of plasminogen to fibrinogen and to the plasminogen receptor on endothelial cells.[26]

Plasma levels of both t-PA and PAI-1 exhibit circadian variations. For example, t-PA activity is lowest in the early morning and highest in the afternoon. Plasma PAI activity peaks in the early morning and passes through a trough in the afternoon. Thus, overall, there is decreased fibrinolytic activity in the morning.[27-30] Differences in patterns have been observed between men and women, suggesting a hormonal influence.[31] Further, PAI activity has been noted to vary secondary to diet, with caffeine-containing beverages possibly enhancing fibrinolytic activity. Conversely, cigarette smoking induces an acute increase in t-PA; this increase in t-PA may deplete normal stores and thus paradoxically decrease fibrinolytic capacity.

From the foregoing discussion, it is evident that the fibrinolytic (plasminogen-plasmin) system plays a vital role in biologic homeostasis. In addition, it has a pivotal role in certain disease states, ranging from atherosclerosis to carcinogenesis.

From a therapeutic standpoint, drugs capable of converting plasminogen to plasmin achieve their lytic effect to a great extent by overwhelming circulating plasmin inhibitors and generating an abundance of plasmin (exogenous fibrinolysis). Circulating plasmin not only produces the desired fibrinolysis but also proceeds to digest circulating fibrinogen. A more desirable situation results in the activation of thrombus-bound plasminogen (endogenous fibrinolysis) by these agents. Thrombus-bound plasminogen is, to a certain extent, protected from circulating inhibitors and thus proceeds with fibrin digestion much more effectively. Current investigations are concentrated on producing agents with a high affinity for thrombus-bound plasminogen and little activation of the circulating zymogen. Clinical experience to date has failed to demonstrate this theoretical benefit. With better understanding of the complexity of the fibrinolytic system, it is possible that these benefits can be realized.

Fibrinolytic Agents

Agents capable of activating the fibrinolytic system can be divided into indirect and direct activators. Indirect activators include a long list of drugs capable of increasing fibrinolytic activity in vivo without direct in vitro activity on plasminogen. The mechanism of action is variable and has not been elucidated for most of these indirect agents.

From a therapeutic standpoint, chronic enhancement of fibrinolytic activity is attractive but of unproved clinical value. Most indirect fibrinolytic drugs lose their effectiveness over time. Such is the case with nicotinic acid and epinephrine. Both cause an abrupt but transient increase in fibrinolytic activity by the release of endothelial plasminogen activator. Thus, long-term administration is of no benefit.

Antidiuretic hormone (ADH) is capable of stimulating the fibrinolytic system at the expense of severe cardiovascular side effects. A more prolonged response without side effects has been observed with a synthetic analog of ADH, desmopressin acetate (DDAVP). Intranasal administration of this analog caused a plasminogen activator response with a half-life of more than 6 hours.[32] The increased fibrinolytic response to DDAVP, however, seems to be clinically insignificant when compared with the endothelial release of factor VIII and other important procoagulant effects, which have been clinically useful in managing patients with certain bleeding diatheses.

Steroids and diguanides (phenformin) are the most promising of these compounds. Stanozolol, for example, is an anabolic steroid capable of producing sustained stimulation of the fibrinolytic system for periods longer than 5 years with daily administration.[33] In a small clinical trial, Jarrett and colleagues treated 16 patients who had chronic recurrent thrombophlebitis with stanozolol.[34] Thirteen patients had no recurrences during short-term treatment (6 weeks). Renewed attacks were seen in five patients after discontinuation of therapy; these attacks were successfully relieved by the readministration of stanozolol and phenformin.

The available evidence on indirect fibrinolytic agents is mostly anecdotal, and the long-term benefits of an enhanced fibrinolytic system are open to speculation. In many cases, the increased fibrinolytic activity occurs in patients whose baseline activity is depressed. In others, no clinical benefit is observed despite a sustained drug effect. In addition, fibrinolytic capacity may be decreased by chronic stimulation, thus rendering the system incapable of adequately responding to a thrombotic stimulus.[10] Certainly, this is an area that requires randomized, controlled, long-term studies to answer important questions about the value of chronic enhancement of fibrinolytic activity in vascular disease.

Thrombolytic Agents

The use of thrombolytic agents has clearly resulted in a significant improvement in the outcome of patients with acute cardiac ischemia or myocardial infarction. It has also resulted in a modification in the treatment algorithm for patients with peripheral arterial occlusion. Although an improved outcome with regard to limb salvage and mortality has not been demonstrated, it is clear that thrombolytic therapy is an important treatment option for patients with vascular occlusive disease. Table 24-1 summarizes the characaeristics of some of the common thrombolytic agents.

FIRST-GENERATION THROMBOLYTIC DRUGS

First-generation thrombolytic agents—namely, streptokinase and urokinase—are very effective at thrombolysis, but their potency is limited by the fact that they are not fibrin specific. They also convert circulating plasminogen to plasmin, but because circulating plasminogen and the plasminogen in thrombus are in equilibrium, the plasminogen in thrombus would be depleted, thus limiting the efficacy of the agent. This has been termed *plasminogen steal* and is thought to reduce clot lysis.

Streptokinase

Streptokinase is a single-chain nonenzymatic protein produced by β-hemolytic streptococci. Its discovery by Tillett and Garner in 1933 revived an interest in fibrinolysis that has spanned the past 7 decades.[35] Early clinical experience was complicated by a multitude of pyogenic and allergic reactions. This prompted manufacturers to refine the drug, achieving the currently purified product and a marked reduction in febrile and allergic reactions.

The mechanism of action of streptokinase is complex. It initially forms an equimolar complex with plasminogen to form a plasminogen activator. Thus, it requires plasminogen as a cofactor and a substrate. The initial reaction is species specific, having excellent affinity for human and cat plasminogen, relatively poor affinity for dog and rabbit plasminogen, and no reaction with bovine proenzyme. Once the activator

TABLE 24–1	Thrombolytic Agents			
	Streptokinase	**Urokinase**	**Tissue Plasminogen Activator**	**Reteplase**
Source	β-hemolytic *Streptococcus*	Fetal renal cell culture	Recombinant DNA technology	Plasminogen activator
Metabolism	Liver	Liver	Liver	Liver
Advantages	Low cost	Direct activator; no allergic reaction	Fibrin-selective direct activator	Plasminogen activator in presence of fibrin
Disadvantages	Allergic reactions; complex mechanism of action	High cost	High cost	High cost
Regional infusion dosage	Low dose: 5000-10,000 U/hr High dose: 30,000-60,000 U/hr	30,000-50,000 U/hr 2000-4000 U/min for 1-2 hr, then 1000-2000 U/min	0.05 -0.1 U/kg/hr	0.5 U/hr IV; no bolus Rate may be adjusted up to 0.75-1.0 U/hr or down to 0.25 U/hr

complex is formed, it is an excellent activator of all mammalian plasminogen. Besides converting uncomplexed plasminogen to plasmin, plasminogen within the activator complex is converted to plasmin, and during this conversion, streptokinase undergoes rapid progressive degradation.

The kinetics of these reactions have been studied in vitro. In vivo, a more complicated series of reactions occurs. Infusion of streptokinase is followed initially by neutralization by circulating antistreptococcal antibodies. The remaining drug then combines with circulating plasminogen to form the activator complex. This then converts uncomplexed plasminogen to plasmin, which combines with any excess free streptokinase, is neutralized by circulating antiplasmins, or binds to preformed fibrin. The last produces the desired effect of thrombolysis. However, when activity is measured, two half-lives are detected—16 minutes and 83 minutes—indicating that these complex interactions have a significant impact on the concentration and activity of the drug.

From the foregoing discussion, it is evident that precise control of thrombolysis is not possible because the dose-response relationship of streptokinase varies from patient to patient. Initially, clinical use was guided by titers of anti-streptococcal antibodies and measurement of the various components or products of the system. This proved impractical, and current practice relies on standardized dosages that achieve the desired effect in the great majority of cases. A potential drawback of this approach is that excess amounts of drug could use most of the circulating plasminogen to form activator complex; this might leave inadequate amounts of zymogen to convert to plasmin. This problem of exceeding plasminogen availability may be important during regional, rather than systemic, administration. Some investigators have combined streptokinase with plasmin administration, resulting in improvements in measured parameters such as plasminogen level, fibrinogen level, and potential fibrinolytic capacity.[36] Similar results are obtained by intermittent rather than continuous infusion of the drug. Unfortunately, the results of these noncontrolled trials have raised doubts about the effectiveness of such regimens. For the average clinician, continuous infusion therapy remains the most practical method of administration.

Streptokinase has largely fallen out of favor, partly because of the immunogenicity of even the refined form, which can result in fever, allergic reactions, and acquired drug resistance. A complex of streptokinase and anisoylated plasminogen streptokinase activator complex (APSAC), or anistreplase, was developed in an attempt to solve some of the problems inherent to streptokinase. Although the concept is theoretically sound, clinical trials were unable to demonstrate any increase in efficacy or any decrease in antigenicity with the administration of APSAC.

Streptokinase is the only thrombolytic agent approved by the U.S. Food and Drug Administration (FDA) for use in peripheral arterial and venous thrombolysis, but it is rare to find it being used for that purpose, for the reasons stated earlier. The newer thrombolytic agents have much better safety profiles and better therapeutic efficacy; therefore, off-label use of these alternative thrombolytic agents is the norm.

Urokinase

Urokinase is a serine protease with direct activator activity; it is normally present in urine as a product of renal tubular cells.

It was originally isolated by MacFarlane and Pilling in 1947.[37] Urokinase is present in varying molecular weights, with variable activity. Original purification was done from urine, yielding small amounts of the enzyme at a considerable cost. Newer production methods use human fetal kidney cell culture.

Urokinase is nonantigenic, and its mechanism of action is much more direct compared with that of streptokinase. Urokinase cleaves plasminogen (its only known protein substrate), by first-order reaction kinetics, to plasmin. It is pH and temperature stable. The lack of circulating neutralizing antibodies and its direct mechanism of action allow for a predictable dose-response relationship. Although allergic reactions are rare, over the last few years a febrile response to drug administration has become more common. It has been suggested that this may be related to interleukins that are still present in recently manufactured drug batches. In the past, when the use of urokinase was less common, aging of the drug actually allowed the interleukins to become inactive. These febrile reactions respond readily to antipyretics. Interestingly, urokinase does not contain any lysine binding sites and therefore does not have any fibrin binding properties.[38] High-affinity receptors for urokinase, however, have been demonstrated in several cell types and have been postulated as a mechanism by which cells can invade the intracellular matrix and play a role in other physiologic and pathologic processes.[39-41]

Urokinase is a serine protease and hydrolyzes synthetic esters containing arginine and lysine. Unlike streptokinase, urokinase directly activates plasminogen by cleaving the Arg560-Val561 "activation bond." The activation of plasminogen by urokinase occurs by proteolysis of its substrate plasminogen. When administered intravenously, urokinase is rapidly removed from the circulation, mainly via hepatic clearance. It has been estimated that the half-life of urokinase in humans is on the order of 14 minutes. Urokinase also reacts with other proteins, including fibrinogen. Urokinase is much more effective in cleaving the susceptible site in plasminogen when it is in the Lys form than in the Glu form. However, the activation reaction of the latter by urokinase may be enhanced by the presence of fibrin.[42] Administration of exogenous plasminogen may also accelerate thrombolysis by urokinase. In an experimental study, urokinase infusion alone was compared with urokinase infusion in clots laced with plasminogen. Lacing with plasminogen resulted in a more rapid restoration of flow. The rate of clot dissolution was also significantly enhanced in the plasminogen-laced thrombi.[3] Therefore, it appears that exhaustion of native plasminogen may be a limiting factor in clot dissolution; thus, the provision of zymogen during thrombolysis may improve the drug's effectiveness.

Controversy exists regarding the actual thrombolytic effect of urokinase when administered in vivo. Experimental studies have suggested exogenous fibrinolysis as the main pathway, with limited activation of plasminogen within the thrombus (endogenous fibrinolysis).[43] In vivo, however, laboratory findings in treated patients have indicated less of a fibrinogenolytic response, suggesting that plasminemia is reduced with urokinase compared with streptokinase administration.[44] This implies a significant endogenous activity. In clinical practice, the results of urokinase therapy have paralleled those achieved with streptokinase, with a decreased incidence of bleeding complications suggested by several investigators.[45-47] Whereas major bleeding complications are seen in 15% to 20% of patients treated with streptokinase, such complications have been reported in only 5% to 10% of patients treated with urokinase. Thus, the benefits observed in laboratory results and the reduced incidence of significant plasminemia with urokinase seem to translate into a decreased incidence of bleeding complications in clinical practice. Although the cost of urokinase remains high compared with that of streptokinase, when complications are taken into account, the cost of therapy for streptokinase and urokinase is comparable.[48]

Residual thromboplastic activity was detected in the early urokinase preparations,[49] and this may account for the initial hypercoagulable state reported by Kakkar and Scully.[50] At present, this does not appear to be a clinically significant problem.

Despite the drug's record of safety and efficacy accrued over the years, the FDA halted the release and use of urokinase, manufactured by Abbott Laboratories, on the grounds of deviations from the FDA's current good manufacturing practices guidelines, developed to prevent the manufacture of unsafe products. The FDA's inspection of Abbott's manufacturing facility in North Chicago in 1998 raised concerns about the neonatal kidney cells that were being used as a source of urokinase.[51,52] They originated from Cali, Colombia, and were obtained through a separate company. The source population was thought to be at high risk for various diseases, including tropical ones, and although there were no documented cases of infectious transmission resulting from urokinase administration, the FDA demurred on the point, stating that any connection between the drug and such cases might have gone unrecognized.

In October 2002, the FDA approved the reintroduction of urokinase to the market after Abbott made significant changes in its quality-control and manufacturing practices. Uruokinase was approved for use in the treatment of pulmonary embolism. Although it has not been approved for use in the peripheral arterial and venous systems, it is likely that, owing to its efficacy and favorable safety profile, most practitioners will revert to using it preferentially, although this remains to be seen. During the time that urokinase was unavailable, increased experience and familiarity were gained with other agents, such as rt-PA and reteplase.[53]

SECOND-GENERATION THROMBOLYTIC DRUGS

Unlike first-generation thrombolytic drugs, which not only act on fibrin but also convert circulating plasminogen to plasmin, second-generation agents are supposed to be fibrin selective. These agents were developed to avoid systemic depletion of circulating fibrinogen and plasminogen and the consequent systemic thrombolytic state; these agents are represented by t-PA, or alteplase, and single-chain u-PA, or pro-urokinase. There is considerable evidence that the plasminogen activator agents are not appreciably fibrin or thrombus specific and that they activate the complement system and damage the cell membranes of platelets and endothelial cells.

Tissue Plasminogen Activator

Tissue plasminogen activator is a naturally occurring enzyme present in all human tissues. Its concentration is variable,

with high levels detected in the uterus and moderate amounts in the heart, skeletal muscles, kidneys, ovaries, lungs, thyroid, pituitary, and lymph nodes. Scant amounts of t-PA are found in the liver, spleen, brain, and testes.[54] It is thought to originate from vascular endothelium, and, with the exception of the liver and spleen, tissue concentration correlates with vascularity.

Isolation and purification of t-PA were initially hampered by inadequate sources and procedures. In 1979, Rijken and associates were successful in obtaining 1 mg of t-PA from 5 kg of human uterine tissue.[55] Recognizing the potential of this drug, investigators have concentrated on other sources.

At present, there are two main sources of t-PA. The Bowes melanoma cell line is uniquely efficient in producing large quantities of t-PA,[56] which was subsequently proved to be identical to uterine t-PA.[57] Another source has emerged from the use of recombinant DNA technology, and efforts in the cloning and expression of the t-PA gene from the melanoma cell line have been successful. Since 1987, when rt-PA was approved for the treatment of acute myocardial infarction, it has been used for peripheral thrombolysis as an alternative to urokinase.

In general, plasminogen activators do not cause clot dissolution directly; they must first find and activate molecules of plasminogen in the vasculature at the site of the clot. t-PA is a direct plasminogen activator. Its main advantage is its high affinity for thrombus-bound fibrin. In addition, the presence of fibrinogen enhances its efficiency in the activation of plasminogen. Two types of t-PA are recognized, with a commercial preparation being a mixture of both types. A single-chain form is cleaved by plasminogen to yield two-chain t-PA. The one- and two-chain forms of t-PA are comparable in activity, with the one-chain form being quickly converted to the two-chain type as lysis proceeds. Most of the circulating t-PA is in the single-chain form. Its selective action promises to produce fewer systemic effects when compared with streptokinase or urokinase.[58] The half-life of t-PA has been estimated to be between 4 and 7 minutes in vivo.[59] With its presumed nonantigenicity and high affinity for fibrin, t-PA theoretically should produce improved clinical results. However, recent randomized trials have failed to demonstrate significant clinical differences from other available agents.

When fibrin-selective agents are used for regional infusion, most of the thrombolytic effect is secondary to fibrin-bound plasminogen. However, the importance of a fresh supply of plasminogen to maintain the fibrin-bound plasminogen pool has been emphasized. Experimental studies have suggested that clot lysis induced by the activation of plasminogen is dependent on clot-associated plasminogen, which in turn depends on the concentration of plasminogen in plasma. Depletion of both contributes to less frequent and less rapid recanalization, which is more noticeable with non–fibrin-selective agents than with fibrin-selective ones, likely the result of the depletion of plasminogen induced by the nonselective agents.[60]

Trials comparing rt-PA with streptokinase in patients with acute coronary thrombosis have failed to establish that this more specific drug is a better thrombolytic agent. Systemic bleeding complications have been similar, despite a milder homeostatic defect by laboratory evaluation in the rt-PA groups.[61] Questions still exist regarding proper dosage to achieve effective local lysis with minimal systemic effects.

Tissue plasminogen activator may also bind and be activated on platelet surfaces.[62] Owing to this binding to platelet receptors, platelets can direct t-PA action on their surface, leading to rapid cleavage of glycoprotein Ib and the loss of platelet binding to von Willebrand's factor. This may explain why concentrations of t-PA achieved early in therapy may inhibit platelet aggregation.

In animal models of thrombolysis, it has been suggested that multiple bolus administrations of t-PA have greater lytic efficacy than equal doses given as a single bolus or a continuous infusion.[63] This may have significant implications for clinical therapy, where protocols requiring continuous infusion of the agent have shown a greater incidence of bleeding complications than protocols in which the drug is administered in bolus form. This may be explained by the accumulation of partially degraded fibrin (X fragments), which may increase the affinity of t-PA for plasminogen by about 17-fold.[7]

In a study in which 17 patients were infused with rt-PA at a rate of 0.1 mg/kg per hour, all patients demonstrated thrombolysis, with 16 showing clinical improvement.[64] More important, there were no systemic complications, with a mean fibrinogen drop of 42% of baseline. The infusion time was 1 to 6 hours, compared with the usual 48 to 72 hours necessary for streptokinase infusion. One patient died from an intracranial hemorrhage during postinfusion heparin therapy. Experience in randomized trials has suggested that a lower dose is just as effective, with a decreased risk of bleeding. The recommended lower dose is 0.05 mg/kg per hour.[65]

Systemic complications may be more related to dose and method of administration with t-PA than with urokinase or streptokinase. It appears that t-PA is more potent and faster than the older agents, perhaps because of its high fibrin affinity. In this regard, t-PA may be ideally suited for intra-arterial administration, because a 4- to 6-hour trial could be followed by timely surgical intervention. In addition, intraoperative use could be a welcome adjunct to surgical embolectomy.

Pro-urokinase

Saruplase, also known as recombinant single-chain urokinase-type plasminogen activator, or pro-urokinase, is a prodrug produced from a naturally occurring physiologic protease.[65] Pro-urokinase is a single-chain polypeptide of 411 amino acids that is converted by plasmin into an active, low-molecular-weight form of urokinase with 276 amino acids.[66] Pro-urokinase functions as a potent plasminogen activator of fibrin-bound plasminogen without requiring extensive systemic conversion to two-chain urokinase. Thus, the entire thrombolytic process is confined to the fibrin clot itself. Administration of pro-urokinase causes decreases in α_2-antiplasmin and fibrinogen and an increase in fibrinogen degradation products. Pro-urokinase is highly effective in the conversion of Lys-plasminogen to plasmin. In contrast, it has little or no activity in the conversion of Glu-plasminogen to plasmin. Because Lys-plasminogen is present in high concentrations in thrombus, this gives pro-urokinase fibrin-specific properties. In addition, plasminogen that is absorbed in thrombus changes its configuration to a pseudo–Lys-plasminogen, which is also attacked by pro-urokinase, converting it to Lys-plasmin. Circulating pro-urokinase is very stable in plasma because of its resistance to plasma inhibitors and ionized calcium.[67]

The fibrin specificities of t-PA and pro-urokinase appear to rely on different mechanisms. Whereas t-PA is fibrin clot binding, the fibrin-selective properties of pro-urokinase are thought to be secondary to its preference for activation of Lys-plasminogen or Lys-like–plasminogen substrate found in thrombus. This effect prolongs its half-life, which has been estimated to be several days. Such a prolonged half-life has theoretical advantages in clinical situations in which prolonged activity is desired. However, in peripheral arterial occlusions, if the regional infusion fails to produce the desired result and the patient must go to the operating room shortly after discontinuation of the infusion, this prolonged effect may be undesirable. At this time, there is no reported experience with such use.

Many of the clinical trials using this drug have been studies of patients with myocardial infarction, where the notable finding was an increased incidence of intracranial hemorrhage (0.9%).[68] The most recent trial was the Prolyse in Acute Cerebral Thromboembolism II (PROACT II) study, which evaluated intra-arterial pro-urokinase for acute ischemic stroke.[69] Early intracranial hemorrhage with neurologic deterioration within 24 hours occurred in 10% of pro-urokinase patients and 2% of control patients. Although it is effective at thrombolysis, the increased bleeding risk has limited its widespread use. A phase II trial evaluating pro-urokinase versus urokinase for thrombolysis of acute peripheral arterial occlusion showed that pro-urokinase had a greater efficacy but an increased risk of bleeding complications at a dose of 8 mg/hour; with a dose of 2 mg/hour, there was a slightly lower rate of thrombolysis, combined with a lower incidence of bleeding complications and fibrinogenolysis.[70]

THIRD-GENERATION THROMBOLYTIC DRUGS

The last few years have seen the development of a new generation of thrombolytic drugs, including mutant molecules of single-chain u-PA and t-PA; chimeric plasminogen activators; conjugates of plasminogen activators with monoclonal antibodies against fibrin, platelets, or thrombomodulin; and plasminogen activators of animal and bacterial origin.[53]

Reteplase

Reteplase is a single-chain deletion mutant of alteplase, consisting of just the kringle-2 and protease domains.[71] Reteplase has a fivefold decrease in fibrin binding and a half-life of 14 to 18 minutes due to the aforementioned structural differences. Reteplase has less binding to endothelium and monocytes compared with t-PA, and this reduced binding results in increased circulating levels in the bloodstream.[72] It catalyzes the cleavage of endogenous plasminogen to generate plasmin. The activation of plasminogen is stimulated in the presence of fibrin and is mediated by the kringle-2 domain.[10,73] Plasmin then degrades the fibrin matrix of the thrombus, thus exerting its fibrinolytic action.

The fact that plasminogen activators in general activate plasminogen molecules in or near the clot allows efficient lysis in small clot burdens such as the coronary circulation. The absolute dependence on a sufficient amount of available plasminogen limits the dose-related efficacy when the clot burden is large. Long, retracted (i.e., organized) clots, such as those in the peripheral arterial circulation, are often deficient in plasminogen. Despite this, plasminogen activators such as reteplase and t-PA are efficacious when delivered through a catheter directly into the thrombus rather than systemically.

Reteplase has increasingly become the thrombolytic agent of choice in the treatment of peripheral vascular occlusion, given the unavailability of urokinase for a few years. Nevertheless, published studies regarding its use in controlled trials are relatively few in number. There are two pilot studies that evaluated the dosing regimen of reteplase in the treatment of myocardial infarction.[74,75] These studies demonstrated that reteplase produced significantly higher TIMI-3 (thromboembolism in myocardial infarction) flow rates at 60 and 90 minutes than did front-loaded alteplase. However, in two subsequent trials—the INJECT[76] and GUSTO III[77] trials—despite the higher TIMI-3 flow rates, this did not translate into a lower mortality in the reteplase-treated patients (7.5% for reteplase vs. 7.2% for alteplase).[15] Reteplase has lower fibrin affinity and thus appears to penetrate thrombus effectively and activate fibrin-bound plasminogen within the clot, resulting in faster clot lysis. Thrombolytics may also cause platelet activation, and this may have been responsible for some of the previously noted lack of efficacy. The addition of glycoprotein IIb/IIIa inhibitors appears to increase the efficacy of thrombolytic agents, as well as speed the lysis.

Tenecteplase

Tenecteplase (TNK-t-PA) is a t-PA mutant in which a threonine molecule ([103]Thr) is replaced by Asn, and the sequence Lys-His-Arg-Arg is changed to Ala-Ala-Ala-Ala. This confers high fibrin selectivity and prolongs the half-life to 15 to 19 minutes. It is very effective in arterial, platelet-rich thrombi and is more resistant to plasminogen activator inhibitor. Although most of the published data regarding tenecteplase have been in relation to acute coronary syndromes, there is increasing experience in peripheral arterial thrombolysis. One group published its experience with continuous tenecteplase infusion in conjunction with glycoprotein IIb/IIIa inhibition with tirofiban for peripheral arterial thrombolysis.[78] The dose of tenecteplase infusion was 0.25 to 0.50 mg/hr, with a mean infusion time of 7.5 hours. Out of 48 patients with iliofemoral arterial thrombosis, complete lysis was achieved in 35 patients (73%). There were no deaths, no intracranial bleeding, and no embolic events. It appears, at least from this study, that lysis time is shorter; however, the longer half-life has implications for surgical intervention, as addressed earlier.

Staphylokinase

Staphylokinase is a plasminogen activator produced by certain strains of *Staphylococcus aureus* and was first described as having fibrinolytic properties in 1948.[79] The gene has been cloned from genomic DNA of a lysogenic strain of *S. aureus*. When exposed to a fibrin clot in human plasma, staphylokinase reacts with plasmin at the clot-plasma interface; this staphylokinase-plasmin complex activates thrombus-bound plasminogen and exerts its fibrinolytic activity. Any plasmin that is liberated from the clot is rapidly inactivated by α_2-antiplasmin. In this manner, plasminogen activation by staphylokinase is confined to the thrombus, and the collateral effects of fibrinogen depletion and serum plasminogen

activation are minimized. Patients treated with staphylokinase do, however, develop neutralizing antibodies, the titers of which can remain elevated for several months.[80]

Immunofibrinolysis

In an attempt to develop fibrin-specific agents, monoclonal antifibrin antibodies have been bonded to urokinase or streptokinase, rendering these agents fibrin selective. These monoclonal antibodies do not appear to cross-react with fibrinogen and thus show a marked increase in in vitro fibrinolysis compared with unmodified activator.[81] The clinical applicability of these agents remains to be determined. They may significantly alter the current approach to the management of thrombotic disease. Nevertheless, repeat therapy would require different monoclonal antibodies to prevent adverse immunologic reactions.

SUMMARY

Most of the clinical experience to date has been with streptokinase, urokinase, and, most recently, t-PA. The effectiveness and complication rates of each of these agents are discussed later in the specific sections dealing with the various clinical entities. Based on the experience to date, streptokinase seems to be a less desirable agent for use in peripheral vascular thrombosis, probably because of its complex mechanism of action, which translates into dosage difficulties and clinical complications.

Bleeding associated with thrombolytic therapy, regardless of the agent used, is most frequent at sites used for cardiac catheterization, arterial blood gas studies, intravenous infusion, or venipuncture. At any invaded site, the vascular endothelium is disrupted, resulting in an inflammatory reaction. The major components of an inflammatory reaction are fibrin and two different cell types that form the hemostatic plug. The fibrin in the hemostatic plug is identical to the fibrin in a pathologic thrombus in freshly (recently) formed thrombi and is much more susceptible to lysis. Thus, if a fibrin-specific thrombolytic agent is infused into the circulation, it will interact with molecularly identical fibrin in both the hemostatic plug and the pathologic thrombus; this brings about dissolution of the hemostatic plug, thereby inducing bleeding. This may be the reason why, in all recently completed studies comparing first- and second-generation thrombolytic agents, there is as much if not more bleeding with the newer, second-generation agents as with the older ones.

The degradation products of fibrinogen or fibrin are the absolute index of the degree of activation of the fibrinolytic system. When there are high levels of these fibrin degradation products, they are easily detected and signify an intense activation of the plasminogen-plasmin proteolytic system. There is good evidence that all the second-generation agents, despite assertions to the contrary, do induce the systemic fibrinolytic system, and this probably explains why the rate of distant hemorrhage is no different from that of first-generation agents.

Although fibrin selectivity has theoretical advantages, the clinical use of fibrin-specific agents has so far failed to demonstrate a significant benefit in various test protocols. Specifically, the rate of bleeding complications with t-PA is no different from that seen with streptokinase when it is used in the treatment of acute myocardial infarction. In fact, a slight increased incidence of intracranial bleeding was seen with t-PA. This may be due to its marked potency compared with other agents currently available. Regional administration of these agents may realize the true benefit of their selective property. In addition to the proper method of infusion (systemic vs. regional), dosage may play an important role in realizing the clinical benefits of a fibrin-specific agent.

Systemic Thrombolytic Therapy

This section discusses systemic thrombolytic therapy for venous and peripheral arterial disease. Treatment of acute coronary thrombosis is purposely omitted.

Although systemic thrombolytic therapy has been used for peripheral arterial occlusions, results have been disappointing, with bleeding complications outweighing the benefits obtained. Local intra-arterial administration prevents some of the systemic complications and is used for peripheral arterial and graft occlusion. Even venous thrombolysis is most effective when catheter directed. Patient selection is probably the most important factor in obtaining good results with either modality.

PATIENT SELECTION

During the course of systemic thrombolytic therapy, a systemic lytic state is achieved in which fibrin is lysed wherever it has been deposited in the body. Thus, hemostatic plugs are as vulnerable as the clot or thrombus for which therapy was initiated. Selection of patients for systemic lytic therapy is based on the presence of an appropriate documented indication (discussed later) and careful evaluation for the presence of contraindications.

Contraindications to systemic therapy are listed in Table 24-2. Absolute contraindications are active internal bleeding and recent (within 2 months) cerebrovascular accident or other intracranial condition. Relative major contraindications include recent (within 10 days) major surgery, trauma, obstetric delivery, organ biopsy, or puncture of a noncompressible vessel; recent gastrointestinal bleed; and severe hypertension. Relative minor contraindications carry a higher risk of complications, but the benefits of therapy may still outweigh the hazards. Peripheral embolization from a central source is a potential hazard of systemic lytic therapy. Therefore, valvular heart disease, atrial fibrillation, and previous history of emboli are relative contraindications to systemic lytic therapy. The presence of a mural thrombus is a relative contraindication to fibrinolytic therapy because of the potential for peripheral embolization due to fragmentation, which could have devastating consequences. In patients with a thrombus in the left side of the heart demonstrable by echocardiography, alternative forms of treatment should be considered. It must be recognized, however, that successful lysis of ventricular thrombi with urokinase has been reported.[82] Severe liver disease affects drug metabolism, making the response unpredictable. During pregnancy, a systemic lytic state may precipitate abruptio placentae or may lead to hypofibrinogenemia in the fetus, with an increased risk of bleeding. Streptokinase is specifically contraindicated in patients with known allergy, previous therapy within 6 months, or recent streptococcal infection.

One of the most devastating complications of fibrinolytic therapy is intracranial hemorrhage. The incidence of this

TABLE 24–2	Contraindications to Systemic Lytic Therapy

Absolute
Active internal bleeding
Recent (<2 mo) cerebrovascular accident
Intracranial pathologic condition

Relative Major
Recent (<10 days) major surgery, obstetric delivery, or organ biopsy
Active peptic ulcer or gastrointestinal disorder
Recent major trauma
Uncontrolled hypertension

Relative Minor
Minor surgery or trauma
Recent cardiopulmonary resuscitation
High likelihood of left heart thrombus (e.g., atrial fibrillation with mitral valve disease)
Bacterial endocarditis
Hemostatic defects (e.g., renal or liver disease)
Pregnancy
Diabetic hemorrhagic retinopathy

Streptokinase
Known allergy
Recent streptococcal infection
Previous therapy within 6 mo

complication is approximatley 1% of treated patients in trials for acute myocardial infarction. The median time between the start of thrombolytic therapy and the onset of clinical signs of intracranial hemorrhage ranges from 3 to 36 hours, with a mean of 16 hours. Mortality is high for this complication, with an estimated mortality of 66%. Factors predictive of intracranial hemorrhage by multivariate logistic regression analysis include oral anticoagulation before admission, body weight less than 70 kg, and age older than 65 years. An increased incidence of intracerebral hemorrhage has been observed in patients receiving higher doses of t-PA. In the Thrombosis in Myocardial Infarction (TIMI) trial,[83] 1.3% of patients receiving 150 mg of t-PA suffered an intracerebral hemorrhage, as opposed to 0.4% of patients receiving 100 mg of the drug. Interestingly, in the TIMI-II trial, patients who received immediate beta blockade as part of their regimen had no incidence of intracerebral hemorrhage when given 100 mg of t-PA, compared with 0.5% in the group that did not receive beta blockade. This was not true, however, for patients treated with 150 mg of t-PA. The mechanism by which beta blockers may protect against intracerebral bleeding has not been established.[84]

In the Surgery versus Thrombolysis for Ischemia of the Lower Extremity (STILE) trial, patients were randomized to thrombolytic therapy with t-PA or urokinase versus surgery for the treatment of lower limb ischemia.[85] When evaluated by an intent-to-treat analysis, the incidence of life-threatening hemorrhage was 5.3% to 5.7%. When analyzed on a per-protocol basis, the incidence of this complication was 7.8% in the thrombolysis group. The incidence was similar in patients treated with t-PA and urokinase; these patients also received aspirin and heparin, which may have added to the risk. However, patients with bleeding complications did not receive more heparin or a higher dose of lytic agent; they appeared to respond differently to the therapy. At the end of the infusion, patients with bleeding complications had a significantly lower fibrinogen level than did patients without hemorrhagic complications (188 mg/dL vs. 310 mg/dL). Measurement of fibrinogen levels, along with the international normalized ratio and partial thromboplastin time (PTT), may be helpful in guiding dose and duration of therapy.

INDICATIONS

Pulmonary Embolism

In 1968, a cooperative, controlled, randomized study to evaluate the use of urokinase in pulmonary embolism was initiated.[86] By 1970, 160 patients were entered and assigned to one of two therapeutic arms. Pulmonary angiography was performed on all patients before and after therapy, with lung scans repeated at 3, 6, and 12 months. The minimal eligibility was occlusion of at least one segmental pulmonary artery on angiography. Excluded from the trial were patients who had had recent operations and those with contraindications to heparin or thrombolytic therapy. Seventy-eight patients received anticoagulants alone (heparin 75 units/pound loading dose, 10 units/pound per hour for 12 hours), and 82 received urokinase (2000 units/pound per hour for 12 hours). Following the 12-hour infusion, all patients received heparin for a minimum of 5 days to maintain a prolonged bleeding time.

The randomization produced a reasonably good balance between the treatment groups. Urokinase therapy resulted in a significantly accelerated resolution of pulmonary emboli at 24 hours, as shown by pulmonary arteriograms, lung scans, and right-sided pressures. No significant differences in mortality or recurrence rates were observed. Patients receiving urokinase tended to respond better if they were younger than 50 years old, the embolus was less than 48 hours old, or the embolus was large, especially if shock was present.

Bleeding complications were significant in both groups (heparin, 27%; urokinase, 45%). This high complication rate is likely the result of demands in the protocol for multiple, frequent invasive procedures, including cutdowns performed for pulmonary angiography. The study group concluded that further studies were needed before specific therapeutic recommendations could be made.

In 1974, the second phase of this cooperative study was reported.[87] This study followed the same guidelines as in phase I, comparing 12 hours of urokinase therapy with 24 hours of urokinase therapy and 24 hours of streptokinase therapy. A group treated with heparin alone was not included because the protocol was almost identical to that in the phase I trial, which showed urokinase to be superior to heparin in clot resolution. Fifty-seven patients were given urokinase (2000 units/pound loading dose, 2000 units/pound per hour for 24 hours), and 61 patients received the same regimen for 12 hours. Fifty-eight patients received streptokinase (250,000 units loading dose, 100,000 units/hour for 24 hours).

As expected, the drop in plasminogen during therapy was steeper for patients receiving streptokinase, but otherwise, the lytic effect was similar. Patients receiving 12 hours of urokinase infusion had nearly equivalent results to those in the phase I trial receiving urokinase. No benefit was seen from extending the urokinase infusion to 24 hours. In patients

with massive embolism, however, the greatest improvement was seen with 24-hour urokinase infusion, although the differences were not statistically significant. Streptokinase and urokinase yielded similar results, with small differences favoring urokinase. The study group concluded that all three regimens were more effective in accelerating the resolution of pulmonary thromboemboli than heparin alone.

One of the major problems with the use of thrombolytic therapy for pulmonary embolism is that these patients usually have major contraindications to thrombolytic therapy. For example, this is the case with pulmonary embolism in a postoperative patient. In 1992, an experience with 13 patients treated for angiographically proven pulmonary embolism within 14 days of surgery was reported.[88] The protocol used urokinase, 2200 units/kg of body weight, injected directly into the clot through a catheter positioned in the pulmonary artery. A continuous infusion at the same dosage was then maintained for up to 24 hours, with the simultaneous administration of heparin at 500 units/hour. The fibrinogen level was maintained at less than 0.2 g/dL. No deaths or bleeding complications were seen, with complete lysis achieved in all patients. This selective therapy for pulmonary embolism may be appropriate for patients in the early postoperative period who suffer a major life-threatening pulmonary embolus.

The long-term results of patients randomized to the Urokinase Pulmonary Embolism Trial (UPET) suggest the clinical importance of resolution of the obstructive process in the pulmonary circulation. Several patients from this study were re-examined 7 years after the original pulmonary embolus. Those assigned initially to thrombolysis had significantly higher pulmonary capillary blood volumes and preservation of the normal pulmonary vasculature response to exercise at 7 years. In contrast, patients who had been treated with anticoagulants alone demonstrated a lower pulmonary capillary blood volume at 1 year and a markedly abnormal increase in pulmonary artery pressure and pulmonary vascular resistance when undergoing exercise testing during right heart catheterization.[89] These data suggest that initial management with thrombolysis can offer improved quality of life years after the event.

More recently, rt-PA has been evaluated in the treatment of acute massive pulmonary embolism. In a multicenter trial, the intravenous administration of rt-PA was compared with intrapulmonary administration in 34 patients with massive pulmonary emboli.[90] All patients were systemically anticoagulated with heparin. The patients received 50 mg of intravenous or intrapulmonary rt-PA over 2 hours, with 22 patients receiving another 50 mg over the subsequent 5 hours. No difference was noted between the intrapulmonary group and the intravenous group, and 7-hour administration was superior to a single infusion of 50 mg over 2 hours. In all groups, up to 38% resolution of the angiographically determined embolism occurred. A decline in the pulmonary arterial pressure was documented in all groups. Fibrinogen levels dropped significantly, and bleeding complications were limited to puncture or operative sites; only four patients required blood transfusions.

In a separate trial, 36 patients with angiographically documented pulmonary emboli received 50 mg of rt-PA over 2 hours, followed by repeat arteriography and, if necessary, an additional 40 mg of rt-PA over 4 hours.[91] Thirty-four of the 36 patients had angiographic evidence of clot lysis, with marked improvement in 24 of the 36. Two bleeding complications occurred, one related to a pelvic tumor and the other 8 days after coronary artery bypass surgery. Again, significant improvement in the clinical condition of these patients was documented.

A randomized, controlled trial of rt-PA versus urokinase in the treatment of acute pulmonary embolism was reported in 1988.[92] Forty-five patients were randomized to 100 mg of rt-PA over 2 hours versus urokinase at systemic doses. At 2 hours, 82% of the rt-PA patients had complete lysis, as opposed to 48% of patients receiving urokinase. Eight of 23 urokinase patients required premature termination of the infusion because of bleeding complications. There was no difference in plasma fibrinogen level or improvement in lung scans between the two groups.

In 1980, the National Institutes of Health Consensus Development Conference concluded that thrombolytic therapy results in greater improvement and normalization of the hemodynamic responses to pulmonary emboli than that observed with heparin alone.[93] Lytic therapy may prevent permanent damage to the pulmonary vascular bed by lysing emboli and restoring the pulmonary circulation to normal. The conference report also stated that although the incidence of bleeding complications was high, contemporary clinical experience suggested an incidence of around 5%, which was certainly within the acceptable range.

The thrombolytic agents currently approved by the FDA for use in the treatment of patients with pulmonary embolism are t-PA, given in a 100-mg dose over 2 hours, and, since 2002, the newly reintroduced urokinase. As stated earlier, there is no evidence of improved survival or outcomes in patients with pulmonary embolism who are hemodynamically stable. Tebbe and colleagues evaluated the efficacy of reteplase, given as two 10-unit boluses 30 minutes apart, compared with t-PA in the 100-mg dose.[94] There was no difference in clinical outcomes, complications, or mortality. The rates of stroke and intracranial hemorrhage were similar. However, reteplase reduced pulmonary vascular resistance more quickly than t-PA did. However, it should be emphasized that there is no level I evidence that thrombolysis for the improvement of pulmonary embolism offers any survival advantage, except in cases of massive embolism with hemodynamic compromise.

In current clinical practice, thrombolytic therapy should be considered in all patients with an established diagnosis of pulmonary embolism, any evidence (clinical or monitoring) of hemodynamic compromise, and no absolute contraindication to systemic lytic therapy. This excludes small pulmonary emboli in a patient who remains clinically stable after the initial episode. In this situation, the benefits of thrombolytic therapy over heparin alone are not clear.

It is important that the diagnosis of pulmonary emboli be well documented. Helical or spiral computed tomography (CT) scans are increasingly being used to detect pulmonary embolism. With current technology, image acquisition can be done in 20 seconds, the equivalent of a single breath-hold. The sensitivity and specificity of helical CT in the diagnosis of acute pulmonary embolism range from 69% to 92% and 86% to 96%, respectively. The validity of CT-angiography in the diagnosis of pulmonary embolism is currently being investigated in a large prospective study named PIOPED II (Prospective Investigation of Pulmonary Embolism Diagnosis II).

If hemodynamic instability precludes pretreatment angiography or imaging, an alternative is to proceed with lytic therapy, which usually results in marked improvement within the hour. Angiography is then performed to help the clinician decide whether to continue therapy. If the angiogram confirms the diagnosis, the drug is continued for 12 to 24 hours, based on the hemodynamic response and the presence or absence of complications or risk factors. Therapy beyond 24 hours does not seem to offer any benefit.

Under these guidelines, a patient who has a large pulmonary embolism *and* evidence of right ventricular dysfunction should be considered for a trial of lytic therapy. Systemic anticoagulation with heparin is critical as soon as the diagnosis is strongly suspected. Pulmonary embolectomy is then reserved for hemodynamically compromised patients who fail lytic therapy or have an absolute contraindication to thrombolytic therapy. Once again, it should be emphasized that thrombolytic therapy has not been shown to affect mortality after pulmonary embolism; its efficacy is reflected in secondary end points, not in survival.

Deep Venous Thrombosis

The goal of therapy for deep venous thrombosis (DVT) is the prevention of pulmonary embolism and of long-term sequelae characterized by the postphlebitic syndrome. Anticoagulation has been highly effective in achieving the former but ineffective in preventing valvular damage and thus avoiding the latter. The incidence of such long-term complications can be as high as 90%.[95]

Several well-controlled, randomized, prospective studies have compared systemic lytic therapy with conventional heparin therapy in the treatment of DVT.[96-100] All concluded that dissolution of DVT with lytic therapy is faster and more complete than that observed with heparin alone. On average, complete lysis was seen in 35% of patients, compared with 4% of those treated with heparin alone. At 3 to 6 months' follow-up, valve function was preserved in 7% of heparin-treated patients, compared with 50% of patients treated with thrombolytic agents. The incidence of pulmonary embolism was similar for both regimens, with no difference in mortality. Bleeding complications averaged 4% and 17% for heparin and lytic therapy, respectively. In one study, phlebography at a mean of 7 months after treatment suggested an improved outcome for patients treated with fibrinolytic agents. Normal venograms were found in 40% of streptokinase-treated patients, compared with 8% of those who had received heparin. Clinical symptoms were related to therapeutic results and previous thrombosis. Longer follow-up was reported by Arnesen and colleagues,[101] who phlebographically evaluated 35 patients at a mean observation period of 6.5 years after they had randomly received streptokinase or heparin. Only seven patients had phlebographically normal veins, and all were in the streptokinase group. On clinical examination, 76% of patients in the streptokinase group had normal legs, compared with 33% of patients in the heparin group. Contrasting results were reported from a small prospective study in which 24 patients with major proximal DVT treated with heparin were compared with 25 patients similarly afflicted and treated with streptokinase.[102] After 2.5 years of follow-up, no major difference in hemodynamic status, as measured by foot volumetry, was seen between the two groups. The authors questioned the validity of treatment with lytic therapy, given its higher complication rate. In all these studies, thrombi older than 3 to 5 days were less likely to respond.

Clinical experience with the use of t-PA in the treatment of DVT is limited. A randomized trial of rt-PA for the treatment of proximal DVT was carried out by Turpie and colleagues.[103] Twenty patients with proximal DVT were randomized to intravenous rt-PA (0.5 mg/kg) or placebo over 4 hours, following initiation of a therapeutic dose of intravenous heparin. Patients were randomized to rt-PA (0.5 mg/kg) or saline over 1 hour if repeat venography within 72 hours did not show complete lysis. Five of 10 patients treated with rt-PA under this protocol showed partial or complete lysis, compared with 1 of 10 patients treated with heparin. A systemic lytic effect was demonstrated by a drop in plasma fibrinogen and α_2-antiplasmin concentration, with positive fibrin degradation split products and elevated euglobulin lysis time. Thus, modest effectiveness was demonstrated in this study, similar to that achieved by urokinase or streptokinase. Long-term follow-up data on these patients are not available. Three other randomized trials have yielded similar results.[104-106]

The concept of lytic therapy for DVT is attractive because it can relieve the obstructive process and may aid in the preservation of valvular function. These two features are established predictors of the development of the post-thrombotic syndrome.[107] The early reports of success with thrombolysis for DVT led to the development of a national multicenter registry for the evaluation of catheter-directed thrombolysis for lower extremity DVT.[108] The early results in 473 patients were published in 1999 and demonstrated that the methods used to deliver the lytic agent (in this case, urokinase) affect the anatomic result. Attempts to lyse the thrombus by a pedal infusion were remarkably unsuccessful, with a failure rate of 80%. In contrast, catheter-directed lysis, with the agent laced directly into the clot, achieved substantial lysis in 83% of cases and complete lysis in 33%. This experience provides a strong argument in favor of abandoning systemic infusion for thrombolysis because the rates of lysis are not improved, but the dose of lytic agent administered is higher with systemic infusion. Major bleeding complications occurred in 11% of patients, most at the puncture site, and mortality was less than 1%. Comerota and colleagues published a report evaluating health-related quality-of-life variables in patients with iliofemoral DVT treated with thrombolysis versus those treated with anticoagulation alone.[109] Patients treated with thrombolysis reported better overall physical functioning, less health distress, less stigma, and fewer post-thrombotic symptoms ($P < 0.05$ for each outcome measure).

It is reasonable to conclude that systemic thrombolytic therapy for DVT is as effective as heparin in preventing pulmonary embolic complications, with the added advantage of faster acute resolution in a significant number of patients. From the available studies, it appears that elimination of the obstructive component of DVT is better achieved with lytic therapy. Whether preservation of valve function is achieved by this more aggressive form of therapy is uncertain. Clearly, with longer follow-up, more patients develop incompetent valves. This may result from minor valve damage that progresses over time to a clinically significant problem. Nevertheless, it is difficult to ignore the significant improvement in the obstructive component of DVT, considering that

the combination of obstruction and valvular incompetence likely results in the most severe form of postphlebitic syndrome. In view of this, should lytic therapy be offered to all patients with DVT? Clearly, the answer is no. When therapy is started more than 5 days after the onset of symptoms, effectiveness is significantly decreased. The incidence of DVT is highest in postoperative patients, women during pregnancy or after childbirth, trauma victims, and patients suffering cerebrovascular accidents or spinal injuries. Lytic therapy is contraindicated in these instances, as well as in septic thrombophlebitis. Prior episodes of thrombophlebitis are likely to have destroyed delicate vein valves, making the benefits of lytic therapy in recurrent attacks uncertain. If clinical evidence of valve competence is present, an attempt to prevent further damage from a recurrent attack and resolve the obstructive component is a reasonable goal. In addition, lytic therapy seems to offer an advantage in more proximal thrombosis (i.e., popliteal vein or higher); thus, treatment of isolated calf thrombi with lytic therapy is of questionable value.

From the foregoing discussion, it is evident that the impact of lytic therapy in DVT is limited. However, patients suffering a first episode who have no contraindications and who receive treatment within 5 days of the onset of symptoms will likely benefit from systemic lytic therapy. As with pulmonary embolism, documentation of the diagnosis is essential before initiating thrombolytic therapy for DVT. It is our practice to obtain a venogram before lytic therapy. Repeat venography to assess the result is not necessary, although it is helpful when the clinical response is uncertain. Noninvasive studies are useful during therapy when an adequate clinical response is observed. The duration of therapy is guided by these studies but is usually no less than 3 days, unless complications require earlier discontinuation of the drug. Therapy beyond 5 days is rarely indicated and suggests resistance to lytic therapy. When using streptokinase, if no improvement is seen within the first 24 to 48 hours or a lytic state (see later) is not documented within this period, a switch to urokinase is recommended.

Phlegmasia cerulea dolens at onset causes massive iliofemoral thrombosis with limb-threatening venous outflow occlusion. Historically, the results of venous thrombectomy have been variable, with a significant incidence of rethrombosis and mortality, although more recent experience has been encouraging.[110,111] A much more compelling argument can be made for the use of thrombolytic therapy in the treatment of phlegmasia cerulea dolens. There is no real consensus on treatment, but the advent of catheter-directed thrombolysis presents an attractive and effective treatment option for this disease, which historically resulted in 20% to 40% mortality and a significant amputation rate in survivors.[112] Patel and colleagues reported on two patients with phlegmasia cerulea dolens who were successfully treated with catheter-directed thrombolytic therapy and stenting, without limb loss.[113] This is one of many case reports that demonstrate the feasibility and efficacy of this approach. Lytic therapy offers an important advantage over surgical thrombectomy, because multiple peripheral thrombi not accessible to the catheter may be dissolved. In addition, a general anesthetic, frequently required for venous thrombectomy, is avoided. Although the experience with thrombolytic therapy in this disease is limited, of 14 reported cases, 13 were judged to have achieved excellent results, with no mortality.[96,114-116]

Axillary Vein Thrombosis

Axillary vein thrombosis (effort thrombosis) usually occurs in young individuals, and its sudden clinical manifestations lead the patient to seek early medical attention. This makes this entity ideally suited for thrombolytic therapy. Anticoagulation rarely leads to resolution and merely arrests the process, allowing for collateral drainage and amelioration of symptoms. This frequently leads to some degree of disability. Catheter-induced axillary subclavian vein thrombosis usually has a more gradual presentation, with slow, progressive occlusion allowing for collateral venous drainage. The clinical presentation aids in the decision whether to offer lytic therapy to a patient with catheter-induced axillary subclavian vein thrombosis. When symptoms develop rapidly over the course of a few days, there is a good probability that the thrombotic material will be sensitive to lytic agents. A combination of infusion through the catheter and in the ipsilateral peripheral vein is most effective. However, if symptoms develop over weeks or months, they tend to be milder in nature and less responsive to fibrinolytic agents. This is likely a result of organization of the thrombotic material.

Both forms of axillary thrombosis have been successfully managed with lytic therapy (Fig. 24-2).[117-119] Either systemic or local low-dose infusion appears to be effective.[117] Local infusion requires that the catheter be lodged in thrombus; otherwise, venous collaterals will decrease its effectiveness. A systemic lytic state is avoided in the majority of patients treated by local infusion.

Once complete resolution of the clot is achieved, repeat venography with the extremity in abduction and external rotation is recommended. If an underlying thoracic outlet compression is identified, surgical correction should be advised. We now perform surgical decompression of the thoracic outlet at the same admission (i.e., after thrombolysis) because we noted no increase in bleeding complications or rethrombosis rates. After thoracic decompression, a repeat venogram is obtained at 2 weeks, and if a stenosis of the vein is identified, balloon dilatation may be successful in avoiding rethrombosis.[117]

Superior Vena Cava Thrombosis

Superior vena cava thrombosis is frequently the result of neoplastic, traumatic, or infectious processes in the mediastinum. In these instances, external compression or inflammation precludes successful resolution of the process with lytic agents. Thrombosis secondary to an indwelling catheter is usually a slow process, allowing for organization and fibrotic replacement of the clot. It is unlikely that this will respond to lytic therapy, and surgical decompression may be an option in these patients. Conversely, patients who develop rapidly progressive symptoms may respond to lytic therapy by means of dissolution of the most recently formed clot, which is likely to be sensitive to lysis.

In about 4% of cases, thrombosis is termed idiopathic. Successful resolution of idiopathic vena cava thrombosis has been reported with systemic thrombolytic therapy.[120]

COMPLICATIONS

Bleeding is the most frequent and important complication of systemic lytic therapy. However, in this day and age, most lytic

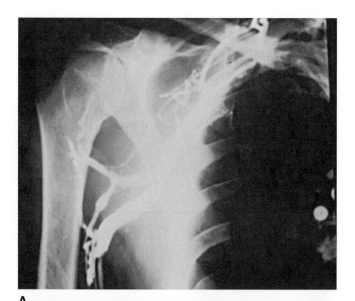

A

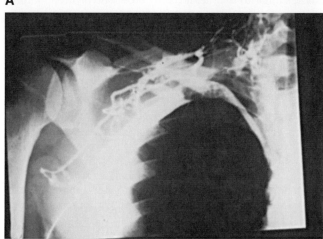

B

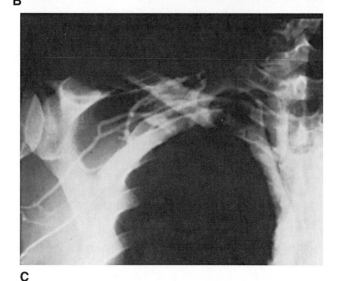

C

FIGURE 24–2 • Venograms of a 28-year-old man with acute onset of pain and swelling in the right upper extremity. *A,* Ascending venogram confirms axillary vein thrombosis. Low-dose streptokinase infusion (10,000 units/hour) was initiated. *B,* Twenty-four hours later, intraluminal thrombus is seen, with patency of the system. *C,* Forty-eight hours later, there is complete resolution of the occlusion.

treatments for peripheral arterial or venous thrombosis are done by catheter-directed techniques rather than by systemic administration of thrombolytics. The major exceptions are thrombolytics for stroke and myocardial infarction, which are administered via a bolus and short-term infusion rather than prolonged infusion. The reported incidence of major bleeding (requiring transfusion or discontinuation of the drug) varies from 7%[121] to as high as 45%.[86] Major bleeding occurs in an average of 15% of cases and correlates with the number and type of invasive procedures during therapy. Duration of therapy also seems to influence the incidence of bleeding.

Two broad categories of bleeding are observed. Superficial bleeding, seen at invasive sites, is frequently controlled with pressure. Avoidance of unnecessary procedures and preservation of an intact vascular system are the best preventive measures. Internal bleeding, usually seen in the gastrointestinal tract or the intracranial space, is frequently the result of poor patient selection. Internal bleeding should be suspected with unexplained drops in hematocrit. As a rule, any change in the neurologic status of a patient receiving fibrinolytic therapy is considered a complication of therapy until proved otherwise. The infusion is discontinued immediately, and appropriate diagnostic and therapeutic measures are instituted.

Superficial bleeding, which is controlled by local measures, can be tolerated in the final stages of therapy. Its occurrence early in the infusion, or any significant bleeding requiring transfusion, should lead to discontinuation of therapy. The hemostatic defect is corrected by the administration of fresh frozen plasma or cryoprecipitate. These two components are rich in fibrinogen and usually result in resolution of the lytic state. ε-Aminocaproic acid administration (plasmin inhibitor) is rarely recommended and carries a significant risk of aggravating the process for which lytic therapy was instituted. Increasing the dose of streptokinase to decrease its proteolytic effect is scientifically correct but unnecessary. It is interesting to note that bleeding tends to occur in the lag period between termination of lytic therapy and anticoagulant administration.[56,122] Thus, heparin administration should be delayed until the thrombin time or PTT is less than twice normal, and it should be initiated without a loading dose.

Laboratory parameters correlate poorly with the risk of bleeding. However, extremely low fibrinogen levels (<20% of baseline) in the presence of an otherwise minor bleeding complication do increase the chances of continued bleeding, requiring cessation of therapy. An alternative is to temporarily discontinue the drug, administer fresh frozen plasma or cryoprecipitate, and restart the infusion several hours later.

Allergic reactions are not infrequent with streptokinase, although most are minor febrile episodes of no clinical consequence. Serious allergic reactions are extremely rare with the current preparations, and the few reported cases have responded well to conventional therapy.[93]

Pulmonary embolism can occur during treatment for DVT. The incidence appears to be similar to that seen with conventional heparin therapy. In the absence of other complications, continuation of lytic therapy is the treatment of choice. If recurrent emboli are observed, discontinuation of the fibrinolytic agent, heparin administration, and placement of a caval filter may be lifesaving.

Intra-arterial Thrombolytic Therapy

The management of acute arterial and graft occlusions by the intra-arterial local administration of fibrinolytic agents has emerged as an occasional alternative and a frequent adjunct to surgical therapy in a selected group of patients. Recently completed prospective, randomized clinical trials have helped establish the role of lytic therapy in the treatment of patients with peripheral vascular disease. Excellent results with low morbidity and mortality are now possible with modern vascular techniques. It is difficult to estimate the impact of intra-arterial lytic therapy based on cases in which surgical management has traditionally been successful.

Emerging from the literature are guidelines that help define the role of intra-arterial lytic therapy. Unquestionably, patient selection is the most important factor in achieving good results with this nonoperative approach. As we gain experience in manipulating the fibrinolytic system, improvements in areas where surgical results are poor may follow.

PATIENT SELECTION

As a rule, intra-arterial fibrinolytic therapy should be considered when the surgical alternative carries a high risk of morbidity or mortality or when the surgical approach has traditionally yielded poor results. In patients with previous multiple vascular reconstructions, lytic therapy may offer an alternative to a difficult and unpredictable surgical intervention. In some cases, it may facilitate such an undertaking, thus serving as a true adjunct to surgical therapy.

In the early experience of intra-arterial fibrinolytic therapy, low doses of the agent were administered close to the thrombus to minimize systemic effects. With a low-dose regimen, dissolution of intra-arterial thrombi is a slow, gradual process, requiring 12 to 72 hours or longer. If this method is chosen, the viability of the ischemic tissues should be ensured. Otherwise, these patients are better managed surgically, because prompt revascularization can be accomplished. Candidates for intra-arterial lytic therapy must be able to tolerate ischemia for the duration of the infusion. However, with a high-dose regimen, restoration of forward flow can often be achieved in 2 to 6 hours; thus, the decision whether to continue fibrinolytic infusion can be made in a timely fashion.

Cumulative retrospective and prospective analysis has helped define guidelines for patient selection. In a prospective study of 80 consecutive patients receiving intra-arterial urokinase for acute (<14 days) ischemia, successful lysis was accomplished in 71% (57 patients).[123] Most of these, however, required additional adjunctive procedures to maintain patency; only 28% of patients avoided the need for additional interventions. Prosthetic graft and native arterial occlusions responded equally well (78% and 72%, respectively), whereas vein graft occlusions were less likely to respond (53%). Diabetics fared significantly worse compared with nondiabetics. Most important, placement of the catheter within the substance of the thrombus and passage of the guidewire through the occlusive process were the best predictors of success. The location of the occlusion influenced the need for adjunctive procedures. Whereas 88% of aortoiliac and 82% of infrainguinal occlusions required adjunctive procedures, only 17% of upper extremity procedures required additional interventions.

TABLE 24–3	Contraindications to Intra-arterial Fibrinolytic Therapy

Absolute
Intolerable ischemia
Active internal bleeding
Cerebrovascular accident within 3 mo
Intracranial pathologic condition

Relative
Recent major surgery or trauma
Minor gastrointestinal bleeding
Severe hypertension
Valvular heart disease
Atrial fibrillation
Endocarditis
Coagulation disorder
Pregnancy
Minor surgery
Severe liver disease
Axillofemoral graft or knitted Dacron graft

Streptokinase
Known allergy
Recent streptococcal infection
Previous therapy within 6 mo

The investigators underscored the importance of patient selection, noting that unsuccessful thrombolysis not only delays revascularization but also increases the risk of bleeding complications.[123]

Absolute and relative contraindications to intra-arterial fibrinolytic therapy are listed in Table 24-3. Approximately 50% of patients receiving low-dose intra-arterial infusion of lytic drugs will develop a systemic lytic state. Thus, patients with active internal bleeding, recent cerebrovascular accidents (within 2 months), or intracranial lesions are not candidates for any form of fibrinolytic therapy.

Relative contraindications represent risk factors associated with a higher incidence of complications. Recent major surgery or trauma significantly increases the risk of bleeding in the presence of a systemic lytic state. Individual judgment is required, but the presence of relative contraindications should not deter the clinician from using regional lytic therapy if significant benefit is anticipated.

Several cases of embolization to the ipsilateral extremity during intra-arterial lytic therapy for occluded axillofemoral grafts have been reported.[123] The length of these grafts makes them unsuitable for lytic therapy, so surgical thrombectomy remains the therapy of choice. Dissolution of the fibrin layer that seals Dacron prostheses can occur with systemic absorption of the drug, leading to oozing through these porous prostheses. Discontinuation of therapy usually results in stabilization of the hematoma by the surrounding capsule.

INDICATIONS

Thrombosis after Percutaneous Angioplasty

Percutaneous angioplasty is frequently performed for stenotic arterial lesions in the iliac and femoral systems. Thrombosis after balloon angioplasty is relatively infrequent, but when it

occurs, local thrombolytic therapy is highly effective in restoring patency. The onset of occlusion is usually within 24 hours of dilatation; thus, the thrombotic material is fresh and highly sensitive to fibrinolysis. The underlying stenosis has been relieved by the angioplasty, and when thrombosis occurs immediately, it is a simple matter to change catheters so that proximal infusion is promptly initiated.

More than 80% of cases of post–balloon dilatation thrombosis can be treated successfully with intra-arterial lytic therapy.[124-126] The duration of therapy is short because the infusion is started early and the thrombotic material is fresh. Thus, thrombectomy of a friable, recently dilated artery can be avoided. If dilatation of an iliac lesion was performed through an ipsilateral puncture, there is a risk of bleeding and pseudoaneurysm formation (Fig. 24-3). If patency was restored by the infusion, repair of the pseudoaneurysm can consist of simple closure of the puncture site without embolectomy.

Native Vessel Occlusion

Acute occlusion of a native artery can be the result of thrombosis secondary to an underlying stenosis or embolization from a central source. In selecting patients for intra-arterial lytic therapy, it is important to attempt to delineate the mechanism of occlusion. Lytic therapy appears to be more effective when applied to peripheral embolization.[123] Whereas 50% to 60% of thrombotic occlusions resolve with thrombolytic therapy, about 80% of embolic occlusions can be effectively lysed. Conversely, surgical management of proximal lower extremity emboli by transfemoral embolectomy is highly successful, with low morbidity and mortality. In addition, some investigators have noted that emboli secondary to atrial fibrillation may have well-organized components and thus be resistant to fibrinolysis.[127] For these reasons, we prefer surgical embolectomy for proximal (iliac, femoral) emboli secondary to atrial fibrillation. If the embolus is secondary to a recent myocardial infarction (i.e., the surgical risk is increased and the embolus is usually fresh clot), intra-arterial fibrinolytic therapy should be considered. It must be kept in mind that the presence of mural thrombus in the ventricle, usually secondary to a recent myocardial infarction, is a relative contraindication to lytic therapy. Although the absence of such findings on echocardiography does not absolutely exclude the possibility, their presence should raise the level of concern about performing lytic therapy.

The management of multiple distal emboli must be individualized, depending on the viability of the extremity and the surgical risk. Intra-arterial lytic therapy is a reasonable option in these patients when the extremity is viable and the anticipated surgical reconstruction difficult. If the ischemia is not well tolerated, we proceed with popliteal exploration, thrombectomy, and, on occasion, intraoperative lytic therapy (discussed later).

The use of local fibrinolytic therapy for thrombotic arterial occlusions should be based on the anticipated difficulty, morbidity, and mortality of the surgical alternative. The success rate of fibrinolytic therapy alone in thrombotic occlusion is variable. Of 25 patients with atherosclerotic occlusion, Risius and associates succeeded in treating 13 (52%); of these 13, only 4 required no further therapy, 3 had successful percutaneous transluminal angioplasty, and the remaining 6 required surgery or distal amputations.[128] Of 40 patients

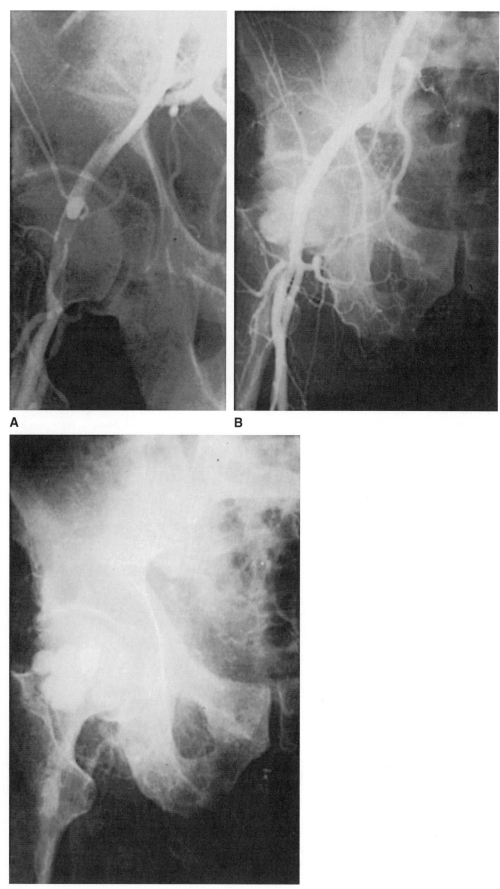

FIGURE 24–3 • This 63-year-old man underwent balloon angioplasty of a right external iliac artery stenosis. *A*, Post-procedure angiogram shows thrombosis of the dilated segment. *B*, After 12 hours of intra-arterial streptokinase, there is complete resolution of the thrombus. *C*, A pseudoaneurysm is evident on angiography. Repair was limited to suture closure of the perforation, with no need for thrombectomy.

with thrombotic occlusions treated by Katzen and colleagues with intra-arterial lytic therapy, 32 (80%) achieved successful outcomes.[125] Successful lysis was achieved by Graor and colleagues in 25 of 45 patients (56%) with thrombotic arterial occlusions.[124] Eighteen of these 25 patients required secondary procedures. Seventy-eight percent of patients whose thrombi were less than 30 days old were successfully lysed, compared with 37% of patients with older occlusions. This trend has been observed by others and confirmed by recently completed randomized, prospective clinical trials (see later).

Careful analysis of the reported series reveals that although the lytic infusion may reestablish patency, additional procedures are often required. If surgical management becomes necessary, this is often simplified because better preoperative planning is possible. Thus, if the ischemia is well tolerated, the anticipated surgical intervention complex, the occlusion fairly recent (within 2 weeks), and the patient at significantly increased surgical risk, thrombolytic therapy seems justified. Based on the reported experience, long-term results depend mainly on whether a correctable lesion is identified and on the location of the occlusion. Larger vessel occlusions resolved by intra-arterial lytic therapy tend to do better, with an expected patency of 60% at 2 years. Similarly treated superficial femoral and popliteal occlusions have a lower long-term patency of about 30% at 2 years.[129] If a correctable lesion is identified and appropriately treated, long-term results are significantly improved. Patencies as low as 20% at 2 years have been reported when no causative lesion was identified.[130]

There are specific instances when surgical intervention has traditionally achieved poor results. Emboli or thrombosis of the popliteal artery with distal clot propagation or multiple tibial emboli carry a risk of amputation of 40%, despite prompt surgical embolectomy.[3,131,132] In patients with a viable extremity at presentation in whom no major runoff vessels are seen on angiography, a trial of local fibrinolytic therapy may improve these results. Surgical correction of the underlying lesion (stenosis or aneurysm) can be performed in a timely fashion. When severe ischemia precludes lytic therapy, we prefer to proceed with popliteal exploration and embolectomy. Intraoperative intra-arterial infusion of lytic agents in an attempt to lyse clots that are inaccessible to the embolectomy catheter may improve the results of embolectomy alone.

Thrombosis or embolization to the renal arteries is a promising area in which thrombolytic therapy may offer significant advantages over surgical intervention (Fig. 24-4). As a complication of myocardial infarction, an embolus to the renal artery carries an inordinate risk with surgical intervention. Capsular collaterals frequently maintain viability of the renal parenchyma to allow sufficient time for success with thrombolytic therapy. The clot material is sensitive to lysis, and the length of the occlusion is short. The reported experience is limited but has been highly successful.[125,133] If a stenosis is uncovered during infusion, percutaneous dilatation or elective surgical repair may be undertaken, as deemed appropriate.

Acute mesenteric artery occlusion has been successfully treated by local intra-arterial streptokinase infusion.[134] In contrast to the kidneys, the bowel is exquisitely sensitive to ischemia and reperfusion. It is difficult to clinically assess the tolerance to ischemia on presentation and during therapy. We have attempted lytic therapy in four patients with emboli to the mesenteric circulation as a complication of acute

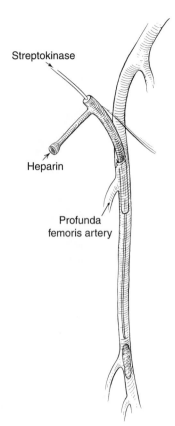

FIGURE 24–4 • Preferred delivery method for intra-arterial lytic therapy for distal lower extremity occlusions. Low-dose heparin is infused through the coaxial system to avoid upstream thrombus.

myocardial infarction. Two patients required laparotomy and bowel resection. In one, no further revascularization was necessary. The other required embolectomy and second-look laparotomy. The third patient had complete resolution of symptoms, avoiding laparotomy altogether (Fig. 24-5). The fourth patient required laparotomy without bowel resection or the need for revascularization. The fourth case underscores the difficulty in clinical follow-up during this type of nonoperative approach. If lytic therapy is elected for acute mesenteric ischemia, any deterioration in the overall clinical status, persistent acidosis, or sepsis mandates emergency exploration. Otherwise, frequent angiographic assessment, as often as every 6 hours, is advisable. Failure to show progress during these intervals should trigger early, rather than delayed, exploration.

Acute Graft Occlusion

Acute occlusion of an arterial graft frequently leads to recurrent symptoms and, on occasion, limb-threatening ischemia. Thrombectomy, with or without revision, achieves excellent results in prosthetic grafts and variable results in autogenous vein grafts.[135] Autogenous vein grafts frequently require extensive revision and replacement. Intra-arterial thrombolytic therapy, in contrast, has been highly unsuccessful in resolving prosthetic graft occlusions. Of 25 patients with prosthetic graft occlusions treated with local lytic therapy by Sussman and coworkers,[123] the treatment was successful in only 6 patients, 5 of whom required surgical correction of the offending lesion. In the 19 failures, amputation followed in 12 patients.

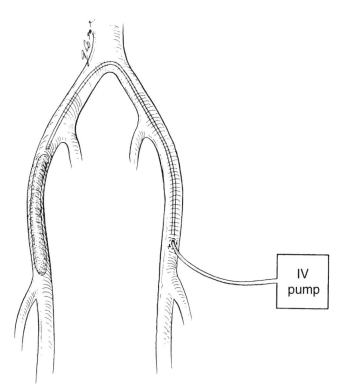

FIGURE 24–5 • Preferred method of intra-arterial lytic therapy for proximal (iliac, common femoral) occlusions. If possible, the catheter tip should be within the thrombus.

In the experience reported by Van Breda and colleagues,[132] among 19 patients with 20 prosthetic graft occlusions, only 4 patients were managed nonoperatively, 2 of whom required percutaneous transluminal angioplasty. Despite this, lytic therapy was considered beneficial because it allowed elective surgery in 12 patients and improvement in the surgical risk in an additional 2 patients. An adjunctive role for lytic therapy was proposed. Although achieving successful lysis in 7 of 10 polytetrafluoroethylene (PTFE) grafts with thrombolytic therapy, Graor and associates noted that surgical revision was required in most of these patients.[124] In view of the excellent results obtained with surgical thrombectomy, one must seriously question the value of thrombolytic therapy in the management of prosthetic graft occlusions.

The results obtained with lytic therapy in the management of occluded autogenous grafts have been somewhat more gratifying. In the experience of Perler and colleagues,[136] occluded vein grafts were more susceptible to lytic therapy than were PTFE grafts. This experience is shared by others.[137] Graor and coworkers,[124] however, observed a similar response between PTFE and vein grafts, reporting a 75% success rate in vein grafts occluded for less than 14 days. Taking into account the variable results with surgical thrombectomy in the management of occluded autologous grafts, a trial of lytic therapy is an attractive alternative if the event is recent. However, in our experience, long saphenous vein grafts to tibial vessels in the lower third of the leg or ankle are less responsive to lytic therapy. This may have to do with limited supplies of plasminogen in these very low-flow grafts. Nevertheless, even in unsuccessful attempts, it is not unusual to find liquefied, thickened blood in the graft at operation, thus minimizing the need for mechanical thrombectomy. The operation may

actually be limited to removal of the most distal occlusive material and revision of an identified lesion. Retrieving an occluded vein graft in these circumstances is possible with minimal mechanical trauma to the endothelium.

We take into account several factors when deciding whether to use lytic therapy for an occluded graft. Certainly, surgical risk must be assessed. Infrequently, surgery is avoided altogether. If delaying surgical intervention allows an improvement of the overall risk, lytic therapy should be considered. If little improvement is expected, it is preferable to proceed with thrombectomy in a timely fashion. When dealing with a prosthetic graft occlusion, thrombectomy remains the therapy of choice. In patients in whom multiple previous reconstructions make a surgical approach less desirable, a trial of lytic therapy is a reasonable option; however, one must realize that the chances of success without eventual surgical correction are low. The management of an occluded vein graft differs, in that the results of surgical thrombectomy are less predictable. Thus, if the ischemia is well tolerated, a trial of lytic therapy may help restore patency of the vein graft. Correction of the causative lesion may then be undertaken without the need for thrombectomy of the graft. This can be accomplished percutaneously if the lesion is less than 0.5 cm long; surgery is preferable for longer lesions. Long-term results of this approach tend to correlate with preocclusion history of the bypass. Grafts that fail within the first year after implantation fare worse than those that have been patent for longer periods. Thus, an early failure of a vein bypass graft in which a complex lesion is identified may be best treated with a new reconstruction if autogenous tissue is available. Failure of a vein graft beyond 1 year may be best treated with a trial of lytic therapy and correction of the causative lesion.

RESULTS OF RANDOMIZED TRIALS

Lower Extremity Ischemia

Despite a multitude of retrospective reviews of the results of thrombolytic therapy in the management of thrombotic complications of peripheral arterial disease, the precise role of this form of therapy could not be clearly established. For this reason, several investigators embarked on prospective, randomized trials comparing surgery to thrombolysis for ischemia of the lower extremities.

The largest trial to date (STILE) randomized 393 patients with native arterial or bypass graft occlusion to either optimal surgical therapy or intra-arterial, catheter-directed thrombolysis with rt-PA or urokinase.[85] Outcomes were analyzed on an intention-to-treat basis to maintain statistical validity. The dosage of rt-PA was 0.05 mg/kg per hour for up to 12 hours; for urokinase, a 250,000-unit bolus injection was followed by 4000 units/minute for 4 hours, then 2000 units/minute for up to 36 hours. End points measured included death, ongoing or recurrent ischemia, major amputation, and major morbidity. Additional end points included reduction in surgical procedure, clinical outcome classification, length of hospitalization, and outcome by duration of ischemia. The randomization produced equivalent groups in terms of risk factors and comorbid conditions. A monitoring committee terminated the study before its anticipated patient recruitment because a significant primary end point occurred in the first interim analysis. Failure or inability to place the catheter in the thrombolytic group occurred in 28% of patients who were randomized, and these were considered treatment failures. A significant benefit of surgical therapy compared with thrombolysis occurred at 30 days, primarily because of a reduction in ongoing or recurrent ischemia. Clinical outcome classification at 30 days was similar. Stratification by duration of ischemia suggested that patients with ischemia of less than 14 days' duration had lower amputation rates with thrombolysis and shorter hospital stays. Patients with ischemia of longer duration (more than 14 days) who were treated surgically had less ongoing or recurrent ischemia and trends toward lower morbidity. At 6 months, there was an improved amputation-free survival in acutely ischemic patients treated with thrombolysis. However, chronically ischemic patients who were treated surgically had lower major amputation rates. Fifty-five percent of patients treated with thrombolysis had a reduction in the magnitude of their surgical procedure. No difference between rt-PA and urokinase was noted, with fibrinogen depletion being a predictor of hemorrhagic complications. The investigators concluded that surgical revascularization of patients with ischemic symptoms of less than 6 months' duration was more effective and safer than catheter-directed thrombolysis. Crossover to surgical treatment from the thrombolytic group probably accounted for the clinical outcomes being similar in both groups at 30 days. Patients with less than 14 days of ischemia who were treated with thrombolysis had an improved amputation-free survival compared with patients who underwent surgical treatment. Of concern was the 28% of patients in the thrombolytic arm who did not receive thrombolytic therapy because of failure to place the catheter within the thrombus. Subsequent analysis revealed that even if these patients were eliminated from the analysis as failures in the thrombolytic arm, the results and conclusions did not change.

Further analysis of those patients in the STILE study who had native, nonembolic arterial thrombosis has been completed.[138] Two hundred thirty-seven patients with lower extremity ischemia due to iliofemoral or superficial femoropopliteal native artery occlusion, with symptomatic deterioration within 6 months, were randomized to either thrombolytic therapy or surgical revascularization. Before randomization, the optimal surgical procedure was determined for subsequent comparison with eventual outcome. For patients randomized to lytic therapy, the catheter could be properly positioned and the lytic agent delivered in 78% of patients; thus, 22% of patients in that group did not receive lytic therapy owing to an inability to position the catheter. A reduction in the subsequent surgical procedure performed occurred in 58% of patients with femoropopliteal occlusions and in 51% of patients with iliofemoral occlusions. Urokinase and rt-PA were equally effective and safe, but lysis time was shorter with rt-PA than with urokinase (8 vs. 24 hours). At 1 year, the incidence of recurrent ischemia was significantly higher in patients treated with thrombolytic therapy than in those treated with surgery (64% vs. 35%). Major amputation rates were also higher in the thrombolytic therapy group, with 10% of patients eventually requiring a major amputation in the thrombolytic arm of the study versus no patients in the surgical arm. Factors associated with poor lytic outcome included femoropopliteal occlusion, diabetes, and presence of critical ischemia. There was no difference in mortality observed at 1 year between the surgical

and lytic therapy groups. The investigators concluded that surgical revascularization for lower extremity native arterial occlusions is more effective and durable than thrombolysis. A reduction in the planned surgical procedure occurred for the majority of patients treated with thrombolysis. However, long-term outcome was inferior, particularly in those patients with femoropopliteal occlusions, diabetes, or critical ischemia.

A prospective, randomized comparison of thrombolytic therapy and operative revascularization in the initial management of acute peripheral arterial ischemia was performed in a single institution and published in 1994.[139] In this study, patients with limb-threatening ischemia of less than 7 days' duration were randomly assigned to intra-arterial, catheter-directed urokinase therapy or operative intervention. If an anatomic lesion was unmasked by the thrombolytic infusion, this was treated with either balloon angioplasty or surgery. Primary end points included limb salvage and survival. A total of 114 patients were randomized; 57 received thrombolytic therapy, and an equal number had surgery. Thrombolytic therapy resulted in dissolution of occluding thrombus in 70% of patients in the lytic group. Cumulative limb salvage was similar in the two treatment groups at 12 months (82%). Cumulative survival, however, was significantly improved in patients randomized to thrombolysis (84% vs. 58% at 12 months). The higher mortality in the surgical arm was primarily due to an increased frequency of in-hospital cardiopulmonary complications. The benefits of thrombolysis appeared to be accomplished without significant differences in the duration of hospitalization and with a modest increase in hospital costs (median, $15,672 vs. $12,253). Intra-arterial thrombolytic therapy was associated with a reduction of in-hospital cardiopulmonary complications and therefore improved patient survival.

Based on these results, and to further elucidate the possible impact of thrombolytic therapy on 1-year survival, a multicenter, randomized, prospective trial comparing thrombolysis and peripheral arterial surgery was carried out.[140] Phase I was designed to be a dose-ranging trial to evaluate the safety and efficacy of three doses of recombinant urokinase in comparison with surgery. Two hundred thirteen patients who had acute lower extremity ischemia of less than 14 days' duration were prospectively randomized to one of two groups. The first group received one of three dosages of recombinant urokinase (2000, 4000, or 6000 IU/minute for 4 hours, then 2000 IU/minute for a maximum of 48 hours). The second group underwent surgical revascularization. Successful thrombolytic therapy was followed by either surgical or endovascular intervention when a lesion responsible for the occlusion was recognized. Follow-up on an intent-to-treat basis was carried out to 1 year. The most effective dosage of recombinant urokinase was found to be 4000 IU/minute. This accomplished complete thrombolysis in 35 of the 49 patients (71%) who were randomized to this dosage in the lytic therapy group. Mean infusion time was 23 hours. Patients who received 2000 IU/minute had a 67% success rate, whereas patients who were randomized to the highest dosage (6000 IU/minute) had a 60% success rate. Hemorrhagic complications were 2%, 13%, and 16% in the 4000-, 2000-, and 6000-IU/minute groups, respectively. When comparing the 4000-IU/minute group with the surgical group, the 1-year mortality rate was similar (14% vs. 16%), and amputation-free survival was not statistically different (75% vs. 65%). Again, patients treated with lytic therapy had a decrease in the planned surgical procedure that was statistically significant. The investigators concluded that recombinant urokinase is most effective at 4000 IU/minute. Thrombolytic therapy and surgical therapy had similar rates of survival and limb salvage.

From the foregoing results, it is evident that in patients with relatively acute ischemia, thrombolytic therapy is an important and effective treatment, with results that compare favorably with those of surgery. Considerable judgment is required in patient selection, which should take into account not only the duration of the ischemia but also the complexity of the anticipated surgical intervention, the presence of contraindications to thrombolytic therapy, and the tolerance of the limb to ischemia. Although the number of vein grafts included in these trials was not sufficient to allow specific recommendations, retrospective information suggests that the long-term outcome of thrombolytic therapy in the management of thrombosed vein grafts is best when the vein graft has failed late (more than 1 year) and when a specific lesion can be identified and corrected after completion of the lytic infusion.

Hemodialysis Access

Thrombosed arteriovenous fistulas can be successfully managed by intragraft administration of fibrinolytic agents. Usually the diagnosis is established early, when the patient notices the absence of a thrill; thus, the thrombotic material is very sensitive to lysis. Administration is by direct puncture because there are no collaterals to dilute the effect of the agent. It is usually best to lace the intragraft thrombus with the lytic agent and then proceed with high-dose intragraft administration. Graor and colleagues were successful in treating 40 of 46 arteriovenous fistulas (87%); PTFE and vein fistulas were equally responsive.[124] Thrombi older than 4 days were less susceptible to lysis (29%). Unfortunately, most patients required surgical revision of the venous anastomosis, and lytic therapy was only a temporizing intervention. In some patients, however, this allowed better preoperative preparation and elective, rather than urgent, operation.

A new method of opening thrombosed grafts is pulse-spray pharmacomechanical thrombolysis, followed by balloon maceration. This allows successful lysis of the graft, but more quickly than with intragraft administration and with a smaller dose of lytic agent. The pulse-spray can be done with heparinized saline or with a thrombolytic agent. A relatively underappreciated but well-documented phenomenon resulting from pulse-spray thrombolysis of clotted hemodialysis access grafts is the development of pulmonary embolism. A prospective, randomized, double-blinded study was conducted to evaluate the incidence of pulmonary embolism following the use of this technique with urokinase versus heparinized saline. Although pulmonary embolism occurred in both groups, as documented by lung perfusion scan, the incidence was 18.2% with urokinase and 64.3% with heparinized saline ($P = 0.04$).[141] All the patients, it should be noted, were asymptomatic.

Many studies have attempted to perform cost-benefit analyses of thrombolysis versus surgical thrombectomy. The most common reason for dialysis graft failure is a lesion, usually neointimal hyperplasia, at the venous anastomosis. The interventional techniques allow thrombolysis and identification of the underlying anatomic lesion. This can be treated with balloon angioplasty, and although this is successful in many cases, surgical revision is usually required at some point in the future.

Acute Stroke

In June 1996, the FDA approved t-PA as a safe and effective treatment for acute stroke, if given within 3 hours of the onset of symptoms.[142] Since then, there has been a proliferation of large clinical trials testing the efficacy of antiplatelet and antithrombotic treatment regimens. The approval of the use of intravenous t-PA was based on the results of the National Institute of Neurological Disorders and Stroke (NINDS) Recombinant Tissue Plasminogen Activator Stroke Study, in which 624 patients with ischemic stroke were treated with 0.9 mg/kg of t-PA within 3 hours of the onset of symptoms.[143] Of the t-PA group, 31% to 50% had complete or near-complete recovery at 3 months, compared with 20% to 38% of the placebo group. This benefit prevailed for 1 year. However, there was a 6.4% incidence of symptomatic brain hemorrhage in the t-PA group, versus 0.6% in the placebo group. The mortality rates were similar between the groups. The presence of a mass effect or a greater severity of initial neurologic deficit presented an increased risk of hemorrhage. The beneficial effect of t-PA was not observed in three other large trials (the European Cooperative Acute Stroke Study I and II and the Alteplase Thrombolysis for Acute Noninterventional Therapy in Ischemic Stroke [ATLANTIS] trial).[144-146] However, patients in these three trials were treated much later (only 14% treated within 3 hours) than those in the NINDS rt-PA study (622 of 624 enrolled within 3 hours, and 48% treated within 90 minutes).

There have been two large randomized trials evaluating intra-arterial thrombolytic therapy for stroke. PROACT II evaluated patients with angiographically documented occlusion of the middle cerebral artery or a first-order branch.[69] By 2 hours, there was partial or complete lysis in 67% of patients in the pro-urokinase group, compared with 18% in the heparin-only group ($P < 0.001$). The primary outcome measure analyzed was the ability to live independently 3 months after the stroke. The percentage of patients able to attain this end point was 40% in the pro-urokinase group and 25% in the heparin group ($P < 0.05$). Intracerebral hemorrhage with neurologic deterioration occurred in 10% of patients in the pro-urokinase group and in 2% in the heparin group ($P = 0.06$). This was the first trial to show a clinical benefit from the use of intra-arterial thrombolysis of a middle cerebral artery occlusion. To date, there are no randomized, controlled trials comparing the efficacy of intravenous versus intra-arterial thrombolytics. It is, however, clear that at this time, thrombolytic therapy for acute ischemic stroke can no longer be considered experimental. It has been shown to have clinical benefit as long as patient selection is strictly in accordance with the criteria set forth in the trials and the NINDS guidelines.

TECHNIQUE

Consideration of thrombolytic therapy should begin before the initial angiographic needle puncture. The approach chosen should maximize access to the occlusion and

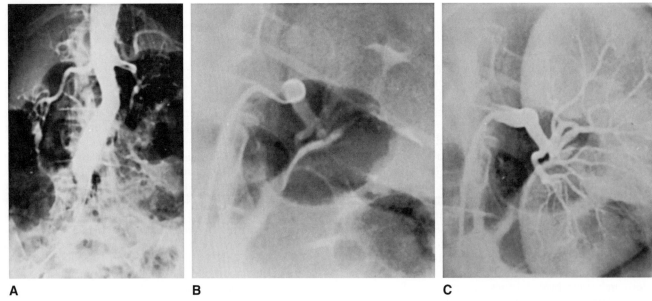

A   **B**   **C**

FIGURE 24–6 • *A*, Aortogram showing left renal artery embolus. *B*, After 1 hour of high-dose intra-arterial urokinase, there is partial clearing and improved perfusion to the left kidney. *C*, Complete clearance of embolus after 3 hours of high-dose intra-arterial urokinase.

minimize morbidity. Arterial punctures distal to the presumed occlusion are avoided. Sites where bleeding may cause serious morbidity (e.g., axillary, translumbar) are avoided. When the suspected occlusion is at a superficial femoral artery or below (strong femoral pulse), we prefer an antegrade ipsilateral puncture (Fig. 24-6). When the suspected occlusion is at the femoral level or above, a contralateral puncture with passage of the catheter around the aortic bifurcation is preferred (Fig. 24-7). Infusions in the upper extremities or aortic branches are carried out through a transfemoral approach. End-hole catheters are used for infusion, with the tip in the thrombus. If this is not possible, there should be no large branches between the catheter tip and the occlusion. When the infusion is at the popliteal level or below, small (3 French) catheters are used through a coaxial system to prevent upstream clot formation (Fig. 24-8). A flush heparin infusion is maintained through the coaxial catheter.

The dosage depends partly on the length and volume of thrombus and the location and clinical importance of the vascular territory. Small-volume, short thrombi in important territories (e.g., renal vessels) are better treated with high-dose infusions aimed at rapid fibrinolysis. Excellent results have been reported using high-dose urokinase (4000 units/minute, followed by 1000 to 2000 units/minute after initial recanalization).[147] Some authors recommend creation of a channel into the thrombus with the angiographic guidewire. In fact, passage of the guidewire through the occlusion is a prognostic indicator of the response to fibrinolytic infusion. Failure to pass the guidewire through the occlusion implies either plaque or well-organized thrombus, which may be resistant to fibrinolysis. Easy passage of the guidewire through the occlusion not only establishes a channel in which the fibrinolytic agent can concentrate but also implies soft, lysable thrombi. The practice of lacing the thrombus with 50,000 units of urokinase, so that the agent is distributed within the thrombus itself, and then retrieving the catheter for infusion is common and seem to be effective. When prolonged infusion

is deemed necessary because of the amount of thrombus, switching to a low-dose regimen (streptokinase 5000 to 10,000 units/hour; urokinase 30,000 to 50,000 units/hour) is appropriate, with angiography carried out within 12 to 16 hours to assess progress. Similarly, if a newer agent such as reteplase is used, a bolus is seldom given. An infusion of 0.5 to 0.75 units/hour is started, and at the next check, the dose is reduced or maintained as appropriate. From the accumulated experience, it appears that bleeding complications correlate most with duration of therapy rather than with total dosage of the agent. High-dose, short-term infusions are better tolerated than long-term, low-dose infusions. Therefore, it is preferable to infuse higher doses of the agent if the duration of therapy can be shortened.

Duration of the infusion is guided by periodic angiographic and clinical monitoring but should rarely exceed 96 hours. When high-dose infusion is used, it is best to keep the patient in the radiology suite and repeat angiography as often as every 30 minutes. For low-dose infusion, the patient is monitored in an intensive care unit, and angiography is repeated daily or more often, depending on the clinical response.

Before initiating therapy, baseline fibrinogen, thrombin time, PTT, and fibrin degradation product measurements are obtained. These are repeated 12 hours after commencing the infusion and then daily. It is expected that the fibrinogen level will drop and fibrin degradation products will become positive. Prolongation of the PTT or thrombin time suggests a systemic lytic state and occurs in about 50% of patients. Although specific parameters do not correlate with the risk of bleeding, presence of a systemic lytic state increases the risk. If good progress is being made by the infusion, a low fibrinogen value (<50% of baseline) or evidence of a lytic state in the absence of bleeding complications is tolerated, and therapy is continued. In the absence of a systemic lytic state when little progress is evident, the dosage is increased and the result reassessed. Therapy should be discontinued if there is

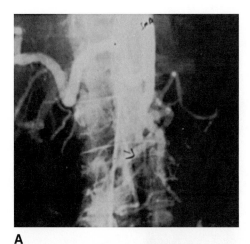

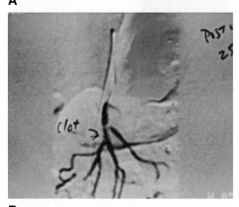

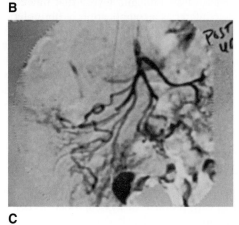

FIGURE 24–7 • *A,* Selective superior mesenteric artery angiogram showing occlusion of the distal tree. *B,* Partial clearing of embolus after 250,000 units of intra-arterial urokinase administered over 1 hour. *C,* Complete resolution of superior mesenteric artery occlusion after 2 hours (500,000 units) of intra-arterial urokinase therapy.

no improvement in any 24-hour interval, persistent or worsening ischemia, or a major bleeding complication.

The administration of heparin during regional thrombolytic therapy is advocated by most investigators. Clearly, in patients with profound ischemia and very low flow in the extremity, and when pericatheter thrombus formation would be significant (e.g., when 3 to 4 cm of the catheter is in a vessel with low or no flow), concomitant heparin administration should be strongly considered. Heparin administration may also be useful in increasing thrombolysis and minimizing the adverse consequences of a potential episode of distal clot migration or embolization. Heparin therapy, however, may increase the incidence and severity of pericatheter bleeding during lytic therapy and may increase the risk of distant bleeding.

Heparin administration is usually through a continuous infusion to maintain a prolonged PTT at 1.5 to 2.0 times control. A bolus infusion before initiation of continuous therapy is used when there is acute, severe ischemia or when low-flow states are identified in the ipsilateral system or around the catheter. When using a coaxial system, a lower dose of heparin may be administered through the larger catheter, usually 500 units/hour. It is important that the PTT not exceed 60 seconds at the time of catheter and sheath removal. Heparin may then be restarted without a bolus.

When emergency surgery is required, the lytic agent is discontinued and fresh frozen plasma is administered if the fibrinogen level is below 100 mg/dL. The half-life of these agents is very short and is usually not a problem in this setting.

COMPLICATIONS

As with any form of lytic therapy, bleeding is the most feared and frequent complication of low-dose fibrinolytic therapy. The risk of major bleeding (requiring cessation of therapy or blood transfusion) ranges from 5% to 15% when appropriate precautions are observed.[124,147] Bleeding is usually related to systemic effects of the drug, and management was discussed earlier in this chapter.

Considering that high-risk patients may be preferentially treated by this nonsurgical approach, the incidence of bleeding with intra-arterial lytic therapy must be considered. The most recent experience indicates that the risk of bleeding correlates more with duration than with total dosage. It is therefore preferable to use higher-dose protocols, especially when a short occlusion is being treated. Although specific coagulation parameters do not correlate with the risk of bleeding, the presence of a systemic lytic state increases this risk. It is important to document whether systemic effects of the drug are present, because such knowledge helps determine the most appropriate course of action. Systemic effects are heralded by a 50% drop in fibrinogen from baseline, a prolongation of the thrombin time to two times normal (or higher), or both. If significant progress is being made, continuation of therapy is warranted, despite systemic fibrinolysis. If no significant improvement is noted within the last interval, reassessment should be made, weighing the risks and benefits of the alternatives.

Treatment of hemorrhagic complications depends on their severity and on the progress made during lytic therapy. A small amount of oozing around the catheter entry site, without hematoma formation during the final stages of the infusion, can be controlled locally, keeping the patient under close observation until therapy is completed. The same situation in the early stages of the infusion, when more than 12 to 24 hours of therapy are anticipated, should lead to discontinuation of the drug. Development of a significant hematoma or bleeding at a remote site warrants cessation of therapy. Fibrinogen should be replaced by the administration of fibrinogen-rich components, such as cryoprecipitate or fresh frozen plasma. This usually suffices because the half-life of both urokinase and streptokinase is short.

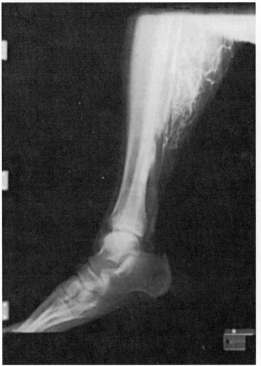 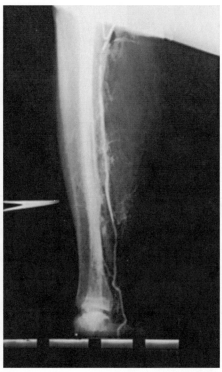

A   **B**

FIGURE 24–8 • *A,* Intraoperative completion angiogram after popliteal embolectomy. Note the absence of runoff vessels to the foot. *B,* Repeat angiogram after intraoperative infusion of streptokinase 60,000 units and heparin 1000 units over 30 minutes through the same catheter used for angiography. Note the remarkable improvement in runoff.

Distal embolization occurs more frequently than is clinically appreciated. Continuation of therapy is preferable, with perhaps a temporary increase in the hourly dose. When severe ischemia is seen as the result of distal emboli, discontinuation of lytic therapy with prompt surgical embolectomy is indicated.

Several cases of embolization to the ipsilateral extremity have been reported during intra-arterial lytic therapy for occlusion of axillofemoral grafts.[124] The length of these grafts makes them unsuitable for lytic therapy; thus, surgical thrombectomy remains the therapy of choice.

Allergic reactions to streptokinase were discussed earlier. Routine administration of 100 mg of intravenous hydrocortisone may prevent some of these reactions and is recommended.

Pseudoaneurysm formation is rare but may occur secondary to bleeding from an arterial puncture site. Surgical repair is recommended.

Intracranial bleeding is a recognized complication of any form of lytic therapy. Any change in the patient's neurologic status during therapy should be viewed as related to the fibrinolytic agent until proved otherwise. Bleeding from an unrecognized intracranial lesion must be ruled out. Lytic therapy should be discontinued while the evaluation is proceeding.

Fatal pulmonary emboli have been reported during intra-arterial fibrinolytic therapy.[126] A possible mechanism for this complication is decreased venous circulation in the ischemic extremity, with clot formation, partial lysis, and eventual pulmonary embolization. This is a rare occurrence. Treatment options include cessation of lytic therapy with heparinization or a switch to systemic intravenous lytic therapy. If the latter is chosen, leaving the intra-arterial catheter in place may decrease the risk of bleeding through the arterial puncture site.

Conversion of an ischemic myocardial infarction into a hemorrhagic infarct as a complication of fibrinolytic therapy has been reported.[126] The relationship between lytic therapy and the few reported cases is unclear. Deterioration of cardiac function in the presence of an acute myocardial infarction during fibrinolytic therapy should lead the clinician to consider this possibility. Therapy should be discontinued until the cause of the cardiac decompensation is determined.

Intraoperative Thrombolytic Therapy

Approximately 30% of lower extremity embolectomies are incomplete, with residual intravascular defects demonstrable by completion angiography.[148] Experimental studies suggest that the true incidence may be as high as 80%.[149] The idea of removing the bulk of thrombus surgically and lysing any remaining defects is attractive from a therapeutic standpoint. Alternatives include repeat embolectomy with the balloon catheter,[150] irrigation in an attempt to flush the residual clot,[151] passage of Dormia catheters,[152] and distal exploration. All these will further injure the endothelium and thus increase its thrombogenicity. Certain endovascular procedures, such as endoscopy, atherectomy, or dilatation, may also temporarily increase the thrombogenicity of these vessels, leading to early thrombosis. Further mechanical manipulation is likely to result in further injury and thus is unlikely to solve the problem. For these reasons, controlled chemical intraoperative fibrinolysis may be a welcome alternative in the treatment of these complications. When dealing with delayed intervention in the presence of a thrombotic process, propagation of clot into the branches of the arterial tree may be problematic.

Once these clots lose their integrity with the parent thrombus, they are difficult to retrieve, and enzymatic dissolution may be the only alternative.

Bleeding complications secondary to intra-arterial fibrinolytic therapy are the result of prolonged infusions necessary to lyse extensive thrombus. The potential for intraoperative or perioperative lytic therapy has been suggested by several investigators.[153-155] Common to all these observations was the lack of bleeding complications. There are several advantages to the intraoperative use of lytic agents when compared with the percutaneous method. First, the bulk of the thrombus has been surgically removed, so less lysis is required. Second, a higher concentration of the agent, with control of inflow (and therefore circulation time), can be accomplished. Finally, infusion within the thrombus or adjacent to it is theoretically unnecessary, and repeat embolectomy with reassessment of the intervention can be done with repeated infusions, as necessary.

In 1985, we reported our initial experience with five patients in whom intraoperative infusions of 20,000 to 100,000 units of streptokinase were successful in restoring adequate circulation to limbs still threatened after embolectomy.[156] We have now extended this experience to 23 infusions in 22 patients.[157] In 17 of these patients, both preinfusion and postinfusion arteriograms were available; improvement following lytic therapy was seen in 13 patients (76%). Only one of these reconstructions rethrombosed in the postoperative period. All four patients without angiographic improvement suffered rethrombosis. Thus, it appears that preinfusion and postinfusion arteriography has prognostic significance, implying that failure to improve after intraoperative infusion of the lytic agent suggests a high likelihood of failure; therefore, alternative methods of reconstruction need to be considered at the time of surgery.

Bleeding is the most feared complication of intraoperative lytic therapy. In our experience, among the 23 patients in whom lytic infusions were carried out intraoperatively, 5 had hematomas. All the hematomas occurred in patients who were fully heparinized postoperatively. Among 12 patients who were not heparinized after surgery, there were no bleeding complications. Thus, bleeding after intraoperative lytic therapy is secondary to aggressive antithrombotic and anticoagulation regimens rather than to the lytic therapy itself.

Clinical experience to date is summarized in Table 24-4.[122,156,158-160] Five additional clinical series have been reported since our initial report. Cohen and colleagues performed 13 bolus infusions of 25,000 to 250,000 units of streptokinase.[122] Eight (61%) of the infusions were successful. Five bleeding complications occurred, one of them resulting in death secondary to retroperitoneal bleeding during aortoiliac reconstruction. This suggests that caution should be exercised when using lytic agents during major abdominal or retroperitoneal surgery. Norem and associates reported their experience with 19 infusions of 50,000 to 200,000 units of streptokinase by bolus injection.[159] They followed the infusion with repeat embolectomy and were able to retrieve

TABLE 24–4	Results of Intraoperative Regional Fibrinolytic Therapy				
Author	No. of Cases	Drug Dose and Method	Successful (%)	Complications	Remarks
Cohen et al[122]	13	SK: 25,000-250,000 U by bolus	61	Five rethromboses; five bleeding complications; one death after retroperitoneal surgery	Two renal infusions, one partly successful; death related to retroperitoneal bleeding
Norem et al[159]	19	SK: 50,000-200,000 U by bolus	100	Two wound hematomas	All patients underwent repeat embolectomy; postoperative heparin in low doses (200-500 U/hr)
Parent et al[160]	28	SK: 50,000-150,000 U by bolus UK: 35,000-150,000 U by bolus	88	Bleeding 11%; compartment syndrome 21%; two deaths	Deaths not related to lytic therapy; bleeding complications in two patients after retroperitoneal surgery
Comerota et al[158]	38	SK: maximum 50,000 U UK: maximum 150,000 U by bolus in 2 patients; isolated limb, UK 1 million U	74	One wound hematoma; five deaths	Deaths not related to lytic agent
Quiñones-Baldrich et al[156]	23	SK: 60,000-100,000 U UK: 250,000-375,000 U plus heparin 1-4 U/mL; gravity infusion over 30 min	74	Six rethromboses; five wound hematomas	All wound hematomas in patients fully heparinized postoperatively

SK, streptokinase; UK, urokinase.

additional thrombus in each instance. Two wound hematomas occurred in the postoperative period. Low doses of heparin (200 to 500 units/hour) were maintained postoperatively. With this regimen, bleeding complications were minimized. In a report from Spain, investigators studied 66 femoropopliteal or distal acute arterial occlusions by means of arteriography and Doppler imaging before and after surgery. Patients were prospectively evaluated after either mechanical thromboembolectomy as a single technique ($n = 35$) or thromboembolectomy plus 250,000 IU of urokinase administered over 30 minutes intra-arterially at completion of the operation ($n = 31$). Intraoperative angiography revealed residual thrombus in 30% of patients and unsuspected arterial lesions in 34%. Recurrence of thrombosis was associated with residual thrombus and amputation. Patients who received the intraoperative thrombolytic infusion had higher ankle-brachial indexes postoperatively than did those who underwent mechanical thromboembolectomy alone. Amputations and the need for distal revascularization were no different between the two groups, although quantitatively, the results were better in the lytic group than in the thromboembolectomy-only group (failure rate, 9.68% vs. 22.86%). There were no bleeding complications with routine intraoperative use of lytic therapy after mechanical thromboembolectomy.

Our preferred technique for intraoperative infusion of fibrinolytic agents consists of a drip infusion of the agent without occlusion of the inflow. Experimental evidence suggests that maintenance of blood flow in the system during administration of fibrinolytic agents enhances their effectiveness. This can be accomplished by insertion of a cannula distal to the arteriotomy after repair of the latter. We prefer urokinase, 250,000 units dissolved in 100 mL of saline, delivered over 30 minutes. On the basis of our original experimental study, we continue to recommend the addition of heparin to the infusate at 1 to 4 units/mL.[149] Preinfusion and postinfusion arteriography is recommended to document the effectiveness of the agent. Failure to show improvement in the postinfusion angiogram suggests a high likelihood of failure and that alternative management should be considered. More recently, the use of isolated limb perfusion with an extracorporeal pump has shown promise in further enhancing the effectiveness of the lytic agent.[161]

Urokinase appears to be a safer agent for intraoperative use. Allergic reactions are not seen. The mechanism of action is direct, and the risk of plasminogen depletion, which may occur with streptokinase, is eliminated. The best method of administration and the appropriate dosage, however, have not been determined. The logistic advantages of bolus infusion are obvious. Nevertheless, a slow infusion has the theoretical advantage of providing a constant amount of the drug while plasminogen is being supplied by the collateral circulation. Bolus infusion, although achieving a high concentration of the agent rapidly, is likely to be washed out, resulting in a very short-lived effect. An experimental study was carried out in our laboratory to further elucidate the best method of infusion. In addition to bolus infusion and slow 30-minute infusion, we included a group of animals in which the limb was isolated with a proximal tourniquet and the artery and vein connected to an extracorporeal pump. Angiographic results were significantly improved with use of the isolated limb perfusion technique with similar doses of urokinase.[161] In addition, maintenance of inflow during the slow infusion

seemed to improve results compared with occluded inflow. However, these differences were not statistically significant, probably due to the number of animals studied. Thus, isolated limb perfusion with extracorporeal pump support of the extremity during revascularization may enhance fibrinolytic activity and improve the efficacy of drug delivery. Clinical experience with this technique to date is promising but limited.

The high selectivity of t-PA for fibrin and the positive early results with relatively short-term infusion suggest that this is a promising agent for intraoperative use. To date, there are no reports of intraoperative use of reteplase.

In summary, we do not hesitate to proceed with an intraoperative fibrinolytic infusion when faced with either residual thrombus inaccessible to the balloon catheter or persistent ischemia after restoration of flow. Although the best method of delivery and most appropriate dosage have not been fully determined, reported clinical experience has allowed guidelines that permit the clinician to obtain the benefits of fibrinolytic infusion in these difficult cases with both safety and efficacy.

REFERENCES

1. Gross R: Fibrinolyse and thrombolyse. Panorama, September 1962, p 4.
2. Malpighi M: De polypo cordis. Opera omnia, p 2. Ludg Batav, 1687, p 311.
3. Morgagni JB: De sedivus et causis morborum per anatomen indagatis, 2nd ed. 1761. Alexander B (trans): The Seats and Causes of Diseases Investigated by Anatomy, vol 3, book 4. London, Millar, 1769.
4. Morawitz P: Über einige postmortale Blutveränderungen. Beitr Chem Physiol Pathol 8:1, 1906.
5. Dastre A: Fibrinolyse dans le sang. Arch Physiol Norm Pathol 5:661, 1893.
6. Astrup T: The haemostatic balance. Thromb Diath Haemost 2:347, 1958.
7. Henkin J, Marcotte P, Yang H: The plasminogen-plasmin system. Prog Cardiovasc Dis 34:135-164, 1991.
8. Kwaan HC: Hematologic aspects of thrombolytic therapy. In Comerota AJ (ed): Thrombolytic Therapy. Orlando, Fla, Grune & Stratton, 1988.
9. Sugiyama N, Iwamoto M, Abiko A: Effects of kringles derived from human plasminogen on fibrinolysis in vitro. Thromb Res 47:459-468, 1987.
10. Wiman B, Lijnen HR, Collen D: On the specific interaction between the lysine-binding sites in plasminogen and complementary sites in α_2-antiplasmin and in fibrinogen. Biochim Biophys Acta 579:142-154, 1979.
11. Lo SK, Ryan TJ, Gilboa N, et al: Role of catalytic and lysine-binding sites in plasmin-induced neutrophil adherence to endothelium. J Clin Invest 84:793-801, 1989.
12. Thorsen S: Differences in the binding to fibrin of native plasminogen and plasminogen modified by proteolytic degradation influence of omega-aminocarboxylic acids. Biochim Biophys Acta 393:55-65, 1975.
13. Rylatt DB, Blake LE, Cottis DA, et al: An immunoassay for human D-dimer using monoclonal antibodies. Thromb Res 31:767, 1983.
14. Burrowes CE: Activation of human prekallikrein by plasmin. Fed Proc 30:451, 1971.
15. Powell JR, Castellino FJ: Amino acid sequence analysis of the asparagine-288 region of the carbohydrate variants of human plasminogen. Biochemistry 22:923-927, 1983.
16. Collen D, Wiman B: Turnover of antiplasmin, the fast-acting plasmin inhibitor of plasma. Blood 53:313-324, 1979.
17. Low DA, Baker JB, Koonce WC: Released protease nexin regulates cellular binding, internalization, and degradation of serine proteases. Proc Natl Acad Sci U S A 78:2340-2344, 1981.
18. Royston D: Review paper: The serine antiprotease aprotinin (Trasylol): A novel approach to reducing postoperative bleeding. Blood Coagul Fibrinolysis 1:55-69, 1990.
19. Verstraete M: Clinical applications of inhibitors of fibrinolysis. Drugs 29:236-261, 1985.
20. Clozel JP, Banken L, Roux S: Aprotinin: An antidote for recombinant tissue-type plasminogen activator (rt-PA) active in vivo. J Am Coll Cardiol 16:507-510, 1990.
21. Kwaan HC: The biologic role of components of the plasminogen-plasmin system. Prog Cardiovasc Dis 34:309-316, 1992.

22. Kirchheimer JC, Wojta J, Christ G, et al: Proliferation of a human epidermal tumor cell line stimulated by urokinase. FASEB J 1:125-218, 1987.

23. Kirchheimer JC, Wojta J, Christ G, et al: Mitogenic effect of urokinase on malignant and unaffected adjacent human renal cells. Carcinogenesis 9:2121-2123, 1988.

24. Rabbani SA, Desjardins J, Bell AW, et al: An aminoterminal fragment of urokinase isolated from a prostate cancer cell line (PC-3) is mitogenic for osteoblast-like cells. Biochem Biophys Res Commun 173:1058-1064, 1990.

25. Juhan-Vague I, Alessi MC, Joly P, et al: Plasma plasminogen activator inhibitor-1 in angina pectoris: Influence of plasma insulin and acute-phase response. Arteriosclerosis 9:362-367, 1989.

26. Wiman B, Hamsten A: Impaired fibrinolysis and risk of thromboembolism. Prog Cardiovasc Dis 34:179-192, 1991.

27. Andreotti F, Davies GJ, Hackett DR, et al: Major circadian fluctuations in fibrinolytic factors and possible relevance to time of onset of myocardial infarction, sudden cardiac death and stroke. Am J Cardiol 62:635-637, 1988.

28. Grimaudo V, Hauert J, Bachmann F, et al: Diurnal variation of the fibrinolytic system. Thromb Haemost 59:495-499, 1988.

29. Angleton P, Chandler WL, Schmer G: Diurnal variation of tissue-type plasminogen activator and its rapid inhibition. Circulation 79:101-106, 1989.

30. Chandler WL, Trimble SL, Loo S-C, Mornin D: Effect of PAI-1 levels on the molar concentrations of active tissue plasminogen activator (t-PA) and t-PA/PAI-1 complex in plasma. Blood 76:930-937, 1990.

31. Urano T, Sumiyoshi K, Nakamura M, et al: Fluctuation of tPA and PAI-1 antigen levels in plasma: Difference in their fluctuation patterns between male and female. J Thromb Res 60:55-62, 1990.

32. Mannucci PM, Rota L: Plasminogen activator response after DDAVP: A clinical fibromycological study. Thromb Res 20:69, 1980.

33. Walker ID, Davidson JF: Long term fibrinolytic enhancement with anabolic steroid therapy: A five year study. In Davidson JF, Rowan RM, Samama MM, Desnoyers PC (eds): Progress in Chemical Fibrinolysis and Thrombolysis, vol 3. New York, Raven Press, 1978, pp 491-500.

34. Jarrett PE, Moreland M, Browse NL: Idiopathic recurrent superficial thrombophlebitis: Treatment with fibrinolytic enhancement. BMJ 1:933, 1977.

35. Tillett WS, Garner RL: The fibrinolytic activity of hemolytic streptococci. J Exp Med 58:485, 1933.

36. Kakkar VV, Sagar S, Lewis M: Treatment of deep vein thrombosis with intermittent streptokinase and plasminogen infusion. Lancet 2:674, 1975.

37. MacFarlane RG, Pilling J: Fibrinolytic activity of normal urine. Nature 159:779, 1947.

38. Lijnen HR, Zamarron C, Blaber M, et al: Activation of plasminogen by pro-urokinase. I. Mechanism. J Biol Chem 261:1253-1258, 1986.

39. Barnathan ES, Kuo A, Rosenfeld L, et al: Interaction of single-chain urokinase-type plasminogen activator with human endothelial cells. J Biol Chem 265:2865-2872, 1990.

40. Behrendt N, Ronne E, Plough M, et al: The human receptor for urokinase plasminogen activator: NH_2-terminal amino acid sequence and glycosylation variants. J Biol Chem 265:6453-6460, 1990.

41. Nykjaer A, Petersen CM, Christensen EI, et al: Urokinase receptors in human monocytes. Biochim Biophys Acta 1052:399-407, 1990.

42. Watahiki Y, Takeda Y, Takeda A: Kinetic analyses of the activation of Glu-plasminogen by urokinase in the presence of fibrin, fibrinogen or its degradation products. Thromb Res 46:9-18, 1987.

43. Feissinger JN, Aiach M, Capron L, et al: Effect of local urokinase on arterial occlusion of lower limbs. Thromb Haemost 45:230, 1981.

44. McNicol GP, Gale SB, Douglas AS: In vitro and in vivo studies of a preparation of urokinase. BMJ 1:909, 1963.

45. Belkin M, Belkin B, Bucknam CA, et al: Intraarterial fibrinolytic therapy: Efficacy of streptokinase versus urokinase. Arch Surg 121:769, 1986.

46. Tennant SN, Dixon J, Venable TC, et al: Intracoronary thrombolysis in patients with acute myocardial infarction: Comparison of the efficacy of urokinase versus streptokinase. Circulation 69:756, 1984.

47. Van Breda A, Katzen BT, Deutsch AS: Urokinase versus streptokinase in local thrombolysis. Radiology 165:109, 1987.

48. Graor RA, Young JR, Risius B, Ruschhaupt WF: Comparison of cost effectiveness of streptokinase and urokinase in the treatment of deep vein thrombosis. Ann Vasc Surg 1:524, 1987.

49. Fletcher AP, Alkjaersig N, Sherry S, et al: The development of urokinase as a thrombolytic agent: Maintenance of a sustained thrombolytic state in man by intravenous infusion. J Lab Clin Med 65:713, 1965.

50. Kakkar VV, Scully MF: Thrombolytic therapy. Br Med Bull 34:191, 1978.

51. Toki N, Sumi H, Sasaki K, et al: Oral administration of high molecular weight urokinase in human subjects and in an experimental dog model. In Davidson JF, Nilsson IM, Astedt B (eds): Progress in Fibrinolysis, vol 5. Edinburgh, Churchill Livingstone, 1981.

52. Ouriel K: Urokinase and the US Food and Drug Administration. J Vasc Surg 30:957-958, 1999.

53. Verstraete M: Third-generation thrombolytic drugs. Am J Med 109:52-58, 2000.

54. Albrechtsen OK: The fibrinolytic agents in saline extracts of human tissues. Scand J Clin Lab Invest 10:91, 1958.

55. Rijken DC, Wijngaards G, Zaal-DeJong M, et al: Purification and partial characterization of plasminogen activator from human uterine tissue. Biochim Biophys Acta 580:140, 1979.

56. Collen D: Human tissue type plasminogen activator: From the laboratory to the bedside [editorial]. Circulation 72:18, 1985.

57. Rijken DC, Collen D: Purification and characterization of the plasminogen activator secreted by human melanoma cells in culture. J Biol Chem 156:7035, 1981.

58. Collen D, Stassen JM, Marafine BJ Jr, et al: Biological properties of human tissue type plasminogen activator obtained by expression of recombinant DNA in mammalian cells. J Pharmacol Exp Ther 231:146, 1984.

59. Sherry S: Tissue plasminogen activator (t-PA): Will it fulfill its promise? N Engl J Med 313:1014, 1985.

60. Stoughton J, Ouriel K, Shortell CK, et al: Plasminogen acceleration of urokinase thrombolysis. J Vasc Surg 19:298-305, 1994.

61. TIMI Study Group: The Thrombolysis in Myocardial Infarction (TIMI) Trial: Phase I findings. N Engl J Med 312:932, 1985.

62. Gao S, Morser J, McLean K, et al: Differential effect of platelets on plasminogen activation by tissue plasminogen activator, urokinase, and streptokinase. Thromb Res 58:421-433, 1990.

63. Klabunde RE, Burke SE, Henkin J: Enhanced lytic efficacy of multiple bolus injections of tissue plasminogen activator in dogs. Thromb Res 58:511-517, 1990.

64. Graor RA, Risius B, Young JR, et al: Peripheral artery and bypass graft thrombolysis with recombinant human tissue type plasminogen activator. Circulation 72(Suppl 3):III-15, 1985.

65. Ross AM: New plasminogen activators: A clinical review. Clin Cardiol 22:165-171, 1998.

66. Stringer KA: Biochemical and pharmacologic comparison of thrombolytic agents. Pharmacotherapy 16:119S-126S, 1996.

67. Pannell R, Gurevich V: Pro-urokinase: A study of its stability in plasma and of a mechanism for its selective fibrinolytic effect. Blood 67:1215-1223, 1986.

68. Tebbe U, Michels R, Adgey J, et al: Randomized, double-blind study comparing saruplase with streptokinase therapy in acute myocardial infarction: The COMPASS Equivalence Trial. Comparison Trial of Saruplase and Streptokinase (COMASS) Investigators. J Am Coll Cardiol 31:487-493, 1998.

69. Furlan A, Higashida R, Wechsler L, et al: Intraarterial prourokinase for acute ischemic stroke. The PROACT II study: A randomized controlled trial. Prolyse in Acute Cerebral Thromboembolism. JAMA 282:2003-2011, 1999.

70. Ouriel K, Kandarpa K, Schuerr DM, et al: Prourokinase versus urokinase for recanalization of peripheral occlusions, safety and efficacy: The PURPOSE trial. J Vasc Interv Radiol 10:1083-1091, 1999.

71. Kohnert U, Randolph R, Verheijen JH, et al: Biochemical properties of the kringle 2 and protease domains are maintained in the refolded t-PA deletion variant BM06.022 by synthetic inhibitors and substrates. Protein Sci 1:1007-1013, 1992.

72. Hajjar KA: The endothelial cell tissue plasminogen activator receptor: Specific interaction with plasminogen. J Biol Chem 266:21962-21970, 1991.

73. Jmazrtin U, Bader R, Bohm E, et al: Boehringer Mannheim 06.22: A novel recombinant plasminogen activator. Cardiovasc Drug Rev 11:299-311, 1993.

74. Smalling RW, Bode C, Kalbfleisch J, et al (for the RAPID investigators): More rapid, complete, and stable thrombolysis with bolus administration of reteplase compared with alteplase infusion in acute myocardial infarction. Circulation 91:2725-2732, 1995.

75. Bode C, Smalling RW, Berg G, et al (for the RAPID II investigators): Randomized comparison of coronary thrombolysis achieved with double-bolus reteplase and front-loaded, accelerated alteplase in patients with acute myocardial infarction. Circulation 94:891-898, 1996.

76. Randomized, double-blinded comparison of reteplase double-bolus administration with streptokinase in acute myocardial infarction (INJECT): Trial to investigate equivalence. International Joint Efficacy Comparison of Thrombolytics. Lancet 346:329-336, 1995.

77. Global Use of Strategies to Open Occluded Coronary Arteries (GUSTO III) investigators: A comparison of reteplase with alteplase for acute myocardial infarction. N Engl J Med 337:1118-1123, 1997.

78. Giugliano RP, Cannon CP, McCabe CH, et al: Lower dose heparin with thrombolysis is associated with lower rates of intracranial hemorrhage: Results from TIMI 10B and ASSENT I. Circulation 96:535, 1997.

79. Lack CH: Staphylokinase: An activator of plasma protease. Nature 161:559-560, 1948.

80. Vanderschueren S, Collen D, Van de Werf F: A pilot study on bolus administration of recombinant staphylokinase for coronary artery thrombolysis. Thromb Haemost 76:541-544, 1996.

81. Bode C, Matsueda G, Haber E: Targeted thrombolysis with a fibrin specific antibody urokinase conjugate. Circulation 72:111-192, 1985.

82. Kremer P, Fiebig R, Tilsner V, et al: Lysis of left ventricular thrombi with urokinase. Circulation 72:112, 1985.

83. Gore JM, Sloan M, Price TR, et al: Intracranial hemorrhage, cerebral infarction, and subdural hematoma after acute myocardial infarction and thrombolytic therapy in the thrombolysis in myocardial infarction study: Thrombolysis in Myocardial Infarction (TIMI), phase II, pilot and clinical trial. Circulation 83:448-459, 1991.

84. Gore JM: Prevention of severe neurologic events in the thrombolytic era. Chest 100(Suppl 4):124S-130S, 1992.

85. STILE investigators: Results of a prospective randomized trial evaluating surgery versus thrombolysis for ischemia of the lower extremity. Ann Surg 220:251-268, 1994.

86. National Heart and Lung Institute Cooperative Study Group: Urokinase Pulmonary Embolism Trial: Phase I results. JAMA 214:2163, 1970.

87. National Heart and Lung Institute Cooperative Study Group: Urokinase-Streptokinase Embolism Trial: Phase II results. JAMA 229:1606, 1974.

88. Molina JE, Hunter DW, Yedlicka JW, Cerra FB: Thrombolytic therapy for postoperative pulmonary embolism. Am J Surg 163:375-381, 1992.

89. Sharma GVRK, Folland ED, McIntyre KM, et al: Long-term hemodynamic benefit of thrombolytic therapy in pulmonary embolic disease [abstract]. J Am Coll Cardiol 15:65A, 1990.

90. Verstraete M, Miller AH, Bounameaux H, et al: Intravenous and intrapulmonary recombinant tissue type plasminogen activator in the treatment of acute massive pulmonary embolism. Circulation 77:353, 1988.

91. Goldhaber SZ, Markis JE, Meyerovitz MF, et al: Acute pulmonary embolism treated with tissue plasminogen activator. Lancet 2:886, 1986.

92. Goldhaber SZ, Kessler CM, Heit J, et al: A randomized controlled trial of recombinant tissue plasminogen activator versus urokinase in the treatment of acute pulmonary embolism. Lancet 2:293-298, 1988.

93. NIH Consensus Development Conference: Thrombolytic therapy in treatment. BMJ 1:1585, 1980.

94. Tebbe U, Graf A, Kamke W, et al: Hemodynamic effects of double bolus reteplase versus alteplase infusion in massive pulmonary embolism. Am Heart J 138:39-44, 1999.

95. Berni GA, Bandyk DF, Zierler RE, et al: Streptokinase treatment of acute arterial occlusion. Ann Surg 198:185, 1983.

96. Arnesen H, Heilo A, Jakobson E: A prospective study of streptokinase and heparin in the treatment of deep vein thrombosis. Acta Med Scand 203:457, 1978.

97. Kakkar VV, Flanc C, Howe CT: Treatment of deep vein thrombosis: A trial of aspirin, streptokinase, and arvin. BMJ 1:806, 1969.

98. Marder VJ, Soulen RL, Atichartakarn V, et al: Quantitative venographic assessment of deep vein thrombosis in the evaluation of streptokinase and heparin therapy. J Lab Clin Med 89:1018, 1977.

99. Porter JM, Seaman AJ, Common HH, et al: Comparison of heparin and streptokinase in the treatment of venous thrombosis. Am Surg 41:511, 1975.

100. Tsapogas MJ, Peabody RA, Wu KT, et al: Controlled study of thrombolytic therapy in deep vein thrombosis. Surgery 74:873, 1973.

101. Arnesen H, Hoiseth A, Ly B: Streptokinase or heparin in the treatment of deep vein thrombosis: Follow-up results of a prospective study. Acta Med Scand 211:65, 1982.

102. Kakkar VV, Lorenz D: Hemodynamic and clinical assessment after therapy for deep vein thrombosis: A prospective study. Am J Surg 140:54, 1985.

103. Turpie GG, Jay RM, Carter CJ, Hirsh J: A randomized trial of recombinant tissue plasminogen activator for the treatment of proximal deep vein thrombosis [abstract]. Circulation 72:193, 1985.

104. Verhaeghe R, Besse P, Bounameaux H, et al: Multi-center pilot study of the efficacy and safety of systemic rt-PA administration in the treatment of deep vein thrombosis of the lower extremities and/or pelvis. Thromb Res 55:5-11, 1989.

105. Goldhaber SZ, Meyerovitz MF, Green D, et al: Randomized controlled trial of tissue plasminogen activator in proximal deep venous thrombosis. Am J Med 88:235-240, 1990.

106. Marder VJ, Brenner B, Totterman S, et al: Comparison of dosage schedules of rt-PA in the treatment of proximal deep vein thrombosis. J Lab Clin Med 119:485-495, 1992.

107. Johnson BF, Manzo RA, Bergelin RO, et al: Relationship between the changes in the deep venous system and the development of the postthrombotic syndrome after an acute episode of lower limb deep vein thrombosis: A one- to six-year follow-up. J Vasc Surg 21:307-312, 1995.

108. Mewissen MW, Seabrook GR, Meissner MH, et al: Catheter-directed thrombolysis for lower extremity deep venous thrombosis: Report of a national multicenter registry. Radiology 211:39-49, 1999.

109. Comerota AJ, Throm RC, Mathias SD, et al: Catheter-directed thrombolysis for iliofemoral deep venous thrombosis improves health-related quality of life. J Vasc Surg 32:130-137, 2000.

110. Alemany J, Marsal T: Early and late results in the surgical treatment of phlegmasia cerulea dolens. Vasc Surg Jul/Aug:271, 1987.

111. Shionoya S, Yamada I, Sakurai T, et al: Thrombectomy for acute deep vein thrombosis: Prevention of postthrombotic syndrome. J Cardiovasc Surg 30:484, 1989.

112. Robinson DL, Teitelbaum GP: Phlegmasia cerulea dolens: Treatment by pulse-spray and infusion thrombolysis. AJR Am J Roentgenol 160:1288-1290, 1993.

113. Patel NH, Plorde JJ, Meissner M: Catheter-directed thrombolysis in the treatment of phlegmasia cerulea dolens. Ann Vasc Surg 12:471-475, 1998.

114. Elliot MS, Immelman EJ, Jeffrey P, et al: The role of thrombolytic therapy in the management of phlegmasia cerulea dolens. Br J Surg 66:422, 1979.

115. Paquet KJ, Popov S, Egli H: Richtlinien und Ergebnisse der konsequenten fibrinolytischen Therapie der Phlegmasia caerulea dolens. Dtsch Med Wochenschr 16:903, 1970.

116. Roberts WM: Some clinical problems in patients undergoing thrombolytic therapy. S Afr Med J 50:243, 1976.

117. Druy EM, Trout HH, Giordano JM, et al: Lytic therapy in the treatment of axillary and subclavian vein thrombosis. J Vasc Surg 2:821, 1985.

118. Rubenstein M, Greger WP: Successful streptokinase therapy for catheter induced subclavian vein thrombosis. Arch Intern Med 140:1370, 1980.

119. Wilson JJ, Lesk D, Newman H: Subclavian-axillary vein thrombosis: Successful treatment with streptokinase. Can Med Assoc J 130:891, 1984.

120. Herrera JL, Wilis SM, Williams TH: Successful streptokinase therapy of acute idiopathic superior vena cava thrombosis. Am Heart J 102:1063, 1981.

121. Elliot MS, Immelman EJ, Jeffrey P, et al: A comparative randomized trial of heparin vs streptokinase in the treatment of acute proximal venous thrombosis: An interim report of a prospective trial. Br J Surg 66:838, 1979.

122. Cohen LH, Kaplan M, Bernhard VM: Intraoperative streptokinase: An adjunct to mechanical thrombectomy in the management of acute ischemia. Arch Surg 121:708, 1986.

123. Sussman B, Dardik H, Ibrahim IM, et al: Improved patient selection for enzymatic lysis of peripheral arterial and graft occlusions. Am J Surg 148:244, 1984.

124. Graor RA, Risius B, Denny KM, et al: Local thrombolysis in the treatment of thrombosed arteries, bypassed grafts, and arteriovenous fistulas. J Vasc Surg 2:406, 1985.

125. Katzen BT, Edwards KC, Albert AS, et al: Low dose direct fibrinolysis in peripheral vascular disease. J Vasc Surg 1:718, 1984.

126. Sicard GA, Schier JJ, Totty WG, et al: Thrombolytic therapy for acute arterial occlusion. J Vasc Surg 2:65, 1985.

127. Taylor LM, Porter JM, Bauer GM, et al: Intraarterial streptokinase infusion for acute popliteal and tibial arterial occlusion. Am J Surg 147:583, 1984.

128. Risius B, Zelch MG, Graor RA, et al: Catheter directed low dose streptokinase infusion: A preliminary experience. Radiology 150:349, 1984.

129. McNamara TO, Bomberger RA: Factors affecting initial and six months patency following high dose intraarterial urokinase thrombolysis. Am J Surg 152:709, 1986.

130. Gardiner GA, Harrington DP, Koltun W, et al: Salvage of occluded arterial bypass grafts by means of thrombolyses. J Vasc Surg 9:426, 1989.

131. Porter JM, Taylor LM: Current status of thrombolytic therapy. J Vasc Surg 2:239, 1985.

132. Van Breda A, Robinson JC, Feldman L, et al: Local thrombolysis in the treatment of arterial graft occlusions. Vasc Surg 1:103, 1984.

133. Cronan JJ, Dorfman GS: Low dose thrombolysis: A non-operative approach to renal artery occlusion. J Urol 130:757, 1983.

134. Pillari G, Doscher W, Fierstein J, et al: Low dose streptokinase in the treatment of celiac and superior mesenteric artery occlusion. Arch Surg 118:1340, 1983.

135. Hargrove WC, Berkowitz HD, Freiman DB, et al: Recanalization of totally occluded femoral popliteal vein grafts with low dose streptokinase infusion. Surgery 92:890, 1982.

136. Perler BA, White RI, Ernst CB, et al: Low dose thrombolytic therapy for infrainguinal graft occlusions: An idea whose time has passed? J Vasc Surg 2:799, 1985.

137. Hargrove WC, Berkowitz HD, Freiman DB, et al: Treatment of acute peripheral arterial and graft thrombosis with low dose streptokinase. Surgery 92:981, 1982.

138. Weaver FA, Comerota AJ, Youngblood M, et al: Surgical revascularization versus thrombolysis for nonembolic lower extremity native artery occlusions: Results of a prospective randomized trial. J Vasc Surg 24:513-523, 1996.

139. Ouriel K, Shortell CK, DeWeese JA, et al: A comparison of thrombolytic therapy with operative revascularization in the initial treatment of acute peripheral arterial ischemia. J Vasc Surg 19:1021-1030, 1994.

140. Ouriel K, Veith FJ, Sasahara AA: Thrombolysis or peripheral arterial surgery: Phase I results. TOPAS investigators. J Vasc Surg 23:64-73, 1996.

141. Kinney TB, Valji K, Rose SC, et al: Pulmonary embolism from pulse-spray pharmacomechanical thrombolysis of clotted hemodialysis grafts: Urokinase versus heparinized saline. J Vasc Interv Radiol 11:1143-1152, 2000.

142. Activase, alteplase recombinant for acute ischemic stroke: Efficacy supplement. Paper presented at Peripheral and Central Nervous System Drug Advisory Committee Meeting, June 1996, Bethesda, Md.

143. National Institute of Neurological Disorders and Stroke rt-PA Stroke Study Group: Tissue plasminogen activator for acute ischemic stroke. N Engl J Med 333:1581-1587, 1995.

144. Hacke W, Kaste M, Fieschi C, et al: Intravenous thrombolysis with recombinant tissue plasminogen activator for acute hemispheric stroke. JAMA 274:1017-1025, 1995.

145. Hacke W, Kaste M, Fieschi C, et al: Randomised, double-blind placebo controlled trial of thrombolytic therapy with intravenous alteplase in acute ischaemic stroke (ECASS II). Lancet 352:1245-1251, 1998.

146. NINDS t-PA Stroke Study Group: Intracerebral hemorrhage after intravenous t-PA for ischemic stroke. Stroke 28:2109-2118, 1997.

147. McNamara TO, Fischer JR: Thrombolysis of peripheral arterial and graft occlusions: Improved results using high dose urokinase. AJR Am J Roentgenol 144:769, 1985.

148. Plecha FR, Pories WJ: Intraoperative angiography in the immediate assessment of arterial reconstruction. Arch Surg 105:802, 1972.

149. Quiñones-Baldrich WJ, Ziomek S, Henderson T, et al: Intraoperative fibrinolytic therapy: Experimental evaluation. J Vasc Surg 4:229, 1986.

150. Satiani B, Gross WS, Evans WE: Improved limb salvage after arterial embolectomy. Ann Surg 118:153-157, 1978.

151. Green RM, DeWeese JA, Rob CG: Arterial embolectomy before and after the Fogarty catheter. Surgery 77:24-33, 1975.

152. Greep JM, Aleman PJ, Jarrett F, Bast TJ: A combined technique for peripheral arterial embolectomy. Arch Surg 105:869-874, 1972.

153. Chaise LS, Comerota AJ, Soulen RL, et al: Selective intraarterial streptokinase therapy in the immediate postoperative period. JAMA 247:2397, 1982.

154. Feissinger JN, Vayssiarirat M, Juillet Y, et al: Local urokinase in arterial thromboembolism. Angiology 31:715, 1980.

155. Tsapogas MJ: The role of fibrinolysis in the treatment of arterial thrombosis: Experimental and clinical aspects. Ann R Coll Surg Engl 24:293, 1964.

156. Quiñones-Baldrich WJ, Zierler RE, Hiatt JC: Intraoperative fibrinolytic therapy: An adjunct to catheter thromboembolectomy. J Vasc Surg 2:319, 1985.

157. Quiñones-Baldrich WJ, Baker JD, Busuttil RW, et al: Intraoperative infusion of lytic drugs for thrombotic complications of revascularization. J Vasc Surg 10:408, 1989.

158. Comerota AJ, White JV, Grosh JD: Intraoperative intraarterial thrombolytic therapy for salvage of limbs in patients with distal arterial thrombosis. Surg Gynecol Obstet 160:283, 1989.

159. Norem RF, Short DH, Kerstein MD: Role of intraoperative fibrinolytic therapy in acute arterial occlusion. Surg Gynecol Obstet 167:87-91, 1988.

160. Parent FN III, Bernhard VM, Pabst TS, et al: Fibrinolytic treatment of residual thrombus after catheter embolectomy for severe lower limb ischemia. J Vasc Surg 9:153, 1989.

161. Quiñones-Baldrich WJ, Colburn MD, Gelabert HA, et al: Isolated limb perfusion with extracorporeal pump increases effectiveness of lysis by urokinase. J Surg Res 57:344-351, 1994.

Questions

1. **Streptokinase and urokinase have which of the following similarities: (1) both are bacterial products, (2) both are enzymes, (3) both are highly fibrin specific, or (4) both are direct fibrinolytic agents?**
   (a) 1, 2, 3
   (b) 1, 3
   (c) 2, 4
   (d) 4
   (e) None of the above

2. **Which of the following statements about increasing the dose of streptokinase to decrease its lytic effect is true?**
   (a) It is indicated when bleeding occurs during therapy
   (b) It is a predictable response
   (c) It is scientifically correct but unnecessary
   (d) It increases the risk of bleeding
   (e) None of the above

3. **Which of the following statements about tissue plasminogen activator is true?**
   (a) It is a nonenzymatic protein
   (b) It has fibrinolytic activity in plasminogen-free media
   (c) It is highly antigenic
   (d) It is mainly an exogenous fibrinolytic activator
   (e) None of the above

4. **Which of the following statements is true of a patient with deep venous thrombosis of the femoral system: he or she (1) is a candidate for lytic therapy if the thrombosis is recent and it is the first episode, (2) may be treated with low-dose local lytic therapy, (3) has about a 50% to 60% chance of failure to clear the clot completely with lytic therapy, or (4) is at higher risk of pulmonary embolism with lytic therapy than with heparin?**
   (a) 1, 2, 3
   (b) 1, 3
   (c) 2, 4
   (d) 4
   (e) None of the above

5. **Which of the following statements about intra-arterial lytic therapy is true?**
   (a) It is initiated with a loading dose
   (b) It is highly effective in graft thrombosis
   (c) It is highly effective in postdilatation thrombosis
   (d) It can be safely administered in patients after a stroke
   (e) It usually prevents a systemic lytic state

6. **What is the dose of urokinase?**
   (a) It is guided by plasminogen levels
   (b) 2000 units/kg per hour without a loading dose
   (c) 2000 units/kg per hour with a loading dose of 2000 units/kg over 10 minutes
   (d) 2000 units/pound per hour
   (e) None of the above

7. **Which of the following statements about pulmonary emboli is true?**
   (a) They may be a complication of lytic therapy
   (b) They require at least 72 hours of systemic lytic therapy to completely resolve
   (c) They can be effectively treated by streptokinase 2000 units/kg per hour
   (d) They should always be treated with systemic thrombolytic therapy
   (e) None of the above

8. **Which of the following statements is true of complications of thrombolytic therapy?**
   (a) They are caused by the antigenicity of the agent
   (b) They are caused by plasminemia
   (c) They are reduced by the avoidance of invasive procedures
   (d) They are sometimes treated by increasing the dose
   (e) All of the above

9. **Which of the following statements is true of intraoperative thrombolytic therapy: it (1) is contraindicated because bleeding results from systemic absorption, (2) may improve the results of incomplete thrombectomy, (3) is done by intravenous administration of the agent, or (4) should include heparin in the infusate?**
   (a) 1, 2, 3
   (b) 1, 3
   (c) 2, 4
   (d) 4
   (e) None of the above

10. **Which of the following statements about streptokinase administration is true?**
    (a) It results in a drop in plasminogen
    (b) It is contraindicated in patients who have received streptokinase any time in the past
    (c) It is more effective than urokinase when given intra-arterially
    (d) It results in a predictable lytic response
    (e) None of the above

Answers

1. d	2. c	3. e	4. b	5. c
6. d	7. a	8. e	9. c	10. a

Thoracic and Lumbar Sympathectomy: Indications, Technique, and Results

Minimally invasive endoscopic technology has rapidly transformed both thoracic and abdominal surgery, and the field of surgical sympathectomy is no exception. For thoracic sympathectomy, the thoracoscopic procedure is now used almost exclusively.[1-6] Laparoscopic[7] and retroperitoneoscopic techniques[8-10] have also been developed for ablation of the lumbar sympathetic chain. Because it is less invasive than open thoracic sympathectomy, the open technique for lumbar sympathectomy is still performed.[10-16] Indications for both thoracic and lumbar sympathectomies have changed during the past decades. Earlier indications such as claudication, uncomplicated Raynaud's syndrome, or scleroderma are not used today. Hyperhidrosis, chronic pain syndrome, Buerger's disease, frostbite, and complicated Raynaud's syndrome with nonhealing digital ulcerations have become the most common indications for surgical sympathectomy.[17-19]

Historical Background

The first cervical sympathectomy was performed by Alexander in 1889 for the treatment of epilepsy.[20] Jabouley suggested sympathetic denervation for vasospastic disorders in 1899,[21] but it was not until 1913 that Leriche introduced periarterial sympathectomy for ischemic lesions caused by vasospasm.[22] The first lumbar sympathectomy was performed by Royle in 1923 to treat a patient with spastic paralysis of the lower limb.[23] The concept of sympathectomy was soon adopted by Diez in Buenos Aires[24] and by Adson and Brown from the Mayo Clinic,[25] who performed lumbar sympathectomies in 1924 and 1925, respectively, to relieve vasospasm of the lower extremities. The less-invasive muscle-splitting retroperitoneal approach was described in 1937 by Pearl.[26] Adson and Brown were the first to perform cervicothoracic sympathectomy in 1929.[27]

Sympathetic denervation for hyperhidrosis was first suggested in 1920 by Kotzareff.[28] Using the single-scope technique, thoracoscopic sympathectomy was popularized by Kux

in Austria as early as 1954.[29] With the advent of endoscopic surgery, both thoracoscopic[1-6] and laparoscopic or retroperitoneoscopic procedures[7-10] have been developed for sympathetic denervation.

Anatomy and Physiology

The peripheral nervous system includes both somatic and autonomic components. The somatic efferent motor nerves control the voluntary striated muscles, and the afferent nerves transmit somatosensory information to the brain. The autonomic nervous system transmits information from the abdominal viscera, smooth and cardiac muscles, and exocrine glands. Autonomic nerves constitute the sympathetic and parasympathetic nervous systems.

ANATOMY

The sympathetic nervous system consists of the central autonomic network, which includes the brainstem, diencephalons, and cortex and of the peripheral sympathetic pathways. The peripheral sympathetic pathway consists of preganglionic and postganglionic neurons. Information from the brainstem and hypothalamus descends through the lateral funiculus of the spinal cord to the preganglionic sympathetic fibers. The preganglionic sympathetic neurons originate in the anteromedial column of the thoracolumbar cord, between T-1 and L-2. These myelinated white nerve fibers travel in the ventral root of the spinal cord to the paravertebral sympathetic ganglia, where they synapse onto the postganglionic unmyelinated gray fibers. It is likely that each preganglionic axon innervates about 10 postganglionic neurons.[30] The postganglionic axons can leave the parasympathetic ganglia at the level of the synapse or can travel up or down in the sympathetic chain before exiting the ganglion via gray rami. The regional activity of the sympathetic chain is the product of reflex arcs between somatic afferent fibers and preganglionic efferent fibers. For sympathetic denervation of the upper limbs, interruption of the sympathetic chain from T-2 to T-4 is required. Although the stellate ganglion has some innervation to the upper limbs, resection of the stellate ganglion results in Horner's syndrome (ptosis, miosis, and enophthalmos). Because of this associated morbidity, the stellate ganglion is not removed surgically. The nerve of Kuntz (Fig. 25-1) is important because it provides direct collaterals from the T-2 and T-3 ganglia to the upper limbs.[31] Resection of the T-2 and T-3 ganglia is therefore thought to be essential to achieve good and durable sympathetic denervation of the arms. The preganglionic fibers may bypass the paravertebral ganglia to synapse with more distal intermediate ganglia or may cross over to innervate the contralateral site as well. Therefore, a "complete" sympathectomy includes division of the preganglionic fibers and excision of the relay T-2 and T-3 ganglia and the intercommunicating fibers (nerve of Kuntz). Several authors advocate T-4 and T-5 resection, especially in patients who undergo the operation for axillary hyperhidrosis.

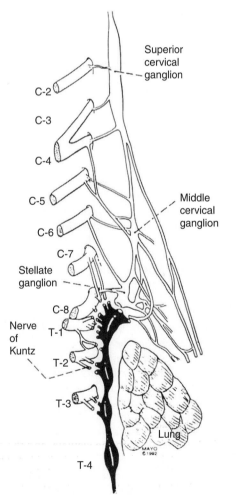

FIGURE 25–1 • Lower cervical and upper thoracic sympathetic chain. Resection of T-2 and T-3 ganglia is essential to achieve effective sympathectomy of the arm. The nerve of Kuntz, originating at the level of T-2, provides direct communicating fibers to the brachial plexus. (From Lowell RC, Gloviczki P, Cherry KJ Jr, et al: Cervicothoracic sympathectomy for Raynaud's syndrome. Int Angiol 12:168-172, 1993.)

It should be mentioned that in addition to the paravertebral ganglia, there is another subtype of peripheral sympathetic ganglia, the prevertebral ganglia. These include the celiac, aortorenal, and superior and inferior mesenteric ganglia located in the abdominal cavity, on top of and around the aorta. These ganglia send postganglionic fibers to the abdominal and pelvic organs.

PHYSIOLOGY

The sympathetic nervous system modifies basal organ functions and mediates the body's response to stress (fright, flight, and fight response). The primary function of the peripheral sympathetic nervous system is to prevent heat loss by reducing blood flow to the skin and subcutaneous tissue of the limbs. The increased activity of the postganglionic sympathetic nerves, mediated by norepinephrine, results in decreased blood flow due to stimulation of the vasoconstrictor fibers innervating the blood vessels; increased sweating is caused by stimulation of the sudomotor fibers innervating the exocrine glands (an activity mediated by acetylcholine, adenosine, and other neuropeptides), and piloerection is mediated through the activity of the pilomotor fibers that innervate the erector pili muscles.[30] The sympathetic system antagonizes the vasodilatory effect of the parasympathetic nerves on arterial resistance vessels, on the cutaneous precapillary sphincters, and on the capacitance venules.

As a result of sympathetic denervation, blood flow to the skin increases, there is loss of sweating and piloerection, and the hands (after thoracic sympathectomy) and feet (after lumbar sympathectomy) become warm, pink, and dry. Sympathectomy also results in decreased pain of the ischemic limb, likely due to an enhanced tolerance to pain stimuli. Pain tolerance is better because of decreased tissue concentration of norepinephrine and because of a reduced spinal augmentation of pain transmission to cerebral centers.[18]

The maximal effect of the sympathectomy is immediate, although vasodilatation will already begin to decrease within a week owing to compensatory mechanisms. Blood flow changes recorded at 6 months following sympathectomy are minimal because of incomplete denervation, regeneration of fibers, and the receptors' hypersensitivity to circulating catecholamines.[18]

Several authors have investigated the effect of sympathectomy on blood flow to the limbs. Cronenwett and Lindenauer found no increase in nutrient capillary perfusion as a result of sympathectomy.[32] Using intradermal xenon clearance, Moore and Hall found increased flow to the cutaneous capillary circulation.[33] Rutherford and Valenta failed to confirm increased muscle flow as a result of sympathectomy.[34] Dalessandri and coworkers, however, described increased collateral circulation in patients who underwent sympathectomy.[35]

It is evident that the effect of sympathectomy on cutaneous blood flow is transient, but this period may be sufficient to heal superficial ulcerations. The more lasting effects of sympathectomy are on sweating, abnormal vasomotor tone, and pain relief.

Thoracic Sympathectomy
INDICATIONS

In a study from the Mayo Clinic, Lowell and colleagues investigated indications for cervicothoracic sympathectomy

TABLE 25–1	Indications and Contraindications for Sympathectomy	
Thoracic Sympathectomy	**Lumbar Sympathectomy**	

Best Indications

Hyperhidrosis	Causalgia
Causalgia	Frostbite
Frostbite	Hyperhidrosis
Raynaud's phenomenon caused by stable arterial occlusions (e.g., traumatic subintimal fibrosis, distal emboli)	Buerger's disease
	Atheroembolism (blue toe syndrome)
Buerger's disease	
Facial blushing	

Acceptable Indications

Raynaud's syndrome with digital ulcerations	Inoperable Buerger's or atherosclerotic arterial occlusions with limited tissue loss
Distal arterial occlusions	Adjunctive to aortofemoral arterial reconstruction
	Rest pain in nondiabetic patient due to small arterial occlusions (e.g., distal Buerger's atherosclerosis, arterial emboli) with or without Raynaud's phenomenon

Contraindications

Uncomplicated Raynaud's disease	Claudication
	Diabetes with neuropathy

Adapted from Rutherford RB: Role of sympathectomy in the management of vascular disease. In Moore WS (ed): Vascular Surgery: A Comprehensive Review, 6th ed. Philadelphia, WB Saunders, 2001.

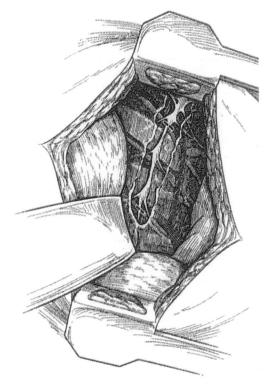

FIGURE 25–2 • Transaxillary mini-thoracotomy through the third intercostal space, performed with resection of a 6-cm-long segment of the third rib. After opening the pleura, the sympathetic chain distal to the stellate ganglion is resected, including the T-2 and T-3 segments. (From Rutherford RB: Atlas of Vascular Surgery. Philadelphia, WB Saunders, 1993.)

in 68 patients.[36] The most frequent indications were atheroembolism, Raynaud's syndrome, causalgia, hand ischemia, reflex sympathetic dystrophy, and Buerger's disease. Today, the most frequent indications for thoracic sympathectomy are hyperhidrosis and causalgia. Additional indications include distal digital occlusion, vasospastic disorders with digital ulcerations that do not respond to medical treatment, Buerger's disease, and frostbite.[1-6,17-19] Recent data indicate a beneficial effect of sympathectomy on facial blushing.[17] Uncomplicated Raynaud's disease and scleroderma are contraindications to cervical sympathectomy (Table 25-1).

TECHNIQUE

Thoracic sympathectomy can be performed using an open surgical technique, via a transaxillary or a cervical approach, or it can be performed thoracoscopically.

Open Surgical Thoracic Sympathectomy

Transaxillary Approach

Patients who undergo the transaxillary approach to the thoracic sympathetic chain are placed in a 90-degree lateral decubitus position with the arm elevated by the surgical assistant or with an arm board. The transverse skin incision is performed

in the axillary fossa, just distal to the axillary hairline, from the anterior to the posterior axillary lines. The dissection is carried down to the third rib, avoiding injury to the long thoracic nerve anteriorly and the subscapular artery and thoracodorsal nerve posteriorly. The pectoralis major muscle is retracted anteriorly, and the latissimus dorsi is retracted posteriorly. A 6-cm-long segment of the third rib is dissected from its periosteum, and it is removed (Fig. 25-2).[37] The pleura is entered, and the thoracic sympathetic chain is dissected in the paravertebral region posteriorly by incising the posterior pleura. The chain is located 1 or 2 cm lateral to the azygos vein. The chain between T-1 and T-5 is sharply dissected, and the sympathetic chain with T-2, T-3, and usually T-4 ganglia is removed. The stellate ganglion should not be removed, and dissection toward the neck should be avoided.

Cervical Approach

The cervical approach to the sympathetic chain is through a supraclavicular skin incision. A 6-cm-long transverse incision is made 2 cm proximal to the clavicle, and the posterior belly of the sternocleidomastoid muscle is divided. The external jugular vein is ligated and divided, and the anterior scalene muscle is divided, carefully retracting the phrenic nerve medially. The subclavian artery is gently retracted caudally, and the stellate ganglion is exposed medial and anterior to the brachial plexus. It usually lies immediately lateral to the vertebral artery (Fig. 25-3).[37] The stellate ganglion is preserved, and dissection is carried down into the thoracic cavity, retracting the pleural dome as much as possible. The T-1, T-2,

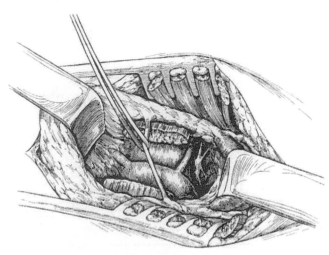

FIGURE 25–3 • Right supraclavicular approach for thoracic sympathectomy. The stellate ganglion is just lateral to the vertebral artery, which is exposed after transaction of the anterior scalene muscle. Note the phrenic nerve on a vessel loop. T-1 to T-3 is resected, gaining further exposure with downward retraction. (From Rutherford RB: Atlas of Vascular Surgery. Philadelphia, WB Saunders, 1993.)

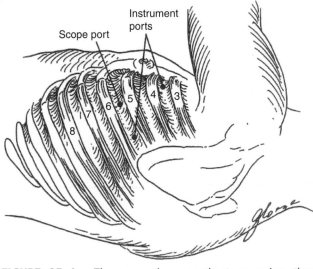

FIGURE 25–4 • Thoracoscopic sympathectomy using three endoscopic ports: two instrument ports in the anterior and posterior axillary line, and one scope port in the midaxillary line. (From Ahn SS, Machleder HI, Concepcion B, Moore WS: Thoracoscopic cervicodorsal sympathectomy: Preliminary results. J Vasc Surg 20:511-519, 1994.)

and T-3 ganglia can usually be removed through this approach. On the left side, the dissection is similar, but care must be taken to avoid injury to the thoracic duct. If injury to the thoracic duct or to one of the larger cervical ducts occurs and leak of chyle is identified, ligation of the duct is warranted to avoid the complications of a chylocutaneous cyst or fistula.

Thoracoscopic Sympathectomy

The technique of thoracoscopic sympathectomy was first described in detail by Kux in 1978 using a single-scope technique.[29] Modern endoscopic instrumentation resulted in significant modifications of the original technique, including the use of multiple ports, as reported in 1994 by Ahn and coauthors (Fig. 25-4).[1] There have been many subsequent modifications, and currently a large number of patients, primarily those with hyperhidrosis, undergo thoracoscopic sympathectomy using one, two, or three endoscopic ports.

An excellent description of uniportal and biportal sympathectomy was presented by Johnson and Patel (Figs. 25-5 and 25-6).[38] The operation is performed under general anesthesia using a double-lumen endotracheal tube for deflation of the ipsilateral lung during the procedure. For bilateral procedures, the patient is positioned supine, with the arms abducted bilaterally. For unilateral procedures, the patient is laid on his or her side.

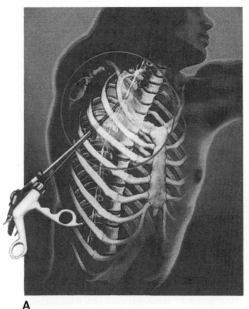

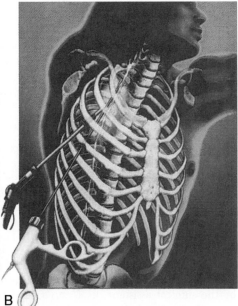

A   B

FIGURE 25–5 • A, Port location and instrument placement for uniportal thoracoscopic sympathectomy. B, Port locations and instrument placement for biportal thoracoscopic sympathectomy. (From Johnson JP, Patel NP: Uniportal and biportal endoscopic thoracic sympathectomy. Neurosurgery 51(5 Suppl):79-83, 2002.)

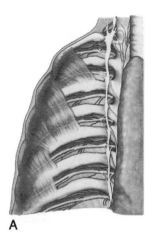
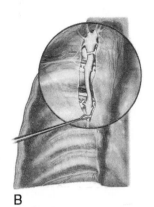

A   **B**

FIGURE 25–6 • *A,* Intrathoracic anatomy (right upper thorax) demonstrating the location of the sympathetic ganglia and chain. *B,* The posterior pleura is incised, and the T-2 and T-3 ganglia rami communicantes at each level are divided. (From Johnson JP, Patel NP: Uniportal and biportal endoscopic thoracic sympathectomy. Neurosurgery 51(5 Suppl):79-83, 2002.)

Standard thoracoscopic instrumentation is used with a 5-mm rigid scope (with a 30-degree right-angle camera), electrocautery, and Harmonic scalpel (Ethicon Endo-Surgery, Inc., Cincinnati, Ohio) for dissection and ablation of the sympathetic ganglia and fibers. The port is placed through the third intercostal space for the uniportal procedure and through the third and fifth spaces for the biportal operation, both in the anterior axillary line (see Fig. 25-5). Some surgeons use three thoracoscopic ports to facilitate retraction of the lung during sympathectomy.[1] The uniportal procedure is performed with the instruments placed through the port beside the endoscope. The sympathetic chain courses over the rib heads just lateral to the vertebral bodies (see Fig. 25-6). The sympathetic chain and ganglia are well visualized through the posterior pleura. The sympathectomy procedure involves incision of the posterior pleura and cauterization of the T-2 and T-3 ganglia, which provide most of the sympathetic innervation to the arm and hand via the nerve of Kuntz.[31] Most authors suggest ablation of the T-4 ganglion as well. On the right side, the azygos vein on the left of the hemiazygos vein may be close to the ganglia and should be avoided. Occasionally, the intercostal veins cross over the sympathetic chain, and injury or cauterization may result in bleeding from these vessels.

RESULTS

Hyperhidrosis

Lesèche and associates recently published the results of 268 thoracoscopic sympathectomies performed in 134 patients.[5] No deaths were reported. There was one conversion to open sympathectomy, and the only complication was in one patient who developed Horner's syndrome. The initial cure rate was 99.2%, and the patient satisfaction rate was excellent, at 97%. The mean follow-up was 44 months, with a late patient satisfaction rate of 91%. Seventy-two percent of the patients complained of compensatory sweating in the area immediately adjacent to the areas without sweating. Twenty-five patients (19%) judged the compensatory sweating to be severe.

Compensatory sweating was not associated with the extent of the sympathectomy.

Zacherl and colleagues reported in 1998 on the long-term results of 630 operations performed in 352 patients.[3] Complications included pneumothorax in 1.3%, Horner's syndrome in 3.8%, and subcutaneous emphysema in 2.1%. The median follow-up was 16 years. Sixty-eight percent of the patients were fully satisfied with the procedure, and 26% were partially satisfied. Permanent cure was obtained in 93% of the patients, although 67% complained of compensatory sweating. Just like other authors, these investigators reported a lower success rate in axillary hyperhidrosis.

Drott and coworkers published a review of the results of thoracic sympathectomy for hyperhidrosis.[6] For palmar hyperhidrosis, the cure rate is almost 100% after thoracoscopic sympathectomy, and the success rate is dependent on resection or ablation of the T-2 ganglion. Compensatory hyperhidrosis is frequent, although avoiding resection of T-3 and T-4 has likely decreased the risk of this complication. The overall satisfaction rate for palmar hyperhidrosis is between 87% and 95%. For axillary hyperhidrosis, the satisfaction rate is much lower (60%), and some surgeons avoid sympathectomy altogether for this complaint. Resection of T-4 and T-5 is frequently required to achieve good results.

Reflex Sympathetic Dystrophy

In patients who have complex regional pain syndrome or reflex sympathetic dystrophy, sympathectomy has been reported to effectively decrease pain. Singh and coworkers reported in 2003 on the long-term results in 42 patients.[39] Thirty-two underwent thoracoscopic and 10 had open cervicothoracic sympathectomy. Early improvement was reported in all patients. There was no morbidity or major early complications. The hospital stay was shorter in the thoracoscopic sympathectomy group, and these patients had a better outcome. These authors did not find preoperative stellate ganglion blockade predictive of postoperative clinical outcome. Because of the obvious benefit of thoracoscopic sympathectomy, they concluded that it is the procedure of choice for patients with complex regional pain syndrome.

Raynaud's Syndrome

Lowell and colleagues from the Mayo Clinic reported on the results of open surgical treatment of 20 patients who underwent cervicothoracic sympathectomies for Raynaud's syndrome.[36] No mortality was reported, but Horner's syndrome was observed in 5 patients (transient in 3 and mild in 2). Three patients had post-sympathectomy neuralgia, 2 patients had phrenic nerve palsy, and 1 patient had pneumothorax. Nineteen of the 20 patients had immediate improvement following surgical treatment. This early benefit, however, disappeared in all patients at 6 months, and the authors concluded that cervicothoracic sympathectomy in patients with uncomplicated Raynaud's syndrome is not recommended.

CONCLUSIONS

The technique of thoracoscopic sympathectomy is currently the operation of choice for patients who need surgical denervation of the thoracic sympathetic chain. If the open technique is necessary in an occasional patient, the best approach is transaxillary. Resection or thoracoscopic ablation of at least the T-2 and T-3 ganglia is necessary to achieve good results with this operation. The best indications for thoracic sympathectomy include hyperhidrosis and causalgia resulting in chronic pain syndrome. Chronic occlusive arterial disease caused by arteritis, such as Buerger's disease or Raynaud's disease with nonhealing superficial ulcerations, is also a good indication for sympathectomy. Preoperative stellate block does not always predict outcome, and complications of the operation include compensatory sweating, Horner's syndrome, and postoperative neuralgia. Compensatory sweating can be such a disabling condition that techniques to reverse the thoracic sympathectomy have been proposed, including reconstruction using nerve grafts and applying clips to the nerves during the first operation—the idea being to remove them later should compensatory sweating develop.

Lumbar Sympathectomy

INDICATIONS

Causalgia, hyperhidrosis, frostbite, Buerger's disease, pain due to atheroembolism (blue toe syndrome), and digital ulcerations are current indications for lumbar sympathectomy.

Patients who have critical limb ischemia but an ankle-brachial index greater than 0.3 have also been suggested as candidates for lumbar sympathectomy. Patients who have claudication or those who have diabetes with diabetic neuropathy should not undergo lumbar sympathectomy.

TECHNIQUE

Open Surgical Lumbar Sympathectomy

The operation is performed with the patient in a semilateral decubitus position (Fig. 25-7). An 8-cm oblique flank incision is made from the tip of the 11th rib either toward the umbilicus or slightly lower, halfway toward the umbilicus and the pubis. The dissection is carried down to the abdominal muscles; the muscles are split along their fibers, and the retroperitoneum is entered. On the right side, the peritoneum with the ureter is retracted medially, and the lumbar sympathetic chain is identified between the inferior vena cava and the psoas muscle (Fig. 25-8). The genitofemoral nerve that lies over the psoas muscle is identified and carefully preserved. On the left side, the sympathetic chain is located between the aorta and the psoas muscle. Care is taken to avoid retractor injury to the aorta, which may cause embolization into the lower limbs, often into the right leg. The sympathetic chain

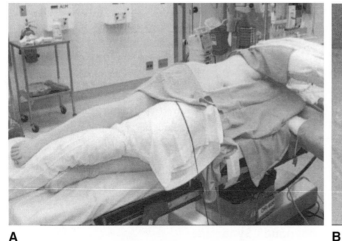

A

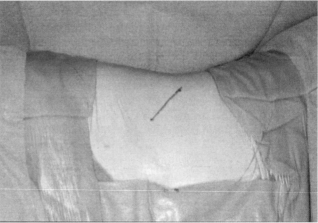

B

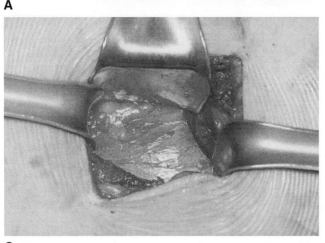

C

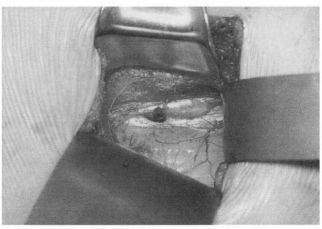

D

FIGURE 25–7 • *A,* Position of the patient on the operating table for right lumbar sympathectomy. *B,* An 8-cm skin incision is made from the tip of the 11th rib toward halfway between the umbilicus and the pubis. *C,* The abdominal muscles are split along their fibers. *D,* Blunt retroperitoneal dissection is made to explore the space between the medial edge of the psoas muscle and the inferior vena cava.

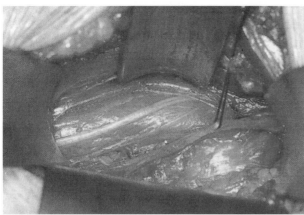

A

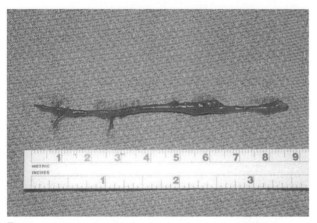

B

FIGURE 25–8 • *A,* The lumbar sympathetic chain is on a black silk thread. Note the genitofemoral nerve over the psoas muscle. *B,* The resected sympathetic chain with L-2, L-3, and L-4 ganglia.

is dissected from the rim of the pelvis all the way up to the level of L-1. Usually, three ganglia (L-2 to L-4) are removed with the intervening sympathetic chain. Frequently, the chain runs under the lumbar vessels, and careful dissection is necessary to avoid injury to these vessels. To avoid sexual dysfunction, L-1 must be preserved in males, and bilateral resection of L-1 ganglia should not be performed at all in young males. After excision of the ganglia and the chain, careful hemostasis is performed, and the muscles, subcutaneous tissue, and skin are closed in layers.

Retroperitoneoscopic Lumbar Sympathectomy

This technique was described in detail by Beglaibter and coauthors, who performed the operation in 27 patients.[10] Balloon dissection of the retroperitoneal space is performed, inserting the balloon through a small incision in the flank. Two ports are used for retraction and dissection (Fig. 25-9).[10] The chain is ablated with excision and electrocautery.

RESULTS

The most frequent early complication of lumbar sympathectomy is post-sympathectomy neuralgia, which has been described in 20% to 50% of patients.[16-18] Paradoxical gangrene is

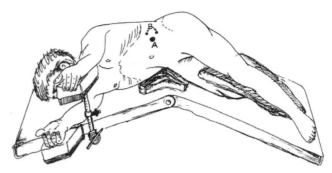

FIGURE 25–9 • Position and port placement for retroperitoneoscopic lumbar sympathectomy. (From Beglaibter N, Berlatzky Y, Zamir O, et al: Retroperitoneoscopic lumbar sympathectomy. J Vasc Surg 35:815-817, 2002.)

usually the result of embolization from the aortoiliac vessels, and careful retraction of the tissues during the operation will prevent this complication. As mentioned earlier, bilateral resection of L-1 sympathetic ganglia may disturb ejaculation or potency.

In 1985, Persson and associates reported on the results of lumbar sympathectomy for ischemic rest pain and ulcers in 37 patients who had inoperable disease.[40] All patients had an ankle-brachial index greater than 0.3. There was no neuropathy, and patients had limited tissue loss. Seventy-eight percent of these patients had long-term pain relief, and only 11% required amputation. In contrast, Fulton and Blakely reported in 1968 that sympathectomy had no effect on amputation in patients with severe distal ischemia.[41] Seventeen unselected patients in their series with advanced arteriosclerosis underwent lumbar sympathectomy; the 70% rate of amputation in these patients discredited the operation. This and other reports caused significant controversy over this operation and decreased its use for critical limb ischemia.

Bandyk and colleagues reported in 2002 on the results of sympathectomy in 73 patients with reflex sympathetic dystrophy.[16] Forty-seven of these patients underwent thoracic sympathectomy, and 37 had lumbar sympathectomy. The authors found that a more than 50% reduction in pain score for more than 2 days after sympathetic block predicted a good response to the operation. No mortality or major morbidity was reported. Transient neuralgia was noted in 20% of the patients after lumbar sympathectomy. Ninety percent of patients reported excellent results at 3 months. At 1 year, 25% still had significant pain relief, and 50% had improvement. Overall patient satisfaction was 77%.

Beglaibter and associates presented the results of 29 retroperitoneoscopic lumbar sympathectomies performed in 27 patients.[10] Twenty-two had ischemia of the lower limb, five because of Buerger's disease, and five patients had severe reflex sympathetic dystrophy. Improvement in symptoms was noted in all patients.

Five patients in the study by Beglaibter and associates had previously undergone computed tomography–guided chemical sympathectomy. Reported complications related to attempts at chemical sympathectomy using phenol or alcohol injections are related to the injection itself and to the effects of the chemicals injected. Ureteral damage, including stricture and necrosis, retroperitoneal abscess formation, and fibrosis have been reported.[42-44]

CONCLUSIONS

Lumbar sympathectomy has the best results in patients who have causalgia, hyperhidrosis, Buerger's disease, and frostbite. Patients with reflex sympathetic dystrophy with confirmed sympathetically mediated pain syndrome can also achieve long-term benefits from this operation. With the advent of lower limb revascularization, the indications for critical limb ischemia have significantly decreased. Good results have been reported with Buerger's disease and in nondiabetic patients with distal atherosclerosis who have rest pain, limited tissue loss, and an ankle-brachial index higher than 0.3. The most frequent complication of the operation is post-sympathectomy neuralgia, which is usually transient and responds well to pain medications. Open lumbar sympathectomy is still preferred by many over the retroperitoneoscopic procedures.

KEY REFERENCES

Bandyk DF, Johnson BL, Kirkpatrick AF, et al: Surgical sympathectomy for reflex sympathetic dystrophy syndromes. J Vasc Surg 35:269-277, 2002.

Claes G: Indications for endoscopic thoracic sympathectomy. Clin Auton Res 13(Suppl 1):I16-I19, 2003.

Johnson JP, Patel NP: Uniportal and biportal endoscopic thoracic sympathectomy. Neurosurgery 51(5 Suppl):79-83, 2002.

Rutherford RB: Atlas of Vascular Surgery. Philadelphia, WB Saunders, 1993.

Schiller Y: The anatomy and physiology of the sympathetic innervation of the upper limbs. Clin Auton Res 13(Suppl 1):I2-I5, 2003.

REFERENCES

1. Ahn SS, Machleder HI, Concepcion B, Moore WS: Thoracoscopic cervicodorsal sympathectomy: Preliminary results. J Vasc Surg 20:511-519, 1994.
2. Kopelman D, Hashmonai M, Ehrenreich M, et al: Upper dorsal thoracoscopic sympathectomy for palmar hyperhidrosis: Improved intermediate-term results. J Vasc Surg 24:194-199, 1996.
3. Zacherl J. Huber ER. Imhof M. et al: Long-term results of 630 thoracoscopic sympathectomies for primary hyperhidrosis: The Vienna experience. Eur J Surg Suppl 580:43-46, 1998.
4. Hashmonai M, Kopelman D, Schein M: Thoracoscopic versus open supraclavicular upper dorsal sympathectomy: A prospective randomised trial. Eur J Surg Suppl 572:13-16, 1994.
5. Lesèche G, Castier Y, Thabut G, et al: Endoscopic transthoracic sympathectomy for upper limb hyperhidrosis: Limited sympathectomy does not reduce postoperative compensatory sweating. J Vasc Surg 37:124-128, 2003.
6. Drott C, Gothberg G, Claes G: Endoscopic transthoracic sympathectomy: An efficient and safe method for the treatment of hyperhidrosis. J Am Acad Dermatol 33:78-81, 1995.
7. Kathouda N, Wattanasirichaigoon S, Tang E, et al: Laparoscopic lumbar sympathectomy. Surg Endosc 11:257-260, 1997.
8. Hourlay P, Vangertruiden G, Verduyckt F, et al: Endoscopic extraperitoneal lumbar sympathectomy. Surg Endosc 9:530-533, 1995.
9. Cheshire NJ, Darzi AW: Retroperitoneoscopic lumbar sympathectomy. Br J Surg 84:1094-1095, 1997.
10. Beglaibter N, Berlatzky Y, Zamir O, et al: Retroperitoneoscopic lumbar sympathectomy. J Vasc Surg 35:815-817, 2002.
11. Mockus M, Rutherford RB, Rosales C: Sympathectomy for causalgia: Patient selection and long-term results. Arch Surg 122:668-672, 1987.
12. Abu Rahma AF, Robinson PA, Powell M, et al: Sympathectomy for reflex sympathetic dystrophy: Factors affecting outcome. Ann Vasc Surg 8:372-379, 1994.
13. Taylor MS: Lumbar epidural sympathectomy for frostbite injuries of the feet. Mil Med 164:566-567, 1999.
14. Olcott C, Eltherington LG, Wilcosky BR, et al: Reflex sympathetic dystrophy: The surgeon's role in management. J Vasc Surg 14:488-492, 1991.
15. Gordon A, Zechmeister K, Collin J: The role of sympathectomy in current surgical practice. Eur J Vasc Surg 8:129-137, 1994.
16. Bandyk DF, Johnson BL, Kirkpatrick AF, et al: Surgical sympathectomy for reflex sympathetic dystrophy syndromes. J Vasc Surg 35:269-277, 2002.
17. Claes G: Indications for endoscopic thoracic sympathectomy. Clin Auton Res 13(Suppl 1):I16-I19, 2003.
18. Rutherford RB: Role of sympathectomy in the management of vascular disease and related disorders. In Moore WS (ed): Vascular Surgery: A Comprehensive Review, 6th ed. Philadelphia, WB Saunders, 2002, pp 365-376.
19. Komori K, Kowasaki K, Okasaki J, et al: Thorascopic sympathectomy for Buerger's disease of the upper extremities. J Vasc Surg 22:344-346, 1995.
20. Alexander W: The Treatment of Epilepsy. Edinburgh, YJ Pentland, 1889, p 228.
21. Jabouley M: Le traitment de quelques troubles trophiques du pied at de la jambes par la denudation de lartere femorale et la distention des nerfs vasculaires. Lyon Med 91:467-468, 1899.
22. Leriche R: De l'elongation et de la section des nerfs perivasculaires dans certains syndromes douloureoux d'origine arterielle at dans quelques troubles trophiques. Lyon Chir 10:378-382, 1913.
23. Royle JP: History of sympathectomy Aust N Z J Surg 69:302-307, 1999.
24. Diez J: Un nuevo metodo de simpatectomia periferica para el tratamiento de las afecciones troficas y gangrenosas de los miembros. Bol Soc Cir Buenos Aires 8:792-806, 1924.
25. Adson AW, Brown GE: Treatment of Raynaud's disease by lumbar rami-section and ganglionectomy and perivascular sympathetic neurectomy of the common iliacs. JAMA 84:1908-1910, 1925.
26. Pearl FL: Muscle splitting extraperitoneal lumbar ganglionectomy. Surg Gynecol Obstet 65:107-112, 1937.
27. Adson AW, Brown GE: Raynaud's disease of the upper extremities: Successful treatment by resection of the sympathetic cervicothoracic and second thoracic ganglion and trunks. JAMA 92:444-449, 1929.
28. Kotzareff A: Resection partielle du tronc sympathetic cervical droit pour hyperhidrose unilaterale (regions faciale, cervicale, thoracique et brachiale droites). Rev Med Suisse Rom 40:111-113, 1920.
29. Kux M: Thoracic endoscopic sympathectomy in palmar and axillary hyperhidrosis. Arch Surg 113:264-266, 1978.
30. Schiller Y: The anatomy and physiology of the sympathetic innervation of the upper limbs. Clin Auton Res 13(Suppl 1):I2-I5, 2003.
31. Kuntz A: Distribution of the sympathetic rami to the brachial plexus: Its relation to sympathectomy affecting the upper extremity. Arch Surg 15:871-877, 1927.
32. Cronenwett JL, Lindenauer SM: Hemodynamic effects of sympathectomy in ischemic canine hind limbs. Surgery 87:417-424, 1980.
33. Moore WS, Hall AD: Effects of lumbar sympathectomy on skin capillary blood flow in arterial occlusive disease. J Surg Res 14:151-160, 1973.
34. Rutherford RB, Valenta J: Extremity blood flow and distribution: The effects of arterial occlusion, sympathectomy and exercise. Surgery 69:332-338, 1971.
35. Dalessandri KM, Carson SN, Tillman P, et al: Effect of lumbar sympathectomy in distal arterial obstruction. Arch Surg 228:1157-1160, 1983.
36. Lowell RC, Gloviczki P, Cherry KJ Jr, et al: Cervicothoracic sympathectomy for Raynaud's syndrome. Int Angiol 12:168-172, 1993.
37. Rutherford RB: Atlas of Vascular Surgery. Philadelphia, WB Saunders, 1993.
38. Johnson JP, Patel NP: Uniportal and biportal endoscopic thoracic sympathectomy. Neurosurgery 51(5 Suppl):79-83, 2002.
39. Singh B, Moodley J, Shaik AS, Robbs JV: Sympathectomy for complex regional pain syndrome. J Vasc Surg 37:508-511, 2003.
40. Persson AV, Anderson L, Rodberg FT Jr: Selection of patients for lumbar sympathectomies. Surg Clin North Am 65:393-403, 1985.
41. Fulton RL, Blakely WR: Lumbar sympathectomy: A procedure of questionable value in the treatment of arteriosclerosis obliterans of the legs. Am J Surg 116:735-744, 1968.
42. Cross FW, Cotton LT: Chemical lumbar sympathectomy for ischemic rest pain: A randomized, prospective controlled clinical trial. Am J Surg 150:341-345, 1985.
43. Redman DR, Robinson PN, Al-Kutoubi MA: Computerized tomography guided lumbar sympathectomy. Anaesthesia 41:39-41, 1986.
44. Heindel W, Ernst S, Manshausen G, et al: CT-guided lumbar sympathectomy: Results and analysis of factors influencing the outcome. Cardiovasc Intervent Radiol 21:319-323, 1998.

Questions

1. Indications for thoracoscopic sympathectomy include all of the following except
   (a) Causalgia
   (b) Hyperhidrosis
   (c) Raynaud's syndrome caused by scleroderma
   (d) Buerger's disease
   (e) Raynaud's phenomenon caused by digital emboli

2. Resection or ablation of which of the following segments of the cervicothoracic chain is recommended to achieve sympathetic denervation of the upper limb?
   (a) Stellate ganglion and T-1
   (b) T-1 and T-2
   (c) T-2 and T-3
   (d) T-3 and T-4
   (e) Stellate ganglion, T-1, and T-2

3. Which of the following is the most frequent complication of T-2 to T-4 sympathectomy?
   (a) Recurrent hyperhidrosis
   (b) Permanent Horner's syndrome
   (c) Chylothorax
   (d) Postoperative neuralgia
   (e) Vasospasm

4. Where are the direct collateral sympathetic fibers to the arm from T-2 and T-3 located?
   (a) Nerve of Herring
   (b) Nerve of Kuntz
   (c) Brachial plexus
   (d) Intercostobrachial nerve
   (e) Prevertebral ganglia

5. Sympathectomy results in all of the following changes in a limb except
   (a) Piloerection
   (b) Decreased sweating
   (c) Decreased pain
   (d) Increased parasympathetic tone
   (e) Increased skin circulation

6. What is the primary function of the sympathetic nervous system?
   (a) Vasodilatation of the arterial resistance vessels
   (b) Closure of the cutaneous precapillary sphincters
   (c) Vasodilatation of the venous capacitance vessels
   (d) Prevention of heat loss by reducing blood flow to the skin and subcutaneous tissue

7. What is the recommended technique for thoracic sympathetic denervation?
   (a) Thoracoscopic sympathectomy
   (b) Transaxillary open sympathectomy
   (c) Supraclavicular cervical sympathectomy
   (d) Percutaneous phenol ablation of T-2 and T-3 ganglia

8. Which of the following is a contraindication for lumbar sympathectomy?
   (a) Digital gangrene
   (b) Diabetic neuropathy
   (c) Frostbite
   (d) Causalgia
   (e) Buerger's disease

9. On the right side, where is the lumbar sympathetic chain located?
   (a) Medial to the psoas muscle
   (b) Medial to the inferior vena cava
   (c) Lateral to the ureter
   (d) Lateral to the genitofemoral nerve
   (e) Just lateral to the aorta

10. Which of the following statements about lumbar sympathectomy is false?
    (a) Transient post-sympathectomy neuralgia is reported in 20 percent of patients
    (b) In patients with chronic pain syndrome, the preoperative response to lumbar sympathetic block predicts good outcome
    (c) Seventy-five percent of patients with reflex sympathetic dystrophy had less pain 1 year after sympathectomy
    (d) Retrograde ejaculation can be avoided by not performing bilateral L-1 sympathectomies
    (e) Percutaneous phenol or alcohol injection is a safe and excellent alternative to open lumbar sympathectomy

Answers

1. c	2. c	3. a	4. b	5. a
6. d	7. a	8. b	9. a	10. e

26

Michael C. Stoner • William A. Abbott

Vascular Grafts: Characteristics and Rational Selection

Most medical historians trace the advent of modern vascular surgery to the work of Carrel,[1] one of four surgeons who have won the Nobel Prize. This work includes a description of autogenous vein grafting in dogs. Since then, both vascular surgeons and scientists have sought superior vascular grafts, with only partial success. Although current synthetic prosthetic grafts yield good results in aortoiliac reconstructive surgery, the best results in peripheral small vessel reconstruction are still achieved with venous autografts. The greater saphenous vein is the conduit of choice for small vessel reconstruction, for it most closely approximates the characteristics of the ideal vascular graft. However, at least 20% of current candidates for infrainguinal reconstruction have insufficient or unsuitable autogenous veins.[2] The saphenous vein may have been used during previous vascular procedures or may be inadequate owing to chronic disease. In these circumstances, the vascular surgeon must be aware of all the graft choices available and the relative advantages and disadvantages of each. Further, although autogenous vein is currently the best conduit, it is not a perfect arterial substitute. It is considered the gold standard, but it is a tarnished one. This gold standard yields 5-year supragenculate and infrageniculate patency rates of approximately 80% and 60%, respectively, as detailed later. A comparison of the major conduits discussed in this chapter is provided in Table 26-1.

This chapter reviews the relevant characteristics of the normal human artery and those of an "ideal" vascular graft, which, unfortunately, does not currently exist. A brief overview of autogenous grafts and the various prosthetic grafts available follows; some conduits that are no longer in use are presented for historical and scientific interest. Some of the more promising research initiatives in vascular graft development are described, and recommendations about the most appropriate grafts for specific procedures are made, based on published results.

The Normal Artery

An artery is much more than the inert conduit it was thought to be until the 1970s. For this reason, prosthetic grafts have

fallen far short of the durability and function of native arteries. The longevity of native arteries in terms of their ability to remain patent and free from occlusive or aneurysmal change is measured in decades, whereas that of prosthetics is generally measured in years. The functional characteristics of large elastic arteries, such as the aorta, differ from those of medium-size muscular arteries, such as the carotid, and these differences must be taken into account when either designing or choosing a prosthetic graft.

An artery is composed of three layers: intima, media, and adventitia (Fig. 26-1). The intima is the inner layer and is composed of endothelium, extracellular matrix, and the internal elastic lamina. The endothelium, in addition to forming a smooth lining, is biologically active; besides its vasoregulatory function, it also modulates the humoral and cellular coagulation systems by imparting a negative (hydrophobic) charge and by actively secreting antithrombotic agents.[3] The vascular endothelial cell is a complex component of the cardiovascular system, with roles as both a mediator and an effector of inflammation, reperfusion, systemic response to injury, and metabolism. The media consists of layers of smooth muscle cells oriented in both longitudinal and circumferential directions that are surrounded by a basal lamina and fibers of collagen and elastin. The media contributes to the strength and durability of the artery; however it is primarily responsible for control over elasticity and vessel diameter. It is also the principal cell involved in arteriosclerosis and secretes a variety of paracrine and hormonal mediators. In addition, vascular smooth muscle cells have been shown to contribute greatly to tissue homeostasis and to the response to a variety of pathologic states. The adventitia, long thought to be an inert, nonfunctional structure, contains the vasa vasorum and a collagenous matrix whose main function is to provide tensile strength to the artery.

Concept of Thromboreactivity

For purposes of this chapter, a *vascular prosthesis* is defined as a man-made or altered device meant to replace a blood vessel. In common vascular surgical usage, the term does not usually

TABLE 26–1	Comparison of Vascular Graft Materials			
Graft	**Femoropopliteal Bypass Patency (%)**	**Femorotibial Bypass Patency (%)**	**Pros**	**Cons**
Autogenous vein	72-82	69-68	Provides best patency	Availability of suitable conduit
Human umbilical vein	53-63	16-50	Improved patency with newer fixation, good compliance match	Problematic surgical characteristics, aneurysm formation
Cryopreserved allograft	23-35	16-34	Compliant biologic conduit	Poor long-term patency
ePTFE	52-60	12-60	Readily available, relative ease of assisted patency	Needle hole bleeding, poor infrapopliteal patency, graft stiffness
ePTFE with distal vein cuff	47-60	49-69	Provides appropriate compliance match at distal anastomosis, patency intermediate between ePTFE and vein	Can be time-consuming or technically difficult. depending on vein and distal vessel
Dacron	57-71	16-34	Readily available with known handling characteristics	Graft porosity, poor infrapopliteal patency, difficult assisted patency

ePTFE, expanded polytetrafluoroethylene.

include living autogenous conduits, such as the saphenous vein. Any prosthesis placed into the arterial system enters a theoretical thromboreactive state that can be defined in terms of intensity and duration. Depending on that state, as well as a number of other host variables (e.g., low flow caused by poor runoff), the graft either remains patent or occludes. Graft thromboreactivity and the parameters that influence it vary over the life of the implant in early (weeks), intermediate (weeks to months), and long-term (years) time frames. Although thromboreactivity is most intense immediately after implantation, in most current prostheses it persists at a low level forever.

Characteristics of an Ideal Prosthetic Graft

A vascular prosthetic graft may be composed of manufactured material, or it may be of biologic (i.e., tissue) origin. An "ideal" vascular prosthetic graft would have characteristics that minimize both the intensity and the duration of the thromboreactive state (Table 26-2). Specifically, such a graft would be impermeable, thromboresistant, compliant, biocompatible, durable, resistant to infection, easy to sterilize, easy to implant, readily available, and cost-effective.[4] This ideal has yet to be achieved.

Impermeability to blood is obviously important, although this characteristic is somewhat at odds with the need for sufficient permeability or porosity to allow graft incorporation and healing. Thromboresistance, the ability of the graft surface to tolerate blood contact without activating platelets or the humoral coagulation cascade, is vital and is related to several factors, including graft surface reactivity with blood, ionic charge, porosity, and compliance relative to that of the adjacent native artery. The physical property of elasticity is critical to graft longevity and function. Compliance, defined as volume change per unit of pressure change, describes this property. Considerable data have shown that compliance and compliance mismatch are important contributors to thrombosis.[5,6] Biocompatibility is necessary because a significant tissue reaction may promote thrombosis, loss of graft integrity, and graft failure. A prosthetic graft must be durable enough to obviate

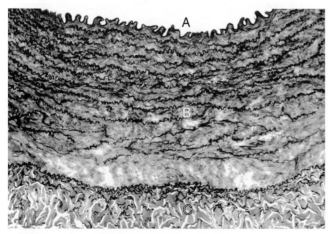

FIGURE 26–1 • Photomicrograph demonstrating arterial wall histology: intima (A), media (B), and adventitia (C).

TABLE 26–2	Characteristics of the Ideal Prosthetic Graft

Impermeable
Thromboresistant
Compliant
Biocompatible
Durable
Resistant to infection
Easy to sterilize
Easy to implant
Readily available
Cost-effective

the need for future replacement owing to degeneration, aneurysm formation, or rupture. Resistance to infection and sterility are necessary to lessen the incidence of graft infection. A graft should also have the handling characteristics—strength, flexibility, suture retention, and ease of suturing—that make it easy to implant. The graft should be readily available for both elective and emergent use. Finally, in this era of increasingly limited health care resources, the graft must be relatively cost-effective, with the cost of the graft measured against the operative time required to implant it, and free from complications that require secondary or revisional intervention.

When considering a prosthetic graft, it is necessary to revisit the autogenous vein as an arterial conduit. Although it is not always possible to use a vein graft in a given clinical situation, when selecting a prosthetic graft, the surgeon must compare outcomes to the gold standard. Accordingly, a review of the vein graft conduit is provided first.

Autogenous Vein Grafts

ANATOMY

The greater saphenous vein, the one most commonly used for arterial reconstruction, consists of a monolayer of endothelium, a basement membrane, a media composed of two layers of smooth muscle cells, and an adventitia, which is the thickest layer of the vein wall (Figs. 26-2 and 26-3).[7] The wall of normal veins is considerably thinner than that of arteries, and although many vein walls are thickened at the time of harvest for bypass grafting, the vein may still be usable as an arterial conduit.

The anatomy of the greater saphenous vein is important to the vascular surgeon, and anatomic variation can affect the success of the vein harvest and its performance as a graft. The greater saphenous vein originates in the dorsum of the foot and ascends anterior to the medial malleolus. It follows a superficial course on the anteromedial aspect of the tibia, and at the level of the knee it lies 8 to 10 cm below the medial edge of the patella.[8] The greater saphenous vein is duplicated in an estimated 8% of patients.[9] Lower extremity veins contain valves, which are more numerous distally and decrease in number proximally. Perforating veins tend to occur in the midthigh at the level of the adductor hiatus, just above the knee joint, and midway between the knee and the ankle.[10]

The lesser saphenous vein runs in a slightly oblique course from behind the lateral malleolus to the popliteal vein. It may be used as an autograft; however, its length and diameter are markedly less than those of the greater saphenous vein.

The cephalic vein is 50 cm long, and although it is often quite thin, it may be an acceptable alternative as an autograft.[11] The same holds true for the basilic vein.[12] In practice, the suitability of a vein for use as a conduit is quite variable and often is not predictable in advance of the operation. The suitability of any autogenous vein is best determined by preoperative venous mapping with duplex scanning.

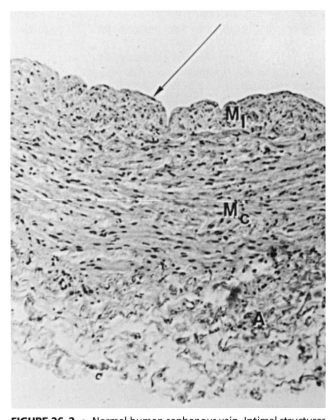

FIGURE 26–2 • Normal human saphenous vein. Intimal structures (*arrow*) include endothelium and scant subendothelial connective tissue. Medial structures are composed of an inner layer of longitudinally arranged smooth muscle (M$_l$) and an outer region of circumferentially oriented smooth muscle (M$_c$). Adventitial structures appear as a loose collection of connective tissue (A) with occasional vasa vasorum. (From Stanley JC, Burkel WE, Lindenauer SM, et al: Biologic and Synthetic Vascular Prostheses. New York, Grune & Stratton, 1982.)

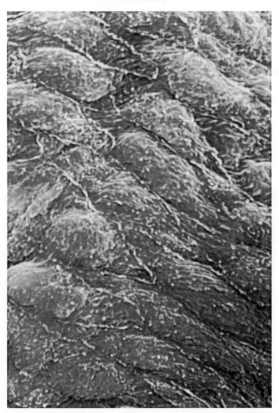

FIGURE 26–3 • Normal vein lumen, showing characteristic endothelial cell surface (SEM, ×30).

ARTERIALIZATION

After implantation as an arterial conduit, autogenous veins undergo morphologic changes in response to the hemodynamic forces of the arterial circulation. These changes begin immediately after implantation, continue over time, and in some cases may become detrimental to the performance of the graft. This process is known as arterialization, and it was originally described by Carrel.[1] In most cases it is a normal and salutary adaptive response of the vein to the new arterial environment. In a small fraction of grafts, it becomes a pathologic response termed intimal hyperplasia. Distinct internal and external elastic laminae appear,[13] and smooth muscle cells migrate into the intima, where they proliferate, hypertrophy, and produce extracellular matrix proteins. In intimal hyperplasia, this process becomes uncontrolled and leads to progressive narrowing of the entire graft, or stenosis. Intimal hyperplasia accounts for a significant percentage of early (within 1 year) graft occlusion.[14,15] Focal hyperplasia is thought to represent an aggravated response to local injury and typically occurs at sites of valve lysis or in perianastomotic regions.[16] Diffuse hyperplasia is poorly understood.

Intimal hyperplasia occurs in approximately 11% to 33% of vein grafts in peripheral arterial reconstructions, with 75% developing within the first year.[17] This problem is being investigated at both the hemodynamic and cellular levels. Data from our laboratory have implicated anastomotic flow disturbances and compliance mismatch in the development of anastomotic neointimal hyperplasia.[18,19] Hyperhomocysteinemia has been shown to be associated with the development of preexisting intimal hyperplasia in veins and subsequent vein graft failure.[20] Clowes and associates investigated the interaction between endothelium and smooth muscle cells at the cellular and cytokine levels and developed a multifactorial theory of smooth muscle cell proliferation.[21]

Because the cause of intimal hyperplasia is poorly understood, no effective prophylactic or treatment measure exists. Several animal studies have shown promise in inhibiting intimal hyperplasia by using external beam irradiation, adenovirus-mediated gene transfer of nitric oxide synthase and other vasoactive peptides, and L-arginine supplementation. Unfortunately, these therapies have had minimal clinical application, and their utility remains to be determined.[22-25]

VEIN HARVEST—SURGICAL TECHNIQUE

Three general methods are used for saphenous vein preparation: the in situ technique, which leaves the vein in its normal anatomic position; the reversed technique, which moves the vein from its native location; and the nonreversed translocation technique, which also moves the vessel from its normal anatomic position but, as with the in situ technique, requires valve lysis. Regardless of the bypass technique used, the technique of vein harvest and preparation affects the performance of the graft. Careful, gentle harvesting and handling increase the early and late patency of vein grafts, whereas vein damage caused by careless technique increases the incidence of early graft failure due to technical problems and late failure due to hyperplastic or degenerative changes in the vein. Endoscopic harvest involves a minimally invasive route and, in well-trained hands, has very good results.[26]

If the in situ or nonreversed translocation technique is used, extreme care must be taken when lysing valves. Several problems can result from improper valve lysis, such as inadvertent injury to the vessel wall. This can lead to perioperative failure from an intimal flap or early failure from neointimal hyperplasia. Missed valves or incomplete lysis of valve leaflets may also cause early graft failure.[20] Even properly lysed valves can develop late focal stenosis.

If the reversed technique is used, limiting the amount of time the graft spends outside the body results in less ischemia to the vein. If necessary, the graft should be kept in a chilled isotonic solution, such as cold autologous heparinized blood.[27]

Vein grafts are susceptible to a number of complications. Aneurysm formation may occur in up to 12% of infrainguinal bypass grafts.[28] Atherosclerosis, which is extremely rare in the venous circulation, may occur in 7% to 15% of transplanted veins,[29] possibly related to smoking and uncontrolled hyperlipidemia.[30] Neointimal hyperplasia, focal stenosis from valve injuries and missed valves, aneurysmal change, and graft atherosclerosis account for a significant number of early and late failures. Careful technique can minimize, but not eliminate, these problems.

RESULTS

Infrainguinal bypass grafts using autogenous vein yield the highest patency rates in the most recent literature. Five-year primary patency rates of 72% to 82% have been reported for femoropopliteal bypass.[2,31,32] For infrapopliteal bypass, 5-year patency rates of 59% to 69% and limb salvage rates of 90% have been reported.[32-34] Interestingly, results do not appear to be significantly different for in situ, reversed, and nonreversed translocation techniques, permitting the decision to be based primarily on anatomic requirements. Primary patency rates with arm and lesser saphenous veins are lower, in the range of 40% to 50% at 5 years, but still considerably higher than those for prosthetic grafts.[35,36] Faries and coworkers demonstrated superior patency and limb salvage with all-autogenous venous conduits versus prosthetics for all permutations of lower extremity grafts.[37] The authors demonstrated a 3-year patency rate of 72.8% and 68.3% for femoropopliteal and femorotibial configurations, respectively. Studies that compare autogenous composite grafts with prosthetic grafts echo these findings.[38] Curi and associates reported a primary assisted patency rate for greater saphenous vein grafts of 57% at 4 years, versus a 45% rate in composite autogenous grafts and a dismal 11% rate in prosthetic lower extremity bypasses.[39] If ipsilateral greater saphenous vein is not available, contralateral saphenous vein is an acceptable alternative and provides superior patency rates.[40] The concern that conduit should be preserved for possible coronary revascularization is unfounded.[41]

Arterial Autografts

Medium-size muscular arteries possess an important characteristic that renders them particularly amenable to autotransplantation as free grafts—their vasa vasorum originate from small arterial branches and remain intact if harvested carefully.[42] For this reason, arterial autografts come closer to the characteristics of the ideal vascular graft than vein grafts do and should be the gold standard. Unfortunately, few arteries are suitable as autografts. In certain situations, common, internal, and external iliac segments may be harvested as a bypass graft and replaced with a prosthetic graft. Alternatively, an occluded iliofemoral segment that has been bypassed can be harvested and, following endarterectomy, used as a bypass conduit. From these sites, segments of graft 10 to 20 cm long may be obtained.[42] The subscapular and epigastric arteries are also viable conduits and can yield very good primary assisted patency rates (82% at 3 years) in distal bypasses, even in the setting of end-stage renal disease.[43]

Arterial autografts are attractive conduits for use in children because their growth rate is proportional to that of the other vessels of the arterial system.[44] They are also particularly advantageous in renal artery reconstruction.[45] Another potential use of arterial autografts is in an infected tissue bed, where a prosthetic graft would not be appropriate because of the danger of graft infection.[45]

The use of splenic artery autografts for extra-anatomic renovascular reconstruction is an accepted and efficacious means of treating renovascular disease.[46] The internal mammary artery is also used in a similar manner; in coronary artery bypass grafts, its patency is superior to that of vein grafts (84% and 53%, respectively, at 10 years), illustrating the better patency rates that can be obtained with arterial autografts.[47]

RESULTS

In properly selected patients, arterial autografts can provide excellent results. In Stoney and colleagues' report of renal revascularization in children, late patency was 100%, grafts were observed to grow normally, and only a single instance of graft dilatation was noted.[48] Cambria and associates, in a review of 52 splenorenal arterial bypass grafts, noted an early and late patency rate of greater than 90% at 5 years.[46]

Allografts

Both arterial and venous allografts were used extensively in the early days of aortic reconstruction[49] for both aneurysmal and occlusive disease. Aortic segments harvested from cadavers were stored in various preservative solutions at 4°C, frozen, or freeze-dried. These grafts suffered from the twin disadvantages of nonviability and tissue antigenicity. Enthusiasm for the use of large vessel allografts waned when reports were published showing a high rate of graft calcification and aneurysm formation.[50,51] As textile grafts for aortic reconstruction became available, the use of allografts all but disappeared. Several authors, however, recommend the use of cadaveric arterial allografts for in situ replacement of infected abdominal aortic grafts[52-55] and for thoracic aortic graft replacement in the presence of endocarditis.[56] Work from our own laboratory shows that cryopreservation actually decreases the rejection of arterial allografts.[57]

Efforts directed at obtaining a useful small vessel allograft have been disappointing. Cadaveric human saphenous vein allografts were implanted in the 1960s in patients with an unsuitable autogenous vein, but follow-up showed poor long-term patency.[58] More recently, cryopreservation of human saphenous vein using dimethyl sulfoxide (DMSO) has resulted in viable vein grafts.[59-61] Unfortunately, viable allografts are antigenic and capable of stimulating a rejection response. Cryopreserved vein allografts are still under investigation, and a phase I study using cryopreserved venous valved segments

to treat chronic venous insufficiency suggests that this may be a therapeutic option in selected individuals.[62]

A recent study confirms previous findings that allograft has a limited role in infrainguinal reconstruction, and the authors recommended the use of this graft only in infected fields when autogenous vein is not available.[63,64] Arterial allografts have also been used for infrainguinal reconstruction; however, they too have relatively poor patency, with primary patency rates of only 23% to 35% at 3 years noted in two studies.[65,66] There is an increasing use of cryopreserved superficial femoral vein grafts for dialysis because they may be more resistant to infection than expanded polytetrafluoroethylene (ePTFE). The role of immunosuppressive drugs and the use of anticoagulation in conjunction with these grafts are still under investigation. In a prospective clinical trial, Carpenter and Tomaszewski found that vein allograft failure was not eliminated by low-dose zidovudine (AZT) immunosuppressive therapy.[67] Unless the results of future studies show a clear advantage of these grafts over existing conduits, their expense may preclude their use.

HUMAN UMBILICAL VEIN ALLOGRAFT

The human umbilical vein (HUV) allograft is of interest because of the relatively large experience surgeons have acquired since it was first implanted more than 40 years ago.[68] Disappointing short-term patency results led to a loss of interest in this graft, but Dardik and colleagues revised it by stabilizing it with glutaraldehyde instead of dialdehyde starch.[69,70] Glutaraldehyde seemingly produces better crosslinking of collagen, resulting in a graft that is purportedly not only stronger but also less antigenic. Following fixation, the graft is encased in a Dacron mesh for added strength, because early animal studies demonstrated a significant incidence of HUV graft dilatation without mesh.[71]

As with other preserved allografts (with the exception of cryopreserved saphenous veins), the HUV graft is not viable after fixation and is essentially a musculocollagenous tube. Thus, any potential advantage of the HUV graft over synthetic prosthetic grafts in terms of late patency is related to the surface characteristics of its inner layer and its compliance.

The majority of HUV graft experience has been in infrainguinal reconstruction. Because autogenous greater saphenous vein is the conduit of choice for these procedures,[2,33] the clinical efficacy of HUV grafts would lie in their ability to provide a better conduit than synthetic grafts for infrainguinal reconstruction in patients for whom autogenous greater saphenous vein is not an option.[2] One factor limiting the potential usefulness of HUV is the greater technical difficulty involved in handling, tunneling, and anastomosing the graft compared with either autogenous vein or other prosthetic grafts.[72] Suturing is tedious owing to the thickness of the graft and because care must be taken to include both the basement membrane and the outer Dacron mesh in the suture line. HUV grafts are also friable and prone to mural dissection if not handled gently.

Results

In 1988, Dardik and colleagues published the largest series of HUV graft experience in a report describing 907 bypasses, half of which were to tibial vessels.[73] Five-year patency rates were 53% for femoropopliteal reconstruction, 26% for femorotibial reconstruction, and 28% for femoroperoneal reconstruction. Several studies demonstrated no significant difference in patency between HUV and ePTFE grafts in infrainguinal reconstruction,[74-77] although two randomized, prospective studies showed superior patency of HUV for femoropopliteal bypasses.[78,79] Published results demonstrating 5-year patency rates of up to 67% confirm the potential utility of HUV grafts.[80] A prospective, randomized study from the Veterans Affairs system demonstrated a 2-year patency rate of 53% in HUV grafts for femoropopliteal reconstruction, intermediate between autogenous and synthetic conduits.[81] The most serious drawback of the HUV graft is its tendency to degenerate. Late graft dilatation and aneurysm formation reportedly occur in up to 57% of HUV grafts (Fig. 26-4).[82-84] Dardik and colleagues recently updated their work to provide information about long-term aneurysm formation.[85] In the last 10 years of the study, no evidence of degeneration was noted, suggesting an improvement in graft usage and technique. Although the incidence of clinically significant aneurysm formation requiring graft salvage or replacement is lower than the previously cited numbers,[86] the problem is still significant enough to make HUV an unacceptable conduit in the opinion of most vascular surgeons.

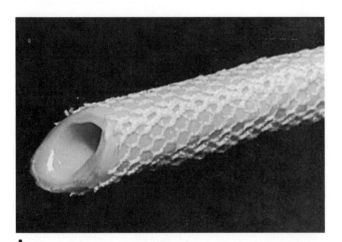

A

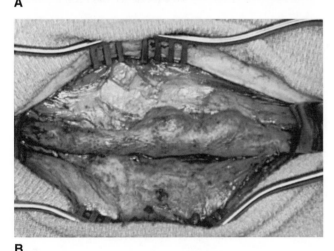

B

FIGURE 26–4 • Human umbilical vein graft with surrounding Dacron mesh before implantation (A) and aneurysmal segment 5 years after implantation (B).

Xenografts

Interest in the use of animal tissue for vascular grafts dates back to the 1950s, when bovine carotid arteries were enzymatically digested with ficin to remove antigenic cellular material and then tanned with dialdehyde starch.[87] This graft was used clinically as a femoropopliteal graft, and over the next decade, considerable experience was gained with it. Unfortunately, its late patency was no better than that of synthetic grafts,[88,89] with 5-year patency rates of 40% to 50% in the above-knee position. The reported incidence of aneurysm formation was 3% to 6%, but it was probably much higher. Infection rates were 3% to 7%.[88] Thus, use of these xenografts in infrainguinal bypasses ceased, although they continued to be somewhat useful in angioaccess for hemodialysis, with high patency and low infection rates.[90] More recent experience with ePTFE for angioaccess has limited the applicability of xenografts for this purpose.[91]

The Solcograft, a bovine carotid artery graft undergoing a totally different chemical fixation process, was developed in Europe.[92] Although its handling properties were excellent and its early results were outstanding, this graft was voluntarily withdrawn from clinical use after a late incidence of aneurysm was noted.[93]

RESULTS

Results with commercially available xenografts have been too poor to recommend their clinical use at this time. Poor patency and graft degeneration continue to plague xenografts. Research into better fixation methods continues, however, because this type of graft offers the real advantage of being a biologic graft in nearly unlimited supply. New grafts of bovine origin preserved using a unique photofixation process are currently under investigation. Short-term results in a canine model undergoing infrainguinal reconstructive procedures show comparable patency to PTFE in the common femoral artery and no evidence of degenerative changes.[94] This approach must await further information.

Synthetic Grafts

The concept of developing grafts from synthetic materials was developed in 1952 when Voorhees,[95] then a surgical resident, observed that a silk thread in the atrium of a dog (being used for another study) was not only tolerated without ill effect but also had become coated with a smooth, intima-like layer. Because of this phenomenon, the investigators speculated that arterial conduits fashioned of synthetic fabric would become similarly coated with a nonthrombogenic pseudointima. The first fabric grafts were made using polymers from the plastics industry. Grafts made of Vinyon-N were implanted into the aortic position in dogs and were found to be well tolerated, patent, and "incorporated," in the sense that they underwent ingrowth of fibroblasts from the surrounding tissue into the interstices of the graft.[95] This laboratory success led to successful implantation in 18 patients.[96]

It soon became apparent that the early textile grafts lost tensile strength over time, and a search was carried out for materials that would maintain strength and be resistant to dilatation. It was imperative that a durable material that allowed for incorporation but not resorption be identified.

Rayon and nylon were tried but were unsatisfactory. Silk, although popular in China, has never been adequately evaluated in the United States. However, two textile grafts, polyethylene terephthalate (polyester or Dacron) and polytetrafluoroethylene (PTFE, or Teflon) were found to retain nearly all their strength long after implantation,[97] and interest was concentrated on these materials. PTFE is no longer available in textile form but is common in its extruded form, which is discussed later.

DACRON (POLYESTER) GRAFTS

Dacron grafts are textile grafts composed of yarn that is either woven or knitted to form the fabric. Braiding was tried but is no longer used for synthetic grafts. Each method imparts different physical characteristics to the fabric. In woven grafts, weaving interlaces threads in both the warp (longitudinally oriented) and the weft (transversely oriented) directions (Fig. 26-5). These grafts are tighter and less porous than knitted grafts and have little stretch in any direction. They are relatively impermeable, fairly stiff, and very strong. They usually do not need preclotting and have little tendency toward late dilatation. They also take longer to become incorporated owing to lower porosity.[98] Traditionally, woven Dacron grafts were recommended when hemostasis without time-consuming preclotting was desirable. The development of impregnated grafts has eliminated these advantages.

Early woven grafts, in addition to being quite stiff, were prone to fraying and actually required heat-sealing of their cut ends to prevent suture pullout. These problems led to the development of knitted grafts, in which the yarn is oriented in either the warp or the weft direction (Fig. 26-6). Knitted grafts are generally more porous than woven grafts; increased porosity is believed to promote faster and more complete healing and incorporation (Fig. 26-7).[97] Knitted grafts also have superior handling characteristics. However, because they are more porous, they require preclotting (instillation of blood into the prosthesis before grafting) to prevent blood loss through the graft. Preclotting seals the interstices of the graft with fibrin and, by coating the lumen of the graft, is thought to render the flow surface less thrombogenic.

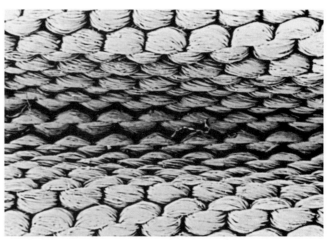

FIGURE 26–6 • Knitted crimped Dacron graft with looped threads forming a continuous chain network (SEM, ×30).

Many modifications to the Dacron prosthesis deserve discussion. Crimping adds flexibility and elasticity to the graft and enables it to be tunneled around bends without kinking. Although crimping imparts better handling characteristics, it also adds the potential disadvantage of greater surface area and an uneven inner graft surface. Many of the advantages of crimping can now be obtained with externally supported rings or coils, which do not interfere with the internal flow surface of the graft.

Another modification is the addition of velour finishes to either or both sides of a Dacron graft. Velour fabrics have loops of yarn extending upward at a right angle to the fabric's surface (Fig. 26-8).[99,100] Velouring was thought to improve the compliance and handling characteristics of Dacron grafts, improve the process of preclotting, and provide for better fibroblast ingrowth. These advantages, however, have not conclusively resulted in better graft patency or durability, so the use of velour finishing is limited.[101]

The latest development is impregnation of the interstices. Impregnation was originally developed to allow bonding of active substances, such as antibacterial agents, to the graft. A by-product of the impregnation process was the realization

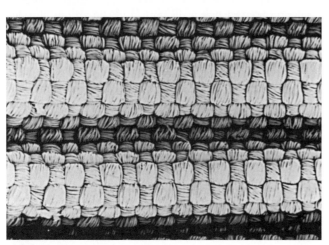

FIGURE 26–5 • Woven crimped Dacron graft with interlaced network of threads (SEM, ×30).

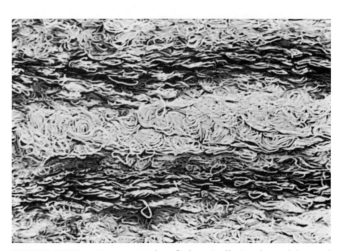

FIGURE 26–7 • Inner capsule of chronically implanted knitted Dacron graft (longitudinal section, ×300).

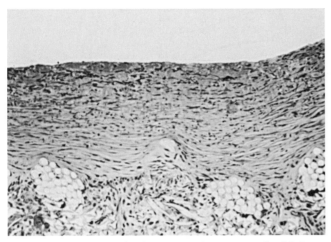

FIGURE 26–8 • Knitted velour crimped Dacron graft with loops of Dacron extending upward from the surface (SEM, ×30).

that knitted Dacron grafts, when coated with a bioresorbable material, maintained their superior handling and incorporation characteristics without the need for preclotting.[102-106] Three different coatings were initially available in the United States—albumin, gelatin, and collagen—although albumin grafts have been withdrawn. Polymer coatings are currently under investigation. The Vantage graft (Boston Scientific, Natick, Mass.), designed for infrainguinal reconstruction, has a light collagen inner surface and a light velour outer surface with microcrimping that provides longitudinal give. The major advantage of these grafts is the time saved in the operating room. In a prospective, randomized trial comparing the long-term performance of the different coating materials in knitted Dacron aortobifemoral prostheses, no significant advantage was seen with any one material. Primary and secondary patency rates at 5 years were 92% and 94% to 98%, respectively.[107] The major disadvantage of these grafts is their expense; they cost approximately twice as much as standard Dacron grafts. This may be a considerable disadvantage in the current economic environment, although most surgeons believe that the operative time saved outweighs this factor. Currently, the overwhelming number of grafts implanted in the Western world are coated or impregnated.

The most common concern about Dacron grafts is dilatation. Knitted grafts are more likely than woven grafts to dilate over time, with increases in size of 23% to 94% reported. The clinical significance of the dilatation is unclear, however.[108] Graft dilatation may be a causative factor in the development of anastomotic aneurysms.[109] For this reason, vascular surgeons should anticipate a dilatation of up to 20% and undersize knitted Dacron grafts accordingly. Monitoring these grafts with periodic imaging studies is also prudent.[110]

Several investigations of antibiotic-coated grafts are under way to determine whether binding antibiotic molecules to the graft or to the coating of impregnated grafts decreases the incidence of graft infection. In a study to determine whether the routine use of antibiotic-bonded gelatin-coated Dacron grafts in extra-anatomic reconstruction decreased the incidence of graft infection, early results showed no significant advantage.[111] Rifampin-coated grafts have demonstrated superior antibacterial characteristics in animal models.[112,113]

Results

Dacron grafts have the highest patency in large vessel reconstruction (e.g., aortoiliac grafts). Late patency rates of 85% to 96% have been reported for aortofemoral reconstruction using Dacron grafts.[114] Patency rates for above-knee femoropopliteal grafts are inferior to those for vein and similar to those for ePTFE, ranging from 57% to 71% in four large studies.[115-118] Patency below the knee is quite poor, as is true for all prosthetic grafts. When used in extra-anatomic vascular reconstruction, assisted primary patency rates of 50% at 5 years have been reported.[119]

EXPANDED POLYTETRAFLUOROETHYLENE GRAFTS

Expanded PTFE is a polymer of carbon and fluorine that was originally developed for industrial use by Gore in 1969.[120] Expanded PTFE is not a textile graft but rather an extruded material that is originally impermeable. After forcible expansion, ePTFE becomes semipermeable (Fig. 26-9), because the resulting material is composed of solid nodes of PTFE with interconnecting fibrils. The micropores lie between the fibrils (Fig. 26-10), and graft porosity is an important determinant of healing. Golden and colleagues showed complete luminal endothelial cell coverage of ePTFE grafts with an internodal distance of 60 μm.[121] Low-porosity (10- to 30-μm) and high-porosity (90-μm) grafts were associated with incomplete or focal endothelial cell loss. PTFE is actually more porous than textile grafts, but permeability to water and blood is less owing to the hydrophobicity of the material.[122] The first clinical application of ePTFE as an arterial bypass graft was reported in 1976,[123] and the graft rapidly gained popularity for many infrainguinal, extra-anatomic, and angioaccess procedures.

Expanded PTFE offers the advantages of strength, resistance to significant dilatation, the ability to be implanted without preclotting, and amenability to thrombectomy with a balloon catheter. Expanded PTFE grafts also have less platelet deposition and decreased activation of the complement cascade, theoretically making the graft less thrombogenic.[124,125] The main disadvantage of ePTFE is its stiffness. The material

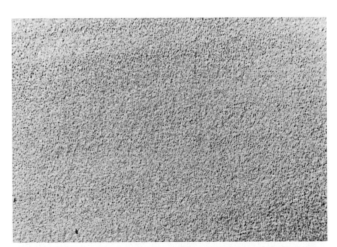

FIGURE 26–9 • Expanded polytetrafluoroethylene graft with a homogeneous surface, characteristic of the extruded manufacturing process (SEM, ×30).

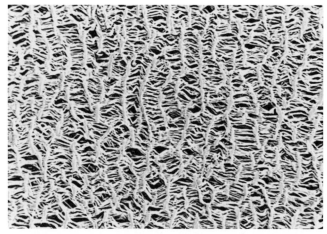

FIGURE 26–10 • Expanded polytetrafluoroethylene (PTFE) graft at a higher magnification (SEM, ×300), revealing circumferentially oriented nodes of PTFE connected by smaller fibrils.

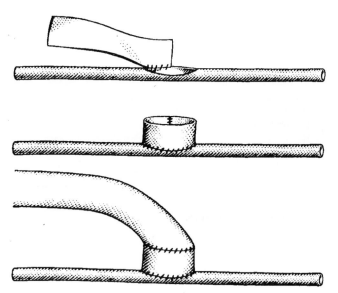

FIGURE 26–11 • Anastomosis of a 6-mm polytetrafluoroethylene graft to a small-caliber artery incorporating an interposition vein cuff. (From Beard JD: Hemodynamics of the interposition vein cuff. Br J Surg 73:823, 1986.)

is less compliant than textile grafts, a characteristic that may contribute to its tendency to form anastomotic aneurysms[6,126,127] and increase the incidence of neointimal hyperplasia, a common cause of late graft failure.[14]

Several modifications of ePTFE grafts have been developed. Thin-walled PTFE grafts still have the outer wrap of solid PTFE but are thinner, allowing for a larger luminal diameter with the same external diameter. They also have better handling characteristics. Stretch PTFE grafts have greater longitudinal elasticity owing to the process of "microcrimping." Stretch grafts are more conformable and forgiving of graft length imprecision. They also result in less needle hole bleeding. No data, however, indicate that either stretch grafts or thin-walled grafts offer superior patency or durability, and they are more expensive than standard ePTFE.[128]

Another common modification consists of externally supporting rings or coils that prevent graft compression. These are particularly helpful when the graft is tunneled across the knee or in extra-anatomic positions. Although rings may be valuable in axillofemoral grafts, the efficacy of external supports has not been definitively documented.[129]

Results

Expanded PTFE initially became popular in femoropopliteal bypass grafts because of reports suggesting that its early patency rates were similar to those of vein grafts above the knee.[123,130] Longer follow-up, however, revealed that the late patency of ePTFE in the above-knee popliteal position was inferior to that obtained with vein.[131] Five-year primary patency rates for above-knee PTFE grafts range from 34% to 69%, with secondary patency rates up to 79% reported.[81,132]

Patency rates for below-knee bypass with ePTFE were more discouraging. One randomized trial comparing saphenous vein and ePTFE for tibial bypasses showed 4-year patency rates of 49% for vein versus 12% for ePTFE.[33] Better results were seen when ePTFE was used for below-knee femoropopliteal bypass in patients with claudication, with primary and secondary patency rates of 58% and 73%, respectively.[132] The poor patency rates of ePTFE grafts used below the knee may be improved with postoperative anticoagulation. In one trial,

a 4-year patency rate of 37% was attained for patients given warfarin postoperatively.[133] The use of vein cuffs (Fig. 26-11) also improves the patency rates of ePTFE grafts to below-knee vessels[134-136] and may be related to a reduction in compliance mismatch or an alteration in the shear stress flow patterns at the distal anastomosis.[5,137] One study showed a 5-year primary patency rate of 58% and a limb salvage rate of 80% for these composite grafts.[138] Several other series concur with this improved primary patency rate.[136,139,140]

Given the poor long-term patency rates of prosthetic material in distal reconstruction, all reasonable routes of autogenous conduit—including arm vein, composite-sequential grafting, short-segment grafting, and combined catheter-directed and surgical therapy—should be considered first. If these options are not available, the use of a synthetic conduit may be considered. Either Dacron or ePTFE is probably appropriate. A prospective, randomized trial comparing a knitted Dacron polyester graft impregnated with collagen with a thin-walled reinforced ePTFE graft to the above-knee popliteal artery showed no statistical difference between groups (62% and 57% 5-year patency rates, respectively). Patency rates in both groups were inferior in patients receiving smaller (5- to 6-mm) grafts and in younger patients who smoked.[118]

Aortic grafts made of ePTFE have seen modest use over the last 10 years. A prospective evaluation of the graft noted an absence of significant graft dilatation or late anastomotic aneurysms.[141] Other authors noted superior patency and lower complication rates with ePTFE aortofemoral grafts,[142-144] although they are not currently accepted as superior to Dacron bifurcated grafts. One group concluded that patency rates were better in smaller vessels with ePTFE and recommended that these grafts be used in patients with small iliac and femoral vessels.[145]

In addition to aortic and infrainguinal reconstruction, common uses for ePTFE include carotid-subclavian, axillofemoral, axilloaxillary, aortorenal, and femorofemoral bypass.[146-148] Expanded PTFE is particularly useful for extra-anatomic tunneling because its relative stiffness makes it resistant to kinking, and its smooth surface is easy to thrombectomize. It is also the material of choice for angioaccess in hemodialysis patients with renal failure, showing surprising resistance to infection.[149,150] Impra has developed a "hooded" graft (Distaflo) designed to improve the laminar flow characteristics at the venous anastomosis. A prospective, nonrandomized study demonstrated significantly better primary and secondary patency rates in patients with critical limb ischemia compared with conventional ePTFE grafts.[151] Finally, ePTFE has been used in reconstruction of the inferior vena cava[152] and in patch angioplasty of the carotid and femoral arteries.

SUMMARY OF RESULTS

Most vascular surgeons believe that there is a role for prosthetic grafts in infrainguinal reconstruction. Prosthetic grafts offer the advantages of shorter operative time and smaller incisions, which may be crucial in selected patients. Patency rates for above-knee femoropopliteal reconstruction with ePTFE grafts range from 38% to 65% in large series, similar to results for Dacron grafts.[116-117,132] Patency rates below the knee are poor but are improved with the addition of an interposition vein cuff at the distal anastamosis[135] or with a hooded modification to the distal graft.[151] In aortofemoral reconstructions, ePTFE and Dacron graft patency rates do not appear to be different, although some data suggest that ePTFE grafts may have a lower incidence of late complications.[141,144] When used for extra-anatomic bypass or hemodialysis access, ePTFE patency rates are similar to those of Dacron. Most surgeons, however, prefer ePTFE in these locations because of the handling characteristics of the graft, its resistance to external compression, and the ease of thrombectomy.[148,153]

Future Concepts

Until recently, the development of a better vascular prosthesis was an active area of research in vascular surgery. However, significant redirection has occurred in regard to endovascular devices, which we believe is shortsighted. The development of new, less thrombogenic prosthetic graft materials (both biologic and synthetic), the modification of existing materials with nonthrombogenic coatings, and the prevention of neointimal hyperplasia are still important unresolved issues (Table 26-3).

ENDOTHELIAL SEEDING

Unfortunately, endothelial cell resurfacing of prosthetic grafts, which occurs partially or completely in many animal models, does not occur in humans except for several centimeters in both directions from the anastomoses of the graft.[154] As yet, no flow surface has been developed that has the antithrombotic properties of endothelium. Endothelial cells in ePTFE-seeded grafts remain functional and have been shown to express factor VIII and thrombomodulin and to activate protein C.[155] In addition, endothelial cell seeding allows the use of biologic-based scaffolds, without thrombogenicity and antigenicity problems.[156]

One avenue that has been pursued is the in vitro seeding of prosthetic grafts with autologous endothelial cells extracted from other tissue beds. Cells were originally harvested

TABLE 26–3	Status of New Developments in Vascular Graft Materials
Concept	**Status**
Endothelial cell seeding	Early clinical trials with coronary and femoropopliteal bypass
Surface-modified grafts	Carbon-impregnated ePTFE in use, active substance modification in experimental models
Polyurethane grafts	Currently in use as angioaccess graft
Fibrocollagenous tubes	Basic feasibility has been demonstrated in animal models
Bioresorbable polymeric grafts	Animal studies suggest role as aortic replacement conduit
Photodynamic fixation	Animal and cell-based models demonstrate modulation of remodeling process
Bioengineered vessel	Experimental, difficult to match native compliance

ePTFE, expanded polytetrafluoroethylene.

mechanically or by enzymatic digestion of adipose tissue.[157] More recently, seeding for prosthetic grafts has been done with endothelial cells cultured from external jugular or cephalic veins[158] or from an immortalized human dermal endothelial cell line.[159] Data in humans have shown that seeded grafts maintain viable endothelial cells and exert an antiplatelet effect not seen in unseeded grafts.[160-162] In a phase II study by Deutsch and colleagues,[158] the 5-year patency rate of an ePTFE graft precoated with fibrin glue was 66% for above-knee grafts and 76% for below-knee grafts, results comparable with those of vein grafts.

Several problems may limit the widespread clinical application of this technology. Methods of obtaining cells in sufficient quantity have not been perfected. Cell culture increases the number of cells available, but seeding may take several weeks—obviously a considerable logistic handicap when grafting for limb salvage or in other emergency situations. In addition, the concept of removing living tissue and transferring it to an in vitro environment introduces the potential for contamination. Implantation techniques are still problematic, with the loss of a significant number of cells when the graft is exposed to flow.[163] Newer methods of improving endothelial cell adherence have been developed that significantly increase the cell retention rate.[164-166] Although clinical applicability is currently limited, early results show this to be a promising technique for the near future.

SURFACE-MODIFIED GRAFTS

The concept of modifying a prosthetic graft with a surface-active substance is not new. Gott and coworkers described the technique of bonding heparin to prosthetic conduits in 1963.[167] Considerable experimental work has been done on the durability of heparin bonding, and studies with animal models have revealed that heparin bonded to ePTFE grafts is not associated with increased intraoperative blood loss[168] and is effective at reducing thrombosis.[169,170] So far, however, heparin bonding has not been clinically effective at preventing prosthetic graft failure. Interest has also focused on the possibility of impregnating thrombolytic substances such as tissue plasminogen activator, which in one study decreased the thrombogenicity, of prosthetic grafts in an animal model.[171] A Biolite or pyrolytic carbon-coated Dacron graft, was shown to enhance endothelial cell growth.[172]

POLYURETHANES

Polyurethanes are a family of synthetic polymers whose compliance closely approximates that of native arteries. They have been under investigation in various forms since 1960.[173] Polyurethanes have compliance characteristics more favorable than those of ePTFE or Dacron, and they are much less thrombogenic, making them potentially attractive for synthetic grafts. Animal studies to date have shown only moderate success, with patency rates not appreciably different from those of other synthetic grafts.[174,175] Durability and structural integrity remain issues, with poly(ester)urethanes and poly(ether)urethanes subject to hydrolytic and oxidative degradation. Short-term results with a second-generation poly(carbonate)urethane graft show that it has improved biodurability.[176] The Vectra graft (Impra) is a vascular access prosthesis made from poly(ether)urethane. The graft has improved porosity and, when used in a dialysis setting, allows for almost immediate postsurgical access.[177] A small-diameter Vectra graft is undergoing clinical trial for coronary artery bypass grafting.

FIBROCOLLAGENOUS TUBES

For several decades, investigators worked on the concept of fibrocollagenous tube formation—that is, an autogenous or heterologous tube formed over a mandrel implanted in a tissue bed. Poor long-term patency and stability with all these conduits suggest that this area is not worthy of further investigation.

A similar avenue, which may be more promising, is the creation of a decellularized allogeneic conduit.[178] The use of cadaveric decellularized arteries could ideally allow for the ingrowth of endothelial cells by either direct extension or seeding. In addition, there is a possibility that genetically modified cells can be delivered on such a conduit. The acellular matrix vascular prosthesis is a new concept that uses a stepwise enzymatic and detergent extraction of arteries, leaving a tissue framework of structural proteins.[179] When used as a coronary artery bypass allograft in canines, these biografts showed no inflammation and minimal cellular repopulation at 6 months.[180] This process is in current clinical use to produce a stentless porcine aortic valve xenograft, with good results.[181]

BIORESORBABLE POLYMERIC GRAFTS

Because the biomechanical effects of the current prosthetic grafts cause a significant number of late graft failures, considerable research has focused on developing a prosthetic graft that would be completely resorbed over time, leaving only autogenous tissue that would be nonantigenic and less thrombogenic. Animal studies have shown that a polyglactin prosthesis made from a polyglycolic acid copolymer is absorbed over several months, leaving a "vessel" consisting of collagen, myofibroblasts, and an endothelium-like surface.[182]

Dilatation and aneurysm formation were problems, however. Short-term results in an animal study with a new copolymer graft of polyglactin and polyhydroxyalkanoate implanted into the thoracic aorta showed no evidence of dilatation, and its mechanical properties approached that of the native artery.[183] Further work with different compounds continues, with the goal of developing a graft that is resistant to intimal hyperplasia and has the physiologic characteristics of native vessels.

PHOTODYNAMIC FIXATION TECHNIQUES

Another area of research interest involves a method of biologic graft fixation by photodynamic treatment. The current unsatisfactory results of biologic prosthetic grafts are the result of graft thrombosis, degeneration, and dilatation. Photodynamic therapy (PDT) is a method of tissue preservation without conventional chemical fixation that may result in a more stable graft. One process involves perfusing an artery with photosensitizing agents such as methylene blue or chloroaluminum sulfonated phthalocyanine, dyes that selectively absorb light energy at a specific wavelength.[184] This process leads to the production of reactive oxygen species, which induce an apoptotic, noninflammatory decellularization of the treated vessel segment.[185,186]

Animal studies have shown that PDT inhibits the development of intimal hyperplasia in the body of vein grafts.[186] Intimal hyperplasia was seen, however, at the anastomoses and was thought to be secondary to proliferating smooth muscle cells from the adjacent native artery. In a clinical study to evaluate the effects of adjuvant endovascular PDT following percutaneous angioplasty of the femoral artery, there was no evidence of thrombosis or restenosis (as determined by duplex ultrasonography) at 6 months.[187] LaMuraglia and coworkers studied PDT-treated allografts in animals and found that PDT inhibited allograft rejection and aneurysmal dilatation.[188] One effect of PDT is that it cross-links proteins in the extracellular matrix, which theoretically may strengthen the vessel. Protein cross-linking also may mask antigenic epitopes of the extracellular matrix, making it a novel technique for the development of a vascular xenograft. In addition, PDT may decrease thrombogenic factors in the endothelial cell.[189] Results of studies investigating the short-term patency and compliance of PDT-treated xenografts are encouraging, and further modifications of this promising technique continue.

BIOENGINEERED BLOOD VESSELS

The poor patency of small-caliber (<4 mm) grafts has stimulated research into the development of bioengineered blood vessels. Huynh and colleagues developed a collagen biomaterial graft derived from porcine intestinal submucosa and bovine collagen that, when implanted into rabbits, serves as a scaffold for infiltration of host smooth muscle and endothelial cells.[190] Short-term results with these grafts show that they are patent and without evidence of thrombosis at 13 weeks. Niklason and associates created a functional artery in vitro by seeding bovine and porcine smooth muscle and endothelial cells on a biodegradable polyglycolic acid scaffold under pulsatile conditions (Fig. 26-12).[191] These bioengineered vessels are histologically similar to native arteries and display contractile responses to serotonin, endothelin-1, and

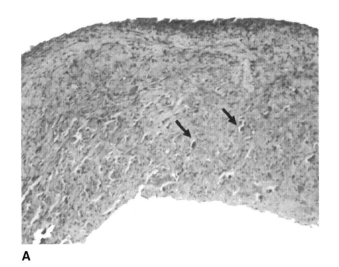

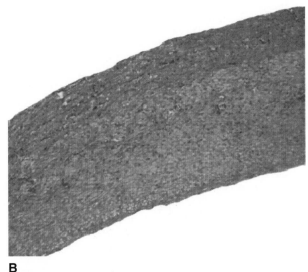

FIGURE 26–12 • Hematoxylin and eosin stain of bioengineered graft. *A,* Autologous porcine vessel before implantation; polymer remnants are indicated *(arrows)*. *B,* Explanted autologous vessel with intact wall structure containing loosely organized smooth muscle cells. The inflammatory response is minimal, and polymer remnants are no longer visible. (From Niklason LE: Functional arteries grown in vitro. Science 284:492, 1999.)

prostaglandin $F_{2\alpha}$. Studies investigating the short-term patency of this promising technique continue.

Current Recommendations

Few absolutes exist in graft selection for a particular reconstruction. In determining the most appropriate graft for an operation, the vascular surgeon must consider the following: the hemodynamic environment (inflow, outflow, blood pressure); the presence of systemic or graft bed infection; and the patient's ability to tolerate lengthy surgery, need for and ability to tolerate chronic anticoagulation, overall health status, and projected life span. These factors must be balanced against the performance characteristics of the various grafts available. For these reasons, a graft that is optimal for one patient may not be the best choice for another. The following general recommendations are applicable in most circumstances.

AORTIC RECONSTRUCTION

Prosthetic large vessel grafts have been implanted into hundreds of thousands of individuals and have shown good patency and durability. The choice of a textile or nontextile synthetic aortic prosthesis depends on several factors.

For operations in which significant hemorrhage, systemic anticoagulation, or extensive dissection is anticipated (e.g., thoracic aortic reconstruction and ruptured abdominal aortic aneurysm repair), a coated or woven Dacron graft or an ePTFE graft may be the best choice, because preclotting is not necessary.

For elective abdominal aneurysm repair, knitted Dacron grafts are routinely used by many surgeons. Standard grafts require preclotting, whereas the coated grafts do not. The newer ePTFE aortic grafts are also a viable choice. As more data become available, the relative resistance of these grafts to dilatation in comparison to textile grafts may be revealed as a significant advantage.

INFRAINGUINAL RECONSTRUCTION

If available, autogenous ipsilateral saphenous vein is clearly the conduit of choice for infrainguinal reconstruction. For infrapopliteal target vessels, the difference in patency between vein and prosthetic conduits is even greater.

Some authors advocate the preferential use of prosthetic conduits when grafting to the above-knee popliteal artery, with the rationale that although the patency of vein may be superior to that of prosthetics, it is not markedly so, particularly for patients with claudication. Many of these patients will die of coronary disease before graft occlusion occurs. Further, those patients requiring additional, more distal peripheral reconstruction or a coronary artery bypass graft would have autogenous vein available.[192-194] Unfortunately, this argument would result in an increased number of total operations and reoperations being performed, a position that is difficult to justify. Certainly, the initial use of prosthetics in selected patients is appropriate.

For all target vessels below the knee, autogenous vein is preferable. When it is not available, the alternative is less attractive. Before the acceptance of ePTFE as a conduit, Dacron grafts were popular in this situation. With no preclotting necessary, ePTFE then became the more popular prosthetic conduit; however, this advantage ceased with the availability of coated grafts. Certainly, in patients without usable veins who are undergoing limb salvage procedures, ePTFE conduits can save the limbs of a third or more of patients, as shown by Veith and associates.[33] The addition of a vein cuff at the distal anastomoses should be considered, especially when using small-diameter (<6 mm) grafts. Considering the cost of rehabilitation and the total cost of primary amputation (similar to distal bypass),[195] the use of a prosthetic graft may be superior to primary amputation in patients with limb-threatening ischemia.

The use of any biologic graft, although intuitively appealing, is currently not justified. HUV allografts were once used in the lower extremity, but because of problems with late degeneration, their use is now rare, despite some data suggesting that their patency may be better in below-the-knee and poor runoff situations.[196] The use of cryopreserved veins should be reserved for limb-threatening ischemia or in infected fields when autogenous vein is not available.

EXTRA-ANATOMIC PROCEDURES

Expanded PTFE has become the graft of choice for most extra-anatomic reconstructions. The advantages in these situations include a lower incidence of hematoma formation from graft leakage and a resistance to kinking.[148,153] Expanded PTFE grafts are also amenable to catheter thrombectomy, an important consideration in axillofemoral or axilloaxillary grafts. Depending on the patient's habitus and the length of the subcutaneous tunnel, externally supported grafts may be helpful.

ANGIOACCESS

For angioaccess in patients receiving hemodialysis in whom arteriovenous fistulas are not feasible or have failed, ePTFE grafts have become the conduit of choice. They are easy to implant, resistant to infection, and amenable to revision and tolerate multiple punctures, with a low incidence of pseudoaneurysm formation.[150]

KEY REFERENCES

Faries PL, Logerfo FW, et al: A comparative study of alternative conduits for lower extremity revascularization: All-autogenous conduit versus prosthetic grafts. J Vasc Surg 32:1080, 2000.

Giglia JS, Ollerenshaw JD, et al: Cryopreservation prevents arterial allograft dilation. Ann Vasc Surg 16:762, 2002.

Halloran BG, Lilly MP, et al: Tibial bypass using complex autologous conduit: Patency and limb salvage. Ann Vasc Surg 15:634, 2001.

Johnson WC, Lee KK: A comparative evaluation of polytetrafluoroethylene, umbilical vein, and saphenous vein bypass grafts for femoral-popliteal above-knee revascularization: A prospective randomized Department of Veterans Affairs cooperative study. J Vasc Surg 32:268, 2000.

Kreienberg PB, Darling RC 3rd, et al: Early results of a prospective randomized trial of spliced vein versus polytetrafluoroethylene graft with a distal vein cuff for limb-threatening ischemia. J Vasc Surg 35:299, 2002.

Neville RF, Tempesta B, et al: Tibial bypass for limb salvage using polytetrafluoroethylene and a distal vein patch. J Vasc Surg 33:266, 2001.

Xue L, Greisler HP: Biomaterials in the development and future of vascular grafts. J Vasc Surg 37:472, 2003.

Yeung KK, Mills JL Sr, et al: Improved patency of infrainguinal polytetrafluoroethylene bypass grafts using a distal Taylor vein patch. Am J Surg 182:578, 2001.

REFERENCES

1. Carrel A, Guthrie CG: Uniterminal and biterminal venous transplantations. Surg Gynecol Obstet 2:226, 1906.
2. Taylor LM, Edwards JM, Porter JM: Present status of reversed vein bypass grafting: Five year results of a modern series. J Vasc Surg 11:193, 1990.
3. Jaff EA: Biology of Endothelial Cells. Boston, Martinus Nijhoff, 1984.
4. Scales JT: Tissue reactions to synthetic materials. Proc R Soc Med 46:647, 1953.
5. Abbott WM, Megerman J, Hasson JE, et al: Effect of compliance mismatch on vascular graft patency. J Vasc Surg 5:376, 1987.
6. Walden R, L'Italien GJ, Megerman J, Abbott WM: Matched elastic properties and successful arterial grafting. Arch Surg :1166, 1980.
7. Milroy CM, Scott DJ, Beard JD, et al: Histologic appearance of the long saphenous vein. J Pathol 159:311, 1989.
8. Gloviczki P, Yao J (eds): Handbook of Venous Disorders, Guidelines of the American Venous Forum. New York, Oxford University Press, 2001, pp 3-11.
9. Thompson H: The surgical anatomy of the superficial and perforating veins of the lower limb. Ann R Coll Surg Engl 61:198, 1979.
10. Shah DM, Chang BB, Leopold PW, et al: The anatomy of the greater saphenous venous system. J Vasc Surg 3:273, 1986.
11. Kakkar VV: The cephalic vein as a peripheral vascular graft. Sug Gynecol Obstet 128:551, 1969.
12. Landry GJ, Moneta GL, et al: Choice of autogenous conduit for lower extremity vein graft revisions. J Vasc Surg 36:238, 2002.
13. Leather RP, Karmody AM: The in situ saphenous vein for arterial bypass. In Staley JC (ed): Biologic and Synthetic Vascular Prostheses. New York, Grune & Stratton, 1982, p 351.
14. Sottiurai VA, Yao JST, Flinn WR, et al: Intimal hyperplasia and neointima: An ultrastructural analysis of thrombosed grafts in humans. Surgery 93:809, 1983.
15. Spray TL, Roberts WC: Fundamentals of clinical cardiology: Changes in saphenous veins used as aortocoronary bypass grafts. Am Heart J 94:500, 1977.
16. Fuchs JCA, Mitchener JS III, Hagen P-O: Postoperative changes in autologous vein grafts. Ann Surg 188:1, 1978.
17. Bandyk DF: Essentials of graft surveillance [review]. Semin Vasc Surg 6:92, 1993.
18. Abbott WM, Wieland S, Austen WG: Structural changes during preparation of autogenous venous grafts. Surgery 76:1031, 1974.
19. Hasson JE, Wiebe DH, Sharefkin JB, Abbott WM: Migration of adult human vascular endothelial cells: Effect of extracellular matrix proteins. Surgery 100:384, 1986.
20. Beattie DK, Sian M, Greenhalgh RM, Davies AH: Influence of systemic factors on pre-existing intimal hyperplasia and their effect on the outcome of infrainguinal arterial reconstruction with vein. Br J Surg 86:1441, 1999.
21. Clowes AW, Clowes MM, Fingerle J, Reidy MA: Regulation of smooth muscle cell growth in injured artery. J Cardiovasc Pharmacol 14:512, 1989.
22. Schafer U, Micke O, Dorszewski A, et al: External beam irradiation inhibits neointimal hyperplasia after injury-induced arterial smooth muscle cell proliferation. Int J Radiat Oncol Biol Phys 42:617, 1998.
23. Shears LL, Kibbe MR, Murdock, AD, et al: Efficient inhibition of intimal hyperplasia by adenovirus-mediated inducible nitric oxide synthase gene transfer to rats and pigs in vivo. J Am Coll Surg 187:295, 1998.
24. Le Tourneau T, Van Belle E, Corseaux D, et al: Role of nitric oxide in restenosis after experimental balloon angioplasty in the hypercholesterolemic rabbit: Effects on neointimal hyperplasia and vascular remodeling. J Am Coll Cardiol 33:876, 1999.
25. Porter KE, Loftus IM, Peterson M, et al: Marimastat inhibits neointimal thickening in a model of human vein graft stenosis. Br J Surg 85:1373, 1998.
26. Jordan WD Jr, Alcocer F, et al: The durability of endoscopic saphenous vein grafts: A 5-year observational study. J Vasc Surg 34:434, 2001.
27. Donaldson MC, Mannick JA, Whittemore AD: Causes of primary graft failure after in situ saphenous vein bypass grafting. J Vasc Surg 15:150, 1992.
28. DeWeese JA, Rob CG: Autogenous venous grafts ten years later. Surgery 82:775, 1977.
29. Stanley JC, Graham LM, Whitehouse WM, et al: Autogenous saphenous vein as an arterial graft: Clinical status. In Stanley JC (ed): Biologic and Synthetic Vascular Prostheses. New York, Grune & Stratton, 1982, p 333.
30. Szilagyi DE, Elliott JP, Hageman JH, et al: Biologic fate of autogenous vein implants as arterial substitutes: Clinical, angiographic and histopathologic observations in femoropopliteal operations for atherosclerosis. Ann Surg 178:232, 1973.
31. Donaldson MC, Mannick JA, Whittemore AD: Femoral-distal bypass with in-situ saphenous vein: Long term results using the Mills valvulotome. Ann Surg 213:457, 1991.
32. Watelet J, Soury P, Menard JF, et al: Femoropopliteal bypass: In situ or reversed vein grafts? Ten-year results of a randomized prospective study. Ann Vasc Surg 11:510, 1997.
33. Veith FJ, Gupta SK, Ascer E, et al: Six year prospective multicenter randomized comparison of autologous saphenous vein and expanded PTFE in infrainguinal reconstruction. J Vasc Surg 3:107, 1986.
34. Luther M, Lepantalo M: Infrainguinal reconstructions: Influence of surgical experience on outcome. Cardiovasc Surg 6:351, 1998.
35. Harward TRS, Coe D, Flynn TC, Seeger JM: The use of arm vein conduits during infrageniculate arterial bypass. J Vasc Surg 3:104, 1986.
36. Calligaro KD, Syrek JR, Dougherty MJ, et al: Use of arm and lesser saphenous vein compared with prosthetic grafts for infrapopliteal arterial bypass: Are they worth the effort? J Vasc Surg 26:919, 1997.
37. Faries PL, Logerfo FW, et al: A comparative study of alternative conduits for lower extremity revascularization: All-autogenous conduit versus prosthetic grafts. J Vasc Surg 32:1080, 2000.
38. Halloran BG, Lilly MP, et al: Tibial bypass using complex autologous conduit: Patency and limb salvage. Ann Vasc Surg 15:634, 2001.
39. Curi MA, Skelly CL, et al: Long-term results of infrageniculate bypass grafting using all-autogenous composite vein. Ann Vasc Surg 16:618, 2002.

40. Chew DK, Owens CD, et al: Bypass in the absence of ipsilateral greater saphenous vein: Safety and superiority of the contralateral greater saphenous vein. J Vasc Surg 35:1085, 2002.
41. Poletti LF, Matsuura JH, et al: Should vein be saved for future operations? A 15-year review of infrainguinal bypasses and the subsequent need for autogenous vein. Ann Vasc Surg 12:143, 1998.
42. Ehrenfeld WK, Stoney RJ, Wylie EJ: Autogenous arterial grafts. In Stanley JC (ed): Biologic and Synthetic Vascular Prostheses. New York, Grune & Stratton, 1982, p 291.
43. Treiman GS, Lawrence PF, et al: Autogenous arterial bypass grafts: Durable patency and limb salvage in patients with inframalleolar occlusive disease and end-stage renal disease. J Vasc Surg 32:13, 2000.
44. Kreitman B, Riberi A, Jimeno MT, Metras D: Experimental basis for autograft growth and viability. J Heart Valve Dis 4:379, 1995.
45. Ehrenfeld WK, Wilbur BG, Olcott CN, et al: Autogenous tissue reconstruction in the management of infected prosthetic grafts. Surgery 85:82, 1979.
46. Cambria RP, Brewster DC, L'Italien GJ, et al: The durability of different reconstructive techniques for atherosclerotic renal artery disease. J Vasc Surg 20:76, 1994.
47. Grondin CM, Campeau L, Lesperance J, et al: Comparison of late changes in internal mammary artery and saphenous vein grafts in two consecutive series of patients 10 years after operation. Circulation 70(Suppl 1):1, 1984.
48. Stoney RJ, DeLuccia N, Ehrenfeld WK, et al: Aortorenal arterial autografts: Long-term assessment. Arch Surg 116:1416, 1981.
49. Gross RE, Hierwitt ES, Bill AH Jr, et al: Preliminary observations on the use of human arterial grafts in the treatment of certain cardiovascular defects. N Engl J Med 239:578, 1948.
50. Szilagyi DE, McDonald RT, Smith RF, et al: Biologic fate of human arterial homografts. Arch Surg 75:506, 1957.
51. Deterling RA, Clauss RH: Long term fate of aortic arterial homografts. J Cardiovasc Surg (Torino) 11:35, 1970.
52. Kieffer E, Bahnini A, Kishas F, et al: In situ allograft replacement of infected infrarenal aortic prosthetic grafts: Results in 43 patients. J Vasc Surg 17:349, 1993.
53. Locati P, Novali C, Socrate AM, et al: The use of arterial allografts in aortic graft infections: A three year experience on eighteen patients. J Cardiovasc Surg 39:735, 1998.
54. Nevelsteen A, Feryn T, Lacroix H, et al: Experience with cryopreserved arterial allografts in the treatment of prosthetic graft infections. Cardiovasc Surg 6:378, 1998.
55. Vogt PR, Brunner-LaRocca HP, et al: Technical details with the use of cryopreserved arterial allografts for aortic infection: Influence on early and midterm mortality. J Vasc Surg 35:80, 2002.
56. Carrel T, Pasic M, Jenni R, et al: Reoperations after operation on the thoracic aorta: Etiology, surgical techniques, and prevention. Ann Thorac Surg 56:259, 1993.
57. Giglia JS, Ollerenshaw JD, et al: Cryopreservation prevents arterial allograft dilation. Ann Vasc Surg 16:762, 2002.
58. Oschner JL, Lawson JD, Eskind SJ, et al: Homologous veins as an arterial substitute: Long term results. J Vasc Surg 1:306, 1984.
59. Selke FW, Meng RC, Rossi NP: Cryopreserved saphenous vein homografts for femoral-distal vascular reconstruction. J Cardiovasc Surg (Torino) 30:836, 1989.
60. Fujtani RM, Bassiouny HS, Gewertz BL, et al: Cryopreserved saphenous vein allogenic homografts: An alternative conduit in lower extremity arterial reconstruction in infected fields. J Vasc Surg 15:519, 1992.
61. Walker PJ, Mitchell RS, McFadden PM, et al: Early experience with cryopreserved saphenous vein allografts as a conduit for complex limb-salvage procedures. J Vasc Surg 18:561, 1993.
62. Dalsing MC, Raju S, Wakefield TW, Taheri S: A multicenter, phase I evaluation of cryopreserved venous valve allografts for the treatment of chronic deep venous insufficiency. J Vasc Surg 30:854, 1999.
63. Farber A, Major K, et al: Cryopreserved saphenous vein allografts in infrainguinal revascularization: Analysis of 240 grafts. J Vasc Surg 38:15, 2003.
64. Martins RS 3rd, Edwards WH, Mulherin JL Jr, et al: Cryopreserved saphenous vein allografts for below-knee extremity revascularization. Ann Surg 219:664, 1994.
65. Albertini JN, Barral X, Branchereau A, et al: Vascular Surgical Society of Great Britain and Ireland: Mid-term results of arterial allograft below-knee bypasses for limb salvage. Br J Surg 86:701, 1999.
66. Harris L, O'Brien-Irr M, et al: Long-term assessment of cryopreserved vein bypass grafting success. J Vasc Surg 33:528, 2001.
67. Carpenter JP, Tomaszewski JE: Immunosuppression for human saphenous vein allograft bypass surgery: A prospective randomized trial. J Vasc Surg 26:32, 1997.
68. Nabseth DC, Wilson JT, Tan B, et al: Fetal arterial heterografts. Arch Surg 81:929, 1960.
69. Dardik H, Baier RE, Meenaghan M, et al: Morphologic and biophysical assessment of long-term human umbilical cord vein implants used as vascular conduits. Surg Gynecol Obstet 154:17, 1982.
70. Dardik H, Ibrahim IM, Dardik I: Modified and unmodified umbilical vein allograft and xenografts employed as arterial substitutes: A morphologic assessment. Surg Forum 26:286, 1975.
71. Dardik I, Dardik H: The fate of human umbilical cord vessels used as interposition arterial grafts in the baboon. Surg Gynecol Obstet 140:567, 1975.
72. Dardik H: Technical aspects of umbilical bypass to the tibial vessels. J Vasc Surg 1:916, 1984.
73. Dardik H, Miller N, Dardik A, et al: A decade of experience with the glutaraldehyde tanned umbilical cord vein graft for revascularization of the lower limb. J Vasc Surg 7:336, 1988.
74. Rutherford RB, Jones DN, Bergentz SE, et al: Factors affecting the patency of infrainguinal bypass. J Vasc Surg 8:236, 1988.
75. Johnson WC, Squires JW: Axillo-femoral (PTFE) and infrainguinal revascularization (PTFE and umbilical vein). J Cardiovasc Surg (Torino) 32:344, 1991.
76. McCollum C, Kenchington G, Alexander C, et al: PTFE or HUV for femoropopliteal bypass: A multicentre trial. Eur J Vasc Surg 5:435, 1991.
77. Alders GJ, Van Vroonhoven TJM: PTFE versus HUV in above-knee femoropopliteal bypass: Six year results in a randomized clinical trial. J Vasc Surg 16:816, 1992.
78. Eickhoff JH, Broome A, Ericsson BF, et al: Four years' results of a prospective randomized clinical trial comparing polytetrafluoroethylene and modified human umbilical vein for below-knee femoropopliteal bypass. J Vasc Surg 6:506, 1987.
79. Aalders FJ, van Vroonhoven TJM: Polytetrafluoroethylene versus human umbilical vein in above-knee femoropopliteal bypass: Six year results of a randomized clinical trial. J Vasc Surg 16:816, 1992.
80. Wengerter K, Dardik H: Biological vascular grafts. Semin Vasc Surg 12:46, 1999.
81. Johnson WC, Lee KK: A comparative evaluation of polytetrafluoroethylene, umbilical vein, and saphenous vein bypass grafts for femoral-popliteal above-knee revascularization: A prospective randomized Department of Veterans Affairs cooperative study. J Vasc Surg 32:268, 2000.
82. Hasson JE, Newton WD, Waltman AC, et al: Mural degeneration in the glutaraldehyde-tanned umbilical vein graft: Incidence and implications. J Vasc Surg 4:243, 1986.
83. Julien S, Gill F, Guidoin R, et al: Biologic and structural evaluation of 80 surgically excised human umbilical vein grafts. Can J Surg 32:101, 1989.
84. Karkow WS, Cranley JJ, Cranley RE, et al: Extended study of aneurysm formation in umbilical vein grafts. J Vasc Surg 4:486, 1986.
85. Dardik H, Wengerter K, et al: Comparative decades of experience with glutaraldehyde-tanned human umbilical cord vein graft for lower limb revascularization: An analysis of 1275 cases. J Vasc Surg 35:64, 2002.
86. Dardik H: Umbilical vein grafts for atherosclerotic lower extremity occlusive disease. In Ernst CB, Stanley JC (eds): Current Therapy in Vascular Surgery. St. Louis, Mosby, 1995, p 484.
87. Rosenberg N, Gaughran ERL, Henderson J, et al: The use of segmental arterial implants prepared by enzymatic modification of heterologous blood vessels. Surg Forum 6:242, 1956.
88. Rosenberg N, Thompson JE, Keshishian JM, et al: The modified bovine arterial graft. Arch Surg 111:222, 1976.
89. Dale WA, Lewis MR: Further experiences with bovine arterial grafts. Surgery 80:711, 1976.
90. Brems J, Castenada M, Garvin PJ: A five year experience with the bovine heterograft for vascular access. Arch Surg 121:941, 1986.
91. Enzler MA, Rajmon T, Lachat M, Largiader F: Long-term function of vascular access for hemodialysis. Clin Transplant 10:511, 1996.
92. Schroder A, Imig H, Peiper U, et al: Results of a bovine collagen vascular graft (Solcograft-P) in infrainguinal positions. Eur J Vasc Surg 2:315, 1988.
93. Guidoin R, Domurado D, Coutue J, et al: Chemically processed bovine heterografts of the second generation as arterial substitutes: A comparative evaluation of three commercial prostheses. J Cardiovasc Surg (Torino) 30:202, 1989.
94. Moazami N, Argenziano M, Williams M, et al: Photo-oxidized bovine arterial grafts: Short-term results. ASAIO J 44:89, 1998.

95. Voorhees AB Jr, Jaretzke AL, Blakemore AH: Use of tubes constructed from Vinyon-N cloth in bridging arterial defects. Ann Surg 135:332, 1952.

96. Blakemore AH, Voorhees AB Jr: The use of tubes constructed from Vinyon-N cloth in bridging arterial defects: Experimental and clinical. Ann Surg 140:324, 1954.

97. Fry WJ, DeWeese MS, Kraft RO, et al: Importance of porosity in arterial prostheses. Arch Surg 88:36, 1964.

98. Snyder RW, Botzko KM: Woven, knitted, and externally supported Dacron vascular prostheses. In Stanley JC (ed): Biologic and Synthetic Vascular Prostheses. New York, Grune & Stratton, 1982, p 485.

99. Lindenauer SM, Weber TR, Miller TA, et al: Velour vascular prosthesis. Trans Am Soc Artifical Internal Organs 20:314, 1974.

100. Hall CW, Liotta D, Ghidoni JJ, et al: Velour fabrics applied to medicine. J Biomed Mater Res 1:179, 1967.

101. Goldman M, McCollum CN, Hawker RJ, et al: Dacron arterial grafts: The influence of porosity, velour, and maturity on thrombogenicity. Surgery 92:947, 1982.

102. Reigel MM, Hollier LH, Pairolero PC, et al: Early experience with a new collagen-impregnated aortic graft. Ann Surg 54:134, 1988.

103. Canadian Multicenter Hemashield Study Group: Immunological response to collagen-impregnated vascular grafts: A randomized prospective study. J Vasc Surg 12:741, 1990.

104. Kottke-Marchant K, Anderson JM, Umennura Y, et al: Effects of albumin coating on the in vitro compatibility of Dacron arterial prostheses. Biomaterials 110:147, 1989.

105. Fleischlag JD, Moore WS: Clinical experience with a collagen-impregnated knitted Dacron vascular graft. Ann Vasc Surg 4:449, 1990.

106. Jones RA, Zieir G, Schoen FJ, et al: A new sealant for knitted Dacron prostheses: Minimally cross-linked gelatin. J Vasc Surg 4:414, 1988.

107. Meister RH, Schweiger H, Lang W: Knitted double-velour Dacron prostheses in aortobifemoral position—long-term performance of different coating materials. Vasa 27:236, 1998.

108. Blumberg RM, Gelfand ML, Barton ED, et al: Clinical significance of aortic graft dilation. J Vasc Surg 14:175, 1991.

109. Claggett GP, Salander JM, Eddleman WL, et al: Dilation of knitted Dacron aortic prostheses and anastomotic false aneurysms: Etiologic considerations. Surgery 93:9, 1983.

110. Nunn DB, Freeman MH, Hodgins PC: Postoperative alterations in size of Dacron aortic grafts: An ultrasonic evaluation. Ann Surg 189:741, 1979.

111. Braithwaite BD, Davies B, Heather BP, Earnshaw JJ: Early results of a randomized trial of rifampicin-bonded Dacron grafts for extra-anatomic vascular reconstruction: Joint Vascular Research Group. Br J Surg 85:1378, 1998.

112. Lehnhardt FJ, Torsello G, et al: Systemic and local antibiotic prophylaxis in the prevention of prosthetic vascular graft infection: An experimental study. Eur J Vasc Endovasc Surg 23:127, 2002.

113. Hernandez-Richter T, Schardey HM, et al: Rifampin and triclosan but not silver is effective in preventing bacterial infection of vascular Dacron graft material. Eur J Vasc Endovasc Surg 26:550, 2003.

114. Szilagyi DE, Smith RF, Elliott JP, et al: Long-term behavior of a Dacron arterial substitute. Ann Surg 162:453, 1965.

115. El-Massry S, Saad E, Sauvage L, et al: Femoropopliteal bypass with externally supported knitted Dacron grafts: A follow-up of 200 grafts for one to twelve years. J Vasc Surg 19:487, 1994.

116. Rosenthal D, Evans D, McKinsey J, et al: Prosthetic above-knee femoropopliteal bypass grafts for intermittent claudication. J Cardiovasc Surg (Torino) 31:462, 1990.

117. Prevec WC, Darling RC, L'Italien GJ, et al: Femoropopliteal reconstruction with knitted non-velour Dacron versus expanded PTFE. J Vasc Surg 16:60, 1992.

118. Abbott WM, Green RM, Matsumoto T, et al: Prosthetic above-knee femoropopliteal bypass grafting: Results of a multicenter randomized prospective trial. Above-Knee Femoropopliteal Study Group. J Vasc Surg 25:19, 1997.

119. Johnson WC, Lee KK: Comparative evaluation of externally supported Dacron and polytetrafluoroethylene prosthetic bypasses for femoro-femoral and axillofemoral arterial reconstructions: Veterans Affairs Cooperative Study #141. J Vasc Surg 30:1077, 1999.

120. Very highly stretched polytetrafluoroethylene and process therefore. U.S. Patent 3,962,153 to WL Gore and Associates, June 8, 1976.

121. Golden MA, Hanson SR, Kirkman TR, et al: Healing of polytetrafluoroethylene arterial grafts is influenced by graft porosity. J Vasc Surg 11:838, 1990.

122. Matsumoto H, Hasegawa T, Fuse K: A renovascular prosthesis for a small caliber artery. Surgery 74:518, 1973.

123. Campbell DC, Brooks DH, Webster MW, et al: The use of expanded microporous polytetrafluoroethylene for limb salvage: A preliminary report. Surgery 79:485, 1976.

124. Senfield NA, Connolly R, Ramberg K, et al: The systemic activation of platelets by Dacron grafts. Surg Gynecol Obstet 166:454, 1988.

125. Shepard AD, Gelfand JA, Callow AD, O'Donnell TF Jr: Complement activation by synthetic vascular prostheses. J Vasc Surg 1:829, 1984.

126. Abbott WM, Cambria RP: Control of physical characteristics (elasticity and compliance) of vascular grafts. In Stanley JC (ed): Biologic and Synthetic Vascular Prostheses. New York, Grune & Stratton, 1982, p 189.

127. Mehigan DG, Fitzpatrick B, Browne HI, Boucher-Hayes DJ: Is compliance mismatch the major cause of anastamotic arterial aneurysms? Analysis of 42 cases. J Cardiovasc Surg (Torino) 26:147, 1985.

128. Gupta SK, Veith FJ, Kram HB, et al: Prospective randomized comparison of ringed and non-ringed PTFE femoropopliteal bypass grafts: A preliminary report. J Vasc Surg 13:162, 1991.

129. Harris JE, Taylor LM, McConnell DB, et al: Clinical results of axillofemoral bypass using externally supported polytetrafluoroethylene. J Vasc Surg 12:416, 1990.

130. Veith FJ, Moss CM, Fell SC, et al: Comparison of expanded PTFE and vein grafts in lower extremity arterial reconstructions. J Cardiovasc Surg (Torino) 19:341, 1978.

131. Archie JP: Femoropopliteal bypass with either adequate ipsilateral reversed saphenous vein or obligatory polytetrafluoroethylene. Ann Vasc Surg 8:475, 1994.

132. Allen BT, Reilly JM, Rubin BG, et al: Femoropopliteal bypass for claudication: Vein vs PTFE. Ann Vasc Surg 10:178, 1996.

133. Flinn WR, Rohrer MJ, Yao JST, et al: Improved long-term patency of infragenicular polytetrafluoroethylene grafts. J Vasc Surg 7:685, 1985.

134. Raptis S, Miller JH: Influence of a vein cuff on polytetrafluoroethylene grafts for primary femoropopliteal bypass. Br J Surg 82:487, 1995.

135. Stonebridge PA, Prescott RJ, Ruckley CV: Randomized trial comparing infrainguinal polytetrafluoroethylene bypass grafting with and without vein interposition cuff at the distal anastomosis: The Joint Vascular Research Group. J Vasc Surg 26:543, 1997.

136. Neville RF, Tempesta B, et al: Tibial bypass for limb salvage using polytetrafluoroethylene and a distal vein patch. J Vasc Surg 33:266, 2001.

137. Zwolak RM, Adams MC, Clowes AW: Kinetics of vein graft hyperplasia: Association with tangential stress. J Vasc Surg 5:126, 1987.

138. Bastounis E, Georgopoulos S, Maltezos C, et al: PTFE-vein composite grafts for critical limb ischaemia: A valuable alternative to all-autogenous infrageniculate reconstructions. Eur J Vasc Endovasc Surg 18:127, 1999.

139. Yeung KK, Mills JL Sr, et al: Improved patency of infrainguinal polytetrafluoroethylene bypass grafts using a distal Taylor vein patch. Am J Surg 182:578, 2001.

140. Kreienberg PB, Darling RC 3rd, et al: Early results of a prospective randomized trial of spliced vein versus polytetrafluoroethylene graft with a distal vein cuff for limb-threatening ischemia. J Vasc Surg 35:299, 2002.

141. Corson JD, Baraniewski HM, Shah DM, et al: Large diameter expanded polytetrafluoroethylene grafts for infrarenal aortic aneurysm surgery. J Cardiovasc Surg (Torino) 31:702, 1990.

142. Avramov S, Petrovic P, Fabri M: Bifurcated grafts (Dacron vs PTFE) in aortoiliac reconstruction: Five years follow-up. J Cardiovasc Surg (Torino) 28:33, 1987.

143. Lord RSA, Nash PA, Raj PT, et al: Prospective randomized trial of polytetrafluoroethylene and Dacron aortic prostheses. I. Perioperative results. Ann Vasc Surg 3:248, 1988.

144. Cintora I, Pearce DE, Cannon JA: A clinical survey of aortobifemoral bypass using two inherently different graft types. Ann Surg 208:625, 1988.

145. Burke PM Jr, Herman JB, Cutler BS: Optimal grafting methods for the smaller abdominal aorta. J Cardiovasc Surg (Torino) 28:420, 1987.

146. Campbell CD, Brooks DH, Siewers RD, et al: Extraanatomic bypass with expanded polytetrafluoroethylene graft. Surg Gynec Obstet 148:525, 1979.

147. Haimov M, Giron F, Jacobson JH II: The expanded polytetrafluoroethylene graft: Three years experience with 362 grafts. Arch Surg 114:673, 1979.
148. Chang JB: Current status of extraanatomic bypasses. Am J Surg 152:202, 1986.
149. Palder SB, Kirkman BL, Whitemore AD, et al: Vascular access for hemodialysis: Patency rates and results of revision. Ann Surg 202:235, 1985.
150. Raju S: PTFE for hemodialysis access: Techniques for insertion and management of complications. Ann Surg 206:666, 1987.
151. Fisher RK, Kirkpatrick UJ, et al: The Distaflo graft: A valid alternative to interposition vein? Eur J Vasc Endovasc Surg 25:235, 2003.
152. Gloviczki P, Pairolero PC, Cherry KJ, et al: Reconstruction of the vena cava and its primary tributaries: A preliminary report. J Vasc Surg 11:373, 1990.
153. Connolly JE, Kwan JHM, Brownell D, et al: Newer developments of extraanatomic bypass. Surg Gynecol Obstet 158:415, 1984.
154. Berger K, Sauvage LR, Rao AM, et al: Healing of arterial prostheses in man: Its incompleteness. Ann Surg 175:118, 1972.
155. Hedeman Joosten PP, Verhagen HJ, Heijnen-Snyder GJ, et al: Thrombomodulin activity of fat-derived microvascular endothelial cells seeded on expanded polytetrafluoroethylene. J Vasc Res 36:91, 1999.
156. Teebken OE, Pichlmaier AM, et al: Cell seeded decellularised allogeneic matrix grafts and biodegradable polydioxanone-prostheses compared with arterial autografts in a porcine model. Eur J Vasc Endovasc Surg 22:139, 2001.
157. Herring M, Gardner A, Glover J: A single-stage technique for seeding vascular grafts with autogenous endothelium. Surgery 84:498, 1978.
158. Deutsch M, Meinhart J, Fischlein T, et al: Clinical autologous in vitro endothelialization of infrainguinal ePTFE grafts in 100 patients: A 9-year experience. Surgery 126:847, 1999.
159. Robinson KA, Candal FJ, Scott NA, Ades EW: Seeding of vascular grafts with an immortalized human dermal microvascular endothelial cell line. Angiology 46:107, 1995.
160. Herring MB, Baughmon S, Glover JL: Endothelium develops on seeded arterial prosthesis: A brief clinical report. J Vasc Surg 2:727, 1985.
161. Ortenwall P, Wadenvick H, Kutti J, et al: Reduction in deposition of indium-111-labeled platelets after autologous endothelial cell seeding of Dacron aortic bifurcation grafts in humans: A preliminary study. J Vasc Surg 6:17, 1987.
162. Ortenwall P, Wadenvick H, Risberg B: Reduced platelet deposition on seeded versus unseeded segments of expanded polytetrafluoroethylene grafts: Clinical observations after a six month follow-up. J Vasc Surg 10:374, 1989.
163. Rosenman JE, Kempczinski RF, Pearce WH, et al: Kinetics of endothelial cell seeding. J Vasc Surg 2:778, 1985.
164. Seeger JM: Improved endothelial cell seeding efficiency with cultured cells and fibronectin coated grafts. J Surg Res 38:641, 1985.
165. Bhattacharya V, McSweeney PA, Shi Q, et al: Enhanced endothelialization and microvessel formation in polyester grafts seeded with CD34+ bone marrow cells. Blood 95:581, 2000.
166. Sugawara Y, Miyata T, Sato O, et al: Rapid postincubation endothelial retention by Dacron grafts. J Surg Res 67:132, 1997.
167. Gott VL, Whiffen JD, Dutton RC: Heparin bonding on colloid in graphite surfaces. Science 142:1927, 1963.
168. Becquemin JP, Riff Y, Kovarsky S, et al: Evaluation of a polyester collagen-coated heparin bonded vascular graft. J Cardiovasc Surg (Torino) 38:7, 1997.
169. Esquivel CO, Bjork C-G, Bergentz S-E, et al: Reduced thrombogenic characteristics of expanded polytetrafluoroethylene and polyurethane arterial grafts after heparin bonding. Surgery 95:102, 1984.
170. Walpoth BH, Rogulenko R, Tikhvinskaia E, et al: Improvement of patency rate in heparin-coated small synthetic vascular grafts. Circulation 98(19 Suppl):II319, 1998.
171. Greco RS, Kim HC, Denetz AP, Harvey RA: Patency of a small vessel prosthesis bonded to tissue plasminogen activator and iloprost. Ann Vasc Surg 9:140, 1995.
172. Bernex F, Mazzucotelli JP, Roudiere JL, et al: In vitro endothelialization of carbon-coated Dacron vascular grafts. Int J Artif Organs 15:172, 1992.
173. Dryer B, Akutsu T, Kolff WJ: Aortic grafts of polyurethane in dogs. J Appl Physiol 15:18, 1960.
174. Geeraert AJ, Callaghan JC: Experimental study of selected small calibre arterial grafts. J Cardiovasc Surg (Torino) 18:155, 1977.
175. Cronenwett JL, Zelenock GB: Alternative small arterial grafts. In Stanley JC (ed): Biologic and Synthetic Vascular Prostheses. New York, Grune & Stratton, 1982, p 595.
176. Edwards A, Carson RJ, Szycher M, Bowald S: In vitro and in vivo biodurability of a compliant microporous vascular graft. J Biomater Appl 13:23, 1998.
177. Glickman MH, Stokes GK, et al: Multicenter evaluation of a polytetrafluoroethylene vascular access graft as compared with the expanded polytetrafluoroethylene vascular access graft in hemodialysis applications. J Vasc Surg 34:465, 2001.
178. Dahl SL, Koh J, et al: Decellularized native and engineered arterial scaffolds for transplantation. Cell Transplant 12:659, 2003.
179. Wilson GJ, Yeger H, Klement P, et al: Acellular matrix allograft small caliber vascular prostheses. ASAIO Trans 36:M340, 1990.
180. Wilson GJ, Courtman DW, Klement P, et al: Acellular matrix: A biomaterials approach for coronary artery bypass and heart valve replacement. Ann Thorac Surg 60(2 Suppl):S353, 1995.
181. O'Brien MF, Gardner MA, Garlick RB, et al: The Cryolife-O'Brien stentless aortic xenograft valve. J Card Surg 13:376, 1998.
182. Greisler HP, Endean ED, Klosak JJ, et al: Polyglactin 910/polydioxanone biocomponent totally resorbable vascular prostheses. J Vasc Surg 7:697, 1988.
183. Shum-Tim D, Stock U, Hrkach J, et al: Tissue engineering of autologous aorta using a new biodegradable polymer. Ann Thorac Surg 68:2298, 1999.
184. Chandrasekar NR, L'Italien G, Warnock DF, et al: Compliance and the effects of photodynamic therapy of arteries. Surg Forum 34:351, 1993.
185. Moore MA, Bohachevsky IK, Cheung DT, et al: Stabilization of pericardial tissue by dye-mediated photooxidation. J Biomed Mater Res 28:611, 1994.
186. LaMuraglia GM, Adili F, Schmitz-Rixen T, et al: Photodynamic therapy of vein grafts: Suppression of intimal hyperplasia of the vein graft but not the anastomosis. J Vasc Surg 21:882, 1995.
187. Jenkins MP, Buonaccorsi GA, Raphael M, et al: Clinical study of adjuvant photodynamic therapy to reduce restenosis following femoral angioplasty. Br J Surg 86:1258, 1999.
188. LaMuraglia GM, Adili F, Schmitz-Rixen T, et al: Photodynamic therapy inhibits experimental allograft rejection: A novel approach for the development of vascular prostheses. Circulation 92:1919, 1995.
189. Fungaloi P, Waterman P, et al: Photochemically modulated endothelial cell thrombogenicity via the thrombomodulin-tissue factor pathways. Photochem Photobiol 78:475, 2003.
190. Huynh T, Abraham G, Murray J, et al: Remodeling of an acellular collagen graft into a physiologically responsive neovessel. Nat Biotechnol 17:1083, 1999.
191. Niklason LE, Gao J, Abbott WM, et al: Functional arteries grown in vitro. Science 284:489, 1999.
192. Edwards JM, Taylor LM, Porter JM: Treatment of failed lower extremity bypass grafts with new autogenous vein bypass grafting. J Vasc Surg 11:136, 1990.
193. Budd JS, Langdon I, Brenan J, Bell PRF: Above-knee prosthetic grafts do not compromise the ipsilateral long saphenous vein. Br J Surg 78:1379, 1991.
194. Brewster DC, LaSalle AJ, Robison JE, et al: Femoropopliteal graft failures: Clinical consequences and success of secondary reconstructions. Arch Surg 118:1043, 1983.
195. Gupta SK, Veith FJ, Ascer E, et al: Cost factors in limb-threatening ischemia due to infrainguinal atherosclerosis. Eur J Vasc Surg 2:151, 1988.
196. Robinson JG, Brewster DC, Abbott WM, Darling RC: Femoropopliteal and tibioperoneal artery reconstruction using human umbilical vein. Arch Surg 118:1039, 1983.

Questions

1. In general, which of the following statements is true of grafts of biologic origin?
   (a) They have patency rates superior to synthetics
   (b) They handle better than synthetics
   (c) They have all had problems with structural degeneration
   (d) b and c
   (e) a, b, and c

2. Coatings added to fabric vascular prostheses do which of the following?
   (a) Improve healing
   (b) Increase resistance to infection
   (c) Decrease overall cost
   (d) All of the above
   (e) None of the above

3. Which of the following statements about autogenous long saphenous vein grafts is true?
   (a) They have ideal performance characteristics
   (b) They never develop aneurysms
   (c) They sometimes occlude due to diffuse intimal hyperplasia
   (d) They achieve superior results when used in situ
   (e) All of the above

4. Which of the following is currently used to impregnate Dacron grafts?
   (a) Gelatin
   (b) Albumin
   (c) Collagen
   (d) a and b
   (e) a and c

5. What is the advantage of using ePTFE rather than Dacron grafts for above-knee femoropopliteal bypass?
   (a) Better patency
   (b) Lower cost
   (c) Less bleeding
   (d) Less anastomotic intimal hyperplasia
   (e) None of the above

6. What is the main disadvantage of ePTFE?
   (a) Stiffness
   (b) High compliance
   (c) High porosity
   (d) High incidence of infection
   (e) Thrombogenic nature

7. Which of the following statements about endothelial cell seeding of grafts is true?
   (a) It has not yet been studied in humans
   (b) It can theoretically use a patient's own endothelial cells
   (c) It is not successful if used with ePTFE grafts
   (d) It provides a temporary population of endothelial cells
   (e) All of the above

8. Which of the following is an investigative therapy for intimal hyperplasia?
   (a) L-Arginine
   (b) Radiation
   (c) Matrix metalloproteinase inhibitors
   (d) None of the above
   (e) All of the above

9. Which of the following statements is true of composite all-autogenous conduits in lower extremity bypass?
   (a) They yield patency rates that approach those of greater saphenous vein
   (b) Use of the basilic vein should be attempted before use of the cephalic vein
   (c) They should be preceded by duplex venous mapping
   (d) a and c
   (e) b and c

10. Which of the following statements about arterial autografts is true?
    (a) Problems with vasoconstriction limit their use
    (b) They are advantageous in pediatric patients
    (c) They are rarely used in cases of visceral revascularization
    (d) They should be avoided in infected tissue beds
    (e) They provide patency rates similar to those of saphenous vein in cases of coronary revascularization

Answers

1. c	2. e	3. c	4. e	5. e
6. a	7. b	8. e	9. d	10. b

27

Larry H. Hollier

Thoracoabdominal Aortic Aneurysms

Since the first successful thoracoabdominal aortic aneurysm (TAAA) repair by Etheredge and associates in 1955,[1] care of the TAAA patient has undergone significant beneficial changes. These improvements have resulted from a refinement of risk assessment, improved diagnostic capabilities, an expansion of anesthetic and intraoperative support, the evolution of surgical techniques, and a multimodality approach to the prevention of perioperative complications.[2,3] Together, these efforts have led to a dramatic reduction in the overall complication rate associated with TAAA repair over more than 40 years. However, TAAA repair remains a formidable procedure associated with serious complications at rates exceeded by few other procedures. Further insight into the cause of these complications, as well as refinements in preoperative assessment, surgical technique, and postoperative care, will allow a continued reduction in the morbidity and mortality associated with TAAA repair.

Classification

Aneurysms of the thoracoabdominal aorta can be classified by their extent and their causes. In 1986, Crawford and colleagues classified TAAAs based on the extent of aortic involvement (Fig. 27-1).[4] This classification can be applied to aortic aneurysms of all causes, including, but not limited to, degenerative or dissected aneurysms or those resulting from Marfan's or Ehlers-Danlos syndrome. Type I aneurysms involve all or most of the descending thoracic aorta and the upper abdominal aorta but do not involve the aorta below the level of the renal arteries. Type II aneurysms involve all or most of the descending thoracic aorta and all or most of the abdominal aorta. Type III aneurysms involve the distal half or less of the descending thoracic aorta and varying segments of the abdominal aorta. Type IV aneurysms involve all or most of the abdominal aorta, including the segment from which the visceral vessels arise.

The Crawford classification has advanced the surgical treatment of TAAA because it permits the standardized reporting of aneurysm extent, allowing the stratification of risk and comparisons among aneurysm types and treatment groups. The Crawford classification has also promoted the evaluation and application of specific treatment modalities based on the extent of TAAA.[5] Similarly, it has allowed a type-specific

determination of neurologic deficit as well as morbidity and mortality associated with TAAA repair (Tables 27-1 and 27-2).

Aortic dissection, whether it develops into an aortic aneurysm or not, has also been classified by numerous authors based on the extent of aortic involvement.[6] The most widely used classification system is that of DeBakey and coworkers (Fig. 27-2),[7] who classified aortic dissection into three basic types related to anatomic and pathologic features. Types I and II involve the ascending aorta, whereas type III involves the descending aorta. Type I and type II dissections are differentiated from each other by the fact that type I dissections extend beyond the aortic arch. DeBakey type III aortic dissections do not involve the ascending aorta or the aortic arch. They can be subdivided into type IIIa (dissecting process limited to the descending thoracic aorta) and type IIIb (dissecting process extending below the diaphragm). A DeBakey type IIIb dissection corresponds to a type I or II TAAA with regard to the extent of aortic involvement by the dissecting process.

Over the past 30 years, a more functional approach to the classification of aortic dissection has emerged (Fig. 27-3). These systems are based on whether the ascending aorta is involved, without regard to the site of the primary intimal tear. If the ascending aorta is involved, the dissection is termed a Stanford type A,[8] Najafi anterior,[9] University of Alabama ascending,[10] or Massachusetts General Hospital proximal[11] aortic dissection. If the ascending aorta is not involved, it may be referred to as a type B, posterior, descending, or distal aortic dissection, respectively (see Fig. 27-3). Combining these five classification systems allows us to see that DeBakey type I and II aortic dissections are synonymous with type A, anterior, ascending, and proximal. These forms of aortic dissection may be associated with complications (cardiac tamponade, acute aortic regurgitation, or coronary artery dissection or occlusion) that require cardiac surgical procedures (ascending aorta replacement, aortic arch replacement, aortic valve replacement or suspension, or coronary artery reimplantation), which are beyond the scope of this chapter. However, DeBakey type IIIa and IIIb aortic dissections, which are synonymous with type B, posterior, descending, and distal aortic dissections, may acutely or chronically degenerate into descending thoracic aortic aneurysms or TAAAs. From the viewpoint of the vascular surgeon, the Stanford

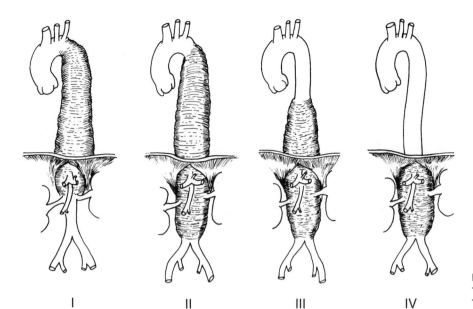

I   II   III   IV

FIGURE 27–1 • Crawford classification of thoracoabdominal aortic aneurysms: types I through IV.

classification is preferred because it is simple yet functional and clearly delineates the surgical approach required.

Aortic dissections that are detected within 14 days of the onset of the process are classified as acute, whereas those diagnosed beyond 2 weeks are termed chronic.[6] Although aortic dissection, whether acute or chronic, may require intervention or surgical treatment for reasons other than aneurysmal expansion, this discussion is limited to aortic dissections that are aneurysmal and involve the descending thoracic or abdominal aorta, or both, thus qualifying as Crawford types I through IV (Table 27-3).

Cause

Atherosclerotic medial degenerative disease (82%) and aortic dissection (17%) together account for nearly all reported cases of TAAA.[12] Marfan's and Ehlers-Danlos syndromes, mycotic aneurysm, and Takayasu's aortitis are less frequent causes. The importance of establishing a proper diagnosis for aneurysmal disease lies in the unique natural history and treatment requirements for each type of TAAA.[13-15]

Patients with nondissecting (including degenerative, Marfan's, Ehlers-Danlos, and others) and dissecting TAAAs have different associated risk factors that influence the natural history, treatment, and long-term survival (Table 27-4). Both groups of patients with TAAAs have a high incidence of associated hypertension. However, patients with degenerative aneurysms tend to have a higher incidence of coronary artery disease, chronic renal insufficiency, cerebrovascular disease, and peripheral vascular disease than do patients with dissecting aneurysms. These patterns of coexistent disease significantly influence the risk of perioperative morbidity (Table 27-5) and mortality (see Table 27-2), as well as the overall risk-benefit ratio of TAAA repair.

TABLE 27–1	Average Incidence of Postoperative Neurologic Deficits by Crawford Classification of Thoracoabdominal Aortic Aneurysms (TAAAs)			
	Type I (%)	Type II (%)	Type III (%)	Type IV (%)
Nondissecting TAAA	13	31	7	4
Dissecting TAAA	20	34	15	11

Modified from Panneton JM, Hollier LH: Nondissecting thoracoabdominal aortic aneurysms: Part I. Ann Vasc Surg 9:503-514, 1995; Panneton JM, Hollier LH: Dissecting descending thoracic and thoracoabdominal aortic aneurysms: Part II. Ann Vasc Surg 9: 596-605, 1995.

TABLE 27–2	Incidence of Operative Mortality Associated with Thoracoabdominal Aortic Aneurysms (TAAAs)*	
	Type of TAAA	
Cause of Mortality	Nondissecting TAAA (Median %)†	Dissecting TAAA (Average %)
Pulmonary complication	38	—
Respiratory failure	—	19
Myocardial infarction	37	—
Cardiac‡	—	44
Renal failure	27	18
Hemorrhage	14	27
Sepsis	19	20
Pulmonary embolism	8	6
Stroke	8	5

*Several series reported multiple causes of death; therefore, the total percentage is less than 100%.

†Median percentages were used owing to the wide variance in reporting of nondissecting TAAA data.

‡Myocardial infarction, low cardiac output, or arrhythmia.

Modified from Panneton JM, Hollier LH: Nondissecting thoracoabdominal aortic aneurysms: Part I. Ann Vasc Surg 9:503-514, 1995; Panneton JM, Hollier LH: Dissecting descending thoracic and thoracoabdominal aortic aneurysms: Part II. Ann Vasc Surg 9:596-605, 1995.

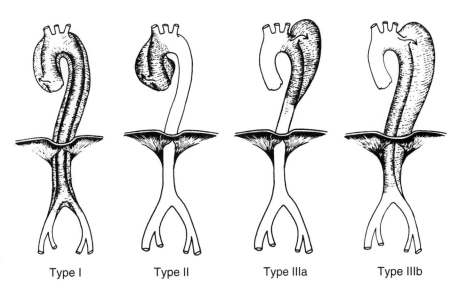

FIGURE 27–2 • DeBakey classification of aortic dissection.

Type I   Type II   Type IIIa   Type IIIb

Natural History

The determination of whether to offer or withhold surgery from a patient diagnosed with a TAAA demands an understanding of the natural history of the aneurysm as well as an assessment of the patient's overall risk for surgery. In 1982, Bickerstaff and coworkers noted a 2-year actuarial survival rate of 28.7% in patients with untreated thoracic and thoracoabdominal aneurysms.[16] In 1986, Crawford and DeNatale published the results of 94 patients with unoperated TAAAs whose cases were followed over a 25-year period.[17] This study, which included a mixture of dissected and nondissected TAAAs, demonstrated a 2-year survival of 24%, with 52% of all deaths resulting from aneurysm rupture. In contrast, in a contemporary review of 605 patients who underwent surgery for TAAA repair, Crawford and coworkers reported a 71% 2-year survival rate.[4]

However, degenerative and dissecting TAAAs differ not only in their causes and associated risk factors but also in their natural history. In the series of Bickerstaff and coworkers,

the 5-year survival for patients with unoperated dissecting aneurysms was 7%, whereas the survival for those with unoperated nondissecting aneurysms was 19.2%; again, rupture was a major cause of death.[16] Cambria and colleagues, in 1995, reported on the natural history of 57 patients with degenerative, nondissecting TAAAs with a 37-month follow-up.[18] In this series, rupture was the second most frequent cause of death, after cardiopulmonary disease. The overall risk of rupture with nonoperative treatment was 12% at 2 years and 32% at 4 years. In patients with aneurysms larger than 5 cm, the risk of rupture increased to 18% at 2 years. The authors reported a repair-free survival rate of 52% at 2 years and 17% at 5 years. In contrast, the authors noted a survival rate of 50% at 5 years after TAAA repair in a contemporary series of patients.

The natural history of acute and chronic aortic dissection should be considered separately, just as the natural history of degenerative and dissecting aortic aneurysms should be. Patients with acute aortic dissection have a higher mortality than those with chronic dissection.[19] Subset analysis of a

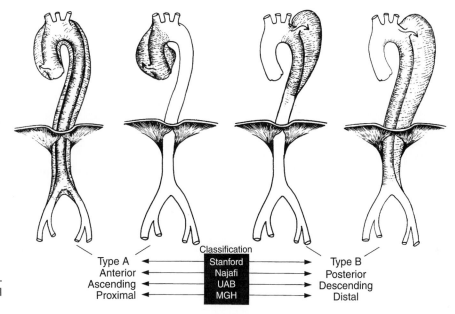

	Classification	
Type A	Stanford	Type B
Anterior	Najafi	Posterior
Ascending	UAB	Descending
Proximal	MGH	Distal

FIGURE 27–3 • Aortic dissection classification systems. MGH, Massachusetts General Hospital; UAB, University of Alabama.

TABLE 27–3	Extent of Aortic Involvement by Crawford Classification of Thoracoabdominal Aortic Aneurysms (TAAAs)			
	Type I (%)	Type II (%)	Type III (%)	Type IV (%)
Nondissecting TAAA	23	23	26	28
Dissecting TAAA	32	48	14	6

Modified from Panneton JM, Hollier LH: Nondissecting thoracoabdominal aortic aneurysms: Part I. Ann Vasc Surg 9:503-514, 1995; Panneton JM, Hollier LH: Dissecting descending thoracic and thoracoabdominal aortic aneurysms: Part II. Ann Vasc Surg 9:596-605, 1995.

mixed population of type B dissecting aneurysms revealed that the percentage of deaths from aortic rupture was 83% in acute type B dissecting aneurysms, as opposed to 56% in chronic type B dissecting aneurysms.[20] Additionally, the 1- and 5-year survival rates of surgically treated patients with acute type B aortic dissection are 56% and 48%, respectively, versus 78% and 59% in surgically treated patients with chronic type B aortic dissection.[19] Further, dissections with a patent false lumen have a higher complication rate than do those with partial or complete thrombosis of the false lumen.[21] High flow rates within a patent false lumen and retrograde flow proximal to the left subclavian artery are also associated with higher complication and mortality rates.[22] These data emphasize the importance of fully assessing the cause and anatomy of a TAAA when determining a patient's treatment plan. The natural history of degenerative TAAA is different from that of both acute and chronic dissecting TAAAs.

TABLE 27–4	Incidence of Risk Factors Associated with Thoracoabdominal Aortic Aneurysms (TAAAs)	
Risk Factor	Nondissecting TAAA (Median %)*	Dissecting TAAA (Average %)
Smoking	80	—
Hypertension	70	83
Coronary artery disease	35	19
Chronic obstructive pulmonary disease	35	25
Visceral occlusive disease	25	—
Chronic renal failure	20	9
Marfan's syndrome	—	6
Congestive heart failure	—	5
Cerebrovascular disease	15	—
Stroke	—	4
Peripheral vascular disease	15	—
Diabetes mellitus	5	3

*Median percentages were used owing to the wide variance in reporting of nondissecting TAAA data.
Modified from Panneton JM, Hollier LH: Nondissecting thoracoabdominal aortic aneurysms: Part I. Ann Vasc Surg 9:503-514, 1995; Panneton JM, Hollier LH: Dissecting descending thoracic and thoracoabdominal aortic aneurysms: Part II. Ann Vasc Surg 9:596-605, 1995.

TABLE 27–5	Incidence of Postoperative Complications Following Thoracoabdominal Aortic Aneurysm (TAAA) Repair	
Complication	Nondissecting TAAA (Average %)	Dissecting TAAA (Average %)
Respiratory insufficiency	32	12
Pulmonary infection	12	—
Tracheotomy	—	9
Renal dysfunction	21	18
Need for dialysis	7	6
Paraplegia/paresis	13	25
Myocardial infarction	11	—
Cardiac*	—	7
Reoperation for bleeding	7	7
Stroke	3	4
Gastrointestinal bleeding	7	3
Pulmonary embolism	—	1

*Myocardial infarction, low cardiac output, or life-threatening arrhythmia.
Modified from Panneton JM, Hollier LH: Nondissecting thoracoabdominal aortic aneurysms: Part I. Ann Vasc Surg 9:503-514, 1995; Panneton JM, Hollier LH: Dissecting descending thoracic and thoracoabdominal aortic aneurysms: Part II. Ann Vasc Surg 9:596-605, 1995.

An evaluation of each individual patient's risk of death from aortic aneurysm rupture compared with his or her operative risk provides the information necessary to devise the best overall treatment plan with the best chance of long-term survival (Table 27-6).

Presentation

Degenerative TAAAs and dissecting type B aortic aneurysms are asymptomatic at the time of diagnosis in 43% and 15% of patients, respectively.[12,23] Although the asymptomatic TAAA may be found during a routine history and physical examination, more commonly, abdominal ultrasonography, computed tomography (CT), or magnetic resonance imaging (MRI) performed during a seemingly unrelated workup reveals an incidental aortic aneurysm.

TABLE 27–6	Late Survival after Thoracoabdominal Aortic Aneurysm (TAAA) Repair	
Survival Time (Yr)	Nondissecting TAAA (%)	Dissecting TAAA (%)
1	80	74
5	61	50
10	33	—

Modified from Panneton JM, Hollier LH: Nondissecting thoracoabdominal aortic aneurysms: Part I. Ann Vasc Surg 9:503-514, 1995; Panneton JM, Hollier LH: Dissecting descending thoracic and thoracoabdominal aortic aneurysms: Part II. Ann Vasc Surg 9:596-605, 1995.

Degenerative TAAAs and dissecting type B aortic aneurysms have a symptomatic presentation in 57% and 85% of patients, respectively.[12,23] The most frequent complaint in both types is pain. As an aneurysm increases in size, it may compress or erode adjacent structures along the course of the aorta, resulting in chest, back, flank, or abdominal pain. Compression of organs and structures adjacent to a large aneurysm can result in a variety of signs and symptoms. Stretching of the recurrent laryngeal nerve may result in hoarseness; left lung or bronchial compression may cause dyspnea, wheezing, cough, or recurrent pulmonary infections; esophageal compression may cause dysphagia; and duodenal stretching from an underlying aneurysm can produce partial small bowel obstruction. Ureteral obstruction may result from an enlarging abdominal or iliac component of a TAAA, especially if the aneurysm has an inflammatory component.[24] Erosion of a large TAAA into the lung, esophagus, duodenum, or renal collecting system may lead to fistula formation, with "herald" or life-threatening hemorrhage in the form of hemoptysis, hematemesis, hematochezia, melena, or hematuria. Erosive fistula formation into the inferior vena cava may appear with an abdominal bruit, widened pulse pressure, edema, and heart failure. Degenerative TAAA may rarely manifest with paralysis resulting from vertebral body erosion with spinal cord compression, spinal artery thrombosis, or embolization.

Dissecting type B aortic aneurysms are more commonly symptomatic than degenerative TAAAs are and may include all previously mentioned presentations. The pain of acute aortic dissection is described as an excruciating ripping or tearing chest or intrascapular pain that may radiate into the flank, abdomen, or legs as the dissection progresses distally. Vascular complications resulting from aortic dissection are not rare and include renal ischemia (12%), visceral ischemia (9%), acute leg ischemia (9%), and paraplegia or paraparesis (3%).

Rupture as a manifestation of TAAA occurs with equal frequency (9%) in both atherosclerotic degenerative and dissecting type B aortic aneurysms.[12,23] TAAAs rupture with equal frequency within the thoracic and abdominal aortic segments.[25] Rarely, rupture occurs into the lung, tracheobronchial tree, or esophagus. Thoracic rupture presents with chest, back, or shoulder pain, whereas abdominal rupture manifests with generalized abdominal, left flank, left shoulder, or back pain. The majority of patients suffering from a ruptured TAAA die outside the hospital. Of patients admitted with rupture, 25% are hypotensive, and 55% suffer a cardiac arrest before operation.[25]

Diagnosis

The modalities available for the diagnosis of and preoperative planning for TAAA include chest radiography, angiography, CT, and transesophageal echocardiography (TEE).

Chest film findings associated with TAAA are typically nonspecific but abnormal in the majority of patients. Findings may be erroneously reported as aortic tortuosity or dilatation; mediastinal widening and displacement of intimal calcifications are less frequently noted (Fig. 27-4). Additionally, chest film findings associated with leaking or ruptured thoracic aortic aneurysms may include pleural effusion or pleural hematoma.

Historically, conventional aortography has been the gold standard for the evaluation of the aorta and its branches.

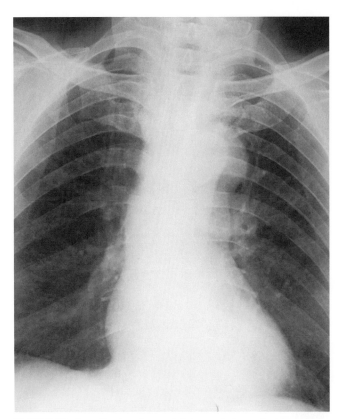

FIGURE 27–4 • Chest radiograph interpreted as a tortuous aorta with a wide mediastinum in a patient with a 9-cm aortic aneurysm.

In that regard, aortography remains the single best study for delineating aneurysm, dissection, or stenosis in aortic branch vessels (Fig. 27-5). However, aortography is the most invasive of all diagnostic techniques, requires nephrotoxic iodinated contrast agents, and does not evaluate nonperfused or thrombosed areas of aortic aneurysms. Therefore, the size and extent of a TAAA may not be fully ascertained using aortography alone.

CT and CT-angiography provide excellent visualization of the aorta, including aneurysm diameter, type and extent of dissection, thrombus characteristics (Fig. 27-6), evidence of aneurysm leak, branch vessel anatomy (Fig. 27-7), venous anatomy and anomalies, and abnormalities of adjacent mediastinal, retroperitoneal, and abdominal organs. Helical or spiral CT, with options for three-dimensional reconstruction, provides additional information about aortic branch vessel anatomy (Fig. 27-8). However, CT-angiography also requires the use of nephrotoxic intravenous contrast agents, and exposures must be appropriately timed with the intravenous bolus to adequately evaluate branch arteries.

MRI, with options for arterial enhancement, three-dimensional reconstruction, and cardiovascular imaging with cine–magnetic resonance angiography (MRA), enables us to define the entire extent of aortic aneurysms and dissections while avoiding nephrotoxic intravenous contrast materials.[26] MRI, MRA, and cine-MRA are user independent, have a large field of view, have multiplane and three-dimensional capabilities, lack ionizing radiation, and do not require critical timing of contrast infusion or image acquisition. The evaluation of aortic branch vessels with magnetic resonance techniques

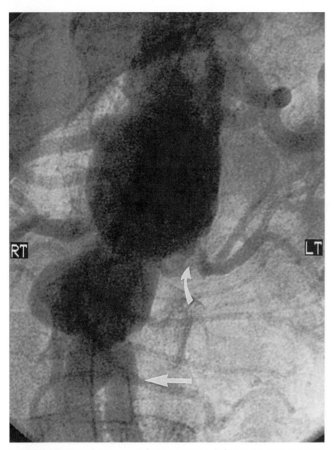

FIGURE 27–5 • Aortogram demonstrating left renal artery stenosis *(curved arrow)* in a patient with a type III thoracoabdominal aortic aneurysm (TAAA) 2 years after infrarenal TAAA repair *(straight arrow)*.

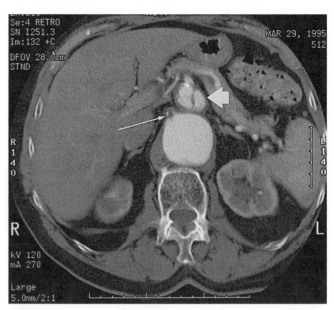

FIGURE 27–7 • Computed tomography angiogram of a thoraco-abdominal aortic aneurysm demonstrating a dissecting aneurysm of the superior mesenteric artery *(thick arrow)* and right renal artery stenosis *(thin arrow)*.

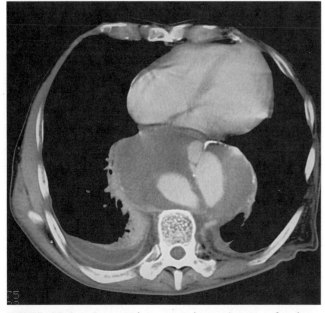

FIGURE 27–6 • Computed tomography angiogram of a large dissecting thoracoabdominal aortic aneurysm with three separately perfused lumens and a circumferential laminated thrombus.

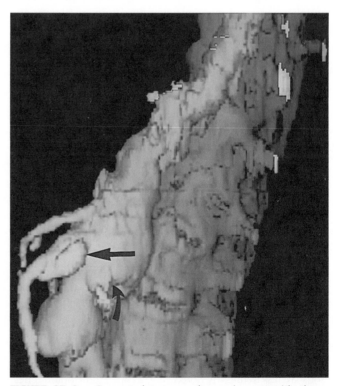

FIGURE 27–8 • Computed tomography angiogram with three-dimensional reconstruction of a thoracoabdominal aortic aneurysm demonstrating a superior mesenteric artery aneurysm *(straight arrow)* and dissection onto the origin of the left renal artery, causing stenosis *(curved arrow)*.

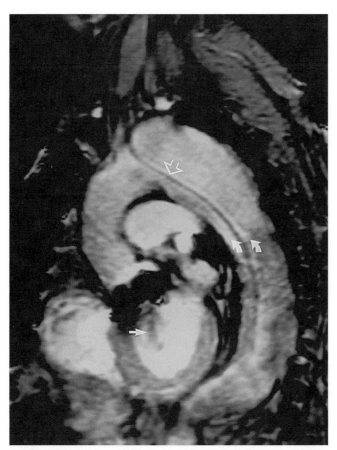

FIGURE 27–9 • Cine–magnetic resonance angiogram of a type B dissection demonstrating perfusion of the true and false lumens *(curved arrows)*, dissection flap *(open arrow)*, and aortic insufficiency *(straight arrow)* in a patient with prior aortic valve replacement.

is generally equivalent to that of CT; however, it is slightly inferior to conventional arteriography. Cine-MRA also has the ability to detect cardiac wall motion abnormalities and valvular disease with nearly as much accuracy as echocardiography (Fig. 27-9). However, magnetic resonance technology has certain limitations. It cannot be offered to patients with implanted electronic devices such as pacemakers, and previously placed metallic surgical clips create artifacts that can obscure anatomic detail. MRI cannot be performed on unstable patients, and mechanical ventilation makes high-quality image acquisition difficult. Patients who suffer from claustrophobia require sedation before undergoing an MRI examination.

TEE can be safely and rapidly performed at the patient's bedside or in the operating room. It provides information on myocardial performance, cardiac valvular function, and the presence of pericardial effusion or tamponade; it also provides excellent anatomic information on the ascending and descending thoracic aorta. It does not require intravenous contrast and can be performed rapidly at a reasonable cost. The disadvantages of TEE include its limitation in visualizing portions of the aortic arch and proximal brachiocephalic vessels and its inability to evaluate the infradiaphragmatic aorta.

In addition to the anatomic assessment of the aneurysm itself, a complete preoperative evaluation of the patient's concomitant risk factors is mandatory for successful outcome

following TAAA repair. After a thorough history and physical examination, routine preoperative studies usually include a baseline chest radiograph; electrocardiogram; arterial blood gases; complete blood count; complete serum chemistry profile, including liver function tests and electrolytes; urinalysis; platelet count; and prothrombin time, partial thromboplastin time, and fibrinogen levels.

All patients undergo thorough cardiac evaluation, including cardiac stress testing to detect possible coronary artery disease and B-mode ultrasonography to assess valvular competence. (Aortic valvular insufficiency is a relative contraindication to proximal clamping of the descending thoracic aorta unless shunt or pump bypass techniques are employed.) If significant coronary artery disease is revealed by stress testing, coronary angiography is performed.

Carotid artery duplex ultrasound scanning is routinely performed as part of the preoperative assessment. Severe carotid artery disease with stenosis greater than 70% diameter reduction is treated by carotid endarterectomy before elective TAAA repair.

Additionally, the patient's nutritional status should be assessed preoperatively. If the patient is found to be in a catabolic state or negative nitrogen balance, attempts should be made to achieve a positive nitrogen balance if this does not delay surgery inappropriately.

Patients found to be fit for surgery undergo preoperative hydration, mechanical bowel preparation, bathing with antimicrobial soap, and type and crossmatching for 6 units of packed red blood cells, 6 units of fresh frozen plasma, and 12 units of platelets.

Treatment

Anesthetic support is critical to the successful performance of TAAA repair. The anesthesiology service is responsible for placement of a double-lumen endotracheal tube with bronchoscopic positioning and assistance with the placement of a Swan-Ganz catheter, radial arterial line, and intrathecal catheter for the drainage of cerebrospinal fluid (CSF) and continuous monitoring of CSF pressure.[2,27] A closed CSF drainage system is used and is manually set at a level of 10 cm H_2O so that CSF will automatically drain as the pressure rises above this level. Additionally, two large-bore central venous catheters are placed for volume infusions, and a high thoracic epidural catheter is placed for perioperative analgesia, attenuation of the catecholamine stress response,[28] enhanced cardioprotection, and hemodynamic stability.[29] TEE is helpful to determine cardiac volume status and intraoperative cardiac valvular function and, most important, to detect myocardial ischemia as evidenced by cardiac wall motion abnormalities.

Distal aortic perfusion techniques have been associated with a decrease in the incidence of serious morbidity and mortality following TAAA repair.[5,30,31] Options available for the performance of distal aortic perfusion include the use of a passive shunt techniques (temporary axillary–to–femoral artery graft, temporary graft–to–iliac artery graft, or Gott shunt) or one of two techniques for pump perfusion (left atrial–to–femoral artery or femoral vein–to–femoral artery bypass). The perfusionist is intimately involved in the performance of the procedure when distal aortic pump perfusion (DAPP) is used. The perfusionist may also be responsible for operating the red blood cell salvage washing and rapid-infusion devices (Cell Saver and R.I.S., Haemonetics Corp., Braintree, Mass.), or this may be a shared responsibility with the anesthesia service. The coordination of the procedure demands frequent communication among the surgical, anesthesia, and perfusion teams.

After the appropriate tubes, lines, and monitoring devices have been placed, the patient is positioned in a right lateral decubitus position, allowing the hips to fall into a near supine position. This provides easy access to the left iliofemoral vessels should that become necessary. The skin is widely prepared with povidone-iodine solution and meticulous placement of adhesive iodinated plastic drapes. The thoracoabdominal incision is made in the fifth intercostal space for a type I or high type II TAAA or in the seventh to ninth intercostal space for type III or type IV TAAA.[2] The abdominal incision is then carried down the midline or paramedian line from the fifth intercostal incision or made obliquely across the abdomen from the seventh to ninth intercostal incision. Additional exposure may be gained by excising a rib or transecting the posterior portion of the rib above and below the intercostal incision. Proper preoperative planning usually prevents the need for a double thoracotomy, which may be associated with an increased risk of postoperative pulmonary complications. The abdominal exposure is continued in a retroperitoneal plane posterior to the left kidney. The diaphragm is divided in a circumferential fashion, with marking sutures placed on the edges of the divided diaphragm to facilitate closure. The crus of the diaphragm is divided to the left of the aorta. The proximal portions of the visceral and renal arteries are identified, and control of the superior mesenteric and renal arteries is obtained to allow these vessels to be snared after placement of selective visceral and renal perfusion catheters. These catheters originate from a Y connection in the arterial perfusion line if pump bypass is used, or from an octopus catheter if side graft perfusion is used (Fig. 27-10); they provide oxygenated blood to the cannulated mesenteric and renal arteries, thus decreasing the overall

ischemic time and subsequent ischemia-related complications. Additional thoracic exposure involves the division of the inferior pulmonary ligament and dissection of the mediastinal pleura overlying the normal aortic segment proximal to the aneurysm.

For type I and type II TAAAs, the proximal clamp may need to be applied on the distal aortic arch between the origin of the left common carotid and left subclavian arteries. Dissection at this level should be performed with great care, protecting the left phrenic, vagus, and recurrent laryngeal nerves. I incorporate the techniques of staged aortic clamping and sequential anastomoses with DAPP during performance of the proximal aortic and intercostal anastomoses. Therefore, an additional segment of mediastinal pleura is dissected overlying a segment of the mid to distal descending thoracic aorta, allowing aortic control at this level as the aneurysm anatomy permits. All intraperitoneal viscera must be carefully retracted medially and to the patient's right, avoiding splenic or pancreatic injury.

Throughout the procedure, and continuing for 3 days postoperatively, CSF is allowed to drain as the pressure rises above 10 cm H_2O. The patient's core temperature is allowed to passively drift down to 32°C to 34°C. Additionally, intravenous steroids, mannitol, and thiopental (or, more frequently, propofol) are administered before aortic clamping.

The distal aortic perfusion technique of choice is the use of Dacron side limbs sutured to the side of the main graft, with one anastomosed to the left iliac artery and the other fitted with octopus cannulas that are used for visceral and renal perfusion (Fig. 27-11). Using staged sequential aortic clamping, the proximal aortic clamp is placed initially, followed by the mid to distal descending thoracic aortic clamp; then the proximal segment of the aneurysm is opened longitudinally. In most instances, no attempt is made to control back-bleeding from intercostal arteries in the opened segment of aorta, because they will be reimplanted after completion of the proximal anastomosis. Autologous shed blood

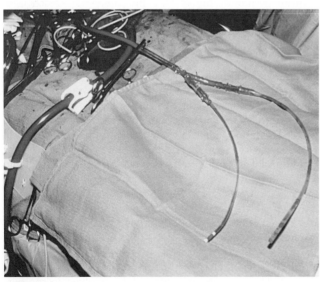

FIGURE 27–10 • Selective perfusion catheters from the divided arterial perfusion line are used with distal aortic pump perfusion to maintain superior mesenteric and renal artery blood flow during visceral aortic reconstruction.

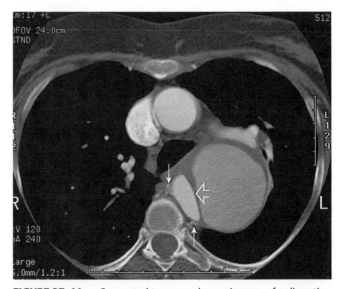

FIGURE 27–11 • Computed tomography angiogram of a dissecting thoracoabdominal aortic aneurysm in which the dissection flap (open arrow) has hidden the orifices of two intercostal arteries (small arrows). The septum should be excised and the intercostal arteries reimplanted or oversewn.

salvaging systems are used to retrieve blood from back-bleeding vessels. The proximal aorta is usually transected to separate it from the adjacent esophagus and thus avoid the development of an aortoesophageal fistula associated with endoaneurysmorrhaphy at this level. Large intercostal arteries in the vicinity of the proximal anastomosis are preserved via incorporation into a posterior tongue of aortic wall as part of an oblique anastomosis. This proximal anastomosis is performed with a properly sized, low-porosity, collagen-impregnated Dacron graft (Hemashield, Meadox, Oakland, N.J.) and sutured with a running 0 polypropylene (Prolene) suture (Ethicon, Summerville, N.J.) on a V7 needle. Felt strip reinforcement of the proximal aortic anastomosis is helpful in obtaining a hemostatic suture line with dissections and friable atheromatous aortic tissue.

After completing the proximal anastomosis, the proximal clamp is moved onto the graft, restoring flow to any reimplanted intercostal arteries, and through the iliac side graft to provide retrograde flow to the visceral segment of the aorta as well as to the lower extremities. The distal aortic clamp is then moved down to the level of the diaphragm, and the distal thoracic aorta is opened. Additional large intercostal arteries are reimplanted as separate cuffs onto the posterior aspect of the graft using the Carrel patch technique. In some cases of aortic dissection, intercostal arteries may be hidden from view by the intimal flap of the dissection (see Fig. 27-11). This flap should be excised and all intercostal arteries exposed so that they can be reimplanted if technically feasible. Occasionally, in extensive or dissecting aneurysms with multiple patent intercostal arteries, two separate cuffs of arteries need to be reimplanted. Each cuff of intercostal arteries is sequentially reperfused by moving the proximal clamp distally on the graft, thus restoring flow to the spinal cord as soon as possible.

Next, an infrarenal portion of aorta or, alternatively, the common iliac arteries are clamped for distal control. The remaining section of the aneurysmal aorta is opened longitudinally, posterior to the orifice of the left renal artery. The orifices of the celiac, superior mesenteric, and renal arteries are inspected. Significant atherosclerotic ostial lesions are treated by endarterectomy. The perfusion cannulas from the octopus catheter are then inserted into the celiac, superior mesenteric, and both renal arteries, and the visceral arteries are perfused by unclamping this side limb (Fig. 27-12). The visceral vessels are then reimplanted into the side of the graft using the Carrel patch technique. Generally, I try to reimplant the celiac, superior mesenteric, and right renal arteries as a single cuff and the left renal artery as a separate cuff; however, if the origins of the renal vessels are closely approximated to the visceral vessels, all can be reimplanted as a single cuff. Occasionally, separate grafts are used to revascularize renal or mesenteric vessels, especially if aortic dissection has extended into the branch vessels.

In patients with aortic dissection, the ostia of the visceral and renal vessels may contain the flap or septum of the dissection process, such that a single-cuff reimplantation of these dissected vessels may lead to perfusion of both a true and a false lumen, risking mesenteric and renal ischemia postoperatively (Fig. 27-13). In these situations, separate grafts can be presutured to the straight aortic graft, allowing independent reimplantation of individual visceral and renal vessels in an end-to-end fashion beyond the point of dissection (Fig. 27-14). After completing the visceral and renal reimplantation,

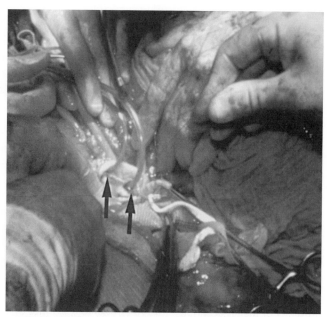

FIGURE 27–12 • Selective visceral perfusion cannulas in the superior mesenteric and right renal arteries *(arrows)* during a type II thoracoabdominal aortic aneurysm repair.

reperfusion of these vascular beds may lead to activation of the complement, cytokine, fibrinolytic promoter, and coagulation cascades, causing hypotension and metabolic acidosis and risking the development of coagulopathy and disseminated intravascular coagulation (DIC). Selective visceral perfusion during the period of visceral aortic reconstruction decreases the period of ischemia to these critical vascular beds and may reduce this risk of ischemia-reperfusion–associated complications. Cambria and coworkers demonstrated that perfusion of the mesenteric bed during aortic cross-clamping resulted in shorter mesenteric ischemia time and a decrease in the rise of end-tidal carbon dioxide following reperfusion of the visceral vessels.[32] The aortic clamp should be released slowly while blood and crystalloid solutions are rapidly infused. Additionally, sodium bicarbonate, mannitol, fresh frozen plasma, and platelets are routinely administered concomitantly with aortic declamping.

Next, the distal aortic anastomosis is performed. Sometimes, this needs to be carried out to the common iliac arteries, as dictated by aneurysm anatomy. Internal iliac artery perfusion should be ensured after completion of the distal anastomosis to decrease the risk of lower spinal cord or lumbosacral nerve root ischemic injury.[33] When cardiac indices and systemic and pulmonary blood pressure have stabilized, protamine is administered based on the activated clotting time to help counteract the anticoagulant effect that may result from mesenteric reperfusion. The approach to distal aortic perfusion should be based on a thorough knowledge of available techniques and individual patient characteristics. I have generally abandoned atriofemoral bypass in favor of Dacron side grafts for iliac and visceral perfusion (Fig 27-15); avoidance of the pump decreases cytokine activation during the procedure and may lessen the postoperative incidence of multisystem organ dysfunction.

After completing each anastomosis, adequate hemostasis must be ensured. Likewise, adequate perfusion to each of the

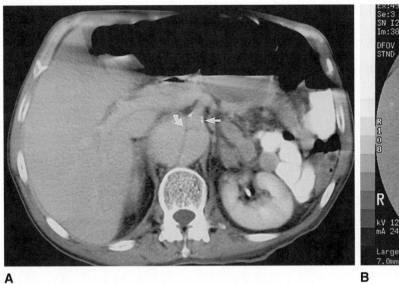 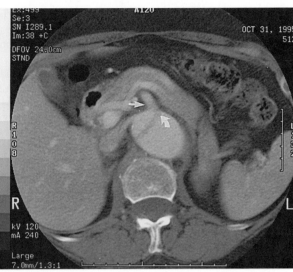

A   **B**

FIGURE 27–13 • Computed tomography scans of two different dissecting thoracoabdominal aortic aneurysms demonstrating the proximity of the dissecting flap *(curved arrows)* to the orifice of the superior mesenteric artery *(straight arrows)*.

branch vessels must be verified. If fibrinolysis is suspected, an infusion of an antifibrinolytic agent is started and continued up to 24 hours postoperatively. The wall of the aneurysm is closed tightly over the entire length of the graft. If coverage is incomplete, a Gore-Tex (W. L. Gore & Associates, Flagstaff, Ariz.) membrane is used to provide full coverage of the aortic graft. This provides tamponade against oozing and prevents graft erosion into adjacent viscera or lung. Fibrin glue may be injected into the space between the graft and the Gore-Tex membrane for additional hemostasis. After achieving hemostasis throughout the operative field, the diaphragm is reapproximated with interrupted mattress sutures. Two chest tubes are used to drain the costophrenic sulcus and the apex of the left chest. Abdominal and retroperitoneal drainage is generally avoided. The chest and abdomen are closed with multiple layers in standard fashion.

The patient is transferred directly to the surgical intensive care unit for close observation.

Postoperative Care

In the immediate postoperative period, maintaining hemodynamic stability and adequate oxygenation decreases the likelihood of tachycardia, myocardial ischemia, stroke, renal failure, or paraplegia. If rewarming is not complete, hypothermia must be corrected with warmed intravenous fluids and inhaled gases and a warming blanket. Blood pressure and cardiac indices are continuously monitored and maintained within the patient's normal preoperative range with crystalloid, colloid, and appropriate blood products. Arterial blood gases, coagulation studies, hemoglobin, and serum electrolytes are frequently monitored and maintained within normal ranges. Inotropic support may be required in the first few hours postoperatively; however, it is discontinued as soon as adequate volume loading has led to hemodynamic stability. The patient is maintained on a low-dose dopamine infusion (2 to 3 µg/kg per minute) to enhance renal vasodilatation for the first 24 to 48 hours, and lactated Ringer's solution is infused at a rate to replace urine output on a milliliter-per-milliliter basis for the first 12 to 24 hours.

The patient is maintained on a ventilator, and weaning is started on the following postoperative day, as dictated by arterial blood gases and evidence of appropriate pulmonary function. Maintenance fluid is decreased daily from the initial rate of 125 mL/hour (plus urinary replacement) to 60 mL/hour by the third postoperative day. Gradual weaning from the ventilator is ideally timed with mobilization of third-space fluid. Furosemide may be given at this point to assist with fluid mobilization and minimize the associated pulmonary congestion. Careful monitoring of serum potassium is important at this time because rapid diuresis may deplete potassium levels and result in cardiac arrhythmias. The chest tubes are removed when drainage has decreased to less than 100 to 200 mL/day, which is generally between the second and fifth postoperative days. CSF pressure monitoring is continued up

FIGURE 27–14 • Operative photograph of separate grafts for individual revascularization of visceral vessels in a patient with aortic dissection.

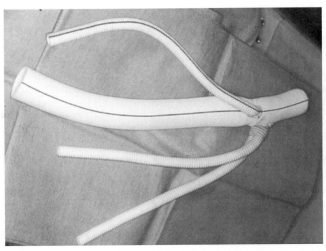

A

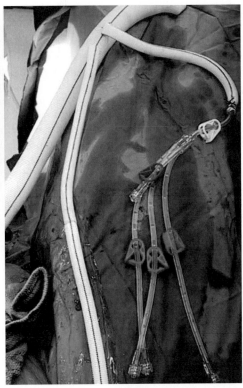

B

FIGURE 27–15 • *A,* Operative photograph of an aortic graft with side limbs attached. *B,* Operative photograph of an aortic graft with side limbs and visceral perfusion cannulas.

to 3 days postoperatively, with pressure maintained at 10 cm H_2O to decrease the risk of delayed-onset neurologic injury. Cephalosporin antibiotics are continued at least until the intrathecal lumbar catheter is removed. Cytoprotective agents or histamine blockers are used for ulcer prophylaxis until the resolution of postoperative ileus, at which time enteral feeding should be started.

Postoperative Complications and Their Prevention

Although it has become a much safer procedure than in years past, TAAA repair is still associated with high complication rates.[34,35] These rates are a reflection of the systemic nature of the arterial diseases affecting the aorta and multiple other organ systems, accounting for a significant incidence of comorbidities. In addition, the procedure itself requires entrance into both the thoracic and the abdominal or retroperitoneal regions, creates an ischemia-reperfusion phenomenon in several organ systems with a risk of cellular injury, may be associated with large fluid shifts and significant blood loss, and is generally associated with a prolonged operative time. Cumulatively, these factors help explain the postoperative complication rates associated with TAAA repair (see Table 27-5). However, the pulmonary, cardiac, renal, neurologic, and hemorrhagic complication rates associated with TAAA repair have consistently improved. A multimodality approach should be taken to the prevention of perioperative morbidity and mortality associated with this procedure.

Evidence of the role of mesenteric ischemia-reperfusion in the development of systemic morbidity after thoracoabdominal aneurysm repair continues to accumulate. The production of proinflammatory cytokines by the mesentery following ischemia-reperfusion has been demonstrated experimentally.[36,37] The mesenteric release of these cytokines results in pulmonary injury in a mouse model.[38] In another series of animal studies, inhibition of certain proinflammatory cytokines (e.g., tumor necrosis factor-α) can attenuate the systemic effects of mesenteric ischemia-reperfusion.[39,40] In the clinical setting, it has been shown that longer periods of mesenteric ischemia lead to higher complication rates following repair of thoracoabdominal aneurysms.[41] Our own experimental studies documented that a longer duration of gut ischemia-reperfusion can significantly increase the incidence of immediate and delayed-onset paraplegia in the rabbit model. Further analysis of the systemic effects of cytokine production by the mesentery after transient ischemia may lead to improvements in outcomes after thoracoabdominal aortic operations.

PULMONARY COMPLICATIONS

Pulmonary insufficiency, need for tracheotomy, and prolonged ventilator dependency are the most common complications associated with TAAA repair. The high incidence of respiratory morbidity is related to the prevalence of preoperative chronic obstructive pulmonary disease, the frequency of tobacco use, the deleterious impact of a thoracophrenolaparotomy on respiratory mechanics, intraoperative lung manipulation and barotrauma, and increased pulmonary microvascular permeability following ischemia-reperfusion.[42,43] Prolonged postoperative ventilator dependency places the patient at increased risk of pneumonia, sepsis, and death. Svensson and collaborators showed a decrease in hospital survival from 98% to 83% and a decreased long-term (12 months) survival from 96% to 71% in patients with postoperative respiratory failure following TAAA repair.[44]

Efforts to minimize the overall pulmonary-related complication rate following TAAA repair should be targeted at the preoperative, intraoperative, and postoperative phases of care. Preoperative pulmonary management includes encouraging the cessation of smoking, antibiotic treatment for any existing bronchitis, bronchodilator treatment, aggressive pulmonary physiotherapy, preoperative instructions in the use of incentive spirometry, and epidural analgesia for postoperative pain relief. Additionally, systemic corticosteroid therapy may be considered for patients with marginal lung function.[45] Intraoperatively, double-lumen tracheal intubation with full collapse of the left lung provides exposure of the descending thoracic aorta and minimizes pulmonary trauma from the combination of lung manipulation, compression, and pulmonary barotrauma, which may result from lung overexpansion following thoracophrenolaparotomy.

The ischemia-reperfusion phenomenon associated with TAAA repair is responsible for local organ injury,[46,47] as well as for injury to remote organs, including the lungs.[42] This injury pattern appears to be a neutrophil-dependent increase in microvascular permeability[48,49] that may be preventable in whole or in part by using free radical scavengers[42] and minimizing the ischemic interval through the use of partial bypass and selective visceral perfusion.[50-52] With the implementation of this pulmonary protocol, including meticulous attention to pulmonary hygiene, Swan-Ganz data, serial blood gas determinations, and transcutaneous oxygen monitoring, gradual weaning from the ventilator is tolerated in the majority of patients, ensuring a successful extubation.

CARDIAC COMPLICATIONS

Cardiac complications are the next most common cause of perioperative morbidity and mortality following TAAA repair. Preoperative cardiac evaluation with resting and stress electrocardiography, as well as stress echocardiography for the assessment of valvular and ventricular function, proves invaluable in stratifying cardiac risk and determining the need for preoperative coronary angiography. Patients with angina, wall motion abnormalities on stress echocardiography, and abnormal redistribution on dipyridamole-thallium scans are at increased risk for perioperative myocardial infarction due to increases in left ventricular afterload associated with thoracic aorta cross-clamping. Anatomic cardiac evaluation in the form of coronary angiography should be performed as indicated based on the findings of the history, physical examination, and functional cardiac evaluation. In elective circumstances, these moderate- and high-risk patients should first undergo myocardial revascularization with percutaneous transluminal coronary angioplasty or coronary artery bypass grafting if they are found to have potentially threatening coronary lesions.

Preoperative evaluation of aortic valvular function should also be part of the cardiac assessment. If the patient has aortic regurgitation, there is an increased risk of acute cardiac dysfunction or even arrest during the procedure due to the increased left ventricular afterload associated with cross-clamping of the thoracic aorta. If valvular dysfunction is noted on preoperative two-dimensional echocardiography, it should be addressed before the thoracoabdominal aortic repair; if this is not feasible, intraoperative precautions need to be taken (such as atriofemoral bypass) to prevent ventricular afterload.

Other measures may also be used to minimize the risk of myocardial ischemia, including preoperative admission to an intensive care unit with Swan-Ganz and arterial monitoring and optimization of myocardial performance using antianginal and inotropic medications. Intraoperative measures recommended to decrease cardiac morbidity include cardiovascular anesthesia, TEE, continued Swan-Ganz and arterial hemodynamic monitoring, and epidural analgesia.[29,45] Additionally, the use of graft bypass during periods of aortic cross-clamping in type I and II TAAA repair can control proximal hypertension and minimize elevations in left ventricular afterload. This is achieved by increasing pump flow rates, so that preoperative pulmonary artery diastolic or left ventricular end-diastolic pressure is maintained during aortic cross-clamping; presuturing a Dacron graft from the aortic replacement graft to the left iliac artery; and initiating flow through this graft after completion of the proximal aortic anastomosis. The resultant left ventricular protection decreases the risk of perioperative myocardial infarction and pulmonary insufficiency.[53] Poldermans and coworkers, in 1999, demonstrated that perioperative beta blockade using bisoprolol also resulted in a significant reduction in cardiovascular morbidity and mortality after vascular surgery in high-risk patients.[54] The combination of temporary partial graft bypass and CSF drainage permits the safe administration of intravenous sodium nitroprusside to control proximal aortic blood pressure, providing additional myocardial protection. Sodium nitroprusside can be given under these circumstances without risking the decrease in spinal cord perfusion pressure that might otherwise result from a steal phenomenon when sodium nitroprusside is given in the absence of distal aortic perfusion.[31,55,56]

RENAL COMPLICATIONS

Patients with preoperative renal insufficiency are at increased risk of operative mortality, postoperative renal dysfunction, neurologic deficits, and late death following TAAA repair.[12,23] Postoperative renal failure is also a significant predictor of early death following TAAA repair. The two major determinants of postoperative renal failure include the extent of preexisting renal dysfunction and the duration of intraoperative renal ischemia.

Existing renal function may be preserved by minimizing or avoiding diagnostic studies requiring nephrotoxic contrast agents and adjusting or replacing medications such as angiotensin-converting enzyme inhibitors, which may exacerbate renal insufficiency. In patients with elevated serum creatinine, MRA can be used to assess aortic anatomy, with selective use of CT-angiography or conventional aortography for the evaluation of specific branch vessel anatomy that is not clearly seen with MRA. Renal artery stenosis should be specifically looked for and treated at the time of TAAA repair. Any contrast studies performed should be preceded by intravenous hydration, mannitol, and furosemide, and consideration should be given to a renal-dose dopamine infusion during and after the procedure. Recent studies suggest that acetylcysteine (Mucomyst, Mucosil) may reduce the incidence of perioperative renal dysfunction.[57]

Serum creatinine levels should be closely monitored following contrast studies, and elective procedures should be delayed until renal function returns to baseline.

Immediate preoperative intravenous volume expansion and intraoperative mannitol administration should precede aortic cross-clamping. Distal aortic perfusion with selective renal perfusion techniques is associated with a decrease in postoperative renal insufficiency,[58] as is renal perfusion using cold (4°C) Collins solution.[59] Postoperatively, low-dose intravenous dopamine at 2 to 3 μg/kg per minute is used as a renal vasodilator until the patient enters a diuretic phase with mobilization of third-space fluid.

NEUROLOGIC COMPLICATIONS

The reported incidence of neurologic injury following TAAA repair averages 13% for extensive nondissecting TAAA and is even higher for dissecting type B TAAA.[12,23] Preoperative variables predictive of neurologic deficit following TAAA repair include prior proximal aortic aneurysm repair and the presence of aortic dissection.[23] Classically, the presence of aortic dissection has been considered a predictor of neurologic morbidity after TAAA repair.[4,23,60,61] However, an analysis of 660 patients by Coselli and colleagues suggested that chronic dissection was not a risk factor for postoperative neurologic deficit.[62] This series emphasized the aggressive reattachment of intercostal and lumbar arteries, selective use of atriodistal bypass, and passive moderate hypothermia. Neurologic complications occurred in 5.5% of patients without dissection and in 5.0% of patients with dissection. Paraplegia occurred in 19% of patients who manifested acute dissection. The authors concluded that acute but not chronic dissection was a risk factor for the development of postoperative neurologic complications.[62] Intraoperative variables predictive of neurologic deficit include the duration of aortic cross-clamping, the extent of aorta replaced, and the oversewing of intercostal arteries. Postoperative hypotension and hypoxia have similarly been shown to consistently place the patient at risk for delayed-onset neurologic deficit.[63,64]

The pathophysiology of neurologic injury following TAAA repair is dictated by the severity of the ischemic insult, the degree of reperfusion injury, and spinal cord neuronal metabolism. A multimodality approach toward the prevention of neurologic injury is targeted at these three variables (Fig. 27-16).

Spinal cord perfusion pressure is equivalent to the difference between the anterior spinal artery pressure and CSF pressure (or venous pressure, whichever is greater).[65] Therefore, maintaining a spinal cord perfusion pressure that minimizes or eliminates ischemia can be achieved by increasing the spinal cord mean arterial pressure, decreasing the CSF pressure, or both. My approach to increasing the spinal cord perfusion pressure includes maintaining a high proximal systolic blood pressure (150 to 170 mm Hg) to maximize collateral blood flow, as well as routinely draining CSF during and after the operative procedure. Additionally, temporary graft bypass provides oxygenated blood flow to unopened portions of the distal aorta, including the lower intercostal, lumbar, and pelvic arteries; the technique of staged clamping and sequential anastomosis is used to perform proximal aortic procedures. I routinely attempt to reimplant all major patent intercostal arteries with either a single-cuff or multicuff Carrel patch technique. Some surgeons have advocated the oversewing of

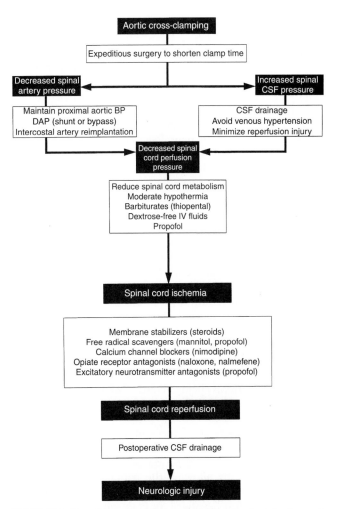

FIGURE 27–16 • Diagram of the cascade of pathophysiologic events leading to neurologic injury *(black boxes)* and the multimodality approach aimed at preventing neurologic injury *(white boxes)* during and after thoracoabdominal aortic aneurysm repair. BP, blood pressure; CSF, cerebrospinal fluid; DAP, distal aortic perfusion; IV, intravenous.

all patent intercostal and lumbar vessels to minimize clamp time and reduce neurologic complications.[60] Most series, however, demonstrate significant reduction in postoperative neurologic deficits when reimplantation of patent intercostal vessels in certain critical regions is performed.[66] Reattachment of patent arteries between the T-8 and L-1 levels appears to be most crucial.[66,67]

Several authors have demonstrated the clinical benefit of CSF drainage to lower the CSF pressure, thus maximizing spinal cord perfusion pressure for any mean arterial blood pressure.[3,27,68] I place an intrathecal catheter at the lumbar level immediately preceding the operation. This catheter is connected to an external drainage system (EDMS, Pudenz-Shulte Medical Corp., Goleta, Calif.), which allows the monitoring of CSF pressure and automatic overflow drainage of CSF whenever the pressure rises above 10 cm H_2O. Similarly, other investigators showed a statistically significant decrease in the incidence of neurologic injury associated with TAAA repair with a combination of DAPP and CSF drainage.[5,31] Safi and associates demonstrated a total neurologic complication rate of 9% for the treatment group (DAPP, moderate hypothermia, and CSF drainage) versus 19% for a control group.[31] Subset analysis demonstrated a 13% neurologic complication rate for patients with type II TAAA in the treatment group, versus 41% in the control group. Further, in patients with aortic clamp times longer than 45 minutes, the neurologic complication rate was 13% in patients treated with the multimodality approach, versus 39% in control patients.[31] A randomized, prospective trial demonstrated significant reduction of neurologic complications with the use of CSF drainage.[69]

The restoration of blood flow to a spinal cord that has suffered any ischemic time risks a reperfusion injury. Many investigators have demonstrated the ability to modulate this reperfusion injury with free radical scavengers, antioxidants, monoclonal antibodies, excitatory neurotransmitter antagonists, opiate receptor antagonists, and calcium channel blockers.[70-76] Our protocol, which attempts to minimize the reperfusion injury, is aimed at eliminating or minimizing the initial ischemic insult. The reperfusion injury is modulated through the administration of steroids to act as membrane stabilizers and the free radical scavenger mannitol before aortic clamping and again before intercostal artery reperfusion. Experimental studies have demonstrated that apoptosis can occur in spinal motor neurons after transient aortic occlusion.[77] Pharmacologic inhibitors of such programmed cell death are currently being investigated. In the future, such agents may be included in the multimodality approach to spinal cord protection.

The last component of the multimodality approach to spinal cord protection is aimed at lowering the neuronal metabolic rate during the period of aortic cross-clamping. This is achieved by allowing the patient's temperature to drift passively to 32°C to 34°C, providing moderate systemic hypothermia that is beneficial for both spinal cord and renal protection. Barbiturate in the form of thiopental sodium has been administered to further decrease the spinal cord metabolic rate; however, the intravenous anesthetic agent propofol is now used in place of thiopental, owing to its ability to reduce central nervous system metabolic requirements for oxygen[78] while maintaining cerebral oxygenation and autoregulation.[79] Further, propofol has been shown to be a free radical scavenger, with excellent central nervous system distribution.[80,81] This may translate into enhanced central nervous system protection from ischemic injury. All intravenous fluids are dextrose-free.[82] I do not recommend the use of local spinal cord cooling through the infusion of cooling solutions into the epidural space, because acute deaths from brainstem infarction have occurred in several centers that used this technique.

HEMORRHAGIC COMPLICATIONS

Perioperative bleeding complications, including coagulopathy and reoperation for bleeding, are associated with significant morbidity and mortality. Reoperation for bleeding is a predictor of early death after TAAA repair. Svensson and colleagues demonstrated a mortality rate of 25% in patients undergoing reoperation for bleeding following TAAA repair.[61] Others have found a mortality rate as high as 58% attributable to perioperative bleeding in patients after TAAA repair.[18] In a review of the literature, the average incidence of reoperation for bleeding after TAAA repair in both dissected and

nondissected aneurysms was 7%. Additionally, hemorrhage as a cause of early death has an incidence of 14% in nondissected and 27% in dissected TAAAs.[12,23] Reoperation for bleeding is also associated with an increased risk of postoperative myocardial infarction and renal failure.[68]

The cause of bleeding associated with TAAA repair is multifactorial. It may be related to the existence of preoperative coagulopathy, inadequate surgical hemostasis, hypothermia, DIC, hemodilution, fibrinolysis, anticoagulation, the use of extracorporeal circulation, or mesenteric ischemia and reperfusion.

Up to 39% of patients with large aortic aneurysms, including TAAAs, have a significant elevation of fibrin split products preoperatively, and 4% of patients have a clinical presentation of DIC with extensive bruising, petechiae, and ecchymosis on physical examination.[83] The cause of preoperative coagulopathy in these patients is the exposed subintima and the aneurysm itself, which result in coagulation factor consumption as well as a subsequent fibrinolysis.[84] The treatment for these patients is aneurysmectomy; however, their preoperative coagulopathy and increased risk of intraoperative bleeding should be appreciated and treated with infusion of platelets and fresh frozen plasma both before and during TAAA repair.

Bleeding complications resulting from improper surgical hemostasis are usually preventable. TAAA repair requires an extensive field of dissection as well as multiple anastomotic suture lines. I use electrocautery for the majority of the dissection and limit it to necessary areas only. Suture lines are usually reinforced with felt strips.

I allow passive moderate hypothermia of 32°C to 34°C to enhance neurologic and renal protection; however, if the temperature continues to drift downward, platelet function and the enzymatic cascades of the coagulation system are negatively affected, placing the patient at risk for hypothermia-associated coagulopathy. I use a warming blanket over the lower limbs during the operative procedure. Additionally, inhalation gases and intravenous fluids are warmed. In the intensive care department, rewarming continues, with the addition of a warm air recirculating blanket.

Besides the preoperative effects on coagulation factors, it has become increasingly clear that supraceliac aortic clamping can itself affect the balance of the coagulation and fibrinolytic systems.[50,51,85] Gertler and coworkers demonstrated a decrease in clotting factors and an increase in fibrinolytic activity after placement of the supraceliac clamp.[86] Illig and colleagues also demonstrated the occurrence of a primary fibrinolytic state soon after supraceliac clamping.[87] Regardless of whether this results from mesenteric ischemia-reperfusion or from hepatic ischemia, with resulting poor clearance of tissue plasminogen activator, it is clear that supraceliac aortic clamping results in an overall state of hypocoagulability and fibrinolysis. Further clinical and experimental studies have demonstrated that mesenteric perfusion during cross-clamping can attenuate this coagulopathy. In addition, the use of antifibrinolytic agents such as aprotinin or ε-aminocaproic acid (Amicar) may be helpful in alleviating the effect of fibrinolysis. Aggressive correction of coagulopathy postoperatively with factor replacement, antifibrinolytics, platelets, and restoration of physiologic temperature is mandatory to avoid reoperation for ongoing bleeding.

The use of extracorporeal circulation for distal aortic perfusion may contribute to the development of hemorrhagic complications. If one elects to use atriofemoral bypass, the use of heparin-coated tubing reduces the amount of systemic heparinization needed and may provide an added margin of safety, as long as the activated clotting time is maintained at longer than 180 seconds. In addition, the heparin-coated circuitry increases the biocompatibility of the extracorporeal circulation system, decreasing the activation of the complement, kininogen, fibrinolytic, and coagulation pathways. The use of heparin-coated circuitry in the performance of femoral vein–to–femoral artery DAPP during TAAA repair has been associated with decreased heparin and protamine requirements, fewer bleeding complications, less bleeding and hemolysis, and reduced transfusion requirements, compared with uncoated circuitry.[30]

Clinical Results

The efficacy of any specific surgical technique is difficult to establish because the current technique has evolved over many years and the various aspects of the procedure have been modified as additional research findings have suggested ways of improvement. Nevertheless, it is useful to tabulate the overall results in a given practice because they provide the surgeon and the patient with a general estimate of risk. Over the past 20 years, I have undertaken the surgical repair of more than 500 TAAAs using routine intercostal reimplantation and CSF drainage as the major effort to reduce neurologic deficit. Tables 27-7 and 27-8 summarize the overall morbidity and mortality associated with TAAA repair, including both elective repair and ruptured aneurysms.

Endovascular Approach to Thoracoabdominal Aortic Aneurysms

The treatment of abdominal aortic aneurysms by endovascular placement of stent-grafts represents a significant advance in the management of these lesions. The technique has undergone rapid improvements since its introduction in 1991. The application of endovascular therapy to thoracic and thoracoabdominal aneurysms has progressed less quickly, owing to a number of anatomic limitations. The need for a 20-mm proximal neck for stent attachment limits the number of lesions that are amenable to endovascular grafting. The use of carotid-subclavian transposition can create a proximal aortic neck of sufficient length to overcome this limitation. In addition, newer devices have bare proximal stents that can be

TABLE 27–8	Occurrence of Neurologic Deficit with Thoracoabdominal Aortic Aneurysms, by Type				
	Type I	Type II	Type III	Type IV	Total
No. of patients	77	139	147	137	500
No. with paraplegia or paraparesis (%)	5 (6.4)	7 (5.0)	7 (4.7)	1 (0.7)	20 (4.0)
No. with deficit at discharge (%)	2 (2.5)	5 (3.6)	2 (1.3)	0	9 (1.8)

placed across the subclavian orifice to improve fixation in the case of shorter proximal necks. The major limitation of stent-grafting for TAAA is the involvement of aortic segments that contain the origins of renal and visceral vessels. The use of composite techniques comprising transabdominal or retroperitoneal replacement of the aneurysmal abdominal aorta followed by placement of a stent-graft to exclude the descending thoracic aneurysm holds promise for expanding the application of this technique to more complex lesions. The inability to reimplant large patent intercostal arteries during endovascular stent-graft placement raises concerns about postoperative paraplegia.

EARLY RESULTS

The earliest devices for excluding thoracic aortic aneurysms were "homemade." Commercially produced stent-grafts designed specifically for TAAA are currently in clinical trials. The results of endovascular stent-grafting for descending thoracic aneurysms in a series of 103 high-risk patients have been published.[88] The authors reported a mortality rate of 9% and an early endoleak rate of 24%. Other major complications included stroke in 7%, paraplegia or paraparesis in 3%, myocardial infarction in 2%, and pulmonary complications in 12% of patients. There was a tendency toward higher paraplegia rates in patients with simultaneous abdominal and descending thoracic aneurysms. The high incidence of stroke was believed to be due to manipulation of catheters and sheaths in and around the aortic arch and its branches. In my own experience with more than 100 thoracic and thoracoabdominal aneurysms, three cases of delayed-onset paraplegia were noted—one on the first postoperative day, one on the fourth postoperative day, and one 6 weeks after operation. Other series have also documented neurologic injury occurring after endovascular repair.[89,90] Interestingly, reversal of neurologic deficits has occurred in some of these patients after instituting temporary CSF drainage.

In my own experience with the endovascular repair of more than 100 thoracic and thoracoabdominal aneurysms, complications such as endoleak and late rupture have been observed. Ongoing experience has uncovered other complications. Delayed-onset back pain has been noted to occur in 8% of cases. In all these cases, complete exclusion of the lesion without evidence of endoleak was demonstrated angiographically. This symptom may be related to muscle ischemia due to intercostal artery thrombosis. The development of clinically significant pleural effusion occurred in 10% of patients, some of whom required thoracentesis; in one

TABLE 27–7	Mortality of Thoracoabdominal Aortic Aneurysms, by Type				
	Type I	Type II	Type III	Type IV	Total
No. of patients	77	139	147	137	500
No. of OR deaths (%)	5 (6.5)	2 (1.4)	2 (1.3)	0	9 (1.8)
No. of 30-day deaths (%)	4 (5.2)	7 (5.0)	9 (6.1)	2 (1.4)	22 (4.4)
Total deaths (%)	9 (11.7)	9 (6.4)	11 (7.4)	2 (1.4)	31 (6.2)

OR, operating room.

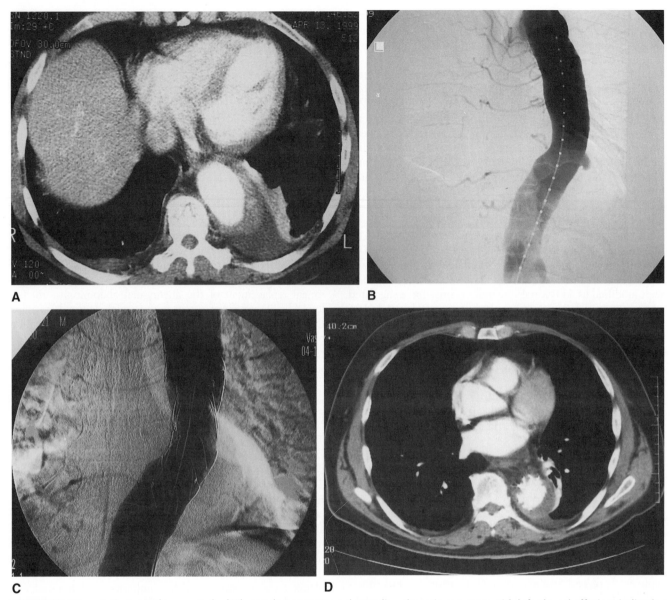

FIGURE 27–17 • *A,* Computed tomography (CT) scan demonstrates a descending thoracic aneurysm with left pleural effusion, indicating a contained rupture. *B,* Preoperative angiogram illustrates penetrating ulcer of the descending thoracic aorta. *C,* Intraoperative angiogram shows exclusion of the aneurysm with a stent-graft. *D,* Postoperative CT scan indicates successful exclusion of the descending thoracic aneurysm without endoleak.

patient, thoracentesis had to be repeated. The cause of this complication is unclear but may represent an inflammatory reaction due to stent compression of the aortic wall. Figure 27-17 demonstrates the case of a man who presented with a contained rupture of a descending thoracic aneurysm. The angiogram showed a penetrating ulcer in the descending aorta, and the CT scan revealed fluid around the aorta, indicating a contained rupture. An intraoperative angiogram and follow-up CT scan demonstrated exclusion of the aneurysm with the stent-graft. As experience with this technology expands, we can expect a larger role for endovascular therapy in thoracic and abdominal aneurysmal disease.

Conclusions

The care of patients with TAAAs has been an evolutionary process in which past techniques have undergone improvement and reapplication and other techniques have been newly introduced or discarded. Although all the complexities of the pathophysiology of TAAA repair are not fully understood, research has greatly improved our knowledge over the past 20 years. Continued research efforts are necessary to provide a more thorough understanding of these processes, enabling us to further refine risk assessment, incorporate useful surgical and perioperative support techniques, and expand the multimodality prevention of perioperative complications. It is hoped that this will allow a further reduction in the morbidity and mortality associated with this most formidable of vascular surgical procedures. Perhaps the ability to treat TAAA from remote access sites using endovascular techniques will lead to improved outcomes, but the applicability of this technology to such complex lesions and its durability have yet to be demonstrated and must await further study.

ACKNOWLEDGMENT

I thank James Green for the original artwork appearing in this chapter.

REFERENCES

1. Etheredge SN, Yee J, Smith JV, et al: Successful resection of a large aneurysm of the upper abdominal aorta and replacement with homograft. Surgery 38:1171-1181, 1955.
2. Hollier LH: Technical modifications in the repair of thoracoabdominal aortic aneurysms. In Greenhalgh RM (ed): Vascular Surgical Techniques. London, WB Saunders, 1989, pp 144-151.
3. Hollier LH, Money SR, Naslund TC, et al: Risk of spinal cord dysfunction in patients undergoing thoracoabdominal aortic replacement. Am J Surg 164:210-214, 1992.
4. Crawford ES, Crawford JL, Safi HJ, et al: Thoracoabdominal aortic aneurysms: Preoperative and intraoperative factors determining immediate and long-term results of operations in 605 patients. J Vasc Surg 3:389-404, 1986.
5. Safi HJ, Bartoli S, Hess KR, et al: Neurologic deficit in patients at high risk with thoracoabdominal aortic aneurysms: The role of cerebral spinal fluid drainage and distal aortic perfusion. J Vasc Surg 20:434-443, 1994.
6. Miller DC: Acute dissection of the descending thoracic aorta. Chest Surg Clin N Am 2:347-378, 1992.
7. DeBakey ME, Henley WS, Cooley DA, et al: Surgical management of dissecting aneurysms of the aorta. J Cardiovasc Surg 49:130-149, 1965.
8. Daily PO, Trueblood HW, Stinson EB, et al: Management of acute aortic dissections. Ann Thorac Surg 10:237-247, 1970.
9. Meng RL, Najafi H, Javid H, et al: Acute ascending aortic dissection: Surgical management. Circulation 64(Suppl 2):II-231-II-234, 1981.
10. Appelbaum A, Karp RB, Kirklin JW: Ascending vs descending aortic dissections. Ann Surg 183:296-300, 1976.
11. Doroghazi RM, Slater EE, DeSanctis RW, et al: Long-term survival of patients with treated aortic dissection. J Am Coll Cardiol 3:1026-11034, 1984.
12. Panneton JM, Hollier LH: Nondissecting thoracoabdominal aortic aneurysms: Part I. Ann Vasc Surg 9:503-514, 1995.
13. Coselli JS, LeMaire SA, Buket S: Marfan syndrome: The variability and outcome of operative management. J Vasc Surg 21:432-443, 1995.
14. Cikrit CF, Miles JH, Silver D: Spontaneous arterial perforation: The Ehlers-Danlos specter. J Vasc Surg 5:248-255, 1987.
15. Hollier LH, Money SR, Creely B, et al: Direct replacement of mycotic thoracoabdominal aneurysms. J Vasc Surg 18:477-485, 1993.
16. Bickerstaff LK, Pairolero PC, Hollier LH, et al: Thoracic aortic aneurysms: A population-based study. Surgery 92:1103-1108, 1982.
17. Crawford ES, DeNatale RW: Thoracoabdominal aortic aneurysm: Observations regarding the natural course of the disease. J Vasc Surg 3:578-582, 1986.
18. Cambria RA, Gloviczki P, Stanson AW, et al: Outcome and expansion rate of 57 thoracoabdominal aortic aneurysms managed nonoperatively. Am J Surg 170:213-217, 1995.
19. Fann JI, Miller C: Basic data underlying clinical decision making: Aortic dissection. Ann Vasc Surg 9:311-323, 1995.
20. Pressler V, McNamara JJ: Thoracic aortic aneurysm: Natural history and treatment. J Thorac Cardiovasc Surg 79:489-498, 1980.
21. Ergin MA, Phillips RA, Galla JD, et al: Significance of distal false lumen after type A dissection repair. Ann Thorac Surg 57:820-825, 1994.
22. Erbel R, Oelert H, Meyer J, et al: Effect of medical and surgical therapy on aortic dissection evaluated by transesophageal echocardiography: Implications for prognosis and therapy. Circulation 87:1604-1615, 1993.
23. Panneton JM, Hollier LH: Dissecting descending thoracic and thoracoabdominal aortic aneurysms: Part II. Ann Vasc Surg 9:596-605, 1995.
24. Pennell RC, Hollier LH, Lie JT, et al: Inflammatory abdominal aortic aneurysms: A thirty year review. J Vasc Surg 2:859-869, 1985.
25. Crawford ES, Hess KR, Cohen ES, et al: Ruptured aneurysm of the descending thoracic and thoracoabdominal aorta. Ann Surg 213:417-426, 1991.
26. Dupuy DE, Hollier LH: Cine magnetic resonance angiography. In Greenhalgh RM (ed): Vascular Imaging for Surgeons. London, WB Saunders, 1995, pp 31-40.
27. McCullough JL, Hollier LH, Nugent M: Paraplegia after thoracic aortic occlusion: Influence of cerebrospinal fluid drainage. Experimental and early clinical results. J Vasc Surg 7:153-160, 1988.
28. Smeets HJ, Kievit J, Dulfer FT, vanKleef JW: Endocrine-metabolic response to abdominal aortic surgery: A randomized trial of general anesthesia versus general plus epidural anesthesia. World J Surg 17:601-606, 1993.

29. Kirno K, Friberg P, Grzegorczyk A, et al: Thoracic epidural anesthesia during coronary artery bypass surgery: Effects on cardiac sympathetic activity, myocardial blood flow and metabolism, and central hemodynamics. Anesth Analg 79:1075-1081, 1994.
30. von Segesser LK, Killer I, Jenni R, et al: Improved distal circulatory support for repair of descending thoracic aortic aneurysms. Ann Thorac Surg 56:1373-1380, 1993.
31. Safi HJ, Hess KR, Randel M, et al: Cerebral spinal fluid drainage and distal aortic perfusion: Reducing neurologic complications in repair of thoracoabdominal aortic aneurysm types I and II. J Vasc Surg 23:223-228, 1996.
32. Cambria RP, Davison JK, Giglia JS, Gertler JP: Mesenteric shunting decreases visceral ischemia during thoracoabdominal aneurysm repair. J Vasc Surg 27:745-749, 1998.
33. Gloviczki P, Cross SA, Stanson AW, et al: Ischemic injury to the spinal cord or lumbosacral plexus after aorto-iliac reconstruction. Am J Surg 162:131-136, 1991.
34. Rectenwald JE, Huber TS, Martin TD, et al: Functional outcome after thoracoabdominal aortic aneurysm repair. J Vasc Surg 35:640-647, 2002.
35. Derrow AE, Seeger JM, Dame DA, et al: The outcome in the United States after thoracoabdominal aortic aneurysm repair, renal artery bypass, and mesenteric revascularization. J Vasc Surg 34:54-61, 2001.
36. Bathe OF, Chow AWC, Phang PT: Splanchnic origin of cytokines in a porcine model of mesenteric ischemia-reperfusion. Surgery 123:79-88, 1998.
37. Tamion F, Richard V, Lyoumi S, et al: Gut ischemia and mesenteric synthesis of inflammatory cytokines after hemorrhagic or endotoxic shock. Am J Physiol 273:G314-G321, 1997.
38. Welborn MB III, Douglas WG, Abouhamze Z, et al: Visceral ischemia-reperfusion injury promotes tumor necrosis factor and interleukin-1 dependent organ injury in the mouse. Shock 6:171-176, 1996.
39. Yao YM, Sheng ZY, Yu Y, et al: The potential etiologic role of tumor necrosis factor in mediating multiple organ dysfunction in rats following intestinal ischemia-reperfusion injury. Resuscitation 29:157-168, 1995.
40. Yao YM, Bahrami S, Redl H, Schlag G: Monoclonal antibody to tumor necrosis factor-α attenuates hemodynamic dysfunction secondary to intestinal ischemia/reperfusion in rats. Crit Care Med 24:1547-1553, 1996.
41. Vermeulen EG, Blankenstein JD, van Urk H: Is organ ischemia a determinant of the outcome of operations for suprarenal aortic aneurysms? Eur J Surg 165:441-445, 1999.
42. Paterson IS, Klausner JM, Goldman G, et al: Pulmonary edema after aneurysm surgery is modified by mannitol. Ann Surg 210:796-801, 1989.
43. Klausner JM, Paterson IS, Mannick JA, et al: Reperfusion pulmonary edema. JAMA 261:1030-1035, 1989.
44. Svensson LG, Hess KR, Coselli JS, et al: A prospective study of respiratory failure after high risk surgery on thoracoabdominal abdominal aorta. J Vasc Surg 14:271-282, 1991.
45. Hallett JW Jr, Bower TC, Cherry KJ Jr, et al: Selection and preparation of high-risk patients for repair of abdominal aortic aneurysms. Mayo Clin Proc 69:763-768, 1994.
46. Murphy ME, Kolvenbach R, Aleksis M, et al: Antioxidant depletion in aortic crossclamping ischemia: Increase of the plasma α-tocopheryl quinone/α-tocopherol ratio. Free Radic Biol Med 13:95-100, 1992.
47. Tan S, Gelman S, Wheat JK, Parks DA: Circulating xanthine oxidase in human ischemia reperfusion. South Med J 88:479-482, 1995.
48. Seekamp A, Mulligan MS: Role of 2 integrins and ICAM-1 in lung injury following ischemia-reperfusion of rat hind limbs. Am J Pathol 143:464-472, 1993.
49. Seekamp A, Mulligan MS, Till GO, Ward PA: Requirements for neutrophil products and L-arginine in ischemia-reperfusion injury. Am J Pathol 142:1217-1226, 1993.
50. Cohen JR, Angus L, Asher A, et al: Disseminated intravascular coagulation as a result of supraceliac clamping: Implications for thoracoabdominal aneurysm repair. Ann Vasc Surg 1:552-557, 1987.
51. Cohen JR, Schroder W, Leal J, Wise L: Mesenteric shunting during thoracoabdominal aortic clamping to prevent disseminated intravascular coagulation in dogs. Ann Vasc Surg 2:261-267, 1988.
52. Kazui M, Andreoni KA, Williams GM, et al: Visceral lipid peroxidation occurs at reperfusion after supraceliac aortic cross-clamping. J Vasc Surg 19:473-477, 1994.
53. Hug HR, Taber RE: Bypass flow requirements during thoracic aneurysmectomy with particular attention to the prevention of left heart failure. J Thorac Cardiovasc Surg 57:203-213, 1969.
54. Poldermans D, Boersma E, Bax JJ, et al: The effect of bisoprolol on perioperative mortality and myocardial infarction in high risk patients undergoing vascular surgery: Dutch Echocardiographic Cardiac Risk Evaluation Applying Stress Echocardiography Study Group. N Engl J Med 341:789-794, 1999.

55. Simpson JI, Eide TR, Schiff GA, et al: Effect of nitroglycerin on spinal cord ischemia after thoracic aortic cross-clamping. Ann Thorac Surg 61:113-117, 1996.

56. Cernaianu AC, Olah A, Cilley JH Jr, et al: Effects of sodium nitroprusside on paraplegia during cross-clamping of the thoracic aorta. Ann Thorac Surg 56:1035-1038, 1993.

57. Tepel M, Giet M, Schwarzfeld C, et al: Prevention of radiographic-contrast-agent-induced reduction in renal function by acetylcysteine. N Engl J Med 343:180-184, 2000.

58. Kazui T, Komatsu S, Yokoyama H: Surgical treatment of aneurysms of the thoracic aorta with the aid of partial cardiopulmonary bypass: An analysis of 95 patients. Ann Thorac Surg 43:622-627, 1987.

59. Gloviczki P, Toomey BJ, Panneton JM: Visceral and spinal cord protection during repair of thoracoabdominal aortic aneurysms: The Mayo Clinic experience. In Weimann S (ed): Thoracic and Thoracoabdominal Aortic Aneurysm. Bologna, Italy, Monduzzi Editore, 1994, pp 189-198.

60. Acher CW, Wynn MM, Hoch JR, et al: Combined use of cerebrospinal fluid drainage and naloxone reduces the risk of paraplegia in thoracoabdominal aneurysm repair. J Vasc Surg 19:236-248, 1994.

61. Svensson LG, Crawford ES, Hess KR, et al: Experience with 1509 patients undergoing thoracoabdominal aortic operations. J Vasc Surg 17:357-370, 1993.

62. Coselli JS, LeMaire SA, Poli de Figueiredo L, Kirby RP: Paraplegia after thoracoabdominal aortic aneurysm repair: Is dissection a risk factor? Ann Thorac Surg 63:28-36, 1997.

63. Moore WM Jr, Hollier LH: The influence of severity of spinal cord ischemia in the etiology of delayed-onset paraplegia. Ann Surg 213:427-432, 1991.

64. Hill AB, Kalman PG, Johnston KW, et al: Reversal of delayed-onset paraplegia after thoracic aortic surgery with cerebrospinal fluid drainage. J Vasc Surg 20:315-317, 1994.

65. Hollier LH: Protecting the brain and spinal cord. J Vasc Surg 5:524-528, 1987.

66. Svennson LG, Hess KR, Coselli JS, Safi HJ: Influence of segmental arteries, extent, and atriofemoral bypass on postoperative paraplegia after thoracoabdominal aortic operations. J Vasc Surg 20:255-262, 1994.

67. Safi HJ, Miller CC III, Carr C, et al: Importance of intercostal artery reattachment during thoracoabdominal aortic aneurysm repair. J Vasc Surg 27:58-66, 1998.

68. Hollier LH, Symmonds JB, Pairolero PC, et al: Thoracoabdominal aortic aneurysm repair: Analysis of postoperative morbidity. Arch Surg 123:871-875, 1988.

69. Coselli JS, LeMaire SA, Schmittling ZC, Koksoy C: Cerebrospinal fluid drainage in thoracoabdominal aortic surgery: Results of a prospective, randomized trial. Semin Vasc Surg 13:308-314, 2000.

70. Granke K, Hollier LH, Zdrahal P, Moore W: Longitudinal study of cerebral spinal fluid drainage in polyethylene glycol-conjugated superoxide dismutase in paraplegia associated with thoracic aortic cross-clamping. J Vasc Surg 13:615-621, 1991.

71. Coles JC, Ahmed SN, Mehta HU, Kaufmann JCE: Role of free radical scavenger in protection of spinal cord during ischemia. Ann Thorac Surg 41:551-556, 1986.

72. Wisselink W, Money SR, Crockett DE: Ischemia-reperfusion injury of the spinal cord: Protective effect of the hydroxyl radical scavenger dimethylthiourea. J Vasc Surg 20:444-450, 1994.

73. Clark WM, Madden KP, Rothlein R, Zivin JA: Reduction of central nervous system ischemic injury by monoclonal antibody to intracellular adhesion molecule. J Neurosurg 75:623-627, 1991.

74. Madden KP, Clark WM, Marcoux FW, et al: Treatment with conotoxin, an "N-type" calcium channel blocker, in neuronal hypoxic-ischemic injury. Brain Res 537:256-262, 1990.

75. Fowl RJ, Patterson RB, Gewirtz RJ, Anderson DK: Protection against postischemic spinal cord injury using a new 21-aminosteroid. J Surg Res 48:597-600, 1990.

76. Yum SW, Faden AI: Comparison of the neuroprotective effects of the N-methyl-D-aspartate antagonist MK-801 and the opiate-receptor antagonist nalmefene in experimental spinal cord ischemia. Arch Neurol 47:277-281, 1990.

77. Sakurai M, Hayashi T, Abe K, et al: Delayed and selective motor neuron death after transient spinal cord ischemia: A role of apoptosis. J Thorac Cardiovasc Surg 115:1310-1315, 1998.

78. Smith I, White PF, Nathanson M, Gouldson R: Propofol: An update on its clinical use. Anesthesiology 81:1005-1043, 1994.

79. Newman MF, Murkin JM, Roach G, et al: Cerebral physiologic effects of burst suppression doses of propofol during nonpulsatile cardiopulmonary bypass: CNS Subgroup of McSPI. Anesth Analg 81:452-457, 1995.

80. Murphy PG, Bennett JR, Myers DS, et al: The effect of propofol anaesthesia on free radical-induced lipid peroxidation in rat liver microsomes. Eur J Anaesthesiol 10:261-266, 1993.

81. Shyr MH, Tsai TH, Tan PP, et al: Concentration and regional distribution of propofol in brain and spinal cord during propofol anesthesia in the rat. Neurosci Lett 184:212-215, 1995.

82. LeMay DR, Neal S, Zelenock GB, D'Alecy LG: Paraplegia in the rat induced by aortic cross-clamping: Model characterization and glucose exacerbation of neurologic deficit. J Vasc Surg 6:383-390, 1987.

83. Fisher DF, Yawn DH, Crawford ES: Preoperative disseminated intravascular coagulation caused by abdominal aortic aneurysm. Arch Surg 118:1252-1255, 1983.

84. Thompson RW, Adams DH, Cohen JR: Disseminated intravascular coagulation caused by abdominal aortic aneurysm. J Vasc Surg 4:184-186, 1986.

85. Godet G, Samama CM, Ankri A, et al: Mécanismes et prédiction des complications hémorragiques au cours de la chirurgie des anévrysmes de l'aorte thoracoabdominale. Ann Fr Anesth Reanim 9:415-422, 1990.

86. Gertler JP, Cambria RP, Brewster DC, et al: Coagulation changes during thoracoabdominal aortic aneurysm repair. J Vasc Surg 24:936-945, 1996.

87. Illig KA, Green RM, Ouriel K, et al: Primary fibrinolysis during supraceliac aortic clamping. J Vasc Surg 25:244-251, 1997.

88. Dake MD, Miller DC, Mitchell RS, et al: The first generation of endovascular stent-grafts for patients with descending thoracic aortic aneurysms. J Thorac Cardiovasc Surg 116:689-704, 1998.

89. Kasirajan K, Dolmatch B, Ouriel K, Clair D: Delayed onset of ascending paralysis after thoracic aortic stent graft deployment. J Vasc Surg 31:196-199, 2000.

90. Greenberg R, Resch T, Nyman U, et al: Endovascular repair of descending thoracic aortic aneurysms: An early experience with intermediate-term follow-up. J Vasc Surg 31:147-156, 2000.

Questions

1. **Which of the following statements about the Crawford classification of thoracoabdominal aortic aneurysms is true?**
   (a) It is based on the extent of aortic involvement
   (b) It applies to degenerative and dissected aneurysms
   (c) It designates thoracoabdominal aortic aneurysms as type I through type IV
   (d) It allows comparisons among aneurysm types and treatment groups
   (e) All of the above

2. **Each of the following classification systems describes aortic dissections except**
   (a) DeBakey
   (b) Crawford
   (c) Stanford
   (d) Najafi
   (e) University of Alabama
   (f) Massachusetts General Hospital

3. **Which of the following is the most common cause of thoracoabdominal aortic aneurysms?**
   (a) Atherosclerotic medial degenerative disease
   (b) Dissection
   (c) Marfan's syndrome
   (d) Ehlers-Danlos syndrome
   (e) Takayasu's aortitis

4. Assign a number (1 = shortest expected survival through 5 = longest expected survival) to each of the following 6-cm thoracoabdominal aortic aneurysms:
   (a) Repaired, nondissecting
   (b) Not operated, nondissecting
   (c) Ruptured
   (d) Repaired, dissecting
   (e) Not operated, acute, dissecting

5. What is the most accurate diagnostic modality for the diagnosis of thoracoabdominal aortic aneurysm?
   (a) Physical examination
   (b) Ultrasonography
   (c) Computed tomography
   (d) Angiography
   (e) Transesophageal echocardiography

6. The preoperative evaluation of patients being considered for thoracoabdominal aortic aneurysm repair should include which of the following systems?
   (a) Respiratory
   (b) Cardiac
   (c) Renal
   (d) Peripheral vascular
   (e) Coagulation
   (f) All of the above

7. Pulmonary complications following thoracoabdominal aortic aneurysm repair may be reduced by which of the following?
   (a) Maximizing preoperative pulmonary function
   (b) Administering epidural anesthesia or analgesia
   (c) Reducing the ischemia-reperfusion phenomenon
   (d) Minimizing pulmonary trauma
   (e) All of the above

8. All of the following modalities are cardioprotective during thoracoabdominal aortic aneurysm repair except
   (a) Epidural anesthesia or analgesia
   (b) Supranormal left ventricular end-diastolic pressures
   (c) Preoperative myocardial revascularization
   (d) Sodium nitroprusside
   (e) Distal aortic perfusion

9. Preoperative renal insufficiency in patients with thoracoabdominal aortic aneurysms is associated with an increased risk of which of the following?
   (a) Operative mortality
   (b) Postoperative renal dysfunction
   (c) Neurologic deficits
   (d) Late death
   (e) All of the above

10. Variables predictive of neurologic deficit following thoracoabdominal aortic aneurysm repair include which of the following?
    (a) Prior proximal aortic aneurysm repair
    (b) Aortic dissection
    (c) Duration of aortic cross-clamping
    (d) Extent of aorta replaced
    (e) Oversewing of intercostal arteries
    (f) All of the above

11. Techniques shown to reduce the incidence of neurologic deficit after thoracoabdominal aortic aneurysm repair include all of the following except
    (a) Cerebrospinal fluid drainage
    (b) Moderate hypothermia
    (c) Distal aortic perfusion
    (d) Reduction of the ischemia-reperfusion phenomenon
    (e) Hyperglycemia

Answers

1. e 2. b 3. a 4. a-5, b-3, c-1, d-4, e-2 5. c
6. f 7. e 8. b 9. e 10. f 11. e

28

Jerry Goldstone

Aneurysms of the Aorta and Iliac Arteries

Aneurysms of the abdominal aorta are common. It is estimated that 1.7 million people have this condition, and 190,000 new cases are diagnosed and more than 50,000 repairs are performed annually in the United States. The incidence (the number of new cases) of this entity has been increasing for more than 3 decades, having tripled since 1970, and is now estimated at between 30 and 66 per 1000 persons. Unfortunately, the age-specific death rate from ruptured aneurysms has also increased. The increased incidence has been noted in the United States as well as other Western countries and is due not only to the aging of the population and improved diagnostic methods but also to an absolute increase in the number of new cases.[1-4] The incidence and prevalence (the number of existing cases) vary, depending on a number of factors, including the population studied; it is lowest in unselected groups and higher in patient groups with other atherosclerotic lesions (Table 28-1).[5-10] In a study at Massachusetts General Hospital, abdominal aortic aneurysms were found in 2% of 24,000 consecutive autopsies.[5] In a more recent autopsy series from Malmö, Sweden, abdominal aortic aneurysms were found in 4.3% of men and 2.1% of women.[6] This last study, as well as others, was performed on an almost entirely white population, and it is known that aneurysms are most common in white males. The prevalence in screening studies from Asian and African countries is much lower, as it is among African and Hispanic Americans (ratio of

white to African American is 3.5:1). The male-female ratio is 4:1 to 5:1 in the 60- to 70-year age group, but beyond age 80 the ratio approaches 1:1. The frequency of aneurysms increases steadily in men older than 55 years, reaching a peak of 5.9% at 80 to 85 years. In women, there is a continuous increase after 70 years of age, reaching a peak of 4.5% at older than 90 years. In community screening programs, the prevalence in men 65 to 74 years old ranges from 2.7% to 3.4%, whereas in elderly hypertensive men and women, the prevalence is 10.7% to 12%.[11,12] The increased incidence noted over the past 3 decades has occurred in both men and women during a time when the incidence of death from coronary artery and other forms of atherosclerosis has been decreasing.

Abdominal aortic aneurysms have a propensity for sudden rupture leading to death. In the United States approximately 15,000 deaths per year are due to abdominal aortic aneurysm, making it the 13th leading cause of death. It is the 10th leading cause of death in men. The importance of this condition is obvious, in that the proportion of elderly in the population is growing, rupture is a highly lethal event, and there is no known effective medical therapy. The only way to reduce the death rate is to identify and treat these lesions before rupture occurs.

There is disagreement about what constitutes an aneurysm, and several formulas have been proposed. The ad hoc committee on reporting standards of the Society for Vascular Surgery and the International Society for Cardiovascular Surgery (North American chapter) defined an *aneurysm* as a permanent localized dilatation of an artery with an increase in diameter of greater than 50% (1.5 times) its normal diameter.[13] However, the normal aortic diameter is variable, depending on several factors, including age, sex, and blood pressure. The aortic diameter increases steadily with age. Thus, the infrarenal aortic diameter in a 75-year-old person can vary from 12.4 mm in a small woman to 27.6 mm in a large man.[14] An aortic diameter of 30 mm should not be called an aneurysm in most people, but this value has been used as the cutoff point for a number of studies on the natural history of small aneurysms. The normal sizes of the aorta in adult males and females are listed in Table 28-2.[14] Generalized dilatation

TABLE 28–1	Incidence of Abdominal Aortic Aneurysms (%)
Category	Incidence
Autopsy	1.5-3.0
Unselected patients screened by ultrasonography	3.2
Selected patients with CAD	5.0
Selected patients with PVD	10.0
Patients with femoral or popliteal aneurysms	50.0

CAD, coronary artery disease; PVD, peripheral vascular disease.

TABLE 28–2	Normal Diameter of Human Aorta*			
	11th Rib	Suprarenal Aorta	Infrarenal Aorta	Aortoiliac Bifurcation
Male	26.9 ± 3.9	23.9 ± 3.9	21.4 ± 3.6	18.7 ± 3.3
Female	24.4 ± 3.4	21.6 ± 3.1	18.7 ± 3.3	17.5 ± 2.5

*All measurements in millimeters, plus or minus standard error. Data from Steinberg CR, Morton A, Steinberg I: Measurement of the abdominal aorta after intravenous aortography in health and arteriosclerotic peripheral vascular disease. AJR Am J Roentgenol 95:703, 1965.

of an arterial segment is frequently present in patients with aneurysms. When the diameter is increased less than 50% above normal, this is termed *ectasia*, whereas *arteriomegaly* represents diffuse enlargement of the arterial tree, but not large enough to meet the definition of aneurysm.[15] Arteriomegaly is an interesting condition that is due to a systemic alteration in the elastic components of the arterial wall. It was seen in about 5% of nearly 6000 patients undergoing arteriography in one series, and there were discrete aneurysms in at least three different locations in about one third of them. All were men who were about 5 years younger than those with solitary aortic aneurysms. In some patients with abdominal aortic aneurysms, the entire aortoiliofemoral arterial tree is arteriomegalic or ectatic. Thus, an aorta of any given diameter may be merely dilated, ectatic, or an aneurysm, depending on the size of the normal aorta above the dilated segment.

Aneurysms of the infrarenal aorta are by far the most common arterial aneurysms encountered in clinical practice. They occur three to seven times more frequently than thoracic aneurysms. Men are affected more than women by a ratio of 4:1.[8] Other aneurysms frequently coexist in patients with aortic aneurysms, including common or internal iliac aneurysms (in 20% to 30% of patients) and femoropopliteal aneurysms (in about 15%). Conversely, popliteal aneurysms are markers of abdominal aortic aneurysms. Aortic aneurysms can be found in about 8% of patients who are diagnosed with a unilateral popliteal aneurysm but in up to 50% of patients who have bilateral popliteal aneurysms. In at least one group of patients with carotid atherosclerosis, there was a 10% incidence of abdominal aortic aneurysm, and in another group of patients with tortuous internal carotid arteries, a 40% incidence of aortic aneurysms was found.[16,17] Overall, multiple aneurysms occur in 3.4% to 13% of patients with thoracic aneurysms in about 12% of those with abdominal aortic aneurysms. Aortic aneurysms are found in 1.5% to 3.0% of ultrasound-screened British men older than 60 years. Aortic aneurysms have also been detected by ultrasound screening in 8.8% of male smokers older than 65 years who have peripheral vascular occlusive disease. Screening appears to be cost-effective in selected patient groups, and considerable efforts are being made by various medical groups, including the American Vascular Association, to conduct public screening programs and advocate for insurance reimbursement for such screening.[18] Because there is a well-recognized familial component to aortic aneurysms, present in about 15% to 25% of cases, screening should be recommended for all first-degree relatives of any patient with this diagnosis.

Cigarette smoking also correlates with the presence of aortic aneurysms, with an 8:1 preponderance of aneurysms in smokers compared with nonsmokers. Hypertension is another common accompanying condition, found in up to 40% of patients with aortic aneurysms. All these associations have implications regarding the cause of aneurysms.

Cause and Pathogenesis of Aortic Aneurysms

There are several well-known but uncommon causes of true abdominal aortic aneurysm, including cystic medial necrosis, dissection, Ehlers-Danlos syndrome, and syphilis. More than 90%, however, are associated with atherosclerosis, which has traditionally been considered the primary cause. Even though aneurysms and occlusive atherosclerosis share most of the same risk factors (e.g., aging, tobacco use, hyperetension, male gender) and atherosclerosis is uniformly present in the wall of aneurysms, this concept has been seriously challenged in recent years by new information that indicates the participation of several factors in addition to atherosclerosis.[19] One observation that casts doubt on atherosclerosis being the sole cause of aortic aneurysms is that most patients with aneurysmal disease do not have occlusive vascular disease involving the aortoiliofemoral segments.[20,21] It has been estimated that no more than 25% of aortic aneurysms are associated with significant occlusive disease.[22] Also, induction of aneurysms in animals fed an atherogenic diet has not been predictable, although regression of experimental atheromas has led to aneurysm formation in monkeys. These plus several other observations have led many investigators to propose that atherosclerosis is either a coincidental or a facilitating process rather than the primary cause. What is becoming clear is that complex biologic processes are responsible for the destruction of the media of the aortic wall that characterizes aneurysms.

Biochemical studies have shown decreased quantities of both elastin and collagen but an increased ratio of collagen to elastin in the walls of aneurysms.[23-26] Elastin fragmentation is the initial structural event, and elastin depletion is complete early in aneurysm development. This has been correlated with the histopathologic features of a thin, dilated wall; replacement and fragmentation of elastin in the media by a much thinner layer of collagen (mostly types I and III); loss of smooth muscle cells; and remodeling of the extracellular matrix. This thinned wall usually contains calcium as well as atherosclerotic lesions, rendering the wall brittle. Laminated thrombus lines the lumen concentrically, resulting in a nearly normal flow channel (Figs. 28-1 to 28-3), but possibly making the inner layers of the aortic wall relatively hypoxic. Aneurysms elongate as they enlarge, causing them to become bowed and tortuous.[21] It is believed that the weakening and fragmentation of the elastic lamellae (elastin) is what permits vessels to lengthen excessively and become tortuous. Thus, failure of elastin to provide sufficient retractive force in the circumferential and longitudinal directions allows for aneurysms' increased diameter and length, respectively.

The aortic wall is made up of lamellar units that consist of collagen (mainly types I and III) and elastin, as well as vascular smooth muscle cells. There are more lamellar units in the thoracic than in the abdominal aorta, and there is a further abrupt decrease below the renal arteries. This is one factor thought to play a role in the predilection for aneurysms

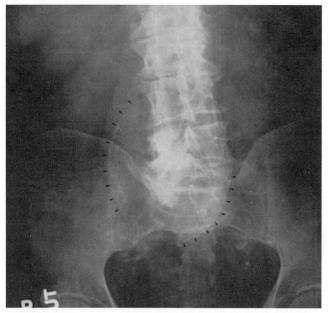

FIGURE 28–1 • Plain abdominal radiograph showing large aortic aneurysm with calcified rim *(arrowheads).*

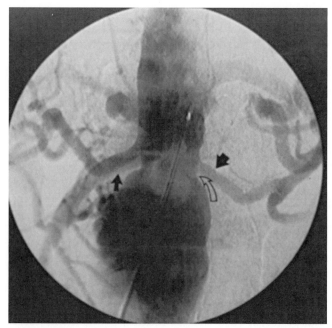

FIGURE 28–2 • Digital subtraction aortogram of large juxtarenal aneurysm. This angled view allows identification of a short infrarenal neck *(open arrow)* and origins of both renal arteries *(dark arrows).*

to develop in the terminal portion of the aorta. Mature elastin and collagen are the major structural proteins responsible for the integrity of the aortic wall. Collagen makes up about 25% of the wall of an atherosclerotic aorta but only 6% to 18% of an aneurysmal aortic wall. In addition, fragmentation of the elastin and the overall thinning of the wall contribute to its weakening.[21] The large loss of elastin is one of the most consistent biochemical and histochemical findings in human aortic aneurysms.[25,26] A chronic inflammatory cell infiltrate is also prominent. A key unresolved question is what triggers this inflammatory reaction and the subsequent chain of events. Many theories have been proposed, including a reaction to mural atherosclerotic plaque or a latent infectious process (such as *Chlamydia pneumoniae* or oral flora).[27-29]

These well-established histologic features have prompted a search for nonatherogenic mechanisms that disrupt collagen and elastin in the aortic wall. Several investigators have found excessive collagenase (MMP-1, -2, -3) activity in the wall of aneurysmal aortas, and others have found increased elastase (MMP-9) activity. These are members of a family of matrix metalloproteases that are now thought to play an essential role in aneurysm formation. MMP-9 is found in abundance in medial smooth muscle cells as well as in inflammatory cells, and increased levels have been found in the aortic wall and serum in up to 50% of patients with aortic aneurysms, but not in those with aortic occlusive disease. These increased serum levels decline to normal after aortic aneurysm repair. Increased activity of other matrix proteases in aneurysmal aortic tissue has also been reported, as has an increased leukocyte-derived elastase in the blood of smokers with aneurysms. Deficiencies in antiproteases, such as several tissue inhibitors of metalloprotease (TIMP) and α_1-antitrypsin, have also been described. The latter is one of the most important natural antagonists to elastase. This may explain the

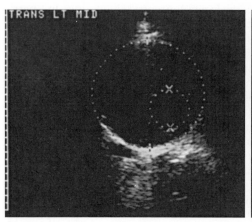

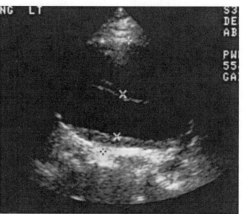

FIGURE 28–3 • *A,* B-mode ultrasound scan showing large aortic aneurysm measuring 74.7 mm in diameter and mural thrombus creating a smaller lumen (26.4 mm) *(transverse view). B,* B-mode ultrasound scan in the same patient showing large aortic aneurysm, mural thrombus, and nearly normal flow channel *(longitudinal view).*

A   **B**

association of aortic aneurysm rupture and chronic obstructive pulmonary disease (emphysema patients with reduced α_1-antitrypsin levels).[30] Another factor is the chronic inflammatory infiltrate that occurs in the outer layers of aneurysmal aortas, consisting of macrophages and T and B lymphocytes. There are also increased levels of cytokines, IgG, and IgM that are not seen in association with aging or with occlusive aortic lesions. These findings may be the explanation for the increased levels of serum inflammatory markers, such as C-reactive protein, found in patients with aneurysms but not in those with occlusive disease. These inflammatory cells and cytokines are believed to interact in some as yet unexplained way with the connective tissue cells and matrix proteins in the pathogenesis of aneurysms.[28,29] Most of the research has focused on the aortic media, but the role of the adventitia in aneurysm formation has recently been investigated. Normally, the adventitia is thought to limit maximal aortic diameter. Topical application of elastase to the adventitia leads to aneurysm formation in experimental animals solely due to degradation of elastin.[31]

Although not all the studies are conclusive, it is now generally agreed that an imbalance between aortic wall proteases and antiproteases is an important factor in the pathogenesis of human abdominal aortic aneurysms. This imbalance causes degradation of extracellular matrix and loss of structural integrity of the aortic wall and is largely responsible for the extensive remodeling of the aorta that occurs during aneurysm formation.

There is also considerable evidence that there is a genetic susceptibility to aortic aneurysm formation.[32,33] Several investigators have discovered genetically linked enzyme deficiencies that are associated with aneurysms in experimental animals. For example, Tilson showed that a deficiency in the copper-containing enzyme lysyl oxidase is the cause of aortic aneurysms in a strain of mice.[34,35] Lysyl oxidase is important in collagen and elastin cross-linking, and this enzyme defect is sex chromosome linked. In addition, several reports of familial clustering of abdominal aneurysms support the notion of a genetic predisposition to this disease.[36-39] Approximately 20% to 29% of patients with abdominal aneurysms have a first-order relative with the same condition.[38] The age- and sex-adjusted increased risk is 11.6 times, according to one report. Female siblings are at particularly high risk. The genetic pattern of increased susceptibility has not been worked out. Available evidence supports both X chromosome–linked and autosomal dominant patterns of inheritance. Among the mutant suspect genes are the type III collagen gene (col3A1) and the fibrillin gene (on chromosome 15). So-called familial aneurysms do not appear to be anatomically or clinically distinguishable from those with no familial pattern, except that they develop earlier in life, have a decreased male-female ratio of 2:1, and appear to have an increased risk of rupture. The clinical implications of these genetic studies, as limited as they are at present, strongly support the screening of first-degree relatives of patients with abdominal aortic aneurysms.

Hemodynamic (mechanical) factors may also contribute to aneurysm development. The abdominal aorta is subjected to large pulsatile stresses as a result of its tapering geometry, relatively increased stiffness, and the reflected pressure waves from the peripheral vessels. Reductions in the number of elastic lamellae and the virtual lack of vasa vasorum in the media of the distal abdominal aorta may also be factors favoring aneurysmal formation in this segment of the arterial tree, making the aorta structurally less capable of handling the increased hemodynamic stresses that occur there.[22]

In summary, contemporary concepts of aortic aneurysm development and growth must incorporate two distinctly different pathophysiologic processes: (1) elastin fragmentation as the critical structural defect required for aneurysm *formation*, and (2) collagen deposition, degradation, and remodeling governing aneurysm *enlargement*. These result in a complex remodeling of the aortic wall. Many other factors, including inflammation, smoking, biomechanical wall stress, and genetic predisposition, interact with these processes to produce the clinical features that are so well recognized. Clearly, aortic aneurysm formation is far more complex than passive dilatation. So, for the present, these aneurysms should be referred to as degenerative or nonspecific rather than atherosclerotic. They account for more than 90% of abdominal aortic aneurysms.

Once an aneurysm develops, regardless of the cause, its enlargement is governed by physical principles, especially Laplace's law. This law describes the relationship among the tangential stress (T) tending to disrupt the wall of a sphere, the radius (R), and the transmural pressure (P): $T = PR$. Thus, for a given transmural pressure, the wall tension is proportional to the radius. Once dilatation of the aorta has started, Laplace's law explains why aortic enlargement is enhanced. It also explains why large aneurysms are more prone to rupture than small ones and why hypertension is an important risk factor for rupture. Using Laplace's law, tripling the aortic radius from 2 to 6 cm results in a more than threefold increase in wall tension, and when this tension exceeds the tensile strength of the collagen in the aortic wall, disruption occurs. Although Laplace's law has long been used as the sole explanation for aneurysm enlargement and rupture, it is, at best, an imperfect explanation. It does not consider the wall thickness, which some investigators now believe is important. In addition, it does not explain why some small aneurysms rupture or why some large ones do not. Also, aneurysms usually do not rupture at the point of greatest diameter, as would be predicted by Laplace's law. Recent studies using finite element analysis have identified wall stress and strain patterns and have shown that in addition to decreased tensile strength, aneurysm walls have increased wall stress, an asymmetrical shape, and a complex radius (actually many radii) of curvature.[27] Wall stress varies with shape and thickness, and the points of maximal stress do not necessarily coincide with the location of maximal diameter. They do, however, correspond closely with the location of rupture. These stress analyses can be done using data derived from contemporary computed tomography (CT) scans and may become a useful method for predicting risk of aneurysm rupture.

Clinical Manifestations

From 70% to 75% of all infrarenal abdominal aortic aneurysms are asymptomatic when first detected.[37] Detection most often occurs during a routine physical examination or during an imaging study performed for some other reason (e.g., upper gastrointestinal series, barium enema, intravenous pyelography, lumbosacral spine radiography, or abdominal CT or ultrasound examination). Occasionally, an aneurysm is first discovered during an unrelated abdominal operation.

Abdominal aortic aneurysms may cause symptoms as a result of rupture or expansion, pressure on adjacent structures, embolization, dissection, or thrombosis.[40,41] Compression of adjacent bowel can cause early satiety and even nausea and vomiting. Because the duodenum crosses in front of the aorta, it is the part of the bowel most frequently compressed. Virtually any type of abdominal, flank, or back pain can be caused by an aneurysm. This fact often leads to delays in diagnosis. Abdominal or back pain is the most common symptom, occurring in up to one third of patients. Large aneurysms can actually erode the spine and cause severe back pain, even in the absence of rupture.

The abrupt onset of severe pain in the back, flank, or abdomen is characteristic of aneurysmal rupture or expansion. It is not certain why pain is produced by an expanding but unruptured (intact) aneurysm. The best explanation is sudden stretching of the layers of the aortic wall, with pressure on adjacent somatic sensory nerves or overlying peritoneum. Tenderness of the palpated aneurysm suggests that abdominal symptoms are arising from the aneurysm, although tenderness by itself is not a reliable indicator of impending rupture. In most surgical series, symptomatic but unruptured aneurysms account for 6% to nearly 40% of cases (average of five series totaling 311 patients: 13.7%). The determination of the timing of surgical treatment is made more difficult in these cases.

Ruptured aneurysms constitute between 20% and 25% of most series. The presence of an aneurysm is known in about 25% to 33% of patients before rupture occurs. The nature of symptoms and their time course vary, depending on the nature of the rupture.[42-44] Small tears of the aneurysmal sac may result in a small leak that temporarily seals with minimal blood loss. This is usually followed within a few hours by frank rupture, which produces a catastrophic medical emergency. Rupture most frequently occurs through the posterolateral aortic wall on the left side into the retroperitoneal space; less commonly, it occurs through the anterior wall into the free peritoneal cavity. The incidence of this latter type of rupture is higher than indicated in most surgical series, because most of these patients die before reaching the hospital. Rarely, an abdominal aortic aneurysm ruptures into the inferior vena cava or one of the iliac veins, producing an aortocaval (or aortoiliac) fistula, or it ruptures into the gastrointestinal tract, producing a primary aortoenteric fistula.

The classic clinical manifestations of ruptured aortic aneurysm consist of mid or diffuse abdominal pain, shock, and a palpable, pulsatile abdominal mass. The pain may be more prominent in the back or flank, or it may radiate into the groin or thigh. Because the most frequent site of rupture is the left posterolateral wall, pain is more commonly felt on the left side. It tends to be severe and steady. The severity of the shock varies from mild to profound, depending on the amount of blood loss. Abdominal distention is common, often preventing palpation of the pulsatile abdominal mass. The duration of symptoms may vary from a few minutes to more than 24 hours. Although aneurysm rupture is usually an acute catastrophic event, it can be contained for prolonged periods. These chronic ruptures have masqueraded as radicular compression, symptomatic inguinal hernia, femoral neuropathy, and even obstructive jaundice. It is thought that chronic contained ruptures eventually progress to free ruptures, and they should be treated surgically on an urgent basis.[45]

The pain of an expanding but intact aneurysm may closely mimic that of a ruptured one. It tends to be severe, constant, and unaffected by position. The signs of hypovolemia are absent because hypotension and shock do not usually occur in the absence of actual rupture.

The diverse and nonspecific nature of the pain caused by expanding and leaking aneurysms all too often leads to errors in diagnosis, delays in finally establishing the correct diagnosis, and catastrophic rupture in the midst of a diagnostic procedure. Occasionally, a patient with a contained rupture arrives in the emergency room with angina pectoris from blood loss and reflex tachycardia and is rapidly transported to a coronary care unit without the abdominal examination that would identify the true cause of the chest pain. Most diagnostic errors such as these are due to failure to palpate the expansile, pulsatile epigastric mass or failure to consider ruptured aneurysm as a possibility.

Diagnostic Methods

Careful physical examination can detect most large aneurysms. Except in thin patients, an abdominal aortic aneurysm must be about 5 cm in diameter to be detectable on a routine physical examination. Thus, aneurysms are seldom palpated in obese patients unless they are large. The reported accuracy in establishing the correct diagnosis by physical examination alone ranges from 30% to 90%. However, even when an aneurysm is detected, determination of its size by palpation is imprecise. Obesity, ascites, and lack of patient cooperation can impair aneurysmal detection by physical examination. Conversely, tumors or cystic lesions adjacent to the aorta, unusual aortic tortuosity, and excessive lumbar lordosis can all lead to a diagnosis of abdominal aortic aneurysm when none is present. The expansile nature of a pulsatile mass is a key element in deciding whether a pulsatile, palpable mass is an aneurysm or a transmitted pulsation.

Although physical examination detects most large aneurysms, more objective methods are necessary to measure size and identify smaller aneurysms. Size determination is especially important because it is the most important predictor of rupture and is often the basis of management decisions. Plain abdominal and lateral spine radiographs can establish the diagnosis of 67% to 75% of abdominal aortic aneurysms by detecting a fine rim of calcium representing the aortic wall (see Fig. 28-1). Unfortunately, accurate determination of maximal aortic size is possible in only about two thirds of these cases. Therefore, a negative or inadequate plain film cannot be relied on to exclude the diagnosis of aortic aneurysm.

IMAGING MODALITIES

Several imaging modalities are now widely available to establish the presence of an aortic aneurysm and accurately determine its size.[46] These include ultrasonography, CT, and magnetic resonance imaging (MRI).

Real-time B-mode ultrasonography is available in most hospitals and clinics and is the imaging method used in the large aneurysm screening and surveillance studies. It employs no ionizing radiation, provides physiologic data as well as structural detail of vessel walls and atherosclerotic plaques, and can accurately measure aneurysm size in longitudinal as well as cross-sectional directions (i.e., it is three-dimensional) (see Fig. 28-3). Compared with intraoperative measurements, ultrasonic measurements are accurate to within ±5 mm. Many studies have documented the ability of B-mode ultrasonography to establish the diagnosis (sensitivity 100%, specificity 95% to 99%) and accurately determine the size of abdominal and peripheral aneurysms.[47-49] Ultrasonography has not been as useful for imaging the thoracic or suprarenal aorta because of the overlying air-containing lung and viscera. Similarly, it has been less reliable in defining the relationship between abdominal aortic aneurysms and the renal arteries. Because ultrasonography can obtain images in longitudinal, transverse, and oblique projections, it can be especially helpful in differentiating a tortuous aorta from an aneurysm.

Ultrasonography requires considerable skill on the part of the technician to obtain a satisfactory image, and interpretation can be difficult. It is important for the image plane to be perpendicular to the axis of the vessel in order to avoid the inaccuracies of oblique measurements. The images are also impaired by obesity, intestinal gas, or barium in the bowel. The overlying bowel gas often interferes with evaluation of the iliac arteries. The major advantages of ultrasonography are its wide availability, painlessness, absence of known side effects, lack of ionizing radiation, relatively low cost, and ability to image vessels in longitudinal as well as cross-sectional planes. The studies can be performed quickly and at the bedside. In addition, the portability of ultrasound machines is advantageous for the emergency room evaluation of suspected ruptured aneurysms. Emergency room ultrasonography can establish the presence of an aneurysm in most cases, but it is not nearly as accurate in demonstrating rupture. These factors make ultrasonography the modality of choice for the initial evaluation of pulsatile abdominal or peripheral masses and for follow-up surveillance of aneurysms to determine any increase in size.

CT employs ionizing radiation to obtain cross-sectional images of the aorta and other body structures. CT images provide reliable information about the size of the entire aorta, including the thoracic portion, so the extent as well as the size of an aneurysm can be accurately measured. Modern CT scanners using helical or spiral technology and an increasing number of detectors possess sufficient spatial resolution to allow precise identification of the celiac, superior mesenteric, renal, and iliac arteries and their relationship to the aneurysm as well as adjacent organs. Major venous structures, including anomalies, can also be identified by CT.[49] The administration of intravenous contrast allows evaluation of the size of the aortic lumen, the amount and location of mural thrombus, and, in the presence of dissection, differentiation of the true lumen from the false lumen (Fig. 28-4). Contrast-enhanced CT scans are also useful for assessing the retroperitoneum and can identify retroperitoneal hematoma (aneurysmal rupture) and the periaortic fibrosis associated with inflammatory aneurysms.[50-53]

CT images are degraded by patient motion and the presence of metallic surgical clips. CT scanning requires more time and is more expensive than ultrasonography, and it provides images in only one (transverse) plane, although three-dimensional reconstructions are now widely available. CT provides more information about other abdominal and retroperitoneal structures than ultrasonography does. One of the most helpful aspects of CT is its ability to define the relationship of an aneurysm to the renal artery origins. Depending on the

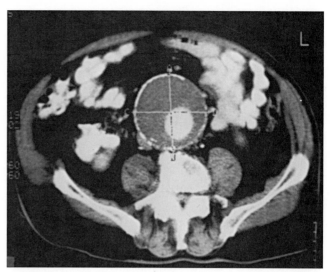

FIGURE 28-4 • Computed tomography scan of the abdomen showing a large, calcified abdominal aortic aneurysm (82.7 mm in diameter).

thickness of each CT slice and the distance between slices, this is not always accurate, especially when there is buckling of the aorta to the extent that the superior border of the aneurysm ascends anterior to the aorta. Many of the limitations of conventional CT scans are avoided by spiral or helical CT scans, which have emerged as an excellent technique to image the abdominal aorta and its branches.[54,55] Scan times are extremely short, and slices as thin as 2 to 3 mm can be obtained. This allows three-dimensional reconstruction of the overlapping cross-sectional images, producing a CT angiogram (Fig. 28-5). Spiral CT is quicker and is associated

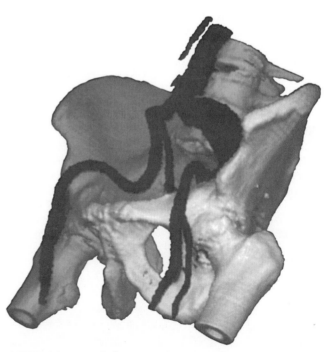

FIGURE 28-5 • Spiral computed tomography scan with three-dimensional reconstruction showing a large left common iliac aneurysm, as viewed from the inferior oblique projection.

with less radiation exposure than aortography, but it requires a relatively large volume of intravenously administered contrast material. Because the reconstructed three-dimensional images can be rotated in space and viewed from any projection, CT-angiography is an excellent method of determining the often complex relationships among the aorta, its branches, and the aneurysm. Non–contrast-enhanced images are useful for determining the degree and location of calcification in the aorta and its branch vessels. Overall, spiral CT scans are currently the most useful imaging method for evaluating the abdominal aorta and have nearly obviated the need for aortography in the evaluation of aneurysmal disease. This technique has also become an almost essential component of the process of determining an aneurysm's suitability for and size of endograft treatment.

MRI has also proved to be a useful modality for the evaluation of aortic diseases (Fig. 28-6).[51,56] MRI employs radiofrequency energy and a strong magnetic field to produce images in longitudinal, transverse, and coronal planes. MRI instruments are not as widely available as ultrasound or CT scanners, and the selection and interpretation of proper scan sequences and images require considerable experience and skill. The spatial resolution has significantly improved, but the presence of metallic surgical clips, cardiac pacemakers, and monitoring equipment makes MRI impossible to perform. Also, these studies are more expensive and require more time than either CT or ultrasonography. Nevertheless, MRI clearly distinguishes arteries and veins from viscera and other surrounding tissue. There is excellent agreement between MRI and ultrasound or CT images in determining aortic diameter, and MRI is better at demonstrating the involvement of branch vessels, especially of the renal arteries. Some authors report visualization of the renal arteries in more than 90% of cases.[51] Other advantages of MRI over CT are the lack of ionizing radiation, the ability to obtain multiplane images (now also available with CT-angiography), and the relatively large image field. In addition, MRI does not require the use of toxic contrast agents to achieve intravascular enhancement; however, paramagnetic contrast agents, such as gadolinium, can improve the imaging of vascular structures.

MRI instruments are able to quantitate blood flow, although this feature is not commonly used clinically, and they can reconstruct images to look like conventional angiograms (magnetic resonance angiography [MRA]).[46] These techniques are becoming routinely available, and magnetic resonance may become the only imaging method necessary for most patients with aortic disease of any type. However, at present, adequate visualization of aortic branch arteries is not achieved as frequently with MRA as with CT-angiography, and a significant number of patients cannot undergo magnetic resonance scanning because of claustrophobia.

Objective documentation of the aortic size should probably be accomplished with one of these imaging modalities in all patients with suspected abdominal aortic aneurysms. Each method can measure the diameter accurately. An initial scan can be used for comparison with subsequent scans to determine aneurysmal enlargement. For routine situations, ultrasonography is probably the method of choice because of its widespread availability, lower cost, and lack of ionizing radiation. When there is suspicion of suprarenal or thoracoabdominal aortic involvement or dissection, MRI or CT is preferable. For preoperative planning in these complex cases, a multiplanar study with three-dimensional reconstruction (CT-angiography, MRA) is usually necessary to clearly delineate the aneurysm, aortic branch vessels, and neighboring structures. This is especially true if treatment by endografting is being considered.

For symptomatic aneurysms, MRI and CT also have the advantage over ultrasonography because of their better ability to identify contained rupture. CT and MRI probably have equal capability to demonstrate unexpected features such as venous anomalies, perianeurysmal fibrosis, and horseshoe kidney, although the ureters are not easily identified by MRI.

AORTOGRAPHY

The limitations of aortography for the diagnosis and evaluation of aortic aneurysms, like those of plain film radiography, are well known. Because mural thrombus (which is nearly always present) tends to reduce the aneurysmal lumen size toward normal, aortography is not a reliable method to determine the diameter of an aneurysm or even to establish its presence. With better imaging methods now routinely available, aortography has little use as a diagnostic method for abdominal aortic aneurysms. However, it may be useful in the preoperative evaluation of some patients with aneurysms.[57,58] It can define the extent of an aneurysm, especially suprarenal and iliac involvement, and also the associated arterial lesions involving renal and visceral vessels, as well as distal occlusive lesions (Table 28-3; see also Fig. 28-2). Although many of these associated lesions are readily detectable and appropriately managed intraoperatively, preoperative identification is useful in planning operative strategy, especially if complex anatomy is suspected. It must be emphasized that aortography used in this way is not a diagnostic study to determine the presence or size of an abdominal aneurysm.

There are risks associated with aortography, including potential renal toxicity from the large contrast volumes that are sometimes required to adequately fill a large aneurysm sac and the branch vessels. In addition, manipulation of a retrograde catheter through the laminated mural thrombus risks distal embolization, and there is always the possibility of local complications at the arterial puncture site through which the

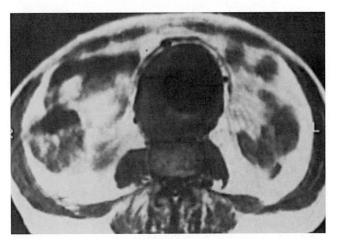

FIGURE 28–6 • Magnetic resonance image of a large abdominal aortic aneurysm showing eccentric mural thrombus and flow channel.

TABLE 28–3	Angiographically Detected Lesions Associated with Abdominal Aortic Aneurysms		
Findings	No. of Patients	Number (n)	Percent
Suprarenal extension	680	46	6.7
Renal stenosis or occlusion	763	138	18.0
Accessory or multiple renal arteries	680	92	13.5
Celiac or superior mesenteric artery stenosis	628	87	13.8
Iliofemoropopliteal stenosis or occlusion	680	298	43.8
Iliofemoropopliteal aneurysm	680	243	34.7

Collected data from Rich NM, Clagett GP, Salander JM, et al: Role of arteriography in the evaluation of aortic aneurysms. In Bergan JJ, Yao JST (eds): Aneurysms: Diagnosis and Treatment. New York, Grune & Stratton, 1982, pp 233-241; Gaspar MR: Role of arteriography in the evaluation of aortic aneurysms: The case against. In Bergan JJ, Yao JST (eds): Aneurysms: Diagnosis and Treatment. New York, Grune & Stratton, 1982, pp 243-254.

angiographic catheter is introduced. The use of digital subtraction angiographic techniques has lessened but not eliminated these risks. Aortography should be performed very selectively in patients with aneurysms for the following indications[59]: (1) clinical suspicion of visceral ischemia, (2) occlusive iliofemoral vascular lesions, (3) severe hypertension or impaired renal function in a patient in whom a concomitant renal artery stenosis would be repaired if discovered, (4) suspicion of a horseshoe kidney, (5) suspicion of suprarenal or thoracoabdominal aneurysm, and (6) presence of femoral or popliteal aneurysms. With the evolution and availability of MRI, MRA, and spiral CT, it is now possible to obtain information similar to that available from aortography, with fewer complications. The introduction of CT scanners with large numbers of detectors allows even faster scans, with improved resolution and better three-dimensional images. Sophisticated three-dimensional reconstructions of CT scans are already available on-line from commercial vendors, making these sophisticated images available to any provider who can transfer the CT data onto a CD or transmit it electronically to the imaging facility.

Risk of Aneurysm Rupture

As noted earlier, the majority of abdominal aortic aneurysms are discovered in asymptomatic patients or during an evaluation for an unrelated problem. Aneurysms are being discovered at a smaller size than when the original studies on their natural history were first published by Estes, Wright, Szilagyi, and others.[60-63] Most aneurysms detected in screening programs are small (<5 cm), and this has led to modifications in our conception of the natural history of these lesions. Even though aneurysms can cause symptoms and serious consequences from thrombosis and distal embolization, rupture is the most important risk, and the size of an aneurysm is the most important factor that determines the risk of rupture.

In general, the risk of rupture correlates directly with size: the larger the aneurysm, the greater the risk of rupture. For example, the yearly risk of rupture for abdominal aortic aneurysms[5,30,63-65] between 4 and 5.4 cm in size is about 0.5% to 1%; this increases to 6.6% for aneurysms between 6 and 7 cm and to 19% for aneurysms larger than 7 cm in diameter.[5,64,65] Calculated as 5-year rupture rates, these figures become 5%, 33%, and 95%, respectively. The steepness of a curve plotting these data increases sharply at a diameter of about 6 cm, which led to earlier recommendations to defer elective aneurysm repair until an aneurysm reached that size. Based on more contemporary data obtained from objective imaging studies, aneurysm rupture risk begins to increase at a diameter of 5 cm, which led to the adoption of this size as the important surgical decision point.[66] However, this recommendation may need to be revised in light of new data.

Two randomized, controlled clinical trials studied survival in patients with asymptomatic abdominal aortic aneurysms that were between 4 and 5.4 to 5.5 cm in diameter: the United Kingdom (UK) Small Aneurysm Trial, published in 1998, and the Veterans Administration–sponsored Aneurysm Detection and Management (ADAM) trial.[67-70] These two trials were quite similar in design, size, and results. The rupture rate for aneurysms in these trials was 0.5% to 1% per year, and neither trial showed a difference in long-term survival, the primary end point, between patients allocated to early operation or ultrasonography or CT surveillance. The 6-year survival in both groups was 64% in the UK trial and about 70% in the ADAM trial. Even though 61% of those randomized to surveillance in both studies ultimately underwent aneurysm operation for enlargement or symptoms, long-term survival was not improved by early operation. Further, delaying operation for these small aneurysms was not associated with increased operative or late mortality. These data are consistent with those from older, nonrandomized studies.[69-71] For example, population-based data from Rochester, Minnesota, showed a mean enlargement rate for aneurysms less than 5 cm in diameter of only 0.32 cm/year, and after 5 years of observation, no aneurysm smaller than 5 cm had ruptured.[72] Rupture risk may be higher in high-risk patients. The ADAM and UK trials enrolled mostly good-risk patients, but in both trials, cohorts were excluded because of refusal or being deemed unfit for elective repair. In both series, there was a higher rupture rate among the ineligible (i.e., high-risk) patients than in those randomized.

Cronenwett and associates showed that chronic obstructive pulmonary disease and systolic hypertension are predictors of increased risk of rupture of small abdominal aneurysms.[30] In a subsequent study, they found that the rate of enlargement of small aneurysms was unpredictable, but either increased systolic or decreased diastolic pressure (i.e., increased pulse pressure) was associated with an increased rate of aneurysm expansion.[73] In this study, there was considerable variability in the rate of aneurysm enlargement, even though the average rate of expansion was 0.4 cm/year in anteroposterior dimensions and 0.5 cm/year in lateral dimensions. Large aneurysms enlarge more rapidly than small ones. Some data suggest that the expansion rate of large aneurysms can be diminished by β-adrenergic blockade (propranolol).[74] Other studies showed that aneurysms are frequently elliptical rather than round and that aneurysmal expansion is initially more rapid in the lateral direction. It is interesting to recall that the most frequent site of aneurysm rupture is in the lateral wall.

In a review of four series, including their own, Cronenwett and coworkers described the outcome of 378 patients with small aortic aneurysms initially treated nonoperatively.[73] After an average follow-up of 31 months, 27% of the patients were alive with intact aneurysms, 29% had died of other causes, 39% had had elective aneurysm operations because the aneurysm diameter reached 5 to 6 cm, and 4% had suffered aneurysm rupture or acute expansion leading to emergency operation. Overall, there was a mean 5-year survival of 54% in these patients, somewhat less than the 6-year survival rates of 64% in the UK trial and 70% in the ADAM trial.[70-74]

In light of these more recent studies, autopsy studies showing high rates of rupture of small aneurysms must be viewed with caution. Some have shown that 23.4% of aneurysms between 4.1 and 5 cm rupture, and the same is true for up to 10% of aneurysms less than 4 cm in diameter.[5] Data such as these have led surgeons to recommend operation for almost all aortic aneurysms in good-risk patients. However, autopsy studies underestimate aneurysm size owing to the lack of a distending blood pressure, and several more recent studies on living patients demonstrate a rupture rate of about 1% per year for aneurysms less than 5 cm in diameter.[5]

There is little debate about the appropriateness of elective aneurysm surgery for patients with large aneurysms (>6 cm in diameter) because of the high risk of rupture and the associated mortality when rupture occurs. This may be especially true in so-called high-risk patients, because most of these patients will die from rupture and not from the conditions that caused them to be considered high risk. Some authors have reported that women have a greater risk of aneurysm rupture at a given size than men; therefore, it has been suggested that women be offered definitive treatment at a smaller aneurysm size than men.

It must be emphasized that although the risk of aneurysm rupture correlates most closely with aneurysm size, and the average rate of aneurysmal enlargement is known (0.4 to 0.5 cm/year), it is impossible to predict when a small aneurysm

may rupture in any given patient.[74] Perhaps the best explanation relates to the fact that aneurysms rupture at points of maximal wall stress, as discussed earlier, and areas of maximal wall stress do not necessarily coincide with areas of maximal diameter.[75,76] Clinical investigations of aneurysm wall stress using finite element analysis of CT-derived data are currently in progress, but for now, diameter remains the best available predictor of risk of aneurysm rupture. And although the harmlessness of a small, asymptomatic abdominal aortic aneurysm is deceptive, coronary artery disease, and not rupture, is the most frequent cause of death in patients with small aneurysms.

Risks of Surgical Treatment

The natural history of untreated abdominal aortic aneurysms is well documented. This is especially true for those aneurysms measuring 5.5 cm or less in diameter. Since the first report of successful surgical resection and graft replacement of an infrarenal aortic aneurysm in 1952, there have been many publications documenting the operative and long-term survival after surgical treatment. There has been a steady improvement in operative results for elective operations. Several large, contemporary series have reported operative mortality rates between 0.9% and 5% for university medical centers and only slightly higher rates for community hospitals.[75-91] The 1.8% operative mortality in the ADAM trial compares favorably with these (Table 28-4). This improvement in surgical results has occurred despite the fact that more patients are being operated on who are older and have more severe comorbid conditions. Preoperative detection and treatment of significant cardiac disease have been important factors.

Operative mortality in this range (<5%) justifies elective repair, even for relatively small aneurysms in good-risk patients.[66] Most of the deaths, even in elective operations, occur in so-called high-risk patients. Chronologic age is not as important as physiologic age in assessing operative risk, so patients should not be denied elective operation based solely on age. Even octogenarians can undergo elective aneurysm surgery with low morbidity and mortality rates.[80]

TABLE 28–4	Operative Mortality and Late Survival of Elective Surgical Treatment of Abdominal Aortic Aneurysm			
Reference	No. of Patients	Mean Age (Yr)	Operative Mortality (%)	Cumulative 5-Year Survival (%)
Levy et al (1966)[84]	100	64	17	34
Szilagyi et al (1966)[62]	401	—	15	49
May et al (1968)[85]	135	—	13	49
Baker and Roberts (1970)[86]	240	63	9	54
Stokes and Butcher (1973)[87]	87	—	3	60
Hicks et al (1975)[88]	225	67	8	60
O'Donnell et al (1976)[89]	63	82	5	70
Crawford et al (1981)[77]	860	66	5	63
Reigel et al (1987)[90]	499	76	3	66
Bernstein and Chan (1984)[64]	123	71	1	72
UK trial (1998)[67]	563	69	5.8	64
ADAM trial (2002)[68]	569	68	1.8	70
Dream trial (2004)[69]	174	69	4.6	Not given

Most vascular surgeons have successfully treated ruptured aneurysms in patients previously rejected for elective operation because they were considered too old.

The major risks for elective abdominal aortic aneurysm resection are similar to those for other major intra-abdominal operations and include adequacy of cardiopulmonary and renal function. High-risk patients are those with unstable angina or angina at rest, cardiac ejection fraction less than 25% to 30%, congestive heart failure, serum creatinine level greater than 3 mg/dL, and pulmonary disease manifested by room air PO_2 of less than 50 mm Hg, elevated PCO_2, or both. A substantial percentage of these high-risk patients dies of ruptured aneurysm and not from the disease that led to their categorization as high risk. With intensive perioperative monitoring and support, aneurysm resection has been carried out even in these high-risk patients, with operative mortality of less than 6% by Hollier and colleagues[92] and others.[74,77,87] Thus, even in high-risk patients, large abdominal aneurysms should be considered for elective treatment if the appropriate support facilities are available. It is in this group, however, that endovascular repair can be expected to offer a significant improvement over standard open aneurysm repair.

The use of endoluminally placed stent-grafts to treat aortic aneurysms has become a clinical reality. More than 62,000 patients have been treated worldwide in this manner.[91] Two stent-graft and deployment systems were approved for general clinical use by the U.S. Food and Drug Administration in 1999, and several others are in various stages of clinical testing. A large number of clinical and experimental studies on this subject have been published, and carefully audited information that includes 3 years of follow-up data is now available. The consistent findings are that 40% to 60% of patients with abdominal aortic aneurysms are anatomically suitable for endoluminal repair, it can be accomplished with mortality rates equal to or lower than those for open surgical repair, and morbidity rates are clearly lower than those of open surgical repair. The length of hospital stay is shortened, and patient satisfaction and surgeon enthusiasm are high. However, there is a small but disturbing incidence of endoleak, failure of the aneurysm sac to shrink, device slippage, device structural failure, and even late aneurysm rupture. Because of these late complications and problems, patients with these implants require close monitoring with CT or other studies every 6 to 12 months indefinitely. Most of the devices in current use are second generation, and continued improvements in ease of insertion, size, and durability can be expected. Because of lingering uncertainties about long-term results, there is no consensus about which patients and which aneurysms are best treated in this manner. For these reasons, at the present time, the indications for endoluminal repair are the same as those for open surgical repair in terms of aneurysm size and expected longevity. This topic is covered in detail in Chapter 22.

In spite of widespread elective aneurysm treatment programs, the incidence of aneurysm rupture has not decreased. A substantial percentage (50%) of patients whose aneurysms rupture die before reaching a medical facility.[69,70] Another 24% arrive at a hospital alive but die before a definitive operation can be performed. Thus, operative mortality figures underestimate the true significance of aneurysmal rupture. The overall mortality from ruptured aneurysms, as reported in two large community-based studies, ranges from 74% to more than 90%.

The operative results for ruptured aneurysms are not nearly as favorable as those for elective aneurysm repair and generally have not improved over the years.[93,94-96] Although there are a few series with better results, overall, nearly 50% of patients die after being operated on for rupture. The nature of the rupture influences the results. Less than 10% of patients presenting in shock with free intraperitoneal rupture survive. In contrast, stable patients with small, contained leaks have a better than 80% survival rate.

The factors contributing to failure in the treatment of ruptured abdominal aortic aneurysm have been reviewed by Hiatt and associates.[93] The four most important factors were failure to perform elective aneurysmectomy in patients with known aneurysms; errors in diagnosing rupture when it occurred, leading to delay in operation; technical errors committed during the operation (all venous injuries); and undue delays in induction of anesthesia. These are all realistically preventable. Other series have also attempted to identify factors leading to death after aortic aneurysm rupture. Repeatedly, delays in performing surgery and the total volume of blood transfused are found to be important.[94,95] Preoperative cardiac arrest, female gender, age 80 years or older, massive blood loss, and ongoing major transfusion requirements were predictors of 90% to 100% mortality in Johansen's series, which included a very efficient transport and resuscitation response.[96] Encouraging early results from the endovascular treatment of ruptures have been reported, with 92% of patients surviving. If these results are sustainable and reproducible, they will represent the most significant advance in the treatment of this highly lethal entity in several decades. Some of the differences in operative mortality among various reports are due in part to inconsistencies in patient categorization or considering all forms of rupture together. Many of these series also fail to separate patients with unruptured but symptomatic aneurysms who undergo emergency operations. The operative morbidity and mortality for this group are intermediate between elective, asymptomatic patients and those with frank rupture, averaging 16% to 19%.[28,72,97] It has been postulated that the reason for this increased mortality is the omission of thorough preoperative evaluation and preparation necessitated by the emergency operation.

Late Survival

It is accepted that the most common cause of death among patients with large abdominal aortic aneurysm is rupture and that elective surgical repair prevents rupture and is associated with excellent perioperative survival rates. Two questions must be answered. What is the long-term outlook for survivors? Is life prolonged by aneurysmectomy? After all, this is the primary objective of the detection and management of this condition. Several long-term studies using life-table methods have revealed 5-year survival rates ranging from 49% to 84% (average 61%) (see Table 28-4).[97-100]

Although these data are far more encouraging than those for the survival of patients not undergoing operation, they do not equal the survival expected for the normal age-matched population. For example, Johnson and coworkers reported a 50% survival of 7.4 years for patients surviving elective operative treatment for abdominal aneurysm,[98] whereas the age-adjusted figure for the U.S. general population was 15.7 years, and that for North Carolina was 14.5 years. These authors could not identify any influence of age on operative mortality, although it affected late mortality, as one would expect. Most of the excess late mortality could be attributed to coronary artery disease. This has led some centers to pursue an aggressive coronary evaluation and treatment protocol before elective aortic aneurysm operations.[101]

Several large surveys have shown that the safety of vascular surgical procedures in patients who have had previous coronary revascularization is comparable to that in patients with no evidence of ischemic cardiac disease, but this has not been evaluated by randomized clinical trials.[102-106] It has been estimated that, based on data from the Canadian Aneurysm Study, aggressive cardiac treatment increases the 5-year survival by only 5% to 10%.[107,108]

Assessment of Cardiac Risk

Approximately 30% to 40% of patients with aortic aneurysms do not have clinically evident coronary artery disease (e.g., no angina pectoris, no history of myocardial infarction, normal electrocardiogram [ECG], normal exercise stress test). However, there is a high prevalence (50%) of angiographically documented severe coronary artery disease in patients in whom coronary disease is clinically suspected (about 50% of the total).[101,106] The prevalence is still 20% in patients in whom the traditional clinical indicators of coronary disease are absent. Coronary artery disease is responsible for at least 50% to 60% of all perioperative and late deaths after operations on the abdominal aorta.[109] The incidence of fatal myocardial infarction after elective abdominal aortic aneurysm surgery has been reported to be as high as 4.7%, and nonfatal infarction occurs in up to 16% of patients.

It is possible to identify high-risk cardiac patients using clinical assessment, exercise stress testing, radionuclide angiography (multiple gated scan), echocardiography, dipyridamole-thallium scanning, continuous portable electrocardiographic Holter monitoring, and coronary angiography.[108,110,111] The problem is deciding which patients need cardiac screening before aneurysm surgery.[112] Clinical factors predictive of increased risk for postoperative cardiac complications include a history of previous myocardial infarction, congestive heart failure, angina pectoris, abnormal preoperative ECG, diabetes mellitus, and advanced age.[110] Dipyridamole-thallium (or dobutamine- or adenosine-thallium) myocardial scanning has replaced exercise stress testing for these elderly patients in many hospitals. It identifies areas of myocardium that are reversibly ischemic and is quite sensitive for identifying patients likely to have perioperative cardiac complications; unfortunately, its specificity is relatively low.[113,114] Determination of left ventricular ejection fraction by radionuclide angiography identifies patients with poor ventricular function. Although an ejection fraction less than 30% has been associated with increased cardiac complications in some series, it does not predict postoperative myocardial infarction or death. Continuous portable ECG monitoring of vascular surgical patients for silent ischemia associated with ST-T segment changes has been shown to correlate with postoperative myocardial infarction in some series, but additional studies are needed to verify the value of this technique. Routine preoperative screening of all aortic aneurysm patients with coronary angiography is not feasible or prudent, even though Hertzer reported a nearly fivefold increase in operative mortality (5.1%) in aneurysm patients with suspected coronary disease, compared with those with no (1.1% mortality) or corrected (0.44% mortality) coronary artery disease.[101,102] Late survival was also better in the groups with no or corrected coronary artery disease. Despite these data, no solid evidence has proved that there is decreased perioperative mortality or increased long-term survival among patients undergoing prophylactic coronary revascularization before aortic aneurysm repair. Further, no single means exists to accurately predict perioperative cardiac risk after aortic aneurysmorrhaphy, but this is currently an area of intensive research.

Each of the modalities discussed has its own usefulness as well as limitations. Older patients with congestive heart failure, active angina pectoris, previous myocardial infarction, or markedly abnormal noninvasive cardiac studies deserve thorough cardiac evaluation before elective aortic aneurysm surgery. Younger patients without overt cardiac disease and with normal ECG readings probably do not need this type of evaluation. The difficult decisions are in patients who fall between these two extremes (about 50% of the total), in whom unexpected coronary events still occur. Because the ultimate objective of a cardiac evaluation is to identify and correct dangerous coronary artery lesions, the results of any subsequent intervention (e.g., coronary artery bypass grafting, percutaneous transluminal angioplasty) in the appropriate hospital must be considered and balanced against the relatively low myocardial infarction rates that can be achieved in patients who do not undergo coronary revascularization. Overall, preliminary myocardial revascularization before aortic aneurysm repair is truly necessary in only about 10% to 20% of patients.

Indications for Abdominal Aortic Aneurysm Repair

The objectives of surgical treatment of abdominal aortic aneurysm are to relieve symptoms (if present), prevent rupture (thereby prolonging life), and restore arterial continuity. These goals are best accomplished when operations are performed electively under optimal conditions. The natural history of unoperated abdominal aortic aneurysms and the excellent results currently achievable with surgical treatment justify an aggressive diagnostic and therapeutic approach.[115] So far, the only way to prevent or delay rupture is surgical treatment.

Emergent operation is indicated for almost all patients with known or suspected rupture, regardless of the size of the aneurysm or age of the patient. There are obvious exceptions to this approach. The coexistence of another fatal illness, such as metastatic cancer, or severe dementia with very poor quality of life may be sufficient reason for choosing a nonoperative approach. Some reports suggest that patients older than 85 years who present in shock should be selected for nonoperative management. Emergent or urgent operation is also indicated for symptomatic aneurysms in the absence of signs of rupture. However, it is frequently impossible to determine whether an aneurysm has in fact ruptured or is just expanding. Although CT and MRI scans can be relied on to detect the presence of periaortic blood in most cases, other more subtle findings, such as a break in the aortic calcium ring, may provide clues to an impending rupture. The absence of these findings should not lead to unnecessary delays in operating, because actual rupture can occur at any time.

Elective aneurysm repair should be recommended for asymptomatic patients with aneurysms 5.5 cm or larger in diameter who are acceptable operative risks and who have an estimated life expectancy of 2 years or more. Elective operation should also be considered for smaller aneurysms, smaller than 5.5 cm in diameter, in good-risk patients, especially if they are hypertensive or live in remote areas where proper medical care would not be readily available should signs and symptoms of rupture develop. Aneurysms between 4 and 5.5 cm in diameter that have shown documented enlargement of more than 0.5 cm in less than 6 to 12 months by serial imaging studies should also be treated surgically. Enlargement at this rate has long been considered a sign of an unstable, changing aortic wall, but there are few if any published data supporting this concept. It is hoped that data from wall stress analyses will become available in the future for use in making surgical decisions. Data from several studies showed that aneurysms in women ruptured at a slightly smaller size than in men, so it may be appropriate to recommend elective repair at around 4.5 to 5 cm in women.

High-risk patients (those who are very old or who have nonreconstructible coronary disease, poor left ventricular function with congestive heart failure, renal failure, or severe obstructive lung disease) with small aneurysms should be observed until the aneurysm becomes symptomatic or large. High-risk patients with large aneurysms require thorough evaluation for the condition that puts them in the high-risk category.[74,92] Frequently, such evaluations fail to substantiate the original degree of presumed risk, and it has been reported that less than 50% of these patients die of the disease for which they were initially denied aneurysm repair. Unfortunately, there is lack of agreement on the definition of these various high-risk categories. It is in these high-risk patients that endoluminal repair may be especially beneficial.

Because of excessively high operative mortality in some very high-risk patients with large abdominal aneurysms, several surgeons have proposed extra-anatomic bypass in conjunction with induced thrombosis of the aneurysm.[116] Thrombosis of the aneurysm, it was argued, would eliminate the risk of rupture, and the extra-anatomic bypass would lower operative mortality by avoiding the risks of a major intra-abdominal operation and aortic cross-clamping. Unfortunately, nonresective therapy has not been as successful as originally hoped. Rupture still occurs in about 20% of patients so treated, and operative mortality exceeds 10%, which is much higher than the mortality reported in similar but highly selected groups of patients subjected to conventional aneurysm operations.[92,117-119] Fortunately, this nonresective form of surgical therapy for abdominal aneurysms is being abandoned, even by some of its earlier proponents. Endoluminal stent-grafting has become the treatment of choice for these very high-risk patients when they have suitable anatomy.

Operative Technique

INCISION AND EXPOSURE

There are three options for the incision for abdominal aortic aneurysm operations: full-length midline, wide transverse, and oblique.

The full-length midline incision provides access to the entire abdominal cavity, including the supraceliac aorta and iliac arteries; it can be made and closed rapidly and involves the fewest limitations. For the treatment of supra- or pararenal aneurysms, medial visceral rotation can be added and usually provides adequate exposure of the entire suprarenal segment of the abdominal aorta. This maneuver involves mobilization, from lateral to medial, of the left colon, spleen, and pancreas in what is normally an avascular plane. Significant splenic injury requiring splenectomy occurs about 25% of the time when this is done, and there is an increased risk of pancreatic injury.

A wide transverse incision extending from flank to flank and curved either above or below the umbilicus, depending on the aortic and iliac pathology, also provides excellent transperitoneal exposure for aortic aneurysm repair and is the preference of many surgeons. It is more time-consuming to create and close than a midline incision and is said to be stronger, although proof of superiority in terms of wound dehiscence is lacking. However, midline incisional hernias occur more frequently after aneurysm repair than after other operations performed through midline incisions, possibly because of the same or similar connective tissue abnormality that is involved in the pathogenesis of aneurysms. Transverse incisions are less painful and therefore interfere less with respiratory function postoperatively because they cut across fewer intercostal nerves.

Both the midline and the transverse incisions offer wide access to the peritoneal cavity and retroperitoneum and their contents. They permit a thorough abdominal exploration that should be performed as a preliminary step in all elective operations, because there is a significant incidence of coexisting pathology, including colon tumors and gallstones.

Retroperitoneal exposure of the aorta can be achieved through an oblique incision extending from the left 11th intercostal space or tip of the 11th rib to the edge of the rectus abdominis muscle.[120-122] The patient is placed in a semilateral position, but with the hips allowed to rotate back to the supine position, which allows access to both femoral arteries. Through this retroperitoneal exposure, the suprarenal aorta can be controlled, if necessary, but access to the right iliac artery is often limited, especially if the aortic aneurysm is large or if there is a large right iliac aneurysm. Among the advantages of the retroperitoneal approach are less postoperative respiratory compromise, lower intravenous fluid volume requirements, less intraoperative hypothermia, a shorter period of postoperative ileus, and avoidance in many cases of the need for postoperative nasogastric intubation. Although the perception is that these patients generally "do better" than those operated on through a midline incision, when the two incisions were compared in prospective studies, no significant important differences were found.[120-122] One major disadvantage of the retroperitoneal approach is that the contents of the peritoneal cavity are not available for inspection, although an opening in the peritoneum can easily be made if necessary. Another is the occurrence of a postoperative flank bulge that can be particularly annoying to some patients. This is probably due to injury to the intercostal nerve in the line of the incision. The retroperitoneal approach loses most of its advantages when there is a retroaortic left renal vein or left-sided cava, because these structures are then in a vulnerable location. Nevertheless, many surgeons prefer this approach for all elective aneurysm operations, and some even use it for ruptured aneurysms that

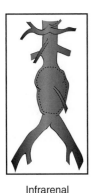
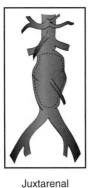
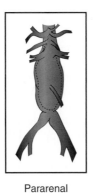
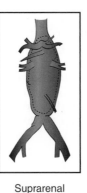
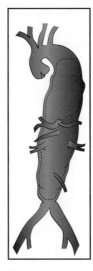

Infrarenal Juxtarenal Pararenal Suprarenal

Thoracoabdominal

FIGURE 28–7 • Morphologic classification of abdominal aortic aneurysms. Aneurysms can be classified according to their relationship to the renal arteries as infrarenal, juxtarenal, pararenal, and suprarenal.

are contained because of the ability to achieve rapid control of the upper abdominal aorta.[123]

The choice of incision is a matter of personal preference. Factors to consider in making this choice include the extent of the aneurysm, the status of the iliac arteries, the degree of obesity and pulmonary disease, previous abdominal operations, the presence and location of stomas, the necessity to inspect intraperitoneal structures (especially in patients with atypical symptoms), and the speed with which aortic control must be attained. The retroperitoneal approach is probably preferable in the presence of an inflammatory aneurysm or horseshoe kidney. Surgeons should be familiar with all three approaches so that they can take advantage of each when appropriate.

Transperitoneal or retroperitoneal exposure of the aorta through small incisions, with or without laparoscopic assistance, has been used successfully to treat aortic aneurysms by several surgical groups. The special instruments, vascular clamps, and retractors necessary to accomplish this have been developed and are being improved. Turnipseed compared 50 patients who had aortic aneurysms or occlusive disease treated via minimal incisions with 50 similar patients treated using a long midline incision. The minimal incision technique was as safe and effective as the standard incision and was associated with shorter intensive care unit and total hospital stay, less morbidity, and reduced costs. It was more cost-efficient than either the standard incision or endoluminal stent-grafting techniques.[124] Completely laparoscopic aneurysm repair has also been performed, and several fairly large series have now been reported, with improving results and reduced operative times.[125] The introduction of robotic devices into this procedure is under investigation.

When midline or transverse incisions are used, the aorta is exposed by a retroperitoneal incision that should be kept slightly to the right of the midline. The duodenum must be carefully reflected laterally, along with the rest of the small bowel. The left renal vein usually marks the cephalad extent of the dissection, unless the aneurysm extends to the renal

arteries (juxtarenal aneurysm) or involves them (pararenal aneurysm) (Fig. 28-7). In either of these situations, suprarenal aortic clamping is necessary, and the left renal vein should be thoroughly mobilized so that it can be retracted cephalad or caudad to facilitate adequate exposure of the pararenal aorta.[126,127] It is sometimes necessary to divide the left renal vein. This is usually well tolerated if the left adrenal and gonadal veins are not ligated, but there is an increased risk of sustained elevation in the serum creatinine level, a temporary reduction of left renal function, and increased retroperitoneal bleeding. Reanastomosis of the transected renal vein avoids these complications but is not always necessary.[128]

Distally, the dissection should avoid the fibroareolar tissue overlying the left common iliac artery in men because it contains branch vessels of the inferior mesenteric artery and the autonomic nerves that control sexual function. If the common iliac arteries are relatively normal (i.e., not aneurysmal, stenotic, or heavily calcified), they can be clamped and a straight tube graft used for the aortic replacement. Significant disease of the common iliac arteries makes a bifurcated graft preferable. Control of the iliac arteries in these situations is best achieved by mobilizing the external and internal iliac arteries and clamping them individually. Particular care must be taken in this location to avoid injury to the accompanying posterior venous structures and to the ureters, which cross anterior to the common iliac bifurcation. Every effort should be made to ensure antegrade perfusion in at least one hypogastric artery to minimize the risk of postoperative ischemia of the left colon as well as buttock claudication. This sometimes requires construction of end-to-side anastomoses between the graft limbs and the external iliac artery when anastomosis to the common iliac is not possible.

Extensive perioperative monitoring is indicated for patients undergoing abdominal aortic aneurysm repair.[74,129] This has contributed significantly to the improved results reported in large series of electively treated patients. Monitoring usually includes continuous recording of the ECG, intra-arterial pressure, body temperature, urine output, and central venous or pulmonary artery pressure. In high-risk patients, especially if the aorta will be cross-clamped above the renal arteries, transesophageal two-dimensional echocardiographic monitoring of left ventricular function may be superior to measurements of pulmonary artery pressure for the evaluation of intravascular volume status.[130] Various blood components should be monitored as well, including arterial oxygen and carbon dioxide content and pH, plasma glucose, electrolytes, and coagulation parameters and factors. Monitoring the clotting system is especially important in ruptured aneurysms and in cases in which large volumes of blood and blood products have been infused or a supraceliac clamp has been used. The use of autotransfusion is routine in some places to minimize the need for homologous blood transfusion. Unfortunately, its use was not found to be cost-effective in randomized trials. For elective operations, patients should be encouraged to donate their own blood for autologous transfusion in the perioperative period.

ANEURYSM REPAIR

Regardless of the extent of the aortic aneurysm, the proximal graft anastomosis should be made as close as possible to the renal arteries to prevent recurrent aortic pathology. The degree of disease in the iliac arteries determines the distal extent of the graft. In some series, up to 80% of patients were successfully treated with a straight tube graft, although in the experience of others, only about one third of patients had suitable anatomy for this approach. There does not appear to be a significant incidence of subsequent iliac aneurysm formation when tube grafts are used in the presence of normal-size or slightly enlarged iliac arteries.

The choice of graft material—polyester (knitted or woven) or expanded polytetrafluoroethylene (PTFE)—is a controversial but relatively unimportant issue. There is no proven superiority of either graft type used for aortic replacement. Most surgeons find knitted grafts easier to handle, and knitted grafts sealed with collagen or gelatin do not require preclotting and are gaining in popularity. For ruptured aneurysms, nonporous grafts are clearly preferable because of savings in time and interstitial blood loss. Many surgeons routinely use woven polyester or expanded PTFE grafts for elective aneurysm repair for the same reason.

Systemic heparin is nearly universally administered during the occlusive phase of elective aneurysm operations, because most surgeons believe that its use provides added protection from distal thrombosis. The distal clamps should be applied before the proximal aortic clamp to prevent distal embolization. The aorta is opened longitudinally and either partially or completely transected at the site of the proximal anastomosis. If there is a very short or no infrarenal neck (juxtarenal aneurysm), temporary proximal aortic clamping above the renal arteries is required to accomplish an adequate infrarenal anastomosis (see Fig. 28-2). This also requires control of the renal arteries to prevent the entrance of embolic debris. The proximal anastomosis can be done with a continuous or interrupted suture technique; the former is quicker. If the aorta is especially weak or friable, the sutures can be supported with Teflon-felt pledgets or strips.

The distal anastomoses can be end to end or end to side, depending on their location and the status of the common and internal iliac arteries. All mural thrombus and atheroma should be débrided from the aneurysm wall. Several studies

have shown a surprisingly high incidence of positive bacterial cultures of this material, ranging from 10% to 40% of patients. The significance of these positive cultures is unknown, but most of them have been due to coagulase-negative *Staphylococcus* species, an organism commonly found in aortic graft infections.[131] Back-bleeding lumbar vessels can be the source of significant blood loss and should be suture-ligated from within the aortic sac. If the inferior mesenteric artery is patent and actively back-bleeding, it can also be ligated within the aneurysm sac, but if back-bleeding is meager, it should be preserved and reassessed after distal flow is reestablished, especially if internal iliac flow is compromised. Reimplantation of the inferior mesenteric artery is relatively easy to perform, when necessary, with use of the Carrel patch technique.

All anastomoses should be constructed with permanent synthetic sutures. Braided polyester and monofilament polypropylene or PTFE are the most commonly used. Theoretical fears about late fracture of polypropylene sutures have not been substantiated in clinical practice. If suprarenal clamping is necessary, the clamp should be moved onto the graft and below the renal arteries as soon as possible to minimize renal ischemia after ensuring that the proximal anastomosis is secure. The distal anastomoses can then be constructed as indicated by the iliac artery disease. It is sometimes easier to control iliac artery back-bleeding by the use of intraluminal balloon catheters and to oversew the common iliac arteries from within the opened aortic, iliac aneurysms, or both. In unusual circumstances, external iliac disease necessitates making the distal anastomosis to the common femoral artery.

Declamping hypotension is now an unusual event in elective aortic aneurysm surgery. It is essential to maintain excellent communication with the anesthesiology team so that depth of anesthesia and blood and fluid replacement can be adjusted in anticipation of lower extremity reperfusion. Even though the graft and native vessels are flushed and back-bled before reestablishing distal flow, it is preferable to reestablish flow first into one hypogastric artery to minimize the chance of distal embolization to the leg. Before abdominal closure, adequacy of lower extremity and left colon perfusion should be ensured by direct inspection or noninvasive instrumentation. The graft should be insulated from the overlying bowel by careful closure of the aneurysm sac over the graft. This is sometimes impossible when the aneurysm is small, and in these situations, rotation of a flap of the aneurysm wall or a vascularized omental pedicle can be used to separate the graft from the duodenum.

It is beyond the scope of this chapter to discuss all the technical details that might be encountered during the surgical treatment of an aortic aneurysm. The principles outlined here are generally applicable in most cases. If additional vascular procedures are required, such as renal or visceral artery reconstruction, appropriate modifications in technique are obviously required.[132] The use of endovascular aortic aneurysm repair seems especially prudent in high-risk patients.[133,134] This is discussed in more detail earlier in this chapter and in Chapter 22.

REPAIR OF RUPTURED ANEURYSM

For ruptured aneurysms, the first priority is to control the hemorrhage by gaining proximal control of the aorta. Resuscitation is best done in the operating room rather than in the emergency department, and it is better to restore blood pressure only to levels sufficient to maintain vital organ function and cerebral perfusion before the induction of anesthesia.[133] It is also better to have the patient prepared and draped, with the surgical team ready to make a rapid entry into the abdomen, before the induction of anesthesia. The induction of anesthesia in these circumstances is often associated with sudden and severe hypotension when the tamponade effects and reflex vasoconstriction are relieved by relaxation of the abdominal wall and the administered anesthetic agents. The practice of proximal balloon occlusion using a catheter inserted via the upper extremity has been reintroduced, largely to avoid this phenomenon. The availability of high-quality digital fluoroscopy in the operating room makes this feasible. If the rupture is contained, proximal aortic control is best achieved at the level of the supraceliac aorta through the lesser omentum. This requires mobilization of the left lobe of the liver and can be far more difficult than anticipated when there is a large hematoma in the mesentery that pushes the upper abdominal viscera cephalad. The hematoma can then be entered and the clamp repositioned distally after the aortic neck is identified. The hematoma usually makes this portion of the dissection relatively easy, but caution must be exercised to avoid injury to major venous structures, which is one of the most common causes of excessive hemorrhage and subsequent death. If there is a free intraperitoneal rupture, the aorta can be quickly compressed at the diaphragm with an assistant's hand or a commercial compression device without formally dissecting this area. An infrarenal clamp or an intraluminal occluding balloon catheter can be substituted as soon as possible. After bleeding is controlled, adequate blood and volume replenishment should be achieved before attempting to restore flow to the lower extremities. Heparin is unnecessary and should be avoided in ruptured aneurysms because bleeding and coagulopathy are frequently associated with the shock, hypothermia, and massive blood loss and replacement that occur. The aggressive use of blood and blood products, including platelets and fresh frozen plasma, is essential for the survival of these patients.[134,135]

Complications of Aortic Aneurysm Repair

Survival after aortic aneurysm surgery was discussed earlier in this chapter. Mortality ranges from 0% to 3% for patients with uncomplicated aneurysms operated on electively to more than 80% for patients with rupture, hypotension, and oliguria. The most frequent cause of death is myocardial dysfunction, usually ischemic in origin. Nonfatal myocardial infarction is also fairly common after even elective aortic aneurysm repair, occurring in 3.1% to 16% (average, 6.9%) of patients in reported series.[8] The varying incidence is due to different criteria used to define myocardial infarction and possibly to different protocols for evaluating and treating coronary artery disease preoperatively.

Several other major complications can occur during or after aortic aneurysm operations. Hemorrhage is a constant threat, most often from injury to iliac or lumbar veins. It can be severe and extremely difficult to control, especially if it involves the left common iliac vein where it passes beneath the right common iliac artery. Extreme care must be taken when mobilizing the iliac arteries, especially if they are aneurysmal, in which case they are more likely to be adherent to the underlying veins. Injury to the left renal vein or one of its tributaries is also associated with brisk bleeding. This is particularly likely when there are venous anomalies such as a retroaortic left renal vein or a circumaortic venous collar. These venous anomalies can usually be identified preoperatively if a CT scan has been obtained. Intraoperatively, they should be suspected when, during cephalad dissection of the aortic neck, either a small or no left renal vein is encountered in its usual location crossing anterior to the aorta. Postoperative hemorrhage can occur in any patient, and hemodynamic instability and evidence of continued blood loss should lead to early re-exploration of the abdomen.

Declamping hypotension is not as frequent or severe a problem as it once was. Better understanding of its physiology, more aggressive management of intravascular volume, and better monitoring and anesthetic techniques have all contributed to the reduction in the incidence and seriousness of this problem. The surgeon can help minimize this condition by giving the anesthesiologist advance notification of plans to restore distal perfusion and then doing it gradually. Despite these precautions, declamping hypotension can still be a serious problem, especially in the setting of a ruptured aneurysm in a cold, hypovolemic patient with poor cardiac performance.

Renal failure is another serious but now infrequent complication. At one time, 3% to 12% of deaths after elective abdominal aortic aneurysm operations and an even higher percentage after emergency operations for rupture were attributable to acute renal failure.[135] Renal failure or less severe degrees of renal impairment can occur even when there is no hypotension and the proximal aortic clamp was infrarenal in location. The cause of renal dysfunction in these situations is poorly understood but is thought to involve reflex renal vasoconstriction and intrarenal redistribution of blood flow. Atheromatous embolization from clamping or manipulation of the perirenal aorta is also a potential contributing factor, as is temporary suprarenal clamping when it is required. Sometimes, the large contrast load of an aortogram or CT scan obtained 1 or 2 days preoperatively can cause renal dysfunction that only becomes apparent postoperatively. Mannitol or loop diuretics are commonly administered before aortic cross-clamping to increase urine output and prevent renal failure. Although this seems reasonable, studies have shown that intraoperative urine volume does not predict postoperative renal function.[136] Renal failure due to acute tubular necrosis is much more common after operations for ruptured aortic aneurysms, occurring in 21% of survivors of operation in one series. Unfortunately, the mortality associated with this complication still ranges from 50% to 70%, despite the use of acute hemodialysis and adequate nutritional support.

Technical injury to the bowel or ureters can cause catastrophic infectious complications involving the newly implanted prosthetic graft. This is most likely to occur when there are adhesions from previous operations or the structures are in an unusual position (e.g., the ureters displaced anteriorly and laterally by the aneurysm). Such injuries should be meticulously repaired and the area irrigated with antibiotic solution. Ureteral injuries should be stented. In some situations, nephrectomy is the safest course to avoid possible graft contamination.

Gastrointestinal complications of a functional nature regularly occur after conventional aortic aneurysm surgery. Ileus is the rule for at least 2 to 3 days after transperitoneal surgery. Typically, gastric and colonic ileus persists longer than small bowel ileus. Nevertheless, the use of nasogastric tubes has not been shown to reduce the incidence of early gastrointestinal dysfunction. Small amounts of liquids can often be safely administered orally beginning on postoperative day 1 or 2. Occasionally, duodenal obstruction persists for longer periods. The presence of hematoma and edema in the vicinity of the proximal anastomosis is thought to contribute to this problem. Postoperative pancreatitis is relatively common, as determined by elevation of the serum amylase level, although clinically apparent pancreatitis is unusual. The pancreas can be injured by retractors, however, and a few patients have serious consequences from these seemingly minor injuries.

The most serious gastrointestinal complication is ischemia of the left side of the colon and the rectum. The incidence of ischemic colitis after aortic reconstruction is about 2% (range, 0.2% to 10%).[137] It is three to four times more common after operations for aortic aneurysm than after operations for occlusive disease, and the incidence is several times higher in patients studied prospectively with colonoscopy after sustaining a ruptured aneurysm. Ligation of a patent inferior mesenteric artery in the presence of inadequate collateral circulation to the sigmoid colon and rectum is thought to be an important pathophysiologic mechanism, but the inferior mesenteric artery is already occluded in the majority of patients with abdominal aneurysms. Improper ligation of the inferior mesenteric artery too far away from the wall of the aneurysm can contribute to this complication by interfering with collateral blood supply to the rectosigmoid.[138] Postoperative hypotension and hemodynamic instability are significant contributory factors. Therefore, it is important to maintain antegrade perfusion in at least one internal iliac artery after arterial reconstruction for aortic aneurysm. Even though most patients with occlusion of both internal iliac arteries and the inferior mesenteric artery have adequate colonic perfusion, postoperative hypotension, bowel distention, and mesenteric vessel compression by hematoma can all contribute to postoperative colonic ischemia.

Postoperative colonic ischemia can involve the mucosa only, which usually causes a transient, mild form of ischemic colitis, or it can involve mucosa and muscularis, which may result in fibrous healing and stricture formation. The most severe and dreaded form is transmural ischemia, which occurs in more than 60% of the reported cases.[139] The clinical manifestations of bowel ischemia depend on its severity. Diarrhea, especially if it is bloody, is one of the earliest manifestations and usually begins within 48 hours of operation. It is an indication for colonoscopy to assess the status of the colonic mucosa. Other findings indicative of bowel gangrene and peritonitis may be present and demand prompt reoperation, resection of all compromised bowel, and creation of appropriate stomas. During bowel resection, efforts should be made to isolate the underlying aortic prosthesis from the surgical field, although this is usually impossible, setting the stage for subsequent prosthetic infection. If the graft becomes grossly contaminated, it should be removed and lower extremity perfusion restored by axillofemoral bypass. Less severe degrees of colonic ischemia can be managed nonoperatively, although subsequent correction of a colonic stricture may be required.

A high index of suspicion of this complication must be maintained to detect and treat it in a timely fashion.

The mortality for postoperative colonic ischemia following aortic aneurysm surgery is about 50% overall but increases to 90% when full-thickness colonic gangrene and peritonitis occur. Preoperative evaluation of the blood supply to the colon and intraoperative assessment of colonic perfusion by Doppler or inferior mesenteric artery back-pressure measurements may help identify patients at highest risk for this disastrous complication so that preventive measures (i.e., inferior mesenteric artery reimplantation) can be taken. Routine inferior mesenteric reimplantation is advocated by some surgeons.

Paraplegia due to spinal cord ischemia, a well-recognized complication of thoracoabdominal aneurysm repair, is a rare event after operations confined to the infrarenal aorta, with only slightly more than 50 cases reported. Szilagyi and coworkers noted an incidence of 0.2% in more than 3000 aortic operations, and it occurred 10 times more frequently in patients with ruptured aneurysms.[140] This suggests that hypotension is a contributing factor in most cases, even though injury to an unusually located arteria magna radicularis (artery of Adamkiewicz) to the spinal cord may be the primary event. Pelvic hypoperfusion associated with internal iliac artery occlusion is an important contributing factor in some patients. This emphasizes again the importance of maintaining perfusion of at least one hypogastric artery. Unfortunately, this complication is not preventable, predictable, or treatable. Although the severity of the clinical manifestations varies and approximately 50% of affected survivors recover some neurologic function, there is a 50% mortality associated with this complication.

Ischemia of the lower extremities can also occur after aortic aneurysm surgery. This may be due to embolization of dislodged mural thrombus or atherosclerotic plaque from the aneurysm itself, thrombosis of a vessel due to distal stasis, creation of an intimal flap, or crushed atherosclerotic plaque. The use of heparin during the occlusive phase of aneurysm repair does not prevent embolic events from occurring but may limit the propagation of thrombus and should prevent the formation of stasis thrombi in the distal vascular beds. Before closing the abdomen, the surgeon must be satisfied with the perfusion status of the lower extremities.

Microembolization can also occur, resulting in small patchy areas of ischemia, usually on the plantar aspect of the feet. Pedal pulses are usually still palpable in this situation. Colloquially, this is known as "trash foot," and if it is recognized intraoperatively, the passage of small balloon catheters can sometimes retrieve at least some of the atheromatous debris. Lumbar sympathectomy may also be beneficial in limiting or preventing full-thickness tissue loss.

An abdominal compartment syndrome has been recognized as an unusual but important cause of renal and respiratory failure, especially after operations for ruptured aneurysms. Manifested by massive abdominal distention, oliguria, and difficulty maintaining adequate ventilation, it is an indication for prompt re-exploration of the abdomen to relieve the intra-abdominal pressure. The usual finding is massive visceral edema, and a deliberate abdominal wall hernia must be created for its treatment. This syndrome may be preventable by mesh-assisted delayed abdominal closure.

Infection involving the prosthetic graft used to restore aortic continuity occurs in from less than 1% to about 6%

of patients. It is more common after treatment of ruptured aneurysms. It may be associated with graft-enteric fistula, which is more common after surgery for aortic aneurysm than after surgery for aortic occlusive disease. These infections usually become manifest months to years after graft implantation and are discussed in detail in Chapter 42.

Unusual Problems Associated with Abdominal Aortic Aneurysms

A number of anatomic and pathologic conditions can complicate the management of abdominal aortic aneurysms and adversely affect the outcome.

VENOUS ANOMALIES

There are several anomalies of the inferior vena cava and left renal vein that are important in aortic surgery. They were found in 2.8% of nearly 1400 aortic operations in one series and are potential sources of serious, unexpected hemorrhage. Many of these can be identified on preoperative CT scans.[141] The inferior vena cava may be entirely on the left side (without situs inversus) or may be duplicated, with one on each side of the aorta. Double vena cava is estimated to occur in up to 3% of patients, but isolated left-sided vena cava occurs in only 0.2% to 0.5%.[142,143] An isolated left-sided vena cava usually crosses obliquely in front of the aorta and may be joined by a short, immobile right renal vein. It can also cross from left to right behind the aorta. These anomalies can be especially troublesome if the aorta is approached retroperitoneally from the patient's left side. These anomalously positioned veins are prone to injury during dissection near the neck of an aortic aneurysm. Sometimes a crossing left inferior vena cava must be divided to enable satisfactory handling of the proximal aortic anastomosis. With a duplicated inferior vena cava, the left-sided one can be ligated if necessary, but care must be taken to ensure that adequate venous drainage of the adrenal gland and left kidney is maintained.

A retroaortic left renal vein, either alone or in association with an anterior vein in the usual location, is another rare anomaly that can lead to exsanguinating hemorrhage if it is injured during dissection or clamping of the aortic neck.[144] The incidence of this anomaly is 1.8% to 2.4% and is the most commonly encountered venous anomaly in some series. As mentioned earlier, when the surgeon cannot find the left renal vein in its usual preaortic location, he or she should assume that it is retroaortic and limit dissection in that area. Great care must be taken when applying the aortic cross-clamp to avoid tearing these posterior veins. If such a vein is injured, transection of the aorta is usually required to expose it well enough to control the bleeding.

Circumaortic venous collar is more common, occurring in up to 8.7% of cases.[145] This anomaly is even more prone to injury because the anterior component can be normal in size, leading the surgeon to disregard the possibility of a second, posterior renal vein.

INFLAMMATORY ANEURYSM

Nearly 5% of abdominal aortic aneurysms are associated with a dense, inflammatory, fibrotic reaction involving the aortic wall and the retroperitoneum that incorporates adjacent structures.[146,147] This appears to be a distinct clinicopathologic entity of uncertain cause, although an autoimmune process has been proposed. It is characterized histologically by marked thickening of the adventitia and media (in contrast to other aortic aneurysms, which have a thinned, attenuated medial layer). Both layers are infiltrated with a prominent acute and chronic inflammatory reaction that includes giant cells. The majority of the inflammatory cells are activated T lymphocytes. The desmoplastic inflammatory reaction involves the duodenum in 90% of cases, the inferior vena cava and left renal vein in more than 50%, and the ureters in about 25%; it can extend above the renal arteries as well as to the iliac arteries.[148] These aneurysms tend to be large, and most patients are symptomatic (pain) in the absence of rupture. In spite of the extremely thickened wall, these aneurysms can and do rupture. A majority of patients have an elevated erythrocyte sedimentation rate of uncertain significance, and many have elevated C-reactive protein levels and have lost weight. The diagnosis can be suspected based on the CT scan, where the periaortic fibrous tissue can easily be seen obliterating tissue planes, and a typical halo effect of this tissue appears after intravenous contrast administration. MRI also shows a characteristic appearance of inflammatory aneurysm consisting of several concentric rings surrounding the aortic lumen. This contrast-enhancing halo represents the highly vascular nature of the inflammatory fibrous tissue. Either of these imaging techniques can establish the presence of an inflammatory aneurysm in a high percentage of cases.

Published reports have pointed out several advantages of the left-sided retroperitoneal approach for these lesions, as discussed earlier, and establishing this diagnosis preoperatively allows the selection of this technique. In cases of ureteric involvement, the ureters are pulled medially and may be obstructed (again, in contrast to other large aneurysms, which tend to push the ureters laterally). At laparotomy, the diagnosis can be immediately established by the unmistakable appearance of a dense, shiny, white, highly vascular reaction in the retroperitoneum, centered over the aortic aneurysm. Once the lesion is recognized, the usual maneuvers of aneurysmorrhaphy should be modified to avoid injury to adherent structures, especially the duodenum. The aorta should be exposed cephalad to the renal vein or at the diaphragm and opened without dissecting the duodenum off the wall. The advantage of the retroperitoneal technique is that the aorta is approached from a lateral direction and the left kidney and renal vein are displaced anteriorly, out of harm's way. The duodenum does not have to be mobilized, and the inflammatory tissue, which is mostly anterior, can mostly be avoided. There have been several reports of successful endovascular repair of inflammatory aneurysm using standard patient selection criteria. With either approach, concomitant ureterolysis is seldom necessary because the inflammatory reaction usually resolves postoperatively. Ureteral catheterization can be a useful adjunct, however, and can help avoid intraoperative ureteral injury. Although the transfusion requirements and operative mortality are slightly higher than for noninflammatory aneurysms, the long-term outlook for these patients is comparable to that for patients with ordinary abdominal aortic aneurysms, and the usual criteria for recommending elective operation should be applied, because these aneurysms can rupture despite their very thick anterior wall.[149]

HORSESHOE KIDNEY

Horseshoe kidney occurs in 1:400 to 1:1000 of the general population. Its association with abdominal aortic aneurysm is rare, but it complicates graft replacement because the kidney mass is usually fused anterior to the aorta, the collecting system and ureters are medially displaced, and there are frequently multiple renal arteries arising from the aorta (including the aneurysmal part), the iliac arteries, or both.[150,151] The renal blood supply is anomalous in 80% of cases and may require some form of surgical correction in most of them.[152] The anomalous fused renal mass is readily apparent on diagnostic imaging studies (CT, MRI, ultrasonography), but preoperative arteriography is essential for the proper evaluation of these renal arteries. The isthmus of a horseshoe kidney seldom needs to be divided (nor should it be), because the aortic graft can be tunneled behind it. If renal arteries arise from the aneurysm, they can be reimplanted into the graft as a Carrel patch. The presence of a horseshoe kidney is another situation in which a left retroperitoneal approach is preferable because it allows easier management of the multiple and accessory renal arteries.

ASSOCIATED INTRA-ABDOMINAL PATHOLOGY AND CONCOMITANT SURGICAL PROCEDURES

Occasionally, there are stenotic atherosclerotic lesions in aortic branches that require surgical correction at the time of aortic aneurysm repair. This most often involves the renal arteries in patients with renovascular hypertension or impaired renal function.[153,154] Rarely, chronic visceral ischemia necessitates concomitant visceral artery repair and aneurysmorrhaphy. In most series, the morbidity and mortality of combined procedures exceed those of elective aneurysm repair alone, so caution is urged in the performance of purely prophylactic procedures in this setting.

Malignant tumors, most of them colonic, are unexpectedly found in 4% to 5% of patients undergoing operation for abdominal aneurysm. They are much more common in patients with aortic aneurysms than in those with aortic occlusive disease. Because operating on the colon converts a clean into a contaminated procedure, with the potential for prosthetic graft infection, the decision regarding how to treat each lesion (aneurysm, colon mass) is not easy. It is sometimes difficult to distinguish colon cancer from inflammatory lesions intraoperatively. In addition, most vascular surgeons do not use a formal bowel preparation for patients undergoing elective aortic aneurysm surgery. For these reasons, unless there are compelling reasons for treating the colon lesion (perforation, obstruction, hemorrhage), the aneurysm procedure should be completed and the colon left alone. The colon lesion can then be properly evaluated and treated postoperatively. Generally, it is possible to perform an elective colon operation sooner after an aortic aneurysm repair than vice versa, especially if there has been a septic complication (common after colon surgery but rare after aortic surgery).

The presence of asymptomatic gallstones is a far more common condition found unexpectedly in 5% to 20% of patients undergoing aortic surgery. Several series have been published attesting to the safety of concomitant cholecystectomy and aortic repair.[155,156] A major impetus for this philosophy is the purported high incidence of postoperative cholecystitis in patients in whom only the aortic pathology is treated. In the series reported by String,[155] there was only one documented late graft infection in 34 patients who underwent combined procedures. However, the follow-up was rather short, especially when one considers the usual long interval between aortic grafting and the first manifestations of graft infection. In addition, the incidence of positive cultures from the bile of patients with cholelithiasis is as high as 33%. As with colon lesions, performance of elective cholecystectomy, which could lead to contamination of a newly implanted aortic prosthesis, should not be performed in conjunction with vascular grafting operations.[156,157] The consequences of infection of the aortic graft are so grave that the risk of performing elective cholecystectomy is unjustified. The advent of laparoscopic cholecystectomy has made this less of an issue because of the relatively benign nature of this procedure, which can be safely performed either shortly before or after aortic aneurysm repair, if necessary.

AORTOCAVAL FISTULA

Abdominal aortic aneurysms can rupture into the inferior vena cava or iliac veins, producing an aortocaval fistula. This occurs in 0.2% to 1.3% of patients with typical, nonspecific abdominal aortic aneurysms.[158,159] The incidence is at least twice as high in cases of ruptured aneurysm. Approximately 5% to 10% of spontaneous aortocaval fistulas occur in conjunction with other entities, such as mycotic aneurysm and Ehlers-Danlos and Marfan's syndromes. The most frequent site of fistulization is the distal aorta at or just above the confluence of the iliac veins. Almost all aortocaval fistulas are symptomatic, and impaired renal function is common. Hemodynamically, there is typically a hyperdynamic, high-output state (tachycardia, decreased diastolic blood pressure, and cardiac dilatation) that can quickly progress to medically refractory congestive heart failure. Abdominal or back pain is present in more than 80% of patients, and most have a palpable mass; 75% have an audible bruit, but only about 25% have a palpable thrill. Venous hypertension can affect the gastrointestinal and urinary tracts as well as the lower extremities, and this is why swollen legs, lower gastrointestinal tract bleeding, and hematuria are common. This often leads to a multitude of diagnostic studies trying to explain these manifestations.

Despite these protean manifestations, the diagnosis of aortocaval fistula is usually not suspected clinically. Aortography is the best diagnostic modality, although the fistulas can sometimes be documented by CT, MRI, or ultrasound scans. The natural history of aortocaval fistula is progressive cardiac decompensation and death. Surgical correction offers the only hope for survival and should be undertaken promptly. A conventional infrarenal aortic aneurysm operation with oversewing of the fistula from within the opened aneurysm sac cures the fistula. Hemodynamic improvement is immediate, and renal function usually recovers rapidly. Nevertheless, reported mortality rates are between 22% and 51%, largely a result of blood loss, cardiac decompensation, and pulmonary embolism.[157]

Mycotic Aortic Aneurysms

A mycotic aneurysm is one of infectious but not necessarily fungal origin. The term *mycotic* is derived from the typically mushroom-shaped false aneurysm of the arterial wall. These aneurysms usually occur when a sufficient quantity of bacterial or septic emboli lodges at a point on the intimal surface of an artery to produce a locally invasive infection that becomes a transmural arteritis. Although this can occur in normal arteries, it more commonly affects large, major atherosclerotic vessels and their branches. Septic emboli can also lodge in the vasa vasorum and initiate the infectious, necrotic process in the arterial wall. A third mechanism is arterial invasion from a septic focus adjacent to a major artery. Traumatic contamination of an artery has replaced endocarditis as the most common cause, often as a result of drug abuse or even arterial catheterization procedures.[160]

In the largest collective review of mycotic aneurysms, the abdominal aorta was the second most frequent site of involvement (31%), exceeded only by the femoral artery (38%).[158] Chan and associates reported 22 mycotic aortic aneurysms out of a series of 2585 patients, an incidence of 0.85%.[161] Coincident with the change in cause, there has been a change in the bacteriology of mycotic aneurysms, with *Salmonella* species declining and *Staphylococcus* species increasing. Together, these are still the most frequently cultured organisms from aortic mycotic aneurysms.[162] The predilection for the infrarenal abdominal aorta probably relates to the frequent occurrence of atherosclerotic plaques in this location.

The triad of abdominal pain, fever, and a pulsatile abdominal mass should suggest the diagnosis of mycotic aneurysm. However, most patients are diagnosed with a nonspecific febrile illness of variable duration, and many do not have a palpable aneurysm. Only about one third have abdominal pain. Leukocytosis is a common finding, but only about 50% have positive blood cultures. Mycotic aneurysms are often detected by CT scans performed for the evaluation of undiagnosed fever. They appear as a mass located on one side of the aorta rather than a circumferential enlargement.[160,162] They enhance with intravenously administered contrast agent, but the significance of this can be difficult to appreciate. Angiography demonstrates the characteristic lobulated saccular aneurysm, which may be multiple and contiguous. These are false aneurysms, contained by compressed periaortic tissue. The aneurysm wall tends to be thin and friable and is associated with contiguous lymphadenopathy and obvious inflammation. Blood clot of varying age is present both within and outside the aneurysmal sac because there is a high incidence of rupture, although it is usually contained. Periaortic abscess may also be present. The opening between the aorta and the aneurysm tends to be irregular or ragged.

Mycotic aneurysms are a fulminant infectious process and must be treated vigorously and promptly.[161,163-165] Control of clinical sepsis does not appear to be necessary before surgical treatment, and delays in operative intervention are associated with aneurysmal rupture. Proper antibiotic therapy must be combined with resection of the infected arterial segments, débridement of all adjacent necrotic tissue, and arterial reconstruction. Control of infection by antibiotics does not prevent rupture of the aneurysm, and excision is mandatory and should be carried out promptly. Many of these aneurysms involve the upper abdominal aorta, where it is not always possible to avoid the use of prosthetic arterial grafts. In situ prosthetic replacement is necessary when renal or visceral perfusion would be compromised by aortic excision. For the infrarenal aorta, if the intraoperative Gram stains are negative and there is no periaortic purulence, in situ prosthetic grafting is also the procedure of choice. It should be followed

with 6 to 8 weeks of specific antibiotic therapy and, in the case of *Salmonella* infections, probably lifelong antibiotics. When there is frank periaortic pus or a positive Gram stain of an infrarenal mycotic aneurysm, management can be aortic débridement and ligation or extra-anatomic bypass and a shorter course of antibiotics or, alternatively, the in situ grafting technique described previously. Recent data tend to favor the in situ method. Using these principles, Chan's group reported an operative survival rate of 86%, with only one recurrent infection.[161]

Iliac Artery Aneurysms

Common iliac artery aneurysms occur in continuity or association with abdominal aortic aneurysms in 16% to 20% of patients. They are very uncommon as isolated lesions, accounting for only 1% to 2% of all aneurysms involving the aortoiliac segments and being identified in only 0.03% of autopsies.[166-170] The cause in the vast majority of cases is the same as that for nonspecific or multifactorial aortic aneurysms; therefore, they occur in association with atherosclerosis in the atherosclerosis-prone age group. However, iliac artery aneurysms can develop during pregnancy in the absence of atherosclerosis, and several other causes have been recognized. Mycotic and traumatic iliac artery aneurysms have been reported, the latter usually after lumbar disk or hip surgery. Other less frequent causes include cystic medial necrosis, dissection, Takayasu's disease, Marfan's and Ehlers-Danlos syndromes, and Kawasaki disease.

Most isolated iliac aneurysms involve the common iliac (70%) or internal iliac (20%) arteries. Isolated external iliac artery aneurysms are extremely rare. Multiple iliac aneurysms occur in the majority of patients, and they are bilateral in about 33%. In the Richardson and Greenfield series, two or more vessels were involved in 67% of patients.[171] Because most occur in association with atherosclerosis, the average age at diagnosis is around 69 years, and the male-female ratio is 7:1. The left and right sides are equally involved.

The clinical presentation of iliac aneurysms is variable and often obscure. Because they are in the pelvis, they are difficult to palpate on physical examination unless they are quite large. The majority, 50% to 67% in recent reviews, are symptomatic even in the absence of rupture. Symptoms are caused mainly by pressure on adjacent pelvic structures (e.g., urinary tract, lower gastrointestinal tract, lumbosacral nerves, pelvic veins).[172] Thus, lower abdominal, flank, and groin pain is common. Because these are not usually symptoms attributable to the arterial system, delays in diagnosis occur frequently. Diagnosis is usually based on an imaging study looking for the cause of the symptoms or for an unrelated condition. Both CT and ultrasonography are highly reliable for these lesions, and there is excellent correlation between CT and ultrasound measurements. As with aortic aneurysms, arteriography documents the presence of most iliac aneurysms but frequently underestimates their size because of the presence of laminated thrombus. Other studies that are occasionally useful in making the diagnosis are barium enema, proctosigmoidoscopy, cystoscopy, and plain radiography films.

Even though iliac artery aneurysms are difficult to detect by routine physical examination, large ones can be palpated on abdominal, rectal, or pelvic examination. Common iliac aneurysms are generally more easily felt abdominally, whereas internal iliac aneurysms are more easily felt rectally.

In most reports, iliac aneurysms tend to be quite large when diagnosed, which probably accounts for the high incidence of symptoms and rupture. In Schuler and Flanigan's collected review, the average size was 8.5 cm, and the incidence of rupture was 51%.[168] In Krupski and coworkers' more recent report, the average size was 5.6 cm, with a 29% rupture rate.[173]

There are no prospective studies of isolated iliac artery aneurysms, but the natural history of large ones appears to be unfavorable. The reported high rate of rupture within a few months of diagnosis probably reflects the aneurysm's large size at the time of discovery. Not surprisingly, operative mortality in patients with ruptured aneurysms ranges from 25% to 56%, with an average of 40%. In contrast, the operative mortality for elective operations is much better, averaging 10% to 11%. The outlook for smaller aneurysms does not appear to be so poor. In Santilli and associates' series of 47 isolated iliac aneurysms, the average size was 2.3 cm, and the only rupture was an aneurysm larger than 5 cm.[174] The average rate of enlargement in that series was 0.12 to 0.26 cm/year, with larger aneurysms expanding at a greater rate than smaller ones. No patient developed symptoms with an aneurysm smaller than 4 cm. These and other data suggest that isolated common iliac aneurysms smaller than 3 cm can be followed with semiannual ultrasound or CT scans, with minimal risk of symptom development or rupture. Aneurysms 3.5 to 4 cm or larger should be repaired, even if asymptomatic. Symptomatic iliac aneurysms should be repaired regardless of size. The same size guidelines should be used for internal and external iliac aneurysms because so few data are available about these uncommon lesions. Common iliac aneurysms associated with aortic aneurysms appear to behave in a similar manner, but it is prudent to deal with aneurysms larger than about 2 to 2.5 cm at the time of aortic aneurysm repair using a bifurcated graft. Smaller iliac artery aneurysms can be left in place with a very low probability that they will enlarge enough to become clinically significant.

The advent of stent-grafts has added another option to the treatment of common iliac aneurysms. The standard treatment is graft replacement, and because the external iliac artery is almost never aneurysmal, the operation can be confined to the abdomen. Bilateral common iliac aneurysms necessitate the use of an aortoiliac bifurcation prosthesis. Small internal iliac aneurysms can be treated with catheter-based techniques by injecting coils and other thrombogenic materials into the aneurysm and its branches. Alternatively, they can be treated by endoaneurysmorrhaphy. They should not be treated by simple ligation of the neck because they will remain pressurized via collaterals, enabling further enlargement.

The long-term prognosis of iliac aneurysms after treatment has not been well documented. Nachbur and colleagues reported a 55% 5-year survival rate for patients with ruptured iliac aneurysms.[175] It is reasonable to expect the survival rates to be similar to those for the treatment of aortic aneurysms.

KEY REFERENCES

Brewster DC, Cronenwett JJ, Hallaett JW Jr, et al: Guidelines for the treatment of abdominal aortic aneurysms: Report of a subcommittee of the Joint Council of the American Association for Vascular Surgery and the Society for Vascular Surgery. J Vasc Surg 37:1106, 2003.

Cambria RP, Brewster DC: Advantages of the retroperitoneal approach for aortic surgery: Fact or fancy? Perspect Vasc Surg 3:52, 1990.

Fillinger MF, Marra SP, Raghavan ML, Kennedy FE: Prediction of rupture risk in abdominal aortic aneurysm during observation: Wall stress versus diameter. J Vasc Surg 37:724, 2003.

Gadowski GR, Pilcher DB, Ricci MA: Abdominal aortic aneurysm expansion rate: Effect of size and beta-adrenergic blockade. J Vasc Surg 19:727, 1994.

Giordano JM, Trout HH: Anomalies of the inferior vena cava. J Vasc Surg 3:924, 1986.

Lederle FA, Wilson SE, Johnson GR, et al: Immediate repair compared with surveillance of small abdominal aortic aneurysms. N Engl J Med 346:1437, 2002.

Rutherford RB, Krupski WC: Current status of open versus endovascular stent-graft repair of abdominal aortic aneurysm. J Vasc Surg 39:1129, 2004.

Santilli SM, Wernsing SE, Lee ES: Expansion rates and outcomes for iliac artery aneurysms. J Vasc Surg 31:114, 2000.

United Kingdom Small Aneurysm Trial participants: Mortality results for randomized controlled trial of early elective surgery or ultrasonographic surveillance for small abdominal aortic aneurysms. Lancet 352:1649, 1998.

United Kingdom Small Aneurysm Trial participants: Long-term outcomes of immediate repair compared to surveillance of small abdominal aortic aneurysms. N Engl J Med 346:1445, 2002.

REFERENCES

1. Lederle FA: Repair of abdominal aortic aneurysms. N Engl J Med 351:1677, 2004.
2. Castelden W, Mercer J: Abdominal aortic aneurysms in western Australia: Descriptive epidemiology and patterns of rupture. Br J Surg 72:109, 1985.
3. Melton L, Bickerstaff L, Hollier LH, et al: Changing incidence of abdominal aortic aneurysms: A population based study. Am J Epidemiol 120:379, 1984.
4. Norman PE, Castleden WM, Hockey RL: Prevalence of abdominal aortic aneurysm in western Australia. Br J Surg 78:1118, 1991.
5. Best VA, Price JF, Fowkes FGR: Persistent increase in the incidence of abdominal aortic aneurysm in Scotland, 1981-2000. Br J Surg 90:1510, 2003.
6. Darling RC, Messina CR, Brewster DC, Ottinger LW: Autopsy study of unoperated aortic aneurysms. Circulation 56(Suppl 2):161, 1977.
7. Bengtsson H, Sonesson B, Bergqvist D: Incidence and prevalence of abdominal aortic aneurysms, estimated by necropsy studies and population screening and ultrasound. Ann N Y Acad Sci 800:1, 1996.
8. Taylor LM, Porter JM: Basic data related to clinical decision-making in abdominal aortic aneurysms. Ann Vasc Surg 1:502, 1980.
9. Graham LM, Zelenock GB, Whitehouse WM, et al: Clinical significance of atherosclerotic femoral artery aneurysms. Arch Surg 155:502, 1980.
10. Vermilion BD, Kimmins SA, Pace WG, Evans WE: A review of 147 popliteal aneurysms with long-term follow-up. Surgery 90:1009, 1981.
11. Bengtsson H, Bergqvist D, Ekberg O, Janzon L: A population based screening of abdominal aortic aneurysms (AAA). Eur J Vasc Surg 5:53, 1991.
12. Scott RAP, Ashton HA, Kay DN: Abdominal aortic aneurysm in 4237 screened patients: Prevalence, development and management over 6 years. Br J Surg 78:1122, 1991.
13. Johnston KW, Rutherford RB, Tilson MD, et al: Suggested standards for reporting on arterial aneurysms. J Vasc Surg 13:452, 1991.
14. Steinberg CR, Morton A, Steinberg I: Measurement of the abdominal aorta after intravenous aortography in health and arteriosclerotic peripheral vascular disease. AJR Am J Roentgenol 95:703, 1965.
15. Hollier LH, Stanson AW, Gloviczki P, et al: Arteriomegaly: Classifications and morbid implications of diffuse aneurysmal disease. Surgery 93:700, 1983.
16. Bengtsson H, Ekberg O, Aspelin P, et al: Abdominal aortic dilatation in patients operated on for carotid artery stenosis. Acta Chir Scand 154:441, 1988.
17. Mukherjee D, Mayberry JC, Inahara T, Greig JD: The relationship of the abdominal aortic aneurysm to the tortuous internal carotid artery: Is there one? Arch Surg 124:955, 1989.
18. Wolfe YG, Otis SM, Schwend RB, Bernstein EF: Screening for abdominal aortic aneurysms during lower extremity arterial evaluation in the vascular laboratory. J Vasc Surg 22:417, 1995.
19. Cohen J: Pathogenesis of aortic aneurysms. Perspect Vasc Surg 3:103, 1990.

20. Tilson DM, Stansel HC: Differences in results for aneurysm vs occlusive disease after bifurcation grafts: Results of 100 elective grafts. Arch Surg 107:1173, 1980.
21. Dobrin PB: Pathophysiology and pathogenesis of aortic aneurysms: Current concept. Surg Clin North Am 69:687, 1989.
22. Zarins CK, Glagov S: Aneurysms and obstructive plaques: Differing local responses to atherosclerosis. In Bergan JJ, Yao JST (eds): Aneurysms: Diagnosis and Treatment. New York, Grune & Stratton, 1982, p 61.
23. Busuttil RW, Abou-Zamzam AM, Machleder HI: Collagenase activity of the human aorta: Comparisons of patients with and without abdominal aortic aneurysms. Arch Surg 115:1373, 1980.
24. Busuttil RW, Heinrich R, Flesher A: Elastase activity: The role of elastase in aortic aneurysm formation. J Surg Res 32:214, 1982.
25. Dobrin PB, Baker WH, Gley WC: Elastolytic and collagenolytic studies of arteries: Implications for the mechanical properties of aneurysms. Arch Surg 119:405, 1984.
26. Cohen J, Mandell C, Chang JB, Wise L: Elastin metabolism of the infrarenal aorta. J Vasc Surg 7:210, 1988.
27. Kurihara N, Inoue Y, Iwai T, et al: Detection and localization of periodontopathic bacteria in abdominal aortic aneurysms. Eur J Vasc Endovasc Surg 28:553, 2004.
28. Louwrens H, Pearce WH: Role of inflammatory cells in aortic aneurysms. In Yao JST, Pearch WH (eds): Aneurysms: New Findings and Treatments. East Norwalk, Conn, Appleton & Lange, 1994, p 11.
29. Dobrin PB, Baumgartner N, Anidjar S, et al: Inflammatory aspects of experimental aneurysms: Effect of methylprednisolone and cyclosporine. Ann N Y Acad Sci 800:74, 1996.
30. Cronenwett JL, Murphy TF, Zelenock GB, et al: Actuarial analysis of variables associated with rupture of small aortic aneurysms. Surgery 98:472, 1985.
31. White JV, Mazzacco SL: Formation and growth of aortic aneurysms induced by adventitial elastolysis. Ann N Y Acad Sci 800:97, 1996.
32. Majumder PP, St Jean PL, Ferrell RE, et al: On the inheritance of abdominal aortic aneurysm. Am J Hum Genet 48:164, 1991.
33. Verloes A, Sakalihasan N, Limet R, Koulischer L: Genetic aspects of abdominal aortic aneurysm. Ann N Y Acad Sci 800:44, 1996.
34. Tilson MD, Seashore MR: Human genetics of the abdominal aortic aneurysm. Surg Gynecol Obstet 158:129, 1984.
35. Tilson MD: Decreased hepatic copper levels: A possible chemical marker for the pathogenesis of aortic aneurysms in man. Arch Surg 117:1212, 1982.
36. Tilson MD: Generalized arteriomegaly: A possible predisposition to the formation of abdominal aortic aneurysms. Arch Surg 116:1030, 1981.
37. Collin J, Walton J: Is abdominal aortic aneurysm familial? BMJ 299:493, 1989.
38. Johansen K, Koepsell T: Familial tendency for abdominal aortic aneurysms. JAMA 256:1934, 1986.
39. Clifton MA: Familial abdominal aortic aneurysms. Br J Surg 64:765, 1977.
40. Szilagyi DE: Clinical diagnosis of intact and ruptured abdominal aortic aneurysms. In Bergan JJ, Yao JST (eds): Aneurysms: Diagnosis and Treatment. New York, Grune & Stratton, 1982, p 205.
41. Sterpetti AV, Feldhaus RJ, Schultz RD, Blair EA: Identification of abdominal aortic aneurysm patients with different clinical features and clinical outcomes. Am J Surg 156:466, 1988.
42. Lawrie GM, Crawford ES, Morris GC Jr, Howell JF: Progress in the treatment of ruptured abdominal aortic aneurysm. World J Surg 4:653, 1980.
43. Rutherford RB, McCroskey BL: Ruptured abdominal aortic aneurysms: Special considerations. Surg Clin North Am 69:859, 1989.
44. Bower TC, Cherry KJ Jr, Pairolero PC: Unusual manifestations of abdominal aneurysms. Surg Clin North Am 69:745, 1989.
45. Moran KT, Persson AV, Jewell ER: Chronic rupture of abdominal aortic aneurysms. Am Surg 55:485, 1989.
46. Goldstone J: Vascular imaging techniques. In Rutherford RB (ed): Vascular Surgery, 3rd ed. Philadelphia, WB Saunders, 1989, p 119.
47. Quill DS, Colgan MP, Summer DS: Ultrasonic screening for the detection of abdominal aortic aneurysms. Surg Clin North Am 69:713, 1989.
48. Bluth EI: Ultrasound of the abdominal aorta. Arch Intern Med 144:377, 1984.
49. Scott RAP, Vardulaki KA, Walker NM, et al: The long-term benefits of a single scan for abdominal aortic aneurysm (AAA) at age 65. Eur J Vasc Endovasc Surg 21:535, 2001.
50. Greatorex RA, Dixon AK, Flower CDR, Pulvertaft RW: Limitations of computed tomography in leaking abdominal aortic systems. BMJ 297:284, 1988.
51. Amparo EG, Hoddick WK, Hricak H, et al: Comparison of magnetic resonance imaging and ultrasonography in the evaluation of abdominal aortic aneurysms. Radiology 154:451, 1985.
52. Clayton MJ, Walsh JW, Brewer WH: Contained rupture of abdominal aortic aneurysms: Sonographic and CT diagnosis. AJR Am J Roentgenol 138:154, 1982.
53. Weinbaum FI, Dubner S, Turner JW, et al: The accuracy of computed tomography in the diagnosis of retroperitoneal blood in the presence of abdominal aortic aneurysm. J Vasc Surg 6:11, 1987.
54. Gomes MN, Davros WJ, Zeman RK: Preoperative assessment of abdominal aortic aneurysm: The value of helical and three-dimensional computed tomography. J Vasc Surg 20:367, 1994.
55. Raptopoulos V, Rosen MP, Kent KC, et al: Sequential helical CT angiography of aorto-iliac disease. AJR Am J Roentgenol 166:1347, 1996.
56. Lee JKT, Ling D, Heiken JP, et al: Magnetic resonance imaging of abdominal aneurysms. AJR Am J Roentgenol 143:1197, 1984.
57. Rich NM, Clagett GP, Salander JM, et al: Role of arteriography in the evaluation of aortic aneurysms. In Bergan JJ, Yao JST (eds): Aneurysms: Diagnosis and Treatment. New York, Grune & Stratton, 1982, p 233.
58. Friedman SG, Kerner BA, Krishnasastry KV, et al: Abdominal aortic aneurysmectomy without preoperative angiography: A prospective study. N Y State J Med 90:176, 1990.
59. Gaspar MR: Role of arteriography in the evaluation of aortic aneurysms: The case against. In Bergan JY, Yao JST (eds): Aneurysms: Diagnosis and Treatment. New York, Grune & Stratton, 1982, p 243.
60. Estes JE Jr: Abdominal aortic aneurysm: A study of 102 cases. Circulation 2:258, 1950.
61. Wright IS, Urdenata E, Wright B: Re-opening the case of the abdominal aortic aneurysm. Circulation 13:754, 1956.
62. Szilagyi DE, Smith RF, De Russo FJ, et al: Contribution of abdominal aortic aneurysmectomy to prolongation of life. Ann Surg 164:678, 1966.
63. Ashton HA, Buxton MJ, Dat NE, et al: The Multicentre Aneurysm Screening Study (MASS) into the effect of abdominal aortic aneurysm screening on mortality in men: A randomized controlled trial. Lancet 360:1531, 2002.
64. Bernstein EF, Chan EL: Abdominal aortic aneurysm in high-risk patients: Outcome of selective management based on size and expansion rate. Ann Surg 200:255, 1984.
65. Lederle FA, Wilson SE, Johnson GR, et al: Rupture rates for large abdominal aortic aneurysms in patients refusing or unfit for elective repair. JAMA 287:2968, 2002.
66. Szilagyi DE, Elliott JP, Smith RF: Clinical fate of the patient with asymptomatic abdominal aortic aneurysm and unfit for surgical treatment. Arch Surg 104:600, 1972.
67. UK Small Aneurysm Trial participants: Mortality results for randomized controlled trial of early elective surgery or ultrasonographic surveillance for small abdominal aortic aneurysms. Lancet 352:1649, 1998.
68. Lederle FA, Wilson SE, Johnson GR, et al: Immediate repair compared with surveillance of small abdominal aortic aneurysms. N Engl J Med 346:1437, 2002.
69. Prinssen M, Verhoeven ELG, Buth JA, et al: A randomized trial comparing conventional and endovascular repair of abdominal aortic aneurysms. N Engl J Med 351:1607, 2004.
70. United Kingdom Small Aneurysm Trial participants: Long-term outcomes of immediate repair compared to surveillance of small abdominal aortic aneurysms. N Engl J Med 346:1445, 2002.
71. Johansson G, Nydahl S, Olofsson P, Swedenborg J: Survival in patients with abdominal aortic aneurysms: Comparison between operative and nonoperative management. Eur J Vasc Surg 4:497, 1990.
72. Nevitt MP, Ballard DJ, Hallett JW Jr: Prognosis of abdominal aortic aneurysms. N Engl J Med 321:1009, 1989.
73. Cronenwett JL, Sargent SK, Wall MH, et al: Variables that affect the expansion rate and outcome of small abdominal aortic aneurysms. J Vasc Surg 11:260, 1990.
74. Gadowski GR, Pilcher DB, Ricci MA: Abdominal aortic aneurysm expansion rate: Effect of size and beta-adrenergic blockade. J Vasc Surg 19:727, 1994.
75. Fillinger MF, Marra SP, Raghavan ML, Kennedy FE: Prediction of rupture risk in abdominal aortic aneurysm during observation: Wall stress versus diameter. J Vasc Surg 37:724, 2003.
76. Raghavan ML, Vorp DA, Federle MP, et al: Wall stress distribution on three-dimensionally reconstructed models of human abdominal aortic aneurysms. J Vasc Surg 31:760, 2000.
77. Crawford ES, Saleh SA, Babb JW III, et al: Infrarenal abdominal aortic aneurysm: Factors influencing survival after operation performed over a 25 year period. Ann Surg 193:699, 1981.

78. Pilcher DB, Davis JH, Ashileoga T, et al: Treatment of abdominal aortic aneurysm in an entire state over $7\frac{1}{2}$ years. Ann J Surg 139:487, 1980.
79. Hertzer NR, Avellone JC, Farrel CJ, et al: The risk of vascular surgery in a metropolitan community. J Vasc Surg 1:13, 1984.
80. Robson AK, Currie IC, Poskitt KR, et al: Abdominal aortic aneurysm repair in the over eighties. Br J Surg 76:1018, 1989.
81. Vasko JS, Spencer FC, Bahnson HT: Aneurysm of the aorta treated by excision: Review of 237 cases followed up to seven years. Am J Surg 105:793, 1963.
82. Cannon JA, Van De Water J, Barker WF: Experience with the surgical management of 100 consecutive cases of abdominal aortic aneurysm. Am J Surg 106:128, 1963.
83. Voorhees AB, McAllister FF: Long term results following resection of arteriosclerotic abdominal aortic aneurysms. Surg Gynecol Obstet 117:355, 1963.
84. Levy JF, Kouchoukos NT, Walker WB, Butcher HR: Abdominal aortic aneurysmectomy: A study of 100 cases. Arch Surg 92:498, 1966.
85. May AG, DeWeese JA, Frank I, et al: Surgical treatment of abdominal aortic aneurysms. Surgery 63:711, 1968.
86. Baker AG, Roberts B: Long-term survival following abdominal aortic aneurysmectomy. JAMA 212:445, 1970.
87. Stokes J, Butcher HR: Abdominal aortic aneurysms: Factors influencing operative mortality and criteria of operability. Arch Surg 107:297, 1973.
88. Hicks GL, Eastland MW, DeWeese JA, et al: Survival improvement following aortic aneurysm resection. Ann Surg 181:863, 1975.
89. O'Donnell TF, Darling RC, Linton RR: Is 80 years too old for aneurysmectomy? Arch Surg 111:1250, 1976.
90. Reigel MM, Hollier LH, Kazmier FJ, et al: Late survival in abdominal aortic aneurysm patients: The role of selective myocardial revascularization on the basis of clinical systems. J Vasc Surg 5:222, 1987.
91. Rutherford RB, Krupski WC: Current status of open versus endovascular stent-graft repair of abdominal aortic aneurysm. J Vasc Surg 39:1129, 2004.
92. Hollier LH, Reigel MM, Kozmier FJ, et al: Conventional repair of abdominal aortic aneurysm in the high-risk patient: A plea for abandonment of nonresective treatment. J Vasc Surg 3:712, 1986.
93. Hiatt JCG, Barker WF, Machleder HI, et al: Determinants of failure in the treatment of ruptured abdominal aortic aneurysms. Arch Surg 119:1264, 1984.
94. Fielding JWL, Black J, Ashton F, Slaney G: Ruptured aortic aneurysms: Postoperative complications and their aetiology. Br J Surg 72:487, 1984.
95. Donaldson MC, Rosenberg JM, Bucknam CA: Factors affecting survival after ruptured abdominal aortic aneurysm. J Vasc Surg 2:564, 1985.
96. Johansen K, Kohler RT, Nicholls SC, et al: Ruptured abdominal aortic aneurysm: The Harborview experience. J Vasc Surg 13:240, 1991.
97. Tambyraja AL, Raza Z, Stuart WP, et al: Does immediate operation for symptomatic non-ruptured abdominal aortic aneurysm compromise outcome? Eur J Vasc Endovasc Surg 28:543, 2004.
98. Johnson G Jr, Gurri JA, Burnham SJ: Life expectancy after abdominal aortic aneurysm repair. In Bergan JJ, Yao JST (eds): Aneurysms: Diagnosis and Treatment. New York, Grune & Stratton, 1982, p 279.
99. Hollier LH, Plate G, O'Brien PC, et al: Late survival after abdominal aortic aneurysm repair: Influence of coronary artery disease. J Vasc Surg 1:290, 1984.
100. Hertzer NR: Fatal myocardial infarction following abdominal aortic aneurysm resection: 343 patients followed 6-11 years postoperative. Ann Surg 190:667, 1980.
101. Hertzer NR: Clinical experience with pre-operative coronary angiography. J Vasc Surg 2:510, 1985.
102. Hertzer NR, Young JR, Bevan EG, et al: Late results of coronary bypass in patients with infra-renal aortic aneurysms: The Cleveland Clinic Study. Ann Surg 205:360, 1987.
103. Crawford ES, Morris GC Jr, Howell JF, et al: Operative risk in patients with previous coronary artery bypass. Ann Thorac Surg 26:215, 1978.
104. Ruby ST, Whittemore AD, Couch NP, et al: Coronary artery disease in patients requiring abdominal aortic aneurysm repair. Selective use of a combined operation. Arch Surg 201:758, 1985.
105. Reul G Jr, Cooley DA, Duncan MJ, et al: The effect of coronary bypass on the outcome of peripheral vascular operation in 1093 patients. J Vasc Surg 3:788, 1986.
106. Bevan EG: Routine coronary angiography in patients undergoing surgery for abdominal aortic aneurysm and lower extremity occlusive disease. J Vasc Surg 3:682, 1986.

107. Johnston KW: Canadian study of the late results of abdominal aortic aneurysm repair. In Yao JST, Pearce WH (eds): Aneurysms: New Findings and Treatments. East Norwalk, Conn, Appleton & Lange, 1994, p 79.
108. Tambyraja AL, Fraser SCA, Murie JA, Chalmers RTA: Quality of life after repair of ruptured abdominal aortic aneurysm. Eur J Vasc Endovasc Surg 28:229, 2004.
109. Blomberg PA, Ferguson IA, Rosengarten DS, et al: The role of coronary artery disease in complications of abdominal aortic aneurysm repair. Surgery 101:150, 1987.
110. Goldman L: Cardiac risks and complications of non-cardiac surgery. Ann Surg 198:780, 1983.
111. Golden MA, Whittemore AD, Donaldson MC, Mannick JA: Selective evaluation and management of coronary artery disease in patients undergoing repair of abdominal aortic aneurysms: A 16-year experience. Ann Surg 212:415, 1990.
112. Cambria RP, Eagle K: Cardiac screening before abdominal aortic aneurysm surgery: A reassessment. Semin Vasc Surg 8:93, 1995.
113. McPhail NV, Ruddy TD, Calvin JE, et al: A complication of dipyridamole-thallium imaging and exercise testing in the prediction of post-operative cardiac complications in patients requiring arterial reconstruction. J Vasc Surg 10:51, 1989.
114. Boucher CA, Brewster DC, Darling RC, et al: Determination of cardiac risk by dipyridamole-thallium imaging before peripheral vascular surgery. N Engl J Med 312:389, 1985.
115. Brewster DC, Cronenwett JJ, Hallett JW Jr, et al: Guidelines for the treatment of abdominal aortic aneurysms: Report of a subcommittee of the Joint Council of the American Association for Vascular Surgery and the Society for Vascular Surgery. J Vasc Surg 37:1106, 2003.
116. Karmody AM, Leather RP, Goldman M, et al: The current position of non-resective treatment for abdominal aortic aneurysm. Surgery 94:591, 1983.
117. Schwartz RA, Nichols WK, Silver D: Is thrombosis of the infrarenal abdominal aortic aneurysm an acceptable alternative? J Vasc Surg 3:448, 1986.
118. Cho SI, Johnson WC, Buch HL Jr, et al: Lethal complications associated with nonresective treatment of abdominal aortic aneurysms. Arch Surg 117:1214, 1982.
119. Inahara T, Beary GL, Mukherjee D, Egan JM: The contrary position to the nonresective treatment for abdominal aortic aneurysm. J Vasc Surg 2:42, 1985.
120. Sicard GA, Allen BJ, Munn JS, Anderson CB: Retroperitoneal vs transperitoneal approach for repair of abdominal aortic aneurysms. Surg Clin North Am 69:795, 1989.
121. Cambria RP, Brewster DC, Abbott WM, et al: Transperitoneal versus retroperitoneal approach for aortic reconstruction: A randomized, prospective study. J Vasc Surg 11:314, 1990.
122. Cambria RP, Brewster DC: Advantages of the retroperitoneal approach for aortic surgery: Fact or fancy? Perspect Vasc Surg 3:52, 1990.
123. Chang BB, Shan DJ, Paty PS, et al: Can the retroperitoneal approach be used for ruptured abdominal aortic aneurysms? J Vasc Surg 11:326, 1990.
124. Turnipseed WD: A less-invasive minilaparotomy technique for repair of aortic aneurysms and occlusive disease. J Vasc Surg 33:431, 2001.
125. Dion Y-M, Gracia CR, Hassen BEK: Totally laparoscopically abdominal aortic aneurysm repair. J Vasc Surg 33:181, 2001.
126. Budden J, Hollier LH: Management of aneurysms that involve the juxtarenal or suprarenal aorta. Surg Clin North Am 69:837, 1989.
127. Allen BT, Anderson CB, Rubin BG, et al: Preservation of renal function in juxtarenal and suprarenal abdominal aortic aneurysm repair. J Vasc Surg 17:948, 1993.
128. AbuRhama AF, Robinson PA: The risk of ligation of the left renal vein in resection of the abdominal aortic aneurysm. SG & O: 173:33, 1991.
129. Goldstone J: Intraoperative monitoring in aortic surgery. In Bergan JJ, Yao JST (eds): Arterial Surgery: New Diagnostic and Operative Techniques. Orlando, Fla, Grune & Stratton, 1988, p 257.
130. Roizen MF, Beaupre PN, Albert RA, et al: Monitoring with two-dimensional transesophageal echocardiography. J Vasc Surg 1:300, 1984.
131. Macbeth GA, Rubin JR, McIntyre KE, et al: The relevance of arterial wall microbiology to the treatment of prosthetic graft infections: Graft infection vs arterial infection. J Vasc Surg 1:754, 1984.
132. Schwarcz TH, Flanigan DP: Repair of abdominal aortic aneurysms in patients with renal, iliac, or distal arterial occlusive disease. Surg Clin North Am 69:845, 1989.
133. Bown MJ, Sutton AJ, Bell PR, Sayers RD: A meta-analysis of 50 years of ruptured abdominal aortic aneurysm repair. Br J Surg 89:174, 2002.

134. Tang T, Lindop M, Munday I, et al: A cost analysis of surgery for ruptured abdominal aortic aneursym. Eur J Vasc Endovasc Surg 26:299, 2003.
135. Patel ST, Korn P, Haser PB, et al: The cost-effectiveness of repairing ruptured abdominal aortic aneurysms. J Vasc Surg 32:247, 2000.
136. Alpert RA, Roizen MF, Hamilton WK, et al: Intraoperative urinary output does not predict postoperative renal function in patients undergoing abdominal aortic revascularization. Surgery 95:707, 1984.
137. Ernst CB, Hagihara PF, Daughorty ME, et al: Ischemic colitis incidence following abdominal aortic reconstruction: A prospective study. Surgery 80:417, 1976.
138. Ernst CB: Prevention of intestinal ischemia following abdominal aortic reconstruction. Surgery 93:102, 1983.
139. Schroeder T, Christofferson JK, Anderson J, et al: Ischemic colitis complicating reconstruction of the abdominal aorta. Surg Gynecol Obstet 160:299, 1985.
140. Szilagyi DE, Hagemen JH, Smith RF, et al: Spinal cord damage in surgery of the abdominal aorta. Surgery 83:38, 1978.
141. Calligaro KD, DeLaurentis DA, Dougherty MJ: Venous anomalies encountered during abdominal aortic surgery. In Caligaro KD, Dougherty MD, Hollie L (eds): Diagnosis and Treatment of Aortic and Peripheral Arterial Aneurysms. Philadelphia, WB Saunders, 1999, p 183.
142. Bartle EJ, Pearce WH, Sun JH, et al: Infrarenal venous anomalies and aortic surgery. J Vasc Surg 6:590, 1987.
143. Giordano JM, Trout HH: Anomalies of the inferior vena cava. J Vasc Surg 3:924, 1986.
144. Brener BJ, Darling C, Frederick PL, et al: Major venous anomalies complicating abdominal aortic surgery. Arch Surg 108:160, 1974.
145. Kunkel JM, Weinstein ES: Preoperative detection of potential hazards in aortic surgery. Perspect Vasc Surg 2:1, 1989.
146. Goldstone J, Malone JM, Moore WS: Inflammatory aneurysms of the abdominal aorta. Surgery 83:425, 1978.
147. Goldstone J: Inflammatory aneurysms of the abdominal aorta. Semin Vasc Surg 1:165, 1988.
148. Crawford JL, Stowe CL, Safitt J, et al: Inflammatory aneurysms of the aorta. J Vasc Surg 2:113, 1985.
149. Pennell RC, Hollier LH, Lie JT, et al: Inflammatory abdominal aortic aneurysms: A thirty year review. J Vasc Surg 2:859, 1985.
150. Conelly TL, McKinnon W, Smith RB III, et al: Abdominal aortic surgery and horseshoe kidney. Arch Surg 115:1459, 1980.
151. Starr DS, Foster WJ, Morris GC Jr: Resection of abdominal aortic aneurysm in the presence of horseshoe kidney. Surgery 89:387, 1981.
152. Hollis HW, Rutherford RB: Abdominal aortic aneurysms associated with horseshoe or ectopic kidneys: Techniques of renal preservation. Semin Vasc Surg 1:148, 1988.
153. Tarazi RY, Hertzer NR, Bevan EG, et al: Simultaneous aortic reconstruction and renal revascularization: Risk factors and late results in 89 patients. J Vasc Surg 5:707, 1987.
154. Stewart MT, Smith RB III, Fulenwider JT, et al: Concomitant renal revascularization in patients undergoing aortic surgery. J Vasc Surg 2:400, 1985.
155. String ST: Cholelithiasis and aortic reconstruction. J Vasc Surg 1:664, 1984.
156. Ouriel K, Ricotta JJ, Adams JT, DeWeese JA: Management of cholelithiasis in patients with abdominal aortic aneurysms. Ann Surg 198:717, 1983.
157. Goldstone J, Effeny DJ: Prevention of arterial graft infection. In Bernhard VM, Towne JB (eds): Complications in Vascular Surgery, 2nd ed. Orlando, Fla, Grune & Stratton, 1985, p 487.
158. Alexander JJ, Imbebo AL: Aorta-vena cava fistula. Surgery 105:1, 1989.
159. Baker WH, Sharzer LA, Ehrenhaft JL: Aortocaval fistula as a complication of aortic aneurysms. Surgery 72:933, 1972.
160. Brown SL, Busuttil RW, Baker JD, et al: Bacteriologic and surgical determinants of survival in patients with mycotic aneurysms. J Vasc Surg 1:541, 1984.
161. Chan FY, Crawford ES, Coselli JS, et al: In situ prosthetic graft replacement for mycotic aneurysms of the aorta. Ann Thorac Surg 47:193, 1989.
162. Parson R, Gregory J, Palmer DL: *Salmonella* infections of the abdominal aorta. Rev Infect Dis 5:227, 1983.
163. Reddy DJ, Lee RE, Oh HK: Suprarenal mycotic aortic aneurysm: Surgical management and follow-up. J Vasc Surg 3:917, 1986.
164. Muller BT, Wegener OR, Grabitz K, et al: Mycotic aneurysms of the thoracic and abdominal aorta and iliac arteries: Experience with anatomic and extra-anatomic repair in 33 cases. J Vasc Surg 33:106, 2001.
165. Scher LA, Brenner BJ, Goldenkranz RJ, et al: Infected aneurysms of the abdominal aorta. Arch Surg 115:975, 1980.
166. Lawrence PF, Lorenzo-Rivero S, Lyon JL: The incidence of iliac, femoral, and popliteal aneurysms in hospitalized patients. J Vasc Surg 22:409, 1995.
167. Brunkwall J, Bergentz SE: Solitary iliac aneurysms. In Yao JST, Pearce WH (eds): Aneurysms: New Findings and Treatments. Norwalk, Conn, Appleton & Lange, 1994, p 459.
168. Schuler JJ, Flanigan DP: Iliac artery aneurysms. In Bergan JJ, Yao JST (eds): Aneurysms: Diagnosis and Treatment. New York, Grune & Stratton, 1982, p 469.
169. Lowry SF, Kraft RO: Isolated aneurysms of the iliac artery. Arch Surg 113:1289, 1978.
170. McCready RA, Pairolero PC, Gilmore JC, et al: Isolated iliac artery aneurysms. Surgery 93:688, 1983.
171. Richardson JW, Greenfield LJ: Natural history and management of iliac aneurysms. J Vasc Surg 8:165, 1988.
172. Marino R, Mooppan UMM, Zein TA, et al: Urologic manifestations of isolated iliac artery aneurysms. J Urol 137:232, 1987.
173. Krupski WC, Selzman CH, Florida R, et al: Contemporary management of isolated iliac aneurysms. J Vasc Surg 28:1, 1998.
174. Santilli SM, Wernsing SE, Lee ES: Expansion rates and outcomes for iliac artery aneurysms. J Vasc Surg 31:114, 2000.
175. Nachbur BH, Inderbitzi RGC, Bär W: Isolated iliac aneurysms. Eur J Vasc Surg 5:375, 1991.

Questions

1. **All of the following are thought to be involved in the pathogenesis of abdominal aortic aneurysms except**
   (a) Heredity
   (b) Atherosclerosis
   (c) Enzyme deficiencies
   (d) Enzyme excess
   (e) Hormones

2. **The incidence of abdominal aortic aneurysm is highest among patients with which of the following?**
   (a) Femoral aneurysm
   (b) Aortoiliac occlusive disease
   (c) Thoracic aortic aneurysm
   (d) Bilateral popliteal aneurysm
   (e) Isolated iliac artery aneurysm

3. **Which of the following statements about the risk of rupture of infrarenal abdominal aortic aneurysms is true?**
   (a) It increases with increasing size of the aneurysm
   (b) It increases with increasing age of the patient
   (c) It is negligible for aneurysms less than 6 cm in diameter
   (d) It is not affected by blood pressure
   (e) It is related to plasma lipoprotein levels

4. **What is the most common cause of late death following surgical treatment of abdominal aortic aneurysms?**
   (a) Renal failure
   (b) Respiratory failure
   (c) Myocardial ischemia
   (d) Graft infection
   (e) Malignancy

5. What is the true mortality for ruptured abdominal aortic aneurysms, including prehospital deaths?
   (a) 15%
   (b) 30%
   (c) 50%
   (d) 60%
   (e) 90%

6. Which of the following is true when the surgeon fails to see the left renal vein during exposure of an abdominal aortic aneurysm?
   (a) The dissection should be extended above the superior mesenteric artery
   (b) The neck of the aneurysm should be thoroughly mobilized
   (c) The inferior mesenteric vein should be carefully preserved
   (d) The left renal vein is probably congenitally absent
   (e) Extra care must be taken during application of the aortic cross-clamp

7. Which of the following statements about aortocaval fistulas is true?
   (a) They are usually infectious in origin
   (b) They are usually symptomatic
   (c) They usually occur just below the left renal vein
   (d) All of the above
   (e) None of the above

8. Which of the following statements about complications of aortic aneurysm repair is true?
   (a) Colon ischemia is associated with a mortality rate of about 50%
   (b) Renal failure does not occur if the aortic cross-clamp is totally infrarenal
   (c) Paraplegia occurs only with suprarenal clamping
   (d) Myocardial dysfunction is now an uncommon cause of postoperative death
   (e) The use of autotransfusion devices has greatly reduced the degree of postoperative hemorrhage

9. All of the following statements about inflammatory aneurysms are true except
   (a) They have thick fibrous walls
   (b) They are frequently associated with abdominal tenderness in the area of the aneurysm
   (c) They require CT scanning for definitive preoperative diagnosis
   (d) They frequently rupture
   (e) They are frequently associated with ureteral obstruction

10. All of the following statements about iliac artery aneurysms are true except
   (a) Asymptomatic aneurysms should be at least 2.5 cm in diameter for repair to be undertaken
   (b) Most are associated with or are an extension of infrarenal abdominal aortic aneurysms
   (c) Most isolated iliac aneurysms manifest symptoms before rupture
   (d) They may be diagnosed by digital examination of the vagina and rectum
   (e) Most can be palpated by abdominal examination

Answers

| 1. e | 2. d | 3. a | 4. c | 5. e |
| 6. e | 7. b | 8. a | 9. d | 10. a |

29

D. Preston Flanigan

Aneurysms of the Peripheral Arteries

Peripheral arterial aneurysms are distinctly less common than aortic aneurysms but can cause significant morbidity. Although these lesions occasionally lead to death, the most common serious complication is end-organ loss or dysfunction. For the purposes of this chapter, peripheral aneurysms include those of the upper extremity arteries distal to and including the subclavian artery, the lower extremity arteries distal to and including the femoral artery, and the extracranial carotid arteries. Mycotic aneurysms affecting these vessels are also included.

Nonmycotic Peripheral Aneurysms

INCIDENCE AND CAUSE

Overall, the most common cause of nonmycotic peripheral aneurysms is atherosclerosis; however, depending on location, this is not true for all peripheral aneurysms. In general, all peripheral aneurysms can be considered rare. In descending order, the relative frequency of these aneurysms is probably popliteal, femoral, subclavian and axillary, and carotid. Reports on distal aneurysms involving the brachial, radial, ulnar, deep femoral, and tibial or peroneal arteries are limited to small series or case reports. Although true aneurysms have been reported in these areas,[1,2] for the most part, forearm and hand aneurysms are secondary to trauma or are mycotic in origin.[3]

Age and sex distribution are dependent on cause. Atherosclerotic aneurysms tend to occur primarily in men older than 50 years. Aneurysms due to trauma are also more common in men but occur at a younger age. Aneurysms secondary to thoracic outlet syndrome are most commonly seen in middle-aged women (75%).

Extracranial Carotid Artery Aneurysms

The rarity of extracranial carotid aneurysms is demonstrated by numerous reports of institutional experience with aneurysm patients. Of 2300 aneurysms reported from Baylor University, only 7 were extracranial carotid aneurysms.[4] In 30 years at Johns Hopkins, only 12 such aneurysms were seen.[5] Only eight carotid aneurysms were noted by Houser and Baker after obtaining 5000 cerebral arteriograms.[6] The largest single series of patients with true extracranial carotid aneurysms was reported by McCollum and coworkers,[7] who saw 37 such aneurysms over a 21-year period. Zhang and associates reported 66 extracranial carotid aneurysms, 28 of which were true, nonmycotic aneurysms.[8]

Currently, the common carotid artery is affected most often, followed by the internal carotid artery. The external carotid artery is rarely involved.[9]

The most common cause of extracranial carotid aneurysms is atherosclerosis. These aneurysms tend to be fusiform and are almost always associated with arterial hypertension. Most of the patients also have evidence of generalized atherosclerosis.[9] Another cause of carotid aneurysm is trauma, both blunt and penetrating.[10] False aneurysms of the carotid artery have occurred after carotid endarterectomy.[11] Rarer causes include cystic medial necrosis, Marfan's syndrome, fibromuscular dysplasia, medial arteriopathy, granulomatous disease, radiation, and congenital defects.[10]

Subclavian and Axillary Artery Aneurysms

Aneurysms of the subclavian and axillary arteries are also rare. In 1982, Hobson and colleagues reviewed the world literature on the subject and found only 195 aneurysms in these locations.[12] This accounts for only 1% of all peripheral aneurysms. Of the 195 cases, 88% involved the subclavian artery. Subclavian and axillary aneurysms are rarely due to atherosclerosis, with this cause accounting for only 15% of the aneurysms. Thoracic outlet syndrome is responsible for the majority of subclavian artery aneurysms (74%), whereas crutch trauma accounts for most axillary aneurysms (54%). Other rarer causes have also been reported (Table 29-1).

Forearm and Hand Aneurysms

True aneurysms in the forearm and hand are quite rare. During a 10-year period, only 10 such patients were treated at the University of Chicago.[2] Half of the true aneurysms in these areas are associated with occupational or recreational trauma. Most forearm and hand aneurysms are false aneurysms secondary to penetrating trauma[3]; most true aneurysms in these locations are secondary to blunt trauma.[13]

TABLE 29–1	Causes of Subclavian and Axillary Aneurysms		
Cause	Subclavian	Axillary	Total
Thoracic outlet syndrome	127	1	128
Crutch trauma	—	13	13
Atherosclerosis	24	5	29
Pseudoaneurysm	5	2	7
Blunt trauma	2	—	2
Fibromuscular dysplasia	—	2	2
Dissection	—	1	1
Other	13	—	13
Total	171	24	195

Data from Hobson RW II, Isreal MR, Lynch TO: Axillo-subclavian arterial aneurysms. In Bergan JJ, Vito JST (eds): Aneurysms. New York, Grune & Stratton, 1982, pp 435-447.

Femoral and Popliteal Artery Aneurysms

Femoral and popliteal artery aneurysms are grouped together because of their similar cause, their similar clinical behavior, and their frequent association.

Aside from trauma and rare degenerative and congenital disorders, femoral and popliteal aneurysms are almost exclusively atherosclerotic in origin.[14,15] Together, these two types of aneurysms account for more than 90% of peripheral aneurysms.[16] Femoral aneurysms may involve the common femoral artery in the groin, but occasionally these aneurysms are limited to the superficial femoral artery in the midthigh. These latter lesions are not unusual and are often seen in patients with arteriomegaly or "aneurysmosis."

Dent and colleagues showed an association between popliteal and femoral aneurysms and other aneurysms of atherosclerotic origin.[17] Most commonly, these associated aneurysms are located in the aortoiliac vessels, but more rarely they involve the renal, splanchnic, and brachiocephalic vessels. Among patients with at least one peripheral aneurysm, 83% had multiple aneurysms. Among patients with a common femoral aneurysm, 95% had a second aneurysm, 92% had an aortoiliac aneurysm, and 59% had bilateral femoral aneurysms. Among patients with a popliteal aneurysm, 78% had a second aneurysm, 64% had an aortoiliac aneurysm, and 47% had bilateral popliteal artery aneurysms.

NATURAL HISTORY

As with aortic aneurysms, peripheral aneurysms may be asymptomatic or may lead to significant complications. Unlike aortic aneurysms, which tend to rupture, peripheral aneurysms most commonly thrombose or give rise to arterial emboli.

Extracranial Carotid Artery Aneurysms

Central neurologic events are very common in these patients. Rhodes and coauthors reported that 13 of the 19 patients with carotid aneurysms reported in the University of Michigan series had amaurosis fugax, transient ischemic attacks, stroke, or vague neurologic symptoms such as dizziness.[9] Most of these symptoms are thought to be secondary to embolization. Cranial nerve compression leads to local neurologic dysfunction and can include facial pain (cranial nerve V), oculomotor

palsies (cranial nerve VI), auricular pain (cranial nerve IX), and hoarseness (cranial nerve X). Horner's syndrome can also occur from compression of the sympathetic chain. As cervical carotid aneurysms enlarge, they can cause dysphagia, cranial nerve compression, and pain. Hemorrhage has also been seen as a complication of these aneurysms; however, rupture is uncommon.

Subclavian and Axillary Artery Aneurysms

Only 10% of patients with known subclavian or axillary aneurysms are asymptomatic.[12] Good natural history studies are not available, probably because of the small number of patients with this problem. Because 90% of patients are symptomatic at the time of presentation, the likelihood of complications eventually occurring in asymptomatic aneurysms appears to be great. The primary complication seen with subclavian and axillary aneurysms is embolization (68%).[12] Thrombosis and rupture are rare but have been reported.[12,18]

Forearm and Hand Aneurysms

The most common presenting signs and symptoms of aneurysms in these areas are mass and pain. Distal embolization occurs in roughly one third of these patients.[2]

Femoral and Popliteal Artery Aneurysms

The natural history of unoperated femoral and popliteal aneurysms shows a high incidence of thromboembolic events. Tolstedt and associates reported a 43% rate of thrombosis in conservatively managed femoral aneurysms,[19] and in Cutler and Darling's series, 47% presented with major complications.[20] In Szilagyi and colleagues' series of popliteal aneurysms, only 32% of those managed conservatively remained without complications at 5 years.[14] Vermilion and colleagues studied 26 popliteal aneurysms for an average of 3 years and demonstrated that 31% of patients suffered limb-threatening complications, with two patients requiring major amputation and two patients left with rest pain.[15] Rupture of femoral or popliteal aneurysms has only rarely been reported. Deep femoral aneurysms are particularly prone to rupture, with rates of 50% being reported.[1] Popliteal aneurysms rupture, on occasion, into the popliteal vein.[21] Less catastrophic complications include pain secondary to tibial nerve compression and popliteal vein thrombosis secondary to popliteal vein compression.

DIAGNOSIS

Most peripheral aneurysms can be diagnosed by simple palpation of the artery in question. More sophisticated studies such as ultrasonography, computed tomography (CT) scans, and arteriography augment the diagnosis and allow for better preoperative planning.

Extracranial Carotid Artery Aneurysms

The most common presentation for carotid aneurysms is a palpable pulsatile, submandibular, lateral neck mass or a mass presenting in the tonsillar fossa. The former presentation is most often seen with common carotid aneurysms, whereas presentation in the tonsillar fossa is more often seen with internal carotid artery aneurysms. Because of the variability in the location of the carotid bifurcation, the presentation is only a rough guide to the artery involved. The differential diagnosis includes linked or redundant carotid arteries, enlarged lymph nodes, salivary gland tumors, branchial cleft cysts, cystic hygromas, and carotid body tumors. When the diagnosis is not clear, CT scanning with contrast injection is usually diagnostic. Arteriography further aids in elucidating the diagnosis and is required for proper preoperative planning. Carotid duplex ultrasound scanning may also be helpful.

Subclavian and Axillary Artery Aneurysms

The most common presenting signs and symptoms are secondary to distal embolization (68%) (Table 29-2). Other signs and symptoms include tissue loss, claudication, pain, and evidence of brachial plexus compression. When the aneurysm is secondary to thoracic outlet syndrome, it often cannot be palpated. Aneurysms secondary to atherosclerosis tend to be larger and are palpable in two thirds of patients at the time of presentation.[18] A bruit may be present in the subclavian fossa or in the axilla. Small, punctate, cyanotic lesions affecting the fingers and palm that are painful and occur suddenly are often present as a result of distal embolization. Rarely, embolization causes large axial artery occlusion. This event usually requires immediate embolectomy but may lead to claudication if the initial ischemia does not precipitate the need for immediate medical attention. With chronic small embolization, the distal radial and ulnar pulses may not be palpable owing to buildup of embolic material. Repeated embolization may be associated with distal digital ulceration or tissue loss and severe pain. Many patients show vague shoulder pain on presentation. Rupture produces severe shoulder pain radiating into the upper arm and lower neck.

When all types of subclavian and axillary aneurysms are considered, only 16% can be palpated.[12] Occasionally, ultrasonography can be applied to diagnose subclavian artery aneurysms, but the bony cage of the thoracic outlet may preclude adequate exposure in some patients. CT scanning can also demonstrate subclavian and axillary aneurysms. However, because in most cases the diagnosis should be suspected on the basis of history and physical examination, arteriography is the most useful test because it is also needed for proper planning of the operative procedure.

Forearm and Hand Aneurysms

Forearm (and especially hand) aneurysms are most often diagnosed by palpation of a pulsatile mass. These aneurysms can also

be diagnosed by ultrasound or CT scanning, but nonpalpable aneurysms are generally found on arteriography in patients being studied for embolization.

Femoral and Popliteal Artery Aneurysms

The diagnosis of femoral and popliteal aneurysms is usually made by palpation. This is particularly easy in the case of femoral aneurysms because of their superficial nature. Popliteal aneurysms are suspected in any patient in whom the popliteal pulse is widened and very easily felt. Diwan and associates, however, found that most femoral and popliteal aneurysms were not detected by physical examination and suggested the routine use of ultrasonography to look for femoral and popliteal aneurysms in men with aortic aneurysms.[22] Femoral and popliteal aneurysms should be considered in any patient with an acute arterial occlusion in the leg or with embolic disease affecting the foot and lower leg. Many popliteal aneurysms are calcified and can be detected by plain radiographs of the popliteal fossa. Both femoral and popliteal aneurysms are easily diagnosed by ultrasonography. CT scanning is particularly accurate in making the diagnosis (Fig. 29-1). Despite the presence of mural thrombus, arteriography usually confirms the diagnosis and is necessary for proper operative planning. The status of the runoff vessels visualized arteriographically is particularly important for patients with popliteal aneurysms.

INDICATIONS FOR OPERATION

Unlike aortic aneurysms, for which size is the main determinant of the need for surgery, the mere presence of a peripheral aneurysm often suggests the need for operative correction. As with aortic aneurysms, the decision to operate on a patient with a peripheral aneurysm must be tempered by the patient's overall medical condition so that the risk of operation is considerably less than the risk of the natural history of the disease.

Extracranial Carotid Artery Aneurysms

The indication for operation in a patient with a cervical carotid artery aneurysm is usually the presence of the aneurysm. Because patients with this condition are rarely seen when asymptomatic, most patients are operated on for the relief of symptoms. The high incidence of cranial nerve compression and central nervous system events in untreated patients (68% in Rhodes and colleagues' series[9]) justifies surgery for

TABLE 29–2	Clinical Findings in Subclavian and Axillary Artery Aneurysms	
Finding	**Number**	**Percent**
Asymptomatic	20	10
Claudication	9	5
Pain	36	18
Brachial plexus palsy	24	12
Tissue loss	20	10
Embolization	136	68

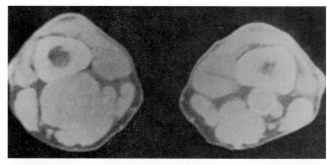

FIGURE 29–1 • Computed tomography scan showing an obvious right popliteal artery aneurysm and a smaller left popliteal artery aneurysm.

asymptomatic carotid aneurysms as well. This finding is common in nearly all reported studies, and the point is not a controversial one.[23-25]

Subclavian and Axillary Artery Aneurysms

Generally, the presence of a subclavian or axillary aneurysm is an indication for surgery. The natural history suggests that these lesions are both life threatening and limb threatening.[18] As is the case with carotid aneurysms, most patients are symptomatic at the time of presentation and have clear indications for surgical intervention. Some controversy exists regarding the small, fusiform, post-stenotic subclavian dilatation often seen with thoracic outlet compression of the subclavian artery. The natural history of this lesion, if not resected at the time of thoracic outlet decompression, is not well established. In the four patients with subclavian artery aneurysms in Pairolero and colleagues' series who had only thoracic outlet decompression, no subsequent thromboembolic events occurred during follow-up.[18]

Femoral and Popliteal Artery Aneurysms

The presence of a femoral or popliteal aneurysm is generally thought to be an indication for surgery. This recommendation is based on the high incidence of thromboembolic complications associated with these lesions, as detailed earlier. Size is generally not used to assess risk from these aneurysms, because even small aneurysms in these locations give rise to serious complications.[26]

TREATMENT

Only two primary objectives exist in the surgical management of peripheral aneurysms: exclusion of the aneurysm and restoration of arterial continuity. In most cases, both objectives can be achieved. In some inaccessible aneurysms, however, exclusion alone must be accepted because restoration of arterial continuity may not be possible.

Extracranial Carotid Artery Aneurysms

The techniques applied to the management of extracranial carotid aneurysms are ligation (or angiographic occlusion), endoaneurysmorrhaphy, resection with primary anastomosis, resection with graft replacement, or stent-grafting.

The preferred treatment is resection with primary anastomosis or graft replacement. Redundancy of the carotid artery is not uncommon when aneurysm is present. In such cases, resection of the aneurysm with mobilization of the carotid artery and primary anastomosis is sometimes quite easily accomplished (Fig. 29-2). This technique is most applicable to internal carotid artery aneurysms. An alternative technique for flow restoration after resection of an internal carotid artery aneurysm is to divide the distal external carotid artery and perform an end-to-end anastomosis between the proximal external carotid and the distal internal carotid arteries. Aneurysms of the external carotid artery are rare and can be resected without the need to restore arterial continuity. Aneurysms of the carotid bifurcation usually require resection with graft replacement between the common and internal carotid arteries. When the internal carotid is redundant,

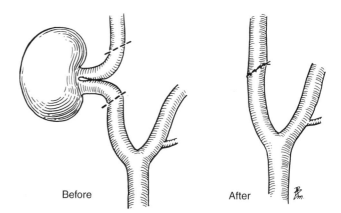

Before   After

FIGURE 29–2 • Method of end-to-end repair of a redundant internal carotid artery after aneurysm resection. (From Trippel OH, et al: Extracranial carotid aneurysms. In Bergen JJ, Yao JST [eds]: Aneurysms. New York, Grune & Stratton, 1982, pp 493-503.)

it can be mobilized and anastomosed end to end to the common carotid artery. In both these latter cases, the external carotid is usually ligated. Aneurysms involving the common carotid artery can usually be treated by resection and primary anastomosis or graft replacement. All these procedures can be performed through a standard neck incision such as that used for carotid endarterectomy.

The need for an indwelling carotid artery shunt is no better understood for aneurysm patients than for patients undergoing carotid endarterectomy. If shunting is desired, it can be accomplished in most patients. In patients undergoing resection with primary anastomosis, a shunt can be inserted into the open ends of the arteries to be anastomosed after opening of the aneurysm. If a graft is to be used, the shunt is placed through the graft before performing any anastomosis and is inserted into the arterial ends after opening of the aneurysm.

Aneurysms that involve the distal cervical internal carotid artery are often inaccessible using standard techniques. In some patients, mandibular subluxation or transection allows application of the previously mentioned methods of repair.[27] Alternative approaches are often required for high internal carotid lesions, however. In some patients, high fusiform aneurysms can be treated by aneurysmorrhaphy using an indwelling shunt for flow continuity and as a method of distal arterial control. In many cases, distal lesions must be treated by ligation or balloon occlusion using angiographic techniques. Unfortunately, acute occlusion of the internal carotid artery in these patients is associated with high neurologic morbidity. Stroke rates from 30% to 60% have been reported after this procedure, with half of those patients dying as a result of the stroke.[10] This degree of morbidity and mortality clearly approaches that associated with the natural history of the disease.

One way to select patients who may safely undergo carotid ligation is to measure carotid stump pressure. This can be done at surgery, but preoperative knowledge of this pressure allows for better operative planning. The carotid stump pressure can also be measured by temporary balloon occlusion at the time of arteriography using an end-hole balloon catheter,[28] or it can be assessed using carotid compression maneuvers during the measurement of ocular pressures using the Gee ocular pneumoplethysmograph.[29] Stump pressures in excess of 70 mm Hg appear to be safe for patients undergoing carotid ligation. Because many strokes that occur after carotid ligation manifest hours to days after the procedure, these patients should be maintained on heparin anticoagulation for 7 to 10 days postoperatively.

When stump pressure measurements indicate that carotid ligation is not safe, the performance of an extracranial-to-intracranial bypass using ipsilateral superficial temporal artery has been suggested.[27] Because this procedure is generally necessary only for high internal carotid lesions, the ipsilateral external carotid artery is usually preserved, thus allowing for adequate inflow into the superficial temporal artery.

More recently, stent-grafts have been used in a few patients. Early results are good, but a larger experience with longer follow-up will be required to determine the appropriateness of this technique.[30,31] In some cases, coil embolization of the external carotid artery may be necessary to allow coverage of the entire aneurysm and to prevent endoleak.[32]

Subclavian and Axillary Artery Aneurysms

The surgical approach to subclavian and axillary aneurysms depends on the cause, size, and location of the aneurysm and the status of the distal circulation. Except in cases of small, asymptomatic subclavian artery aneurysms secondary to thoracic outlet (for which thoracic outlet decompression alone may be adequate), the aneurysm should be excluded and arterial continuity restored if possible. Proximal and distal ligation of these aneurysms has been reported. Although tissue loss does not usually occur after this procedure, claudication is not uncommon.[18]

When a symptomatic or large asymptomatic subclavian aneurysm is present as a result of thoracic outlet syndrome, repair of the aneurysm should be accompanied by thoracic outlet decompression. Although this combined technique has been reported through an axillary approach, I prefer the supraclavicular approach; this allows for safe control of the artery, although the thoracic outlet decompression is more involved. Hobson and colleagues recommended performing the aneurysm repair through the supraclavicular approach combined with a transaxillary approach to the first rib.[12]

Atherosclerotic and traumatic distal subclavian artery aneurysms or pseudoaneurysms can be managed with a supraclavicular approach. When the aneurysm is proximal enough so that proximal control cannot be safely obtained through this approach, a median sternotomy (right side) or a left-sided thoracotomy (left side) is needed, usually in combination with the supraclavicular approach. Midsubclavian lesions can often be managed through a supraclavicular approach with medial clavicular resection.

Primary anastomosis is usually not possible, and graft replacement is required. This is most commonly performed as an interposition graft using either saphenous vein or prosthetics. Prosthetics are more commonly used because of the size of the subclavian artery. The vertebral artery should be preserved when possible. In patients with a dominant contralateral vertebral artery, this may not be necessary.

High-risk patients with proximal aneurysms who are considered too frail to undergo a major procedure can be treated with distal ligation and axilloaxillary bypass. Alternatively, stent-grafting can be applied to carefully selected high-risk patients, but long-term results are not yet known.[33-35]

Management of axillary artery aneurysms can often be accomplished through the axillary approach. In many patients, proximal control must be obtained through an infraclavicular approach. With more proximal lesions or lesions involving both the subclavian and the axillary arteries, a combined supraclavicular and infraclavicular approach must be used. Aneurysms involving the axillary artery are often intimately involved with the cords of the brachial plexus, and resection may be hazardous. When symptoms of brachial plexus compression are present, resection and interposition grafting may be indicated. For smaller lesions, however, proximal and distal ligation combined with bypass can be performed, thus avoiding dissection around the brachial plexus.

When subclavian and axillary aneurysms are complicated by embolization and ischemia, revascularization of the arm may be required in combination with aneurysm repair. This is usually accomplished by autogenous vein bypass proximal to the aneurysm to the most appropriate distal artery. In this situation, the aneurysm can be either ligated, if appropriate, or resected.

Forearm and Hand Aneurysms

Aneurysms of the forearm arteries can be treated by ligation if the remaining vessels provide adequate collateral circulation to the hand. More often, however, vein interposition grafting is performed because it is simple to accomplish. Aneurysms of vessels in the hand tend to be less well collateralized, and vein graft repair is usually necessary.[2]

Femoral and Popliteal Artery Aneurysms

The treatment of femoral artery aneurysms is usually resection and graft interposition. Because of the size of the common femoral artery, a prosthetic graft is preferred. When the deep femoral artery is involved, the graft may be sewn end to end to the superficial femoral artery, and the origin of the deep femoral artery implanted into the side of the graft. When femoral aneurysms are being treated concomitantly with an inflow or outflow procedure, it is still best, in most cases, to replace the common femoral artery with an interposition graft. Inflow or outflow grafts are then anastomosed to the interposition graft in an end-to-side fashion (Fig. 29-3). Repair of

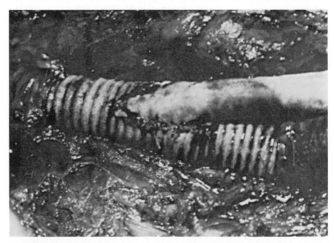

FIGURE 29–3 • Concomitant repair of femoral aneurysm followed by prosthetic femoropopliteal bypass.

deep femoral artery aneurysms is dictated by the patency of the superficial femoral artery and by how distal the aneurysm's location is in the artery. Approximately 50% of deep femoral aneurysms can be safely ligated, and 50% require the reestablishment of arterial continuity.[1]

Superficial femoral and popliteal aneurysms are preferably bypassed rather than resected. In most cases, this means an above-knee to below-knee bypass using autogenous vein through a medial approach. In some patients, the popliteal aneurysm may extend proximally into the superficial femoral artery. In these patients, the proximal anastomosis can be made to the common femoral artery or, more commonly, to the midsuperficial femoral artery proximal to the adductor canal.

Reports have been published on the use of femoropopliteal stent-grafts for the elective treatment of popliteal aneurysms.[36,37] Stent-grafts have also been used successfully in the treatment of ruptured popliteal aneurysms.[38]

When extensive embolization leading to obliteration of the outflow tract of the popliteal artery has occurred, popliteal-to-tibial or popliteal-to-peroneal bypass is required. This should be performed using autogenous vein.

When popliteal aneurysms are large enough to cause symptomatic compression of the surrounding nerve and vein, consideration should be given to resection of the aneurysm with interposition grafting. The risk of damage to these structures is greater, but if this is not done, many patients remain symptomatic postoperatively. This procedure is best performed through a posterior approach, as long as both anastomoses are within the limitations of the operative field.

When patients show severe ischemia due to thromboembolic complications of popliteal artery aneurysms, the degree of arterial occlusion is often so great that no outflow vessel is patent. Many of these patients, especially those presenting late, also have thrombosis of the microcirculation. In such patients, bypass is often not possible or is subject to a high failure rate owing to poor runoff. The use of preoperative or intraoperative thrombolytic therapy provides patent runoff in most of these patients, thereby allowing for successful bypass.[39] In patients at especially high surgical risk, thrombolytic therapy alone has been used with success.[40,41]

RESULTS OF THERAPY

Because most patients with peripheral aneurysms do not have occlusive disease, the results of reconstructive vascular procedures are usually excellent. In some cases, however, embolization from the aneurysm can lead to obliteration of some or all of the outflow tract, leading to poor results.

Extracranial Carotid Artery Aneurysms

The small number of patients included in reports assessing the results of surgical therapy for carotid aneurysms makes the calculation of morbidity and mortality statistics somewhat unreliable. Most reports, however, indicate that these procedures can be performed with safety. In Rhodes and colleagues' series from Michigan, 1 of 19 aneurysm operations resulted in a stroke, which was thought to be due to intraoperative embolization.[9] No operative death occurred. Excision of large and distal aneurysms is associated with an increased incidence of cranial nerve injury. Long-term results are sparse, but when reported, they have been excellent. All investigators agree

that the results of surgery are vastly superior to the natural history of the disease.[9,10,23-25] Long-term results for carotid aneurysm repair using stent-grafts are not yet available.

Subclavian and Axillary Artery Aneurysms

The results of surgery for subclavian and axillary aneurysms are similar to those for upper extremity reconstruction for occlusive disease.[18,42] Pairolero and colleagues showed that 18 of 18 patients undergoing aneurysm resection with restoration of arterial continuity retained patent reconstructions during an average 9.2-year follow-up.[18] This is most likely due to the lack of distal occlusive disease. Patients with obliteration of the radial and ulnar arteries, however, have a high failure rate following arm revascularization.[42] This latter point further emphasizes the need for early surgical intervention in these patients. Primary and secondary patency rates as high as 89% and 100% have been reported at 29 months for stent-graft repair of subclavian artery aneurysms.[34]

Forearm and Hand Aneurysms

Both ligation in the presence of adequate collateral circulation and vein graft repair are quite successful in the treatment of forearm and hand aneurysms. Clark and associates reported 100% patency at 7 years for vein graft repairs in the forearm and hand.[2]

Femoral and Popliteal Artery Aneurysms

When femoral and popliteal aneurysms are treated before complications arise, the results are excellent. The 18 asymptomatic patients with femoral aneurysms in Cutler and Darling's series all had excellent early and late results (no graft occlusions).[20] However, of the 45 symptomatic patients with femoral aneurysms, 4 had amputations, and 17 remained symptomatic despite therapy. In Lilly and colleagues' series of 48 popliteal aneurysms, the 5-year patency rate for reconstructions for asymptomatic lesions was 91%, compared with 54% for symptomatic lesions.[43] These differing results were directly related to the status of the tibial runoff vessels. In a series of 51 popliteal aneurysms reported by Shortell and colleagues, results were dependent on the clinical presentation and the status of the runoff vessels.[44] Patients presenting with limb-threatening ischemia had a graft patency rate of 69% at 1 year, whereas all electively performed grafts were patent at 1 year. After 3 years, runoff dictated patency; grafts with good runoff had a patency rate of 89%, whereas poor runoff was associated with a 3-year patency rate of only 30%. Numerous, more recent reports of large series of popliteal aneurysms have confirmed these earlier results.[39,45-48]

Because of the vastly inferior results of therapy once thromboembolic complications have occurred, attention has focused on the reestablishment of runoff preoperatively through the use of thrombolytic therapy.[39] Although no prospective, randomized studies have been carried out, most reports indicate good success in improving runoff and suggest improved limb salvage when preoperative thrombolytic therapy is employed. Varga and coworkers performed a retrospective, multicenter study of 200 popliteal aneurysms and concluded that intra-arterial thrombolytic therapy clearly improves preoperative runoff in patients with limb-threatening ischemia.[39]

Hoelting and associates described 24 patients with acute ischemia secondary to popliteal artery aneurysm thrombosis.[40] Nine patients were treated with preoperative thrombolysis and underwent successful bypass. Six of these patients achieved complete lysis. For three patients, lysis was incomplete but established sufficient runoff so that successful bypass could be performed. These authors also reviewed the literature and demonstrated an amputation rate of approximately 27% in 455 patients treated with bypass alone, compared with approximately 20% in 14 patients in whom only thrombolytic therapy was used.[40] However, in 30 patients in whom thrombolytic therapy was combined with bypass, no limb was lost. Varga and colleagues suggested that thrombolysis is of value in restoring distal runoff before bypass in the presence of limb-threatening ischemia but not in elective situations.[39]

Treatment of popliteal artery aneurysms with stent-grafts has been successful technically, but patency is considerably less than that achieved with bypass. Tielliu and coauthors reported a 15-month patency rate of 74% for 23 popliteal aneurysms treated with stent-grafting.[49]

Dawson and colleagues compared operative and nonoperative approaches to 71 popliteal aneurysms.[50] Thromboembolic complications developed in 57% of unoperated asymptomatic popliteal aneurysms over a mean follow-up period of 5 years. In aneurysms studied a full 5 years, the complication rate was 74%. In comparison, operated patients had graft patency and limb salvage rates of 64% and 95%, respectively, at 10-year follow-up. These authors also found a high risk of subsequent aneurysm development in these patients. At 5-year follow-up, 32% of patients had developed additional aneurysms, and at 10 years, 49% had new aneurysms.

These reports strongly support the early surgical treatment of asymptomatic femoral and popliteal aneurysms and underscore the need for careful follow-up of these patients for the development of new aneurysms.

Mycotic Aneurysms

Mycotic aneurysms are considered separately because they generally have a different cause, affect arteries in a different distribution, require different treatment, and have poorer outcomes than bland aneurysms. Despite the term, mycotic aneurysms are considered to be any true or false aneurysm that is infected.

CAUSE

Numerous classifications for mycotic aneurysms have been proposed and are nicely described by Moore and Malone[51] and Wilson and colleagues.[52] Patel and Johnston indicated that the source of infection must be either endogenous or exogenous.[53] Endogenous sources include embolism, septicemia, or direct extension; exogenous sources include trauma and iatrogenic injury. They further suggested that classifications be based on the preexisting status of the artery: normal, atherosclerotic, aneurysmal, or prosthetic. Any classification must consider these factors.[53]

Normal axial arteries are seldom infected primarily, but clumps of bacteria or fungi may lodge in smaller vessels and cause transmural necrosis and aneurysm formation. Normal larger arteries can be infected, however, by organisms lodging in the vasa vasorum. Arteries that are diseased with atherosclerosis or aneurysms, as well as prosthetic grafts, are subject to local invasion by circulating organisms. The process is similar to that described earlier, in that infection leads to arterial wall weakening and subsequent aneurysm formation. Infection may spread to arterial walls from outside the vessel through direct contact with abscesses, wound infections, salivary glands, and the like. Exogenous sources of arterial infections include diagnostic and therapeutic catheterizations, penetrating trauma, and drug abuse. Graft infections may also lead to infected pseudoaneurysm formation, usually as a result of disruption of an anastomosis.

Mycotic aneurysms have been reported in essentially all arteries, and their location is determined primarily by their cause. Those secondary to bacterial endocarditis favor the superior mesenteric artery, followed by the aorta and femoral arteries. Mycotic aneurysms that occur after trauma mostly commonly involve the extremities, whereas those caused by infection of preexisting atherosclerotic aneurysms commonly affect the aorta and the femoral and popliteal arteries. Those secondary to atherosclerosis alone involve the aorta and superficial femoral arteries as well as other common atherosclerotic sites. Those secondary to catheters and drug abuse involve the brachial, radial, and, most commonly, femoral arteries. For unknown reasons, *Salmonella* species favor the infrarenal aorta.

The organisms most commonly involved in mycotic aneurysms differ, depending on the source of the organism. When bacterial endocarditis is the source, *Streptococcus* and *Staphylococcus* prevail. *Salmonella*, *Staphylococcus*, and *Escherichia coli* are the most common organisms causing mycotic aneurysms secondary to bacteremia. Mycotic aneurysms secondary to direct extension of infections are predominantly caused by *Salmonella*, *Staphylococcus*, *Mycobacterium*, and fungi.[51] *Staphylococcus aureus* and *E. coli* are the most common organisms seen in mycotic aneurysms secondary to trauma (all types).[54]

In the preantibiotic era, most mycotic aneurysms were secondary to bacterial endocarditis and syphilis. Today, most mycotic aneurysms are probably secondary to trauma (including drug abuse, surgery, and arterial catheterization). This change is most likely due to the use of antibiotic therapy for endocarditis, the significant decrease in the prevalence of syphilis, the increasing use of diagnostic catheterization, the increase in violent trauma, and widespread drug abuse. In my experience, these forces have made common femoral artery mycotic aneurysms the most common type currently encountered.

NATURAL HISTORY

Once established, the natural course of a mycotic aneurysm is to enlarge and eventually rupture in most known cases. Occasionally, spontaneous thrombosis may occur, with resolution of the septic process; however, the thrombosed aneurysm may serve as a continuing septic focus. Septic emboli arising from aneurysms are not uncommon and can lead to miliary abscesses and septic arthritis.

DIAGNOSIS

Patients with mycotic aneurysms may show catastrophic illness or insidious disease. Most patients have some combination of

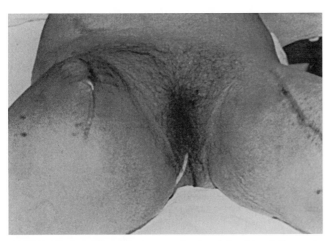

FIGURE 29–4 • Mycotic aneurysm in the right side of the groin with overlying skin necrosis and imminent rupture.

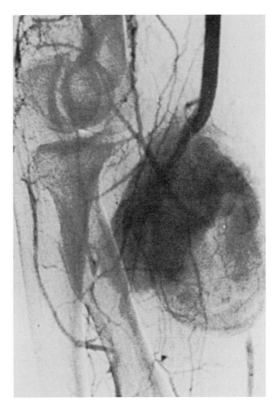

FIGURE 25–5 • Arteriogram of a mycotic popliteal artery aneurysm.

fever, malaise, weight loss, chills, night sweats, pain, leukocytosis, positive downstream blood cultures, and elevated sedimentation rate. A history of trauma or a recent infectious disease usually exists. When the aneurysm is superficial, as most peripheral aneurysms are, it can be palpated in 90% of patients.[55] The aneurysm may appear bland but more commonly shows signs of erythema, warmth, and tenderness. Particularly large aneurysms may also show skin necrosis and risk of imminent rupture (Fig. 29-4). Petechial lesions in the skin may be seen distal to the aneurysm when embolization has occurred. Many patients show rupture on presentation.

The diagnosis of mycotic aneurysm is often deduced by combining the history and physical examination findings with test findings. In some patients, the history and physical examination may be sufficient (see Fig. 29-4; this patient had a retained polyester chimney left attached to her right femoral artery after removal of an intra-aortic balloon catheter). In other patients, the diagnosis is made by the finding of sepsis and an aneurysm in a patient in whom no other septic focus can be found.

Ultrasound and CT scans can be used to visualize mycotic aneurysms. CT scans have the advantage of being able to clearly demonstrate surrounding fluid or gas, a finding consistent with infection. Gallium scans and radioactively tagged white cell scans are usually positive with mycotic aneurysms. Arteriography is usually required for preoperative planning, except in emergency situations, and usually demonstrates a saccular aneurysm or pseudoaneurysm (Fig. 29-5).

TREATMENT

The indication for treatment of a mycotic aneurysm is its presence. Antibiotic therapy, guided by culture results when available, should be used in all patients. Antibiotics alone are not sufficient, and surgical removal of the mycotic aneurysm is required in nearly all cases. Basic surgical principles dictate that all infected tissue must be removed and that adequate circulation must remain or be provided, when possible.

Extracranial Carotid Artery Mycotic Aneurysms

As noted earlier, cervical carotid aneurysms are rare, and cervical carotid mycotic aneurysms are extremely rare. In 1988, Jones and Frusha reviewed the English literature and found only 23 bacteriologically proven cases.[56] In 1991, Jebara and colleagues noted an additional four cases.[57]

Treatment of these lesions requires complete excision of the artery under antibiotic coverage and débridement of all infected tissue. Vascular reconstruction should be avoided, if possible, because reconstruction in an infected field yields less than optimal results.[58] Patients should be selected for arterial ligation based on carotid stump pressure as described earlier. Heparin should be continued for 7 to 10 days postoperatively when ligation is employed. If ligation is not safe, reconstruction using autogenous vein is the treatment of choice. In Jones and Frusha's review, the overall mortality rate was 23%. The mortality rate was 27% in the ligation group, compared with 11% in the grafted group. Extracranial-intracranial bypass has not been reported in these patients.

Subclavian and Axillary Artery Mycotic Aneurysms

Mycotic aneurysms in this area are also quite rare and are usually the result of trauma or drug abuse. The approach to the subclavian artery depends on the size and on the distal and proximal extent of the aneurysm, as described for bland aneurysms in this location. Complete excision of the aneurysm may be too risky in view of the proximity of the brachial plexus and subclavian vein. Successful treatment with arterial ligation and incision and drainage of the aneurysm has been reported.[59] Proximal subclavian artery ligation usually does not lead to the need for revascularization.

Axillary mycotic aneurysms are usually palpable. The management principles for subclavian mycotic aneurysms generally apply to axillary lesions as well. Axillary artery ligation may be associated with a greater risk of ischemia, however, and extra-anatomic bypass may be required in some patients. This can usually be performed in clean tissue planes about the shoulder using autogenous vein.

Forearm and Hand Mycotic Aneurysms

Treatment of mycotic aneurysms in these areas follows the general guidelines for other mycotic aneurysms. Arterial ligation with aneurysm excision is generally all that is required. In the rare situation in which distal ischemia might occur, autogenous revascularization in clean planes is required.

Femoral and Popliteal Artery Mycotic Aneurysms

The treatment of infected groin aneurysms has evolved through several stages. Although most of these lesions are secondary to trauma or drug abuse, the same management principles apply to mycotic groin aneurysms from other causes. Several options are available, including remote bypass followed by aneurysm resection; aneurysm resection followed by remote bypass, if needed; aneurysm resection alone; or aneurysm resection with in situ reconstruction.

Initial obturator bypass followed by aneurysm resection usually requires the use of prosthetic material, because most of these patients are drug addicts whose saphenous veins have been destroyed. Reddy and colleagues showed that this approach was associated with a 100% graft infection rate in drug addicts.[54] In other patients in whom vein is available, this approach is preferred. Buerger and Feldman reported that revascularization is not effective in reducing the amputation rate after aneurysm resection in drug addicts (17% in their series) and may occasionally be a fatal approach.[60] In their series, the same amputation rate was achieved without any deaths when aneurysm excision and ligation alone were used.

Reddy and colleagues obtained a similar amputation rate (19%) with excision and ligation.[54] They reported that excision and ligation of only one of the three femoral arteries in the groin can be performed without limb loss, but that when the common femoral artery is involved, thus necessitating the ligation of all three vessels, the amputation rate is very high. As an alternative in these latter patients, they suggested that immediate autogenous vein reconstruction with sartorius muscle flap coverage be used when adequate débridement can be performed to control sepsis. Using this approach, they reported a 9% amputation rate without mortality. Reddy and colleagues found that even in drug addicts, satisfactory saphenous vein usually exists in the thigh for femoral artery reconstruction. Benjamin and coworkers reported successful treatment of mycotic aneurysms using deep leg veins when larger-sized conduits were required.[61] Ligation and excision with postoperative observation to assess the need for subsequent revascularization did not yield satisfactory results in the Reddy series.[54]

Mycotic aneurysms involving the popliteal artery are uncommon, and few guidelines are provided in the vascular surgical literature. In my experience, aneurysm excision with in situ autogenous interposition grafting has worked well. Most of these patients have normal tibial artery runoff, facilitating long-term patency, and the readily available soft tissue coverage afforded by the muscles in the popliteal space facilitates healing of the surgical wound without complications.

KEY REFERENCES

Dent TL, Lindenaur SM, Ernst CE, et al: Multiple arteriosclerotic arterial aneurysms. Arch Surg 105:338, 1972.

Greenberg R, Wellander E, Nyman U, et. al: Aggressive treatment of acute limb ischemia due to thrombosed popliteal aneurysms. Eur J Radiol 28:211-218, 1998.

Hobson RW II, Isreal MR, Lynch TO: Axillo-subclavian arterial aneurysms. In Bergan JJ, Vito JST (eds): Aneurysms. New York, Grune & Stratton, 1982, pp 435-447.

Lilly MP, Flinn WR, McCarthy WJ, et al: The effect of distal arterial anatomy on the success of popliteal aneurysm repair. J Vasc Surg 7:653, 1988.

Pairolero PC, Walls JT, Payne WS, et al: Subclavian-axillary artery aneurysms. Surgery 90:757, 1981.

Reddy DJ, Smith RF, Elliot JP, et al: Infected femoral artery false aneurysms in drug addicts: Evolution of selective vascular reconstruction. J Vasc Surg 3:718, 1986.

Rhodes EL, Stanley JC, Hoffman CL, et al: Aneurysms of extracranial carotid arteries. Arch Surg 111:339, 1976.

Szilagyi DE, Schwartz RL, Reddy DJ: Popliteal arterial aneurysms: Their natural history and management. Arch Surg 116:724, 1981.

Tolstedt GE, Radke HM, Bell JW: Late sequelae of arteriosclerotic femoral aneurysms. Angiology 12:601, 1961.

Vermilion ED, Kinunmns SA, Pace WC, et al: A review of one hundred forty-seven popliteal aneurysms with long-term follow-up. Surgery 90:1009, 1981.

REFERENCES

1. Tait WF, Vohra RK, Carr HMI, et al: True profunda femoris aneurysms: Are they more dangerous than other atherosclerotic aneurysms of the femoropopliteal segment? Ann Vasc Surg 5:92-95, 1991.
2. Clark FT, Mass DP, Bassiouny HS, et al: True aneurysmal disease in the hand and upper extremity. Ann Vasc Surg 5:276-281, 1991.
3. Flinn WR, Yao JST, Bergan JJ: Aneurysms of secondary and tertiary branches of major arteries. In Bergan JJ, Yao JST (eds): Aneurysms. New York, Grune & Stratton, 1982, pp 449-467.
4. Beall AC, Crawford ES, Cooley DA, et al: Extracranial aneurysms of the carotid artery: Report of seven cases. Postgrad Med 32:93, 1962.
5. Reid MR: Aneurysms in the Johns Hopkins Hospital. Arch Surg 12:1, 1926.
6. Houser OW, Baker HL Jr: Fibromuscular dysplasia and other uncommon diseases of the cervical carotid artery: Angiographic aspects. Am J Roentgenol Radium Ther Nucl Med 104:201, 1968.
7. McCollum CH, Wheeler WG, Noon GP, et al: Aneurysms of the extracranial carotid artery: Twenty-one years' experience. Am J Surg 137:196, 1979.
8. Zhang Q, Duan SJ, Xin XW, et al: Management of extracranial carotid artery aneurysms: 17 years' experience. Eur Endovasc Surg 18:162-165, 1999.
9. Rhodes EL, Stanley JC, Hoffman CL, et al: Aneurysms of extracranial carotid arteries. Arch Surg 111:3, 1976.
10. Goldstone J: Aneurysms of the extracranial carotid artery. In Rutherford RB (ed): Vascular Surgery. Philadelphia, WB Saunders, 1984, pp 1279-1287.
11. Ehrenfeld WK, Hays RJ: False aneurysm after carotid endarterectomy. Arch Surg 104:288, 1972.
12. Hobson RW II, Isreal MR, Lynch TO: Axillo-subclavian arterial aneurysms. In Bergan JJ, Vito JST (eds): Aneurysms. New York, Grune & Stratton, 1982, pp 435-447.
13. Gray RJ, Stone WM, Fowl RJ, et al: Management of true aneurysms distal to the axillary artery. J Vasc Surg 28:606, 1998.
14. Szilagyi DE, Schwartz RL, Reddy DJ: Popliteal arterial aneurysms: Their natural history and management. Arch Surg 116:724, 1981.

15. Vermilion ED, Kinunmns SA, Pace WC, et al: A review of one hundred forty-seven popliteal aneurysms with long-term follow-up. Surgery 90:1009, 1981.

16. Evans WE, Vermilion ED: Popliteal and femoral aneurysms. In Rutherford RB (ed): Vascular Surgery. Philadelphia, WB Saunders, 1984, pp 814-827.

17. Dent TL, Lindenaur SM, Ernst CE, et al: Multiple arteriosclerotic arterial aneurysms. Arch Surg 105:338, 1972.

18. Pairolero PC, Walls JT, Payne WS, et al: Subclavian-axillary artery aneurysms. Surgery 90:757, 1981.

19. Tolstedt GE, Radke HM, Bell JW: Late sequelae of arteriosclerotic femoral aneurysms. Angiology 12:601, 1961.

20. Cutler BS, Darling RC: Surgical management of arteriosclerotic femoral aneurysms. Surgery 74:764, 1973.

21. Reed MIC, Smith EM: Popliteal aneurysm with spontaneous arteriovenous fistula. J Cardiovasc Surg 32:482-484, 1991.

22. Diwan A, Sarkar R, Stanley JC, et al: Incidence of femoral and popliteal artery aneurysms in patients with abdominal aortic aneurysms. J Vasc Surg 31:863-869, 2000.

23. Faggioli G, Freyrie A, Stella A, et al: Extracranial internal carotid artery aneurysms: Results of a surgical series with long-term follow-up. J Vasc Surg 23:587-595, 1996.

24. Rosset E, Roche PH, Magnan PE, et al: Surgical management of extracranial internal carotid artery aneurysms. Cardiovasc Surg 2:567-572, 1994.

25. Coffin O, Maiza D, Galateau-Salle F, et al: Results of surgical management of internal carotid artery aneurysm by the cervical approach. Ann Vasc Surg 11:482-490, 1997.

26. Poirier NC, Verdant A: Popliteal aneurysm: Surgical treatment is mandatory before complications occur. Ann Chir 50:613-618, 1996.

27. Stoney RJ, Qvarfordt PC: Accessible and inaccessible aneurysms of the extracranial carotid artery. In Moore WS (ed): Surgery for Cerebrovascular Disease. New York, Churchill Livingstone, 1987, pp 567-577.

28. Mathis JM, Barr J, Yonas H, et al: Temporary balloon test occlusion of the internal carotid artery: Experience in 500 cases. AJNR Am J Neuroradiol 16:749-754, 1995.

29. Gee W, Mehigan JT, Wylie EJ: Measurement of collateral cerebral hemispheric blood pressure by ocular pneumoplethysmography. Am J Surg 130:121, 1975.

30. Beregi JP, Prat A, Willoteaux S, et al: Covered stents in the treatment of peripheral arterial aneurysms: Procedural results and midterm follow-up. Cardiovasc Intervent Radiol 22:13-19, 1999.

31. Hurst RW, Haskal ZJ, Bagley LJ, et al: Endovascular stent treatment of cervical internal carotid artery aneurysms with parent vessel preservation. Surg Neurol 50:313-317, 1998.

32. Mukherjee D, Roffi M, Yadov JS: Endovascular treatment of carotid artery aneurysms with stent grafts. J Invasive Cardiol 14:260-272, 2002.

33. Szeimies U, Kueffer G, Stoeckelhuber B, et al: Successful exclusion of subclavian aneurysms with covered nitinol stents. Cardiovasc Intervent Radiol 21:246-249, 1998.

34. Hilfiker PR, Razavi MK, Kee ST, et al: Stent-graft therapy for subclavian artery aneurysms and fistula: Single-center mid-term results. J Vasc Interv Radiol 11:578-584, 2000.

35. Baudier JF, Justesen P, Astrup M, et al: Endovascular treatment of subclavian artery aneurysm. Ugeskr Laeger 161:1774-1775, 1999.

36. Muller-Hulsbeck S, Link J, Schwarzenberg H, et al: Percutaneous endoluminal stent and stent-graft placement for treatment of femoropopliteal aneurysms: Early experience. Cardiovasc Intervent Radiol 22:96-102, 1999.

37. van Sambeek MR, Gussenhoven EJ, van der Lugt A, et al: Endovascular stent-grafts for aneurysms of the femoral and popliteal arteries. Ann Vasc Surg 13:247-253, 1999.

38. Ihlberg LH, Roth WD, Alback NA, et al: Successful percutaneous endovascular treatment of a ruptured popliteal artery aneurysm. J Vasc Surg 31:794-797, 2000.

39. Varga ZA, Locke-Ednunds JC, Baird RN, et al: Multicenter study of popliteal aneurysms. J Vasc Surg 20:171-177, 1994.

40. Hoelting T, Paetz B, Richter GM, et al: The value of preoperative lytic therapy in limb-threatening acute ischemia from popliteal artery aneurysm. Am J Surg 168:227-231, 1994.

41. Greenberg R, Wellander E, Nyman U, et al: Aggressive treatment of acute limb ischemia due to thrombosed popliteal aneurysms. Eur J Radiol 28:211-218, 1998.

42. Gross WS, Flanigan DP, Kraft RO, et al: Chronic upper extremity ischemia: Etiology, manifestations, and treatment. Arch Surg 84:417, 1978.

43. Lilly MP, Flinn WR, McCarthy WJ, et al: The effect of distal arterial anatomy on the success of popliteal aneurysm repair. J Vasc Surg 7:653, 1988.

44. Shortell CK, DeWeese JA, Ouriel IC, Green EM: Popliteal artery aneurysms: A 25 year experience. J Vasc Surg 14:771-779, 1991.

45. Sarcina A, Bellosta R, Luzzani L, Agrifoglio G: Surgical treatment of popliteal artery aneurysm: A 20-year experience. J Cardiovasc Surg (Torino) 38:347-354, 1997.

46. D'Angelo F, Gatti S, Pace M, et al: Aneurysm of the popliteal artery: A case contribution of a 15-year surgical experience. Minerva Cardioangiol 44:499-509, 1996.

47. Davidovic LB, Lotina SI, Kostie DM, et al: Popliteal artery aneurysms. World J Surg 22:812-817, 1998.

48. Duffy ST, Colgan MP, Sultan S, et al: Popliteal aneurysms: A ten year experience. Eur J Vasc Surg 16:218-222, 1998.

49. Tielliu IF, Verhoeven EL, Prins TR, et al: Treatment of popliteal artery aneurysms with the Hemobahn stent-graft. J Endovasc Ther 10:111-116, 2003.

50. Dawson I, van Bockel H, Brand R, Terpstra JL: Popliteal artery aneurysms: Long-term follow-up of aneurysmal disease and results of surgical treatment. J Vasc Surg 13:398-407, 1991.

51. Moore WS, Malone JM: Mycotic aneurysms. In Bergan JJ, Yao JST (eds): Aneurysms. New York, Grune & Stratton, 1982, pp 581-595.

52. Wilson SE, Van Wagenen P, Passaro E Jr: Arterial infection. Curr Probl Surg 15:1-89, 1978.

53. Patel S, Johnston KW: Classification and management of mycotic aneurysms. Surg Gynecol Obstet 144:691, 1977.

54. Reddy DJ, Smith RF, Elliot JP, et al: Infected femoral artery false aneurysms in drug addicts: Evolution of selective vascular reconstruction. J Vasc Surg 3:718, 1986.

55. Anderson CE: Mycotic aneurysms. In Rutherford RB (ed): Vascular Surgery. Philadelphia, WB Saunders, 1984, pp 835-847.

56. Jones TR, Frusha JD: Mycotic cervical carotid artery aneurysms: A case report and review of the literature. Ann Vasc Surg 2:373, 1988.

57. Jebara VA, Acar C, Dervanian P, et al: Mycotic aneurysms of the carotid arteries: Case report and review of the literature. J Vasc Surg 14:215-219, 1991.

58. Howell HS, Baruraao T, Craziano J: Mycotic cervical carotid aneurysm. Surgery 81:357, 1977.

59. Miller CM, Sangiuolo P, Schanzer H: Infected false aneurysms of the subclavian artery: A complication in drug addicts. J Vasc Surg 1:684, 1984.

60. Buerger F, Feldman AJ: Infected groin aneurysms from heroin addiction. In Bergan JJ, Yao JST (eds): Aneurysms. New York, Grune & Stratton, 1982, pp 643-655.

61. Benjamin ME, Cohn EJ Jr, Purtill WA, et al: Arterial reconstruction with deep leg veins for the treatment of mycotic aneurysms. J Vasc Surg 30:1004-1015, 1999.

Questions

1. **Subclavian artery aneurysms are most commonly caused by which of the following?**
   (a) Atherosclerosis
   (b) Thoracic outlet syndrome
   (c) Fibromuscular dysplasia
   (d) Trauma

2. **What is the most common complication of subclavian artery aneurysms?**
   (a) Rupture
   (b) Pain secondary to nerve compression
   (c) Embolization
   (d) Thrombosis

3. **Most carotid artery aneurysms are identified because of which of the following?**
   (a) Rupture of the aneurysm
   (b) Mass in the neck
   (c) Neurologic complications
   (d) Swishing sound heard in the patient's ipsilateral ear

4. **Which of the following statements is true regarding femoral and popliteal artery aneurysms?**
   (a) These aneurysms should be repaired only when they become very large and cause pain from adjacent nerve compression
   (b) These aneurysms are rarely associated with other peripheral aneurysms
   (c) These aneurysms are particularly dangerous because of a high incidence of distal embolization or aneurysm thrombosis
   (d) Long-term results of the surgical treatment of these aneurysms are not dependent on the degree of arterial occlusive disease distal to the aneurysm

5. **What is the most common cause of peripheral aneurysms?**
   (a) Atherosclerosis
   (b) Infection
   (c) Trauma
   (d) Connective tissue disorders

6. **Which of the following peripheral aneurysms is most likely to rupture?**
   (a) Popliteal
   (b) Carotid
   (c) Deep femoral
   (d) Axillary

7. **For a patient with ischemia secondary to thrombosis of a popliteal artery aneurysm and occlusion of the popliteal outflow tract, what is the best initial treatment?**
   (a) Thrombolytic therapy
   (b) Thrombectomy and bypass
   (c) Observation
   (d) Sympathectomy

8. **What is the most common cause of mycotic aneurysms?**
   (a) Trauma
   (b) Bacterial endocarditis
   (c) Direct extension of adjacent infection
   (d) Food poisoning

9. **Which of the following statements about popliteal aneurysms is true?**
   (a) They are frequently bilateral
   (b) They are commonly associated with abdominal aortic aneurysms
   (c) They rarely rupture
   (d) All of the above

10. **Which of the following statements about carotid artery aneurysms is true?**
    (a) They most commonly involve the internal carotid artery
    (b) They are more common than subclavian artery aneurysms
    (c) They require surgical repair in most patients
    (d) None of the above

Answers

1. b	2. c	3. c	4. c	5. a
6. c	7. a	8. a	9. d	10. c

30

James C. Stanley • Louis M. Messina • Gerald B. Zelenock

Splanchnic and Renal Artery Aneurysms

Splanchnic Artery Aneurysms

Aneurysms of the visceral branches of the abdominal aorta are being recognized with increasing frequency. More than 3700 splanchnic and renal artery aneurysms have been described in the English-language literature, and more than half of them have been reported in the past 25 years. Splanchnic aneurysms are approximately three times more common than renal aneurysms. These aneurysms are best addressed individually because of the marked variability in their biologic character and clinical importance.

Splanchnic artery aneurysms are an uncommon but important vascular disease (Table 30-1). Nearly 22% of these aneurysms appear as surgical emergencies, including 8.5% that result in the patient's death. The major splanchnic vessels involved with these macroaneurysms, in decreasing order of frequency, are the splenic; hepatic; superior mesenteric; celiac; gastric and gastroepiploic; jejunal, ileal, and colic; pancreaticoduodenal and pancreatic; and gastroduodenal arteries.

The clinical manifestations of splanchnic artery aneurysms have become well defined during the past 3 decades.[1-10] The treatment of certain aneurysms has changed in recent years. Endovascular therapy has become widespread and provides an alternative to conventional surgical therapy, although long-term follow-up is lacking and disparate results have been reported, with early success rates ranging from less than 60% to greater than 90%.[11-13] Nevertheless, treatment of many splanchnic artery aneurysms remains open operative therapy. The cause, presentation, and management of aneurysms affecting each of the splanchnic arteries deserve separate comment.

SPLENIC ARTERY ANEURYSMS

Splenic artery aneurysms account for 60% of all reported splanchnic artery aneurysms.[10,14] The frequency of splenic artery aneurysms in the general population approaches the 0.78% incidence noted in nearly 3600 consecutive abdominal arteriographic studies performed for reasons other than suspected aneurysmal disease.[14] Women are nearly four times more likely than men to have these aneurysms.

Three distinct, preexisting conditions are suspected to contribute to the development of splenic artery aneurysms. First is medial fibrodysplasia, usually a cause of hypertension secondary to renal artery involvement. Blood pressure elevations in these patients may also contribute to aneurysm formation. Coexistence of renal artery medial fibrodysplasia and splenic artery aneurysms has been identified only in women. Approximately 2% of women with renal artery medial fibrodysplasia have splenic artery aneurysms. Second are the deleterious effects on elastic vascular tissue of increased splenic blood flow and the altered levels of reproductive hormones that accompany repeated pregnancies. Approximately 40% of women harboring these aneurysms are grand multiparas, having completed six or more pregnancies. Third, portal hypertension with splenomegaly is associated with splenic artery macroaneurysms in nearly 10% of patients.[14-16] This may reflect the greater splenic blood flow velocities[17,18] as well as elevated estrogen activity associated with cirrhosis. There has been an increased recognition of these aneurysms in patients subjected to orthotopic liver transplantation.[19-21] Aneurysms are more common in female than male liver transplant patients, and they appear to be directly related to the severity of the patient's antecedent portal hypertension.[21]

Although certain splenic artery aneurysms exhibit arteriosclerotic disease, the typical advanced arteriosclerotic calcific changes in many aneurysms are more likely a secondary event rather than a primary etiologic process. Inflammatory disease, such as chronic pancreatitis and penetrating trauma, are less common causes of these aneurysms. Splenic microaneurysms are usually associated with generalized vasculitis, such as polyarteritis nodosa, and are of less clinical importance than extraparenchymal macroaneurysms.

Most splenic artery aneurysms associated with arterial fibrodysplasia, multiple pregnancies, or portal hypertension are saccular and occur at vessel branchings (Fig. 30-1). These are true aneurysms, not false aneurysms. At arterial branchings, discontinuities exist in the internal elastic lamina of normal vessels, and subsequent degenerative effects involving elastic tissue (e.g., during pregnancy) are apt to produce aneurysmal changes at these sites. Aneurysms unrelated to portal hypertension are multiple 20% of the time. In patients with portal hypertension severe enough to lead to liver transplantation, these aneurysms are multiple 90% of the time.[21] In contrast, splenic artery aneurysms associated with pancreatitis usually involve the main splenic artery and tend to be solitary (Fig. 30-2).

TABLE 30–1	Distribution of Splanchnic Artery Aneurysms		
Aneurysm Location	**Frequency within Splanchnic Circulation (%)**	**Male-Female Ratio**	**Contributing Factors**
Splenic artery	60.0	1:4	Medial degeneration, arterial fibrodysplasia, multiple pregnancies, portal hypertension, chronic pancreatitis with arterial erosion by pseudocysts
Hepatic artery	20.0	2:1	Medial degeneration, blunt and penetrating liver trauma, infection related to intravenous substance abuse
Superior mesenteric artery	5.5	1:1	Infection related to bacterial endocarditis, often associated with nonhemolytic streptococci and, more recently, with intravenous substance abuse; medial degeneration
Celiac artery	4.0	1:1	Medial degeneration
Gastric and gastroepiploic arteries	4.0	3:1	Periarterial inflammation, medial degeneration
Jejunal, ileal, and colic arteries	3.0	1:1	Medial degeneration, connective tissue diseases
Pancreaticoduodenal, pancreatic, and gastroduodenal arteries	1.5	4:1	Pancreatitis-related arterial necrosis and arterial erosion by pseudocysts (60% of gastroduodenal and 30% of pancreaticoduodenal artery aneurysms), flow-related medial degeneration (with celiac artery occlusion)

Curvilinear or signet-ring calcifications in the left upper quadrant on radiographs are often evidence of a splenic artery aneurysm. However, diagnosis usually results from arteriographic demonstration of the aneurysm during studies undertaken for some other disease state. Ultrasonography, computed tomography (CT), CT arteriography, and magnetic resonance imaging are useful in recognizing these lesions and are often helpful in identifying bleeding aneurysms.[10,22] These noninvasive studies are particularly valuable for following size changes in asymptomatic aneurysms.

Left upper quadrant or epigastric pain occurs in a minority of individuals with splenic artery aneurysms, although some form of abdominal discomfort affected approximately 20% of patients in an early report.[14] In a 1996 review of 83 cases that included many single case reports, 46% of patients had abdominal pain, and 25% presented in shock.[5] However, it is important to note that individual case reports are often spectacular and are unlikely to be representative of the usual patient's clinical course.

Initial bleeding from a ruptured splenic artery aneurysm may be contained within the lesser sac. Eventually, free hemorrhage into the peritoneal cavity occurs and causes vascular collapse. This "double-rupture" phenomenon is often referred to in discussions of splenic artery aneurysms but is, in fact, relatively uncommon. Pancreatitis-related aneurysms are often a source of intestinal hemorrhage after erosion of a pseudocyst

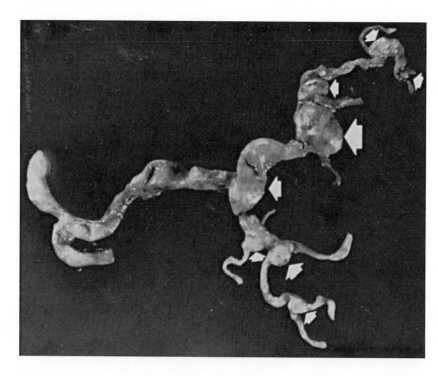

FIGURE 30–1 • Multiple splenic artery aneurysms *(arrows)* occurring at each bifurcation of the distal artery in a grand multipara. (From Stanley JC, Thompson NW, Fry WJ: Splanchnic artery aneurysms. Arch Surg 101:689-697, 1970.)

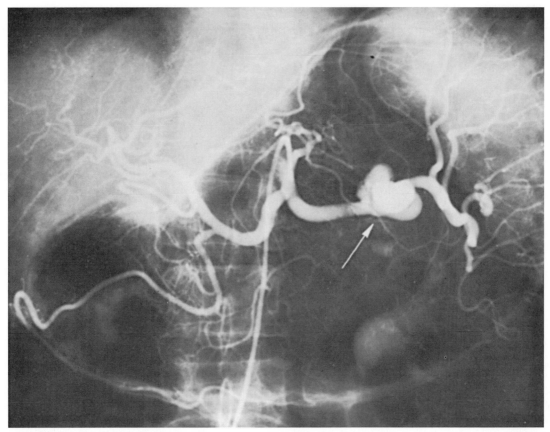

FIGURE 30–2 • Solitary splenic artery aneurysm affecting the midportion of the vessel *(arrow)*, caused by arterial erosion from a pancreatic pseudocyst in an alcoholic patient. (From Stanley JC, Frey CF, Miller TA, et al: Major arterial hemorrhage: A complication of pancreatic pseudocysts and chronic pancreatitis. Arch Surg 111:435-440, 1976.)

into an adjacent artery and subsequently into the stomach or pancreatic ductal system.[23-27] Arteriovenous fistula formation from rupture of a splenic artery aneurysm into the adjacent splenic vein is a rare but recognized cause of gastrointestinal hemorrhage from esophageal varices due to left-sided portal hypertension.[28]

The risk of splenic artery aneurysm rupture is related to its cause (Table 30-2). Rupture of bland aneurysms occurs in less than 2% of cases.[14] Contrary to earlier misconceptions, rupture is just as likely to occur with a calcified aneurysm, in a normotensive patient, or in the very elderly. Bland aneurysms in liver transplant recipients appear to be nearly twice as likely to rupture as those in other patients,[19,21] and the mortality following rupture of a splenic artery aneurysm in a liver transplant patient exceeds 50%.[29]

Nearly 95% of aneurysms first recognized during pregnancy rupture.[30-33] Maternal mortality in these cases approaches 70%, and fetal mortality exceeds 75%. However, these figures are misleading, in that most women develop aneurysms during the course of repeated pregnancies. Although the reported rupture rate during pregnancy is very high, most splenic artery aneurysms in pregnant women are likely to go unrecognized without rupture. Nevertheless, splenic artery aneurysms diagnosed during pregnancy, even though asymptomatic, represent a serious potential threat to the health of the mother and the fetus.

The operative mortality from rupture of a bland splenic artery aneurysm was 25% in the past.[7] Thus, it would seem prudent to undertake elective operative intervention for asymptomatic splenic artery aneurysms, when the risk of operative death is less than 0.5%. This latter figure represents the product of the 25% operative mortality and the 2% rupture rate of bland aneurysms. Even if the mortality rate accompanying rupture is greater, elective intervention should be undertaken only in good-risk patients.

Splenectomy for splenic artery aneurysms was the most common form of surgical therapy in the past.[5,10,14] With contemporary recognition of the immunologic benefits of splenic preservation, even in the aged, simple ligature obliteration or excision of these aneurysms is preferable to splenectomy.[34] This is clearly appropriate in the management of most proximal and many extraparenchymal distal splenic artery aneurysms. In select cases, this may be undertaken by a laparoscopic approach.[35,36]

Certain inflammatory splenic artery aneurysms embedded in the pancreas are best treated by distal pancreatectomy. Other aneurysms, especially false aneurysms associated with pseudocyst erosion into the adjacent artery, are most easily treated initially by incising the aneurysmal sac and ligating the entering and exiting vessels.[26] Pancreatic resection in the latter cases depends on the degree of associated pancreatic inflammation and the general condition of the patient.[37]

Percutaneous transcatheter embolization of splenic artery aneurysms is often a preferred alternative to open operative intervention.[2,38-40] Careful follow-up of endovascular-treated patients is mandatory. Splenic infarction and late rupture are

TABLE 30–2	Rupture of Splanchnic Artery Aneurysms			
Aneurysm Location	Frequency of Reported Rupture (%)	Site of Rupture	Mortality with Rupture (%)	Usual Treatment Options
Splenic artery	2 (bland aneurysms)	Intraperitoneal within lesser sac; intragastric with pancreatitis-related inflammatory aneurysms	Bland and unassociated with pregnancy: 25 During pregnancy: 70 maternal, 75 fetal	Splenectomy; aneurysm exclusion or excision without splenectomy; transcatheter aneurysm obliteration
Hepatic artery	20	Intraperitoneal and biliary tract with equal frequency	35	Aneurysmectomy with or without hepatic artery reconstruction; hepatic territory resection; transcatheter aneurysm obliteration
Superior mesenteric artery	Uncommon (thrombosis more common)	Intraperitoneal and retroperitoneal	50	Aneurysmectomy with superior mesenteric artery reconstruction; ligation if collateral circulation is adequate
Celiac artery	13	Intraperitoneal	50	Aneurysmectomy with celiac artery reconstruction; ligation if circulation is adequate
Gastric and gastroepiploic arteries	90	Intraperitoneal: 30 Intestinal tract: 70	70	Aneurysm excision with involved gastric tissue; ligation if extramural
Jejunal, ileal, and colic arteries	30	Intestinal tract common; intraperitoneal uncommon	20	Aneurysm excision with involved intestine; ligation if extramural
Pancreatico-duodenal, pancreatic, and gastroduodenal arteries	Inflammatory: 75 Noninflammatory: 50	Intestinal tract: 85 Intraperitoneal: 15	50	Aneurysm ligation within false aneurysms (pseudocyst related); pancreatic resection; ligation if extrapancreatic; transcatheter aneurysm obliteration

concerns, as is nondurable obliteration of the aneurysm or coil migration and erosion into the adjacent viscera.[41,42] Stent-graft exclusion of an aneurysm with maintenance of splenic artery flow can be used in select cases.[43-45]

HEPATIC ARTERY ANEURYSMS

Hepatic artery aneurysms account for 20% of all reported splanchnic artery aneurysms,[10,46,47] although they appear to be more common in contemporary practice.[5] Men are twice as likely to be affected as women, although gender differences appear to be less significant in more recent times.[5,48] More than a third of patients with these aneurysms have other splanchnic artery aneurysms.[49] Nontraumatic and nonmycotic aneurysms are most often discovered during the sixth decade of life.

Certain facts regarding the cause of hepatic artery aneurysms are noteworthy. With increasing societal violence, both penetrating and blunt liver injuries have led to a marked increase in the number of reported traumatic aneurysms. In fact, nearly 50% of recently reported hepatic artery aneurysms were false aneurysms of intrahepatic arterial branches.[5] Most of these represent small pseudoaneurysms diagnosed by CT studies in motor vehicle accident patients subjected to emergent scanning. Iatrogenic false aneurysms secondary to open biliary tract and pancreatic operative trauma are rare but well recognized[50]; false aneurysms associated with percutaneous and therapeutic biliary tract procedures are slightly

more common.[5] Arteriosclerosis represents a secondary event rather than an actual cause of these aneurysms. Mycotic aneurysms associated with sepsis related to intravenous drug abuse and endocarditis are another contemporary factor. Surprisingly, nearly 17% of hepatic artery aneurysms reported from 1985 to 1995 were associated with liver transplantation.[5] Connective tissue arteriopathies, such as periarteritis nodosa, have also been incriminated as a cause of occasional macroaneurysms involving the hepatic vessels.[51] Hepatic artery aneurysms are usually solitary; they are extrahepatic in nearly 80% of cases and intrahepatic in 20%. In general, these aneurysms are fusiform when less than 2 cm in diameter and saccular when larger (Fig. 30-3).

Most hepatic artery aneurysms are asymptomatic and are discovered incidentally during arteriography, CT, or ultrasonography for other illnesses.[5,52,53] Nontraumatic hepatic artery aneurysms are occasionally symptomatic, in which case they characteristically produce right upper quadrant and epigastric pain. Acute expansion of hepatic artery aneurysms can cause severe abdominal discomfort, similar to that of pancreatitis. Large aneurysms may cause obstructive jaundice.[54] However, most hepatic artery aneurysms are too small to compress the biliary ducts. These lesions rarely manifest as pulsatile abdominal masses. Trauma-related aneurysms, because of the very nature of abdominal injury, are often associated with pain.

The reported incidence of rupture of hepatic artery aneurysms in contemporary times is close to 20%, but the

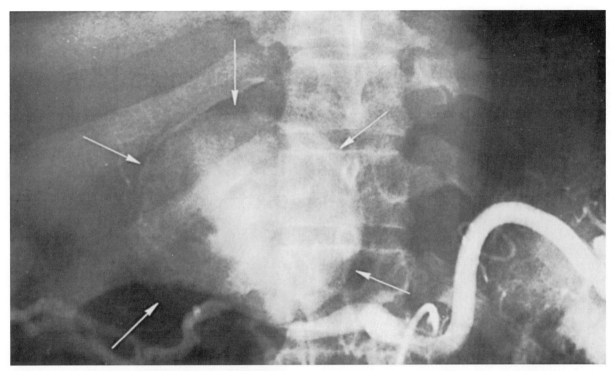

FIGURE 30–3 • Large hepatic artery aneurysm *(arrows)* affecting the proximal artery in a patient with an underlying connective tissue disorder. (From Stanley JC, Whitehouse WM Jr: Aneurysms of splanchnic and renal arteries. In Bergan JJ, Yao JST [eds]: Surgery of the Aorta and Its Body Branches. New York, Grune & Stratton, 1979, pp 497-519.)

true incidence may be considerably less. Reported overall mortality rates attending aneurysm rupture are approximately 35%, although recent experience suggests that mortality is lower.[5] Bleeding from ruptured hepatic artery aneurysms occurs equally into the biliary tract and into the peritoneal cavity. In the case of the former, hemobilia is often evident, manifested by biliary colic, hematemesis, and jaundice.[55,56] Chronic gastrointestinal hemorrhage is an uncommon but recognized sequela of aneurysm rupture into the biliary tract. Intraperitoneal bleeding is usually associated with false aneurysms caused by periarterial inflammatory processes eroding into the hepatic vessels.

Common hepatic artery aneurysms are generally treated by aneurysmectomy or aneurysm exclusion, without arterial reconstruction.[5,46] Simple ligation is usually undertaken if temporary occlusion of the aneurysmal artery does not cause obvious hepatic ischemia. The extensive arterial collateral circulation to the liver and the ability of the portal venous flow to increase usually provide adequate liver blood flow despite interruption of the proximal hepatic artery. If compromised liver blood flow becomes apparent after hepatic artery occlusion, direct vascular reconstruction must be undertaken with a prosthetic or autologous graft. Hepatic ischemia is most likely to accompany treatment of aneurysms involving the more distal hepatic artery, and casual ligation of extrahepatic branches to control bleeding from intrahepatic aneurysms may cause liver necrosis.[46] Because of this complication, hepatic territory resection for intrahepatic aneurysms may be necessary in select patients.

Percutaneous transcatheter obliteration of hepatic artery aneurysms with balloons, coils, or thrombogenic particulate matter is a reasonable and often preferred alternative to open surgical intervention.[5,38,50,57-59] It is recognized that transcatheter embolization may be only transiently successful, and repeated embolization or eventual surgical therapy may be required to adequately treat these patients.[47,60] Transcatheter thrombin injection[61] and endograft exclusion of select aneurysms may prove useful in carefully chosen patients.[62,63]

SUPERIOR MESENTERIC ARTERY ANEURYSMS

Aneurysms of the proximal superior mesenteric artery are the third most common splanchnic artery aneurysm, accounting for 5.5% of these lesions.[14] Men are affected nearly twice as often as women.[5] Mycotic aneurysms secondary to bacterial endocarditis are a common lesion affecting this vessel.[5,64] Nonhemolytic streptococci and a variety of pathogens associated with intravenous substance abuse account for these latter lesions. Although infectious aneurysms were common in the past, they are encountered less often in contemporary practice.[65] Superior mesenteric artery aneurysms may also be related to medial degeneration, periarterial inflammation, and trauma. Arteriosclerosis, when present, is considered a secondary event rather than an etiologic process. Superior mesenteric artery aneurysms are usually recognized during arteriographic studies for other diseases. The majority of reported superior mesenteric artery aneurysms are asymptomatic.[5] In other patients, abdominal pain varies from mild to severe and, in many cases, is suggestive of intestinal angina.

Superior mesenteric artery aneurysm rupture is unusual,[66] and aneurysmal dissection is uncommon.[67] Gastrointestinal hemorrhage associated with these aneurysms usually reflects their acute occlusion and bleeding from areas of intestinal infarction.[7] The unique location of these aneurysms near the origins of the inferior pancreaticoduodenal and middle colic arteries effectively isolates the distal mesenteric circulation should aneurysmal dissection or occlusion occur. Profound intestinal ischemia occurs in this setting because the usual collateral networks from the adjacent celiac and inferior mesenteric arterial circulations are lost.

Aneurysmectomy or simple ligation of vessels entering and exiting a superior mesenteric artery aneurysm may necessitate intestinal revascularization by means of an aortomesenteric graft or some other bypass. However, this has been accomplished infrequently. Because of the potential for graft infection if bowel ischemia is present, autologous vein grafts are favored over prosthetic conduits for these reconstructions.

Ligation of superior mesenteric artery aneurysms without arterial reconstruction has proved possible in certain cases,[5,10] especially for aneurysms associated with prior arterial obstruction and development of an adequate collateral circulation to the midgut structures.[10] Surprisingly, ligation and aneurysmorrhaphy are the most common means of managing these lesions.[66,68-70] Doppler documentation of blood flow along the intestine's antimesenteric border assists in establishing the adequacy of collateral vessels in these circumstances.

Endovascular placement of a stent-graft has appeal for selected superior mesenteric artery aneurysms,[71,72] although infection and thrombosis may compromise this treatment. Obliteration of these aneurysms by coils or direct thrombin injection may be preferred in high-risk patients with discrete aneurysm necks.[65,73]

CELIAC ARTERY ANEURYSMS

Celiac artery aneurysms account for 4% of all splanchnic artery aneurysms.[10] Men and women appear to be equally affected.[74] Half the celiac artery aneurysms encountered before 1950 had an infectious cause, although such lesions are decidedly uncommon today.[75,76] More recently, most aneurysms are associated with medial defects. Aortic aneurysms affect nearly 20% of these patients, and nearly 40% have other splanchnic aneurysms.[74] Arteriosclerosis is a frequent finding, but, as in the case of other splanchnic artery aneurysms, it is considered a secondary process. Celiac artery aneurysms are usually saccular, affecting the distal trunk of this vessel (Fig. 30-4), with some evolving from poststenotic dilatations caused by preexisting occlusive disease or median arcuate ligament entrapment of the proximal celiac artery.

Most contemporary celiac artery aneurysms are asymptomatic or are associated with vague abdominal discomfort.[5,74] Antemortem diagnosis usually results when these aneurysms are recognized as incidental findings during ultrasonography, angiography, or CT for other diseases. Rupture reportedly occurs in 13% of these aneurysms and carries a mortality of 50%.[74] In contrast to this more contemporary experience are previously published rupture rates of greater than 80%.[77] Celiac artery aneurysm rupture usually causes life-threatening intraperitoneal hemorrhage. Aneurysmal rupture rarely occurs into the gastrointestinal tract.

Operative treatment of all celiac artery aneurysms is recommended, unless prohibitive surgical risks exist. Most nonruptured aneurysms can be treated through an abdominal approach, although in the presence of acute expansion or rupture, a thoracoabdominal incision may be favored. Aneurysmectomy with arterial reconstruction of the celiac

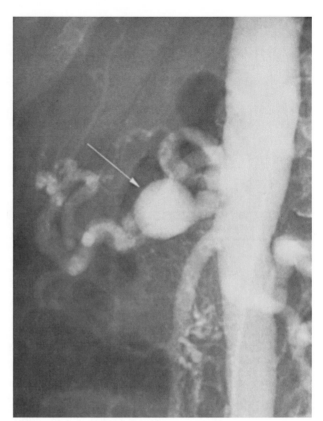

FIGURE 30–4 • Celiac artery aneurysm *(arrow)* affecting the distal trunk of the vessel. (From Whitehouse WM Jr, Graham LM, Stanley JC: Aneurysms of the celiac, hepatic, and splenic arteries. In Bergan JJ, Yao JST [eds]: Aneurysms: Diagnosis and Treatment. New York, Grune & Stratton, 1981, pp 405-415.)

trunk is the preferred surgical therapy. However, aneurysm exclusion with ligation of entering and exiting branches can be performed in select patients.[5,74,78,79] If simple ligature is undertaken, the foregut collateral blood flow to the liver must be sufficient to prevent liver necrosis. If such is not the case, hepatic revascularization is mandatory. An aortoceliac or aortohepatic artery bypass under these circumstances is usually undertaken with an autologous vein or prosthetic graft. In contemporary reports, successful outcomes of surgical therapy are greater than 90%.[74]

Endovascular treatment of celiac artery aneurysms is unattractive because of the need to occlude the hepatic, splenic, and left gastric arteries, and perhaps the inferior phrenic arteries, to obliterate the aneurysm. Nevertheless, glue-embolic occlusion of a false aneurysm, approached through the gastroduodenal artery, has been reported.[80]

GASTRIC AND GASTROEPIPLOIC ARTERY ANEURYSMS

Gastric and gastroepiploic artery aneurysms account for 4% of splanchnic artery aneurysms.[10] Gastric artery aneurysms are 10 times more common than gastroepiploic artery aneurysms. Men are three times more likely than women to have these aneurysms. The majority of these lesions affect patients older than 50 years. Most of these aneurysms are solitary and are acquired as a result of either periarterial inflammation or medial degeneration. Arteriosclerosis, when present, is a secondary accompaniment of these lesions.

Surprisingly, few gastric or gastroepiploic artery aneurysms are asymptomatic when initially recognized.[10,81] In fact, these perigastric aneurysms usually present as emergencies without preceding symptoms.[10,82,83] Rupture occurred in more than 90% of reported cases, with gastrointestinal bleeding being twice as common as intraperitoneal hemorrhage. Aneurysm rupture may be catastrophic, as emphasized by the reported 70% mortality of such an event.[7]

Surgical treatment of gastric and gastroepiploic artery aneurysms does not involve vascular reconstructive surgery.[10,81] Intramural gastric aneurysms require excision with the involved portion of the stomach. Extramural aneurysms should be treated by arterial ligation alone, with or without aneurysm excision. In select cases, laparoscopic resection may be appropriate.[84] Gastric and gastroepiploic artery aneurysms are usually very small, and a search for them is often tedious if they have not been localized preoperatively by arteriographic studies.[7,26]

JEJUNAL, ILEAL, AND COLIC ARTERY ANEURYSMS

Aneurysms of the jejunal, ileal, and colic arteries account for 3% of splanchnic artery aneurysms.[10] They are usually recognized in patients older than 60 years, with men and women affected equally. Solitary aneurysms are reported in 90% of cases. Acquired medial defects are responsible for most lesions; arteriosclerosis, present in 20% of these aneurysms, is considered a secondary event rather than a causative process. Multiple aneurysms tend to evolve as a result of infected emboli associated with subacute bacterial endocarditis,[85] or they result from periarteritis nodosa or other connective tissue diseases.[86]

Most reported aneurysms are symptomatic, with the majority exhibiting abdominal pain.[5,87] Nevertheless, many aneurysms are undoubtedly asymptomatic and are recognized as incidental findings during arteriography for gastrointestinal bleeding (Fig. 30-5).[88] Although the majority of reported intestinal branch aneurysms have ruptured, actual rupture rates are probably close to 30%. Aneurysms of ileal branches are more apt to rupture, with jejunal branch aneurysm rupture being relatively rare.[89] Rupture is associated with a mortality of approximately 20% and is frequently a cause of gastrointestinal hemorrhage.[10] Rupture into the small bowel mesentery or the mesocolon, as well as into the free peritoneal cavity, is uncommon. Operations for extraintestinal aneurysms usually entail arterial ligation, with or without aneurysmectomy. Intramural aneurysms or those associated with bowel infarction necessitate resection of the involved segment of intestine. In selected patients, transcatheter embolization may be undertaken, but intestinal necrosis with acute perforation or later stricture formation is a recognized complication of such therapy.[90] Aneurysms of the inferior mesenteric artery are quite rare, and knowledge of their clinical importance is anecdotal at best.[5,91]

PANCREATICODUODENAL, PANCREATIC, AND GASTRODUODENAL ARTERY ANEURYSMS

Pancreatic and pancreaticoduodenal artery aneurysms account for 2%, and gastroduodenal artery aneurysms represent an

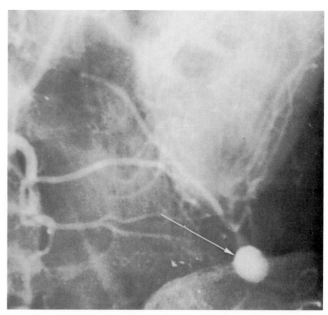

FIGURE 30–5 • Ileal artery branch aneurysm *(arrow).* (From Stanley JC, Whitehouse WM Jr: Aneurysms of splanchnic and renal arteries. In Bergan JJ, Yao JST [eds]: Surgery of the Aorta and Its Body Branches. New York, Grune & Stratton, 1979, pp 497-519.)

additional 1.5%, of all splanchnic artery aneurysms.[10] Men are four times as likely as women to have pancreaticoduodenal and gastroduodenal artery aneurysms, with gender differences being more notable in the former than the latter aneurysms. Most patients with these lesions are older than 45 years. In general, these peripancreatic aneurysms are the most difficult splanchnic artery aneurysms to treat.[26,92-97]

The most common cause of these aneurysms is pancreatitis-related vascular necrosis or vessel erosion by an adjacent pancreatic pseudocyst (Fig. 30-6). Medial degenerative and traumatic lesions are less common, and arteriosclerosis is invariably a secondary process. Isolated non–pancreatitis-related pancreaticoduodenal artery aneurysms are most likely to evolve as an apparent consequence of excessive blood flow within these arteries, functioning as collateral vessels in patients having celiac artery stenosis.[98-102] Although less well recognized, gastroduodenal artery aneurysms may develop for the same reason in cases of superior mesenteric artery stenosis.[103]

The vast majority of patients with these aneurysms experience epigastric pain and discomfort.[6,10] This may be due to underlying pancreatic disease, in that approximately 50% of gastroduodenal and 30% of pancreaticoduodenal artery aneurysms are related to pancreatitis. Arteriography is necessary to confirm the existence of these lesions. CT and magnetic resonance imaging are of increasing importance in recognizing these aneurysms and are helpful in detecting the presence of rupture or associated pancreatic lesions.

Gastroduodenal and pancreaticoduodenal aneurysm rupture has been described in more than half of reported cases, affecting 75% of inflammatory and 50% of noninflammatory lesions.[5,10,100] Bleeding usually occurs into the stomach, biliary tract, or pancreatic ductal system. Hemorrhage into the peritoneal cavity is less common, occurring in approximately 15% of these aneurysms. Overall, mortality rates with rupture approach 25% but may be as high as 50% in the case of true pancreaticoduodenal artery aneurysms.[5]

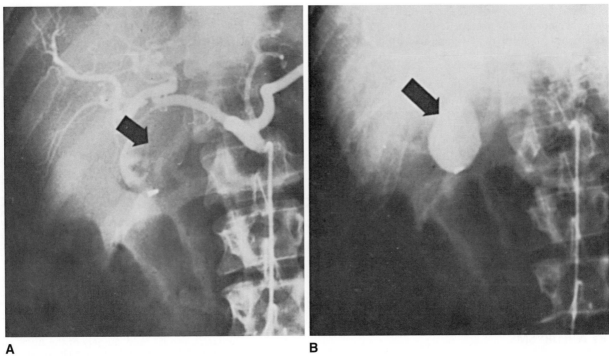

A   B

FIGURE 30–6 • Gastroduodenal aneurysm *(arrow)* associated with arterial erosion by an adjacent infected pancreatic pseudocyst. *A,* Early-phase selective celiac arteriogram. *B,* Late-phase arteriogram with contrast collection in the false aneurysm *(arrow).*

Operative intervention is mandatory in all but the highest-risk patients with gastroduodenal, pancreaticoduodenal, or pancreatic arterial aneurysms.[5,26,92,93,104,105] Surgical treatment of pancreatitis-related false aneurysms is often accomplished by arterial ligation from within the aneurysmal sac rather than extra-aneurysmal arterial ligation. Extensive dissection about the pancreas in this setting is hazardous. If a pancreatic pseudocyst or abscess has eroded into an artery and caused a false aneurysm, some form of drainage procedure may need to accompany ligature control of the affected vessel. Concurrent or later pancreatic resection, including distal pancreatectomy or pancreaticoduodenectomy, may be the safest therapy in select patients.[26,106]

Transcatheter embolization and electrocoagulation have been employed in very high-risk patients to ablate certain aneurysms.[107-111] Thrombin injections may serve as an effective means of occluding small aneurysms.[112,113] Unfortunately, rebleeding and late aneurysmal rupture can occur with these therapies and restrict their universal use.[99,114] However, in critically ill patients who are unstable, endovascular occlusion of the bleeding aneurysm may be an appropriate lifesaving measure, followed by a later definitive open resection. In those patients with coexistent celiac artery occlusion, the aneurysmal artery may be part of an important collateral vessel, and simple operative ligature or transcatheter embolic occlusion may result in foregut ischemia and should be undertaken cautiously.

Renal Artery Aneurysms

Renal artery aneurysms represent an uncommon vascular disease (Table 30-3). Controversy continues concerning their clinical importance.[115-125] This relates, in part, to the fact that complications of these aneurysms have been overestimated in spectacular case reports rather than relying on population-based experiences.[125,126] Discussion of these lesions must take into consideration the differences between true aneurysms and dissections of the renal artery.

TRUE RENAL ARTERY ANEURYSMS

The incidence of true renal artery aneurysms approaches 0.1%, a figure derived from the 0.09% frequency of these lesions in approximately 8500 patients subjected to arteriographic studies for nonrenal disease.[124] Women are slightly more likely than men to have renal artery aneurysms.[118] However, when aneurysms in patients having renal arterial dysplasia are excluded, there is no gender predilection. That the right renal artery is more likely than the left to develop aneurysms may reflect the fact that dysplastic disease is known to affect the right renal artery more commonly.[124] Most renal artery aneurysms are saccular (Fig. 30-7). Seventy-five percent are located at first- or second-order renal artery bifurcations. Intraparenchymal aneurysms occur in less than 10% of cases. Most aneurysms have diameters less than 1.5 cm.

Renal artery aneurysms are usually caused by a medial degenerative process. In many instances, this may be a manifestation of systemic medial fibroplasia (Fig. 30-8).[118,119,124] Arteriosclerosis, evident by hemorrhage, calcium deposition, collections of cholesterol, and necrotic cellular debris within a matrix of fibrous tissue, affects a third of these aneurysms. However, similar changes affecting the adjacent renal artery are very uncommon, and the former findings are thought to represent a secondary event rather than a primary process. Importantly, arteriosclerosis in some but not all aneurysms in the same patient suggests a nonarteriosclerotic cause of these lesions.[118,124] Microaneurysms secondary to necrotizing arteritides, such as polyarteritis nodosa, are a third type of

TABLE 30–3		**Renal Artery Aneurysms**			
Lesion	**Male-Female Ratio**	**Contributing Factors**	**Frequency of Reported Rupture (%)**	**Mortality with Rupture (%)**	**Treatment Options**
Renal artery aneurysm	1:1.2	Medial degeneration, arterial fibrodysplasia, hypertension	3 (bland aneurysms)	Bland aneurysms:10 During pregnancy: 50 maternal, 75 fetal	Aneurysmectomy with renal artery reconstruction; transcatheter aneurysm obliteration (intraparenchymal lesions); nephrectomy for ruptured aneurysms
Renal artery dissection	10:1	Blunt abdominal trauma, intra-arterial catheterization, medial degeneration	Uncommon (thrombosis more common)	Undefined	Renal artery reconstruction; nephrectomy for irreparable renal ischemia

true aneurysm.[127] These latter aneurysms often thrombose with the passage of time.

The majority of renal artery aneurysms are asymptomatic.[124] Some authors have suggested that few of these aneurysms ever cause serious clinical complications.[119,125,126] Nevertheless, aneurysmal expansion or renal infarction from dislodged thrombus may occasionally account for pain and hypertension attributed to these lesions. Hematuria and abdominal bruits, when present, are unlikely to be related to aneurysmal disease.

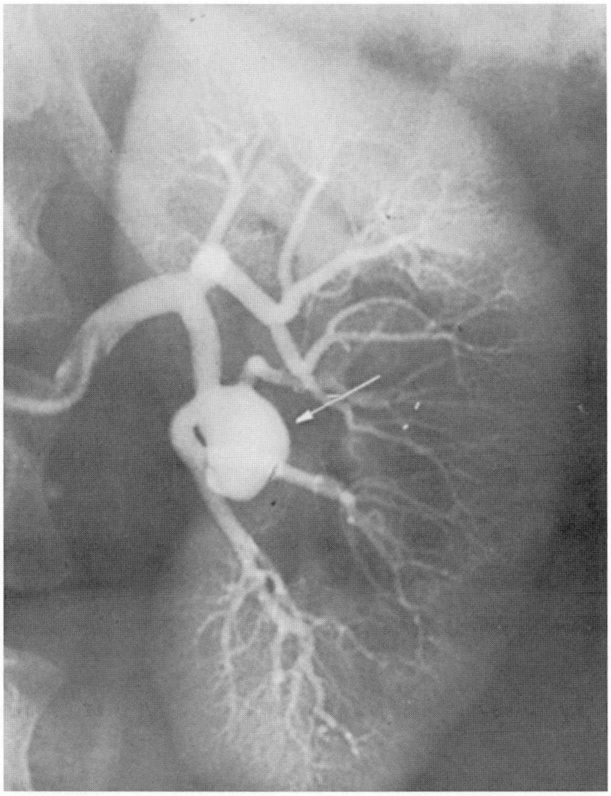

Similarly, because they are small, very few aneurysms present as pulsatile masses.

Rupture represents the most serious complication of renal artery aneurysms.[128] Such an event is likely to affect less than 3% of cases.[118] Mortality with rupture was reported to be approximately 10% in the past but appears to be less common today. However, loss of the kidney is almost inevitable with aneurysm rupture. It has been suggested that aneurysms less than 1.5 cm in diameter, calcified aneurysms, and those occurring in normotensive patients are not likely to rupture, but this has not proved to be the case.

Renal artery aneurysm rupture during pregnancy is an exception to the otherwise non–life-threatening nature of these lesions.[129-133] Rupture in this setting does not appear to be related to patient age, presence of hypertension, or parity. Aneurysm rupture in pregnancy can cause nearly 75% fetal mortality and 50% maternal mortality.[132] Surprisingly, the

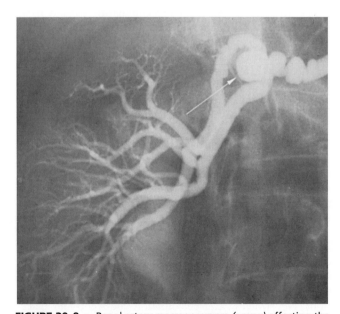

FIGURE 30–7 • Saccular renal artery aneurysm (arrow) occurring at a segmental branching. (From Stanley JC, Whitehouse WM Jr: Renal artery macroaneurysms. In Bergan JJ, Yao JST [eds]: Aneurysms: Diagnosis and Treatment. New York, Grune & Stratton, 1981, pp 417-431.)

FIGURE 30–8 • Renal artery macroaneurysm (arrow) affecting the primary bifurcation of a vessel exhibiting medial fibrodysplasia. (From Stanley JC, Whitehouse WM Jr: Renal artery macroaneurysms. In Bergan JJ, Yao JST [eds]: Aneurysms: Diagnosis and Treatment. New York, Grune & Stratton, 1981, pp 417-431.)

affected kidney can be salvaged in nearly 20% of surviving women.

The association between renal artery aneurysms and elevated arterial blood pressure is controversial.[118,123,134-137] Most agree that hypertension contributes to aneurysm progression, but there is no consensus on the converse. Nevertheless, treatment of certain aneurysms is associated with an improvement in the patient's hypertension, and it is difficult to ignore the potential cause-and-effect relation.[118] It is possible that aneurysmal thrombus may embolize or propagate and occlude a distal artery, thereby producing renal ischemia and renovascular hypertension.[121,124] Extensive atheromatous disease within large aneurysmal sacs may predispose to such thromboembolic events, but even small nonarteriosclerotic aneurysms may be the cause of embolism-related cortical ischemia. Aneurysmal compression, or twisting and narrowing of adjacent arteries, has been proposed as an additional cause of renovascular hypertension, but this is very uncommon. However, intrinsic stenotic disease adjacent to an aneurysm, which is not always evident on preoperative arteriograms, may be a cause of secondary hypertension in these patients. Determination of renal-systemic renin indices in hypertensive patients with isolated renal artery aneurysms may better define the presence or absence of renin-mediated blood pressure elevation.[118]

Indications for the operative treatment of renal artery macroaneurysms have been widely dicussed.[117,118,124] Certainly, all symptomatic patients with suspected aneurysmal expansion should be subjected to operation. Similarly, aneurysms coexisting with functionally important renal artery stenoses are best treated operatively. Because of the potential for catastrophic rupture during pregnancy, operative therapy is recommended for all aneurysms in women of childbearing age who might conceive in the future. An aneurysm diameter greater than 1.5 cm is a relative indication for elective operation, but only when undertaken by an experienced vascular surgeon.

Surgical therapy is directed at eliminating the aneurysm without loss of the kidney or compromise of normal renal blood flow.[118,121,124,138] An exception is the management of ruptured aneurysms, when kidney salvage may be impossible and nephrectomy may be the only logical therapy.[128,132] Large aneurysms of the main renal artery can often be excised with simple primary repair of the artery. Excision of smaller aneurysms may necessitate an angioplastic vein patch arterial closure or implantation of the involved artery into an adjacent uninvolved artery. Partial nephrectomy may be necessary when treating intraparenchymal aneurysms. In situ renal artery reconstruction with autogenous saphenous vein or internal iliac artery grafts is preferred for aneurysms associated with functionally important stenoses. In select cases, ex vivo repairs are appropriate.[139,140]

Intraparenchymal renal artery aneurysms and occasional aneurysms of the extrarenal arteries can be treated by transcatheter embolization.[121,141] However, endovascular exclusion of most extraparenchymal renal artery aneurysms is not possible because of their usual location at arterial bifurcations. Nevertheless, coil embolization and stent-graft placement may carry less risk than an open procedure in select patients.[141-143] These patients and those not subjected to operation must be followed carefully with serial CT scanning or arteriography. Particular efforts should be directed toward controlling hypertension in all patients not subjected to surgical therapy.

RENAL ARTERY DISSECTIONS

Isolated dissections of the renal arteries are classified as those due to blunt abdominal trauma or intraluminal catheter-induced injury and those occurring spontaneously.[144,145] All forms of dissection may be associated with false aneurysm formation (Fig. 30-9). Men are 10 times more likely than women to exhibit dissection of the renal artery.[146] The right renal artery is affected much more often than the left. This may be due to increased arterial stretching because of the greater ptosis of the right kidney. Approximately one third of renal artery dissections are bilateral.

Two primary mechanisms contribute to renal artery dissection caused by blunt abdominal trauma. The first is displacement of the kidney during deceleration, with marked stretching of the vascular pedicle. In these circumstances, fracture of the intima, which is the least elastic arterial wall component, leads to subintimal dissection. The second relates to direct trauma of the renal artery over the unyielding posteriorly located vertebral body, with medial hemorrhage and false aneurysm formation.

Catheter-based diagnostic renal arteriography is an uncommon cause of dissection. In one large series, only four renal artery dissections were encountered among more than 11,000 abdominal arteriographic examinations, including more than 2200 selective diagnostic renal arteriograms.[144] Therapeutic interventions with balloon angioplasty are often associated with dissection. Most of these dissections are inconsequential, but if they appear to compromise the renal circulation, they are usually easily treated with stent placement.

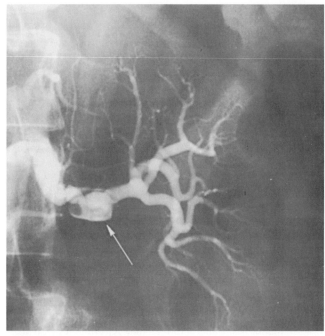

FIGURE 30–9 • Renal artery dissection with associated false aneurysm *(arrow)*. (From Gewertz BL, Stanley JC, Fry WJ: Renal artery dissections. Arch Surg 112:409-414, 1977.)

Spontaneous dissections affect the renal arteries more than any other muscular artery. They are usually related to coexistent arteriosclerotic and fibrodysplastic renovascular disease. Spontaneous dissections are more common with the latter, being reported in 0.5% of patients with renal artery dysplasia.[144] Spontaneous dissections usually extend within the outer media. This is in contrast to the subintimal and inner medial location of traumatic dissections. In some instances, spontaneous dissections are attributed to rupture of abnormal vasa vasorum. Dissecting mural hematomas may contribute to vessel wall ischemia and further aneurysmal changes. Spontaneous renal artery dissections most often originate in the proximal renal artery and terminate at a first-order branching.

Pain, hematuria, and elevated blood pressure are frequent manifestations of acute renal artery dissection, regardless of the cause.[144] Chronic dissections are often associated with compromised renal function and renovascular hypertension. Delayed arterial rupture is very rare. An incorrect initial clinical diagnosis occurs in nearly 60% of patients with renal artery dissection.[144] Intravenous urography, often with tomography, may be useful in establishing the presence of renal ischemia in these cases, but the accuracy of this study is limited. Because prompt diagnosis may improve the outcome of surgical therapy, intravenous urography should be deferred in favor of prompt arteriography.

Criteria for the arteriographic diagnosis of renal artery dissection include (1) luminal irregularities, with aneurysmal dilatation or saccular dissections associated with segmental stenosis; (2) the predilection of dissections to extend distally to the first renal artery bifurcation; (3) cuffing at branchings, causing a "rolled-down sock" appearance; and (4) variable degrees of reversibility documented by serial studies.

Kidney preservation is of prime importance in patients with renal artery dissection, particularly because renal artery disease involves the contralateral kidney in half the patients exhibiting spontaneous dissection.[144] Arterial reconstruction using autogenous saphenous vein or hypogastric artery may be complex, and ex vivo repairs are appropriate in select cases.

Traumatic renal artery dissections associated with blunt injuries usually necessitate emergent arterial reconstruction. Delayed repair is necessary when hypertension persists or renal function deteriorates. Some physicians take a cautious, nonsurgical approach toward managing traumatic dissections because operation in the acute setting often results in nephrectomy. Treatment of traumatic lesions using an endovascular stent has appeal but still remains an unproven therapy.[147] All spontaneous renal artery dissecting aneurysms should be subjected to surgical therapy once hemodynamically significant stenoses or occlusions are recognized as causing renovascular hypertension or a deterioration in renal function.[144,146]

KEY REFERENCES

Eckhauser FE, Stanley JC, Zelenock GB, et al: Gastroduodenal and pancreaticoduodenal artery aneurysms: A complication of pancreatitis causing spontaneous gastrointestinal hemorrhage. Surgery 88:335-355, 1980.

Graham LM, Stanley JC, Whitehouse WM Jr, et al: Celiac artery aneurysms: Historical (1745-1949) versus contemporary (1950-1984) differences in etiology and clinical importance. J Vasc Surg 2:757-764, 1985.

Henke PK, Cardneau JD, Welling TH, et al: Renal artery aneurysms: A 35-year clinical experience with 252 aneurysms in 168 patients. Ann Surg 234:454-463, 2001.

Larson RA, Solomon J, Carpenter JP: Stent graft repair of visceral artery aneurysms. J Vasc Surg 36:1260-1263, 2002.

Lumsden AB, Mattar SG, Allen RC, et al: Hepatic artery aneurysms: The management of 22 patients. J Surg Res 60:345-350, 1996.

de Perrot M, Berney T, Deleaval J, et al: Management of true aneurysms of the pancreaticoduodenal arteries. Ann Surg 229:416-420, 1999.

Reilly LM, Cunningham CG, Maggisano R, et al: The role of arterial reconstruction in spontaneous renal artery dissection. J Vasc Surg 14:468-479, 1991.

Shanley CJ, Shah NL, Messina LM: Common splanchnic artery aneurysms: Splenic, hepatic and celiac. Ann Vasc Surg 10:315-322, 1996.

Shanley CJ, Shah NL, Messina LM: Uncommon splanchnic artery aneurysms: Pancreaticoduodenal, gastroduodenal, superior mesenteric, inferior mesenteric and colic. Ann Vasc Surg 10:506-515, 1996.

Stanley JC, Fry WJ: Pathogenesis and clinical significance of splenic artery aneurysms. Surgery 76:889-909, 1974.

REFERENCES

1. Busuttil RW, Brin BJ: The diagnosis and management of visceral artery aneurysms. Surgery 88:619-630, 1980.
2. Carr SC, Pearce WH, Vogelzang RL, et al: Current management of visceral artery aneurysms. Surgery 120:627-633, 1996.
3. Graham JM, McCollum CH, DeBakey ME: Aneurysms of the splanchnic arteries. Am J Surg 140:797-801, 1980.
4. Rokke O, Sondenaa K, Amundsen SR, et al: Successful management of eleven splanchnic artery aneurysms. Eur J Surg 163:411-417, 1997.
5. Shanley CJ, Shah NL, Messina LM: Common splanchnic artery aneurysms: Splenic, hepatic and celiac. Ann Vasc Surg 10:315-322, 1996.
6. Shanley CJ, Shah NL, Messina LM: Uncommon splanchnic artery aneurysms: Pancreaticoduodenal, gastroduodenal, superior mesenteric, inferior mesenteric and colic. Ann Vasc Surg 10:506-515, 1996.
7. Stanley JC, Thompson NW, Fry WJ: Splanchnic artery aneurysms. Arch Surg 101:689-697, 1970.
8. Stanley JC, Wakefield TW, Graham LM, et al: Clinical importance and management of splanchnic artery aneurysms. J Vasc Surg 3:836-840, 1986.
9. Wagner WH, Allins AD, Treiman RL, et al: Ruptured visceral artery aneurysms. Ann Vasc Surg 11:342-347, 1997.
10. Zelenock GB, Stanley JC: Splanchnic artery aneurysms. In Rutherford RB (ed): Vascular Surgery, 5th ed. Philadelphia, WB Saunders, 2000, pp 1369-1382.
11. Carmeci C, McClenathan J: Visceral artery aneurysms as seen in a community hospital. Am J Surg 179:486-489, 2000.
12. Gabelmann A, Gorich J, Merkle EM: Endovascular treatment of visceral artery aneurysms. J Endovasc Ther 9:38-47, 2002.
13. Pilleul F, Dugougeat F: Transcatheter embolization of splanchnic aneurysms/pseudoaneurysms: Early imaging allows detection of incomplete procedure. J Comput Assist Tomogr 26:107-112, 2002.
14. Stanley JC, Fry WJ: Pathogenesis and clinical significance of splenic artery aneurysms. Surgery 76:889-909, 1974.
15. Lee PC, Rhee RY, Gordon RY, et al: Management of splenic artery aneurysms: The significance of portal and essential hypertension. J Am Coll Surg 189:483-490, 1999.
16. Puttini M, Aseni P, Brambilla G, et al: Splenic artery aneurysms in portal hypertension. J Cardiovasc Surg 23:490-493, 1982.
17. Nishida O, Moriyasu F, Nakamura T, et al: Hemodynamics of splenic artery aneurysm. Gastroenterology 90:1042-1046, 1986.
18. Ohta M, Hashizume M, Ueno K, et al: Hemodynamic study of splenic artery aneurysm in portal hypertension. Hepatogastroenterology 41:181-184, 1994.
19. Ayalon A, Wiesner RH, Perkins JD, et al: Splenic artery aneurysms in liver transplant patients. Transplantation 45:386-389, 1988.
20. Bronsther O, Merhav H, Van Thiel D, et al: Splenic artery aneurysms occurring in liver transplant recipients. Transplantation 52:723-756, 1991.
21. Kobori L, van der Kolk MJ, de Jong KP, et al: Splenic artery aneurysms in liver transplant patients: Liver Transplant Group. J Hepatol 27:890-893, 1997.
22. Martin KW, Morian JP Jr, Lee JK, et al: Demonstration of a splenic artery pseudoaneurysm by MR imaging. J Comput Assist Tomogr 9:190-192, 1985.
23. de Vries JE, Schattenkerk ME, Malt RA: Complications of splenic artery aneurysm other than intraperitoneal rupture. Surgery 91:200-204, 1982.
24. Harper PC, Gamelli RL, Kaye MD: Recurrent hemorrhage into the pancreatic duct from a splenic artery aneurysm. Gastroenterology 87:417-420, 1984.
25. Stabile BE, Wilson SE, Debas HT: Reduced mortality from bleeding pseudocysts and pseudoaneurysms caused by pancreatitis. Arch Surg 118:45-51, 1983.

26. Stanley JC, Frey CF, Miller TA, et al: Major arterial hemorrhage: A complication of pancreatic pseudocysts and chronic pancreatitis. Arch Surg 111:435-440, 1976.

27. Wager WH, Cossman DV, Treiman RL, et al: Hemosuccus pancreaticus from intraductal rupture of a primary splenic artery aneurysm. J Vasc Surg 19:158-164, 1994.

28. Brothers TE, Stanley JC, Zelenock GB: Splenic arteriovenous fistula: Review of the literature with four new case reports. Int Surg 80:189-194, 1995.

29. Gaglio PJ, Regenstein F, Slakey D, et al: α-1 Antitrypsin deficiency and splenic artery aneurysm rupture: An association? Am J Gastroenterol 95:1531-1534, 2000.

30. Angelakis EJ, Bair WE, Barone JE, et al: Splenic artery aneurysm rupture during pregnancy. Obstet Gynecol 48:145-148, 1993.

31. MacFarlane JR, Thorbjarnason B: Rupture of splenic artery aneurysm during pregnancy. Am J Obstet Gynecol 95:1025-1037, 1966.

32. O'Grady JP, Day EJ, Toole AL, et al: Splenic artery aneurysm rupture in pregnancy: A review and case report. Obstet Gynecol 50:627-630, 1977.

33. Vassalotti SB, Schaller JA: Spontaneous rupture of splenic artery aneurysm in pregnancy: Report of first known antepartum rupture with maternal and fetal survival. Obstet Gynecol 30:264-268, 1967.

34. Taylor JL, Woodward DA: Splenic conservation and the management of splenic artery aneurysm. Ann R Coll Surg Engl 69:179-180, 1987.

35. Arca MJ, Gagner M, Beniford BT, et al: Splenic artery aneurysms: Methods of laparoscopic repair. J Vasc Surg 30:184-188, 1999.

36. Hashizume M, Ohta M, Ueno K, et al: Laparoscopic ligation of splenic artery aneurysm. Surgery 113:352-354, 1993.

37. de Perrot M, Buhler L, Schneider PA, et al: Do aneurysms and pseudo-aneurysms of the splenic artery require different surgical strategy? Hepatogastroenterology 46:2028-2032, 1999.

38. Baker KS, Tisnado J, Cho SR, et al: Splanchnic artery aneurysms and pseudoaneurysms: Transcatheter embolization. Radiology 163:135-159, 1987.

39. McDermott VG, Shlansky-Goldberg R, Cope C: Endovascular management of splenic artery aneurysms and pseudoaneurysms. Cardiovasc Intervent Radiol 17:179-184, 1994.

40. Waltman AC, Luers PR, Athanasoulis CA, et al: Massive arterial hemorrhage in patients with pancreatitis: Complementary roles of surgery and transcatheter occlusive techniques. Arch Surg 121:439-443, 1986.

41. Takahashi T, Shimada K, Kobayashi N, et al: Migration of steel-wire coils into the stomach after transcatheter arterial embolization for a bleeding splenic artery pseudoaneurysm: Report of a case. Surg Today 31:458-462, 2001.

42. Wholey MH, Chamorro HA, Rao G, et al: Splenic infarction and spontaneous rupture of the spleen after therapeutic embolization. Cardiovasc Radiol 1:249-253, 1978.

43. Arepally A, Dagli M, Hofmann LV, et al: Treatment of splenic artery aneurysm with use of stent-graft. J Vasc Interv Radiol 13:631-633, 2002.

44. Brountozos EN, Vagenas K, Apostolopoulou SC, et al: Pancreatitis-associated splenic artery pseudoaneurysm: Endovascular treatment with self-expandable stent-grafts. Cardiovasc Intervent Radiol 26:88-91, 2003.

45. Yoon H-K, Lindh M, Uher P, et al: Stent-graft repair of a splenic artery aneurysm. Cardiovasc Intervent Radiol 24:200-203, 2001.

46. Iseki J, Tada Y, Wada T, et al: Hepatic artery aneurysm: Report of a case and review of the literature. Gastroenterol Jpn 18:84-92, 1983.

47. Guida PM, Moore SW: Aneurysm of the hepatic artery: Report of five cases with a brief review of the previously reported cases. Surgery 60:299-310, 1966.

48. Lumsden AB, Mattar SG, Allen RC, et al: Hepatic artery aneurysms: The management of 22 patients. J Surg Res 60:345-350, 1996.

49. Abbas MA, Fowl RJ, Stone WM, et al: Hepatic artery aneurysm: Factors that predict complications. J Vasc Surg 38:41, 2003.

50. Otah E, Cushin BJ, Rozenblit GN, et al: Visceral artery pseudoaneurysms following pancreaticoduodenectomy. Arch Surg 137:55-59, 2002.

51. Parangi S, Oz MC, Blume RS, et al: Hepatobiliary complications of polyarteritis nodosa. Arch Surg 126:909-912, 1991.

52. Athey PA, Sax SL, Lamki N, et al: Sonography in the diagnosis of hepatic artery aneurysms. AJR Am J Roentgenol 147:725-727, 1986.

53. Kibbler CC, Cohen DL, Cruicshank JK, et al: Use of CAT scanning in the diagnosis and management of hepatic artery aneurysm. Gut 26:752-756, 1985.

54. Lal RB, Strohl JA, Piazza S, et al: Hepatic artery aneurysm. J Cardiovasc Surg 30:509-513, 1989.

55. Harlaftis NN, Akin JT: Hemobilia from ruptured hepatic artery aneurysm: Report of a case and review of the literature. Am J Surg 133:229-232, 1977.

56. Stauffer JT, Weinman MD, Bynum TE: Hemobilia in a patient with multiple hepatic artery aneurysms: A case report and review of the literature. Am J Gastroenterol 84:59-62, 1989.

57. Kadir S, Athansoulis CA, Ring EJ, et al: Transcatheter embolization of intrahepatic arterial aneurysms. Radiology 134:335-339, 1980.

58. Okazaki M, Higashihara H, Ono H, et al: Percutaneous embolization of ruptured splanchnic artery pseudoaneurysms. Acta Radiol 32:349-354, 1991.

59. Thibodeaux LC, Deshmukh RM, Hearn AT, et al: Management options for hepatic artery aneurysms. Ann Vasc Surg 9:285-288, 1995.

60. Salam TA, Lumsden AB, Martin LG, et al: Nonoperative management of vascular aneurysms and pseudoaneurysms. Am J Surg 164:215-219, 1992.

61. Patel JV, Weston MJ, Kessel DO, et al: Hepatic artery pseudoaneurysm after liver transplantation: Treatment with percutaneous thrombin injection. Transplantation 75:1755-1757, 2003.

62. Bürger T, Halloul Z, Meyer F, et al: Emergency stent-graft repair of a ruptured hepatic artery secondary to local postoperative peritonitis. J Endovasc Ther 7:324-327, 2000.

63. Larson RA, Solomon J, Carpenter JP: Stent graft repair of visceral artery aneurysms. J Vasc Surg 36:1260-1263, 2002.

64. Friedman SG, Pogo GJ, Moccio CG: Mycotic aneurysm of the superior mesenteric artery. J Vasc Surg 6:87-90, 1987.

65. Stone WM, Abbas M, Cherry KJ, et al: Superior mesenteric artery aneurysms: Is presence an indication for intervention? J Vasc Surg 36:234-237, 2002.

66. Blumenberg RM, David D, Skovak J: Abdominal apoplexy due to rupture of a superior mesenteric artery aneurysm: Clip aneurysmorrhaphy with survival. Arch Surg 108:223-226, 1974.

67. Cormier F, Ferry J, Artru B, et al: Dissecting aneurysms of the main trunk of the superior mesenteric artery. J Vasc Surg 15:424-430, 1992.

68. DeBakey ME, Cooley DA: Successful resection of mycotic aneurysm of superior mesenteric artery: Case report and review of the literature. Am Surg 19:202-212, 1953.

69. Geelkerken RH, van Bockel JH, de Roos WK, et al: Surgical treatment of intestinal artery aneurysms: Eur J Vasc Surg 4:563-567, 1990.

70. Olcott C, Ehrenfeld WK: Endoaneurysmorrhaphy for visceral artery aneurysms. Am J Surg 133:636-639, 1977.

71. Appel N, Duncan JR, Schuerer DJE: Percutaneous stent-graft treatment of superior mesenteric and internal iliac artery pseudoaneurysms. J Vasc Interv Radiol 14:917, 2003.

72. Cowan S, Kahn MB, Bonn J, et al: Superior mesenteric artery pseudo-aneurysm successfully treated with polytetrafluoroethylene covered stent. J Vasc Surg 35:805-807, 2002.

73. Hama Y, Iwasaki Y, Kaji T, et al: Coil compaction after embolization of the superior mesenteric artery pseudoaneurysm. Eur Radiol 12:S189-S191, 2002.

74. Graham LM, Stanley JC, Whitehouse WM Jr, et al: Celiac artery aneurysms: Historical (1745-1949) versus contemporary (1950-1984) differences in etiology and clinical importance. J Vasc Surg 2:757-764, 1985.

75. Stone WM, Abbas MA, Gloviczki P, et al: Celiac arterial aneurysms. Arch Surg 137:670-674, 2002.

76. Werner K, Tarasoutchi F, Lunardi W, et al: Mycotic aneurysm of the celiac trunk and superior mesenteric artery in a case of infective endocarditis. J Cardiovasc Surg 32:380-383, 1991.

77. Shumacker HB Jr, Siderys H: Excisional treatment of aneurysm of celiac artery. Ann Surg 148:885-889, 1958.

78. Hertzer NR, Mullally PH: Celiac artery aneurysmectomy with hepatic artery ligation. Arch Surg 104:337-339, 1972.

79. Parfitt J, Chalmers RTA, Wolfe JHN: Visceral aneurysms in Ehlers-Danlos syndrome: Case report and review of the literature. J Vasc Surg 31:1248-1251, 2000.

80. Schoder M, Cejna M, Langle F, et al: Glue embolization of a ruptured celiac trunk pseudoaneurysm via the gastroduodenal artery. Eur Radiol 10:1335-1337, 2000.

81. Funahashi S, Yukizane T, Yano K, et al: An aneurysm of the right gastroepiploic artery. J Cardiovasc Surg 38:385-388, 1997.

82. Jacobs PP, Croiset van Ughelen FA, Bruyninckx CM, Hoefsloot F: Haemoperitoneum caused by a dissecting aneurysm of the gastroepiploic artery. Eur J Vasc Surg 8:236-237, 1994.

83. Witte JT, Hasson JE, Harms BA, et al: Fatal gastric artery dissection and rupture occurring as a paraesophageal mass: A case report and literature review. Surgery 107:590-594, 1990.

84. Uchikoshi F, Sakamoto T, Imabunn S, et al: Aneurysm of the right gastroepiploic artery: A case report of laparoscopic resection. Cardiovasc Surg 1:550-551, 1993.

85. Trevisani MF, Ricci MA, Michaels RM, et al: Multiple mesenteric aneurysms complicating subacute bacterial endocarditis. Arch Surg 122:823-824, 1987.

86. Selke FW, Williams GB, Donovan DL, et al: Management of intra-abdominal aneurysms associated with periarteritis nodosa. J Vasc Surg 4:294-298, 1986.

87. Sarcina A, Bellosta R, Magnaldi S, et al: Aneurysm of the middle colic artery: Case report and literature review. Eur J Vasc Endovasc Surg 20:198-200, 2000.

88. Bleichrodt RP, Smulders TAE, Schreuder F, et al: Aneurysms of the jejunal artery. J Cardiovasc Surg 25:376-377, 1984.

89. Diettrich NA, Cacioppo JC, Ying DPW: Massive gastrointestinal hemorrhage caused by rupture of a jejunal branch artery aneurysm. J Vasc Surg 8:187-189, 1988.

90. Naito A, Toyota N, Ito K: Embolization of a ruptured middle colic artery aneurysm. Cardiovasc Intervent Radiol 18:56-58, 1995.

91. Graham LM, Hay MR, Cho KJ, et al: Inferior mesenteric artery aneurysms. Surgery 97:158-163, 1985.

92. Eckhauser FE, Stanley JC, Zelenock GB, et al: Gastroduodenal and pancreaticoduodenal artery aneurysms: A complication of pancreatitis causing spontaneous gastrointestinal hemorrhage. Surgery 88:335-355, 1980.

93. Gadacz TR, Trunkey D, Kieffer RF: Visceral vessel erosion associated with pancreatitis: Case reports and a review of the literature. Arch Surg 113:1438-1440, 1978.

94. Gangahar DM, Carveth SW, Reese HE, et al: True aneurysm of the pancreaticoduodenal artery: A case report and review of the literature. J Vasc Surg 2:741-742, 1985.

95. Spanos PK, Kloppedal EA, Murray CA: Aneurysms of the gastroduodenal and pancreaticoduodenal arteries. Am J Surg 127:345-348, 1974.

96. Taheri SA, Mueller G: Surgical approach and review of literature on gastroduodenal aneurysm: A case report. Angiology 36:895-898, 1985.

97. Verta MJ Jr, Dean RH, Yao JST, et al: Pancreaticoduodenal artery aneurysms. Ann Surg 186:111-114, 1977.

98. Chiou AC, Josephs LG, Menzoian JO: Inferior pancreaticoduodenal artery aneurysm: Report of a case and review of the literature. J Vasc Surg 17:784-789, 1993.

99. de Perrot M, Berney T, Deleaval J, et al: Management of true aneurysms of the pancreaticoduodenal arteries. Ann Surg 229:416-420, 1999.

100. Iyomasa S, Matsuzaki Y, Hiei K, et al: Pancreaticoduodenal artery aneurysm: A case report and review of the literature. J Vasc Surg 22:161-166, 1995.

101. Quandalle P, Chambon JP, Marache P, et al: Pancreaticoduodenal artery aneurysms associated with celiac axis stenosis: Report of two cases and review of the literature. Ann Vasc Surg 4:540-545, 1990.

102. Suzuki K, Kashimura H, Sato M, et al: Pancreaticoduodenal artery aneurysms associated with celiac axis stenosis due to compression by medial arcuate ligament and celiac plexus. J Gastroenterol 33:434-438, 1998.

103. Gouny P, Fukui S, Aymard A, et al: Aneurysm of the gastroduodenal artery associated with stenosis of the superior mesenteric artery. Ann Vasc Surg 8:281-284, 1994.

104. Coll DP, Ierardi R, Kerstein MD, et al: Aneurysms of the pancreaticoduodenal arteries: A change in management. Ann Vasc Surg 12:286-291, 1998.

105. Granke K, Hollier LH, Bowen JC: Pancreaticoduodenal artery aneurysms: Changing patterns. South Med J 83:918-921, 1990.

106. Pitkaranta P, Haapiainen R, Kivisaari L, et al: Diagnostic evaluation and aggressive surgical approach in bleeding pseudoaneurysms associated with pancreatic pseudocysts. Scand J Gastroenterol 26:58-64, 1991.

107. Carr JA, Cho JS, Shepard AD, et al: Visceral pseudoaneurysms due to pancreatic pseudocysts: Rare but lethal complications of pancreatitis. J Vasc Surg 32:722-730, 2000.

108. Nyman U, Svendsen P, Jivegard L, et al: Multiple pancreaticoduodenal aneurysms: Treatment with superior mesenteric artery stent-graft placement and distal embolization. J Vasc Interv Radiol 11:1201-1205, 2000.

109. Mandel SR, Jaques PF, Mauro MA, et al: Nonoperative management of peripancreatic arterial aneurysms: A 10-year experience. Ann Surg 205:126-128, 1987.

110. Thakker RV, Gajjar B, Wilkins RA, et al: Embolization of gastroduodenal artery aneurysm caused by chronic pancreatitis. Gut 24:1094-1098, 1983.

111. Vujic I, Anderson MC, Meredith HC, et al: Successful embolization of the dorsal pancreatic artery to control massive upper gastrointestinal hemorrhage. Ann Surg 46:184-186, 1980.

112. McIntyre TP, Simone ST, Stahlfield KR: Intraoperative thrombin occlusion of a visceral artery aneurysm. J Vasc Surg 36:393-395, 2002.

113. Manazer JR, Monzon JR, Dietz PA, et al: Treatment of pancreatic pseudoaneurysm with percutaneous transabdominal thrombin injection. J Vasc Surg 38:600-602, 2003.

114. Lina JR, Jaques P, Mandell V: Aneurysm rupture secondary to trans-catheter embolization. AJR Am J Roentgenol 132:553-556, 1979.

115. Bastounis W, Pikoulis E, Georgopoulos S, et al. Surgery for renal artery aneurysms: A combined series of two large centers. Eur Urol 33:22-27, 1998.

116. Bulbul MA, Farrow GA: Renal artery aneurysms. Urology 40:124-126, 1992.

117. Dzinich C, Gloviczki P, McKusick MA, et al: Surgical management of renal artery aneurysm. Cardiovasc Surg 1:243-247, 1993.

118. Henke PK, Cardneau JD, Welling TH, et al: Renal artery aneurysms: A 35-year clinical experience with 252 aneurysms in 168 patients. Ann Surg 234:454-463, 2001.

119. Henriksson C, Lukes P, Nilson AE, et al: Angiographically discovered, non-operated renal artery aneurysms. Scand J Urol Nephrol 18:59-62, 1984.

120. Hubert JP Jr, Pairolero PC, Kazmier FJ: Solitary renal artery aneurysm. Surgery 88:557-565, 1980.

121. Hupp T, Allenberg JR, Post K, et al: Renal artery aneurysm: Surgical indications and results. Eur J Vasc Surg 6:477-486, 1992.

122. Lumsden AB, Salam TA, Walton KG: Renal artery aneurysm: A report of 28 cases. Cardiovasc Surg 4:185-189, 1996.

123. Martin RS III, Meacham PW, Ditesheim JA, et al: Renal artery aneurysm: Selective treatment for hypertension and prevention of rupture. J Vasc Surg 9:26-34, 1989.

124. Stanley JC, Rhodes EL, Gewertz BL, et al: Renal artery aneurysms: Significance of macroaneurysms exclusive of dissections and fibrodysplastic mural dilations. Arch Surg 110:1327-1333, 1975.

125. Tham G, Ekelund L, Herrlin K, et al: Renal artery aneurysms: Natural history and prognosis. Ann Surg 197:348-352, 1983.

126. Henriksson C, Bjorkerud S, Nilson AE, et al: Natural history of renal artery aneurysm elucidated by repeated angiography and pathoanatomical studies. Eur Urol 11:244-248, 1985.

127. Smith DL, Wernick R: Spontaneous rupture of a renal artery aneurysm in polyarteritis nodosa: Critical review of the literature and report of a case. Am J Med 87:464-467, 1989.

128. Schorn B, Falk V, Dalichau H, et al: Kidney salvage in a case of ruptured renal artery aneurysm: Case report and literature review. Cardiovasc Surg 1345:134-136, 1997.

129. Cohen JR, Shamash FS: Ruptured renal artery aneurysms during pregnancy. J Vasc Surg 6:51-59, 1987.

130. Cohen SG, Cashdan A, Burger R: Spontaneous rupture of a renal artery aneurysm during pregnancy. Obstet Gynecol 39:897-902, 1972.

131. Dayton B, Helgerson RB, Sollinger HW, et al: Ruptured renal artery aneurysm in a pregnant uninephric patient: Successful ex vivo repair and autotransplantation. Surgery 107:708-711, 1990.

132. Lacroix H, Bernaerts P, Nevelsteen A, et al: Ruptured renal artery aneurysm during pregnancy: Successful ex situ repair and autotransplantation. J Vasc Surg 33:188-190, 2001.

133. Schoon IM, Seeman T, Niemand D, et al: Rupture of renal arterial aneurysm in pregnancy. Acta Chir Scand 154:593-597, 1988.

134. Reiher L, Grabitz K, Sandmann W: Reconstruction for renal artery aneurysm and its effect on hypertension. Eur J Endovasc Surg 20:454-456, 2000.

135. Cummings KB, Lecky JW, Kaufman JJ: Renal artery aneurysms and hypertension. J Urol 109:144-148, 1973.

136. Ruberti U, Miani S, Scorza R, et al: Aneurysms of the renal artery. Int Angiol 6:407-414, 1987.

137. Soussou ID, Starr DS, Lawrie GM, et al: Renal artery aneurysm: Long-term relief of renovascular hypertension by in situ operative correction. Arch Surg 114:1410-1415, 1979.

138. Mercier C, Piquet P, Piligian F, et al: Aneurysms of the renal artery and its branches. Ann Vasc Surg 1:321-327, 1986.

139. Bugge-Asperheim B, Sdal G, Flatmark A: Renal artery aneurysm: Ex vivo repair and autotransplantation. Scand J Urol Nephrol 18:63-66, 1984.

140. Dubernard JM, Martin X, Gelet A, et al: Aneurysms of the renal artery: Surgical management with special reference to extracorporeal surgery and autotransplantation. Eur Urol 11:26-30, 1985.

141. Centenera LV, Hirsch JA, Choi IS, et al: Wide-necked saccular renal artery aneurysm: Endovascular embolization with the Guglielmi detachable coil and temporary balloon occlusion of the aneurysm neck. J Vasc Interv Radiol 9:513-516, 1998.

142. Bui BT, Oliva VL, Leclerc G, et al: Renal artery aneurysm: Treatment with percutaneous placement of a stent-graft. Radiology 195:181-182, 1995.

143. Karkos CD, D'Souza SP, Thompson GJ, et al: Renal artery aneurysm: Endovascular treatment by coil embolization with preservation of renal blood flow. Eur J Vasc Endovasc Surg 19:214-216, 2000.

144. Gewertz BL, Stanley JC, Fry WJ: Renal artery dissections. Arch Surg 112:409-414, 1977.

145. Reilly LM, Cunningham CG, Maggisano R, et al: The role of arterial reconstruction in spontaneous renal artery dissection. J Vasc Surg 14:468-479, 1991.

146. Edwards BS, Stanson AW, Holley KE, et al: Isolated renal artery dissection: Presentation, evaluation, management and pathology. Mayo Clin Proc 57:564-571, 1982.

147. Mali WP, Geyskes GG, Thalman R: Dissecting renal artery aneurysm: Treatment with an endovascular stent. AJR Am J Roentgenol 153:623-614, 1989.

Questions

1. Which of the following represents the reported ranking of splanchnic artery aneurysms in order of decreasing frequency?
   - (a) Splenic, hepatic, superior mesenteric, celiac
   - (b) Hepatic, splenic, celiac, superior mesenteric
   - (c) Intestinal, celiac, hepatic, splenic
   - (d) Splenic, hepatic, celiac, superior mesenteric

2. Which of the following statements about splenic artery aneurysms is true?
   - (a) They are more common in women than men
   - (b) They tend to be saccular and occur at vessel branchings
   - (c) They may exhibit a "double-rupture" phenomenon
   - (d) All of the above

3. Which of the following statements about hepatic artery aneurysms is true?
   - (a) They account for 20% of reported splanchnic artery aneurysms
   - (b) They often appear with obstructive jaundice
   - (c) They rupture in 20% of reported cases, with an approximately 50% mortality rate accompanying rupture
   - (d) They are twice as likely to rupture into the biliary tract as into the peritoneal cavity

4. Which of the following statements about aneurysms of the superior mesenteric artery is true?
   - (a) They are the fifth most common splanchnic artery aneurysm, accounting for 2.5% of all such aneurysms
   - (b) They are commonly mycotic in origin
   - (c) They affect women twice as often as men
   - (d) They rupture in 12% of reported cases

5. Which of the following statements about celiac artery aneurysms is true?
   - (a) They are best treated by simple ligation with or without aneurysmectomy
   - (b) They are rarely diagnosed before rupture in contemporary practice
   - (c) Mortality is 50% when they rupture
   - (d) They are more likely to affect women than men

6. Which of the following statements about jejunal, ileal, and colic artery aneurysms is true?
   - (a) They are most commonly due to atherosclerosis
   - (b) They occur most commonly in women
   - (c) When multiple, they tend to be associated with subacute bacterial endocarditis or periarteritis nodosa
   - (d) They carry a 30% risk of rupture

7. Which of the following statements about renal artery aneurysms is true?
   - (a) They are demonstrated in 0.1% of patients undergoing angiography for nonrenal indications
   - (b) They tend to be fusiform and occur at branchings of the main renal artery
   - (c) They are usually caused by atherosclerosis
   - (d) They cause hypertension in approximately 80% of cases

8. Which of the following statements about ruptured renal artery aneurysms is true?
   - (a) They usually appear with hematuria
   - (b) They carry a mortality approaching 10%
   - (c) They are most commonly treated by arterial reconstruction
   - (d) They are more likely to occur with noncalcified than calcified lesions

9. Renal artery aneurysms may be associated with hypertension due to which of the following?
   - (a) Depulsatile blood flow beyond the aneurysm
   - (b) Common compression of adjacent veins
   - (c) Intrinsic stenotic disease adjacent to the aneurysm
   - (d) Contralateral release of renal renin

10. Which of the following statements about spontaneous dissection of the renal artery is true?
    - (a) It is a rare form of arterial dissection
    - (b) It occurs most often in women
    - (c) It is bilateral in a third of cases
    - (d) It rarely requires surgical therapy

Answers

1. d	2. d	3. a	4. b	5. c
6. c	7. a	8. b	9. c	10. c

31

Michael Belkin • Anthony D. Whittemore •
Magruder C. Donaldson • John A. Mannick

Aortoiliac Occlusive Disease

Arteriosclerotic occlusive disease of the abdominal aorta and iliac arteries is a common cause of ischemic symptoms in the lower extremities of middle-aged and elderly patients in the Western world. Although not as common as occlusive disease of the femoropopliteal arterial system, with which it may be combined, aortoiliac occlusive disease may be more disabling because of the greater number of muscle groups subjected to diminished perfusion. The initial manifestation of occlusive disease of the distal aorta or iliac arteries is intermittent claudication with symptoms involving muscles of the thigh, hip, and buttock, as well as the calf. Because the calf muscles are usually the only muscle groups affected by intermittent claudication caused by superficial femoral artery occlusion, the involvement of more proximal muscles in the symptom complex may help distinguish aortoiliac occlusive disease from femoropopliteal occlusive disease. Unfortunately, a sizable minority of patients with aortoiliac disease complain only of calf claudication. In addition to claudication, male patients with aortoiliac occlusive disease may complain of difficulty in achieving and maintaining an erection because of inadequate perfusion of the internal pudendal arteries. The Leriche syndrome in males consists of the manifestations of aortoiliac occlusive disease and includes claudication of the muscles of the thigh, hip, and buttock; atrophy of the leg muscles; impotence; and diminished femoral pulses.[1]

Aortoiliac occlusive disease per se is rarely the cause of ischemia at rest or ischemic tissue loss, except by embolization. The collateral circulation that develops around the occlusive process in the aorta and iliac arteries is usually rich and sufficient to supply the lower extremities with adequate quantities of arterial blood to ensure good resting tissue perfusion. However, arteriosclerotic plaques in the aorta and iliac arteries may cause the so-called blue toe syndrome (i.e., microembolization of arteriosclerotic debris to the terminal vessels in the foot).[2-5] Such symptoms may occur in a patient who otherwise appears to have adequate distal arterial supply, including, in some instances, palpable pedal pulses. Under these circumstances, a search must be made by angiography for a proximal source of microembolization.

When aortoiliac occlusive disease is combined with femoropopliteal occlusive disease—a finding more common in elderly patients—resting ischemia may result.[6] As in any

arterial system, tandem lesions in the arteries supplying the extremities are more significant than single lesions.

The risk factors for aortoiliac occlusive disease are those for atherosclerosis in general and include cigarette smoking, hypertension, elevated serum cholesterol, and diabetes.[7-18] In our experience, patients reporting symptoms of claudication caused by aortoiliac occlusive disease are on average nearly a decade younger than those complaining of claudication from superficial femoral artery occlusion. However, patients with ischemia at rest from the combination of aortoiliac and femoropopliteal occlusive disease are generally in the seventh decade of life and are not notably younger than those who develop ischemic rest pain from femoropopliteal disease.

The initial lesions of aortoiliac occlusive disease usually begin at the terminal aorta and the proximal portions of the common iliac arteries or at the bifurcations of the common iliac arteries (Fig. 31-1). The lesions then progress proximally and distally. Approximately 33% of the patients we have operated on for symptomatic aortoiliac disease have had disease at the origin of the deep femoral arteries in the groin, and more than 40% have had superficial femoral artery occlusions. The natural history of aortoiliac occlusive disease is one of slow progression.[19,20] The ultimate anatomic result of aortoiliac atherosclerosis is variable but may lead to occlusion of the distal abdominal aorta, with progression of the thrombus up to the level of the renal arteries (Fig. 31-2). Although occlusion of the terminal aorta, once it occurs, may remain stable for years, it does not always have a benign course, as indicated in the report by Starrett and Stoney.[21] They observed that more than one third of patients with aortic occlusion went on to show thrombosis of the renal arteries over a period of 5 to 10 years (Fig. 31-3). However, Reilly and colleagues later suggested that the renal arteries remain patent; no instances of thrombosis occurred in 21 patients followed up with arteriography after a mean of 27.7 months.[22]

Variants in the pattern of aortoiliac occlusive disease occur, including relatively circumscribed occlusive lesions of the midabdominal aorta described in early middle-aged women who are heavy cigarette smokers (Fig. 31-4). Although the upper abdominal aorta is ordinarily spared in patients with aortoiliac occlusive disease, a minority of such patients have

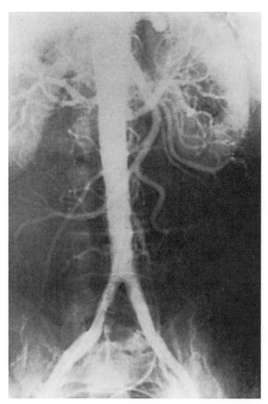

FIGURE 31–1 • The earliest manifestations of aortoiliac occlusive disease are evident in the terminal aorta and proximal common iliac vessels.

marked involvement of this aortic segment, with occlusive disease at the origins of the major visceral vessels and renal arteries (Fig. 31-5).

Diagnosis

The diagnosis of aortoiliac occlusive disease is ordinarily easily made on the basis of the patient's symptoms. Complaints of high claudication, with or without accompanying sexual dysfunction in males, certainly suggest this disease process. Claudication symptoms, however, must be distinguished from symptoms of nerve root irritation caused by spinal stenosis or intervertebral disk herniation, which may be associated with activity and relieved by sitting or lying down in some individuals.[23] These patients can ordinarily be distinguished quite easily from patients with true claudication by the fact that their symptoms are produced as much by standing still as by walking and by the typical sciatic distribution of the pain.

A patient with intermittent claudication due to aortoiliac disease ordinarily has lower extremities that appear healthy and well perfused at rest, although the muscles may be somewhat atrophic from disuse. Diminished or even absent femoral pulses are often a principal clue to the level of the occlusive process. Bruits heard in the groins can also call attention to proximal occlusive lesions. However, stenotic lesions at the origins of the superficial or deep femoral arteries can also cause femoral bruits. Easily palpable pedal pulses at rest may be found in patients with severe claudication from

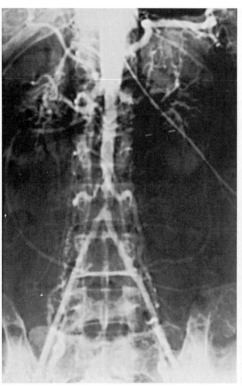

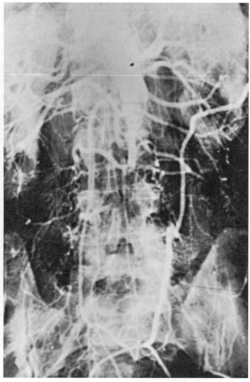

FIGURE 31–2 • Aortoiliac occlusive disease results in a variable degree of collateralization, shown as a discrete channel from a lumbar to the deep iliac circumflex artery (A) and as a multiplicity of small vessels that supply the hemorrhoidal and gluteal arteries that reconstitute the femoral vessels via iliac and femoral circumflex arteries (B).

A   **B**

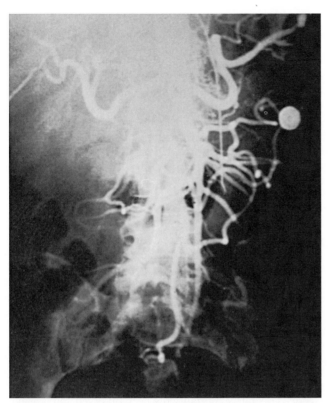

FIGURE 31–3 • The end result of aortoiliac occlusive disease consists of total aortic thrombosis, which may include the origins of the renal arteries.

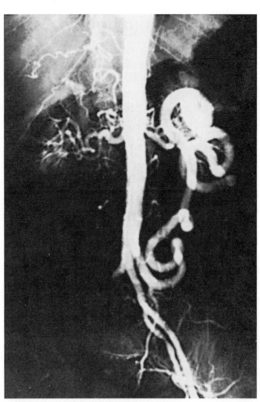

FIGURE 31–5 • A large meandering mesenteric artery associated with total superior mesenteric artery celiac occlusion, renal artery stenosis, complete occlusion of the right common iliac artery, and distal left external iliac stenoses with a single patent hypogastric artery. End-to-side proximal anastomosis may best preserve both mesenteric and pelvic circulation.

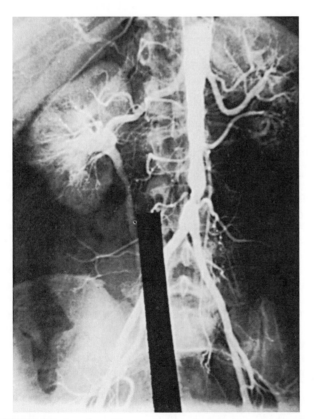

FIGURE 31–4 • Aortoiliac occlusive disease may consist of a short-segment circumferential lesion, especially common in younger women. Such a lesion may be amenable to localized endarterectomy.

aortoiliac occlusive disease, even when the femoral pulses are barely discernible. This reflects the rich collateral circulation that is ordinarily present in such patients.

Segmental Doppler pressures at all levels in the lower extremity are ordinarily lower than the brachial pressure. If no accompanying superficial femoral occlusive disease exists, no impressive gradient occurs between the high thigh pressure and the ankle pressure; however, disabling symptoms may occur in patients with aortoiliac disease who have resting ankle pressures in the near-normal range and a normal ankle-brachial pressure index. Thus, in evaluating these patients, repeating the pressure measurements after a period of graded exercise is often wise.[24] A marked fall in ankle pressure immediately after exercise occurs if the patient's symptoms are caused by significant aortoiliac occlusive disease. More sophisticated Doppler waveform analysis or the use of a pulse-volume recorder may reveal patterns suggestive of proximal occlusive lesions.[25-27] We have found, however, that resting and postexercise Doppler pressure measurements are satisfactory for the evaluation of the majority of patients.

The indications for surgery in symptomatic aortoiliac occlusive disease are disabling claudication and ischemia at rest manifested by rest pain in the foot, ischemic ulceration, or pregangrenous skin changes. Patients with aortoiliac disease and ischemia at rest ordinarily have accompanying femoropopliteal disease unless the ischemic lesions are the result of microemboli, as noted earlier.

Preoperative Evaluation

Preoperative evaluation of a patient with aortoiliac occlusive disease includes a careful evaluation of any accompanying cardiac and pulmonary disease. In our experience, approximately 40% of patients with symptomatic aortoiliac occlusive disease have clear-cut clinical and electrocardiographic evidence of coronary artery disease. Symptomatic unstable coronary artery disease in such individuals clearly demands investigation, including cardiac catheterization and coronary angiography in many cases. If coronary artery reconstruction is indicated, this procedure should be done first and the aortoiliac occlusive disease repaired as a second procedure. Patients with mild or stable coronary artery disease can ordinarily undergo aortoiliac reconstruction without great risk. Elderly patients with severe cardiopulmonary disease who are not good candidates for coronary artery reconstruction are probably best managed by extra-anatomic bypass procedures of lesser magnitude than formal aortoiliac or aortofemoral reconstruction. Patients with severe restrictive pulmonary disease may require a period of preoperative preparation that includes bronchodilators, broad-spectrum antibiotics, and abstinence from cigarette smoking.

Angiography has historically played a major role in the preoperative evaluation of patients with symptomatic aortoiliac disease and can generally be performed by the retrograde Seldinger technique using the femoral approach.[28] When this is not possible, studies by the translumbar or transaxillary route are performed.[29,30] The goal of the radiographic examination is to provide views of the entire abdominal aorta in two planes to demonstrate unexpected lesions of the celiac axis or superior mesenteric artery origins, to provide anteroposterior and oblique views of the pelvis to define any iliac artery lesions in more than one plane, and to demonstrate possible lesions at the origins of the deep femoral arteries. Views should also be obtained of the vessels in the thighs, at the knees, and in the calves to demonstrate associated femoropopliteal occlusive disease and the quality of the runoff. At the time of angiography, obtaining pull-back pressures across iliac artery lesions of doubtful significance is a useful technique because it can demonstrate whether such lesions are likely to interfere with flow. Measurements should be taken at rest and after papaverine injection or during a period of reactive hyperemia after tourniquet ischemia to mimic the hemodynamic situation that occurs during exercise.[31] Intra-arterial digital subtraction angiography has become quite useful for evaluation of the aortoiliac arterial segment. This technique's advantages include the use of very small amounts of contrast medium and good resolution of the vessels studied.

Increasing experience with magnetic resonance arteriography has documented a high degree of accuracy for the evaluation of infrainguinal arterial occlusive disease.[32] Although the accurate diagnosis of aortoiliac disease often proved problematic with earlier technology, results have continued to improve.[33] In most patients, detailed pathologic anatomy, sufficient for planning either percutaneous or surgical therapy, can be obtained from magnetic resonance arteriography. More recently, high-speed spiral computed tomography angiography with contrast enhancement has offered an additional imaging modality.

Percutaneous balloon therapy with or without stenting has supplanted surgical reconstruction as the most common therapy for aortoiliac occlusive disease. The recent TransAtlantic Inter-society Consensus (TASC) document delineated which patients are best served by percutanous versus surgical therapy.[34] It is generally believed that TASC types A and B lesions (focal, short-segment lesions, unilateral or bilateral) are best treated with endovascular techniques. Conversely, TASC type D lesions (long-segment occlusions and diffuse, severe long-segment disease, particularly bilateral) are best treated with open surgery. Intermediate TASC type C lesions can be appropriately treated with either technique but are increasingly being treated initially with percutaneous approaches.

Aortofemoral Bypass Graft

Over the past 2 decades, the aortofemoral bypass graft has remained the gold standard for the treatment of severe symptomatic aortoiliac occlusive disease. This procedure's 30-day operative mortality rate of 5% to 8% in the early 1970s has been reduced in our own experience to less than 2% over the past 15 years, a level consistent with reports from other surgeons and similar to that observed in patients undergoing elective abdominal aortic aneurysm repair.[35-41] Arterial insufficiency of the lower extremities is a manifestation of a systemic process that results in clinically evident coronary artery disease in approximately 50% of these patients.[42-44] Reduced operative mortality has been observed and is associated with a concomitant reduction in the number of early cardiac deaths. The improved perioperative management of patients with diseased hearts has resulted from a number of factors, including selective employment of preliminary cardiac surgery for certain individuals, sophisticated pharmacologic management of the damaged myocardium, and more precise perioperative fluid management tailored to the individual patient's myocardial reserve.[41]

SURGICAL TECHNIQUE

The knitted Dacron prosthesis is the standard graft material used by most surgeons with experience in aortoiliac reconstruction. This material, usually impregnated with collagen or gelatin, may provide a more stable pseudointima than woven prostheses do.[45,46] An important factor contributing to improved results has undoubtedly been recognition of the critical role of the deep femoral artery in providing sustained patency of the aortofemoral graft limb.[35,38,47,48] The current practice of extending the distal anastomosis down over the origin of the deep femoral artery to ensure an adequate outflow tract has been widely accepted and is important in patients with tandem superficial femoral occlusions and in patients with stenosis of the deep femoral origin. We have found, however, that if extensive profundaplasty or endarterectomy is necessary, this vessel is better closed with an autogenous tissue patch of saphenous vein or endarterectomized superficial femoral artery than attempting to make a long deep femoral patch with the distal end of an aortofemoral prosthesis.[47]

The incidence of graft infection has been minimized with preoperative and intraoperative antibiotics.[35,49-51] Aortoenteric fistulas can be prevented by closure of retroperitoneal tissue and the posterior parietal peritoneum over the graft and proximal suture line to prevent erosion of the graft into the duodenum.[35,52,53] The abandonment of silk sutures in favor of

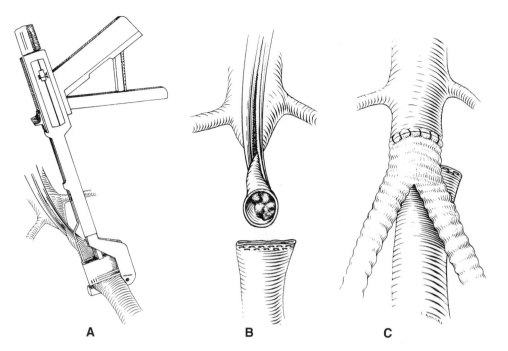

FIGURE 31–6 • End-to-end proximal anastomosis for aortofemoral reconstruction can be initiated with the infrarenal aortic cross-clamp placed in an anteroposterior direction, with minimal dissection as close to the origin of the renal arteries as possible. The aorta is then stapled or occluded with a second clamp just proximal to the origin of the inferior mesenteric artery *(A)*. After transection of the infrarenal aorta and complete thrombo-endarterectomy of the proximal infrarenal aortic cuff *(B)*, end-to-end anastomosis is completed with continuous 3-0 polypropylene sutures *(C)*.

A   **B**   **C**

permanent prosthetic suture material has undoubtedly helped reduce the incidence of false aneurysm formation.

A good deal of controversy remains over the proper method of performing the proximal anastomosis of an aortobifemoral graft.[35,54,55] Most surgeons favor the end-to-end technique of proximal anastomosis, with transection of the aorta between clamps about 1 to 2 inches below the renal arteries and over-sewing or stapling of the distal end (Fig. 31-6). This permits an endarterectomy or thrombectomy of the proximal aortic stump under direct vision before constructing the anastomosis. It also has the advantage of not requiring flow to be reestablished in the more distal aorta, where arteriosclerotic plaque and mural thrombus may have been loosened by application of the distal clamp. This may avoid intraoperative emboli to the lower extremities.

Some authors claim that the end-to-end technique reduces the incidence of aortoduodenal fistulas because the end-to-end anastomosis does not project anteriorly, as does an end-to-side aortofemoral reconstruction. Unfortunately, the controlled studies that are available do not substantiate that the results of the end-to-end technique are significantly superior to those of the end-to-side technique. Therefore, our position is that the end-to-end technique is probably more appropriate for those patients who will not suffer any hemo-dynamic disadvantage from interruption of forward flow in the abdominal aorta. This technique also appears to be desir-able for patients who have already suffered complete aortic occlusion. The end-to-side technique (Fig. 31-7) is reserved for individuals who would lose perfusion of an important hypogastric or inferior mesenteric artery if forward flow in the aorta were sacrificed at the time of surgery.[54] Arteriographic studies in patients with indications for an end-to-side anasto-mosis are shown in Figures 31-5 and 31-8.

Although aortofemoral reconstruction has the potential to restore potency to males with sexual dysfunction because of inadequate hypogastric artery perfusion,[54,55] surgical dis-section in the area of the terminal aorta and proximal left

common iliac artery can also cause difficulty with both erection and ejaculation by interfering with the autonomic nervous plexus, which sweeps over these vessels.[56] When performing aortofemoral bypass grafting, we therefore confine the dissection of the aorta to the area between the renal arteries and the inferior mesenteric artery. The aorta is exposed anteriorly and laterally, without distorting the vessel, to avoid embolization of arteriosclerotic debris. After sys-temic heparinization, the distal clamp is placed proximal to the inferior mesenteric artery; then the aorta is cross-clamped below the renal arteries, where the aortic wall is likely to be considerably less diseased. The aorta is divided transversely, and the distal end is beveled and oversewn.

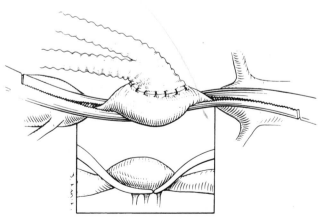

FIGURE 31–7 • End-to-side proximal anastomosis for aortofemoral reconstruction is required to preserve antegrade pelvic perfusion when retrograde perfusion from distal femoral anastomoses is doubtful. The infrarenal aorta is occluded proximal to the origin of the inferior mesenteric artery and just distal to the origin of the renal arteries. After longitudinal arteriotomy and thorough thromboendarterectomy, if required, the anastomosis is constructed using continuous polypropylene sutures.

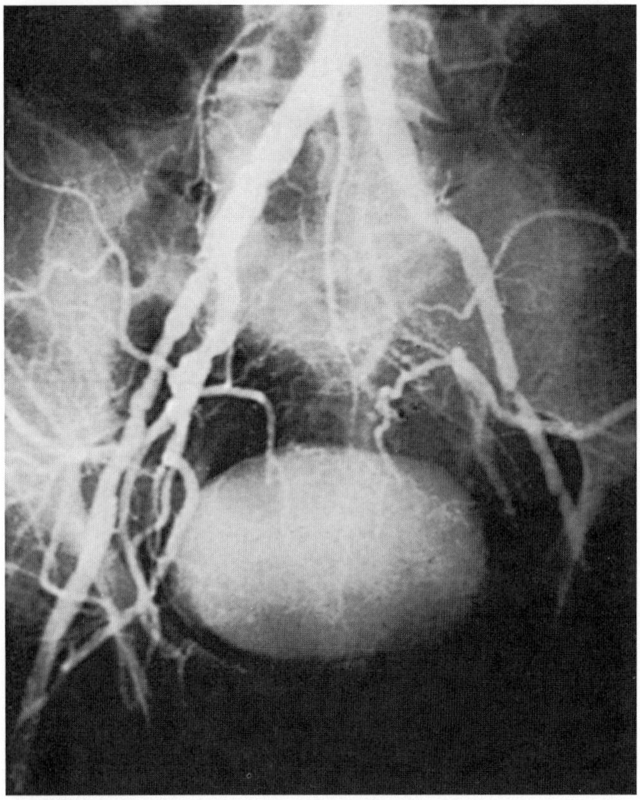

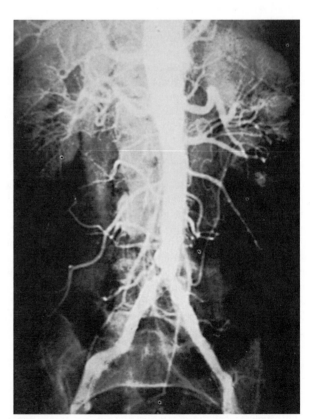

FIGURE 31–8 • Diffuse aortoiliac disease with left hypogastric occlusion and minimal left pelvic collateralization may warrant end-to-side proximal anastomosis to preserve the right hypogastric system.

Despite significant advances in laparoscopic general surgery, applications of this new technique to vascular surgery have been few. However, several authors have applied laparoscopic techniques to aortofemoral reconstruction. Whether performed completely via the laparoscopic approach or through limited incisions with laparoscopy-assisted dissection, the procedure has proved to be time-consuming and technically challenging.[57,58] As the technology evolves and intracorporeal anastomotic techniques are refined, however, the role of laparoscopic aortofemoral bypass will expand and become clearer.

In patients with well-localized aortoiliac lesions, aortoiliac endarterectomy may be a suitable option. This operation, even in the hands of enthusiasts, is now confined to patients whose disease ends distally near the bifurcation of the common iliac arteries (Fig. 31-9; also see Fig. 31-4).[35] Endarterectomy of the external iliac artaery is tedious and unrewarding for most surgeons. At present, little evidence suggests that endarterectomy is superior to a properly performed aortofemoral bypass graft in terms of early or late results. In our practice, aortoiliac endarterectomy is confined to a minority of individuals who appear to have principally aortic disease with little involvement of the iliac arteries. This group of patients characteristically consists of early middle-aged women with occlusive disease of the midabdominal aorta that ends at the aortic bifurcation or in the proximal portions of the common iliac arteries. We avoid aortoiliac endarterectomy in males because of concerns about interfering with the autonomic nerves at the terminal aorta and proximal left common iliac artery.

In the case of an end-to-side anastomosis, the longitudinal aortotomy is placed high, up near the renals in the more normal aorta, and great care is taken to remove all loose debris and mural thrombus from the lumen in the excluded aortic segment. At completion of an end-to-side anastomosis, attention is also given to adequate back-flushing of all loosened debris and clot from the distal aorta before forward flow is reestablished. In performing either type of proximal anastomosis, a short stem of a graft is sutured to the aorta with a running suture of 3-0 polypropylene. Knitted Dacron prostheses are invariably used; the size is selected so that the limb diameter corresponds to the diameter of the patient's common femoral arteries. The average prosthesis size used for males is 14 × 7 mm or, in larger individuals, 16 × 8 mm. For females, the most commonly used sizes are 12 × 6 mm and 14 × 7 mm. After completion of the proximal anastomosis, the limbs are tunneled retroperitoneally into the groins. On the left, the tunnel ordinarily passes beneath the sigmoid mesentery and ureter and into the groin in a rather lateral channel that avoids trauma to the nerve plexuses at the terminal aorta. On the right, the tunnel is made along the course of the right common iliac artery beneath the ureter. In the groins, end-to-side anastomoses are fashioned in the distal common femoral artery with 5-0 polypropylene. The anastomoses are carried down into the deep femoral arteries for a short distance if there is any evidence of incipient stenosis of the origins of these vessels or if the superficial femorals are occluded. The end of the graft thus acts as a patch, widening the orifice of the deep femoral artery.

FIGURE 31–9 • Aortoiliac occlusive disease with significant lesion confined to the origin of the right common iliac artery, amenable to either local endarterectomy or percutaneous transluminal angioplasty.

RESULTS

Initial aortobifemoral graft limb patency rates approach 100%, and the 5-year patency is greater than 80% in a number of reports.[35,36,38,59,60] Long-term patency has also improved to an anticipated 75% at 10 years.[35] A number of refinements of operative technique may be responsible for the low incidence of graft limb thrombosis in recent years. The more prevalent use of the aortobifemoral graft as opposed to aortoiliac bypass or extended aortoiliofemoral endarterectomy has negated the effect of unsuspected or progressive atherosclerosis in the external iliac vessels. Meticulous avoidance of graft limb redundancy and an awareness of the desirability of compatibility between the diameter of the graft limb and that of the vessel into which it is implanted have also probably helped maintain long-term patency.

Our results with aortofemoral bypass grafting are illustrated in Figure 31-10. The 5-year cumulative patency of 86% is comparable with that reported in a number of other studies.[35,36,38,59] Thirty-day operative mortality was slightly less than 1%. This low mortality rate undoubtedly reflects careful patient selection as well as improved operative management and anesthetic technique. However, because aortoiliac occlusive disease is rarely life threatening (although it may be limb threatening), we prefer to treat high-risk patients with procedures of lesser magnitude.

Although most authors have reported excellent patency rates after aortofemoral bypass, several subgroups with inferior results have been identified. Younger patients and those with small aortas are more vulnerable to late graft failure. A study of aortofemoral reconstructions in 73 patients younger than 50 years documented a 50% primary patency rate 5 years after bypass.[55] In that study, patients with aortas less than 1.8 cm wide had significantly lower patency rates (6-year patency of 20%) than did those with aortas larger than 1.8 cm (6-year patency of 60%). Similarly, we have documented lower patency rates in younger patients: 5-year patency rates were only 66% in patients younger than 50 years, compared with 87% for 50- to 60-year-olds and 96% for those older than 60.[61] Younger patients also had significantly smaller aortas, corroborating the influence of aortic size on long-term outcomes. There were no significant differences in patency rates for patients operated on for limb salvage versus claudication, and no significant differences between the genders.

Although the excellent graft patency rates for aortofemoral bypass grafts do not necessarily reflect functional results, approximately 95% of patients are initially rendered asymptomatic or improved; after 5 years, about 80% remain in this category.[38,59] A study from the United Kingdom indicated that among patients fully employed before aortobifemoral bypass, 85% returned to full employment an average of 4 months after surgery, and more than 50% of those not previously employed returned to work after bypass.[62] Other studies have documented a more sobering functional outcome after successful aortofemoral arterial reconstruction. One study, employing the SF-20 questionnaire, found that after aortobifemoral bypass, patients had decrements in physical and role function and general health perception similar to those of patients with congestive heart failure or recent myocardial infarction.[63] Clearly, more functional outcome analysis is necessary after the treatment of aortoiliac occlusive disease.

The 5-year cumulative survival rate for patients undergoing aortofemoral bypass grafting remains some 14% lower than that anticipated for a normal age-corrected population. However, nearly 80% survive 5 years, whereas less than 50% survive 10 years.[43]

CONCOMITANT DISTAL RECONSTRUCTION

When patients have threatened limb loss from a combination of aortoiliac and femoropopliteal occlusive disease, repair of the proximal or inflow lesions is necessary to salvage the extremity. However, whether concomitant distal reconstruction, such as femoropopliteal bypass, should be performed at the time of the initial operation is not always clear. Results reported in the literature and our own experience suggest that in the majority of patients with ischemia at rest caused by combined aortoiliac and femoropopliteal disease, repair of the aortoiliac occlusive disease and restoration of normal perfusion to the deep femoral arteries achieve limb salvage in the vast majority (probably 80%) of patients.[48,64] However, in patients who have extensive tissue necrosis of the skin of the forefoot or heel, particularly individuals with diabetes, restoration of pulsatile flow in the foot may be necessary to achieve healing. Under these circumstances, we believe that a combination of both proximal and distal reconstructive procedures may be necessary at the initial operation. The combined procedure has the disadvantage of increasing the operating time and surgical trauma in a group of patients who are likely to be elderly with a high incidence of coronary artery disease; however, with modern anesthetic management and a two-team operative approach, this combined reconstruction can be performed safely and within a reasonable time.

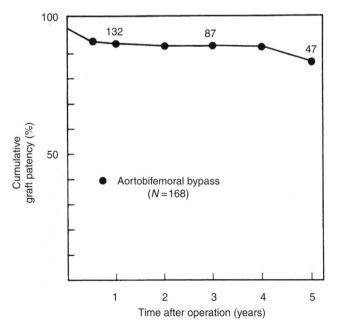

FIGURE 31–10 • For 168 aortobifemoral graft limbs inserted in 84 consecutive patients, the 5-year cumulative patency was 86%.

Alternatives for High-Risk Patients

Although transabdominal arterial reconstruction for aortoiliac occlusive disease can be performed successfully, with low morbidity and mortality, in many patients, less extensive procedures may be preferable in patients who are high risks for major surgery under general anesthesia. In such patients, distal aortic and proximal iliac occlusions can be treated by axillofemoral bypass grafts, which are discussed later.[65-69] If the occlusive disease is limited to one common, or external, iliac artery, alternatives to axillofemoral bypass are warranted in poor-risk individuals; use of the patent iliac system as the origin for a bypass permits a shorter graft segment and affords better long-term patency. The femorofemoral bypass is an example of such a procedure.[70] However, an anatomically similar procedure, the iliofemoral graft, has received little attention in the literature.

ILIOILIAC AND ILIOFEMORAL BYPASS GRAFTS

We reviewed our experience with 94 patients undergoing ilioiliac or iliofemoral bypass grafting from 1982 to 1992. Poor-risk patients, particularly those with severe cardiopulmonary impairment, who had no important occlusive disease in the aorta or in the proximal segment of at least one common iliac artery were considered for reconstruction using a patent common or external iliac artery for the proximal anastomosis (see Fig. 31-5). The iliac site for anastomosis has several technical advantages, including exposure through an oblique, suprainguinal, "renal transplant" incision, which is technically simple, even in obese patients. The graft is more deeply placed and therefore more cushioned than in the femorofemoral position. Ilioilial grafts are shorter than femorofemoral grafts, and no disturbance of inguinal lymph nodes or lymphatics occurs. The femoral artery on the donor side is left undisturbed for later use as the origin for a distal bypass, if indicated.

The mean age of the 94 patients undergoing ilioiliac or iliofemoral bypass was 60 years, and 26% had diabetes mellitus.

Forty-one percent had clear-cut clinical and electrocardiographic evidence of coronary artery disease, and 43% had significant hypertension. Fifty-eight percent of the patients were operated on for claudication, and 42% for limb salvage. Twenty-three patients had ilioilial grafts, and 91 patients had iliofemoral grafts. Fifty-seven iliounifemoral grafts and 14 iliobifemoral grafts were performed.

In patients subjected to iliac artery reconstruction, the patent iliac segment was exposed extraperitoneally through a curvilinear incision parallel to and above the inguinal ligament, identical to the approach for renal transplantation. Limited iliac endarterectomy was necessary in a few instances. Separate vertical groin incisions were made to expose the common femoral arteries. For ilioiliac bypass, symmetrical incisions were made to expose the iliac vessels, and the graft was positioned in the retroperitoneum (Fig. 31-11A). The grafts to the femoral arteries were placed under the inguinal ligament (Fig. 31-11B and C). For patients undergoing bilateral iliofemoral reconstruction, the crossover limb was placed from the iliofemoral graft retroperitoneally in the iliac fossa or, in a few cases, subcutaneously to the contralateral femoral artery (see Fig. 31-11C).

The 30-day operative mortality for these procedures was zero. The 4-year cumulative patency for the ilioiliac grafts (23 limbs) was 96%, and that for the iliofemoral grafts (91 limbs) was 72%. The 4-year patency for iliobifemoral grafts (28 limbs) was 72%, and that for iliounifemoral grafts (63 limbs) was 71% (Fig. 31-12). When both the superficial and deep femoral arteries were patent, the cumulative patency rate for iliofemoral grafts was higher (85%) at 4 years than when only the deep femoral artery was patent (62%). Demonstration of a statistically significant difference in late patency between aortofemoral grafts and iliofemoral grafts was not possible, although the aortofemoral grafts had numerically superior 4- and 5-year patencies. We thus believe that the iliofemoral bypass is an adequate substitute for aortofemoral bypass in certain elderly and poor-risk individuals who have proximal occlusive disease confined largely to the external iliac arteries or to one iliac system.

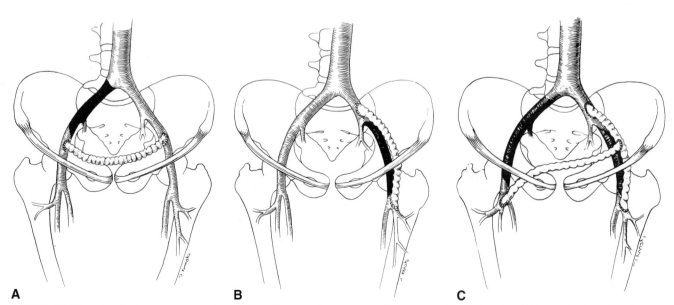

A　　　　　　　　**B**　　　　　　　　**C**

FIGURE 31–11 • A patent common or external iliac artery may be used as a donor vessel for ilioiliac (A), iliofemoral (B), or iliobifemoral (C) bypasses in appropriate patients who would otherwise require axillofemoral reconstruction.

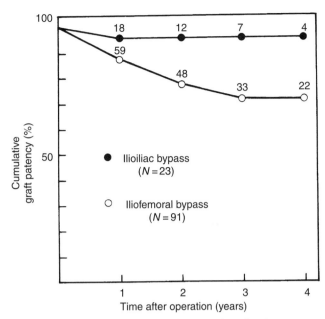

FIGURE 31–12 • Using a patent iliac vessel as the donor artery, the 4-year cumulative graft patency for 23 ilioiliac grafts was 96%, whereas the patency for 91 iliofemoral graft limbs was 72%.

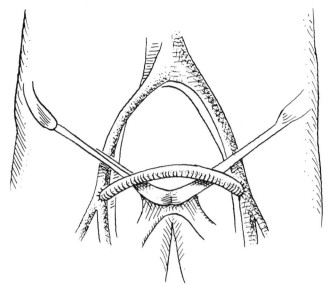

FIGURE 31–13 • The femorofemoral bypass graft is illustrated, with the preferred C configuration of the subcutaneous tunnel constructed well above the pubis.

FEMOROFEMORAL BYPASS GRAFT

In patients whose occlusive disease is confined to one iliac artery and whose aorta and contralateral iliac system are free of hemodynamically significant lesions, the femorofemoral bypass is often used. One of the most common current indications for femorofemoral bypass is for patients undergoing aortounifemoral repair of aortic aneurysms necessitating contralateral revascularization. Brief and coworkers,[71] Plecha and Pories,[72] Vetto,[70] and our own group[68] demonstrated that these operations yield quite satisfactory long-term results (60% to >80% 5-year patency). Failure of these grafts because of progressive worsening of proximal atherosclerosis has been uncommon. Such worsening may be retarded by increased flow through the donor iliac system, which is required to supply both of the lower extremities with blood. Berguer and coworkers reported experimental support for this hypothesis by demonstrating in animals that intimal hyperplasia correlates inversely with blood flow and shear stress.[73] However, experimental results yielding the opposite conclusion have also been reported.[74]

The femorofemoral graft is particularly applicable to high-risk patients because it can be performed easily under epidural or spinal anesthesia. The two common femoral arteries are exposed through short vertical groin incisions. The groin incisions are connected by a subcutaneous suprapubic tunnel created by blunt dissection on the deep fascia. We prefer to have the graft form a **C** configuration, with the anastomoses placed in the distal common femoral arteries and the graft traveling proximally up through the suprapubic tunnel and down to the opposite common femoral artery (Fig. 31-13). In our experience with femorofemoral bypass, 60% of patients were operated on for limb salvage and 40% for disabling claudication. The average age of these patients was 61 years. Forty-one percent had clinical evidence of coronary

artery disease, 33% were diabetic, and 44% had significant hypertension. The 5-year cumulative graft patency was 80% (Fig. 31-14). Although the difference in late patency rates for femorofemoral and aortofemoral bypass is not statistically significant in our hands, femorofemoral bypass is slightly inferior numerically.

The reasonably good long-term results, the ease of performance, and the low morbidity associated with femorofemoral bypass suggest that it might logically be employed in good-risk as well as poor-risk patients who have proximal occlusive disease confined to one iliac arterial segment. Although it is difficult to argue against this point of view, the

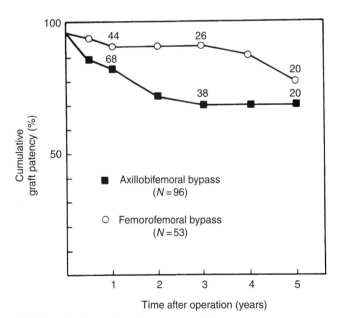

FIGURE 31–14 • The 4-year cumulative graft patency for 53 femorofemoral grafts was 80%, and the patency for 48 axillobifemoral grafts (96 limbs) was 70%.

fact that the groins have been operated on and the common femoral arteries dissected during the performance of a femorofemoral graft makes an aortobifemoral reconstruction in such individuals technically more difficult if progression of proximal disease causes a return of symptoms or late failure of the femorofemoral bypass. Therefore, in good-risk patients with evidence of arteriosclerotic disease in the aorta or in the patent iliac system, we often recommend aortobifemoral bypass at the outset in an attempt to avoid possible future reoperation.

AXILLOFEMORAL BYPASS GRAFT

In very elderly and high-risk patients who are in danger of limb loss from a combination of aortoiliac and femoropopliteal occlusive disease and whose proximal occlusive lesions involve the aorta and proximal iliac arteries, the axillofemoral bypass graft is a logical alternative to aortoiliac reconstruction or primary amputation. Extra-anatomic reconstruction may also prove useful for patients with multiple prior abdominal procedures, multiple adhesions, or previous pelvic irradiation. Intra-abdominal sepsis, sometimes resulting from an infected aortic graft, is another common indication. If an axillofemoral graft is chosen for such individuals, a bifemoral graft is preferred to a unifemoral one, because several reports, beginning with that of LoGerfo and colleagues,[67] showed that the axillobifemoral graft has a decidedly better 5-year cumulative patency.[69] The probable reason for this finding is that the axillobifemoral graft has approximately double the flow rate in its axillary limb as the axillounifemoral graft.

In constructing an axillobifemoral graft, the first portion of the axillary artery is exposed by an incision placed beneath the clavicle on the side selected for the proximal anastomosis (Fig. 31-15). We ordinarily split the pectoralis major and divide the pectoralis minor muscle to provide better operative exposure and more space for the graft as it emerges from the axilla into the subcutaneous plane. The common femoral arteries are exposed through bilateral short groin incisions.

A DeBakey tunneling instrument can then be passed from the infraclavicular incision laterally to a subcutaneous plane in the midaxillary line. The curve in the tunneler is used to direct the tunnel anteriorly above the iliac crest and then in front of the inguinal ligament into the ipsilateral groin incision. An externally supported Dacron or polytetrafluoroethylene prosthesis, usually 8 mm in diameter, is attached to the tunneling instrument and drawn back through the tunnel into the axillary incision for anastomosis with the first portion of the axillary artery. A side limb is attached to the graft in the ipsilateral groin incision just proximal to the anastomosis with the common femoral artery. The side limb is then passed through a subcutaneous suprapubic tunnel into the opposite groin in a manner similar to that used for a femorofemoral graft.

Because neither the thoracic nor the abdominal cavity is "entered" when an axillofemoral graft is performed, this procedure usually does not interfere with the patient's ability to breathe, cough, or take oral feedings. On the first postoperative day, most patients are ambulatory and on a regular diet. From 1982 to 1992, we performed axillobifemoral grafts electively in 48 poor-risk patients for symptomatic aortoiliac occlusive disease. All but two of these patients were operated on for limb salvage necessitated by a combination of

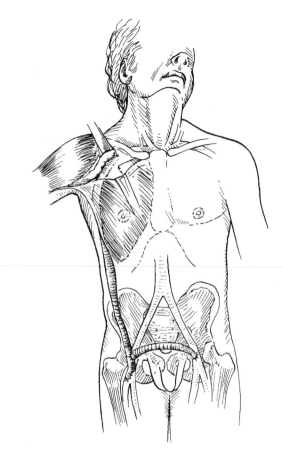

FIGURE 31–15 • Subcutaneous axillobifemoral bypass graft completed with proximal anastomosis to the right axillary artery, right distal anastomosis to the common and deep femoral arteries, and extension of the prosthesis with a side limb to the left common femoral artery.

far-advanced aortoiliac and femoropopliteal disease. The 5-year cumulative graft patency in this group of patients was 70% (see Fig. 31-14). Although this figure is not completely discouraging, it is statistically significantly inferior to the results achieved with aortofemoral bypass grafting during the same period. We therefore believe that axillofemoral grafts should be offered only to poor-risk individuals in danger of limb loss and should not be used for the treatment of symptoms of claudication alone.

When axillofemoral grafts do fail, they can frequently be reopened by thrombectomy under local anesthesia if the patient presents promptly after graft thrombosis has occurred. About 25% of grafts thrombectomized in this fashion go on to long-term patency.[67] Thus, the functional results achieved with axillobifemoral grafting may be somewhat better than the 70% graft patency figure indicates.

Patency rates associated with axillofemoral reconstruction range from a low of 30% to a high of 85%.[75-77] The reasons for this extraordinary variability can be explained in large part by patient selection, indication, and status of the outflow vessels. Extra-anatomic reconstruction for nonocclusive disease, such as in patients with intra-abdominal sepsis or an infected aneurysm repair, achieves better patency rates than does operation primarily for occlusive disease. Patients with claudication fare better than those requiring limb salvage because of inherent outflow restriction in the latter group. In similar fashion, patients who undergo simultaneous distal femoropopliteal reconstruction show better results than those whose infrainguinal disease is not addressed. Finally, in some series, axillobifemoral grafts sustain a significantly better 5-year patency rate than do unilateral reconstructions. Flow through the descending axillary limb in bilateral reconstructions is twice that of axillounilateral grafts, perhaps explaining the improvement in some series. Other investigators have found no significant difference between bilateral and unilateral reconstructions, again probably reflecting patient selection and status of outflow.

Some of the most favorable results were reported by Harris and colleagues in 1990.[76] They achieved an 85% patency rate after 4 years in a group of 76 patients, 26% of whom were operated on for nonocclusive disease, 20% of whom underwent simultaneous outflow reconstruction, and all of whom had axillobifemoral grafts. This series was also carried out in a single institution using a technique that had been standardized for many years. Similar excellent 5-year patency and limb salvage rates of 74% and 89%, respectively, were reported by Passman and colleagues.[78] These authors believe that more liberal application of the axillobifemoral bypass is warranted. In contrast, a less favorable patency rate (29%) was reported by Donaldson and colleagues for 72 patients managed in several institutions by a group of 30 surgeons operating on patients with predominantly occlusive disease.[75] Finally, many authors have reported secondary patency rates, either exclusively or in addition to primary rates, which further confuses the statistics. These series clearly show that the secondary patency rate is significantly better than the primary, attesting to the fact that up to 25% of axillobifemoral grafts require subsequent thrombectomy to maintain patency.

DESCENDING THORACIC AORTA–TO–FEMORAL ARTERY BYPASS

The descending thoracic aorta may be used as an inflow source for bypass to the femoral arteries.[79,80] Although seldom indicated as a primary procedure, this bypass offers a durable alternative after aortic failure, aortic graft infection, or other problems that necessitate avoidance of the abdominal aorta. We generally expose the thoracic aorta through a sixth or seventh interspace incision. A 10-mm synthetic graft is tunneled through the diaphragm at the posterior pleural reflection and down through the retroperitoneal space to the left groin. We usually make a small lateral flank incision to facilitate safe tunneling through the retroperitoneum. The descending thoracic aorta is generally of good quality and is usually clampable with a partially occluding clamp. The procedure is completed with a femorofemoral bypass. Relatively few reports focusing on this procedure are available in the literature. McCarthy and colleagues achieved a 100% 4-year patency rate with 21 thoracic aorta–to–femoral artery bypasses,[79] whereas Criado and Keagy reported an 83% 6- to 8-year secondary graft patency rate.[80]

PERCUTANEOUS TRANSLUMINAL ANGIOPLASTY

Percutaneous catheter dilatation of atheromatous vascular stenoses was introduced by Dotter and Judkins in 1963.[81] However, this technique did not become widely applied until

Gruntzig designed and developed the double-lumen balloon catheter for percutaneous transluminal angioplasty in the early 1970s. In the Gruntzig technique, the balloon catheter is inserted into a stenotic arterial region with the Seldinger technique and expanded to a fixed diameter. In one of Gruntzig's original reports in 1977, percutaneous dilatation was attempted in 41 patients with isolated iliac artery stenosis and proved to be initially successful in 90%.[82]

Early success is not necessarily sustained, as evidenced by the lower 50% to 60% 5-year success rate reported by Johnston and coworkers among 684 iliac angioplasties carried out in Toronto between 1978 and 1986.[83] If initial technical failures are excluded, however, success rates improve by 10% to 15%, as confirmed in a randomized, prospective, multicenter trial reported by Wilson and coworkers.[84] This study demonstrated that successful results were sustained for 3 years in 73% of dilated iliac lesions, not significantly different from the 82% success rate observed with conventional surgery. Success rates for percutaneous transluminal angioplasty are maximal when the procedure is performed for claudication resulting from common iliac stenosis with excellent runoff (75%); they are minimal when it is carried out for critical ischemia caused by external iliac occlusion with poor runoff (19%).

This technique has been very useful in the initial management of patients with symptomatic short-segment iliac stenoses (see Fig. 31-9). High-risk patients with appropriate lesions can be palliated effectively without the need for anesthesia and major surgery. Even in good-risk patients, percutaneous transluminal angioplasty has an advantage as an initial therapy for symptomatic lesions, in that it does not jeopardize a future surgical approach to the aorta or iliac arteries if the angioplasty ultimately fails.

The application of intraluminal stents has increased the number of iliac lesions amenable to balloon angioplasty. Whether employed secondarily to correct a technically inadequate angioplasty (e.g., a dissection of residual stenosis) or primarily to open a long-segment occlusion, stents have increased the technical success rates of percutaneous angioplasty. A review of 230 iliac Palmaz stent placements in 184 patients followed up with angiography at 6 months confirmed an 86% 4-year primary patency rate.[85] Most restenotic lesions were successfully treated with follow-up angioplasty.

The cost-effectiveness of a successful procedure is unquestionable, because patients may be discharged from the hospital on the day of or the day after dilatation. Despite the increasing enthusiasm for percutaneous therapy, it has not been shown to offer superior long-term benefit when compared with aggressive risk factor modification and exercise. Selection for intervention is best individualized, based on the degree of patient disability, risk of intervention, and pathologic anatomy.

REFERENCES

1. Leriche R, Morel A: The syndrome of thrombotic obliteration of the aortic bifurcation. Ann Surg 127:193, 1948.
2. Crane C: Atherothrombotic embolism to lower extremities in arteriosclerosis. Arch Surg 94:96, 1967.
3. Karmody AM, Powers SR, Monaco VJ, et al: "Blue toe" syndrome. Arch Surg 111:1263, 1976.

4. Moldveen-Geronimus M, Merriam JC Jr: Cholesterol embolization: From pathological curiosity to clinical entity. Circulation 35:946, 1967.

5. Williams GM, Harrington D, Burdick J, White RI: Mural thrombus of the aorta. Am Surg 194:737, 1981.

6. Brewster DC, Perier BA, Robison JG, et al: Aortofemoral graft for multilevel occlusive disease: Predictors of success and need for distal bypass. Arch Surg 117:1593, 1982.

7. Ballantyne D, Lawrie TDV: Hyperlipoproteinemia and peripheral vascular disease. Clin Chim Acta 47:269, 1973.

8. Cox FC, Rifking B, Robinson J, et al: Primary hyperlipoproteinaemias in myocardial infarction. In Peeters H (ed): Protides of the Biological Fluids, vol 19. New York, American Elsevier, 1972, p 279.

9. Doyle JT, Dawber TR, Kannel WB, et al: The relationship of cigarette smoking to coronary heart disease: The second report of the combined experience of the Albany, NY, and Framingham, Mass, studies. JAMA 190:886, 1964.

10. Greenhalgh RM, Rosengarten DS, Mervant I, et al: Serum lipids and lipoproteins in peripheral vascular disease. Lancet 2:947, 1971.

11. Kannel WB, Castelli WP, Gordon T, et al: Serum cholesterol lipoproteins and the risk of coronary heart disease. Ann Intern Med 74:1, 1971.

12. Kannel WB, Dawber TR, Friedman GD, et al: Risk factors in coronary artery disease. Ann Intern Med 61:888, 1964.

13. Oberman A, Harlan WR, Smith M, et al: The cardiovascular risk: Associated with different levels and types of elevated blood pressure. Minn Med 52:1283, 1969.

14. Paterson D, Slack J: Lipid abnormalities in male and female survivors of myocardial infarction and their first degree relatives. Lancet 1:393, 1972.

15. Paul O: Physical inactivity: The associated cardiovascular risk. Minn Med 52:1327, 1969.

16. Sirtori CR, Biasi G, Vercellio G, et al: Diets, lipids and lipoproteins in patients with peripheral vascular disease. Am J Med Sci 268:325, 1974.

17. Strong JP, Eggen DA: Risk factors and atherosclerotic lesions. In Jones RJ (ed): Atherosclerosis: Proceedings of the Second International Symposium. New York, Springer-Verlag, 1970, p 355.

18. Vogelberg KH, Berchtold P, Berger H, et al: Primary hyperlipoproteinemias as risk factors in peripheral artery disease documented by arteriography. Atherosclerosis 22:271, 1975.

19. Boyd AM: The natural course of arteriosclerosis of the lower extremities. Proc R Soc Med 55:591, 1962.

20. Imparato AM, Kim G, Davidson T, et al: Intermittent claudication: Its natural course. Surgery 78:795, 1975.

21. Starrett RW, Stoney RJ: Juxta-renal aortic occlusion. Surgery 76:890, 1974.

22. Reilly LM, Sauer L, Weinstein ES, et al: Infrarenal aortic occlusion: Does it threaten renal perfusion or function? J Vasc Surg 11:216, 1990.

23. Karayannacos PE, Yashon D, Vasko JS: Narrow lumbar spinal canal with "vascular" syndromes. Arch Surg 111:803, 1976.

24. Raines JK, Darling RC, Both J, et al: Vascular laboratory criteria for the management of peripheral vascular disease of the lower extremities. Surgery 79:21, 1976.

25. Darling RC, Raines JK, Brener BJ, et al: Quantitative segmental pulse volume recorder: A clinical tool. Surgery 72:873, 1972.

26. Winsor T, Sibley AE, Fisher EK, et al: Peripheral pulse contours in arterial occlusive disease. Vasc Dis 5:61, 1968.

27. Yao JST: Haemodynamic studies in peripheral arterial disease. Br J Surg 57:761, 1970.

28. Seldinger SE: Catheter replacement of needle in percutaneous arteriography: New technique. Acta Radiol 39:368, 1953.

29. Plug MH, Westra D: Complications in catheterization of the axillary artery. Radiol Clin Biol 42:510, 1973.

30. McAfee JG, Wilson JKV: A review of the complications of translumbar aortography. AJR Am J Roentgenol 75:956, 1956.

31. Udoff EJ, Barth KH, Harrington DP, et al: Hemodynamic significance of iliac artery stenosis: Pressure measurements during angiography. Radiology 132:289, 1979.

32. Itoch M, Tullis MJ, Kennell TW, et al: Use of magnetic resonance angiography for the preoperative evaluation of patients with infrainguinal arterial occlusive disease. J Vasc Surg 23:792, 1996.

33. Baum RA, Rutter CM, Quinn SF, et al: Multicenter trial to evaluate vascular magnetic resonance angiography of the lower extremity. JAMA 274:875, 1995.

34. Dormandy JA, Rutherford RB: Management of peripheral artery disease (PAD). TASC Working Group. TransAtlantic Inter-Society Consensus (TASC). J Vasc Surg 31:S1-S296, 2000.

35. Brewster DC, Darling RC: Optimal methods of aortoiliac reconstruction. Surgery 84:739, 1978.

36. Crawford ES, Bomberger RA, Glaeser DH, et al: Aortoiliac occlusive disease: Factors influencing survival and function following reconstructive operation over a twenty-five-year period. Surgery 90:1055, 1981.

37. DeBakey ME, Crawford ES, Cooley DA, et al: Surgical considerations of occlusive disease of the abdominal aorta and iliac and femoral arteries: Analysis of 803 cases. Am Surg 148:306, 1958.

38. Malone JM, Moore WS, Goldstone J: The natural history of bilateral aortofemoral bypass grafts for ischemia of the lower extremities. Arch Surg 110:1300, 1975.

39. Moore WS, Caferata HT, Hall AD, et al: In defense of grafts across the inguinal ligament: An evaluation of early and late results of aortofemoral bypass grafts. Ann Surg 168:207, 1968.

40. Perdue GD, Long WD, Smith RB III: Perspective concerning aortofemoral arterial reconstruction. Ann Surg 173:940, 1971.

41. Whittemore AD, Clowes AW, Hechtman HB, et al: Aortic aneurysm repair: Reduced operative mortality associated with maintenance of optimal cardiac performance. Ann Surg 192:414, 1980.

42. Kannel WB, Skinner JJ Jr, Schwartz MJ, et al: Intermittent claudication: Incidence in the Framingham study. Circulation 41:857, 1970.

43. Malone JM, Moore WJ, Goldstone J: Life expectancy following aortofemoral arterial grafting. Surgery 81:551, 1977.

44. McAllister FF: The fate of patients with intermittent claudication managed non-operatively. Am J Surg 132:593, 1976.

45. Cooley DA, Wukasch DC, Bennett JG, et al: Double velour knitted Dacron grafts for aortoiliac vascular replacements. Paper presented at Vascular Graft Symposium, National Institutes of Health, Nov 5, 1976, Bethesda, Md.

46. Yates SG, Barros D'Sa AA, Berger K, et al: The preclotting of porous arterial prosthesis. Ann Surg 188:611, 1978.

47. Malone JM, Goldstone J, Moore WS: Autogenous profundaplasty: The key to long-term patency in secondary repair of aortofemoral graft occlusion. Ann Surg 188:817, 1978.

48. Morris GC Jr, Edwards W, Cooley DA, et al: Surgical importance of profunda femoris artery. Arch Surg 82:32, 1961.

49. Kaiser AB, Clayson KR, Mulherin JL, et al: Antibiotic prophylaxis in vascular surgery. Ann Surg 188:283, 1978.

50. Lindenaver SM, Fry WJ, Schaub G, et al: The use of antibiotics in the prevention of vascular graft infections. Surgery 62:487, 1967.

51. Szilagyi DE, Smith RF, Elliott JP, et al: Infection in arterial reconstruction with synthetic grafts. Ann Surg 176:321, 1972.

52. Knox GW: Peripheral vascular anastomotic aneurysms. Ann Surg 183:120, 1976.

53. Stoney RJ, Albo EJ, Wylie EJ: False aneurysms occurring after arterial grafting operations. Am J Surg 110:153, 1965.

54. Pierce GE, Turrentine M, Stringfield S, et al: Evaluation of end-to-side v end-to-end proximal anastomosis in aortobifemoral bypass. Arch Surg 117:1580, 1982.

55. Valentine RJ, Hansen ME, Myers SI, et al: The influence of sex and aortic size on late patency after aortofemoral revascularization in young adults. J Vasc Surg 21:296, 1995.

56. Van Schaik J, van Baaleen JM, Visser MJT, et al: Nerve-preserving aortoiliac reconstruction surgery: Anatomical study and surgical approach. J Vasc Surg 33:983, 2001.

57. Ahn SS, Hiyama DT, Rudkin GH, et al: Laparoscopic aortobifemoral bypass. J Vasc Surg 26:128, 1997.

58. Said S, Mall J, Peter F, Muller JM: Laparoscopic aortofemoral bypass grafting: Human cadaveric and initial clinical experiences. J Vasc Surg 29:639, 1999.

59. Mozersky DJ, Summer DS, Strandness DE: Long-term results of reconstructive aortoiliac surgery. Am J Surg 123:503, 1972.

60. Whittemore AD, Mannick JA: The ischemic leg. In McLean LD (ed): Advances in Surgery. St. Louis, Mosby-Year Book, 1981, p 293.

61. Reed AB, Conte MC, Donaldson MC, et al: The impact of patient age and aortic size on the results of aortobifemoral bypass grafting. J Vasc Surg 37:1219, 2003.

62. Waters KJ, Proud G: Return to work after aortofemoral bypass surgery. BMJ 2:556, 1977.

63. Scheider JR, McHorney CA, Malenka DJ, et al: Functional health and well-being in patients with severe atherosclerotic peripheral vascular occlusive disease. Ann Vasc Surg 7:419, 1993.

64. Royster TS, Lynn R, Mulcare RJ: Combined aortoiliac and femoropopliteal occlusive disease. Surg Gynecol Obstet 143:949, 1976.

65. Blaisdell FW, Hall AD, Lim RC Jr, et al: Aortoiliac substitution utilizing subcutaneus grafts. Ann Surg 172:775, 1970.

66. Eugene J, Goldstone J, Moore WS: Fifteen year experience with subcutaneous bypass grafts for lower extremity ischemia. Ann Surg 186:177, 1977.

67. LoGerfo FW, Johnson WC, Carson JD, et al: A comparison of the late patency rates of axillobilateral femoral and axillounilateral femoral grafts. Surgery 81:33, 1977.

68. Maini BS, Mannick JA: Effect of arterial reconstruction on limb salvage. Arch Surg 113:1297, 1978.

69. Mannick JA, Williams LE, Nabseth DC: The late results of axillofemoral grafts. Surgery 68:1038, 1970.

70. Vetto RM: The treatment of unilateral iliac artery obstruction with a transabdominal, subcutaneous, femorofemoral graft. Surgery 52:342, 1962.

71. Brief DK, Brener FJ, Alpert J, Parsonnet V: Cross-over femorofemoral grafts followed up five years or more. Arch Surg 110:1294, 1975.

72. Plecha FR, Pories WJ: Extra-anatomic bypasses for aortoiliac disease in high risk patients. Surgery 80:480, 1976.

73. Berguer R, Higgins RF, Reddy DJ: Intimal hyperplasia: An experimental study. Arch Surg 115:332, 1980.

74. Towne JB, Quinn K, Salles-Cunha S, et al: Effect of increased arterial blood flow on localization and progression of atherosclerosis. Arch Surg 117:1469, 1982.

75. Donaldson MC, Louras JC, Bucknam CA: Axillofemoral bypass: A tool with a limited role. J Vasc Surg 3:757, 1986.

76. Harris EJ, Taylor LM, McConnell DB, et al: Clinical results of axillobifemoral bypass using externally supported polytetrafluoroethylene. J Vasc Surg 12:416, 1990.

77. Martin D, Katz SG: Axillofemoral bypass for aortoiliac occlusive disease. Am J Surg 180:100, 2000.

78. Passman MA, Taylor LM, Moneta GL, et al: Comparison of axillofemoral and aortofemoral bypass for aortoiliac occlusive disease. J Vasc Surg 23:263, 1996.

79. McCarthy WJ, Mesh CL, McMillan WD, et al: Descending thoracic aorta-to-femoral artery bypass: Ten years' experience with a durable procedure. J Vasc Surg 17:336, 1993.

80. Criado E, Keagy BA: Use of the descending thoracic aorta as an inflow source in aortoiliac reconstruction: Indications and long term procedure. Ann Vasc Surg 8:38, 1994.

81. Dotter CT, Judkins MD: Transluminal treatment of arteriosclerotic obstruction: Description of a technique and a preliminary report of its application. Circulation 30:654, 1964.

82. Gruntzig A: Die perkutane transluminale Rekanalisation chronischer Arterienverschlüsse mit einer neuen Dilatationstechnik. Baden-Baden, Germany, G Witzstrock Verlag, 1977.

83. Johnston KW, Rae M, Hogg-Johnston SA, et al: Five year results of a prospective study of percutaneous transluminal angioplasty. Ann Surg 206:403, 1987.

84. Wilson SE, Wolf GL, Cross AP, et al: Percutaneous transluminal angioplasty versus operation for peripheral arteriosclerosis. J Vasc Surg 9:1, 1989.

85. Henry M, Amor M, Ethevenot G, et al: Palmaz stent placement in iliac and femoropopliteal arteries: Primary and secondary patency in 310 patients with 2-4-year follow-up. Radiology 197:167, 1995.

Questions

1. **Symptoms of the Leriche syndrome include all of the following except**
   (a) Claudication of the thigh and buttock
   (b) Rest pain of the feet
   (c) Impotence
   (d) Diminished femoral pulses

2. **Blue toe syndrome is usually characterized by which of the following?**
   (a) Severe claudication symptoms
   (b) Absence of distal palpable pulses
   (c) Palpable pedal pulses
   (d) Severe tibial artery occlusive disease

3. **Which of the following statements is true of patients with isolated aortoiliac occlusive disease?**
   (a) They generally do not suffer from ischemic rest pain
   (b) They often have relatively normal ankle-brachial indices at rest
   (c) They frequently have palpable pedal pulses
   (d) All of the above
   (e) None of the above

4. **Advantages of the end-to-end technique for proximal anastomosis of an aortobifemoral bypass graft include all of the following except**
   (a) Decreased incidence of aortoduodenal fistula
   (b) More complete endarterectomy of the proximal aortic stump
   (c) More complete preservation of pelvic blood flow
   (d) Decreased incidence of distal atheroemboli

5. **The end-to-side technique for aortobifemoral bypass grafts is preferred in patients with which of the following?**
   (a) Extremely calcified infrarenal aortas
   (b) Occluded inferior mesenteric arteries
   (c) Common iliac artery occlusions
   (d) External iliac artery occlusions

6. **Reported results of aortobifemoral bypass surgery suggest which of the following?**
   (a) 5-year cumulative patency rates greater than 80%
   (b) Poor patency rates for patients with small (<1.8-cm) aortas
   (c) Significant decrements in physical and social role function despite successful bypass
   (d) All of the above

7. **Reported results of aortobifemoral bypass surgery suggest which of the following?**
   (a) Younger patients enjoy superior long-term results
   (b) Aorta size is not a major predictor of long-term outcome
   (c) Results are relatively equal between the genders
   (d) Superficial femoral artery outflow is an important predictor of long-term patency

8. **Success rates for percutaneous transluminal angioplasty of the iliac arteries are better for which of the following?**
   (a) Common iliac rather than external iliac lesions
   (b) Patients with claudication rather than rest pain
   (c) Stenotic rather than occlusive lesions
   (d) All of the above

9. Which of the following statements about the use of intraluminal stents for iliac angioplasty is true?
   (a) It should be performed as an adjunct for all iliac angioplasty
   (b) It should be reserved for only technical failures of primary balloon angioplasty
   — (c) It has increased the number of iliac lesions amenable to balloon angioplasty
   (d) It has had no significant impact on the primary patency of iliac angioplasty

10. Concomitant inflow and infrainguinal revascularization is indicated in which of the following situations?
    (a) In all patients with complete superficial femoral artery occlusion
    (b) For patients with severe rest pain
    — (c) For patients with extensive tissue necrosis
    (d) For diabetics

Answers

1. b	2. c	3. d	4. c	5. d
6. d	7. c	8. d	9. c	10. c

32

Evan C. Lipsitz • Frank J. Veith

Femoral, Popliteal, and Tibial Occlusive Disease

Arteriosclerosis may involve the femoral arteries; the popliteal artery; any of the infrapopliteal arteries, including their terminal branches; or any combination of these arteries. This involvement generally begins early in adult life and progresses slowly to the point where a flow-reducing stenosis or occlusion may occur in one or more of the arteries below the inguinal ligament. As the average age of the population increases, the number of individuals with hemodynamically significant infrainguinal arteriosclerosis also increases. This chapter deals with the present status of treatment for arteriosclerotic occlusive disease of the femoral, popliteal, and tibial arterial systems.

Obviously, this disease is associated in varying degrees with arteriosclerotic involvement elsewhere in the body, and this fact must always be considered when making therapeutic decisions regarding affected patients. This consideration should guide the surgeon to less extensive interventions or operations that maintain function rather than ones that restore a normal circulation. The generalized and slowly progressive nature of the disease process and the imperfect results of all interventional treatments should also deter attempts to treat asymptomatic or minimally disabling arteriosclerotic occlusive lesions of the lower extremities. In the management of the increasingly common entity of infrainguinal arteriosclerosis, diagnostic and therapeutic restraint and the desire to minimize risks and avoid doing harm must be paramount principles if the disease is not producing major functional impairment or tissue necrosis. If, however, there is substantial threat of limb loss as a result of the disease process, aggressive intervention for both diagnosis and treatment is justified, despite the advanced age and generally poor condition of the affected population.

Clinical Presentation

The reserve of the human arterial system is enormous. Hemodynamically significant stenoses or major artery occlusions can exist in the infrainguinal arterial tree with no or only minimal symptoms. This is particularly true if collateral pathways are normal or the patient's activity level is limited by coronary arteriosclerosis or other disease processes. Accordingly, the most common manifestation of a short segmental occlusion of the superficial femoral artery, the most common site of major arteriosclerotic involvement below the inguinal ligament, is mild intermittent claudication. Similarly, this lesion is often totally asymptomatic, as is usually the case if only one or two tibial arteries are occluded without other significant lesions. Thus, the usual patient with severe, disabling intermittent claudication or tissue necrosis has multiple sequential occlusions or so-called combined segment disease, with hemodynamically significant lesions at the aortoiliac level and the superficial femoral and popliteal levels, or lesions at one or both of these levels combined with severe infrapopliteal disease.[1]

Staging

Patients with hemodynamically significant infrainguinal arteriosclerosis can be classified into one of five stages, depending on their clinical presentation (Table 32-1). Patients in stages III and IV are those whose limbs are imminently threatened, although some patients with mild ischemic rest pain may remain stable for many years, and an occasional patient with a small patch of gangrene or an ischemic ulcer experiences healing with aggressive local wound care and close observation. With the exception of these few patients, invasive diagnostic procedures such as angiography are easily justified for those with stages III and IV disease, which is usually associated with disease at several levels.

Rest pain as an isolated symptom in patients with infrainguinal arteriosclerosis can be difficult to evaluate unless it is accompanied by other findings. Many patients with significant arterial lesions have pain at rest from causes other than arteriosclerosis, such as arthritis or neuritis. Such pain is not improved by a revascularization procedure. Significant ischemic rest pain must be associated not only with decreased pulses but also with other objective manifestations of ischemia such as atrophy, decreased skin temperature compared with

TABLE 32–1	Staging of Infrainguinal Arteriosclerosis with Hemodynamically Significant Stenosis or Occlusions	
Stage	**Presentation**	**Invasive Diagnostic and Therapeutic Intervention**
0	No signs or symptoms	Never justified
I	Intermittent claudication (present after walking <1 block), no physical changes	Usually unjustified
II	Severe claudication (present after walking <½ block), dependent rubor, decreased temperature	Sometimes justified but not always necessary; may remain stable
III	Rest pain, atrophy, cyanosis, dependent rubor	Usually indicated but may do well for long periods without revascularization
IV	Nonhealing ischemic ulcer or gangrene	Usually indicated

the contralateral extremity, marked rubor, and relief of pain with dependency. In some patients with rest pain of complex origin, a noninvasive laboratory and angiographic evaluation may be necessary before the predominant cause of the symptom can be determined and appropriate treatment instituted. Not every patient with pain at rest and decreased pulses is a candidate for angiography and arterial bypass. Some of these patients experience relief through appropriate treatment of comorbid conditions such as gout or osteoarthritis. Others can be well managed with simple analgesics and reassurance that the limb is not in jeopardy. Such reassurance generally suffices for patients with stage I disease and those with stage II disease who are elderly (older than 80 years) or at high risk because of intercurrent disease or atherosclerotic involvement of other organs such as the heart, kidneys, or brain.

This conservative approach to patients with stage I involvement from infrainguinal arteriosclerosis is becoming increasingly widespread, albeit not universally so.[2] Conservatism appears to be clearly justified by the numerous reports of the benignancy and slow progression of stage I disease.[3-5] Without treatment, 10% to 15% of patients in stage I improve over 5 years, and 60% to 70% do not progress over the same period. The 10% to 15% who do worsen are, in our opinion, best treated with a primary operation or other therapeutic intervention *after* their disease progresses. We further believe that this conservative approach to stage I disease is justified by the greater surgical difficulty encountered when a procedure for claudication fails in the early or remote postoperative period and the patient then has a threatened limb—a situation we have seen all too frequently.

The fact that some patients in stage II and a few in stage III or IV may remain stable and be easily managed without intervention for protracted periods of 1 or more years justifies a cautiously conservative nonoperative approach to selected patients in these stages. This often requires frequent visits to the physician so that the patient and the progress of ischemia can be assessed. This conservative approach is particularly indicated if the patient is elderly and is a poor surgical risk from both a systemic and a local point of view, such as an octogenarian with intractable congestive heart failure in whom a difficult distal small vessel bypass would be required to alleviate stage III signs and symptoms. Close observation is often the preferred management for such patients for several months or even years; however, we do not hesitate to revascularize these patients when their rest pain becomes intolerable or when they develop a small progressive patch of gangrene.[1,6]

Threshold for Therapy

The relative simplicity of percutaneous balloon angioplasty alone or in combination with other newer endovascular treatments (atherectomy devices, stents, and endovascular grafts) has prompted some physicians to recommend a lowering of the therapeutic threshold for the treatment of infrainguinal atherosclerosis. Some surgeons, radiologists, and particularly cardiologists new to the peripheral vascular field and armed with these new techniques and devices have used them routinely to treat stage I and even stage 0 disease detected incidentally during physical examination or coronary arteriography. This practice should be condemned at this time, for many reasons. Most important, the mid- and long-term results of these newer treatments are totally unknown. Even if they are immediately successful, they can initiate a healing process in the artery that may cause late failure or, worse, an acceleration of the occlusive process and, ultimately, net harm to the patient. Therefore, patients are subjected to risks that they may not fully appreciate. Practitioners should not treat these relatively early, minimally symptomatic lesions before more is known about these new high-tech treatments. Although they are exciting and interesting to patients and physicians alike, and although they may prove to be safe and effective, this has not yet been shown. Accordingly, there is no justification for lowering the threshold for intervening in patients with infrainguinal arteriosclerosis. This fact should be clearly communicated to patients to offset the unjustified marketing efforts of uninformed practitioners.

Differential Diagnosis

Intermittent claudication, or pain brought on by exertion and relieved by rest, is a fairly distinct symptom and usually a manifestation of arteriosclerotic occlusive disease. Mild calf claudication can be produced by a significant stenotic lesion in the iliac, superficial femoral, or popliteal arteries. An occasional patient describes claudication as a sense of heaviness, weakness, or fatigue in the limb without pain, and such patients may be mistakenly diagnosed as having neuromuscular disorders. Sometimes claudication-like symptoms can be produced by lesions compressing the lower spinal cord or cauda equina.[7,8] Such pseudoclaudication is most often produced by spinal stenosis and can easily be suspected when peripheral pulses are normal. Occasionally, neurologic problems coexist with arterial occlusive disease, making an exact determination of the cause of the patient's symptoms a difficult challenge for the neurologist and the vascular surgeon. In such circumstances, angiography and computed tomography or magnetic resonance imaging of the lumbar spine and myelography may be necessary.

Some of the difficulties encountered in differentiating pain at rest from true ischemic rest pain have already been discussed. Similar difficulties can be encountered in determining the primary cause of ulcerating lesions in the ankle region and on the foot. The typical venous ulcer occurs in a setting of chronic venous disease, is associated with stasis changes and normal arterial pulses, is usually relatively painless, and heals with elevation and compressive measures. The typical arterial or ischemic ulcer is far more painful and is associated with other manifestations of ischemia. It usually has a more necrotic base and is located at an area of chronic pressure or trauma, such as over the malleoli or the bunion area. Both conditions may be improved by hospitalization, bed rest, and local care. The differential diagnosis is difficult only when chronic venous and arterial disease coexist. Venous evaluations, including duplex scanning, plethysmography, and sometimes venography in addition to arteriography, may be required to completely evaluate these patients. In some patients, the primary cause of the ulcer can be determined only when arterial reconstruction produces healing after a period of intense conservative management has failed to do so.

When a patient has a gangrenous (black) or pregangrenous (blue) toe, several causes other than progression of chronic arteriosclerotic occlusive disease must be considered. Local infection can be the sole or a major contributing cause of a toe lesion. This is particularly common in diabetics. If foot pulses or noninvasive tests of arterial function are normal, the gangrenous condition can be presumed to result from local arterial or arteriolar thrombosis secondary to infection. Radical local excision and drainage of all involved tissue plus antibiotics usually results in a healed foot. Diagnosis is more difficult when infection coexists with arterial occlusive disease. Noninvasive studies and arteriography are usually required to determine whether the treatment should consist of excision and drainage alone or in combination with an arterial reconstruction. Decision making under these conditions is among the most difficult tasks in vascular surgery.

Black or blue toes may also occur as the result of embolic processes. Such emboli may originate from the heart, a proximal (thoracic, abdominal, or popliteal) aneurysm, or any proximal atherosclerotic lesion. In the last circumstance, small cholesterol, platelet, or fibrin emboli may lodge in interosseous or digital arteries. Peripheral pedal pulses may be normal, and spontaneous improvement of the resulting blue toe often occurs. This sequence of events has been termed the "blue toe syndrome," and its pathogenesis is thought to be analogous to that of transient ischemic attacks from atherosclerotic disease at the carotid bifurcation.[9] If a single dominant arterial lesion can be identified by noninvasive means or angiography (or both), it should be treated by endarterectomy or, more commonly, by an appropriate bypass. However, in our experience, identifying a single lesion in the arterial tree of these patients is difficult, and we usually operate only after a patient has experienced multiple embolic episodes.

When ischemia develops suddenly, the possibility of a major embolus from the heart or a proximal aneurysm must

be considered. In such circumstances, angiography is indicated even if limb viability is not in question, because major emboli should be removed as soon as they are identified. In the last several decades, with the significant improvements made in the prevention and treatment of rheumatic heart disease, the majority of patients we have evaluated with major arterial emboli and acute occlusions have had them superimposed on extensive arteriosclerosis. Even with angiography, which we employ routinely in such cases, the diagnosis and treatment of embolic disease are difficult, and the results imperfect.[10] The only certain diagnostic feature of embolic occlusion is multiplicity. Further, the location of the embolus may be atypical, and the vascular surgeon treating a presumed embolus in the presence of extensive arteriosclerosis must be prepared to perform an extensive arterial reconstruction or bypass even if the operation is undertaken soon after the acute event.[10]

Because of these facts and because acute thrombosis sometimes cannot be differentiated in any way from an embolus, complete preoperative angiography should be performed in any patients with suspected embolic occlusion of the lower extremity who may have significant arteriosclerosis. Exploration of the distal popliteal artery is usually the best surgical approach in patients with severe ischemia due to an acute occlusion of the popliteal or distal superficial femoral arteries,[11] although use of intra-arterially administered lytic agents may have significant therapeutic advantages in the management of acute thromboembolic occlusions of native lower extremity arteries, especially those with some underlying atherosclerosis.[12] Moreover, the care and surgical treatment of such patients should be undertaken only by an experienced vascular surgeon. A more complete discussion of the management of acute thromboembolic arterial occlusions appears in Chapter 40.

Patient Evaluation

LOCAL FACTORS AND PHYSICAL EXAMINATION

As already indicated, the findings on physical examination of the involved extremity contribute to the staging of the atherosclerotic process and provide a rough guide to whether diagnostic or therapeutic intervention is justified and needed. Physical findings such as discoloration, swelling, erythema, and localized tenderness can provide evidence of the presence and extent of infection in the involved foot. As a general rule, the extent of infection and necrosis deep to the skin is greater than one might expect from an examination of the skin. Re-examination after a short period of soaking to soften the epidermis and dried exudate may be helpful in revealing purulent collections and subcutaneous necrosis. Exploration of suspicious areas can sometimes be carried out without anesthesia if the patient has diminished sensation from diabetic neuropathy. If not, such exploration and necessary débridement should be performed in the operating room under appropriate anesthesia.

A thorough initial examination of a patient with suspected infrainguinal arterial disease is required and is helpful in ascertaining the nature and extent of previous arterial surgery and ipsilateral saphenous vein harvest, as well as evidence of associated chronic disease. In evaluating an ischemic limb, particular attention must be given to careful inspection of the heel and between the toes, where unsuspected ischemic ulcers or infection may be present. A flashlight is extremely helpful in this regard. The uninvolved extremity must also be examined carefully. Because of the symmetry of atherosclerosis, the opposite extremity may harbor unsuspected ischemic lesions. Moreover, findings such as coolness and bluish discoloration are far more meaningful if they are asymmetrical, because cool, dusky extremities are sometimes present without significant arterial disease.

Pulse examination in the lower extremities of a patient with suspected ischemia is extremely important. It requires considerable experience and must be performed with care. The strength of a pulse as assessed by an experienced examiner is a valuable semiquantitative assessment of the arterial circulation at that level. Pulses are graded from 0 to 4+, and a pulse cannot be described as "plus or minus" or "questionable"; the latter indicates an incomplete examination. A 0 pulse cannot be felt. A 1+ pulse is definitely present but definitely diminished. Both 2+ and 3+ are normal intensities, and 4+ is an abnormally strong pulse, as with an aneurysm or aortic insufficiency. If a pulse is 2+ on one side and 3+ on the opposite side, the 2+ is a decreased pulse, and arterial pressure at that site is probably diminished (unless the 3+ pulse is due to an aneurysm).

In examining a patient with diminished pulses, counting the pulse to an assistant who is palpating the patient's radial pulse helps ensure that the examiner is not feeling his or her own pulse or spurious muscular activity. Before one describes a pulse as being absent, considerable time and effort must be expended, and ectopic localization of pulses, such as the lateral tarsal artery pulse, must be done. In this era of frequent noninvasive arterial tests, the value of a carefully performed and recorded pulse examination cannot be overemphasized. An accurate pulse examination predicts both the pattern of infrainguinal disease and the treatment required to relieve the symptoms. It also provides a basis for comparison if disease progression occurs.

For example, if a patient with a gangrenous toe lesion has a pedal pulse, local treatment without reconstructive arterial surgery is almost always the correct approach to achieve a healed foot. If a patient with an ischemic foot lesion has a normal popliteal pulse but no pedal pulses, some form of infrapopliteal or small vessel bypass is almost always the correct approach. If a patient with an ischemic foot lesion has a normal ipsilateral femoral pulse without distal pulses, some form of infrainguinal arterial reconstruction, preferably a femoropopliteal bypass, is the correct approach. If such a patient has a diminished femoral pulse, often with an associated bruit, some form of proximal arterial reconstruction or angioplasty above the inguinal ligament is almost certainly required.

SYSTEMIC FACTORS

Systemic factors that are important in a patient who is a candidate for interventional treatment for infrainguinal arteriosclerosis include all those in the history, physical examination, and routine laboratory tests that might indicate major organ failure. Most important are heart disease, diabetes, renal disease, hypertension, chronic pulmonary disease, and atherosclerotic involvement of the cerebral circulation. All these intercurrent diseases, if present, require appropriate

medical management before, during, and after diagnostic and therapeutic interventions so that risks are minimized. A detailed discussion of this management is beyond the scope of this chapter. However, because all patients with infrainguinal arteriosclerosis also have some degree of coronary involvement, and because myocardial infarction is the principal cause of operative as well as late mortality in this group of patients, some details of cardiac evaluation and management should be mentioned.

Evidence of myocardial ischemia and congestive heart failure should be sought. Noninvasive cardiac stress tests after exercise or the infusion of intravenous agents such as dipyridamole or dobutamine may be useful for screening. If marked abnormalities or severe angina pectoris is present, some patients should be subjected to coronary arteriography and aortocoronary bypass before treatment of the limb ischemia. Patients with recent myocardial infarctions and those in congestive heart failure should have a Swan-Ganz catheter inserted and have their fluid and volume replacement optimized before, during, and after operation on the basis of appropriate cardiac output and pressure measurements.[13] Renal function must be monitored repetitively after any angiographic procedure, because transient renal failure is common. If it is detected and appropriately treated, however, this is almost always reversible and is rarely a serious problem.

NONINVASIVE VASCULAR LABORATORY TESTS

Although the nature and value of noninvasive laboratory tests are discussed in depth in Chapter 14, several relevant points should be made here regarding their role in patients with infrainguinal arteriosclerosis. In the early stages, when interventional measures are not required, segmental arterial pressures and pulse-volume recordings provide an objective and semiquantitative assessment of the circulation and help confirm the diagnosis made by the history and physical examination, including a careful pulse examination. These tests also provide a baseline for future comparison and serve as a rough index of the localization of occlusive lesions and the degree of ischemia in the foot. However, the correlation is not absolute. Flat ankle and forefoot wave tracings with ankle pressures less than 35 mm Hg may not be associated with foot lesions or serious symptoms. In addition, decreased thigh waveforms and pressures may be entirely due to disease below the inguinal ligament as well as aortoiliac disease. The differentiation between these two types of lesions can be made only by femoral pulse examination and direct pressure measurements. The exact localization and definition of these lesions can be accomplished using duplex scanning, and there has been a great deal of interest in planning infrainguinal revascularization on the basis of duplex arterial mapping alone,[14,15] but angiography, often in two planes, may be necessary. In some circumstances, screening duplex arterial mapping supplemented by limited intraoperative arteriography provides an excellent road map and also minimizes contrast administration, cost, and preoperative hospitalization. We have been using this approach with increasing frequency, with good results.

Noninvasive testing can be extremely helpful in predicting when a toe amputation or local procedure on the foot has virtually no chance of healing. A flat-line forefoot tracing with an ankle pressure below 50 mm Hg indicates that a toe amputation or other foot operation for an ischemic lesion will not heal without prior revascularization. Because these tests do not evaluate the severity or extent of infection, the opposite is not always true. Good forefoot pulse waves and ankle pressures do not guarantee the healing of foot operations, although they suggest that healing will occur if infection can be eliminated. There is also a gray zone of intermediate values, in which case noninvasive tests are of limited value and a therapeutic trial of a local foot procedure is justified and appropriate.

ANGIOGRAPHIC EVALUATION

As in other areas of vascular surgery, proper high-quality arteriography is essential to make the most accurate diagnosis of infrainguinal arteriosclerosis, to determine whether a therapeutic intervention is possible and justified by its risk, and to plan the optimal form of intervention.[5] Adequate arteriography also defines the localization and extent of arteriosclerotic involvement in the infrarenal aorta and iliac arteries, although for optimal accuracy, it may have to be supplemented by direct pressure measurements taken at the time of arteriography or operation.

To provide adequate information, the arterial tree from the renal arteries to the forefoot should be well visualized in continuity, preferably by the transfemoral route. Oblique views may be required to completely visualize the origin and proximal portion of the deep femoral artery. Good preoperative distal artery visualization is, in our opinion, the key to performing optimal bypass surgery on arteries in the foot and lower leg. Reactive hyperemia, digitally augmented views, and delayed films may be necessary to achieve the necessary visualization. Although others have advocated intraoperative arteriography to achieve this end,[16] we have found it less effective and rarely necessary. Magnetic resonance angiography can provide preoperative evaluation of patent distal leg and foot arteries without the need for dye injection and arterial catheterization.[17,18] Although this technique is becoming more widely available, it is expensive and of variable quality in different centers.[19]

Saphenous venography and, more recently, duplex ultrasonography are also helpful in planning long bypasses.[20,21] They may show a vein defect preoperatively and thereby spare the patient and the surgeon the needless effort of harvesting a saphenous vein that cannot be used. These techniques are particularly indicated in patients who have undergone prior bypasses, because many of these patients have had their veins used or inadvertently injured at their first operation. However, neither method is totally accurate, and surgical exploration is the only way to assess vein quality with certainty.

Treatment: Principles, Procedures, and Judgment Issues

In general, our approach, which is detailed in subsequent paragraphs, represents the most aggressive effort for limb salvage in patients with severe infrainguinal arteriosclerosis. Patients who have ischemic foot lesions or pain but who can be treated successfully by aortofemoral, femorofemoral, or axillofemoral bypass alone are excluded from the following discussion, even though many of them have infrainguinal arteriosclerosis in addition to their more proximal disease.

GENERAL CONSIDERATIONS

According to our aggressive approach to patients whose limbs are threatened because of infrainguinal arteriosclerosis, limb salvage should be considered and attempted if feasible, unless gangrene extends into the deeper tissues of the tarsal region of the foot or the patient has severe organic mental syndrome with inability to ambulate, communicate, or provide self-care.[1,6] Patients in the latter categories should undergo primary below- or above-knee amputation. Primary above-knee amputation should also be employed if a patient with foot gangrene is unable to stand or walk because of long-standing severe flexion contractures.

MEDICAL CONSIDERATIONS

As expected, these patients have a high incidence of other arteriosclerotic manifestations, and more than 60% have diabetes mellitus.[6] The mean age is older than 70 years, and the number of patients older than 80 years is rapidly increasing. Many have suffered documented myocardial infarctions, some are in uncompensated congestive heart or renal failure, some have had myocardial infarctions within 3 weeks of presentation,[6,22] and some have concurrent carcinomas.[2]

The general plan of medical management is to achieve maximal improvement of cardiac, renal, and diabetic status before proceeding with arteriographic examination and operation. In some instances, the urgency of the ischemic situation, coupled with progressive infection in the foot, makes it necessary to perform the angiographic examination and intervention before ideal medical control can be achieved. In these patients, the decision to proceed is made jointly by the surgeon, the internist, and the patient. Almost without exception, age, medical status, incurable malignancy, and a contralateral amputation are not considered absolute contraindications to arterial reconstruction.[1,6]

SURGICAL CONSIDERATIONS AND CRITERIA FOR RECONSTRUCTIBILITY

Femoropopliteal Bypass

Patients whose limbs are clearly threatened and who have undergone arteriographic examination should have femoropopliteal bypass when the superficial femoral or popliteal artery is occluded and the patent popliteal artery segment distal to the occlusion has luminal continuity, on arteriographic examination, with any of its three terminal branches. This is true even if one or more of these branches ends in an occlusion anywhere in the leg. Even if the popliteal artery segment into which the graft is to be inserted is occluded distally, femoropopliteal bypass to this isolated segment may be the procedure of choice in selected patients.[23] If the isolated popliteal segment is less than 7 cm long or if extensive gangrene or infection is present in the foot, a femoral-to-popliteal-to-distal artery bypass, or sequential bypass, is sometimes performed in one or two stages.[24,25] All femoropopliteal bypasses can be classified on the basis of their relationship to the knee joint and runoff from the popliteal artery, as determined radiographically by previously described criteria.[25] However, all angiographic evaluations of popliteal runoff are imperfect and correlated in only a limited way with outflow resistance and bypass patency.[26]

Infrapopliteal Bypass

Bypasses to arteries beyond the popliteal (small vessel or tibial bypasses) are performed only when femoropopliteal bypass is not deemed possible or appropriate, according to the foregoing criteria. These small vessel bypasses are performed to the posterior tibial, the anterior tibial, or the peroneal arteries, in that order of preference. A tibial artery is generally used only if its lumen runs without obstruction into the foot, although short vein bypasses to isolated tibial artery segments and other disadvantaged outflow tracts have been performed and have remained patent over 4 years.[27-30] A peroneal artery is usually used if it is continuous with one or two of its terminal branches, which then run into the foot. Absence of a plantar arch and vascular calcification are not considered contraindications to a reconstruction.[6,27,28] Some patients require a bypass to an artery or arterial branch in the foot.[1,6 27-30] Very few patients fail to have an artery in their leg or foot that meets these requirements; therefore, less than 1% of our patients are now considered unreconstructible on the basis of angiographic findings.[1]

With both femoropopliteal and small vessel bypasses, a stenosis of less than 50% of the diameter of the vessel is acceptable at or distal to the site chosen for the distal anastomosis. Although every effort is made to find the most disease-free segment of artery to use for the distal anastomosis, this may be tempered by the advisability of using the most proximal patent segment possible to shorten the length of the bypass. For example, we believe that a mildly diseased proximal popliteal artery should be used for a distal anastomosis in preference to a nondiseased distal popliteal artery.

The common femoral artery has generally been used as the site of origin for all bypasses to the popliteal and more distal arteries. However, since 1976, we have also used the superficial femoral, popliteal, or tibial arteries as inflow sites when these vessels were relatively undiseased or vein length was limited.[27,31,32] The superficial femoral and popliteal arteries are now used preferentially if possible—that is, if no proximal luminal stenosis exists in excess of 40% of the cross-sectional diameter.

Axillopopliteal Bypass

Axillopopliteal bypass is used only when amputation is imminent and a more standard arterial reconstruction is not feasible because of groin infection, previous operative scarring, or extensive bilateral arteriosclerotic involvement of the iliac and femoral arterial systems.[33,34]

Profundaplasty

Endarterectomy of the origin and proximal portion of the deep femoral artery is most valuable for salvaging threatened limbs when it is combined with some form of inflow operation, such as an aortofemoral or axillofemoral bypass.[35] As an isolated procedure in patients whose limbs are threatened because of infrainguinal arteriosclerosis, we have found profundaplasty to be of little value. Perhaps it is occasionally justified as the sole procedure if the patient has rest pain without necrosis and a tight stenosis or occlusion of the deep femoral artery with a demonstrable pressure gradient across the lesion at operation. In practice, we have used a short vein bypass to the distal deep femoral artery more frequently than an isolated profundaplasty.

GRAFT MATERIAL AND TYPE

Autologous Saphenous Vein versus Polytetrafluoroethylene Grafts

Until 1976, reversed autologous saphenous vein (ASV) grafts were clearly the graft material of choice, with a variety of polyester fabric grafts serving as alternatives if the vein was unavailable. Tubular expanded polytetrafluoroethylene (PTFE) grafts became available in 1976 and were initially used only when ipsilateral saphenous vein was unavailable or unusable. Promising early and intermediate results with this material in femoropopliteal bypasses[36-38] prompted liberalization of the indications for its use in this operation to include patients whose probable life expectancy was less than 3 years. Some surgeons, after adequately analyzing their results, still advocate the preferential use of PTFE grafts for femoropopliteal bypass to the above-knee segment.[39]

In 1986, we and our colleagues completed a cooperative, randomized, prospective study comparing ASV with PTFE grafts in all infrainguinal bypass operations.[40,41] ASV and PTFE grafts were compared in 845 infrainguinal bypass operations, 485 to the popliteal artery and 360 to infrapopliteal arteries. Life-table primary patency rates for randomized PTFE grafts to the popliteal artery paralleled those for randomized ASV grafts to the same level for 2 years and then became significantly different (4-year patency of 68% ± 8% [± standard error] for ASV, vs. 47% ± 9% for PTFE; $P < 0.025$). Four-year patency differences were not statistically significant for randomized above-knee grafts (61% ± 12% for ASV, vs. 38% ± 13% for PTFE; $P < 0.25$), but they were for randomized below-knee grafts (76% ± 9% for ASV, vs. 45% ± 11% for PTFE; $P < 0.05$). Four-year limb salvage rates after bypasses to the popliteal artery for critical ischemia did not differ for the two types of randomized grafts (75% ± 10% for ASV, vs. 72% ± 10% for PTFE; $P < 0.025$). Although primary patency rates for randomized PTFE grafts and obligatory PTFE grafts to the popliteal artery were significantly different ($P < 0.025$), 4-year limb salvage rates were not (70% ± 10% vs. 68% ± 20%; $P < 0.25$). Primary patency rates at 4 years for infrapopliteal bypasses with randomized ASV grafts were significantly better than those with randomized PTFE grafts (49% ± 10% vs. 12% ± 7%; $P < 0.001$). Three-and-one-half-year limb salvage rates for infrapopliteal bypasses with both randomized grafts (57% ± 10% for ASV and 61% ± 10% for PTFE) were better than those for obligatory infrapopliteal PTFE grafts (38% ± 11%; $P < 0.01$). These results fail to support the routine preferential use of PTFE grafts for either femoropopliteal or more distal bypasses. However, this graft may be used preferentially in selected poor-risk patients for femoropopliteal bypasses, particularly those that do not cross the knee. In addition, although every effort should be made to use autologous vein for infrapopliteal bypasses, a PTFE distal bypass is a better option than a primary major amputation. Reports have shown improved results for femorotibial bypasses using PTFE grafts with or without distal anastomotic vein patches. The best reported primary patency rates of these grafts at 5 years with a distal anastomotic vein patch are 54% ± 10%.[42] A study of distal PTFE grafts without a distal vein patch reported 5-year secondary patency rates of 43% ± 10% and limb salvage rates of 66% ± 8%.[43] Others have reported their experience with precuffed PTFE grafts and found no difference in patency or limb salvage rates when compared with PTFE grafts with a vein cuff.[44]

Although we believe that PTFE grafts are currently the best alternative arterial prosthetic if the ipsilateral ASV is not available for femoropopliteal bypass or if no vein is available for infrapopliteal bypass, other grafts have been used with some success. The tanned umbilical vein graft has received the greatest attention, and patency rates similar to those of PTFE grafts have been reported in both the femoropopliteal and infrapopliteal positions.[45] A number of randomized comparisons of the two grafts have been completed. However, many of these studies were flawed or yielded inconclusive differences. In addition, reports of a high incidence of aneurysmal degeneration occurring in umbilical vein grafts after even a few years are worrisome and suggest that this graft be used with caution, even though the manufacturers have strengthened the external polyester fabric mesh.[46]

Another alternative prosthetic that may have some usefulness in infrainguinal bypasses is the polyester fabric graft. A 1992 retrospective study by Pevec and colleagues suggested that these grafts can have excellent results when used as a femoropopliteal conduit.[47] In addition, externally supported grafts may be useful for infrapopliteal bypasses.[48] Polyester fabric and PTFE grafts have been compared in a randomized, prospective fashion as conduits for femoropopliteal bypasses to arterial segments above the knee.[49] At 5 years, no significant difference was evident in primary or secondary patency rates.

At present, use of any new prosthetic grafts in preference to ipsilateral ASV is clearly wrong until appropriate randomized, prospective studies comparing the prosthetic graft with vein have been completed. Many surgeons succumb to the temptation to use a prosthetic graft preferentially. We believe that this temptation must be resisted and encourage randomized study of all promising new prosthetic grafts before they are used preferentially. Sixty percent to 80% of patients have a usable vein if a real effort is made to find it.[17,50] In the remaining 20% to 40% of patients, however, use of a prosthetic graft is far better than an unwise attempt to use a small (<3 mm in distended diameter), fibrotic, or otherwise inadequate autologous vein.[50-53] These considerations should be kept in mind when evaluating an "all-autologous policy" for infrainguinal bypass procedures.[54] As more and more secondary operations become necessary to save limbs, the percentage of patients who do not have an adequate autologous vein conduit will increase. In such patients, a prosthetic (PTFE) graft yields better results than ill-advised use of a poor or intrinsically diseased vein.

In Situ versus Reversed Saphenous Vein Grafts

The in situ saphenous vein graft was described as an infrainguinal arterial conduit by Hall in 1962.[55] It has several theoretical advantages over the more commonly used reversed saphenous vein graft, although the technique is demanding and requires elimination of all venous valves and occlusion of branches. Leather and coworkers devised methods for rendering the venous valves incompetent,[56] and the Albany group[57] and Gruss and coworkers[58] of Germany popularized the use of in situ vein grafts for infrainguinal arterial reconstructions.

Recently, a number of claims have been made regarding the superiority of in situ vein grafts to reversed vein grafts, particularly for tibial and peroneal bypasses. Although better endothelial preservation may be possible with in situ veins, and although they may offer advantages when long bypasses with small veins are required, superior patency rates in comparable situations have never been proved. Comparisons using historical controls are not valid.

In a multicenter, prospective, randomized comparison of in situ and reversed vein grafts that we and our colleagues carried out,[59] no significant differences were evident in the primary patency, secondary patency, and limb salvage rates between the two groups. Moreover, many of the striking results that can be accomplished with in situ vein grafts can also be successfully accomplished with reversed vein grafts.[27] This includes the use of small-caliber veins to disadvantaged outflow tracts (Figs. 32-1 to 32-3). In addition, many patients who have autologous vein suitable for an ectopic reversed vein graft do not have a vein suitable for an in situ graft. Patients with no remaining major superficial vein in the ipsilateral lower extremity but with a good vein in the opposite leg or an arm are one example. Thus, until the superiority of in situ grafts is clearly documented by adequately controlled studies, we will adhere to the belief that the technical perfection of the operation and the surgical team's commitment to the goal of limb salvage are far more important in achieving

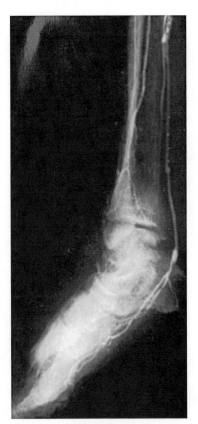

FIGURE 32–1 • Arteriogram performed on a patient 3 years after posterior tibial–to–posterior tibial bypass. The plantar arch is incomplete. (From Veith FJ, Ascer E, Gupta SK, et al: Tibiotibial vein bypass grafts: A new operation for limb salvage. J Vasc Surg 2:552-557, 1985.)

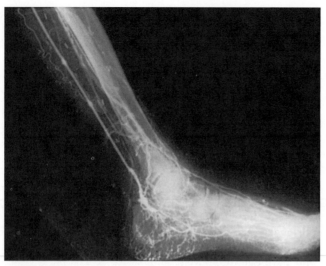

FIGURE 32–2 • Intraoperative arteriogram after bypass from the tibioperoneal trunk to the posterior tibial artery at its bifurcation in the foot. Note the small size of the vein graft and the intact plantar arch. (From Veith FJ, Ascer E, Gupta SK, et al: Tibiotibial vein bypass grafts: A new operation for limb salvage. J Vasc Surg 2:552-557, 1985.)

good results than whether the vein graft is in the reversed or in situ position.

Taylor and colleagues published their results with infrainguinal reversed vein bypasses and claimed that reversed vein grafts were better than in situ grafts.[60] However, more than

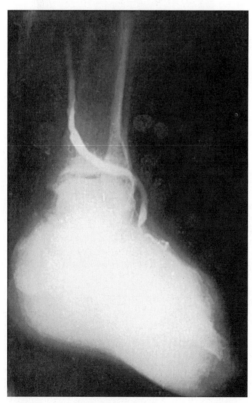

FIGURE 32–3 • Postoperative arteriogram after bypass to the lateral tarsal artery, which appears to end in a total occlusion. There is also no patent plantar arch. (From Veith FJ, Ascer E, Gupta SK, et al: Tibiotibial vein bypass grafts: A new operation for limb salvage. J Vasc Surg 2:552-557, 1985.)

20% of their patients were operated on for indications other than limb salvage. Thus, their claims of the superiority of reversed vein grafts are based on data without comparable, concurrent controls—the same defect that they noted in the reports of others who claimed that the in situ technique gave superior results. Thus, the question of which type of vein graft is better remains an unanswered one that requires further study. We noted extremely poor late patency rates for long reversed vein grafts less than 3.5 mm in diameter and short vein grafts less than 3 mm in diameter.[52,53] Because similar poor patency has not been reported in small-diameter in situ grafts,[61] the in situ technique may be superior in patients whose vein is less than 3 mm in distended diameter.

Upper Extremity Veins

The cephalic and basilic veins from the upper extremities have been advocated for use as a graft when lower extremity autologous vein is unavailable. Although the work of Schulman and Bradley and many others suggests that arm veins are inferior to the saphenous vein in infrainguinal bypasses, other observations indicate that the cephalic vein can be used with good success in lower extremity arterial reconstructions.[62-65] However, arm veins are more thin walled and more difficult to work with than the saphenous vein. Moreover, in our experience, arm veins may have fibrotic, recanalized segments from previous trauma and venipunctures. When several healthy segments are joined to form a composite graft, poorer patency results. This is due in part to intrinsic disease in the venous conduit. Intraoperative angioscopy is very useful in evaluating these veins,[66] so that severely diseased segments that may appear normal on external inspection can be discarded. In addition, aggressive surveillance is necessary to discover and potentially correct the vein graft lesions that more commonly develop in these conduits.[54]

On this basis and because of the high degree of symmetry in infrainguinal arteriosclerosis, we believe that use of a prosthetic graft in the femoropopliteal position is presently justified if the ipsilateral saphenous vein is unsuitable or unavailable. However, for infrapopliteal bypasses, every effort should be made to find usable autogenous vein. In this regard, lesser saphenous veins, accessory saphenous veins, and veins from the opposite thigh and upper extremities may all be useful, and we use them in that order of preference.

OPERATIVE TECHNIQUE

All operations are performed with the patient under light general, spinal, or epidural anesthesia. Care is taken to protect the opposite heel by placing a small pillow under the Achilles tendon. The arterial blood pressure is monitored by a radial artery catheter. Surgical techniques are detailed elsewhere[34,37,67] and illustrated in Figures 32-4 and 32-5. Vessels are occluded with a minimum of force and distortion. We have found tourniquet occlusion, as recommended by Bernhard and colleagues,[68] to be very useful during the creation of the distal and sometimes proximal anastomoses. Anastomoses are meticulously constructed with continuous 6-0 polypropylene sutures, with particular care to take small, evenly spaced bites of all layers of the vessel wall and to exclude all adventitia from the anastomotic lumen. Intraoperative angiographic examination is performed after most small vessel bypasses,

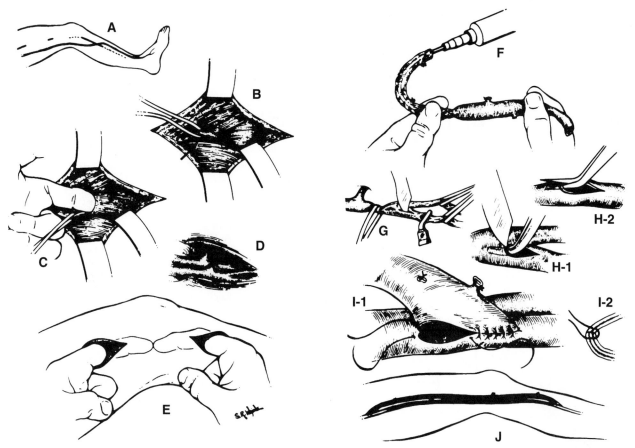

FIGURE 32–4 • Small vessel bypass in the upper and middle thirds of the leg. This can be performed to the tibioperoneal trunk, the posterior tibial artery, or the peroneal artery using a medial approach below the knee joint to gain access to these vessels. The anterior tibial artery requires an additional anterior incision (shown in Fig. 32-5). *A*, Heavy lines show the position of the incisions required to perform bypasses from the femoral artery to the tibioperoneal trunk or the peroneal or posterior tibial arteries in the upper third of the leg. The upper incision provides access to the common or superficial femoral artery. The above-knee incision allows tunneling under the sartorius muscle and along the course of the popliteal vessels behind the knee. The dashed extension to the lower incision provides access to the posterior tibial and peroneal arteries in the middle third of the leg. If the saphenous vein is to be used, all incisions should be placed over the vein, as shown by the double line, and access to deeper structures can be obtained when needed by raising thick flaps. *B*, The below-knee incision is opened through the skin, subcutaneous fat, and deep fascia of the popliteal space. The gastrocnemius muscle is retracted posteriorly. The more superficial popliteal vein is encircled with a Silastic loop to facilitate dissection of the underlying popliteal artery *(arrow)*, which can be seen disappearing deep to the fibers of the soleus muscle. *C*, A finger or right-angle clamp is placed deep to the soleus muscle before cutting it at its origin from the fibrous band that attaches to the back of the tibia. This exposes the origin of the anterior tibial artery and its accompanying vein or veins. *D*, Division of these veins allows further retraction of overlying veins and exposure of the tibioperoneal trunk and its terminal branches. *E*, Tunnels are fashioned by finger dissection. *F*, Details of vein preparation using a long (6-inch) cannula to permit the vein to be distended in segments so that leaks can be controlled and recanalized segments can be detected. *G*, Elevation of the arteries by Silastic vessel loops and the beginning of the scalpel incision in the artery. In this view, only the taut Silastic loops are required to control bleeding, except for the posterior tibial artery, which also has a microvascular clip applied to it. *H*, Placement of a mosquito clamp to facilitate extension of the initial opening in the artery (1). Alternatively, a microvascular scissors may be used to extend the arteriotomy if the vessel is thin walled and normal (2). *I*, Details of the anastomotic suturing, which is begun at the distal end and continued to the midportion of each side of the anastomosis of the artery and the saphenous vein graft. Equal bites of all layers of each vessel are included in each stitch, which is always placed under direct vision. *J*, Completed graft in place. If more distal exposure of the posterior tibial or peroneal arteries is required, further separation of the soleus muscle from the posterior surface of the tibia and its overlying muscles provides access to the neurovascular bundles. Careful dissection of the veins, with ligation of crossing branches, provides access to the more deeply placed arteries. These can be dissected free, taking great care to preserve all branches, so that an appropriate segment of artery can be elevated and controlled to perform the distal anastomosis. (From Veith FJ, Gupta SK: Femoral-distal artery bypasses. In Bergan JJ, Yao JST [eds]: Operative Techniques in Vascular Surgery. New York, Grune & Stratton, 1980, pp 141-150.)

but it is used only if special problems are encountered after a femoropopliteal bypass. Although many vascular surgeons think of completion angiography as a panacea, it is not. Defects can be overlooked or not visualized because the proximal portion of the reconstruction is not included on the film. Moreover, "pseudodefects" may be visualized, prompting

further time-consuming, needless, and potentially harmful manipulation.[69] Intraoperative fluoroscopy is a very useful adjunct to infrainguinal bypass surgery.[70] After introduction of a small diagnostic catheter, the graft, both anastomoses, and the runoff vessels can be carefully evaluated in multiple planes with minimal contrast material, enhancing the accuracy

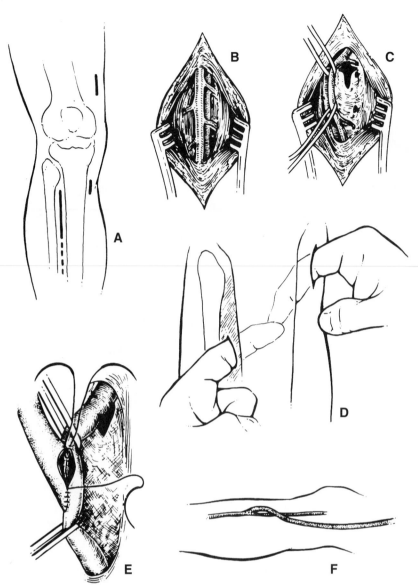

FIGURE 32–5 • Bypass to the anterior tibial artery in the upper and middle thirds of the leg. *A*, This requires an anterolateral incision in the leg midway between the tibia and fibula over the appropriate segment of patent artery. Additional small medial incisions are required for tunneling. *B*, The anterior incision is carried through the deep fascia, and the fibers of the anterior tibial muscle and the long extensors of the toes are separated to reveal the neurovascular bundle. Mobilization of accompanying veins, with division of branches, allows visualization of the anterior tibial artery, which can then be carefully mobilized. *C*, After the artery is freed, it is elevated and retracted, along with the accompanying veins, by Silastic loops. This permits further posterior dissection, which allows the interosseous membrane to be visualized and incised in a cruciate fashion. *D*, Careful blunt finger dissection from this anterior approach and from the popliteal fossa via the medial incision facilitates the creation of a tunnel without injuring the numerous veins in the area. Alternatively, the tunnel for the bypass may be placed lateral to the knee in a subcutaneous plane. *E*, By elevating the anterior tibial artery, a meticulous distal anastomosis can be constructed, as already described. *F*, The resulting graft in place. (From Veith FJ, Gupta SK: Femoral-distal artery bypasses. In Bergan JJ, Yao JST [eds]: Operative Techniques in Vascular Surgery. New York, Grune & Stratton, 1980, pp 141-150.)

of the study.[71] In addition, intraoperative duplex scanning can be used to evaluate the hemodynamics of the arterial tree and bypass graft immediately after completion of the procedure.[72] Both techniques allow prompt diagnosis and correction of any problems.

BYPASSES TO ANKLE OR FOOT ARTERIES

For many years, our group has advocated the effectiveness of performing bypasses to arteries near the ankle or in the foot in patients who have no usable patent artery for distal bypass insertion at a more proximal level.[6,27] With adequate preoperative arteriography, these very distal arteries can usually be visualized if they are patent. Indeed, visualizing such arteries and using them for bypass insertion have been major factors in reducing the proportion of patients whose arterial disease is so distal that they are considered unsuitable for an attempt at limb salvage or inoperable. Although our advocacy of these very distal perimalleolar and inframalleolar bypasses was at first greeted with skepticism, these procedures are now being

performed and advocated widely. Excellent results have been reported for perimalleolar and inframalleolar bypasses to major arteries.[27,28,31] In addition, bypasses to the plantar and tarsal branches of pedal arteries can be successfully performed (Fig. 32-6; see also Figs. 32-1 to 32-3).[29,30]

PERIOPERATIVE AND POSTOPERATIVE DRUG TREATMENT

All patients receive prophylactic antibiotic treatment with 1 g of cefazolin preoperatively and postoperatively, if necessary. Vancomycin 1 g, adjusted for renal function, may be given in cases of penicillin allergy. All receive 100 to 150 units/kg of heparin during periods of vascular occlusion, and adequate anticoagulation is ensured by following activated clotting times intraoperatively.

Based on the experimental observations of Oblath and colleagues,[73] all patients receive perioperative antiplatelet therapy. This generally consists of 325 mg of aspirin given one to three times daily, with or without the addition of a more

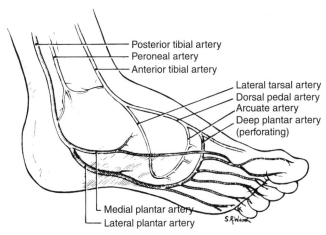

FIGURE 32–6 • Named arteries in the ankle region and foot. Any of the main arteries or their branches, if patent, can be approached surgically and used as the distal outflow for a limb salvage bypass. (From Ascer E, Veith FJ, Gupta SK: Bypasses to plantar arteries and other tibial branches: An extended approach to limb salvage. J Vasc Surg 8:434-441, 1988.)

potent agent, such as clopidogrel. Therapy is begun 48 hours before operation and continued for several weeks.[74] After this period, one of these drugs, usually aspirin, is continued indefinitely if possible.

MANAGEMENT OF FOOT LESIONS

Approximately 75% of our patients have gangrenous or necrotic foot or toe lesions.[1,6] Small (<2 cm²), uninfected gangrenous lesions on the toe or foot are not treated. Larger gangrenous lesions and any area of infection associated with necrosis is usually extensively débrided at the end of any arterial reconstruction. These débridements often require excision of one or more toes and frequently consist of a partial (medial or lateral) transmetatarsal amputation. An attempt is made to excise enough bone so that overhanging skin and soft tissue are present. These wounds are usually left open, and drying of the soft tissues is prevented by placing a normal saline wet dressing on the wound. Subsequent débridement of foot lesions is often required on the ward or in the operating room. This is performed to remove all infected or necrotic tissue and exposed cartilage without regard for anatomic landmarks.

Performing multiple secondary operative procedures is sometimes necessary, particularly in diabetic patients, to achieve a healed foot. Skin grafts are used to cover large cutaneous defects but are placed only when the wound is rendered entirely clean and granulating by débridement and frequent dressing changes. In some patients, particularly those with extensive foot gangrene or infection and a femoropopliteal bypass inserted into an isolated popliteal artery segment, achieving healing at the metatarsal or even tarsal level is impossible, and below-knee amputation is required even though the bypass is patent. In some similar instances, foot healing has been obtained by performing a secondary bypass to an artery distal to the popliteal segment.[25] However, in an occasional patient with extensive infection and necrosis, a healed foot cannot be obtained, even with straight-line arterial flow into the pedal arteries. This is particularly common in patients with end-stage renal disease and diabetes.[75]

REOPERATION

Host patients whose bypasses thrombose in the first month after operation undergo reoperation. The techniques employed have been described in detail elsewhere.[76]

Intraoperative fluoroscopy is a very useful adjunct to the performance of graft and arterial thrombectomy and for complete evaluation of the graft inflow and outflow vessels.[70,77] It significantly improves intraoperative evaluation and surgical manipulations compared with static intraoperative angiography.

Vein grafts that fail immediately after operation usually require interposition of a segment of PTFE or total replacement with this material,[78] although in our experience, an occasional thrombectomized vein graft remains patent if no causative lesion is present.

Patients whose bypasses thrombose after the first postoperative month are considered for aggressive reoperation, and femoral angiography is usually performed; however, patients are subjected to reoperation only if the bypass failure is associated with a renewed threat to limb viability. If the patient's original operation was performed elsewhere and details of the first operation are not known or the distal anastomosis is at or below the knee joint, a totally new bypass is usually performed. This is best accomplished using a variety of unusual approaches that permit access to infrainguinal arteries via unscarred, uninfected tissue planes.[76,78,79] These approaches include a direct approach to the distal two thirds of the deep femoral artery (Figs. 32-7 and 32-8),[80,81] lateral approaches to the popliteal artery above and below the knee,[82] and medial

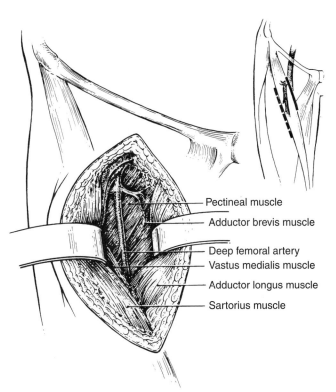

Pectineal muscle
Adductor brevis muscle
Deep femoral artery
Vastus medialis muscle
Adductor longus muscle
Sartorius muscle

FIGURE 32–7 • Incisions and anatomy for direct approaches to the distal two thirds of the deep femoral artery. (From Nunez A, Veith FJ, Collier P, et al: Direct approach to the distal portions of the deep femoral artery for limb salvage bypasses. J Vasc Surg 8:576-581, 1988.)

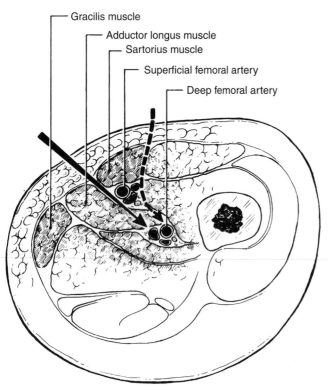

FIGURE 32–8 • Cross-sectional anatomy for direct approaches to the distal two thirds of the deep femoral artery. (From Nunez A, Veith FJ, Collier P, et al: Direct approach to the distal portions of the deep femoral artery for limb salvage bypass. J Vasc Surg 8:576-581, 1988.)

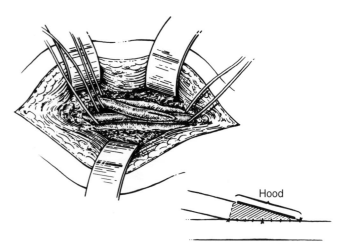

FIGURE 32–9 • Technique for a reoperation in which graft salvage will be attempted. Control of the artery proximal and distal to the anastomosis must be obtained. The opening in the graft is placed so that the interior of the anastomosis can be visualized.

or lateral approaches to all three of the infrapopliteal arteries. In addition to permitting dissection in virginal tissue planes, these unusual access routes facilitate the use of shorter grafts, which enable the surgeon to use the patient's remaining segments of good vein when his or her ipsilateral greater saphenous vein has been used or injured by the primary operation.

If the surgeon elects to salvage an old PTFE graft, which may be appropriate if the original distal anastomosis was above the knee and the patient's veins are poor, as determined by venography or duplex ultrasonography, appropriate surgical techniques are critical to obtaining a favorable outcome.[76,79] The prior distal incision is opened, and the distal end of the graft, the distal anastomosis, and the proximal and distal artery are dissected free. The graft is opened with a longitudinal incision to within a few millimeters of its distal tip (Fig. 32-9). The graft is then thrombectomized by passage of balloon catheters, best performed under fluoroscopic control.[71] This technique allows the evaluation of the contour of the thrombectomy balloon for a potential lesion and its location. In addition, catheter-wire techniques can be used to advance a thrombectomy catheter safely in patients in whom this is difficult to do.

Thrombus is gently removed from the distal anastomosis under direct vision, and balloon catheters are passed proximally and distally in the artery using extreme gentleness and care. If no disease or defect is seen within the anastomotic lumen, the opening in the graft is closed, and a complete fluoroscopic evaluation of the inflow, graft, and outflow vessels is performed. If no lesion is found, the operation is terminated.

If intimal hyperplasia or other disease is noted at or just distal to the anastomosis, the opening in the graft is extended across its toe and down the artery to a point beyond the disease. A patch graft is placed to close this opening, and a completion study is performed. If graft thrombosis has resulted from progression of arteriosclerosis proximal or distal to an anastomosis, an appropriate graft extension is constructed after removing all clot. Failed below-knee PTFE femoropopliteal and small vessel bypasses can be similarly managed but are probably best treated by performance of an entirely new bypass, preferably with vein and using previously undissected arteries, if possible. Thrombolytic therapy can be used to salvage a thrombosed graft, but its role in the treatment of these patients is still under evaluation. Early results suggest that lysis of a prosthetic graft leads to only a 25% 6-month patency rate after the intervention.[83] If a treatable lesion is found, the results are better, with a 6-month patency rate of 80%.[83]

Patients presenting with a threatened limb and multiple failed bypasses present special challenges. For many years, our policy has been to avoid amputation in patients with imminent limb threat by making further attempts at limb revascularization, even when patients have failed two or more previous bypasses.[1] One might suspect that patients undergoing a lower extremity bypass after two or more previous failures would have a poorer outcome on the basis of disease severity and progression and the difficulties associated with reoperation. Difficulties encountered with these multiple reoperations include complicated redo dissections, increased risk of subsequent graft or wound infection, lack of a suitable autogenous conduit, and the need for more proximal or distal inflow or more distal outflow. We and others have reviewed our experiences with patients requiring multiple reoperations for limb-threatening ischemia to assess the effect of an increasing number of procedures on patency and limb salvage rates.[84-87] These studies demonstrate that the likelihood of success of repetitive limb revascularization is unrelated to the number of previous failures and that there is no incrementally higher failure rate with each successive bypass. These results, coupled with 3- to 5-year limb salvage rates from 50% to 70% in patients who otherwise would have required amputation, lend support to aggressive use of limb revascularization even after two or more failed bypasses.

FAILING GRAFTS

Intimal hyperplasia, progression of proximal or distal disease, or lesions within the graft itself can produce signs and symptoms of hemodynamic deterioration in patients with a prior arterial reconstruction without producing concomitant thrombosis of the bypass graft.[88-90] We refer to this condition as a "failing graft" because, if the lesion is not corrected, graft thrombosis will almost certainly occur.[89] The importance of this failing graft concept lies in the fact that many difficult lower extremity revascularizations can be salvaged for protracted periods by relatively simple interventions if the lesion responsible for the circulatory deterioration and diminished graft blood flow can be detected before graft thrombosis occurs.

We have been able to detect more than 250 failing grafts and correct the lesions before graft thrombosis occurred. The majority of these grafts were vein grafts, but nearly half were prosthetic grafts.[91] Invariably the corrective procedure is simpler than the secondary operation required if the bypass goes on to thrombose. Some lesions responsible for the failing state can be remedied by percutaneous transluminal angioplasty (PTA), although many require a vein patch angioplasty, a short bypass of a graft lesion, or a proximal or distal graft extension. Some of the transluminal angioplasties of these lesions fail and require a second reintervention; others remain effective in correcting the responsible lesion, as documented by arteriography more than 2 to 5 years later. If the failing graft is a vein bypass, detection of the failing state permits accurate localization and definition of the responsible lesion by arteriography and salvage of any undiseased vein. In contrast, if the graft is permitted to thrombose, the responsible lesion may be difficult to identify; the vein may be difficult or impossible to thrombectomize; and the patient's best graft, the ipsilateral greater saphenous vein, may have to be sacrificed, rendering the secondary operation even more difficult and more likely to fail, with associated limb loss. Most important, the results of reinterventions for failing grafts, in terms of both continued cumulative patency and limb salvage rates, have been far superior to the results of reinterventions for grafts that have thrombosed and failed.[89-92]

This difference in results, together with the ease of reintervention for failing grafts, mandates that surgeons performing infrainguinal bypass operations monitor their patients closely in the postoperative period and indefinitely thereafter. Ideally, noninvasive laboratory tests, including duplex studies, should be performed with similar frequency.[92] If the patient has any recurrence of symptoms or the surgeon detects any change in the peripheral pulse or other manifestations of ischemia, the circulatory deterioration must be confirmed by noninvasive modalities and urgent arteriography. If a lesion is detected and is identified as the cause of the failing state, it is corrected urgently by PTA or operation. Surgical reconstruction is the treatment of choice for failing vein graft lesions,[93-95] but single lesions less than 1.5 cm long with grafts more than 3 mm in diameter yield reasonable results after successful PTA.[95] The role of stents and atherectomy devices for these lesions is still under investigation.

ROLE OF ANGIOPLASTY

Opinions regarding the usefulness of angioplasty differ considerably, and its exact role in the treatment of infrainguinal arteriosclerosis is still debated. Experience suggests that with appropriate patient selection and in skilled hands, the complication rate is low. Moreover, when complications or failure of PTA do occur, they can generally be well treated by relatively simple surgical procedures with little if any increased patient morbidity or mortality.[96] The role of angioplasty can be expected to increase with ongoing improvements in endovascular techniques and devices, especially in the treatment of high-risk patients.[97] Additionally, the anatomic lesions considered amenable to treatment with angioplasty (TASC type A lesions) will likely expand and include some long-segment occlusions (TASC type D lesions).[98]

Traditionally, the results of balloon angioplasty in the crural vessels have been poor. However, the increasing use of lower-profile guidewires, balloons, and stents has facilitated the treatment of smaller-caliber vessels throughout the body, including the popliteal and tibial vessels. Whether the use of these 0.014- and 0.018-inch systems will improve the long-term results of balloon angioplasty in the lower extremities remains to be seen.[99,100] Owing to the relatively poor long-term results with balloon angioplasty with stainless steel stents, self-expanding nitinol stents have been used, with some early success, in the femoropopliteal segment. However, their ultimate role and long-term benefit remain unproved.[101,102]

On this basis, we presently attempt PTA on any patient with sufficiently severe disease and ischemia (usually stage III or IV) to warrant intervention and in whom the procedure is deemed suitable. Patients with stage III or IV ischemia who have a hemodynamically significant segmental iliac stenosis and infrainguinal arteriosclerosis generally have PTA, with or without stent placement, of the iliac lesion as their first therapeutic intervention. If PTA is unsuccessful, a bypass to the femoral level is performed. If PTA is successful, further arterial intervention, usually some form of infrainguinal bypass, is performed only if the ischemia is unrelieved and a healed foot cannot be obtained. We do not hesitate to perform a bypass distal to an iliac artery treated by PTA, and subsequent experience has borne out the effectiveness of this approach.[1,6,103,104]

PTA is also used as the primary therapeutic intervention in patients without hemodynamically significant iliac artery disease who have a short (<5-cm) segmental stenosis of the superficial femoral or popliteal artery, if this lesion is judged hemodynamically significant on the basis of pulse examination or noninvasive testing. In slightly less than half of our cases treated by angioplasty, some form of direct arterial surgery has also been required, usually for bypass of a second lesion distal to the one successfully treated by angioplasty.[1,6] PTA has also been effective in the treatment of stenotic lesions in tibial arteries and stenoses developing in or proximal or distal to a still-functioning vein or PTFE graft.[1,89,105] The use of atherectomy, stents, and endovascular grafts for infrainguinal disease has been less promising but is still under evaluation.[106,107]

Cutting balloons have been used with some success in a variety of settings, including primary angioplasty of native arteries and angioplasty for the treatment of failing vein bypasses and arteriovenous access graft stenoses.[108] These balloons have three or four longitudinally arranged microtomes along their length. The balloons are designed to produce an effective dilatation of very fibrotic lesions and a more uniform dilatation of the vessels by creating microfractures of the plaque and reducing the incidence of irregular plaque fractures and dissections, especially those extending beyond the treated segment. On a similar theoretical basis, cryoplasty balloons have been used in the hope of creating a more uniform and stable vessel dilatation, also with encouraging preliminary results.[109] In this technique, an angioplasty balloon is filled with nitrous oxide and simultaneously both dilates and cools the plaque and vessel wall. This has the theoretical advantage of producing a more uniform dilatation by creating microfractures of the plaque due to freezing, which leads to more uniform vessel dilatation and reduces the risk of a larger dissection. There is also reduction in vessel wall recoil due to loss of elasticity, which may decrease the need for stent placement in conjunction with angioplasty. Finally, the method is believed to reduce the subsequent development of neointimal hyperplasia and extensive remodeling of the vessel wall.

Subintimal angioplasty for the treatment of total occlusions has recently gained popularity and is being used at a growing number of centers. Promising results have been reported, and although it was initially evaluated in the femoropopliteal segment, the application of subintimal angioplasty has expanded to include the iliac and crural arteries as well.[110-114] The procedure is performed by using a guidewire to create a subintimal dissection plane that begins proximal to the origin of the occlusion, crosses the occlusion in the subintimal plane, and then reenters the patent, native lumen distal to the occlusion (Fig. 32-10). This recanalized segment is then balloon dilated, creating a new lumen in the subintimal space. The technique does not require the use of stents, which are placed only in the event of a flow-limiting dissection or other significant abnormality. When this technique is carefully applied, bypass options are preserved in the setting of either procedural failure or subsequent reocclusion. Although the reported patency rates following subintimal angioplasty are less than those for bypass surgery, the corresponding limb salvage rates have been excellent.[115] This fact, coupled with the minimally invasive nature of the procedure, has made it an attractive option in the treatment of lower extremity ischemia, especially in high-risk patients.

Results of Treatment

Arteriosclerotic involvement is generally less, in terms of both extent and multiplicity of lesions, in patients with intermittent claudication than in those who have a threatened limb. Not surprisingly, short-term and long-term patency results of infrainguinal arterial bypasses performed for intermittent claudication are generally better than those done for limb salvage, and this difference has been documented by virtually every author who evaluated results on the basis of operative indications.[50,116] Because we believe that femoropopliteal bypass should rarely be performed for intermittent claudication and that the other infrainguinal bypasses should never be performed for this indication alone, we restrict our discussion of results to operations performed because of severe ischemic rest pain, a nonhealing ulcer, or gangrene. However, femoropopliteal bypasses for truly disabling claudication are justified by their good results and low risk rate,[2] provided the patient is informed of the risks

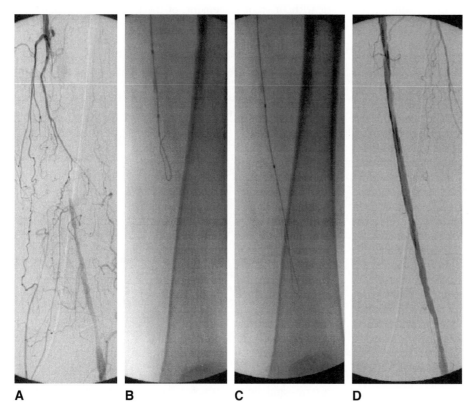

FIGURE 32–10 • Subintimal angioplasty. *A,* Preprocedure occlusion of the superficial femoral artery (SFA). *B* and *C,* Advancement of wire with a wide loop through the subintimal plane. *D,* Postprocedure completion angiogram showing a patent, recanalized SFA.

A   B   C   D

of intervention. In our experience, when patients are so informed, they usually opt for a trial of noninterventional treatment before considering other options.

Results of infrainguinal bypasses clearly vary with the training, technical skill, and commitment of the surgeon. These operations are demanding and should be performed only by surgeons who do them regularly and, more important, who have the skill and commitment to reoperate successfully should a bypass fail in the early or late postoperative period. In deciding whether these operations and an aggressive approach to limb salvage are, in fact, justified in a given setting, vascular surgeons should continually examine their own results to determine whether they are good enough to justify the continued application of these sometimes difficult operations in these often brittle patients.

OPERATIVE MORTALITY

The 30-day mortality for all patients undergoing infrainguinal arterial reconstructions for threatened limbs ranges from 2% to 6%.[1,6,76,117] Operative mortality is slightly greater for infrapopliteal and axillopopliteal bypasses than for femoropopliteal bypasses, probably because the former operations are required in patients with more advanced generalized as well as lower extremity disease. The principal cause of death from these operations is myocardial infarction.

These low operative mortalities contrast with the high late-death rates reflected in Figure 32-11, which shows that only 48% of all patients who had arterial reconstructions were alive 5 years later. Almost all late deaths were unrelated to the original operation; most were attributed to concurrent arteriosclerotic events, chiefly myocardial infarction. These findings again reflect the advanced stage of generalized arteriosclerosis present in these patients.

LIMB SALVAGE

When the aggressive approach already outlined for the management of patients whose limbs are threatened by infrainguinal arteriosclerosis was used, and when only those

patients who had organic mental syndrome and extensive local gangrene were excluded, 96% of patients underwent arteriographic examination.[6] Ninety-four percent of patients who underwent arteriography were suitable candidates for some form of arterial revascularization procedure. With recent technical advances, only 1% to 2% of patients undergoing arteriography do not have some patent distal artery suitable for use in an attempt at revascularization, and most of these are patients who underwent previous failed operations.[1]

Immediate Limb Salvage

Defined as relief of ischemia and healing of ischemic lesions for 1 month after the first revascularization procedure, immediate limb salvage was achieved in 86% of patients in whom revascularization was possible.[6] This immediate limb salvage rate was calculated by subtracting from the number of patients who could undergo revascularization procedures those patients who died or whose arterial reconstructive operation or angioplasty failed irretrievably within 1 month of the primary procedure and those patients who required major amputations despite a successful revascularization procedure. Multiple local operations and prolonged hospitalizations were required to achieve foot healing in 7% of our patients. Heel and forefoot gangrene did not preclude ultimate limb salvage, although they could, if extensive, contribute to the need for prolonged periods of hospitalization. Even when the initial procedure to achieve limb salvage failed immediately, the involved extremity could often be saved by promptly performing some secondary procedure.[1,6,90] This was particularly common if PTA was technically unsuccessful or failed to improve the arterial supply to the foot.[1,6,96]

Late Limb Salvage

The cumulative limb salvage rates for all patients having arterial reconstructive operations are shown in Figure 32-12. Sixty-six percent of the patients who survived 5 years after a reconstructive arterial operation below the inguinal ligament for limb salvage had an intact limb up to that time. The limb

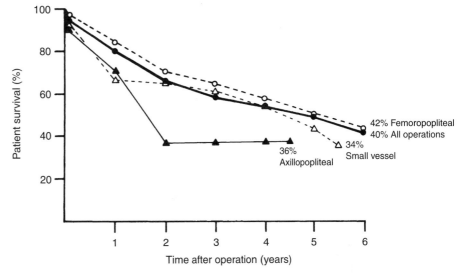

FIGURE 32–11 • Cumulative life-table patient survival rates after 318 femoropopliteal, 204 small vessel (infrapopliteal), and 29 axillopopliteal bypasses. Fifty-two percent of all patients undergoing all reconstructive arterial operations for limb-threatening infrainguinal arteriosclerosis died within 5 years. (From Veith FJ, Gupta SK, Samson RH, et al: Progress in limb salvage by reconstructive arterial surgery combined with new or improved adjunctive procedures. Ann Surg 194: 386-400, 1981.)

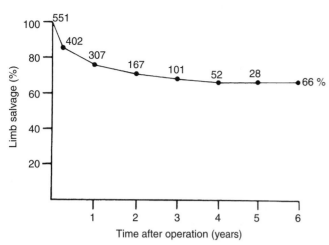

FIGURE 32–12 • Cumulative life-table limb salvage rates of all patients undergoing reconstructive arterial operations for limb-threatening infrainguinal arteriosclerosis. The number at each point indicates the number of patients observed with intact limbs for that length of time. (From Veith FJ, Gupta SK, Samson RH, et al: Progress in limb salvage by reconstructive arterial surgery combined with new or improved adjunctive procedures. Ann Surg 194:386-400, 1981.)

salvage rates were better after femoropopliteal bypass than after a small vessel bypass or an axillopopliteal bypass ($P < 0.25$) (Fig. 32-13). Even though all operations were performed because the limb was threatened, limb salvage rates (see Fig. 32-12) could not be equated with bypass patency rates (Fig. 32-14). In some patients, gangrene and infection had been healed by the original operation, and the limb remained intact when the bypass thrombosed; moreover, in many instances when the limb was rethreatened, bypass patency could be restored by appropriate reoperation. This was particularly common if the original procedure was a femoropopliteal bypass.[76] Conversely, limb salvage rates could be lower than bypass patency rates if a major amputation was required despite a patent arterial reconstruction, which is most common in patients with end-stage renal disease.[75]

PATENCY OF ARTERIAL RECONSTRUCTIVE OPERATIONS

Older cumulative life-table patency rates for reconstructive arterial operations are shown in Figure 32-14. More recent patency rates have improved somewhat and continue to be significantly better for femoropopliteal bypasses than for small vessel or axillopopliteal bypasses ($P < 0.01$). Our small vessel bypass patency rate was not affected by age, sex, hypertensive or diabetic status, or previous ipsilateral bypass. In contrast to reports from other groups, an incomplete plantar arch, a heavily calcified bypass insertion site, an unusable saphenous vein, and a very low ankle pressure did not preclude long-term success, although these factors were associated with a somewhat higher early failure rate.[1,6]

Several reports have documented better late limb salvage and bypass patency results than those presented. Although some of these apparently better results may reflect more refined surgical and management techniques, these more optimistic reports generally included only patients operated on by a particular surgical technique, such as reversed vein bypass or in situ vein bypass. Because these techniques, although ideal, are not applicable to all patients with a threatened lower extremity, the older statistics are probably still representative of the overall results that can be achieved in an entire group of patients undergoing lower limb arterial reconstruction to save an extremity. Moreover, some articles with favorable late bypass patency results are actually reporting secondary patency figures that are achievable with a more aggressive policy of detecting failing bypasses and reintervening, and some reports include results on substantial numbers of patients undergoing operation for intermittent claudication. Thus, although the results may be real, much of the success may be due to patient selection and differences in the methods of reporting or analyzing results.

REOPERATIONS

Our policy of performing a graft thrombectomy on all thrombosed small vessel and axillopopliteal bypasses, if and when the thrombosis is associated with a threat to the limb, has not

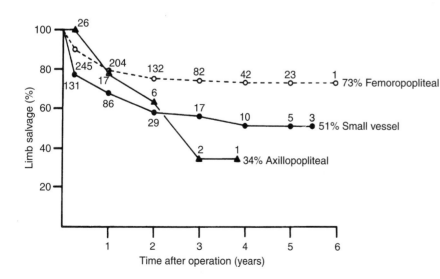

FIGURE 32–13 • Cumulative life-table limb salvage rates of 318 femoropopliteal, 204 small vessel (infrapopliteal), and 29 axillopopliteal bypasses performed for limb-threatening infrainguinal arteriosclerosis. The number at each point indicates the number of patients observed with intact limbs for that length of time. (From Veith FJ, Gupta SK, Samson RH, et al: Progress in limb salvage by reconstructive arterial surgery combined with new or improved adjunctive procedures. Ann Surg 194:386-400, 1981.)

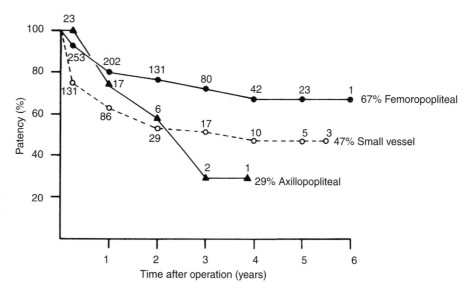

FIGURE 32–14 • Cumulative life-table patency rates of 318 femoropopliteal, 204 small vessel (infrapopliteal), and 29 axillopopliteal bypasses performed for limb-threatening infrainguinal arteriosclerosis. The number at each point indicates the number of grafts observed to be patent for that length of time. (From Veith FJ, Gupta SK, Samson RH, et al: Progress in limb salvage by reconstructive arterial surgery combined with new or improved adjunctive procedures. Ann Surg 194:386-400, 1981.)

resulted in any operative deaths but has generally been unrewarding. The majority of these reoperated grafts rethrombosed within a few days, weeks, or months. In occasional instances (approximately 10% of cases), patency was restored and persisted more than 3 years.

Thus, our present policy for the treatment of failed small vessel bypass if the limb is rethreatened is to perform an entirely new bypass to another unoperated segment of an infrapopliteal artery. Our results with such secondary small vessel bypasses have not differed greatly from those of primary procedures, although others have not had a similar experience.

The results of aggressive reoperation for failed vein and nonvein femoropopliteal bypasses have been surprisingly good.[1,6,76,84,90,118] In our series of 318 femoropopliteal bypasses, 13 failed during the first month after operation, and all were treated by reoperation. One postoperative death and two late deaths occurred among the patients with patent bypasses, 3 and 14 months after operation. Eight of the 10 other bypasses were patent for 2 to 44 months (mean, 25 months). The ninth patient had a viable limb 26 months after the original operation, although the graft subsequently rethrombosed, and the 10th patient also had a viable limb 4 months after the original operation, although her graft reoccluded 2 months after reoperation.

Thirty-nine of our femoropopliteal bypasses failed more than 1 month after operation and were considered for aggressive reoperation. A conservative approach to a failed bypass that did not place the limb in jeopardy was justified by the continued viability for 2 to 72 months of all eight limbs in this category. Reoperation was performed in the remaining 31 patients with threatened limbs. In 28 patients, bypass patency was reestablished for at least 2 months. In 20 patients, graft patency persisted until death or the present. The range of patency after reoperation in this group of 20 patients is 2 to 48 months, with a mean of longer than 17 months, although 7 patients required a secondary reoperation to maintain bypass patency and limb viability. Sixteen grafts have remained open more than 1 year after reoperation. Only 8 of the 39 patients in whom late graft occlusion occurred ultimately required a major amputation, and in all but two

instances this could be successfully performed below the knee. One of the 31 patients died within 1 month of the reoperation.

The sustained effectiveness of appropriate reoperations when femoropopliteal bypasses for limb salvage fail in the early or late postoperative period is illustrated by Figure 32-15, which shows that reoperation increased overall patency rates by 15% at 5 years. When the same calculations were applied to 440 cases with longer periods of follow-up, this difference between primary and secondary patency rates at 5 years fell to 8%. Limb salvage rates are, of course, similarly increased by effective reoperations. The efficacy of such reoperations in maintaining durable patency is further shown by the cumulative life-table 4- to 6-year patency rate of 56% for our

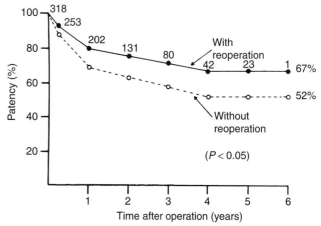

FIGURE 32–15 • Cumulative life-table patency rates of 318 femoropopliteal bypasses performed for limb salvage. The upper curve was calculated without regard to whether a reoperation was required to maintain patency. The lower curve was calculated on the basis of time to first bypass occlusion, even if reoperation restored patency. The number at each point indicates the number of grafts observed to be patent for that length of time. (From Veith FJ, Gupta SK, Samson RH, et al: Progress in limb salvage by reconstructive arterial surgery combined with new or improved adjunctive procedures. Ann Surg 194:386-400, 1981.)

44 femoropopliteal bypasses requiring reoperation for thrombosis. Limb salvage rates were even higher. Similar patency rates and limb salvage rates have also been achieved by Whittemore and colleagues,[90] who employed reoperations in the management of a group of patients with failed vein femoropopliteal bypasses and threatened limbs. Whittemore's group, our group, and many other groups have found that the detection of failing reconstructions before graft thrombosis has occurred permits simpler corrective measures to be used and results in much better long-term graft patency and limb salvage rates.[78,88-91,95,119]

Although Craver and colleagues showed many years ago that reoperation for early postoperative thrombosis of femoropopliteal vein grafts was associated with poor long-term patency rates,[120] we found that this is not the case with PTFE bypasses above the knee,[76] and Whittemore and associates reported similar protracted successes after reoperation for failure of saphenous vein femoropopliteal grafts.[90] Appropriate use of intraoperative angiography and other technical details of these reoperations are important in achieving the reported good results. In both series, surgical clot removal from thrombosed vein and PTFE grafts sometimes allowed these conduits to be used effectively for protracted periods if all other lesions encroaching substantially on the lumen were corrected or bypassed.[76,90]

LYTIC AGENTS

A number of reports have advocated the use of intra-arterially administered streptokinase, urokinase, and tissue plasminogen activator to restore patency to thrombosed infrainguinal grafts. Although these agents may ultimately prove to be useful to treat failed grafts and to detect the cause of failure, PTA or surgical graft revision is almost always required to correct the lesion causing thrombosis. In patients with acute ischemia and a closed graft, urokinase has been used successfully, as in other patients with acute ischemia.[12] Early reports suggest that these agents can restore patency in 70% to 90% of grafts, but short-term results are very poor if a treatable lesion is not found.[89] Moreover, the long-term efficacy of such combined procedures remains to be demonstrated, and in most patients, a totally new bypass may be the best treatment for a thrombosed graft that is associated with limb-threatening ischemia.

ARTERIOGRAPHIC OUTFLOW CHARACTERISTICS OF THE POPLITEAL ARTERY

With significant numbers of patients now receiving follow-up for 5 years or more, patency rates of femoropopliteal bypasses inserted into popliteal artery segments that appeared to be occluded at both ends on arteriograms were not significantly different from those of bypasses inserted into popliteal arteries that appeared to be continuous with one or more of their main terminal branches. These results support the use of femoropopliteal bypass to isolated segments of the popliteal artery in selected patients.[25,121] This appears to be true even when the absence of a usable saphenous vein makes it necessary to use a PTFE graft. A major disadvantage is the high incidence of continued threat to the limb despite a patent bypass. This is particularly common if extensive gangrene or infection is present in the foot.[25] In such circumstances,

a femoral-to-popliteal-to-small vessel bypass, or sequential bypass, is indicated, and the most distal portion of this complex bypass is best performed with autologous vein if it is available in any of the patient's extremities.[24,25,122,123]

RELATIONSHIP BETWEEN ANASTOMOSIS POSITION AND PATENCY

In our hands, femoropopliteal bypass patency was not significantly influenced solely by the position of the distal anastomosis relative to the knee joint. This was true with both PTFE and vein grafts. Other patient-related factors are probably more important in determining patency than the location of the popliteal anastomosis. These factors are not controlled in any study comparing above-knee and below-knee results, thereby rendering the comparisons meaningless in terms of selecting the best level to use if the popliteal artery is patent both above and below the knee in a given patient.

AMPUTATION LEVEL

When major amputation was required after a revascularization procedure, every effort was made to perform it below the knee. This was possible in all 18 patients who required amputation despite a patent bypass, in 90% of patients who required a major amputation when a femoropopliteal bypass occluded, in 69% of patients requiring major amputation after a failed small vessel bypass, and in 30% of major amputations required after thrombosis of an axillopopliteal bypass.[6] The operative mortality rate for these secondary amputations was 4%.

Cost-Benefit Analysis of Aggressive Efforts at Limb Salvage

Our results indicate that more than 98% of patients whose limbs are threatened because of infrainguinal arteriosclerosis have a distribution of occlusive and stenotic arterial lesions that is suitable for reconstructive arterial surgery, which can relieve the ischemia at least partially and salvage the limb. The results also show that immediate limb salvage is possible in more than 85% of the patients in whom revascularization is possible, with an operative mortality rate of less than 4% and a low morbidity rate despite the frequent existence of local and systemic factors that might have precluded attempts at revascularization and limb salvage in the past. These factors include advanced age, recent congestive heart failure or myocardial infarction, concurrent malignancy, extensive forefoot or heel gangrene, contralateral amputation, isolated popliteal artery segment, absence of usable saphenous vein, and presence of a popliteal pulse with three-vessel occlusive disease in the upper, middle, and lower thirds of the leg. In the last circumstance, a bypass to a target artery at the ankle or foot level may still be feasible.

The fact that limbs can now be saved in such circumstances is of interest. Alone, it does not mean that limb salvage attempts, which may require multiple operations and prolonged periods of hospitalization to obtain a healed foot, are justified in this group of patients, whose life expectancy is known to be poor. The question is, does the cost-benefit ratio make such attempts at limb salvage worthwhile in these patients?

This is a difficult question to answer with certainty because the answer depends, in part, on one's philosophy and perspective and on subjective factors such as quality of life and the ability to live and function independently. However, certain objective parameters are relevant. Among these are the durability of limb salvage in surviving patients and the longevity of these patients. Figure 32-11 is an index of patient longevity, and Figure 32-12 is a measure of the durability of limb salvage in surviving patients. Of the 48% of patients who survived 5 years after operation, two thirds retained their limb at least that long. Of every 100 patients who underwent operation, 68 lived at least 1 year after operation with an intact limb, and 54 lived at least 2 years with a viable, usable extremity. Moreover, of the 52% of patients who died within 5 years, an average of 88% (81% to 95%) retained the salvaged limb until they died (Fig. 32-16). We and almost all our patients believe that these benefits outweigh the risks and costs of an aggressive attempt at limb salvage, even if this attempt entails a lengthy period of hospitalization with several operative procedures to achieve a healed foot. Similar conclusions have been reached by Reichle and Tyson,[117] Maini and Mannick,[124] and Perdue,[125] Bartlett,[84] and Auer[126] and their colleagues in their analyses of patients with limb-threatening ischemia.

A case can also be made for performing a primary below-knee amputation in some or all of these patients. Although relatively rapid rehabilitation may be achieved with such a procedure,[127,128] our experience has shown that older, poor-risk patients do not ambulate easily or quickly with a below-knee prosthesis.[129] Such patients may never walk, and if they do, they may require 2 or 3 months of institutional training to learn. For some patients, limb salvage offers the only opportunity for them to care for themselves, maintain their independence, and avoid permanent admission to an institution. Further, in many patients, the opposite limb soon becomes threatened because of the symmetry of the disease process, and salvage of at least one limb is critical for the patient to maintain independence. Finally, the point has been made that unsuccessful attempts at limb salvage result in a high incidence of loss of the knee.[50,128,130] Our data fail

to confirm this, except after failed axillopopliteal bypass, a procedure performed in patients with the most advanced disease. Thus, we believe that limb salvage should be attempted if suitable vessels for revascularization are present, unless the patient has severe organic mental syndrome or gangrene and infection proximal to the midfoot.

The dollar cost of an aggressive approach to limb salvage is high, with a mean cost of $19,000 for femoropopliteal bypass and $29,000 for small vessel bypass. These figures include all physician, hospital, and rehabilitation costs, including those of reoperations. In contrast, the mean total cost of below-knee amputation, which in 26% of our patients resulted in failed rehabilitation and a need for chronic institutional care or professional assistance at home, was $27,000. Thus, limb salvage surgery is expensive, but no more so than the less attractive alternative of amputation.[131] In the new climate of efforts to reduce medical expenses, many of these patients are being treated successfully with significantly shorter hospital stays and decreased costs.

New Developments

Clearly, all the principles and practices outlined thus far describe our present attitudes toward the treatment of a complex disease process. As we have pointed out, many of these attitudes are controversial. More important, they are all in a state of constant evolution. As more data and newer methods become available, our attitudes and those of others interested in the problems of femoral, popliteal, and tibial arteriosclerosis will change. In this section we describe some of the new developments that have the greatest likelihood of leading to future therapeutic improvements.

DIAGNOSTIC TECHNIQUES

Noninvasive arterial evaluations, including duplex scanning,[72] magnetic resonance angiography,[17,18] and helical computed tomography scanning, are rapidly improving and may become the initial diagnostic modality for patients with aortoiliac and infrainguinal aneurysmal and occlusive disease, but further refinements are needed before these techniques can replace diagnostic arteriography. Intravascular ultrasonography is another diagnostic modality being developed to better assess the extent of arterial disease and to evaluate immediate results after interventions.[132-134]

ENDOVASCULAR DEVICES

Angioplasty has been used successfully for the treatment of stenotic iliac lesions, and the results have improved further with the use of intravascular stents.[135] The role of infrainguinal angioplasty has been limited but is increasing. To date, the use of stents has not significantly improved results. However, stents are being used for selected lesions in the femoral and popliteal arterial segments. Atherectomy has been used successfully in the coronary circulation, but the results for infrainguinal disease have been very poor thus far.[136,137] New devices are currently being evaluated in the hope of improving these results.[138]

A further development is the use of endovascular grafts. These have been used for the treatment of a variety of arterial lesions, with early success.[139] The role of these evolving techniques in the treatment of infrainguinal disease is still unclear.

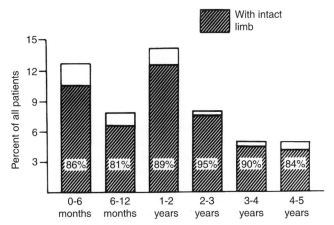

FIGURE 32–16 • Percentage of all patients who underwent limb salvage attempts and died in the various intervals after operation. The crosshatched areas indicate the proportion of these patients who died without losing their previously threatened limbs. (From Veith FJ, Gupta SK, Samson RH, et al: Progress in limb salvage by reconstructive arterial surgery combined with new or improved adjunctive procedures. Ann Surg 194:386-400, 1981.)

Whether covering the treated segment with a covered stent will improve long-term results remains to be seen.[140]

TIBIAL AND PEDAL BYPASSES

Since 1981, because of some of the promising results already discussed, we have been evaluating other procedures to simplify or extend the limits of operability for limb salvage. Some of these procedures show sufficient promise to deserve mention.

Tibiotibial bypasses are an extension of our concept of using more distal arteries as bypass origins than were previously thought optimal.[31] All these distal origin procedures allow shorter segments of saphenous vein to be used, shorten the operative time, avoid dissection in obese or infected groins, and may have superior patency. We have now performed more than 80 distal vein bypasses to the lower third of the leg or foot using the infrapopliteal (tibial) arteries as inflow sites.[27,28] Many of these grafts remained patent more than 4 years, despite their insertion into isolated tibial artery segments and the fact that they were performed with saphenous veins 2.5 to 3 mm in smallest diameter (see Figs. 32-1 to 32-3).

Small vessel bypasses to blind tibial artery segments have been performed in some patients facing imminent amputation. These operations have been done in patients in whom no other procedures were possible because of the arterial anatomy or local infection in the foot. Again, vein grafts were used. Several of these bypasses have remained patent more than 2 years, and many otherwise unsalvageable limbs have been saved.[27]

Use of heavily calcified tibial arteries for distal bypass insertion sites has been possible with a variety of techniques that include crushing of the involved artery and intraluminal occlusion to permit incision and suture placement. Acceptable early and midterm patency has resulted.[6] Small vessel bypasses to plantar and tarsal arterial branches can be achieved in patients with patent pedal arches, with acceptable long-term patency and excellent limb salvage results.[29,30,141]

MINIMALLY INVASIVE TECHNIQUES

Less invasive techniques are being developed for the performance of in situ and reversed saphenous vein bypasses. The use of long flexible valvulotomes, angioscopic visualization,[142,143] coil occlusion techniques for side branches,[144,145] and endoscopic subcutaneous vein dissection and harvesting[146] may allow the performance of these lower extremity bypasses through smaller incisions, allowing diminished pain, fewer local complications, and decreased hospital stays for some patients.

INTRAOPERATIVE TECHNIQUES

The intraoperative use of fluoroscopy has added a new dimension to the options of the vascular surgeon. Diagnostic arteriography can be performed before and after a bypass procedure. Graft and arterial thrombectomies can be performed using catheter-guidewire techniques to improve success and safety.[71] The greater saphenous vein can be evaluated for in situ bypasses. Proximal and distal arterial lesions can be treated using balloon angioplasty,[147] with or without the addition of intravascular stents. And finally, fluoroscopy allows the performance of complex procedures, such as endovascular grafting, that require the combined use of interventional and standard surgical techniques.[139] Angioscopy, duplex scanning, and intravascular ultrasonography are also being used to improve the results of intraoperative procedures.

PHARMACOLOGIC ADJUNCTS

Some of the most promising developments in the treatment of lower extremity occlusive disease have come in the area of pharmacologic adjuncts. The addition of the antiplatelet agent clopidogrel, a glycoprotein IIb/IIIa inhibitor, has had a major impact on the treatment of cerebral, cardiac, and peripheral vascular disease. In a subgroup analysis of patients with peripheral arterial disease, clopidogrel conferred an overall risk reduction of 24% compared with aspirin.[148] Clopidogrel has been widely adopted for monotherapy as well as in conjunction with aspirin for the prevention of vascular events. This is especially true for patients undergoing either percutaneous or open peripheral interventions.

The statin medications are now being evaluated more thoroughly for their impact on peripheral vascular disease and interventions to treat this condition. One recent study found that there was no difference in primary patency, limb salvage, or survival at 2 years between patients taking a statin and those not taking a statin. However, univariate and multivariate analyses showed that patients on statins had both higher primary revised (94% ± 2% vs. 83% ± 5%) and higher secondary (97% ± 2% vs. 87% ± 4%) graft patency rates at 2 years.[149] In this study, the risk of graft failure was found to be 3.2 times greater for patients not taking statins. Perioperative cholesterol levels were reported for less than half the patients, but these were not found to be statistically different between the groups.

Greater attention is also being given to the overall optimal medical regimen for patients undergoing infrainguinal bypass. There is good evidence that angiotensin-converting enzyme inhibitors, cholesterol-lowering statin drugs, and antiplatelet agents have significant beneficial effects in patients with systemic atherosclerosis. It has been suggested that patients undergoing bypass procedures may be underprescribed with regard to cardioprotective medications. A recent analysis of more than 300 infrainguinal bypass procedures found that factors independently associated with increased graft patency included statin drug use, male sex, and adherence to a graft surveillance protocol; factors associated with decreased amputation rates were statin drug use and ongoing graft surveillance.[150] Decreased mortality was observed in patients adhering to a graft surveillance protocol, whereas increased mortality was seen in patients with congestive heart failure and end-stage renal disease on hemodyalysis. Life-table analysis showed that in terms of medications, only angiotensin-converting enzyme inhibitors were associated with lower mortality. There was a trend toward lower mortality with aspirin, and although no effect was seen with beta blockers, the authors stated that the numbers were likely too small and the follow-up too brief to document any effect because the majority of patients were already taking these medications.

KEY REFERENCES

Ascer E, Veith FJ, Gupta SK: Bypasses to plantar arteries and other tibial branches: An extended approach to limb salvage. J Vasc Surg 8:434-441, 1988.

Aulivola B, Pomposelli FB: Dorsalis pedis, tarsal and plantar artery bypass. J Cardiovasc Surg (Torino) 45:203-212, 2004.

Bartlett ST, Olinde AJ, Flinn WR, et al: The reoperative potential of infrainguinal bypass: Long-term limb and patient survival. J Vasc Surg 5:170-179, 1987.

Dormandy JA, Rutherford RB: Management of peripheral artery disease (PAD). TASC Working Group. TransAtlantic Inter-Society Consensus (TASC). J Vasc Surg 31:S1-S296, 2000.

Lipsitz EC, Veith FJ, Ohki T: The value of subintimal angioplasty in the management of critical lower extremity ischemia: Failure is not always associated with a rethreatened limb. J Cardiovasc Surg (Torino) 45:231-237, 2004.

Lipsitz EC, Veith FJ, Wain RA: Digital fluoroscopy as a valuable adjunct to open vascular operations. Semin Vasc Surg 16:280-290, 2003.

Veith FJ, Gupta SK, Ascer E, et al: Six year prospective multicenter randomized comparison of autologous saphenous vein and expanded polytetrafluoroethylene grafts in infrainguinal arterial reconstructions. J Vasc Surg 3:104-114, 1986.

Veith FJ, Gupta SK, Ascer E, et al: Improved strategies for secondary operations on infrainguinal arteries. Ann Vasc Surg 4:85-93, 1990.

Veith FJ, Gupta SK, Wengerter KR, et al: Changing arteriosclerotic disease patterns and management strategies in lower limb-threatening ischemia. Ann Surg 212:402-414, 1990.

Wengerter KR, Veith FJ, Gupta SK: Influence of vein size (diameter) on infrapopliteal reversed vein graft patency. J Vasc Surg 11:525-531, 1990.

REFERENCES

1. Veith FJ, Gupta SK, Wengerter KR, et al: Changing arteriosclerotic disease patterns and management strategies in lower limb-threatening ischemia. Ann Surg 212:402-414, 1990.

2. Donaldson MC, Mannick JA: Femoropopliteal bypass grafting for intermittent claudication: Is pessimism warranted? Arch Surg 115:724-727, 1980.

3. Boyd AM: The natural course of arteriosclerosis of the lower extremities. Proc R Soc Med 55:591-593, 1962.

4. Coran AG, Warren R: Arteriographic changes in femoropopliteal arteriosclerosis obliterans: A five year follow-up study. N Engl J Med 274:643-645, 1966.

5. Imparato AM, Kim GE, Davidson T, Crowley JG: Intermittent claudication: Its natural course. Surgery 78:795-797, 1975.

6. Veith FJ, Gupta SK, Samson RH, et al: Progress in limb salvage by reconstructive arterial surgery combined with new or improved adjunctive procedures. Ann Surg 194:386-401, 1981.

7. Goodreau JJ, Greasy JK, Flanigan DP, et al: Rational approach to the differentiation of vascular and neurogenic claudication. Surgery 84:749-757, 1978.

8. Kavanaugh GJ, Svien HJ, Holman CB, Johnson RM: "Pseudoclaudication" syndrome produced by compression of the cauda equina. JAMA 206:2477-2481, 1968.

9. Karmody AM, Powers SR, Monaco VJ, Leather RP: Blue toe syndrome: An indication for limb salvage surgery. Arch Surg 111:1263-1268, 1976.

10. Haimovici HC, Moss CM, Veith FJ: Arterial embolectomy revisited. Surgery 78:409-411, 1975.

11. Gupta SK, Samson RH, Veith FJ: Embolectomy of the distal part of the popliteal artery. Surg Gynecol Obstet 153:254-258, 1981.

12. Ouriel K, Shortell CK, DeWeese JA, et al: A comparison of thrombolytic therapy with operative revascularization in the initial treatment of acute peripheral arterial ischemia. J Vasc Surg 19:1021-1030, 1994.

13. Whittemore AD, Clowes AW, Hechtman HB, Mannick JA: Aortic aneurysm repair: Reduced operative mortality associated with maintenance of optimal cardiac performance. Ann Surg 192:414-420, 1980.

14. Ascher E, Mazzariol F, Hingorani A, et al: The use of duplex ultrasound arterial mapping as an alternative to conventional arteriography for primary and secondary infrapopliteal bypasses. Am J Surg 178:162-165, 1999.

15. Wain RA, Berdejo GL, Del Valle WN, et al: Can duplex scan arterial mapping replace contrast arteriography as the test of choice before infrainguinal revascularization? J Vasc Surg 29:100-107, 1999.

16. Flanigan DP, Williams LR, Keifer T, et al: Prebypass operative arteriography. Surgery 92:627-633, 1982.

17. Owen RS, Carpenter JP, Baum RA, et al: Magnetic resonance imaging of angiographically occult runoff vessels in peripheral arterial occlusive disease. N Engl J Med 326:1577-1581, 1992.

18. Carpenter JP, Owen RS, Baum RA, et al: Magnetic resonance angiography of peripheral runoff vessels. J Vasc Surg 16:807-815, 1992.

19. Hoch JR, Tullis MJ, Kennell TW, et al: Use of magnetic resonance angiography for the pre-operative evaluation of patients with infrainguinal arterial occlusive disease. J Vasc Surg 23:792-800, 1996.

20. Sapala JA, Szilagyi DE: A simple aid in greater saphenous phlebography. Surg Gynecol Obstet 140:265-266, 1975.

21. Veith FJ, Moss CM, Sprayregen S, Montefusco CM: Preoperative saphenous venography in arterial reconstructive surgery of the lower extremity. Surgery 85:253-255, 1979.

22. Rivers SP, Scher LA, Gupta SK, Veith FJ: Safety of peripheral vascular surgery after recent myocardial infarction. J Vasc Surg 11:17-35, 1967.

23. Mannick JA, Jackson BT, Coffman JD: Success of bypass vein grafts in patients with isolated popliteal artery segments. Surgery 61:17-35, 1967.

24. Flinn WR, Flanigan DP, Verta MJ, et al: Sequential femoral-tibial bypass for severe limb ischemia. Surgery 88:357-365, 1980.

25. Veith FJ, Gupta SK, Daly V: Femoropopliteal bypass to the isolated popliteal segment: Is polytetrafluoroethylene graft acceptable? Surgery 89:296-303, 1981.

26. Ascer E, Veith FJ, Morin B, et al: Components of outflow resistance and their correlation with graft patency in lower extremity arterial reconstructions. J Vasc Surg 1:817-825, 1984.

27. Veith FJ, Ascer E, Gupta SK, et al: Tibiotibial vein bypass grafts: A new operation for limb salvage. J Vasc Surg 2:552-557, 1985.

28. Lyon RT, Veith FJ, Marsan BU, et al: Eleven-year experience with tibiotibial bypass: An unusual but effective solution to distal tibial artery occlusive disease and limited autologous vein. J Vasc Surg 20:61-69, 1994.

29. Ascer E, Veith FJ, Gupta SK: Bypasses to plantar arteries and other tibial branches: An extended approach to limb salvage. J Vasc Surg 8:434-441, 1988.

30. Sanchez LA, Schwartz ML, Veith FJ: Bypass surgery into plantar vessels: An effective extension of limb salvage surgical techniques. Perspect Vasc Surg 7:47-55, 1994.

31. Veith FJ, Gupta SK, Samson RH, et al: Superficial femoral and popliteal arteries as inflow site for distal bypasses. Surgery 90:980-990, 1981.

32. Wengerter KR, Yang PM, Veith FJ, et al: A twelve-year experience with the popliteal-to-distal artery bypass: The significance and management of proximal disease. J Vasc Surg 15:143-151, 1992.

33. Gupta SK, Veith FJ, Ascer E, et al: Five year experience with axillopopliteal bypass for limb salvage. J Cardiovasc Surg 26:321-324, 1985.

34. Veith FJ, Moss CM, Daly V, et al: New approaches in limb salvage by extended extraanatomic bypasses and prosthetic reconstructions to foot arteries. Surgery 84:764-774, 1978.

35. Towne JB, Bernhard VM, Rollins DL, Baum PL: Profundaplasty in perspective: Limitations in the long-term management of limb ischemia. Surgery 90:1037-1046, 1981.

36. Campbell CD, Brook DH, Webster MW, et al: Expanded micro-porous polytetrafluoroethylene as a vascular substitute: A two-year follow-up. Surgery 85:177-183, 1979.

37. Gupta SK, Veith FJ: Three year experience with expanded polytetrafluoroethylene arterial grafts for limb salvage. Am J Surg 140:214-217, 1980.

38. Veith FJ, Moss CM, Fell SC, et al: Comparison of expanded polytetrafluoroethylene and autologous saphenous vein grafts in high risk arterial reconstructions for limb salvage. Surg Gynecol Obstet 147:749-752, 1978.

39. Quiñones-Baldrich WJ, Busuttil RW, Baker JD, et al: Is the preferential use of polytetrafluoroethylene grafts for femoropopliteal bypass justified? J Vasc Surg 8:219-228, 1988.

40. Bergan JJ, Veith FJ, Bernhard VM, et al: Randomization of autogenous vein and polytetrafluoroethylene grafts in femoral-distal reconstruction. Surgery 92:921-930, 1982.

41. Veith FJ, Gupta SK, Ascer E, et al: Six year prospective multicenter randomized comparison of autologous saphenous vein and expanded polytetrafluoroethylene grafts in infrainguinal arterial reconstructions. J Vasc Surg 3:104-114, 1986.

42. Taylor RS, Loh A, McFarland RJ, et al: Improved technique for polytetrafluoroethylene bypass grafting: Long-term results using anastomotic vein patches. Br J Surg 79:348-354, 1992.

43. Parsons RE, Suggs WD, Veith FJ, et al: Polytetrafluoroethylene bypasses to infrapopliteal arteries without cuffs or patches: A better option than amputation in patients without autologous vein. J Vasc Surg 23:347-356, 1996.

44. Panneton JM, Hollier LH, Hofer JM: Multicenter randomized prospective trial comparing a pre-cuffed polytetrafluoroethylene graft to a vein cuffed polytetrafluoroethylene graft for infragenicular arterial bypass. Ann Vasc Surg 18:199-206, 2004.

45. Dardik H, Baier RE, Meenaghan M, et al: Morphologic and biophysical assessment of long term human umbilical cord vein implants used as vascular conduits. Surg Gynecol Obstet 154:17-26, 1982.

46. Cranley JJ, Karkow WS, Hafner CD, Flanagan LD: Aneurysmal dilatation in umbilical vein grafts. In Bergan JJ, Yao JST (eds): Reoperative Arterial Surgery. Orlando, Fla, Grune & Stratton, 1986, pp 343-358.

47. Pevec WC, Darling RC, L'Italien GJ, Abbott WM: Femoropopliteal reconstruction with knitted non-velour Dacron vs expanded polytetrafluoroethylene. J Vasc Surg 16:60-65, 1992.

48. Kenney AD, Sauvage LR, Wood SJ, et al: Comparison of noncrimped, externally supported (EXS) and crimped, nonsupported Dacron prosthesis for axillofemoral and above knee femoropopliteal bypasses. Surgery 92:931-946, 1982.

49. Green RM, Abbott WM, Matsumoto T, et al: Prosthetic above knee femoropopliteal grafting: Five year results of a randomized trial. J Vasc Surg 31:417-425, 2000.

50. Szilagyi DE, Hageman JH, Smith RF, et al: Autogenous vein grafting in femoropopliteal atherosclerosis: The limits of its effectiveness. Surgery 86:836-851, 1979.

51. Szilagyi DE, Smith RF, Elliot JP, Hageman JH: The biologic fate of autogenous vein implants as arterial substitutes: Clinical, angiographic and histopathologic observations in femoropopliteal operations for atherosclerosis. Ann Surg 178:232-244, 1973.

52. Wengerter KR, Gupta SK, Veith FJ, et al: Critical vein diameter for infrainguinal arterial reconstructions. J Cardiovasc Surg (Torino) 28:109, 1987.

53. Wengerter KR, Veith FJ, Gupta SK: Influence of vein size (diameter) on infrapopliteal reversed vein graft patency. J Vasc Surg 11:525-531, 1990.

54. Kent KC, Whittemore AD, Mannick JA: Short-term and mid-term results of an all autologous tissue policy for infrainguinal reconstruction. J Vasc Surg 9:107-114, 1989.

55. Hall KV: The great saphenous vein used "in-situ" as an arterial shunt after extirpation of the vein valves. Surgery 51:492-495, 1962.

56. Leather RP, Shah DM, Karmody AM: Infrapopliteal bypass for limb salvage: Increased patency and utilization of the saphenous vein used "in situ." Surgery 90:1000-1008, 1981.

57. Leather RP, Shah DM, Chang BB, et al: Resurrection of the in situ vein bypass: 1000 cases later. Ann Surg 205:435-442, 1988.

58. Gruss JD, Bartels D, Vargas H, et al: Arterial reconstruction for distal disease of the lower extremities by the in situ vein graft technique. J Cardiovasc Surg (Torino) 23:231-234, 1982.

59. Wengerter KR, Veith FJ, Gupta SK, et al: Prospective randomized multicenter comparison of in situ and reversed vein infrapopliteal bypasses. J Vasc Surg 12:189-199, 1991.

60. Taylor LM, Edward JM, Porter JM: Present status of reversed vein bypass: Five year results of a modern series. J Vasc Surg 11:207-215, 1990.

61. Towne JB, Schmidt DD, Seabrook GR, Bandyk DF: The effect of vein diameter on early patency and durability of in situ bypass grafts. J Cardiovasc Surg (Torino) 30:64, 1989.

62. Schulman ML, Bradley MR: Late results and angiographic evaluation of arm veins as long bypass grafts. Surgery 92:1032-1041, 1982.

63. Harris RW, Andros G, Dulana LB, et al: Successful long-term limb salvage using cephalic vein bypass grafts. Ann Surg 200:785-794, 1984.

64. Londrew GL, Bosher LP, Brown PW, et al: Infrainguinal reconstruction with arm vein, lesser saphenous vein and remnants of greater saphenous vein: A report of 257 cases. J Vasc Surg 20:451-457, 1994.

65. Sesto ME, Sullivan TM, Hertzer NR, et al: Cephalic vein grafts for lower extremity revascularization. J Vasc Surg 15:543-549, 1992.

66. Stonebridge PA, Miller AM, Tsoukas A, et al: Angioscopy of arm vein infrainguinal bypass grafts. Ann Vasc Surg 5:170-175, 1991.

67. Veith FJ, Gupta SK: Femoral-distal artery bypasses. In Bergan JJ, Yao JST (eds): Operative Techniques in Vascular Surgery. New York, Grune & Stratton, 1980, pp 141-150.

68. Bernhard VM, Boren CH, Towne JB: Pneumatic tourniquet as a substitute for vascular clamps in distal bypass surgery. Surgery 87:709-713, 1980.

69. Marin ML, Veith FJ, Panetta TF, et al: A new look at intraoperative completion arteriography: Classification and management strategies for intraluminal defects. Am J Surg 166:136-140, 1993.

70. Lipsitz EC, Veith FJ, Wain RA: Digital fluoroscopy as a valuable adjunct to open vascular operations. Semin Vasc Surg 16:280-290, 2003.

71. Marin ML, Veith FJ, Panetta TF, et al: A new look at intraoperative completion arteriography: Classification and management strategies for intraluminal defects. Am J Surg 166:136-140, 1993.

72. Bandyk DF, Kaebnick, Bergamini TM, et al: Hemodynamics of in situ saphenous vein arterial bypass. Arch Surg 123:477-482, 1988.

73. Oblath RW, Buckley FO, Green RM, et al: Prevention of platelet aggregation and adherence to prosthetic vascular grafts by aspirin and dipyridamole. Surgery 84:37-44, 1978.

74. Creager MA: Results of the CAPRIE trial: Efficacy and safety of clopidogrel. Clopidogrel versus aspirin in patients at risk of ischemic events. Vasc Med 3:257-260, 1998.

75. Sanchez LA, Goldsmith JG, Rivers SP, et al: Limb salvage surgery in end stage renal disease: Is it worthwhile? J Cardiovasc Surg (Torino) 33:344-348, 1992.

76. Veith FJ, Gupta SK, Ascer E, et al: Improved strategies for secondary operations on infrainguinal arteries. Ann Vasc Surg 4:85-93, 1990.

77. Parsons R, Marin ML, Veith FJ, et al: Fluoroscopically assisted thromboembolectomy: An improved method for treating acute occlusions of native arteries and bypass grafts. Ann Vasc Surg 10:201-210, 1996.

78. Sanchez LA, Suggs WD, Marin ML, et al: The merit of polytetrafluoroethylene extensions and interposition grafts to salvage failing infrainguinal vein bypasses. J Vasc Surg 23:329-335, 1996.

79. Veith FJ, Ascer E, Nunez A, et al: Unusual approaches to infrainguinal arteries. J Cardiovasc Surg (Torino) 28:58, 1987.

80. Nunez A, Veith FJ, Collier P, et al: Direct approach to the distal portions of the deep femoral artery for limb salvage bypasses. J Vasc Surg 8:576-581, 1988.

81. Bertucci WR, Marin MD, Veith FJ: Posterior approach to the deep femoral artery. J Vasc Surg 29:741-744, 1999.

82. Veith FJ, Ascer E, Gupta SK, Wengerter KR: Lateral approach to the popliteal artery. J Vasc Surg 6:119-123, 1987.

83. McNamara TO, Bomberger RA: Factors affecting initial and 6-month patency rates after intraarterial thrombolysis with high-dose urokinase. Am J Surg 152:709-711, 1986.

84. Bartlett ST, Olinde AJ, Flinn WR, et al: The reoperative potential of infrainguinal bypass: Long-term limb and patient survival. J Vasc Surg 5:170-179, 1987.

85. De Frang RD, Edwards JM, Moneta GL, et al: Repeat leg bypass after multiple prior bypass failures. J Vasc Surg 19:268-277, 1994.

86. George SM Jr, Klamer TW, Lambert GE Jr: Value of continued efforts at limb salvage despite multiple graft failures. Ann Vasc Surg 8:332-336, 1994.

87. Lipsitz EC, Veith FJ, Rhee SJ, et al: Is repetitive bypass justified after multiple previous failures: When is enough enough? Vascular 12 (Suppl. 2):109, 2004.

88. O'Mara CS, Flinn WR, Johnson ND, et al: Recognition and surgical management of patent but hemodynamically failed arterial grafts. Ann Surg 193:467-476, 1981.

89. Veith FJ, Weiser RK, Gupta SK, et al: Diagnosis and management of failing lower extremity arterial reconstructions. J Cardiovasc Surg (Torino) 25:381-384, 1984.

90. Whittemore AD, Clowes AW, Couch NP, Mannick JA: Secondary femoropopliteal reconstruction. Ann Surg 193:35-42, 1981.

91. Sanchez L, Gupta SK, Veith FJ, et al: A ten-year experience with one hundred fifty failing or threatened vein and polytetrafluoroethylene arterial bypass grafts. J Vasc Surg 14:729-738, 1991.

92. Bandyk DF, Cata RF, Towne JB: A low flow velocity predicts failure of femoro-popliteal and femoro-tibial bypass grafts. Surgery 98:799-809, 1985.

93. Perler BA, Osterman FA, Mitchell SE, et al: Balloon dilatation vs surgical revision of infrainguinal autogenous vein graft stenoses: Long term follow-up. J Vasc Surg 14:729-738, 1991.

94. Whittemore AD, Donaldson MC, Polak JF, Mannick JA: Limitations of balloon angioplasty for vein graft stenosis. J Vasc Surg 14:340-345, 1991.

95. Sanchez LA, Suggs WD, Marin ML, et al: Is percutaneous balloon angioplasty appropriate in the treatment of graft and anastomotic lesions responsible for failing vein bypasses? Am J Surg 168:97-101, 1994.

96. Samson RH, Sprayregen S, Veith FJ, et al: Management of angioplasty complication, unsuccessful procedures and early and late failures. Ann Surg 199:234-240, 1984.

97. Nasr MK, McCarthy RJ, Hardman J, et al: The increasing role of percutaneous transluminal angioplasty in the primary management of critical limb ischaemia. Eur J Vasc Endovasc Surg 23:398-403, 2002.

98. Dormandy JA, Rutherford RB: Management of peripheral artery disease (PAD). TASC Working Group. TransAtlantic Inter-Society Consensus (TASC). J Vasc Surg 31:S1-S296, 2000.

99. Silva MB Jr, Bohannon WT, Santana D: Technical note on renal angioplasty and stenting: New developments that facilitate its performance. Vascular 12:42-50, 2004.

100. Parsons RE, Suggs WD, Lee JJ, et al: Percutaneous transluminal angioplasty for the treatment of limb threatening ischemia: Do the results justify an attempt before bypass grafting? J Vasc Surg 28:1066-1071, 1998.

101. Vogel TR, Shindelman LE, Nackman GB, Graham AM: Efficacious use of nitinol stents in the femoral and popliteal arteries. J Vasc Surg 38:1178-1184, 2003.

102. Jahnke T, Voshage G, Muller-Hulsbeck S, et al: Endovascular placement of self-expanding nitinol coil stents for the treatment of femoropopliteal obstructive disease. J Vasc Interv Radiol 13:257-266, 2002.

103. Alpert JR, Ring EJ, Freiman DB, et al: Balloon dilatation of iliac stenosis with distal arterial surgery. Arch Surg 115:715-717, 1980.

104. Kadir S, Smith GW, White RI Jr, et al: Percutaneous transluminal angioplasty as an adjunct to the surgical management of peripheral vascular disease. Ann Surg 195:786-795, 1982.

105. Bandyk DF, Johnson BL, Gupta AK, Esses GE: Nature and management of duplex abnormalities encountered during infrainguinal vein bypass grafting. J Vasc Surg 24:430-436, 1996.

106. Ahn SS, Concepcion B: The current status of peripheral atherectomy. Eur J Vasc Endovasc Surg 10:133-135, 1995.

107. Lampmann LE: Stenting in the femoral superficial artery: An overview. Eur J Radiol 29:276-279, 1999.

108. Kasirajan K, Schneider PA: Early outcome of "cutting" balloon angioplasty for infrainguinal vein graft stenosis. J Vasc Surg 39:702-708, 2004.

109. Fava M, Loyola S, Polydorou A, et al: Cryoplasty for femoropopliteal arterial disease: Late angiographic results of initial human experience. J Vasc Interv Radiol 15:1239-1243, 2004.

110. Bolia A: Percutaneous intentional extraluminal (subintimal) recanalization of crural arteries. Eur J Radiol 28:199-204, 1998.

111. London NJ, Srinivasan R, Naylor AR, et al: Subintimal angioplasty of femoropopliteal artery occlusions: The long-term results. Eur J Vasc Surg 8:148-155, 1994.

112. Lipsitz EC, Ohki T, Veith FJ, et al: Does subintimal angioplasty have a role in the treatment of severe lower extremity ischemia? J Vasc Surg 37:386-391, 2003.

113. Vraux H, Hammer F, Verhelst R, et al: Subintimal angioplasty of tibial vessel occlusions in the treatment of critical limb ischaemia: Mid-term results. Eur J Vasc Endovasc Surg 20:441-446, 2000.

114. Bolia A, Fishwick G: Recanalization of iliac artery occlusion by subintimal dissection using the ipsilateral and the contralateral approach. Clin Radiol 52:684-687, 1997.

115. Lipsitz EC, Veith FJ, Ohki T: The value of subintimal angioplasty in the management of critical lower extremity ischemia: Failure is not always associated with a rethreatened limb. J Cardiovasc Surg (Torino) 45:231-237, 2004.

116. DeWeese JA, Robb CG: Autogenous venous grafts ten years later. Surgery 82:775-784, 1977.

117. Reichle FA, Tyson R: Comparison of long-term results of 364 femoropopliteal or femorotibial bypasses for revascularization of severely ischemic lower extremities. Ann Surg 182:449-455, 1975.

118. Boontje AH: Occlusion of femoropopliteal bypasses (Biograft). J Cardiovasc Surg (Torino) 25:385-390, 1984.

119. Sanchez LA, Suggs WD, Veith FJ, et al: Is surveillance to detect failing polytetrafluoroethylene bypasses worthwhile? Twelve-year experience with ninety-one grafts. J Vasc Surg 18:981-990, 1993.

120. Craver JM, Ottinger LW, Darling RC, et al: Hemorrhage and thrombosis as early complications of femoropopliteal bypass grafts: Causes, treatment and prognostic implications. Surgery 74:839-845, 1973.

121. Davis RC, Davies WT, Mannick JA: Bypass vein grafts in patients with distal popliteal artery occlusion. Am J Surg 129:421-425, 1975.

122. DeLaurentis DA, Friedman P: Arterial reconstruction above and below the knee: Another look. Am J Surg 121:392-397, 1971.

123. Edwards WS, Gerety E, Larkin J, Hoyt TW: Multiple sequential femoral tibial grafting for severe ischemia. Surgery 80:722-728, 1976.

124. Maini BS, Mannick JA: Effect of arterial reconstruction on limb salvage: A ten-year appraisal. Arch Surg 113:1297-1304, 1978.

125. Perdue GD, Smith RB, Veazey CR, Anslery JD: Revascularization for severe limb ischemia. Arch Surg 115:168-171, 1980.

126. Auer AI, Hurley JJ, Binnington HB, et al: Distal tibial vein grafts for limb salvage. Arch Surg 118:597-602, 1983.

127. Hobson RW, Lynch TG, Jamil Z, et al: Results of revascularization and amputation in severe lower extremity ischemia: A five-year clinical experience. J Vasc Surg 2:205-213, 1985.

128. Stoney RJ: Ultimate salvage for the patients with limb-threatening ischemia: Realistic goals. Am J Surg 136:228-232, 1978.

129. Suggs WD, Yuan JG, Parsons RE, et al: Functional outcome after infrainguinal bypass: A justification for limb salvage surgery. Paper presented at the Peripheral Vascular Surgery Meeting, June 7-8, 1996, Chicago.

130. Ramsburgh SR, Lindenauer SM, Weber IR, et al: Femoropopliteal bypass for limb salvage surgery. Surgery 81:453-458, 1977.

131. Gupta SK, Veith FJ, Samson RH, et al: Cost analysis of operations for infrainguinal arteriosclerosis. Circulation 66(Suppl 2):II-9, 1982.

132. Tabbara M, White R, Cavaye D, Kopchock G: In vivo comparison of intravascular ultrasonography and angiography. J Vasc Surg 14:496-504, 1991.

133. Waller BF, Pinkerton CA, Slack JD: Intravascular ultrasound: A histological study of vessels during life: The new "gold standard" for vascular imaging. Circulation 85:2305-2310, 1992.

134. Van Sambeek MRHM, Qureshi A, Van Lankeren W, et al: Discrepancy between stent deployment and balloon size used assessed by intravascular ultrasound. Eur J Vasc Endovasc Surg 15:57-61, 1998.

135. Palmaz JC, Laborde JC, Rivera FJ, et al: Stenting of the iliac arteries with the Palmaz stent: Experience from a multicenter trial. Cardiovasc Intervent Radiol 15:291-297, 1992.

136. Myers KA, Denton MJ, Devine TJ: Infrainguinal atherectomy using the transluminal endarterectomy catheter: Patency rates and clinical success for 144 procedures. J Endovasc Surg 1:61-70, 1994.

137. Collaborative Rotablator Atherectomy Group (CRAG): Peripheral atherectomy with the Rotablator: A multicenter report. J Vasc Surg 19:509-515, 1994.

138. Zeller T, Frank U, Burgelin K, et al: Initial clinical experience with percutaneous atherectomy in the infragenicular arteries. J Endovasc Ther 10:987-993, 2003.

139. Marin ML, Veith FJ, Cynamon J, et al: Initial experience with transluminally placed endovascular grafts for the treatment of complex vascular lesions. Ann Surg 222:449-469, 1995.

140. Bray PJ, Robson WJ, Bray AE: Percutaneous treatment of long superficial femoral artery occlusive disease: Efficacy of the Hemobahn stent-graft. J Endovasc Ther 10:619-628, 2003.

141. Aulivola B, Pomposelli FB: Dorsalis pedis, tarsal and plantar artery bypass. J Cardiovasc Surg (Torino) 45:203-212, 2004.

142. White GH, White RA, Kopchok GE: Intraoperative video angioscopy compared to arteriography during peripheral vascular operations. J Vasc Surg 6:488-495, 1987.

143. White GH, White RA, Kopchok GE, Wilson SE: Angioscopic thromboembolectomy: Preliminary observations with a recent technique. J Vasc Surg 7:318-325, 1988.

144. Rosenthal D: Improved endovascular techniques for in situ vein bypass. In Veith FJ (ed): Current Critical Problems in Vascular Surgery, vol 6. St. Louis, Quality Medical Publishing, 1994, pp 130-132.

145. Rosenthal D, Arous EJ, Friedman SG, et al: Endovascular-assisted versus conventional in situ saphenous vein bypass grafting: Cumulative patency, limb salvage, and cost results in a 39-month multicenter study. J Vasc Surg 31:60-68, 2000.

146. Lumsden AB, Eaves FF: Subcutaneous, video-assisted saphenous vein harvest. Perspect Vasc Surg 7:43-55, 1994.

147. Fogarty TJ, Chin A, Shoor PM, et al: Adjunctive intraoperative arterial dilatation: Simplified instrumentation technique. Arch Surg 116:1391-1398, 1981.

148. CAPRIE Steering Committee: A randomised, blinded, trial of clopidogrel versus aspirin in patients at risk of ischaemic events (CAPRIE). Lancet 348:1329-1339, 1996.

149. Abbruzzese TA, Havens J, Belkin M, et al: Statin therapy is associated with improved patency of autogenous infrainguinal bypass grafts. J Vasc Surg 39:1178-1185, 2004.

150. Henke PK, Blackburn S, Proctor MC, et al: Patients undergoing infrainguinal bypass to treat atherosclerotic vascular disease are underprescribed cardioprotective medications: Effect on graft patency, limb salvage, and mortality. J Vasc Surg 39:357-365, 2004.

Questions

1. **Which of the following statements concerning arterial emboli is generally not true?**
   (a) The only certain way to diagnose an embolic occlusion is the demonstration that the occlusive process is multifocal
   (b) Emboli are often associated with moderate or severe atherosclerosis
   (c) The treatment of emboli is generally simple, and results are almost uniformly good
   (d) Angiography is usually indicated for lower extremity emboli
   (e) Emboli can be effectively removed even after several days

2. **Bypasses to arteries below the popliteal artery should be performed for limb salvage with PTFE grafts in which of the following circumstances?**
   (a) When no acceptable autologous vein is present in the involved lower extremity
   (b) Only when no autologous vein is available in any of the patient's four extremities
   (c) In no circumstances
   (d) Only to the posterior tibial artery
   (e) None of the above

3. **True or false: Heavily calcified, incompressible tibial arteries are unsuitable for use in limb salvage arterial bypasses.**

4. **True or false: Studies have clearly shown that in situ vein bypasses are uniformly superior to reversed vein bypasses.**

5. **True or false: The standard arteriogram for femoropopliteal occlusive disease should visualize all arteries from the renals to the forefoot.**

6. **Preferential use of PTFE grafts for above-knee femoropopliteal bypass is justified in patients whose life expectancy is less than**
   (a) 1 year
   (b) 2 years
   (c) 3 years
   (d) 4 years
   (e) None of the above

7. **When is bypass to a tibial artery at the ankle level or in the foot indicated for disabling intermittent claudication?**
   (a) Always
   (b) Almost never
   (c) Almost always
   (d) Frequently
   (e) Never

8. **True or false: Toe amputation or foot débridement should never be combined with arterial revascularization.**

9. **True or false: The presence of pedal pulses is evidence of sufficiently good circulation in the foot that a toe amputation for infection is likely to heal.**

10. **True or false: In patients with a failed infrainguinal bypass and a rethreatened limb, there is a poor chance of saving the foot by performing a secondary revascularization.**

Answers

1. c	2. b	3. false	4. false	5. true
6. b	7. b	8. false	9. true	10. false

33

Kimberley J. Hansen • K. Todd Piercy • Richard H. Dean

Management of Renovascular Disease

Historical Background

RENOVASCULAR HYPERTENSION

Goldblatt defined a causal relationship between renovascular disease and hypertension through his innovative work published in 1934,[1] but Bright of Guy's Hospital, London, first called attention to a potential association between hypertension and renal disease 100 years earlier.[2] Bright observed that patients with "dropsy" and albuminuria during life had shrunken kidneys and an enlarged heart (cardiac hypertrophy) at autopsy. He suggested that the altered quality of the blood so affected the small circulation as to render greater action necessary to force the blood through the terminal divisions of the vascular system.

Although Bright failed to recognize the relationship between increased blood pressure and cardiac hypertrophy, his observations stimulated many theories. Among them was Traube's speculation that elevated blood pressure led to increased myocardial work and subsequent hypertrophy.[3] Based on Bright's observations and subsequent hypotheses, several investigators described experimental models intended to re-create the clinical lesions observed in the kidney and heart. In 1879, Growitz and Israel produced acute occlusion of one renal artery and performed contralateral nephrectomy to decrease functioning renal mass.[4] Although these investigators created what they thought was cardiac hypertrophy in some animals, elevated blood pressures occurred in none.

Lewinski might well have predated Goldblatt's observations had his experiments included blood pressure measurements.[5] In 1880, he reported that 6 of 25 dogs developed cardiac hypertrophy after partial constriction of the renal arteries. In 1905, Katzenstein created hypertension in dogs by producing partial occlusion of the renal arteries, although complete occlusion after torsion of the renal pedicle did not produce elevated blood pressures.[6] Katzenstein demonstrated that the elevated pressures returned to normal when constricting rubber bands were removed. However, he mistakenly concluded that the blood pressure changes were not related to a chemically mediated mechanism. In 1898, Tigerstedt and Bergman published the landmark description of a renal pressor substance in rabbits, a crude extract they termed "renin."[7] Although their work was confirmed in 1911

by Senator,[8] these and other investigators did not consider renin central to the pathogenesis of hypertension.

In 1934, Goldblatt demonstrated that constriction of the renal artery produced atrophy of the kidney and hypertension in the dog.[1] As a clinical pathologist, Goldblatt noticed that extensive vascular disease was often present at autopsy in patients with hypertension and was frequently severe in the renal arteries. In his own words: "Contrary, therefore, to what I had been taught, I began to suspect that the vascular disease comes first and, when it involves the kidneys, the resultant impairment of the renal circulation probably, in some way, causes elevation of the blood pressure."[1] Goldblatt's elegant experiments introduced a new era by demonstrating that renal artery stenosis could produce a form of hypertension corrected by nephrectomy.

Leadbetter and Burkland, in 1938, described the first successful treatment of this correctable form of hypertension.[9] They cured a 5-year-old child with severe hypertension by removal of an ischemic ectopic kidney. The photomicrographs published from that renal artery specimen were the first documentation of a renovascular origin of hypertension. In subsequent years, numerous patients were treated by nephrectomy, based on the findings of hypertension and a small kidney on intravenous pyelogram. Smith reviewed 575 such cases in 1956 and found that only 26% of patients were cured of hypertension by nephrectomy.[10] This led him to suggest that nephrectomy should be limited to strictly urologic indications.

In 1954, Freeman performed an aortic and bilateral renal artery thromboendarterectomy in a hypertensive patient, which resulted in resolution of the hypertension.[11] This first cure of hypertension by renal revascularization, in combination with the widespread use of aortography, was followed by enthusiastic reports describing blood pressure benefit after renal revascularization.[12-15] Nevertheless, by 1960, it became apparent that renal revascularization in hypertensive patients with renal artery stenosis was associated with a beneficial blood pressure response in fewer than half of individuals. These clinical results fostered general pessimism regarding the value of operative renal artery reconstruction for the treatment of hypertension.

Contemporary operative management of renovascular hypertension began with the introduction of tests of functional significance. Split renal function by Howard and Connor,[16]

Stamey and associates,[17] Page and Helmes,[18] and others[19-21] identified the role of the renin-angiotensin system in blood pressure control, thus describing the pathophysiology of renovascular hypertension. After accurate assays for plasma renin activity became available, physicians could accurately predict which renal artery lesion was producing renovascular hypertension.

RENOVASCULAR RENAL INSUFFICIENCY

Until the current era, the pathophysiology and management of renovascular disease focused solely on hypertension; however, contemporary reports have emphasized the relationship between renovascular disease and renal insufficiency.[22-30]

The term *ischemic nephropathy* has been adopted to recognize this relationship. By definition, ischemic nephropathy describes the presence of severe occlusive disease of the extraparenchymal renal artery in combination with excretory renal insufficiency. In 1962, Morris and associates reported on eight azotemic patients with global renal ischemia who experienced improved blood pressure and renal function after renal revascularization.[31] Novick, Libertino, and Dean and their groups found a similar beneficial functional response when bilateral renal lesions were corrected in azotemic patients.[24,25,27,28] These early reports and the reports that followed suggested that ischemic nephropathy could mediate renal insufficiency that was rapidly progressive, contributing to end-stage renal disease. In this chapter, diagnostic studies and methods of management for renovascular disease (RVD), renovascular hypertension (RVH), and ischemic nephropathy are reviewed.

Pathology

Occlusive lesions of the renal artery can be divided into two main categories: atherosclerosis and fibromuscular dysplasia. Atherosclerosis of the renal artery is not unique. The pathogenesis parallels atherosclerotic lesions elsewhere, with cholesterol-rich lipid deposition and intimal thickening. Later, this atheroma may undergo central degeneration and even calcification. Atheromas typically occur at or near the renal artery ostium (Fig. 33-1). This ostial lesion reflects aortic atheroma that spills over into the renal artery orifice. Most commonly, these lesions are found on the left and account for about 70% of patients with RVH. Like atherosclerosis elsewhere, angiographic findings that are pathognomonic for a hemodynamically significant lesion include post-stenotic dilatation and the presence of collateral vessels. Often, there is simultaneous angiographic involvement of the abdominal aorta and its bifurcation. Most commonly, the renal artery lesion is only one manifestation of generalized atherosclerosis.

Fibromuscular dysplasia of the renal artery encompasses a variety of hyperplastic and fibrosing lesions of the intima, media, or adventitia. They are most frequently seen in young women. This is of no predictive value, however, because fibrodysplastic lesions can be found at any age and in either sex. Medial fibroplasia is the most common lesion, accounting for 85% of dysplastic lesions. The right renal artery is more commonly affected than the left, but bilateral involvement is present in the vast majority of patients. The basic cause of medial fibroplasia remains unknown, but its frequent

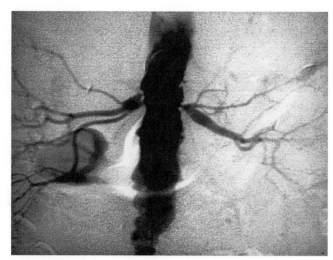

FIGURE 33–1 • Arteriogram showing typical appearance of ostial atherosclerotic renal artery stenosis. Aortic atheroma spills over into the renal artery to create stenosis.

occurrence in multiple arteries suggests a systemic arteriopathy. It often involves long segments of the renal artery and its branches, producing a characteristic "string-of-beads" appearance angiographically. Embryologic variations, hormonal influences, autoimmune mechanisms, and even recurrent trauma during youth have been suggested as possible causative factors. None of these explanations is adequate, however, and the supporting evidence remains mostly conjectural.

Based on the angiographic appearance of fibromuscular disease, several methods of categorization have been suggested. To establish a uniform terminology, Harrison and McCormack combined their experience and developed a classification of these lesions correlating the histologic and angiographic appearance.[32] Depending on the layer predominantly involved, lesions may be categorized as intimal, medial, or adventitial (Fig 33-2). Clinically, however, it may be difficult to segregate individual lesions into one of these categories. The most common variety of fibromuscular dysplasia is medial fibroplasia (85%) with mural microaneurysms (Fig. 33-3). Less commonly, the dysplastic lesions may present as a single mural stenosis (see Fig. 33-2) consistent with intimal fibroplasia (5%). Perimedial dysplasia (10%) demonstrates the same gender predilection and arterial septa as medial fibroplasia; however, mural microaneurysms are absent.

Pathophysiology

The kidney, because of its influence on circulating plasma volume and on the modulation of vasomotor tone, is a dominant site of blood pressure regulation. To examine the pathophysiology of RVH, a review of the normal homeostatic activities of the kidney in blood pressure regulation is appropriate.

RENIN-ANGIOTENSIN-ALDOSTERONE SYSTEM

The renin-angiotensin-aldosterone system is a complex feedback mechanism that normally acts to maintain a stable blood pressure and blood volume under varying conditions. Richly innervated modified smooth muscle cells located

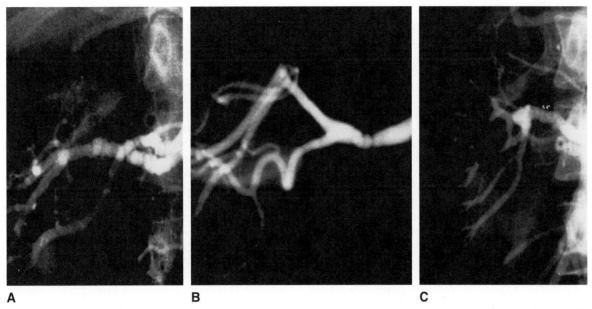

FIGURE 33–2 • Angiographic appearance of fibromuscular dysplasia: alternating septa and mural microaneurysms of medial fibroplasia *(A),* focal stenosis of intimal fibroplasia *(B),* and fine septa without microaneurysms characteristic of perimedial dysplasia *(C).*

along the afferent arterioles in juxtaposition to the renal glomerulus (juxtaglomerular apparatus) are sensitive monitors of perfusion pressure. Diminished perfusion pressure stimulates these cells to release renin, a proteolytic enzyme. Renin interacts with angiotensinogen, an α-globulin manufactured in the liver, to produce angiotensin I. Angiotensin I, an inactive and labile decapeptide, is converted to the potent vasoconstrictor angiotensin II by angiotensin-converting enzyme, which is abundant in the lungs and other tissues. In addition to its potent vasoconstrictor properties, angiotensin II, through its conversion to angiotensin III, also increases blood pressure by stimulating aldosterone release from the zona glomerulosa of the adrenal cortex. This, in turn, increases plasma volume by increasing sodium and water resorption in the renal tubules. Through these actions of angiotensin II and III, blood pressure, plasma volume, and plasma sodium content are increased. In addition, the adjacent cells of the distal convoluted tubule (macula densa) may play a role by acting as sensors of sodium concentration in the distal tubules and exerting a positive

feedback mechanism on renin release. As these mechanisms increase perfusion pressure in the juxtaglomerular cells, further renin production and release are suppressed, and blood pressure is modulated within a narrow range.

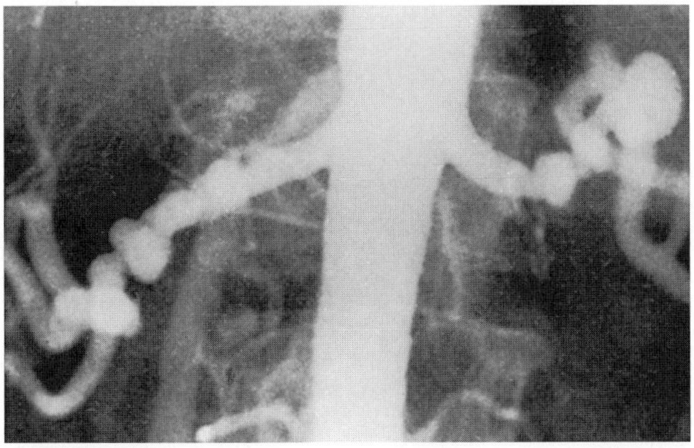

Potentially, two forms of hypertension may be produced by hemodynamically significant RVD: renin-dependent hypertension and volume-dependent hypertension. Through the mechanisms just described, decreased perfusion activates the renin-angiotensin-aldosterone axis of vasoconstriction and volume expansion. Current information regarding the nature of RVH suggests that a functionally significant unilateral renal artery stenosis activates the angiotensin II–mediated increase in peripheral resistance and blood pressure as well as the aldosterone-mediated volume expansion. When the contralateral renal artery and kidney are normal, the feedback mechanisms in the normal kidney produce a natriuresis and compensatory reduction in circulating plasma volume. In this scheme, an angiotensin II–vasoconstrictive source of hypertension is created.

In contrast, when the contralateral renal artery or kidney is also diseased, this compensatory diuresis is lost and volume expansion occurs, producing an angiotensin-aldosterone–mediated, volume-dependent hypertension. Modification of renal perfusion by renal revascularization can effectively diminish or abolish the underlying mechanism producing either of these varieties of RVH.

It would be simplistic to think that these factors provide a complete description of all the mechanisms activated by the onset of renal hypoperfusion. In the clinical context, however, the pathophysiology of renal hypertension can be characterized by a sustained elevation in peripheral vascular resistance that is mediated by the activation of both the renin-angiotensin and the sympathetic nervous systems and their concomitant contribution to vascular endothelial dysfunction. Although the contribution of increased renin secretion and angiotensin II production is a sustaining stimulus for the hemodynamic and hormonal response, the actions of angiotensin II on the vascular endothelium may play the

FIGURE 33–3 • Arteriogram demonstrating typical "string-of-beads" appearance of medial fibroplasia with fine septa and microaneurysm.

biggest role in sustained blood pressure elevation. Both the renin-angiotensin and the sympathetic nervous systems appear to act in concert to regulate the integrated hormonal response that operates to regulate sodium and potassium balance and arterial pressure.

It is well accepted that RVH is caused by increased activity of the renin-angiotensin system produced initially by hypersecretion of renin from the juxtaglomerular apparatus of the ischemic kidney. However, as hypertension evolves into a chronic stage, adaptive cardiovascular changes may become an essential mechanism for the maintenance of elevated blood pressure and peripheral vascular resistance. The effect of hypertension on precapillary resistant vessels triggers a myogenic response that is evidenced by the combination of hypertrophy and hyperplasia of the vascular smooth muscle.[33,34] This augments vascular reactivity to pressor agents. There is also evidence that renin may be trapped in structural elements of the vascular wall.[35] Local production of angiotensin II by tissue renin-angiotensin systems may contribute to the remodeling of resistance vessels.[36] Angiotensin-converting enzyme exists in the plasma membrane of vascular endothelial and smooth muscle cells. Thus, the necessary components for the production of angiotensin II may be found in both vascular and cardiac tissue. In the chronic phases of the hypertension process, hypersecretion of renin from the ischemic kidney may be less important than increased production of vascular angiotensin II as the mechanism that sustains the elevation in arterial pressure.

The pathophysiology of renovascular renal insufficiency (i.e., ischemic nephropathy) is incompletely understood.[37] The earliest clinical reports suggested a "glomerular filtration failure" based on hypoperfusion of the kidney,[38] but the molecular basis for ischemic nephropathy is poorly characterized. Like RVH, the renin-angiotensin system likely contributes to ischemic nephropathy through its paracrine effects—intrarenal angiotensin peptides increase efferent arteriolar tone.[39] In the presence of a pressure-reducing renal artery lesion, this paracrine effect increases glomerular capillary pressure to support glomerular filtration. In contrast to these positive effects, angiotensin peptides have also been shown to promote tubulointerstitial injury in the presence of a renal artery lesion.[40] This observation is supported by the induction of transforming growth factor-β and interstitial platelet-derived growth factor-β, which are associated with increased extracellular matrix and interstitial fibrosis.[41-44] Disruption of the tubular cell cytoskeleton and the loss of tubular membrane polarity have also been suggested. Besides these potentially reversible contributors to excretory renal insufficiency, an atherosclerotic renovascular lesion can also be a source of atheroemboli.[45] The inability to distinguish potentially reversible ischemic nephropathy from irreversible renal parenchymal disease has enormous clinical importance. Recovery of renal function after renovascular intervention has proved to be the strongest predictor of dialysis-free survival.[23,26]

Prevalence of Renovascular Hypertension and Ischemic Nephropathy

RVH is generally thought to account for 5% to 10% of the hypertensive population. Tucker suggested an even lower prevalence.[46] Likewise, Shapiro and colleagues suggested that

the identification and successful operative treatment of RVH in patients older than 50 years are so unlikely that diagnostic investigation for a correctable cause in that group should be undertaken only when hypertension is severe and uncontrollable.[47] Estimates of the prevalence of hypertension in the United States from all causes range from 60 to 80 million people, and hypertension may be present in 25% to 30% of the adult population.

The actual contribution of RVD to hypertension or renal insufficiency has been uncertain because the population-based prevalence of RVD was unknown. Past prevalence estimates of RVD were extrapolated from case series, autopsy examinations, or angiography obtained to evaluate diseases of the aorta or peripheral circulation.[31,48-54] Recently, the population-based prevalence of RVD has been estimated for participants in the Cardiovascular Health Study (CHS) sponsored by the National Heart, Lung, and Blood Institute. The CHS is a longitudinal, prospective, population-based study of coronary heart disease and stroke in elderly men and women. This study showed that hemodynamically significant RVD was present in 6.8% of this elderly, free-living cohort.[55] Multivariate analysis demonstrated that increasing participant age ($P = 0.028$; odds ratio [OR], 1.44; 95% confidence interval [CI], 1.03 to 1.73) and increasing systolic blood pressure at baseline ($P = 0.007$; OR, 1.44; 95% CI, 1.10 to 1.87) were significantly and independently associated with the presence of RVD. Moreover, renal insufficiency was associated with RVD, but only when renal artery disease coexisted with significant hypertension. Contrary to historical assumptions, RVD demonstrated no significant relationships with gender or ethnicity.[55]

Like in the general population, the incidence of RVH is undoubtedly low when all patients with hypertension are considered. Because RVH tends to produce relatively severe hypertension, its prevalence in the large population of mildly hypertensive patients (diastolic blood pressure < 105 mm Hg) is probably negligible. In contrast, however, it is a frequent cause of hypertension in the smaller group of patients with severe hypertension. In our experience, the presence of severe hypertension at the two extremes of life carries the highest probability of its being RVH. Our review of the causes of hypertension in 74 children admitted for diagnostic evaluation over a 5-year period showed that 78% of the children younger than 5 years had a correctable renin-dependent cause (Table 33-1).[56] In 1996, our center screened 629 hypertensive adults older than 50 years for RVD (Table 33-2). Overall, 25% of subjects demonstrated significant renal artery disease. However, 52% of those older than 60 years

TABLE 33–1	Classification of Hypertension in 74 Children by Age			
	0-5 Yr	**6-10 Yr**	**11-15 Yr**	**16-20 Yr**
Total no. of children	9	9	29	27
Essential hypertension	1	5	24	21
Correctable hypertension	8 (89%)	4 (44%)	5 (17%)	6 (22%)

From Lawson JD, Boerth RK, Foster JH, et al: Diagnosis and management of renovascular hypertension in children. Arch Surg 112:1307, 1977.

TABLE 33–2	Results of Renal Duplex Sonography in 629 New Hypertensive Adults		
	Renal Vascular Disease		
	Present (%)	*Absent (%)*	**Total (%)**
All patients	154 (24)	475 (76)	629 (100)
< 60 yr + DBP ≥ 110 mm Hg	98 (52)	91 (48)	189 (30)
DBP ≥ 110 mm Hg + SCr ≥ 2.0 mg/dL	53 (71)	22 (29)	75 (12)

DBP, diastolic blood pressure; SCr, serum creatinine.
From Deitch JS, Hansen KJ, Craven TE, et al: Renal artery repair in African-Americans. J Vasc Surg 26:465-473, 1997.

whose diastolic pressure was greater than 110 mm Hg had significant renal artery stenosis or occlusion. When serum creatinine was elevated in conjunction with this age and blood pressure, 71% of subjects demonstrated hemodynamically significant RVD.

Based on these data, the probability of finding RVH correlates with patient age, the severity of hypertension, and the presence of associated renal insufficiency. Accordingly, the search for RVD should be directed toward the subset of patients at the extremes of age who have severe hypertension, especially when it is associated with renal insufficiency. The reader should keep in mind, however, that the severity of hypertension is based on its level without medication and does not refer to the difficulty of medical control.

Characteristics of Renovascular Hypertension

Because of the small proportion of RVH among the entire hypertensive population, many reports have focused on the value of demographic factors, physical findings, and screening tests to discriminate between essential hypertension and RVH. Most frequently cited as discriminate factors suggesting the presence of RVH and a need for further study are recent onset of hypertension, young age, lack of family history of hypertension, and presence of an abdominal bruit. The most complete study comparing the clinical characteristics of patients with RVH to those with essential hypertension was the Cooperative Study of Renovascular Hypertension.[57] In that study, the prevalence of certain clinical characteristics in 339 patients with essential hypertension was compared with their prevalence in 175 patients with RVH secondary to atherosclerotic lesions (91 patients) and fibromuscular dysplasia (84 patients). Although the prevalence of several characteristics was significantly different in RVH compared with essential hypertension, none of the characteristics had sufficient discriminant value to be used to exclude patients from further diagnostic investigation for RVH. Certainly, the finding of an epigastric bruit in a young white female with malignant hypertension is strongly suggestive of a renovascular origin of the hypertension. The absence of such criteria, however, does not exclude the presence of RVH, and such criteria should not be used to eliminate patients from further diagnostic study.

In a review of the first 200 patients with RVH treated in our center, 64% had family histories of hypertension, 46% had no audible abdominal bruit, and ages ranged from 5 to 80 years (mean, 56 years).[58] Because RVH can be secondary to any of several diseases affecting the renal artery, and because each of these diseases has its own clinical characteristics, the use of demographic or physical findings such as age, abdominal bruit, and duration of hypertension to exclude patients from study inappropriately excludes some patients with RVH from further evaluation. Therefore, the decision to undertake diagnostic study should be based on the severity of hypertension. Mild hypertension has a minimal chance of being renovascular in origin. In contrast, the more severe the hypertension, the higher the probability that it is from a correctable cause. With this in mind, we evaluate all adult patients with diastolic blood pressures greater than 105 mm Hg who would be considered for intervention to evaluate for a renovascular lesion as a correctable origin of hypertension. Children are evaluated when their blood pressure exceeds the 95th percentile for height and age.[59]

Diagnostic Evaluation

The selection and appropriate sequence of diagnostic studies in patients with suspected RVD are still ill defined. The general evaluation of all hypertensive patients should include a careful medical history, physical examination, serum electrolyte and creatinine determination, and electrocardiography. Electrocardiography is important to gauge the extent of secondary myocardial hypertrophy or associated ischemic heart disease. Serum electrolyte and serial serum potassium determinations can effectively exclude patients with primary aldosteronism if potassium levels are greater than 3.0 mg/dL. One must remember, however, that hypokalemia is often due to salt-depleting diets and previous diuretic therapy. Finally, estimation of renal function is mandatory. Preexisting renal disease may reduce renal function and cause hypertension. Conversely, renal dysfunction may reflect ischemic nephropathy.

SCREENING STUDIES

Identification of a noninvasive screening test that accurately identifies all patients with RVD that may warrant interventional management remains an elusive goal. Prior methods such as peripheral plasma renin activity, rapid-sequence intravenous pyelography, and saralasin infusion have been abandoned. Screening studies are basically of two types: functional studies or anatomic studies. Of the functional type, isotope renography continues to be proposed as a valuable screening test, yet the methods employed are continually modified with the hope of improving its sensitivity and specificity. The newest versions of isotope renography consist of renal scans performed before and after the administration of an inhibitor to angiotensin I–converting enzyme. Of these, only captopril renal scanning has gained widespread use and acceptance as a screening tool. Anatomic screening studies include renal duplex sonography and arteriography.

Captopril Renal Scanning

To understand the basis of captopril renal scanning, one must consider some of the features of renal physiology and the

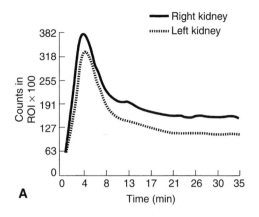

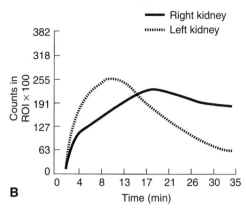

FIGURE 33–4 • Captopril renal scintigraphy before *(A)* and after *(B)* captopril administration demonstrates the positive finding of a time delay in reaching peak radioactivity after captopril. ROI, region of interest.

importance of the renin-angiotensin system in the maintenance of homeostasis. Glomerular filtration is governed partially by the relative tone of the afferent and efferent arterioles. During periods of reduced blood pressure recognized by the juxtaglomerular apparatus (e.g., proximal renal artery stenosis), increased renin is released, which ultimately leads to an increase in the level of intrarenal angiotensin II. Angiotensin II acts predominantly to constrict the efferent arteriole to maintain renal glomerular perfusion pressure and filtration. When an angiotensin I–converting enzyme inhibitor such as captopril is given in this circumstance, an acute reduction in the amount of angiotensin II occurs. This leads to a reduction in constriction of the efferent arteriole and a decrease in the glomerular filtration rate (GFR). Captopril renal scanning is composed of a baseline renogram and a repeat renogram obtained after a dose of captopril. A test is considered positive when a normal baseline scan becomes abnormal after captopril administration—that is, when the time to peak activity increases to more than 11 minutes or when a normal glomerular filtration ratio between the two sides increases to greater than 1.5:1 (Fig. 33-4). In experienced hands, this study is reported to be highly reliable.[60] Unfortunately, it is less reliable when significant parenchymal disease is present. For that reason, we do not rely on its results to eliminate RVD in azotemic patients.

Renal Duplex Sonography

Through continued improvements in probe design and duplex sonographic technology, imaging and Doppler shift interrogation of deep abdominal vasculature have been introduced as screening methods to identify and quantify visceral and renal artery occlusive disease. We have evaluated the role of duplex sonography as an initial surface screening test, as an intraoperative study to confirm the technical success of reconstructive procedures, and as a postoperative surveillance method to follow progression of disease and stability of reconstructions.[59,61-64]

Technically successful studies, defined as a complete main renal artery interrogation from aortic origin to renal hilum, can be obtained in almost 95% of cases. These results are ensured by proper patient preparation and method of examination. Details of the conduct of the procedure are covered elsewhere.[61]

The criteria for identifying renal artery stenosis by renal duplex sonography are given in Table 33-3. Assuming that renal artery peak systolic velocity (PSV) varies with the degree of renal artery stenosis and aortic PSV (i.e., inflow), most authors have advocated using the ratio of renal artery PSV to aortic PSV (the renal-aortic ratio) to define critical renal artery stenosis.[65-68] In contrast, we have found no relationship between renal artery PSV and aortic PSV in the presence or absence of disease (Fig. 33-5). Focal renal artery PSV of 1.8 m/second or more in combination with distal post-stenotic turbulence correlates highly with the angiographic presence of diameter-reducing renal artery stenosis of 60% or greater.[61] In 122 kidneys with single renal arteries and renal angiography for comparison, renal duplex sonography correctly identified 67 of 68 kidneys with normal arteries or less than 60% renal artery stenosis, and 35 of 39 kidneys with 60% to 99% renal artery stenosis. All 15 renal artery occlusions were correctly identified by failure to obtain a Doppler-shifted signal from an imaged renal artery. Using this method and these criteria for interpretation, renal duplex sonography was 93% sensitive and 98% specific.

Renal Angiography

Controversy continues over the use of aortography and renal angiography in the routine screening of hypertensive individuals. Some believe that these methods should be reserved for select groups of patients. We do not share this view and proceed with angiography in the circumstances summarized earlier.

TABLE 33–3	Doppler Velocity Criteria for Significant Stenosis and Occlusion	
Defect	**Criteria**
<60% diameter-reducing RA defect	RA-PSV from entire RA < 1.8 m/sec
≥60% diameter-reducing RA defect	Focal RA-PSV ≥ 1.8 m/sec and distal turbulent velocity waveform
Occlusion	Doppler-shifted signal from RA B-scan image
Inadequate study for interpretation	Failure to obtain Doppler samples from entire main RA

RA, renal artery; RA-PSV, renal artery peak systolic velocity.
From Hansen KJ, Tribble RW, Reaves SW, et al: Renal duplex sonography: Evaluation of clinical utility. J Vasc Surg 12:227-236, 1990; Motew SJ, Cherr GS, Craven TE, et al: Renal duplex sonography: Main renal artery versus hilar analysis. J Vasc Surg 32:462-471, 2000.

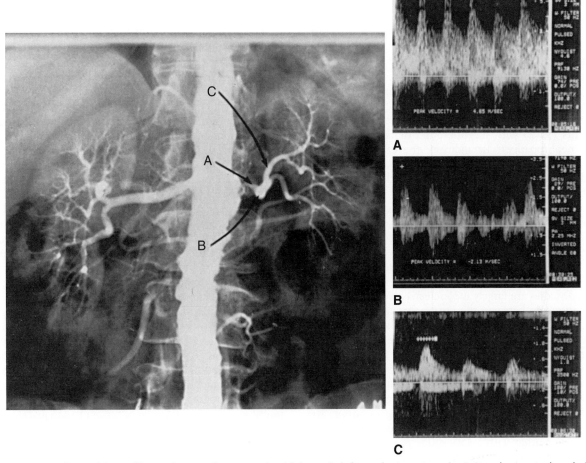

FIGURE 33–5 • Radiographic cut-film angiogram demonstrating high-grade left renal artery stenosis. *A*, Doppler spectral analysis at the site of stenosis demonstrating focal increase in renal artery peak systolic velocity (RA-PSV; 4.6 m/second). *B*, Distal spectral analysis demonstrating turbulent waveform and decreased RA-PSV with irregular spectral envelope and spontaneous bidirectional signals. *C*, Spectral analysis several vessel diameters distal to stenosis demonstrating return of nearly normal waveform.

Details of performing angiography to evaluate aortic and branch disease are addressed elsewhere. Currently, intra-arterial digital subtraction angiography is used to evaluate the majority of patients. The fact that angiography in patients with severe renal insufficiency, especially those with concomitant diabetes mellitus, can aggravate renal failure is widely recognized. Nevertheless, we believe that this risk is justified in patients with severe or accelerated hypertension and in those with positive renal duplex sonography results. In these circumstances, the potential benefit derived from the identification and correction of a functionally significant renovascular lesion exceeds the risk of contrast exposure. In addition, the use of carbon dioxide and gadolinium as alternatives may reduce the risk of nephrotoxicity.[69,70]

Because the mortality and the morbidity of contrast nephropathy leading to dialysis dependence are high, measures to protect renal function during angiography should be taken. Conventional contrast agents have iodine incorporated into their structure to absorb x-ray photons, thereby achieving visualization of the vasculature. The nephrotoxicity of such iodinated contrast agents has been recognized for many years. The principal site of contrast-induced nephrotoxicity is the renal tubule from transient regional renal ischemia, whereas the effect on glomerular function appears

to be mild.[71,72] It was thought that the ionization and high osmolarity of early contrast agents may have contributed to their nephrotoxicity. Nonionic contrast agents (e.g., iohexol) are now available that provide comparable absorption of x-ray photons but are significantly less charged than traditional agents. It was hoped that the reduced ionic nature would decrease their nephrotoxicity, but the occurrence of severe adverse renal events did not differ between ionic and nonionic contrast media in a large randomized clinical trial.[73]

Renal nephrotoxicity after exposure to ionic agents occurs most commonly in patients with preexisting renal insufficiency (3.3 relative risk) alone or in combination with diabetes mellitus, especially juvenile-onset diabetes.[73] Other risk factors such as dehydration, volume of contrast used, and simultaneous exposure to other nephrotoxins contribute to the likelihood of acute contrast nephrotoxicity.[74] Other risk factors include multiple myeloma and heavy proteinuria. Overall, the incidence of acute renal dysfunction following contrast angiography varies from zero to 10%, although these estimates are skewed by several studies that included only juvenile diabetics. In one study, hospital-acquired nephropathy occurred in 12% of patients.[75] In patients with normal renal function, however, the incidence of contrast nephropathy is only 1% to 2%.[76] The impact of diabetes on the risk of acute renal failure following angiography appears to be dependent on the type of diabetes and the magnitude of secondary diabetic nephropathy.

Type 1 diabetics appear to be more susceptible to contrast-induced acute renal failure than type 2 diabetics.[77,78] Harkonen and Kjellstrand found that 20 of 26 patients (76%) with a prestudy serum creatinine level greater than 2 mg/dL who underwent excretory urography developed acute renal failure.[77] Weinrauch and associates reported that acute renal failure following coronary angiography developed in 12 of 13 patients (92%) with juvenile-onset diabetes and severe diabetic nephropathy.[79] In addition, the cause of chronic renal insufficiency appears to affect recovery from contrast-induced acute renal failure. Whereas both diabetic and nondiabetic patients with renal insufficiency are at increased risk for contrast-induced acute renal failure, diabetics appear to recover less often and are at greater risk of permanent dependence on dialysis as a consequence of contrast-induced acute renal failure.[77-79]

Specific measures to minimize the risk of contrast-induced acute renal failure remain controversial, and the results from controlled studies are largely inconclusive. Nevertheless, the basic relationship between the use of contrast material and the risk of contrast nephropathy appears to be related to the amount of time the kidney is exposed to the contrast material. For this reason, maximizing urine flow rate during and immediately after angiography and limiting the quantity of contrast agent used are important considerations. Maximal urine flow rate should be achieved by preliminary intravenous hydration of the patient. Studies that examined the optimal preparation of patients with renal insufficiency indicated that hydration with 0.45% saline provides better protection against acute decline in renal function associated with radiocontrast agents than does hydration with 0.45% saline plus mannitol or furosemide.[80] Recent evidence suggests that administration of sodium bicarbonate before contrast exposure may significantly reduce renal dysfunction.[81]

By scavenging reactive oxygen species, acetylcysteine may protect against contrast-induced nephrotoxicity. Tepel and colleagues studied patients with chronic renal dysfunction who required nonionic contrast for computed tomography.[82] They documented a significant reduction in serum creatinine with the use of oral acetylcysteine and hydration compared with placebo and hydration.

Although further study is needed to better define the role of acetylcysteine during aortography, we administer two oral doses of acetylcysteine (600 mg) before and after these studies in patients at high risk for contrast nephropathy. We routinely admit any patient at risk for contrast nephropathy 12 hours before angiography for intravenous hydration at 1.5 mL/kg per hour. The patient receives two 600-mg oral doses of acetylcysteine immediately before angiography and a bolus of intravenous fluid (3 to 5 mL/kg) with or without sodium bicarbonate. Finally, intravenous hydration is continued for 4 to 6 hours, and two additional doses of acetylcysteine are administered after completion of the study.

Although attempts to calculate a safe upper limit of contrast material have met with some success, no definitive limit currently exists. Even small doses (30 to 60 mL) may induce renal failure in patients with extreme renal insufficiency (GFR $\leq$ 15 mL/minute). Conversely, more than 300 mL of contrast material may be safely administered to other patients

with no risk factors for acute renal failure.[83] Our practice is to limit the quantity of nonionized contrast agent to less than 50 to 75 mL in patients with a significant reduction in GFR (<20 to 30 mL/minute). If additional contrast material is required to complete the vascular evaluation, we postpone further study and approach the total evaluation in a sequential manner. In almost all instances, digital subtraction techniques have been useful in limiting the quantity of contrast material required. We have found that a single midstream aortic injection, using 10 to 20 mL of low-osmolar, nonionic contrast material and digital subtraction, provides images approaching the quality of prior conventional cut-film studies.

Adjuncts or alternatives to angiography are appropriate in many instances. In addition to the use of digital subtraction techniques, carbon dioxide gas can be used for angiography with minimal renal risk.[84] Because it offers limited detail, carbon dioxide angiography is often used to identify the site of disease, which is then better defined with conventional contrast agents. Other alternatives to conventional angiography that reduce or eliminate the risk of nephrotoxicity include the use of gadolinium as a contrast agent for angiography,[69,70] magnetic resonance angiography,[85] and abdominal ultrasonography with visceral or renal artery duplex sonography.

Finally, high-dose loop diuretics, angiotensin-converting enzyme inhibitors, and angiotensin II receptor antagonists are held for at least 72 hours before aortic reconstruction or exposure to arterial contrast agents. Selective beta blockers and calcium channel blockers are substituted when necessary.[86]

Both aortography and selective renal angiography using multiple projections may be necessary to adequately examine the entire renal artery. The proximal third of the left renal artery usually courses anteriorly, the middle third transversely, and the distal third posteriorly, whereas the right renal artery arises from the anterior aorta and then pursues a more consistent posterior course. Lesions in the renal artery that are coursing anteriorly or posteriorly are frequently not seen or may appear insignificant in an anteroposterior aortogram. Oblique aortography or oblique selective renal angiography projects these portions of the vessels in profile and reveals

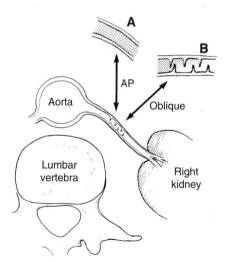

FIGURE 33–6 • Graphic illustration of how the septa of medial fibroplasia can be missed. When the vessel is viewed with an anteroposterior (AP) arteriogram (A), the septa are masked by the overlying dye column. In the oblique projection (B), the septa are demonstrated because they are parallel to the direction of the x-ray.

the stenosis. Figure 33-6 illustrates how the delicate septal lesions of fibromuscular dysplasia may be unrecognizable or appear insignificant in the anteroposterior projection, whereas in the oblique projection the true severity is demonstrated.

FUNCTIONAL STUDIES

Two tests, renal vein renin assays and split renal function studies, have proved valuable in confirming the functional significance of renal artery stenosis. Neither has great value, however, when severe bilateral disease or disease in the renal artery supplying a single kidney is present. In these circumstances, the decision for operation is based on the severity of hypertension and the degree of renal insufficiency. Further, urologically performed split renal function studies are no longer done in any center studying patients with RVH. Therefore, the reader is referred to earlier texts describing their use.[87,88]

Renal Vein Renin Assays

When a unilateral obstructive renal artery lesion is found by renal angiography, its functional significance should be evaluated. Most centers now rely solely on renal vein renin assays (RVRAs) to establish the diagnosis of RVH. The unfortunate consequence of this trend is that one must presume that all patients with RVH have lateralizing RVRAs. Results of the evaluation of this study in our center underscore the fallacy of this presumption. Many factors can affect the RVRA; if these are not properly managed, erroneous results may occur.

The effect of antihypertensive medications and unrestricted sodium intake on renin release, and thereby the RVRA, is widely recognized. Many antihypertensive medications, especially those that function through β-adrenergic blockade, suppress renin output and can lead to false nonlateralization of the RVRA. Before one can presume that no drug is interfering with the release of renin, all such medications must be withheld for at least 5 days—preferably, 2 weeks—before the RVRA. Similar effects on renin levels are seen when sodium intake is not restricted. For this reason, the patient must be on no more than a 2-g sodium diet for at least 2 weeks before the study. The preparation of patients for RVRA in our center is summarized in Table 33-4.

The technical aspects of performing the RVRA cannot be overemphasized. The left renal vein contains not only renal venous effluent but also adrenal, gonadal, and lumbar venous effluent. Misplacement of the venous catheter into the origin of one of the nonrenal branches or sampling in the proximal renal vein, where a mixture from these other sources is present, may dilute the renin activity coming from the kidney.

TABLE 33-4	Patient Preparation for Renal Vein Renin Assay

1. Chronic salt restriction (2-g-sodium diet daily)
2. Discontinue all antihypertensive drugs except diuretics and calcium channel for at least 5 days before the study
3. Oral furosemide (40 mg) diuresis the night before the study
4. Nothing by mouth for 8 hr before the study
5. Strictly flat bed rest for 4 hr before and during the study
6. Prestudy sedation with intramuscular diazepam (5 mg)

This leads to erroneously low measurements of renin activity and produces a false interpretation of the RVRA.

The time of sampling the two renal veins for renin activity is also a potential source of error in the RVRA. In studies performed with a single catheter, several minutes may elapse between sampling the two renal veins as the catheter is switched from one side to the other. Further, catheter manipulation and patient discomfort may affect renin release. Not surprisingly, when a single catheter is employed, both false-positive and false-negative renal vein renin ratios are common.

Several methods of stimulating renin release have been suggested. These include tilting the patient to the upright posture during the study, stimulation with intravenous hydralazine hydrochloride, and nitroprusside stimulation. Although all these methods increase renin release, they also increase false-positive determinations and reduce the reliability of the RVRA to unacceptable levels.

Vaughan and colleagues stressed the importance of expressing the RVRA in relation to the systemic renin activity rather than simply evaluating the ratio of renin activity between the two renal veins.[89] In patients with RVH secondary to unilateral renal artery stenosis, one should find hypersecretion of renin from the ischemic kidney and suppression of renin secretion from the normal kidney. Through application of this hypothesis, Stanley and Fry showed a statistically significant difference in the renal-systemic renin indices in patients who were cured of RVH by operation compared with those who were only improved.[90] Although this method has appeal as a predictor of the extent of benefit, its value in patients with bilateral renal artery lesions is limited. Because both lesions may be producing RVH, both this method and renal vein renin ratios have less validity as predictors of response to operation. If one bases the decision for operative management solely on whether absolute cure is expected, many patients with severe hypertension who would benefit from its reduction to a mild, easily controlled level would be excluded from consideration as operative candidates. Therefore, this method of RVRA interpretation should be considered only as an additional predictive tool and not as an alternative to the evaluation of renal vein renin ratios.

RVRAs also may be inaccurate in patients with accessory or segmental renal artery stenosis if renal venous sampling is limited to the main renal vein. Because recognition of renin hypersecretion depends on sampling the ischemic areas of the kidneys, selective segmental venous sampling must be done in these patients. When segmental sampling is required, the renin activity from the segment sampled is compared with the simultaneously collected contralateral main renal vein sample to calculate the renal vein renin ratio.

Management Options

The question of what constitutes the best method of management for patients with RVH or ischemic nephropathy is unanswerable. There are no prospective, randomized trials that compare all available treatment options. In the absence of level I data, advocates of medical management, percutaneous transluminal angioplasty (PTA), or operative intervention cite selective clinical data to support their particular views.

A majority of the medical community evaluates patients for RVH only when medications are not tolerated or hypertension

TABLE 33–5	**Frequency of Severe Deterioration in Parameters of Renal Function during Drug Therapy**				
Parameter	**No. of Patients Monitored**	**Mean Follow-up (mo)**	**Failure Event**	**Number Affected**	**Percentage Affected**
Renal length	38	33	≥10% decrease	14	37
Serum creatinine	41	25	≥100% increase	2	5
Glomerular filtration rate or creatinine clearance	30	19	≥50% decrease	1	3

From Dean RH, Kieffer RW, Smith BM, et al: Renovascular hypertension. Arch Surg 116:1408, 1981.

remains severe and poorly controlled. The study by Hunt and Strong remains the most informative study available to assess the comparative value of medical therapy and operation.[91] In this nonrandomized study, the results of operative treatment in 100 patients were compared with the results of drug therapy in 114 similar patients. After 7 to 14 years of follow-up, 84% of the operated group was alive, compared with 66% of the drug therapy group. Of the 84 patients alive in the operated group, 93% were cured or significantly improved, compared with only 21% of the surviving patients in the drug therapy group. Death during follow-up was twice as common in the medically treated group as in the operated group, resulting in differences that were statistically significant in patients with either atherosclerosis or fibromuscular dysplasia of the renal artery.

Additional prospective data regarding medical therapy for RVH suggest that a decrease in kidney size and renal function may occur despite satisfactory blood pressure control. Dean and colleagues reported the results of serial renal function studies performed on 41 patients with RVH (i.e., hypertension and positive functional studies) secondary to atherosclerotic renal artery disease who were randomly selected for nonoperative management (Table 33-5).[92] In 19 patients, serum creatinine levels increased between 25% and 120%. GFRs dropped between 25% and 50% in 12 patients, and 14 patients lost more than 10% of renal length. In 4 patients, a significant stenosis progressed to total occlusion. Overall, 17 patients (41%) had deterioration of renal function or loss of renal size that led to operation, and 1 patient required removal of a previously reconstructible kidney. Of the 17 patients in whom renal function deteriorated, 15 had acceptable control of blood pressure during the period of nonoperative observation. This experience suggests that progressive decline of renal function in medically treated patients with atherosclerotic RVD and RVH occurs despite medical blood pressure control.

The detrimental changes that may occur during medical therapy alone are often cited as supporting evidence for intervention for all renovascular lesions. It should be emphasized, however, that the only prospective angiographic data were obtained from patients with *proven* RVH (i.e., high-grade renal artery stenosis with severe hypertension and positive physiologic studies).[92] Accordingly, these data should not be applied to asymptomatic patients. Our indications for interventional management include all patients with severe, difficult-to-control hypertension.[55,58] This includes patients with complicating factors such as branch lesions and extrarenal atherosclerotic disease, including those with associated cardiovascular disease that would be improved by blood pressure reduction. Moreover, young patients whose hypertension is moderate, who have no associated end-organ disease, and who have an easily correctable atherosclerotic or dysplastic main renal artery lesions are also candidates for operative intervention. The chance of curing moderate hypertension is quite good in such patients, and it remains to be proved that medical blood pressure control is equivalent to the cure of hypertension. Finally, no evidence exists that age, type of renovascular lesion (whether atherosclerotic or dysplastic), duration of hypertension, or presence of bilateral lesions accurately estimate the likelihood of successful surgical management. Consequently, the presence or absence of these factors should not be used as determinants of intervention.

Operative Techniques

A variety of operative techniques have been used to correct renal artery stenoses. From a practical standpoint, three basic operations are most frequently used: aortorenal bypass, thromboendarterectomy, and reimplantation. Bypass is most versatile. Endarterectomy has particular application to artificial atherosclerosis, especially when renal-type arteries are involved. When the renal artery is sufficiently redundant, reimplantation is technically easiest and has particular application in children (Fig. 33-7).

Antihypertensive medications are reduced during the preoperative period to the minimum necessary for blood pressure control. Frequently, patients requiring large doses of multiple medications for control have significantly reduced requirements while hospitalized and on bed rest. If continued therapy is required, vasodilators (e.g., nifedipine) in combination with selective β-adrenergic blockers (e.g., atenolol) are the drugs of choice. There is little effect on hemodynamics when these agents are combined with anesthesia. If the patient's diastolic blood pressure exceeds 120 mm Hg, the pressure must be brought under control, and operative treatment must be postponed until this is accomplished. If blood pressure is difficult to control, we may transfer the patient to the intensive care unit, where intravenous nitroprusside therapy with continuous intra-arterial monitoring of blood pressure is instituted for 24 hours before operation. Similarly, if the patient has a significant history of heart disease, pulmonary artery wedge pressure and cardiac performance are monitored to maintain optimal cardiac hemodynamics and recognize and correct adverse changes before they become clinically significant.

Certain measures and maneuvers are applicable to almost all renal artery operations. Mannitol, 12.5 g, is administered intravenously early in the operation. Just before renal artery cross-clamping, heparin, 100 units/kg, is given intravenously, and systemic anticoagulation is verified by activated clotting time.

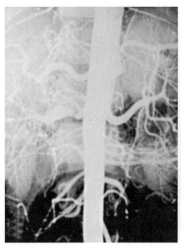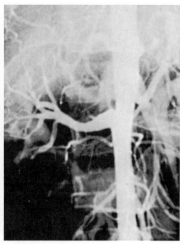

A   **B**

FIGURE 33-7 • Preoperative *(A)* and postoperative *(B)* arteriograms in a 5-year-old child who underwent right renal artery reimplantation.

Protamine is rarely required for the reversal of heparin at the end of the reconstruction.

MOBILIZATION AND DISSECTION

Through a midline xiphoid-to-pubis incision, the posterior peritoneum overlying the aorta is incised longitudinally, and the duodenum is reflected to the patient's right to expose the left renal artery (Fig. 33-8). By extending the posterior peritoneal incision to the left along the inferior border of the pancreas, an avascular plane behind the pancreas can be entered to expose the entire renal hilum on the left (Fig. 33-9).

This exposure is of special significance when distal lesions must also be managed. The left renal artery lies behind the left renal vein. In some cases, the vein can be retracted cephalad to expose the artery; in other cases, caudal retraction of the vein provides better access. Usually, the gonadal and adrenal veins, which enter the left renal vein, must be ligated and divided to facilitate exposure of the artery. Frequently, a lumbar vein enters the posterior wall of the left renal vein, and it can be avulsed easily unless special care is taken while mobilizing the renal vein. The proximal portion of the right renal artery can be exposed through the base of the mesentery by ligating two or more pairs of lumbar veins and retracting the left renal vein cephalad and the vena cava to the patient's right. However, the distal portion of the right renal artery is best exposed by mobilizing the duodenum and right colon medially (Fig. 33-10). Then the right renal vein is mobilized and usually retracted cephalad to expose the artery.

When bilateral renal artery lesions are to be corrected, and when correction of a right renal artery lesion or bilateral lesions is combined with aortic reconstruction, we modify these exposure techniques. First, we extend the base of the mesentery exposure to allow complete evisceration of the entire small bowel and the right and transverse portions of the colon; in this exposure, the posterior peritoneal incision begins with division of the ligament of Treitz and proceeds along the base of the mesentery to the cecum and then up the lateral gutter to the foramen of Winslow (Fig. 33-11). Second, we extend the incision to the left along the inferior border of the pancreas to enter a retropancreatic plane, thereby exposing the aorta to a point above the superior mesenteric artery. Through this modified exposure, simultaneous bilateral

renal endarterectomies, aortorenal grafting, or renal artery attachment to the aortic graft can be performed with wide visualization of the entire area.

One other technique that we sometimes use is to partially divide both diaphragmatic crura as they pass behind the renal arteries to their paravertebral attachment. By partially dividing the crura, the aorta above the superior mesenteric artery is easily visualized and can be mobilized for suprarenal cross-clamping.

AORTORENAL BYPASS

Three types of graft are usually available for aortorenal bypass: autologous saphenous vein, autologous hypogastric artery, and synthetic prosthesis. The decision of which graft to use depends on a number of factors. We use the saphenous vein preferentially. However, if it is small (<4 mm in diameter) or sclerotic, the hypogastric artery or a synthetic prosthesis may be preferable. A thin-walled, 6-mm polytetrafluoroethylene graft is satisfactory when the distal renal artery is of large caliber.

When an end-to-side renal artery bypass is used, the anastomosis between the renal artery and the graft is done first. Silastic slings can be used to occlude the renal artery distally. This method of vessel occlusion is especially applicable to this procedure. In contrast to vascular clamps, these slings are essentially atraumatic to the delicate renal artery. The absence of clamps in the operative field is also advantageous. Further, when tension is applied to the slings, they lift the vessel out of the retroperitoneal soft tissue for more accurate visualization.

The length of the arteriotomy should be at least three times the diameter of the renal artery to guard against late suture line stenosis. A 6-0 or 7-0 monofilament polypropylene suture material is employed with loop magnification.

After the renal artery anastomosis is completed, the occluding clamps and slings are removed from the artery, and a small bulldog clamp is placed across the vein graft adjacent to the anastomosis. The aortic anastomosis is then done. First, an ellipse of the anterolateral aortic wall is removed, and then the anastomosis is performed. If the graft is too long, kinking of the vein and subsequent thrombosis may result. If any element of kinking or twisting of the graft occurs

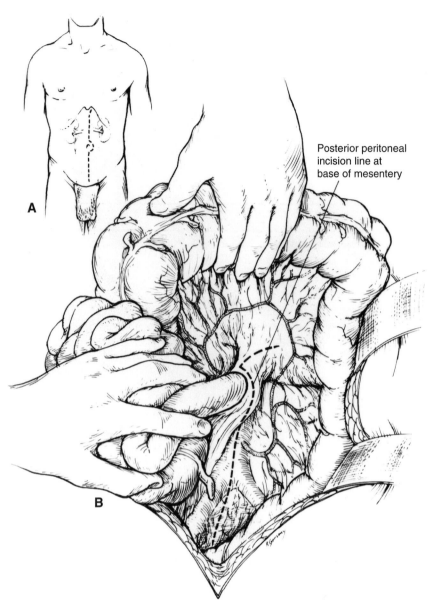

Posterior peritoneal incision line at base of mesentery

FIGURE 33–8 • *A*, Skin incision. *B*, Exposure of the aorta and left renal hilum through the base of the mesentery. Extension of the posterior peritoneal incision to the left, along the inferior border of the pancreas, provides entry to an avascular plane behind the pancreas. This allows excellent exposure of the entire left renal hilum as well as the proximal right renal artery. (From Benjamin ME, Dean RH: Techniques in renal artery reconstruction: Part I. Ann Vasc Surg 10: 306-314, 1996.)

after both anastomoses are completed, the aortic anastomosis should be taken down and redone after appropriate shortening or reorientation of the graft. In most instances, an end-to-end anastomosis between the graft and the renal artery provides a better reconstruction. This is especially true for combined aortorenal reconstruction. In this circumstance, the renal artery graft is attached to the Dacron aortic graft before its insertion. After the aortic graft is attached and flow is restored to the distal extremities, the renal artery can be transected and attached to the end of the saphenous vein graft without interrupting aortic flow.

THROMBOENDARTERECTOMY

Thromboendarterectomy is used only for atherosclerotic renal artery stenosis. It is not applicable in fibromuscular disease. Transaortic endarterectomy of bilateral main renal artery lesions has been strongly advocated by Wylie and colleagues (Fig. 33-12).[93] In this procedure, the proximal aortic clamp must usually be placed above the superior mesenteric artery. If it is placed below this artery, it seriously compromises the

exposure of the orifices of the renal arteries. Visualization of the distal end of the renal artery endarterectomy is facilitated by inversion of the renal artery into the aorta. Alternatively, a transrenal endarterectomy uses a transverse aortotomy, carrying the incision across the stenoses and into each renal artery. By this method, the entire endarterectomy can be performed under direct vision with Dacron patch closure.

EXTRA-ANATOMIC BYPASS

Extra-anatomic procedures have become increasingly popular as an alternative method of renal revascularization for high-risk patients.[94] We do not believe that these procedures are equivalent to direct reconstructions, but they are useful in a highly select subgroup of high-risk patients.

Hepatorenal Bypass

A right subcostal incision is usually used to perform the hepatorenal bypass. The hepatoduodenal ligament is incised, and the common hepatic artery both proximal and distal to the

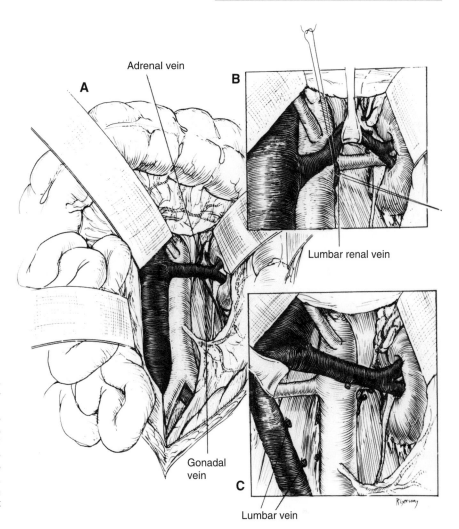

Adrenal vein

B

Lumbar renal vein

Gonadal
vein

Lumbar vein

C

FIGURE 33–9 • *A,* Exposure of the proximal renal arteries through the base of the mesentery. *B,* Mobilization of the left renal vein by ligation and division of the adrenal, gonadal, and lumbar renal veins allows exposure of the entire left renal artery to the hilum. *C,* Two pairs of lumbar vessels have been ligated and divided to allow retraction of the vena cava to the right, providing adequate exposure of proximal renal artery disease. (From Benjamin ME, Dean RH: Techniques in renal artery reconstruction: Part I. Ann Vasc Surg 10:306-314, 1996.)

gastroduodenal artery origin is encircled. Next, the descending duodenum is mobilized by Kocher's maneuver, the inferior vena cava is identified, the right renal vein is identified, and the right renal artery is encircled where it is found, either immediately cephalad or caudad to the renal vein (Fig. 33-13).

A greater saphenous vein graft is usually used to construct the bypass. The hepatic artery anastomosis of the vein graft can be placed at the site of the amputated stump of the gastroduodenal artery or proximal to this branch when it must be saved as a collateral for gut perfusion. After completion of this anastomosis, the renal artery is transected and brought anterior to the vena cava for anastomosis end to end to the graft.

Splenorenal Bypass

Splenorenal bypass can be performed through a midline or a left subcostal incision. The posterior pancreas is mobilized by reflecting the inferior border cephalad. When the retropancreatic plane has been entered, the splenic artery can be mobilized from the left gastroepiploic artery to the level of its branches. The left renal artery is exposed as described earlier. After the splenic artery has been completely mobilized, it is divided distally, spatulated, and anastomosed end to end to the transected renal artery (Fig. 33-14).

EX VIVO RECONSTRUCTION

Ex vivo management is necessary in patients with fibromuscular dysplasia and aneurysms or stenoses involving renal artery branches; patients with fibromuscular dysplasia, renal artery dissection, and branch occlusion; patients with congenital arteriovenous fistulas of renal artery branches requiring partial resection; and patients with degeneration of previously placed grafts to the distal renal artery. Several methods of ex vivo hypothermic perfusion and reconstruction are available. A midline xiphoid-to-pubic incision is used for most renovascular procedures and is preferred when autotransplantation of the reconstructed kidney or combined aortic reconstructions are to be performed. An extended flank incision made parallel to the lower rib margin and carried to the posterior axillary line is used for complex branch renal artery repairs and is our preferred approach for ex vivo reconstructions without autotransplantation. The ureter is always mobilized but left intact, and an elastic sling or noncrushing clamp is placed around it to prevent collateral perfusion, inadvertent rewarming, or continued blood loss through the ureteric collaterals.

After the kidney is mobilized and the vessels divided, the kidney is placed on the abdominal wall and perfused with a renal preservative solution. Continuous perfusion during the period of total renal ischemia is possible with complex

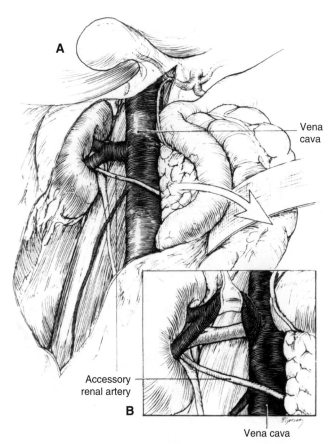

FIGURE 33–10 • *A,* Not uncommonly, an accessory right renal artery arises from the anterior aorta and crosses anterior to the vena cava. *B,* The right renal vein is typically mobilized superiorly for exposure of the distal right renal artery. (From Benjamin ME, Dean RH: Techniques in renal artery reconstruction: Part I. Ann Vasc Surg 10:306-314, 1996.)

perfusion pump systems and may be superior for prolonged renal preservation during storage periods. However, simple intermittent flushing with a chilled preservative solution provides equal protection during the shorter periods (2 to 3 hours) required for ex vivo dissection and complex renal artery reconstructions. For intermittent flushing, we refrigerate the preservative overnight, add the additional components (Table 33-6) immediately before use to make up 1 L of solution, and hang the chilled (5°C to 10°C) solution on an intravenous stand to provide gravitational perfusion pressure of at least 2 m. Five hundred milliliters of solution is flushed through the kidney immediately after its removal from the renal fossa. If arterial exposure is adequate, the vein may be left intact, controlled with an atraumatic clamp and a small venotomy made for the egress of perfusate. Regardless whether the vein is divided or left intact, as each anastomosis is completed, an additional 150 to 200 mL of solution is flushed through the kidney, a procedure that also shows any leaks at the suture line.

Surface hypothermia is used to maintain constant hypothermia during ex vivo renal artery reconstruction. Our method of surface hypothermia consists of the following steps. We place two 1-L bottles of normal saline solution in ice slush overnight. When we remove the kidney, we place it in a watertight plastic sheet from which excess saline solution can be suctioned away and place laparotomy pads over the

kidney, keeping it cool and moist by a constant drip of the chilled saline solution. With this technique, we can maintain renal core temperatures of 10°C to 15°C throughout the period of ischemia.

When both renal artery and renal vein have been divided, we do not believe that autotransplantation to the iliac fossa is necessary for most ex vivo reconstructions, even though it is an accepted method for reattachment of the ex vivo reconstructed renal artery. Autotransplantation of the reconstructed kidney to the iliac fossa was adapted from renal transplant surgeons, with no thought given to the significant difference between the two patient populations. Reduction in the magnitude of the operative exposure, manual palpation of the transplanted kidney, potential use of irradiation for episodes of rejection, and ease of removal when treatment of rejection has failed are all historical and practical reasons for placing the transplanted kidney into the recipient's iliac fossa, but none of these advantages apply to patients requiring ex vivo reconstruction.

Rather, the factors most important in this patient population are related to improving the predictability of permanent patency after revascularization. Because many ex vivo procedures are performed in relatively young patients, the durability of operation should be measured in terms of decades. For this reason, attaching the kidney to the iliac arterial system within or below sites that are highly susceptible to significant atherosclerotic occlusive disease subjects the repaired vessels to disease that may, in time, threaten their patency. Further, subsequent management of peripheral vascular disease may be complicated by the presence of the autotransplanted kidney. Finally, if the kidney is replaced in the renal fossa and the renal artery graft is properly attached to the aorta at a proximal infrarenal site, the result should mimic that of the standard aortorenal bypass and thus carry a high probability of technical success and long-term durability.

For replacement of the kidney in its original site, Gerota's capsule must be opened during mobilization. Before transection of the renal vein begins, a large vascular clamp is placed to partially occlude the vena cava where it is entered by the renal vein. An ellipse of vena cava containing the entrance site of the renal vein is then excised, and the kidney is removed for ex vivo perfusion and reconstruction (Fig. 33-15). When the distal renal artery–graft anastomoses are completed and the kidney is replaced in its bed, the ellipse of vena cava is reattached. This technique protects against stenosis of the renal vein anastomosis as a result of technical error. The renal artery graft is then attached to the aorta in the standard manner.

NEPHRECTOMY

Nephrectomy is a procedure that should be limited to a subgroup of patients with RVH in whom the kidney responsible for the hypertension has nonreconstructible vessels and negligible residual excretory function. In these circumstances, nephrectomy can be of benefit because it controls hypertension without diminishing overall excretory function. In all other circumstances in which significant residual excretory function is present, the price of nephrectomy (loss of functioning renal mass) is greater than the potential benefit. This extreme conservatism with regard to nephrectomy is based on the knowledge that more than 35% of patients with atherosclerotic lesions

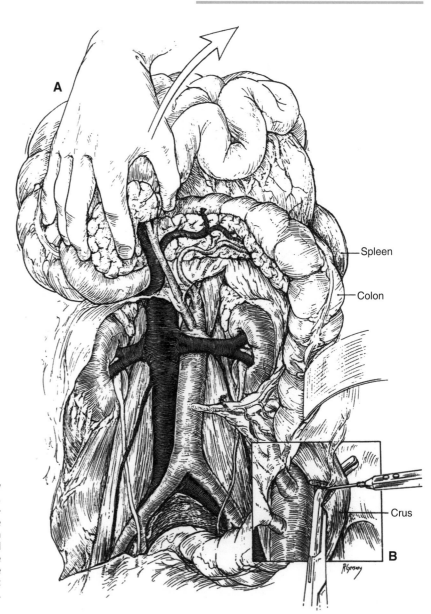

FIGURE 33–11 • *A,* For bilateral renal artery reconstruction combined with aortic repair, extended exposure can be obtained with mobilization of the cecum and ascending colon. The entire small bowel and right colon are then mobilized to the right upper quadrant and placed onto the chest wall. *B,* Division of the diaphragmatic crura exposes the origin of the mesenteric vessels. (From Benjamin ME, Dean RH: Techniques in renal artery reconstruction: Part I. Ann Vasc Surg 10:306-314, 1996.)

develop severe contralateral lesions during follow-up. Such lesions place the patient at risk for clinically severe renal failure and recurrent hypertension. This risk is even more important in children, because 50% of those who initially show a unilateral lesion subsequently develop contralateral disease.

Effect of Operation on Hypertension

Most of the controversy surrounding the role of open surgical treatment of RVH relates to the morbidity and mortality associated with operation, the frequency of technical failure, and the low rate of a favorable blood pressure response to operation. Certainly, the literature documents the fact that poorly performed operations in poorly selected patients seldom result in a blood pressure benefit. Current results of operative intervention in centers experienced with the management of RVD, however, underscore the high rate of long-term patency and benefit to both blood pressure and renal function.

Although our cumulative experience spans more than 40 years and includes the operative management of more than 1500 patients, a review of the results of a recent series of 500 consecutive atherosclerotic patients exemplifies current experience.[23] The evolution of the patient population seeking treatment is shown by comparing this group with 122 patients reported more than 30 years ago (Table 33-7).

Among patients with nonatherosclerotic RVD, 92% had a beneficial hypertension response, but only 43% were considered cured, a lower cure rate than that reported in the earlier surgical series.[30,95] This difference may be explained by the number of older patients, the number of patients with uncorrected contralateral lesions, and the duration of hypertension in many of these patients with nonatherosclerotic RVD. In contrast to the blood pressure results obtained in the entire group, patients younger than 45 years who had all anatomic renal artery lesions corrected and who had been hypertensive for less than 5 years had a cure rate of 68% and an improvement rate of 32%. This response rate is comparable with results from earlier reports.

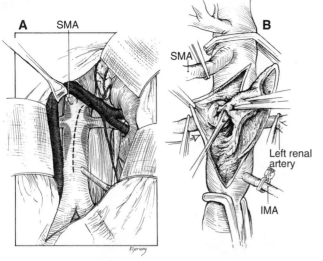

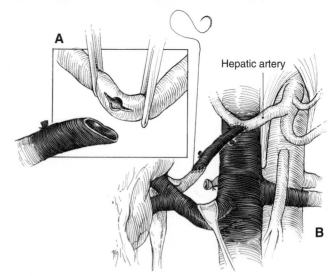

FIGURE 33–12 • Exposure for a longitudinal transaortic endarterectomy is through the standard transperitoneal approach. The duodenum is mobilized from the aorta laterally in standard fashion or, for more complete exposure, the ascending colon and small bowel are mobilized. *A,* Dotted line shows the location of the aortotomy. *B,* The plaque is transected proximally and distally, and with eversion of the renal arteries, the atherosclerotic plaque is removed from each renal ostium. The aortotomy is typically closed with a running 4-0 or 5-0 polypropylene suture. IMA, inferior mesenteric artery; SMA, superior mesenteric artery. (From Benjamin ME, Dean RH: Techniques in renal artery reconstruction: Part I. Ann Vasc Surg 10:306-314, 1996.)

FIGURE 33–13 • The reconstruction is completed using a saphenous vein interposition graft between the side of the hepatic artery *(A)* and the distal end of the transected right renal artery *(B).* (From Benjamin ME, Dean RH: Techniques in renal artery reconstruction: Part II. Ann Vasc Surg 10:409-414, 1996.)

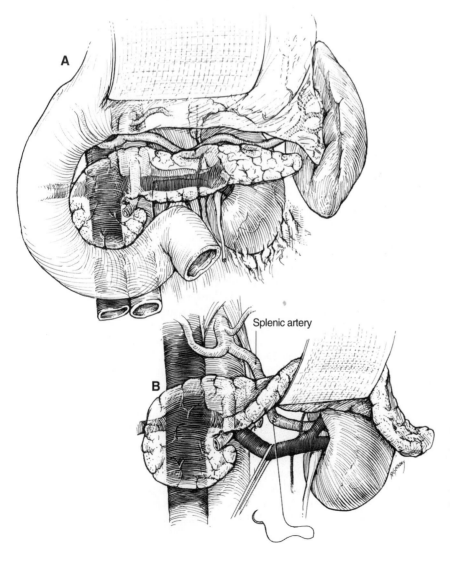

FIGURE 33–14 • *A,* Exposure of the left renal hilum in preparation for splenorenal bypass. The pancreas has been mobilized along its inferior margin and retracted superiorly. *B,* The transected splenic artery is anastomosed end to end to the transected left renal artery. A splenectomy is not routinely performed. (From Benjamin ME, Dean RH: Techniques in renal artery reconstruction: Part II. Ann Vasc Surg 10:409-414, 1996.)

TABLE 33–6	Electrolyte Solutions* for Ex Vivo Repair			
Composition		**Ionic Concentration**		
Component	Amount (g/L)	Electrolyte	Concentration (mEq/L)	**Additives to 930 mL of Solution at Time of Use**
K_2HPO_4	7.4	Potassium	115	50% dextrose: 70 mL
KH_2PO_4	2.04	Sodium	10	Sodium heparin: 2000 units
KCl	1.12	Phosphate (HPO_4^{2-})	85	
$NaHCO_3$	0.84	Phosphate ($H_2PO_4^-$)	15	
		Chloride	15	
		Bicarbonate	10	

*Electrolyte solution for kidney preservation supplied by Travenol Labs, Inc., Deerfield, Ill.

Although operation was accomplished in the nonatherosclerotic RVD group without death and with minimal morbidity (8.5%), the operative (3.1%) and follow-up (17.1%) mortality among 500 patients with atherosclerotic RVD was high. Blood pressure benefit (i.e., cured and improved) was observed in 85% of patients, although only 12% of patients were cured (i.e., normotensive off all medications). Patients who benefited from operation had an average decrease of almost 60 mm Hg systolic pressure and 25 mm Hg diastolic pressure (Table 33-8). However, only patients who were cured demonstrated a significant and independent increase in survival free from adverse cardiovascular events (Fig. 33-16).

Effect of Renal Revascularization on Renal Function

Little information is available regarding the incidence, prevalence, or natural history of ischemic nephropathy. Nevertheless, circumstantial evidence suggests that it may be a more common cause of progressive renal failure in the atherosclerotic age group (55 years or older) than previously recognized. In a 1988 report, 73% of end-stage renal disease patients were in the atherosclerotic age group.[96] In a report by Mailloux and colleagues,[97] a presumed renovascular cause of end-stage renal disease increased in frequency from 6.7% for the period 1978 to 1981 to 16.5% for the period 1982 to 1985. The median age at onset of end-stage renal disease for that group was the oldest of all groups, falling in the seventh decade of life.

To improve our understanding of ischemic nephropathy, we undertook a retrospective review of data collected during a 42-month period from 58 consecutive patients with ischemic nephropathy who were admitted to our center for operative management.[98] We examined the rate of decline in their renal function during the period before intervention and the impact of operation on their outcome. Their ages ranged from 22 years

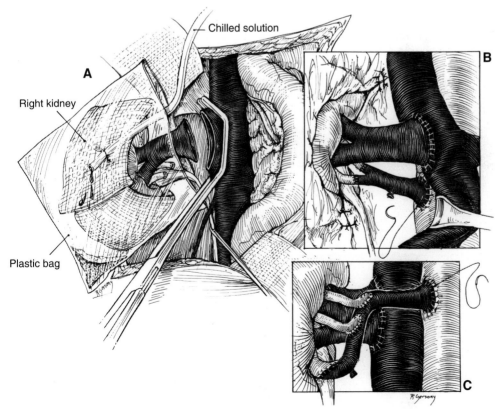

FIGURE 33–15 • Renal reconstruction requiring longer than 40 to 45 minutes of warm renal ischemia is facilitated by cold perfusion techniques. A, An ellipse of the vena cava containing the renal vein origin is excised by placement of a large, partially occluding clamp. After ex vivo branch repair, the renal vein can be reattached without risk of anastomotic stricture. B, The kidney is repositioned in its native bed after ex vivo repair. Gerota's fascia is reattached to provide stability to the replaced kidney. Arterial reconstruction can be accomplished via end-to-end anastomoses (as in B). C, Alternatively, reconstruction is occasionally performed with a combination of end-to-end and end-to-side anastomoses. If exposure is adequate, the renal vein can be controlled but left intact with a small venotomy for egress of perfusate. (From Benjamin ME, Dean RH: Techniques in renal artery reconstruction: Part II. Ann Vasc Surg 10: 409-414, 1996.)

TABLE 33–7	Comparison of Surgical Experience over Time	
	1961-1972	**1987-1999**
No. of patients	122	500
Mean age (yr)		
NAS RVD	33	38
AS RVD	50	65
Duration of hypertension (yr)		
NAS RVD	4.6	11.2
AS RVD	5.1	10.0
Renal artery disease (%)		
NAS RVD	35	21
AS RVD	65	79
Renal artery repair (%)		
Unilateral	80	59
Bilateral	20	41
Combined*	13	39
Ischemic nephropathy (%)		
Not dependent on dialysis	8	49
Dependent on dialysis	0	8
Graft failure (%)	16	3
Hypertension response (%)		
NAS RVD		
Cured	72[†]	43
Improved	24[†]	49
AS RVD		
Cured	53[†]	12
Improved	36[†]	73

*Combined aortic repair for occlusive or aneurysmal disease.
[†]Excluding technical failures.
AS, atherosclerotic; NAS, nonatherosclerotic; RVD, renovascular disease.
Data for 1961-1972 adapted from Foster JH, Dean RH, Pinkerston JA, et al: Ten years experience with the surgical management of renovascular hypertension. Ann Surg 177:755-766, 1973. Data for 1987-1999 from Hansen KJ, Staff SM, Sands RE, et al: Contemporary surgical management of renovascular disease. J Vasc Surg 16:319-333, 1992; Cherr GS, Hansen KJ, Craven TE, et al: Surgical management of atherosclerotic renovascular disease. J Vasc Surg 35:236-245, 2002.

to 79 years (mean, 69 years). Based on serum creatinine values, immediate preoperative estimated GFR ranged from 0 to 46 mL/minute (mean, 23.85 ± 9.76 mL/minute). Patients with at least three sequential measurements for the calculation of estimated GFR changes during the 6 months before operation ($n = 50$) and the first 12 months after operation ($n = 32$) were used to describe the preoperative rate of decline in estimated GFR and the impact of operation on this decrease in the operative survivors. In addition, comparative analyses of data from patients with unilateral versus bilateral lesions and patients classified as having improvement in estimated GFR versus no improvement after operation were performed. Comparison of the immediate preoperative and immediate postoperative estimated GFRs for the entire group showed significant improvement in response to operation (see Fig. 33-16). Likewise, the rate of deterioration in estimated GFR for the total group was improved after operation (Fig. 33-17). A similar improvement in the rate of deterioration in estimated GFR was seen in the subgroup of patients who had an immediate improvement in response to operation (Fig. 33-18).

From this review, we found that the site of disease (unilateral or bilateral), the anatomic status of the distal renal artery, and the rate of deterioration in renal function were significant predictors of a beneficial effect on renal function. Conversely, unilateral disease, absence of severe hypertension, and diffuse branch vessel occlusive disease were negative predictors of such benefit.

The data presented in this retrospective review argue that ischemic nephropathy is a rapidly progressive form of renal insufficiency. The effect of renal revascularization on renal function, however, was heterogeneous. Nevertheless, the frequency of both retrieval of renal function and slowing the rate of its deterioration during follow-up was gratifying and encourages continued study of the role of operation in properly selected patients.

Recently, we reviewed the functional response to operation in more than 200 consecutive hypertensive patients treated for ischemic nephropathy.[26] Overall, two thirds of

TABLE 33–8	Blood Pressure Response to Operation for Renal Artery Atherosclerosis in 472 Patients				
Response	**No. of Patients (%)**	**Preoperative Blood Pressure (mm Hg)**	**Postoperative Blood Pressure (mm Hg)**	**No. of Preoperative Medications**	**No. of Postoperative Medications**
Cured	57 (12)	195 ± 35 103 ± 22	$137 \pm 16*$ $78 \pm 9*$	2.0 ± 1.1	$0 \pm 0*$
Improved	345 (73)	205 ± 35 107 ± 21	$147 \pm 21*$ $81 \pm 11*$	2.8 ± 1.1	$1.7 \pm 0.8*$
Failed	70 (15)	182 ± 30 87 ± 13	$158 \pm 28*$ $82 \pm 12†$	2.0 ± 0.9	2.0 ± 0.9
All	472 (100)	201 ± 35 104 ± 22	$148 \pm 22*$ $81 \pm 11*$	2.6 ± 1.1	$1.6 \pm 0.9*$

*$P < 0.0001$ compared with preoperative value.
[†]$P = 0.001$ compared with preoperative value.
Blood pressure and medications are mean $\pm$ standard deviation.
From Cherr GS, Hansen KJ, Craven TE, et al: Surgical management of atherosclerotic renovascular disease. J Vasc Surg 35:236-245, 2002.

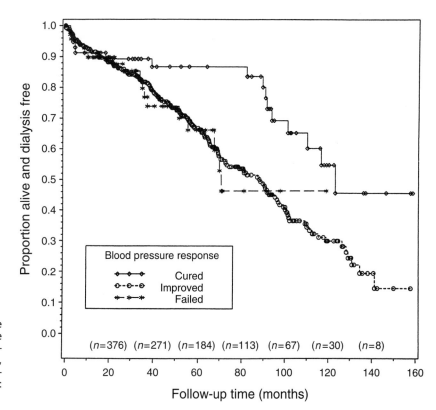

FIGURE 33–16 • Product limit estimates of time to death or dialysis according to blood pressure response to operation for atherosclerotic renovascular disease (N = 472). (From Cherr GS, Hansen KJ, Craven TE, et al: Surgical management of atherosclerotic renovascular disease. J Vasc Surg 35: 236-245, 2002.)

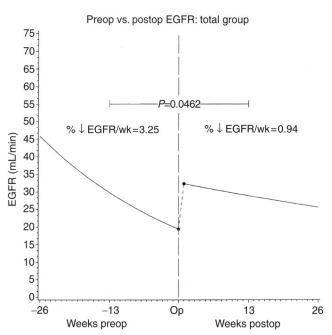

FIGURE 33–17 • Graphic depiction of the percentage deterioration of estimated glomerular filtration rate (EGFR) per week for the entire group during the 6 months before (n = 50) and after (n = 32) operation (Op). The immediate effect of operation on the EGFR is also depicted. The P values for differences are determined using the t test for unpaired data. Note the improvement in the slope of decline in EGFR after operation.

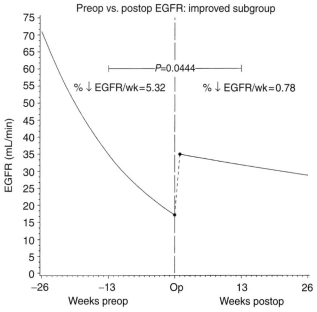

FIGURE 33–18 • Graphic depiction of the percentage deterioration of estimated glomerular filtration rate (EGFR) per week during the 6 months before (n = 23) and after (n = 25) operation (Op) in the improved group of patients (i.e., those who had at least a 20% improvement in EGFR following operation). The immediate effect of operation on EGFR in this improved group is also depicted. The P values for differences are determined using the t test for unpaired data. Note the improvement in the slope of decline in EGFR after operation in this group.

TABLE 33–9	Renal Function Response versus Preoperative Serum Creatinine (SCr)			
Renal Function Response	**Preop SCr 1.8-2.9 mg/dL**	**Preop SCr ≥ 3.0 mg/dL**	**Dialysis Dependent**	**Total**
Improved (%)	52	59	75	58
No change (%)	39	33	25	35
Worse (%)	9	8	—	7

From Hansen KJ, Cherr GS, Craven TE, et al: Management of ischemic nephropathy: Dialysis-free survival after surgical repair. J Vasc Surg 32:472-482, 2000.

patients had early improvement in excretory renal function (i.e., ≥20% increase in estimated GFR), and three quarters of dialysis-dependent patients were permanently removed from dialysis after operation (Table 33-9). When estimated survival was stratified to renal function response, only patients who were improved demonstrated increased dialysis-free survival. Patients who were unchanged or worse had nearly identical rates of follow-up death or eventual dialysis dependence (Fig. 33-19). Hypertension response in this subgroup with ischemic nephropathy had no apparent effect on survival (Fig. 33-20).

Our experience demonstrates the potential benefit of operation on both GFR and its rate of deterioration in a subset of patients. Nevertheless, the risk associated with operation is not inconsequential. This risk and the rate of survival must be placed in context with the probability of survival without operation. In a study of the duration of survival after the institution of dialysis, Mailloux and coworkers found that end-stage renal disease caused by uncorrected RVD was associated with the most rapid rate of death during follow-up.[97] In their study, patients with RVD had a median survival after the initiation of dialysis of only 27 months and a 5-year survival rate of only 12%. In our patients who progress to dialysis dependence, median survival has been 16.5 months.[26]

These findings equate with a death rate in excess of 20% per year. In this regard, we reported our experience with 20 patients who were dialysis dependent at the time of operation. No operative deaths occurred in this group, and 16 (80%) were rendered free of dialysis postoperatively.[99] Their life-table estimate of survival is shown in Figure 33-19. Survival in those rendered dialysis independent was excellent. Those not freed from dialysis by operation had a death rate during follow-up similar to those in Mailloux's group[97] who were not submitted to operation.

This experience underscores two important points. In the contemporary patient population with ischemic nephropathy, severe hypertension is the clinical characteristic favoring a correctable renovascular cause for renal insufficiency. However, renal function response after operation is the key determinant of dialysis-free survival. Only patients with an incremental increase in function are spared eventual dialysis. Although patients whose renal function is unchanged are frequently considered "preserved," these data suggest that such patients progress to death or dialysis dependence at a pace equivalent to that of patients who are worse after surgery. Most important, the results argue that a carefully controlled, prospective, randomized trial comparing operation with balloon angioplasty and medical therapy is necessary to confirm the value of operation in patients with controlled hypertension. Only through this method can we accurately clarify the role of intervention in dialysis-free survival among patients with ischemic nephropathy.

Late Follow-up Reconstructions

From our experience with the operative management of RVH, 1- to 23-year follow-up sequential angiography of 198 reconstructions is available for evaluation. Ten grafts developed suture line or midgraft stenoses requiring revision from 1 to 8 years after the initial operation (Fig. 33-21). Four patients had graft occlusions during follow-up and probably represent missed graft stenoses that progressed to occlusion. Three grafts required correction of aortic anastomotic false aneurysms in Dacron prostheses in two patients 8 and 20 years postoperatively. The remaining grafts (88%) had no untoward changes and continued patency during follow-up.

Five saphenous vein grafts and two hypogastric autografts underwent aneurysmal dilatation. Only one of these, a hypogastric autograft, required replacement (Fig. 33-22). The remaining six stabilized, and the patients remained cured of hypertension. Aneurysmal dilatation of autogenous grafts (vein or artery) has occurred only in young children in our experience. This suggests that the saphenous vein in young patients is particularly susceptible to this phenomenon. For this reason, we prefer the normal hypogastric artery as the

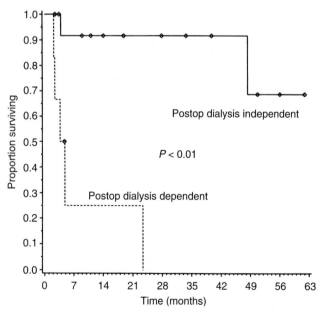

FIGURE 33–19 • Product limit estimate of patient survival according to dialysis status after operation for dialysis-dependent ischemic nephropathy (N = 20). (From Hansen KJ, Thomason RB, Craven TE, et al: Surgical management of dialysis-dependent ischemic nephropathy. J Vasc Surg 21:197-211, 1995.)

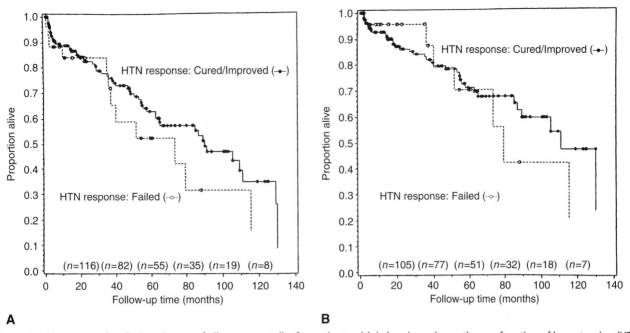

FIGURE 33–20 • *A,* Product limit estimates of all-cause mortality for patients with ischemic nephropathy as a function of hypertension (HTN) response to operation. *B,* Product limit estimates of cardiovascular or renal mortality for patients with ischemic nephropathy as a function of hypertension response to operation. Hypertension response did not affect the rate of death or cardiovascular death. (From Hansen KJ, Cherr GS, Craven TE, et al: Management of ischemic nephropathy: Dialysis-free survival after surgical repair. J Vasc Surg 32:472-482, 2000.)

conduit of choice for this group. In the two instances of autogenous arterial graft aneurysmal degeneration, fibromuscular dysplasia of the donor hypogastric artery was identified in retrospective microscopic evaluation.

Follow-up angiography and renal duplex sonography showed progression of mild to moderate contralateral RVD in 38% of patients. This is most important in children, as 7 of 15 with fibromuscular dysplasia had bilateral involvement.[56] In only three of these seven children was the contralateral disease evident at the time of initial evaluation and

operation; in the remaining four, the development and progression of contralateral disease were documented subsequently. This occurrence of contralateral stenosis has led us to perform nephrectomy in children only if blood pressure is uncontrollable and revascularization is impossible. Because the longest follow-up was only 10 years, the true incidence of subsequent contralateral disease in children is unknown.

Although the failure of operative repairs is infrequent, the dialysis-free survival of patients with failed repairs is decreased. Figure 33-23 compares patients requiring secondary

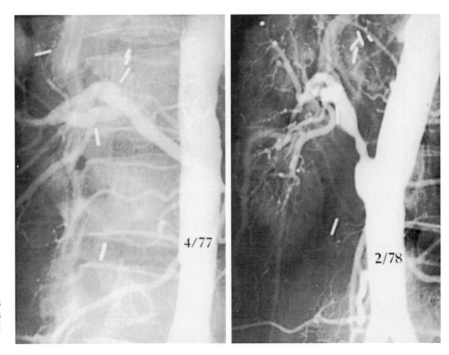

FIGURE 33–21 • Postoperative arteriograms showing fibrous narrowing of the saphenous vein graft secondary to subendothelial fibroblastic proliferation.

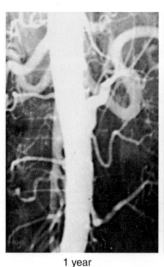
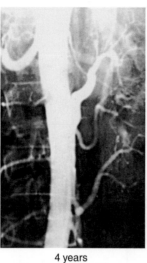
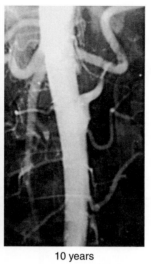

1 year   4 years   10 years

FIGURE 33–22 • Sequential follow-up arteriograms of a 10-year-old child who underwent a hypogastric autograft to the left renal artery and an iliac vein autograft to the superior mesenteric artery. Ultimately, both grafts required replacement.

intervention with patients having only primary renovascular repair. Patients requiring secondary intervention demonstrated a significant and independent increased risk of eventual dialysis dependence (relative risk [RR], 12.6; CI, 4.5 to 34.9; $P < 0.001$) and decreased dialysis-free survival (RR, 2.4; CI, 1.1 to 5.4; $P = 0.035$). Whether failed balloon angioplasty with or without stenting demonstrates similar associations with eventual dialysis dependence is not known.

Effect of Blood Pressure Response on Long-Term Survival

The rationale for the management of hypertension of any cause is to decrease long-term cardiovascular morbidity and improve event-free survival. Consequently, we reviewed the

outcome of 71 patients who underwent operative management of RVH 15 to 23 years previously.[100] Complete follow-up was available in 66 of the 68 patients who survived operation. Comparison of the initial blood pressure response after operation (1 to 6 months postoperatively) with the blood pressure status at the time of death or current date (up to 23 years later) showed that the effect of operative treatment is maintained over long-term follow-up (Fig. 33-24). In those patients who required repeat renovascular operation for recurrent RVH during follow-up, the majority of the operations were performed for the management of contralateral lesions that had progressed to functional significance (i.e., produced RVH).

Assessment of the effect of blood pressure response on late survival produced results that are not surprising. Although

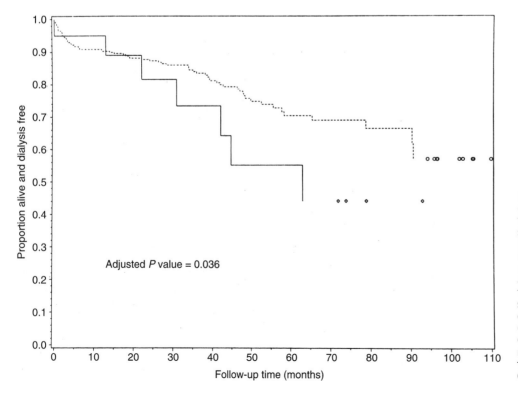

Adjusted *P* value = 0.036

FIGURE 33–23 • Product limit estimates of dialysis-free survival for 20 patients requiring a secondary renal artery operation (*solid line*) and 514 patients having primary renal artery repair only (*broken line*) with adjusted *P* values. Operative failure was associated with a significant and independent decrease in dialysis-free survival. (From Hansen KJ, Deitch JS, Oskin TC, et al: Renal artery repair: Consequences of operative failures. Ann Surg 227: 678-690, 1998.)

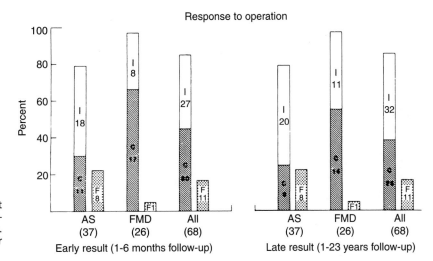

FIGURE 33–24 • Comparison of initial benefit and late blood pressure response in the different types of lesions treated in the 1960s. AS, arteriosclerotic lesion; FMD, fibromuscular dysplasia.

the subgroup of nonresponders was small, they experienced a significantly more rapid death rate during follow-up than did those patients who had a positive blood pressure response to operation (Fig. 33-25). This confirms the validity of the premise that inadequate management of RVH leaves the patient at higher risk of early death from cardiovascular events. The presence of angiographically diffuse atherosclerosis at the time of evaluation and operation was predictive of a more rapid rate of death during follow-up (Fig. 33-26).

This difference in subsequent death rate was present even though a comparison between patients with diffuse atherosclerotic disease and those with focal atherosclerotic disease was undertaken only in patients experiencing a significant blood pressure response. In view of the suggestion by some physicians that the presence of diffuse disease precludes a high rate of blood pressure response to operation, we stress

that no significant difference occurred in the frequency of response between the focal (80%) and diffuse (77%) groups in this study. In addition, although the presence of diffuse disease was associated with a more rapid death rate, it does not preclude the probability of a longer survival in this subgroup compared with a similar group of patients who either did not undergo operation or received no blood pressure benefit from such intervention. Further, if one considers that diffuse disease is only a later stage of focal disease, it is not surprising that the end point of clinically significant disease—namely, death from cardiovascular events—arrives sooner when one begins follow-up or removes a risk factor that causes its acceleration later in its natural history.

In contrast, the contemporary group of 500 atherosclerotic patients managed at our center did not demonstrate improved event-free survival in association with beneficial

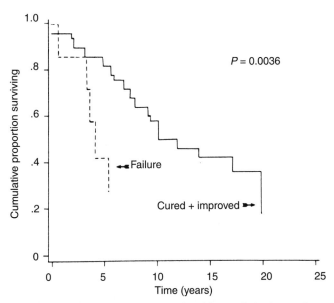

FIGURE 33–25 • Kaplan-Meier life-table analysis for patients treated in the 1960s, showing survival by response to operation in 37 arteriosclerotic patients (deaths from cardiovascular causes). These observations differ significantly from those in the contemporary population with atherosclerotic renovascular disease (see Fig. 33-16).

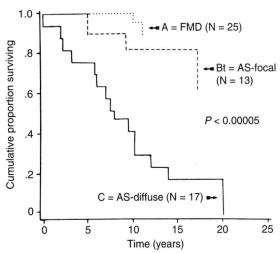

FIGURE 33–26 • Kaplan-Meier life-table analysis of survival of patients who benefited from operation by type and stage of disease, with 55 patients cured or improved from the 1960s (deaths from cardiovascular causes). AS-diffuse, diffuse atherosclerosis; AS-focal, focal atherosclerosis; FMD, fibromuscular dysplasia.

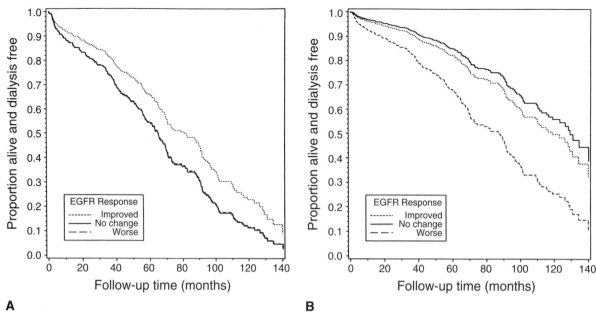

FIGURE 33–27 • Predicted dialysis-free survival according to postoperative renal function response for patients with a preoperative estimated glomerular filtration rate (EGFR) of 25 mL/min/m² (25th percentile) or 39 mL/min/m² (median value). The interaction between preoperative EGFR and renal function response for dialysis-free survival was significant and independent. (From Cherr GS, Hansen KJ, Craven TE, et al: Surgical management of atherosclerotic renovascular disease. J Vasc Surg 35:236-245, 2002.)

blood pressure response to operation (Fig. 33-27).[101] As noted earlier, only atherosclerotic patients cured (i.e., normotensive without medications) have demonstrated increased survival. Although there are a number of possible explanations for this observed difference, renal function response among contemporary patients demonstrated a significant and independent association with follow-up survival. Global renal disease treated with complete renal artery repair after rapid decline in renal function provided the best opportunity for improved glomerular filtration. Patients whose renal function was unimproved or worse remained at increased risk for eventual dialysis dependence. In the contemporary population, progression to dialysis dependence was the single strongest risk factor for follow-up death.

Percutaneous Transluminal Angioplasty

The introduction of PTA as an alternative interventional modality by Gruntzig and colleagues in 1978 led to a new era in the management of patients with renal artery stenosis.[102] This technique employs the principle of coaxial dilatation of the vessel by inflation of a balloon-tipped catheter introduced across the stenotic renal artery lesion. The stenotic lesion is disrupted and, by stretching the vessel wall itself, portions of the media are disrupted as well, leaving the vessel diameter greater than it was before dilatation. The increased luminal diameter is created primarily by disruption of the intima and the atherosclerotic or fibrodysplastic lesion and by dilatation of the less diseased arterial wall. Early reports of the results of this technique showed that stenotic renal arteries could often be dilated successfully, with immediate improvement in hypertension in patients with RVH.

By reviewing the reported experience with PTA and observations from the operative management of unsuccessful

PTA, one can formulate indications for the preferential use of each procedure in the treatment of RVH. Reported experience with PTA of medial fibroplasia shows early results similar to those of open surgical repair. Beneficial blood pressure responses have been reported to be as high as 100% after PTA in properly selected patients, and although vessel perforation, hemorrhage, and branch occlusions have been reported, their incidence is less than 5%.[103] One would anticipate that such complications would be most likely in patients with diffuse fibromuscular dysplasia affecting both the distal main renal artery and its branches. When the procedure is performed by an experienced interventionalist, the cure rate after PTA of fibromuscular dysplasia ranges from 37% to 51%.[104] We believe that fibromuscular dysplasia involving the branch level is best managed primarily by an open operative approach and that PTA should be reserved for the subgroup of patients with medial fibroplasia limited to the main renal artery.

Stenotic lesions occurring in children are usually discrete narrowings and therefore appear to be ideal for PTA. However, the stenotic area is commonly a congenital hypoplasia of the entire vessel wall and is composed predominantly of elastic tissue. When such a hypoplastic vessel is submitted to PTA, the original diameter returns after dilatation or, if the vessel has been overdistended, rupture of the vessel wall is likely. Therefore, we believe that PTA is an inappropriate method of intervention in children with renal artery stenosis and that lifelong success is best achieved by operative correction.

Finally, a review of series reporting results with PTA for atherosclerotic lesions illustrates the frequency of failure with this lesion as well. An early report by Miller and colleagues in 1985 noted that only 45% of ostial and mixed lesions were improved after 6 months[105]; Sos and colleagues reported only a 14% benefit rate when bilateral ostial lesions were treated.[104] These results show that PTA alone has little value in the treatment of this type of lesion; one must accept the

| TABLE 33–10 | Results after Primary Renal Artery Stent Placement for Ostial Atherosclerotic Renal Artery Stenosis |

Reference	No. of Patients with Ostial Lesions	No. of Patients with Renal Dysfunction	Renal Function Response (%)			Hypertension Response (%)			Restenosis (%)
			Improved	Unchanged	Worse	Cured	Improved	Failed	
Rees et al (1991)[107]	28	14	36	35	29	11	54	36	39
Hennequin et al (1994)[113]	7	2	0	50	50	0	100	0	43
Raynaud et al (1994)[116]	4	3	0	33	67	0	50	50	33
MacLeod et al (1995)[115]	22	13	15	85	N/R	0	31	69	20
van de Ven et al (1995)[120]	24	N/R	33	58	8	0	73	27	13
Blum et al (1997)[109]	68	20	0	100	0	16	62	22	17
Rundback et al (1998)[118]	32	32	16	53	31	N/R	N/R	N/R	26
Fiala et al (1998)[110]	21	9	0	100	0	53	N/R	47	65
Tuttle et al (1998)[119]	129	74	16	75	9	2	46	52	14
Gross et al (1998)[112]	30	12	55	27	18	0	69	31	12
Rodriguez-Lopez et al (1999)[117]	82	N/R	No change in mean SCr			13	55	32	26
van de Ven et al (1999)[121]	40	29	17	55	28	15	43	42	14
Baumgartner et al (2000)[108]	21	N/R	33	42	25	43		57	20
Giroux et al (2000)[111]	34	23	70	N/R	30	53	N/R	47	N/R
Lederman et al (2001)[114]	286	106	8	78	14	70		30	21
Totals	828	337	15	69	16	5	58	37	21

N/R, not reported; SCr, serum creatinine.

risks of cholesterol embolization, vessel thrombosis, and loss of renal function for only a minimal chance of prolonged benefit.

Endoluminal stenting of the renal artery as an adjunct to PTA was first introduced in the United States in 1988 as part of a multicenter trial.[106] During this same period, the Palmaz stent and Wallstent were being used in Europe. Currently, no stent has Food and Drug Administration approval for renal use in this country. However, the most common indications for their use appear to be (1) elastic recoil of the vessel immediately after angioplasty, (2) renal artery dissection after angioplasty, and (3) restenosis after angioplasty. With 263 patients entered, results from the multicenter trial demonstrated cure or improvement of hypertension in 61% of patients at 1 year. At follow-up of less than 1 year, angiographic restenosis occurred in 32.7% of patients.

Recognizing the poor immediate success of PTA alone for ostial atherosclerosis, some have advised the primary placement of endoluminal stents for these lesions.[107] Table 33-10 summarizes single-center reports on renal function and angiographic follow-up after treatment of ostial atherosclerosis by PTA in combination with endoluminal stents.[107-121] These studies differ with regard to criteria for ostial lesions, evaluation of the clinical response to intervention, and parameters for significant restenosis. Despite these differences, these cumulative results provide the best available estimates of early hypertension response, change in renal function, and primary patency. From these data, immediate technical success was observed in 99% of patients, and beneficial blood pressure response (cured and improved) was observed in 63%. However, only 15% of

patients with renal insufficiency demonstrated improved excretory renal function, while 16% of patients were worse after intervention. During angiographic follow-up ranging from 5.8 to 16.4 months, restenosis was observed in 21% of patients.

Based on available data, PTA with endoluminal stenting of ostial atherosclerosis appears to yield blood pressure, renal function, and anatomic results that are inferior to contemporary surgical results.[58,110,118] Moreover, no studies to date have examined long-term renal function results or dialysis-free survival after either primary or secondary PTA with or without stents. For these reasons, we believe that open operative repair remains the initial treatment of choice for patients with ostial renal artery atherosclerosis when hypertension is present in combination with renal insufficiency.

To summarize, experience with the liberal use of PTA has helped clarify its role as one of the therapeutic options in the treatment of RVH, but the data now accumulated argue for its selective application. In this regard, PTA of nonorificial atherosclerotic lesions and medial fibroplasia limited to the main renal artery yields results comparable with those of operation if performed by persons experienced in the technique. In contrast, the use of PTA for the treatment of congenital stenotic lesions, fibrodysplastic lesions involving renal artery branches, and ostial atherosclerotic lesions in association with ischemic nephropathy is associated with inferior results and with increased risk of complications. We believe that operation remains the initial treatment of choice for patients in these groups, although the type of interventional therapy for RVD must always be individualized.

REFERENCES

1. Goldblatt H: Studies on experimental hypertension. J Exp Med 59:346, 1934.
2. Bright R: Cases and observations illustrative of renal disease accompanied with the secretion of albuminous urine. Guy's Hosp Rep 1:388, 1836.
3. Traube L: Über den zusammenhang von herz und nieren krankheiten. In Hirschwald A (ed): Gesammelte Beiträge zur Pathologie und Physiologie, vol 2. Berlin, 1871, p 290.
4. Growitz P, Israel O: Experimentelle Untersuchung über den Zusammenhand zwischen Nierenerkrangung und Herzhypertrophie. Arch Pathol Anat 77:315, 1879.
5. Lewinski L: Über den Zusammenhang zwischen Nierenschrumpfung and Herzhypertrophie. Z Klin Med 1:561, 1880.
6. Katzenstein M: Experimenteller Beitrag zur Erkenntmis der bei Nephritis auftretenden Hypertrophie des linken Herzens. Virchows Arch 182:327, 1905.
7. Tigerstedt R, Bergman PG: Niere und Kreislauf. Skand Arch Physiol 8:223, 1898.
8. Senator H: Über die Beziehungen des Nierenkreislaufs zum arteriellen Blutdruck und über die Ursachen der Herzhypertrophie bei Nierenkrankheiten. Z Klin Med 72:189, 1911.
9. Leadbetter WFG, Burkland CE: Hypertension in unilateral renal disease. J Urol 39:611, 1938.
10. Smith HW: Unilateral nephrectomy in hypertensive disease. J Urol 76:685, 1956.
11. Freeman N: Thromboendarterectomy for hypertension due to renal artery occlusion. JAMA 157:1077, 1954.
12. DeCamp PT, Birchall R: Recognition and treatment of renal arterial stenosis associated with hypertension. Surgery 43:134-151, 1958.
13. Morris GC Jr, Cooley DA, Crawford ES, et al: Renal revascularization for hypertension: Clinical and physiological studies in 32 cases. Surgery 48:95-110, 1960.
14. Abelson DS, Haimovici H, Hurwitt ES, Seidenberg B: Splenorenal arterial anastomoses. Circulation 14:532-539, 1956.
15. Luke JC, Levitan BA: Revascularization of the kidney in hypertension due to renal artery stenosis. AMA Arch Surg 79:269-275, 1959.
16. Howard JE, Connor TB: Use of differential renal function studies in the diagnosis of renovascular hypertension. Am J Surg 107:58-66, 1964.
17. Stamey TA, Nudelman IJ, Good PH, et al: Functional characteristics of renovascular hypertension. Medicine (Baltimore) 40:347-394, 1961.
18. Page IH, Helmes OM: A crystalline pressor substance (angiotensin) resulting from the reaction between renin and renin activator. J Exp Med 71:29, 1940.
19. Bruan-Memendez E, Fasciolo JC, Lelois LF, et al: La substancia hypertensora de la sangre del rinon, isquemiado. Rev Soc Argent Biol 15:420, 1939.
20. Lentz KE, Skeggs LT Jr, Woods KR, et al: The amino acid composition of hypertensin II and its biochemical relationship to hypertensin I. J Exp Med 104:183-191, 1956.
21. Tobian L: Relationship of juxtaglomerular apparatus to renin and angiotensin. Circulation 25:189-192, 1962.
22. Bengtsson U, Bergentz SE, Norback B: Surgical treatment of renal artery stenosis with impending uremia. Clin Nephrol 2:222-229, 1974.
23. Cherr GS, Hansen KJ, Craven TE, et al: Surgical management of atherosclerotic renovascular disease. J Vasc Surg 35:236-245, 2002.
24. Dean RH, Lawson JD, Hollifield JW, et al: Revascularization of the poorly functioning kidney. Surgery 85:44-52, 1979.
25. Dean RH, Englund R, Dupont WD, et al: Retrieval of renal function by revascularization: Study of preoperative outcome predictors. Ann Surg 202:367-375, 1985.
26. Hansen KJ, Cherr GS, Craven TE, et al: Management of ischemic nephropathy: Dialysis-free survival after surgical repair. J Vasc Surg 32:472-481, 2000.
27. Libertino JA, Zinman L: Revascularization of the poorly functioning and nonfunctioning kidney. In Novick AC, Stratton RA (eds): Vascular Problems in Urologic Surgery. Philadelphia, WB Saunders, 1982, p 173.
28. Novick AC, Pohl MA, Schreiber M, et al: Revascularization for preservation of renal function in patients with atherosclerotic renovascular disease. J Urol 129:907-912, 1983.
29. Scoble JE, Maher ER, Hamilton G, et al: Atherosclerotic renovascular disease causing renal impairment—a case for treatment. Clin Nephrol 31:119-122, 1989.
30. Zinman L, Libertino JA: Revascularization of the chronic totally occluded renal artery with restoration of renal function. J Urol 118:517-521, 1977.
31. Morris GC Jr, Debakey ME, Cooley DA: Surgical treatment of renal failure of renovascular origin. JAMA 182:609, 1962.
32. Harrison EG Jr, McCormack LJ: Pathologic classification of renal arterial disease in renovascular hypertension. Mayo Clin Proc 46:161-167, 1971.
33. Folkow B: Physiological aspects of primary hypertension. Physiol Rev 62:347-504, 1982.
34. Pipinos II, Nypaver TJ, Moshin SK, et al: Response to angiotensin inhibition in rats with sustained renovascular hypertension correlates with response to removing renal artery stenosis. J Vasc Surg 28:167-177, 1998.
35. Swales JD, Abramovici A, Beck F, et al: Arterial wall renin. J Hypertens Suppl 1:17-22, 1983.
36. Appel RG, Bleyer AJ, Reavis S, Hansen KJ: Renovascular disease in older patients beginning renal replacement therapy. Kidney Int 48:171-176, 1995.
37. Textor SC, Tarazi RC, Novick AC, et al: Regulation of renal hemodynamics and glomerular filtration in patients with renovascular hypertension during converting enzyme inhibition with captopril. Am J Med 76:29-37, 1984.
38. Dzau VJ, Re R: Tissue angiotensin system in cardiovascular medicine: A paradigm shift? Circulation 89:493-498, 1994.
39. Hricik DE, Browning PJ, Kopelman R, et al: Captopril-induced functional renal insufficiency in patients with bilateral renal-artery stenoses or renal-artery stenosis in a solitary kidney. N Engl J Med 308:373-376, 1983.
40. Kobayashi S, Ishida A, Moriya H, et al: Angiotensin II receptor blockade limits kidney injury in two-kidney, one-clip Goldblatt hypertensive rats with special reference to phenotypic changes. J Lab Clin Med 133:134-143, 1999.
41. Eddy AA: Molecular insights into renal interstitial fibrosis. J Am Soc Nephrol 7:2495-2508, 1996.
42. Johnson RJ, Alpers CE, Yoshimura A, et al: Renal injury from angiotensin II-mediated hypertension. Hypertension 19:464-474, 1992.
43. Kim S, Ohta K, Hamaguchi A, et al: Contribution of renal angiotensin II type I receptor to gene expressions in hypertension-induced renal injury. Kidney Int 46:1346-1358, 1994.
44. Maschio G, Alberti D, Janin G, et al: Effect of the angiotensin-converting-enzyme inhibitor benazepril on the progression of chronic renal insufficiency: The Angiotensin-Converting-Enzyme Inhibition in Progressive Renal Insufficiency Study Group. N Engl J Med 334:939-945, 1996.
45. Scoble JE: Atherosclerotic nephropathy. Kidney Int Suppl 71:S106-S109, 1999.
46. Tucker RM: Frequency of surgical treatment for hypertension in adults at the Mayo Clinic from 1973 through 1975. Mayo Clin Proc 52:549-555, 1977.
47. Shapiro AP, Perez-Stable E, Scheib ET, et al: Renal artery stenosis and hypertension: Observations on current status of therapy from a study of 115 patients. Am J Med 47:175-193, 1969.
48. Choudhri AH, Cleland JG, Rowlands PC, et al: Unsuspected renal artery stenosis in peripheral vascular disease. BMJ 301:1197-1198, 1990.
49. Holley KE, Hunt JC, Brown AL Jr, et al: Renal artery stenosis: A clinical-pathologic study in normotensive and hypertensive patients. Am J Med 37:14-22, 1964.
50. Metcalfe W, Reid AW, Geddes CC: Prevalence of angiographic atherosclerotic renal artery disease and its relationship to the anatomical extent of peripheral vascular atherosclerosis. Nephrol Dial Transplant 14:105-108, 1999.
51. Schwartz CJ, White TA: Stenosis of renal artery: An unselected necropsy study. BMJ 5422:1415-1421, 1964.
52. Valentine RJ, Clagett GP, Miller GL, et al: The coronary risk of unsuspected renal artery stenosis. J Vasc Surg 18:433-439, 1993.
53. Wachtell K, Ibsen H, Olsen MH, et al: Prevalence of renal artery stenosis in patients with peripheral vascular disease and hypertension. J Hum Hypertens 10:83-85, 1996.
54. Wilms G, Marchal G, Peene P, Baert AL: The angiographic incidence of renal artery stenosis in the arteriosclerotic population. Eur J Radiol 10:195-197, 1990.
55. Hansen KJ, Edwards MS, Craven TE, et al: Prevalence of renovascular disease in the elderly: A population-based study. J Vasc Surg 36:443-451, 2002.
56. Lawson JD, Boerth R, Foster JH, Dean RH: Diagnosis and management of renovascular hypertension in children. Arch Surg 112:1307-1316, 1977.
57. Simon N, Franklin SS, Bleifer KH, Maxwell MH: Clinical characteristics of renovascular hypertension. JAMA 220:1209-1218, 1972.

58. Hansen KJ, Starr SM, Sands RE, et al: Contemporary surgical management of renovascular disease. J Vasc Surg 16:319-330, 1992.

59. Update on the 1987 Task Force Report on High Blood Pressure in Children and Adolescents: A working group report from the National High Blood Pressure Education Program. National High Blood Pressure Education Program Working Group on Hypertension Control in Children and Adolescents. Pediatrics 98:649-658, 1996.

60. Meier GH, Sumpio B, Black HR, Gusberg RJ: Captopril renal scintigraphy—an advance in the detection and treatment of renovascular hypertension. J Vasc Surg 11:770-776, 1990.

61. Hansen KJ, Tribble RW, Reavis SW, et al: Renal duplex sonography: Evaluation of clinical utility. J Vasc Surg 12:227-236, 1990.

62. Hansen KJ, O'Neil EA, Reavis SW, et al: Intraoperative duplex sonography during renal artery reconstruction. J Vasc Surg 14:364-374, 1991.

63. Hudspeth DA, Hansen KJ, Reavis SW, et al: Renal duplex sonography after treatment of renovascular disease. J Vasc Surg 18:381-388, 1993.

64. Motew SJ, Cherr GS, Craven TE, et al: Renal duplex sonography: Main renal artery versus hilar analysis. J Vasc Surg 32:462-469, 2000.

65. Barnes RW: Utility of duplex scanning of the renal artery. In Bergan JJ, Yao JST (eds): Arterial Surgery: New Diagnostic and Operative Techniques. Orlando, Fla, Grune & Stratton, 1988, pp 351-366.

66. Kohler TR, Zierler RE, Martin RL, et al: Noninvasive diagnosis of renal artery stenosis by ultrasonic duplex scanning. J Vasc Surg 4:450-456, 1986.

67. Norris CS, Pfeiffer JS, Rittgers SE, Barnes RW: Noninvasive evaluation of renal artery stenosis and renovascular resistance: Experimental and clinical studies. J Vasc Surg 1:192-201, 1984.

68. Taylor DC, Kettler MD, Moneta GL, et al: Duplex ultrasound scanning in the diagnosis of renal artery stenosis: A prospective evaluation. J Vasc Surg 7:363-369, 1988.

69. Hammer FD, Goffette PP, Malaise J, Mathurin P: Gadolinium dimeglumine: An alternative contrast agent for digital subtraction angiography. Eur Radiol 9:128-136, 1999.

70. Rieger J, Sitter T, Toepfer M, et al: Gadolinium as an alternative contrast agent for diagnostic and interventional angiographic procedures in patients with impaired renal function. Nephrol Dial Transplant 17:824-828, 2002.

71. Donadio C, Tramonti G, Lucchesi A, et al: Tubular toxicity is the main renal effect of contrast media. Ren Fail 18:647-656, 1996.

72. Larson TS, Hudson K, Mertz JI, et al: Renal vasoconstrictive response to contrast medium: The role of sodium balance and the renin-angiotensin system. J Lab Clin Med 101:385-391, 1983.

73. Rudnick MR, Goldfarb S, Wexler L, et al: Nephrotoxicity of ionic and nonionic contrast media in 1196 patients: A randomized trial. The Iohexol Cooperative Study. Kidney Int 47:254-261, 1995.

74. Barrett BJ: Contrast nephrotoxicity. J Am Soc Nephrol 5:125-137, 1994.

75. Hou SH, Bushinsky DA, Wish JB, et al: Hospital-acquired renal insufficiency: A prospective study. Am J Med 74:243-248, 1983.

76. Parfrey PS, Griffiths SM, Barrett BJ, et al: Contrast material-induced renal failure in patients with diabetes mellitus, renal insufficiency, or both: A prospective controlled study. N Engl J Med 320:143-149, 1989.

77. Harkonen S, Kjellstrand CM: Exacerbation of diabetic renal failure following intravenous pyelography. Am J Med 63:939-946, 1977.

78. Shieh SD, Hirsch SR, Boshell BR, et al: Low risk of contrast media-induced acute renal failure in nonazotemic type 2 diabetes mellitus. Kidney Int 21:739-743, 1982.

79. Weinrauch LA, Healy RW, Leland OS Jr, et al: Coronary angiography and acute renal failure in diabetic azotemic nephropathy. Ann Intern Med 86:56-59, 1977.

80. Solomon R, Werner C, Mann D, et al: Effects of saline, mannitol, and furosemide to prevent acute decreases in renal function induced by radiocontrast agents. N Engl J Med 331:1416-1420, 1994.

81. Merten GJ, Burgess WP, Gray LV, et al: Prevention of contrast-induced nephropathy with sodium bicarbonate: A randomized controlled trial. JAMA 291:2328-2334, 2004.

82. Tepel M, van der Giet M, Schwarzfeld C, et al: Prevention of radiographic-contrast-agent-induced reductions in renal function by acetylcysteine. N Engl J Med 343:180-184, 2000.

83. Cigarroa RG, Lange RA, Williams RH, Hillis LD: Dosing of contrast material to prevent contrast nephropathy in patients with renal disease. Am J Med 86:649-652, 1989.

84. Seeger JM, Self S, Harward TR, et al: Carbon dioxide gas as an arterial contrast agent. Ann Surg 217:688-697, 1993.

85. Goyen M, Ruehm SG, Debatin JF: MR-angiography: The role of contrast agents. Eur J Radiol 34:247-256, 2000.

86. Bonventre JV: Mechanisms of ischemic acute renal failure. Kidney Int 43:1160-1178, 1993.

87. Dean RH, Rhamy RK: Split renal function studies in renovascular hypertension. In Stanley JC, Ernst CB, Fry WJ (eds): Renovascular Hypertension. Philadelphia, WB Saunders, 1984, p 135.

88. Dean RH: Renovascular hypertension. Curr Probl Surg 22:1-67, 1985.

89. Vaughan ED Jr, Buhler FR, Laragh JH, et al: Renovascular hypertension: Renin measurements to indicate hypersecretion and contralateral suppression, estimate renal plasma flow, and score for surgical curability. Am J Med 55:402-414, 1973.

90. Stanley JC, Fry WJ: Surgical treatment of renovascular hypertension. Arch Surg 112:1291-1297, 1977.

91. Hunt JC, Strong CG: Renovascular hypertension: Mechanisms, natural history and treatment. Am J Cardiol 32:562-574, 1973.

92. Dean RH, Kieffer RW, Smith BM, et al: Renovascular hypertension: Anatomic and renal function changes during drug therapy. Arch Surg 116:1408-1415, 1981.

93. Wylie EJ, Perloff DL, Stoney RJ: Autogenous tissue revascularization technics in surgery for renovascular hypertension. Ann Surg 170:416-428, 1969.

94. Moncure AC, Brewster DC, Darling RC, et al: Use of the splenic and hepatic arteries for renal revascularization. J Vasc Surg 3:196-203, 1986.

95. Foster JH, Dean RH, Pinkerton JA, Rhamy RK: Ten years experience with the surgical management of renovascular hypertension. Ann Surg 177:755-766, 1973.

96. Eggers PW: Effect of transplantation on the Medicare end-stage renal disease program. N Engl J Med 318:223-229, 1988.

97. Mailloux LU, Bellucci AG, Mossey RT, et al: Predictors of survival in patients undergoing dialysis. Am J Med 84:855-862, 1988.

98. Dean RH, Tribble RW, Hansen KJ, et al: Evolution of renal insufficiency in ischemic nephropathy. Ann Surg 213:446-455, 1991.

99. Hansen KJ, Thomason RB, Craven TE, et al: Surgical management of dialysis-dependent ischemic nephropathy. J Vasc Surg 21:197-209, 1995.

100. Dean RH, Krueger TC, Whiteneck JM, et al: Operative management of renovascular hypertension: Results after a follow-up of fifteen to twenty-three years. J Vasc Surg 1:234-242, 1984.

101. Hansen KJ, Deitch JS, Oskin TC, et al: Renal artery repair: Consequence of operative failures. Ann Surg 227:678-689, 1998.

102. Gruntzig A, Kuhlmann U, Vetter W, et al: Treatment of renovascular hypertension with percutaneous transluminal dilatation of a renal-artery stenosis. Lancet 1:801-802, 1978.

103. Tegtmeyer CJ, Kellum CD, Ayers C: Percutaneous transluminal angioplasty of the renal artery: Results and long-term follow-up. Radiology 153:77-84, 1984.

104. Sos TA, Pickering TG, Sniderman K, et al: Percutaneous transluminal renal angioplasty in renovascular hypertension due to atheroma or fibromuscular dysplasia. N Engl J Med 309:274-279, 1983.

105. Miller GA, Ford KK, Braun SD, et al: Percutaneous transluminal angioplasty vs surgery for renovascular hypertension. AJR Am J Roentgenol 144:447-450, 1985.

106. Rees CR: Renovascular interventions. Paper presented at the 21st Annual Meeting of the Society of Cardiovascular and Interventional Radiology, 1996.

107. Rees CR, Palmaz JC, Becker GJ, et al: Palmaz stent in atherosclerotic stenoses involving the ostia of the renal arteries: Preliminary report of a multicenter study. Radiology 181:507-514, 1991.

108. Baumgartner I, von Aesch K, Do DD, et al: Stent placement in ostial and nonstial atherosclerotic renal arterial stenoses: A prospective follow-up study. Radiology 216:498-505, 2000.

109. Blum U, Krumme B, Flugel P, et al: Treatment of ostial renal-artery stenoses with vascular endoprostheses after unsuccessful balloon angioplasty. N Engl J Med 336:459-465, 1997.

110. Fiala LA, Jackson MR, Gillespie DL, et al: Primary stenting of atherosclerotic renal artery ostial stenosis. Ann Vasc Surg 12:128-133, 1998.

111. Giroux MF, Soulez G, Therasse E, et al: Percutaneous revascularization of the renal arteries: Predictors of outcome. J Vasc Interv Radiol 11:713-720, 2000.

112. Gross CM, Kramer J, Waigand J, et al: Ostial renal artery stent placement for atherosclerotic renal artery stenosis in patients with coronary artery disease. Cathet Cardiovasc Diagn 45:1-8, 1998.

113. Hennequin LM, Joffre FG, Rousseau HP, et al: Renal artery stent placement: Long-term results with the Wallstent endoprosthesis. Radiology 191:713-719, 1994.

114. Lederman RJ, Mendelsohn FO, Santos R, et al: Primary renal artery stenting: Characteristics and outcomes after 363 procedures. Am Heart J 142:314-323, 2001.

115. MacLeod M, Taylor AD, Baxter G, et al: Renal artery stenosis managed by Palmaz stent insertion: Technical and clinical outcome. J Hypertens 13:1791-1795, 1995.
116. Raynaud AC, Beyssen BM, Turmel-Rodrigues LE, et al: Renal artery stent placement: Immediate and midterm technical and clinical results. J Vasc Interv Radiol 5:849-858, 1994.
117. Rodriguez-Lopez JA, Werner A, Ray LI, et al: Renal artery stenosis treated with stent deployment: Indications, technique, and outcome for 108 patients. J Vasc Surg 29:617-624, 1999.
118. Rundback JH, Gray RJ, Rozenblit G, et al: Renal artery stent placement for the management of ischemic nephropathy. J Vasc Interv Radiol 9:413-420, 1998.
119. Tuttle KR, Chouinard RF, Webber JT, et al: Treatment of atherosclerotic ostial renal artery stenosis with the intravascular stent. Am J Kidney Dis 32:611-622, 1998.
120. van de Ven PJ, Beutler JJ, Kaatee R, et al: Transluminal vascular stent for ostial atherosclerotic renal artery stenosis. Lancet 346:672-674, 1995.
121. van de Ven PJ, Kaatee R, Beutler JJ, et al: Arterial stenting and balloon angioplasty in ostial atherosclerotic renovascular disease: A randomised trial. Lancet 353:282-286, 1999.

Questions

1. Which test is most sensitive for the identification of all hypertensive patients who might have renovascular hypertension?
   (a) Isotope renography
   (b) Rapid-sequence intravenous pyelography
   (c) Arteriography
   (d) Peripheral plasma renin activity

2. Which finding is most accurate in confirming the presence of renovascular hypertension?
   (a) Demonstration of collaterals by renal arteriography
   (b) Lateralization (1.5:1) of renal venous renin assays
   (c) Absence of function on rapid-sequence intravenous pyelography
   (d) Elevation of peripheral plasma renin activity
   (e) Presence of severe renal artery stenosis in a patient with hypertension

3. What endogenous pressor substance causes elevation of blood pressure in patients with renovascular hypertension?
   (a) Angiotensinogen
   (b) Renin
   (c) Angiotensin I
   (d) Prostaglandin E$_2$
   (e) Atrial natriuretic factor

4. Which of the following factors is most predictive of renal function retrieval by renal revascularization?
   (a) Low volume with hypoconcentration of creatinine in urine from the affected kidney
   (b) Normal intrarenal vessels on arteriography
   (c) Hyperconcentration of nonreabsorbable solutes in the urine of the affected kidney
   (d) Normal glomeruli and tubules on microscopic evaluation of renal biopsy
   (e) None of the above

5. Which operative technique is never an acceptable method for treatment of an orificial renal artery occlusion?
   (a) Thromboendarterectomy
   (b) Saphenous vein aortorenal bypass
   (c) Synthetic graft aortorenal bypass
   (d) Renal artery reimplantation
   (e) None of the above

6. In terms of long-term durability, which material is best for renal revascularization in children?
   (a) Normal saphenous vein
   (b) Expanded polytetrafluoroethylene
   (c) Normal hypogastric artery
   (d) Polyester
   (e) None of the above

7. What is the apparent incidence of progressive loss of renal function in kidneys of patients treated medically for renovascular hypertension secondary to atherosclerotic renal artery stenosis?
   (a) Less than 10%
   (b) 10% to 20%
   (c) Greater than 30%
   (d) Greater than 60%
   (e) Greater than 80%

8. What technical success rate is acceptable when performing renal revascularization?
   (a) Less than 50%
   (b) 50% to 70%
   (c) 70% to 80%
   (d) 80% to 90%
   (e) Greater than 95%

9. Which factor most frequently determines the likelihood of long-term maintenance of initially successful blood pressure reduction by operative management of renovascular hypertension?
   (a) Graft material used for aortorenal bypass
   (b) Progression of contralateral disease
   (c) Development of stenosis of graft anastomosis
   (d) Development of new lesions beyond the bypass in the kidney operated on
   (e) None of the above

10. What is the most important determinant of dialysis-free survival following operative treatment for ischemic nephropathy?
    (a) Blood pressure response
    (b) Renal function response
    (c) Number of functioning kidneys
    (d) Failure of operative renal artery repair
    (e) b and d

Answers

1. c	2. b	3. e	4. c	5. e
6. c	7. c	8. e	9. b	10. e

34

Lewis B. Schwartz • James F. McKinsey •
Brian Funaki • Bruce L. Gewertz

Visceral Ischemic Syndromes

Although the causal relationship between acute mesenteric vascular occlusion and intestinal gangrene had been known for centuries, it was not until 1895 that the first successful case of preoperative recognition and treatment by intestinal resection was reported by Elliott.[1] Recognition of the chronic form soon followed, with the term *angina abdominis* applied by Goodman to illustrate the similarities to the newly described *angina pectoris*.[2] Indisputable evidence was provided in 1936 by Dunphy,[3] a surgical resident at the Peter Bent Brigham Hospital in Boston, who described the clinical course of a 47-year-old man with weight loss and periumbilical pain out of proportion to the findings on physical examination. The patient died suddenly in the hospital, and postmortem examination revealed chronic mesenteric disease with fresh thrombus completely occluding the celiac trunk. Dunphy reviewed 12 other deaths from mesenteric vascular occlusion and found an antecedent history of chronic recurrent abdominal pain in seven.

The first successful reports of mesenteric revascularization appeared in 1958.[4] In that year, Shaw and Maynard from the Massachusetts General Hospital reported two cases of superior mesenteric artery (SMA) thrombosis superimposed on atherosclerotic occlusive disease. Both patients were treated by SMA thromboendarterectomy and survived. The surgeons made the astute observation that although the responsible atherosclerotic lesions involved all three mesenteric arteries, they were confined to the proximal segments, such that vascular reconstruction was technically feasible.[4]

Since that time, intestinal ischemic disorders have been recognized as uncommon but clinically important causes of abdominal pain. Although their incidence is estimated at only a few cases per 100,000 population, their lethal nature requires vigilance and a high index of clinical suspicion to avoid catastrophe. This chapter reviews the pathophysiology, clinical presentation, and treatment of intestinal ischemic disorders.

Vascular Anatomy

The mesenteric circulation consists primarily of three branches of the abdominal aorta (Fig. 34-1): the celiac axis, the SMA, and the inferior mesenteric artery (IMA).

Their multiple branch points and interconnections form such a rich anastomotic network that compromise of two of the three major arteries is usually required for the development of chronic ischemic symptoms. Knowledge of the normal and variant anatomy is essential for surgical diagnosis and revascularization.

CELIAC AXIS

The celiac axis supplies the stomach, liver, spleen, portions of the pancreas, and the proximal duodenum. It originates from the ventral portion of the abdominal aorta, near the level of T-12 to L-1, between the diaphragmatic crura. Its origin is encased in the median arcuate ligament, a dense, fibrous portion of the central posterior diaphragm draped across the aortic hiatus. In most patients, the celiac axis branches soon after its origin into the common hepatic, splenic, and left gastric arteries. In 1% of cases, the SMA arises from the celiac axis as well, forming a common celiomesenteric trunk.

The hepatic artery is usually the first branch of the celiac axis. It may also arise from the SMA (the so-called replaced right hepatic artery) in about 12% of cases. Additional variants include the replaced common hepatic artery (about 2.5%) and direct origin of the common hepatic artery from the aorta (about 2%). The common hepatic artery gives rise to the right gastric artery and the gastroduodenal artery, which further divides into the right gastroepiploic and superior pancreaticoduodenal arteries. The remaining proper hepatic artery gives rise to the cystic, right hepatic, and left hepatic arteries, which serve the gallbladder, the right and caudate hepatic lobes, and the middle and left hepatic lobes, respectively.

The second branch of the celiac axis is the splenic artery. Its first named branch is the dorsal pancreatic artery, supplying the posterior body and tail of the pancreas. Just before entering the splenic hilum, the splenic artery gives rise to the left gastroepiploic artery and multiple short gastric arteries, providing blood flow to the gastric fundus.

The final branch of the celiac axis is the left gastric artery. It courses cephalad and to the left to supply the gastric cardia and fundus along the lesser curvature of the stomach, joining centrally with the right gastric artery from the hepatic artery.

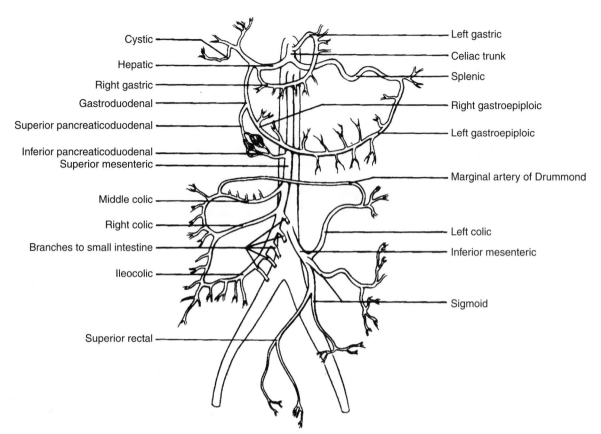

FIGURE 34–1 • The mesenteric circulation. (From Schwartz LB, Davis RD Jr, Heinle JS, et al: The vascular system. In Lyerly HK, Gaynor JW Jr [eds]: The Handbook of Surgical Intensive Care, 3rd ed. St. Louis, Mosby Year Book, 1992, p 287.)

In approximately 12% of the population, the left hepatic artery originates from the left gastric artery.

SUPERIOR MESENTERIC ARTERY

The SMA arises from the aorta just distal to the celiac axis at the level of L-1 to L-2. It passes behind the neck of the pancreas, in front of the uncinate process, and over the third portion of the duodenum. Its first branch, the inferior pancreaticoduodenal artery, courses superiorly to join the superior pancreaticoduodenal artery (from the gastroduodenal) and forms the most proximal collateral pathway with the celiac axis. The central branches of the SMA supply the midgut from the ligament of Treitz to the midtransverse colon. These include the middle colic (serving the proximal two thirds of the transverse colon), right colic (mid- and distal ascending colon), and ileocolic (distal ileum, cecum, appendix, and proximal ascending colon).

INFERIOR MESENTERIC ARTERY

The IMA arises from the left side of the aorta 8 to 10 cm distal to the SMA at the level of L-3. It travels caudad and to the left before dividing into the left colic and sigmoid arteries. The IMA supplies the distal third of the transverse colon, the descending and sigmoid colons, and the proximal rectum. It has anastomotic communications with the left branch of the middle colic from the SMA and with portions of the middle and inferior rectal arteries from the internal iliac.

COLLATERAL CIRCULATION

The mesenteric circulation has a redundant collateral network that serves to maintain perfusion even with compromise of the proximal main channels. The celiac axis and SMA communicate primarily via the superior and inferior pancreaticoduodenal arteries (via the gastroduodenal artery). The SMA and IMA communicate via the centrally located arch of Riolan (often referred to as the meandering mesenteric artery), as well as by the multiple communications at the periphery of the colon called the marginal arteries of Drummond. In addition to these collateral pathways, muscular branches of the aorta may contribute to intestinal perfusion, including the lumbar intercostal arteries, internal mammary arteries (via the deep epigastric arteries), middle sacral artery, and internal iliac arteries (via collaterals between the inferior and superior rectal arteries). Because of this plentiful collateral network, it is understandable that in most instances of gradual occlusion, at least two of the three major mesenteric orifices must be blocked to produce the clinical syndromes of chronic intestinal ischemia. In contrast, sudden occlusion of one widely patent vessel can cause acute ischemia because collaterals may be underdeveloped.

Acute Ischemia

PATHOPHYSIOLOGY

There are four primary causes of acute mesenteric ischemia (AMI): embolization to the SMA (roughly 50% of all cases), thrombosis of a preexisting atherosclerotic lesion at the origin of the vessel (20%), nonocclusive mesenteric ischemia (20%), and mesenteric venous thrombosis (10%).[5,6] In earlier series, the phenomenon of nonocclusive mesenteric ischemia was not well appreciated and was frequently misdiagnosed as acute venous occlusion. For example, Cokkinis reported in 1935 that acute mesenteric venous thrombosis accounted for the majority of cases of AMI.[7]

Other unusual arteriopathies, such as Takayasu's arteritis, fibromuscular dysplasia, and polyarteritis nodosa, may first present with intestinal ischemia. Isolated dissections of the SMA also have been reported,[8] although the more common mechanism is extension of dissections of the descending thoracic aorta into the SMA and celiac axis.[9,10]

If untreated, intestinal ischemia commonly leads to intestinal infarction. Tissue loss may result from both hypoxia during flow interruption and reperfusion injury once intestinal arterial blood flow is restored. Reperfusion injury is principally mediated by activation of the enzyme xanthine oxidase and the recruitment and activation of circulating polymorphonuclear neutrophils (PMNs).[11,12] In the presence of oxygen and hypoxanthine (a by-product of adenosine triphosphate metabolism), xanthine oxidase produces oxygen-derived free radicals that cause severe local tissue injury through lipid peroxidation, membrane disruption, and increased microvascular permeability.[13] PMNs are attracted to reperfused tissue by the local secretion of cytokines (tumor necrosis factor-α, interleukin-1, platelet-derived growth factor) by ischemic endothelium.[14-16] Subsequent rolling, adherence, and activation of the PMNs in the microcirculation result in the secretion of myeloperoxidase, collagenases, and elastases that can further injure the already ischemic and vulnerable tissue.[17-19] Activation of the inflammatory cascade may also have systemic effects, with cardiac, pulmonary, and other organ system dysfunction.[20]

ACUTE MESENTERIC ARTERIAL EMBOLISM

Most mesenteric arterial emboli originate from left atrial or ventricular mural thrombi or cardiac valvular lesions. These thrombi are usually associated with cardiac dysrhythmias such as atrial fibrillation or hypokinetic regions from previous myocardial infarctions. The majority of mesenteric emboli lodge in the SMA because of its high basal flow and near-parallel course to the abdominal aorta. Only 15% of SMA emboli remain impacted at the origin of the vessel. The majority of emboli progress distally 3 to 10 cm to the tapered segment of the SMA just past the origin of the middle colic artery (Fig. 34-2). A substantial fraction (10% to 15%) of mesenteric emboli are associated with concurrent emboli to another arterial bed.[21] Intestinal ischemia due to embolic arterial occlusion can be compounded by reactive mesenteric vasoconstriction, which further reduces collateral flow and aggravates the ischemic insult.

ACUTE MESENTERIC ARTERIAL THROMBOSIS

Thrombosis of the SMA or the celiac axis is usually associated with preexisting arterial lesions. When carefully questioned, many of these patients have histories consistent with chronic mesenteric ischemia (CMI), including postprandial pain, weight loss, "food fear," bloating, and early satiety. By far, the

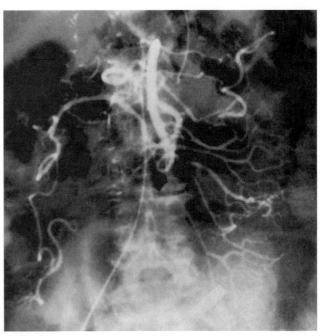

FIGURE 34–2 • Anteroposterior view of the aorta revealing embolic occlusion of the proximal superior mesenteric artery (SMA). Note the normal-appearing proximal jejunal arterial branches and then an abrupt cutoff of the SMA. (From McKinsey JF, Gewertz BL: Acute mesenteric ischemia. Surg Clin North Am 77:307-318, 1997.)

most common underlying lesion is an atherosclerotic plaque that slowly progresses to a critical stenosis over years, until the residual lumen suddenly thromboses during a period of low flow. Unlike embolic occlusions, thrombosis of the SMA generally occurs flush with the aortic origin of the vessel.

As noted previously, an unusual cause of AMI is aortic dissection involving the origins of the visceral vessels. The intimal flap of the dissection can exclude, compress, or extend into the visceral vessels, resulting in acute thrombosis. The symptoms of bowel ischemia may be masked by the pain associated with the aortic dissection, leading to a delay in diagnosis and treatment. AMI following coronary artery bypass grafts is very rare but highly lethal, with mortality rates as high as 70%. As would be expected, ischemia occurs in patients with severely stenotic mesenteric vessels that occlude during the nonpulsatile perfusion of extracorporeal bypass.[22,23]

NONOCCLUSIVE MESENTERIC ISCHEMIA

Mesenteric ischemia unassociated with anatomic arterial or venous obstruction can occur during periods of low cardiac output. Such low-flow states can result from cardiac failure, sepsis, or administration of α-adrenergic agents or digitalis compounds. Although less common, mesenteric vasospasm can also follow elective revascularization procedures for chronic SMA occlusion, in which case vasoconstriction of small and medium-size vessels is precipitated by early enteral feeding.[24] The older mean age of the population has produced a group of people with severe medical problems at risk for this type of mesenteric ischemia. The diagnosis is made at the time of angiography. Radiographic criteria suggesting the diagnosis include (1) narrowing of the origins of multiple branches of the SMA; (2) alternate dilatation and narrowing of the intestinal branches—the "string-of-sausages" sign; (3) spasm of the mesenteric arcades; and (4) impaired filling of the intramural vessels.[25] The mortality of this specific subset of patients is relatively high regardless of treatment, owing to the serious underlying medical conditions and the frequent delay in diagnosis.[26]

MESENTERIC VENOUS THROMBOSIS

Mesenteric venous thrombosis (MVT) refers to thrombosis of the veins draining the intestine (inferior mesenteric, superior mesenteric, splenic, and portal veins). The obstruction in venous return leads to edema, distention, and eventual infarction of affected segments. Primary MVT is idiopathic, although given the improved understanding of predisposing conditions, the number of patients in this category is diminishing. Patients in whom a causative factor is identified are said to have secondary MVT. These factors include myriad clinical syndromes, including trauma, surgery, cancer, cirrhosis, pancreatitis, dehydration, and increasingly recognized hypercoagulable syndromes such as polycythemia vera, thrombocytosis, protein C and S deficiency, antithrombin III deficiency, antiphospholipid antibody syndrome, and factor V Leiden mutation (activated protein C resistance).[27]

Patients with MVT have a somewhat different presentation from those who have ischemia due to arterial obstruction; the onset of symptoms may be insidious and the findings more subtle. Pain out of proportion to the physical examination is still an essential feature. The test of choice to confirm the diagnosis is contrast-enhanced computed tomography (CT), although duplex scanning and magnetic resonance imaging (MRI) are gaining popularity. Thrombus is located in the superior mesenteric vein in 70% of patients, with portal and inferior mesenteric vein thrombus found in about 30%.[28]

Symptomatic acute MVT is a lethal disease, with a 30-day mortality of about 25% and a 3-year survival of 35%.[28] Patients with evidence of chronic thrombosis fare somewhat better, because collateral venous channels form to augment intestinal venous drainage.

CLINICAL PRESENTATION AND DIAGNOSIS

AMI can appear precipitously with decompensation over hours or insidiously with progression over days. Classic symptoms of AMI include sudden abdominal pain out of proportion to the physical examination, with gut emptying at the onset of pain. The subacute pattern of mesenteric ischemia is characterized by a more gradual development of vague abdominal signs and symptoms. These include less intense and nonspecific abdominal pains with nausea, vomiting, and changes in bowel habits. The abdomen may become distended but still have active bowel sounds.

Predictably, physical signs intensify as the syndrome progresses. In the early phases, signs of peritoneal irritation such as abdominal guarding and rebound are absent. As the bowel becomes more ischemic, necrosis progresses from the mucosal layers to the seromuscular layers. After full-thickness bowel infarction, the abdomen is often grossly distended, with absent bowel sounds and exquisite tenderness to palpation. Bowel infarction can impart a feculent odor to the breath.

Ancillary laboratory evaluations often reveal an increase in hemoglobin and hematocrit, consistent with hemoconcentration. There is a marked leukocytosis with a predominance of immature white blood cells (left shift). Although no specific laboratory findings are diagnostic, serum levels of amylase, lactic dehydrogenase, creatine phosphokinase, and alkaline phosphatase, singly or severally, are often elevated, along with a metabolic acidosis with a persistent base deficit.[29] Unfortunately, most of these abnormalities do not develop until after bowel necrosis has occurred.

Plain abdominal radiographs are used to exclude other potential causes of abdominal pain rather than confirm the diagnosis of AMI. In fact, completely normal plain abdominal films are seen in more than 25% of patients with mesenteric ischemia.[30] Subtle signs of AMI on plain abdominal films include a dynamic ileus and distended air-filled loops of bowel. Bowel wall thickening from submucosal edema or hemorrhage can be prominent, especially in cases of acute MVT. In advanced stages, pneumatosis of the bowel wall and portal vein gas portend an extremely poor prognosis.

Barium contrast evaluations of the upper and lower gastrointestinal tracts are contraindicated because residual intraluminal contrast material can limit visualization of the mesenteric vasculature during diagnostic angiography. On the rare occasion when barium studies are performed in a patient with the gradual development of abdominal pain, the submucosal edema and hemorrhage of intestinal ischemia are manifest by thickening of the bowel wall, strictures, or ulcerations.

Duplex ultrasonography may be of some benefit in visualizing flow in the SMA and celiac axis. With expert technical assistance, these tests can document proximal stenoses in the SMA or celiac axis or complete occlusion of these vessels.[31] In newer series, color Doppler ultrasonography has been shown to be a valuable screening tool for AMI; it is far more specific than clinical evaluation alone.[32,33] Unfortunately, a significant percentage of patients at risk for mesenteric ischemia have dilated air-filled loops of bowel that make ultrasonography difficult if not impossible.

CT of the abdomen and pelvis can delineate subtle changes consistent with subacute bowel ischemia such as focal or segmental bowel wall thickening.[34] Thrombus within the mesenteric veins or the lack of opacification of the veins after intravenous contrast administration is often seen in MVT.[35] Nonenhancement of the arterial vasculature with timed intravenous contrast injections can be noted in acute mesenteric arterial thrombosis or embolization. CT scans can also vividly demonstrate pneumatosis or portal vein gas.

Advances in contrast-enhanced and cine phase magnetic resonance angiography have allowed better visualization of the visceral vasculature and may, in the future, have a more important role in the diagnosis of AMI.[36] Specifically, when MRI is coupled with magnetic resonance oximetry, both anatomic and physiologic information regarding the mesenteric circulation can be obtained.[37]

Despite these aforementioned developments, the definitive diagnostic study remains mesenteric angiography. Angiography requires multiple views for adequate assessment of the vessels at risk. The origins of the celiac axis and the SMA can be visualized only by lateral views, whereas the more distal celiac axis and SMA distributions are best viewed through anteroposterior projections. Selective cannulation of the origins of the celiac axis and SMA is often required to completely define the anatomy and pathophysiology. Thorough aortography is also needed to evaluate potential inflow and outflow sites for bypass grafts, as well as to clarify the extent and location of other atherosclerotic lesions in the iliac artery and the IMA.

In patients suffering from nonocclusive ischemia, angiography usually reveals multiple areas of narrowing and irregularity in major branches. The small and medium-size arterial branches may be decreased or absent, and the vasculature is diffusely pruned, with an absent submucosal "blush." In MVT, selective angiograms may demonstrate reflux of contrast material back into the aorta owing to extremely slow flow and heightened outflow resistance. A prolonged arterial phase with accumulation of contrast and thickened bowel walls is also characteristic. In extreme cases, angiographic contrast may extravasate into the bowel lumen, indicative of active bleeding. The definitive diagnosis of MVT is made during the venous phase; either a filling defect is noted within the portal vein or, in more severe cases, the entire venous phase is absent.

TREATMENT OPTIONS

Initial treatment of patients with AMI includes volume resuscitation, correction of acidosis, and administration of appropriate antibiotics. Heparin anticoagulation should be started immediately to prevent further propagation of thrombus. A urinary catheter, as well as a peripheral arterial catheter, should be placed for monitoring intravascular volumes and hemodynamic status. A nasogastric tube should be placed to decrease the chance of aspiration.

Mesenteric angiography should be performed immediately. As noted earlier, such studies are diagnostic and have the potential to be therapeutic in selected cases. In highly selected patients with an early diagnosis of SMA embolus unassociated with bowel necrosis, some authors have advocated a trial of thrombolytic therapy.[38,39] Such treatment should be strictly limited to patients with abdominal pain for less than 8 hours' duration without signs of peritoneal irritation. If lysis is not evident within 4 hours of commencing high-dose thrombolytic therapy, or if peritoneal signs develop, the infusion should be discontinued and immediate surgical exploration performed.

An increasing number of case reports have detailed the use of percutaneous angioplasty to dilate significant atherosclerotic plaques of the SMA that are unmasked by thrombolytic therapy.[40-42] Owing to the variable angle of the origin of the SMA from the aorta, placement and removal of the angioplasty catheter and stent placement may be more difficult than for lower extremity angioplasties.[10] Restenosis rates range from 25% to 50% in the limited series reported to date.[40,41]

When an aortic dissection involves the origin of one or more of the visceral vessels, endovascular repairs have been attempted through stent placement[43,44] and balloon fenestration of the dissection septum.[45] Although such minimally invasive treatments are quite attractive, they are currently limited by the frequently rapid onset of ischemic symptoms, inability to gain access to the dissection channel, or the need for surgical repair of an associated aortic aneurysm.

Irrespective of cause, most patients with acute arterial occlusion require early surgical exploration and reestablishment of mesenteric flow to prevent or minimize bowel infarction. A generous midline incision should be made and the extent of mesenteric ischemia and necrosis assessed. If the entire small bowel is frankly gangrenous, enterectomy with lifelong hyperalimentation is the only option. In many instances, patient preferences and family consultation may argue for simple abdominal closure with terminal pain relief as a more appropriate choice. If bowel infarction is not profound, surgical revascularization should be performed.

To achieve adequate exposure, the transverse colon is retracted superiorly, and the fourth portion of the duodenum is mobilized to the ligament of Treitz. The SMA is identified by palpation of the root of the mesentery. If the cause of mesenteric ischemia is an embolus, a more proximal SMA pulse is often noted. The SMA is encircled at or just distal to the level of obstruction (Fig. 34-3A), and a transverse arteriotomy is made. Balloon-tipped embolectomy catheters are inserted retrograde, and the embolus is extracted (Fig. 34-3B).

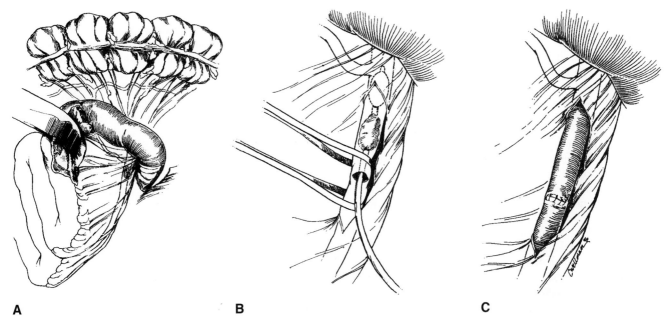

A   **B**   **C**

FIGURE 34–3 • *A,* Mobilization of the transverse colon and duodenum to expose the superior mesenteric artery. *B,* Balloon-tipped catheter extraction of a mesenteric embolus through a transverse arteriotomy. *C,* Primary closure of the arteriotomy without stricture. (From McKinsey JF, Gewertz BL: Acute mesenteric ischemia. Surg Clin North Am 77:307-318, 1997.)

Embolectomy catheters should also be passed distally to ensure that no fragmentation of the clot or discontinuous thrombosis has occurred. Transverse arteriotomies are closed primarily with interrupted fine monofilament sutures to ensure that the vessel is not stenosed (Fig. 34-3C). If a longitudinal arteriotomy is required, closure is best accomplished with a vein patch. Appropriately selected longitudinal arteriotomies can also be used for distal anastomoses of bypass grafts if thrombectomies are unsuccessful in obtaining arterial inflow.

When flow is restored, the bowel is reinspected for persistent regions of ischemia. Segments that previously demonstrated equivocal viability may improve with revascularization, and resection may be avoided; lengths of bowel that are obviously nonviable must be removed. Bowel continuity can be restored primarily, or stomas may be exteriorized if the patient is unstable. In most instances, a second-look operation should be performed at 24 to 36 hours to assess the cumulative effects of reperfusion. Planning for this re-exploration allows the surgeon to minimize the amount of bowel resected primarily and to ensure that the final bowel anastomoses are performed with viable bowel.

The management of SMA thrombosis due to underlying atherosclerotic lesions is more challenging because simple surgical thrombectomy is unlikely to be durable.[46] The proximal SMA should be opened through a longitudinal arteriotomy. If thrombectomy is temporarily successful, an intra-arterial shunt is placed while the exposures needed for definitive revascularization are performed. The longitudinal arteriotomy in the SMA can serve as the distal anastomotic site for both antegrade bypasses originating in the supraceliac aorta and retrograde bypasses from the infrarenal aorta or iliac vessels. If there is a high likelihood of bowel resection, an autologous conduit should be used for the bypass.

In syndromes of nonocclusive ischemia, the primary therapy is selective arterial administration of vasodilating agents such as papaverine. Such treatment must be coupled with the cessation of α agonists or other vasoconstrictors. Heparin should also be administered to prevent thrombosis in the cannulated vessel, but the drug must be infused through a peripheral intravenous catheter to avoid precipitation when mixed with papaverine. If a patient demonstrates signs of continued bowel ischemia or necrosis, as evidenced by rebound tenderness or guarding, surgical exploration is required. All necrotic bowel should be resected while arterial infusions of vasodilators continue. The room temperature should be elevated and the bowel kept in moist laparotomy pads to minimize vasoconstriction during exploration. Most patients should undergo a second-look operation in 24 to 48 hours to reassess bowel viability.

The surgical treatment of MVT is restricted to fluid resuscitation, correction of any underlying coagulopathy, and resection of nonviable bowel. Unfortunately, venous thrombectomy is of limited durability and has not proved effective in most instances. The extent of bowel resection should be generous, and repeat exploratory laparotomy is often required to ensure that adequate bowel resection has been performed. Because many patients succumb despite these measures, a more aggressive stance toward early surgical thrombectomy or fibrinolysis has been advocated by some.[47,48] The risks of these maneuvers are considerable, however, and intervention should be reserved for patients who do not improve with conventional therapy.

Although the detection of frankly necrotic bowel is not difficult, the determination of viability in marginally perfused bowel is more challenging. Simple indicators of viability include visible peristalsis as well as a pink and normal color of the serosa. Along with palpation of the distribution of the SMA for arterial pulsations, Doppler ultrasonography can be used to further evaluate arterial signals within the vascular arcades. If any question remains, the bowel should be reassessed at a minimum of 30 minutes after revascularization. Administration of intravenous fluorescein followed by illumination with a Wood's ultraviolet light will confirm perfusion of the bowel. The primary limitation of fluorescein is that it is eventually absorbed in fat; therefore, it can be administered only once before it diffuses throughout all tissue and loses its specificity. Unfortunately, no combination of tactics is sufficiently sensitive or specific for error-free evaluation of bowel viability.[49]

Long-term patient outcomes after acute intestinal ischemia are strongly dependent on the timeliness of diagnosis, the underlying lesion, and the associated cardiovascular status. In a comprehensive report by Klempnauer and colleagues of 90 patients suffering from intestinal ischemia, 31 patients survived and were discharged from the hospital.[50] Cumulative 5-year survival was about 50% (16 of 31). Mortality was greatest during the first year after the incident. The worst survival (20% at 5 years) was seen in patients who suffered mesenteric arterial thrombosis, and the best survival was seen in patients with emboli or nonocclusive ischemia (about 70%). Only one patient who survived the first episode of arterial thrombosis died because of recurrent bowel ischemia. Remarkably, 8 of the 15 surviving patients returned to work.

Chronic Mesenteric Ischemia

In contrast to the varied causes of AMI, CMI is a result of end-stage atherosclerosis in more than 90% of cases. Risk factors parallel those of atherosclerosis in general, including a positive family history, smoking, hypertension, and hypercholesterolemia. Interestingly, in most series, there is a slight female preponderance, and nearly 50% of patients have a history of prior cardiovascular surgery.[51] Nonatherosclerotic causes of CMI include thrombosis associated with thoracoabdominal aneurysm, aortic coarctation, aortic dissection, mesenteric arteritis, fibromuscular dysplasia, neurofibromatosis, middle aortic syndrome, Buerger's disease, and extrinsic celiac artery compression by the median arcuate ligament.

CLINICAL PRESENTATION

The sine qua non of CMI is postprandial abdominal pain. It is characteristically dull and crampy, occurring primarily in the epigastrium or midabdomen. The discomfort results from activation of visceral afferent nerves that respond to distention and ischemia but that poorly localize pain. The pain occurs 15 to 45 minutes after eating, with increasing severity according to the size and nature of the meal. The temporal relationship between pain and food ingestion often leads to "food fear," another classic but not invariable complaint.

Weight loss is the second classic symptom of CMI. Although malabsorption can contribute to malnutrition in severe cases, most weight loss is simply due to the patient's fear of eating. Many patients become so emaciated that they undergo extensive evaluations for occult neoplasms.

Other, less common symptoms of CMI include diarrhea, nausea and vomiting, and constipation. The variability in signs and symptoms is due in part to the region of the gut affected. Foregut ischemia (celiac axis distribution) is usually accompanied by nausea, vomiting, and bloating, whereas midgut ischemia (SMA) causes classic postprandial abdominal pain and weight loss. The infrequent findings of constipation, occult blood in the stool, and ischemic colitis on colonoscopic biopsy may signify hindgut (IMA) involvement. The lack of specificity of the signs and symptoms of this syndrome often leads to a delay in diagnosis, and it is common for affected patients to have undergone myriad interventions, including antacid or antireflux therapy, cholecystectomy, hysterectomy, and adhesiolysis.

The findings on physical examination are also nonspecific, but the astute clinician can recognize several clues indirectly suggesting the diagnosis. Unexplained weight loss and emaciation alone should arouse suspicion of the syndrome. Manifestations of atherosclerosis in other vascular beds are common, including a cervical or peripheral bruit, decreased peripheral pulses, and signs of chronic lower extremity ischemia. An abdominal bruit can be heard in up to 70% of affected patients.

DIAGNOSIS

Routine laboratory evaluation is rarely helpful, although malnutrition may be accompanied by hemoconcentration, immunoincompetence, hypoalbuminemia, hypoproteinemia, or hypocholesterolemia. Tests for panmalabsorption, such as stool fat content, D-xylose tolerance, or vitamin B_{12} absorption, may be positive but are nonspecific. Plain abdominal films may reveal aortic or arterial calcification, suggesting mesenteric atherosclerosis. Additional imaging studies, such as endoscopy, gastrointestinal contrast examination, and CT, rarely establish the diagnosis but are useful in excluding more common clinical syndromes.

Ultrasonography has added a new dimension to the diagnostic evaluation of patients with suspected CMI. The ability to screen patients with chronic abdominal pain without incurring the risk of contrast arteriography has been a significant advance in the identification of affected patients. Predictive values in excess of 80% have been documented using peak systolic velocity criteria of greater than 275 cm/second for the SMA and greater than 200 cm/second for the celiac axis.[52,53] The test is highly operator dependent, however, and independent confirmation of accuracy is necessary for each noninvasive vascular test laboratory employing this technique.

For positive or equivocal ultrasound examinations, diagnostic arteriography is required for more exact lesion localization and for planning revascularization. A complete examination consists of both anteroposterior and lateral aortic views, as well as selective injections of the celiac axis, SMA, and IMA (Fig. 34-4). Occlusion of two or three of the main trunks is generally required for development of the CMI syndrome (Fig. 34-5). Significant mesenteric occlusive disease combined with the development of large collateral vessels is essentially pathognomonic (Fig. 34-6). Celiac axis occlusion by the median arcuate ligament is also readily

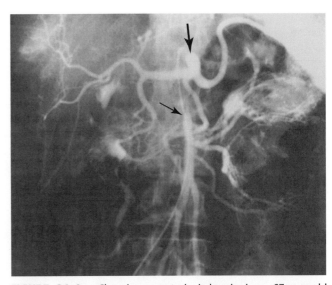

FIGURE 34-4 • Chronic mesenteric ischemia in a 67-year-old woman who had undergone antrectomy, vagotomy, and cholecystectomy and who presented with nausea, vomiting, and a 40-pound weight loss. Anteroposterior arteriogram with direct celiac injection shows critical stenosis of the celiac axis *(thick arrow)* and distal reconstitution of an occluded superior mesenteric artery *(thin arrow)*. (From Schwartz LB, Gewertz BL: Chronic mesenteric arterial occlusive disease: Clinical presentation and diagnostic evaluation. In Perler BA, Becker GL [eds]: Vascular Intervention: A Clinical Approach. New York, Thieme Medical, 1998, p 522).

demonstrated by contrast arteriography and may be responsible for CMI in younger patients[54] (Fig. 34-7).

More recent developments in CT and image processing have allowed such detailed reconstructions of the visceral aortic branches that catheter-based arteriography may become unnecessary in many cases. As demonstrated in Figures 34-8 and 34-9, identification of a highly calcified plaque at the SMA origin prompted contrast-enhanced CT reconstruction. Significant orificial lesions with post-stenotic dilatation of both the celiac axis and the SMA were demonstrated in this patient with symptoms of CMI and a large abdominal aortic aneurysm.

TREATMENT OPTIONS

Because there is no effective medical therapy for CMI, its treatment is focused on the mechanical relief of occlusive lesions and restoration of blood flow. Percutaneous transluminal mesenteric angioplasty with or without intraluminal stenting is now being employed more frequently[27,55] (Fig. 34-10). Early results have been encouraging, with technical success in up to 80% of cases and relief of symptoms and weight gain in the majority. Although restenosis has historically been problematic, occurring in 30% to 50% of early cases, improved techniques and stent placement have produced results comparable to those of surgical revascularization.

One of the largest experiences with angioplasty of mesenteric vessels was recently reported by the Cleveland Clinic's vascular and interventional group.[56] They performed a retrospective, nonrandomized but contemporaneous review of 28 patients undergoing endovascular treatment and compared their demographics and outcomes with those of 85 patients undergoing operative revascularization. Patients treated with

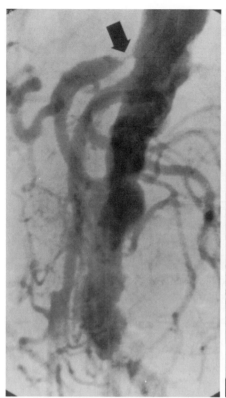
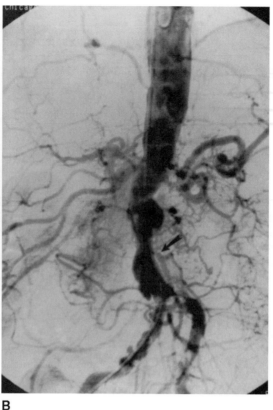

A   **B**

FIGURE 34–5 • Chronic mesenteric ischemia in a 78-year-old woman who had undergone coronary artery bypass and carotid endarterectomy and who presented with claudication, a 30-pound weight loss, and postprandial pain. *A,* Lateral aortogram shows critical celiac axis stenosis *(arrow)*. *B,* Anteroposterior aortogram shows severe infrarenal aortic disease and critical inferior mesenteric artery stenosis *(arrow)*. (From Schwartz LB, Gewertz BL: Intestinal ischemic disorders. In Yao JST, Pearce WH [eds]: Modern Trends in Vascular Surgery. Stamford, Conn, Appleton & Lange, 1999, pp 347-367.)

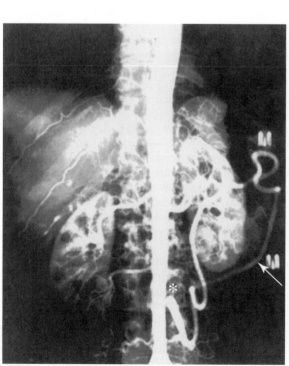
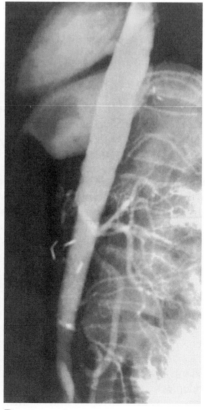

A   **B**

FIGURE 34–6 • Chronic mesenteric ischemia in a 67-year-old woman with postprandial abdominal pain and a 30-pound weight loss. *A,* Anteroposterior aortogram (early phase) shows occlusion of the celiac axis and superior mesenteric artery (SMA), along with critical stenosis of the inferior mesenteric artery (IMA) origin *(asterisk)*. Note the presence of a meandering mesenteric artery *(arrow)*. *B,* Lateral aortogram demonstrating occlusion of both the celiac and superior mesenteric arteries at the orgin. (From Schwartz LB, Gewertz BL: Chronic mesenteric arterial occlusive disease: Clinical presentation and diagnostic evaluation. In Perler BA, Becker GL [eds]: Vascular Intervention: A Clinical Approach. New York, Thieme Medical, 1998, p 521.)

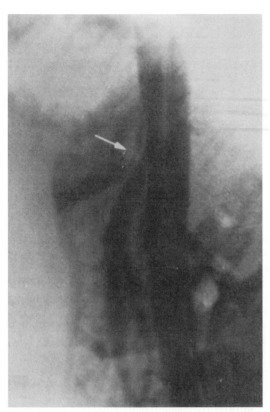

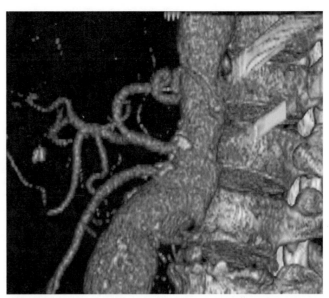

FIGURE 34–9 • Contrast-enhanced reconstruction of computed tomography scan confirms the hemodynamic significance of orificial lesions of the celiac axis and superior mesenteric artery. Note the detail of the distal vessels on the image, allowing operative planning.

FIGURE 34–7 • Median arcuate compression syndrome. Lateral aortogram in a 27-year-old woman with postprandial abdominal cramping, bloating, and occasional nausea and vomiting. Note the compression of the celiac axis and superior mesenteric artery *(arrow)*. Her twin sister had similar complaints and arteriographic findings. (From Bech F, Loesberg A, Rosenblum J, et al: Median arcuate ligament compression syndrome in monozygotic twins. J Vasc Surg 19:935, 1994.)

angioplasty were slightly older (68 vs. 62 years) and experienced a higher incidence of clinically important coronary artery disease (68% vs. 33%). Postprocedural complications were similar, with 11% mortality in the endovascular group and 8% mortality in the operated patients. Interestingly,

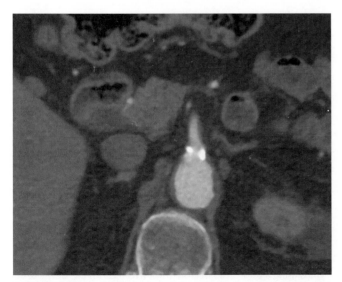

FIGURE 34–8 • Calicific plaque is noted at the origin of the superior mesenteric artery.

although patency at 3 years was comparable, patients undergoing operative repair experienced more durable relief of symptoms, with complete cure in approximately 90% of operative patients at 3 years, compared with 65% of those treated with angioplasty.

In our recent experience with angioplasty for these lesions, we found it to have considerable utility in very high-risk or debilitated patients in whom operative approaches might be perilous. Failure of angioplasty to relieve symptoms either initially or in the long term is experienced in roughly 20% of patients. These failures are usually due to inadequate revascularization as well as progressive occlusive disease in other untreated vessels. Perhaps the most likely cause of failure is the simple fact that, despite appropriate visceral stenotic lesions, the symptoms were not related to mesenteric occlusive disease.

Surgical revascularization remains the most durable treatment for CMI. Early reports emphasized single-vessel reconstruction using autologous vein and a retrograde approach with bypass grafts originating from the infrarenal aorta.[57,58] Although this procedure avoids supraceliac aortic dissection and clamping, the geometry of a retrograde bypass is theoretically unfavorable, with the potential for compression by the overlying abdominal viscera. In the modern era, antegrade bypass using grafts originating in the supraceliac aorta has become the preferred surgical technique.[59]

Proper patient selection for mesenteric revascularization is critical to optimize results. Other common gastrointestinal disorders should be excluded and the diagnosis of CMI ascertained. Concurrent extracranial carotid and coronary artery disease should be detected and treated appropriately. Medical or percutaneous treatment for myocardial ischemia is preferred, because patients with CMI are at increased risk for intestinal infarction during and after coronary artery revascularization.

Although hypoproteinemia with serum albumin of less than 3 mg/dL frequently accompanies CMI, postponement of

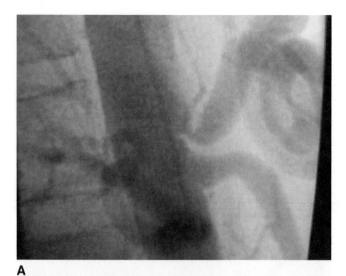

A

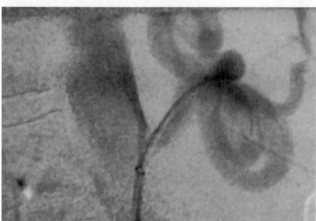

B

FIGURE 34–10 • *A,* Severe stenosis of the celiac axis in a patient with foregut ischemic symptoms. *B,* Successful angioplasty with stent placement despite angulation of the artery origin.

operative therapy to nourish the patient is rarely helpful. The risk of intestinal infarction during the preoperative period is significant and is often associated with catastrophic results. In patients with life-threatening malnutrition, consideration should be given to endovascular therapy as a temporizing measure before surgical reconstruction.

ANTEGRADE BYPASS

Aortic-celiac-mesenteric bypass is best performed through a transperitoneal approach. After a thorough exploration of the abdomen, attention is directed toward exposure of the distal thoracic aortic inflow source. This portion of the aorta is usually spared from atherosclerosis. The triangular ligament of the left lobe of the liver is divided, and moist laparotomy packs are inserted to protect the liver parenchyma. Although exposure is greatly facilitated by the use of self-retaining retractor systems, care should be taken to avoid excessive force. The lesser sac is entered by division of the gastrohepatic ligament. The esophagus is retracted to the left, and final aortic exposure is achieved by division of the diaphragmatic crura and median arcuate ligament. This allows isolation of 8 to 10 cm of the distal thoracic aorta without division of the diaphragm.

The mesenteric arterial branches are identified next. The origin of the celiac axis is already substantially exposed during the aortic dissection. Dissection along its length is continued until a soft patent distal target is appreciated (usually within the distal celiac axis before its branching). Following this, the operative field is temporarily shifted to the midabdomen by lifting and superiorly displacing the transverse colon. The small bowel and the fourth portion of the duodenum are retracted to the right. The SMA is palpated in the small bowel mesentery as the vessel courses from the retroperitoneum at the inferior margin of the pancreas. The peritoneal membrane is incised, and a suitable segment is isolated. Blunt dissection is used to develop a tunnel behind the pancreas on the left side of the aorta.

Intravenous heparin (100 units/kg) and mannitol (25 g) are administered. A longitudinal incision is made in the aorta, and additional arterial wall is removed as needed. A bifurcated Dacron or polytetrafluoroethylene graft (typically 14×7 mm) is delivered to the field. Proximal aortic followed by distal celiac axis anastomosis is performed, and the viscera are reperfused. SMA anastomosis is performed last, after the second limb of the graft is tunneled beneath the pancreas (Fig. 34-11). An alternative but equally effective technique involves sequential bypass using a single 8-mm Dacron graft[59-61] (Fig. 34-12).

RETROGRADE BYPASS

Mesenteric bypass grafts originating from the infrarenal aorta or iliac arteries (retrograde bypass) were the first techniques

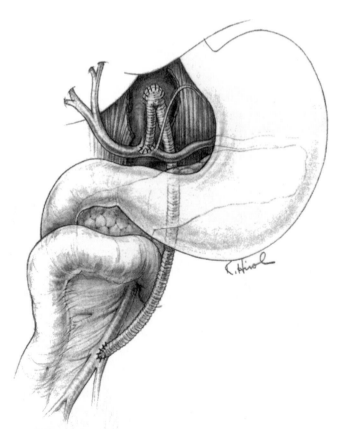

FIGURE 34–11 • Aorta–carotid artery–superior mesenteric artery bypass using a bifurcated Dacron graft. (From Zarins CK, Gewertz BL: Atlas of Vascular Surgery. New York, Churchill Livingstone, 1989, p 109.)

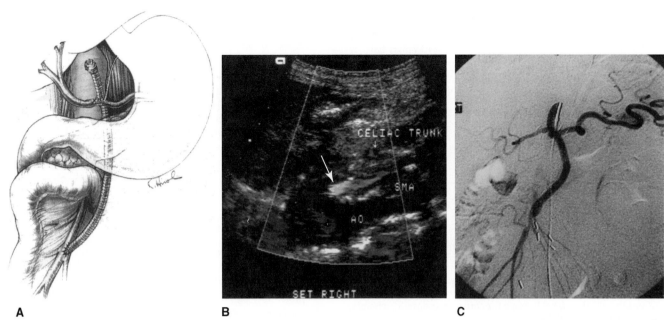

FIGURE 34–12 • Sequential aorta–celiac axis–superior mesenteric artery bypass using an 8-mm Dacron graft. *A,* Drawing of the reconstruction. *B,* Postoperative duplex scan with color-flow mapping shows a patent bypass graft *(large arrow)* from the aorta (AO) to the celiac trunk and superior mesenteric artery (SMA). *C,* Postoperative angiogram shows patent sequential reconstruction. (Modified from Zarins CK, Gewertz BL: Atlas of Vascular Surgery. New York, Churchill Livingstone, 1989, p 109; and Moawad J, McKinsey JF, Wyble CW, et al: Current results of surgical therapy for chronic mesenteric ischemia. Arch Surg 132:616, 1997.)

used in surgical correction of mesenteric arterial lesions.[6] This approach offers the advantages of limited dissection and avoidance of supraceliac aortic occlusion. Despite these features, retrograde bypass has been used less frequently in recent years. Results from a number of clinical series suggest (but do not prove) that retrograde bypass is less durable than its antegrade counterpart.[62,63] This is presumed to be due to the tendency for SMA grafts to kink or twist when the viscera are returned to their normal anatomic positions. Although the use of stiffer prosthetic conduits and meticulous technique can improve the orientation of these reconstructions, retrograde bypass should be considered a third option to be used only if antegrade bypass and aortomesenteric endarterectomy are not feasible. Specific indications for retrograde bypass currently include (1) emergency revascularization in patients undergoing laparotomy for AMI, (2) inaccessible supraceliac aorta due to previous surgery or subphrenic inflammation, (3) severe cardiac disease with contraindications to supraceliac aortic occlusion, and (4) the need for simultaneous infrarenal aortic and mesenteric revascularization.

Retrograde mesenteric bypass begins with exposure of the most proximal suitable segment of the SMA as it exits from beneath the pancreas. The more proximal the anastomosis in the SMA, the less likely it is that kinking will occur, because the graft will lie geometrically parallel to the aorta. The mesentery is then returned to its normal position as the graft is pulled taut to lie adjacent to the aorta. A soft portion of the aorta or iliac artery is located, and the proximal anastomosis is performed; a fair amount of tension must be maintained on the graft to avoid laxity and kinking when the abdomen is closed (Fig. 34-13).

Access to the celiac axis is problematic with this approach; therefore, celiac revascularization is usually performed via

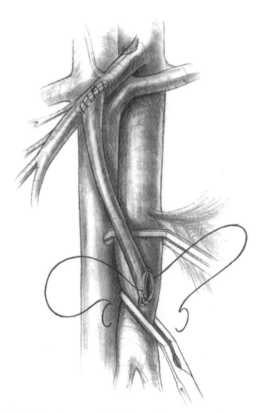

FIGURE 34–13 • Retrograde infrarenal aorta–superior mesenteric artery bypass using autologous vein. (From Zarins CK, Gewertz BL: Atlas of Vascular Surgery. New York, Churchill Livingstone, 1989, p 107.)

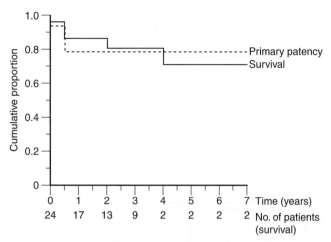

FIGURE 34–14 • Symptom-free survival (*n* = 24) and primary patency (*n* = 19) in patients undergoing surgical revascularization for chronic mesenteric ischemia. Calculation was done using the life-table method. Number of patients per interval is shown at the bottom. (Modified from Moawad J, McKinsey JF, Wyble CW, et al: Current results of surgical therapy for chronic mesenteric ischemia. Arch Surg 132:616, 1997.)

anastomosis to the common hepatic artery or, less commonly, the splenic artery. The common hepatic anastomosis (distal anastomosis) is performed in an end-to-side fashion at 90 degrees. After the Kocher maneuver, the graft can be tunneled behind the duodenum and head of the pancreas, en route to the infrarenal aorta. In this position, torsion and kinking are minimized. When the less robust splenic artery is used, grafts are tunneled behind the tail of the pancreas and anterior to the left renal vein.

OUTCOMES OF SURGICAL TREATMENT

A review of collected series of the surgical treatment of CMI during the 1980s and 1990s reveals an overall operative mortality rate of 6%, with 20% of patients sustaining major complications.[64] Although documentation of nearly 500 cases appears in the literature, most of these represent small case series, and the rarity of the syndrome implies that few institutions have extensive experience. Most clinicians agree that recurrence is less likely if more than one vessel is revascularized. This concept was first championed by Robin and colleagues,[48] who noted differential recurrence rates corresponding to the number of vessels treated. Subsequent reports confirmed this finding,[65,66] making complete revascularization the standard.

Although many clinicians report excellent symptomatic relief after surgical revascularization for CMI, only a few have rigorously examined graft patency.[59,67,68] McMillan and coworkers used duplex scans and arteriography to document graft patency in 25 patients undergoing mesenteric bypass.[67] Their series included 16 patients treated for CMI and 9 treated for AMI, in whom the perioperative morbidity was predictably higher. Considering the 22 patients who survived for more than 1 month, graft patency after a mean of 35 months was 89%. The success rates of retrograde and antegrade grafts were indistinguishable, as were the outcomes of prosthetic and autogenous vein reconstructions. It was noted that two of the three patients experiencing occluded grafts were

asymptomatic, emphasizing that patency cannot be inferred from clinical criteria alone.

Expected results in the modern era are typified by the University of Chicago experience with 24 consecutive patients undergoing mesenteric revascularization over a 10-year period.[59] All patients had significant SMA involvement, and 21 also had lesions of the celiac axis. Seventeen antegrade and seven retrograde bypasses were performed. Calculated 5-year primary patency, documented by duplex scans, arteriography, or both, was 78%; 5-year patient survival by life-table analysis was 71% (Fig. 34-14).

REFERENCES

1. Elliot J: The operative relief of gangrene of intestine due to occlusion of the mesenteric vessels. Ann Surg 1:9-23, 1895.
2. Goodman EH: Angina abdominis. Am J Med Sci 155:524-528, 1918.
3. Dunphy JE: Abdominal pain of vascular origin. Am J Med Sci 192:109-113, 1936.
4. Shaw RS, Maynard EP III: Acute and chronic thrombosis of the mesenteric arteries associated with malabsorption. N Engl J Med 258:874-878, 1958.
5. Kairaluoma MI, Karkola P, Heikkinen D, et al: Mesenteric infarction. Am J Surg 133:188-193, 1977.
6. Stoney RJ, Cunningham CG: Acute mesenteric ischemia. Surgery 114:489-490, 1993.
7. Cokkinis A: Mesenteric Venous Occlusion. London, Bailliere, Tindall, 1935.
8. Vignati PV, Welch JP, Ellison L, Cohen JL: Acute mesenteric ischemia caused by isolated superior mesenteric artery dissection. J Vasc Surg 16:109-112, 1992.
9. Cambria RP, Brewster DC, Gertler J, et al: Vascular complications associated with spontaneous aortic dissection. J Vasc Surg 7:199-209, 1988.
10. Chopra PS, Grassi CJ: Superior mesenteric artery angioplasty with the TEG wire: Usefulness and technical difficulties. J Vasc Interv Radiol 3:523-526, 1992.
11. Parks DA, Granger DN: Ischemia-induced vascular changes: Role of xanthine oxidase and hydroxyl radicals. Am J Physiol 245:G285-G289, 1983.
12. Parks DA, Granger DN: Contributions of ischemia and reperfusion to mucosal lesion formation. Am J Physiol 250:G749-G753, 1986.
13. Del Maestro RF, Bjork J, Arfors KE: Increase in microvascular permeability induced by enzymatically generated free radicals. I. In vivo study. Microvasc Res 22:239-254, 1981.
14. Ali MH, Schlidt SA, Hynes KL, et al: Prolonged hypoxia alters endothelial barrier function. Surgery 124:491-497, 1998.
15. Marcus BC, Wyble CW, Hynes KL, Gewertz BL: Cytokine-induced increases in endothelial permeability occur after adhesion molecule expression. Surgery 120:411-416, 1996.
16. Marcus BC, Hynes KL, Gewertz BL: Loss of endothelial barrier function requires neutrophil adhesion. Surgery 122:420-426, 1997.
17. Korthuis RJ, Anderson DC, Granger DN: Role of neutrophil-endothelial cell adhesion in inflammatory disorders. J Crit Care 9:47-71, 1994.
18. Korthuis RJ, Granger DN: Reactive oxygen metabolites, neutrophils, and the pathogenesis of ischemic-tissue/reperfusion. Clin Cardiol 16:119-126, 1993.
19. Sisley AC, Desai T, Harig JM, Gewertz BL: Neutrophil depletion attenuates human intestinal reperfusion injury. J Surg Res 57:192-196, 1994.
20. Tullis MJ, Brown S, Gewertz BL: Hepatic influence on pulmonary neutrophil sequestration following intestinal ischemia-reperfusion. J Surg Res 66:143-146, 1996.
21. Kaleya RN, Sammartano RJ, Boley SJ: Aggressive approach to acute mesenteric ischemia. Surg Clin North Am 72:157-182, 1992.
22. Schutz A, Eichinger W, Breuer M, et al: Acute mesenteric ischemia after open heart surgery. Angiology 49:267-273, 1998.
23. Klempnauer J, Grothues F, Bektas H, Wahlers T: Acute mesenteric ischemia following cardiac surgery. J Cardiovasc Surg (Torino) 38:639-643, 1997.
24. Gewertz BL, Zarins CK: Postoperative vasospasm after antegrade mesenteric revascularization: A report of three cases. J Vasc Surg. 14:382-385, 1991.
25. Siegelman SS, Sprayregen S, Boley SJ: Angiographic diagnosis of mesenteric arterial vasoconstriction. Radiology 112:533-542, 1974.

26. Deehan DJ, Heys SD, Brittenden J, Eremin O: Mesenteric ischaemia: Prognostic factors and influence of delay upon outcome. J R Coll Surg Edinb 40:112-115, 1995.

27. Schwartz LB, Gewertz BL: Mesenteric ischemia. Surg Clin North Am 77:275-507, 1997.

28. Rhee RY, Gloviczki P, Mendonca CT, et al: Mesenteric venous thrombosis: Still a lethal disease in the 1990s. J Vasc Surg 20:688-697, 1994.

29. Graeber GM, Cafferty PJ, Reardon MJ, et al: Changes in serum total creatine phosphokinase (CPK) and its isoenzymes caused by experimental ligation of the superior mesenteric artery. Ann Surg 193:499-505, 1981.

30. Smerud MJ, Johnson CD, Stephens DH: Diagnosis of bowel infarction: A comparison of plain films and CT scans in 23 cases. AJR Am J Roentgenol 154:99-103, 1990.

31. Harward TR, Smith S, Seeger JM: Detection of celiac axis and superior mesenteric artery occlusive disease with use of abdominal duplex scanning. J Vasc Surg 17:738-745, 1993.

32. Danse EM, Van Beers BE, Goffette P, et al: Diagnosis of acute intestinal ischemia by color Doppler sonography: Color Doppler sonography and acute intestinal ischemia. Acta Gastroenterol Belg 59:140-142, 1996.

33. Danse EM, Laterre PF, Van Beers BE, et al: Early diagnosis of acute intestinal ischaemia: Contribution of colour Doppler sonography. Acta Chir Belg 97:173-176, 1997.

34. Klein HM, Lensing R, Klosterhalfen B, et al: Diagnostic imaging of mesenteric infarction. Radiology 197:79-82, 1995.

35. Rosen A, Korobkin M, Silverman PM, et al: Mesenteric vein thrombosis: CT identification. AJR Am J Roentgenol 143:83-86, 1984.

36. Li KC: MR angiography of abdominal ischemia. Semin Ultrasound CT MR 17:352-359, 1996.

37. Li KC: Magnetic resonance angiography of the visceral arteries: Techniques and current applications. Endoscopy 29:496-503, 1997.

38. McBride KD, Gaines PA: Thrombolysis of a partially occluding superior mesenteric artery thromboembolus by infusion of streptokinase. Cardiovasc Intervent Radiol 17:164-166, 1994.

39. Rivitz SM, Geller SC, Hahn C, Waltman AC: Treatment of acute mesenteric venous thrombosis with transjugular intramesenteric urokinase infusion. J Vasc Interv Radiol 6:219-223, 1995.

40. Hallisey MJ, Deschaine J, Illescas FF, et al: Angioplasty for the treatment of visceral ischemia. J Vasc Interv Radiol 6:785-791, 1995.

41. Levy PJ, Haskell L, Gordon RL: Percutaneous transluminal angioplasty of splanchnic arteries: An alternative method to elective revascularisation in chronic visceral ischaemia. Eur J Radiol 7:239-242, 1987.

42. VanDeinse WH, Zawacki JK, Phillips D: Treatment of acute mesenteric ischemia by percutaneous transluminal angioplasty. Gastroenterology 91:475-478, 1986.

43. Slonim SM, Nyman UR, Semba CP, et al: True lumen obliteration in complicated aortic dissection: Endovascular treatment. Radiology 201:161-166, 1996.

44. Yamakado K, Takeda K, Nomura Y, et al: Relief of mesenteric ischemia by Z-stent placement into the superior mesenteric artery compressed by the false lumen of an aortic dissection. Cardiovasc Intervent Radiol 21:66-68, 1998.

45. Slonim SM, Nyman U, Semba CP, et al: Aortic dissection: Percutaneous management of ischemic complications with endovascular stents and balloon fenestration. J Vasc Surg 23:241-251, 1996.

46. Whitehill T, Rutherford R: Acute mesenteric ischemia caused by arterial occlusions: Optimal management to improve survival. Semin Vasc Surg 3:149-155, 1990.

47. Poplausky MR, Kaufman JA, Geller SC, Waltman AC: Mesenteric venous thrombosis treated with urokinase via the superior mesenteric artery. Gastroenterology 110:1633-1635, 1996.

48. Robin P, Gurel Y, Lang M, et al: Complete thrombosis of mesenteric vein occlusion with recombinant tissue-type plasminogen activator. Lancet 1:1391, 1988.

49. Ballard JL, Stone WM, Hallett JW, et al: A critical analysis of adjuvant techniques used to assess bowel viability in acute mesenteric ischemia. Am Surg 59:309-311, 1993.

50. Klempnauer J, Grothues F, Bektas H, Pichlmayr R: Long-term results after surgery for acute mesenteric ischemia. Surgery 121:239-243, 1997.

51. Schwartz LB, Gewertz BL: Chronic mesenteric arterial disease: Clinical presentation and diagnostic evaluation. In Perla BA, Becker GJ (eds): Vascular Intervention: A Clinical Approach. New York, Thieme Medical, 1998, pp 517-524.

52. Moneta GL, Lee RW, Yeager RA, et al: Mesenteric duplex scanning: A blinded prospective study. J Vasc Surg 17:79-84, 1993.

53. Nicoloff AD, Williamson K, Moneta GL, et al: Duplex ultrasonography in evaluation of splanchnic artery stenosis. In Schwartz LB, Gewertz BL (eds): Mesenteric Ischemia. Philadelphia, WB Saunders, 1997, pp 339-355.

54. Bech F, Loesberg A, Rosenblum J, et al: Median arcuate ligament compression syndrome in monozygotic twins. J Vasc Surg 19:934-958, 1994.

55. Allen RC, Martin GH, Rees CR, et al: Mesenteric angioplasty in the treatment of chronic intestinal ischemia. J Vasc Surg 24:415-421, 1996.

56. Kasirajan K, O'Hara PJ, Gray BH, et al: Chronic mesenteric ischemia: Open surgery versus percutaneous angioplasty and stenting. J Vasc Surg 33:63-71, 2001.

57. Hildebrand HD, Zierler RE: Mesenteric vascular disease. Am J Surg 139:188-192, 1980.

58. Crawford ES, Morris GC Jr, Myhre HO, Roehm JO Jr: Celiac axis, superior mesenteric artery, and inferior mesenteric artery occlusion: Surgical considerations. Surgery 82:856-866, 1977.

59. Moawad J, McKinsey JF, Wyble CW, et al: Current results of surgical therapy for chronic mesenteric ischemia. Arch Surg 132:613-618, 1997.

60. Wolf YG, Berlatzky Y, Gewertz BL: Sequential configuration for aorto-celiac-mesenteric bypass. Ann Vasc Surg 11:640-642, 1997.

61. Geroulakos G, Tober JC, Anderson L, Smead WL: Antegrade visceral revascularisation via a thoracoabdominal approach for chronic mesenteric ischaemia. Eur J Vasc Endovasc Surg 17:56-59, 1999.

62. Rapp JH, Reilly LM, Qvarfordt PG, et al: Durability of endarterectomy and antegrade grafts in the treatment of chronic visceral ischemia. J Vasc Surg 3:799-806, 1986.

63. Johnston KW, Lindsay TF, Walker PM, Kalman PG: Mesenteric arterial bypass grafts: Early and late results and suggested surgical approach for chronic and acute mesenteric ischemia. Surgery 118:1-7, 1995.

64. Schwartz LB, Moawad J, Gewertz BL: Mesenteric ischemia. In Corson JD, Williamson RN (eds): Surgery. London, Mosby-Year Book, 2001, pp 4.141-14.6.

65. Zelenock GB, Graham LM, Whitehouse WM Jr, et al: Splanchnic arteriosclerotic disease and intestinal angina. Arch Surg 115:497-501, 1980.

66. McAfee MK, Cherry KJ Jr, Naessens JM, et al: Influence of complete revascularization on chronic mesenteric ischemia. Am J Surg 164:220-224, 1992.

67. McMillan WD, McCarthy WJ, Bresticker MR, et al: Mesenteric artery bypass: Objective patency determination. J Vasc Surg 21:729-740, 1995.

68. Kihara TK, Blebea J, Anderson KM, et al: Risk factors and outcomes following revascularization for chronic mesenteric ischemia. Ann Vasc Surg 13:37-44, 1999.

Questions

1. **What is the incidence of a "replaced right hepatic artery" arising from the SMA rather than the celiac axis?**
   (a) 2%
   (b) 5%
   (c) 12%
   (d) 20%
   (e) 40%

2. **What is the most common site of origin of a mesenteric embolus?**
   (a) Midthoracic aorta
   (b) Left ventricle
   (c) Aortic valve
   (d) Supraceliac aorta
   (e) Pelvic veins (paradoxical embolus)

3. **Nonocclusive mesenteric ischemia is associated with all of the following except**
   (a) Digitalis toxicity
   (b) Low cardiac output
   (c) Administration of β-adrenergic agents
   (d) Sepsis
   (e) Inotropic administration

4. **What is the most common cause of mesenteric venous thrombosis?**
   (a) Leukemia
   —(b) Hypercoaguable states
   (c) Intra-abdominal abscess
   (d) Primary portal hypertension
   (e) Pancreatic cancer

5. **What is the most common location for a clinically significant acute embolic obstruction of the mesenteric circulation?**
   (a) Origin of the celiac axis
   (b) Origin of the SMA
   (c) Origin of the IMA
   —(d) Mid-SMA just distal to the origin of the middle colic artery
   (e) None of the above

6. **What is the most common location for a clinically significant chronic obstruction of the mesenteric circulation?**
   (a) Origin of the celiac axis
   ⌐ (b) Origin of the SMA
   (c) Origin of the IMA
   (d) Mid-SMA just distal to the origin of the middle colic artery
   (e) None of the above

7. **What is the best clinical indicator of the presence of acute intestinal ischemia?**
   (a) Severe leukocytosis
   —(b) Severe abdominal pain without rebound tenderness
   (c) Acidosis
   (d) Atrial fibrillation
   (e) Hyperamylasemia

8. **All of the following statements about angioplasty for mesenteric vascular disease are true except**
   (a) The immediate failure rate is less than 5%
   (b) The periprocedural mortality is lower than that for operative therapy
   (c) Percutaneous transluminal angioplasty is useful in ischemia related to aortic dissection
   (d) Durability (defined as relief of symptoms) is less than that with operative repair
   (e) Stenting has improved patency

9. **What is the principal advantage of antegrade mesenteric bypass versus retrograde bypass for chronic mesenteric ischemia?**
   (a) Lower operative mortality
   (b) Higher blood flow in grafts
   (c) Allows use of autogenous conduits
   (d) Avoids potential kinking of grafts
   (e) Lower cardiac stress

10. **What is the most reliable sign or symptom when making the clinical diagnosis of chronic mesenteric ischemia?**
    (a) Postprandial pain
    (b) Weight loss
    (c) Melena
    (d) Postprandial vomiting
    (e) Hypoalbuminemia

Answers

1. c	2. b	3. c	4. b	5. d
6. b	7. b	8. b	9. d	10. a

35

Wesley S. Moore

Extracranial Cerebrovascular Disease: The Carotid Artery

Historical Review

The development of surgery on the extracranial cerebrovascular circulation was dependent on three principal factors: (1) recognition of the pathologic relationship between extracranial cerebrovascular disease and subsequent cerebral infarction, (2) the introduction of cerebral angiography to identify lesions before the patient's death, and (3) the development of vascular surgical techniques that could be applied to the extracranial vessels once the anatomic patterns of disease were understood and described.

The earliest report linking cervical carotid artery disease to stroke is credited to Savory,[1] who in 1856 described a young woman with left monocular symptoms in combination with a right hemiplegia and dysesthesia. Postmortem examination demonstrated an occlusion of the cervical portion of the left internal carotid artery, along with bilateral subclavian artery occlusions. In 1875, Gowers reported a similar case,[2] and subsequent reports of individual cases were made by Chiari in 1905,[3] Guthrie and Mayou in 1908,[4] and Cadwater in 1912.[5] By 1914, Hunt,[6] in an important publication, emphasized the relationship between extracranial carotid artery disease and stroke. He also described the phenomenon of intermittent cerebral symptoms associated with partial occlusion and used the term *cerebral intermittent claudication* as a characterizing analogy. Hunt also pointed out that the clinicopathologic observations in patients with stroke were hampered by the fact that routine autopsies did not include examination of the cervical carotid arteries (as is often the case today because of the desire to maintain access to the external carotid artery for the mortician). He emphasized that no examination of cerebral infarction can be considered complete without examination of the neck vessels.[6]

The next major step in the evolution of the management of extracranial cerebrovascular disease came with the development of carotid angiography by Moniz in 1927.[7] By 1937, Moniz and colleagues had described four cases of internal carotid occlusion diagnosed by angiography.[8] In 1938, Chao and colleagues added two more cases,[9] and by 1951, Johnson and Walker had collected from the world literature a total of 101 cases of occlusion of the cervical carotid artery diagnosed by angiography.[10] In spite of these early observations, the medical world was still slow to appreciate the relationship between extracranial cerebrovascular disease and cerebral symptoms, as emphasized by the fact that when cerebral angiography came into common use for neurologic diagnosis in the 1950s and 1960s, only the intracranial vessels were included on films. The area of the carotid bifurcation was seldom looked at. By the late 1950s, patients with hemiplegia were still commonly diagnosed as having a middle cerebral artery thrombosis, without considering the carotid bifurcation as a source of the problem.

The next major steps in the evolution of understanding came from reports by Fisher in 1951 and 1954.[11,12] Fisher re-emphasized the relationship between extracranial arterial occlusive disease and cerebral symptoms. He also pointed out that the lesion could be either total occlusion or stenosis. His most important observation, however, was that the disease was often quite localized to a short segment of the carotid artery, and he predicted that surgical correction might be possible if patients could be identified in the early stages of the clinical syndrome. Fisher stated, "It is even conceivable that some day vascular surgery will find a way to bypass the occluded portion of the artery during the period of ominous fleeting symptoms. Anastomosis of the external carotid artery or one of its branches with the internal carotid artery above the area of narrowing should be feasible."

The surgical phase of understanding and managing extracranial cerebrovascular disease probably began in 1951, but it was not reported in the literature until 1955. This early report by Carrea and colleagues from Buenos Aires described their experience with the management of a patient with carotid artery stenosis.[13] They resected the diseased internal carotid artery and performed an anastomosis between the external carotid artery and the distal internal carotid, as predicted earlier by Fisher. In 1953 Strully and coworkers attempted a thromboendarterectomy of a totally thrombosed internal carotid artery.[14] This was unsuccessful, but the authors suggested that thromboendarterectomy should be technically feasible before thrombosis, as long as the internal carotid artery is patent distally. The first carotid endarterectomy was probably performed by DeBakey and colleagues in an operation done on August 7, 1953, but it was not actually written up until 1959 and then reviewed in 1975.[15,16] The report that was most important in calling the world's attention to the feasibility of carotid artery reconstruction came from Eastcott and associates,[17] who published their experience in the *Lancet* in November 1954. Their operation was performed on May 19, 1954, on a patient who was having hemispheric transient ischemic attacks (TIAs) with demonstrable disease at the carotid bifurcation; they used direct, end-to-end anastomosis between the common carotid artery and the internal carotid artery distal to the atherosclerotic lesion.

Although operations on the carotid artery were in the early phase of development, surgical attack was also considered feasible on occlusive lesions of the major arch vessels. In 1956, Davis and colleagues reported their experience with endarterectomy of the innominate artery performed on a patient on March 20, 1954.[18] In 1957, Warren and Triedman reported the second case.[19]

By this time, the stage was set for the explosive development of an aggressive surgical approach to managing extracranial cerebrovascular disease as a means of preventing or treating cerebral infarction.

Thompson,[20] in his 1996 Willis lecture, related in great detail the history of surgery to prevent stroke. Those interested in the definitive history will be rewarded by reading this excellent paper.

Natural History of Extracranial Arterial Occlusive Disease

Therapy aimed at the prevention of cerebral infarction must be compared with the natural history of the disease process. The prognosis of a patient with extracranial arterial occlusive disease differs, depending on the presence or absence of symptoms. When a permanent neurologic deficit is present, the outlook worsens, thus underscoring the importance of prevention. A thorough understanding of the natural history of the disease is essential to formulating a rational and effective therapeutic program. The physician needs to be familiar with the expected results of each available option. This implies that no one alternative is applicable to all situations and that individualization is the key to effective prevention.

In the United States, approximately 500,000 people suffer a first stroke each year. In 200,000 of these cases, death follows, but at any one time, about 1 million stroke victims are alive and disabled. In 1976, the annual direct and indirect cost of stroke was estimated at $7,363,784,000.[21] Nearly 30 years later, with inflation and the accelerating cost of medical care, this cost has probably quadrupled. The incalculable morbidity of the affected individual adds further to the magnitude of this problem. Prevention remains the most plausible alternative.

The initial mortality of an ischemic stroke ranges from 15% to 33%.[22-24] Survivors remain at an inordinately high risk of subsequent stroke, estimated between 4.8% and

20% per year.[25,26] This implies that half of patients will experience a second event within 5 years.[23,27,28] The average recurrent stroke rate reported in the literature is between 6% and 12% each year. The most common cause of death in patients with extracranial arterial occlusive disease is myocardial infarction (MI). In an analysis of 535 stroke victims, however, the leading cause of death was recurrent stroke, as opposed to the expected myocardial mortality.[26]

Since 1973, public health statistics have documented an accelerating decline in stroke mortality.[29] This has led to the erroneous assumption that a decline has also occurred in stroke incidence, which is not the case.

In 1989, Wolf and colleagues reported the epidemiologic data from the Framingham Study to the 14th International Joint Conference on Stroke and Cerebral Circulation.[30] They reviewed the experience from three successive decades, beginning in 1953. A decline in stroke fatality in both men and women was observed. However, the 10-year prevalence of stroke actually rose, and the incidence of stroke in men rose from 5.7% to 7.6% to 7.9%, without any apparent change in women. The authors postulated that falling case fatality rates might have resulted from changes in diagnostic criteria, a lessening in stroke severity, or improved care of stroke patients.

Harmsen and colleagues reviewed the stroke incidence and fatality in Göteborg, Sweden, between 1971 and 1987.[31] They noted that the stroke incidence remained the same during that interval, but the stroke fatality rate declined in both sexes. This was more marked for intracerebral hemorrhage and subarachnoid hemorrhage than for infarction. They concluded that the decline in stroke fatality rates might have been related to a decrease in smoking or better management of blood pressure. They could not explain why no corresponding decline in stroke incidence occurred.

Finally, Modan and Wagener examined the epidemiologic aspects of stroke based on death certificate information available from the National Center for Health Statistics' compressed mortality file for all 50 states and the District of Columbia for the period 1968 to 1988.[32] They noted a decline in stroke mortality that continued through the 1970s and 1980s, whereas morbidity remained constant and possibly even increased. They noted similar morbidity and mortality rates in both sexes. They concluded that the observed decrease in stroke mortality rates resulted from improved survival rather than a decline in incidence.[32]

A variety of reasons for the decline in stroke mortality have been postulated, including the more aggressive treatment of hypertension. No one has suggested that the decline of stroke mortality might be related to the increasing use of carotid endarterectomy, as illustrated in Figure 35-1. Although this is not proof of a relationship, a possible relationship cannot be discounted.

Two clinical syndromes deserve special emphasis because of their dismal natural history. *Stroke in evolution*, also known as progressing stroke or incomplete stroke, is an acute neurologic deficit of modest degree that within hours or days progresses to a major cerebral infarct. This can happen in a sequential series of acute exacerbations or in a pattern of waxing and waning signs and symptoms over hours or days, with incomplete recovery eventually leading to a major fixed neurologic deficit. *Crescendo transient ischemic attacks* is the pattern that allows complete recovery between ischemic events,

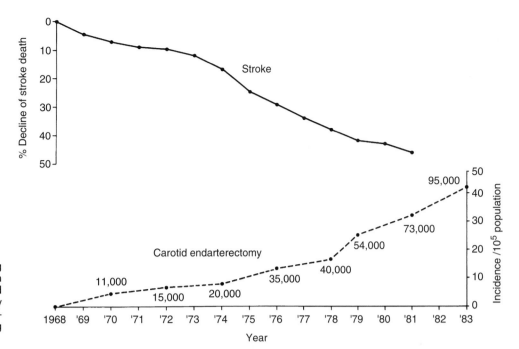

FIGURE 35–1 • The declining incidence of stroke-related death from 1968 to 1981 is compared with the accelerated frequency with which carotid endarterectomy was performed during the same period.

suggesting repeated frequent embolization from a point arterial source in the affected territory.

In a review of the literature, Mentzer and colleagues identified 263 reported cases of stroke in evolution managed conservatively.[33] Twenty-three percent had complete resolution or mild neurologic deficit on follow-up. Sixty-two percent had a moderate to severe deficit in the early recovery phase. The overall mortality was 14.5%. In their own series, 26 patients with stroke in evolution were treated conservatively. Mortality was 15%, but, more important, 66% suffered moderate to severe permanent neurologic deficits, with only five patients recovering completely or experiencing only mild neurologic dysfunction. These results are compared with a series of 17 patients operated on emergently for stroke in evolution. None of these patients had worsening of the preoperative neurologic deficit, four (24%) remained unchanged, and 12 (70%) had complete recovery.[33]

In 1972, Millikan reviewed the natural history of patients with progressing stroke.[34] Of 204 patients, 12% were normal at 14 days, 7% had developed moderate to severe neurologic deficits, and 14% had died. Thus, stroke in evolution treated conservatively carries a poor prognosis. More than half of patients develop a severe permanent neurologic deficit within a few days of the onset, and around 15% die as a result. Only 10% to 20% recover full or partial neurologic function.[34]

Patients who experience TIAs are also at a higher risk of developing a stroke. In the Mayo Clinic population study,[35] 118 patients with TIAs were monitored as a control group without therapy. The stroke rates at 1, 3, and 5 years were 23%, 37%, and 45%, respectively. Most permanent deficits occurred during the first year. This represents a 16-fold increased risk of stroke compared with an age- and sex-adjusted population. The Oxfordshire project reported an actuarial risk of stroke during the first year after the onset of TIAs to be 11% to 16%.[36] For each subsequent year, the rate

was 5% to 9% per year. Some series have reported lower figures,[37,38] but the average reported in the literature is on the order of 30% to 35% at 5 years, or 10% the first year and 6% each year thereafter.

Finally, Toole,[39] in his Willis lecture, reminded us that cerebral infarction in TIA patients goes unrecognized by either patient or physician surprisingly often. These lesions are now identified by better neuroimaging techniques, and one question is whether TIAs are actually small strokes.[39] If a TIA is actually a small stroke, the implied benignity of TIAs must be re-examined, and it may be equally important to prevent TIAs. This consideration is further strengthened by the observations of Grigg and colleagues,[40] who correlated cerebral infarction and atrophy as a function of TIAs and percentage of stenosis. They graded carotid stenosis in symptomatic patients from A (no stenosis) to E (occlusion). In patients with amaurosis fugax, the incidence of cerebral infarction rose from 2% in patients with stenosis grades A, B, and C to 40% in grade D and 58% in grade E. The incidence of atrophy increased in parallel, from 10% in grade A to 30% in grade E.

The natural history of asymptomatic patients with significant extracranial or arterial occlusive disease is difficult to predict accurately. Most studies that have addressed this problem used the presence of a cervical bruit as the sole criterion for inclusion. This inevitably includes patients without significant occlusive disease and omits others without cervical bruit but with high-risk lesions in the extracranial circulation.

As noninvasive studies develop, detection of hemodynamically significant lesions in the carotid system improves. Kartchner and McRae monitored for a mean of 24 months 1130 patients who either were asymptomatic or had nonhemispheric symptoms.[41] Of 303 patients with hemodynamically significant lesions, 11.9% had strokes at 2 years. The group with negative noninvasive studies had a much lower stroke rate, on the order of 3% over the same follow-up period. Busuttil and colleagues noted an unfavorable trend toward higher stroke rates in asymptomatic patients with hemodynamically significant lesions in the carotid bifurcation.[42]

In a report by Roederer and colleagues,[43] 167 asymptomatic patients with cervical bruits were monitored with serial duplex scanning regardless of the degree of stenosis at the time of presentation. During follow-up, 10 patients became symptomatic. The development of symptoms was accompanied by disease progression in 80% of patients. By life-table analysis, the annual rate of symptom occurrence was 4%; however, the presence of progression graded at 80% stenosis was highly correlated with the development of either total occlusion of the internal carotid artery or new symptoms. Thus, 89% of the symptoms were preceded by progression of the lesion to greater than 80% stenosis. Progression of a lesion to more than 80% stenosis was an important warning sign, because it carried a 35% risk of ischemic symptoms or internal carotid occlusion within 6 months and a 46% risk at 12 months. Conversely, only 1.5% of the lesions that remained at less than 80% stenosis developed such a complication. These data suggest that careful follow-up with repeated noninvasive evaluation is of great assistance in determining the appropriate management of asymptomatic carotid lesions.[43]

In an analysis of 294 asymptomatic and nonhemispheric patients submitted to cerebrovascular testing, Moore and colleagues found a 15% stroke incidence during the first 2 years in patients with greater than 50% stenosis.[44] In contrast, there was a 3% stroke incidence at 2 years in patients with 1% to 49% stenosis. The difference was found to be statistically significant ($P < 0.05$). The 5-year cumulative stroke incidence was 21% with greater than 50% stenosis, 14% with 1% to 49% stenosis, and 9% in patients with no noninvasive evidence of carotid artery disease.

Chambers and Norris monitored a group of 500 asymptomatic patients with noninvasive studies and clinical evaluation.[45] They identified two high-risk groups: those with stenosis greater than 75%, and those who showed disease progression between studies. For patients with greater than 75% stenosis, the 1-year neurologic event rate (TIA and stroke) was 22%. The 1-year stroke rate alone was 5%. In a later publication,[46] the authors continued to note that neurologic events correlated with an increasing percentage of stenosis as well as disease progression between test intervals. In the study viewed over 5 years, the annual average neurologic event rate was 10% to 15%, with the highest event rate occurring within the first year of diagnosis. Finally, the incidence of silent cerebral infarction as documented by computed tomography (CT) was studied in the same patient population. The authors noted a 10% incidence of cerebral infarction among patients with mild (35% to 50%) stenosis, 17% with moderate (50% to 75%) stenosis, and 30% in patients with severe (>75%) stenosis. The authors concluded that silent cerebral infarction might be an indication for carotid endarterectomy in asymptomatic patients.[47]

Although the natural history of asymptomatic carotid stenosis remains controversial, studies using serial noninvasive cerebrovascular testing have concluded that an increased risk of stroke exists ipsilateral to a 50% or greater carotid artery stenosis. These lesions appear to carry a risk of subsequent stroke on the order of 4% per year. In addition, progression of the disease carries an even higher risk of stroke, with lesions causing greater than 80% stenosis carrying a 35% risk of subsequent symptoms or carotid occlusion at 2 years.

Other studies have suggested that the composition of the plaque influences the stroke risk of carotid artery lesions. In one analysis, 297 patients with carotid stenosis greater than 75% at the time of initial study were at higher risk than peers without significant narrowing or development of symptoms ipsilateral to the lesion.[48] Even those patients with less than 75% stenosis were at greater risk if the associated plaque was less organized (i.e., soft). This was determined by B-mode ultrasonography, which was used to classify plaques as dense, calcified, or soft. A definite trend toward higher risk was seen in plaques of lower density. Only 10% of those patients with calcified plaque in significantly stenotic vessels developed symptoms, whereas 92% of patients with soft plaques and tight stenosis developed symptoms within the first 3 years of follow-up.[48] The morphology of the atherosclerotic plaque, as documented by B-mode ultrasonography, is emerging as one of the more important factors associated with embolic potential and stroke risk. Two studies have concluded that a heterogeneous plaque carries an increased risk of stroke and is a variable independent from carotid stenosis alone.[49,50]

The embolic potential of ulcerated carotid lesions has been well documented.[51-53] Patients who experience symptoms from these lesions probably have the same prognosis as patients with occlusive lesions. Whether the former patient group responds more favorably to platelet antiaggregants remains to be determined. Moore and coworkers first pointed out that asymptomatic patients with significant ulceration in a carotid plaque in the absence of stenosis appear to be at higher risk of stroke.[54] In a subsequent report, they expanded their series to 153 patients with asymptomatic nonstenotic ulcerative lesions in the carotid bifurcation. Patients with deep (grade B) or complex (grade C) ulcerations received follow-up and were found to have a stroke rate of 4.5% and 7.5% each year, respectively.[55] Other reports have suggested a similar stroke risk for complex ulcerations in the carotid bulb. However, a much lower stroke risk was reported for deep ulcerations, with no significant added risk of stroke observed in these patients. Controversy still exists about deep ulcerations without complex morphology. However, agreement exists that complex ulcerations in the carotid bulb do increase the risk of stroke in asymptomatic patients.[56]

The presence of an asymptomatic hemodynamically significant stenosis may increase the risk of stroke during major surgery. Kartchner and McRae reported their experience with 234 patients, 41 of whom had evidence of significant carotid artery stenosis by oculoplethysmography.[57] Seven postoperative strokes developed in the group with positive criteria (17%), whereas postoperative cerebral infarction developed in 2 of 192 patients (1%) with negative noninvasive studies. The mechanisms of stroke and the territory involved were not specifically reported. This high incidence of permanent neurologic deficits led the authors to conclude that prophylactic carotid endarterectomy should be considered in patients with hemodynamically significant carotid stenosis who are undergoing a major cardiovascular procedure.[57]

Other series have reported results to the contrary.[58-61] Using noninvasive vascular evaluation and, in one series, angiography, patients with 50% or greater stenosis in the carotid bifurcation were compared with patients who had lesser degrees of stenosis undergoing cardiovascular surgery.

No increased incidence of perioperative strokes was found in patients with positive criteria. Most of these investigators, however, excluded preocclusive stenosis in their considerations. Lesions causing 90% or greater stenosis were excluded from these series and were subjected to prophylactic endarterectomy before cardiovascular operation.

Cardiac surgeons have long been concerned about the presence of carotid stenosis in patients who will be undergoing bypass with a decrease in pump perfusion pressure, believing that a corresponding and unacceptable drop in cerebral blood flow will occur. In fact, the opposite occurs. Von Reutern and colleagues used transcranial Doppler ultrasonography to study middle cerebral artery blood flow before and during cardiopulmonary bypass in patients with and without carotid artery disease.[62] Surprisingly, middle cerebral artery blood flow actually increased during cardiopulmonary bypass. Although the increase was not as great in patients with carotid artery disease, it was clearly an increase over baseline. This observation should dispel concern about the potential drop in cerebral blood flow in patients with carotid stenosis while on the pump.

Patients with a combination of severe carotid stenosis and symptomatic coronary artery disease represent a cohort that is at high risk of death, MI, and stroke. Brener and colleagues carried out an extensive literature review that examined complications associated with different treatment strategies.[63] Patients who underwent staging with carotid endarterectomy first had a high cardiac morbidity and mortality. Patients who had coronary bypass first had a higher stroke morbidity. The data suggested that combined or simultaneous coronary artery bypass grafting and carotid endarterectomy might reduce overall morbidity and mortality. However, evidence from retrospective reviews was not sufficiently compelling to make a definitive recommendation.[63] Consensus exists that this is an appropriate topic for a prospective, randomized trial.

The natural history of extracranial arterial occlusive disease cannot be complete without a consideration of the natural history of frequently associated conditions such as coronary artery disease, hypertension, and diabetes. MI remains the most frequent cause of death in these patients. Including these variables in the equation when one is formulating a treatment plan for a particular patient is therefore important. The goal of therapy should be the prevention of a permanent neurologic deficit. When deciding on the most effective way to achieve this, one must consider the life expectancy of the patient and the inherent risk of each particular form of therapy.

Pathology of Extracranial Arterial Occlusive Disease

The pathology of cerebrovascular disease of extracranial origin can be divided into flow-restrictive lesions and lesions with embolic potential. Each of these can be further subdivided into occlusive and aneurysmal lesions. All entities that have been described as etiologic in extracranial disease fall within these categories.

ATHEROSCLEROSIS

By far the most common lesion found in patients with extracranial cerebrovascular disease is an atherosclerotic plaque in the carotid bifurcation. This can produce symptoms

by reducing blood flow to the hemisphere supplied or, more commonly, by releasing embolic material. Emboli can be made up of clot, platelet aggregates, or cholesterol debris.

The carotid bifurcation appears to be susceptible to the development of atherosclerotic plaques.[64] Frequently, severe changes at the carotid bifurcation occur with minimal or no changes present in the common or internal carotid artery.[65] Several investigators have proposed conflicting theories based on hemodynamic observations in various models. High shear stress and fluctuations in shear stress,[66] disordered or turbulent flow, flow separation, and high and low flow velocity have all been implicated.[67-70] Which of these mechanisms is responsible for plaque formation is not known. Zarins and colleagues used a model of the human carotid bifurcation under steady flow and compared its hemodynamics with those of cadaver specimens.[71] They concluded that carotid lesions localize in regions of low flow velocity and flow separation rather than in regions of high velocity and increased shear stress. They used their model to explain the propensity of the outer wall of the carotid sinus opposite the flow divider to develop atherosclerotic plaques (Fig. 35-2). This may have further clinical implications, in that an enlarged carotid bulb after endarterectomy may create a region of reduced flow velocity and increased boundary layer separation, which may favor recurrent plaque deposition.

Once the initial intimal injury is produced by these forces, platelet deposition, smooth muscle cell proliferation, and the slow accumulation of lipoproteins are involved in the reparative process (Fig. 35-3). These eventually lead to plaque formation, which further alters the hemodynamics of the system and favors further injury.

The contribution of platelets to atheroma development may take several forms.[72] Platelets may adhere to one another, to the diseased vessel, or both. This can lead to thrombus formation. This process may narrow the vessel lumen, or the thrombus

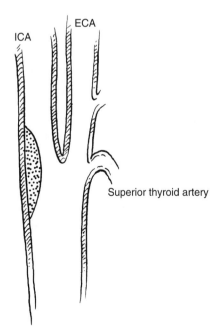

FIGURE 35–2 • The common carotid artery bifurcation, the most common site for atherosclerotic plaque deposition, is located on the wall opposite the divider. ECA, external carotid artery; ICA, internal carotid artery.

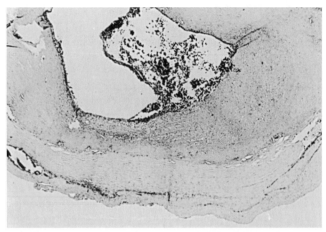

FIGURE 35–3 • Microscopic section of an atherosclerotic plaque removed from the carotid bifurcation. Notice the fibrointimal proliferation with cholesterol cleft formation. Thrombotic material is adherent to the luminal surface of the plaque.

may dislodge, resulting in distal embolization. Vasoactive substances stored in granules within the platelet may be released, causing vasospasm and further contributing to compromise of the arterial lumen. The platelets' interaction with collagen, exposed in an injured intima, may include elaboration of a smooth muscle growth factor that can lead to intimal thickening. The activation of enzymes in platelets, by their contact with collagen, initiates the production of highly active prostaglandins. The production of thromboxane A_2 represents the final common pathway of platelet response to diverse stimuli.[73] This substance is a potent stimulant of platelet aggregation and a powerful vasoconstrictor and is believed to be important in the pathophysiology of plaque formation or the development of symptoms from an already established atheroma.

Hemorrhage into a plaque may also play a significant role in the development of symptoms from an atherosclerotic lesion. Imbalances in wall tension secondary to asymmetrical deposition of plaques can lead to sudden plaque fracture and intraplaque hemorrhage.[74] These can lead to sudden expansion of the atheroma, with acute restriction of flow or breakdown of the intimal surface and concomitant embolization. An alternative mechanism for sudden intraplaque hemorrhage may be related to an increase in neovascularity within the plaque substance. Hypertension may be responsible for precipitating rupture of neovascular vessels, leading to intraplaque hemorrhage and expansion.[75] This process may be responsible for a large number of symptomatic lesions. In a prospective evaluation of 79 atheromatous plaques removed from 69 patients undergoing carotid endarterectomy, 49 of 53 (92.5%) symptomatic patients had evidence of intramural hemorrhage.[76] In contrast, only 7 of 26 (27%) asymptomatic patients showed recent or acute intraplaque hemorrhage. Rupture of an atherosclerotic plaque with intraluminal release of atheromatous debris has also been correlated with acute stroke and internal carotid occlusion in an autopsy study.[77]

FIBROMUSCULAR DYSPLASIA

Fibromuscular dysplasia is a nonatherosclerotic process that affects medium-size arteries. It was first described in the carotid artery in 1964,[78] and since then it has been recognized as a cause of cerebrovascular symptoms.[79] It may also affect the intracranial arteries, and around 30% of patients with cervical involvement have associated intracranial aneurysms.[80] Up to 65% of patients have bilateral disease,[80] and 25% have associated atherosclerotic changes.[81]

Four histologic types of fibromuscular dysplasia have been described[82]:

1. *Intimal fibroplasia* accounts for about 5% of cases and affects both sexes equally. It usually appears as long tubular stenoses in young patients and as focal stenoses in older patients. It results from an accumulation of irregularly arranged subendothelial mesenchymal cells with a loose matrix of connective tissue. Medial and adventitial structures are always normal.

2. *Medial hyperplasia* is a rare form of the disease that produces focal stenoses. The intima and adventitia remain normal, whereas the media shows excess smooth muscle.

3. *Medial fibroplasia* is the most common pattern of fibromuscular dysplasia, accounting for most, if not all, internal carotid artery involvement. It may appear as a focal stenosis or multiple lesions with intervening aneurysmal outpouchings. Histologically, the disease is limited to the media, with replacement of smooth muscle by compact fibrous connective tissue. The inner media may show an accumulation of collagen and ground substance separating disorganized smooth muscle cells. Gradation of these changes correlates with the severity of the lesion. Mural dilatations and microaneurysms are common.

4. *Perimedial dysplasia* is characterized by the accumulation of elastic tissue between the media and adventitia. It affects renal arteries and is associated with macroaneurysms.

Fibromuscular dysplasia preferentially affects long arteries with few primary branches. Hormonal effects on medial tissue, mechanical stresses on the vessel wall, and unusual distribution of the vasa vasorum in these arteries seem to play a causative role.[82] Some experimental evidence[83] and the fact that women are most commonly affected (92% of cases)[81] support a possible role of hormones in this process. In the appropriate hormonal environment, the normal paucity of vasa vasorum in long, nonbranching arterial segments such as the extracranial carotid artery and the renal artery may predispose to mural ischemia and initiation of the fibroplastic process. Experimental evidence supports this concept.[84]

The exact cause of symptoms is controversial. Thromboembolism from clot, platelets, or both; decreased flow due to a critical stenosis or a series of noncritical narrowings; intracranial involvement, with or without aneurysm formation; and hypertension have been implicated.[81]

COILS AND KINKS

Coils and kinks of the extracranial system on occasion have been associated with fibromuscular dysplasia.[81] More commonly, these are due to embryologic events and changes that occur in the aging process. Neurologic manifestations from these anomalies have been reported in children[85] and in adults.[86-88] Embryologically, the internal carotid artery is derived from the third aortic arch and the dorsal aortic root. In the early stages of development, a normally occurring kink is straightened as the heart and great vessels descend in the mediastinum. Failure of this process may account for the occurrence of coils and loops in children and for its bilaterality in about 50% of cases.[88]

In adults, kinking of the extracranial vessels is almost always associated with atherosclerosis. In the aging process, loss of elasticity of the vessel wall occurs, which, in combination with lateral stresses, causes elongation between fixed points—the skull and the thoracic inlet. This produces bowing, with the eventual formation of coils and kinks. Between 5% and 16% of patients submitted for angiographic evaluation have coiling or kinking of one of the extracranial vessels.[86,88] Kinking of the artery is more likely to produce symptoms due to either flow reduction or concomitant plaque formation with distal embolization. Kinking is considered to be an angle of less than 90 degrees between arterial segments (Fig. 35-4). Flow restriction is unlikely to exist in the absence of this configuration. This acute angulation is more likely to occur when the head is turned to the ipsilateral side.[85] In other cases, contralateral rotation, neck flexion, and extension may exaggerate the abnormality, leading to markedly reduced flow. A history of TIAs associated with head motion should lead the clinician to suspect the presence of a kink. Abnormal pulsations in the neck, sometimes suggesting an aneurysmal dilatation, may be present on physical examination. Secondary arteriosclerotic changes may occur because of abnormal flow patterns that predispose to plaque formation and ulceration, accounting for the development of neurologic symptoms. Rarely is the vertebral circulation affected by a kink.[86]

ANEURYSMS

Aneurysms of the carotid artery can cause neurologic symptoms by several mechanisms. Thrombosis and rupture are rare, but embolization is a frequent event.[89] Pressure on cranial nerves can be seen when expansion is rapid, but more frequently this is associated with acute dissection.

Most extracranial aneurysms are secondary to atherosclerosis. Internal elastic lamina disruption and medial thinning are frequent histologic findings.[90] Two types of aneurysms are recognized: fusiform and saccular. Fusiform aneurysms are more common; they are frequently bilateral and are associated with other arterial aneurysms. Saccular aneurysms are often unilateral and tend to involve the common or internal carotid arteries more often. They may also have a congenital, degenerative, or traumatic origin.[91] Atherosclerotic aneurysms of the extracranial circulation are almost always associated with hypertension.[90]

Trauma is a frequent cause of carotid aneurysms. These are usually saccular and most commonly result from blunt rather than penetrating injury. Hyperextension and rotation of the neck cause compression of the internal carotid artery on the transverse process of the atlas.[92] An intimal injury is produced that frequently leads to thrombosis, but it may also produce aneurysmal dilatation.[90]

Mycotic aneurysms are rare. Syphilis and peritonsillar abscess were once common causes of these aneurysms.[93] *Staphylococcus aureus* is currently the predominant responsible organism.

False aneurysms of the carotid artery may form after penetrating injury, but the most frequent cause is previous carotid surgery. They are more common after patch closure of the artery than after primary closure.[89] Disruption of the suture line by infection, suture failure, and technical error are believed to be responsible for their formation. False aneurysms can expand, thrombose, rupture, or lead to distal embolization. The diagnosis of false aneurysm is an indication for surgical repair.

Acute dissection of the carotid artery with or without aneurysm formation is another cause of neurologic events resulting from abnormalities in the extracranial circulation. It can occur secondary to atherosclerosis, fibromuscular dysplasia, or cystic medial necrosis.[94] A history of trauma may or may not be present. On gross inspection, a sharply demarcated transition between the normal color and size of the carotid artery and the dark blue, cylindrical dilatation in the dissected segment is noted.[95] More commonly, the internal carotid artery is affected, and frequently the end of the dissection is not surgically accessible. A double lumen is usually present, with the dissection occurring in the outer layers of the media. Smooth muscle cells are widely separated, and degeneration and fragmentation of the internal elastic membrane occur.[95] The most frequent presentation is a sudden onset of temporal headache or cervical pain associated with a neurologic or visual deficit or Horner's syndrome. Acute expansion may cause compression of cranial nerves IX, X, XI, or XII, with concomitant dysfunction.[94] Horner's syndrome is thought to be secondary to disruption of periadventitial sympathetic fibers. The carotid artery is far more frequently affected than the vertebral artery. Only a few cases of the latter have been reported, with involvement of the segment between C-1 and C-2 noted consistently.[94]

TAKAYASU'S ARTERITIS

In 1908, Takayasu described ocular changes in a 21-year-old woman with nonspecific arteritis.[96] These consisted of a peculiar capillary flush, with rustlike arteriovenous anastomoses around the papilla and blindness due to cataracts. Similar cases were later described with the absence of pulses in the arm. Since then, Takayasu's arteritis has been recognized as a cause of neurologic symptoms secondary to a nonspecific inflammatory process of unknown cause segmentally affecting the aorta and its main branches. The end result of this process is constriction or occlusion of, and occasional aneurysm formation in, the affected vessels secondary to marked fibrosis and thickening of the arterial wall.[97] Originally thought to be rare in the Western Hemisphere, many cases of atypical coarctations of the aorta and other unusual lesions of its main branches are now well recognized as Takayasu's arteritis. This explains the many eponyms given to this syndrome.[98]

Four varieties of the disease are recognized.[99] In type 1, involvement is localized to the aortic arch and its branches. Type 2 does not have arch involvement; the lesions are confined to the descending and abdominal aorta. Type 3 has features of both, and type 4 describes any of the first three types plus involvement of the pulmonary artery. In a retrospective study of 107 patients, 84% were female, and 80% were aged 11 to 30 years.[99]

Two phases of the disease are recognized. In the acute or prepulseless stage, systemic symptoms of a nonspecific nature are present. Skin rash, fever, myalgia, arthralgia, pleuritis, generalized weakness, and other nonspecific symptoms develop, making the diagnosis difficult. These may resolve and go unrecognized by the patient or physician until months or years later, when the second, or occlusive, stage evolves. Then, symptoms of obstruction of the main aortic branches develop. These lesions are not easily managed by endarterectomy. This makes bypass surgery the treatment of choice.

Other forms of arteritis, specifically giant cell arteritis, can cause neurologic symptoms because of extra- or intracranial involvement. These patients are older than those with Takayasu's arteritis, and both sexes appear to be equally affected.[98] Systemic symptoms are usually present. Tenderness over the carotid artery or other affected areas may occur.[100]

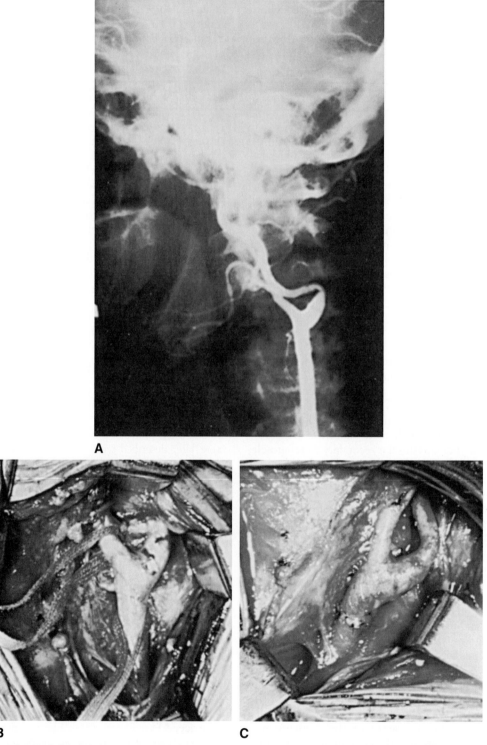

A

B   **C**

FIGURE 35–4 • *A,* Selective left carotid arteriogram demonstrating a kink of the internal carotid artery. Note the angulation of less than 90 degrees and the paucity of contrast material beyond the kink. *B,* Operative appearance of the internal carotid artery kink. *C,* Operative appearance of the internal carotid artery after connection of the kink by mobilization and segmental resection of the common carotid artery. The carotid bifurcation is pulled down, and an end-to-end anastomosis is constructed.

The histologic picture is characteristic, with changes confined to the media, where a large number of giant cells interspersed with lymphocytes are seen. Early diagnosis is important, because corticosteroid therapy may abort the latter stages of the process.[100]

RADIATION THERAPY INJURY

External cervical radiation therapy is now recognized as a cause of accelerated atherosclerotic changes in the extracranial circulation. Experimentally, atherosclerotic lesions similar to the naturally occurring ones can be produced in the abdominal aorta in dogs by x-ray and electron beam radiation.[101] Injury to the endothelial cell, ground substance, elastic lamina, and smooth muscle appears to alter the vessel wall, increasing its permeability to circulating lipids and impairing its ability to repair elastic tissue, leading to the formation of a plaque characterized by fibrosis, fatty infiltration, and intimal destruction.[102] These changes may occur months to years after completion of therapy. Lesions occur in locations unusual for atherosclerosis (Fig. 35-5). Blowout of the affected carotid artery may occur, but this is more frequent when surgery is combined with radiation in treating cervical malignancies. Hyperlipidemia and hypercholesterolemia appear to predispose patients receiving radiation therapy to the development of these accelerated changes.[103] Endarterectomy of the affected segments is difficult but can be carried out safely.[102,104]

Moritz and colleagues reported their experience with 53 patients who had undergone radiation therapy to the neck an average of 28 months earlier and compared them with a control group of 38 patients who had not had radiation.[105] Thirty percent of the radiated group had moderate to severe lesions of the carotid bifurcation, as detected by duplex scanning, in contrast to only 6% of the control group. Five patients in the radiated group were symptomatic. The authors concluded that patients who receive carotid radiation should undergo periodic follow-up duplex scanning of the carotid arteries.

RECURRENT CAROTID STENOSIS

Recurrent carotid stenosis has been reported to occur in 1% to 21% of cases[106-111] and may yield an incidence of hemodynamically significant stenosis as high as 32% after 7 years.[106] This can lead to neurologic symptoms by producing emboli or restricting flow. The most common lesion developing within the first 2 years after surgery is myointimal fibroplasia. Histologically, a concentric lesion occurs, with no calcium or lipid deposits. A dense accumulation of collagen and mucopolysaccharides surrounds cellular elements. These substances are produced by the myointimal cell in the normal healing process. Their accelerated production seems to be responsible for the development of the fibroplastic lesion leading to luminal stenosis. An endarterectomy plane is almost impossible to develop.

The morphologic characteristics of the early (<2 years) restenosis suggest a lower risk of stroke when compared with arteriosclerotic lesions of a similar degree.[112] In addition, regression of stenosis documented by noninvasive tests has been reported. Thus, controversy exists over the management

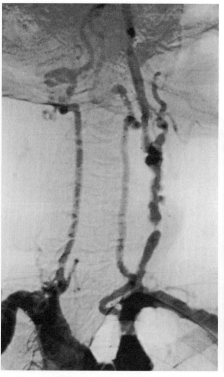
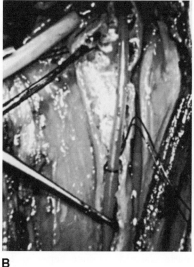
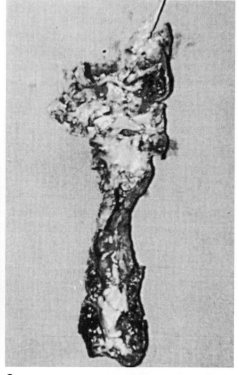

A **B** **C**

FIGURE 35–5 • *A,* Arch angiogram demonstrating carotid artery disease secondary to external cervical radiation. Note complete occlusion of the right common carotid artery. Multiple stenoses are in the left common carotid artery, an unusual site for primary atherosclerosis. *B,* Operative appearance of the lesion secondary to external radiation. *C,* Intimectomy specimen of the lesion produced by external cervical radiation.

of early recurrent stenosis after carotid endarterectomy.[113] In the asymptomatic stage, a restenosis documented by successive noninvasive testing should lead the surgeon to consider surgical intervention if progression to greater than 80% of the diameter occurs. Recurrent symptoms are certainly an indication for reoperation unless a different cause is suspected. Interestingly, Bernstein and colleagues showed an inverse correlation between greater than 50% recurrent stenosis and late stroke and death.[114] Their data suggested that patients with early recurrent stenosis had a better long-term prognosis than those who did not develop recurrent stenosis.

When a stenotic lesion develops more than 2 years after carotid endarterectomy, atherosclerosis is usually the cause. Injury to the vessel by vascular clamps may play a role. Elevated serum cholesterol has a statistically significant association with recurrent carotid stenosis.[107]

These lesions probably carry the same stroke risk as primary arteriosclerotic lesions in the carotid bifurcation. Recommendation for reoperation is thus based on the known risk factors of similar primary arteriosclerotic lesions.

Some investigators have suggested that patch closure at the time of the initial carotid endarterectomy may prevent recurrent stenosis. Several prospective, randomized studies, either completed or in progress, suggest a lower incidence of restenosis with the use of patch angioplasty.[108,115-118] The most compelling argument in favor of patch closure comes from a prospective study by Abu Rahma and colleagues.[119] The authors identified 74 patients with bilateral carotid stenoses in need of bilateral operation. One side was closed primarily, and the opposite side was closed with patch angioplasty. In this manner, demographic and patient characteristics were controlled. The incidence of ipsilateral stroke for primary closure was 4%, versus 0% for patch closure. In the primary closure group, there was a 22% incidence of recurrent stenosis, versus 1% in the patch group ($P < 0.003$). There was an 8% incidence of internal carotid artery occlusion with primary closure, versus 0% with patch closure. Restenosis requiring reoperation occurred in 14% of the primary closure group and in 1% of the patch group. In a life-table analysis, the 24-month freedom from recurrence was 75% in the primary closure group, versus 98% in the patch group.[119] A significant benefit of patch angioplasty appears to be a reduction in technical end point problems. Therefore, patching may be equally important in preventing occurrence and recurrence. The same objective can be achieved by preventing or correcting technical errors at the time of operation when they are identified by completion angiography. Data obtained from experimental hemodynamic studies suggest that an enlarged bulb following patch closure of an endarterectomy site may predispose to areas of low shear stress and therefore recurrent disease. For this reason, it is important not to overenlarge the bulb when using a patch. Overenlargement may be responsible for a higher incidence of recurrence after vein patch angioplasty (9%) versus prosthetic patch angioplasty (2%). However, both were superior to primary closure (34%) in a randomized study.[120]

The benefit of patch closure was also seen in a retrospective analysis of other data from the Asymptomatic Carotid Atherosclerosis Study (ACAS). The study examined the incidence of recurrence for three time intervals: within 3 months of operation (residual disease), 3 to 18 months (myointimal hyperplasia), and 18 to 60 months (recurrent atherosclerosis).

The use of patch angioplasty reduced the overall risk of restenosis from 21.2% to 7.1%.[121] Factors associated with early recurrence include an incomplete intimectomy, the use of distal tacking sutures, female sex, continued cigarette smoking, and primary closure of an anatomically small internal carotid artery.[122-124]

Many clinicians routinely prescribe aspirin preoperatively as well as postoperatively, in the hope that embolic events from platelet aggregates can be reduced or eliminated. The rationale is that aspirin will reduce the incidence of myointimal hyperplasia by reducing platelet adhesion or aggregation and interfering with the platelet release reaction. Unfortunately, the carotid artery, like other areas subjected to arterial reconstruction, has not been shown to benefit. A prospective, randomized, placebo-controlled trial failed to show any benefit of aspirin in preventing early carotid restenosis.[125]

CAROTID BODY TUMORS

Vascular surgeons are frequently called on to remove carotid body tumors because of their intimate adherence to the carotid bifurcation and the possible need to clamp, resect, graft, or otherwise repair the carotid artery during the course of resecting the tumor from the neck.

The carotid body is made up of chemoreceptor cells surrounded by a vascular stroma. Carotid body tumors are true neoplasms that arise from chemoreceptor cells. The tumors have an extremely rich blood supply, which makes their surgical removal both difficult and hazardous. Biopsy of a carotid body tumor is absolutely contraindicated because of the risk of uncontrollable hemorrhage. Immunohistochemical studies suggest that the tumor cells are capable of synthesizing several different neural endocrine substances, yet these tumors seldom have a pathologic endocrine function.

Most carotid body tumors are benign and usually cause problems because of enlargement and compression of adjacent neural or vascular structures. The cranial nerves that can be involved include IX, X, XI, and XII, with associated dysfunction related to the distribution of those nerves. Carotid body tumors, on occasion, can exhibit malignant behavior. Malignancy can be determined only when there is evidence of lymph node or distant metastases. It is not possible to differentiate a benign from a malignant tumor based on histologic examination alone.

Pathogenetic Mechanisms of Transient Ischemic Attacks and Cerebral Infarction

In reviewing the mechanisms for TIA and cerebral infarction, emphasis is placed on those events related to disease in the extracranial vessels. Hemorrhagic stroke is excluded. Cerebral ischemic events related to hypertension and cardiac emboli are briefly reviewed because of their importance in the differential diagnosis and workup of symptomatic patients. Finally, from a pathogenetic standpoint, the difference between TIA and fixed deficit is a matter of degree, duration, and presence of actual infarction. The mechanisms of occurrence are essentially the same. Therefore, for purposes of discussion, we use the general inclusive term *ischemic event.*

ARTERIAL THROMBOSIS

When an atherosclerotic plaque expands to produce a critical reduction in blood flow, the vessel ultimately undergoes thrombosis. In the case of the internal carotid artery, if this column of thrombus stops at the ophthalmic artery and remains stable, and if collateral circulation is sufficient via the circle of Willis, the thrombotic event may be entirely asymptomatic (Fig. 35-6). If the thrombus propagates beyond the ophthalmic artery to occlude the middle cerebral artery (Fig. 35-7), or if small thrombi rather than a thrombotic column form and are subsequently carried to the intracranial vessels by continuous blood flow (Fig. 35-8), the patient experiences cerebral symptoms that can vary from transient ocular or hemispheric events to a profound hemiplegia, depending on the extent of propagated thrombus or embolus. In addition, if the collateral circulation to the circle of Willis is poor, the sudden loss of flow through a diseased internal carotid artery may incite a precipitous drop in flow to the hemisphere, resulting in ischemic infarction as a consequence of inadequate proximal blood flow.

FLOW-RELATED ISCHEMIC EVENTS

Although flow-related ischemia used to be considered the most common cause of transient ischemic events, it is actually a rather rare occurrence. Transient drops in hemispheric blood flow or the development of a chronic low-flow state can be responsible for nonspecific symptoms of lightheadedness, presyncope, or intellectual deterioration.[1,126] It must also be recognized that other, nonvascular causes of these symptoms exist and are probably more frequent.

The collateral blood flow to the brain, via the circle of Willis, is an extremely efficient system. Multiple patients

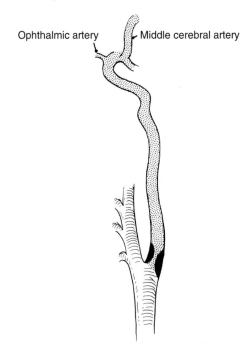

FIGURE 35–7 • Thrombus secondary to an occlusive atherosclerotic lesion of the internal carotid artery progresses beyond the ophthalmic artery to involve the middle cerebral artery.

have been described who had bilateral internal carotid artery occlusion, perhaps combined with occlusion of the vertebral artery, but were totally asymptomatic from a central neurologic point of view. Experience obtained performing carotid endarterectomy under local anesthesia has shown that only about 10% of patients experience neurologic symptoms when

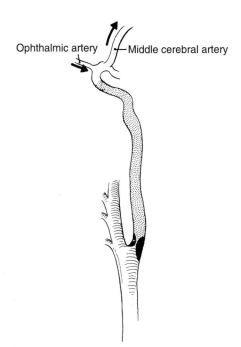

FIGURE 35–6 • Thrombus occurring distal to an occlusive lesion of the internal carotid artery. Note that the column of thrombus stops short of the ophthalmic artery, and patency of the middle cerebral artery is maintained.

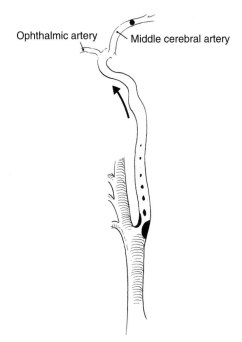

FIGURE 35–8 • Emboli released from a plaque strategically placed at the origin of the internal carotid artery can pass into the middle cerebral artery and lodge in the terminal branch. This results in either a temporary or a permanent neurologic deficit in the distribution appropriate to the arterial occlusion.

the carotid artery is clamped.[53] This 10% may have symptoms on the basis of compromised blood flow when the stenosis progresses or goes on to complete occlusion. Another circumstance that can produce symptoms of global ischemia is simultaneous stenosis or occlusion in more than one extracranial vessel—for example, a carotid occlusion on one side combined with a high-grade stenosis in the contralateral carotid artery. Under these circumstances, transient drops in blood pressure, perhaps posturally related, can produce either global or focal ischemic symptoms. Rarely, patients with unilateral carotid occlusion may have a downstream vascular bed that is marginally perfused. Postural changes under these circumstances can also produce focal ischemia and result in a flow-related TIA. Under these conditions, a patient would be a good candidate for extracranial-to-intracranial bypass grafting.

Flow-restricting lesions in the vertebral arteries or in major vessels proximal to the vertebral origin, such as the innominate or subclavian artery, can produce symptoms related to hypoperfusion in the posterior circulation. One of the most dramatic anatomic observations is the so-called subclavian steal syndrome. If a stenosis or occlusion of the subclavian artery is present proximal to the vertebral artery takeoff, the pressure drop distal to the obstruction causes its branches to serve as sources of collateral blood flow by reversing the normal flow direction. The branches now contribute to the flow of the main trunk rather than receiving flow from the proximally affected artery. The vessels that contribute to collateral blood flow of the distal subclavian artery by reversing flow include the vertebral artery. Under these circumstances, the vertebral artery not only is deprived of the usual antegrade flow but also actually siphons off blood flow from the basilar artery circulation because of flow reversal. This siphoning off of blood may be entirely without symptoms if abundant sources of inflow from the other vertebral artery or from the anterior circulation exist. Conversely, if the opposite vertebral artery is small or occluded, a deficiency in basilar artery flow may be present that results in symptoms of basilar artery insufficiency. These symptoms may first appear or become exaggerated if the demand for flow in the affected subclavian artery increases, such as results from active exercise of the arm (Fig. 35-9).

CEREBRAL EMBOLI

The most common causes of cerebral ischemic events are embolic phenomena, primarily arterial in origin and secondarily from cardiac sources. The emboli of arterial origin occur as a consequence of morphologic change present on the luminal surface of a critical artery.[52,53,127,128] These changes most often are associated with atheromatous plaques but can also occur with other lesions such as fibromuscular dysplasia. When an irregular surface produces turbulence, a stimulus for platelet aggregation is present. If the platelet aggregates become large enough and embolize to an important vessel in the brain, symptoms occur. If the platelet aggregates break up quickly from mechanical forces or from the effect of arterial prostacyclin, the symptoms are transient. If the embolic fragment persists, however, it can lead to focal infarction (Fig. 35-10).

An atherosclerotic plaque may undergo central degeneration or softening. When this occurs, bleeding into the plaque substance may also occur, leading to sudden plaque expansion with intraluminal rupture,[49,75,110,129] or the plaque may

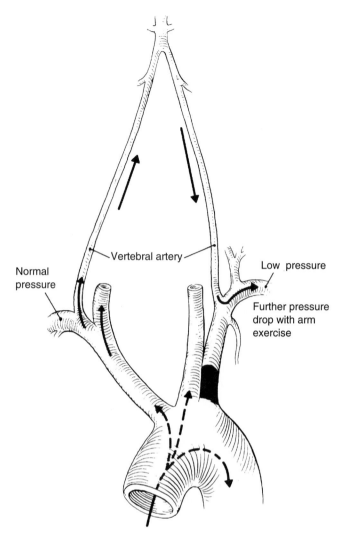

FIGURE 35–9 • Mechanism of the subclavian steal syndrome. Note the occlusion in the origin of the left subclavian artery. This produces a pressure gradient with reversal of blood flow in the left vertebral artery, producing a siphoning or steal from the basilar artery.

spontaneously rupture into the lumen, discharging its contents into the arterial stream. The plaque contents consist of degenerative atheromatous debris, including various mixtures of cholesterol crystals, calcific material, or thrombotic remnants. If the atherosclerotic plaque is located at a critical point, such as the origin of the internal carotid artery, considerable likelihood exists that embolic atheromatous fragments will be carried to important vascular beds of the brain, producing either transient or permanent neurologic events (Fig. 35-11). These events are considered primary embolic events of atherosclerotic plaque origin.

After the plaque has ruptured, a defect is left behind that is called an ulcer (Fig. 35-12). Further primary emboli can continue to escape from the raw ulcerated surface, or the ulcer itself may serve as a focal point for thrombus or platelet aggregate material to form. These platelet or thrombotic aggregates may secondarily dislodge, owing to blood flow turbulence, and embolize to the brain (Fig. 35-13). Thus, the embolic material from an atherosclerotic plaque can consist of atheromatous debris, platelet aggregates, or blood clot.

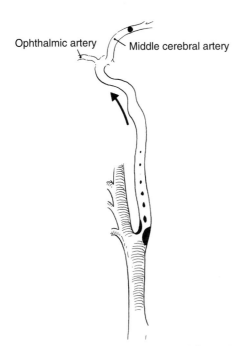

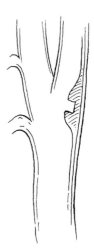

FIGURE 35–10 • Embolic fragment in the middle cerebral artery. If this persists, it will lead to focal infarction. If the fragment breaks up and distributes itself through the microcirculation, the ischemic event will be transient.

The emboli of arterial origin can be primary, occurring with plaque rupture or on thrombogenic arterial plaque surfaces,[128,130] or secondary, having developed within ulcerative lesions from previous plaque rupture.[131]

Embolic events may produce dramatic focal neurologic events that are immediately appreciated by the patient, or the embolic fragments may travel to more silent areas of

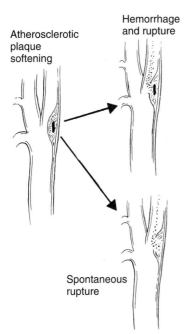

FIGURE 35–11 • Atherosclerotic plaque undergoing central softening. Spontaneous hemorrhage may occur into the center of the plaque, producing rupture and discharge of embolic fragments, or the plaque may spontaneously rupture as a result of hydrostatic forces, releasing necrotic embolic debris.

FIGURE 35–12 • Following evacuation of an atherosclerotic plaque, a defect or ulcer is left behind.

the brain, in which case the results are more subtle and appreciated on a chronic basis, such as cerebral atrophy or multi-infarct dementia.[132,133] The use of transcranial Doppler ultrasonography has provided more objective evidence of emboli from carotid plaques by discerning discrete noise as an embolic particle passes a point of Doppler insonation.[134] Finally, the occurrence of TIAs in a hemisphere distal to a carotid occlusion raises the question of the importance of decreased flow to arterial border zones. Experimental data have demonstrated that emboli originating from a contralateral carotid artery can cross through the circle of Willis and produce focal infarcts in the hemisphere distal to a carotid occlusion.[135] Thus, the contralateral patent carotid artery should always be considered a possible source of emboli when a patient with a carotid occlusion begins to experience symptoms in the hemisphere distal to the occlusion.

Emboli can also occur from cardiac sources, which include aortic valvular disease, mitral valve prolapse, cardiac arrhythmias, and mural thrombus after MI. More recently, atherosclerotic plaques of the ascending aorta, as seen with transesophageal echocardiography, have been identified as another source of cerebral embolization.[136-138]

LACUNAR INFARCTION

Focal areas of cerebral necrosis occurring in the basal ganglia, internal capsule, or pons have been described as a consequence of end-vessel occlusive disease involving the lenticulostriate or thalamoperforating arteries. The underlying cause is related to uncontrolled hypertension, and the resulting neurologic deficit is often clinically identified as a pure motor or pure sensory stroke.[139] Although descriptions of this phenomenon date back to the early 1900s, its current understanding is based on the efforts and writings of Fisher.[140]

The clinical picture may often be confused with arterial-arterial emboli, in that antecedent TIAs may have occurred. The differential diagnosis is best made by the very focal neurologic deficit seen clinically and the typical anatomic location seen on the CT scan of the brain. Evidence now shows that the so-called lacunae may, in fact, be the consequence of emboli of arterial origin.[141-144] Thus, symptoms and imaging of a deep white matter infarct do not rule out atheromatous plaque from the carotid bifurcation as a cause of the event.

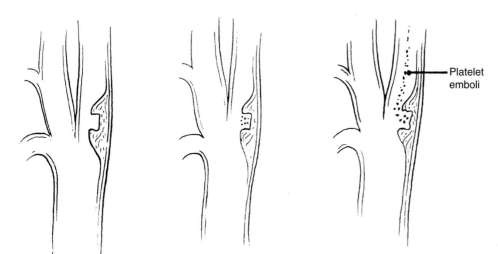

Platelet
emboli

FIGURE 35–13 • The ulcerated lesion within an atheromatous plaque can serve as a nidus for platelet aggregation or thrombotic material. These aggregates can secondarily embolize from the ulcer crypt.

Clinical Syndromes of Extracranial Arterial Occlusive Disease

Extracranial arterial occlusive disease may result in varying symptoms or may be completely asymptomatic. A thorough history must be obtained, because this alone can provide clues to the specific nature of the event. Often, one discovers the existence of symptoms that the patient has been ignoring. A complete review of symptoms is mandatory, because this may alter the therapeutic alternatives available. Risk factors for atherosclerosis should be specifically recorded.

Patients can be classified into three categories: asymptomatic patients, patients with TIAs, and patients with cerebral infarction. In asymptomatic patients, a hemodynamically significant lesion or a nonocclusive ulcerated arteriosclerotic plaque in the extracranial circulation may be discovered in the absence of transient or permanent neurologic symptoms. The presence or absence of a bruit in the cervical area should not be a criterion for inclusion in this category. It should be recorded as a general marker of a patient at high risk for atherosclerosis.[145]

In an analysis of 1287 patients with cervical bruits, less than one third of the carotid lesions with bruits proved to be hemodynamically significant by noninvasive criteria.[41] The fact that significant lesions can occur in the absence of a bruit and vice versa is important. The available data on the natural history of asymptomatic bruits cannot be applied to patients with these lesions. This group of patients is usually discovered by angiography while studying other conditions or by noninvasive studies carried out because of the presence of a bruit or for screening before major surgical procedures. Because of what is known about the natural history of these lesions, as discussed later, therapeutic intervention in the asymptomatic stage may be beneficial.

The two categories of symptomatic patients with extracranial arterial occlusive disease are discussed separately.

TRANSIENT ISCHEMIC ATTACKS

General Considerations

TIAs are defined as temporary focal neurologic deficits lasting no more than 24 hours, with complete recovery. The event is caused by ischemia in the territory of the brain supplied by a particular artery or branch. Because of its territorial nature, symptoms tend to be stereotyped. Clinically, symptoms are of sudden onset and without aura, and resolution is often quick. Disappearance of symptoms ordinarily takes only a few minutes.[146] When symptoms last longer than 6 hours, a permanent abnormality is more likely, although it may not be clinically detectable.[147] The frequency of attacks is variable. The patient may experience only one episode or multiple attacks, with variable symptom-free intervals. The most common cause of these transient territorial deficits is extracranial arterial occlusive lesions. The pathology of these lesions has already been discussed. Other important causes in the differential diagnosis include heart disease; hematologic disorders such as systemic lupus erythematosus, hyperglobulinemia, polycythemia, and sickle cell disease; disseminated intravascular coagulation; subacute bacterial endocarditis; paroxysmal embolism; and several rare connective tissue disorders such as pseudoxanthoma elasticum and Ehlers-Danlos syndrome.[147] Migraine, especially when associated with transient neurologic deficit, can be confused with a TIA. A history of migraine in the family, the throbbing quality of the headache, and its occurrence on recovery from the neurologic deficit can be helpful in the differential diagnosis.

An important concept when evaluating patients with symptoms suggestive of TIA is that the symptoms secondary to emboli from a point source such as the extracranial circulation are the same with every attack. In contrast, patients whose emboli are from the heart tend to have variable symptoms.

Because only about 9% of patients with TIAs are seen by a physician during an attack,[148] the history remains the main factor in establishing the diagnosis. In this regard, family members may be extremely helpful.

Two important syndromes deserve mention. Occasionally, a patient experiences frequent repeated attacks of a specific neurologic deficit with no interval allowing time for complete recovery. If the deficit is the same with each attack and no deterioration in function is seen, this is known as crescendo TIAs. If progressive deterioration is seen with each successive attack, a stroke in evolution may be present. In any case, evaluation must proceed on an emergency basis. If a surgically correctable lesion is present and the neurologic deficit is not dense (no loss of consciousness or dense hemiparesis), serious consideration should be given to proceeding with emergency operation.

Carotid Artery Transient Ischemic Attacks

Manifestations of a transient ischemic episode in the territory of the carotid artery include deficits in areas supplied by the anterior and middle cerebral arteries. In older individuals, both anterior and posterior cerebral arteries may be supplied by one carotid artery.[147]

Ischemia in a cerebral hemisphere often produces contralateral symptoms. Motor dysfunction can include weakness, paralysis, or clumsiness of one or both limbs contralateral to the affected hemisphere. Sensory alterations include numbness, loss of sensation, or paresthesia in the opposite side of the face or in one or both limbs. When a patient is examined during an attack, this sensory loss may not be objectively demonstrable.[148]

Ninety-five percent of patients have a dominant left hemisphere. Both receptive aphasia and motor aphasia can occur. When the former is present, the patient or family may interpret it as confusion. Dysarthria may occur as a function of TIA in the nondominant hemisphere, but when it is the sole symptom, vertebrobasilar TIA is more likely. Other functional deficits of the nondominant side include inattention to the patient's own person and environment on the contralateral side.[147] Loss of function of these areas may also be interpreted as confusion.

Transient visual loss (amaurosis fugax) or blurring of vision in the ipsilateral eye is one of the most reliable symptoms of carotid artery TIAs.[149] This may be described as a curtain coming down (altitudinal) or as quadrant field defects. Conjugate eye deviation, as occurs in seizures or completed strokes, is not seen. Homonymous hemianopsia in combination with any of the above-mentioned symptoms suggests carotid TIAs. This is the result of ischemia in the area of the optic radiation emanating from the optic chiasm. This produces loss of vision in the ipsilateral temporal visual field and the contralateral nasal visual field. When TIAs occur secondary to carotid artery disease, these visual field defects are usually limited to a quadrant corresponding to the distribution of the optic radiation. When hemianopsia is complete, it cannot be distinguished from a vertebrobasilar TIA.[147]

Ischemic optic neuropathy is characterized by blindness and is associated with giant cell arteritis in about 10% of cases. In the other 90% of cases, it has been labeled idiopathic. Berguer found a significant correlation between extracranial occlusive disease and idiopathic optic neuropathy.[150] In fact, of 20 symptomatic eyes examined, significant extracranial arterial occlusive disease was found in 12 (60%). An embolic mechanism was suggested as the cause of the optic nerve infarct. A more severe form is seen in patients with very severe extracranial disease, usually occlusion on one side and a high degree of stenosis on the other. These patients develop an ischemic ophthalmopathy characterized by neovascularization of the iris. The term *rubeosis* has been used to characterize this entity. This suggests that patients with idiopathic optic neuropathy that is not secondary to giant cell arteritis should undergo extracranial vascular evaluation.[150]

Convulsions can occur but are more suggestive of a completed or hemorrhagic stroke. When sensory or motor symptoms are present, they appear all at once, without a march suggestive of focal seizure activity.[147] A combination of symptoms may have more diagnostic reliability than a single symptom alone. In right carotid artery TIA, the combination of ipsilateral visual loss and any contralateral arm symptoms has an increased relationship. In left carotid TIA, diagnostic reliability is increased when language disturbance is combined with right face or extremity weakness or sensory loss.[149]

Altered consciousness or syncope can occur, but it is rarely the only symptom and is more often associated with other disorders, such as cardiac arrhythmias.[147] Other symptoms that make the initial evaluation difficult are dizziness, amnesia, or confusion and impaired vision with alteration in consciousness. These, without other more specific symptoms, cannot be considered manifestations of TIAs, because they occur most often with other illnesses.

Vertebrobasilar System Transient Ischemic Attacks

Transient ischemia of the area of the brain supplied by the vertebrobasilar system can occur due to flow restriction or emboli from lesions in the vertebral or basilar arteries. Emboli from other sources may also affect this system.

An occlusive lesion at the origin of the subclavian artery can cause vertebrobasilar symptoms as the affected arm is exercised and reversal of flow occurs in the vertebral circulation. This subclavian steal is often accompanied by exertional pain in the arm of the affected side.[147]

Alternating hemipareses, hemisensory symptoms in repetitive attacks, and bilateral circumoral sensory symptoms associated with unilateral arm or leg weakness or ataxia are highly suggestive of vertebrobasilar TIAs. Symptoms may change from one side to the other with different attacks and may even involve all four limbs at one time. Drop attacks, or falling precipitously to the ground without premonitory symptoms, occur in less than 4% of patients.[149] In this syndrome, loss of consciousness is absent or so brief that the patient remembers striking the ground, a feature not present in syncope or seizure.[147]

Equilibratory gait or postural disturbance not associated with vertigo can occur. Complete or partial loss of vision in both homonymous fields or homonymous hemianopsia alone is highly suggestive. Vertigo alone, when not associated with other specific symptoms, should not be considered indicative of TIA. When it occurs in clear relationship to focal weakness of the face, arm, or leg or to ataxia or persistent diplopia, the existence of TIA is likely. Tinnitus is not a feature of vertebrobasilar TIA and is suggestive of labyrinthine vertigo. Single occurrences of bilateral visual blurring, dysarthria, hoarseness, diplopia, dysphasia, confusion, hiccups, vomiting, loss of consciousness, and vital sign alteration may be manifestations of vertebrobasilar TIAs. These symptoms have so many other causes, however, that the diagnosis is uncertain unless they occur in combination or with additional signs of focal brainstem or posterior hemisphere dysfunction.

CEREBRAL INFARCTION

A completed cerebral infarction with or without a clinically apparent neurologic deficit can be another manifestation of extracranial arterial occlusive disease. The specific deficits that are clinically detectable are the same as those discussed earlier as manifestations of TIAs.

Accurately estimating the percentage of strokes that are secondary to lesions in the extracranial circulation is difficult. Available studies differ in terms of population, criteria for diagnosis, and therapeutic approach; thus, the estimates range from 15% to 52%.[151,152] Extracranial vascular lesions play a major role in the occurrence of cerebral infarction. Approximately 50% of these events are preceded by TIAs, thus providing a clue to diagnosis.[153]

Lacunar infarcts, emboli from a cardiac source, intracerebral or intracranial bleeding, and some hematologic disorders should be included in the differential diagnosis of the cause of stroke. Cerebrospinal fluid examination, electroencephalography (EEG), echocardiography, Holter monitoring, and brain CT are helpful adjuncts. Angiography should be considered, because noninvasive studies do not exclude ulcerative lesions in the extracranial circulation that may be responsible for the embolic infarction.

Identification of a cause of the stroke is essential, because these patients remain at high risk of developing a subsequent cerebral infarction.

Role of the Vascular Laboratory

The role of the vascular laboratory in the evaluation of patients with suspected cerebrovascular disease has been disputed by some and perhaps misused by others. However, it has an increasingly important role, and this section reviews its current application. The vascular laboratory is covered in detail in Chapter 14.

ASYMPTOMATIC PATIENTS

Patients without symptoms may come to our attention as possible candidates for extracranial cerebrovascular disease because of the presence of one or more associated risk factors (cigarette smoking, hypertension, diabetes mellitus, coronary artery disease, or peripheral vascular disease) or by the presence of a bruit heard over the carotid artery bifurcation. In the past, the occurrence of a preocclusive carotid stenosis could be ascertained only by carotid angiography, but the incidence of finding a significant lesion by angiographic screening was only 20% to 30%. That means that 70% of the suspect population was subjected to costly and needless hospitalization, plus the risk and discomfort of angiography. Currently, the presence or absence of a hemodynamically significant lesion can be ascertained by the vascular laboratory in an inexpensive, noninvasive manner with an accuracy of greater than 95%.

SYMPTOMATIC PATIENTS

Patients may show territorial neurologic events typical of carotid artery or vertebrobasilar disease, or they may have symptoms that are entirely nonspecific or atypical. In the case of a patient with nonspecific symptoms, such as "dizzy spells," these symptoms may be related to global ischemic events as a consequence of decreased blood flow associated with multiple extracranial occlusive lesions, or they may be due to myriad disorders unrelated to cerebrovascular disease. The vascular laboratory serves as an effective screen for these patients, avoiding many negative and hence useless angiograms.

Angiography used to be considered mandatory for the workup of symptomatic patients. This is no longer true. Duplex scanning in a qualified laboratory can provide definitive information necessary for both medical and surgical management. For this reason, carefully performed duplex scanning has become a critical part of the evaluation of symptomatic patients. Contrast angiography is now reserved for patients whose symptoms are not explained by findings on duplex scans.

In addition, the preoperative baseline data from the vascular laboratory are extremely helpful in following patients immediately after operation as well as in the late follow-up period. A conversion from a positive to a negative test after operation is expected. If this does not occur, a technical problem is suggested that may require investigation and management. Also, an abnormal study 6 months or a year after surgery in a patient who had a normal study after operation alerts the surgeon to the possibility of recurrent stenosis, often before the onset of symptoms. Finally, the importance of obtaining baseline data on the opposite, asymptomatic carotid artery should not be overlooked. Late strokes that occur in patients who have undergone successful carotid endarterectomy are most often related to the side not operated on. Early identification of progression on the contralateral side permits earlier intervention to prevent contralateral stroke.

Brain Scans and Angiography

The advent of CT and magnetic resonance imaging (MRI) has been a benefit in the evaluation of patients with cerebrovascular disease and has virtually eliminated the use of radionuclide scanning. Intracranial space-occupying lesions such as neoplasms, vascular malformations, or subdural hematomas enter into the differential diagnosis of patients with even the most convincing symptoms of transient cerebral ischemia. CT and MRI are quick, noninvasive means of ruling out other abnormalities during the patient workup.

A patient who presents with a TIA may have actually suffered a small cerebral infarction. CT or MRI can identify an unsuspected cerebral infarction and establish a baseline status before operation. The advance knowledge that a small infarction exists is helpful with respect to intraoperative and postoperative management.

Although head scanning may not be a routine part of the preoperative workup, it should become a standard part of the evaluation of symptomatic patients. MRI is replacing CT in some centers. It does not require ionizing radiation or contrast material. It can identify acute cerebral infarction sooner than CT and can image smaller infarcts than CT. Finally, new acquisition programs have enabled the use of magnetic resonance techniques to reconstruct cervical and intracranial arterial anatomy, so-called magnetic resonance angiography (MRA).

Those patients with a clinically overt cerebral infarction should have CT or MRI to document the infarct size and to differentiate between ischemic and hemorrhagic infarction. A hemorrhagic infarction is promptly visible on the CT scan, whereas an ischemic infarction may take several days of evolution before its low-density character is visualized. CT scan data are necessary to determine the proper timing of operation after acute stroke in patients who have had a good neurologic recovery. In fact, of 245 patients with persistent neurologic deficits seen by Dosick and colleagues,[154] 171 were found to have negative CT scans. Appropriate carotid lesions were found in 110 (64%) of this group. All 110 patients underwent carotid endarterectomy within 14 days of the initial onset of their neurologic deficits. The perioperative morbidity was 0.9%. These investigators concluded that angiography and carotid endarterectomy can be safely performed when indicated in patients with negative CT scans within the first 2 weeks after a prolonged neurologic deficit.

EEG has generally not been considered helpful in the workup of patients with cerebrovascular disease, with the exception of ruling out seizure disorder in the differential diagnosis. However, a new application of cerebral electrical activity, so-called computerized brain mapping, is of value. This modality uses 32 electrodes (rather than the 16 used with EEG) arranged over both hemispheres. The data are digitized and color-coded. The information is computer-analyzed, and hard-copy integrated data are generated. In a report comparing CT, MRI, and brain mapping, brain mapping was more sensitive in identifying small areas of cortical dysfunction.[155]

Aortocranial angiography was once the cornerstone of diagnosis in the workup of patients with suspected cerebrovascular disease. Today, however, *the angiogram is a preoperative study* and should not be ordered unless the patient and surgeon are prepared to proceed promptly with operation. Angiography has no role as a routine database item unless the information obtained is going to be used for therapeutic decision making. Noninvasive studies are now sophisticated enough for diagnosis. The angiogram should be used to confirm the presence of a surgically accessible lesion and a satisfactory distal vascular bed.

The extent of angiographic visualization required for proper evaluation in patients with cerebrovascular disease is controversial. The options include (1) visualization of the aortic arch and extracranial vessels in two oblique views, (2) selective injection of both common carotid arteries in anteroposterior and lateral projections to obtain both extracranial and intracranial carotid visualization, (3) combined arch and selective carotid angiography, (4) the addition of subclavian-vertebral angiography for both extracranial and intracranial visualization, (5) digital intravenous or intra-arterial subtraction angiography, and (6) no angiography at all, relying solely on noninvasive testing.

Although aortocranial angiography remains the gold standard for identifying both extracranial and intracranial cerebrovascular disease, an increasing number of institutions around the world are electing to forgo angiography, provided that noninvasive preoperative testing is of diagnostic quality and correlates with the patient's clinical presentation. Noninvasive testing, primarily carotid duplex scanning, perhaps supplemented with information from MRA or CT-angiography, can clearly identify patients with carotid bifurcation disease. MRA or CT may be more accurate in defining the percentage of stenosis than data from contrast angiography; the contrast angiogram almost inevitably underestimates the percentage of stenosis. Noninvasive testing cannot accurately define carotid ulceration independent of carotid stenosis, but even with angiography, the definition of carotid ulceration is limited. The correlation between the preoperative angiogram and inspection of the plaque at the time of operation was analyzed in the first 540 patients entered into the North American Symptomatic Carotid Endarterectomy Trial (NASCET).[156] The sensitivity and specificity for detecting ulcerated plaques was 45.9% and 74.1%, respectively. The positive predictive value for identifying an ulcer was 71.8%. Thus, even the gold standard of angiography is imperfect in diagnosing ulceration. One possible explanation is that the ulceration may be filled with thrombus when the angiogram is obtained.

The routine preoperative use of angiography has been questioned in the literature. This remains a controversial issue, but the practice has clearly increased in those centers that have validated, certified vascular laboratories.[157]

The benefit of performing carotid endarterectomy without angiography is that angiography carries a significant risk in patients with extracranial arterial occlusive disease. In the ACAS,[158,159] the neurologic morbidity and mortality was 1.2% for angiography alone. This is almost equal to the risk of operation. Although some express the opinion that this complication rate was abnormally high, all patients had been prescreened with ultrasonography and had documented hemodynamically significant lesions. Therefore, this represents a select, high-risk group of patients for angiography. With improved techniques of imaging the carotid bifurcation, there has been increasing acceptance of noninvasive imaging as a substitute for preoperative angiography in patients scheduled for carotid endarterectomy. This change in opinion began with the use of improved-quality duplex scanning, and it continues with the use of MRA. Finally, recognizing the limitations of both of these techniques, some suggest combining duplex scanning and MRA for preoperative assessment. When there is clear agreement between the two techniques, this appears to be a safe substitute for contrast angiography; however, when conflicting information is obtained, when the noninvasive study is unsatisfactory, or when the clinical picture is unexplained by noninvasive imaging, the selective use of contrast angiography is clearly indicated.[157,160-170]

Surgical Considerations and Technique

ANESTHESIA AND HEMODYNAMIC MONITORING

Patients about to undergo cerebrovascular surgery are probably best managed under general anesthesia. Although some surgeons still prefer to do carotid endarterectomy under local or cervical block anesthesia,[171] general anesthesia has the advantage of reducing the cerebral metabolic demand of the brain and increasing cerebral blood flow. General anesthesia also provides good airway control, reduced patient anxiety, and a quiet surgical field.

Intraoperative blood pressure control and oxygenation are particularly critical during periods of arterial clamping. These parameters are best monitored with an arterial line, usually placed in the radial artery. The judicious use of nitroprusside or vasopressors by the anesthesiologist to maintain blood pressure in the patient's optimal physiologic range is of paramount importance.

Two primary options are available to monitor cerebral perfusion, which might be required during trial clamping of the carotid artery before a decision to use an internal shunt.

These options are the measurement of internal carotid artery back-pressure[172,173] and the intraoperative use of EEG.[174] Although controversy exists as to which is more effective, excellent results have been reported with both techniques. EEG with CT brain mapping is a sensitive and accurate means of identifying patients who require shunting.[155,175] Another technique, that of somatosensory evoked potentials, has been investigated and does not appear to be as sensitive as EEG.[176] Finally, proponents of no monitoring exist; some advocate the routine use of an intraluminal shunt,[177] and others advocate routine operation without a shunt but done in an expeditious manner.[178,179] The literature currently supports either selective shunting based on clinical and monitoring criteria or routine shunting. The consensus is that either of these techniques provides a safe operation with the best outcome.[180,181]

The argument in favor of selective shunting is as follows: because only 15% of patients actually require an intraluminal shunt, as judged by observations during operations carried out under local anesthesia, why expose the other 85% of patients to the risks of an internal shunt, which include (1) possible air or atheroma embolisms, (2) scuffing or dissection of distal intima, (3) difficulty with end-point visualization, and (4) risk of leaving an intimal flap that may lead to thromboembolic complications? The arguments in favor of the routine use of an intraluminal shunt are that, with routine use, operator facility with the technique is increased and there is less likelihood of complications, and the intraluminal shunt acts as a stent, which can aid in the closure of the internal carotid portion of the arteriotomy.

The criteria for mandatory shunting based on back-pressure measurement, as originally described by Moore and colleagues,[172,173] include a prior cerebral infarction on the side of operation (regardless of back-pressure value) or no prior cerebral infarction but a back-pressure of 25 mm Hg or less in a patient who is otherwise neurologically intact. The EEG criteria for shunt use include a loss of amplitude or slowing of rhythm during trial clamping of the carotid artery.

CAROTID BIFURCATION ENDARTERECTOMY

Indications

The indications for carotid endarterectomy have undergone considerable review and analysis. Data based on retrospective reviews, results of prospective, randomized trials, and committee discussions based on expert opinion have been brought together to define the current indications for carotid endarterectomy.[182-184]

More recently, the Stroke Council of the American Heart Association convened a consensus conference on the indications for carotid endarterectomy. These two reports constitute the most up-to-date agreement concerning indications.[185,186] The ad hoc committee recognized four categories: (1) proven—the strongest indication, usually supported by results of prospective, randomized trials; (2) acceptable but not proven—a good indication for operation supported by promising but not scientifically certain data; (3) uncertain—data insufficient to define the risk-benefit ratio; and (4) proven inappropriate—current data adequate to show that the risk of surgery outweighs any benefit.

The recommendations are further stratified by the symptomatic or asymptomatic status of the patient. Finally, the risk of operation based on the comorbid condition of the patient and the individual surgeon's track record is taken into account. Based on this classification, the general indications for carotid endarterectomy can be classified as follows, for symptomatic good-risk patients with a surgeon whose surgical morbidity and mortality rate is less than 6%:

A. Proven indications
  1. One or more TIAs in the last 6 months and carotid stenosis greater than or equal to 70%
  2. Mild stroke with carotid stenosis greater than or equal to 70%
B. Acceptable but not proven indications
  1. TIAs in the past 6 months and stenosis of 50% to 69%
  2. Progressive stroke and stenosis greater than or equal to 70%
  3. Mild or moderate stroke in the past 6 months and stenosis of 50% to 69%
  4. Carotid endarterectomy ipsilateral to TIAs and stenosis greater than or equal to 70%, combined with required coronary bypass grafting
C. Uncertain indications
  1. TIAs with stenosis less than or equal to 50%
  2. Mild stroke with stenosis less than or equal to 50%
  3. Symptomatic acute carotid thrombosis
D. Proven inappropriate indications
  1. Moderate stroke with stenosis less than or equal to 50%, not receiving aspirin
  2. Single TIA, stenosis less than or equal to 50%, not receiving aspirin
  3. High-risk patient with multiple TIAs, stenosis less than or equal to 50%, not receiving aspirin
  4. High-risk patient, mild or moderate stroke, stenosis less than or equal to 50%, not receiving aspirin
  5. Global ischemic symptoms with stenosis less than or equal to 50%
  6. Acute internal carotid dissection, asymptomatic, receiving heparin

For asymptomatic good-risk patients treated by a surgeon whose surgical morbidity-mortality rate is less than 3%, the indications for carotid endarterectomy are as follows:

A. Proven indications: stenosis greater than or equal to 60% (following ACAS publication)
B. Acceptable but not proven indications: none defined
C. Uncertain indications: high-risk patient or surgeon with a morbidity-mortality rate greater than 3%, combined carotid-coronary operations, or nonstenotic ulcerative lesions
D. Proven inappropriate indications: operations with a combined stroke morbidity-mortality rate greater than or equal to 5%

The Stroke Council of the American Heart Association has updated this report and reaffirmed the indications.[187]

Technique

After the induction of satisfactory anesthesia and the placement of appropriate access and monitoring lines, the patient is positioned supine on the operating table with the head turned away from the side of operation. The neck is moderately extended on the shoulders. The head of the table is flexed about 10 degrees to reduce venous pressure, which minimizes bleeding.

I prefer a longitudinal incision placed along the anterior border of the sternocleidomastoid muscle and centered over the carotid bifurcation. This incision can be extended proximally to the sternal notch for more proximal exposure of the common carotid artery and distally to the mastoid process for extensive exposure of the internal carotid artery, when needed. The dissection plane is maintained along the anterior border of the sternocleidomastoid muscle, which permits anterior mobilization of the tail of the parotid gland rather than the bloody division of its substance, with risk of a salivary fistula. The sternocleidomastoid muscle is mobilized off the carotid sheath, and self-retaining retractors are placed. The jugular vein is visualized through the carotid sheath, and the sheath is open along the anterior border of the vein. The vein is mobilized until the large tributary, the common facial vein, is identified. The common facial vein, when present, is a relatively constant landmark for the carotid bifurcation. The common facial vein is divided between ligatures. In the case of a high carotid bifurcation, particular care must be taken to make sure that the hypoglossal nerve is not lurking behind the common facial vein, because this may lead to its inadvertent injury. Once the common facial vein is divided, the jugular vein can be mobilized laterally off the carotid bifurcation, providing excellent exposure. The vagus nerve usually lies in the posterior portion of the carotid sheath, but on occasion it may spiral anteriorly. Particular care must be taken to watch for this anomalous course to avoid nerve injury. Another anomaly is the occasional presence of a nonrecurrent laryngeal nerve that comes directly off the vagus on the way to innervate the vocal cord. This nerve can cross anterior to the carotid artery and may be mistaken for part of the ansa hypoglossi, resulting in mistaken division and cord paralysis. This anomaly most often occurs on the right side of the neck, but it has also been seen on the left side.

The common carotid artery is mobilized for a sufficient length to get proximal to the atheromatous lesion, as well as to provide sufficient length in case an internal shunt is required. When the dissection approaches the area of the carotid bifurcation, it may be necessary to inject a local anesthetic in the area to block the nerve to the carotid body to prevent or reverse reflex bradycardia. The external and internal carotid arteries are then mobilized for a sufficient length to get completely beyond the atheromatous plaque to a point where the vessels are completely normal circumferentially. When mobilizing the internal carotid artery, particular care must be taken to avoid injury to the hypoglossal nerve (Fig. 35-14).

In the case of a high bifurcation or an extensive lesion, mobilizing the internal carotid artery for its maximum extracranial length may be necessary. Several maneuvers are available to gain additional length. The first and most important maneuver is to extend the skin incision all the way up to the mastoid process, with complete mobilization of the sternocleidomastoid muscle toward its tendinous insertion on the mastoid process. Care must be taken to avoid injury to the spinal accessory nerve (cranial nerve XI), which enters the substance of the sternocleidomastoid muscle at that level. The posterior belly of the digastric muscle comes into view. This muscle can be mobilized anteriorly or, if necessary, divided with impunity, giving additional exposure of the internal carotid artery. If further exposure is needed, the limiting structures are the styloid process and the ramus of

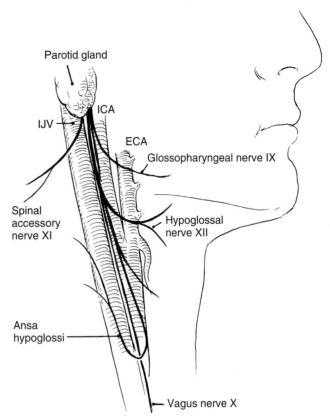

FIGURE 35-14 • Anatomic relationship between the carotid bifurcation and the cranial nerves in the neck. Note the intimate relationship between the hypoglossal nerve and the upper portion of the internal carotid artery (ICA). ECA, external carotid artery; IJV, internal jugular vein.

the mandible. The styloid process, after suitable preparation, can be divided with bone rongeurs, and the mandible can be displaced anteriorly. Techniques have also been described for dividing the ramus of the mandible to gain additional exposure, but I have not found this maneuver necessary.

Once the carotid artery has been sufficiently mobilized, 5000 units of heparin are administered systemically.

The decision whether to shunt the patient can be made using EEG or back-pressure criteria. If back-pressure is selected, a 22-gauge needle is connected to rigid pressure tubing and hooked up to an arterial pressure transducer. The tubing is flushed with saline, and a 0 pressure level is obtained adjacent to the carotid bifurcation. The needle is carefully bent at a 45-degree angle and inserted into the common carotid artery so that the axis of the distal needle is parallel to the axis of the artery and lies freely within the lumen. The free carotid artery pressure is measured and compared with the radial artery pressure to ensure an accurate reading. When the patient's blood pressure is stable and at the optimal level, the common carotid artery is clamped proximal to the needle, and the external carotid artery is also clamped, thus permitting the reading of the internal carotid artery back-pressure (Fig. 35-15). If the back-pressure is greater than 25 mm Hg, the internal carotid artery is clamped and the needle withdrawn. If the pressure is less than 25 mm Hg, the clamps on the common and external carotid arteries are temporarily removed, the needle is withdrawn, and preparations are made for the use of an internal shunt.

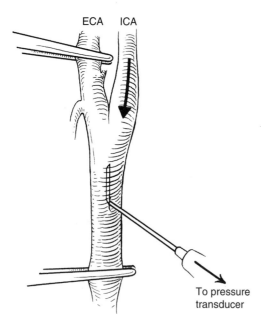

FIGURE 35–15 • Technique of measuring the internal carotid artery (ICA) back-pressure. Note the needle placement and needle angulation to maintain the tip of the needle in an axial plane with the common carotid artery. A disease-free portion of the common carotid artery is chosen for arterial puncture. ECA, external carotid artery.

With the common, external, and internal carotid arteries clamped, an arteriotomy is made on the lateral portion of the common carotid artery with a No. 11 blade and is extended toward the plaque and up the internal carotid artery with Potts scissors. The arteriotomy is extended as far as necessary up the internal carotid artery to get beyond the plaque and to expose relatively normal artery. An intimectomy plane is then established between the diseased intima and the internal elastic lamina, attempting to leave the circular medial fibers attached to the arterial adventitia. This facilitates getting a clean distal end point. The proximal end point is obtained by sharply dividing the plaque. The intimectomy surface is copiously irrigated with heparinized saline solution to allow the visualization of all bits of debris and facilitate their removal.

The arteriotomy can be closed primarily, but overwhelming evidence now indicates better results with patch angioplasty closure. Evidence suggests that female patients, patients with small internal carotid arteries, and patients who continue to smoke are at increased risk of recurrent carotid stenosis.[122,123] The use of patch angioplasty in these patients may reduce the risk of recurrent stenosis. Trial results indicate that routine use of a prosthetic patch results in the lowest rates of peripheral complications and recurrent stenosis.[119-121] Patch angioplasty should be routinely used when the indication for operation is recurrent stenosis.

Flow is established first to the external and then to the internal carotid artery. I recommend the use of routine completion angiography. There is a 5% to 8% incidence of unsuspected technical errors associated with carotid endarterectomy, and these are best documented with completion angiography.[188,189] Completion angiography is used primarily to identify technical errors involving the internal carotid artery; however, intimal flaps in the external carotid artery occur more commonly

and are erroneously considered to be of no consequence. We reported three cases of postoperative stroke secondary to intimal flaps in the external carotid artery: clot formed, propagated in a retrograde direction, and then embolized up the internal carotid artery.[190] For this reason, we advocate correction of intimal flaps of the external as well as the internal carotid artery.

An alternative to completion angiography is the use of intraoperative duplex scanning. Lipski and colleagues reported that the incidence of residual disease and perioperative neurologic complications was statistically significantly reduced in patients who had completion duplex scanning compared with a control group who did not undergo completion imaging.[191] Further, the use of completion duplex scanning identified technical problems and led to their prompt correction in 9 of 39 patients.

INTERNAL CAROTID ARTERY DILATATION

Indications

Internal carotid artery dilatation is uniquely applicable to fibromuscular dysplasia of the carotid artery. It is a major technical advance in simplifying the surgical correction of this lesion.

Technique

The carotid bifurcation is exposed in the usual manner. The internal carotid artery is exposed for its maximal length so that dilatation can be carried out under visual and palpable control. Heparin is administered systemically, and the artery is clamped. A vertical arteriotomy, approximately 1 cm long, is made in the carotid bulb, adjacent to the internal carotid artery. Coronary artery dilators are introduced and gently passed toward the base of the skull. I usually start with a 2-mm dilator and progress at 0.5-mm increments to a 4-mm dilator. The surgeon has a sensation of intraluminal septal "popping" as the dilator is passed to the base of the skull. Back-bleeding is allowed to occur after each passage to allow tissue fragments to be washed out and prevent embolization (Fig. 35-16). On completion, the arteriotomy is closed, blood flow is restored, and a completion angiogram is obtained to ensure adequate dilatation.

Alternatively, intraoperative balloon angioplasty of the affected segment of the internal carotid artery may be carried out. This technique is probably safer because traction injury to the intima is avoided. The intraoperative use of balloon angioplasty, through an open arteriotomy, avoids the possibility of forward embolization from the angioplasty site. After the balloon angioplasty is completed, vigorous back-bleeding of the vessel is allowed, to retrieve any debris loosened by the dilatation. As with progressive dilatation of the vessel, completion angiography is highly recommended to ensure an adequate technical result. I do not favor percutaneous balloon dilatation of fibromuscular dysplastic segments of the extracranial vessels.

On occasion, the surgeon may not be sure that the dilator has been advanced fully to the base of the skull. Under these circumstances, obtaining a plain x-ray film with the dilator in place and comparing that film with the preoperative angiogram to ensure that the dilator has been passed sufficiently far distally is helpful.

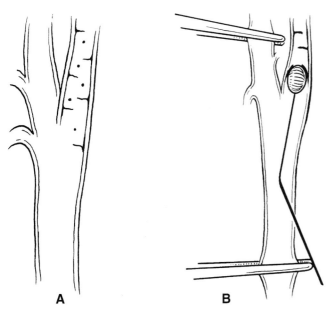

FIGURE 35–16 • *A,* Septated lesion of fibromuscular dysplasia. This kind of irregularity leads to symptoms from platelet aggregation and embolization. *B,* A coronary dilator is introduced through a small arteriotomy and advanced up the internal carotid artery. The olive tip of the dilator disrupts the small septa of the fibromuscular dysplastic segment. With an open arteriotomy, back-bleeding flushes any residual intimal segments or platelet aggregates.

CORRECTION OF KINKING OF THE INTERNAL CAROTID ARTERY

Indications

This procedure is indicated for symptomatic kinking of the internal carotid artery and excessive redundancy of the internal carotid artery after mobilization of that vessel for endarterectomy.

Technique

Redundancy of the internal carotid artery can be corrected in a variety of ways, including (1) resection of the redundant internal carotid artery with an end-to-end anastomosis, (2) division of the internal carotid artery with reimplantation onto the proximal common carotid artery, and (3) resection of a segment of the common carotid artery, thus permitting the redundant internal carotid artery to straighten when the carotid bifurcation is brought down for an end-to-end anastomosis (Fig. 35-17).

In my experience, the easiest repair is resection of a segment of the common carotid artery, because the anastomosis is the easiest to perform. This requires mobilization of the external carotid artery to move the entire bifurcation proximally.

EXTERNAL CAROTID ENDARTERECTOMY

Indications

External carotid endarterectomy is indicated in the case of TIAs from embolization or flow reduction and for the correction of significant stenosis or ulceration before extracranial-to-intracranial bypass grafting.

Technique

The carotid bifurcation is dissected out in the usual manner. The internal carotid artery distal to the obstructed plaque is carefully examined because, on occasion, the vessel may still be patent, thus permitting a standard endarterectomy to be performed, with restoration of blood flow to the internal carotid artery. If the internal carotid artery is confirmed to be occluded, it is divided flush with the carotid bifurcation. An arteriotomy is positioned on the posterolateral aspect of the common carotid artery so that its distal extension passes through the divided orifice of the internal carotid artery and onto the external carotid artery, beyond the atherosclerotic plaque in that vessel. An endarterectomy is then performed. The arteriotomy may be closed primarily, leaving a smooth, tapered transition from the common carotid to the external carotid artery (Fig. 35-18). If the external carotid artery is particularly small, use of a patch may be necessary and is probably preferable. The patch may be of prosthetic material, a vein, or a segment of the occluded internal carotid artery that has been resected and opened. This serves nicely as an autogenous arterial patch.

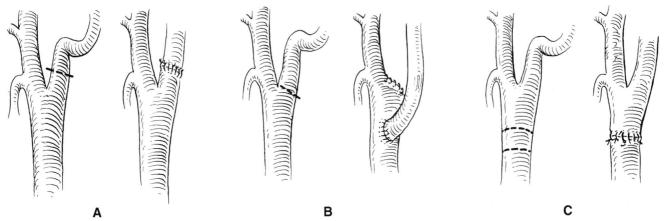

FIGURE 35–17 • *A,* A kink of the internal carotid artery can be repaired by segmental resection of the redundant portion of the artery and direct end-to-end anastomosis. *B,* The redundant internal carotid artery can be straightened by dividing it at its origin and moving it proximally to the common carotid artery for end-to-side anastomosis. *C,* The kinked internal carotid artery can be straightened by mobilization of the carotid bifurcation, resection of a segment of the common carotid artery, and direct end-to-end anastomosis, resulting in straightening of the kinked vessel.

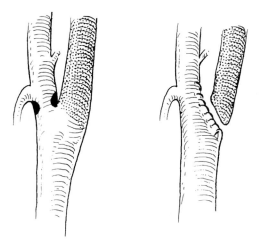

FIGURE 35–18 • External carotid endarterectomy can be performed by removing the occluded internal carotid artery and continuing the arteriotomy past the stenotic lesion. This permits endarterectomy under direct vision and primary closure, leaving a smooth taper between the common and external carotid arteries.

RESECTION OF CAROTID BODY TUMOR

The initial approach for exposing a carotid body tumor is the same as that for exposing the carotid bifurcation for endarterectomy. Once the sternomastoid muscle is fully mobilized and the carotid sheath is exposed, the initial maneuver is the circumferential mobilization of the common carotid artery proximal to the tumor mass. When mobilizing the common carotid artery, the vagus nerve should also be identified. After the artery is circumferentially mobilized, the dissection is carried cephalad, with careful separation of the vagus nerve from the artery. As the dissection approaches the area of the carotid bifurcation, the dissection plane, in the periadventitial tissue, continues on the lateral aspect of the bifurcation, on the outer aspect of the internal carotid artery. Once the common facial vein is identified, it can be circumferentially mobilized, clamped, divided, and ligated. This permits the jugular vein to be separated from the carotid bifurcation and the tumor mass. The dissection continues on the lateral aspect of the internal carotid artery. Once the internal carotid artery can be safely circumferentially mobilized above the tumor mass, this maneuver is completed. Care is taken to identify, protect, and mobilize the 12th cranial nerve. Dissection is now carried down on the medial aspect of the internal carotid artery, separating the tumor mass from that vessel until the area of the carotid bifurcation is encountered. At this point, the external carotid artery can be carefully mobilized for proximal control. The rich blood supply to the tumor mass is derived from branches of the external carotid artery. In the case of a relatively small tumor, 1 cm or less, it may be possible to separate the tumor mass from the trunk of the external carotid artery by dividing the individual branches that come off the artery and feed the tumor. This can be done until the tumor mass is fully mobilized and excised. More commonly, however, it will be necessary to excise the tumor mass with the entire external carotid artery. Once the external carotid artery is fully mobilized, it can be clamped, divided, and ligated. This will help control the blood supply inflow to the tumor mass. The outer margins of the tumor are then carefully circumferentially mobilized

around the pseudocapsule of the tumor mass. Branches of the external carotid artery are divided as they exit the tumor mass. Once the tumor mass is fully circumferentially mobilized, it can be removed.

In the case of a very large tumor, the mass may, on occasion, encircle and intimately adhere to the internal carotid artery. In this rare instance, the carotid bifurcation may have to be resected with the tumor, and a graft must be placed between the common and internal carotid arteries to restore blood flow. It is my practice to always anticipate this possibility and have the patient monitored with EEG, placed before the operation, to determine whether a shunt will be required or temporary clamping can be used before sewing in an interposition graft. Although a vein graft can be used for this purpose, it is my experience that a thin-walled polytetrafluoroethylene (PTFE) graft offers better long-term patency.

Postoperative Care

The first 12 hours are the most critical in managing a patient after cerebrovascular reconstruction. In addition to the usual care required for a patient recovering from general anesthesia, the most important factors are observation of the patient's neurologic status, blood pressure control (either hypotension or hypertension must be appropriately treated), and close wound observation. An expanding hematoma should be identified early and the patient promptly returned to the operating room.

Although intensive care monitoring used to be routine, now only a small percentage of patients actually require an intensive care unit. The majority of patients can be sent to a regular room if they are neurologically intact and hemodynamically stable in the recovery room. Most patients can be safely discharged the next morning. This method of case management has reduced hospital costs.[192-194]

Our practice is to resume antiplatelet drugs. One adult aspirin per day is recommended. If this is not tolerated, dipyridamole (Persantine) or clopidogrel (Plavix) can be used. The rationale for the continued use of antiplatelet drugs is to prevent platelet aggregation and embolization from the new intimectomy site, as well as to serve as prophylaxis in the case of residual, unoperated atherosclerotic plaques in other critical cerebral vessels.

Complications after Carotid Endarterectomy

Few vascular operations are as well tolerated as uncomplicated carotid endarterectomy. The operative trauma, blood loss, and recovery period are minimal after a successful reconstruction. Unfortunately, the benefits of the procedure, especially in asymptomatic patients, can be negated by a high complication rate. The justification for surgical repair requires that the morbidity of the procedure be kept to a minimum. Possible intraoperative and postoperative complications, their prevention, and their management are discussed.

INTRAOPERATIVE COMPLICATIONS

One of the most important steps in the prevention of intraoperative problems is adequate preoperative preparation of the patient. Hypertensive patients should have their blood pressure well controlled before the procedure. Patients must be well hydrated, especially if an angiographic procedure has been done within 24 to 48 hours or if they have been on chronic diuretic therapy. Their myocardial status must be ascertained by careful history, electrocardiography, and other studies as indicated. The use of nitrates during the procedure should be considered in patients with coronary artery disease.

Intraoperative monitoring includes electrocardiographic and frequent or continuous blood pressure readings. I routinely use an intra-arterial line to obtain continuous readouts and promptly recognize fluctuations in the patient's blood pressure. The use of Swan-Ganz catheters should be considered in selected patients.

Hypertension and Hypotension

Hypertension and hypotension are frequent during and immediately after carotid endarterectomy. Bove and colleagues found significant hypertension in 19% and hypotension in 28% of 100 consecutive patients undergoing carotid endarterectomy and reported a 9% incidence of neurologic deficits in this group, as opposed to no neurologic morbidity in normotensive patients.[195] This fact, plus the deleterious effects on myocardial function, underscores the importance of early recognition and immediate treatment of extremes of blood pressure. Taking into account the minimal trauma and blood loss that occur during carotid endarterectomy, other factors must play a role in the development of this fluctuation. Some investigators have found a significant increase in the incidence of this problem in chronically hypertensive patients not well controlled preoperatively.[196] The interference with the baroreceptor mechanisms at the carotid sinus may contribute to postoperative blood pressure fluctuations. The postendarterectomy bulb, which is now distensible, may also play a role.[197] Increased cerebral renin production during carotid cross-clamping has been implicated in the development of postendarterectomy hypertension.[198] In a retrospective study of 100 patients, we found a correlation between the use of halogenated fluorocarbon general anesthesia and the development of postendarterectomy hypertension.[199] In a subsequent study, we demonstrated a correlation between cranial norepinephrine levels in jugular venous blood, but not renin, and the development of postoperative hypertension.[200]

Bradycardia during carotid manipulation usually responds to the local injection of 0.5% lidocaine (Xylocaine) in the soft tissues around the nerve to the carotid sinus. Failure of this maneuver to restore a normal heart rate and blood pressure should be followed by immediate investigation and correction of other possible causes. Ranson and colleagues suggested that an uncorrected preoperative deficit in intravascular volume is a critical factor in the development of hypotension and bradycardia.[201] Blocking the reflex arch by the administration of atropine sulfate while volume deficits are corrected frequently returns the blood pressure to within normal limits. If no response is seen after this, the use of vasoconstrictor agents should be considered, and they should be routinely available for immediate administration. Use of these drugs can be deleterious to myocardial function in the presence of hypovolemia.[147,202] My preference is the use of dopamine hydrochloride titrated by an infusion pump.

Hypertension during or after endarterectomy should also be promptly treated. My preference is to use sodium nitroprusside

by infusion pump. It is usually started when the systolic blood pressure is above 160 mm Hg in normotensive patients and above 180 mm Hg in chronically hypertensive patients. It is titrated to keep the systolic levels between 140 and 160 mm Hg, respectively. In any case, diastolic pressure is kept below 100 mm Hg. The need for intravenous antihypertensive therapy usually lasts less than 24 hours. In patients with essential hypertension, oral medications are restarted within that period.

Technical Complications

Technical problems during the procedure can be avoided by careful dissection and adherence to a proven established routine. The occurrence of intimal flaps at the distal end point of the endarterectomized segment usually results from incomplete removal of the plaque or too deep a plane of dissection in the media. Several steps must be taken to ensure that no distal intimal flap develops. Careful angiographic assessment and gentle palpation of the internal carotid artery reveal the distal end of the plaque. The arteriotomy should be carried beyond this point. If a shunt is to be inserted, this becomes critical.[203] Only in this manner can the lesion be completely removed under direct vision. As the endarterectomy is carried distally in the internal carotid artery, the most superficial plane in the media that allows complete removal of the plaque should be chosen. In this manner, a tapered end is almost always encountered, and tacking sutures are virtually never required. The use of intraoperative completion angiograms is encouraged so that distal end-point defects can be recognized and corrected before completion of the procedure.

Emboli during or after carotid endarterectomy are probably the most frequent cause of neurologic deficits seen after the procedure. Intraoperatively, these can occur during artery mobilization or shunt insertion or after arteriotomy closure. Care should be taken during the distal insertion of the shunt so that it is done beyond the end of the lesion, as previously mentioned. Failure to do this results in fragmentation of the plaque, with embolization or elevation and wrinkling of the intima. Allowing the shunt to back-bleed freely ensures adequate position and removal of all air. I prefer proximal insertion with the shunt fully clamped so that slow, careful release allows immediate reclamping if any air or debris is seen flowing through the shunt.

After the endarterectomy is completed, the area should be free of any loose fragments. Careful irrigation with heparinized saline ensures this. Before completion of the arteriotomy closure, the internal, external, and common carotid arteries should be allowed to bleed freely. Flow should be established to the external carotid artery first to ensure that any debris present goes to this system.

Emboli in the immediate postoperative period in the absence of an intimal flap or other technical error are likely to be from fibrin and platelet aggregates formed in the endarterectomized segment. Antiplatelet agents such as aspirin or dextran 40 may prevent such occurrences.

Occasionally, once the procedure is completed, one finds that a kink is now present in the endarterectomized portion of the internal carotid artery. If the angle between the segments is less than 90 degrees, flow restriction may occur, and disturbances that promote recurrent stenosis are likely. Many times, this can be anticipated when an elongated or coiled artery is present before the endarterectomy. I do not feel comfortable when this situation develops, and in severe cases, I prefer to correct the problem by an angioplastic procedure. My preference is resection of a segment of the common carotid artery with pull-down and primary anastomosis (see Fig. 35-17C). Ligation and division of the external carotid artery are rarely required, because dissection of the trunk and main branches allows sufficient mobility to correct the kink. Ligation and division of the nerve of Hering and surrounding bifurcation tissues are always necessary.

A carotid–cavernous sinus fistula is a feared complication of embolectomy with balloon catheters of the internal carotid artery. On the rare occasion when it is necessary, several maneuvers should be attempted before the use of balloon catheters. The clot should be carefully separated from the intima and gently pulled down. The internal carotid back-pressure is sometimes helpful in this process, and shunting the external circulation may make a difference, allowing extraction of the clot. If the use of balloon catheters is necessary, they should never be inserted beyond the proximal intracranial portion of the artery, and the use of force is condemned. Although perforating the carotid artery intracranially with the balloon catheter is possible, the most common mechanism of injury that creates a carotid–cavernous sinus fistula is that of traction with the balloon catheter. This shearing force creates a transverse tear in the portion of the intracranial carotid that is intimately adherent to the cavernous sinus and fixed to the petrous portion of the skull. Therefore, traction on the inflated balloon catheter should be gentle. Fluoroscopic guidance may be helpful. Failure of these maneuvers makes abandonment of the procedure mandatory and requires consideration of an extracranial-to-intracranial bypass.

Cranial Nerve Injury

Peripheral cranial nerve injury is another source of morbidity after carotid endarterectomy. In a prospective analysis, Hertzer and colleagues found a 16% incidence of cranial nerve dysfunction after this procedure.[204] Only 60% of injuries were symptomatic. The rest would have gone unnoticed by the patient or physician had further detailed examination been omitted. A similar overall incidence was found by Evans and colleagues on clinical grounds,[205] but when speech pathologists were added as part of the evaluation team, the incidence increased to 39%, mostly related to superior laryngeal and recurrent laryngeal nerve dysfunction. The great majority of these deficits were temporary, and when evaluation was repeated in 6 weeks, the incidence was between 1% and 4%. These injuries can be avoided with careful dissection, the principle being to stay in the plane of the artery and to be familiar with the anatomy of the area, including well-recognized anomalies (Fig. 35-19).

The hypoglossal nerve is almost always visualized during carotid endarterectomy. It can be seen descending along the course of the internal carotid, then crossing the external carotid in a more superficial plane. Mobilization of this nerve is necessary only when a high bifurcation is present or when the lesion extends high in the internal carotid artery. This is accomplished by careful division of small veins that tent the nerve downward. A branch of the external carotid to the sternocleidomastoid muscle is frequently present and requires division.

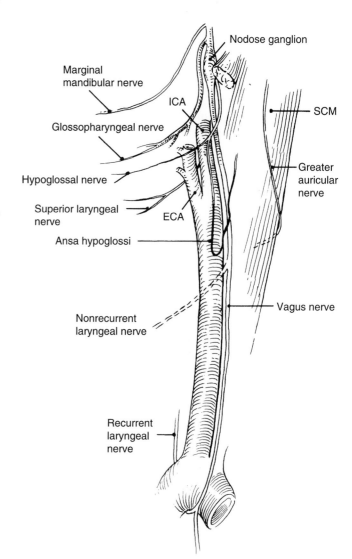

FIGURE 35–19 • Surgical anatomy and relationship of structures encountered during exposure of the carotid bifurcation. ECA, external carotid artery; ICA, internal carotid artery; SCM, sternocleidomastoid muscle.

The ansa hypoglossi can frequently be retracted medially, but on occasion it requires division as it comes off the hypoglossal nerve. Traction or retractor injury to the hypoglossal nerve should be avoided. Clinically, the deficit is manifested by deviation of the tongue to the ipsilateral side. Speech, deglutition, and mastication problems have been reported.[204]

The spinal accessory nerve is rarely seen during this dissection, but on high dissections it may be seen entering the sternocleidomastoid muscle superiorly. It can be left attached and retracted with the muscle, but care should be taken not to compress it with the retractor.

The vagus nerve is always seen, usually posterolateral to the carotid artery, between the latter and the jugular vein. On occasion, it lies anteromedial to the artery. Keeping the dissection close to the artery prevents injury to this nerve. The recurrent laryngeal nerve usually lies within the trunk of the vagus at this level, but a nonrecurrent laryngeal nerve on occasion traverses posterior to the common carotid artery. Injury to these structures can be asymptomatic or manifested by hoarseness, but hoarseness in the postoperative period is due to vocal cord paresis in about half of patients.[204] This underscores the importance of laryngoscopic examination in reaching a specific diagnosis. The asymptomatic injury gains significance when bilateral staged reconstructions are planned, in which case routine laryngoscopic visualization of the vocal cords is highly recommended. Detection of a paralyzed vocal cord mandates delaying the procedure until recovery is complete. If vocal cord paralysis is permanent, appropriate precautions should be taken to avoid bilateral injury, and perioperative airway management should be given special consideration.

The superior laryngeal nerve leaves the inferior ganglion of the vagus (nodose ganglion) and courses behind the internal carotid artery, bifurcating into an internal and an external branch. The internal branch is sensitive to the larynx, and the external innervates the inferior constrictor and cricothyroid muscles. The latter is responsible for the quality of voice, specifically the higher pitches. Injury to the external laryngeal nerve can be avoided by keeping the dissection close to the arterial wall, specifically when controlling the superior thyroid artery.

The glossopharyngeal nerve is usually not seen in the dissection but can be injured when dissections are carried high, especially those requiring division of the digastric muscles.[206,207] This nerve courses posterior to the high portion of the internal carotid artery and can be injured with the application of a vascular clamp that includes tissues other than the artery itself. Again, dissection close to the arterial wall is the key to prevention. Clinically, the dysfunction is evident when tasks requiring oral pharyngeal muscle activity, mostly deglutition, are examined. Horner's syndrome may be produced by injury to the ascending sympathetic fibers in the area of the glossopharyngeal nerve.

The cervical branch of the facial nerve lies beneath the platysma, inferior to the angle of the jaw. In some patients, this nerve sends branches to the mandibular branch, and its injury produces sagging of the ipsilateral corner of the lower lip. The marginal mandibular branch can itself be injured when the incision is carried too close to the jaw. Both of these injuries can be prevented by curving the upper portion of the incision toward the mastoid process.[203] Self-retaining retractors should be carefully placed in this area.

The greater auricular nerve courses deep to the platysma over the sternocleidomastoid muscle at an angle toward the ear in the upper portion of the dissection. Its division should be avoided but is frequently necessary in high dissections. Numbness of the earlobe is the usual consequence, although, surprisingly, some patients have no complaints after its deliberate division.

The parotid gland lies in the superior portion of the incision anterior to the sternocleidomastoid muscle. Again, curving the incision toward the mastoid process prevents injury in high dissections. Troublesome bleeding and the risk of a parotid fistula can be prevented by this maneuver.

POSTOPERATIVE COMPLICATIONS

On completion of an operation done under general anesthesia, the patient is awakened in the operating room. A gross neurologic examination is performed. If no deficit is found, the patient is transferred to the recovery room, where a more detailed examination is performed.

Stroke is the most feared complication of carotid endarterectomy. In experienced hands, this occurs in between 1% and 3% of patients, depending on the indication for the procedure.[208] Most of the low rates of stroke have been reported from specialized centers. Unfortunately, pooled data from community surveys have shown rates of combined stroke morbidity and mortality ranging from 6.5% to 21%.[209-211] Because carotid endarterectomy is a prophylactic operation employed to prevent stroke, these higher complication rates erase most benefits and are clearly unacceptable. A committee of the Stroke Council of the American Heart Association reviewed this problem and set standards for upper acceptable limits of stroke and death as a function of indication for operation. Thus, for patients undergoing carotid endarterectomy for asymptomatic carotid stenosis, the combined operative stroke morbidity and mortality should not exceed 3%; for TIA as an indication, 5%; for prior stroke as an indication, 7%; and for recurrent carotid stenosis, 10%.[212] A mechanism for individual surgeon audit was described and recommended.

TIAs in the first postoperative week have been reported with a frequency as high as 8%. When a neurologic deficit is found on awakening the patient, the main question to be resolved is the patency of the internal carotid artery. If a completion angiogram is obtained and no abnormalities are seen, the event is likely to be embolic, and immediate reoperation would be of no benefit. If no angiographic data are available, patency of the vessel should be assessed by noninvasive means.[213] If occlusion is suggested, immediate reoperation may reverse the deficit.[214] If the vessel appears patent by noninvasive tests, the surgeon needs to determine whether the emboli occurred during the operation or whether a source is now present in the operated segment. This is also the case in a patient who is neurologically intact and develops an event in the ipsilateral hemisphere hours or days after surgery. Once patency is evidenced by noninvasive means, immediate angiography is indicated. Reoperation is necessary if a significant defect or any clot is present. Otherwise, conservative therapy with anticoagulation, antiplatelet agents, or both is warranted. This excludes a patient experiencing repeated or progressive neurologic events, in whom immediate reoperation should be considered. Other factors inevitably influence the decision to reoperate or observe the patient. The difficulty of the initial reconstruction, the patient's general status, and the availability and reliability of ancillary facilities affect this difficult decision (Fig. 35-20).

Mortality after carotid endarterectomy has declined significantly as the incidence of postoperative stroke has diminished. Pulmonary problems, renal insufficiency, and sepsis are extremely unusual complications owing to the nature of this procedure. MI remains the most frequent cause of death in the early postoperative period, more so in patients with suspected coronary artery disease.[215] Because of this, preoperative assessment is of paramount importance. Postoperatively, electrocardiographic monitoring for the first 24 hours and a 12-lead electrocardiographic tracing should be obtained. Any suspicion of a myocardial event should be investigated and treated aggressively.

Wound infections after carotid endarterectomy are extremely rare. Routine use of prophylactic antibiotics for 24 hours during the perioperative interval is recommended.

Taking into account that the procedure is done under full heparinization and that many patients have received platelet

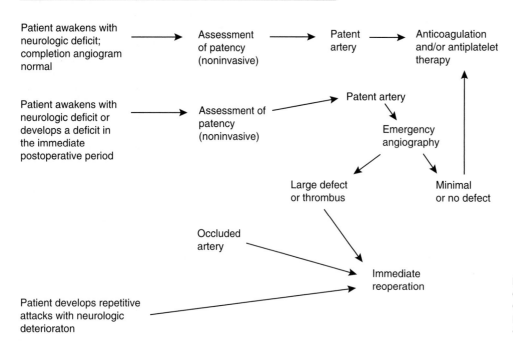

FIGURE 35–20 • Algorithm that can be applied to the management of a patient who awakens with a postoperative neurologic deficit after carotid endarterectomy.

antiaggregates preoperatively, the incidence of wound bleeding is low. In Thompson's personal series,[208] reoperation for this problem was required in 0.7% of 1022 patients.

Large cervical hematomas may form, and reoperation and drainage should be strongly considered in an otherwise stable patient. The routine use of a Silastic drain may reduce the incidence of this complication. Rarely does bleeding occur from the suture line. More often, a diffuse ooze is present, requiring reversal of anticoagulation. In any case, drainage of the hematoma and correction of its cause prevent chronic draining wounds, infection, and the rare occurrence of pseudoaneurysm formation. The last is more frequent when closure is performed with a patch.[208]

Headache after carotid endarterectomy is not unusual. It may be associated with a neurologic deficit, in which case a CT scan should be performed. In the majority of cases, however, it runs a self-limited course and is probably related to altered autoregulatory dysfunction of the cerebral circulation. The use of propranolol (Inderal) has been effective in treating troublesome headache.

Complications after carotid endarterectomy may be prevented by careful patient preparation, meticulous technique, and adherence to a rational, well-established routine. An uneventful operation is the best way to effectively change the natural history of extracranial arterial occlusive disease.

Results of Surgical Treatment for Extracranial Arterial Occlusive Disease

The most frequently performed operation for extracranial arterial occlusive disease is endarterectomy of the carotid bifurcation. As experience is gained with this procedure, results have improved, and in experienced hands it can be done with morbidity and mortality rates well below the Stroke Council guidelines. When recommending this procedure, the results of the particular surgeon or institution should be considered, because a higher morbidity and mortality may negate any beneficial effects of surgery.

The first multi-institutional study that compared surgical and medical treatment in a prospectively randomized fashion came from the joint study on extracranial arterial occlusion,[216] in which 1225 symptomatic patients with extracranial arterial occlusive disease were randomly allocated to receive either medical or surgical therapy. Long-term survival of as long as 42 months was better in surgically treated patients with unilateral carotid stenosis who were experiencing TIAs or cerebral infarction with minimal residual deficit. The neurologic morbidity in 316 patients who were identified as having hemispheric TIAs as an indication for inclusion in the study was evaluated. The incidence of cerebral infarction at 42 months was reduced in the surgical group. Recurrent TIAs or cerebral infarction usually affected the side not operated on in the surgical patients, in contrast to the medically treated group, in whom neurologic events occurred chiefly in the distribution of the symptomatic artery at the time of randomization. The differences were statistically significant. The combined postoperative morbidity and mortality in the surgically treated group was around 8%, which is considered high by today's standards. This may have affected the results of this study in favor of medical therapy.

The preoperative neurologic status of the patient affects the immediate postoperative results. Asymptomatic patients fare better than patients with TIAs, and the latter have lower morbidity than patients with completed strokes. Rothwell and colleagues reviewed 25 studies and performed a meta-analysis.[217] The combined perioperative risk of death and stroke was 3% to 3.5% in asymptomatic patients, compared with 5.18% for symptomatic patients. These differences were consistent across all studies and indicate that operation on asymptomatic patients is safest. In fact, late results may be similarly affected. Bernstein and colleagues reported a series of 456 carotid endarterectomies monitored for 1 to 11 years, with an average follow-up of 45.3 months.[218] Asymptomatic patients who were operated on had a 1.6% incidence of TIAs and a 3.2% incidence of stroke on late follow-up. Those operated on because of TIAs had a 19.5% and 5.2% incidence of recurrent TIAs and stroke, respectively. Patients with a permanent neurologic deficit preoperatively had a 7.9% incidence of TIAs, and 11% developed a stroke on late follow-up.

Similar results were reported by Hertzer and Arison in 329 patients monitored for a minimum of 10 years after carotid endarterectomy.[219] The cumulative incidence of stroke by the life-table method was 24% at 10 years after operation. Only 10% of patients sustained strokes that clearly involved the ipsilateral cerebral hemisphere. Hypertension, preoperative stroke as an indication, and patients with recognized contralateral carotid stenosis had a much higher incidence of stroke on long-term follow-up. Contralateral hemispheric strokes occurred in 36% of patients with uncorrected contralateral lesions, compared with 8% of those who had elective bilateral reconstruction. This difference was statistically significant. Patients undergoing elective myocardial revascularization had a significant increase in long-term survival when compared with patients with uncorrected coronary artery disease. These results suggest that the annual incidence of late stroke, specifically involving the cerebral hemisphere ipsilateral to the previous carotid repair, is 1.1%, a figure within the expected range for the normal population. Stroke in the subset of patients with bilateral carotid arterial disease was five times more common in the contralateral than in the ipsilateral cerebral hemisphere.

Therefore, staged contralateral endarterectomy should be seriously considered in patients with documented but otherwise asymptomatic advanced contralateral carotid stenosis.[219]

Analysis of the available surgical series with long-term follow-up reveals that a successfully performed carotid endarterectomy places the patient at a significantly lower risk of stroke. The results of the various surgical series are summarized in Table 35-1, according to the indications for operation.[220-229] Asymptomatic patients have a 1.2% per year stroke risk, including perioperative morbidity and mortality. Patients whose indication for endarterectomy is TIAs have an initial perioperative morbidity and mortality of about 3%, with a long-term risk of stroke of 2% per year. Patients whose indication for operation is cerebral infarction have a higher perioperative morbidity, averaging about 5%. Long-term results suggest that these patients have an annual stroke rate of approximately 4% per year. The average recurrence of TIAs is on the order of 8% to 10% at 5 years for all indications. These results represent a clear improvement over the natural history of the disease, including the use of antiplatelet drugs; however, they underscore the importance of maintaining the operative stroke rate at acceptable levels for the various indications. A higher figure negates the early and late beneficial results of surgical therapy.

The results of carotid endarterectomy for nonhemispheric symptoms are less predictable. In a series of 107 patients

TABLE 35-1 Results of Carotid Endarterectomy According to the Indication for Operation

Indication	Author	No. of Patients	Follow-up	Operative Morbidity (%)	Operative Mortality (%)	Recurrent TIAs, Ipsilateral (%)	Stroke Ipsilateral (%)	Stroke Contralateral (%)
Asymptomatic	Thompson et al[177]	132	55.1 mo	0	1.2	0.75	4.7*	NS
	Sergeant et al[220]	43	6.48 mo	2.3	2.3	0	0	0
	Moore et al[221]	72	6-180 mo	0	0	2.7	5.6†	2.7
	Bernstein et al[222]	87‡	43 mo	NS§	0	NS	6.3‖	NS
	Hertzer and Arison[219]	126	10-14 yr	NS	NS	NS	9¶	7¶
	Lord[223]	226	30-144 mo	2.6	1.1	NS	0.4	1.1
TIA	Bernstein et al[222]	370**	12-132 mo	NS	0	19.5††	5.2	NS
	DeWeese et al[224]	103	60-mo minimum	6.0	0.97	18.4‡‡	7.7§§	10.6
	Thompson et al[225]	293	Up to 156 mo	2.7	1.4	16.3	4.7	0.6
	Takolander et al[226]	142	5-yr actuarial	4.9	1.8	14.7	6.5	4.0
	Hertzer and Arison[219]	123	10-14 yr	NS	NS	NS	6¶	9¶
Stroke	Thompson et al[225]	217	Up to 156 mo	5.0	7.4		8.2	NS
	Eriksson et al[227]	55	21-mo avg	3.7	3.7		3.8	NS
	Bardin et al[228]	127	56-mo avg	3.9	3.1		20	NS
	Takolander et al[226]	60	5-yr actuarial	4.9	5.9	11.6‖	10	NS
	McCullough et al[229]	50	41-mo avg	3.4	1.7		3.3	NS
	Hertzer and Arison[219]	80	10-14 yr	NS	NS	NS	6¶	13

*Side of stroke not specified; three strokes were fatal.
†Two patients suffered transient postoperative deficits with complete recovery.
‡Number of procedures; exact number of patients not specified.
§Perioperative stroke rate of 3% in the entire series of 370 patients.
‖Side of neurologic event not specified; risk of stroke at 5 years by life-table analysis.
¶Does not include perioperative strokes.
**Total number of patients in series, including TIA patients.
††Territory affected not specified.
‡‡Includes patients with nonterritorial symptoms.
§§Includes operative morbidity.
NS, not specified; TIA, transient ischemic attack.

subjected to carotid endarterectomy, the initial perioperative morbidity and mortality were similar to those in patients with specific indications for operation. Carotid endarterectomy was successful in ameliorating symptoms in patients with nonhemispheric symptoms who had greater than 60% diameter reduction of the carotid artery and classic symptoms of vertebrobasilar insufficiency.[230] The same series of 61 patients was updated by Ricotta and colleagues.[231] They compared the results of their cohort of patients with nonhemispheric symptoms to the remainder of their series. Follow-up lasted a mean of 42.3 months. The perioperative stroke rate was 4.9%. Survival was 85.3% at 3 years and 64.9% at 5 years. Stroke-free survival was 77.1% at 3 years and 63.4% at 5 years. During follow-up, 11 patients (18%) developed recurrent nonhemispheric symptoms. These results were not different from the cohort of 553 patients. The authors concluded that carotid endarterectomy provided long-term benefit in this group of patients.

The use of cerebral angiography can also be very helpful in selecting patients. The presence of a posterior communicating artery suggests that the anterior circulation may be a major contributor to the vertebrobasilar system. Its presence suggests that removal of a hemodynamically significant lesion in the carotid territory would be beneficial in alleviating posterior circulation systems.

In the absence of significant extracranial carotid artery disease, direct vertebral artery reconstruction is the procedure of choice for patients with vertebrobasilar system lesions secondary to extracranial occlusive disease. The results of direct vertebral artery reconstruction have been good, although the experience is not as extensive as that with carotid artery surgery. In a series of 109 vertebral artery operations, Imparato reported an operative mortality of 3%.[232] Other complications included temporary hemidiaphragm paralysis and Horner's syndrome. Two thromboses of the reconstruction occurred; there were no perioperative strokes. Long-term follow-up revealed a stroke incidence of 1.5% per year of follow-up. No controlled series on the natural history of these patients is available for comparison.

The experience with external carotid revascularization is limited; therefore, long-term results are not available. In a series of 42 external carotid artery reconstructions, O'Hara and colleagues reported no early morbidity or mortality when the operation was limited to external carotid endarterectomy and patch angioplasty.[233] When the procedure was combined with bypass to the external carotid artery or with an extracranial-to-intracranial bypass, however, a 33% incidence of stroke was observed. No neurologic symptoms occurred in 25 patients (60%) during follow-up ranging from 1 to 72 months (mean, 27 months). These authors concluded that external carotid endarterectomy can be performed with acceptable risks and long-term effectiveness. When the reconstruction involves bypass to the external carotid artery or extracranial-to-intracranial bypass, a higher operative risk can be expected. A similar note of caution was expressed by Halstuk and colleagues,[234] describing 49 external carotid revascularization procedures performed in 36 patients. Indications included ipsilateral TIAs, amaurosis fugax, and a preparatory procedure in anticipation of extracranial-to-intracranial bypass. Twenty patients had preoperative strokes. Twenty-nine patients underwent unilateral external carotid endarterectomy, with the remaining patients undergoing other procedures in

TABLE 35–2	Effect of Perioperative Use of Aspirin		
Time after Operation	Complication	CEA with ASA, No. of Patients (%)	CEA without ASA, No. of Patients (%)
1 wk	Stroke	0	7 (6)
30 days	Stroke	2 (1.7)	11 (9.6)
6 mo	Stroke	2 (1.7)	11 (9.6)
30 days	Mortality	0.8	4.3
6 mo	Mortality	3-4	6

ASA, acetylsalicylic acid; CEA, carotid endarterectomy.

addition to the external revascularization. The incidence of postoperative stroke within 8 days of external carotid revascularization was 13.8%. One operative death occurred, for a mortality rate of 2.7%. Long-term follow-up ranging from 1 to 75 months (mean, 29 months) revealed a 14.2% incidence of late neurologic ischemic events. Three of these were TIAs, one was a reversible ischemic neurologic deficit, and one patient had a stroke 50 months after his initial operation. These results suggest caution in recommending external carotid artery surgery, especially when the revascularization will involve more than just endarterectomy with patch closure.

The perioperative use of aspirin in patients undergoing carotid endarterectomy reduces the risk of stroke and death up to 6 months. Lindblad and associates carried out a prospective, randomized trial comparing carotid endarterectomy in patients with and without aspirin.[235] Their results are summarized in Table 35-2.

Current Status of Prospective, Randomized Trials

In spite of the fact that retrospective data analysis clearly demonstrates the superiority of carotid endarterectomy over medical management with respect to stroke prevention, a number of well-meaning critics point out that retrospective data analysis can be misleading. Retrospective studies compare surgical results with available natural history data. The natural history of a particular disease process can change, often for the better, making the basis of comparison invalid. Likewise, retrospective reviews are often performed in centers of excellence, where surgical complication rates may be lower than the actual risk of operation in the community. For this reason, several prospective, randomized trials were initiated in North America and Europe. The objective of these trials was to scientifically evaluate the efficacy (or lack thereof) of carotid endarterectomy in preventing stroke for a variety of indications when compared with a true control group. The trials can generally be categorized into two major classifications: asymptomatic and symptomatic carotid artery disease.

Three asymptomatic trials have completed their data acquisition and reported results: the Veterans Administration Asymptomatic Carotid Stenosis Study, ACAS, and the European Asymptomatic Carotid Surgery Trial. Three symptomatic trials have been completed: NASCET, the Medical Research Council European Carotid Surgery Trial (ECST), and the Veterans Administration Symptomatic Trial.

ASYMPTOMATIC TRIALS

Veterans Administration Asymptomatic Carotid Stenosis Study

Ten Veterans Administration (VA) medical centers entered into a prospective, randomized trial designed to test the hypothesis that carotid endarterectomy plus best medical management (aspirin and risk factor control) would result in fewer TIAs than treatment with best medical management alone. The design of the study was published in 1986.[236] Angiography was performed in 713 patients, 3 of whom (0.4%) sustained a neurologic deficit.[237]

A total of 444 patients were randomized over a 54-month interval. In the surgical group, 211 carotid endarterectomies were performed; these patients also received aspirin therapy. In the medical group, 233 patients were treated with aspirin alone. The study spanned a total of 8 years. The 30-day mortality rate for the surgery group was 1.9%, and the incidence of stroke was 2.4%. The combined stroke and mortality rate was 4.3%.[238]

The data analysis demonstrated that all neurologic events (stroke, TIA, amaurosis fugax) in any distribution (including the study artery), combined with deaths, totaled 30 in the carotid endarterectomy group, which represented 14.2% of that population. For the patients treated medically, a total of 55 events occurred, for an event rate of 23.6%. This difference was statistically significant ($P < 0.006$). When the data were analyzed for deaths plus ipsilateral events only, a total of 21 events occurred in the carotid endarterectomy group, for an incidence of 10%; in contrast, there were 46 events in the medically treated group, for an incidence of 19.7%. Once again, this difference was statistically significant ($P < 0.002$). Although the study was not designed to look at stroke alone, this was done retrospectively. A total of 10 strokes occurred in the carotid endarterectomy group ipsilateral to the study artery, for an incidence of 4.7%. A total of 20 strokes occurred in the study artery distribution in the medically treated group, for an incidence of 8.6%. This difference fell just short of statistical significance ($P = 0.056$), probably because of the small sample size. There was no difference in survival rate between the surgically and medically treated groups. This is not surprising, because the major cause of death in this patient group is MI, and prevention of stroke is unlikely to have a beneficial effect on reducing fatal MI. This lack of difference in survival between the surgically and medically treated groups should not be considered a negative factor when interpreting data results, because the objective of operation is to maintain the patient stroke free during his or her remaining lifetime.[239]

Asymptomatic Carotid Atherosclerosis Study

The ACAS, sponsored by the National Institutes of Health (NIH), was the largest multicenter (34 centers), North American, prospective, randomized trial of surgery for asymptomatic carotid stenosis. It tested the hypothesis that carotid endarterectomy plus aspirin and risk factor control would result in fewer TIAs, strokes, and deaths than aspirin and risk factor control alone.

The design of the study was published in 1989.[240] Initially, 1500 patients were to be randomized, with TIA as an end point. After criticism of the VA study, the protocol was amended to have stroke and death as the end points. The Data Safety and Monitoring Committee of the NIH gave permission to increase the sample size from 1500 to 1800 patients.

In December 1994, the committee called a halt to the study and informed the investigators, and subsequently the public, that an end point had been reached in favor of carotid endarterectomy.[241] The full report was published in *JAMA*.[158] A total of 1662 patients with diameter-reducing lesions of 60% or greater (as measured by angiography using the North American method; see later) were randomly allocated to receive carotid endarterectomy plus best medical management, including aspirin; the control group received best medical management alone. After a mean follow-up of 2.7 years (4657 patient-years of observation), the aggregate risk over 5 years for ipsilateral stroke, any perioperative stroke, and death was 5.1% for surgical patients and 11% for patients treated medically. The results of surgery, including perioperative morbidity and mortality, reduced the risk of death and stroke by 5.9% absolutely and yielded a 53% risk reduction. This difference was highly significant.

The beneficial effect of surgery in asymptomatic patients was due in large part to the low 30-day perioperative stroke morbidity and mortality. Before the study began, the surgical management committee for ACAS established criteria to audit surgeons who wished to participate in the study.[242] Validation of the audit method was possible on conclusion of the study. Among 825 patients randomized to surgery, the stroke morbidity and mortality rate within 30 days of randomization was 2.3%. However, this included a stroke morbidity and mortality of 1.2% for preoperative angiography. Because of the intent-to-treat design, the angiographic complications were credited to surgery. Of the 724 patients who actually had carotid endarterectomy, mortality was 0.14%, and the stroke rate was 1.38%. Thus, the true 30-day stroke morbidity and mortality rate was 1.52%.[159]

Asymptomatic Carotid Surgery Trial

A group of European investigators, headed by a team from the United Kingdom, embarked on yet another trial. However, included in their trial were methods designed to try to identify a higher-risk group of patients.[243] The investigators reported their results in 2004 in the *Lancet*.[244] A total of 3128 asymptomatic patients with carotid artery stenoses of 70% or greater, as measured by ultrasonography, were entered into the trial from 1993 through 2003. The patients were equally randomized between immediate carotid endarterectomy and indefinite deferral of operation.

The 30-day risk of stroke or death in the surgical group was 3.1%. When analyzing the 5-year results of the two groups, the stroke risk, excluding perioperative events, was 3.8% in the surgical group, versus 11% in the nonsurgical group ($P < 0.0001$). Half the stroke events were disabling or fatal. If perioperative events were included, the 5-year stroke rate in the two groups was 6.4% versus 11.8% ($P < 0.0001$). Comparing fatal or disabling strokes, the event rate was 3.5% in the surgical group versus 6.1% in the nonsurgical group. The investigators found that the results were significant for both men and women when analyzed separately. The authors concluded that, in asymptomatic patients 75 years of age or younger with a diameter-reducing stenosis of 70% or greater as measured by ultrasonography, immediate carotid endarterectomy reduced the net stroke risk by half, from about 12% in the control group to 6% (including a 3% perioperative hazard) in the surgical group. Further, half of the 5-year benefit involved disabling or fatal strokes.[244]

SYMPTOMATIC TRIALS

North American Symptomatic Carotid Endarterectomy Trial

The NASCET is a large prospective trial designed to test the hypothesis that symptomatic patients (those with TIA or prior mild stroke) with ipsilateral carotid stenosis (30% to 99%) have fewer fatal and nonfatal strokes after carotid endarterectomy than do patients treated with medical management alone, including aspirin. Investigators anticipated that approximately 3000 patients would be randomly allocated to receive either medical or surgical management and monitored for a minimum of 5 years. The NASCET was also stratified to study two subsets of patients as a function of the degree of carotid occlusive disease: those with 70% to 99% stenosis, and those with more moderate lesions ranging from 30% to 69% stenosis.[245] Included in the design of the trial and required by the granting institution (NIH) was the establishment of an oversight committee that was responsible for reviewing the results of the data from time to time and calling a halt to the study if a clear difference was observed between the two groups.

On February 25, 1991, a clinical alert was issued by the oversight committee, which reported that a clear difference had developed between the two groups, indicating that carotid endarterectomy was superior to medical management in the high-grade stenosis category (70% to 99%). No clear difference had yet occurred in the moderate stenosis group (30% to 69%), and the latter continues to enter patients for randomization.

In the high-grade stenosis category, 295 patients received medical management and 300 patients received surgical management. Sixteen of the medically treated patients (5.4%) actually crossed over to surgery, but because of the "intent-to-treat" design, these patients continued to be analyzed as if they were managed medically, in spite of their operations. Crossovers become important if the group that patients are leaving is in fact a disadvantaged group, as is the case in this study.

The 30-day operative morbidity and stroke mortality rate for patients managed surgically was 5%. The analysis at the end of 18 months of follow-up, which led the oversight committee to halt this arm of the study, was as follows: In the surgical group, a 7% incidence of fatal and nonfatal strokes occurred (including perioperative morbidity and mortality). In the medical group, a 24% incidence of fatal and nonfatal strokes occurred. The difference was highly statistically significant ($P < 0.001$). This represents an absolute risk reduction of 17% in favor of surgical management and a relative risk reduction of 71% with surgical management versus medical management at the end of 18 months.

A surprising finding occurred when the mortality rates were analyzed. To date, no study had shown that carotid endarterectomy patients enjoy greater longevity than those treated medically. However, at the end of 18 months, the mortality rate among the medically treated group was 12%,

in contrast to 5% for the surgically treated group. Once again, this difference was statistically significant ($P < 0.01$). This indicates a relative mortality risk reduction of 58% in favor of carotid endarterectomy. Further analysis demonstrated that for every 10% increase in stenosis between 70% and 99%, a progressive increase occurred in morbidity and mortality in the control group.[230,246]

The NASCET investigators reported their results in the moderate stenosis group (30% to 69%) in 1998.[247] They demonstrated a beneficial effect of surgery in the 50% to 69% stenosis group but not in those patients with less than 50% stenosis. The 30-day mortality and disabling stroke rate was 2.7%, and the nondisabling stroke rate was 4%, for a total of 6.7%. The 5-year rate for ipsilateral stroke in the surgical group was 15.7%, compared with 22% for patients treated medically. Thus, 15 patients would need to undergo carotid endarterectomy to prevent one stroke over a 5-year interval.

Medical Research Council European Carotid Surgery Trial

The ECST was a large multicenter trial of symptomatic patients with carotid artery disease that was carried out over a 10-year period and reported at approximately the same time as the NASCET. It confirmed NASCET's results reported to date. A total of 2518 patients were randomized over 10 years, providing a mean follow-up of 3 years. This trial stratified the data into three groups: mild stenosis (10% to 29%), moderate stenosis (30% to 69%), and severe stenosis (70% to 99%). In the mild stenosis category, no apparent benefit was evident for carotid endarterectomy compared with the risk of operation. However, in the severe stenosis category, a highly significant benefit in favor of operation was evident. Carotid endarterectomy, in spite of a 7.5% risk of death and stroke in the perioperative interval, resulted in a sixfold reduction in subsequent strokes over a 3-year interval. This difference was highly statistically significant ($P < 0.0001$).[248]

One interesting and important difference has come to light between NASCET and ECST: they have different methods of measuring carotid stenosis. In the European method,

$$\% \text{ Stenosis} = (1 - R/B) \times 100$$

where R is minimal residual lumen diameter through the stenosis, and B is the projected diameter of the carotid bulb. This cannot actually be visualized because it is occupied by plaque. Therefore, an imaginary line is drawn to outline what is believed to be the bulb.

NASCET uses a method common in North America and first described in the VA asymptomatic trial. In this method,

$$\% \text{ Stenosis} = (1 - R/D) \times 100$$

where D is the diameter of the normal internal carotid artery where the walls become parallel.

The result of this difference is most apparent for moderate stenosis, for which the European method appears to greatly overestimate the percentage of stenosis. Eliasziw and colleagues compared the same angiograms using the European and North American methods.[249] Their findings are partly summarized in Table 35-3.

Because the ECST found significant benefit of carotid endarterectomy in patients with stenosis of 60% to 90%, this corroborated the results in the NASCET moderate

TABLE 35–3	Comparison of Carotid Stenosis Estimated by European and North American Methods

Percent Stenosis, European	Percent Stenosis, North American
60	18
70	40
80	61
90	80

Data from Eliasziw M, Smith RF, Singh N, et al: Further comments on the measurements of carotid stenosis from angiograms. Stroke 25:2445-2449, 1994.

stenosis group. The ECST reported no benefit of surgery in the 30% to 69% group as measured by the European method. This is not surprising, because a 69% ECST stenosis is only a 40% stenosis as measured by the North American method.[250]

Veterans Administration Symptomatic Trial

The VA symptomatic trial was a prospective, randomized trial designed to test the hypothesis that patients with greater than 50% ipsilateral internal carotid artery stenosis who were experiencing symptoms (including transient cerebral ischemia and mild stroke) would have fewer neurologic events (including cerebral infarction and crescendo TIAs) in the vascular distribution of the study artery after carotid endarterectomy plus best medical management than those receiving best medical management alone. This study was just getting under way when the results of the ECST and NASCET were reported, which led to its being halted earlier than anticipated. Nonetheless, 189 patients with symptomatic carotid stenoses were randomly allocated to receive either medical or surgical management. When the results were analyzed with a mean follow-up of 11.9 months, 7.7% of the patients randomized to surgical care had experienced stroke or crescendo TIAs during the perioperative or follow-up interval. In contrast, those patients randomized to medical management alone experienced a 19.4% incidence of stroke or crescendo TIAs. This difference was statistically significant ($P = 0.01$). The benefit of operation became apparent within 2 months of randomization.[251]

Alternatives to Surgical Therapy

The pathophysiology involved in the development of a stroke from an extracranial lesion has been discussed. The rationale for current medical therapy evolved from an attempt to alter the factors responsible for the development of symptoms secondary to extracranial arterial occlusion. At present, two forms of therapy are considered mainstays in the medical management of this disease: antiplatelet agents and anticoagulation.

Any form of therapy aimed at stroke prevention must include the control of commonly associated conditions such as hypertension, diabetes, arrhythmias, and coronary artery disease. Cigarette smoking is also a major independent risk factor for the development of carotid bifurcation disease and stroke.[252-254] Any medical approach to stroke risk reduction must begin by advising the patient to stop smoking.

Anticoagulation, mainly with warfarin sodium (Coumadin), has been evaluated in several reports in an attempt to determine whether its use significantly alters the natural history of extracranial arterial lesions. Baker and associates reported a randomized, prospective study in patients with TIAs who were treated with Coumadin.[255] On follow-up, those treated with anticoagulation had a significant reduction in the number of TIAs when compared with control patients. A favorable trend for fewer strokes was noted in the treated group, although the difference in the incidence of cerebral infarction between treated and control patients was not statistically significant.

A reduction in stroke rate was observed in a retrospective study in the community of Rochester, Minnesota, regarding the use of anticoagulants to treat cerebral ischemia.[35] In this study, the net probability of having a stroke within 5 years was around 20% for those patients treated with anticoagulants. Although this compares favorably with the probability in untreated controls (40%), it represents a significant risk when compared with other available therapies.

Two reports from Sweden also showed a reduction in the development of TIAs and strokes in patients treated with anticoagulants. The study by Link and colleagues showed a higher incidence of stroke when anticoagulants were discontinued; thus, long-term therapy was recommended.[256] In the second study, by Terent and Anderson,[257] patients treated with anticoagulants showed an increased mortality rate, and serious bleeding complications were seen in this group. Finally, a meta-analysis of 16 randomized studies of anticoagulation failed to show any benefit in patients suffering from TIA or ischemic stroke compared with untreated control groups. However, evidence suggests that patients with thrombosis in evolution may benefit from anticoagulation.[258]

The available evidence indicates that although the incidence of stroke and recurrent TIAs is reduced in patients treated with anticoagulants, it remains high compared with other available therapies. The need for long-term administration, with the concomitant increased risk of complications, makes anticoagulant therapy less desirable.

Antiplatelet agents, mainly aspirin, have been advocated for use in patients with extracranial arterial occlusive disease. The rationale for this therapy is based on evidence that platelets play a major role in the pathophysiology of this disease. At present, seven double-blind, randomized, prospective studies have compared the use of platelet antiaggregants with placebo in treating patients with cerebral ischemia secondary to extracranial atherosclerosis. In the Canadian Cooperative Study Group,[259] 585 patients who evidenced cerebral ischemia of extracranial origin were prospectively randomized into four treatment regimens. Each regimen was taken four times daily and consisted of a 200-mg capsule of sulfinpyrazone plus placebo, a placebo tablet plus 325 mg of aspirin, both active drugs, or both placebos. Follow-up from 12 to 57 months revealed no statistically significant reduction in TIAs, stroke, or death among patients on sulfinpyrazone. Aspirin reduced the risk for continuing ischemic episodes, stroke, or death by 19%. When analysis was restricted to stroke or death alone, the risk reduction increased to 31%, and when male patients were analyzed separately, the reduction was even higher. No statistically significant differences in stroke or death rate were found among female patients taking any of the four regimens. Based on this observation, the probability of stroke in men taking aspirin was in excess of 5% each year, and in women it was higher than 8% each year.[260] Platelet antiaggregants reduce the incidence of stroke in patients with extracranial lesions. The question still remains whether this reduction equals that achieved by other therapies.

In 1972, a double-blind, randomized, prospective trial of aspirin versus placebo was started in several American centers and continued for 37 months.[261] Sixty percent of these patients had operable lesions in the extracranial territory. The treatment group received 625 mg of aspirin twice daily. At 6 months' follow-up, a statistically significant difference in favor of aspirin was seen when death, cerebral or retinal infarction, and TIAs were grouped together. When each group was considered separately, the difference did not achieve statistical significance. Patients for whom a decision was made to proceed with endarterectomy were also assigned to a randomized, double-blind trial of aspirin during the postoperative period. The results of this trial constitute a separate report.[262] Life-table analyses of these end points at 24 months did not reveal a statistically significant difference in favor of aspirin. When non–stroke-related deaths were eliminated, a significant difference in favor of aspirin emerged. A favorable trend was also noted when the occurrence of TIAs within the first 6 months of follow-up was taken into consideration. In the placebo group, eight brain infarcts occurred among eight patients, reaching an end point in the first 24 months. Eight patients also reached an end point in the aspirin group; however, only two of these suffered a neurologic event.

These two studies showed a favorable trend toward a reduction in the stroke rate among patients receiving aspirin as treatment for symptomatic lesions in the extracranial circulation. In the first, aspirin was used as the principal form of therapy, whereas in the second, aspirin was an adjunct to surgical therapy. The absolute level of cases with an unfavorable outcome in the surgically treated group was about one fifth the percentage of unfavorable outcomes among those treated medically (2% in the surgically treated group, versus 11.3% in the medically treated group). This difference may reflect the independent favorable effect of surgery.

Two other studies have evaluated the use of aspirin in a randomized, controlled, prospective fashion. In a study from France,[263] 604 patients with arteriothrombotic cerebral ischemic events referable to the carotid or vertebrobasilar circulation were entered in a double-blind, randomized clinical trial comparing aspirin 1 g/day, aspirin 1 g/day plus dipyridamole 225 mg/day, and placebo. A comparison of the placebo and aspirin groups showed a significant reduction ($P < 0.05$) of cerebral infarction in the aspirin group. Overall, 66 patients in the entire group suffered cerebral infarction during the trial. This corresponds to a cumulative stroke rate for the placebo group of 18% and a rate of 10.5% for each of the aspirin groups. No significant difference in the aspirin plus dipyridamole group was found. Thus, the incidence of stroke per year was on the order of 6% for placebo versus 3% for the treatment groups. This represents, again, a 50% reduction in stroke risk. In the dipyridamole-aspirin trial in cerebral ischemia, the American-Canadian Cooperative Study Group found no difference in the stroke risk in patients receiving aspirin or aspirin plus dipyridamole for the prevention of stroke during long-term follow-up.[264] Interestingly, the stroke rate in patients treated with either aspirin or aspirin plus dipyridamole was about 20% at 5 years. This yields a 4% per year stroke risk, which is not dissimilar to the lower rates reported in natural history studies.

In 1983, a Danish cooperative study comparing the outcomes of patients with extracranial occlusive disease treated with aspirin or placebo was reported.[265] No favorable influence of aspirin in the prevention of ischemic attacks could be determined. Unfortunately, only 203 patients were monitored, which is probably an insufficient number to achieve any statistically valid data. This study has been criticized and probably suffers from type II statistical error.[266]

The objective of any treatment regimen for carotid artery disease should be the reduction of stroke risk. Although each of the prospective, randomized trials of antiplatelet agents showed a trend toward stroke risk reduction, none achieved statistical significance with regard to that parameter. Only when the end points of TIA, stroke, and nonfatal and fatal MI were lumped together did a statistically significant benefit in favor of aspirin emerge. Individual studies lacked sufficient numbers of patients to show a reduction of stroke risk in favor of aspirin; however, in a meta-analysis combining the patients from the various series, the best that could be shown was a 15% stroke risk reduction in favor of aspirin, and this still failed to achieve statistical significance.[267]

The antiplatelet drug ticlopidine hydrochloride was compared with aspirin in a multicenter, prospective, randomized trial of 3069 patients with recent transient or mild persistent focal cerebral or retinal ischemia.[268] The 3-year event rate for nonfatal stroke or death from any cause was 17% for ticlopidine and 19% for aspirin. The rates of fatal and nonfatal stroke at 3 years were 10% for ticlopidine and 13% for aspirin. The authors concluded that ticlopidine was somewhat more effective than aspirin in preventing stroke in their study population but that the risks of side effects were greater.

Failures of antiplatelet therapy in the treatment of symptomatic carotid artery disease have been reported.[269] Caution should be used in patients who receive platelet antiaggregants as primary therapy for this disease. Partial disappearance of their symptoms should be considered a failure and alternative forms of treatment considered. Patients who experience complete relief of symptoms should be monitored carefully with annual noninvasive studies. Progression of the lesion may be obscured because of suppression of symptoms by the therapy. In a review of 27 aspirin failures requiring urgent operation,[269] 12 of the surgical specimens showed fresh hemorrhage in the atherosclerotic plaque. Whether this was induced or aggravated by aspirin could not be concluded. This incidence of fresh hemorrhage in an endarterectomy specimen appears to be high when compared with the findings in elective cases. Finally, good evidence suggests that aspirin is of no benefit to asymptomatic patients with respect to subsequent neurologic events. Cote and colleagues carried out a prospective, randomized trial in asymptomatic patients with carotid stenosis of at least 50%.[270] One hundred patients received aspirin, and 184 patients received placebo. The median follow-up was 2.3 years. The annual rates for vascular events were 11% in the placebo group and 10.7% in the aspirin group.

A 1995 report described the use of lovastatin in an attempt to modify carotid plaques.[271] In patients who were in the 60th to 90th percentiles of low-density lipoprotein cholesterol levels, lovastatin appeared to slow the rate of plaque progression. No evidence existed of plaque regression.

In conclusion, the available forms of medical management produce a reduction in the stroke rate in patients with significant atherosclerotic lesions of the extracranial circulation. This reduction does not appear to be as significant as that achieved by successful carotid endarterectomy. Medical treatment for symptomatic extracranial arterial disease should thus be reserved for patients with limited life expectancy or unidentified or surgically inaccessible lesions or for those who are poor surgical candidates.

New and Controversial Topics in Cerebrovascular Disease

CAROTID ENDARTERECTOMY FOR ACUTE STROKE

Emergent operation after acute stroke was used early in the history of endarterectomy. Because of several reports indicating a risk of converting an ischemic cerebral infarction into a hemorrhagic one, this procedure was abandoned. In reviewing these reports, it is possible to identify several types of patients who experienced such complications, including those with massive cerebral infarctions and in obtunded states, those in whom an attempt was made to open an occluded internal carotid artery several days to weeks after thrombosis, and those with severe, inadequately controlled hypertension.[272]

Later evidence suggested improved results if carotid artery surgery is delayed for at least 5 weeks after the acute event. Of 49 carotid endarterectomies done for acute cerebral infarction, 27 were performed within 5 weeks and 22 were done between 5 and 20 weeks after the acute neurologic event. The latter group showed no morbidity or mortality, whereas patients undergoing early operation had an 18.5% incidence of new postoperative neurologic deficits. The authors concluded that an unstable situation during the early phase of stroke contraindicated endarterectomy. No details about the degree of preoperative neurologic deficit or later recovery were available.[273] Following these guidelines, Dosick and colleagues noted a 21% incidence of recurrent stroke during the 4- to 60-week observation interval.[154] This led the authors to select their patients on the basis of CT scans, proceeding with surgery if the scans were negative. In their series, 110 patients underwent early endarterectomy after a persistent neurologic deficit with negative CT scans. No patient suffered a neurologic deficit in the territory of the operated artery, and no patient died. Whittemore and colleagues reported a similar experience in 28 patients with small, fixed neurologic deficits undergoing endarterectomy an average of 11 days after the onset of symptoms.[274] There was one postoperative death in this small group of patients and no new perioperative neurologic deficits. The authors recommended proceeding with endarterectomy early in this select group of patients with small cerebral infarcts.

In general, surgical intervention during the acute phase of a stroke is contraindicated. If the patient has a dense neurologic deficit, loss of consciousness, or cardiovascular instability, clearly surgery is not indicated. However, if the patient has a mild to moderate deficit and is fully conscious and otherwise stable, carotid endarterectomy of the responsible lesion can be undertaken soon after the patient has reached a plateau in recovery. This may be days or weeks after the onset of the event. In the small group of patients in whom a clinically unstable lesion exists, manifested by crescendo TIAs or stroke in evolution, emergent endarterectomy should be strongly considered.

CRESCENDO TRANSIENT ISCHEMIC ATTACKS AND STROKE IN EVOLUTION

Crescendo TIAs and stroke in evolution used to be considered contraindications to operation. I initially reported my experience with a select group of patients with stroke in evolution or crescendo TIAs who were acutely studied with angiography. If an unstable condition such as a free-floating thrombus or a propagating thrombus in the presence of a distally patent internal carotid artery was identified, the patient was taken promptly to the operating room. The net result in a series of approximately 25 patients was no deaths and a return to essentially normal neurologic status, in contrast to the natural history of stroke in evolution, which has an approximately 80% expected mortality.[275]

A similar experience was reported by Mentzer and colleagues with 17 patients operated on emergently for stroke in evolution.[33] None had worsening of the preoperative neurologic deficit, four (24%) remained unchanged, and 12 (70%) had complete recovery. One death occurred, for a 6% operative mortality. This compared favorably with a parallel nonrandomized group of 26 patients with stroke in evolution treated conservatively. The medical group had 15% mortality, but more important, 17 patients (66%) suffered moderate to severe permanent neurologic deficits. This report also presented the collated operative results from 90 cases in the literature. After successful endarterectomy, 55% were improved, 25% had no change, and 10% were worse. A 10% mortality for the collated experience was reported. Thus, surgical intervention in the presence of stroke in evolution carries a significantly increased risk of both perioperative stroke and death. However, the results of surgical therapy are considerably better than the natural history of the untreated condition. A specific goal for surgical intervention must be identified by preoperative angiography. Indications for emergent endarterectomy include the presence of an unstable condition such as a free-floating thrombus or propagating thrombus in the presence of a distally patent internal carotid artery. It is highly recommended that CT be used to exclude other associated conditions that could appear to be stroke in evolution.

More recently, a derivative report from the VA symptomatic trial identified crescendo TIAs as a surgical imperative.[276]

POSSIBLE DELETERIOUS EFFECT OF ANTIPLATELET DRUGS

In patients with asymptomatic carotid bifurcation plaques or with minimal plaques and TIAs who are treated with antiplatelet drugs, there have been reports of progression—more rapid than expected—of the atheromatous lesion to near-total occlusion. Operation at that time indicated a high degree of intraplaque hemorrhage. Thus, antiplatelet drugs may precipitate intraplaque hemorrhage and a rapid progression of the lesion.[269] A subsequent report compared plaque histopathology with the preoperative use of antiplatelet drugs. Those patients taking antiplatelet drugs had an 80.1% incidence of multiple intraplaque hemorrhages, in contrast to a 19.7% incidence of intraplaque hemorrhage in patients not receiving antiplatelet drugs.[277]

CAROTID BALLOON ANGIOPLASTY AND STENTING

Carotid balloon angioplasty with stenting is being used with increasing frequency in many centers worldwide. Initially, anecdotal reports provided conflicting data with regard to safety and efficacy. The first large series was reported by

Dietrich and colleagues.[278] Between April 1993 and September 1995, 110 nonconsecutive patients underwent treatment using balloon angioplasty and stenting in accord with an approved protocol in a single institution. It is important to note that 72% of the patients in this series were asymptomatic and, therefore, represented the lowest risk group. There were seven periprocedural (in-hospital) strokes, for an incidence of 6.4%, and there were two in-hospital deaths, for an incidence of 1.8%; thus, the combined in-hospoital stroke morbidity and mortality was 8.2%. Two patients undergoing stented angioplasty went on to occlusion within 30 days. The same year, Roubin and colleagues reported their experience with 74 patients undergoing placement of 210 stents in 152 vessels.[279] They had one death and nine in-hospital strokes, for a periprocedural stroke morbidity and mortality of 14%.

These and several other anecdotal reports prompted a multidisciplinary group of physicians to write an editorial expressing concern about the proliferation of this procedure without proof of its safety or efficacy. They recommended that a prospective trial comparing stented balloon angioplasty with carotid endarterectomy be carried out.[280] Several retrospective comparative studies of carotid endarterectomy and carotid angioplasty with stenting have also been reported. Jordan and colleagues compared percutaneous transluminal angioplasty (PTA) with stenting in 107 patients in their institution with 166 carotid endarterectomies done concurrently.[281] The 30-day combined stroke morbidity and mortality for PTA and stenting was 9.3%, versus 3.6% for carotid endarterectomy. In evaluating the late results (>30 days), including such items as amaurosis, recurrent stenosis, TIA, minor stroke, major stroke, and death, the combined adverse event rate for PTA with stenting was 18.7%, versus 6.6% for carotid endarterectomy. These same authors also did a cost comparison and found that the total cost for carotid endarterectomy was $21,670 per patient, whereas carotid angioplasty with stenting cost $30,140.

Several prospective, randomized trials have also reported their results. In a European trial, largely from centers in the United Kingdom, the 30-day results were a combined stroke and death rate of 9.9% for carotid angioplasty and 9.8% for carotid endarterectomy.[282] Nehler and colleagues attempted to do a single-institution prospective, randomized trial,[283] but the trial was stopped after only 17 patients were entered into the study. Ten carotid endarterectomies were performed without death or stroke; however, five strokes occurred during the course of seven angioplasties.

There were also several industry-sponsored trials. The first of these was the Schneider Wallstent trial, whose results were presented at the 26th International Stroke Conference in February 2001.[284] The 2-day periprocedural stroke and death rate was 7.5% in the stent group and 1.8% in the carotid endarterectomy group; the 30-day stroke and death rate was 12.1% in the stent group and 4.5% in the carotid endarterectomy group; and the primary adverse event rate at the end of 1 year was 12.1% in the stent group and 3.6% in the carotid endarterectomy group. The authors concluded that carotid angioplasty and stenting are not equivalent to carotid endarterectomy.

The trials up to this point had been done without cerebral antiembolism devices. Several devices have since been introduced, and most contemporary trials are now being done in conjunction with their use. The most influential industry-sponsored trial to date has been the SAPPHIRE study, sponsored by Johnson and Johnson/Cordis.[285] Both 30-day and 1-year data have been reported, and based on these reports, the Food and Drug Administration has given conditional approval for the J&J stent and antiembolism device for use in high-risk patients. The trial randomized 159 patients to stent–balloon angioplasty with cerebral protection versus 151 carotid endarterectomies. All these procedures were carried out in what was defined as a high-risk patient group. The authors compared a number of parameters, including death and stroke in the postprocedure interval. They also added nonfatal MI, which included both Q-wave and non–Q-wave MI. Interestingly, there was no difference in the death and stroke rate with angioplasty and stenting versus carotid endarterectomy. However, there was a major, statistically significant difference in the incidence of MI in the two groups. The MI rate in the carotid endarterectomy group was 7.9%, wheres in the angioplasty and stenting group it was 2.5%. When comparing all patients, both symptomatic and asymptomatic, the combined death, stroke, and MI rate was 5.8% in the stent group and 12.6% in the carotid endarterectomy group. This difference reached statistical significance in favor of angioplasty and stenting for high-risk patients. The difference held at the end of 1 year, when the major adverse event rate was 11.9% in the stent group and 19.9% in the carotid endarterectomy group (P = 0.048).

The only independently funded study is CREST (Carotid Revascularization Endarterectomy vs. Stent Trial). It is funded by the NIH, with some financial contribution from Guidant with regard to administrative support and training in the use of the Guidant stent and the Guidant antiembolism device. The trial is ongoing, and the results of the randomization will be unknown for several years. However, during the lead-in phase of the trial, the data associated with carotid angioplasty and stenting among the participating centers were reported.[285] Among symptomatic patients, the 30-day morbidity and mortality rate was 5.5%; for asymptomatic patients, it was 2.8%. These results compared very well with the surgical series in the NASCET and ACAS.

In conclusion, current data suggest that the combination of carotid angioplasty and stenting has reached clinical equipoise with carotid endarterectomy. The early results justify a well-designed prospective, randomized trial that is independently funded and carefully monitored. We anticipate that the CREST results will definitively determine whether the technique of carotid angioplasty and stenting with cerebral protection is equivalent to, better than, or worse than carotid endarterectomy.

ASYMPTOMATIC CAROTID ULCERATION

Not uncommonly, a large, nonstenotic, ulcerative lesion in a contralateral carotid artery is discovered incidentally when the ipsilateral symptomatic carotid artery is being studied by angiography. Whether to operate on this ulcerative lesion is a common question. My colleagues and I carried out two retrospective reviews of patients with identified nonstenotic ulcerative lesions that were monitored without treatment. We observed that medium and large ulcerative lesions carried a significant stroke risk, usually not preceded by warning TIAs.[54] In the most recent study, the risk of stroke in patients with large ulcerative lesions being monitored expectantly was approximately 7.5% each year of follow-up after initial identification.[55] I currently recommend that medium grade B and large grade C ulcers, when identified incidentally, undergo prophylactic repair.

TANDEM LESIONS

Not uncommonly, one discovers a stenosis of the origin of the internal carotid artery in conjunction with a significant lesion of the carotid siphon. The question often raised is whether operating on the carotid artery alone is justified if the siphon lesion is larger than the artery lesion. Several reports now indicate that even though tandem lesions exist, the embolic potential of the atherosclerotic plaque at the carotid bifurcation greatly outweighs the thrombotic or embolic risk of the lesion in the carotid siphon.[287] My practice is to operate on the carotid bifurcation lesion in symptomatic patients in spite of the presence of a siphon lesion.[288] A retrospective review compared the perioperative morbidity, mortality, and late results in patients undergoing carotid endarterectomy with and without angiographically documented intracranial arterial occlusive disease. There was no difference between the two groups. The perioperative stroke rate was 1.9% versus 1.8%; mortality was 0.5% versus 0.7%; and the 3-, 5-, and 10-year stroke rates were 93% versus 92%, 87% versus 90%, and 79% versus 85%, respectively.[289]

COMBINED CAROTID AND CORONARY OCCLUSIVE DISEASE

The carotid-coronary area is particularly controversial, and treatment depends on whether symptoms exist in either vascular bed. In patients with symptomatic coronary artery disease in whom an asymptomatic carotid stenosis is found, it is difficult to know whether the carotid artery should be fixed first, followed by coronary artery bypass; whether both lesions should be fixed simultaneously; or whether surgery for the carotid artery lesion should be put off until after coronary artery bypass. The literature is controversial on this subject, and I continue to individualize treatment, depending on which lesion appears to be more critical. For example, if a patient has triple coronary artery disease with unstable angina and an asymptomatic carotid stenosis, I usually recommend that the coronary artery surgery be performed first and that the carotid lesion be evaluated after recovery. Conversely, if a patient has relatively stable angina and symptomatic carotid artery disease or a preocclusive (<90%) stenosis, operating on the carotid artery first and then managing the coronary artery lesions a few days later may be wise. Finally, if a patient has both symptomatic carotid artery disease and unstable angina, a simultaneous, combined approach would be justified.

INTELLECTUAL TESTING AND IMPROVEMENT WITH CAROTID ENDARTERECTOMY

After carotid endarterectomy, patients and their families often report that the patient appears intellectually brighter and is able to carry out tasks that have been alien for quite some time. Numerous attempts have been made to quantitate this intellectual improvement, usually without success. We must be careful not to regard intellectually impaired patients

as routine candidates for carotid endarterectomy, because the majority of these patients are suffering from organic brain disease rather than compromised blood flow.

EXTRACRANIAL-TO-INTRACRANIAL BYPASS GRAFTING

The technical ability to connect an extracranial arterial branch such as the temporal artery to a cortical branch of the middle cerebral artery has been developed over the past 15 years. To determine whether extracranial-to-intracranial (EC-IC) bypass surgery would benefit patients with symptomatic atherosclerotic disease of the internal carotid artery, an international randomized trial was begun in 1977 and completed in 1982.[290] In that study, 1377 patients with recent hemispheric strokes, retinal infarction, or TIAs who had narrowing or occlusion of the ipsilateral carotid artery or middle cerebral artery were randomized: 714 were assigned to best medical care, and 663 were assigned to surgery. In the latter group, an EC-IC arterial bypass was performed, with a patency rate on long-term follow-up of 96%. The 30-day surgical mortality was 6.6%, with a stroke morbidity of 2.5%. Nonfatal and fatal strokes on long-term follow-up occurred both more frequently and earlier in patients treated with EC-IC bypass. Survival analysis comparing the two groups demonstrated a similar lack of benefit from surgery. Reduction in the number of TIAs was noted in 77% of the surgical patients. An almost equal number (80%) of the medical patients also showed a reduction or disappearance of TIAs. In all parameters studied, EC-IC bypass failed to improve the results of medical therapy. The large number of patients with long-term follow-up, the uniformity of the disease process in the population studied, the randomization method (which produced a balanced treatment group), the presence of complete and accurate records of all entry and event dates, and the achievement of effective anastomosis with acceptably low morbidity and mortality suggest that this conclusion is not only statistically powerful but also clinically significant.

MAGNETIC RESONANCE ANGIOGRAPHY

In the continuing quest to find a substitute for invasive contrast angiography, the use of MRI of the vascular system has been developed: so-called magnetic resonance angiography. Various computer programs for postprocessing of magnetic resonance images to delineate the vascular system are under active development. To date, excellent imaging of the cervical and intracranial vessels has been achievable. However, several limitations of MRA have been identified. In several instances, the image suggested total occlusion, whereas contrast angiograms showed a patent vessel with a string sign. MRA also tends to overestimate the percentage stenosis, making minimal lesions look like hemodynamically significant lesions. Finally, MRA cannot delineate surface irregularity or ulceration.[291-293]

KEY REFERENCES

Abu Rahma AF, Robinson PA, Saiedy S, et al: Prospective randomized trial of bilateral carotid endarterectomies: Primary closure versus patching. Stroke 30:1185-1189, 1999.

Chervu A, Moore WS: Carotid endarterectomy without angiography: Personal series and review of the literature. Ann Vasc Surg 8:296-302, 1994.

Dixon S, Pais SO, Raviola C, et al: Natural history of nonstenotic, asymptomatic ulcerative lesions of the carotid artery: A further analysis. Arch Surg 117:1493, 1982.

Eastcott HHG, Pickering GW, Rob C: Reconstruction of internal carotid artery in a patient with intermittent attacks of hemiplegia. Lancet 2:994-996, 1954.

Executive Committee for the Asymptomatic Carotid Atherosclerosis Study: Endarterectomy for asymptomatic carotid artery stenosis. JAMA 273:1421-1428, 1995.

Halliday A, Mansfield A, Marro J, et al: Prevention of disabling and fatal strokes by successful carotid endarterectomy in patients without recent neurological symptoms: Randomized control trial. Lancet 363:1491-1502, 2004.

Moore WS, Barnett HJ, Beebe ME, et al: Guidelines for carotid endarterectomy: A multidisciplinary consensus statement from the ad hoc committee, American Heart Association. Stroke 26:188-201, 1995.

Moore WS, Hall AD: Importance of emboli from carotid bifurcation in pathogenesis in cerebral ischemia attacks. Arch Surg 101:708, 1970.

Moore WS, Kempczinski RF, Nelson JJ, Toole JF: Recurrent carotid stenosis: Results of this asymptomatic carotid atherosclerosis study. Stroke 29:2018-2025, 1998.

North American Symptomatic Carotid Endarterectomy Trial collaborators: Beneficial effect of carotid endarterectomy in symptomatic patients with high-grade carotid stenosis. N Engl J Med 325:445-453, 1991.

Thompson JE: The evolution of surgery for the treatment and prevention of stroke: The Willis lecture. Stroke 27:1427-1434, 1996.

REFERENCES

1. Savory WS: Case of a young woman in whom the main arteries of both upper extremities and of the left side of the neck were throughout completely obliterated. Med Chir Trans Lond 39:205-219, 1856.
2. Gowers WR: On a case of simultaneous embolism of central retinal and middle cerebral arteries. Lancet 2:794, 1875.
3. Chiari M: Ueber das Verhalten des tei lungs-winkels der Carotis communis bei der Endarteritis chronica deformans. Verh Dtsch Ges Pathol 9:326-330, 1905.
4. Guthrie LG, Mayou S: Right hemiplegia and atrophy of left optic nerve. Proc R Soc Med 1:180, 1908.
5. Cadwater WB: Unilateral optic atrophy and contralateral hemiplegia consequent on occlusion of the cerebral vessels. JAMA 59:2248, 1912.
6. Hunt JR: The role of the carotid arteries in the causation of vascular lesions of the brain, with remarks on certain special features of the symptomatology. Am J Med Sci 147:704-713, 1914.
7. Moniz E: L'encéphalographie artérielle: Son importance dans la localisation des tumeurs cérébrales. Rev Neurol (Paris) 2:72-90, 1927.
8. Moniz E, Lima A, de Lacerda R: Hémiplégies par thrombose de la carotide interne. Proc Med 45:977-980, 1937.
9. Chao WH, Kwan ST, Lyman RS, et al: Thrombosis of the left internal carotid artery. Arch Surg 37:100-111, 1938.
10. Johnson HC, Walker AE: The angiographic diagnosis of spontaneous thrombosis of the internal and common carotid arteries. J Neurosurg 8:631-659, 1951.
11. Fisher M: Occlusion of the internal carotid artery. Arch Neurol Psychiatry 65:346-377, 1951.
12. Fisher M: Occlusion of the carotid arteries. Arch Neurol Psychiatry 72:187-204, 1954.
13. Carrea R, Molins M, Murphy G: Surgical treatment of spontaneous thrombosis of the internal carotid artery in the neck: Carotid-carotideal anastomosis: Report of a case. Acta Neurol Latinoam 1:71-78, 1955.
14. Strully KJ, Hurwitt ES, Blankenberg HW: Thromboendarterectomy for thrombosis of the internal carotid artery in the neck. J Neurosurg 10:474-482, 1953.
15. DeBakey ME, Crawford ES, Cooley DA, et al: Surgical considerations of occlusive disease of innominate, carotid, subclavian, and vertebral arteries. Ann Surg 149:690-710, 1959.
16. DeBakey ME: Successful carotid endarterectomy for cerebrovascular insufficiency: Nineteen-year follow-up. JAMA 233:1083, 1975.
17. Eastcott HHG, Pickering GW, Rob C: Reconstruction of internal carotid artery in a patient with intermittent attacks of hemiplegia. Lancet 2:994-996, 1954.
18. Davis JB, Grove WJ, Julian OC: Thrombic occlusion of the branches of the aortic arch, Martorell's syndrome: Report of a case treated surgically. Ann Surg 144:124-126, 1956.
19. Warren R, Triedman LJ: Pulseless disease and carotid artery thrombosis. N Engl J Med 257:685-690, 1957.
20. Thompson JE: The evolution of surgery for the treatment and prevention of stroke: The Willis lecture. Stroke 27:1427-1434, 1996.
21. Adelman SM: Economic impact. In McDowell FM (ed): Report on the National Survey of Stroke (American Heart Association Monograph No. 75). Stroke 12:1, 1981.
22. Mohr JP, Caplan LR, Meski JW, et al: The Harvard Cooperative Stroke Registry: A prospective registry. Neurology 28:754, 1978.
23. Sacco RL, Wolf PA, Kannel WB, McNamara PM: Survival and recurrence following stroke: The Framingham Study. Stroke 13:290, 1982.
24. Soltero I, Lin K, Cooper R, et al: Trends in mortality from cerebrovascular diseases in the United States, 1960 to 1975. Stroke 9:549, 1978.
25. Enger E, Boysen S: Long-term anticoagulant therapy in patients with cerebral infarction: A controlled clinical study. Acta Med Scand Suppl 438:1-61, 1965.
26. Robinson RW, Demirel M, LeBeau RJ: Natural history of cerebral thrombosis: 9-19 year follow-up. J Chronic Dis 21:221, 1968.
27. Schmidt EV, Smirnov VE, Ryabova VS: Results of the seven-year prospective study of stroke patients. Stroke 19:942-949, 1988.
28. Swedish Cooperative Study: High-dose acetylsalicylic acid after cerebral infarction. Stroke 18:325-334, 1987.
29. Klag MJ, Whelton PK, Seidler AJ: Decline in US stroke mortality: Demographic trends and antihypertensive treatment. Stroke 20:14-21, 1989.
30. Wolf PA, O'Neal A, D'Agostino RB, et al: Declining mortality, not declining incidence of stroke: The Framingham Study. Stroke 20:29, 1989.
31. Harmsen P, Tsipogianni A, Wilhelmsen L: Stroke incidence rates were unchanged, while fatality rates declined, during 1971-1987 in Göteborg, Sweden. Stroke 23:1410-1415, 1992.
32. Moden B, Wagener DK: Some epidemiologic aspects of stroke: Mortality/morbidity trends, age, sex, race, socioeconomic status. Stroke 23:1230-1236, 1992.
33. Mentzer RM Jr, Finkelmeier BA, Crosby JK, Wellons HA Jr: Emergency carotid endarterectomy for fluctuating neurologic deficits. Surgery 89:60, 1981.
34. Millikan CH: Discussion. In McDowell FH, Brennan RW (eds): Cerebral Vascular Diseases (Transactions of the Eighth Princeton Conference on Cerebral Vascular Disease). New York, Grune & Stratton, 1973, p 209.
35. Whisnant JP, Matsumoto M, Elveback LR: The effects of anticoagulant therapy on the prognosis of patients with transient cerebral ischemic attacks in a community: Rochester, Minnesota, 1965-1969. Mayo Clin Proc 48:844, 1973.
36. Dennis M, Bamford J, Sandercock P, Warlow C: Prognosis of transient ischemic attacks in the Oxfordshire Community Stroke Project. Stroke 21:848-853, 1990.
37. Hass WK, Jonas S: Caution falling rock zone: An analysis of the medical and surgical management of threatened stroke. Proc Inst Med 33:80, 1980.
38. Loeb C, Priano A, Albana C: Clinical features and long-term follow-up of patients with reversible ischemic attacks. Acta Neurol Scand 57:471, 1978.
39. Toole JF: The Willis lecture: Transient ischemic attacks, scientific method, and new realities. Stroke 22:99-104, 1991.
40. Grigg MJ, Papadakis K, Nicolaides AN, et al: The significance of cerebral infarction and atrophy in patients with amaurosis fugax and transient ischemic attacks in relation to internal carotid artery stenosis: A preliminary report. J Vasc Surg 7:215-222, 1988.
41. Kartchner MM, McRae LP: Noninvasive evaluation and management of the asymptomatic carotid bruit. Surgery 82:840, 1977.
42. Busuttil RW, Baker JD, Davidson RK, Machleder HI: Carotid artery stenosis: Hemodynamic significance and clinical course. JAMA 245:1438, 1981.
43. Roederer GO, Langlois YE, Jager KA, et al: The natural history of carotid arterial disease in asymptomatic patients with cervical bruits. Stroke 15:605-613, 1984.
44. Moore DJ, Miles RD, Gooley NA, Summer DS: Non-invasive assessment of stroke risk in asymptomatic and non-hemispheric patients with suspected carotid disease: Five year follow-up of 294 unoperated and 81 operated patients. Ann Surg 202:491-504, 1985.
45. Chambers BR, Norris JW: Outcome in patients with asymptomatic neck bruits. N Engl J Med 315:860-865, 1986.
46. Norris JW, Zhu CZ, Bornstein NM, Chambers BR: Vascular risks of asymptomatic carotid stenosis. Stroke 22:1485-1490, 1991.
47. Norris JW, Zhu CZ: Silent stroke and carotid stenosis. Stroke 23:483-485, 1992.

48. Johnson JM, Kennelly MM, Decesare D, et al: Natural history of asymptomatic carotid plaque. Arch Surg 120:1010-1012, 1985.
49. Langsfeld M, Gray-Weale AC, Lusby RJ: The role of plaque morphology and diameter reduction in the development of new symptoms in asymptomatic carotid arteries. J Vasc Surg 9:548-557, 1989.
50. Sterpetti AV, Schultz RD, Feldhaus RJ, et al: Ultrasonographic features of carotid plaque and the risk of subsequent neurologic deficits. Surgery 104:652-660, 1988.
51. Madison FE, Moore WS: Ulcerated atheroma of the carotid artery: Arteriographic appearance. AJR Am J Roentgenol 107:530, 1969.
52. Moore WS, Hall AD: Ulcerated atheroma of the carotid artery: A cause of transient cerebral ischemia. Am J Surg 116:237, 1968.
53. Moore WS, Hall AD: Importance of emboli from carotid bifurcation in pathogenesis in cerebral ischemia attacks. Arch Surg 101:708, 1970.
54. Moore WS, Boren C, Malone JM, et al: Natural history of nonstenotic asymptomatic ulcerative lesions of the carotid artery. Arch Surg 113:1352, 1978.
55. Dixon S, Pais SO, Raviola C, et al: Natural history of nonstenotic, asymptomatic ulcerative lesions of the carotid artery: A further analysis. Arch Surg 117:1493, 1982.
56. Harward TRS, Kroener JM, Wickbom IG, et al: Natural history of asymptomatic ulcerative plaques of the carotid bifurcation. Am J Surg 146:208, 1983.
57. Kartchner MM, McRae LP: Guidelines for non-invasive evaluation of asymptomatic carotid bruits. Clin Neurosurg 28:418-428, 1981.
58. Barnes RW, Liebman PR, Marszalek PP, et al: Natural history of asymptomatic carotid disease in patients undergoing cardiovascular surgery. Surgery 90:1075-1083, 1981.
59. Breslau PJ, Fell G, Ivey TD, et al: Carotid arterial disease in patients undergoing coronary artery bypass operations. J Thorac Cardiovasc Surg 82:765-767, 1981.
60. Furlan AJ, Craciun AR: Risk in stroke during coronary artery bypass graft surgery in patients with internal carotid artery disease documented by angiography. Stroke 16:797-799, 1985.
61. Turnipseed WD, Berkoff HA, Belzer FO: Post-operative stroke in cardiac and peripheral vascular disease. Ann Surg 192:365-368, 1980.
62. Von Reutern G-M, Hetzel A, Birnbaum D, Schlosser V: Transcranial Doppler ultrasonography during cardiopulmonary bypass in patients with severe carotid stenosis or occlusion. Stroke 19:674-680, 1988.
63. Brener BJ, Hermans H, Eisenbud D, et al: The management of patients requiring coronary bypass and carotid endarterectomy. In Moore WS (ed): Surgery for Cerebrovascular Disease, 2nd ed. Philadelphia, WB Saunders, 1996, pp 278-287.
64. Schwartz CJ, Mitchell JRA: Observations on localization of arterial plaques. Circ Res 11:63, 1962.
65. Heath D, Smith P, Harris P, Winson M: The atherosclerotic human carotid sinus. J Pathol 110:49, 1973.
66. Caro CG, Fitzgerald JN, Schroter RC: Atheroma and arterial wall shear: Observation, correlation and proposal of a shear-dependent mass transfer mechanism for atherogenesis. Proc R Soc Lond B Biol Sci 117:109, 1971.
67. Balasubramanian K, Giddens DP, Maybon RS: Steady flow at the carotid bifurcation. In Schneck DJ (ed): Biofluid Mechanics, vol 6. New York, Plenum Press, 1980, p 475.
68. Ferguson GG, Roach MR: Flow conditions at bifurcations as determined in glass models with reference to the focal distribution of vascular lesions. In Bergel DH (ed): Cardiovascular Fluid Dynamics, vol 2. New York, Academic Press, 1972.
69. Fox JA, Hugh AE: Static zones in the internal carotid artery: Correlations with boundary layer separation and stasis in mobile flows. Br J Radiol 43:370, 1976.
70. LoGerfo FW, Nowak MD, Quist WC, et al: Flow studies in a model carotid bifurcation. Arteriosclerosis 1:235, 1981.
71. Zarins CK, Giddens DB, Glagov S: Atherosclerotic plaque distribution and flow velocity profiles in the carotid bifurcation. In Bergan JJ, Yao JST (eds): Cerebrovascular Insufficiency. New York, Grune & Stratton, 1982, p 19.
72. Salzman EW: Platelet-vessel interactions in cerebrovascular disease: The role of prostaglandins in cerebrovascular insufficiency. In Bergan JJ, Yao JST (eds): Cerebrovascular Insufficiency. New York, Grune & Stratton, 1983, p 31.
73. Meyers KM, Seachord CL, Holmsen H, et al: The dominant role of thromboxane formation in secondary aggregation of platelets. Nature 282:331, 1979.
74. Born BGR: Arterial thrombosis and its prevention. In Hayase S, Murao S (eds): Proceedings of the Eighth World Congress of Cardiology, Tokyo. Amsterdam, Excerpta Medica, 1978, p 81.
75. Fryer JA, Myers PC, Appleberg M: Carotid intraplaque hemorrhage: The significance of neovascularity. J Vasc Surg 63:341-349, 1987.
76. Lusby RJ, Ferrell LD, Wylie EJ: The significance of intraplaque hemorrhage in the pathogenesis of carotid arteriosclerorosis. In Bergan JJ, Yao JST (eds): Cerebrovascular Insufficiency. New York, Grune & Stratton, 1983, p 41.
77. Ogata J, Masuda J, Yutani C, Yamguchi T: Rupture of atheromatous plaque as a cause of thrombotic occlusion of stenotic internal carotid artery. Stroke 21:1740-1745, 1990.
78. Palubinskas AJ, Ripley HR: Fibromuscular hyperplasia in extrarenal arteries. Radiology 82:451, 1964.
79. Patman RD, Thompson JE, Talkington CM, et al: Natural history of fibromuscular dysplasia of the carotid artery. Stroke 1:135, 1980.
80. Osborn AG, Anderson RE: Angiographic spectrum of cervical and intracranial fibromuscular dysplasia. Stroke 8:617, 1977.
81. Effeney DJ, Ehrenfeld WK, Stoney RJ, et al: Fibromuscular dysplasia of the internal carotid artery. World J Surg 3:179, 1979.
82. Stanley JC, Gewertz BL, Bove EL, et al: Arterial fibrodysplasia: Histopathologic character and current etiologic concepts. Arch Surg 110:561, 1975.
83. Ross R, Klebanoff SJ: Fine structural changes in uterine smooth muscle and fibroblasts in response to estrogen. J Cell Biol 32:155, 1967.
84. Nakata Y: An experimental study on the vascular lesions caused by obstruction of the vasa vasorum. Jpn Circ J 31:275, 1967.
85. Sarkari NBS, Palms JM, Bickerstaff ER: Neurological manifestations associated with internal carotid loops and kinks in children. J Neurol Neurosurg Psychiatry 33:194, 1973.
86. Metz H, Murray-Leslie RM, Bannister RG, et al: Kinking of the internal carotid artery in relation to cerebrovascular disease. Lancet 1:424, 1961.
87. Quattlebaum JK Jr, Upson ET, Neville RL: Strokes associated with elongation and kinking of the internal carotid artery. Ann Surg 150:824, 1959.
88. Vannix RS, Joergenson EJ, Carter R: Kinking of the internal carotid artery: Clinical significance and surgical management. Am J Surg 134:82, 1977.
89. Busuttil RW, Davidson RK, Foley KT, et al: Selective management of extracranial carotid arterial aneurysms. Am J Surg 140:85, 1980.
90. Rhodes EL, Stanley JC, Hoffman GL, et al: Aneurysms of extracranial carotid arteries. Arch Surg 111:339, 1976.
91. Kaupp HA, Haid SP, Jurayj MN, et al: Aneurysms of the extracranial carotid artery. Surgery 72:946, 1972.
92. Boldrey E, Maass L, Miller E: The role of atlantoid compression in the etiology of internal carotid thrombosis. J Neurosurg 13:127, 1956.
93. Smith RF, Szilagyi DE, Colville JM: Surgical treatment of mycotic aneurysms. Arch Surg 85:663, 1962.
94. Bradac GB, Kaernbach A, Bolk-Weischedel D, Finck GA: Spontaneous dissecting aneurysm of cervical cerebral arteries: Report of six cases and review of the literature. Neuroradiology 21:149, 1981.
95. Ehrenfeld WK, Wiley EJ: Spontaneous dissection of the internal carotid artery. Arch Surg 111:1294, 1976.
96. Takayasu M: Case with unusual changes of the central vessels of the retina. Acta Soc Ophthalmol Jpn 12:554, 1908.
97. Nasu T: Pathology of pulseless disease: Systematic study and critical review of 21 autopsy cases reported in Japan. Angiology 14:225, 1962.
98. Lande A, Berkmen YM: Aortitis: Pathologic, clinical and arteriographic review. Radiol Clin North Am 14:219, 1976.
99. Lupi-Herrera E, Sanchez-Torres G, Marcushamer J, et al: Takayasu's arteritis. Clinical study of 107 cases. Am Heart J 93:94-103, 1977.
100. Hamrin B, Jousson N, Landberg T: Involvement of large vessels in polymyalgia arteritica. Lancet 1:1193, 1965.
101. Lindsay S, Entenman C, Ellis EE, Geraci CL: Aortic arteriosclerosis in the dog after localized aortic irradiation with electrons. Circ Res 10:61, 1962.
102. Silverberg GD, Britt RH, Goffinet DR: Radiation-induced carotid artery disease. Cancer 41:132, 1978.
103. McCready RA, Hyde GL, Bevins BA, et al: Radiation-induced arterial injuries. Surgery 93:306-312, 1983.
104. Levinson SA, Close MB, Ehrenfeld WK, Stoney RJ: Carotid artery occlusive disease following external cervical irradiation. Arch Surg 107:395-397, 1973.
105. Moritz MW, Higgins RF, Jacobs JR: Duplex imaging and incidence of carotid radiation injury after high-dose radiotherapy for tumors of the head and neck. Arch Surg 125:1181-1183, 1990.
106. DeGrotte RD, Lynch JG, Jamil Z, Hobson RW II: Carotid restenosis: Long term non-invasive follow-up after carotid endarterectomy. Stroke 18:1031-1036, 1987.

107. Hertzer NR, Martinez BD, Benjamin SP, Beven EG: Recurrent stenosis after carotid endarterectomy. Surg Gynecol Obstet 149:360-364, 1979.

108. Hertzer NR, Beven EG, O'Hara PJ, Krajewski LP: A prospective study of vein patch angioplasty during carotid endarterectomy. Ann Surg 206:628-635, 1987.

109. Lees CD, Hertzer NR: Postoperative stroke and late neurologic complications after endarterectomy. Arch Surg 116:1561, 1981.

110. Stoney RJ, String ST: Recurrent carotid stenosis. Surgery 80:705-710, 1976.

111. Zierler RE, Bandyk DF, Thiele BL, Strandness DE Jr: Carotid artery stenosis following endarterectomy. Arch Surg 117:1408-1415, 1982.

112. O'Donnell TF Jr, Callew AD, Scott G, et al: Ultrasound characteristics of recurrent carotid disease: Hypothesis explaining the low incidence of symptomatic recurrence. J Vasc Surg 2:26-41, 1985.

113. Nicholls SC, Phillips DJ, Bergelin RO, et al: Carotid endarterectomy: Relationship of outcome to early restenosis. J Vasc Surg 2:375-381, 1985.

114. Bernstein EF, Torem S, Dolley RB: Does carotid restenosis predict an increased risk of late symptoms, stroke, or death? Ann Surg 212:629-636, 1990.

115. Awad IA, Little JR: Patch angioplasty in carotid endarterectomy—advantages, concerns, and controversies. Stroke 20:417-422, 1989.

116. Curley S, Edwards WS, Jacob TP: Recurrent carotid stenosis after autologous tissue patching. J Vasc Surg 6:350-354, 1987.

117. Eikelboom BC, Ackerstaff RGA, Hoeneveld H, et al: Benefits of carotid patching: A randomized study. J Vasc Surg 7:240-247, 1988.

118. Lord RSA, Raj TB, Stary DL, et al: Comparison of saphenous vein patch, polytetrafluoroethylene patch, and direct arteriotomy closure after carotid endarterectomy. Part 1. Perioperative results. J Vasc Surg 9:521-529, 1989.

119. Abu Rahma AF, Robinson PA, Saiedy S, et al: Prospective randomized trial of bilateral carotid endarterectomies: Primary closure versus patching. Stroke 30:1185-1189, 1999.

120. Abu Rahma AF, Robinson PA, Saiedy S, et al: Prospective randomized trial of carotid endarterectomy with primary closure and patch angioplasty with saphenous vein, jugular vein, and polytetrafluoroethylene: Long-term follow-up. J Vasc Surg 27:222-232, 1998.

121. Moore WS, Kempczinski RF, Nelson JJ, Toole JF: Recurrent carotid stenosis: Results of this asymptomatic carotid atherosclerosis study. Stroke 29:2018-2025, 1998.

122. Salvian A, Baker JD, Machleder HI, et al: Cause and noninvasive detection of restenosis after carotid endarterectomy. Am J Surg 146:29-34, 1983.

123. Gelabert HA, El-Massry S, Moore WS: Carotid endarterectomy with primary closure does not adversely affect the rate of recurrent stenosis. Arch Surg 129:648-654, 1994.

124. Petrik PV, Gelabert HA, Moore WS, et al: Cigarette smoking accelerates carotid artery intimal hyperplasia in a dose-dependent manner. Stroke 26:1409-1414, 1995.

125. Hansen F, Lindblad B, Persson NH, Bergqvist D: Can recurrent stenosis after carotid endarterectomy be prevented by low-dose acetyl salicylic acid? A double blind, randomized and placebo-controlled study. Eur J Vasc Surg 7:380-385, 1993.

126. Crawford ES, De Bakey ME, Blaisdell FW, et al: Hemodynamic alteration in patients with cerebral arterial insufficiency before and after operation. Surgery 48:76, 1960.

127. Gunning AJ, Pickering GW, Robb-Smith AHT, Russell RR: Mural thrombosis of the internal carotid artery and subsequent embolism. Q J Med 33:155-195, 1964.

128. Hertzer NR, Beven EG, Benjamin SP: Ultramicroscopic ulcerations and thrombi of the carotid bifurcation. Arch Surg 112:1394-1402, 1977.

129. Imparato AM, Riles TS, Gorstein F: The carotid bifurcation plaque: Pathology findings associated with cerebral ischemia. Stroke 10:238-245, 1979.

130. Edwards JH, Kricheff II, Riles T, Imparato A: Angiographically undetected ulceration of the carotid bifurcation as a cause of embolic stroke. Radiology 132:369-373, 1979.

131. Sterpetti AV, Hunter WJ, Schultz RD: Importance of ulceration of carotid plaque in determining symptoms of cerebral ischemia. J Cardiovasc Surg (Torino) 32:154-158, 1991.

132. Loeb C, Gandolfo C, Bino G: Intellectual impairment and cerebral lesions in multiple cerebral infarcts. Stroke 19:560-565, 1988.

133. Zukowski AJ, Nicolaides AN, Lewis RJ, et al: The correlation between carotid plaque ulceration and cerebral infarction seen on CT scan. J Vasc Surg 1:782-786, 1984.

134. Siebler M, Sitzer M, Steinmetz H: Detection of intracranial emboli in patients with symptomatic extracranial stroke 23:1652-1654, 1992.

135. Tietjen GE, Futrell N, Garcia JH, Millikan C: Platelet emboli in rat brain cross when the contralateral carotid artery is occluded. Stroke 22:1053-1058, 1991.

136. Amarenco P, Cohen A, Baudrimont M, Bousser MG: Transesophageal echocardiographic detection of aortic arch disease in patients with cerebral infarction. Stroke 23:1005-1009, 1992.

137. Amarenco P, Cohen A, Tzourio C, et al: Atherosclerotic disease of the aortic arch and the risk of ischemic stroke. N Engl J Med 331:1474-1479, 1994.

138. Stone DA, Hawke MW, La Monte M, et al: Ulcerated atherosclerotic plaques in the thoracic aorta are associated with cryptogenic stroke: A multiphase transesophageal echocardiographic study. Am Heart J 130:105-108, 1995.

139. Mohr JP: Lacunes. Stroke 13:3-11, 1982.

140. Fisher CM: Pure motor hemiplegia of vascular origin. Arch Neurol 13:30-44, 1965.

141. Pullicino P, Nelson RF, Kendall BE, Marshall J: Small deep infarcts diagnosed on computed tomography. Neurology 30:1090-1096, 1980.

142. Bladin PF, Berkovic SF: Striatocapsular infarction: Large infarcts in the lenticulostriate arterial territory. Neurology 34:1423-1430, 1984.

143. Bamford JM, Warlow CP: Evolution and testing of the lacunar hypothesis. Stroke 19:1074-1082, 1988.

144. Horowitz DR, Tuhrim S, Weinberger JM, Rudolph SJ: Mechanisms in lacunar infarction. Stroke 23:325-327, 1992.

145. Heyman A, Wilkinson WE, Heyden S, et al: Risk of stroke in asymptomatic persons with cervical arterial bruits: A population study in Evans County, Georgia. N Engl J Med 302:838, 1980.

146. Heyman A, Leviton A, Millikan CK, et al: XI. Transient focal cerebral ischemia: Epidemiological and clinical aspects. Stroke 5:277, 1974.

147. Reinmuth OM: Transient ischemic attacks. Curr Neurol 1:166, 1978.

148. Price TR, Gotshall RA, Poskanzer DC, et al: Cooperative study of hospital frequency and character of transient ischemic attacks. VI. Patients examined during an attack. JAMA 238:2512, 1977.

149. Futty DE, Conneally M, Dyker ML, et al: Cooperative study of hospital frequency and character of transient ischemic attacks. V. Symptom analysis. JAMA 238:2386, 1977.

150. Berguer R: Idiopathic ischemic syndrome of the retina and optic nerve and their carotid origin. J Vasc Surg 2:649-653, 1985.

151. Mohr JP: Transient ischemic attacks and the prevention of stroke. N Engl J Med 299:93, 1978.

152. Pessin MS, Duncan GW, Mohr JP, Poskanzer DC: Clinical and angiographic features of carotid transient ischemic attacks. N Engl J Med 296:358, 1977.

153. Yatsu SM, Coull BM: Stroke. Curr Neurol 3:159, 1981.

154. Dosick SM, Whalen RC, Gale SS, Brown OW: Carotid endarterectomy in the stroke patient: Computerized axial tomography to determine timing. J Vasc Surg 2:214-219, 1985.

155. Ahn SS, Jordan SE, Nuwer MR, et al: Compared electroencephalographic topographic brain mapping: A new and accurate monitor of cerebral circulation and function for patients having carotid endarterectomy. J Vasc Surg 8:247-254, 1988.

156. Strefler JY, Eliasziw M, Fox AJ, et al: Angiographic detection of carotid plaque ulceration: Comparison with surgical observations in a multicenter study [North American Symptomatic Carotid Endarterectomy Trial]. Stroke 25:1130-1132, 1994.

157. Moore WS, Ziomek S, Quiñones-Baldrich WJ, et al: Can clinical evaluation and noninvasive testing substitute for arteriography in the evaluation of carotid artery disease? Ann Surg 208:91-94, 1988.

158. Executive Committee for the Asymptomatic Carotid Atherosclerosis Study: Endarterectomy for asymptomatic carotid artery stenosis. JAMA 273:1421-1428, 1995.

159. Moore WS, Young B, Baker WH, et al: Surgical results: A justification of the surgeon selection process for the ACAS Trial. J Vasc Surg 23:323-328, 1996.

160. Blackshear WM, Connar RG: Carotid endarterectomy without angiography. J Cardiovasc Surg (Torino) 23:477, 1982.

161. Sandmann W, Hennerici M, Nullen H, et al: Carotid artery surgery without angiography: Risk or progress? In Greenhalgh RM, Rose FC (eds): Progress in Stroke Research II. London, Pitman, 1983, pp 447-461.

162. Ricotta JJ, Holen J, Schenk E, et al: Is routine angiography necessary prior to carotid endarterectomy? J Vasc Surg 1:96-102, 1984.

163. Crew JR, Dean M, Johnson JM, et al: Carotid surgery without angiography. Am J Surg 148:217-220, 1984.

164. Walsh J, Markowitz I, Kerstein MD: Carotid endarterectomy for amaurosis fugax without angiography. Am J Surg 152:172-174, 1986.

165. Marshall WG, Kouchoukos NT, Murphy SF, Pelate C: Carotid endarterectomy based on duplex scanning without preoperative arteriography. Circulation 78(Suppl 1):I-1-I-5, 1988.

166. Gelabert HA, Moore WS: Carotid endarterectomy without angiography. Surg Clin North Am 70:213-223, 1990.

167. Ranaboldo C, Davies J, Chant A: Duplex scanning alone before carotid endarterectomy: A five-year experience. Eur J Vasc Surg 5:415-419, 1991.

168. Wagner WH, Treiman RL, Cossman DV, et al: The diminishing role of diagnostic arteriography in carotid artery disease: Duplex scanning as definitive preoperative study. Ann Vasc Surg 5:105-110, 1991.

169. Gertler JP, Cambria RP, Kistler JP, et al: Carotid surgery without arteriography: Non-invasive selection of patients. Ann Vasc Surg 5:253-256, 1991.

170. Chervu A, Moore WS: Carotid endarterectomy without angiography: Personal series and review of the literature. Ann Vasc Surg 8:296-302, 1994.

171. Connolly JE: Carotid endarterectomy in the aware patient. Am J Surg 150:159, 1985.

172. Moore WS, Hall AD: Carotid artery back pressure. Arch Surg 99:702, 1969.

173. Moore WS, Yee TM-I, Hall AD: Collateral cerebral blood pressure: An index of tolerance to temporary carotid occlusion. Arch Surg 106:520, 1973.

174. Baker JD, Glueklich B, Watson CW, et al: An evaluation of electroencephalographic monitoring for carotid surgery. Surgery 78:787-794, 1975.

175. Elmore JR, Eldrup-Jorgensen J, Leschey WH, et al: Computerized tomographic brain mapping during carotid endarterectomy. Arch Surg 125:734-738, 1990.

176. Kearse LA Jr, Brown EN, McPeck K: Somatosensory evoked potentials sensitivity relative to electroencephalography for cerebral ischemia during carotid endarerectomy. Stroke 23:498-505, 1992.

177. Thompson JE, Patman RD, Talkington CM: Asymptomatic carotid bruit: Long term outcome of patients having endarterectomy compared with unoperated controls. Ann Surg 188:308, 1978.

178. Baker WM, Dorner DB, Barnes RW: Carotid endarterectomy: Is an indwelling shunt necessary? Surgery 82:321, 1977.

179. Whitney DG, Kahn EM, Estes JW, Jones CE: Carotid surgery without a temporary indwelling shunt: 1917 consecutive procedures. Arch Surg 115:1393-1399, 1980.

180. Archie JP Jr: Technique and clinical results of carotid stump back-pressure to determine selective shunting during carotid endarterectomy. J Vasc Surg 13:319-327, 1991.

181. Halsey JH Jr: Risks and benefits of shunting in carotid endarterectomy. Stroke 23:1583-1587, 1992.

182. Matchar DB, Goldstein LB, McCory DC, et al: Carotid endarterectomy: A literature review and ratings of appropriateness and necessity. Rand GRA-05, 1992.

183. Moore WS, Mohr JP, Najafi H, et al: Carotid endarterectomy: Practice guidelines. Report of the ad hoc committee to the joint council of the Society for Vascular Surgery and the North American Chapter of the International Society for Cardiovascular Surgery. J Vasc Surg 15:469-479, 1992.

184. Moore WS: Current status of carotid endarterectomy for stroke prevention. West J Med 159:37-43, 1993.

185. Moore WS, Barnett HJ, Beebe HG, et al: Guidelines for carotid endarterectomy. A multidisciplinary consensus statement from the Ad Hoc Committee, American Heart Association. Stroke 26:188-201, 1995.

186. Moore WS, Barnett HJ, Beebe HG, et al: Guidelines for carotid endarterectomy: A multidisciplinary consensus statement from the Ad Hoc Committee, American Heart Association. Circulation 91:566-579, 1995.

187. Biller J, Feinberg WM, Lastaldo JE, et al: Guidelines for carotid endarterectomy: A statement for health care professionals from a special writing group of the Stroke Council, American Heart Association. Stroke 29:554-562, 1998.

188. Blaisdell FM, Lim R Jr, Hall AD: Technical results of carotid endarterectomy: Arteriographic assessment. Am J Surg 114:239, 1967.

189. Gaspar MR, Movius HJ, Rosental JJ: Routine intraoperative arteriography in carotid artery surgery. J Cardiovasc Surg (Torino) Spec No: 477-481, 1973.

190. Moore WS, Martello JY, Quiñones-Baldrich WJ, Ahn SS: Etiologic importance of the intimal flap of the external carotid artery in the development of post-carotid endarterectomy stroke. Stroke 21:1497-1502, 1990.

191. Lipski DA, Bergamini TM, Garrison RN, Fulton RL: Intraoperative duplex scanning reduces the incidence of residual stenosis after carotid endarterectomy. J Surg Res 60:317-320, 1996.

192. O'Brien MS, Ricotta JJ: Conserving resources after carotid endarterectomy: Selective use of the intensive care unit. J Vasc Surg 14:796-800, 1991.

193. Hoyle RM, Jenkins JM, Edwards WH Sr, et al: Case management in cerebral revascularization. J Vasc Surg 20:396-401, 1994.

194. Hirko MK, Morasch MD, Burke K, et al: The changing face of carotid endarterectomy. J Vasc Surg 23:622-627, 1996.

195. Bove EL, Fry WJ, Gross WS, Stanley JC: Hypotension and hypertension as consequences of baroreceptor dysfunction following carotid endarterectomy. Surgery 85:633-637, 1979.

196. Towne JB, Bernard VM: The relationship of postoperative hypertension to complications following carotid endarterectomy. Surgery 88:375, 1980.

197. Angell-James JE, Lumley JSP: The effects of carotid endarterectomy on the mechanical properties of the carotid sinus and carotid sinus nerve activity in atherosclerotic patients. Br J Surg 61:805, 1974.

198. Smith BL: Hypertension following carotid endarterectomy: The role of cerebral renin production. J Vasc Surg 1:623-627, 1984.

199. Skydell JL, Machleder HI, Baker JD, et al: Incidence and mechanism of post-carotid endarterectomy hypertension. Arch Surg 122:1153-1155, 1987.

200. Ahn SS, Marcus DR, Moore WS: Post-carotid endarterectomy hypertension: Associated with elevated cranial norepinephrine. J Vasc Surg 9:351-360, 1989.

201. Ranson JHC, Imparato AM, Clauss RH, et al: Factors in the mortality and morbidity associated with surgical treatment of cerebrovascular insufficiency. Circulation 39(Suppl 1):I269-I274, 1969.

202. Riles TL, Koppleman I, Imparato AM: Myocardial infarction following carotid endarterectomy: A review of 683 operations. Surgery 85:249, 1979.

203. Matsumoto GH, Cossman D, Callow AD: Hazards and safeguards during carotid endarterectomy: Technical consideration. Am J Surg 133:485, 1977.

204. Hertzer NR, et al: A prospective study of the incidence of injury to the cranial nerve during carotid endarterectomy. Surg Gynecol Obstet 151:781, 1980.

205. Evans WE, Mendelowitz DS, Liapis C, et al: Motor speech deficit following carotid endarterectomy. Am Surg 196:461-464, 1982.

206. Bryant MF: Complications associated with carotid endarterectomy. Am Surg 42:665, 1976.

207. Verta MJ Jr, Applebaum EL, McCluskey DA, et al: Cranial nerve injuring during carotid endarterectomy. Ann Surg 185:192-195, 1977.

208. Thompson JE: Complications of endarterectomy and their prevention. World J Surg 3:155, 1979.

209. Brott T, Thalinger K: The practice of carotid endarterectomy in a large metropolitan area. Stroke 15:950-955, 1984.

210. Brott TG, Labutta RJ, Kempczinski RF: Changing patterns in the practice of carotid endarterectomy in a large metropolitan area. JAMA 225:2609-2612, 1986.

211. Easton JD, Sherman DG: Stroke and mortality rate in carotid endarterectomy: 228 consecutive operations. Stroke 8:565-568, 1977.

212. Beebe HG, Clagett GP, DeWeese JA, et al: Assessing risk associated with carotid endarterectomy. Stroke 20:314-315, 1989.

213. Sundt TM Jr, Houser DW, Sharbrough FW, Messick JM Jr: Carotid endarterectomy: Results, complications, and monitoring techniques. Adv Neurol 16:97, 1977.

214. Kwaan JHM, Connelly JE, Sharefkin JB: Successful management of early stroke after carotid endarterectomy. Ann Surg 190:676, 1979.

215. Hertzer NR, Lees CD: Fatal myocardial infarction following carotid endarterectomy: 335 patients followed 6-11 postoperative years. Ann Surg 194:212-218, 1981.

216. Bauer RB, Meyer JS, Fields WS, et al: Joint study of extracranial arterial occlusion. III. Progress report of controlled study of long-term survival in patients with and without operation. JAMA 208:509-518, 1969.

217. Rothwell PM, Slattery J, Warlow CP: A systematic comparison of the risks of stroke and death due to carotid endarterectomy for symptomatic and asymptomatic stenosis. Stroke 25:266-269, 1996.
218. Bernstein EF, et al: Influence of preoperative factors on late neurologic events after carotid endarterectomy. In International Vascular Symposium Programs and Abstracts. New York, Macmillan, 1981, p 460.
219. Hertzer NR, Arison R: Cumulative stroke and survival ten years after carotid endarterectomy. J Vasc Surg 2:661-668, 1985.
220. Sergeant PT, Derom F, Berzsenyi G, et al: Carotid endarterectomy for cerebrovascular insufficiency: Long-term follow-up of 141 patients followed for up to 16 years. Acta Chir Belg 79:309-316, 1980.
221. Moore WS, Boren C, Malone JM, et al: Asymptomatic carotid stenosis: Immediate and long term results after prophylactic endarterectomy. Am J Surg 138:228, 1979.
222. Bernstein EF, Humber PB, Collins GM, et al: Life expectancy and late stroke following carotid endarterectomy. Ann Surg 198:80, 1983.
223. Lord RSA: Later survival after carotid endarterectomy for transient ischemic attacks. J Vasc Surg 1:512, 1984.
224. DeWeese JA, Rob CG, Satran R, et al: Results of carotid endarterectomy for transient ischemic attacks—five years later. Ann Surg 178:258-264, 1973.
225. Thompson JE, Austin BJ, Patman RD: Carotid endarterectomy for cerebrovascular insufficiency: Long-term results in 592 patients followed up to 13 years. Ann Surg 172:663, 1970.
226. Takolander RJ, Bergentz SE, Ericsson BF: Carotid artery surgery in patients with minor stroke. Br J Surg 70:13, 1983.
227. Eriksson SE, Link H, Alm A, et al: Results from eighty-eight consecutive prophylactic carotid endarterectomy in cerebral infarction and transitory ischemic attacks. Acta Neurol Scand 63:209, 1981.
228. Bardin JA, Bernstein EF, Humber PB, et al: Is carotid endarterectomy beneficial in prevention of recurrent stroke? Arch Surg 117:1401, 1982.
229. McCullough JL, Mentzer RM, Harman PK, et al: Carotid endarterectomy after a completed stroke: Reduction in long term neurologic deterioration. J Vasc Surg 2:7, 1985.
230. Ouriel K, et al: Carotid endarterectomy for nonhemispheric symptoms: Predictors of success. J Vasc Surg 1:331-345, 1984.
231. Ricotta JJ, O'Brien MS, DeWeese JA: Carotid endarterectomy for non-hemisphere ischemia: Long-term follow-up. Cardiovasc Surg 2:561-566, 1994.
232. Imparato AM: Vertebral arterial reconstruction: A nineteen year experience. J Vasc Surg 2:626-634, 1985.
233. O'Hara PJ, Hertzer NR, Beven EG: External carotid revascularization: Review of a ten year experience. J Vasc Surg 2:709-714, 1985.
234. Halstuk KS, Baker WH, Littooy FN: External carotid endarterectomy. J Vasc Surg 1:398-402, 1984.
235. Lindblad B, Persson NH, Takolander R, Bergqvist D: Does low-dose acetylsalicylic acid prevent stroke after carotid surgery? A double-blind, placebo-controlled randomized trial. Stroke 24:1125-1128, 1993.
236. Veterans Administration: A Veterans Administration Cooperative Study: Role of carotid endarterectomy in asymptomatic carotid stenosis. Stroke 17:534-539, 1986.
237. Hobson RW, Song IS, George AM, Weiss DG: Results of arteriography for asymptomatic carotid stenosis. Stroke 20:135, 1989.
238. Towne JB, Weiss DG, Hobson RW: First phase report of cooperative Veterans Administration asymptomatic carotid stenosis study—operative morbidity and mortality. J Vasc Surg 11:252-259, 1990.
239. Hobson RW, Weiss DG, Fields WS, et al: Efficacy of carotid endarterectomy for asymptomatic carotid stenosis. N Engl J Med 328:221, 1993.
240. Asymptomatic Carotid Artery Stenosis Group: Study design for randomized prospective trial of carotid endarterectomy for asymptomatic atherosclerosis. Stroke 20:844-849, 1989.
241. Clinical advisory: Carotid endarterectomy for patients with asymptomatic internal carotid artery stenosis. Stroke 25:523-524, 1994.
242. Moore WS, Vescera CL, Robertson JT, et al: Selection process for surgeons who wished to participate in the Asymptomatic Carotid Atherosclerosis Study. Stroke 22:1353-1357, 1991.
243. Halliday AM, Thomas D, Mansfield A: The Asymptomatic Carotid Surgery Trial (ACST): Rationale and design. Eur J Vasc Surg 8: 703-710, 1994.
244. Halliday A, Mansfield A, Marro J, et al. Prevention of disabling and fatal strokes by successful carotid endarterectomy in patients without recent neurological symptoms: Randomized control trial. Lancet 363:1491-1502, 2004.
245. North American Symptomatic Carotid Endarterectomy Trial (NASCET) Steering Committee: North American Symptomatic Carotid Endarterectomy Trial: Methods, patient characteristics, and progress. Stroke 22:711-720, 1991.
246. North American Symptomatic Carotid Endarterectomy Trial collaborators: Beneficial effect of carotid endarterectomy in symptomatic patients with high-grade carotid stenosis. N Engl J Med 325:445-453, 1991.
247. Barnett MJM, Taylor DW, Eliasziw M, et al: Benefit of carotid endarterectomy in patients with symptomatic moderate or severe stenosis. N Engl J Med 339:1415-1425, 1998.
248. European Carotid Surgery Trialists' Collaborative Group: MRC European Carotid Surgery Trial: Interim results for patients with severe (70-99%) or with mild (0-29%) carotid stenosis. Lancet 337: 1235-1243, 1991.
249. Eliasziw M, Smith RF, Singh N, et al: Further comments on the measurements of carotid stenosis from angiograms. Stroke 25:2445-2449, 1994.
250. Endarterectomy for moderate symptomatic carotid stenosis: Interim results from the MRC European Carotid Surgery Trial. Lancet 347:1591-1593, 1996.
251. Maybert MR, Wilson SE, Yatsu F, et al: Carotid endarterectomy and prevention of cerebral ischemia in symptomatic carotid stenosis. JAMA 266:3289, 1991.
252. Wolf PA, D'Agostino RB, Kannel WB, et al: Cigarette smoking as a risk factor for stroke: The Framingham Study. JAMA 259:1025-1029, 1988.
253. Whisnant JP, Homer D, Ingall TJ, et al: Duration of cigarette smoking is the strongest predictor of severe extracranial carotid artery atherosclerosis. Stroke 21:707-714, 1990.
254. Dempsey RJ, Moore RW: Amount of smoking independently predicts carotid artery atherosclerosis severity. Stroke 23:693-696, 1992.
255. Baker RN, Schwartz WS, Rose AS: Transient ischemic strokes: A report of a study of anticoagulant therapy. Neurology 16:841, 1964.
256. Link H, Lebram G, Johansson I, Radberg C: Prognosis in patients with infarction and TIA in carotid territory during and after anticoagulant therapy. Stroke 10:529, 1979.
257. Terent A, Anderson B: The outcome of patients with transient ischemic attacks and stroke treated with anticoagulants. Acta Med Scand 208:359, 1980.
258. Jonas S: Anticoagulant therapy in cerebrovascular disease: Review and meta-analysis. Stroke 19:1043-1048, 1988.
259. Canadian Cooperative Study Group: A randomized trial of aspirin and sulfinpyrazone in threatened strokes. N Engl J Med 299:53, 1978.
260. Whisnant JP: The Canadian trial of aspirin and sulfinpyrazone in threatened strokes. Am Heart J 99:129, 1980.
261. Fields WS, Lemak NA, Frankowski RF, Hardy RJ: Controlled trial of aspirin in cerebral ischemia. Stroke 8:301, 1977.
262. Fields WS, et al: Controlled trial of aspirin in cerebral ischemia. Part 2. Surgical group. Stroke 9:309, 1978.
263. Bousser MD, et al: AICLA controlled trial of aspirin and dipyridamole in the secondary prevention of arteriothrombotic cerebral ischemia. Stroke 14:5-14, 1983.
264. American-Canadian Cooperative Study Group: Persantine-aspirin trial in cerebral ischemia. Part 2. End point results. Stroke 16:405, 1985.
265. Sorenson PS, Pedersen H, Marquardsen J, et al: Acetylsalicylic acid in the prevention of stroke in patients with reversible cerebral ischemic attacks: A Danish cooperative study. Stroke 14:15-22, 1983.
266. Dyken ML: Editorial. Stroke 14:2-4, 1983.
267. Sze PC, Reitman D, Pincus MM, et al: Antiplatelet agents in the secondary prevention of stroke: Meta-analysis of the randomized control trials. Stroke 19:436-442, 1988.
268. Hass WK, Easton D, Adams MP Jr, et al: A randomized trial comparing ticlopidine hydrochloride with aspirin for the prevention of stroke in high-risk patients. N Engl J Med 321:501-507, 1989.
269. Carson SN, et al: Aspirin failure in symptomatic arteriosclerotic carotid artery disease. Surgery 90:1084, 1981.
270. Cote R, Battista RM, Abrahamowicz M, et al: Lack of effect of aspirin in asymptomatic patients with carotid bruits and substantial carotid narrowing. Ann Intern Med 123:649-655, 1995.
271. Probstfield JL, Magrite SE, Byington RP, et al: Results of the primary outcome measure and clinical events from the Asymptomatic Carotid Artery Progression Study. Am J Cardiol 76:47C-53C, 1995.
272. Wylie EJ, Hein MF, Adams JE: Intracranial hemorrhage following surgical revascularization for treatment of acute strokes. J Neurosurg 21:212-215, 1964.

273. Giordano JM, et al: Timing carotid arterial endarterectomy after stroke. J Vasc Surg 2:250, 1985.

274. Whittemore AD, Ruby ST, Couch NP, et al: Early carotid endarterectomy in patients with small fixed neurologic deficits. J Vasc Surg 1:795, 1984.

275. Goldstone J, Moore WS: Emergency carotid artery surgery in neurologically unstable patients. Arch Surg 111:1284, 1976.

276. Wilson SE, Mayberg MR, Yatsu F, Weiss DG: Crescendo transient ischemic attacks: A surgical imperative. J Vasc Surg 17:49-55, 1993.

277. Abu Rahma AF, Boland JP, Robinson P, Delanio R: Antiplatelet therapy and carotid plaque hemorrhage and its clinical implications. J Cardiovasc Surg 31:66-70, 1990.

278. Dietrich EB, Ndiaye M, Reid DB: Stenting in the carotid artery: Initial experience in 110 patients. J Endovasc Surg 3:42-46, 1996.

279. Roubin GS, Yadev S, Iyer SS, Vitek J: Carotid stent-supported angioplasty: A neurovascular intervention to prevent stroke. Am J Cardiol 78:8-12, 1996.

280. Beebe MG, Archie JP, Baker WH, et al: Concern about safety of carotid angioplasty. Stroke 27:197-198, 1996.

281. Jordan WD, et al: Cost comparison of balloon angioplasty and stenting versus endarterectomy for the treatment of carotid artery stenosis. J Vasc Surg 27:16-24, 1998.

282. Endovascular versus surgical treatment in patients with carotid stenosis in the Carotid and Vertebral Artery Transluminal Angioplasty Study (CAVATAS): A randomised trial. Lancet 357:1729-1737, 2001.

283. Nehler AR, et al: Randomized study of carotid angioplasty and stenting versus carotid endarterectomy: A stopped trial. J Vasc Surg 28:326-334, 1998.

284. Alberts MJ: Result of a multicenter prospective randomized trial of carotid artery stenting vs. carotid endarterectomy. Stroke 32:328, 2001.

285. Yadav JS, Wholey MH, Kuntz RE, et al: Protected carotid-artery stenting versus endarterectomy in high-risk patients. N Engl J Med 351:1493-1501, 2004.

286. Hobson RW, Howard VJ, Roubin GS, et al: Carotid artery stenting is associated with increased complications in octogenarians: 30-day stroke and death rates in the CREST lead-in phase. J Vasc Surg 40:1106-1111, 2004.

287. Schuler JJ, et al: The effect of carotid siphon stenosis on stroke rate, death, and relief of symptoms following elective carotid endarterectomy. Surgery 92:1058-1067, 1982.

288. Moore WS: Does tandem lesion mean tandem risk in patients with carotid artery disease? J Vasc Surgery 7:454-455, 1988.

289. Mackey WC, O'Donnell JF Jr, Callow AD: Carotid endarterectomy in patients with intracranial vascular disease: Short-term risk and long-term outcome. J Vasc Surg 10:432-438, 1989.

290. EC/IC Bypass Study Group: Failure of extracranial-intracranial arterial bypass to reduce the risk of ischemic stroke: Results of an international randomized trial. N Engl J Med 313:1191-1200, 1985.

291. Wilkerson DK, Keller I, Mezich R, et al: The comparative evaluation of three-dimensional magnetic resonance for carotid artery disease. J Vasc Surg 14:803-811, 1991.

292. Mattle HP, Kent KC, Adelman RR, et al: Evaluation of the extracranial carotid arteries: Correlation of magnetic resonance angiography, duplex ultrasonography, and conventional angiography. J Vasc Surg 13:838-845, 1991.

293. Wiles TS, Eidelman EM, Litt AW, et al: Comparison of magnetic resonance angiography, conventional angiography, and duplex scanning. Stroke 23:341-346, 1992.

Questions

1. **What is the most common cause of perioperative neurologic deficit after carotid endarterectomy?**
   (a) Thrombosis of the repair
   (b) Lack of cerebral perfusion
   (c) Tandem lesions in the carotid system
   (d) Low cardiac output
   (e) None of the above

2. **Carotid endarterectomy for asymptomatic disease (1) is a proven indication for stenosis of 60% or greater, as documented by angiography; (2) carries the lowest perioperative morbidity and mortality; (3) should be considered when progression to 80% stenosis is documented; (4) may prevent stroke, which is the most common initial manifestation of asymptomatic carotid disease. Which of the preceding statements is (are) true?**
   (a) 1, 2, 3
   (b) 1, 3
   (c) 2, 4
   (d) 4
   (e) 1, 2, 3, and 4

3. **Which of the following statements about tandem lesions in the intracranial carotid system is true?**
   (a) They carry a similar stroke risk compared with a carotid bifurcation lesion
   (b) They carry a lower stroke risk than a similar extracranial bulb lesion
   (c) They carry a higher stroke risk than a similar extracranial bulb lesion
   (d) They should deter the surgeon from recommending bifurcation endarterectomy
   (e) They are more frequently the source of symptoms when combined intra- and extracranial disease is present

4. **With regard to fibromuscular dysplasia: (1) it is best described as an atherosclerotic process affecting medium-size arteries; (2) 30% of patients with cervical involvement may have intracranial aneurysms; (3) medial hyperplasia is the most common type affecting the carotid system; (4) it most commonly affects women, suggesting a hormonal factor. Which of the preceding statements is (are) true?**
   (a) 1, 2, 3
   (b) 1, 3
   (c) 2, 4
   (d) 4
   (e) None

5. **Which of the following statements about kinks of the carotid artery is true?**
   (a) They are frequently the cause of cerebrovascular symptoms
   (b) They may be congenital
   (c) They never cause symptoms
   (d) They frequently require excision and grafting for repair
   (e) They are rarely associated with atherosclerosis

6. **Transient ischemic attacks (1) carry a 40% risk of stroke over 5 years when secondary to extracranial arterial occlusive disease; (2) are always secondary to platelet emboli; (3) may be a manifestation of lacunar infarction; (4) as a manifestation of cardiac emboli, are usually stereotyped, with similar symptoms with each occurrence. Which of the preceding statements is (are) true?**
   (a) 1, 2, 3
   (b) 1, 3
   (c) 2, 4
   (d) 4
   (e) 1, 2, 3, and 4

7. Which of the following statements about the use of an internal shunt during carotid endarterectomy is true?
   (a) It is necessary in approximately 50% of patients
   (b) It can be predicted based on angiographic findings
   (c) It carries no added risk
   (d) All of the above
   (e) None of the above

8. Which of the following statements about external carotid endarterectomy is true?
   (a) It carries significant risks when combined with extracranial-intracranial bypass
   (b) It rarely requires patch closure
   (c) It frequently relieves amaurosis but rarely relieves hemispheric TIAs
   (d) All of the above
   (e) None of the above

9. Stroke in evolution (1) may be a manifestation of lacunar infarction; (2) suggests an unstable process requiring urgent evaluation and therapy; (3) has a 10% mortality with surgical therapy; (4) should be treated with prompt medical therapy in view of the increased risk of surgery. Which of the preceding statements is (are) true?
   (a) 1, 2, 3
   (b) 1, 3
   (c) 2, 4
   (d) 4
   (e) None

10. With regard to carotid endarterectomy for acute stroke: (1) the risks of surgical intervention during the acute phase of a stroke are high, so surgery is never indicated; (2) if a CT scan done within 12 hours of the event is negative, endarterectomy can be safely performed; (3) level of consciousness, hypertension, and severity of the deficit should not influence the timing of surgical intervention; (4) if the patient shows continual recovery without deterioration, endarterectomy can be safely performed once a plateau has been reached. Which of the preceding statements is (are) true?
    (a) 1, 2, 3
    (b) 1, 3
    (c) 2, 4
    (d) 4
    (e) None

Answers

1. e	2. e	3. b	4. c	5. b
6. b	7. e	8. a	9. a	10. d

36

Ramon Berguer

Surgical Reconstruction of the Supra-aortic Trunks and Vertebral Arteries

The supra-aortic trunks (SATs) are the branches of the aortic arch that ascend through the mediastinum and terminate short of the carotid bifurcation and the origin of the vertebral arteries. These trunks carry the entire blood supply to the head and upper extremities. The vertebrobasilar system is composed of the two vertebral arteries, the basilar artery, and their branches to the brainstem, cerebellum, and occipital lobes.

The three most common variants in the anatomy of the SATs have implications in terms of the technique chosen for their reconstruction. These variants are a shared ostium (16%) or a common origin (8%) for the innominate and left common carotid arteries, a left vertebral artery with a separate origin from the aortic arch (6%), and a right retroesophageal subclavian artery (0.5%). A separate origin of the left vertebral artery is associated with an abnormally high (C-4 or C-5) entry of this artery into the transverse foramina of the cervical spine. A retroesophageal right subclavian artery is associated with a thoracic duct that empties on the right jugulosubclavian confluent, a nonrecurrent right inferior laryngeal nerve, and, in approximately half these patients, a right vertebral artery originating from the low right common carotid artery or a common carotid trunk giving origin to both common carotid arteries.

Through the mechanisms of low flow or atheroembolization, occlusive disease of the SATs may cause symptoms in any of the territories supplied: the hemispheric (carotid) territory, the posterior (vertebrobasilar) territory, and, in the case of proximal subclavian disease, the upper extremity. Vertebral artery occlusive disease may restrict inflow into the basilar artery, resulting in vertebrobasilar ischemia. This is more likely if compensatory flow from the carotid system is not available due to an internal carotid occlusion or a minute or absent posterior communicating artery.

The SATs are involved by atherosclerosis in the fifth or sixth decade of life. This results in the development of plaques that may obstruct flow or embolize (atheroembolism). Aneurysmal atherosclerotic disease of the SATs is rare. In some places, the SATs are a common site for Takayasu's arteritis, usually in younger individuals. Traumatic and mycotic aneurysms of the SATs are uncommon but life-threatening conditions.

The incidence of atherosclerotic disease is lower in the SATs than in the internal carotid and vertebral arteries. Nevertheless, the extensive study of extracranial arterial disease reported in 1968 by Hass and colleagues showed that one third of patients undergoing arteriography had a severe lesion involving one or more of the SATs.[1] The morphology of atherosclerotic lesions of the SATs is not as well defined as that of the plaques found in the internal carotid artery. This is partly due to the fact that for years the SATs were not routinely visualized during arteriography of the cerebral vessels. In addition, they are difficult to image by ultrasound techniques, which provide valuable morphologic information in other areas such as the carotid bifurcation. Because we have limited knowledge of the natural history of these lesions, our surgical indications are based partly on inferences. In addition, SAT lesions are often found in individuals who already have concomitant disease of the carotid or vertebral arteries—a situation that confuses the identification of the offending lesion. Stenosing lesions of the SATs usually appear at their origin from the aortic arch and often involve more than one artery. Plaques located in the ostia of the SATs are often continuous with atheroma that extends over the dome of the aortic arch.

Outlining SAT lesions by arteriography requires an arch injection, preferably in two oblique projections (right and left posterior oblique). If circumstances permit, the arteriographic study should also include selective injections of both common carotid and subclavian arteries (four-vessel arteriogram). The high incidence of concomitant carotid and vertebral artery lesions makes it mandatory to outline the extra- and intracranial cerebrovascular supply when evaluating a patient for cerebrovascular symptoms.

Vertebrobasilar ischemia may be caused by poor inflow through the carotid and vertebral arteries, reversal of blood flow in a vertebral artery caused by a proximal subclavian artery occlusion (subclavian steal), reversal of right carotid and vertebral artery flow from an innominate artery occlusion, and embolization from the proximal subclavian or vertebral arteries.

Symptoms of Occlusive Disease of the Supra-aortic Trunks

Patients with occlusive disease of the SATs may show symptoms of carotid, vertebrobasilar, and upper extremity arterial ischemia. Although there is no pathologic evidence to support this view, it has traditionally been taught that in patients with disease of the SATs, cerebral symptoms are due to low flow rather than atheroembolization.. This concept runs contrary to clinical evidence that suggests that the mechanisms of cerebral ischemia from disease of the SATs are similar to those from atheroma of the carotid bifurcation. In stenosing lesions of the subclavian artery, both mechanisms—low flow and embolization—are observed.

Obliteration of the SATs is suggested by absent pulses in the neck (subclavian, carotid) or arm (axillary, brachial) on one or both sides and by the recording of unequal or abnormally low pressures in the upper extremities. Waveforms recorded by Doppler tracings are dampened in arteries whose origins are stenosed or occluded. Bruits may or may not be present. In patients with subclavian steal, a pulse lag may be felt between the radial arteries of the two arms or, more precisely, a pulse wave delay of greater than 30 msec may be measured by simultaneously recording both brachial artery waveforms.[2] Claudication of the arm and digital artery embolization may be present in subclavian artery disease. A computed tomography scan of the brain is an essential part of the workup of patients with disease of the SATs. It may reveal clinically unsuspected cerebral infarctions.[3]

In symptomatic vertebral (or basilar) artery occlusive disease, the patient may have any combination of the following symptoms: dizziness, vertigo, diplopia, perioral numbness, blurred vision, tinnitus, ataxia, bilateral sensory deficits, and drop attacks. The mechanism that triggers the symptom (e.g., standing up, rotating the neck) must be sought when evaluating these patients. Patients with orthostatic hypotension have vertebrobasilar symptoms when they stand abruptly after sitting or lying down. Blood pressure measurements taken immediately after they stand up and experience symptoms shows a drop in systolic pressure greater than 20 mm Hg. This mechanism is particularly common in diabetic patients with sympathetic paralysis and loss of venomotor tone because a substantial amount of blood is pooled in their legs on standing.

The presence of vertebrobasilar ischemia related to turning of the neck suggests osteophytic compression on the vertebral arteries or inner ear disease. In general, in patients with labyrinthine disorders, symptoms appear with brief, head-shaking motions. Patients who develop symptoms by extrinsic compression of the vertebral arteries usually require a few seconds with the neck rotated maximally in a particular direction to develop symptoms. In addition to orthostatism and osteophytic compression, other conditions are capable of causing vertebrobasilar ischemia and must be ruled out. Dissection of a vertebral artery is accompanied by neck pain. In these patients, the symptoms of brain ischemia may be due to critical compromise of the true lumen of the vertebral artery by an intramural dissecting hematoma or thromboembolization from the distal reentry point of the dissection. A number of medical conditions also present with symptoms of vertebrobasilar ischemia; among the most common are inappropriate antihypertensive medication, cardiac arrhythmia, anemia, brain tumor, and subclavian steal.

Indications for Surgery

No morphologic database exists for atherosclerotic lesions of the SATs comparable to that available for internal carotid artery disease. We know from arteriograms and postmortem studies that the SATs are less frequently involved by atherosclerotic disease than is the carotid bifurcation. We generally do not have the ability to use ultrasonography to study the composition of SAT plaques, and the specimens obtained at operation are few because most interventions to reconstruct the SATs are bypasses rather than endarterectomies. The few specimens available for pathologic study show degenerative features similar to those seen in carotid plaques: surface thrombus, ulceration, and intraplaque hemorrhage. One may reasonably infer that the same pathologic mechanisms operate in both carotid artery plaques and SAT lesions. Until more precise information becomes available, it seems sensible to use criteria similar to those applicable to carotid disease to determine treatment guidelines. These criteria, however, must be tempered by the fact that the risk of surgical reconstruction of the SATs is higher than that of carotid endarterectomy.

Indications for surgical repair of SAT lesions are (1) lesions encroaching on more than 70% of the SAT diameter, or plaques with ulceration or surface irregularities in patients with appropriate symptoms (ipsilateral carotid or vertebrobasilar); (2) the same lesions plus ipsilateral internal carotid disease for which an endarterectomy is indicated (the operation should correct both); (3) the same lesions plus a nonacute ipsilateral hemispheric infarction (overt or silent); and (4) preocclusive lesions (>90% cross-sectional area loss) in asymptomatic patients who are good surgical risks and have more than 5 years of life expectancy. This last indication is arbitrary albeit reasonable.

The primary indication for reconstructing a vertebral artery is to treat vertebrobasilar ischemia. Severe occlusive disease of the vertebral artery may be found in individuals who have no symptoms of vertebrobasilar ischemia. Conversely, many systemic causes of vertebrobasilar ischemia are not related to vertebral artery disease. Therefore, the decision to reconstruct a vertebral artery must be based on a strong anatomic and clinical presumption that the symptom (vertebrobasilar ischemia) is secondary to the anatomic lesion (occlusive disease of the vertebral arteries).

Vertebrobasilar ischemia may be due to stenosis or occlusion of the vertebral or basilar arteries, restricting flow in the territory supplied by these arteries. This is the so-called low-flow (or hemodynamic) mechanism. These patients often have repetitive transient ischemic attacks triggered by positional or postural mechanisms. Although their risk for stroke is lower than that in patients with carotid disease, they may suffer serious traumatic injuries due to loss of balance. Ischemia of the vertebrobasilar territory may also be due to microembolization (atheroemboli). Contrary to prevalent views in the neurologic literature, about one third of vertebrobasilar ischemic episodes are caused by atheroembolization from plaques or mural lesions of the vertebral arteries.[4] Patients with embolic symptoms are at high risk for infarctions of the brainstem, cerebellum, and occipital lobes. The mechanism here is microembolization from the irregular surface or from the core of a plaque in the proximal subclavian or vertebral arteries or from a lesion in the wall of the vertebral artery secondary to repetitive trauma from an osteophyte or intramural dissection.

In patients with low-flow symptoms of ischemia in the vertebrobasilar territory, the surgical indication rests on the assumption that the basilar artery is not receiving adequate inflow from the vertebral arteries.

Because two vertebral arteries usually supply the basilar artery, the presence of a normal vertebral artery contraindicates an operation on the opposite artery, regardless of its anatomic condition (in patients with low-flow symptoms). A vertebral artery of normal caliber emptying into a basilar artery is enough to supply the basilar territory. This means that for a lesion in the vertebral arteries to be considered significant, it must be severe (>75% stenosis) and the opposite vertebral artery must be equally diseased, hypoplastic, or absent.

My approach to a patient with low-flow vertebrobasilar ischemia is first to determine whether any other clinical condition (e.g., orthostatism, arrhythmia) capable of producing these symptoms is present. If so, it should be corrected. If symptoms persist after treatment, an arteriogram is indicated. If the arteriogram shows a lesion that fulfills the anatomic criteria listed previously and the operation appears to be technically feasible, a reconstruction of the vertebral artery is indicated.

In patients with vertebrobasilar ischemic symptoms secondary to embolization, the indication for surgery rests on demonstration of the emboligenic lesion, regardless of the condition of the opposite vertebral artery. The criteria of bilateralism and degree of severity that apply to low-flow lesions are irrelevant when considering treatment for atheroembolic disease.

Reconstruction of the Supra-aortic Trunks

The main decision involved in reconstruction of the SATs is whether to do the repair through the chest or through the neck. Cervical repairs are traditionally done by means of a bypass from a suitable donor vessel to the diseased one. Most of these bypasses run transversely either between vessels on the same side of the neck (carotid and subclavian) or across the neck (remote bypasses). Bypass procedures between the ipsilateral carotid and subclavian arteries are largely being superseded by transposition procedures that provide the advantage of a single arterial anastomosis without the need

for a saphenous vein graft or a prosthetic tube. Transthoracic or axial repairs require a partial or total sternotomy for a direct approach to these vessels. The lesions are rarely dealt with by endarterectomy and are almost always corrected with a bypass from the ascending aorta.

The choice between transthoracic (axial) and cervical (transverse) repairs can be made using the following general guidelines. Axial repairs are preferred in younger patients who have innominate artery lesions or multiple lesions (usually innominate and left common carotid). They are also the natural choice for patients in whom a simultaneous coronary bypass operation is indicated. In patients with atherosclerotic disease of the SATs and coronary arteries, repairing concomitant severe lesions of the first segment of the left subclavian artery is advisable even if this stenosis is asymptomatic. This repair permits a later myocardial revascularization using the left internal mammary artery.

Cervical repairs are preferred in older patients, in those who are at high risk of thoracotomy, and in those who have had previous transsternal procedures. Cervical repair is the choice for all single arterial lesions (other than those of the innominate artery).

CERVICAL REPAIRS

In the early 1970s, techniques for revascularization of the SATs consisted of a transverse bypass between a donor and a recipient (diseased) artery. The insertion of a bypass between the carotid and subclavian arteries, although described in 1957,[5] did not become popular until the 1970s. These bypasses were between the midsegment of the carotid artery and the second (retroscalene) segment of the subclavian artery. In some cases, the carotid artery acted as the donor vessel, and the bypass corrected a blockage of the first portion of the subclavian artery. In others, the subclavian artery was the donor vessel to bypass a proximal common carotid artery lesion. In subclavian-carotid bypasses, when the anastomosis to the carotid artery is of the end-to-side type, there is always the possibility of a source of proximal embolization (from the diseased proximal common carotid artery) or of extension of the proximal thrombus across the end-to-side anastomosis. Because of this, I advocate an end-to-end anastomosis (see later) into the common carotid artery.

Carotid-subclavian bypasses became the standard operation for the correction of subclavian steal syndrome in the 1970s. When use of the carotid as the donor vessel was not advisable (because it was the only patent carotid artery or because of disease in the proximal common carotid artery), correction of subclavian steal was achieved with bypasses between both subclavian arteries or both axillary arteries. These remote bypasses became known as *extra-anatomic* operations. Although they offer the advantages of avoiding a thoracotomy and carrying a lower operative mortality, they have lower long-term patency rates than those achieved by axial or shorter reconstructions. These remote bypasses are constructed with the graft crossing the neck in front of the sternum, giving a poor cosmetic result and subjecting them to external compression. Most significantly, bypasses in this anterior, low-neck location may interfere with an eventual tracheostomy and certainly with a midsternotomy that might be required for coronary revascularization later on.

Many of the cervical bypasses done in the 1970s used saphenous vein as the preferred graft material. There was fear of embolization from the "neointima" of prosthetic tubes and doubts about their long-term patency. Saphenous veins also presented specific problems, however. They were not always available, and gross mismatches in caliber often occurred between the vein and the recipient arteries. Additionally, the length required for remote bypasses led to the possibility of axial rotation or compression or kinking of the vein graft with rotation of the neck. Because of these difficulties, many surgeons explored the use of prosthetic substitutes for arterial bypass in the neck. The reported results indicate that polytetrafluoroethylene (PTFE) grafts are preferable to saphenous vein for bypasses in the neck; they provide a good-caliber match, and their patency rates are excellent,[5] probably as a result of the high flow rates usually measured in these arteries.

Anatomic Indications

Innominate Artery Occlusion or Stenosis

A variety of cervical techniques are available to correct flow deficits caused by innominate artery stenosis or occlusion. Subclavian-subclavian and axilloaxillary bypasses can supply the right carotid artery through retrograde flow into the proximal subclavian or axillary arteries. Carotid-carotid bypasses are technically feasible, but for the correction of severe innominate artery disease, they represent an unnecessary risk because both carotid systems will likely be severely hypotensive during the proximal anastomosis of the bypass to the donor left common carotid artery (unless shunted).

If the innominate artery lesion is suspected to be embolizing—or if it exhibits a grossly irregular surface or large ulcerations—the distal innominate artery should be ligated (excluded) at the completion of the remote bypass procedure. This may not be possible using a supraclavicular approach. A complex solution is an end-to-end anastomosis between the proximal subclavian artery and the proximal right common carotid artery, with ligation of the proximal carotid stump and then revascularization of the middle or distal third of the right subclavian through a remote bypass from the other side of the neck. I prefer axial reconstructions (see later) for all innominate artery lesions.

Common Carotid Artery Occlusion or Stenosis

The common carotid artery can be revascularized by means of a subclavian-carotid bypass from the ipsilateral subclavian artery, with the distal anastomosis being performed end to end to avoid embolization from the diseased proximal common carotid artery. When the entire carotid system on one side is not visualized on the arteriogram, one must consider the possibility that the carotid bifurcation is patent, with retrograde flow from the external carotid artery perfusing the internal carotid artery antegradely. Delayed subtraction films may show this late opacification, but duplex imaging is the best way to show patency of the carotid bifurcation and this peculiar combination of retrograde (external carotid) and antegrade (internal carotid) flow. In these patients, atheromatous plaque is usually found at the origin of the internal carotid artery, necessitating endarterectomy before performing the distal anastomosis. The traditional means of constructing a distal anastomosis for a graft at the level of the carotid bifurcation is with an end-to-side junction (an onlay patch), with or without a concomitant endarterectomy of the carotid

bulb (Fig. 36-1). This end-to-side anastomosis is functionally transformed into an end-to-end junction by ligation of the common carotid artery below the anastomosis, in the soft segment created by endarterectomy of the distal portion of the common carotid artery. I employ a different technique for the distal anastomosis (Fig. 36-2): after amputation of the distal common carotid artery, the carotid bulb is either opened posteriorly or everted for endarterectomy (type 2 eversion). The oblique or round cross section of the carotid bifurcation allows a simple end-to-end anastomosis to the bypass arising from the subclavian artery.

If the stenosing lesion of the common carotid artery is located at its origin and its distal two thirds are free of disease, transposing the midportion of the common carotid artery to the subclavian artery is a better solution than a subclavian-carotid bypass. It requires only one anastomosis and no prosthesis. At times, a thrombosed common carotid artery with a patent bifurcation can be thrombectomized after dividing it low in the neck and doing an eversion endarterectomy up to the bifurcation. The distal portion of the endarterectomy is terminated under direct vision through the standard arteriotomy used for a conventional carotid endarterectomy. After endarterectomy, the common carotid artery is reimplanted into the second portion of the subclavian artery. Subclavian-carotid bypass and transposition of the carotid into the subclavian are easier on the right side, where the subclavian artery is more accessible.

In those cases in which the ipsilateral subclavian artery is not a suitable donor vessel, a common carotid artery lesion can be corrected by means of a carotid-carotid bypass. This operation is traditionally done by placing a bypass between both carotids in front of the airway. I prefer to use a shorter retropharyngeal route (see later in this chapter).

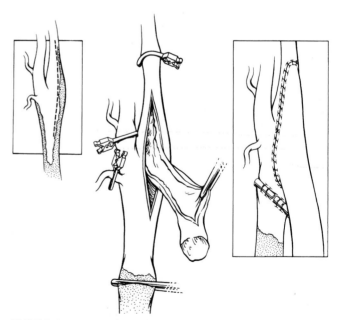

FIGURE 36–1 • Traditional method of anastomosing the distal limb of a graft to the carotid bifurcation following endarterectomy of the latter. Occlusion of the common carotid artery immediately below the anastomosis transforms it into a functional end-to-end junction *(inset, right)*.

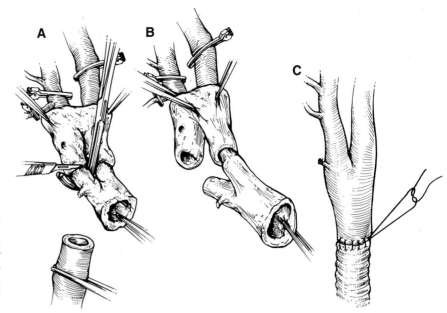

FIGURE 36–2 • My preference for anastomosing the graft to the carotid bifurcation is an eversion endarterectomy followed by an end-to-end anastomosis. *A,* Eversion of the external carotid after exposing the flow divider in the plaque. *B,* Eversion of the internal carotid component of the plaque. *C,* Anastomosis of the graft to everted bifurcation.

Subclavian Artery Occlusion

Reconstruction of the proximal subclavian artery is done (1) to correct a symptomatic subclavian steal, (2) to correct an emboligenic lesion of the proximal subclavian, (3) to revascularize the subclavian before an internal mammary transposition to the coronary arteries, or (4) to transpose the left subclavian to the left common carotid artery before extending a thoracic stent-graft across its origin. Carotid-subclavian bypass is a proven operation to revascularize the subclavian artery. If the subclavian lesion has been the source of embolization, the prevertebral subclavian artery must be ligated at the time of the bypass. My preference for the last 15 years has been to use a direct transposition of the subclavian artery (prevertebral portion) to the common carotid artery. Although this operation is slightly more complex than the bypass, it involves only one anastomosis, excludes the diseased proximal subclavian artery, and does not require a graft.

Techniques

Carotid-Subclavian or Subclavian-Carotid Bypass and Carotid (or Subclavian) Transposition

The approach is through a supraclavicular incision dividing the clavicular head of the sternocleidomastoid muscle. The dissection is first lateral to the jugular vein, which is retracted medially. The prescalene fat pad is entered, and the anterior scalene muscle is exposed. The subclavian artery is isolated beneath the anterior scalene (second portion) or lateral to it (third portion) if a bypass is planned. In the first case, the phrenic nerve is isolated from the surface of the anterior scalene, and the subclavian artery is exposed after division of this muscle. The site chosen for anastomosis of the bypass is usually lateral to the thyrocervical trunk. Alternatively, the subclavian artery can be exposed in the third segment, between the brachial plexus and the anterior scalene muscle, with partial division of the latter.

The dissection is then moved medial to the jugular vein, and the common carotid artery is exposed. A suitable site is selected for the anastomosis of the graft to the carotid artery. In the case of a carotid-subclavian bypass for subclavian steal, the vein graft or prosthetic tube is anastomosed to the side wall of the carotid artery and then passed under the jugular vein into proximity with the subclavian artery (Fig. 36-3). Both anastomoses are end to side.

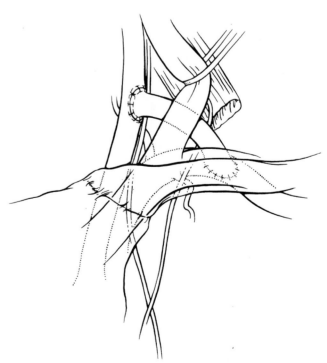

FIGURE 36–3 • Carotid-subclavian bypass graft tunneled under the jugular vein.

If the bypass is intended to revascularize the common carotid artery, the subclavian artery anastomosis is done first; the graft is then tunneled under the jugular vein and anastomosed end to end to the common carotid artery or to its bifurcation (Fig. 36-4), ligating the proximal carotid stump. Another alternative is to do an end-to-side anastomosis to the common carotid artery and ligate the common carotid artery immediately proximal to the anastomosis, which makes it functionally an end-to-end junction. The proximal exclusion is necessary to avoid embolization from the proximal common carotid artery or extension of the thrombus into the distal common carotid artery.

I seldom use the bypass technique between the carotid and subclavian arteries, and only in cases of common carotid artery occlusion and in patients with a left internal mammary artery–coronary anastomosis. Transposing one of these arteries into the other is a more elegant surgical solution (Fig. 36-5), in that only one artery-to-artery anastomosis is required. The long-term patency rates for carotid-subclavian transposition are superb. The drawbacks are the greater technical difficulty and the possibility of mediastinal bleeding from improper handling of the stump of the left subclavian artery. The transposition operation is particularly easy when the common carotid artery is the one being transposed; once freed, the common carotid, which has no branches, moves about the neck with ease. Translocation of the subclavian artery into the common carotid artery may be difficult on the left side, where the subclavian artery may have a deep location or the vertebral artery may have a low origin. When this low origin

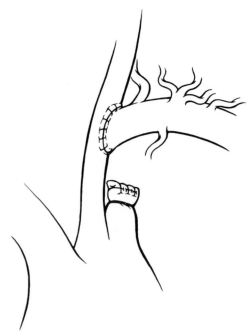

FIGURE 36–5 • Transposition of the left subclavian artery to the left common carotid artery.

interferes with good proximal control of the short first portion of the subclavian, I divide the vertebral artery at its origin and the subclavian artery low in the neck (but distal to the stump of the vertebral artery). The subclavian artery is transposed to the common carotid artery and, separately, the vertebral artery is transposed into either of the two vessels.

When transposing the subclavian artery to the common carotid artery, care must be taken to ensure proper position of the vertebral artery when the subclavian is brought into apposition to the common carotid before the anastomosis. Excessive length of the vertebral artery, once the subclavian artery is freed and moved upward, may cause kinking of this vessel and thrombosis. Although some authors have written that division of the left internal mammary artery facilitates the transposition, this is not so; it is an unwise maneuver that negates the possibility of a later myocardial revascularization using the internal mammary artery.

Subclavian-Subclavian Bypass

There is hardly any indication for this operation. The incision is supraclavicular on both sides, and the second or third portions of the subclavian are approached in the manner described earlier. The tunnel connecting the two subclavian arteries is made behind the sternocleidomastoid muscle, staying as low as possible to protect the graft behind the upper edge of the manubrium. Care is taken to avoid any axial rotation of the graft when tunneling across the neck.

Axilloaxillary Bypass

This too is an operation in search of an indication. The axillary arteries are exposed between the sternal and clavicular heads of the pectoralis major. Removal of part or all of the pectoralis minor from the coracoid process improves exposure of the axillary artery. The graft is tunneled under the sternal part of the pectoralis major and through presternal subcutaneous

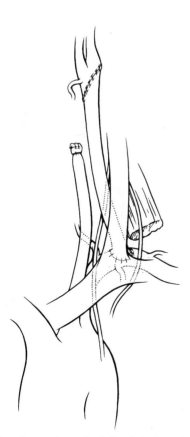

FIGURE 36–4 • Bypass from the left subclavian artery to the left carotid bifurcation.

tissue into the opposite axillary artery. Both anastomoses are end to side.

Carotid-Carotid Bypass

This technique is used to revascularize a common carotid artery whose origin in the mediastinum is involved by disease. One carotid acts as the donor vessel to the other. Because exposure of the common carotid arteries is a reasonably simple procedure, carotid-carotid bypass is a good technique to revascularize one common carotid trunk when the other one is healthy and the ipsilateral subclavian artery is not a suitable donor vessel. The bypass between both common carotid arteries lies low in the midline, partially hidden by the upper edge of the manubrium. Although these grafts make a rather lengthy loop and take off from the donor site at an oblique angle, their patency rate is excellent, provided the donor vessel is free of disease. These bypasses are sometimes cosmetically poor and, as mentioned previously, the grafts run a lengthy trajectory to link two vessels that are only four finger-breadths apart anatomically. I prefer to tunnel the bypass across the neck through the retropharyngeal space (Fig. 36-6), which is a shorter and straighter path. The tunnel for the bypass is behind the pharynx and in front of the prevertebral lamina. This space is loose and easily admits an 8-mm prosthesis without any pharyngeal compression.[6]

The distance between both carotids in the retropharyngeal space is short enough that it permits the direct reimplantation of one carotid into the other without a graft (Fig. 36-7). This procedure has the disadvantage of requiring clamping of both common carotid arteries simultaneously, and because of this, it is one of the few instances in which the protection of a shunt may be required to perfuse a clamped (donor) common carotid artery.

AXIAL REPAIRS

Endarterectomy was the first technique reported for reconstruction of the innominate artery,[7] and it was later formally

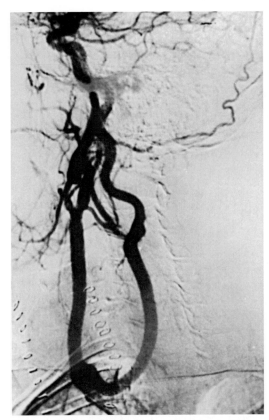

FIGURE 36–7 • Direct transposition of the left carotid artery to the right common carotid artery using the retropharyngeal route. (From Berguer R: The short retropharyngeal route for arterial bypasses across the neck. Ann Vasc Surg 1:127-129, 1986.)

described and perfected by Carlson and colleagues.[8] Innominate endarterectomy has the appeal of being an "anatomic" reconstruction that avoids the need for a prosthesis (Fig. 36-8), but I have abandoned this technique because of safety concerns. Its main drawback is the difficulty of clamping the origin of the innominate artery without occluding the left common carotid artery or damaging the plaque that may be present about the ostium of either. A common origin of the innominate and left common carotid arteries is found in 17% of individuals. The left common carotid is a branch of the innominate in another 8% of individuals. In either case, a clamp placed to exclude the origin of the innominate artery would result in bilateral hemispheric ischemia. When an innominate endarterectomy is done in a patient who has a common ostium for the innominate and left common carotid arteries, a temporary shunt from the ascending aorta to the left common carotid artery is mandatory. With innominate endarterectomy, it is also difficult to achieve a satisfactory termination of the endarterectomy in the aortic wall, where tacking sutures are often required. Finally, about half the patients with symptomatic innominate artery stenosis have severe lesions of either the left common carotid or left subclavian artery. These concomitant lesions are not suited for endarterectomy using the transsternal approach.

Rather than endarterectomy, I prefer to use a bypass from the ascending aorta to correct innominate artery and other associated lesions that may be present. The technique of bypass from the ascending aorta was introduced by DeBakey and associates.[9]

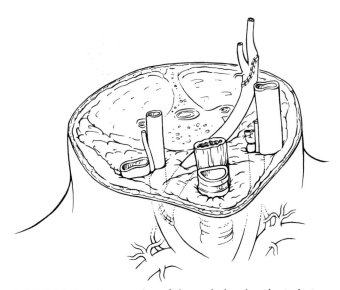

FIGURE 36–6 • Cross section of the neck showing the trajectory of a carotid-carotid bypass through the retropharyngeal space.

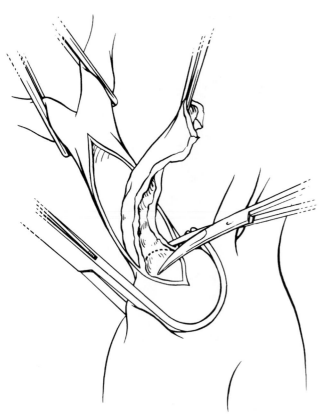

FIGURE 36–8 • Endarterectomy of the innominate artery ends proximally at the level of the aortic arch. The intima of the latter is later affixed to the endarterectomized wall of the innominate artery by a continuous monofilament suture to avoid dissection of the arch when flow is reestablished.

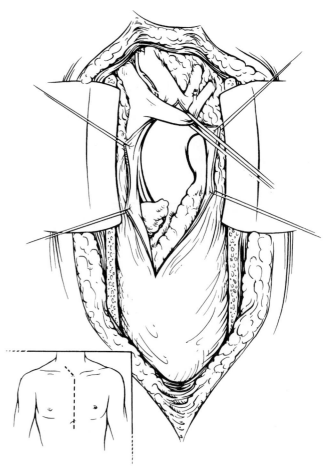

FIGURE 36–9 • Exposure of the ascending aorta and anterior supra-aortic trunks through the traditional full sternotomy (*inset* shows the skin incision).

Technique

Midsternotomy

Traditionally, the anterior mediastinal arteries (innominate and right common carotid) are approached through a midsternotomy (Fig. 36-9). The sternotomy is prolonged through a short incision that follows the right anterior edge of the sternocleidomastoid muscle to expose and obtain control of the proximal right common carotid and right subclavian arteries. After dividing the sternum, the innominate vein is dissected, and the thymic veins are ligated. The thymus is separated through its midline and preserved, to be used as tissue interposed between the graft and the sternum at the time of closure. The ascending aorta is approached below the innominate vein after opening the pericardial sac. The dissection continues over the origin of the innominate artery and onto its bifurcation. During dissection of the innominate bifurcation, care is taken not to injure the recurrent nerve near the origin of the right subclavian artery.

Partial Midsternotomy

In 1991, after being confronted with a poorly executed midsternotomy, it became apparent to me that approaching the ascending aorta and the anterior trunks did not require complete splitting of the sternum. Since then, I have approached the anterior SATs with a partial sternotomy, splitting only the upper three sternal segments (Fig. 36-10). The manubrium is sewn down to the third intercostal space, where a small notch

is made laterally with the oscillating saw. This facilitates a subperiosteal fracture at this site when the sternal spreader is used. Dissection of the brachiocephalic vein and thymus and exposure of the ascending aorta follow the same steps described for the full sternotomy. The advantages of this partial midsternotomy are that the chest cage remains intact and stable in its lower half, postoperative pain is noticeably reduced, and the chance of sternal instability is minimal.

Bypass from the Ascending Aorta

If the intent is to replace the innominate artery with a bypass (Fig. 36-11), the first inch of the right subclavian and right common carotid arteries are exposed. More often, however, one and sometimes both carotid bifurcations need to be exposed to be revascularized. The carotid bifurcation in this case is exposed through the standard neck incision used for carotid endarterectomy. After isolating the proximal right subclavian and common carotid arteries, an appropriate prosthetic tube is selected for the bypass. I use an 8- to 10-mm PTFE or Dacron fabric tube that matches the caliber of the innominate artery, requires only a moderate amount of aortic wall to be excluded, and does not occupy much space in the anterior mediastinum.

The proximal end of the prosthesis is beveled. Safe exclusion clamping of the ascending aorta requires the use of a nitroglycerin drip to reduce the systolic pressure to 110 mm Hg.

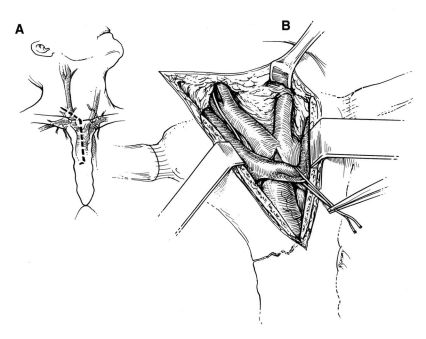

FIGURE 36–10 • Skin incision *(A)* and exposure *(B)* obtained through a partial sternotomy.

The exclusion clamp is placed on the proximal aorta (Fig. 36-12). With the clamp secured, the aorta is opened, and the beveled end of the graft is anastomosed to the ascending aortotomy with continuous 4-0 polypropylene sutures. Before unclamping and to avoid air embolization, the patient is momentarily placed in the Trendelenburg position, and the proximal anastomosis is vented and tested. If it is found to be satisfactory, a clamp is placed immediately above the anastomosis, and the table is returned to the horizontal position.

The patient is then systemically heparinized. Occluding clamps are placed first in the proximal right carotid and subclavian arteries and in the proximal portion of the innominate artery. The innominate artery is divided proximal to its bifurcation and prepared for anastomosis. The bypass graft, which is placed over the brachiocephalic vein, is cut to appropriate length and anastomosed to the innominate artery with continuous 5-0 polypropylene sutures. The graft and the distal vessels are bled before completing the anastomosis, and

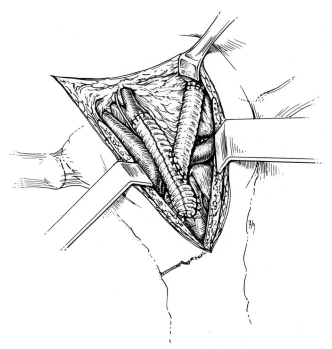

FIGURE 36–11 • Ascending aorta–to–innominate and left common carotid artery bypass completed through a partial sternotomy.

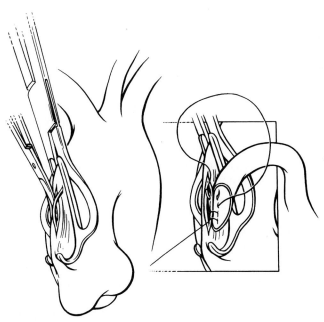

FIGURE 36–12 • Exclusion clamping of the ascending aorta and anastomosis of the main prosthesis to the aortotomy.

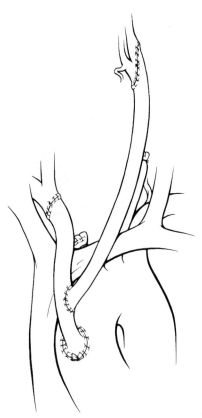

FIGURE 36–13 • Common pattern for revascularization of the anterior supra-aortic trunk: the main prosthesis (10 mm) replaces the innominate artery, and an 8-mm side branch supplies the left carotid system.

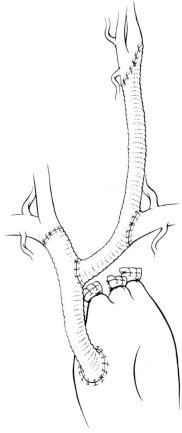

FIGURE 36–14 • Revascularization of all three supra-aortic trunks completed by transposing the left subclavian artery to the prosthesis that replaces the left carotid system.

flow is reestablished first into the right subclavian artery and then into the right common carotid artery. The proximal stump of the innominate artery is closed with a continuous double running suture.

In cases in which additional arteries need to be revascularized (usually the left common carotid), an additional 8-mm PTFE or Dacron side branch is anastomosed at an appropriate angle to the 10-mm main prosthesis after the proximal suture line is completed (Fig. 36-13). Any anticipated side branches are added before the distal anastomosis is done to avoid having to reclamp the innominate portion of the bypass after establishing flow through it. With the side branch anastomosed and excluded, one can perfuse the right carotid and vertebral arteries while constructing the left carotid anastomosis. In multiple replacements of the SATs (Fig. 36-14), the main bypass is the one supplying the right-sided trunk (innominate, right carotid, right subclavian). From this trunk emerge the branches supplying the left carotid or left subclavian artery or both.

RESULTS AND COMPLICATIONS OF RECONSTRUCTION OF THE SUPRA-AORTIC TRUNKS

Transthoracic reconstructions are generally done in younger patients with multiple-vessel involvement. Cervical repairs are done in older patients who are less likely to tolerate a thoracotomy and in patients with single-vessel disease of the common carotid or proximal subclavian arteries.

Any comparison of the results of the thoracic and cervical approaches must be done with reticence because of the differences between the two groups of patients. In addition to age and anatomic extent of disease, other considerations affect the choice of the approach, such as pulmonary function, previous coronary artery bypass surgery, and life expectancy.

A review of my experience with SAT reconstruction from 1982 to 1998 encompassed 282 cases—182 cervical repairs and 100 transthoracic repairs (Table 36-1). The most frequent indication for cervical repair in my practice is single-trunk disease (carotid or subclavian artery) or a history of myocardial revascularization. All innominate artery lesions are operated on through the chest.

Reported operative mortality for transthoracic repair ranges from 3% to 19%,[10,11] with most authors reporting series of 20 to 40 patients; some smaller series reported no mortality.[11] Increasing experience, refinement in anesthesia and perioperative care, and better patient selection have

TABLE 36–1	Morbidity and Mortality of Repair of the Supra-aortic Trunks		
Approach	**No. of Patients**	**TIA or Stroke (%)**	**Deaths (%)**
Cervical	182	3.8	0.5
Thoracic	100	8.0	8.0

TIA, transient ischemic attack.

reduced the mortality of transthoracic repair from 10% to 5% in reports from the Baylor group[11,12] and from 10% to 3.8% between the first and second halves of my experience.[13]

Reported mortality for cervical repairs is lower than that for thoracic repairs, between 0% and 4%. In my series, the morbidity from stroke and transient ischemic attack in patients undergoing cervical repair was 3.8%.[14] Patients undergoing cervical repair are some of the highest-risk patients among those with cerebrovascular disease; many have had previous myocardial revascularization procedures or are limited by restrictive pulmonary disease.

The higher morbidity in my earlier series of cervical reconstructions dropped significantly as experience was gained, leading to improved techniques and better patient selection. Over the last 14 years, a change in operative techniques has led to a reduction in operative complications and an increase in patency rates. Whereas 15 years ago I did subclavian-carotid and carotid-subclavian grafts for single-vessel disease, today most of these reconstructions are direct transpositions of one vessel to the other. The patency rate for cervical transposition procedures in my series was 100% after 5 years.[14]

Likewise, the techniques for transthoracic reconstruction have been refined and extended. Partial sternotomy is now my standard approach. Endarterectomy of the innominate artery is no longer performed. I try to extend the revascularization of the SATs to the left subclavian artery in patients who are likely candidates for future myocardial revascularization. With these refinements and changes in patient selection criteria in the latter half of my experience (1988 to 1998), the combined mortality and morbidity of cervical and transthoracic repair has been the same (3.8%). Table 36-1 shows the incidence of stroke and death following cervical and transthoracic repair in the entire series.

The most frequent and serious complication reported after either cervical or transthoracic repair of the SATs is myocardial infarction.[15,16] The second most frequent complication is stroke, which may develop during the operation or 3 to 4 days afterward. A delayed stroke may be hemorrhagic and is likely related to hyperperfusion and regional hypertension. In my experience, stroke has been a more frequent complication than myocardial infarction. Perioperative strokes are more common in patients with multiple intra- and extracranial involvement.[11] Some postoperative strokes may be due to technical flaws resulting in distal embolization or to prolonged clamp ischemia times. The latter can be managed with the usual cerebral protection methods. I routinely use intravenous dexamethasone before clamping, controlled heparin activity (activated clotting time), and—in patients with extensive and multiple disease—mild superficial hypothermia. I do not use shunts for SAT repair, with the rare exception noted under the description of carotid-carotid bypass.

Technical problems may cause peri- or postoperative bleeding, which can be severe and life threatening. Suture line bleeding, aortic wall tears from clamp or suture injury, and bleeding from an innominate artery stump may result in serious perioperative bleeding and severe tension hemothorax. Postoperative graft thrombosis and infections are rare.

The long-term outcome of these patients is largely determined by the progress of their coronary atherosclerotic disease. For patients undergoing cervical and transthoracic repairs, the 10-year survival is 50%.[16-18] Myocardial infarction is the most common cause of death (80%).

The long-term patency of these reconstructions is excellent.[17] Cumulative primary patency rates at 10 years are 82% and 88% for cervical and thoracic repairs, respectively.[13,14] Transpositions have the best patency rate (100% at 5 years in my series) of all cervical repairs. Saphenous veins fare worse than synthetics when used for SAT reconstruction; axial rotation, caliber mismatches, kinking, and intimal hyperplasia probably account for this.

In conclusion, cervical reconstruction is indicated in patients who have had previous myocardial revascularization and in those with single lesions of the common carotid or subclavian arteries. In this last group, my preference is to use transposition techniques between the carotid and the subclavian and, if the midline needs to be crossed, a retropharyngeal bypass. Reconstructive techniques using short (retropharyngeal) bypasses or no bypasses at all (transpositions) have outstanding patency rates, in contrast to the poor patency rates reported for conventional extra-anatomic bypasses. The transthoracic approach is favored for patients with multiple-vessel disease. SAT reconstruction may be done in conjunction with coronary artery bypass grafts. This approach should be confined to centers with experience in these techniques, where the operative mortality is similar to that obtained in cervical repairs.[17]

Reconstruction of the Vertebrobasilar System

The indications for vertebral artery reconstruction were discussed earlier. The vertebral artery is generally reconstructed at two levels: in its proximal segment for stenosing disease of its ostium, and in its distal segment (above C-2) for compression or thrombosis or a source of embolization from the intraspinal segment of this artery.

RECONSTRUCTION OF THE PROXIMAL VERTEBRAL ARTERY

Although the first reconstructions of the vertebral arteries were endarterectomies,[19-22] this technique is seldom used today. Vertebral artery bypass was advocated in the 1970s.[23] Today, most proximal vertebral artery lesions are dealt with by transposition of the artery into the neighboring common carotid artery[24-26] (Fig. 36-15). The appeal of this operation is that it consists of one artery-to-artery anastomosis and does not require a vein graft (needed for bypass) or extensive dissection of the subclavian artery (needed for endarterectomy).

The operation is done through a supraclavicular incision. The approach is between the bellies of the sternocleidomastoid muscles. The vertebral artery is isolated below the vertebral vein, dissected from its origin up to the point where it disappears under the longus colli, and freed from the overlying sympathetic ganglion or crossing sympathetic fibers. After clearing the adventitia of the chosen transposition site in the posterolateral wall of the common carotid artery, the patient is heparinized and the vertebral artery is divided above the stenotic area, suture-ligating its proximal stump. The distal segment of the artery is swung into the common carotid artery (Fig. 36-16). Using an aortic punch, a small arteriostomy is made in the common carotid wall to which the vertebral artery is anastomosed in end-to-side fashion using 6-0 or 7-0 polypropylene sutures and an open-type anastomosis.

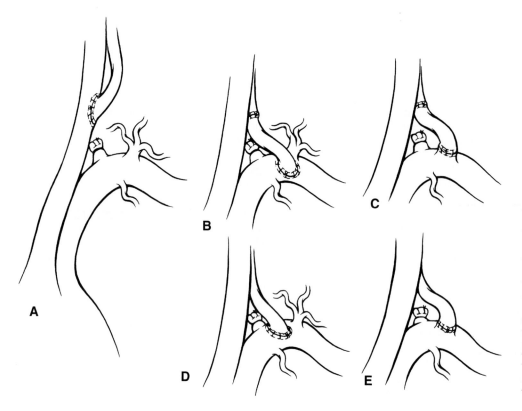

FIGURE 36–15 • Common techniques for reconstruction of the proximal vertebral artery. *A,* Transposition of the proximal vertebral artery to the common carotid artery. *B,* Bypass from the subclavian to the proximal vertebral artery. *C,* Subclavian-vertebral bypass originating in the amputated stump of the thyrocervical trunk. *D,* Transposition of the vertebral artery to another subclavian site. *E,* Transposition of the vertebral artery to the stump of the thyrocervical trunk.

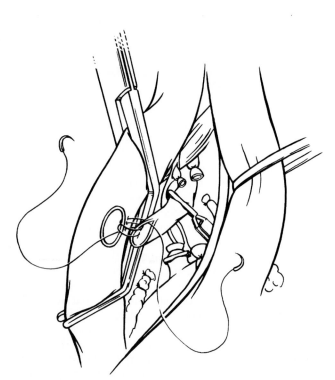

FIGURE 36–16 • Technique for transposition of the left vertebral artery to the left common carotid artery. The thoracic duct has been double ligated. The proximal vertebral artery stump has been clipped and suture-ligated. The sympathetic chain, left intact, is now seen behind the vertebral artery as the latter is brought close to the common carotid artery for anastomosis.

In a few cases, this technique is not possible. The most frequent reason is a contralateral common or internal carotid artery occlusion or an abnormally short first segment of the vertebral artery entering the cervical spine through the transverse process of C-7 rather than C-6. If the opposite common or internal carotid artery is occluded, clamping the remaining ipsilateral common carotid artery to transpose the vertebral artery to it carries severe risk of brain ischemia. In this situation, a subclavian-to-vertebral artery bypass is preferred. If the vertebral artery is too short to be brought easily to the common carotid artery wall, it can also be bypassed from the subclavian artery using a saphenous vein graft.[22,23] The bypass originates from the subclavian artery lateral to the thyrocervical trunk and is anastomosed end to end to the vertebral artery below the longus colli muscle. This procedure does not require any type of shunting. The most frequent complications from proximal vertebral artery dissection and transposition are partial Horner's syndrome from manipulation (or injury) of the intermediate sympathetic ganglion overlying the vertebral artery and an occasional lymphocele from injury to, or failed ligature of, the main or accessory thoracic ducts.

RECONSTRUCTION OF THE DISTAL VERTEBRAL ARTERY

Regardless of the level between C-6 and C-2 where the external compression or occlusive process occurs, the distal vertebral artery is reconstructed at the space between the C-1 and C-2 transverse processes (Fig. 36-17). This is the widest gap

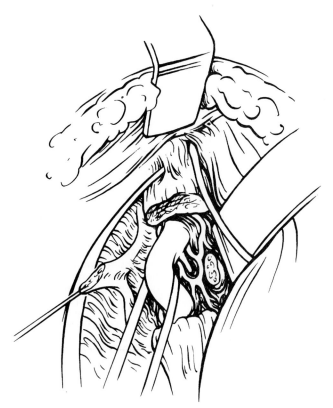

FIGURE 36–17 • Exposure of the vertebral artery between the transverse processes of C-1 and C-2. The anterior ramus of the C-2 nerve has been divided, and its anterior end is retracted with a stay suture. The artery has been dissected away from the surrounding vertebral plexus, which is now seen behind it.

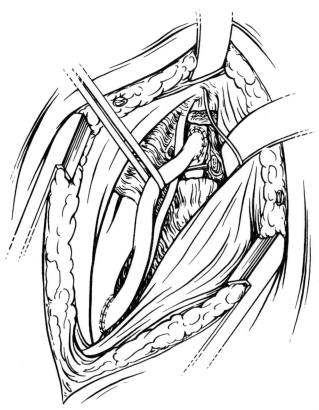

FIGURE 36–18 • Completed common carotid–to–distal vertebral artery bypass graft. A metal clip occludes the distal vertebral artery immediately below the anastomosis, making it function as an end-to-end junction.

between transverse processes in the neck and is also the segment where the vertebral artery is often maintained patent by collaterals from the occipital artery when the proximal segment of the artery is occluded.[24-26]

The operation is done through an incision similar to that used for carotid endarterectomy. Exposure of the vertebral artery at this level requires dissecting posterior to the jugular vein and identifying the spinal accessory nerve and the levator scapulae muscle. The levator is cut, exposing the transverse course of the anterior ramus of the C-2 nerve. The artery lies below the ramus and is perpendicular to it. The ramus is cut, and the artery is exposed. Dissection of the vertebral artery may be made difficult by the plexus of veins that surrounds it.

Once the artery is isolated, it can be reconstructed in several ways. The most common reconstruction is a bypass from the common carotid artery to the distal vertebral artery immediately below the transverse process of C-1 using autogenous vein (Fig. 36-18). This requires dissection of the common carotid below the bifurcation and the availability of a saphenous vein with a caliber approximating that of the vertebral artery. Once the end-to-side anastomosis of the vein graft to the vertebral artery is completed, the latter is ligated immediately below the anastomosis to avoid embolization from its proximal segment.

Another alternative is to use the external carotid artery (or, in rare cases, the occipital artery) to revascularize the distal

vertebral artery (Fig. 36-19). The external carotid is skeletonized and transposed below the jugular vein, anastomosing it end to end to the distal vertebral artery. The appeal of this procedure is that it does not require clamping of the internal carotid supply and that the caliber match between the distal external carotid artery and the vertebral artery is usually good. This choice obviously requires that the external carotid artery and the carotid bifurcation be free of atherosclerotic disease. I use this type of operation most often in individuals who have external compression or occlusion of the vertebral artery by osteophytes during neck rotation. These patients are generally younger and free of disease in the carotid bifurcation.

A third solution is transposing the distal segment of the vertebral artery to the neighboring internal carotid artery by means of an end-to-side anastomosis. This, again, has the appeal of a limited dissection and no need for a vein graft. The shortcoming is that one needs to clamp the internal carotid artery for the end-to-side anastomosis. This technique should not be used in patients in whom the opposite internal carotid artery is severely diseased or occluded.

A few patients have extrinsic compression or disease of the vertebral artery above the level of C-1. In these patients, the reconstruction is done in the distalmost segment of the extracranial vertebral artery before it penetrates the dura mater as it courses over the lamina of the atlas (the pars atlantica). The approach is posterior through a racquet-shaped incision (Fig. 36-20) with the patient in the park-bench position.

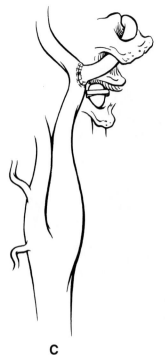

FIGURE 36–19 • Alternative methods for reconstruction of the distal vertebral artery. *A,* External carotid transposition to the distal vertebral artery. *B,* Occipital artery transposition to the distal vertebral artery. *C,* Transposition of the distal vertebral artery to the distal internal carotid artery.

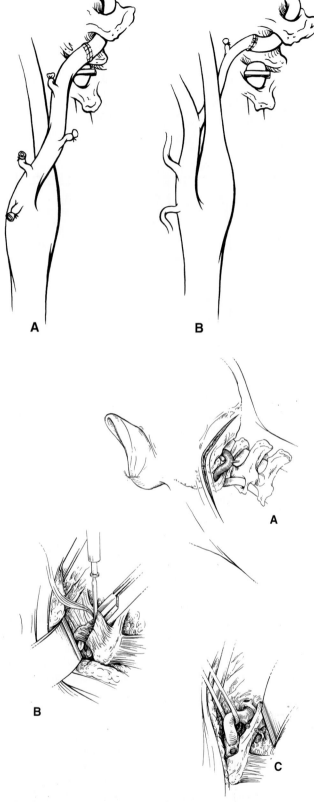

FIGURE 36–20 • *A,* Incision to approach the suboccipital segment of the vertebral artery. *B,* Division of the obliquus capitis superior. *C,* The looped vertebral artery is lifted from the underlying lamina of C-1. A descending muscular branch has been ligated and divided. (From Berguer R: Revascularization of the vertebral arteries. In Nyhus LM, Baker RJ, Fischer JE [eds]: Mastery of Surgery. Boston, Little, Brown, 1996.)

The semispinalis, splenius, and longus capitis muscles are cut, and the sternomastoid is de-inserted from the mastoid process. The transverse process of C-1 is identified, and the obliquus capitis superior muscle is cut. The artery rests on the posterior lamina of the atlas, covered by a dense plexus of veins and tethered by one or two muscular branches, which are divided. The vein bypass is anastomosed end to side. The distal cervical internal carotid artery can be isolated after dissecting away the vagus and hypoglossal nerve trunks, which, in this posterior approach, overlie the internal carotid artery. The bypass is anastomosed end to side to the distal cervical internal carotid artery (Fig. 36-21). In some patients, the vertebral artery pathology is extrinsic bony compression of the artery between the occipital ridge and the posterior lamina of C-1. In this situation, once the vertebral artery is dissected (using the suboccipital approach described here), laminectomy of C-1 eliminates the compression. Unless there is demonstrable damage to the wall of the vertebral artery by the bony impingement, a bypass is not needed.

RESULTS AND COMPLICATIONS OF RECONSTRUCTION OF THE VERTEBRAL ARTERIES

The risks and patency rates of vertebral artery operations are different for proximal and distal repairs.[26] Proximal reconstructions are technically easier. Distal reconstructions are more demanding and lengthier procedures. My colleagues and I reported on 252 proximal vertebral artery reconstructions with a combined mortality and morbidity of 0.9%.[26] No stroke or death occurred in 159 patients undergoing only a proximal vertebral artery reconstruction. The only morbidity and mortality occurred in patients undergoing simultaneous carotid and vertebral artery reconstruction. The cumulative secondary patency rate for proximal reconstructions was 92% at 10 years.

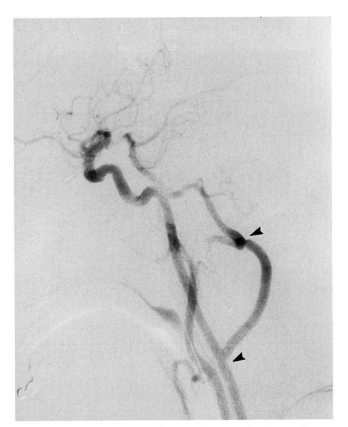

FIGURE 36–21 • Postoperative arteriogram showing a bypass from the cervical internal carotid artery to the suboccipital vertebral artery *(arrowheads)* before its entry into the foramen magnum.

In 117 distal vertebral reconstructions, the combined mortality and morbidity was 3.4%, four times higher than that for proximal repairs. Kieffer and colleagues reported 2.4% mortality.[27] Refinements in patient selection and surgical safeguards in the last 12 years have reduced the combined morbidity and mortality rates for proximal (0%) and distal (1.3%) vertebral reconstructions.

Postoperative thrombosis of a proximal reconstruction is rare. I have seen this complication in 3 of 252 cases (1.2%). In all three cases, a short vertebral artery (entering at C-7) could not be repaired by a standard vertebral-to-carotid transposition, and a subclavian-vertebral or carotid-vertebral bypass was done. In one case, tension at the anastomotic line, and in two others, a kink of the interposition vein graft, resulted in postoperative thrombosis. All patients underwent reoperation and thrombectomy, and the technical flaw was corrected. These three reoperations were recorded as patent at 3, 5, and 7 years postoperatively. Other complications of proximal reconstruction are an occasional lymphocele and a partial Horner's syndrome from manipulation of or injury to the lower cervical sympathetics. In one case of distal reconstruction, the spinal accessory nerve was damaged.

Postoperative thrombosis is more frequent following operations on the distal vertebral artery. I have seen it in 4 of 117 distal reconstructions (3.4%). The causes were faulty anastomoses or inadequate vein grafts. Thrombectomy and replacement with a new graft reestablished patency in two of the four failures.

Presenting symptoms of vertebrobasilar ischemia were relieved in 83% of patients.[22,25] Among survivors, the 5-year rate of protection from stroke was 97%.

REFERENCES

1. Hass WK, Fields WS, North RR, et al: Joint study of extracranial arterial occlusion. II. Arteriography, techniques, sites, and complications. JAMA 203:961-968, 1968.
2. Berguer R, Higgins RF, Nelson R: Noninvasive diagnosis of reversal of vertebral flow. N Engl J Med 301:1349-1351, 1980.
3. Berguer R, Hodakowski GT, Sieggren M, Lazo A: The silent brain infarction in carotid surgery. J Vasc Surg 3:442-447, 1986.
4. Caplan L, Tettenborn B: Embolism in the posterior circulation. In Berguer R, Caplan L (eds): Vertebrobasilar Arterial Disease. St. Louis, Quality Medical, 1992.
5. Lyons C, Gailbraiter G: Surgical treatment of atherosclerotic occlusion of the internal carotid artery. Ann Surg 146:487-494, 1957.
6. Berguer R: The short retropharyngeal route for arterial bypass across the neck. Ann Vasc Surg 1:127-129, 1986.
7. David JB, Grove WJ, Julian OC: Thrombotic occlusion of the branches of the aortic arch, Martorell's syndrome: Report of a case treated surgically. Ann Surg 144:124-126, 1956.
8. Carlson RE, Ehrenfeld WK, Stoney RJ, Wylie EJ: Innominate artery endarterectomy: A 16-year experience. Arch Surg 112:1389-1393, 1977.
9. DeBakey ME, Morris GC, Jordan GL, et al: Segmental thrombo-obliterative disease of branches of aortic arch. JAMA 166:988, 1958.
10. Brewster DC, Moncure AC, Darling RC, et al: Innominate artery lesions: Problems encountered and lessons learned. J Vasc Surg 2:99-112, 1985.
11. DeBakey ME, Crawford ES, Cooley DA, et al: Surgical considerations of occlusive disease of the innominate, carotid, subclavian and vertebral arteries. Ann Surg 149:690-710, 1959.
12. Thompson BW, Read RC, Campbell GS: Operative correction of proximal blocks of the subclavian or innominate arteries. J Cardiovasc Surg (Torino) 21:125-130, 1980.
13. Berguer R, Morasch MD, Kline RA, et al: Cervical reconstruction of the supra-aortic trunks: A 16-year experience. J Vasc Surg 29:239-248, 1999.
14. Berguer R, Morasch MD, Kline RA: Transthoracic repair of innominate and common carotid artery disease: Immediate and long-term outcome for 100 consecutive surgical reconstructions. J Vasc Surg 27:34-42, 1998.
15. Criado FJ: Extrathoracic management of aortic arch syndrome. Br J Surg 69(Suppl):S45-S51, 1982.
16. Crawford ES, Stowe CL, Powers RW Jr: Occlusion of the innominate, common carotid, and subclavian arteries: Long term results of surgical treatment. Surgery 94:781, 1983.
17. Zelenock GB, Cronenwett JL, Graham LM, et al: Brachiocephalic arterial occlusions and stenoses: Manifestations and management of complex lesions. Arch Surg 120:370-376, 1985.
18. Vogt DP, Hertzer NR, O'Hara PJ, et al: Brachiocephalic arterial reconstruction. Ann Surg 196:541-552, 1982.
19. Moore WS, Malone JM, Goldstone J: Extrathoracic repair of branch occlusions of the aortic arch. Am J Surg 132:249-257, 1976.
20. Cate WR, Scott HW: Cerebral ischemia of central origin: Relief by subclavian vertebral artery thromboendarterectomy. Surgery 45:19, 1959.
21. Imparato AM, Lin JPT: Vertebral artery reconstruction: Internal plication and vein patch angioplasty. Ann Surg 166:213-221, 1967.
22. Natali J, Maraval M, Kieffer E: Surgical treatment of stenosis and occlusion of the carotid and vertebral arteries. J Cardiovasc Surg (Torino) 13:4-15, 1972.
23. Berguer R, Bauer RB: Vertebral artery reconstruction: A successful technique in selected patients. Ann Surg 193:441, 1981.
24. Roon AJ, Ehrenfeld AJ, Cooke PB, et al: Vertebral artery reconstruction. Am J Surg 138:29-36, 1980.
25. Berguer R: Distal vertebral artery bypass: Technique, the "occipital connection" and potential uses. J Vasc Surg 2:621, 1985.
26. Berguer R, Flynn LM, Kline RA, Caplan L: Surgical reconstruction of the extracranial vertebral artery: Management and outcome. J Vasc Surg 31:9-18, 2000.
27. Kieffer E, Rancurel G, Richard T: Reconstruction of the distal cervical vertebral artery. In Berguer R, Bauer RB (eds): Vertebrobasilar Arterial Occlusive Disease. New York, Raven Press, 1984, pp 265-289.

Questions

1. In a patient with a retroesophageal right subclavian artery, which of the following associated anomalies are expected or likely to occur: (1) nonrecurrent right inferior laryngeal nerve; (2) thoracic duct emptying on the right side; (3) common trunk as the origin of both common carotid arteries; (4) right vertebral artery arising from the right common carotid artery; (5) left vertebral artery arising from the left common carotid artery?
    (a) 1, 3, 4, 5
    (b) 2, 3, 4, 5
    (c) 1, 2, 3, 4
    (d) 1, 2, 3, 4, 5

2. What is the most efficient operation to correct a severe stenosis of the origin of a vertebral artery?
    (a) Subclavian–to–vertebral artery autogenous vein bypass
    (b) Transposition of the vertebral artery to the common carotid artery
    (c) Endarterectomy and patch of the origin of the vertebral artery
    (d) Balloon angioplasty of the stenotic origin

3. Vertebrobasilar ischemia may be the result of which of the following: (1) a hemodynamically significant lesion of the vertebral artery; (2) a hemodynamically significant lesion of the basilar artery; (3) microembolization from a vertebral artery lesion; (4) microembolization from a subclavian artery plaque; (5) microembolization from a dissected vertebral artery?
    (a) 1, 3, 4, 5
    (b) 1, 3, 5
    (c) 1, 2, 5
    (d) 1, 2, 3, 4, 5

Answers

1. c   2. b   3. d

37

Samuel S. Ahn • Toshifumi Kudo

Thoracic Outlet Syndrome and Vascular Disease of the Upper Extremity

Thoracic Outlet Syndrome

Thoracic outlet syndrome (TOS) is defined as symptomatic compression of the neurovascular bundle at the thoracic outlet. This syndrome can take three main forms—neurogenic, venous, and arterial—depending on the specific structures compressed. Most patients with TOS have neurologic symptoms, although vascular problems may be present. This chapter reviews the history and the current etiologic, diagnostic, and therapeutic theories concerning TOS and its treatment.

HISTORY

TOS is still a controversial subject with respect to its diagnosis, conservative management, and surgical treatment. The concept of the disease and the anatomic structures focused on have changed over the centuries. In 1821, Cooper noted that subclavian artery thrombosis was due to compression by a cervical rib.[1] This compression became known as *cervical rib syndrome*. From 1920 to 1931, the scalene muscles, first rib, and congenital ligaments became the focus to explain neurovascular compression in the thoracic outlet region.[2-4] Then, the term *scalenus anticus syndrome* became popular, and an association with trauma was described.[5,6] The *costoclavicular syndrome*, compression between the clavicle and first rib, was described in 1943.[7] Peet and colleagues introduced the term *thoracic outlet syndrome* in 1956,[8] and Rob and Standeven proposed the term *thoracic outlet compression syndrome* in 1958.[9] More recent studies have emphasized histologic abnormalities indicating scalene muscle fibrosis in TOS patients.[10,11]

Over the years, various surgical approaches have been proposed. Coote performed a cervical rib resection in 1861.[12] Murphy performed a first rib resection in 1908.[13] Because of the high nerve complication rate associated with this procedure, the first scalenectomy was performed by Adson and Coffey in 1927,[14] but it was realized that division of the muscle alone eventually led to reattachment of the muscle fibers and

scarring, causing recurrent symptoms. Clagett reintroduced the first rib resection with a posterior approach in 1962.[15] In 1966, Roos described the transaxillary approach for first rib resection,[16] which is less invasive and more cosmetic and has become one of the standard approaches. In the late 1960s, an approach using an infraclavicular incision alone was described.[17] However, this approach produced a large, cosmetically unpleasant scar and, more importantly, provided only limited exposure posteriorly. Sanders and coworkers reintroduced scalenectomy for the treatment of recurrent TOS after first rib resection and post-traumatic TOS in 1979.[18] For the purpose of total decompression, Atasoy introduced a combined approach, a transaxillary first rib resection and transcervical anterior and middle scalenectomy, in 1996.[19]

INCIDENCE AND DEMOGRAPHICS

The incidence of TOS is reported to be approximately 0.3% to 2% in the general population.[19,20] The most common age range is 25 to 40 years. Patients in their teens as well as octogenarians have also been diagnosed with TOS, although rarely. Women are more commonly affected than men, with a female-male ratio of 4:1.

ANATOMY

A knowledge of the complex anatomy of the thoracic outlet is crucial to understanding the pathogenesis of TOS and making the diagnosis. The thoracic outlet is defined as the musculoskeletal structures surrounding three important structures: subclavian artery, subclavian vein, and brachial plexus. This triangle is formed by the anterior scalene muscle, middle scalene muscle, and first rib (Fig. 37-1). The subclavian artery arises from the upper mediastinum, passes behind the anterior scalene muscle, and arches over the first rib. It therefore courses through the scalene triangle, which is bordered by the anterior and middle scalene muscles and has the first rib as its floor.

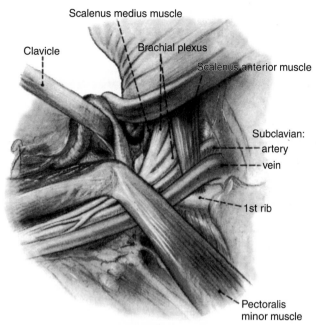

Scalenus medius muscle

Clavicle

Brachial plexus

Scalenus anterior muscle

Subclavian:
— artery
— vein

1st rib

Pectoralis minor muscle

FIGURE 37–1 • Anatomic dissection showing the anatomy at the thoracic outlet. The cadaver's head is turned to the left, and the clavicle is reflected laterally. (From Machleder HI [ed]: Vascular Disorders of the Upper Extremity, 3rd ed. Mt. Kisco, NY, Futura Publishing, 1998.)

The nerve roots (C-5 to T-1) of the brachial plexus, after exiting the intervertebral foramina, unite to form the upper (C-5 and C-6), middle (C-7), and lower (C-8 and T-1) trunks of the brachial plexus. They lie posterior, lateral, and superior to the subclavian artery and travel through the scalene triangle with the artery, with the lower trunk having a close relationship with the artery. The subclavian vein follows a similar course but, in contrast to the subclavian artery and brachial plexus, does not traverse the scalene triangle. It courses anterior to the insertion of the anterior scalene muscle on the first rib, outside the scalene triangle, and runs inferior and lateral to the subclavius tendon and costocoracoid ligament. All three structures then follow a similar course, passing under the clavicle and subclavius muscle and beneath the pectoralis minor near its insertion into the coracoid process and giving off several branches before entering the upper arm. Throughout their course, the neuromuscular structures are confined by various myofascial coverings.

Three main spaces in the thoracic outlet region are potentially responsible for compression of the neurovascular structures as they travel to the upper extremity: scalene triangle, costoclavicular space, and retro–pectoralis minor space. The scalene triangle is the most common site of nerve compression. Its contents are the brachial plexus and subclavian artery. The costoclavicular space, bordered by the clavicle and the first rib, is distal to the scalene triangle. It is traversed by all three structures: artery, vein, and nerve. The retro–pectoralis minor space is formed by the coracoid process and the insertion of the pectoralis minor, and by the ribs posteriorly. It is outside the thoracic outlet area and is less important in TOS. The brachial plexus may be compressed or tethered around the coracoid process with arm abduction or elevation.

In addition to the brachial plexus, two nerves in this area are surgically important. The phrenic nerve, a motor nerve to the diaphragm, arises primarily from C-4 and usually receives branches from C-3 and C-5. It travels on the anterior surface of the anterior scalene muscle, crossing lateral to medial. Because of this anatomic relationship, it is vulnerable to injury during scalenectomy. Thirteen percent of the population has a double phrenic nerve.[21] The long thoracic nerve arises primarily from C-6 and usually receives branches from C-5 and C-7. It courses through or just posterior to the middle scalene muscle and then descends over the first rib to reach the serratus anterior muscle. Injury to the nerve results in winging of the scapula.

Another surgically important structure is the thoracic duct, which empties into the left subclavian vein and is susceptible to operative injury resulting in troublesome lymphatic leakage.

CAUSE

The cause of neurogenic TOS is hypothesized to be a combination of osseous changes, soft tissue abnormalities, trauma, and inflammation—in other words, congenital predisposing anatomic structures and acquired extrinsic factors that may produce further compression of the neurovascular structures in the thoracic outlet area. In vascular TOS, the cause of arterial TOS is usually a bony abnormality—a cervical rib or a rudimentary first rib. Primary venous TOS is generally due to the costoclavicular ligament and subclavius muscle compressing the subclavian vein. It is important to consider the interaction between the neurovascular structures and the surrounding bony and muscular framework as a dynamic rather than a static process to understand the pathogenesis of TOS. Tumor can also be the cause of TOS; 1% to 2% of patients presenting with TOS have underlying tumor at the thoracic outlet in our series (unpublished data).

Osseous Changes

Cervical ribs, present since birth, are regarded as predisposing factors. They have an incidence of 0.5% to 1.5% in the general population[22-24]; approximately 50% are bilateral,[25,26] and there is a female-male ratio of 2:1. Most are asymptomatic,[27] but they are found with increasing prevalence in patients with TOS, reportedly occurring in 4% to 11% of patients who undergo TOS decompression surgery.[23,28,29] The size of the cervical rib may vary. They often have rudimentary or incomplete ossification, with a fibrous band extending from the tip and inserting on the first rib (Fig. 37- 2). Complete cervical ribs often insert on the first rib and occasionally are accompanied by an area of hyperostosis or even a fairly well-developed joint structure (Fig. 37-3). The brachial plexus is stretched over the cervical rib or accompanying fibrous bands, which produces compression, usually in the lower trunk.[30] Other osseous factors predisposing a patient to symptomatic TOS include a long transverse process of C-7, first rib fracture, bifid first rib, and malunion of the clavicle. Poor posture with anterior displacement[31] and saggy or droopy shoulders are also included in this category. It should be noted that the presence of a radiographically observed anatomic anomaly is not always necessary for the diagnosis.

Soft Tissue Abnormalities

Congenital fibromuscular bands and ligaments are observed in a majority of patients with neurogenic TOS.[30] Some authors

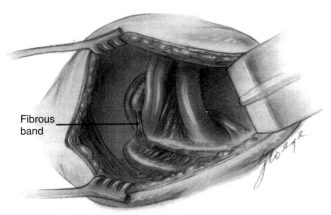

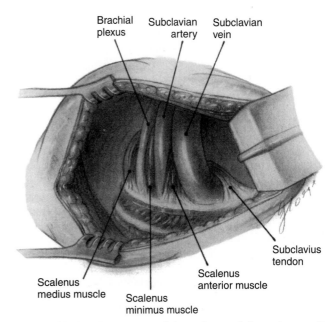

FIGURE 37–2 • View of a fibrocartilaginous band from the tip of the right-sided seventh cervical transverse process from the transaxillary surgical approach. This abnormality can compress the brachial plexus and subclavian artery, causing symptoms identical to those resulting from a cervical rib. The fibrocartilaginous band commonly occurs with an elongated C-7 transverse process and represents partial formation of a cervical rib. (From Makhoul RG, Machleder HI: Developmental anomalies at the thoracic outlet: An analysis of 200 consecutive cases. J Vasc Surg 16:534-545, 1992.)

FIGURE 37–4 • Appearance of the scalenus minimus abnormality from the transaxillary surgical approach. (From Makhoul RG, Machleder HI: Developmental anomalies at the thoracic outlet: An analysis of 200 consecutive cases. J Vasc Surg 16:534-545, 1992.)

report anomalous bands or ligaments found at the time of surgery in more than 80% of their patients.[32,33] These bands and ligaments have been present since birth and are categorized into nine different types.[30,34]

Scalene muscles are the most important structures that cause upper extremity symptoms. Congenital or acquired scalene muscle changes may be observed. One anatomic variation is the smallest scalene muscle (scalenus minimus) originating from the transverse process of the C-7 vertebra, interdigitating between the subclavian artery and the brachial plexus, inserting in conjunction with the anterior scalene muscle on the first rib, and producing further compression (Fig. 37-4). The role of the smallest scalene muscle has previously been underappreciated, but our review of 185 patients undergoing TOS surgery revealed that it was a prevalent (68.1%) and clinically significant marker for contralateral TOS surgery (unpublished data).

Another variation is a narrow scalene triangle, which may play a significant role in the development of TOS symptoms.[35] The anatomic relationship between the scalene angle and the brachial plexus—the nerve roots emerging from the apex of the scalene triangle (a higher anatomic region)—may also contribute to symptoms.[35] A hypertrophied subclavius muscle may be a factor in TOS as well.

Trauma

In addition to anatomic predispositions, trauma has been implicated as a precipitating factor for symptomatic TOS. Typical major trauma includes whiplash injuries of the neck[36] and blows to the shoulders resulting in acute hyperextension injury, often occurring during motor vehicle accidents. Some reports note that about 80% of TOS patients have symptoms precipitated by trauma to the neck and shoulder girdle area.[37,38] Stress injury, caused by repetitive motion or specific occupational activities over a prolonged period (e.g., continual abduction of the arms or excessive computer use), can also lead to TOS. Even upper extremity injury can cause TOS. Trauma causes spasm, inflammation, edema, and swelling, followed by scarring and fibrosis; this leads to increased muscle thickness, narrow interscalene spaces, and, eventually, compression of the neurovascular structures during contraction. The onset of symptoms may be delayed by days to weeks or even months.[35] Significant histologic muscle fiber changes have been demonstrated in the scalene muscles of patients with neurogenic TOS.[10,11]

PATHOLOGY

Studies focusing on the histochemical and morphometric analysis of the anterior scalene muscle have opened a new area of investigation into the causes of neurovascular compression at the thoracic outlet.[10,11] This research has been particularly useful in demonstrating the changes that occur in

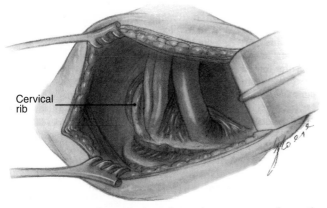

FIGURE 37–3 • View of thoracic outlet structures from the transaxillary surgical approach. The brachial plexus and subclavian artery are compressed and displaced by a right-sided cervical rib. This cervical rib articulates in the center of the first thoracic rib. (From Makhoul RG, Machleder HI: Developmental anomalies at the thoracic outlet: An analysis of 200 consecutive cases. J Vasc Surg 16:534-545, 1992.)

post-traumatic neurogenic TOS and often appear in the absence of obvious structural abnormalities.

Vertebrate skeletal muscle is composed of several distinctive muscle fiber types, each having different morphologic, metabolic, and contractile characteristics that are distinguishable by specific histochemical staining methods. Despite a high degree of specialization, these fibers retain the capacity to accommodate changes in demand and patterns of stimulation, responding with alterations in basic biochemical elements.

Human skeletal muscle usually comprises predominantly type 2, quick-reacting fibers, which have a low oxidative enzyme capacity. A smaller percentage of slow tonic-contracting type 1 fibers, characterized by a greater oxidative capacity, is present. These latter fibers (type 1) are common to postural muscle groups. Anterior scalene muscle demonstrates type 1 fiber predominance, which indicates that this muscle has a uniquely structured fiber composition to sustain protracted periods of tonic contraction.

Striking increases in type 1 fiber composition and selective hypertrophy of the type 1 fiber system occur in patients with post-traumatic TOS. The anterior scalene muscle in these patients demonstrates an extraordinary adaptive transformation and recruitment response in the type 1 fiber system, possibly reflecting chronic increased tone or motor neuron stimulation. It seems likely that in post-traumatic TOS, stretch injury to the muscle initiates a response of muscle contraction or denervation and reinnervation, compromising the scalene triangle (between the anterior and middle scalene muscles) and constricting the brachial plexus, which both accentuates and perpetuates the neurovascular compressive phenomenon.

CLINICAL PRESENTATION

The signs and symptoms of TOS are representative of the neurovascular structures involved in compression: the brachial plexus and the subclavian artery and vein. Symptoms may develop spontaneously or following trauma of a type that causes chronic muscle spasm in the neck or shoulder region. Presenting symptoms span a broad range of severity, from mild to disabling. Some patients report the onset of symptoms after a cervical injury or motor vehicle accident. More commonly, the onset of neurogenic symptoms is insidious; they may be mild and intermittent at first and are generally ignored by the patient. The symptoms gradually increase in frequency and severity, followed by progression that affects job, sleep, or activities of daily living. Patients may experience upper extremity pain, paresthesia, and numbness. Headache, neck pain, chest pain, and almost any upper extremity complaint may be attributable to TOS. Patients with vascular TOS may have a sudden onset.

Neurologic Symptoms

Neurologic symptoms caused by thoracic outlet compression of the brachial plexus predominate in 94% to 97% patients.[37,39] The symptoms of neurogenic TOS are basically the same as those of nerve compression in other regions of the body: pain, paresthesia, tingling sensation, and weakness for peripheral nerves; and Raynaud's syndrome, temperature change, and color change for autonomic nerves. Typically, two patterns of brachial plexus compression have emerged. Lower plexus (C-8 and T-1) involvement is regarded as more common than

upper plexus (C-5 and C-6) involvement. However, the picture is often mixed.[40]

Lower brachial plexus thoracic outlet compression usually causes sensory disturbance to the ulnar nerve distribution. Patients complain of pain and paresthesias in the medial (ulnar) aspect of the arm from the axilla, through the brachial area and the forearm, down to the hand (the fourth and fifth fingers). Ulnar-innervated muscles include the hypothenar, interosseous, and deep flexors of the ring and little finger. Pain in the anterior or posterior shoulder region and the side or back of the neck radiating into the occipital or mastoid area of the skull is also characteristic.[41]

Patients with upper plexus TOS usually present with symptoms in the forearm and upper arm, rather than the hand. Upper plexus TOS also produces pain in the side of the neck that radiates upward to the ear and may even include the mandible, face, temple, and occipital regions, with hemicranial headaches.[40] The pain radiates posteriorly to the rhomboid area, anteriorly across the clavicle into the upper pectoral region, laterally through the trapezius and deltoid muscle areas, and down the outer arm.[41] Compression of the upper trunk may cause evidence of C-5 to C-7 nerve root involvement or sensory disturbance to the median nerve distribution.[42]

Brachial plexus compression can cause subjective coldness of the hand, even pallor, which may be mistakenly interpreted as arterial insufficiency or complex regional pain syndrome type I (reflex sympathetic dystrophy). In more advanced cases, weakness of the hand and loss of dexterity of the fingers frequently develop.[22] The lateral thenar muscles are most severely affected. In late cases there is muscle atrophy, impaired use of the arm without paralysis, or even a "claw" hand.

TOS can present with headache as the primary component. Occipital and orbital headaches that radiate forward are common. In contrast, frontal headaches are not due to TOS. Surgical decompression of the thoracic outlet can be effective in treating TOS-related headaches. In our review of 227 TOS patients, the prevalence of headache was 41%, and the primary and secondary success rates of TOS surgery for relieving headache were found to be 52.7% and 75.2%, respectively, at 1 year, using life-table analysis (unpublished data).

Venous Symptoms

Venous TOS is less common than neurogenic TOS and accounts for 2% to 3% of cases.[21,39] Venous obstruction produces swelling, edema, cyanosis, and discomfort of the arm that is aggravated with exercise. Patients may have a sudden onset of symptoms due to subclavian vein thrombosis. The natural clinical course is protracted, with continued disability. Collateral venous circulation develops over time and may be evident as distended superficial veins of the shoulder and chest. Vigorous activity is often difficult in the presence of chronic subclavian vein occlusion.

Arterial Symptoms

Arterial involvement is the least common form of presentation, constituting 1% to 2% of cases.[21,39] These patients present with signs of ischemia: pain, pallor, pulselessness, and coolness of the affected side. They often experience fatigue of the arm with exercise and ischemic claudication, particularly with the arm elevated. Ischemic ulcers on the hand or gangrenous fingertips may occur due to thrombosis or embolization. This indicates severe narrowing or aneurysm of the subclavian artery. Retrograde embolization to the brain circulation can occur. In our series, 1.5% of all surgical TOS patients (43% of arterial TOS patients) presented with vertebrobasilar stroke (unpublished data).

Exacerbating Factors

Symptoms are typically exacerbated with increased arm activity and elevation, particularly overhead, abducted, and externally rotated arm positions. Common activities such as combing the hair, reaching or working with the arms overhead, or even driving a car with the hands on top of the steering wheel can bring on symptoms. With prolonged use of the upper extremities, patients may describe feelings of tiredness, weakness, or heaviness and note relief with lowering the arms. The paresthesias are often nocturnal, awakening the patient with a feeling of numbness or, more commonly, pain. Sleep disturbance is common. Heavy work during the day may be followed by misery at night.

DIAGNOSIS

The diagnosis of TOS is still controversial, because objective findings are few. No single clinical or objective test has been accepted as definitively establishing the diagnosis. The overall clinical evaluation is critical, because the diagnosis of TOS is usually based on patient history, subjective complaints, and findings on physical examination. The workup begins with a thorough history, including onset of symptoms, any exacerbating or alleviating factors, history of trauma, and complaints in the head, neck, shoulder, and upper extremity.

PHYSICAL EXAMINATION

The physical examination should not be limited to testing for TOS. It should focus on all the patient's problems and be geared toward ruling out more common causes of symptoms in the upper extremity, such as cervical stenosis, carpal tunnel syndrome, or cubital tunnel syndrome. After a general examination, attention is turned to the neck, shoulder, and upper extremities, especially to the intrinsic muscles of the hand and the distribution of sensory changes. Both extremities need to be examined, whether or not they are symptomatic.

Patients with obvious venous or arterial TOS may have a much clearer clinical picture and objective findings than those with neurogenic TOS.

Inspection and Palpation

The initial examination of the upper extremity should begin with inspection and palpation for discoloration, such as blanching, cyanosis, or gangrene; muscle atrophy; abnormal fingernail and hair growth; and temperature, moisture, and pulse. A note should be made of abnormal distention of veins, which could be collateral vessels, particularly around the shoulder. The symmetry and positional change of the vessels should be noted.[43] Muscle atrophy, particularly in the hypothenar, is not common, but not rare, in TOS. The hands should be examined at the same time and compared with each other.

The supra- and infraclavicular areas should be examined by palpation. In patients with TOS, there is often tenderness to compression over the anterior scalene muscle. Reduced sensation to light touch may be present in the involved fingers. Peripheral pulsation and blood pressure should be examined in both arms. A difference in blood pressure between the two arms of more than 20 mm Hg suggests blockage of the arterial circulation.

Allen's test is useful for evaluating the integrity of the palmar arch; however, it is generally not helpful in diagnosing TOS.

Auscultation

Auscultation should begin in the supraclavicular fossa bilaterally. It should then be performed with the stethoscope just beneath the middle third of the clavicle beginning with the arm in the neutral position and then gradually bringing it up into the abducted and externally rotated position. This is done while palpating the radial pulse. If obliteration of the radial pulse occurs, the stethoscope should be moved laterally in the infraclavicular area, then medially in the supraclavicular area, to detect bruits and a site of compressive occlusion. Because blood flow may be totally obliterated at the thoracic outlet, the maneuver should be performed slowly so as not to overlook bruits.[43]

Muscle Strength Test

Because muscle weakness can be one of the objective findings of TOS, the strength of all muscle groups of the arm should be tested. Patients may have weakness of the shoulder girdle muscles (deltoid), biceps, and triceps in cases of upper plexus compression (C-5 to C-7) and weakness of the intrinsic muscles of the hands in lower plexus compression (C-8 to T-1). Note that most TOS patients (85% to 90%) have combined symptoms of upper and lower plexus compression.[40] The patient is asked to make a ring with the thumb (the thenar muscle innervated by the median nerve) and the little finger (the hypothenar muscle innervated by the ulnar nerve) against resistance. The interosseous muscles are tested using the interdigital card test and spreading the fingers apart against resistance. Grip strength should be measured by dynamometry.

Provocative Clinical Tests

Positional and pressure maneuvers that increase pressure on the nerve may be used to elicit symptoms and make a clinical diagnosis. The patient should complain of reproduction of symptoms in the correct nerve distribution. However, these results should be interpreted carefully. Obliteration of a peripheral pulse or even the production of symptoms during the examination does not necessarily mean pathology; this may occur in normal individuals. These tests should be used to supplement other physical, radiographic, or historical findings that point to the diagnosis. These provocative tests (pressure, position, and Tinel) should also be performed at the common distal sites of nerve compression in the upper extremity to determine any concomitant sites of nerve compression that may be present and contributing to the patient's symptoms.[23]

TINEL'S SIGN. Tinel's sign (distal tingling on percussion) should be considered positive if the patient complains of a radiating tingling sensation in the arm when tapping over the brachial plexus at the supraclavicular area.

ADSON'S TEST. Adson's test is performed by holding the patient's arm down while the head is turned toward the affected side with slight cervical extension.[14] The radial pulse is evaluated when the patient inspires deeply. This maneuver may narrow the scalene triangle, compressing the subclavian artery and brachial plexus. It should be considered positive when the radial pulse is obliterated or diminished or symptoms are reproduced.

ABDUCTION AND EXTERNAL ROTATION TEST AND WRIGHT'S HYPERABDUCTION TEST. The abduction and external rotation (AER) test requires abducting the arms to 90 degrees in external rotation, which rotates the clavicle and subclavius muscle posteriorly and inferiorly. Wright's hyperabduction test is performed with the shoulders hyperabducted to 180 degrees and rotated externally while turning the head away from the affected side.[44] Symptoms caused by a narrow interscalene space are aggravated by abduction of the extremity because the nerves are pushed up against the tight, narrow area, increasing pressure on them. Deep inspiration with breath-holding may accentuate an ambiguous response. The patient is checked for any change in pulse and any symptoms in the arm. The test should be considered positive when the radial pulse is obliterated or diminished or if symptoms, such as weakness, tiredness, and numbness in the arm and paresthesia in the fingers, are reproduced. The duration of these provocative tests should not exceed 2 minutes and preferably should last only 1 minute. Care must be taken to avoid misdiagnosing an ulnar nerve neuropathy at the elbow.

ELEVATED ARM STRESS TEST. The elevated arm stress test (EAST, or Roos' test) requires the shoulders to be abducted and externally rotated 90 degrees and the elbows flexed 90 degrees with rapid opening and closing of the hands.[30] This test is performed for up to 3 minutes, as long as the patient has no complaint. Reproduction of symptoms, such as fatigue, cramping, pain, or paresthesia, within 3 minutes is considered a positive test.

LABORATORY TESTS

Electrophysiologic Tests

Because the majority of the symptoms of TOS are caused by neural compression, a variety of electrophysiologic tests have been proposed for the objective diagnosis of TOS. However, because compression is positional and intermittent, and electrophysiologic change may occur in late cases,[41] these tests have a low level of sensitivity for TOS diagnosis.[19] A positive electrophysiologic study confirms the clinical diagnosis of TOS, but a negative finding does not exclude its presence. These tests may also be useful in the differential diagnosis of more peripheral nerve lesions, such as median nerve compression at the carpal tunnel or ulnar nerve compression at the cubital tunnel or Guyon's canal.

ELECTROMYOGRAPHY. In most TOS patients, sensory function is involved. Because electromyography evaluates motor nerve function, findings are usually normal.

NERVE CONDUCTION VELOCITY. The typical findings of nerve conduction studies in patients with TOS are as follows: normal sensory and low-amplitude motor responses in the median nerve region; low-amplitude sensory and relatively low- or normal-amplitude responses in the ulnar nerve region.[19,45]

F-WAVE RESPONSES. When a peripheral nerve is stimulated percutaneously and the centrally propagated (antidromic) impulse reaches the motor neuron in the spinal cord, some of the impulses will be reflected back down the axon in an orthodromic direction. This "reflected" potential is called an F wave.[46] In some settings, quantitative measurements can enhance the sensitivity of this electrophysiologic response.[47]

SOMATOSENSORY EVOKED POTENTIALS. Progress has been made in facilitating the objective evaluation of neurogenic TOS by recording somatosensory evoked potentials across the brachial plexus and in the supraclavicular fossa and cervical spinal cord.[48,49] The most characteristic abnormality found in patients with neurogenic TOS is a reduction in the amplitude of the ulnar nerve response at the N9 electrode, or Erb's point, or the brachial plexus recording electrode, whereas the median somatosensory evoked potential is normal. This dampening of the N9 amplitude can be accentuated, or the potential completely ablated, by placing the arm in the abducted and externally rotated position, which is the most symptomatic position for patients with TOS.

Anatomic Studies

PLAIN RADIOGRAPHY. Plain radiographs of the cervical spine and shoulder should be obtained in all patients being evaluated for TOS to identify bony or other abnormalities that might be the cause of compression, including cervical disk disease, an abnormal first rib, a cervical rib, elongated C-7 transverse processes, or shoulder pathology. Cervical ribs and long transverse processes at C-7 may be the origin of radiolucent congenital bands to the first thoracic rib.[22,41] Patients with a low-lying shoulder girdle have a narrow costoclavicular space.

A chest radiograph should be obtained to rule out the presence of Pancoast's tumor at the apex of the lung.

COMPUTED TOMOGRAPHY AND MAGNETIC RESONANCE IMAGING. Computed tomography (CT) scanning is not conclusively diagnostic in TOS patients. Brantigan and Roos claimed that a high-speed multidetector CT study with contrast is a promising technique because spatial resolution is much better than with magnetic resonance imaging (MRI), and the study is faster.[41] Individual muscles can be visualized and peeled back using computer techniques.

MRI has also been proposed for the diagnosis of TOS because of its better visualization of soft tissues; fibrous bands and brachial plexus deviation have been shown.[50] Using special sequences, Collins and others have performed detailed studies of the thoracic outlet with a high degree of accuracy in diagnosing TOS compression.[51] These tests are helpful to confirm compression, but it should be noted that such compression may not necessarily be the cause of the patient's symptoms. MRI is also useful to rule out other causes, such as tumor. Impaired venous flow at the thoracic outlet can be demonstrated by MRI without contrast medium.

ARTERIOGRAPHY. Angiography is not indicated in patients with neurologic symptoms alone. Positional arterial obstruction can usually be confirmed by simple physical examination. Arteriography should be reserved for patients in whom arterial

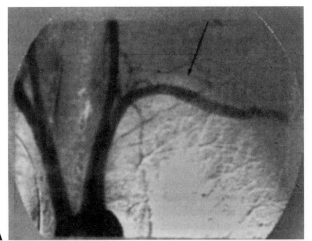

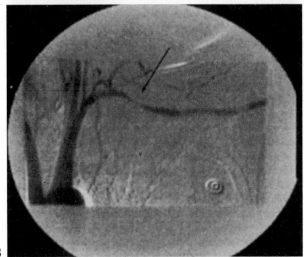

FIGURE 37–5 • Digital intravenous axillosubclavian angiogram obtained in the supine *(A)* and sitting *(B)* positions to demonstrate thoracic outlet compressive changes *(arrows)*, which are often seen only in the sitting position.

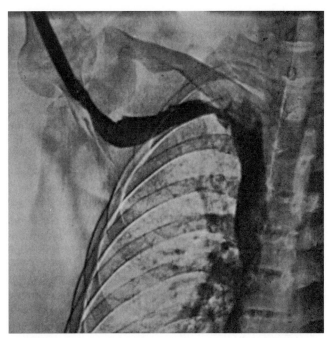

FIGURE 37–6 • Typical venographic picture of axillosubclavian compression at the thoracic outlet that eventually leads to thrombosis and an acute clinical presentation. Note that the right upper extremity is hyperabducted.

involvement is suspected by clinical findings: an infraclavicular or supraclavicular bruit, absent radial pulse, significant blood pressure difference between arms (>20 mm Hg), limb ischemia, suspicion of embolization, or pulsating paraclavicular mass.

In patients with arterial thoracic outlet compression, arteriography and venography in the upper extremities should be performed in the neutral position, with the arm at the patient's side, and in the stress position, with the upper arm at right angles to the chest. The use of digital intravenous angiography, which allows the patient to be radiographed in the sitting position, demonstrates a much higher yield of arterial compression lesions, correlating much more closely with the clinical findings (Fig. 37-5). We often perform the positional exposures with the patient's hand behind the head. If this is not done, many of the compressive abnormalities at the thoracic outlet are missed.

Venography. Venography is indicated if venous involvement is suspected. Venograms with the patient's arm in various positions can show intermittent occlusion or complete occlusion with collateralization (Fig. 37-6). Magnetic resonance angiography is also being used for that purpose.[41] Early venography combined with catheter-directed thrombolysis is indicated in a patient with acute occlusion of the

axillosubclavian vein, an acutely swollen upper extremity, or when the possibility of Paget-Schroetter syndrome exists.

Provocative Tests (Scalene Muscle Block)

A newer test with high sensitivity and specificity for the diagnosis of neurogenic TOS is the electromyogram-guided selective scalene block. The method and results have been reported by Jordan and Machleder.[52] Anesthetic blocks of the anterior scalene muscle have been used as a method of diagnosing and confirming TOS and for predicting which patients may benefit from surgical decompression.[28] When a local anesthetic agent is injected into the anterior scalene muscle and paralyzes it temporarily, the patient's symptoms caused by compression are relieved for a few hours to a few days. However, the standard technique of using surface landmarks often results in inadvertent somatic and sympathetic block because there is no reliable way to verify needle tip localization.[19]

Jordan and Machleder reported that electrophysiologic guidance facilitates accurate needle tip placement in the performance of anterior scalene muscle blocks.[47,52] A Teflon-coated 25-gauge hypodermic needle, bared at the tip, is advanced through the sternocleidomastoid muscle. Electromyographic activity is monitored as the needle is advanced through the tissue layers; the anterior scalene muscle can be activated with lateral neck bending against resistance and with deep inspiration. In most patients, a twitch of the scalene muscles is visible with electrical stimulation. The patient is asked whether pain is produced and whether insertion at this depth produces pain that is similar in quality and location to the usual pain experienced. After an injection of 2 mL of 2% lidocaine into the anterior scalene muscle, the arm is placed into a stress position and exercised for 1 minute; the patient is then asked to rate the pain. Attempts to activate the anterior scalene muscle are performed again with lateral neck movement and with deep inspiration, but only distant motor action potentials can be identified. Electrical stimulation can no longer produce a visible twitch of the scalene muscles. A positive test occurs if the patient has greater than 50% improvement in the elevated arm stress pain score after anesthetic injection of the anterior scalene muscle compared with a baseline examination. The results of these blocks correlate with surgical outcomes; a positive result predicts a good outcome to surgical decompression. Note that the absence of pain relief does not exclude the presence of TOS, as long as the patient has symptoms and clinical findings.

DIFFERENTIAL DIAGNOSIS

Failure to make the correct diagnosis or to appreciate the presence of other problems is a major concern in the treatment of patients with TOS.[53] It is not uncommon for TOS to coexist with other conditions; in particular, lung tumors, cardiac disease, and psychiatric disorders should be considered, as well as cervical spine, neurologic, and musculoskeletal disorders.

Cervical Spine Disorders

Neurovascular compression of the cervical spine can cause intermittent pain and tenderness in the neck and back of the head, often radiating down the arm in the radial nerve distribution. Provocative maneuvers include head turning with tilting back and the Spurling test (pressing the forehead downward), which can reproduce symptoms. MRI of the cervical spine is useful for the diagnosis.

Neurologic Disorders

A double-crush syndrome may be present in TOS patients, which refers to two coexisting entrapment syndromes—commonly, carpal tunnel syndrome or cubital tunnel syndrome combined with brachial plexus compression.[54,55] If surgical intervention is necessary, the more peripheral entrapment should be treated first.

CUBITAL TUNNEL SYNDROME (ULNAR NERVE ENTRAPMENT AT THE ELBOW). The ulnar nerve originates from the C-8 to T-1 nerve routes and supplies motor branches to the flexor carpi ulnaris and the medial half of the flexor digitorum profundus. It can be entrapped as it courses through the ulnar groove behind the medial condyle of the humerus. Its compression at the elbow produces tingling pain, with paresthesias and numbness in the ulnar distribution (the last two fingers) but few symptoms in the shoulder and neck. The presence of medial forearm numbness can also help delineate TOS from ulnar neuropathy, because that area is innervated by the medial antebrachial cutaneous nerve (lower cord of brachial plexus; C-8 and T-1 nerve roots). Electrophysiologic tests are useful for the diagnosis.

CARPAL TUNNEL SYNDROME. Carpal tunnel syndrome is caused by compression of the median nerve by the carpal ligament at the wrist. Because it is a pure median neuropathy, the first three fingers are involved predominantly, delineating it from TOS. Carpal tunnel syndrome typically produces symptoms that originate in the hand and radiate up the arm, in contrast to TOS, which produces pain in the neck and shoulder that moves down to the hand. Tinel's sign elicited by tapping the volar wrist crease and Phalen's test (wrist

flexion) are helpful in making the diagnosis. Confirmation is achieved with electrodiagnostic studies that show delayed nerve conduction across the wrist.

Musculoskeletal Disorders

SHOULDER PATHOLOGY. Inflammation or tears of the tendons around the shoulder cause reduced shoulder range of motion and tenderness at the biceps and rotator cuff tendons. MRI is helpful in making the diagnosis.

COMPLEX REGIONAL PAIN SYNDROME. Complex regional pain syndrome (CRPS) is a neuropathic pain disorder that involves dysfunction of the peripheral and central nervous systems.[56,57] It may develop after trauma. CRPS type I (without a definable nerve lesion) and type II (with a definable nerve lesion) were formerly known as reflex sympathetic dystrophy and causalgia, respectively. CRPS is clinically characterized by sensory (burning, spontaneous pain, allodynia, hyperalgesia), autonomic (edema, sweating abnormalities, change in skin color or temperature), and motor (muscle weakness, postural or action tremor, decreased range of motion, muscle spasms, dystonia) disturbances. In chronic stages, trophic changes such as abnormal nail growth, increased or decreased hair growth, fibrosis, thin glossy skin, and osteoporosis may be present. Patients with CRPS commonly suffer from psychological dysfunction (depression, anxiety, phobia).

CONSERVATIVE MANAGEMENT

In general, conservative treatment should be tried initially in every patient with TOS except for those with severe, long-standing symptoms and those with obvious neurologic signs, ischemic symptoms, or venous obstruction.[19] It includes education and instruction, several types of physical therapy modalities, and medication.

Education

Patient education is important to encourage compliance with treatment. The purpose of treatment and its expected benefits should be understood. Even a simple explanation of the syndrome and reassurance may satisfy some patients. A review of factors that exacerbate or relieve symptoms and previous successful or unsuccessful treatment is valuable. In some cases, modification of activities of daily living or work habits can help the patient's symptoms, particularly the avoidance of repetitive activities, overhead work, and weight lifting. A slower work pace with frequent short breaks should be emphasized. Many individuals experience sleep disturbances. These patients should be instructed how to rest and protect the cervical spine at night to avoid irritating positions. Obesity, breast hypertrophy, and general physical condition may contribute to symptoms in some patients.

Posture

Most patients with TOS have subtle or obvious posture deformities. Forward-flexed postures exacerbate TOS symptoms.[23,58] A postural assessment, including the spine, should be performed initially.[59,60] Rebalance and strengthening of the muscular and skeletal system, particularly the cervicoscapular muscles, can correct poor posture, which helps relax the neck muscles and decompress the brachial plexus. Good posture should be maintained when sitting, standing, and walking.[59]

Exercise

The home program is initially directed toward range-of-motion exercises and stretching exercises for scalene muscles and other tight muscles. Then it can gradually strengthen the shoulder girdle muscles, including the trapezius, rhomboids, and levator scapulae muscles.[19,28] Elevating the arms above 90 degrees abduction should be avoided. It may take more than 2 to 3 months for symptomatic improvement to occur.

Medication

Patients can get relief from various medications, including analgesics, muscle relaxants, nonsteroidal anti-inflammatory drugs, and antidepressants. Pain clinics and biofeedback can be recommended for pain relief. Edema control with compressive garments, elevation, and retrograde massage is beneficial if swelling is present. Most patients are helped by conservative treatment and can manage their lives and tolerate their discomfort without surgery. If the symptoms have improved enough so that the patient can live with them, conservative therapy should be continued.

SURGICAL CONSIDERATIONS AND TECHNIQUE

Indications

The goal of surgery is to decompress the neurovascular structure at the thoracic outlet space. If there are vascular complications, direct approaches to the subclavian artery and vein should be considered, as well as decompression. Surgical procedures are directed toward a variety of normal and abnormal structures, including the anterior and middle scalene muscles (two sides of the scalene triangle), the first rib, the cervical rib, fibrous bands, and ligaments. Besides confirming the diagnosis and ruling out more common causes of symptoms in the upper extremity, indications for surgery include (1) failure of conservative management and physical therapy after several months; (2) completion of treatment of all associated conditions; (3) disability in terms of work, recreation, or daily activities; and (4) vascular complications. Kashyap and colleagues reviewed some of the advantages and disadvantages of different surgical approaches.[61]

Transaxillary Rib Resection and Partial Scalenectomy

This approach was originally described by Roos in 1966 and is arguably the most common approach used for thoracic outlet decompression.[16] First rib resection is recommended mainly for the lower type of TOS with C-8 to T-1 root symptoms.[19] Supraclavicular scalenectomy is applicable in patients with the upper type of TOS involving C-5 to C-7 roots[40] or in those with recurrence after first rib resection, thought to be due to scarring of the scalenes.[62] In our practice, the surgical strategy for neurogenic TOS is (1) transaxillary first rib resection and subtotal lower scalenectomy as a primary procedure and (2) completion scalenectomy with a supraclavicular approach for patients with recurrent symptoms who need surgery.

Technique

The patient is placed in the semisupine lateral position (45 to 60 degrees) with a soft axillary roll placed under the dependent axilla. The ipsilateral arm, neck, chest wall, and axilla are prepared. The arm is covered with a sterile cotton stockinette, wrapped with a gauze bandage, and then placed in a sterile arm holder for retraction. Retraction of the arm to the contralateral side and upward provides better visualization of the neurovascular structures in the axillary tunnel. However, it is important to avoid overzealous arm retraction with this approach, and occasional intermittent release of traction prevents arm ischemia or brachial plexus injury.

A transverse incision is made just below the hair-bearing area in the axilla between the pectoralis major and latissimus dorsi muscles (Fig. 37-7). The incision is deepened in the subcutaneous tissue until the chest wall is reached. The thoracoepigastric vein should be divided for adequate exposure. The brachiointercostal nerve may also have to be sacrificed to gain adequate exposure. A tissue plane deep to the axillary fascia and on top of the serratus anterior is bluntly dissected superiorly and anteriorly through loose areolar tissue. The highest thoracic artery, a branch from the axillary artery penetrating the first intercostal space, should be identified, ligated, and divided to avoid troublesome bleeding. Using further blunt dissection with a sponge-tipped hemostat, the loose tissue is cleared to identify the first rib. The subclavian vein, anterior scalene muscle, subclavian artery, brachial plexus, and middle scalene muscle are carefully dissected (see Fig. 37-7). The phrenic nerve anterior to the anterior scalene muscle must be identified and carefully protected. It is necessary to lift the arm carefully to facilitate the exposure. To avoid serious injury, the blade of the retractor must not apply traction to the nerve roots or the brachial plexus.

Once the anterior scalene muscle is dissected and the vessels are free, a right-angled clamp placed under the muscle elevates it away from other structures as the muscle is divided with scissors as far from the first rib as possible. The smallest scalene muscle, if it exists, is divided off Sibson's fascia and the C-7 transverse process. The middle scalene muscle is dissected and divided with scissors at the highest level feasible,

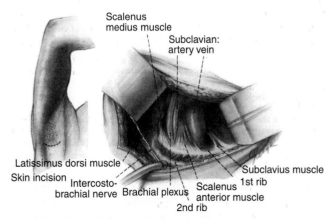

FIGURE 37-7 • View of thoracic outlet structures from the transaxillary approach to first rib resection. (From Machleder HI [ed]: Vascular Disorders of the Upper Extremity, 2nd ed. Mt. Kisco, NY, Futura Publishing, 1989.)

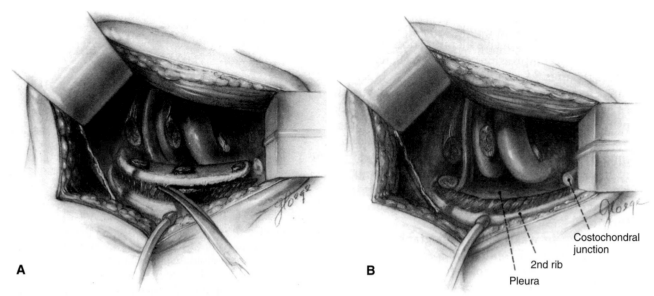

FIGURE 37–8 • Steps in transaxillary first rib resection. *A,* Division of subclavius, anterior scalene, and middle scalene tendons, as well as initial incision of the intercostal muscle. *B,* Relationship of structures after removal of the first rib.

with a right-angled clamp placed to hook the muscle. The long thoracic nerve posterior to the middle scalene muscle must be identified and carefully protected. The first rib resection is performed in an extraperiosteal fashion, except in areas where the vein or artery may be adherent to the periosteum and prone to tearing, where subperiosteal dissection is required. The intercostal muscle is pushed away by blunt dissection with a periosteal elevator (Fig. 37-8A). The first rib is then freed circumferentially by the periosteal elevator and a blunt-tip right-angled clamp anteriorly and posteriorly. With a Roos nerve protector shielding the C-8 and T-1 nerve roots, an angled bone-cutting instrument is carefully placed on the posterior neck of the rib and applied to cut the rib posteriorly. The subclavius tendon is divided sharply to the sternal joint space with a scalpel under direct vision, with careful protection of the vein. The rib is then divided anteriorly with a Bethune rib shear. The rib is thus detached and removed from the field (Fig. 37-8B). A large-angled bone rongeur is used to trim the anterior remaining end of the rib to the sternal joint. The posterior stump of the first rib is further truncated close to the transverse process using a box-shaped bone cutter. Any sharp bony fragments must be identified with visual inspection or palpation and removed. Any additional soft tissue bands crossing the brachial plexus nerve roots are sought and carefully divided. The remaining anterior and middle scalene muscles are trimmed further until the stumps are above the neurovascular bundle.

A drainage tube connected with closed suction is brought out through a separate stab wound below the incision. After closure of the subcutaneous tissue, the skin is closed using monofilament polypropylene suture with plastic surgery technique.

During the performance of this operation, adequate lighting and visualization need to be maintained because of the configuration and depth of the operative field. Cautery must not be used after reaching the first rib for fear of injuring the neurovascular structures.

Advantages and Limitations

This approach allows rapid exposure of the first rib without much manipulation of the subclavian vessels or brachial plexus. The incision itself is cosmetically appealing and allows for rapid recovery, and most patients leave the hospital on the first postoperative day. Many groups have used this procedure with short- and long-term success.[40,63,64] A cervical rib can be dealt with through the axillary approach.

The drawbacks of this approach are directly related to the operative view. Visualization is through a long axillary tunnel that must be adequately lighted to prevent injury, which occurs most commonly to the axillary vein or T-1 nerve root.[65] A supplementary light source from a headlight is indispensable, and we have found that a fiber-optic lighted retractor is paramount for the safe conduct of this operation. Congenital fibromuscular bands are sometimes hidden from view because they are most often medial and superior to the first rib and obscured by the neurovascular bundle.

In patients with arterial complications, an associated upper dorsal sympathectomy can be added easily. However, satisfactory exposure of the subclavian-axillary artery and its reconstruction are technically daunting.

Supraclavicular Scalenectomy with or without Rib Resection

Procedures performed through a supraclavicular approach include anterior and middle scalenectomy alone or combined with first rib resection.

Technique

This anterior approach to the thoracic outlet requires that the patient be placed supine. An incision is made in the supraclavicular area approximately 1 to 2 cm above and parallel to the clavicle between the internal and external jugular veins. Subplatysmal flaps are constructed, and the clavicular head of the sternocleidomastoid must be divided. The internal jugular vein is retracted medially, and if one is operating on the left side, the thoracic duct is carefully identified and may be ligated. The scalene fat pad must be reflected laterally or superiorly to arrive at the anterior scalene muscle. Coursing on the antero-medial surface of the anterior scalene muscle is the phrenic nerve, which must be carefully dissected free of the muscle and protected without undue tension. Then the muscle is transected at a low point, with care to avoid injuring the underlying subclavian artery. A simple scalenectomy has been advocated by some and requires division of the muscle close to its origin at the cervical transverse processes.[66,67] However, many advocate completion of the decompression by removing the first rib as well. Rib resection requires mobilization of the brachial plexus and division of the middle scalene muscle (Figs. 37-9 and 37-10). The long thoracic nerve exits in the posterolateral aspect of the middle scalene muscle and indicates the lateral margin of muscle division. Even after division of the scalenes, the operative wound should be palpated to identify any remaining fibrous or muscular bands causing compression. If a cervical rib is present, it will be found within the fibers of the middle scalene muscle. An extraperiosteal first rib resection is performed and requires detachment of the intercostal muscles at the inferior aspect of the first rib.[68] A subperiosteal resection of the rib may allow easier separation of the intercostals and less bleeding; however, reossification in the periosteal bed may lead to recurrent symptoms. Division of the first rib posteriorly is done as close to the transverse process as possible and requires gentle retraction of the brachial plexus anteromedially. After separation of the pleura and subclavian vessels from the first rib periosteum with blunt dissection, the rib is divided as anteriorly as possible, with retraction and separation of the subclavian vein and artery. The anterior division of the first rib has proved problematic in some patients, and some authors recommend a routine infraclavicular counterincision for rib division close to the costochondral junction, which is usually required for venous TOS.[69]

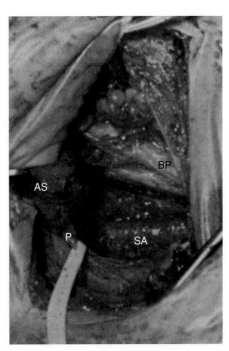

FIGURE 37–10 • Operative view of transcervical approach after resection of anterior scalene muscle. AS, anterior scalene muscle stump; BP, brachial plexus; P, phrenic nerve; SA, subclavian artery.

Advantages and Limitations

The main advantages of the supraclavicular approach are an excellent view of the structures in the thoracic outlet, with wide exposure and the ability to perform arterial reconstruction if necessary. Cervical ribs or prolonged transverse processes are easily removed with this approach.[70] Long-term success in correcting compressive symptoms has been documented.[71,72]

This approach requires the dissection and mobilization of the phrenic nerve, brachial plexus, and long thoracic nerve, which leads to its major disadvantage—the risk of nerve damage caused by traction injury or transection of these structures.[65] This approach is also limited for venous TOS.

Combined Approach

Technique

This approach requires the patient to be placed in the lateral decubitus position for the transaxillary approach and then moved to the supine position for the supraclavicular approach. Once the first rib resection is complete, the anterior and middle scalenectomy can be performed easily because most of the distal insertions were already released from the first rib during resection.

Advantages and Limitations

The transaxillary approach allows removal of the first rib in a safe and expeditious manner, and the supraclavicular approach allows complete scalenectomy and arterial reconstruction. The combination of both procedures allows complete decompression of the thoracic outlet and correction of the arterial source of embolization in one setting. This approach can be used in selected patients but is not needed for most patients with TOS.[73,74]

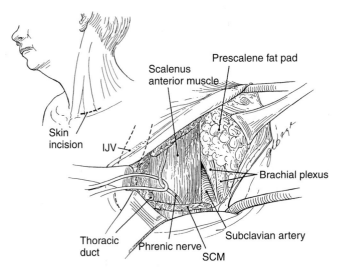

FIGURE 37–9 • Transcervical approach to scalenectomy for relief of thoracic outlet compression syndrome. The relationship of major surrounding anatomic structures is depicted. IJV, internal jugular vein; SCM, sternocleidomastoid muscle. (From Machleder HI, Moll FL: In Trout HH 3rd, DePalma RG [eds]: Reoperative Vascular Surgery. New York, Marcel Dekker, 1987.)

Posterior Approach

Technique

This approach requires a posterior periscapular incision, with division of the trapezius muscle and elevation of the scapula. With superior retraction, the thoracic outlet can be reached and the first rib freed from the surrounding structures. In Clagett's original description,[15] the rib is essentially removed subperiosteally, but then as much periosteum is removed as necessary to prevent bony regeneration.

Advantages and Limitations

Experience with this approach indicates that it may play a role in a few selected patients needing exposure of the proximal brachial plexus roots, particularly at the intraforaminal level.[75] Patients with prior anterior irradiation and tissue fibrosis who require exposure of the thoracic outlet or those requiring reoperations for TOS may also benefit from this approach.

This approach has not been widely accepted because of the relatively high morbidity compared with other surgical options. The incision and posterior dissection lead to considerable postoperative pain and shoulder disability. Further, visualization of the anterior structures is difficult, and arterial reconstruction is impossible with this approach.

POSTOPERATIVE CARE

An upright chest radiograph is performed in the recovery room to detect pneumothorax or phrenic nerve injury. A large pneumothorax may need transthoracic aspiration, but small air collections usually resolve spontaneously. Pain medication should be prescribed. Most patients leave the hospital on the first postoperative day. The closed suction drain is usually removed in the outpatient clinic once the total amount of lymphatic fluid discharge is less than 30 mL per 24 hours. Showering with sutures in place is allowed once drain sites are closed. Patients are encouraged to use the affected side to perform activities of daily living and to begin a home exercise program (arm exercises at least three to four times a day) starting on day 1. These exercises help prevent a "frozen" shoulder. Heavy lifting (>5 pounds) should be avoided until 3 to 4 weeks after surgery. We see patients for a follow-up visit within 2 weeks after surgery. Many patients return to work in 4 to 6 weeks. Sutures with plastic surgery technique should be removed 3 to 4 weeks postoperatively to prevent hypertrophic scars and keloids. Typically, patients undergoing surgery have had symptoms for a long time, and even after decompression surgery, they often have some residual or intermittent symptoms of dysesthesia, numbness, or other tolerable symptoms that may need ongoing attention.

SURGICAL COMPLICATIONS

Vascular, nervous, and lymphatic injuries can occur from decompression surgery for TOS.

Pneumothorax

Intraoperative pneumothorax occurs once the pleura is torn during the rib resection. It has been reported in up to one third of cases, being the most common complication of first rib resection.[53] However, the condition usually resolves spontaneously or by transthoracic aspiration without a chest tube. A closed suction drain is now used routinely and usually eliminates the need for a chest tube.

Nerve Injuries

Brachial plexus injury, either temporary or permanent, represents one of the most serious complications. This occurs as a result of excessive and prolonged traction of the arm in the transaxillary approach. Occasional intermittent release of arm traction is important during surgery. Another cause is inadvertent nerve traction during exposure of the scalene muscle or the first rib in the supraclavicular approach. Direct operative injury may also occur; the lower plexus (C-8 and T-1) is more commonly injured because it is in close proximity to the posterior end of the first rib. This injury is major and usually permanent. The motor deficit includes the long flexors of the fingers and the intrinsic muscles of the hand, although the sensory deficit involves only the small finger in the hand and the medial side of the forearm.[53] In large series, the incidence of permanent brachial plexus is less than 1% with each approach.[37,40,66]

The phrenic nerve, based on its relationship with the anterior scalene muscle, is prone to injury during scalenectomy, particularly with supraclavicular approach. The nerve should be carefully defined, using a nerve stimulator if necessary, before anterior scalenectomy. It should then be kept within a vessel loop. Although most injuries are temporary, they may take months to resolve. In patients with bilateral TOS requiring operation on the contralateral side, it is essential to ensure that phrenic nerve paresis has completely resolved before a second operation. If not, it may result in complete diaphragmatic paralysis and severe ventilatory incapacity.[76]

Long thoracic nerve injury can occur during middle scalenectomy. The nerve should be identified before excising the muscle. Traction injury to the long thoracic nerve may result in a winged scapula, although this is usually transient. Division of the nerve results in a permanent winged scapula.

The intercostobrachial nerve usually originates from the second intercostal nerve. It appears under the second rib in the midaxillary line, at the midpoint of the transaxillary wound. Injury to this nerve results in temporary or permanent numbness or paresthesias on the medial aspect of the arm. It is often sacrificed deliberately to allow better exposure of the thoracic outlet structures.

Injury to the Subclavian Artery and Vein

Vascular injury in the transaxillary approach may be difficult to visualize, because the exposure is very deep and limited, and the rib or the muscle may hide the injury. If the field becomes bloody, it is prudent to pack the operative field for a few minutes rather than proceeding. Most injuries are small initially. After tamponade of the vessel or removal of the rib, vessel repair can proceed. Another incision may be necessary to control the artery proximally if the bleeding is major.

Lymphatic Leakage

The thoracic duct usually empties into the venous system at the junction of the left subclavian vein and the internal jugular vein. However, the anatomy may be variable; there may be double ducts or significant branches.[77] Injury to the thoracic duct can occur in the supraclavicular approach on the left side. It is rare through the transaxillary approach or on the right side. The duct should be controlled with a suture or a vascular clip to prevent chylothorax.

RESULTS OF SURGICAL TREATMENT FOR NEUROGENIC THORACIC OUTLET SYNDROME

Decompression surgery for TOS has few standard objective criteria for evaluation, and most postoperative results are reported with a subjective grading of success that relies on the patient's response to treatment. Functional outcome is an important parameter, as is improvement of symptoms. Thus, the patient's ability to return to the same job provides a good index of operative success.

We define primary success as either 50% or more improvement on the ipsilateral side of the operation or the patient's return to preoperative work status without the need for an additional ipsilateral procedure. Secondary success is similarly defined following an additional ipsilateral procedure. We reviewed our recent 9-year experience of 254 primary first rib resections with partial scalenectomy via a transaxillary approach, followed by 80 secondary operations for recurrent symptoms using the supraclavicular scalenectomy in 185 patients.[78] The initial success rate at 2 months was 86.6% for primary procedures. Life-table analysis revealed that the primary success rates were 46.9% at 18 months, 37.6% at 36 months, and 36.0% at 72 months. The secondary success rates were 71.7% at 18 months, 58.9% at 36 months, and 49.1% at 72 months (Fig. 37-11). In evaluating these results, length of follow-up is a crucial factor, because recurrent TOS usually occurs within 18 months after the initial surgery; 90% and 65% of failures occurred within 18 months of primary and secondary success, respectively. Thus, reports with short-term follow-up may mask the overall success rate of the procedures performed.

In the literature, reported results were similar to our results. Improvement of neurogenic TOS symptoms may be noticed shortly after surgery, sometimes immediately.[19] The initially high percentage of improvement generally decreases after a few years.[19] When comparing different approaches, Sanders' review of the surgical results for TOS showed some interesting data.[79] Transaxillary, supraclavicular, infraclavicular, posterior, and transpleural first rib resection, as well as scalenectomy and combined rib resection, all had similar success rates. Additionally, in Sanders and coworkers' own series, which included transaxillary first rib resection, anterior and middle scalenectomy, and combined scalenectomy and rib resection, the 3- to 5-year success rate—with *success* being defined as enough symptomatic improvement for the patient to believe that the surgery was worthwhile—was approximately the same, and the overall improvement was 70% using life-table methods.[37,80]

One of the main causes of recurrent TOS is scar tissue formation around the brachial plexus and subclavian vessels, which follows nerve decompression operations anywhere in the body during the healing process. To minimize the effect of scar tissue and give early mobility to the brachial plexus and subclavian vessels, patients should be instructed to perform active range-of-motion exercises beginning the day after surgery, as mentioned earlier.

The most significant variable reported is the cause of the TOS. Occupational repetitive stress injuries were reported to be associated with poor outcome following TOS surgery.[28] Other studies have found that preoperative depression[81] and surgeries for some other compression syndrome, such as carpal or cubital tunnel syndrome, were associated with a worse outcome.

In recurrent TOS patients, symptoms may develop several weeks or months after the primary surgery. After 2 years, symptoms of recurrence occur less frequently.[82] In Sanders and colleagues' series of 134 operations in 97 patients for recurrent TOS using the transaxillary and transcervical approach over 22 years, the 84% initial success rate dropped to 59% at 1 to 2 years, 50% at 3 to 5 years, and 41% at 10 to 20 years.[62]

VASCULAR THORACIC OUTLET SYNDROME

Venous Thoracic Outlet Syndrome (Paget-Schroetter Syndrome)

Spontaneous, or effort-related, thrombosis of the axillosubclavian vein is a disabling disorder of young, otherwise healthy individuals. This type of thrombosis was described independently more than 100 years ago by Paget in England and Von Schroetter in Germany—hence, Paget-Schroetter syndrome.[83] With subsequent investigations, it is now understood that despite the apparent spontaneous nature of the event, there is an underlying chronic venous compressive anomaly at the thoracic outlet plus repetitive trauma (Figs. 37-12 and 37-13). The subclavius muscle tendon can be demonstrated to be the site of obstruction in many cases in which intermittent obstruction is present but has not yet led to thrombosis. Physical findings include obvious arm swelling and dilated collateral veins in the shoulder girdle region. Venography confirms the diagnosis. Pulmonary embolism from axillosubclavian vein thrombosis has been well documented,[84,85] and deaths from pulmonary embolism from these sources have been recorded in the surgical literature.[85] Studies of relatively large groups of patients have shown the value of immediate

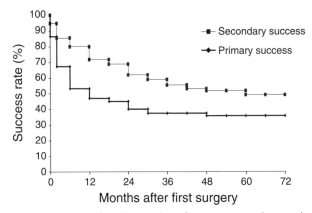

FIGURE 37–11 • Life-table analysis for primary and secondary clinical success rates after transaxillary first rib resection with partial scalenectomy followed by supraclavicular scalenectomy. Note that 90% and 65% of failures occur within 18 months of primary and secondary success, respectively. (From Altobelli GG, Kudo T, Haas BT, et al: Thoracic outlet syndrome: Pattern of clinical success following surgical decompression. J Vasc Surg 42:111–117, 2005.)

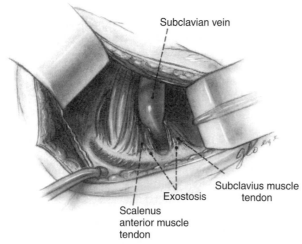

FIGURE 37–12 • Typical Paget-Schroetter abnormality. Hypertrophy of the subclavius tendon and associated exostoses are seen at the subclavius and anterior scalene insertions to the first rib (visualized from the transaxillary surgical approach). The vein is compressed in the most medial area of the thoracic outlet. (From Kunkel JM, Machleder HI: Treatment of Paget-Schroetter syndrome: A staged multidisciplinary approach. Arch Surg 124:1153-1158, 1989.)

catheter-directed thrombolytic therapy with urokinase followed by a period of anticoagulation to allow the acute phlebitic process to subside. Patients are then treated by transaxillary first rib resection to relieve the external compression. In patients with long-standing compression of the vein, stricture and fibrosis may result. This can be treated with transvenous balloon angioplasty after the external compressive elements have been removed. With this course of therapy, an excellent functional result can be expected.[86-88] Although studies have validated the staged, multidisciplinary approach, there have been reports of successful immediate surgical decompression following thrombolytic therapy; however,

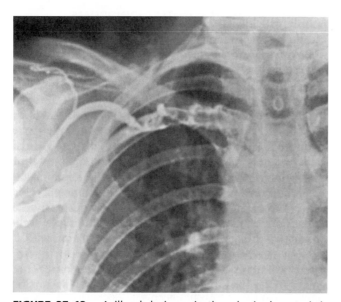

FIGURE 37–13 • Axillosubclavian vein thrombosis characteristic of Paget-Schroetter syndrome or the effort thrombosis variant of thoracic outlet compression syndrome. Note the collateral vessels and intraluminal thrombus.

these cases are insufficient in number to result in a publication available for general review.[88]

Arterial Thoracic Outlet Syndrome

The earliest lesion of arterial TOS is usually simple stenosis of the vessel lumen, which can spontaneously reverse after thoracic outlet decompression. However, long-standing, repeated compression of the subclavian artery may eventually result in post-stenotic dilatation and aneurysm formation with chronic inflammation. The most common cause is the presence of bony abnormalities (complete or incomplete cervical rib, elongated C-7 transverse process, or malunion following fracture of the clavicle or first rib).[89,90] In addition, isolated congenital bands, hypertrophic anterior scalene muscles, and physiologic drooping of the shoulder girdle can lead to arterial entrapment. The consequences range from relatively minor microembolic events to major vessel thromboembolic complications resulting in potentially limb-threatening ischemia.

Even when TOS has been recognized, the arterial manifestations may be overlooked because of the belief that nerve compression is causing the patient's symptoms.[91] As a result, the appropriate diagnosis may not be made until obvious ischemic changes of the upper extremity occur. Factors such as unilateral involvement, a predominant distribution in the hands and digits, and the absence of any underlying vascular disorders suggest artery-to-artery embolization. The diagnosis may be suggested by a pulsatile mass, subclavian artery bruit, atrophic skin changes, gangrene or ulcerations of the fingertips, history of fractured clavicle or ribs, and decreased blood pressure in the affected extremity. Duplex scan imaging of the vascular system at the subclavian artery can be useful. Transfemoral arteriography of the entire upper extremity vascular system, including positional views, should be used in any patient suspected of having arterial thoracic outlet compression.

Options for the surgical treatment of vascular TOS consist of (1) management of ischemia of the extremity, (2) decompression, (3) repair of the arterial lesion, and (4) dorsal sympathectomy. Surgical thrombectomy or catheter-based thrombolysis should be done after diagnostic angiography in the operating room. Usually, decompression surgery, including rib resection and scalenectomy, should be performed later to reduce the risk of hemorrhage. Vessels with aneurysmal changes or post-stenotic dilatation more than 2 cm should be resected and reconstructed with autogenous saphenous vein or synthetic prosthesis using the supraclavicular approach with an infraclavicular incision. An arterial lesion less than 2 cm can be left alone, and only rib resection and scalenectomy should be performed using the transaxillary approach. Dorsal sympathectomy can be performed through the axillary incision or under thoracoscopic guidance.[92,93] Increased cutaneous perfusion and improved pain threshold can be observed. Generally, excellent outcomes can be expected with timely diagnosis and treatment.[89,90]

Vascular Disease of the Upper Extremity

The upper extremities are subject to a variety of unique intrinsic arterial and venous disorders, as well as the peripheral manifestations of systemic collagen vascular diseases. Patients developing arterial insufficiency of the upper extremities generally demonstrate one of three different clinical patterns: (1) attacks of Raynaud's disease symptoms, (2) digital ischemia and gangrene, or (3) crampy pain with exercise, often referred to (with disregard for the word origin) as claudication. The initial examination of the upper extremity should begin with inspection, palpation, and auscultation. Noninvasive vascular testing, such as segmental systolic pressure measurement with Doppler flow detector, digital plethysmography, and duplex scan, can be used to further document the disorder.

AFFLICTIONS OF THE MAJOR VASCULAR STRUCTURES

About 50% of cases of acute arterial insufficiency of the upper extremity are secondary to embolization; of the remainder, 25% are the result of primary arterial thrombosis and 25% are iatrogenic in origin, including arterial blood pressure monitoring, sampling of arterial blood gases, and creation of an arteriovenous fistula for dialysis. Brachial artery catheterization is a well-documented cause of upper extremity ischemia.[94] Trauma to the brachial vessels generally carries a poor prognosis secondary to the commonly associated nerve injury (Fig. 37-14). When signs of ischemia accompany an upper extremity fracture, fracture reduction should be done as a primary maneuver, and reassessment of arterial integrity should be done promptly. Takayasu's arteritis should be considered, particularly in a relatively young female patient.

The vast majority of embolic arterial occlusions in the upper extremity are of cardiac origin, but brachiocephalic aneurysmal disease occasionally results in embolic episodes. The diagnosis of upper extremity ischemia is quite straightforward. The triad of symptoms—pain, paresthesias, and pallor—is generally

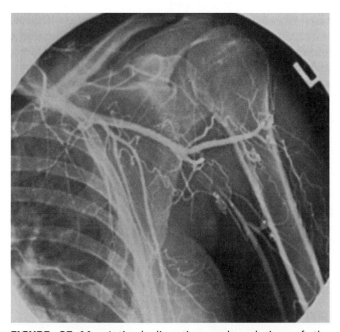

FIGURE 37–14 • Intimal dissection and occlusion of the axillobrachial artery at the level of the brachial plexus cords. This lesion is best repaired by reverse vein grafting, with care being taken to avoid entrapment of brachial plexus elements.

accompanied by a loss of radial and ulnar pulse and diminished segmental pressures on noninvasive testing. Diagnostic and therapeutic measures must be prompt in episodes of acute upper extremity embolization. It has been documented that patients treated within 12 hours of the embolic episode have excellent long-term results.[95,96] Two modes of therapy may produce satisfactory results: the immediate administration of continuous intravenous heparin with careful monitoring of the thromboplastin time, and embolectomy with careful observation for the development of compartment syndrome. High-dose local infusion of urokinase (250,000 units of urokinase dissolved in 100 mL of normal saline over 30 minutes) by a transarterial catheter has been effective in the lysis of intra-arterial thrombi.[97] This technique can be used intraoperatively to more effectively remove thrombotic material from the very vasoactive vessels of the upper extremities. If there is any clinical or radiographic evidence of vasospasm, 30 mg of papaverine can be infused via the same catheter.[98] Experience has also been accumulating on the use of recombinant tissue-plasminogen activator.[99]

SMALL VESSEL OCCLUSION IN THE UPPER EXTREMITY

The collagen vascular diseases manifest themselves by deposition of immune complexes in the intimal and subintimal surfaces of small vessels. Additionally, obliterative, proliferative processes characterize diseases such as scleroderma and diabetes. Scleroderma is the most common entity manifesting with digital ischemia. The fact that digital ischemia may precede systemic manifestations of these diseases adds to the difficulty of the initial diagnosis and emphasizes the need for a logical approach, which may have to be repeated during the evolution of the patient's disease.[100,101] The response to cigarette smoking, particularly in men suspected of suffering from Buerger's disease, is characteristic in this group of patients. The presence of digital gangrene in a young patient without evidence of atherosclerosis or aneurysmal disease, and particularly in the presence of normal upper extremity segmental pressures, should lead one to suspect a generalized collagen vascular disease. The process of gangrene in the fingers is quite different from that of necrosis, which is a wet suppurative process. Fingertip gangrene is more often a process of desiccation and mummification. Serologic tests are the basis of the diagnostic workup in these patients. Plain radiographs of the hands are also indicated. Evidence of skin atrophy and shiny tenseness or calcinosis of the skin are also valuable diagnostic findings. In cases in which skin biopsy is performed, immunofluorescence staining is extremely helpful. Specific arteriographic findings of collagen vascular diseases have been well documented: bilateral lesions; arterial obstruction without calcification; absence of atherosclerotic changes; smooth narrowing of the arterial lumen; total arterial occlusion or a stringlike appearance; multiple lesions, predominantly in the forearm and hand; less collateral circulation, giving a winding, corkscrew appearance; and small, attenuated terminal digital branches having the appearance of a "tree root."[102] Arteriography is also useful in excluding proximal lesions, although it rarely demonstrates specific changes characteristic of certain types of arteritis (Fig. 37-15). Medical management includes avoidance of cold exposure, use of gloves, discontinuation of tobacco use, and medication such as nifedipine, which is useful in relieving arterial spasm and associated digital ischemia.

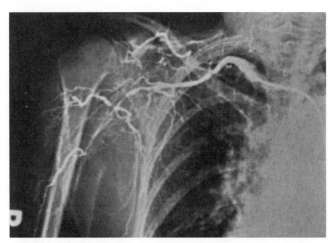

FIGURE 37-15 • Typical pattern of axillosubclavian arterial occlusive disease seen in giant cell arteritis.

Raynaud's disease is a vasospastic condition. Although associated with the collagen diseases, it can also be idiopathic. The chief symptom is a peculiar blanching and cyanosis of the fingertips due to profound vasoconstriction of the capillary beds caused primarily by exposure to cold and aggravated by the use of tobacco and caffeine. The diagnosis is confirmed by arteriography. Intra-arterial injection of 25 mg tolazoline (Priscoline) during arteriography relieves the spasm momentarily and elucidates the spastic process. Initial treatment is with calcium channel blockers, such as nifedipine 30 to 60 mg daily. Surgical treatment is a dorsal sympathectomy, often performed by a thoracoscopic approach.

ARTERIOGRAPHY

Arteriography can be useful in the diagnosis and assessment of vascular disorders of the upper extremity. The transfemoral route is preferred, particularly to enable visualization of the proximal aortic vessels and to avoid the need to traverse a potentially diseased axillosubclavian vessel. Proximal aneurysmal dilatation and atherosclerotic occlusive disease, as well as thrombosis and ulcerating plaques, are generally well identified radiographically. Proximal subclavian occlusion with subclavian steal phenomenon and retrograde flow in the vertebral artery is easily demonstrated. This lesion should be suspected whenever there is a pressure discrepancy greater than 20 mm Hg in the contralateral brachial artery pressure.

Magnification views of the hand during arteriography, particularly if augmented by hand cooling or warming, or injection of intra-arterial vasodilating drugs, such as papaverine or nitroglycerin, can differentiate between Raynaud's phenomenon, which is generally associated with segmental occlusions, and Raynaud's disease, which is generally identifiable only by vasospastic hypersensitivity. The angiographic characteristics of arterial vasospasm are marked delay in flow, a threadlike appearance, and tapered areas of occlusion relieved by the injection of vasodilating drugs or hand warming.

IATROGENIC VENOUS INSUFFICIENCY OF THE UPPER EXTREMITY

Although thoracic outlet compression can lead to axillosubclavian vein thrombosis, the vast majority of venous occlusive processes result from trauma or iatrogenic injury. Long-term intravenous alimentation, upper extremity intravenous access for therapy, or procedures such as central venous pressure monitoring and Swan-Ganz monitoring may result in axillosubclavian thrombotic episodes. It is important to recognize that chronic axillosubclavian vein thrombosis may be an indolent and relatively silent process and is seldom associated with symptoms in the upper extremity. Whenever this problem has been looked at prospectively, however, the incidence of venous thrombosis in the major upper extremity veins approaches 25%. Heparin therapy rarely leads to lysis but may prevent extension of thrombosis with removal of cannulas. Thrombolytic therapy with streptokinase or recombinant tissue plasminogen activator may prove efficacious. Reports of successful surgical therapy by either thrombectomy or interposition grafting do not demonstrate any superiority over conservative management, and the failure rate is sufficiently high that enthusiastic recommendation of surgical intervention cannot be supported.

KEY REFERENCES

Atasoy E: Thoracic outlet compression syndrome. Orthop Clin North Am 27:265-303, 1996.

Durham JR, Yao JS, Pearce WH, et al: Arterial injuries in the thoracic outlet syndrome. J Vasc Surg 21:57-70, 1995.

Jordan SE, Machleder HI: Diagnosis of thoracic outlet syndrome using electrophysiologically guided anterior scalene blocks. Ann Vasc Surg 12:260-264, 1998.

Machleder HI: Evaluation of a new treatment strategy for Paget-Schroetter's syndrome. J Vasc Surg 17:305-317, 1993.

Machleder HI, Moll F, Verity MA: The anterior scalene muscle in thoracic outlet compression syndrome: Histochemical and morphometric studies. Arch Surg 121:1141-1144, 1986.

Novak CB, Mackinnon SE: Thoracic outlet syndrome. Orthop Clin North Am 27:747-762, 1996.

Oates SD, Daley RA: Thoracic outlet syndrome. Hand Clin 12:705-718, 1996.

Sanders RJ, Haug CE, Pearce WH: Recurrent thoracic outlet syndrome. J Vasc Surg 12:390-400, 1990.

Sanders RJ, Pearce WH: The treatment of thoracic outlet syndrome: A comparison of different operations. J Vasc Surg 10:626-634, 1989.

Urschel HC Jr, Razzuk MA: Neurovascular compression in the thoracic outlet: Changing management over 50 years. Ann Surg 228:609-617, 1998.

REFERENCES

1. Cooper A: An exostosis. In Cooper, Cooper, Travers (eds): Surgical Essays, 3rd ed. London, 1821, p128.
2. Law AA: Adventitious ligaments simulating cervical ribs. Ann Surg 72:497-499, 1920.
3. Bramwell E, Dykes HB: Rib pressure and the brachial plexus. Edinburgh Med J 27:65, 1927.
4. Telford ED, Stopford JSB: Vascular complications of cervical rib. Br J Surg 18:557, 1931.
5. Ochsner A, Gage M, Debakey M: Scalenus anticus syndrome. Am J Surg 28:669-695, 1935.
6. Naffziger HC, Grant WT: Neuritis of the brachial plexus mechanical in origin: The scalenus origin. Surg Gynecol Obstet 67:722-729, 1938.
7. Falconer MA, Weddell G: Costoclavicular compression of the subclavian artery and vein. Lancet 2:539-543, 1943.
8. Peet RM, Henriksen JD, Anderson TD, Martin GM: Thoracic outlet syndrome: Evaluation of a therapeutic exercise program. Mayo Clin Proc 31:281-287, 1956.
9. Rob CG, Standeven A: Arterial occlusion complicating thoracic outlet compression syndrome. BMJ 2:709-712, 1958.
10. Machleder HI, Moll F, Verity MA: The anterior scalene muscle in thoracic outlet compression syndrome: Histochemical and morphometric studies. Arch Surg 121:1141-1144, 1986.
11. Sanders RJ, Jackson CG, Banchero N, Pearce WH: Scalene muscle abnormalities in traumatic thoracic outlet syndrome. Am J Surg 159:231-236, 1990.

12. Coote H: Exostosis of the left transverse process of the seventh cervical vertebra surrounded by blood vessels and nerves: Successful removal. Lancet 1:360-361, 1861.

13. Murphy T: Brachial neuritis caused by pressure of first rib. Aus Med J 15:582-585, 1910.

14. Adson AW, Coffey JR: Cervical rib: A method of anterior approach for relief of symptoms by division of the scalenus anticus. Ann Surg 85:839-857, 1927.

15. Clagett OT: Presidential address: Research and prosearch. J Thorac Cardiovasc Surg 44:153-166, 1962.

16. Roos DB: Transaxillary approach to first rib resection to relieve thoracic outlet syndrome. Ann Surg 163:354-358, 1966.

17. Gol A, Patrick DW, McNeel DP: Relief of costoclavicular syndrome by infraclavicular removal of first rib: Technical note. J Neurosurg 28:81-84, 1968.

18. Sanders RJ, Monsour JW, Gerber WF, et al: Scalenectomy versus first rib resection for treatment of the thoracic outlet syndrome. Surgery 85:109-121, 1979.

19. Atasoy E: Thoracic outlet compression syndrome. Orthop Clin North Am 27:265-303, 1996.

20. Lascelles RG, Schady W: The thoracic outlet syndrome. In Vinken PJ, Bruyn GW, Klawans HL (eds): Handbook of Clinical Neurology, vol 7. New York, Elsevier Science, 1987, pp 119–131.

21. Sanders RJ, Roos DB: The surgical anatomy of the scalene triangle. Contemp Surg 35:11-16, 1989.

22. Leffert RD: Thoracic outlet syndromes. Hand Clin 8:285-297, 1992.

23. Novak CB, Mackinnon SE: Thoracic outlet syndrome. Orthop Clin North Am 27:747-762, 1996.

24. Felson B: A review of 30,000 normal chest roentogenograms. In Felson B (ed): Chest Roentgenology. Philadelphia, WB Saunders, 1973, p 494.

25. Pollack EW: Surgical anatomy of the thoracic outlet syndrome. Surg Gynecol Obstet 150:97-103, 1980.

26. Adson WA: Surgical treatment for symptoms produced by cervical ribs and the scalenus anticus muscle. Surg Gynecol Obstet 85:687-700, 1947.

27. Sanders RJ, Hammond SL: Management of cervical ribs and anomalous first ribs causing neurogenic thoracic outlet syndrome. J Vasc Surg 36:51-56, 2002.

28. Sanders RJ: Thoracic Outlet Syndrome: A Common Sequela of Neck Injuries. Philadelphia, JB Lippincott, 1991.

29. Oates SD, Daley RA: Thoracic outlet syndrome. Hand Clin 12:705-718, 1996.

30. Roos DB: Congenital anomalies associated with thoracic outlet syndrome: Anatomy, symptoms, diagnosis, and treatment. Am J Surg 132:771-778, 1976.

31. Stockstill JW, Harn SD, Strickland D, Hruska R: Prevalence of upper extremity neuropathy in a clinical dentist population. J Am Dent Assoc 124:67-72, 1993.

32. Thomas GI, Jones TW, Stavney LS, Manhas DR: The middle scalene muscle and its contribution to the thoracic outlet syndrome. Am J Surg 145:589-592, 1983.

33. Qvarfordt PG, Ehrenfeld WK, Stoney RJ: Supraclavicular radical scalenectomy and transaxillary first rib resection for the thoracic outlet syndrome: A combined approach. Am J Surg 148:111-116, 1984.

34. Brantigan CO, Roos DB: Etiology of neurogenic thoracic outlet syndrome. Hand Clin 20:17-22, 2004.

35. Sanders RJ, Hammond SL: Etiology and pathology. Hand Clin 20:23-26, 2004.

36. Kai Y, Oyama M, Kurose S, et al: Neurogenic thoracic outlet syndrome in whiplash injury. J Spinal Disord 14:487-493, 2001.

37. Sanders RJ, Pearce WH: The treatment of thoracic outlet syndrome: A comparison of different operations. J Vasc Surg 10:626-634, 1989.

38. Liu JE, Tahmoush AJ, Roos DB, Schwartzman RJ: Shoulder-arm pain from cervical bands and scalene muscle anomalies. J Neurol Sci 128:175-180, 1995.

39. Sellke FW, Kelly TR: Thoracic outlet syndrome. Am J Surg 156:54-57, 1988.

40. Roos DB: The place for scalenectomy and first-rib resection in thoracic outlet syndrome. Surgery 92:1077-1085, 1982.

41. Brantigan CO, Roos DB: Diagnosing thoracic outlet syndrome. Hand Clin 20:27-36, 2004.

42. Wood VE, Ellison DW: Results of upper plexus thoracic outlet syndrome operation. Ann Thorac Surg 58:458-461, 1994.

43. Machleder HI: The initial clinical examination. In Machleder HI (ed): Vascular Disorders of the Upper Extremity, 3rd ed. Armonk, NY, Futura Publishing, 1998, pp 3-13.

44. Wright IS: The neurovascular syndrome produced by hyperabduction of the arms. Am Heart J 29:1-19, 1945.

45. Wilbourn AJ: Thoracic outlet syndromes. Neurol Clin 17:477-497, 1999.

46. Machleder HI: Thoracic outlet compression syndromes. In Callow AD, Ernst CB (eds): Vascular Surgery. Stamford, Conn, Appleton & Lange, 1995, pp 235-265.

47. Jordan S, Machleder HI: Electrodiagnostic evaluation of patients with painful syndromes affecting the upper extremity. In Machleder HI (ed): Vascular Disorders of the Upper Extremity, 3rd ed. Armonk, NY, Futura Publishing, 1998, pp 137-153.

48. Machleder HI, Moll F, Nuwer M, Jordan S: Somatosensory evoked potentials in the assessment of thoracic outlet compression syndrome. J Vasc Surg 6:177-184, 1987.

49. Siivola J, Pokela R, Sulg I: Somatosensory evoked responses as a diagnostic aid in thoracic outlet syndrome (a postoperative study). Acta Chir Scand 149:147-150, 1983.

50. Panegyres PK, Moore N, Gibson R, et al: Thoracic outlet syndromes and magnetic resonance imaging. Brain 116:823-841, 1993.

51. Collins JD, Shaver ML, Disher AC, Miller TQ: Compromising abnormalities of the brachial plexus as displayed by magnetic resonance imaging. Clin Anat 8:1-16, 1995.

52. Jordan SE, Machleder HI: Diagnosis of thoracic outlet syndrome using electrophysiologically guided anterior scalene blocks. Ann Vasc Surg 12:260-264, 1998.

53. Leffert RD: Complications of surgery for thoracic outlet syndrome. Hand Clin 20:91-98, 2004.

54. Upton AR, McComas AJ: The double crush in nerve entrapment syndromes. Lancet 2:359-362, 1973.

55. Askin SR, Hadler NM: Double-crush nerve compression in thoracic-outlet syndrome. J Bone Joint Surg Am 73:629-630, 1991.

56. Stanton-Hicks M, Janig W, Hassenbusch S, et al: Reflex sympathetic dystrophy: Changing concepts and taxonomy. Pain 63:127-133, 1995.

57. Wasner G, Schattschneider J, Binder A, Baron R: Complex regional pain syndrome: Diagnosis, mechanisms, CNS involvement and therapy. Spinal Cord 41:61-75, 2003.

58. Leffert RD: Thoracic outlet syndrome. J Am Acad Orthop Surg 2:317-325, 1994.

59. Crosby CA, Wehbe MA: Conservative treatment for thoracic outlet syndrome. Hand Clin 20:43-49, 2004.

60. Walsh MT: Therapist's management of brachial plexopathies. In Hunter JM, Mackin EJ, Callahan AD (eds): Rehabilitation of the Hand and Upper Extremity, 5th ed. Philadelphia, Mosby, 2002, pp 742-761.

61. Kashyap VS, Ahn SS, Machleder HI: Thoracic outlet neurovascular compression: Approaches to anatomic decompression and their limitations. Semin Vasc Surg 11:116-122, 1998.

62. Sanders RJ, Haug CE, Pearce WH: Recurrent thoracic outlet syndrome. J Vasc Surg 12:390-400, 1990.

63. Makhoul RG, Machleder HI: Developmental anomalies at the thoracic outlet: An analysis of 200 consecutive cases. J Vasc Surg 16:534-545, 1992.

64. Urschel HC Jr, Razzuk MA: Neurovascular compression in the thoracic outlet: Changing management over 50 years. Ann Surg 228:609-617, 1998.

65. Melliere D, Becquemin JP, Etienne G, Le Cheviller B: Severe injuries resulting from operations for thoracic outlet syndrome: Can they be avoided? J Cardiovasc Surg 32:599-603, 1991.

66. Cheng SW, Reilly LM, Nelken NA, et al: Neurogenic thoracic outlet decompression: Rationale for sparing the first rib. Cardiovasc Surg 3:617-624, 1995.

67. Fantini GA: Reserving supraclavicular first rib resection for vascular complications of thoracic outlet syndrome. Am J Surg 172:200-204, 1996.

68. Sanders RJ, Raymer S: The supraclavicular approach to scalenectomy and first rib resection: Description of technique. J Vasc Surg 2:751-756, 1985.

69. Robicsek F, Eastman D: "Above-under" exposure of the first rib: A modified approach for the treatment of thoracic outlet syndrome. Ann Vasc Surg 11:304-306, 1997.

70. Luoma A, Nelems B: Thoracic outlet syndrome: Thoracic surgery perspective. Neurosurg Clin N Am 2:187-226, 1991.

71. Hempel GK, Shutze WP, Anderson JF, Bukhari HI: 770 Consecutive supraclavicular first rib resections for thoracic outlet syndrome. Ann Vasc Surg 10:456-463, 1996.

72. Thomas GI, Jones TW, Stavney LS, Manhas DR: Thoracic outlet syndrome. Am Surg 44:483-495, 1978.

73. Cina C, Whiteacre L, Edwards R, Maggisano R: Treatment of thoracic outlet syndrome with combined scalenectomy and transaxillary first rib resection. Cardiovasc Surg 2:514-518, 1994.

74. Urschel HC Jr, Razzuk MA: Upper plexus thoracic outlet syndrome: Optimal therapy. Ann Thorac Surg 63:935-939, 1997.

75. Dubuisson AS, Kline DG, Weinshel SS: Posterior subscapular approach to the brachial plexus: Report of 102 patients. J Neurosurg 79:319-330, 1993.

76. Thompson RW, Petrinec D, Toursarkissian B: Surgical treatment of thoracic outlet compression syndromes. II. Supraclavicular exploration and vascular reconstruction. Ann Vasc Surg 11:442-451, 1997.

77. Langford RJ, Daudia AT, Malins TJ: A morphological study of the thoracic duct at the jugulo-subclavian junction. J Craniomaxillofac Surg 27:100-104, 1999.

78. Altobelli GG, Kudo T, Haas BT, et al: Thoracic outlet syndrome: Pattern of clinical success following surgical decompression. J Vasc Surg 42:111-117, 2005.

79. Sanders RJ: Results of the surgical treatment for thoracic outlet syndrome. Semin Thorac Cardiovasc Surg 8:221-228, 1996.

80. Sanders RJ, Hammond SL: Supraclavicular first rib resection and total scalenectomy: Technique and results. Hand Clin. 20:61-70, 2004.

81. Axelrod DA, Proctor MC, Geisser ME, et al: Outcomes after surgery for thoracic outlet syndrome. J Vasc Surg 33:1220-1225, 2001.

82. Atasoy E: Recurrent thoracic outlet syndrome. Hand Clin 20:99-105, 2004.

83. Hughes ESR: Venous obstruction in the upper extremity (Paget-Schroetter's syndrome). Int Abstr Surg 88:89217, 1949.

84. Monreal M, Lafoz E, Ruiz J, et al: Upper-extremity deep venous thrombosis and pulmonary embolism: A prospective study. Chest 99:280-283, 1991.

85. Hingorani A, Ascher E, Lorenson E, et al: Upper extremity deep venous thrombosis and its impact on morbidity and mortality rates in a hospital-based population. J Vasc Surg 26:853-860, 1997.

86. Machleder HI: Effort thrombosis of the axillosubclavian vein: A disabling vascular disorder. Compr Ther 17:18-24, 1991.

87. Machleder HI: Evaluation of a new treatment strategy for Paget-Schroetter's syndrome. J Vasc Surg 17:305-317, 1993.

88. Machleder HI: Thrombolytic therapy and surgery for primary axillosubclavian vein thrombosis: Current approach. Semin Vasc Surg 9:46-49, 1996.

89. Cormier JM, Amrane M, Ward A, et al: Arterial complications of the thoracic outlet syndrome: Fifty-five operative cases. J Vasc Surg 9:778-787, 1989.

90. Durham JR, Yao JS, Pearce WH, et al: Arterial injuries in the thoracic outlet syndrome. J Vasc Surg 21:57-70, 1995.

91. Patton GM: Arterial thoracic outlet syndrome. Hand Clin 20:107-111, 2004.

92. Ahn SS, Ro KM: Thoracoscopic sympathectomy. Ann Vasc Surg 12:509-514, 1998.

93. Ahn SS, Wieslander CK, Ro KM: Current developments in thoracoscopic sympathectomy. Ann Vasc Surg 14:415-420, 2000.

94. Machleder HI, Sweeney JP, Barker WF: The pulseless arm after brachial artery catheterization. Lancet 1:407-409, 1972.

95. Kofoed H, Hansen HJ: Arterial embolism in the upper limb. Acta Chir Scand Suppl 47:113-115, 1976.

96. Savelyev BS, Zatevakhin II, Stephanov NV: Arterial embolism of the upper limbs. Surgery 81:367-375, 1977.

97. Chaise LS, Comerota AJ, Sonlen RL, et al: Selective intraarterial streptokinase therapy in the immediate postoperative period. JAMA 247:2397-2400, 1982.

98. Quiñones-Baldrich WJ, Baker JD, Busuttil RW, et al: Intraoperative infusion of lytic drugs for thrombotic complications of revascularization. J Vasc Surg 10:408-417, 1989.

99. Cejna M, Salomonowitz E, Wohlschlager H, et al: rt-PA thrombolysis in acute thromboembolic upper-extremity arterial occlusion. Cardiovasc Intervent Radiol 23:218-223, 2001.

100. Fan PT, Davis JA, Somer T, et al: A clinical approach to systemic vasculitis. Semin Arthritis Rheum 9:248-304, 1980.

101. Fauci AS, Hanes BF, Katz P: The spectrum of vasculitis: Clinical, pathologic, immunologic and therapeutic considerations. Ann Intern Med 89:660-676, 1978.

102. Rivera R: Roentgenographic diagnosis of Buerger's disease. Cardiovasc Surg 14:40-46, 1973.

Questions

1. **Allen's test is useful in evaluating which of the following?**
   (a) Thoracic outlet compression
   (b) Presence of cervical rib
   (c) Integrity of palmar arch
   (d) Digital blood flow
   (e) Acute effort thrombosis

2. **The thoracic outlet is bounded by which of the following structures? (More than one may be correct.)**
   (a) Medial border of sternum
   (b) First thoracic rib
   (c) Clavicle
   (d) Subclavian artery
   (e) Subclavius tendon

3. **The thoracic outlet is traversed by which of the following structures? (More than one may be correct.)**
   (a) Subclavian artery
   (b) Brachial plexus
   (c) Anterior scalene muscle
   (d) Pectoralis major tendon
   (e) Middle scalene muscle

4. **Digital gangrene is not associated with which of the following?**
   (a) Buerger's disease
   (b) Vasculitis
   (c) Raynaud's disease
   (d) Arterial thoracic outlet syndrome
   (e) Paget-Schroetter disease

5. **Digital plethysmographic tracings are most apt to be misinterpreted secondary to which of the following?**
   (a) Cuff malfunction
   (b) Transducer malfunction
   (c) Segmental arterial occlusions
   (d) Changes in sympathetic activity
   (e) Poor light

6. **Which of the following is a common cause of prominent right-sided supraclavicular pulsation?**
   (a) Common carotid aneurysm
   (b) Subclavian aneurysm
   (c) Subclavian tortuosity or elongation
   (d) Innominate artery aneurysm
   (e) Mycotic aneurysm

7. **Effort thrombosis of the subclavian vein is often associated with which of the following?**
   (a) Straining at bowel movement
   (b) Hypercoagulation syndrome
   (c) Thoracic outlet compression syndrome
   (d) Calcinosis cutis, Raynaud's phenomenon, sclerodactyly, and telangiectasia (CRST syndrome) or scleroderma
   (e) Collagen vascular disease in general

8. **What is the correct course when peripheral pulses are absent following fracture-dislocation of the humerus?**
   (a) Arteriography should be done promptly before reduction
   (b) Arterial exploration should be done at the fracture site as the first step
   (c) Fracture reduction should be followed by arterial re-evaluation
   (d) Sympathetic block should be performed immediately
   (e) Pulses should be rechecked in about 1 hour, before fracture manipulation

9. Diagnosis of thoracic outlet syndrome has to fulfill which of the following criteria?
   (a) Symptoms referable to the thoracic outlet neurovascular bundle
   (b) Compression of the neurovascular bundle at the thoracic outlet space
   (c) Symptoms related to compression
   (d) No other explanation for symptoms
   (e) All of the above

10. When diagnosing neurogenic thoracic outlet syndrome, the single best test to determine if symptoms are related to the compression of the neurovascular bundle at the thoracic outlet is which of the following?
   (a) Magnetic resonance angiography
   (b) Magnetic resonance venography
   (c) An electrophysiologic test, such as electromyogram or somatosensory evoked potential test
   (d) EMG-guided scalene muscle stimulation and block test
   (e) Provocative Adson's or abduction and external rotation test

Answers

1. c	2. b, c, e	3. a, b	4. e	5. d
6. c	7. c	8. c	9. e	10. d

38

Robert S. Bennion • Samuel E. Wilson

Hemodialysis and Vascular Access

Direct access to the vascular system for the delivery of medications and for the removal of life-threatening endogenous or exogenous chemicals from the circulation is one of the foundations of modern clinical practice. In broad terms, vascular access includes any form of cannulation of arteries or veins. This chapter reviews the historical aspects; provides a practical consideration of percutaneous cannulation, autogenous fistulas, and internal arteriovenous fistulas; and discusses the prevention of complications and the outcome for each type of vascular access.

Temporary access to the venous system for the infusion of drugs or the transfusion of blood products has been in fairly common practice for well over 300 years. Sir Christopher Wren, the great 17th-century English architect, is generally credited with developing an instrument for intravenous therapy in 1656, which was used for injecting drugs (opium and crocus metallorum) into the veins of dogs.[1] It consisted of a cannula, made from a goose quill, with a pointed tip, which permitted penetration of the skin and underlying vein. In 1663, Robert Boyle described and published Wren's experiments and was the first person to extend intravenous infusions to humans, using prison inmates in London as subjects.[2]

The development of long-term cannulation of the circulatory system, however, was spurred by the introduction of a practical hemodialysis machine by Kolff in the mid-1950s.[3] Initial enthusiasm for hemodialysis was blunted by the major technical problems associated with the need for repeated vascular access. Having to perform a cutdown on the artery and vein for each dialysis session, and then ligate these vessels at the termination of each procedure, essentially limited early hemodialysis to short-term therapy for acute renal failure. In 1960, the development of the Scribner arteriovenous shunt afforded relatively safe long-term access to the circulation,[4] and repeated hemodialysis for the treatment of chronic renal failure became a reality.

As shown in Figure 38-1, the number of individuals requiring vascular access for hemodialysis continues to rise. By the end of 2001, there were more than 400,000 people in the United States with end-stage renal disease (ESRD) from all causes, including nearly 100,000 who had just been diagnosed that year.[5] In what appears to be an ongoing trend, during the 10 years between 1992 and 2001, the number of patients on

hemodialysis doubled.[5] Figure 38-2 demonstrates the number of vascular access device insertions during the same 10-year period.[5] It is interesting to note the decrease in the number of access grafts inserted and the increase in the number of arteriovenous fistulas constructed during this time. These changes are in line with the recent guidelines favoring fistulas published by the National Kidney Foundation's Kidney Disease Outcomes Quality Initiative.[6]

Short-term Hemodialysis Access

The external arteriovenous shunt described by Quinton and colleagues in 1960 consisted of a loop of silicone rubber tubing lying on the volar aspect of the forearm connecting two cannulas placed in the radial artery and a nearby wrist vein (Fig. 38-3).[4] Although quickly and widely adopted as a practical means of providing access in chronic renal failure patients, three major disadvantages to the long-term use of external shunts became apparent: (1) high risk of infection because of the likelihood of bacterial contamination at the tubing's entrance sites in the skin, (2) frequent clotting due to the

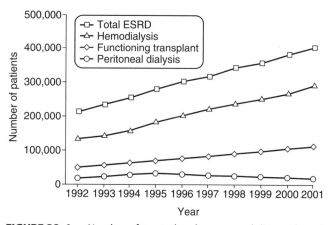

FIGURE 38–1 • Number of treated end-stage renal disease (ESRD) patients in the United States by treatment modality, 1992 to 2001. (Modified from US Renal Data System: USRDS 1999 Annual Data Report. Bethesda, Md, National Institutes of Health, National Institute of Diabetes and Digestive and Kidney Diseases, April 1999.)

Fistulas and grafts

Percutaneous catheter

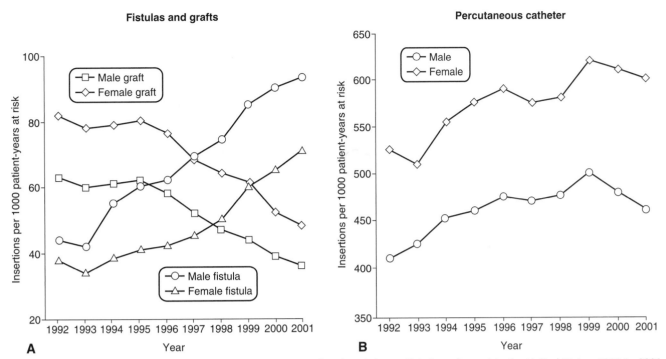

A   Year

B   Year

FIGURE 38–2 • Number of primary vascular access procedures for chronic hemodialysis performed in the United States, 1992 to 2001. (Modified from Owings MF, Lawrence L: Detailed diagnoses and procedures: National Hospital Discharge Survey, 1997. Vital Health Stat 13 145:1-157, 1999.)

small diameter of the silicone rubber and intravenous conduits, and (3) restriction of the patients' daily activities, such as bathing, by the external appliance and the extra care necessary to prevent dislodgment or infection. Consequently, patency rates of external shunts were very low.[7]

Although acute hemodialysis was once carried out primarily with external shunts, these have now been replaced by percutaneously placed central venous catheters.[8] This technique allows preservation of the vascular sites best suited for later construction of subcutaneous arteriovenous fistulas. The usual

indications for hemodialysis by percutaneous venipuncture are (1) acute renal failure in which only a short course of dialysis is required; (2) immediately after surgery, while awaiting maturation of an internal fistula in patients with chronic renal failure; (3) patients with poorly functioning transplants who have thrombosed arteriovenous fistulas; (4) patients needing urgent transfer from peritoneal dialysis; and (5) treatment of poisoning.

Short-term dialysis needs are met through the percutaneous introduction of a catheter into a major vein (Fig. 38-4). The catheters are usually introduced by the Seldinger technique over a guidewire and are commonly left in place for a week; with care, they can last up to several months.[9] The catheter may be changed over a guidewire every 10 to 20 days, and the catheter tip cultured; any drainage from the cutaneous entry

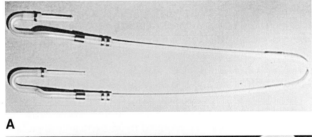

A

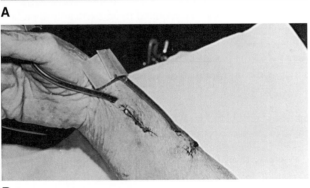

B

FIGURE 38–3 • *A,* Scribner shunt apparatus. *B,* Radiocephalic Scribner shunt in place.

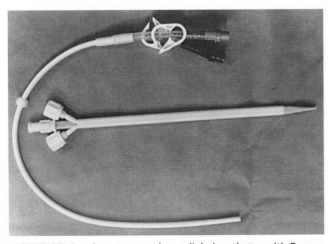

FIGURE 38–4 • Percutaneous hemodialysis catheter with Dacron cuff and oval dilator and sheath.

site is also routinely cultured. Depending on the clinical demands, either single-catheter dialysis with pulsatile flow or double-catheter dialysis with continuous flow may be elected. The latter is usually chosen when urgent and aggressive hemodialysis is necessary, because this is 20% to 30% more efficient than single-catheter dialysis. Thrombosis is prevented by continuous low-dose heparin infusion or an intermittent injection of heparin every 12 hours. Stable patients may be given the option of going home with the catheter in place and receiving intermittent heparin injections for outpatient dialysis. Interestingly, patients with these catheters in place have a 40% incidence of moderate to severe ipsilateral subclavian vein stenosis on angiography, whereas no stenosis was found in a control group of patients without a recent history of central venous catheters in the subclavian vein.[10] Placement of the catheter in the internal jugular vein is associated with less stenosis. Avoiding placement of a percutaneous access line ipsilateral to a planned permanent access site would be prudent.

Central venous catheters are usually placed via the internal jugular or subclavian vein into the superior vena cava; this involves the usual danger of a percutaneous puncture of a major vein.[11] The inferior vena cava may also be used; however, because of the danger of pelvic venous thrombosis, the catheter should not be left in place for a prolonged period. Although the incidence of catheter sepsis is generally low, one series reported a 28% incidence of infection in catheters left in position more than 4 weeks.[12]

Long-term use of percutaneous vascular access is becoming a more common form of chronic hemodialysis in patients with no other site for hemodialysis. Using a silicone dual-lumen catheter with a Dacron cuff, a 65% 1-year catheter survival rate and an 18.5-month median length of catheter use were achieved.[13] Although thrombotic complications occurred in 46% of patients, the use of thrombolytic therapy was successful in restoring catheter function more than 95% of the time. Catheter exit site infection in 21% of patients and bacteremia in 12% of patients were the other principal complications.

Autogenous Arteriovenous Fistula

The autogenous arteriovenous fistula, usually constructed by joining the cephalic vein to the radial artery at the level of the wrist or in the mid forearm, remains the most dependable type of long-term vascular access. One long-term prospective study demonstrated a useful patency rate for first-time fistulas of 90% at 1 year and more than 75% at 4 years.[14] In addition, revision of a failing fistula can extend its longevity. An autogenous arteriovenous fistula may be unsatisfactory, however, in patients (especially those with diabetes) with advanced atherosclerotic changes extending into the radial artery or in patients whose veins are too small, fragile, or thin walled for repeated needle punctures.

RADIOCEPHALIC ARTERIOVENOUS FISTULA

The subcutaneous autogenous arteriovenous fistula was initially described by Brescia and coworkers in 1966.[15] Readily accepted by nephrologists and surgeons, the Brescia-Cimino fistula, constructed of the patient's own vessels, largely overcomes the disadvantages of infection and early clotting found with external arteriovenous fistulas. After formation of the fistula, arterial pressure is transmitted directly into the contiguous

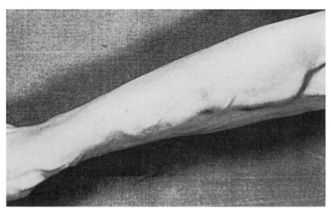

FIGURE 38–5 • View of dilated forearm veins following construction of a Brescia-Cimino radiocephalic fistula.

veins, resulting in dilatation and development of a hypertrophied muscular wall (Fig. 38-5). This "arterialization" of the veins may take up to 6 weeks before vessels of sufficient size and wall thickness have developed to tolerate repeated venipuncture. During this postoperative period, hemodialysis may be accomplished using internal jugular or subclavian cannulation.

Our technique is as follows. Before operation, the veins, preferably in the nondominant arm, are distended and examined using a sphygmomanometer with the cuff applied to the upper arm and inflated to below the systolic pressure level to produce venous engorgement. All suitably sized veins are marked with an indelible pen. This is done so that if the fistula of choice fails immediately after construction, these markings can aid the surgeon in identifying other possible fistula sites. The ulnar and radial artery pulses are palpated, and if there is any uncertainty about their adequacy, the systolic pressure in each is measured with a Doppler probe. Determining beforehand, using Allen's test, that the ulnar artery can support the circulation of the hand is advantageous to prevent symptomatic steal. The patient makes a fist and the examiner applies digital compression to the wrist, occluding both arteries; this is followed by pallor of the elevated and opened hand. Release of compression over the ulnar artery returns the hand's appearance to normal if the blood supply is sufficient. In addition to visual inspection, many surgeons perform duplex examination of both arms to find the most suitable veins.

Local infiltration anesthesia using 0.5% to 1% lidocaine is usually satisfactory for construction of autogenous arteriovenous fistulas in the forearm or antecubital fossa. Although general anesthesia may be required in an extremely apprehensive or potentially uncooperative patient, a report on the effect of different types of anesthesia on blood flow during construction of a fistula showed that general anesthesia significantly decreases mean arterial blood pressure compared with local infiltrative anesthesia or regional block.[16] In addition, brachial plexus block (supraclavicular approach) significantly increases brachial artery blood flow compared with local anesthesia. If available, an axillary block is an ideal anesthetic for vascular work in the forearm.

The arm is prepared with povidone-iodine, abducted at a right angle from the body on an arm board, and aseptically draped. The surgeon and instrument nurse are seated comfortably. An oblique or longitudinal incision is made midway between the radial artery and the cephalic vein. An adjacent

4- to 5-cm length of cephalic vein is dissected free of surrounding subcutaneous tissue. Its tributaries are ligated, freeing it further so that it lies adjacent to the radial artery without kinking or twisting. A 2- to 3-cm length of the radial artery, found under the deep fascia of the forearm, is also isolated from surrounding structures. The distal cephalic vein is divided, and its proximal segment is approximated to the radial artery in an end-to-side fashion using 6-0 monofilament suture and magnifying glasses.

Four different anastomotic connections of artery and vein have been used (Fig. 38-6), and each has its advantages and disadvantages:

1. *Side-to-side anastomosis*, with a fistula opening approximately 1 cm long, was the first procedure used. Technically, this is an easy anastomosis to construct and produces the highest fistula blood flow.[17] It is also the most likely fistula to be associated with venous hypertension of the hand.[18] This complication is moderated by the presence of venous valves that prevent reversal of venous blood flow in the hand, at least in the early months.

2. *Arterial end–to–vein side anastomosis* minimizes turbulence and distal steal of blood but results in slightly lower fistula flows and is subject to twisting of the artery during construction.

3. *Vein end–to–arterial side anastomosis* also decreases turbulence if constructed properly and results in the highest proximal venous flow with minimal distal venous hypertension.[19] It is more technically difficult to construct than the side-to-side fistula, and fistula flow overall is somewhat less. Most surgeons prefer this anastomosis because of the absence of vascular complications. If a branch vein is present, opening the inner aspect of the Y creates a generous oval patch to join to the side of the radial artery.

4. *End-to-end anastomosis* produces the least distal arterial steal and venous hypertension but has the lowest fistula flow of the four configurations.[20]

Proximal and distal control of the two vessels is gained by application of small vascular clamps or a fine silicone rubber sling. The vessels are anastomosed in the desired configuration with 6-0 polypropylene sutures, with knots placed outside the lumen. One must ensure that when approximating the artery and vein, spiral rotation of these vessels does not occur. Before the anastomosis is finally closed, a check is made by gently passing a coronary artery dilator to detect any stenosis. Hydrostatic dilatation with heparin-treated saline of a marginally small vein may aid in maintaining early patency.[21] Any bleeding from the anastomotic site should first be controlled by simple pressure with a gauze swab for several minutes. Too hasty a resort to suture repair is liable to produce further bleeding sites and narrowing of the anastomosis.

Upon conclusion, the artery and vein should lie without twists or kinks. A thrill should be easily felt over the fistula and propagated for a moderate distance along the proximal venous channel. A transmitted pulse without a thrill suggests an outflow obstruction or a clotted fistula. In this case, the proximal vein may be probed and inflated with a Fogarty catheter (avoiding intimal damage by not inflating the balloon during manipulation of the catheter) or carefully dilated with bougies. If these maneuvers do not produce a strong thrill and the fistula is technically satisfactory, construction of the fistula at another, more proximal site should be considered. On occasion, however, the appearance of a bruit and thrill is delayed until the veins dilate and blood flow increases, especially when no outflow obstruction can be demonstrated.

After the operation, the patient is sent home and asked to keep the arm elevated for 24 hours and not to sleep on the arm. Avoidance of constricting dressings, sphygmomanometer cuffs, and tight clothing is mandatory. Any swelling usually resolves over subsequent weeks. At least 4 to 6 weeks must elapse before the fistula will be ready for hemodialysis. Puncturing the vessels before they are arterialized is often associated with hematoma formation, because the dilated veins are thin walled during the first few weeks.[18] Although exercise of the forearm by squeezing a rubber ball to increase fistula flow and promote maturation of the arterialized veins has been advocated by some,[21] others have reported that it has no benefit.[22]

REVERSE ARTERIOVENOUS FISTULA

The internal reverse arteriovenous fistula is a method first used to salvage a failing fistula[23] (Fig. 38-7). This type of access procedure involves a side-to-side brachial artery–to–basilic vein anastomosis, thereby reversing blood flow into the superficial median antecubital and ulnar veins and providing an additional site for a hemodialysis fistula in patients whose forearm vessels have been exhausted surgically. The primary requisite for the procedure is the presence of a 4- to 5-cm segment of antecubital vein.

Two technical points are emphasized in this procedure for reversing the flow in the forearm veins. First, the valves in the forearm veins just distal to the level of the anastomosis must be ruptured with a blunt probe via a basilic venotomy; however, because of the previous venous arterialization, these valves are often incompetent and require minimal instrumentation. Second, in carrying out rupture of the valves, care must be taken

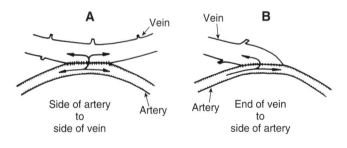

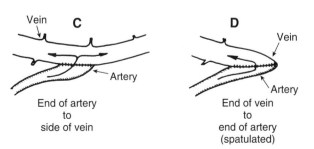

FIGURE 38–6 • Four anastomotic options for autogenous arteriovenous fistula construction.

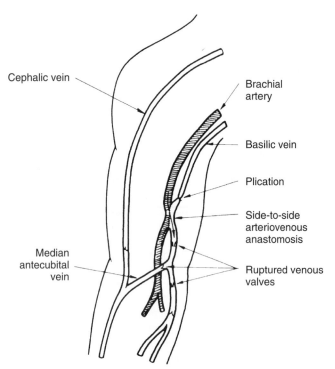

FIGURE 38–7 • Reversed autogenous arteriovenous fistula.

not to injure the deep brachial veins, because these eventually represent the major route of venous return in the arm, and damage to them may result in venous hypertension. First described in 1979, this procedure has limited application today.

BRACHIOBASILIC AND BRACHIOCEPHALIC ARTERIOVENOUS FISTULAS

Brachiobasilic (with vein transposition) and brachiocephalic arteriovenous fistulas may be used to achieve upper extremity vascular access after failure of a more distal extremity arteriovenous fistula or because the forearm vessels are inadequate.

Patency rates of 80% at 3 years demonstrate the usefulness of these areas for chronic hemodialysis vascular access.[24]

The brachiobasilic fistula (Fig. 38-8C) is constructed by initially identifying the basilic vein just anterior to the medial epicondyle of the humerus and then mobilizing the vein proximal to the axilla. Care must be taken during mobilization to avoid injuring the cutaneous nerves to the forearm, which lie adjacent to the vein. The vein is divided in the antecubital fossa and relocated in a subcutaneous tunnel running down the anterior aspect of the arm. The proximal end of the vein remains in continuity with the axillary vein. The brachial artery is isolated in the antecubital fossa, and the end of the relocated vein is anastomosed to the anterior aspect of the artery in an end-to-side fashion at this level, using a 1-cm arteriotomy.

Construction of the brachiocephalic fistula (Fig. 38-8B) is technically easier. The cephalic vein already lies in a superficial position on the anterolateral aspect of the arm, so there is no need for repositioning. The vein is mobilized a sufficient distance proximal to the antecubital fossa to secure a tension-free end-to-side anastomosis. To prevent steal, a branch of the cephalic vein—for example, the median cubital vein—can be used for the anastomosis.

Vascular Grafts (Bridge Fistulas)

Successful long-term management of chronic renal failure frequently means that the patient outlives the usefulness of several serially constructed vascular access routes. When an autogenous arteriovenous fistula is no longer feasible, the use of a prosthetic conduit to form a bridge arteriovenous fistula is the best alternative. Arteriovenous grafts can be placed between almost any suitably sized superficial artery and vein. After implantation, these easily palpable conduits can be readily punctured by a needle; however, if possible, this should be delayed for about 2 weeks until the prosthesis has been incorporated into the patient's subcutaneous tissue. Early puncture without careful hemostasis after needle removal may result in leaking of blood from the puncture site and formation of a perigraft hematoma.[25]

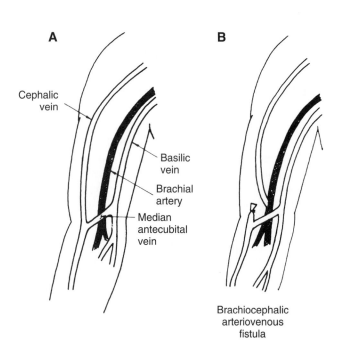
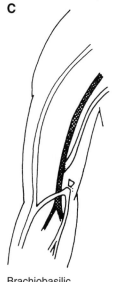

FIGURE 38–8 • Normal anatomy (A) and brachiocephalic (B) and brachiobasilic (C) autogenous arteriovenous fistulas.

The prosthetic material selected for the conduit in an arteriovenous bridge fistula is anastomosed end to side to the recipient artery and vein. If the two anastomoses are situated close to each other, the conduit takes on a U-shaped configuration; if they are separated by some distance, the conduit may lie straight or in a gentle curve. The conduit courses subcutaneously, allowing an adequate length for hemodialysis access.

SITES FOR ARTERIOVENOUS PROSTHETIC FISTULAS

Bridge arteriovenous fistulas can be constructed at almost any location where suitably sized arteries and veins are surgically accessible. For patient comfort, ease of handling during hemodialysis, and safety, however, the majority are constructed in the upper extremity or occasionally in the thigh.

In the upper extremity, bridge arteriovenous fistulas can be satisfactorily constructed between the radial artery and an antecubital fossa vein, between the brachial artery (in the antecubital fossa before its branching) and either the adjacent cephalic or basilic vein (U-configuration loop), and between the brachial artery and the axillary vein (Fig. 38-9). Construction of an upper extremity bridge fistula is often more technically demanding than the creation of a femoral fistula, and its long-term patency is not as high.[26,27] This is generally attributed to the larger vessels and greater blood flow in the thigh. The risk of infection and distal limb ischemia is less in fistulas constructed in the upper extremity,[25] however, and this is the preferred site. Patients with claudication or an ankle arterial pressure less than 80% of that at the wrist may not

be suitable for thigh fistulas because the proximal steal of blood through the fistula is likely to increase ischemia in the leg.[28] Therefore, upper extremity fistulas are particularly well suited for elderly patients with significant atherosclerosis in the lower extremities. Obese patients in whom perspiration or dermatitis involving the groin skinfolds may increase the likelihood of infection should have an arm fistula. Incontinence is a relative indication for implantation of the graft in the upper thigh.

The arterial anastomosis in the lower extremity should be to the superficial femoral artery, immediately proximal to either the adductor canal or its more cephalad portion (Fig. 38-10A). If the superficial femoral artery is occluded, the common femoral artery may be used (Fig. 38-10B), with the understanding that if it becomes infected and ligation is subsequently necessary, leg ischemia may ensue. At times, patency of a short segment, including the origin of the superficial femoral artery, can be reestablished and used for the arterial anastomosis. The venous anastomosis is made to the proximal saphenous, common, or superficial femoral vein.

Traditionally, the site selected for the initial placement of an arteriovenous bridge fistula was in the forearm, from the distal radial artery to the cephalic or basilic vein in the antecubital fossa.[29] The graft was anastomosed in an end-to-side fashion to the distal radial artery, tunneled along the lateral aspect of the forearm, and then anastomosed end to side to the largest vein in the antecubital fossa. In positioning the graft, one had to ensure that the patient's arm would rest comfortably when receiving hemodialysis.

Today, more common vascular access sites in the upper extremity include brachiocephalic or brachiobasilic loop fistulas in the forearm and brachioaxillary fistulas in the upper arm. Loop fistulas placed in the forearm allow a large area of graft to be available for needle puncture, whereas the brachioaxillary fistula, which curves over the lateral aspect of the upper arm, has several sites for venous anastomosis on the axillosubclavian segment. Upper extremity loop grafts have also been found to have significantly higher patency rates at all time intervals than do straight upper extremity grafts.[30] Upper extremity procedures can be performed using an axillary nerve block or local infiltration anesthesia.

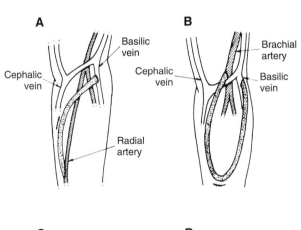

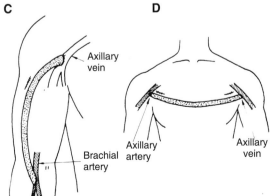

FIGURE 38–9 • Upper extremity bridge arteriovenous fistulas.

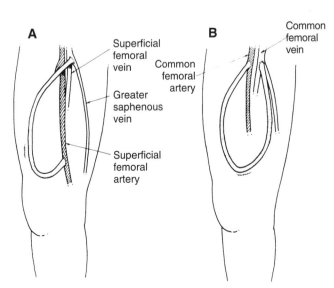

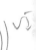

FIGURE 38–10 • Lower extremity bridge arteriovenous fistulas.

Arteriovenous bridge fistulas in the thigh are usually constructed with the patient under a spinal or general anesthetic, although in cooperative patients, a local infiltration technique can be used. Placing the arterial origin of the conduit just proximal to the adductor canal portion of the superficial femoral artery is often advisable so that if a vascular complication should cause occlusion of the artery, adequate collateral channels will provide filling of the popliteal segment. The end-to-side arterial anastomosis should be oblique, and the graft should leave the artery at an angle to minimize turbulence. The venous anastomosis is also performed in an end-to-side fashion and as obliquely as possible. This is to counteract any purse-string effect of the suture, as well as buildup of fibrin and fibrous tissue at the venous anastomosis, which commonly causes late graft thrombosis. A vascular steal phenomenon, with reversal of flow in the distal superficial femoral artery, is common in bridge fistulas in the lower extremity and can lead to symptoms of limb ischemia.[31] Fortunately, most patients with steal do not have symptoms, because dialysis patients are often fairly inactive.

The femorosaphenous bridge fistula is curved subcutaneously over the lateral aspect of the thigh and anastomosed to the proximal saphenous vein. The caudal portion of the saphenous vein may be ligated to prevent retrograde venous flow, although venous hypertension in the lower extremity is not a problem with a patent iliofemoral system. Another lower extremity access configuration is the loop fistula placed in the groin from the common femoral or very proximal superficial femoral artery to the femoral vein. The high blood flow rate (>1000 mL/minute) can lead to a significant increase in cardiac output. The possibility of limb loss in the event of infectious complications and the increased risk of infection make this site less desirable.[31]

With the longer survival of chronic hemodialysis patients, the surgeon may be asked to evaluate a patient who requires vascular access but whose extremity access sites have all been expended. In this circumstance, a more central location, such as a bridge arteriovenous fistula placed between the axillary artery on one side and the axillary vein on the other side, has been used successfully.[32] The grafts are of fairly large diameter, so they are easy to cannulate; flow is reported to be excellent, and despite the location of the access site on the anterior chest wall, patients adapt promptly.[23] The major drawback of central access sites is that when complications occur, they are serious and more difficult to manage.

MATERIALS FOR PROSTHETIC ARTERIOVENOUS BRIDGE GRAFTS

Both biologic and prosthetic materials have been used in the creation of arteriovenous bridge fistulas for hemodialysis since this modality was introduced in 1969.[33] Although saphenous vein, bovine heterografts, human umbilical vein, cryopreserved homografts, and Dacron velour grafts have all been tried during the last 3 decades, only expanded polytetrafluoroethylene (PTFE) grafts have had an extended period of observation.

Since its initial introduction as an alternative material for the creation of arteriovenous bridge fistulas in 1976,[34] expanded PTFE has become the most commonly used material. Much of its popularity stems from the fact that it is easy to handle, requires no preclotting, is widely available, has a long shelf life, and has relatively high patency rates with secondary revisions. PTFE bridge fistulas are consistently reported to have 12-month secondary patency rates of over 70%,[35] and in a large comparative clinical study comprising 187 graft placements, 36-month patency rates of PTFE grafts were significantly greater than those of bovine heterografts (62% vs. 24%).[36] Forty-eight-month patency rates of 43% to 60% have been reported.[37,38] However, multiple procedures for revision are usually required to maintain patency, with one study reporting an average of one operation for revision required every 1.1 years (range, 1 to 16 revisions per graft).[39]

Thrombosis of the conduit is a relatively common event in PTFE bridge fistulas, with figures ranging from 7% to 55%.[37,38] Most, however, are easily dealt with by thrombectomy and outflow revision, and some respond to simple Fogarty balloon catheter embolectomy alone.[38] Infection of PTFE fistulas is not uncommon, with one report of 80 fistulas monitored for 30 months showing an overall incidence of infection of 19%, with 67% of these infections occurring during the initial 4 months of use.[40] Of the infected fistulas, 73% required excision, and the remainder were treated successfully with antibiotics. The most common type of graft infection today occurs at needle puncture sites. Pseudoaneurysm at needle puncture sites develops in approximately 5% of fistulas.[37]

It is interesting to note that one study demonstrated that the overall patency rates of PTFE bridge fistulas with multiple secondary procedures are not significantly less than those of arteriovenous fistulas, although the arteriovenous fistulas require fewer revisions (Fig. 38-11).[41]

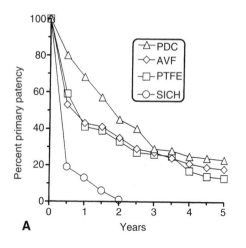

A

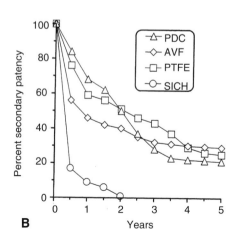

B

FIGURE 38–11 • Primary *(A)* and secondary *(B)* patency rates of peritoneal dialysis catheters (PDC), arteriovenous fistulas (AVF), polytetrafluoroethylene grafts (PTFE), and surgically implanted dual-lumen central venous hemodialysis catheters (SIHC). (Modified from Hodges TC, Fillinger MF, Zwolek RM, et al: Longitudinal comparison of dialysis access methods: Risk factors for failure. J Vasc Surg 26:1009-1014, 1997.)

Pediatric Vascular Access

Maintenance of chronic vascular access in children is a formidable task for vascular surgeons, with their small vessels being a major limiting factor. Although many of the principles and techniques are the same as for adults, certain aspects of the placement of long-term central venous catheters for total parenteral nutrition (discussed later) and the creation of hemodialysis access sites are sufficiently different to warrant discussion.

Dialysis (either hemodialysis or peritoneal dialysis) with subsequent renal transplantation is the preferred therapeutic regimen for ESRD in children. Transplantation is usually attempted as quickly as possible, because in general, children tolerate dialysis poorly; they frequently develop severe growth retardation (not reversible by transplantation), failure of maturation, renal osteodystrophy, and psychosocial problems.[42,43] In addition, long-term hemodialysis is, at best, difficult in children younger than 10 years and is extremely difficult in those younger than 5 years.

Short-term hemodialysis in children may be performed in a variety of ways with good results. Newborn or premature infants can be dialyzed via direct cannulation of the umbilical vessels using a 5 or 8 French catheter. Single-cannula hemodialysis may be used in older children in whom the superior or inferior vena cava has been cannulated by either the Seldinger technique or direct venous cutdown.[43] Another method in an older child involves placement of an indwelling brachial artery catheter and a large-bore central venous catheter via the external jugular vein to separate inflow and return and provide the hemodialysis return with a large-bore egress route.[44]

Long-term vascular access for hemodialysis in children weighing less than 20 kg may be accomplished by placement of a central venous catheter inserted as described previously.[44] In addition, creation of an autogenous arteriovenous fistula between the brachial artery at the elbow and an antecubital vein using microsurgical techniques has been done in children weighing between 10 and 23 kg, with excellent results.[45,46]

For long-term hemodialysis access in children weighing more than 30 kg, an internal form of access, either autogenous fistula or bridge fistula, should be attempted. For children weighing between 20 and 30 kg, the type of access attempted must be individualized according to the size of their vessels. A Brescia-Cimino autogenous arteriovenous fistula may be created in children weighing more than 30 kg without much difficulty, and with patency rates of approximately 80% at 12 months. The use of microsurgical techniques enhances the patency rate, especially in children with small vessels.[46] Bridge fistulas of PTFE have also been employed in children, with acceptable patency rates.

The usual types of complications and their rates of occurrence with both autogenous and bridge fistulas in children approximate those in adults. However, one of the most common complications of hemodialysis in small children is convulsions, occurring in up to 30% of patients.[47] This is probably due to two factors: the use of overly efficient dialysis, and the greater sensitivity of children to changes in osmolality. Convulsions can probably be avoided by tightly regulating the efficiency of the dialysis procedure based on the child's body weight.

One major disadvantage of the use of internal vascular access fistulas in children is the physical and psychological pain of repeated needle punctures, which may require much time and counseling to overcome.

Vascular Access Complications

INFECTION

Infection causes 10% of all deaths in dialysis patients, exceeded only by cardiovascular disease.[48] Many of the systemic infections encountered in these patients are direct complications of infection at the site of hemodialysis access. Two large dialysis centers found an incidence of 0.11 septic episodes per patient-dialysis-year related specifically to the vascular access site.[49] This represented more than 73% of the total number of septic episodes encountered.

The elevated rate of sepsis associated with hemodialysis vascular access sites is partially due to the deficient immune defense mechanisms in patients with chronic renal failure and the consequent increase in infection risk.[50] The bacterial phagocytic and killing ability of polymorphonuclear leukocytes also decreases by nearly 50% in patients with chronic renal failure.[51] Lymphocytes in chronic renal failure exhibit suppressed cellular immunity, and inhibition of lymphocyte transformation, which is unaffected by dialysis, has been detected.[52] In addition, the serum of uremic animals contains a nondialyzable inhibitor of the mixed lymphocyte reaction, which is probably a glycoprotein and distinct from either α-macroglobulin or immune complexes.[53] The actual ability of the animal to produce antibodies when antigen-stimulated, however, does not appear to be depressed in chronic renal failure.[54]

In addition to alterations in host defense mechanisms, other factors contribute to the increased propensity of patients on long-term hemodialysis to develop infection. Poor healing of surgical wounds is a recognized consequence of renal failure and may result in wound infections. Measurement of the bacterial colonization rate of patients receiving hemodialysis revealed that 62% of these patients carried *Staphylococcus aureus* in their oro- or nasopharynx or on the skin, and 65% of those patients with positive cultures developed infections in their hemodialysis access sites.[55] Further, 30% of the dialysis staff carried *S. aureus*, whereas only 11% of normal controls had positive cultures. In the same study, more than 70% of all infections encountered were caused by *S. aureus*. Strict antisepsis is the best means to prevent *S. aureus* colonization and reduce the risk of vascular access site infection.[56]

Although infection of an autogenous arteriovenous fistula is unusual, it can occur. Repeated puncture of the fistula may result in formation of a hematoma that can subsequently become infected by skin microflora. In addition, the anastomotic site of the fistula itself may become infected, resulting in an endovasculitis with subsequent septicemia and metastatic abscess formation. Treatment generally consists of therapeutic courses of appropriate antibiotic agents coupled with local measures such as drainage of a perifistula abscess from an infected hematoma. Rarely, the fistula anastomosis may have to be dismantled and the vessels ligated in the presence of an infection-induced anastomotic pseudoaneurysm.

Bridge fistulas placed for vascular access are susceptible to multiple sources of infection. Contamination from skin flora may occur during implantation and is more frequent when the fistula is placed in the thigh than when it is located in the upper extremity. In part, this is caused by the greater difficulty in preparing a sterile surgical field on the medial thigh and inguinal skinfold.[57,58] Direct inoculation of the graft by needle puncture through inadequately prepared skin also occurs, as well as inoculation of hematomas, resulting in perigraft abscess formation.

The type of material in bridge fistulas also affects the infection rate, with autogenous saphenous vein fistulas demonstrating few, if any, infections and biologic conduits (human umbilical vein graft, bovine heterograft) being particularly susceptible to aggressive infections; synthetic conduits are also susceptible to infection by low-virulence organisms.[59] The newly implanted prosthesis is particularly susceptible to infection; however, tissue incorporation and neointima formation confer increased resistance to infection.[60] A 2-week delay in initiating hemodialysis using bridge fistulas allows tissue incorpo-ration of the prosthesis and development of a neointima. Disruption of an infected bridge fistula anastomosis (Fig. 38-12) may occur at any time during the course of a prosthetic infection and does not appear to be influenced by incorporation.[59]

Treatment of an established infection of a conduit is excision of the prosthetic material. Attempts at in situ sterilization using antibiotics or povidone-iodine irrigation have not been reliably successful. A possible exception to this would be infection surrounding an autogenous saphenous vein prosthesis, for which treatment with antibiotics has been reported.[61] After excision of the infected access site, several days should elapse before placing a new access, for control of any associated bacteremia.

Regimens aimed at preventing this complication should always be practiced, including perioperative antibiotic administration. Randomized, prospective, double-blind studies have consistently shown the protective role of perioperative antibiotics in vascular surgery.[62,63] This was confirmed in a study of vascular access surgery, in which the perioperative use of a cephalosporin in a randomized, double-blind setting resulted in a significant decrease in postoperative wound infection rates, including cellulitis.[64] Vancomycin is very effective in the prevention of vascular access graft infections, especially in the pediatric population.[65] In addition, the use of aseptic technique by the dialysis staff and the patient is required to prevent infection at the site of hemodialysis access.

THROMBOSIS

The most frequent complication encountered in vascular access surgery is thrombosis of the fistula or shunt. The likelihood of thrombosis depends on multiple factors, including the type of shunt or fistula constructed, the site of the arteriovenous anastomosis, the prosthetic material used, and the adequacy of the patient's vessels. Thrombosis at the access site may occur at any time after construction. Early thrombosis, usually defined as occurring within the first month, is generally due to technical factors, whereas late thrombosis, occurring after a month, is usually caused by continuing trauma to the access site by needle puncture, outflow stenosis, or external pressure.

Lack of adequate venous runoff is the primary cause of early failure of distal access sites.[66] In the operating room, this can be recognized soon after completion of the final anastomosis by the absence of pulse, bruit, or palpable thrill. Ascertaining the patency and adequate diameter of the runoff vessel by use of a Fogarty embolectomy catheter or coronary artery dilators can guard against this setback. Narrowing of the lumen of the artery or vein during construction or catching the back wall of the vessel while suturing can result in immediate clotting. Thrombosis in the early postoperative period may also be due to compression of the fistula by a hematoma. This can result from inadequate hemostasis during the procedure or early puncture of the fistula, with subsequent extravasation of blood (Fig. 38-13). Excessive pressure over the needle puncture site after a hemodialysis run may also result in fistula thrombosis. In each of these situations, early re-exploration, with evacuation of any hematoma and thrombectomy of the fistula, often

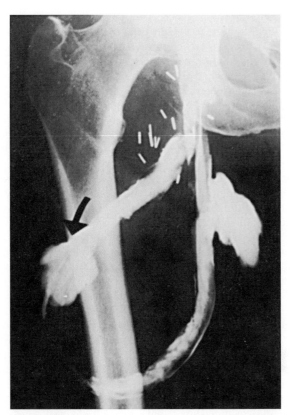

FIGURE 38-13 • Angiogram demonstrating extravasation of blood and hematoma formation *(arrow)* following too early use of a bridge fistula.

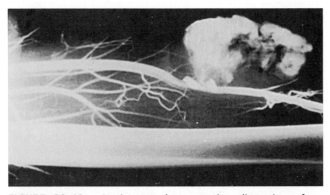

FIGURE 38-12 • Angiogram demonstrating disruption of an infected bridge fistula anastomosis.

results in salvage of the fistula.[67] Interventional radiology may be helpful in dissolving thrombosis with lytic therapy and improving outflow by transluminal angioplasty and stenting.

Thrombosis of a vascular access fistula may be due to repeated trauma from needle punctures, with subsequent fibrosis and narrowing. In synthetic bridge fistulas, a needle-induced flap tear of the prosthetic wall can cause late thrombosis.

Outflow obstruction due to stenosis at the site of venous anastomosis is a relatively frequent cause of thrombosis in older bridge fistulas and may be heralded by a gradual increase in the venous return pressure measured during hemodialysis. The combination of forceful pulsation throughout the fistula and a loud bruit at the venous end strongly suggests the development of outflow obstruction, which can be confirmed by angiography or duplex scanning (Figs. 38-14 and 38-15). True vessel aneurysmal dilatation from repeated needle punctures has also been reported as a major cause of late thrombosis in autogenous fistulas.[66] In addition, cigarette smoking significantly increases the likelihood of thrombosis and late occlusion of arteriovenous fistulas and should be avoided if at all possible.[68]

Fistula thromboses were treated successfully by thrombectomy, restoring flow in more than 80% of fistulas in one report.[69] This same study, however, indicated that approximately 70% of successfully thrombectomized fistulas reclotted within 6 months. This was thought to be due to unsuspected anatomic lesions and technical imperfections, which can be demonstrated with angiography.[70] Aggressive outflow revision, directed by angiography at the time of thrombectomy, has resulted in 6-month patency rates greater than 70%.[69]

Because elevated venous return pressure during dialysis is a very sensitive indicator of significant venous stenosis,[71,72] we strongly recommend some type of imaging of the fistula as soon as an elevation in venous return pressure is noted. Although fistula angiography remains the gold standard, noninvasive methods of assessing fistula flow are more convenient. Doppler ultrasound examination of the fistula can diagnose partial or complete thrombosis, aneurysmal dilatation, or perifistula hematoma with exceptional accuracy.[73,74] Today, ultrasound imaging should probably be the initial investigative technique in cases of suspected fistula malfunction. If recognized before thrombosis, venous runoff stenosis can often be corrected with percutaneous transluminal dilatation, with patency rates of 91% at 1 year and 57% at 2 years being reported.[75]

If acute thrombosis has already occurred, fibrinolytic agents may be successful in clearing the fistula of thrombus. In one series employing streptokinase, 52% of thrombosed fistulas were restored to function without surgical intervention, and another 21% had restoration of flow but required surgical correction of an underlying problem thereafter.[76] Another group was successful in restoring function in more than 65% of cases using urokinase.[77] The use of fibrinolytic agents in this manner appears to be most successful when the cause of failure is thrombosis secondary to hypotension or excessive compression of fistula puncture sites after dialysis. Fistula failure associated with excessive proliferation of neointima does not respond nearly as well and usually requires surgical revision.

In an effort to improve on the thrombogenic tendency of vascular access fistulas, prophylaxis against thrombosis has been attempted, with mixed results. One investigative group reported a highly significant reduction in fistula thrombotic episodes with low-dose aspirin therapy (160 mg/day).[78]

FIGURE 38–14 • Angiogram demonstrating stenosis near a venous anastomosis.

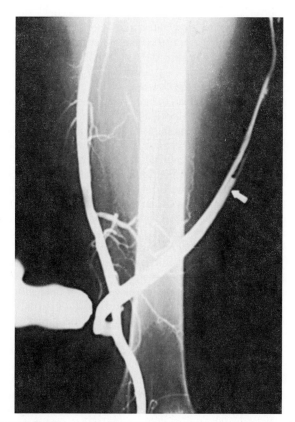

FIGURE 38–15 • Angiogram showing partially occluding thrombus (*arrow*) in a lower extremity bridge fistula.

Another group reported the successful establishment and maintenance of arteriovenous fistulas in nonuremic individuals by the use of aspirin and low-dose heparin therapy.[79] The use of oral pentoxifylline was found to significantly decrease access thrombosis in patients receiving long-term hemodialysis in one report, but this agent is not commonly used today.[80]

HEMODYNAMIC COMPLICATIONS

The three principal hemodynamic complications of an arteriovenous fistula are congestive heart failure; peripheral vascular insufficiency, or steal phenomenon; and venous hypertension. The physiologic responses associated with an arteriovenous fistula for hemodialysis include a decrease in total systemic vascular resistance; an increase in cardiac output, with increases in heart rate and, somewhat later, stroke volume; an increase in venous pressure and venous return to the heart; and reversal of flow in the artery distal to the site of the fistula when the diameter of the fistula opening exceeds the diameter of the feeding artery.[19,20,81] In addition, a significant decrease in subcutaneous tissue oxygen tension to levels less than 30 mm Hg occurs.[82]

Depending on the diameter of the arteriovenous communication and the size of the artery feeding it, the venous return to the heart from an arteriovenous fistula increases proportionately. This leads to a variable increase in cardiac output and work of the heart, which can be significant enough to lead to cardiomegaly and congestive heart failure. Fistula flow as low as 20% to 25% of the resting cardiac output has resulted in heart failure.[83] Because the mean blood flow rate through distal (radiocephalic) upper extremity autogenous or bridge fistulas has been measured in one report as 242 ± 89 mL/minute, high-output heart failure is unusual but does occur.[84,85] In the same report, resting flow rates from more proximal upper extremity fistulas based on the brachial artery were noted to more than double, averaging 641 ± 111 mL/minute. Similarly, bridge fistulas placed in the thigh arising from the superficial femoral artery had resting flow rates of 592 ± 134 mL/minute. Therefore, congestive heart failure is much more likely to result from a more proximally located fistula.

Initial blood flow through an autogenous arteriovenous fistula for hemodialysis is too low to cause heart failure, except in patients who already have severely compromised cardiac function.[85] With dilatation of the venous outflow system, shunted blood flow through the fistula can increase greatly. One group of investigators, using echocardiographic evaluation of cardiac performance, suggested that creation of any hemodialysis vascular access fistula causes a significant time-related cardiac decompensation compared with normal controls.[86] Echocardiographic assessment may also be useful preoperatively to identify patients with poor contractility, as manifested by changes in the mean velocity of fiber shortening, ejection fraction, and left ventricular or septal wall hypertrophy.[87] Abnormal studies may warn the clinician of a propensity toward future development of heart failure and lead to creation of the smallest and, if possible, most distal arteriovenous fistula compatible with adequate access.

When congestive heart failure arises from a high-flow arteriovenous fistula, operative correction is possible. Although revision of the fistula by narrowing the arterial anastomosis or construction of a completely new fistula may

be done to correct the problem, the simplest corrective procedure is banding of the existing fistula by suturing a small cuff (1 cm wide) of synthetic material (Dacron, PTFE) around the prosthesis of a bridge fistula or the main venous outflow tract of an autogenous fistula. An electromagnetic flowmeter is placed around the vein proximal to the fistula and banding cuff, and continuous flow is recorded. When the fistula flow is within the range of 300 to 400 mL/minute, the banding cuff is securely sutured.

Patients who are identified preoperatively as being at risk for access-induced congestive heart failure (e.g., elderly patients or those with existing cardiac dysfunction) and who require a bridge fistula should have either a tapered or a stepped graft placed. The diameter of the arterial end of these grafts is 4 mm, so that when they are placed in the patient (with the smaller end anastomosed to the artery), flow through the graft is somewhat reduced, thereby lessening the risk of congestive heart failure.

Arterial insufficiency, or steal syndrome, in patients with vascular access for hemodialysis was originally described as occurring in Brescia-Cimino fistulas with side-to-side anastomoses because of reversed blood flow in the distal radial artery.[88] An area of very low resistance is formed on the venous portion of the anastomosis so that the blood flow tends to course through the palmar arch from the ulnar to the radial side and steals flow from the muscles and soft tissues of the palm and fingers.[89] The syndrome is characterized by pain on exertion of the musculature of the hand, and the hand often appears cold, clammy, and pale. Severely symptomatic radial artery steal is rare, with one large study reporting only 8 of 444 patients who had 516 Brescia-Cimino fistulas constructed for hemodialysis (1.6%) developing significant steal symptoms,[90] although up to 80% of patients with Brescia-Cimino fistulas have mild, asymptomatic arterial steal documented by a significant decrease in thumb blood pressure.[91] Steal syndrome has also been described in 6.4% of 357 patients with upper extremity bridge fistulas, one third of whom required fistula ligation to preserve function of the hand, whereas the other two thirds were successfully managed with surgical narrowing of the arterial side of the fistula.[92] Surgical correction of radial steal from a side-to-side autogenous fistula has been accomplished by ligation of the radial artery immediately distal to the fistula, which converts the side-to-side anastomosis to an arterial end-to-side anastomosis.[89]

Arterial insufficiency has also been noted with the use of bridge fistulas in both the upper extremity[25] and the lower extremity[28] as a result of steal from the high-flow fistulas. When steal becomes symptomatic with bridge fistulas, restriction of arterial inflow (by placing a clip on the graft at the arterial end) to decrease fistula flow often causes these patients to become asymptomatic.[26] Very rarely, the entire fistula may have to be dismantled, or, if this is the only route for access, arterial ligation with distal revascularization using saphenous vein bypass results in restoration of satisfactory perfusion ("DRIL" procedure).

Arterialization of the venous system proximal to an arteriovenous fistula results in venous hypertension and, if the venous valves are incompetent, retrograde venous flow. Noted most frequently with side-to-side Brescia-Cimino fistulas and, to a lesser extent, reverse arteriovenous fistulas, retrograde venous hypertension is marked by distal extremity

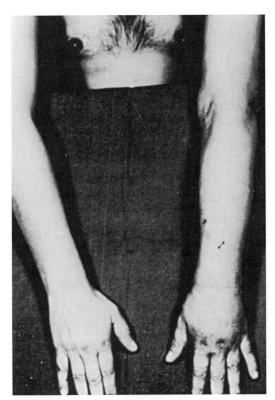

FIGURE 38–16 • Left upper extremity edema caused by venous hypertension from a Brescia-Cimino fistula.

edema, distention of superficial veins, and pigmentation of the skin (Fig. 38-16). Ulceration and neuralgias can also occur in long-standing cases.[93,94] Surgical correction is obtained by ligation of the vein immediately distal to the fistula, converting the side-to-side anastomosis of the Brescia-Cimino fistula to a functional venous end-to-side anastomosis, and converting the bridge fistula to a functional end-to-end anastomosis.

INTIMAL HYPERPLASIA

Progressive venous stenosis occurring as a consequence of vascular access fistula placement is a recurring problem leading to thrombosis and multiple revisions or replacement of fistulas in patients requiring long-term hemodialysis. Indeed, it is the main drawback associated with prosthetic conduits. Although the stenosis may be related to the technical performance of the anastomosis, it is mainly attributable to chronic changes known to occur in the runoff veins of arteriovenous fistulas. The development of intimal myointimal hyperplasia may result from focal endothelial trauma caused by the shearing effect of blood flow at the site of the venous anastomosis.[95,96] In addition, venous hypertension in the runoff vessels of an arteriovenous fistula causes intimal lipid deposition, further compounding the situation.[97] Segmental stenosis of autogenous fistulas and bridge fistulas constructed using biologic conduits has also been noted to occur from fibrosis and intimal hyperplasia secondary to the trauma of repeated needle punctures.[98]

Surgical correction of the stenotic area may be accomplished by patch angioplasty at the site of an anastomosis, by placing an extension of the graft around a long stenotic area, or by locating the venous anastomosis in a new vein. The use of percutaneous transluminal balloon angioplasty has been advocated for dilatation of stenotic segments in failing arteriovenous fistulas and shunts.[75] Using the Seldinger technique to gain access to the fistula, a double-lumen dilator catheter is placed at the site of the stenosis under fluoroscopic control, and the stenosis is dilated twice for 30 seconds each time. Before catheter removal, an angiogram is obtained, and the dilatation is repeated if greater than 30% residual stenosis is present. Using this technique, an initial success rate of 95% has been achieved.[75] Patency, however, is shorter than that achieved by surgical outflow correction.

ANEURYSM FORMATION

Aneurysmal dilatation of bridge fistula conduits depends on the material used. True aneurysm formation occurs primarily in biologic materials (saphenous vein, bovine heterograft, human umbilical vein graft) and has been attributed to degeneration over time of the graft material itself.[25] Early PTFE grafts were also prone to true aneurysm formation from nodal fracture and a gradual stretching of the PTFE fibrils[99]; however, with an increase in the wall thickness of PTFE grafts, this is no longer a problem. Excessive aneurysmal enlargement of the fistula is best treated by parallel placement of a new conduit of synthetic material. Pseudoaneurysm formation secondary to trauma at the site of needle punctures can occur with any of the materials used for bridge fistulas (Fig. 38-17). If no infection is apparent, treatment consists of local suture repair of the defect in the graft material. Somewhat larger defects may require excision of the defect and the interposition

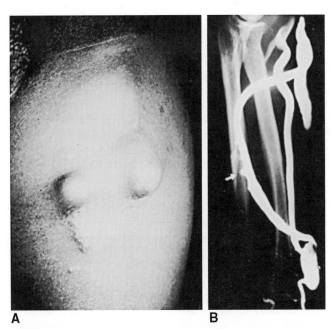

A   B

FIGURE 38–17 • *A,* Pseudoaneurysm formation at needle puncture sites of a hemodialysis fistula. *B,* Angiogram demonstrating multiple pseudoaneurysms *(arrow)* at needle puncture sites of a bridge fistula.

of a small segment of new graft material. Aneurysms are unsightly but may be safely observed unless skin breakdown or thrombosis occurs.

CENTRAL VENOUS OCCLUSION

Occlusion of the axillosubclavian veins or the superior vena cava in patients undergoing hemodialysis for ESRD via percutaneous catheters is a common occurrence. Over time, a central dialysis catheter can injure the endothelium of the large vein, resulting in thrombus formation, fibrosis, and eventually total occlusion. Nearly 5% of patients undergoing chemotherapy by peripherally placed central venous access devices developed symptomatic axillosubclavian vein thrombosis[100]; it is likely that more were asymptomatic. In dialysis patients, the proportion of symptomatic patients is increased to 12% because of the augmentation of venous flow in the upper extremity.[101] After catheter insertion, the time to development of thrombosis can be short, with venograms detecting partial thrombus formation in 30% and complete occlusion in 6% of patients by 6 weeks; 10% of patients had total occlusion by 12 weeks.[102]

The diagnosis of central venous occlusion is suspected on clinical grounds by swelling of the entire upper extremity, particularly if there is a rapid onset of edema after arteriovenous correction in that extremity. Subcutaneous collateral vein formation, venous aneurysms, and skin breakdown are often seen later. Dialysis personnel may report increased recirculation or elevated venous return pressure, but, somewhat surprisingly, most arteriovenous fistulas and access grafts continue to function even with central vein occlusion. Confirmation can be obtained with greater than 90% reliability using duplex ultrasonography, which detects occlusion by imaging the thrombus and showing an absence of spontaneous flow, no respiratory phasic flow, and an incompressible vein with increased collaterals.[103]

Initial treatment for acute central venous thrombosis is anticoagulation to prevent clot extension and potential pulmonary embolus. For most patients, clot lysis followed by percutaneous transluminal angioplasty and stenting is the first method to consider. Initial success can be expected in more than 75% of patients, with resumption of successful dialysis in more than 50%.[101] Cumulative patency rates of 70% at 2 years can be expected after salvage in this manner, although patency seems to decline rapidly thereafter.[104] If intervention is unsuccessful in a symptomatic patient, relocation of the access site may eliminate symptoms if there is a well-developed collateral circulation. A surgical approach is possible in selected patients with a limited segment of occlusion. The surgical options include transposition of the internal jugular vein to the axillary vein ("turndown" procedure), axillary-to-jugular PTFE bypass, and crossover bypass using a PTFE graft to the other axillary vein. The first technique has been used successfully in appropriate anatomic occlusions; however, there is minimal experience with the other two methods.

Because central venous catheters cannot be avoided entirely in hemodialysis, prevention of potential problems should be actively pursued. Techniques include limiting the duration of indwelling percutaneous catheters to approximately 6 weeks whenever possible and minimizing the use of Dacron-cuffed, tunneled, long-term catheters. A subclavian vein catheter has a higher incidence of thrombosis than one laced through the

internal jugular vein, although thrombosis associated with this insertion site certainly occurs. It is important to position the tip of the catheter in the superior vena cava at the right atrial junction because there is an increase in axillosubclavian vein thrombosis when the catheter tip resides in the brachiocephalic or subclavian vein. Patients who have had a catheter in place for more than 3 weeks should have routine screening duplex ultrasonography of the axillosubclavian veins performed before a permanent access site is chosen.

Vascular Access for Total Parenteral Nutrition or Chemotherapy

The use of surgically created arteriovenous fistulas to obtain vascular access for reasons other than hemodialysis is of interest. Several reports have found that chronic total parenteral nutrition (TPN) can be administered using arteriovenous fistulas that remain patent up to 7 years.[105,106] The advantages are a very low incidence of infection and longevity of the access site. The primary disadvantage is that the patient must undergo a significant operation to establish vascular access. The use of an autogenous arteriovenous fistula for the delivery of chemotherapeutic agents has also been advocated.[107,108] Bridge arteriovenous fistulas have been used; however, one series reported a significantly higher complication rate for bridge fistulas compared with Silastic right atrial catheters (48% vs. 19%) for chemotherapy use.[109]

Despite these reports on the use of arteriovenous fistulas for chemotherapy and TPN, the more common method used to deliver these therapeutic modalities is a chronic indwelling central venous catheter. For a number of years, the accepted method for central venous cannulation involved percutaneous catheterization with a polyethylene catheter. The propensity of percutaneously placed polyethylene catheters to develop infection and thrombosis and the inherent danger of the technique used to place these catheters led to the development of specialized large-bore catheters that are less reactive and less thrombogenic.

The Broviac[110] and Hickman[111] central venous catheters are made of soft, radiopaque material; they are 90 cm long and have a small Dacron felt cuff 30 cm from the external end. The only difference is that the Broviac catheter has an internal diameter of 1 mm, and the Hickman catheter's internal diameter is 1.6 mm. Each catheter consists of a relatively thin-walled intravascular segment and a thicker-walled extravascular portion. A smaller, pediatric-sized Broviac catheter is also available, as are double-lumen catheters in various sizes. These catheters are placed via direct venous cutdown into the cephalic (Fig. 38-18), external jugular, or greater saphenous vein, and the extravascular portion of the catheter is tunneled through the subcutaneous tissue to separate the skin exit site from the venotomy site. Fibrous tissue ingrowth into the Dacron cuff located in the subcutaneous tunnel serves to anchor the catheter and presents an effective barrier to the migration of microorganisms from the skin into the venous system along the outer surface of the catheter. For further protection against infection, some catheters have an additional cuff positioned in the subcutaneous tunnel between the Dacron cuff and the skin exit site. As a consequence, the sepsis rate with these catheters is relatively low.[112,113]

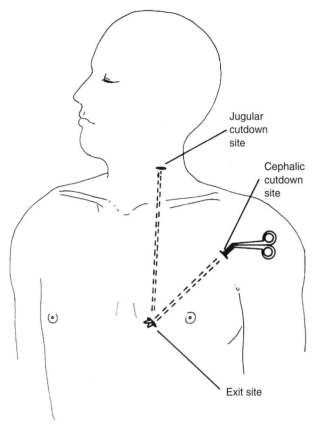

FIGURE 38–18 • Position of subcutaneous tunnel exit site for an upper body Broviac or Hickman catheter.

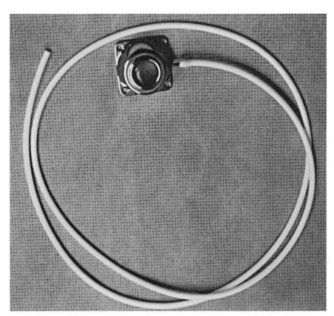

FIGURE 38–19 • Implantable port showing the reservoir with a self-sealing septum and the silicone catheter.

Innovations in central venous access include the introduction of the Groshong catheter and implantable ports. Unlike either the Hickman or the Broviac catheter, the Groshong catheter has no clamps, comes without the hub attached, and possesses a unique two-way valve. This valve is designed to remain closed when the catheter is not in use, and it opens either outward for fluid infusion or inward for blood draws. This design requires significantly less maintenance by either the patient or the health care worker, with only a single 5-mL saline flush being recommended once a week when the catheter is not in use. One group has suggested that less frequent flushings are needed if a heparinized saline solution is used.[114]

Implantable ports (Fig. 38-19) are central venous access devices that consist of a subcutaneously implantable reservoir containing a self-sealing septum that can withstand more than 2000 needle punctures. They are connected to a silicone rubber catheter with an internal diameter ranging from 1 to 1.6 mm. The reservoir body, which can be constructed of plastic, stainless steel, or titanium, is placed in a subcutaneous pocket over the anterior chest or abdomen in an easily palpable location and is accessed with a Huber needle for either blood withdrawal or drug delivery. These implantable ports have the advantage of requiring little daily care and therefore interfere less with the patient's normal activities. Also, implantable ports have a catheter-related sepsis rate of 3% and a 1% incidence of thrombosis, compared with a 15% rate of catheter-related sepsis and a 22% incidence of thrombosis in external central venous catheters.[115] A prospective comparison demonstrated that external shunts have 0.13 exit site infections and 0.03 bacteremic episodes per 100 catheter-days, compared with

0.06 pocket infections and 0 bacteremic episodes per 100 catheter-days for implantable ports.[116]

A newer subcutaneous port is the peripherally inserted central catheter line shown in Figure 38-20. A polyurethane catheter is placed via an antecubital vein and threaded into the superior vena cava. Its primary advantage is ease of insertion; the procedure can be performed at the bedside.

The placement of any central venous catheter for TPN or chemotherapy is always considered an elective, sterile, operative procedure. Thus, hypovolemia and any electrolyte abnormalities should be corrected before catheter placement.

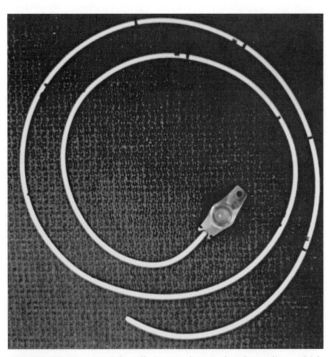

FIGURE 38–20 • Peripherally inserted central catheter line, which is placed via an antecubital vein.

Adequate lighting, instruments, assistance, and aseptic techniques are absolute prerequisites for the safe insertion of the catheter. The internal jugular vein is preferred for long-term patency and may be located with Doppler imaging. In patients requiring long-term central venous catheterization who have had numerous previous catheters placed, preoperative duplex ultrasonography or venography may be required to verify the patency of the vena cava (superior or inferior), the subclavian or iliac vein, or their tributaries.

In most hospitals, Broviac or Hickman catheter insertion is performed in the controlled environment of the operating suite, where radiography or fluoroscopy is available to confirm the proper position of the catheter tip before skin closure. The cutdown site is then selected. For the cephalic vein cutdown, the skin incision is made just inferior to the coracoid process in the area of the deltopectoral groove. For the external jugular vein approach, a transverse midcervical incision is made over the vein. When the greater saphenous vein is used, a longitudinal incision over the vein and just distal to the inguinal ligament is employed.

After dissection verifies patency and adequate size of the selected vein, a subcutaneous tunnel is made from the cutdown site to a cutaneous exit site medial to either the breast (if a cephalad central vein is chosen) or the anterior abdominal wall (if a caudad vein is used). A small stab wound is made at the cutaneous exit site, and the catheter is drawn through the tunnel until the Dacron cuff resides 2 to 4 cm inside the tunnel. The catheter is then shortened so that the tip just reaches the right atrium from the upper body or about the level of the renal veins from the lower body. The catheter is filled with heparin-treated saline by syringe. The vein is ligated distally, and the catheter is introduced through a small venotomy, advanced to its full length, and aspirated with the attached syringe. If dark venous blood does not return, the catheter is either kinked or misplaced, and it should be withdrawn and advanced again. A proximal ligature around the vein secures the catheter in place. Radiographic verification of proper catheter tip position should always be obtained before wound closure (Fig. 38-21). The catheter is fixed to the skin at the exit site with a monofilament suture, which is removed 7 to 14 days later, after fibrous ingrowth into the Dacron cuff has occurred. Povidone-iodine

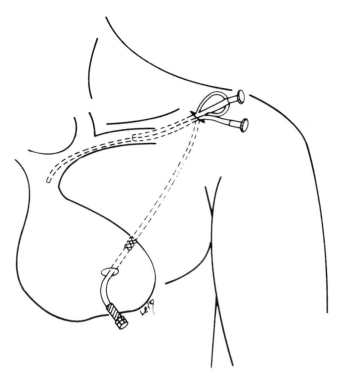

FIGURE 38–22 • Placement of a Silastic catheter by percutaneous subclavian venipuncture.

ointment and a sterile dressing are applied to the exit site, and the loop of redundant catheter is taped to the body wall. The catheter may be either heparin-locked or immediately connected to an intravenous infusion set.

Once they are properly inserted and positioned, Broviac and Hickman catheters have been left in place for more than 1 year, with an average duration of more than 2 months.[112,113] Because of the chronic nature of the underlying diseases in patients who require long-term catheterization, multiple insertions were necessary in 13% of patients in one study.[112] The primary complications of Broviac and Hickman catheter use are sepsis, thrombosis, and dislodgment of the catheter; in two series comprising 199 catheter placements, these complications occurred in 12%, 5%, and 3.5% of cases, respectively.[112,113] Central vein thrombosis as a result of long-term catheterization can also occur, but infrequently.

An alternative technique for the placement of Broviac and Hickman catheters involving direct venipuncture has been reported.[112] With this technique, two small (<1 cm) skin incisions are made at the proposed venous entry site and skin exit site, and a subcutaneous tunnel is created between them. The catheter is brought through the tunnel until the Dacron cuff lies 2 to 4 cm within the tunnel. The chosen vein is then punctured through the vein entry incision as if for placement of a central venous pressure line. A guidewire is inserted through the needle, thus allowing the needle to be removed. A vein dilator and peel-away sheath are placed over the guidewire, and once they are in place, the guidewire and dilator are removed. The Broviac or Hickman catheter is introduced into the vein through the peel-away sheath, and the sheath is withdrawn and peeled apart, leaving the catheter in place. Radiographic verification of catheter position is obtained, and wound closure and catheter care are performed as for standard Broviac or Hickman catheter placement (Fig. 38-22).[23]

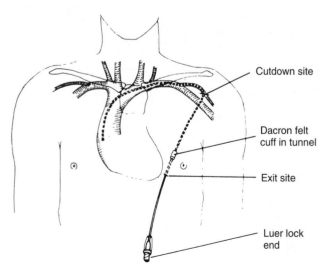

Cutdown site

Dacron felt cuff in tunnel

Exit site

Luer lock end

FIGURE 38–21 • Correct position of a Broviac or Hickman catheter placed via the cephalic vein.

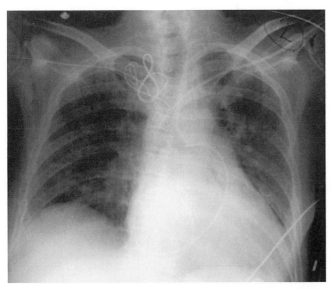

FIGURE 38–23 • Coiled percutaneously inserted central catheter.

Although malposition of the catheter (Fig. 38-23) is the most common complication of direct venipuncture,[117] any of the complications seen with standard central venous catheter placement are possible because of the relatively blind nature of the technique. These include pneumohemothorax, arterial laceration or perforation, arteriovenous fistula formation, brachial plexus or other nerve injury, air or catheter embolism, and lymphatic fistula formation.[11]

KEY REFERENCES

Hodges TC, Fillinger MF, Zwolak RM, et al: Longitudinal comparison of dialysis access methods: Risk factors for failure. J Vasc Surg 26:1009–1019, 1997.

National Kidney Foundation: K/DOQI Clinical Practice Guidelines for Vascular Access. Update 2000. Am J Kidney Dis 37:S137–S181, 2001.

REFERENCES

1. Garrison FH: An Introduction to the History of Medicine, 4th ed. Philadelphia, WB Saunders, 1929, p 273.
2. Wheatley HB: The Diary of Samuel Pepys, vol 2. New York, Random House, 1966, p 426.
3. Kolff WJ: The first clinical experience with the artificial kidney. Ann Intern Med 62:609-619, 1965.
4. Quinton WE, Dillard D, Scribner BH: Cannulation of blood vessels for prolonged hemodialysis. Trans Am Soc Artif Intern Organs 6:104-113, 1960.
5. US Renal Data System: USRDS 2003 Annual Data Report. Bethesda, Md, National Institutes of Health, National Institute of Diabetes and Digestion and Kidney Diseases, December 2003.
6. National Kidney Foundation: K/DOQI Clinical Practice Guidelines for Chronic Kidney Disease: Executive Summary. New York, National Kidney Foundation, 2002.
7. Ishihara AM, Meyers CH: Longevity of arteriovenous shunts for hemodialysis. Ann Surg 168:281-286, 1968.
8. Harder F, Landmann J: Trends in access surgery for hemodialysis. Surg Annu 16:135-149, 1984.
9. Dunn J, Nylander W, Richie R: Central venous dialysis access: Experience with a dual-lumen, silicone rubber catheter. Surgery 102:784-789, 1987.
10. Surratt RS, Picus D, Hicks ME, et al: The importance of preoperative evaluation of the subclavian vein in dialysis planning. AJR Am J Roentgenol 156:623-625, 1991.
11. Herbst CA: Indications, management and complications of percutaneous subclavian catheters: An audit. Arch Surg 113:1421-1425, 1978.
12. Giacchino JL, Geis WP, Wittenstein BH, Gandhi VC: Recent trends in vascular access. Am Surg 48:501-504, 1982.
13. Moss AH, Vasilakis BS, Holley JL, et al: Use of a silicone dual-lumen catheter with a Dacron cuff as a long-term vascular access for hemodialysis patients. Am J Kidney Dis 16:211-215, 1990.
14. Reilly DT, Wood RFM, Bell PRF: Prospective study of dialysis fistulas: Problem patients and their treatment. Br J Surg 69:549-553, 1982.
15. Brescia MJ, Cimino JE, Appel K, Hurwich BJ: Chronic hemodialysis using veni-puncture and a surgically created arteriovenous fistula. N Engl J Med 275:1089-1092, 1966.
16. Monquet C, Bitker MO, Bailliart O, et al: Anesthesia for creation of a forearm fistula in patients with endstage renal failure. Anesthesiology 70:909-914, 1989.
17. Johnson G: Local pathophysiology of an arteriovenous fistula. In Swam KG (ed): Venous Surgery in the Lower Extremity. St. Louis, Warren H. Greene, 1975, pp 41-50.
18. Bennion RS, Williams RA: The radiocephalic fistula. Contemp Dial 3:12-16, 1982.
19. Anderson CB, Etheridge EE, Harter HR, et al: Local blood flow characteristics of arteriovenous fistulas in the forearm for dialysis. Surg Gynecol Obstet 144:531-533, 1977.
20. Johnson G, Dart CH, Peters RM, Steele F: The importance of venous circulation in arteriovenous fistula. Surg Gynecol Obstet 123:995-1000, 1966.
21. Mindich BP, Levowitz BS: Enhancement of flow through arteriovenous fistula. Arch Surg 111:195-196, 1976.
22. Moran MR, Enriquez AA, Boyero MR, et al: Hand exercise effect in maturation and blood flow of dialysis arteriovenous fistulas. Angiology 35:641-644, 1984.
23. Giacchino JL, Geis WP, Buckingham JM, et al: Vascular access: Long-term results, new techniques. Arch Surg 114:403-409, 1979.
24. Bender MHM, Bruyninckx CMA, Gerling PGG: The brachiocephalic elbow fistula: A useful alternative angioaccess for permanent hemodialysis. J Vasc Surg 20:808-813, 1994.
25. Wilson SE, Stabile BE, Williams RA, Owens ML: Current status of vascular access techniques. Surg Clin North Am 62:531-551, 1982.
26. Owens ML, Stabile BE, Gahr JE, Wilson SE: Vascular grafts for hemodialysis: An evaluation of sites and materials. Dial Transplant 8:521-525, 1979.
27. Rohr MS, Browder W, Freutz GD, McDonald JC: Arteriovenous fistulas for long-term dialysis: Factors that influence fistula survival. Arch Surg 113:153-155, 1978.
28. Fee HJ, Golding AL: Lower extremity ischemia after femoral arteriovenous bovine shunts. Ann Surg 183:42-45, 1976.
29. Humphries AL, Nesbit RP, Carnana RJ, et al: Thirty-six recommendations for vascular access operations: Lessons learned from our first thousand operations. Am Surg 47:145-151, 1981.
30. Rizzuti RP, Hale JC, Burkart TE: Extended patency of expanded polytetrafluoroethylene grafts for vascular access using optimal configuration and revisions. Surg Gynecol Obstet 166:23-27, 1988.
31. Wilson SE, Hillman M, Owens ML: Hemodynamic effects of bovine femorosaphenous fistula. Dial Transplant 6:84-89, 1977.
32. Garcia-Rinaldi R, Von Koch L: The axillary artery to axillary vein bovine graft for circulatory access. Am J Surg 135:265-268, 1978.
33. May J, Tiller D, Johnson J, et al: Saphenous-vein arteriovenous fistula in regular dialysis treatment. N Engl J Med 280:770, 1969.
34. Haimor M, Burrows L, Schanzer H, et al: Experience with arterial substitutes in the construction of vascular access for hemodialysis. J Cardiovasc Surg (Torino) 21:149-154, 1980.
35. Baker LD, Johnson JM, Goldfarb D: Expanded polytetrafluoroethylene (PTFE) subcutaneous arteriovenous conduit: An improved vascular access for chronic hemodialysis. Trans Am Soc Artif Intern Organs 22:382-387, 1976.
36. Sabanayagam P, Schwartz AB, Soricelli RR, et al: A comparative study of 402 bovine heterografts and 225 reinforced expanded PTFE grafts as AVG in the ESRD patient. Trans Am Soc Artif Intern Organs 26:88-92, 1980.
37. Munda R, First MR, Alexander JW, et al: Polytetrafluoroethylene graft survival in hemodialysis. JAMA 249:219-222, 1983.
38. Palder SB, Kirkman RL, Whittemore AD, et al: Vascular access for hemodialysis: Patency rates and results of revisions. Ann Surg 202:235-239, 1985.
39. Schuman ES, Gross GF, Hayes JF, Standage BA: Long-term patency of polytetrafluoroethylene graft fistulas. Am J Surg 155:644-646, 1988.
40. Bhat DJ, Tellis VA, Kohlberg WI, et al: Management of sepsis involving expanded polytetrafluoroethylene grafts for hemodialysis access. Surgery 87:445-450, 1980.

41. Hodges TC, Fillinger MF, Zwolak RM, et al: Longitudinal comparison of dialysis access methods: Risk factors for failure. J Vasc Surg 26:1009-1019, 1997.
42. Offner G, Aschendorff C, Hoyer PF, et al: End stage renal failure: 14 years' experience of dialysis and renal transplantation. Arch Dis Child 63:120-126, 1988.
43. Gibson TC, Dyer DP, Postlethwaite RJ, Gough DCS: Vascular access for acute hemodialysis. Arch Dis Child 62:141-145, 1987.
44. Hiatt JR, Busuttil RW: A method for vascular access in small children. Surgery 93:343-344, 1983.
45. Kinnaert P, Janssen F, Hall M: Elbow arteriovenous fistula (EAVF) for chronic hemodialysis in small children. J Pediatr Surg 18:116-119, 1983.
46. Bourquelot P, Wolfeler L, Lamy L: Microsurgery for haemodialysis distal arteriovenous fistulae in children weighing less than 10 kg. Proc Eur Dial Transplant Assoc 18:537-541, 1981.
47. Nevins TE, Kjellstrand CM: Hemodialysis for children: A review. Int J Pediatr Nephrol 4:155-169, 1983.
48. Jacobs C, Brunner SP, Chantler C, et al: Combined report on regular dialysis and transplantation in Europe. Proc Eur Dial Transplant Assoc 14:3-69, 1977.
49. Dobkin JF, Miller MH, Steigbigel NH: Septicemia in patients on chronic hemodialysis. Ann Intern Med 88:28-33, 1978.
50. Peresesuschi G, Blum M, Aviram A, Spirer ZH: Impaired neutrophil response to acute bacterial infection in dialyzed patients. Arch Intern Med 141:1301-1302, 1981.
51. Salant DJ, Glover AM, Anderson R, et al: Depressed neutrophil chemotaxis in patients with chronic renal failure on dialysis and after renal transplantation. J Lab Clin Med 88:536-545, 1976.
52. Hurst KS, Saldhana LF, Steinberg SM, et al: The effects of varying dialysis regimens on lymphocyte transformation. Trans Am Soc Artif Intern Organs 21:329-334, 1975.
53. Raskova J, Morrison AB, Shea SM, Raska K: Humoral inhibitors of the immune response in uremia. II. Further characterization of an immunosuppressive factor in uremic serum. Am J Pathol 97:277-290, 1979.
54. Nelson J, Ormrod DJ, Wilson D, Miller TE: Host immune status in uraemia. III. Humoral response to selected antigens in the rat. Clin Exp Immunol 42:234-240, 1980.
55. Kirmani N, Tuazon CU, Murry HW, et al: *Staphylococcus aureus* carriage rate of patients receiving long-term hemodialysis. Arch Intern Med 138:1657-1659, 1978.
56. Kaplowitz LG, Comstock JA, Landwehr DM, et al: Prospective study of microbial colonization of the nose and skin and infection of the vascular access site in hemodialysis patients. J Clin Microbiol 26:1257-1262, 1988.
57. Morgan AP, Knight DC, Tilney NL, Lazaris JM: Femoral triangle sepsis in dialysis patients: Frequency, management, and outcome. Ann Surg 191:460-464, 1980.
58. Wilson SE, Van Wagenen P, Passaro S: Arterial infection. Curr Probl Surg 15:1-89, 1978.
59. Bennion RS, Wilson SE, Williams RA: Vascular prosthetic infection. Infect Surg 1:45-55, 1982.
60. Moore WS, Swanson RJ, Compagna G, et al: Pseudointimal development and vascular prosthesis susceptibility to bacteremic infection. Surg Forum 25:250-251, 1974.
61. Ehrenfield WK, Wilbur BG, Olcott CN, Stoney RJ: Autogenous tissue reconstruction in the management of infected prosthetic grafts. Surgery 85:82-92, 1979.
62. Kaiser AB, Clayson DR, Mulherin JL, et al: Antibiotic prophylaxis in vascular surgery. Ann Surg 188:283-289, 1978.
63. Pitt HA, Postier RG, MacGowen WAL, et al: Prophylactic antibiotics in vascular surgery. Ann Surg 192:356-364, 1980.
64. Bennion RS, Hiatt JR, Williams RA, Wilson SE: A randomized, prospective study of perioperative antimicrobial prophylaxis for vascular access surgery. J Cardiovasc Surg (Torino) 26:270-274, 1985.
65. Fivush BA, Bock GH, Guzzetta PC, et al: Vancomycin prevents polytetrafluoroethylene graft infections in pediatric patients receiving chronic hemodialysis. Am J Kidney Dis 5:120-123, 1985.
66. Raju S: PTFE grafts for hemodialysis access: Techniques for insertion and management of complications. Ann Surg 206:666-673, 1987.
67. Bell DD, Rosental JJ: Arteriovenous graft life in chronic hemodialysis: A need for prolongation. Arch Surg 123:1169-1172, 1988.
68. Griffin PJA, Davies F, Salaman JR, Coles GA: Effects of smoking on long term patency of arteriovenous fistulas. BMJ 286:685-686, 1983.
69. Bone GE, Pomjzl MJ: Management of dialysis fistula thrombosis. Am J Surg 138:901-906, 1979.
70. Glanz S, Bashist B, Gordon DH, et al: Angiography of upper extremity access fistulas for dialysis. Radiology 143:45-52, 1982.
71. Gain JS, Fowler PR, Steinberg AW, et al: Use of the fistula assessment monitor to detect stenoses in access fistulae. Am J Kidney Dis 17:303-306, 1991.
72. Choudhury D, Lee J, Elivera HS, et al: Correlation of venography, venous pressure, and hemoaccess function. Am J Kidney Dis 25:269-275, 1995.
73. Ritgers SE, Garcia-Valdez C, McCormick JT, Posner MP: Noninvasive flow measurement in expanded polytetrafluoroethylene grafts for hemodialysis access. J Vasc Surg 3:635-642, 1986.
74. Weber M, Kuhn FP, Quintes W, et al: Sonography of arteriovenous fistulae in hemodialysis patients. Clin Nephrol 22:258-261, 1984.
75. Gmelin E, Winterhoff R, Rinast E: Insufficient hemodialysis access fistulas: Late results in treatment with percutaneous balloon angioplasty. Radiology 171:657-660, 1989.
76. Zeit RM, Cope C: Failed hemodialysis shunts: One year of experience with aggressive treatment. Radiology 154:353-356, 1985.
77. Mangiarotti G, Canavese C, Thea A, et al: Urokinase treatment for arteriovenous fistulae declotting in dialyzed patients. Nephron 36:60-64, 1984.
78. Harter HR, Burch JW, Majerus PW, et al: Prevention of thrombosis in patients on hemodialysis by low-dose aspirin. N Engl J Med 301:577-579, 1979.
79. Flye MW, Mundinger GH, Schulz SC, et al: Successful creation of arteriovenous fistulas in nonuremic patients with heparin and aspirin therapy. Am J Surg 142:759-763, 1981.
80. Radmilovic A, Boric Z, Naumovic T, et al: Shunt thrombosis prevention in hemodialysis patients—a double-blind, randomized study: Pentoxifylline vs placebo. Angiology 38:499-505, 1987.
81. Johnson G, Blythe WB: Hemodynamic effects of arteriovenous shunts used for hemodialysis. Ann Surg 171:715-721, 1970.
82. Jensen JA, Goodson WH, Omachi RS, et al: Subcutaneous tissue oxygenation falls during hemodialysis. Surgery 101:416-421, 1987.
83. Ahern DJ, Maher JF: Heart failure as a complication of hemodialysis arteriovenous fistula. Ann Intern Med 77:201-204, 1972.
84. Anderson CB, Codd JR, Graff RA, et al: Cardiac failure and upper extremity arteriovenous dialysis fistulas. Arch Intern Med 136:292-297, 1976.
85. Anderson CB, Etheridge EE, Harter HR, et al: Blood flow measurements in arteriovenous dialysis fistulas. Surgery 81:459-461, 1977.
86. Riley SM, Blackstone EH, Sterling WA, Diethelm AG: Echocardiographic assessment of cardiac performance in patients with arteriovenous fistulas. Surg Gynecol Obstet 146:203-208, 1978.
87. Von Bibra H, Castro L, Autenieth G, et al: The effects of arteriovenous shunts on cardiac function in renal dialysis patients: An echocardiographic evaluation. Clin Nephrol 9:205-209, 1978.
88. Storey BG, George CRP, Stewart JOH, et al: Embolic and ischemic complications after anastomosis of radial artery to cephalic vein. Surgery 66:325-327, 1969.
89. Bussell JA, Abbott JA, Lim RC: A radial steal syndrome with arteriovenous fistula for hemodialysis. Ann Intern Med 75:387-394, 1971.
90. Haimov M: Vascular access for hemodialysis. Surg Gynecol Obstet 141:619-625, 1975.
91. Duncan H, Ferguson L, Faris I: Incidence of the radial steal syndrome in patients with Brescia fistula for hemodialysis: Its clinical significance. J Vasc Surg 4:144-147, 1986.
92. Odland MD, Kelly PH, Ney AL, et al: Management of dialysis-associated steal syndrome complicating upper extremity arteriovenous fistulas: Use of intraoperative digital photoplethysmography. Surgery 110:664-670, 1991.
93. Knezevic W, Mastaglia FL: Neuropathy associated with Brescia-Cimino arteriovenous fistulas. Arch Neurol 41:1184-1186, 1984.
94. Wood ML, Reilly GD, Smith GT: Ulceration of the hand secondary to a radial arteriovenous fistula: A model for varicose ulceration. BMJ 287:1167-1168, 1983.
95. Bond MG, Hotstetler JR, Karayannocas PE, et al: Intimal changes in arteriovenous bypass grafts: Effects of varying the angle of implantation at the proximal anastomosis and of producing stenosis in the distal runoff artery. J Thorac Cardiovasc Surg 71:907-916, 1976.
96. Telles D, Weinstein P: Intimal cellular response to microvascular anastomosis. Scanning Microsc 3:227-234, 1980.
97. Stehbens WE, Karmody AM: Venous atherosclerosis associated with arteriovenous fistulas for hemodialysis. Arch Surg 110:176-180, 1975.
98. Mennes PA, Gilula LA, Anderson CB, et al: Complications associated with arteriovenous fistulas in patients undergoing chronic hemodialysis. Arch Intern Med 138:1117-1121, 1978.

99. Owens ML, Shinaberger JH, Wilson SE, Wang SMS: Aneurysmal enlargement of e-PTFE fistulas. Dial Transplant 7:692-694, 1978.

100. Deppe G, Kahn ML, Malviya VK, et al: Experience with the PAS-PORT venous access device in patients with gynecologic malignancies. Gynecol Oncol 62:340-343, 1996.

101. Criado E, Marston WA, Jaques PF, et al: Proximal venous outflow obstruction in patients with upper extremity arteriovenous dialysis access. Ann Vasc Surg 8:530-535, 1994.

102. Horne MK, May DJ, Alexander HR, et al: Venographic surveillance of tunneled venous access devices in adult oncology patients. Ann Surg Oncol 2:174-178, 1995.

103. Koksoy C, Kuzu A, Kutlay J, et al: The diagnostic value of colour Doppler ultrasound in central venous catheter related thrombosis. Clin Radiol 50:687-689, 1995.

104. Kalman PG, Lindsay TF, Clarke K, et al: Management of upper extremity central venous obstruction using interventional radiology. Ann Vasc Surg 12:202-206, 1998.

105. Engels JGL, Skotincki SH, Buskens FGM, van Tougeren JHM: Home parenteral nutrition via arteriovenous fistulae. JPEN J Parenter Enteral Nutr 7:412-414, 1983.

106. Havill JH, Blair RD: Home parenteral nutrition using shunts. JPEN J Parenter Enteral Nutr 8:321-324, 1984.

107. Wobbes T, Slooff MJH, Lichtendahl DHE, et al: The radiocephalic fistula as vascular access for chemotherapy. World J Surg 7:532-535, 1983.

108. Wobbes T, Slooff MJH, Sleijfer DT, et al: Five years' experience in access surgery for polychemotherapy: An analysis of results in 100 consecutive patients. Cancer 52:978-982, 1983.

109. Raaf JH: Results from use of 826 vascular access devices in cancer patients. Cancer 55:1312-1321, 1985.

110. Broviac JW, Cole JJ, Scribner BH: A silicone rubber atrial catheter for prolonged parenteral alimentation. Surg Gynecol Obstet 136:602-606, 1973.

111. Hickman RO, Buckner CD, Clift RA, et al: A modified right atrial catheter for access to the venous system in bone marrow transplant recipients. Surg Gynecol Obstet 148:871-875, 1979.

112. Thomas JH, MacArthur RI, Pierce GE, Hermreck AS: Hickman-Broviac catheters: Indications and results. Am J Surg 140:791-796, 1980.

113. Weber TR, West KW, Grosfeld JL: Broviac central venous catheterization in infants and children. Am J Surg 145:791-796, 1983.

114. Bedini AV, Tavecchio L, Bonalumi MG, et al: Reliability of prolonged infusion in cancer chemotherapy with the Groshong central venous catheter. Reg Cancer Treat 3:232-234, 1990.

115. Greene FL, Moore W, Strickland G, McFarland J: Comparison of a totally implantable device for chemotherapy (Port-A-Cath) and long-term percutaneous catheterization (Broviac). South Med J 81:580-585, 1988.

116. Ross MN, Haase GM, Poole MA, et al: Comparison of totally implanted reservoirs with external catheters as venous access devices in pediatric oncologic patients. Surg Gynecol Obstet 167:141-144, 1988.

117. Stellato WE, Gauderer MW, Cohen AM: Direct central vein puncture for silicone rubber catheter insertion: An alternative technique for Broviac catheter placement. Surgery 90:896-899, 1981.

Questions

1. **After construction of a radiocephalic autogenous fistula, which configuration is associated with the lowest incidence of venous hypertension?**
   - (a) Arterial side–to–vein side anastomosis
   - (b) Vein end–to–arterial side anastomosis
   - (c) Arterial end–to–vein side anastomosis
   - (d) Brachiobasilic side-to-side anastomosis
   - (e) None of the above

2. **The highest 2-year patency rate in vascular access procedures has been achieved with which of the following?**
   - (a) PTFE bridge fistulas
   - (b) Autogenous saphenous vein bridge fistulas
   - (c) Scribner shunts
   - (d) Autogenous radiocephalic fistulas
   - (e) Percutaneous double-lumen Silastic catheters

3. **Early postoperative hemodynamic changes that may be encountered soon after construction of a proximally located, high-flow arteriovenous fistula for hemodialysis include all of the following except**
   - (a) Increased stroke volume
   - (b) Reversal of flow in the distal artery when the fistula opening exceeds the diameter of the feeding artery
   - (c) Increased cardiac output
   - (d) Increased heart rate
   - (e) Decreased total systemic resistance

4. **Which of the following is not a complication of percutaneous subclavian central venous catheterization?**
   - (a) Hemopneumothorax
   - (b) Catheter embolism
   - (c) Brachial plexus injury
   - (d) Lymphatic fistula formation
   - (e) All are possible complications

5. **Correction of localized venous runoff stenosis can be accomplished by all of the following except**
   - (a) Patch angioplasty of the outflow anastomosis
   - (b) Extension bypass graft to a more proximal vein
   - (c) Percutaneous transluminal dilatation
   - (d) Relocation of the venous anastomosis to an adjacent vein
   - (e) Directed thrombolytic therapy with double catheters

6. **Which of the following is a characteristic of venous runoff stenosis?**
   - (a) It may be related to the shearing effect of blood flow on intima at the anastomotic site or compliance mismatch
   - (b) It develops as early as 6 months after graft placement
   - (c) It is most often seen after construction of prosthetic arteriovenous fistulas
   - (d) It manifests as an increase in venous return pressure during dialysis
   - (e) All of the above

7. **The potential benefits of implantable ports over percutaneous central venous catheters for the delivery of chemotherapy include all of the following except**
   - (a) Lower catheter-related sepsis rate
   - (b) Lower incidence of thrombosis
   - (c) Does not require heparinization
   - (d) Requires little daily care
   - (e) Interferes less with the patient's normal activities

8. **Vascular access in children weighing less than 10 kg may be reliably accomplished by each of the following except**
   (a) Percutaneous central vein catheterization
   (b) Forearm PTFE bridge fistula
   (c) Creation of a brachial artery–to–antecubital vein autogenous fistula
   (d) Direct cannulation of umbilical vessels if the patient is a newborn
   (e) Placement of an external arteriovenous shunt

9. **Increased risk of infection in a prosthetic arteriovenous graft for hemodialysis can be related to all of the following except**
   (a) Poor aseptic technique during needle puncture
   (b) High colonization rate of dialysis patients and dialysis staff with *Staphylococcus aureus*
   (c) Decreased chemotactic response of polymorphonuclear leukocytes in uremia
   (d) Decreased bacterial phagocytosis in uremic patients
   (e) All of the above

10. **With regard to thrombosis of the axillosubclavian vein after percutaneous dialysis catheter placement, which of the following is correct?**
    (a) Diagnosis can be made reliably only with venography
    (b) It is most often seen after internal jugular placement
    (c) It is not a source of pulmonary emboli
    (d) It may be treated with percutaneous transluminal dilatation and stent in many patients
    (e) It occurs only after the catheter has been in place for more than 3 months.

Answers

1. b	2. d	3. a	4. e	5. e
6. e	7. c	8. b	9. e	10. d

39

Malcolm O. Perry • Frederic S. Bongard

Vascular Trauma

Trauma is a leading cause of death in the United States. More males younger than 18 years old die from handgun injuries than from car crashes, communicable diseases, or drugs.[1] Many victims have multiple injuries involving major vascular structures. Those who survive are frequently incapacitated due to amputation or dysfunction caused by associated soft tissue and neural injuries.

In most situations, serious injury can be ascertained with little difficulty. Multiple wounds are challenging and require careful planning, organization, and integration of resources. The basic principles of resuscitation should always assume priority.

Cause

Major vascular wounds can occur in any environment, but the greatest incidence is in urban areas, where violence is endemic. Penetrating injury is more common than blunt trauma; most penetrating wounds are caused by knives and bullets. Incidental wounds may be inflicted by shards of glass or pieces of metal during motor vehicle accidents or industrial mishaps (Table 39-1).[2]

Among penetrating injuries, stab wounds are more common than gunshot wounds. However, because such injuries are not as deep or widespread, they are less likely to produce severe vascular wounds and often can be treated by simple débridement and ligation of superficial vessels. Deeper structures are often spared when small knives are used. These knife wounds may be meant to punish rather than to kill, and the point is extended in such a way that only a small laceration results. Gunshot wounds usually penetrate deeply and often involve the trunk or thorax as well as the extremities; they are more likely to produce serious vascular and visceral wounds. The vessels of the extremities are most often involved, because they are longer and may be injured during attempts at self-defense (Table 39-2).[2]

Mechanisms of Injury

Most penetrating injuries are caused by low-velocity agents, which means that the damage is largely confined to the wound tract. Low-velocity bullets and knives usually cause punctures, lacerations, and contusions to structures in their path. Complete vessel transection is likely with bullet wounds. The concussive effects of higher-velocity missiles produce widespread damage. The cavitation caused by a high-velocity bullet (1500 to 3000 feet/second) may even damage a vessel remote from the wound tract. This occurs when the blast cavity collapses, causing a suction effect that draws structures into the wound. These structures may include bits of skin, clothing, or dirt particles, increasing the possibility of infection.

A high-velocity bullet or metal fragment can produce a great deal of tissue damage. The kinetic energy (KE) of a bullet is proportional to its mass (m) and the square of its velocity (v) ($KE = \frac{1}{2} mv^2$). Hence, high-velocity bullets (such as from a .458 Winchester), which are also fairly heavy, have the highest wounding potential. When the bullet strikes tissue, it dissipates its energy rapidly. Fast-moving bullets that yaw and tumble on impact (dumdum bullets) cause large amounts of damage because they lose virtually all their energy as they pass through the target. Such destructive effects may not be

TABLE 39–1	Relationship Between Mechanism of Injury and Location				
Mechanism of Injury	**Head/Neck**	**Thorax**	**Abdomen**	**Arms**	**Legs**
Gunshot wound	11	10	16	50	45
Stab wound	27	13	34	94	15
Motor vehicle accident	14	15	12	11	22
Fall	6	1	0	3	3
Other	4	0	1	3	1
Total	62	39	63	161	86

Data from 411 patients seen over a 9-year period in a level I trauma center.
From Bongard F, Dubrow T, Klein S: Vascular injuries in the urban battleground: Experience at a metropolitan trauma center. Ann Vasc Surg 4:415-418, 1990.

TABLE 39–2	Distribution of Vascular Injuries
Location of Injury	**No. of Injuries**
Head and Neck Vessels	***n = 62***
Carotid	13
Jugular vein	7
External jugular vein	10
Multiple arteries	5
All other	27
Thoracic Vessel	***n = 39***
Aorta	11
Innominate/subclavian artery	9
Subclavian vein	2
Innominate/subclavian vein	2
Pulmonary vessels	2
All other	13
Abdominal Vessels	***n = 63***
Aorta	3
Inferior vena cava/hepatic veins	23
Celiac/mesenteric arteries	19
Portal/splenic veins	3
Renal arteries	3
Iliac arteries	7
All other	5
Upper Extremity Vessels	***n = 161***
Axillary arteries/veins	18
Brachial arteries/veins	55
Radial/ulnar arteries	64
Palmar/digital arteries	12
All other	12
Lower Extremity Vessels	***n = 86***
Common femoral arteries	8
Superficial femoral arteries	24
Femoral veins	3
Saphenous veins	4
Popliteal arteries/veins	20
Tibial arteries/veins	5
All other	22

Data from 411 patients seen over a 9-year period in a level I trauma center; all causes included. From Bongard F, Dubrow T, Klein S: Vascular injuries in the urban battleground: Experience at a metropolitan trauma center. Ann Vasc Surg 4:415-418, 1990.

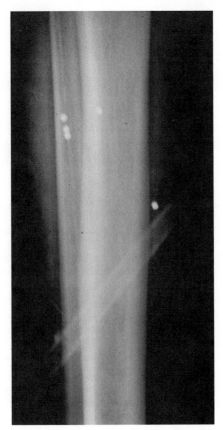

FIGURE 39–1 • Plain radiograph shows shotgun pellet emboli to the tibial arteries. The wound is in the ipsilateral superficial femoral artery.

suspected on initial inspection; only a small entrance wound may be present, yet interior damage is widespread, and extensive débridement is required if tissue necrosis and invasive sepsis are to be avoided.

Special problems are encountered from close-range shotgun blasts. Although the muzzle velocity of a shotgun pellet is similar to that of a .22-caliber rifle bullet (approximately 1200 feet/second), the damage inflicted by multiple pellets is usually widespread, and the shotshell wadding and bits of clothing carried into the wound greatly enhance the possibility of infection. As with high-velocity wounds, close-range shotgun blasts often cause a great deal more damage to interior structures than is apparent from inspection of the entry sites in the skin. Shotgun pellets may embolize in both the arterial and venous systems. Distal ischemia may result from the embolization of a single pellet. Plain films of the distal extremity should be obtained to exclude this possibility (Fig. 39-1).

Motor vehicle accidents continue to increase in frequency and complexity as traffic density grows and automobiles get smaller. These accident victims commonly have multiple injuries that often include fractures and dislocations. Direct trauma to major vessels can occur, but in many cases the vascular injury is the result of a fracture. This is especially common with fractures near the joints, where the vessels are relatively fixed and vulnerable to shear forces. Posterior dislocations of the knee are particularly likely to injure the relatively immobile popliteal artery and vein.[3,4]

The bending and sudden fracture of large, heavy bones such as the femur or the tibia release tremendous forces. Damage to soft tissue and neurovascular structures is frequently extensive, and the effects on these tissues are quite similar to those produced by the cavitation associated with high-velocity bullet wounds (Fig. 39-2). Remote vascular injuries can occur, but after the bones fall back into a near-normal position, the magnitude of the injury forces may not be appreciated, and the severity of damage is often underestimated. Evaluation of these patients is particularly difficult because of extensive soft tissue and bony deformity.

General Principles

DIAGNOSIS

Clinical and Imaging Features

Physical examination is the single most important step in the evaluation of a patient with a suspected vascular injury.

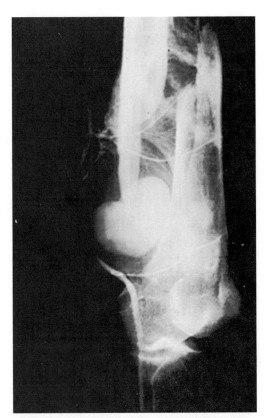

FIGURE 39–2 • Spiral fracture of the femur causing extensive damage to the soft tissues of the thigh and puncture of the superficial femoral artery.

Complete disruption of a major vessel, regardless of mechanism, typically results in a distal pulse deficit. When the injury is due to a blunt mechanism, destruction of surrounding soft tissue may also disturb collateral pathways to the extent that distal ischemia is pronounced. When a penetrating mechanism is responsible, significant ischemia may follow injury to the common femoral or superficial femoral arteries. Severe ischemia of the upper extremity is unusual after penetrating injuries unless the brachial artery is completely transected.

The physical signs of arterial trauma are divided into two groups, hard and soft. Hard signs include severe external hemorrhage, an expanding hematoma, a palpable thrill, a continuous murmur, and any of the classic findings of acute ischemia known as the six Ps: pain, pallor, pulselessness, paresthesia, poikilothermy, and paralysis. When sufficient collateral flow is present around the injury, a pulse deficit may be present in the absence of ischemia. Recent studies suggest that the incidence of vascular injury requiring surgical repair in the absence of any sign is very small. Certain high-risk groups exist, however, and mandate further evaluation. These include patients with gunshot injuries to the calf, forearm, antecubital fossa, medial or posterior thigh, or medial or posterior arm. Extended follow-up in these patients has been limited, and the incidence of late complications such as pseudoaneurysm formation is still undefined. Physical examination alone after blunt trauma has also been advocated, but because of the frequency of associated soft tissue destruction, further evaluation of patients with abnormal pulse examinations after these injuries is mandatory.

Proximity of a penetrating injury to a major vascular structure constitutes the most common soft sign of injury. Other soft signs include a small nonpulsatile and nonexpanding hematoma, an ipsilateral neurologic deficit, or a history of prehospital hemorrhage or shock.

Although weak or absent pulses beyond a suspected vascular wound are fairly common, pulses may be normal in up to 20% of operatively proven arterial injuries.[5] The pulse wave is a pressure wave that reaches velocities of 7 to 13 m/second. This wave may be transmitted beyond intimal flaps, through limited areas of fresh soft clot, or via the large collateral vessels; thus, it may be detectable distal to a significant arterial injury. The flow wave of blood has a velocity of 40 to 50 cm/second and is distinct from the pulse wave. Physical examination must take these facts into account. Wounds of arteries crossing the shoulder or the pelvis, areas with rich collateral circulation, are more likely to be associated with distal pulses. Moreover, injuries of arteries such as the deep femoral or deep brachial do not disturb distal pulses. Major venous wounds are not exposed by examination of pulses; the only finding in these patients may be hematomas or persistent bleeding. In the case of an acute traumatic arteriovenous (AV) fistula, abnormal distention of the veins is noted, along with a bruit or murmur and thrill over the injury.

The detection of Doppler signals and the measurement of distal arterial systolic blood pressure by this or other techniques is helpful, but the specificity of these tests is influenced by the same hemodynamic features that govern distal pulses. Subtle abnormalities are common, but relatively normal values are also observed, compromising the reliability of these methods for excluding vascular wounds. They are useful adjuncts and serve as an extension of the physical examination, but they may be misleading.

Wounds of the deep femoral or deep brachial artery do not alter distal pulses or distal limb blood pressure measurements. Likewise, an injury of a single tibial artery may not change the ankle-brachial index. In questionable cases, duplex ultrasound tests may expose the injury or detect false aneurysms or AV fistulas. In the absence of other indications for surgical exploration, these adjunctive methods can provide helpful information about possible injuries to large arteries.[6,7] Color-flow duplex ultrasonography may also be helpful in screening for occult venous injuries.[8]

Injuries of the heart and great vessels present special diagnostic problems because of their inaccessibility to clinical examination. Table 39-3 lists those clinical features that suggest the presence of significant intrathoracic vascular injuries. Hemopneumothorax or mediastinal bleeding is common with penetrating injuries of the chest, even without injuries of a major artery. Initially, the patient may be stable and appear to have only minor parenchymal lung damage, until sudden

TABLE 39–3	Clinical Features Suggesting Injuries of the Great Vessels
Cardiac arrest	
Persistent shock	
Cardiac tamponade	
Wide mediastinum	
Recurring hemothorax	

hemodynamic collapse occurs. Preoperative identification of such severe injuries is important, permitting the surgeon to prepare for the possibility of major vascular reconstruction of the heart or great vessels. Many patients benefit from preoperative arteriography if they are sufficiently stable to permit the delay required for such studies.

Computed tomography (CT) is very useful in the initial evaluation of patients with multiple injuries, especially those caused by blunt trauma. Injuries to parenchymal intra-abdominal organs, hematomas, and displacement of other structures may be seen clearly by CT scanning, thus validating the need for operative exploration. Negative studies are of less value in excluding injuries, but a positive study offers a compelling reason to proceed with surgery. The CT scan is now advocated by some as a screening technique for angiography in patients at risk of thoracic aortic disruption after blunt trauma. Because only one third of patients with this injury have any abnormal physical findings on presentation, a high index of suspicion is required. Numerous findings on chest radiographs may be suggestive of thoracic aortic disruption (see Table 35-3), but none is specific. The incidence of false-negative CT scans is probably low when thin (5-mm) cuts are taken.[9] Recently, helical CT scanning has received attention as a diagnostic modality among victims of blunt trauma with a widened mediastinum on the initial chest film. A prospective series of 112 blunt trauma patients with 9 aortic ruptures found helical CT accurate in diagnosing 8 of them.[10] The false-negative reading was in a patient who had a brachiocephalic injury. The authors suggested that all high-risk patients (those with high-speed deceleration injuries) undergo helical CT scanning, irrespective of chest radiographic findings; however, the true accuracy of helical CT needs to be studied further. Magnetic resonance imaging (MRI) promises to be of more value than CT scanning; the delineation of structures is much clearer, and the detection of even minor abnormalities should be possible.

Arteriography

In the management of trauma, preoperative arteriography is used to exclude the need for surgery, to expose a suspected injury not otherwise detectable, and to plan an operation (Table 39-4). In a study of 183 patients with penetrating injuries of the extremities, the validity and usefulness of arteriography were established.[11] In those with penetrating injuries of the arms and legs, all had arteriograms and were operated on regardless of the arteriographic findings. One false-negative examination and 28 false-positive examinations were encountered. The study concluded that high-grade biplane arteriography offers reliable, but not infallible, evidence regarding the presence or absence of arterial injuries.

TABLE 39–4	Indications for Preoperative Arteriography

Blunt trauma with fractures
Penetrating injuries to the chest
Cervical injuries—base of skull and thoracic inlet (zones I and III)
Assessment of multiple pellet wounds
Injuries to forearm or leg

Particular problems are encountered with preoperative arteriography in the assessment of injuries of the great vessels near the arch of the aorta, where obtaining good biplane films is difficult because of overlapping images.

Studies have shown a low yield when arteriograms are obtained only because the wound is near a major artery. A study by Weaver and colleagues described 157 patients with penetrating extremity injuries in whom the path of the penetrating object was judged to be in proximity to a major neurovascular bundle.[12] None of the patients had pulse deficits, nerve deficits, hematoma, history of hemorrhage or hypotension, bruit, fracture, major soft tissue injury, or delayed capillary refill. Angiographic abnormalities were demonstrated in 17 patients (11%); 4 abnormalities were major (3%), and 13 (8%) were minor. In a group of 216 patients with significant physical findings, the authors found injuries in 65 (30%); 22 (10%) of the injuries were major. The majority of injuries identified by arteriography in otherwise asymptomatic patients are small intimal deficits, pseudoaneurysms, or occlusions of "noncritical" vessels. A careful physical examination usually determines the need for arteriograms.[13] Frykberg and colleagues described 366 penetrating extremity wounds in 310 patients.[14] Twenty-three patients required surgical intervention; 21 of these patients (91.3%) were initially diagnosed solely by physical examination, each producing at least one hard sign. Unfortunately, patients with no findings or only soft signs were observed during a short hospital stay (without angiography) and were presumed to harbor no injury if signs did not manifest before discharge, making the true predictive accuracy of a negative physical examination difficult to assess. Among the patients with no abnormal findings initially, two required surgery during the period of inpatient observation. For patients who are hemodynamically stable with no indications for surgical exploration, delaying arteriography is often acceptable, rather than obtaining emergency studies in the middle of the night. Careful observation is required until the tests are completed and precise treatment is initiated. Noninvasive tests may help separate these patients from those who require expedient surgery.

When firm indications for operation are present, arteriograms may be unnecessary; any untoward delay is undesirable and, in some situations, may be dangerous. If the patient is unstable, further evaluation is best performed in the operating room, using the routine commonly employed for the management of patients with leaking abdominal aortic aneurysms. The patient is taken directly to the operating room, and further assessment is performed while preparations for surgery are under way. If sudden cardiovascular collapse occurs, immediate operation can begin, and control of bleeding can be achieved rapidly. Such a patient should not be sent to the radiology department for study nor admitted to an intensive care unit if unstable, because an emergency operation may be required at any time.

The experience with computed tomography-angiography (CTA) has been reviewed by several centers. As with any new modality, early reports must be scrutinized to ensure the use of appropriate controls. In the case of CTA, only formal angiography can serve as such a standard. Reports citing clinical outcome to validate CTA findings must be regarded with extreme caution.

CTA has gained popularity primarily for imaging the thoracic aorta and the extracranial cerebral vasculature.

TABLE 39–5	Angiographic Grading of Blunt Carotid Injuries
Grade	**Finding**
I	Irregularity of vessel wall or dissection/intramural hematoma < 25% luminal stenosis
II	Intramural thrombosis or raised intimal flap
	Small arteriovenous fistula or dissection/intramural hematoma ≥ 25% luminal narrowing
III	Pseudoaneurysm
IV	Vessel occlusion
V	Transection or hemodynamically significant arteriovenous fistula

From Biffl WL, Moore EE, Offner PJ, et al: Blunt carotid arterial injuries: Implications of a new grading scale. J Trauma 47:845-853, 1999.

A study by Biffl and coworkers compared the results of CTA and formal angiography in 46 patients who had sustained blunt cervical injury.[15] Of the 23 who had normal CTA results, 7 (30%) had cerebrovascular injuries demonstrated on formal angiography. Of the 23 with abnormal CTA examinations, 8 had normal results on formal angiography. The overall sensitivity of CTA was 68%, the specificity was 67%, the positive predictive value was 65%, and the negative predictive value was 70%. When the authors examined the types of lesions missed, they found that the greatest false-negative rate for CTA was in those patients who had grade I lesions (Table 39-5).[15]

The experience in penetrating carotid and vertebral injuries is also limited, but the sensitivity and specificity of CTA in these injuries may be higher. At present, it is difficult to assess the overall accuracy of CTA for the diagnosis of cerebrovascular injuries. Prudence dictates caution when CTA is used as the only diagnostic study, especially in symptomatic patients and those at risk for other injuries.

PRIORITIES AND RESUSCITATION

The management of trauma requires a rapid but thorough evaluation. Many of these patients have associated injuries (Table 39-6), and priorities must be set. Initial attention to the airway, breathing, and control of bleeding takes precedence. A dangerous situation exists when the patient has achieved cardiopulmonary stability via compensatory mechanisms and then suddenly deteriorates. Collapse is sudden, and irreversible shock may occur. This is particularly true in older patients whose compensatory mechanisms may be unable to deal with even relatively minor injuries.

TABLE 39–6	Associated Injuries in Trauma Patients	
Injury		**Incidence (%)**
Significant vein		34
Major nerve		18
Separate artery		7
Lung, abdominal viscera		39
Shock		36

Once an airway is secured and control of external bleeding has been obtained, vital signs are assessed, an overall evaluation is made, and proper priorities are set. Baseline studies are recorded, and a rapid physical examination is performed to be certain that all injuries are identified and emergency measures completed. The patient must be fully undressed so that unsuspected injuries in seemingly uninvolved parts of the body can be uncovered. A carefully performed and well-documented peripheral neurologic examination (sensory and motor) of the involved extremity is critical before surgical intervention is undertaken.

Fluid and blood requirements in the injured patient are often impressive, and adequate intravenous access lines are needed. Large catheters are placed into an uninjured upper extremity whenever possible. Peripheral venous cutdowns are preferable to central venous access. Hypovolemic patients have collapsed central veins, which are difficult to cannulate. Misguided and persistent attempts at subclavian venous access can result in a pneumothorax or laceration of nearby arteries. When selecting veins for the administration of intravenous fluids, the possibility of injury to the vein proximal to the site of insertion of the line must be considered, because it may be necessary to clamp that vein to control bleeding. One line is committed to fluid replacement and another to drug administration and anesthetic manipulations. If hemorrhage is severe, large volumes of blood must be infused rapidly. Venous autografts may be needed for vascular repair; preserving the saphenous or cephalic vein in an uninjured extremity is often prudent. The treatment of shock takes priority, however, and these veins may be needed for resuscitation.

A combination of a balanced salt solution, such as lactated Ringer's solution, and blood is chosen for resuscitation. Trauma and shock cause shifts of fluid from the interstitial to the intravascular space. This fluid is best replenished with a balanced salt solution followed by blood as required. Blood should be replaced with type- and crossmatched units when possible. Type-specific and O-negative blood can be used until crossmatched transfusions are available. It is wise not to overtransfuse these patients, especially if chest trauma or cardiac disease is present.

Often, arterial lines and Swan-Ganz catheters are helpful if the patient is hemodynamically unstable and does not respond to resuscitation as anticipated. A radial artery catheter inserted in a patient who has a normal Allen's test (which demonstrates connection of the radial and ulnar artery through the palmar arch) is safe and useful. The radial artery catheter should not be irrigated with large amounts of fluid, because a thrombus in the catheter can be dislodged and scatter multiple emboli throughout the hand. The line is kept open with a continuous infusion of minute amounts of heparinized saline (1000 units of heparin in 1 L normal saline). The brachial artery should not be chosen for continuous in-line monitoring if other sites are accessible, because brachial artery lines are associated with high complication rates related to thrombosis and embolization.

WOUND PROTECTION

During the initial treatment of patients with serious injuries, a tendency exists to overlook the problem of wound care. Because the incidence of infection and subsequent complications may be directly related to contamination of wounds at the time of resuscitation, injuries should be protected, and all undamaged tissue should be conserved for future use in covering repaired vessels. When a patient has multiple wounds, the use of several incisions may be required, especially if fractures and other injuries are present. If incisions are poorly placed, intervening tissues may be devitalized, important collateral vessels may be divided unnecessarily, and final coverage of the vessels may be difficult to secure. Wound care is an extremely important part of initial management, especially if extensive soft tissue damage is present, as occurs with close-range shotgun wounds and motor vehicle accidents. Preservation of potentially viable soft tissue is extremely important in victims of trauma because it provides both venous and arterial collaterals around the area of injury. Remote bypass grafts to restore flow may be required because of heavy contamination of the initial wounds. Exploratory incisions should be placed to preserve areas for the use of subcutaneous grafts. Meticulous care in creating and handling these incisions is essential to avoid secondary infections.

Most trauma surgeons use prophylactic antibiotics in these situations. Second-generation cephalosporins are often chosen and are begun when the patient is initially examined. Customarily, they are continued while central lines are in place, or as long as specific indications exist for antibiotic therapy. The patient's tetanus immunization status should not be overlooked.

ANTICOAGULATION

Although regional or systemic anticoagulation is used during the course of many vascular operations while major arteries and veins are temporarily occluded, administering systemic heparin to trauma patients is not generally recommended unless there is an isolated vascular injury. Distal clot propagation is a problem in such patients, especially in the face of hypotension. Thrombosis can convert an initially manageable situation into one with risk of tissue loss. Nevertheless, systemic anticoagulation in patients with multiple injuries (especially injuries of the central nervous system, eyes, and bones) carries an unacceptably high risk. Expeditious surgery rather than systemic anticoagulation is preferred.[5,16]

Operative Management

ANESTHESIA, POSITIONING, AND INCISIONS

During preparation for surgery, the selection of anesthetic agent is important, especially in patients who are already hypotensive. The cardiodepressant action of some anesthetic agents should be kept in mind as the operation begins. Careful positioning of the neck during induction of anesthesia is necessary to avoid dislodging clots from injured vessels in the neck. Of great importance is care in positioning the patient to avoid aggravating cervical spine injuries. Most patients are placed supine in the anatomic position, thus affording access to the chest, the abdomen, and all four extremities. If the surgeon needs to enter the left chest only (for repair of a single injury of the subclavian artery), the right lateral decubitus position is preferable.

Vertical exploratory incisions are desirable because they can be extended easily and, in the extremities, parallel the neurovascular bundles. Midline abdominal incisions can be extended into the chest as a median sternal splitting incision.

Vertical incisions along the anterior sternocleidomastoid muscle used to expose the carotid and jugular vessels can also be extended into a median sternal incision if injuries are present in the root of the neck.[17] Transverse incisions generally limit flexibility and are not recommended.

CONTROL OF BLEEDING

External hemorrhage is best controlled with direct digital pressure. If the wound is not bleeding, not disturbing it during early resuscitation is best, and no attempt should be made to remove foreign bodies or to evacuate clots until surgical control is possible. Penetrating objects that are still in the wound must be protected during transport and should not be removed until the patient is in the operating room and proximal and distal control of major arteries has been obtained. No attempt should be made to clamp vessels blindly before formal exploration in the appropriate environment. When fatal hemorrhage appears imminent, the wound can be extended and vascular clamps applied under direct vision.

After penetrating trauma, emergency room thoracotomy may be lifesaving. Closed cardiac massage for hypovolemic shock may not be effective, and open massage is often required. An aggressive approach is warranted in these infrequent situations. A team of experienced surgeons is required if these maneuvers are to be successful.[18] Resuscitative thoracotomy is generally ineffective after blunt trauma, and its use is discouraged in these situations.

Once the surgical plan has been established, the injuries are approached directly through vertical incisions. If the hematoma is large, it is often advisable to expose the vessels proximally and gain control in an area where the artery and vein can be clearly visualized. In extremities with multiple distal wounds and large hematomas, exposure of the vessels can be difficult, and placing an orthopedic tourniquet around the extremity proximal to the injury may be prudent. If severe bleeding is encountered before direct control of the artery is achieved, the tourniquet can be quickly inflated, thus arresting the hemorrhage while precise identification and control are obtained. A good alternative for lower extremity injuries, especially those involving the proximal femoral vessels, is to obtain inflow control at the external iliac artery. This is accomplished by creating a flank incision and approaching the iliac artery through the retroperitoneum; the artery can then be identified easily and the bleeding controlled within several minutes. If necessary, an assistant can apply direct digital pressure over the bleeding vessel while iliac control is obtained.

Proximal control is best achieved by using soft vascular tapes, latex tubing, or vascular clamps. These measures, combined with adequate suction and direct pressure with fingers or sponge sticks, are usually satisfactory to control hemorrhage while the injuries are identified and vascular clamps are applied.

Once the injury has been exposed, clots should be evacuated carefully and the extent of the injury examined. Every effort should be made to avoid fragmenting and dislodging clots or extending the damage to the vessel. This is particularly important in patients who have atherosclerosis and fragile arteries. In some cases, using a Foley or Fogarty catheter with an attached three-way stopcock may be necessary to control hemorrhage. The catheter is inserted into the wound, inflated, and gently retracted until bleeding stops. It is left in place until precise proximal and distal control is obtained. Repairs are not begun until all hemorrhage is arrested and the extent of associated injuries is assessed. Pausing at this point to ascertain that there is no persistent bleeding is wise. Resuscitation should be essentially complete before definitive repair of noncritical structures is begun. Organs such as the kidneys and liver are more susceptible to hypoxia than others, and the repair of major vessels supplying them should be undertaken first. Such prioritization of injuries is one of the basic tenets of trauma surgery.

In the past few years, the staged laparotomy for multiply injured patients has received a great deal of attention.[19,20] Because injuries can be extensive, it is often unwise to attempt definitive repair on initial exploration. An example is a gunshot victim with a liver injury, iliac artery disruption, and small bowel enterotomies.[21] A reasonable approach would be repair of the iliac artery, oversewing of the small bowel injuries, and packing of the liver. A scheduled return to the operating room 24 to 48 hours later can accomplish definitive repair. The advantage of such an approach is that it permits repair or control of the most significant injuries while temporizing the others. This minimizes hypothermia, reduces coagulopathy, and allows better physiologic resuscitation. Such staged laparotomy should be employed when a constellation of injuries exists that would require extensive repair and resection.

BASIC TECHNIQUES

The selection of suture materials for repair of major vessels is largely the preference of the operating surgeon, but a recent tendency is to select less reactive plastic sutures instead of the braided cardiovascular silk sutures that were popular in the past. Silk sutures handle well, and although they are not permanent (most of their tensile strength is gone in 6 months), this is not a major drawback in primary repairs because the approximated vessel ends heal to each other. Nonreactive monofilament plastic sutures are less likely to harbor bacteria than are braided sutures and may reduce the risk of postoperative infection. They are often chosen by vascular surgeons despite their relative stiffness and lack of pliability. Satisfactory results are obtained with all such materials, but polypropylene and Dacron are more popular than others.

The vessels are repaired by the usual vascular techniques. Continuous over-and-over sutures are quite effective and can be used in almost all vessels. In small vessels (< 4 mm diameter), using interrupted sutures may be prudent to ensure intima-to-intima coaptation, although magnification has shown that continuous sutures are just as effective, even in small arteries, when placed properly. Small vessels may be sewn end to end more easily if they are transected obliquely or spatulated to obtain a larger suture line, which also means less chance of subsequent stenosis.

Tangential lacerations of larger vessels can be successfully treated by lateral suture repair using standard vascular surgical techniques. Débridement is important in the management of vascular injuries, and it is best to refrain from making a firm decision about the type of repair until débridement has been concluded. Most civilian vascular wounds are inflicted by knives or low-velocity missiles, and wide débridement is generally not required. With most bullet wounds, débriding only the amount of vessel that appears to be injured is sufficient. With high-velocity gunshot wounds, the injury often extends beyond that which is immediately visible to the naked eye, and approximately 5 mm of vessel beyond the apparent damage should be removed.

Smaller vessels can rarely be repaired by lateral suture techniques and require either patch-graft angioplasty or, more commonly, resection and end-to-end anastomosis. The most commonly injured vessels (femoral and brachial) can usually be mobilized to permit resection of approximately 1 cm and still allow a satisfactory end-to-end anastomosis. If the extent of the injury is such that an end-to-end anastomosis cannot be accomplished without tension, interposing a suitable autograft is better than accepting an improper repair performed under tension. The saphenous vein is usually chosen for such autografts in medium-size and small vessels of the extremities, but the hypogastric artery, external iliac artery, and other arterial autografts may be used as necessary. When the injury involves a lower extremity, the saphenous vein should be harvested from the contralateral leg. The ipsilateral vein should be left in situ because an unexpected injury of the deep venous system leaves the saphenous vein as the only significant pathway for venous return. An arterial autograft is likely more resistant to invasive infection than are other types of prosthetic grafts.[22] When heavy bacterial contamination has occurred, arterial autografts are favored.

Studies suggest that the disruption caused by infection is not unfavorably influenced by the presence of plastic prostheses, particularly polytetrafluoroethylene (PTFE) grafts. Further, these plastic substitutes may be used even when bacterial contamination is present. This opinion is not shared by all vascular surgeons, and most use autogenous tissue if available in the appropriate size.[23] In the aortoiliac system, plastic prostheses are used when extensive damage is present, because large autografts are not available. If bacterial contamination is heavy, such as with combined aortic and colonic injuries, oversewing the major vascular injuries and constructing remote subcutaneous prosthetic bypass grafts on a temporary basis may be the best option until healing is complete. Axillofemoral and femorofemoral grafts are often selected in these circumstances to avoid placing the repaired arteries in heavily contaminated areas.

ASSESSMENT OF REPAIR IN THE OPERATING ROOM

In most cases, vascular repair is followed by the immediate return of pulsatile flow. In patients who are incompletely resuscitated, hypotensive, cold, and vasoconstricted, it may be difficult to determine clinically whether the repair is satisfactory. A sterile Doppler probe is useful in documenting distal patency in such circumstances. Angiograms should be obtained in all cases to assess the adequacy of the repair and the patency of the distal runoff bed.[24]

In the postoperative period, if any question exists regarding the adequacy of flow, an arteriogram is needed. The sine qua non for viability of the extremity is continued perception of light touch and adequate intrinsic motor function. Any deterioration is a compelling reason to obtain an arteriogram, regardless of skin color, temperature, presence or absence of pulses, or limb blood pressure.[5]

Management of Specific Problems

BRACHIOCEPHALIC ARTERIAL INJURIES

Most wounds of the cervical vessels are caused by penetrating trauma. The common carotid artery is usually involved, the left more often than the right. Associated wounds of the pharynx, esophagus, and trachea may also be present, thus increasing the likelihood of bacterial contamination. The neurologic deficit associated with some of these injuries presents a unique and often perplexing problem. The outcome in most patients appears to be directly related to the extent of the initial neurologic insult, unless a technical misadventure occurs.[24,25]

Carotid Injuries

Carotid injuries are divided into three groups for evaluation and repair. The first and largest group contains those patients with common or internal carotid artery wounds but no neurologic deficit. Group 2 includes those who have mild neurologic deficits, and group 3 includes those who have severe neurologic deficits (coma, hemiplegia).[25]

The results of several large studies strongly support surgical repair of all carotid artery injuries in patients who have either no neurologic deficit or only a mild deficit. Thus, all patients in groups 1 and 2 would undergo repair of isolated carotid artery injuries. This decision is easy when the arterial injury is bleeding actively, but it may be more difficult when the patient shows complete carotid artery occlusion and no neurologic symptoms.[26] In such a situation, technical problems encountered during surgery could conceivably produce brain damage, although in the reported experience, this has been rare.[27] The risk does exist, however, and careful neurologic and arteriographic studies are required to assess the danger accurately before operation is undertaken in these patients. Even an artery depicted as being completely occluded by arteriography may be open at operation. MRI can be of great assistance in determining whether flow is present in a vessel. This may be helpful in patients suspected of having a hyperextension injury in which the internal carotid artery is forcibly stretched over the transverse process of C-3 and the body of C-2 (a mechanism of injury that predisposes to thromboembolic events). Until a neurologic problem appears, little evidence of carotid artery injury is usually present (Fig. 39-3).

Preoperative Evaluation

The basic management of penetrating trauma to the neck is straightforward: wounds that pierce the platysma require exploration. Dividing penetrating wounds of the neck into three zones, as suggested by Monson and colleagues,[28] is helpful. Zone III extends from the base of the skull to the angle of the mandible, zone II from the angle of the mandible to 1 cm above the head of the clavicle, and zone I from 1 cm below the head of the clavicle to include the rest of the thoracic outlet. Ascertaining whether injuries in zones I and III have damaged major vascular structures may be difficult with clinical examination alone. Preoperative arteriography is extremely important if these patients are hemodynamically stable. Patients with penetrating injuries in zone II who have no neurologic deficit but require surgery may undergo surgery without arteriography, although preoperative arteriography is helpful in localizing the injury.

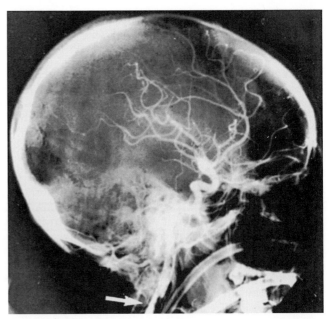

FIGURE 39-3 • Area of the internal carotid artery damaged by hyperextension trauma *(arrow)*.

Signs and symptoms suggesting arterial injury in the extremities apply equally to the neck, but unfortunately, these arteries may not be accessible for examination, especially after blunt trauma (Fig. 39-4). The clinical features of blunt trauma to the carotid artery are summarized in Table 39-7.[29] Few signs

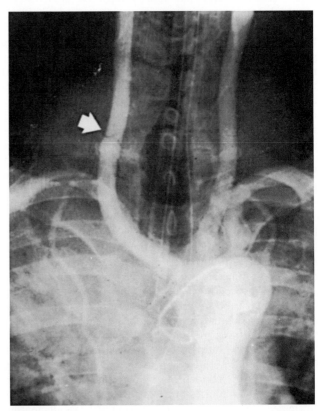

FIGURE 39-4 • Steering wheel injury *(arrow)* during an automobile accident caused pulmonary contusions and a fracture of the right common carotid artery. A graft was required to replace this section of the vessel.

TABLE 39–7	Clinical Features of Blunt Trauma to Carotid Arteries

Hematoma of lateral neck
Horner's syndrome
Transient ischemic attack
Lucid interval
Limb paresis in an alert patient

From Jernigan WR, Gardner WC: Carotid artery injuries due to closed cervical trauma. Trauma 11:429, 1971.

of injury may be present, because less than half of patients have local evidence of blunt trauma. Arteriography should be used liberally after blunt and penetrating trauma to the neck and thoracic outlet.

Aerodigestive injuries frequently accompany carotid artery trauma, especially with penetrating mechanisms. The surgeon must be vigilant to detect and treat these injuries, which can result in devastating complications if not addressed early. Endoscopy should include examination of the oropharynx, trachea, and esophagus. This is followed by esophagography with water-soluble media and, subsequently, barium. When aerodigestive injuries are present, the incision and repair strategy is critical to protect the vascular repair from gross contamination.

Operative Management

Patients who have carotid artery injuries and continued prograde flow are candidates for surgical repair. A patient who has complete occlusion of the internal carotid artery as a result of blunt trauma, is not bleeding, and has a severe neurologic deficit manifested by coma or hemiplegia is probably best treated nonoperatively. If operation is required for other reasons, the internal carotid artery can be ligated.[27] Complete removal of thrombus in these situations is often difficult, and residual clot may embolize and worsen the neurologic deficit.[30]

Vascular control and repair are performed as described in the preceding sections. Standard techniques are used, and every effort is made to avoid thromboembolic complications; precise suture and graft techniques are essential. As shown in Figure 39-5, the external carotid artery may be used to repair the internal carotid artery in certain circumstances. If lateral repair is not possible, a saphenous vein graft or an arterial autograft may be interposed, as shown in Figure 39-6. If the back-pressure from the internal carotid artery is less than 70 mm Hg, or if back-bleeding is scanty, the use of an intraluminal shunt is a satisfactory method to maintain cerebral blood flow while repairs are being completed.

A recent review of routine radiographic examination of patients sustaining blunt cerebrovascular injuries based its conclusions on injury grade. Grade I injuries were those with internal irregularity; grade II had dissection, flap, or thrombosis; grade III showed pseudoaneurysm formation; grade IV injuries were occlusions; and grade V were complete transections (see Table 39-5). The majority of carotid and vertebral arteries with grades IV and V lesions were unchanged 7 to 10 days after injury, whereas 57% of grade I and 8% of grade II injuries had healed, allowing cessation of therapy. Eight percent of grade I and 43% of grade II lesions had progressed to pseudoaneurysm formation, requiring intervention. Significantly, the

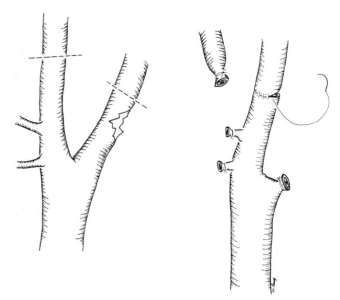

FIGURE 39–5 • If the internal carotid artery cannot be repaired directly, the external carotid artery can be mobilized and used as a substitute graft.

authors found no difference in healing or lesion progression based on whether the patient was treated with heparin, received antiplatelet therapy, or was left untreated. However, heparin may improve neurologic outcome in those with ischemic deficits and may prevent stroke in asymptomatic patients.[15]

Endovascular stent management has been reported with increasing regularity in the trauma literature. Although the series are generally small and the follow-up times comparatively short, there is an evolving trend toward the use of covered

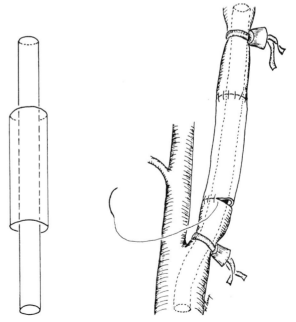

FIGURE 39–6 • When injuries of the internal carotid artery are associated with low back-pressure (<70 mm Hg) or scanty back-bleeding, a saphenous vein graft can be placed over the temporary inlaying shunt as the repair is completed.

stent-grafts, especially in patients with anatomically restrictive lesions or those in whom anticoagulation would be excessively risky.[31,32] Although some authors have already concluded that endovascular repair of both spontaneous and traumatic internal carotid artery dissections is a safe alternative to conventional surgery, long-term follow-up (75 years) must still be evaluated.[33] Presently, cautious optimism is warranted for endovascular stenting for such lesions in properly selected patients who are neurologically intact.

Postoperative Care

Although any vascular repair is susceptible to bleeding, bleeding is unusual unless multiple injuries or coagulation defects are present. Drains are not usually employed in isolated vascular wounds. However, in selected patients with cervical injuries, drains may be used for 12 to 24 hours to prevent the accumulation of blood, which may cause a compressing hematoma beneath the relatively rigid cervical fascia. Patients are carefully monitored for the appearance of neurologic deficits. Neurologic symptoms usually require arteriography or duplex ultrasonography to evaluate the status of the repair and to assess the possibility of cerebral thromboembolism. Postoperative carotid artery occlusion rarely occurs, but if it does, the patient should be returned immediately to the operating room for thrombectomy, correction of any technical errors, and reestablishment of flow. In these situations, a delay to perform arteriography is not recommended. Thrombosis and the emergence of a stroke require immediate surgery. Expeditious restoration of flow is often successful in preventing permanent neurologic problems.

Injuries of Vessels of the Root of the Neck

Injuries of vessels in zone I (thoracic outlet) are difficult to evaluate because they may be obscure. Operative exposure of the wound without proximal control can lead to fatal hemorrhage. If a penetrating wound in zone I is thought to have injured the great vessels, proximal control via a middle sternal splitting incision is recommended before exposing the wound. Similarly, if, during the course of cervical exploration through an incision along the anterior sternocleidomastoid muscle border, bleeding, hematoma, or blood staining of the carotid sheath in the depths of the wound at the root of the neck is encountered, an immediate sternal splitting incision should be made to control the great vessels of the arch.[18] All the vessels of the arch, with the exception of the left subclavian artery, can be reached easily through this approach; if necessary, the incision can be extended into the second or third interspace, or a separate left thoracotomy incision can be made to control the left subclavian artery. Because of its intrapleural location, the proximal left subclavian artery is best approached through an anterolateral thoracotomy. Although this incision facilitates proximal control, the more distal extrapleural portions cannot be reached. A supraclavicular incision is added for this purpose. Although many authors speak of the "open book" created when a median sternotomy connects an anterolateral thoracotomy to a supraclavicular incision, we have found that the approach does not open easily and typically results in multiple posterior rib fractures.

Repairs of these arteries are performed in the same fashion as described in the preceding sections. In most cases, backpressure in the innominate or left common carotid artery

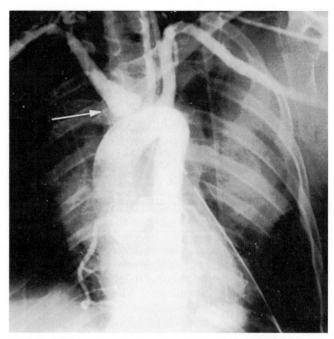

FIGURE 39–7 • A load of lumber fell on this young man and produced lung contusions and a wide mediastinum, which prompted the arteriogram. Note the nearly avulsed innominate artery (arrow).

exceeds 70 mm Hg. Temporary shunting techniques are not required if the patient's blood pressure is maintained within a normal range. Prosthetic grafts are needed more often for repair of the great vessels of the arch, because autografts of this size are usually not available (Fig. 39-7).

Several small series have reported the use of endovascular stents for the acute management of blunt thoracic aortic injuries. It is difficult to evaluate these studies because of the variation among traumatic lesions and associated injuries. Specifically, the time between injury and stent placement tends to be longer than that associated with traditional open operative management. One of the larger studies reported a mean time after injury of 5 months.[34] As with other endovascular series, long-term follow-up is limited. Reported procedural and short-term complications include hematoma at the access site (groin) and partial or complete coverage of nearby vessels, including the subclavian and iliac arteries.[35,36] Neurologic complications are rare. At this time, the use of covered stent-grafts should be approached with cautious optimism until long-term results become available.

INJURIES OF THE ABDOMINAL AORTA AND ITS BRANCHES

Almost all major vascular injuries in the abdomen are caused by penetrating trauma, usually gunshot wounds. Associated gastrointestinal injuries are common. This is a lethal combination, especially if multiple vascular wounds are present. Less than half of these patients survive.[18,37]

Diagnosis

In a hypotensive patient with a penetrating wound of the abdomen, the usual signs and symptoms of vascular injury can be expected, but because the arteries are inaccessible for examination, indirect evidence of injury assumes more importance. Although abdominal distention from the accumulation of blood can occur, massive retroperitoneal bleeding can be hidden, and little blood may be present in the peritoneal cavity. This may occur with knife wounds that enter from the back, particularly if the blade passes between two of the lower ribs. Such a wound may appear benign. Moreover, pulse deficits and limb ischemia, if present, are difficult to interpret in hypotensive patients. Because of the severity of most of these injuries, little time is available for protracted examination and diagnostic studies. The need for surgical exploration is obvious.

Plain radiographs, CT scans, "one-shot" intravenous pyelograms, and arteriograms all may be useful. Even if a vascular wound is not detected, such studies can expose other problems that require surgical correction. Abdominal paracentesis or lavage can document intraperitoneal bleeding, but false-negative results do occur, especially in the face of severe pelvic fractures.[38]

Hematuria should alert the surgeon to the possibility of a renovascular injury. If a patient shows microscopic hematuria and has not been in shock, the chance of a significant renovascular injury being present is very small, and additional evaluation is not indicated. However, if microscopic hematuria is accompanied by severe hypotension, or if gross hematuria is present, further evaluation is required, usually in the form of an intravenous contrast-enhanced CT scan. If kidney function is normal, with no apparent parenchymal or collecting system dysfunction, hospitalization and observation are acceptable. If kidney function is impaired or absent, or if parenchymal disruption is present, renal arteriography is indicated. If the major renal vascular architecture is intact, observation is sufficient, with repeated studies. If vascular wounds are present or collecting system disruption is diagnosed, surgical correction is required.

Operative Management

Hemodynamically unstable patients are taken immediately to the operating room; preparations for surgery are completed as necessary diagnostic maneuvers are finished and interpreted. The operating team is scrubbed and ready to intervene in the event of sudden collapse.[18] This may occur upon induction of anesthesia, when the tamponading effect of the tensed abdominal musculature is lost due to the use of paralytic agents.

The abdomen is opened through a long midline incision, a rapid exploration is performed, and attention is directed toward the major vessels. If a bleeding wound can be seen and exposed easily, it is controlled with vascular clamps. This is often the case with isolated wounds of the branches of the visceral arteries. Injuries of the aorta, especially the supraceliac aorta and that part containing the origins of the visceral branches (zones I and II as described by Lim and colleagues),[37] usually require a supraceliac clamp to control bleeding. This part of the aorta is approached through the gastrohepatic ligament, and the aorta is freed from the left crus of the diaphragm with finger dissection. Only the front and sides are mobilized to permit the placement of a long straight or slightly curved vascular clamp directly across the aorta in an anteroposterior plane. Temporary aortic occlusion at this level allows more rapid and precise exposure of wounds of the lower aorta and its branches. Control through a left thoracotomy may be required if the supraceliac approach is impractical or fails.

Infrarenal aortic wounds (Lim zone III) usually can be approached directly through the root of the mesentery using the usual methods for elective aortic operations. Wounds in the center of the mesenteric root often involve the pancreas and duodenum and can damage the major veins located there. A combination of aortic and major venous wounds is often lethal, and control of large venous injuries in this area is difficult to achieve.

When exposure of midaortic wounds is difficult because of obscuring hematomas, brisk bleeding, or multiple organ damage, mobilization of the left colon, spleen, and pancreas can allow the surgeon to reach the aorta and its branches. Reflection of the ascending colon and duodenum exposes the vena cava and aorta from the right side.

Once the vascular wounds are controlled, priorities of repair are set. Blood flow should be restored to the kidneys and liver first, because these organs are most sensitive to hypoxia. The intestine and the lower extremities can tolerate longer periods of ischemia. Repairs rarely require more than an hour to complete.

The method of vascular reconstruction is dictated by the nature of the wound. Usually, resection and end-to-end anastomosis are adequate for the aortic branches, unless tissue loss is extensive and interposition grafts are needed. Aortic wounds caused by knives and low-velocity gunshot wounds occasionally can be repaired with simple suturing; more extensive damage mandates patch angioplasty or grafting. Plastic prostheses are customarily needed to reconstruct the aortoiliac tree.

Large bowel penetration resulting in heavy bacterial soilage in association with aortic wounds presents special problems. Autogenous tissue repairs may succeed in some of these cases, but occasionally even arteries that are simply oversewn break down later because of infection. Severe contamination is an indication to restore blood flow to the lower extremities via a remote bypass rather than by aortoiliac grafting. Axillofemoral and femorofemoral subcutaneous grafts are favored. Sewing the two common iliac arteries together may be possible, thus using one axillofemoral graft to perfuse both legs. This avoids placing a prosthetic graft into an abdominal cavity with heavy bacterial contamination. Careful closure of oversewn arterial stumps (aortic and iliac especially) is essential. The closed ends are covered and protected by pedicle flaps of the greater omentum. Antibiotics are continued until all wounds are healed and all intravenous catheters are removed. Once healing is completed, restoration of normal vascular architecture can be considered.

Blunt renal artery injuries are being reported with increasing frequency, largely owing to the availability and routine use of CT scans.[39] To this end, case reports have emerged reporting the use of endovascular stents for repair.[40] Although the preliminary results are encouraging, stenting must be approached with caution. It is likely that endovascular techniques are most appropriate in patients with blunt renal artery injuries and multiple concomitant injuries, in whom extended open exploration and repair are relatively contraindicated.[40]

INJURIES OF THE ARTERIES OF THE EXTREMITIES

Femoral arteries are among the most frequently injured vessels, constituting approximately 20% of all arterial injuries. Acute ligation of the common femoral artery results in an amputation rate of approximately 50%—only slightly less than that noted after acute occlusion of the popliteal artery. Large veins and important nerves are found within the femoral triangle, making associated injuries of these structures common.

Popliteal artery injuries are especially difficult problems, and failure to repair them results in limb loss in almost two thirds of patients.[41] Penetrating wounds are usually easily diagnosed because virtually all create pulse deficits and, frequently, ischemia of the lower extremity. Patients with blunt trauma often show more difficult problems upon evaluation. Posterior dislocations of the knee, for example, are very likely to injure the popliteal artery. As Lefrac,[4] Dart and Braitman,[3] and others have indicated, these patients should have preoperative arteriography. Lefrac reported that of 152 patients with knee dislocations, 28% sustained popliteal artery injuries; half of these patients eventually lost the limb.[4] Overlooking an unstable knee during the examination of a patient who has multiple injuries is very easy. Although popliteal artery injuries caused by fracture-dislocations are usually easily identified because of a pulse deficit and, in most cases, ischemia, inexperienced examiners may assume that spasm is at fault. This can be a serious error that ultimately results in limb loss. Preoperative arteriography is important and may be the only way to ascertain the extent of the injury.[24]

Preoperative Preparation

Many of these patients have lost a great deal of blood by the time they are examined. Resuscitation should proceed in an aggressive and orderly manner before surgery. Stabilization of fractures should be performed early. This is easier if the patient is taken directly to the operating room, especially if he or she is hemodynamically unstable. Many surgeons favor the use of external techniques for bone stabilization to avoid introducing foreign bodies into the area of potential vascular repair. However, both internal fixation and external fixation have been used successfully. Temporary stabilization is essential during early care to prevent further damage.

Operative Management

As with other vascular wounds, general anesthesia is usually required for operative repair. The opposite extremity is prepared so that if vascular autografts are required, the contralateral saphenous vein will be available. With concomitant femoral or popliteal vein injuries, one may wish to preserve the ipsilateral saphenous vein in case more serious venous injuries cannot be repaired. Repairing concomitant popliteal vein injuries is especially important if the saphenous vein is damaged.[41]

Rich and Spencer presented compelling reasons for repair of the popliteal vein as well as the artery, pointing out that the incidence of thromboembolic events is approximately 13% after vein repair but is more than 50% after ligation.[42] These authors and Snyder and colleagues[41] also suggested that continued popliteal artery patency is enhanced by simultaneous repair of popliteal vein injuries.

In most situations, the wounds are approached through the same medial vertical incision used for elective surgery.

Proximal and distal control can be difficult to obtain when the patient is prone and the vessels are approached posteriorly through the popliteal space.

The basic techniques of repair are those used in other vascular surgery. Damaged tissue is resected, and an end-to-end anastomosis with careful intimal coaptation is constructed. Popliteal arteries are especially vulnerable to injury by a vascular clamp, and soft noncrushing instruments are best for temporary occlusion. If the injury is in an atherosclerotic artery, controlling the bleeding by inserting an intraluminal catheter may be more suitable, thus avoiding wall damage that might predispose to immediate thrombosis or enhance the subsequent progress of the atheromatous disease.

For patients who have sustained blunt trauma and multiple fractures, initial repair of the popliteal artery and vein may be necessary. The vascular surgeon remains in attendance while final stabilization of the fractures is obtained by either internal or external fixation. In situations in which ischemia is not present, such as the case of a superficial femoral artery occlusion, completing the orthopedic repairs first may be practical. Once the bone is stabilized, constructing an arterial repair of the proper length and tension is easier. If the foot is ischemic and extensive orthopedic repairs are required, temporary inlaying shunts can be placed in the popliteal artery and vein. These decisions should be made through consultation between the vascular surgeon and the orthopedic surgeon; both should be in attendance during bony repair to avoid disruption of the vascular suture lines.

Postoperatively, patency of the repair is usually apparent by the immediate reappearance of pedal pulses. If there is any question about the adequacy of the repair, or if distal thromboembolism appears likely, operative arteriography is indicated. Failure to restore pulses is usually a technical problem and is seldom caused by persistent spasm.

TIBIAL ARTERY INJURIES

Injuries to the tibial arteries present a difficult problem because, in most cases, they do not result in severe ischemia unless two of the three arteries are damaged. In patients who have penetrating trauma but otherwise do not require operative exploration, and if only one tibial artery is occluded and no bleeding is present, such an injury can be accepted without repair. Arteriographic survey of these patients is essential to determine whether a significant problem is present. In the absence of other indications, exploration of a tibial artery injury would be performed only if it were bleeding or if arteriography revealed an AV fistula or false aneurysm.

FALSE ANEURYSMS AND ARTERIOVENOUS FISTULAS

Complications of vascular injuries such as thrombosis, delayed bleeding, AV fistulas, and false aneurysms are more likely to occur, and are much more difficult to manage, if the injury is not treated promptly. False aneurysms and AV fistulas can occur immediately after the injury; bleeding occurs into a cavity that is confined by surrounding tissue, and a hematoma forms (sometimes false aneurysms are called pulsating hematomas). Although spontaneous regression of AV fistulas and false aneurysms can occur, the studies of Shumacker and Wayson demonstrated that this is unlikely.[43] Less than 3% of AV fistulas and less than 6% of false aneurysms heal spontaneously.

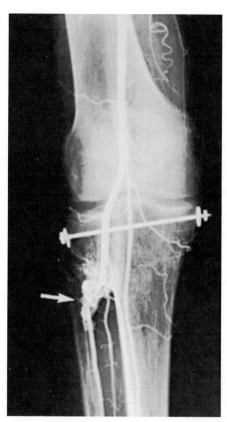

FIGURE 39–8 • Arteriovenous fistula of the anterior tibial artery and vein *(arrow).* Orthopedic repairs were completed previously, without knowledge of the vascular wound.

These lesions resolve only when they thrombose, and thrombosis of major arteries is not tolerated without unacceptable ischemia. Because spontaneous regression is unlikely, and because most AV fistulas and false aneurysms increase in size and complexity with the passage of time, operative repair becomes much more difficult if surgery is delayed. Increasing edema, inflammation, and expansion of the lesion slowly encroach on and involve surrounding neurovascular structures, making repair more difficult (Fig. 39-8).

A false aneurysm is the result of an incomplete injury that permits continued bleeding from a laceration. Transection of an artery is customarily followed by retraction and clotting and, in the case of small vessels, cessation of bleeding. Contiguous tangential wounds of arteries and veins may develop into AV fistulas, even acutely.

The most apparent clinical feature of a false aneurysm is a pulsatile mass that is associated with either an acute or a chronic penetrating wound. A murmur may be heard over the mass because the tangential laceration of the artery permits the escape of blood into the surrounding tissues, ultimately forming a tamponading clot. Although the physical diagnosis is usually easy when the mass is located in the extremities, arteriography is important to ascertain the exact number and location of the involved vessels and to plan the operative repair properly.

An AV fistula may be associated with a false aneurysm, or a clean endothelial channel may form in a chronic AV fistula. In some cases, very little inflammation may be present about the lesion, although the entrance of high-pressure arterial blood flow into the veins produces varicosities if the veins are thin walled and fragile. Occasionally, false aneurysms and AV fistulas are combined.

The Nicoladoni-Branham sign can be elicited in some patients with AV fistulas. Digital occlusion of the fistula results in a slowing of the heart rate because of the reduction of flow into the right atrium. A continuous, machinery-like murmur usually occurs over the fistula, and there may be evidence of venous hypertension and adjacent varicosities. When the shunt is large, ischemia of the distal extremity may result from shunting of large amounts of arterial blood into the low-pressure venous system. On rare occasions, large traumatic AV fistulas between the aorta and the vena cava cause florid heart failure as a result of the recirculation of enormous amounts of blood. Emergency operations may be required to treat congestive heart failure.

Large AV fistulas produce relentless enlargement of the feeding vessels and an increase in the number and complexity of the veins in the drainage system. The arteries become elongated and tortuous, and their walls become thinner. Spontaneous rupture is unusual, but trauma can lead to dangerous hemorrhage.

Mural thrombosis within the system occurs occasionally. Intravascular coagulation can cause bleeding tendencies as clotting factors are depleted. Such complications should be identified and corrected before surgical repair is undertaken.

Initial surgical treatment of identified arterial injuries reduces the incidence of delayed traumatic AV fistulas and false aneurysms. Only those injuries that were missed on the initial examination and were not immediately apparent will become large enough to develop symptoms. These are clearly few in number when appropriate repair is undertaken after the initial trauma.

Preoperative arteriography of AV fistulas and false aneurysms is an important step for operative planning because the lesion may be much more extensive than it appears clinically. This is especially true of deep-seated lesions involving the root of the neck, the cervical vessels, or the abdominal vessels. Even in the extremities, these lesions can be formidable. Before entering them, proximal and distal control of major arteries and veins must be achieved. In the extremities, this can be facilitated by the use of a proximal pneumatic orthopedic tourniquet. In other areas, careful dissection remote from the area of the AV fistula is required to gain control before the lesion is entered (Fig. 39-9).

For nonessential small vessels involved with a false aneurysm or AV fistula, ligation may be satisfactory. For major muscular arteries, however, repair is indicated. This is performed in the usual fashion once the vessels are controlled and identified. With large false aneurysms, the most expedient method generally involves obtaining proximal and distal control without entering the immediate area of the pseudoaneurysm. Once the vessels are clamped, the aneurysm is opened and feeding branches are controlled from within the aneurysm sac by using intraluminal occlusion catheters (such as a Fogarty catheter with an attached three-way stopcock) or special balloon occlusion catheters designed for this purpose. Repair is then completed in the usual fashion. This often requires only lateral arteriorrhaphy, because most false aneurysms result not from complete transection of the artery but from a tangential laceration that does not permit the vessel to retract and clot. If lateral repair is not possible without undue narrowing, patch-graft angioplasty may be performed. Resection and anastomosis, with appropriate graft interposition, are also used for repair.

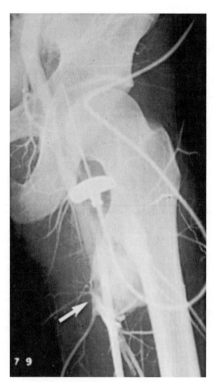

FIGURE 39–9 • This large false aneurysm of the deep femoral artery *(arrow)* was diagnosed only by arteriography.

The postoperative care of these patients is similar to that provided after the repair of other arterial lesions. The pulses be monitored, and neuromuscular function of the extremity must be tested to ascertain that the repair remains patent.

Intraluminal endovascular techniques are now being used to place stent-grafts across traumatic AV fistulas and pseudo-aneurysms. Although most reports include only a few patients, increased expertise is being gained rapidly.[44] Percutaneous stent placement is guided by either angiography or intravascular sonography, and duplex ultrasonography is used postoperatively to assess patency and graft position. Although deployed in a number of locations, the most practical use of these techniques appears to be where traditional operative exposure is difficult to obtain, such as the axillosubclavian system (Fig. 39-10).[45] Experience with these devices has generally been limited to case reports, although some small series have been reported.[46,47] Initial success rates appear to be favorable, but conclusions about long-term results cannot be made because such series admix acute and chronic patients and those with iatrogenic and traumatic causes.[46] Some of the reported disadvantages of endovascular management of these injuries include fatigue of the materials, the need for a large introducer, failure of molding of the stent-graft to the arterial wall (especially in rapidly tapering or tortuous vessels), and wrinkling at its ends.[47,48] Additional stents may be required at the ends of the graft. Intimal hyperplasia and the need for subsequent angioplasty have also been reported.[47] At present, the use of such endovascular techniques should be reserved for anatomically difficult lesions. Prospective trials are required before they can be recommended routinely, even for larger vessels such as the thoracic aorta.[49] Close postprocedure follow-up is required to ensure patency and maintenance of stent integrity.

MINIMAL (NONOCCLUSIVE) VASCULAR INJURY

In conjunction with the trend away from routine angiography for suspected extremity injuries, some have begun to question the need to repair "minimal" vascular injuries.[50] Many of these injuries, although occurring in major or critical arteries, consist of intimal fractures, small pseudoaneurysms, mural stenoses, and small AV fistulas (Fig. 39-11). Based on the fact that arteries punctured and dilated for vascular access usually heal without incident, the need to repair all vascular injuries is being examined. The nonocclusive lesions involved vary somewhat among authors, but typical angiographic findings include intimal defects (eccentric irregularities of the contrast column adjacent to the arterial wall), intimal flaps (non–flow-limiting injuries that appear as a longitudinal band of decreased contrast concentration extending across the lumen), pseudoaneurysms (usually <0.5 cm), arterial stenoses, and small AV fistulas.[50,51]

A number of series have reported good outcomes in patients with minimal injuries treated nonoperatively. Unfortunately, in many of these studies, the duration of follow-up was limited to either inpatient observation or a few clinic visits.[50,51] Although some of the studies have more longitudinal information, the natural history of these untreated lesions is not well defined. Pseudoaneurysms seem to have the greatest propensity to thrombose or expand and require the closest follow-up when treated nonoperatively. Small intimal flaps and defects probably have a better prognosis. AV fistulas that enlarge can usually be treated with endovascular techniques such as embolization. Tufaro and coworkers questioned the wisdom of the nonoperative approach in their experience with seven patients treated for "minor" intimal flaps.[52] All the patients were monitored after the initial injury with repeat ankle-brachial index measurements for up to 48 hours before discharge. Six of the seven returned with acute onset of pain or paresthesias. Identified abnormalities included thrombosis, pseudoaneurysms, and an AV fistula, all of which required surgery. In an experimental canine model reported by Neville and colleagues,[53] intimal flaps with stenosis greater than 75% were at high risk of thrombosis, even though they were not initially occlusive after formation.

The long-term outcome of minimal vascular injuries is precarious. Clearly, a difference exists between injuries caused by the low-velocity, directed punctures produced by an angiography needle and those caused by a knife or bullet. Associated soft tissue and venous trauma in the latter group clearly contributes to outcome. Nonoperative management should be elected only in those patients whose lesions are clearly nonocclusive and who will return regularly for evaluation. The duration of such follow-up is still uncertain but should last at least several years and should include duplex sonography.

INJURIES OF THE INFERIOR VENA CAVA

Wounds of the inferior vena cava are among the most lethal vascular injuries.[54] One in every 50 gunshot wounds and 1 in every 300 knife wounds of the abdomen injure the vena cava. Because of the serious nature of these injuries, one third of patients die before they reach the hospital, and half of the remainder die during their hospitalization. Most deaths during treatment are caused by bleeding, because of the difficulty of controlling injuries of the large veins, but many patients

Pretreatment   Postdeployment

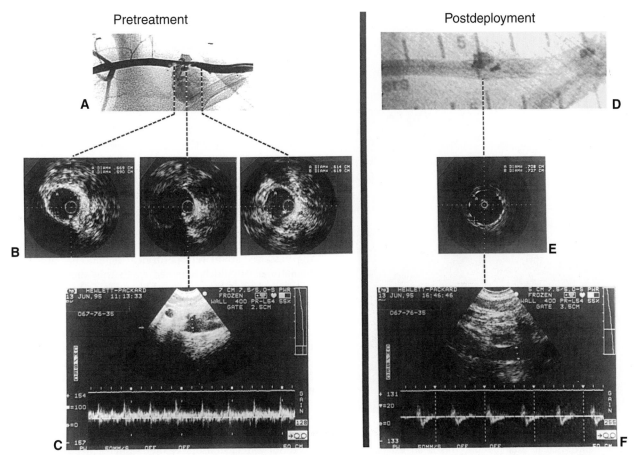

FIGURE 39–10 • Composite photograph of the pretreatment and post-treatment images acquired during intravascular ultrasound-guided deployment of an endoluminal graft to treat an arteriovenous (AV) fistula of the right axillary artery caused by a gunshot injury. Intravascular ultrasound images acquired at the beginning of the procedure revealed the dimensions of the proximal and distal artery and the length of the injury to the vessel. A corresponding duplex gray-scale surface ultrasound image of the lesion taken before beginning the intervention demonstrates the AV connection. The postdeployment angiogram demonstrates complete isolation and exclusion of the AV fistula, which is confirmed by the intravascular ultrasound inspection and postprocedure gray-scale surface duplex image of the device. (From White RA, Donayre CE, Walot I, et al: Preliminary clinical outcome and imaging criterion for endovascular prosthesis development in high risk patients with aortoiliac and traumatic arterial lesions. J Vasc Surg 24:556-571, 1996.)

also have associated injuries. As described by Perry,[5] 79% of patients with penetrating trauma causing inferior vena cava wounds had injuries of other retroperitoneal structures that adversely affected survival. The renal vein, portal vein, and aorta are vulnerable to these injuries, as are the colon, liver, pancreas, and duodenum. Table 39-8 lists those injuries often associated with vena cava wounds.

The cause of the vena cava injury affects mortality (Table 39-9). Patients who have blunt trauma and shotgun injuries are more likely to die than are those who have stab wounds, especially if the injury is located in the upper part of the vena cava (Table 39-10).

Most patients, when initially examined, have an obviously serious injury manifested by hypotension and occasional abdominal distention. Few laboratory results are of diagnostic value, except perhaps the presence of hematuria or gastrointestinal bleeding, which suggests the presence of other injuries. Routine radiographic studies of the chest and abdomen are recommended if the patient is stable, but except for inferior venacavography, these tests are rarely specific. The predictors of high mortality are summarized in Table 39-11.

Operative Management

Most patients can be managed with a midline abdominal incision from the xiphoid to the pubis. In some instances, thoracotomy may be required if a suprarenal caval injury is present. The chest should be prepared in case the incision must be extended into the thorax.

A rapid abdominal exploration usually exposes major vascular injuries; this allows the surgeon to establish priorities of repair. Controlling the bleeding initially, completing the resuscitation, and then assigning priorities is preferable. Control of retroperitoneal bleeding may require direct pressure with fingers or sponge sticks while the vein is exposed and the vascular clamps are placed. Use of vascular clamps before adequate mobilization of the vena cava virtually guarantees additional iatrogenic injury. Sponge sticks should be used until exposure is adequate.

The suggestion has been made that some retroperitoneal injuries do not need to be explored unless they are expanding or pulsatile, but this has not been our experience. In a study of 110 patients with penetrating caval injuries, the size of the

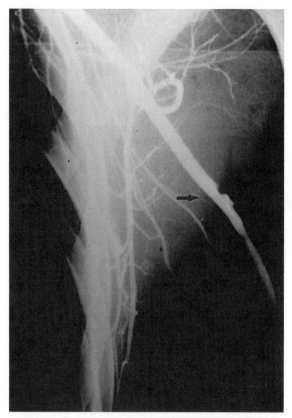

FIGURE 39–11 • Enlargement of an angiogram obtained after a gunshot wound to the left axilla. The patient had a normal ipsilateral neurovascular examination. This is an example of a nonocclusive "minimal" vascular injury (*arrow* points to the intimal defect).

hematoma did not predict the injury.[5] Moreover, three fourths of the patients had an associated injury of some kind. In contrast, pelvic hematomas caused by fractures are not opened unless specific injuries have been identified by arteriography or other studies. Bleeding from cancellous pelvic bones is often profuse and difficult to control. Hemorrhage from pelvic fractures is best diagnosed preoperatively by CT scan, which reveals a contained retroperitoneal hematoma. When these patients undergo surgery for other indications,

TABLE 39–8	Injuries Associated with 110 Inferior Vena Cava Injuries
Location of Injury	**No. of Injuries**
Aorta, iliac artery	13
Major splanchnic vessel	26
Renal artery or vein	20
Liver	46
Duodenum	27
Kidney	21
Pancreas	18
Spleen	10
Colon	27
Other	21

From Perry MO: Management of Acute Vascular Injuries. Baltimore, Williams & Wikins, 1981.

TABLE 39–9	Mortality from Inferior Vena Cava Injuries by Mechanism of Injury		
Injury	**No. of Patients**	**No. Died**	**Mortality (%)**
Bullet	74	24	32
Shotgun pellets	8	6	75
Stab wound	15	2	13
Blunt trauma	13	11	85
Total	110	43	39

From Perry MO: Management of Acute Vascular Injuries. Baltimore, Williams & Wikins, 1981.

the hematoma should not be entered because the resulting hemorrhage is extremely difficult to control.[55] These injuries are best managed by radiographic embolization of the bleeding vessels. Lateral retroperitoneal hematomas and central hematomas should be opened when they are expanding or pulsatile. Inflow control should be obtained before entering the hematoma. All central hematomas after penetrating injury should be explored.

Simple lacerations or punctures can be repaired by venorrhaphy and tangential repair. If the wound is large, a partially occluding clamp may be placed about it and the lesion oversewn with a continuous suture. In patients who have anterior and posterior injuries of the vena cava, repair of the posterior wound may be effected by rotation of the cava (perhaps requiring ligation of lumbar veins) and direct suture. In some instances, the anterior caval wound can be enlarged and the posterior wall laceration repaired from the inside under direct vision.[38]

Transections of the vena cava can usually be repaired by end-to-end vascular techniques, although the vena cava does not permit loss of a long segment. If the cava is severely lacerated, if multiple wounds are present that require complicated grafts, or if repair poses a prohibitive risk in a patient with multiple injuries, ligation of the infrarenal cava is acceptable. This is rarely necessary, however.

Wounds at or above the renal veins are difficult to expose and carry a higher mortality; more than half these patients die.[54] If bleeding from behind the liver is encountered and cannot be easily identified as coming from a laceration of the anterior cava below the caudate lobe, other maneuvers may be needed. Division of the supporting ligaments permits the liver to be displaced medially a considerable distance, and, in some people, adequate exposure can be obtained for primary repair of the cava.[16,56] Sudden interruption of the inferior vena

TABLE 39–10	Mortality from Inferior Vena Cava Injuries by Location		
Location	**No. of Patients**	**No. Died**	**Mortality (%)**
Above renal veins	20	11	55
At renal veins	22	13	59
Below renal veins	52	15	29
Bifurcation	16	4	25
Total	110	43	39

From Perry MO: Management of Acute Vascular Injuries. Baltimore, Williams & Wikins, 1981.

TABLE 39–11	Predictors of High Mortality after Vena Cava Injuries

History
  Blunt trauma
Resuscitation
  Admission blood pressure < 70 mm Hg
  Failure to respond to volume resuscitation
  Preoperative cardiac arrest
  Need for emergency room thoracotomy
Operative findings
  Retrohepatic caval injury
  Associated cardiac or aortic injury
  Severe liver injury
  Multiple-organ or vascular injuries
  Severe central nervous system injury

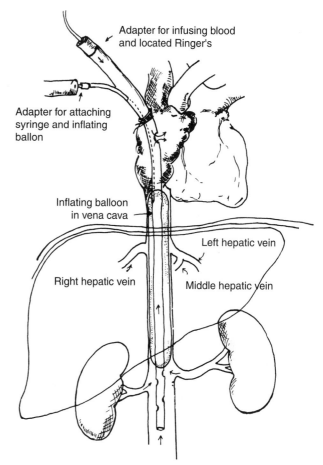

FIGURE 39–13 • Madding-Kennedy intracaval shunt. (Redrawn from Madding GF, Kennedy PA: Trauma to the Liver. Philadelphia, WB Saunders, 1971.)

cava blood flow returning to the heart may result in cardiac arrest. Temporary caval occlusion should be approached cautiously, with careful monitoring of blood pressure and heart rate. If extensive suprarenal caval injuries are seen after mobilization of the liver, or if two or three hepatic veins are involved in the injury, employing an intracaval shunt as described by Schrock and colleagues may be necessary[57] (Fig. 39-12). A 38 French Tygon shunt with appropriate openings can be inserted by the transatrial technique, although McClelland and associates described a method using an infrarenal caval shunt.[38] In most situations, this technique is not required, because adequate mobilization permits temporary occlusion and repair. If an intracaval shunt is used, the balloon shunt described by Madding and Kennedy may be the simplest to use for these procedures[56] (Fig. 39-13).

Concomitant repair of hepatic vein injuries is easier in these situations if an intracaval shunt is in place, but one of the hepatic veins may be safely ligated if repair is not possible.

These vena cava repairs can usually be completed within 30 minutes, a period of ischemia that is well tolerated by the normothermic liver. Almost inevitably, hypothermia occurs with these injuries because of the infusion of large amounts of blood and electrolyte solutions. Further regional hypothermia for liver protection may be induced by irrigating the liver directly with a saline solution at 4°C. This offers additional protection if prolonged liver ischemia occurs during caval repair (and especially if temporary hepatic artery occlusion is required).

In patients with isolated wounds of the inferior vena cava below the renal veins, direct suture is usually effective, and complications are few; operative mortality is approximately 11%. However, in our experience, 67% of patients with a vena cava injury associated with one or more major vessel injuries had a fatal outcome. All the patients with inferior vena cava wounds at or above the renal veins had associated injuries, usually to the liver or bowel and occasionally to the pancreas, stomach, or colon. Mortality is very high in this group of patients regardless of the cause of injury, but mortality

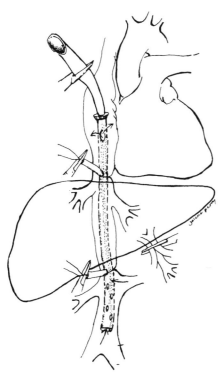

FIGURE 39–12 • Transatrial intracaval shunt in place. (Redrawn from Schrock T, Blaisdell FW, Mathewson C Jr: Management of blunt trauma to the liver and hepatic veins. Arch Surg 96:698, 1968.)

TABLE 39–12	Mortality from Inferior Vena Cava Injuries by Type of Hemorrhage		
Type of Hemorrhage	**No. of Patients**	**No. Died**	**Mortality (%)**
Active bleeding	45	34	76
Tamponade	62	9	15
Not specified	3	0	0
Total	110	43	39

From Perry MO: Management of Acute Vascular Injuries. Baltimore, Williams & Wikins, 1981.

is especially high if the vena cava is injured as a result of blunt trauma or a shotgun blast and is actively bleeding at the time of surgery (Table 39-12).

Late thromboembolic phenomena are uncommon, although few studies have described serial inferior venacavograms. Most patients with isolated vena cava wounds do not have recurrent thrombosis or thromboembolic phenomena. These data strongly suggest that repair of the vena cava is an effective procedure and is associated with fewer problems than is ligation.

REFERENCES

1. California Wellness Foundation: Fact Sheet, Feb 12, 1995.
2. Bongard F, Dubrow T, Klein S: Vascular injuries in the urban battleground: Experience at a metropolitan trauma center. Ann Vasc Surg 4:415-418, 1990.
3. Dart CH, Braitman HE: Popliteal artery injury following fracture or dislocation at the knee. Arch Surg 112:969-973, 1977.
4. Lefrac EA: Knee dislocation. Arch Surg 111:1021, 1976.
5. Perry MO: Management of Acute Vascular Injuries. Baltimore, Williams & Wilkins, 1981.
6. Lynch J, Johansen KH: Can Doppler pressure measurement replace "exclusion" arteriography in the diagnosis of arterial trauma? Ann Surg 214:737-741, 1991.
7. Bynoe RP, Miles WS, Bell RM, et al: Noninvasive diagnosis of vascular trauma by duplex ultrasonography. J Vasc Surg 14:346-352, 1991.
8. Gagne P, Cone JB, McFarland D, et al: Proximity penetrating extremity trauma: The role of duplex ultrasound in the detection of occult venous injuries. J Trauma 39:1152-1163, 1995.
9. Morgan PW, Goodman LR, Aprahamian C, et al: Evaluation of traumatic aortic injury: Does dynamic contrast-enhanced CT play a role? Radiology 182:661-666, 1992.
10. Demetriades D, Gomez H, Velmahos G, et al: Routine helical computed tomographic evaluation of the mediastinum in high-risk blunt trauma patients. Arch Surg 133:1084-1088, 1998.
11. Snyder WH III, Thal ER, Bridges RA, et al: The validity of normal arteriography in penetrating trauma. Arch Surg 113:424-426, 1978.
12. Weaver FA, Yellin AE, Bauer M, et al: Is arterial proximity a valid indication for arteriography in penetrating extremity trauma? Arch Surg 125:1256-1260, 1990.
13. Reid JDS, Weigelt JA, Thal ER, et al: Assessment of proximity of a wound to major vascular structures as an indication for arteriography. Arch Surg 128:942-946, 1988.
14. Frykberg ER, Dennis JW, Bishop K, et al: The reliability of physical examination in the evaluation of penetrating extremity trauma for vascular injury: Results at one year. J Trauma 31:502-511, 1991.
15. Biffl WL, Ray CE Jr, Moore EE, et al: Treatment-related outcomes from blunt cerebrovascular injuries: Importance of routine follow-up arteriography. Ann Surg. 235:699-706, 2002.
16. Rich N, Spencer F: Vascular Trauma. Philadelphia, WB Saunders, 1978, p 75.
17. Flint LM, Snyder WH, Perry MO, Shires GT: Management of major vascular injuries in the base of the neck. Arch Surg 106:407-413, 1973.
18. Mattox KL, McCollum WB, Beall AC, et al: Management of penetrating injuries of the suprarenal aorta. J Trauma 15:808-815, 1975.
19. Moore EE, Burch JM, Francoise RJ, et al: Staged physiologic restoration and damage control surgery. World J Surg 22:1184-1190, 1998.
20. Hirshberg A, Walden R: Damage control for abdominal trauma. Surg Clin North Am 77:813-820, 1997.
21. Carillo EH, Spain DA, Wilson MA, et al: Alternatives in the management of penetrating injuries to the iliac vessels. J Trauma 44:1024-1029, 1998.
22. Ehrenfeld WK, Wilbur BG, Olcott CN, Stoney RJ: Autogenous tissue reconstruction in the management of infected prosthetic grafts. Surgery 85:82-92, 1979.
23. Bongard FS, White GH, Klein SR: Management strategy of complex extremity injuries. Am J Surg 158:151-155, 1989.
24. Bongard FS: Management strategy for combined vascular and orthopedic injuries. Perspect Vasc Surg 3:8-30, 1991.
25. Thal ER, Snyder WH, Hays RJ, Perry MO: Management of carotid artery injuries. Surgery 76:955-962, 1974.
26. Yamada S, Kindt GW, Youmans JR: Carotid artery occlusion due to nonpenetrating injury. J Trauma 7:333-342, 1967.
27. Liekweg WG, Greenfield LJ: Management of penetrating carotid injury. Ann Surg 188:587-592, 1978.
28. Monson DO, Saletta JD, Freeark RJ: Carotid-vertebral trauma. J Trauma 9:987, 1969.
29. Jernigan WR, Gardner WC: Carotid artery injuries due to closed cervical trauma. Trauma 11:429-435, 1971.
30. Perry MO, Snyder WH, Thal ER: Carotid artery injuries caused by blunt trauma. Ann Surg 192:74-77, 1980.
31. Wyers MC, Powell RJ: Management of carotid injuries in a hostile neck using endovascular grafts. J Vasc Surg 39:1335-1339, 2004.
32. Biffl WL, Moore EE, Offner PJ, et al: Blunt carotid and vertebral arterial injuries. World J Surg 25:1036-1043, 2001.
33. Assadian A, Senekowitsch C, Rotter R, et al: Long-term results of covered stent repair of internal carotid artery dissections. J Vasc Surg 40:484-487, 2004.
34. Meites G, Conil C, Rousseau H, et al: Indication of endovascular stent grafts for traumatic rupture of the thoracic aorta. Ann Fr Anesth Reanim 23:700-703, 2004.
35. Uzieblo M, Sanchez LA, Rubin BG, et al: Endovascular repair of traumatic descending thoracic arotic disruptions: Should endovascular therapy become the gold standard? Vasc Endovasc Surg 38:331-337, 2004.
36. Dunham MB, Zygun D, Petrasek P, et al: Endovascular stent grafts for acute blunt aortic injury. J Trauma 56:1173-1178, 2004.
37. Lim RC, Trunkey DD, Blaisdell FW: Acute abdominal aortic injury. Arch Surg 109:706, 1974.
38. McClelland RN, Canizaro PC, Shires GT: Repair of hepatic venous, intrahepatic vena caval and portal venous injuries. Major Probl Clin Surg 3:146-153, 1971.
39. Bruce LM, Croce MA, Santaniello JM, et al: Blunt renal artery injury: Incidence, diagnosis, and management. Am Surg 67:550-554, 2001.
40. Lee JT, White RA: Endovascular management of blunt traumatic renal artery dissection. J Endovasc Ther 9:354-358, 2002.
41. Snyder WH, Watkins WL, Bone GE: Civilian popliteal artery trauma: An eleven year experience with 83 injuries. Surgery 85:101, 1979.
42. Rich N, Spencer F: Venous injuries. In Vascular Trauma. Philadelphia, WB Saunders, 1978, p 156.
43. Shumacker HB, Wayson EE: Spontaneous care of aneurysms and arteriovenous fistulas with some notes on intravascular thrombosis. Am J Surg 79:532, 1950.
44. Marin ML, Veith FJ, Panetta TF, et al: Transluminally placed endovascular stented graft repair for arterial trauma. J Vasc Surg 20:466-472, 1994.
45. White RA, Donayre CE, Walot I, et al: Preliminary clinical outcome and imaging criterion for endovascular prosthesis development in high-risk patients with aortoiliac and traumatic arterial lesions. J Vasc Surg 24:556-571, 1996.
46. Parodi JC, Schonholz C, Ferreira LM, Bergan J: Endovascular stent-graft treatment of traumatic arterial lesions. Ann Vasc Surg 13:121-129, 1999.
47. Sanchez LA, Veith FJ, Ohki T, et al: Early experience with the Corvita endoluminal graft for treatment of arterial injuries. Ann Vasc Surg 13:151-157, 1999.
48. Patel AV, Marin ML, Veith FJ, et al: Endovascular graft repair of penetrating subclavian artery injuries. J Endovasc Surg 3:382-388, 1996.
49. Rousseau H, Soula P, Perreault P, et al: Delayed treatment of traumatic rupture of the thoracic aorta with endoluminal covered stent. Circulation 99:498-504, 1999.
50. Stain SC, Yellin AE, Weaver FA, et al: Selective management of nonocclusive arterial injuries. Arch Surg 124:1136-1141, 1989.
51. Frykberg ER, Crump JM, Dennis JW, et al: Nonoperative observation of clinically occult arterial injuries: A prospective evaluation. Surgery 109:85-96, 1991.

52. Tufaro A, Arnold T, Rummel M, et al: Adverse outcome of nonoperative management of intimal injuries caused by penetrating trauma. J Vasc Surg 20:656-659, 1994.
53. Neville RF, Hobson RW 2nd, Watanabe B, et al: A prospective evaluation of arterial intimal injuries in an experimental model. J Trauma 31:669-675, 1991.
54. Graham JM, Mattox KL, Beall AC, DeBakey ME: Traumatic injuries of the inferior vena cava. Arch Surg 113:413-418, 1978.
55. Klein SR, Bongard FS, Mehringer CM: Management strategy of vascular injuries associated with pelvic fractures. J Cardiovasc Surg (Torino) 33:349-357, 1992.
56. Madding GF, Kennedy PA: Trauma to the Liver. Philadelphia, WB Saunders, 1971.
57. Schrock T, Blaisdell FW, Mathewson C Jr: Management of blunt trauma to the liver and hepatic veins. Arch Surg 96:698, 1968.

Questions

1. **A 20-year-old man has a stab wound of the right groin near the common femoral artery. Arterial bleeding occurred initially, but now a 2- by 2-cm hematoma overlies the vessels. Which of the following protocols is preferred?**
   (a) Immediate exploration in the operating room
   (b) Arteriogram with runoff films
   (c) B-mode sonogram
   (d) Hospitalization and observation for a few days

2. **Arterial injuries as a result of blunt trauma are especially likely with which of the following injuries?**
   (a) Shoulder dislocation
   (b) Posterior knee dislocation
   (c) Midfemoral shaft fracture
   (d) Clavicular fracture

3. **A 25-year-old man is admitted because of a bullet wound of the right flank. He is not in shock and has no hematuria or gastrointestinal bleeding. At exploration, a moderate collection of blood overlies the aorta and inferior vena cava above the bifurcation. What should be done now?**
   (a) If the colon and small bowel are intact, nothing
   (b) Exposure and exploration of the right kidney
   (c) Arteriogram on the table
   (d) Exploration of midline hematoma

4. **A 22-year-old man is admitted with a gunshot wound to the right groin. His leg is pulseless and cool. At exploration, he is found to have extensive soft tissue destruction and a 3-cm defect in the superficial femoral artery. He is hemodynamically stable during the exploration. What is the best strategy at this time?**
   (a) Replace the missing segment with an appropriately sized PTFE graft
   (b) Replace the missing segment with ipsilateral saphenous vein
   (c) Replace the missing segment with contralateral saphenous vein
   (d) Ligate the proximal and distal ends of the vessel and plan reoperation as indicated if the limb becomes ischemic

5. **A 17-year-old boy incurred a penetrating wound of his left medial thigh during a motor vehicle accident. When examined, he had no ischemia, but moderate swelling surrounded the wound. A continuous murmur was heard in this area. Which of the following clinical features is least likely to be present?**
   (a) Nicolodani-Branham sign
   (b) Tachycardia
   (c) Empty veins
   (d) Decreased ankle blood pressure

6. **What is the best course of treatment for the patient in question 5?**
   (a) Admit him for observation, awaiting resolution
   (b) Observe him and measure the ankle-brachial index every 4 hours
   (c) Schedule MRI of the legs
   (d) Admit him for arteriography

7. **A patient presents with a gunshot wound of the right medial thigh near the course of the superficial femoral artery. Distal pulses are normal, but a murmur is heard over the injury site. Which of the following treatment options is most appropriate?**
   (a) Admit the patient for observation with serial ankle-brachial index measurements
   (b) Perform duplex ultrasonography as an outpatient
   (c) Explore immediately with on-table angiography
   (d) Admit for angiography

8. **Which of the following "minimal" vascular injuries has the highest incidence of subsequent complications?**
   (a) Intimal flap
   (b) Stenosis
   (c) Intimal defect
   (d) Pseudoaneurysm

9. **Which of the following is true with regard to injuries of the inferior vena cava?**
   (a) Infrarenal injuries carry the best chance for survival
   (b) Posterior injuries usually do not need to be explored
   (c) Posterior injuries cannot be repaired through an anterior venotomy
   (d) Pulmonary emboli occur frequently after repair

10. **Concomitant tibial bone fractures causing transection of the popliteal vein and artery should be treated by which of the following?**
    (a) Immediate external fixation and stabilization of the tibia
    (b) Initial traction and internal fixation with arterial repair
    (c) Repair of the vein and artery and internal fixation of bones
    (d) Exploration and repair of the artery

Answers

1. a	2. b	3. d	4. c	5. c
6. d	7. d	8. d	9. a	10. c

40

Niren Angle • William J. Quiñones-Baldrich

Acute Arterial and Graft Occlusion

Acute limb ischemia resulting from a native vessel or graft occlusion remains one of the most common and potentially devastating problems in vascular surgery. The consequences of acute limb ischemia are dependent on the speed and accuracy of diagnosis and treatment. Timely recognition of acute limb ischemia is difficult, however, because its presentation can range from subtle to dramatic. Vascular specialists—and ideally, every physician—must be aware of the different manifestations of acute limb ischemia so that appropriate diagnostic and therapeutic measures can be instituted. A delay in diagnosis and treatment results in increased morbidity and mortality.

There are two distinct phases in the physiology of acute vascular and graft occlusion—ischemia and reperfusion—which can have grave and distinct consequences for patients. The longer the period of ischemia, the more likely it is that the tissue deprived of flow will not be viable. Reperfusion of ischemic tissue can have both local and systemic effects, the latter in the form of hemodynamic instability and remote organ injury. In the last 30 years, a tremendous amount of insight has been gained through laboratory research and clinical observation, but unfortunately, there is no evidence that this has resulted in any dramatic reduction in morbidity and mortality. Vascular surgeons must be acutely aware of the pathophysiology of ischemia and reperfusion, because knowledge of this phenomenon has profound consequences for management and patient outcome.

This chapter focuses on the causes, pathophysiology, clinical manifestations, and medical and surgical management of patients with acutely ischemic limbs. Ischemia may be secondary to native artery occlusion from thrombosis or embolism, or the patient may have thrombosis from a previous vascular reconstruction. Although the clinical presentation may be similar, the cause and management of these two entities are different and thus are considered separately. Acute cerebral ischemia and visceral ischemia are addressed in other chapters in this book.

Pathophysiology

The ultimate consequence of ischemia is the progressive depletion of high-energy substrate owing to lack of oxygen delivery to the tissue and subsequent conversion to anaerobic metabolism. The balance between supply and demand determines the magnitude and speed of the depletion of the cellular energy compounds. Different tissues have different rates of metabolism, and the consequences of interrupted or decreased blood flow are different based on the duration of ischemia. Tissues such as the heart and brain extract oxygen maximally at rest; thus, any increase in their oxygen demand can be met only by an increase in blood flow. Tissues such as the kidneys and skeletal muscles do not extract oxygen maximally at rest; thus, an increase in metabolic demand is compensated for by greater tissue extraction of oxygen and an increase in blood flow.

Oxygen demand is a function of metabolic activity, so one potential therapeutic intervention is to reduce tissue metabolism. For example, efforts to limit ischemic myocardial infarct size concentrate on reducing metabolic demand by unloading the heart during the critical recovery phase through the use of beta blockers and afterload-reducing agents. The brain, in contrast, is exquisitely sensitive to ischemia because it is incapable of significantly reducing its metabolic demand. Adjunctive measures, such as therapeutic cooling or the use of barbiturates, are used to reduce basal metabolism, thus reducing the consequences of ischemia after an ischemic brain injury.

In an extremity, tissues differ in their ability to tolerate ischemia, reflecting their basal metabolic demand. Skin and subcutaneous tissue are relatively resistant to ischemia. Conversely, peripheral nerve has been shown by Chervu and colleagues to be exquisitely sensitive to ischemia and reperfusion, with prolonged functional deficits demonstrable after 3 hours of ischemia.[1] The prior impression that peripheral nerve was relatively resistant to ischemia might have been a reflection of the lack of dramatic morphologic changes under microscopic examination.

Skeletal muscle makes up the majority of tissue mass in the extremities. It is relatively tolerant of ischemia owing to its slow resting metabolic rate, stores of glycogen, and high-energy phosphate bonds in the form of creatine phosphate, as well as its ability to function by anaerobic glycolysis.

In the clinical situation, the supply side of this equation is variable and largely depends on the location of the vascular occlusion, the rapidity with which such occlusion developed, and the presence of collateral circulation before the occlusion. Thus, a specific ischemic interval has variable effects, depending on all these parameters. The concept of a safe period of ischemia beyond which the viability of the tissue is unlikely cannot be substantiated. Thus, other parameters must be used in the assessment of an ischemic extremity. In experimental animals, measurement of contractile function is much more reliable than time as a predictor of ischemic injury.[2]

When tissues are injured by ischemia or anoxia, their ability to control the metabolism of oxygen is compromised.[3] For some time, the cell can continue cellular functions by drawing on stored adenosine triphosphate (ATP). If the rate of metabolism is slowed, the energy sources can be replenished by anaerobic glycolysis or by the use of stored energy sources such as creatine. With a longer duration of ischemia, energy stores are depleted, and ATP is metabolized to adenosine diphosphate (ADP) and eventually to adenosine monophosphate (AMP). The cell is unable to sustain cellular functions, and transmembrane gradients cannot be maintained. The cell membrane becomes compromised, and there is a net cellular calcium influx.

Reperfusion or reoxygenation causes increased oxygen free radical production, associated tissue injury, and functional impairment. Injured tissues may produce superoxide radicals by various mechanisms, not necessarily involving neutrophils. Isolated organ preparations that are perfused with buffer, in the absence of neutrophils, still produce abundant free radicals. In tissues containing abundant xanthine dehydrogenase, ischemia results in massive catabolism of the adenine nucleotide pool owing to the low energy status of the tissue. Adenosine is broken down to inosine, and then to hypoxanthine, which accumulates.[4] Approximately 10% of a tissue's xanthine dehydrogenase exists as xanthine oxidase; ischemia induces proteolytic conversion, resulting in a marked increase in xanthine oxidase, which accumulates within the cell. This results in an abundance of the superoxide-producing xanthine oxidase and its substrate hypoxanthine. On reintroduction of the second substrate, molecular oxygen, during reperfusion, a burst of superoxide is produced.

There is great variability among species and among tissues with regard to the amount of xanthine dehydrogenase or xanthine oxidase present.[5,6] Reperfused organs are dramatically protected by inhibitors of xanthine oxidase or by superoxide dismutase (SOD).[7,8] McCord and colleagues used the rabbit heart as a model of the xanthine oxidase–deficient human heart and found that enzyme-inhibiting doses of allopurinol do not protect the heart, but SOD does.[9] This finding implies the existence of xanthine oxidase–independent mechanisms of free radical production, most likely resulting from ischemic changes to the mitochondria.[10] Oxygen radical injury has been demonstrated in most tissues subjected to ischemia and reperfusion.[11] Reperfusion results in lipid peroxidation and destruction of cellular membrane integrity.[12] Although reperfusion injury to ischemic muscle is mediated by superoxide and hydroxyl radicals, the source of these free radicals is not known; however, the xanthine oxidase pathway in skeletal muscle is of questionable clinical significance.[13]

Administration of free radical scavengers during the time of reperfusion has been advocated, with the goal of retrieving injured skeletal muscle.[14] Potential sources of these radicals are present in other cellular components, and specifically in white blood cells that may be resident in the tissues during the ischemic period or introduced during the early phases of reperfusion. The ischemia may result in upregulation of the CD11b/CD18 integrin complex, which is necessary for neutrophil-endothelial cell adhesion to occur.[15,16] Leukocyte accumulation in reperfused muscle was demonstrated by Rubin and coworkers.[17]

After reperfusion, a significant "leak" develops in the tissues, resulting in edema and macromolecule extravasation. It appears that hypoxia induces the upregulation of hypoxia-inducible factor (HIF-1), which then leads to upregulation of the potent pro-angiogenic molecule vascular endothelial growth factor (VEGF). VEGF is also known as vascular permeability factor (VPF) and mediates endothelial cell permeability. When reperfusion occurs, the stage is set for endothelial permeability, and it is easy to see how this contributes to tissue edema and subsequent compartment hypertension.

Acute occlusion results in a series of events, each of which potentiates the ischemic insult and amplifies the injury. The thrombus can propagate to involve and occlude collateral side branches. The ischemic tissues accumulate fluid and swell, leading to compression of the vascular channels within a fascial compartment. This results in endothelial swelling and luminal narrowing, with subsequent microvascular obstruction.

An additional feature of reperfusion injury is the "no-reflow" phenomenon. Reperfusion injury also results in other changes—besides direct free radical injury—that cause progressive microcirculatory obstruction. There is some evidence that leukocyte-capillary plugging impairs the reflow process.[18] This leads to an increase in resistance, which has been found to correlate with the extent of tissue damage after a brief period of ischemia.[19] Leukocyte adhesion to the venules and leukocyte extravasation[20] are both operative in tissue injury after ischemia-reperfusion. These two mechanisms can lead to increased permeability of the microvascular endothelial barrier, which has been shown to be a mechanism of ischemia-reperfusion injury after prolonged ischemia.[21,22] Additionally, ischemia-reperfusion results in endothelial swelling, which itself can lead to capillary closure, exacerbating the damage done by leukocyte plugging.[23] Thus, the no-reflow phenomenon prevents nutrient delivery, in spite of the restoration of blood flow, and prolongs the ischemic injury. Another study using a model of 3 hours of ischemia and 2 hours of reperfusion demonstrated that the loss of capillary perfusion associated with the ischemia-reperfusion injury was the consequence of macromolecular leakage and resultant tissue edema, not leukocyte-capillary plugging.[24] Elimination of white blood cells from the initial perfusate was of no advantage in an experimental model of ischemia and reperfusion of skeletal muscle.[25] The role of the leukocyte in the no-reflow phenomenon is therefore uncertain. In our laboratory, we have observed that this process becomes more prevalent with longer periods of ischemia. Whereas muscles that are ischemic for 1 to 3 hours are easily reperfused without evidence of the no-reflow phenomenon, muscles subjected to 5 hours or more of ischemia demonstrate this phenomenon in up to 40% to 50% of specimens.[26]

Blood is a non-Newtonian fluid, the rheology of which takes on special significance in this phenomenon. The energy required to reestablish movement of the blood after it has stopped flowing is proportional to the third power of the red blood cell mass and the second power of the fibrinogen content.[27] The concept of "opening pressure" may therefore be important in the early phases of reperfusion.

Thus, two major components appear to be responsible for reperfusion injury. Initially, the ischemic period results in the depletion of glycogen stores and stores of high-energy substrate. At some point, molecular oxygen is introduced into this milieu, and the superoxide anion and other free radicals are produced. This phase of reperfusion has been dealt with experimentally by administering a xanthine oxidase inhibitor, allopurinol; by administering free radical scavengers[14,28]; by leukocyte depletion[29]; and by controlling the rate of reperfusion[30]—all with varying degrees of success. The second major component is the no-reflow phenomenon, which prolongs the ischemic component at the cellular level.

Reperfusion, especially after prolonged ischemia, leads to changes in vasomotor tone and responsiveness and to an increase in microvascular permeability, with resultant tissue edema. It has been hypothesized that the alteration in vasomotor tone is due to a reduction in nitric oxide (NO) levels. NO diffuses freely through the cell membrane into the surrounding smooth muscle and initiates a cascade of events culminating in smooth muscle relaxation.[31] At the same time, it diffuses into the luminal side of the endothelium, where it helps prevent platelet aggregation and adhesion to vessel walls.[32] Huk and colleagues demonstrated that ischemia results in a significant depletion of tissue NO.[33] Administration of the substrate L-arginine can significantly decrease superoxide production and increase the accumulation of NO, resulting in protection from vasoconstriction.[33] In another model of ischemia-reperfusion, pentoxifylline, a xanthine-derived phosphodiesterase inhibitor, was shown to reduce reperfusion-associated membrane injury, suppress leukocyte adhesion, and improve hindlimb flow.[34]

After acute occlusion of an artery, the clinical presentation depends in large part on the presence or absence of collateral circulation. This, in turn, depends on the preexistence of occlusive arterial disease and the site of occlusion. After the initial event, ischemia may be aggravated by proximal or distal thrombus propagation, or both. This impairs collateral circulation, further aggravating the process. This fragmentation may also produce intermittent improvement and worsening, depending on its severity and location. Venous thrombosis may accompany acute extremity ischemia, usually as a secondary event due to the low flow and thrombogenicity of the system. This further aggravates the ischemic process and may complicate revascularization.

Reperfusion of ischemic tissue can result in striking and sometimes lethal effects on remote organ function. The release from ischemic tissue of cytokines such as tumor necrosis factor-α, interleukin-1β, platelet-activating factor (PAF), prostaglandins such as thromboxanes, and leukotrienes can cause profound perturbations in hemodynamics and organ injury (e.g., acute lung injury). However, a more immediate systemic effect, one that can be lethal in severe cases, was described by Haimovici and termed the "myonephropathic-metabolic syndrome."[35] It is similar to the deleterious effects seen in crush injury. Upon restoration of flow, acidic blood enters the systemic circulation, capable of causing an abrupt and lethal metabolic acidosis. Some authorities recommend the administration of bicarbonate during the early phase of reperfusion in anticipation of this problem. Ischemic muscle that is not salvageable can leak enough potassium to produce acute hyperkalemia. This problem can be compounded by acute renal insufficiency due to myoglobinuria. Anticipation of this problem helps avoid or at least minimize its consequences.

Insulin and glucose cause potassium to shift into cells and should be used to treat the hyperkalemia. Myoglobin precipitates in the renal tubules at a pH of less than 5.8, so alkalization of the urine by the administration of bicarbonate or ammonium chloride is important to prevent acute tubular necrosis as a result of myoglobinuria. In addition, a vigorous rate of fluid administration is vital.

The pathophysiologic changes underlying acute ischemia and reperfusion are not yet completely understood, but the years have brought a blossoming of research and insights in the field. Our current understanding suggests that the quality and content of the initial perfusate are important for achieving optimal results, representing a promising area of clinical research.

Cause

The cause of acute limb ischemia, whether native vessel or vascular graft occlusion, can be grouped broadly into two distinct categories: thrombosis and embolism (Table 40-1). In addition, it is important to recognize that arterial dissection, whether spontaneous or iatrogenic (e.g., during endovascular intervention), may manifest as acute limb ischemia. Although older reports suggested that embolic disease is far more common,[36,37] more recent series suggest that thrombotic occlusions outnumber embolic occlusions by a 6:1 ratio.[38] Thrombosis in native vessels or grafts is usually due to an underlying lesion in the conduit itself, whereas an embolus tends to lodge in an otherwise healthy vessel, originating from another site. Bypass graft thrombosis occurs more frequently than native arterial occlusion.

ACUTE ARTERIAL OCCLUSION

Embolism

Most emboli to the lower extremities originate in the heart, with 60% to 70% of patients having underlying myocardial disease.[39] This is most common after a myocardial infarction, because the dyskinetic portion of the heart serves as a reservoir of stagnant blood and site of thrombus formation. Mural thrombi can occur within hours to weeks after a myocardial infarction.[40] An embolus may be the first manifestation of a silent myocardial infarction. In addition, arrhythmias may predispose to atrial thrombus formation.

Peripheral arterial embolism is much more consequential, because there are usually few collateral vessels to the affected bed. Arterial embolism commonly lodges at vessel bifurcations, obstructing flow into two parallel channels. The upper extremities are less commonly affected than the lower extremities. Common sites of emboli are the femoral bifurcation, iliac artery bifurcation, and tibioperoneal trunk. Emboli to the visceral vessels account for 7% to 10% of recognized emboli. Whereas rheumatic disease has significantly declined in incidence, embolization from prosthetic cardiac valves now occurs more frequently, with an increasing segment of the population receiving prosthetic valves and living longer. Chronic anticoagulation is essential, because the risk of recurrent peripheral embolization is significant. Atrial myxomas can also present as a peripheral embolus of either the tumor or the clot organized around the tumor. Bacterial endocarditis remains an important consideration in a young patient with a peripheral embolus without any underlying risk factors.

TABLE 40–1　Causes of Acute Arterial Ischemia

Embolism	Hypercoagulable states	Drug abuse
Heart	Vascular grafts	Inhalation of cocaine
Atherosclerotic heart disease	Progression of disease	Intra-arterial administration
Coronary artery disease	Intimal hyperplasia	Drug toxicity
Acute myocardial infarction	Mechanical	Contaminant microembolization
Arrhythmia	***Trauma***	***Outflow Venous Occlusion***
Valvular heart disease	Penetrating	Compartment syndrome
Rheumatic	Direct vessel injury	Phlegmasia
Degenerative	Indirect injury	***Low-Flow States***
Congenital	Missile emboli	Cardiogenic shock
Bacterial	Proximity	Hypovolemic shock
Prosthetic	Blunt	Drug effect
Artery-to-artery	Intimal flap	Mesenteric
Aneurysm	Spasm	Digoxin
Atherosclerotic plaque	Iatrogenic	H_2 blockers
Idiopathic	Intimal flap	
Paradoxical embolus	Dissection	
Thrombosis	Presence of medical device	
Atherosclerosis	Space-occupying thrombosis	
Low-flow states	Clot propagation	
Congestive heart failure	External compression	
Hypovolemia		
Hypotension		

Patients with deep venous thrombosis and an acute arterial occlusion should be investigated for the presence of a patent foramen ovale, which can produce a paradoxical embolism. Other rare causes of embolization from a central origin include tumor invasion of the intrathoracic vessels or direct arterial invasion with concomitant tumor or thrombus embolization.[41]

Proximal aneurysms frequently harbor thrombus that can embolize. The most common are abdominal and popliteal artery aneurysms. Atherosclerotic plaque can embolize and cause acute ischemia, particularly from the arch of the aorta or the descending thoracic aorta.[42] This may result in acute ischemia of the lower extremities (Fig. 40-1) or the viscera or may even cause a stroke if the atheromatous plaque originates from the arch itself. Emboli to the lower extremities may manifest in a variety of ways. In its most dramatic presentation, a microembolus can produce acute ischemia of a toe, leading to gangrene. This is referred to as the blue toe syndrome. Blue toes should prompt a search for a proximal source of embolization in either the heart or the proximal vasculature.

Thrombosis

Thrombosis usually occurs in the setting of an underlying lesion in the blood vessel. It represents the final stage in the progression of atherosclerotic arterial disease. One of the most common sites of vessel occlusion is the superficial femoral artery at the adductor canal. Although atherosclerotic disease has been noted to occur equally along the entire femoral artery, the occlusion tends to occur preferentially at the adductor canal.[43] It has been hypothesized that the normal process of arterial enlargement in response to atheroma deposition is blunted at the adductor canal, thus explaining its preferential involvement.

The progression from a mild atherosclerotic lesion to thrombosis begins with the deposition of lipids in the intima of the artery. A lipid-calcium core is then developed. Initially, there is a fibrous cap that shields the lipid-rich core from the vessel lumen. A subsequent stimulus such as macrophage infiltration, activation of matrix metalloproteinases, or release of other proteases results in disruption of the cap. Exposure of the underlying core is then postulated to result in accelerated thrombosis.[44] It may indeed be the case that the thickness of the cap is more predictive of the risk of occlusion than is the degree of stenosis as determined by arteriography.

The ongoing process of atherosclerosis and thrombus formation is slow, allowing a gradual development of symptoms, probably owing to the development of collaterals. However, propagation of thrombus can also occur quite rapidly and may require immediate attention. The distinction between a thrombus and an embolus is important, because the therapy for each is different. A low-flow state in the presence of an underlying diseased intima can induce rapid thrombosis. This is important to keep in mind in the general management of an elderly patient. Hemodynamics should be optimized and attention paid to subtle manifestations of increasing ischemia.

Thrombosis may be secondary to hypercoagulable conditions. These constitute a long list of factors that predispose to thrombosis in an otherwise unaffected arterial segment. Heparin-induced thrombosis is an important cause, usually recognized by a significant drop in the platelet count during heparin therapy and the occurrence of a thrombotic event. When not recognized in a timely fashion, this may lead to limb- or life-threatening complications.[45,46] Most other hypercoagulable states are properly treated with heparin (with concomitant administration of fresh frozen plasma for antithrombin III deficiency), with intervention indicated by the severity of the ischemia. Malignancy may be an important

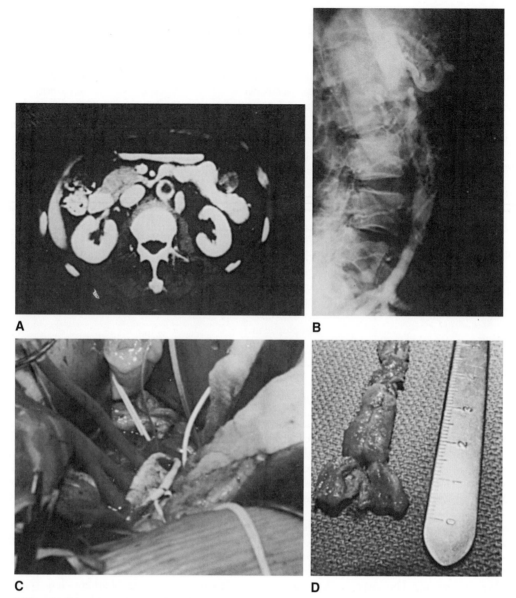

FIGURE 40–1 • A 72-year-old woman presented with bilateral acute and distal ischemic rest pain of both lower extremities secondary to microembolization. *A,* Computed tomography scan with intravenous contrast shows an intraluminal defect in the abdominal aorta. *B,* Lateral aortogram demonstrates an intraluminal defect starting at the level of the superior mesenteric artery. *C,* Operative view of the infrarenal aorta with temporary control of lumbar arteries, bilateral renal artery control with vessel loops, and supraceliac aortic cross-clamping. *D,* Operative specimen after complete abdominal aortic thrombectomy. Angioscopy was helpful in assessing the completeness of the suprarenal portion of the embolectomy.

underlying cause in elderly individuals with a hypercoagulable condition.[47] Chemotherapy may actually temporarily aggravate the process and lead to arterial embolism or thrombosis.[48]

Traumatic injury of an axial artery may lead to immediate thrombosis, disruption, or embolization. Penetrating trauma may disrupt an artery, thus causing acute extremity ischemia. Embolization of a missile has been reported and must be kept in mind in a patient with a remote penetrating injury who develops acute extremity ischemia.[49] Injuries due to proximity are usually seen with high-velocity missiles and are secondary to intimal disruption of the adjacent artery. Blunt trauma may cause acute arterial obstruction secondary to intimal disruption of the adjacent artery, intimal flap, or, on occasion, spasm due to a large expanding hematoma. Blunt trauma to an extremity may cause fractures, with associated

arterial injury. This is most commonly seen with supracondylar fractures of the upper extremity, where the brachial artery is in intimate relationship with the humerus. In the lower extremity, fractures of the distal femur and posterior knee dislocations, with or without tibial plateau fractures, are most commonly associated with arterial injury. These may range from complete disruption of the artery to intimal tears and fractures, leading to secondary thrombosis (Fig. 40-2). Ascribing severe distal extremity ischemia to spasm without appropriate arteriographic evaluation is to be condemned and may lead to unnecessary tissue loss. Comparing distal pressures obtained by Doppler examination of the involved and uninvolved extremities has been suggested as an accurate means of determining which patients need arteriography. In a review of 509 consecutive patients with isolated upper or

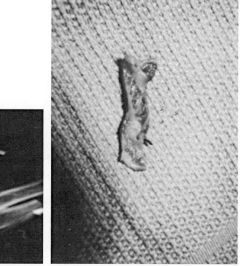
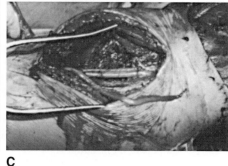

A   **B**   **C**

FIGURE 40–2 • A 27-year-old patient involved in a motorcycle accident presented with a fracture of the left humerus. *A,* Arteriogram shows complete occlusion of the midbrachial artery and fracture of the distal third of the humerus. *B,* Operative specimen shows spiral disruption of the intima with thrombosis. *C,* Operative appearance of the segmental vein interposition repair. Note that complete transection of the median nerve accompanied this injury and was the major cause of morbidity.

lower extremity penetrating injury, Weaver and colleagues found that only pulse deficit or an ankle-brachial index less than 1.0 was a predictor of significant arterial injury.[50]

Acute aortic dissection may occasionally appear with acute limb ischemia. Patients are usually hypertensive and complain of severe chest and back pain. Arteriography before intervention is of utmost importance to establish the diagnosis and assess visceral ischemia. On occasion, a patient is taken to the operating room having been misdiagnosed with an embolic occlusion to a limb, only to discover an aortic dissection when passage of the Fogarty catheter fails to go beyond the occlusion or does not retrieve clot or induce blood flow. The artery itself may appear friable, with easy separation of the intima through the medial plane. The inner layers of the vessel may be retrieved by the Fogarty catheter, thus compounding the problem. Failure to establish the proper diagnosis may prove fatal.

With the increased use of percutaneous endovascular techniques, iatrogenic arterial trauma is acquiring importance as a cause of acute extremity ischemia. This is usually secondary to intimal flaps, dissection, or thrombosis and frequently requires operative therapy. Treatment may prove difficult in patients with preexisting peripheral vascular disease. Although arteriography may be omitted in a young patient without occlusive disease, it is highly recommended when preexisting disease may mandate a complex vascular reconstruction to reestablish circulation. The presence of a medical device within the arterial system, in and of itself, may cause significant extremity ischemia. Intra-aortic balloon pumps may lead to ipsilateral or contralateral extremity ischemia secondary to clot around the device, embolization, or thrombosis. The clinical manifestations are usually aggravated because of the low-flow state necessitating the device. Temporizing with heparinization is a reasonable alternative if it is anticipated that the intra-aortic balloon will be removed

within the next few hours. Otherwise, construction of an extra-anatomic bypass distal to the balloon insertion site may be limb-saving.

Hand ischemia secondary to a radial artery line is usually the result of inadequate preinsertion evaluation. Performance of the Allen test before insertion of an arterial line in the upper extremity to document the integrity of the palmar arch is an underemphasized maneuver. Failure to do this procedure inevitably results in patients experiencing hand ischemia because of interruption of radial artery flow. Removal of the radial artery cannula may result in improvement, with an occasional patient requiring operative intervention.

External compression secondary to either tourniquet or cast application to an extremity is an important preventable cause of acute extremity ischemia. Patients with peripheral vascular disease undergoing orthopedic procedures should be managed with caution; subcutaneous collateral vessels serving to irrigate the distal extremity are most susceptible to external compression and, because of the rheology of stagnant blood, may require higher pressures to spontaneously open once they are collapsed. Emergency reconstructions in these patients may prove difficult because of the orthopedic device and preexisting peripheral vascular process. These patients are best evaluated before the orthopedic intervention so that appropriate recommendations can be made, the tourniquet avoided altogether, and the intervention facilitated if a complication occurs.

Accidental intra-arterial administration of illicit drugs can lead to devastating extremity ischemia secondary to toxicity of the drug itself or to contaminant microembolization. Treatment is usually supportive, and tissue loss is common.

Occlusion of venous outflow of an extremity may be secondary to compartment syndrome. This syndrome may be seen after revascularization following prolonged ischemia, trauma, or any other process that increases compartment pressures.

As the pressure in a fascial compartment increases, venous outflow is impeded, thus producing a further increase in compartment pressures. If this process is left unchecked, arterial inflow is restricted, leading to nerve and muscle ischemia. Early fasciotomy can be limb-saving. Outflow occlusion secondary to venous thrombosis is rare but should be recognized in a markedly swollen and painful extremity. As the venous thrombotic process progresses, arterial inflow is impeded, leading to limb-threatening ischemia (phlegmasia). Treatment alternatives include heparinization, thrombolytic therapy, and venous thrombectomy, singly or in combination.

Extreme low-flow states, usually seen in patients with cardiogenic or hypovolemic shock, can lead to extremity ischemia, especially in those with preexisting peripheral vascular disease. This process is aggravated by vasoactive drugs, which are frequently needed to support the patient. Correction of the hemodynamic derangement is the primary goal, with intervention reserved for patients with persistent ischemia. Heparinization may be of benefit, preventing thrombosis in these poorly perfused extremities.

VASCULAR GRAFT FAILURE

Early and late failures of arterial reconstructions can be caused by the same processes discussed in the section on acute arterial occlusion. In addition, processes specifically involving the graft and either the inflow or outflow vascular bed influence the performance of these reconstructions.

For purposes of this discussion, the causes of autogenous and prosthetic graft failure are examined separately. In addition, we limit the scope of these discussions to lower extremity bypasses. Infection is an important cause of vascular graft failure and is discussed at length elsewhere in this text. Here, it suffices to say that autogenous reconstructions are more resistant to infection and, in fact, may be used as an alternative to a prosthetic implant in the presence of infection.[51] Acute infection of an autogenous graft usually requires graft replacement through uninvolved tissue. Chronic late-occurring infections of prosthetic grafts may be appropriately treated with autogenous reconstruction in the same bed. Exceptions are necrotizing infections caused by organisms such as *Pseudomonas* and *Salmonella*.

Autogenous Reconstructions

Autogenous reconstruction of the lower extremities is usually seen in infrainguinal bypasses, where reversed, nonreversed, or in situ saphenous vein is used. Early failures of such reconstructions are usually secondary to technical defects that are best avoided by the liberal use of angiography, duplex scanning, or another modality at the completion of the original operation to document the technical success of the repair. Early failure may also be secondary to a defect in the graft, usually the result of previous episodes of superficial phlebitis, which may have led to sclerotic changes in a segment of the vein.[52] Additionally, injury may be caused at the time of harvest or preparation. Preservation of endothelial function should be the goal and is best accomplished by careful technique, avoiding trauma to the vein. Distention of the graft should be accomplished gently, preferably using heparinized blood. Alternatively, distention may be accomplished by the arterial pressure itself, after connecting the graft in its proximal

anastomosis. One of the potential advantages of the in situ technique is that it minimizes the degree of ischemia suffered by the vein graft. Other causes of early failure include external compression or kinks, the latter avoided by ensuring that there are no twists in the vein (either in situ or reversed). Marking the proximal and distal ends of the veins before mobilization may help accomplish this with minimal effort. Tunnels performed anatomically for autogenous grafts may produce external compression on the vein. This can be identified on completion angiography by the effacement of the contrast during injection. Subcutaneous tunnels may have an advantage in this regard, with the additional benefit of being readily accessible if revision becomes necessary.

In situ saphenous vein bypasses may also fail acutely secondary to residual arteriovenous (AV) fistulas or inadequate valve lysis. Residual AV fistulas do not lead to clinical symptoms in most instances. On occasion, however, they manifest with limb edema out of proportion to that expected. They can be readily diagnosed on physical examination by the presence of a murmur over the fistula. Inadequate valve lysis can manifest as an early or late failure due to stenosis of the segment. The use of angioscopy has been suggested by some as a means of ensuring complete valve lysis in preparation of the in situ graft. Alternatively, these problems can be identified on continuous-wave Doppler examination by a change in signal quality, implying high velocities through the segment. Completion angiography also detects these defects and avoids early failure.[53]

Intimal hyperplasia of either the proximal or distal anastomosis, or of the vein graft itself, continues to be the most frequent cause of late failure of autogenous infrainguinal reconstructions.[54] These lesions tend to occur within the first year after implantation and are rare beyond 2 years. In a series of 109 primary femoropopliteal bypasses, failure within the first 30 days resulted primarily from technical or judgmental errors. Stenotic lesions developing within the vein graft were noted to be the most common cause of failure within the first year. Progression of distal disease was the leading cause of failure after 2 years.[55] Thus, the time when failure occurs aids in determining the cause.

Other lesions may affect autogenous vein grafts' long-term performance. Aneurysmal dilatation is rare. When it occurs, it threatens the patency of the bypass, usually by either thrombosis or distal embolization. Stenotic lesions may develop at the inflow or outflow portion of the aneurysm, usually secondary to a kink. Rupture is rare. Repair is indicated when the lesion threatens patency of the reconstruction.

Prosthetic Reconstructions

Failure of prosthetic vascular reconstructions differs from autogenous grafts in that intrinsic graft problems are extremely unusual. With the exception of the umbilical vein graft, aneurysmal dilatation is usually not seen. Prosthetic graft stenoses are usually the result of external compression or twists during implantation. Externally supported grafts may avoid some of these problems. Kinking of the outflow popliteal artery in above-knee femoropopliteal bypass has been described and may account for some failures of above-knee reconstructions.[56] By far, the most common cause of failure within the first 2 years after implantation of a prosthetic infrainguinal reconstruction is progression of distal disease. In a review of 111 failures of polytetrafluoroethylene (PTFE) infrainguinal bypasses over a 10-year period, 64% of failures occurred within the first year; 56% were due to either severity or progression of the distal disease. Progression occurred in 25% of cases and was most commonly seen as progression of iliac disease in patients operated on to relieve claudication or as thrombosis of an inflow reconstruction in limb salvage patients. Only 8% of cases had isolated intimal hyperplasia as a cause of failure, although half the patients with progression of distal disease had some degree of intimal hyperplasia at the distal anastomosis.[57]

Infection is a rare but important cause of failure of infrainguinal prosthetic reconstructions. When it occurs, graft excision with alternative revascularization, when indicated, is the preferred treatment.

If, after a thorough search for the cause of early failure, none is identified, a hypercoagulable condition should be suspected. A history of superficial or deep thrombophlebitis, prior bypass failure, or other thrombotic events suggests this origin. Identification of the specific abnormality is important in directing management. From a clinical standpoint, however, heparin is generally the treatment of choice, with the exception of heparin-induced thrombosis and supplementation of antithrombin III in deficient patients. Identification of heparin-induced thrombosis is of paramount importance to avoid continued thrombotic events. Serial platelet counts during heparin therapy are most helpful, with confirmation of the diagnosis by in vitro platelet aggregation studies. Although most commonly seen in the early postoperative period, hypercoagulable conditions may play a role in early failure during the first few months after surgery. Because of prosthetic grafts' initial thrombogenicity, some patients show acute thrombosis, and no identifiable cause for failure can be determined. These patients may benefit from long-term anticoagulation.[58]

Another important and increasingly frequent condition is acute thrombosis and occlusion of one limb of an endovascular aortic stent-graft. This may occur due to kinking in an unsupported graft or disease progression distal to the iliac artery attachment site; in some cases, the reason is not clear. Thrombolysis is the preferred treatment if the limb is not severely ischemic. If the limb is imminently threatened, prompt restoration of flow requires graft thrombectomy or extra-anatomic bypass, such as femorofemoral bypass. If thrombectomy is performed, we insist that it be done under live fluoroscopy of the proximal attachment site to ensure that traction of the thrombectomy catheter does not result in migration or displacement of the endograft. A completion arteriogram is essential, and if a distal stenosis is discovered, angioplasty or stenting may be appropriate.

Clinical Manifestations

ACUTE ARTERIAL OCCLUSION

The clinical manifestations of acute extremity ischemia vary, depending on the level and severity of the obstruction and, most important, the adequacy of collateral circulation. The latter is mostly dependent on the presence or absence of concomitant arterial occlusive disease and, to a lesser degree, location of the occlusion. In obtaining a history, one should determine the functional status of the extremity before the event. Patients with no history of claudication or previous vascular reconstruction are most likely affected by peripheral embolization.

Physical examination of a patient with an acutely ischemic extremity is of utmost importance in planning appropriate management. Examination of the contralateral extremity may provide clues as to the preischemic status of the involved extremity.

Acute occlusion of an otherwise normal, noncollateralized artery leads to the classic manifestations of acute extremity ischemia: pulselessness, pain, pallor, paresthesia, and paralysis (the five Ps). Certainly, the disappearance of a previously palpable pulse or the absence of a pulse in a patient with these symptoms and normal pulses in the opposite extremity is pathognomonic of an acute arterial occlusion. The presence or severity of these manifestations depends on the severity of the ischemia.

In addition to the disappearance of the pulse, an arterial occlusion may cause tenderness over the affected artery. This is usually proximal to the ischemic changes. The ischemic manifestations are usually most severe one joint distal to the level of obstruction. The classic example is the patient with foot ischemia with a relatively well-perfused calf secondary to an embolus to the level of the trifurcation of the popliteal artery.

Pain is the most common manifestation of an acute arterial occlusion. Characteristically, it is severe and progressive, with the most distal part of the extremity affected early. As the ischemia progresses, however, sensory deficits may ensue that mask the pain, confusing the inexperienced clinician. The pain is slowly replaced by a feeling of numbness, which denotes progression of the ischemic progress and demands immediate attention.

Pallor is one of the initial manifestations of acute ischemia. The extremity rapidly develops a waxy appearance secondary to complete emptying and vasospasm of the arterial circulation. With progression, however, this is replaced by mottling, secondary vasodilatation, and stagnant circulation in the capillary bed. Blanching of these mottled areas with application of digital pressure denotes a retrievable capillary bed. Once the mottled areas become nonblanching, a manifestation of capillary sludging, early gangrene is likely. This represents advanced ischemia. Without revascularization, this leads to blistering of the skin with further discoloration; as water is lost, desiccation occurs, with changes typical of dry gangrene.

Paralysis and sensory deficits are usually late manifestations of severe ischemia. Because of the lack of nutrient flow, skeletal muscle and nerve dysfunction leads to the patient's inability to move the extremity. As the energy stores within the muscle decrease, inability to relax the muscles leads to rigor, a sign of far-advanced ischemia. Large sensory nerve fibers are responsible for pressure, deep pain, and temperature sensations that may be maintained until ischemia is advanced. Proprioception and light touch are usually lost early. A careful sensory examination may help the clinician estimate the severity of ischemia. Palpation of the muscle groups may denote tenderness initially, but as the ischemia progresses, the muscles may become hard (rigor), a sign of skeletal muscle death. Even with prompt revascularization, functional impairment is likely, limb loss often occurs, and systemic effects of revascularization are a major risk. Revascularization at this late stage is likely to fail, with systemic manifestations of such an undertaking profound and sometimes lethal. This has led some authors to suggest that ischemia of this severity and duration is best treated with systemic anticoagulation, allowing demarcation of the extremity and early amputation.[59]

VASCULAR GRAFT OCCLUSION

The clinical manifestations of vascular graft occlusion also vary widely. The indication for the original intervention influences the presentation, with patients operated on for disabling claudication usually manifesting recurrent symptoms, and patients operated on for limb salvage presenting with limb-threatening ischemia. In the former group, however, when late occlusions occur, the patient may show limb-threatening ischemia. The cause of failure influences the clinical presentation. We analyzed the pattern and causes of primary failure of PTFE grafts in a series of patients operated on for claudication; when failure was due to progression of proximal or distal disease, patients most commonly presented with limb-threatening ischemia.[57] Of 14 patients initially operated on for severe claudication whose grafts failed because of progression of distal occlusive disease, 12 manifested severe limb-threatening ischemia. Similarly, 50% of patients operated on for claudication whose grafts failed due to progression of disease in the inflow arterial segment manifested limb-threatening ischemia, whereas the rest manifested recurrent claudication. Thus, most patients operated on for limb salvage manifest limb-threatening ischemia upon failure of the reconstruction; patients with claudication manifest recurrent claudication unless significant progression of disease occurs in the inflow or outflow segments.

When the cause of failure is graft related, which most commonly occurs with autogenous grafts, clinical manifestations are usually similar to the original presentation and indication for the reconstruction. This is particularly true within the first 12 to 18 months after reconstruction. Beyond that time, other factors, mainly progression of disease, influence the clinical presentation of the failed vascular graft.

After healing of the affected area, a small number of patients whose initial indication for reconstruction was limb-threatening ischemia (specifically, those with tissue loss) may exhibit failure of the reconstruction and perhaps symptoms of claudication without clinical symptoms of severe ischemia. This is evident in most series of infrainguinal reconstructions, where limb salvage figures are almost universally higher than primary patency rates. Most of these patients do not require intervention; their symptoms can be managed conservatively with control of risk factors and exercise.

More recently, the concept of the failing (rather than failed) vascular graft has been emphasized, with several series documenting improved results when intervention occurs while the graft is still patent. Clinical manifestations of failing grafts include diminished pulses, recurrent symptoms of claudication, or failure of areas of tissue loss in the foot to heal completely after an initial period of rapid healing. Most commonly, however, failing grafts have no clinical manifestations; therefore, it behooves the physician to identify these cases by noninvasive means. Serial ankle-brachial indexes are not sensitive enough to predictably detect a failing graft.[60] The most important mode of identification is duplex scanning by insonating the entire graft and identifying areas of stenosis that lead to increased velocities in that segment. In addition, average velocity throughout the graft may decrease over time, again suggesting that the graft may be failing. Although cutoff points for velocities have been proposed, these are not sensitive enough to be completely reliable. Although most grafts with velocities higher than 45 cm/second continue to have long-term patency, grafts below this cutoff point do not necessarily fail, nor does a demonstrable lesion appear on arteriography. Additional duplex scan criteria to detect failing grafts have been proposed and include diameter reduction and peak and end-systolic velocities.[61-63] This is specifically evident in very distal reconstructions at the ankle, where the outflow bed may not allow for velocities in this range throughout the graft. Nevertheless, experience has shown excellent long-term results without the need for further interventions.

Initial Evaluation

ACUTE ARTERIAL OCCLUSION

The morbidity and mortality of an acute arterial occlusion largely depend on the overall medical condition of the patient, the degree of ischemia of the extremity at presentation, and the promptness of management. All three aspects must be carefully evaluated and documented. In general, prompt revascularization should be the goal after stabilization and control of coexistent medical conditions in patients showing an acute ischemic extremity.

At clinical presentation, the majority of patients with acute arterial occlusion of an extremity have atherosclerotic heart disease, which must be addressed before any intervention. An acute myocardial infarction must be excluded by appropriate clinical and laboratory evaluations. Although its presence does not preclude surgical intervention, it mandates appropriate maneuvers, such as placement of a Swan-Ganz catheter or arterial line to minimize the morbidity and mortality associated with surgical intervention. Stabilization of hemodynamics is of primary importance, including correction of arrhythmias, replenishment of circulating volume, and establishment of an adequate urine output.

The history gives the clinician clues about the status of the extremity before the acute arterial occlusion. Patients with an identifiable source of an embolus, without a history of claudication or previous vascular reconstruction, and with a normal contralateral extremity are likely suffering from embolization. Patients with no identifiable source of an embolus; with a history of peripheral vascular disease, claudication, or previous vascular reconstruction; and with physical findings in the opposite limb suggestive of peripheral vascular disease likely have an arterial thrombosis. The importance of differentiating between these two processes is evident when one considers their management. Whereas patients with embolization are appropriately managed by thrombectomy, patients with preexisting vascular disease usually require a much more involved vascular reconstruction. Careful preoperative planning may make an important difference in outcome. A history of a previous embolic event is present in up to one third of patients with an embolus, and nearly three fourths have a history of atrial fibrillation. In contrast, only 4% of patients with an acute thrombotic occlusion have a history of atrial fibrillation.[64] Symptoms tend to be much more acute in patients with an embolic occlusion, with a fairly well-established area of demarcation. Patients with a thrombotic occlusion are likely to show less severe symptoms and a larger area of transition.

Heparinization of patients presenting with an acutely ischemic extremity is well established. In general, at least 10,000 units of intravenous heparin is recommended to establish immediate and complete anticoagulation. The goal is to prevent proximal and distal thrombus propagation and distal thrombosis. In general, patients experience an almost immediate improvement in their symptoms, likely secondary to the anti-inflammatory effects of heparin. Clearly, patients with a history of heparin-induced thrombosis should be excluded from this recommendation. Patients with associated traumatic injuries or other systemic diseases that may present an unacceptable bleeding risk are not candidates for systemic heparinization; they may receive local instillation of a dilute heparin solution in the vascular bed during operative therapy.

Once the patient has been stabilized and adequate anticoagulation accomplished, a decision regarding preoperative arteriography should be made. The desirability of arteriography is increased in patients with preexisting vascular disease or reconstruction. If the patient can tolerate the ischemia, preoperative arteriography may be extremely helpful in elucidating the cause and planning the proper surgical approach. Arteriography should be omitted, however, if it will significantly delay revascularization. Alternatively, operative arteriograms can be obtained at the time of intervention. A patient whose history and physical examination are suggestive of an embolus may be properly handled without arteriography. If arteriography is undertaken, typically the outflow vascular bed is not well visualized, and the time necessary for this study prolongs the ischemia without adding useful information. When the differentiation between an embolic and a thrombotic event cannot be made, or when the cause is uncertain, arteriography is appropriate. A sharp cutoff with a crescent-shaped (meniscus sign) occlusion in an otherwise normal artery is suggestive of an embolus. Multiple filling defects are also suggestive of an embolic occlusion. The location of the occlusion may also be helpful, with emboli tending to lodge in areas of bifurcations (Fig. 40-3). Clot propagation following either an embolic or a thrombotic event may make this distinction difficult, however.

Doppler examination of the extremity can be most helpful in determining patency of the distal outflow tract. In patients with an embolic occlusion, its presence is reassuring, because it implies an open distal tree and, therefore, a retrievable situation. In a patient with preexisting vascular disease, Doppler examination may help identify the most suitable distal bed for bypass reconstruction. Doppler examination of the venous system may disclose an otherwise unsuspected venous thrombosis.

Patients with concomitant injuries, such as fractures or dislocations, should have prompt restitution of blood volume and restoration of adequate blood pressure. Stabilization of the extremity is essential to prevent further injury and, on occasion, to restore distal circulation. Life-threatening injuries should take precedence over limb-threatening injuries. The use of temporary arterial shunts in these circumstances may help preserve the limb.

VASCULAR GRAFT OCCLUSION

The initial evaluation of a patient presenting with a prosthetic graft occlusion is influenced by the clinical presentation. Patients showing recurrent claudication may be evaluated electively. Anticoagulation is not indicated in these patients. Intervention is indicated only in those whose claudication is disabling. Patients with limb-threatening ischemia, in contrast, are best evaluated on an urgent basis because some nonoperative treatments (including thrombolytic therapy) are most effective within a short time after thrombosis. In most

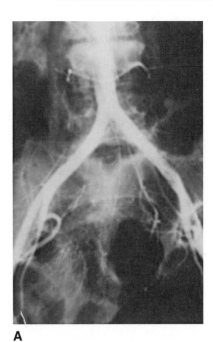

A

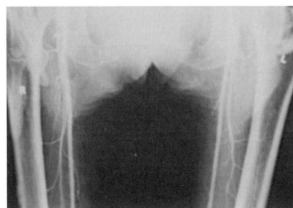

B

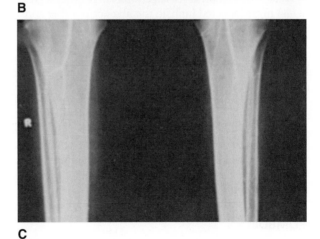

C

FIGURE 40–3 • Arteriogram of a 67-year-old woman who presented with acute left lower extremity ischemia. *A,* Left iliac filling defect at the level of the bifurcation, typical of an embolus. Some fragmentation has occurred, with filling defects also involving the distal external iliac and proximal common femoral arteries. The patient had flow around this embolus to produce a normal femoral pulse. *B,* Open superficial femoral and deep femoral system without evidence of significant atherosclerotic disease. *C,* Evidence of distal fragmentation of the embolus, with occlusion of the posterior tibial and peroneal arteries. Successful embolectomy was carried out through a combined transfemoral and infrapopliteal approach.

instances, the initial management is similar to that of patients with acute ischemia secondary to native vessel occlusion.

Patients with indications for intervention (disabling claudication or limb-threatening ischemia) due to failure of a previous vascular reconstruction are best evaluated with thorough arteriography. This study should include both inflow and outflow systems, with an attempt to establish the cause of failure. Herein lies one of the main advantages of thrombolytic therapy in the initial management of a failed infrainguinal reconstruction. Although both early and long-term results remain unclear when compared with those of surgical intervention, thrombolytic therapy in most instances identifies the cause of failure, allowing directed intervention.

Examination of the patient should include not only the presence or absence and quality of pulses in the involved extremity but also alternative inflow sites and, most important, availability of autogenous tissue for secondary reconstruction. Experience within the last 15 years suggests that patients requiring secondary bypasses after failure of an infrainguinal reconstruction are best managed with a new autogenous reconstruction. In addition to physical examination, duplex scanning of the remaining venous segments may be of benefit, if properly performed. This examination should be performed either with a proximal tourniquet applied to distend the vein or with the patient semierect. Failure to do so usually results in an underestimate of the size and quality of available veins.

Treatment

The principal goal of intervention is the retrieval of ischemic tissue and limb salvage—anatomic and functional. Revascularization of an acutely ischemic limb can be accomplished by one of two techniques: surgical thrombectomy or thrombolysis. The decision to treat by operative thrombectomy versus thrombolysis is largely based on the degree of ischemia in the affected limb, in the absence of other considerations that may be relative or absolute contraindications.

The advantage of thrombolysis is the avoidance of surgical morbidity, particularly in a reoperative field. It also can unmask a lesion that may have caused the arterial occlusion. The disadvantage is that, in most cases, thrombolysis takes 24 to 48 hours; this kind of time is not available for limbs with severe, advanced ischemia. After lysis, a stenosis may be discovered that requires operative intervention. The advantage of operative thrombectomy is rapid restoration of flow. One can and should obtain a completion arteriogram to ensure complete clearance of thrombus and identification of anatomic defects.

THROMBOLYSIS

Thrombolytic therapy is an attractive alternative in patients with acute limb ischemia. This modality, however, should be reserved for patients with clearly viable extremities and should be performed in centers that are familiar with the use and complications of thrombolytic agents. In patients with prior multiple vascular reconstructions, thrombolytic therapy may facilitate recognition of the causative lesion, with either percutaneous or surgical correction done in a timely fashion. When ischemia is severe, however, thrombolytic therapy,

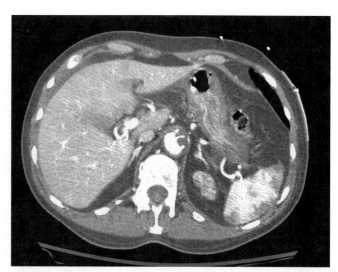

FIGURE 40–4 • Computed tomography scan of the distal thoracic aorta in a patient with acute left lower extremity ischemia. Note the prominent thrombus present in the aortic lumen, the most likely source of the embolism.

especially when carried out by inexperienced clinicians, may delay revascularization and increase tissue loss.

An additional and critical consideration is the physical makeup of the lesion responsible for the acute ischemia. It is a mistake to consider all acute occlusions as being composed primarily of thrombus. The source may be atrial myxoma, aortic atheroembolism, or tumor thrombus. Figure 40-4 is the computed tomography scan of a patient who presented with severe acute ischemia of the left leg. The left femoral pulse was absent, and operative thrombectomy was performed. The femoral artery was found to be obstructed by an organized, rubbery embolus that could not be fragmented, even with forceps. Subjecting a lesion like this to lysis would have resulted in failure; more important, critical time would have been wasted, allowing ongoing ischemia of the lower extremity.

The technique of thrombolysis has undergone significant modifications since the description by McNamara and colleagues.[65] The thrombolytic agent is now infused through multiple side-hole catheters, allowing more efficient delivery of the agent into a longer segment of the thrombus. The original protocol, confirmed by multiple trials, used urokinase at a dose of 4000 IU/minute for 4 hours, decreasing to 2000 IU/minute until the thrombus was fully dissolved. Urokinase was subsequently removed from the market by the Food and Drug Administration for reasons unrelated to its safety or efficacy. It has now been reintroduced, but while it was unavailable, experience was gained with alternative thrombolytics such as tissue plasminogen activator (t-PA) and reteplase. It is clear that these agents, used in appropriate dose regimens, have an equivalent efficacy and a comparable safety profile.

Patient Selection

An acute native vessel occlusion or graft occlusion can be treated initially with thrombolytic therapy. This allows restoration of flow while simultaneously providing an opportunity to discover the underlying lesion that may have precipitated the thrombosis. Figure 40-5 is an arteriogram of a patient with

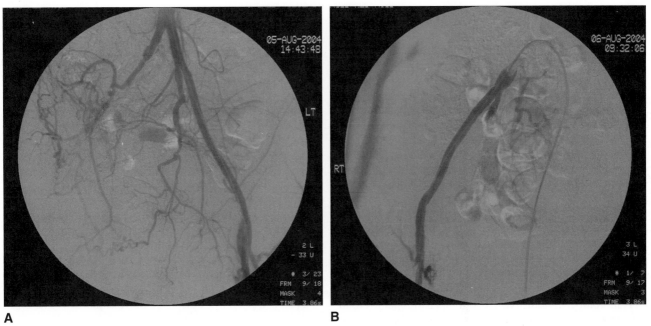

A   **B**

FIGURE 40–5 • *A,* Arteriogram of a 60-year-old woman who had undergone an iliofemoral bypass for chronic right external iliac artery occlusion and presented with the acute onset of severe right leg claudication. *B,* After an overnight infusion of reteplase, the graft was successfully opened. No underlying stenosis was identified.

acute thrombosis of an iliofemoral bypass graft. The patient had some mild sensory deficits, but the limb was not severely ischemic. An overnight infusion of reteplase at 0.5 U/hour resulted in complete lysis, and no underlying lesion was found.

A number of multicenter trials have reported data that may help clarify which patients are best treated with thrombolysis. The study of Surgery or Thrombolysis for the Ischemic Lower Extremity (STILE) compared two thrombolytic agents, recombinant t-PA (rt-PA) and urokinase, with primary surgery for lower extremity symptoms of less than 6 months' duration.[66] The primary end point was a composite outcome index including various factors such as ongoing ischemia, death or major amputation, severe hemorrhage, and wound complications. This study was terminated prematurely by the safety committee at the first interim analysis because of poorer results in the thrombolysis groups, primarily due to a higher rate of recurrent or ongoing ischemia. Amputation and mortality were no different between groups.

The Thrombolysis or Peripheral Arterial Surgery (TOPAS) trial randomized patients with acute limb ischemia of various causes to treatment with recombinant urokinase or immediate operation.[67] There were no statistically significant differences between the thrombolysis group and the surgery group with regard to the primary end point of amputation-free survival at 6 months. The authors concluded that the thrombolysis group required, on average, fewer surgical procedures than the surgical group—a conclusion that is hardly surprising, given that the surgery group was randomized to operation upon entry into the trial. In an accompanying editorial, Porter pointed out that the study was flawed with regard to its designated primary end points, amputation-free survival and mortality.[68] Thirty-two patients (12.5%) in the thrombolysis group had major bleeding, including intracranial hemorrhage in four patients, one of whom died. It must

be concluded that thrombolytic therapy is not benign, does not offer any significant outcome benefits compared with surgery, and should be used selectively.

Over time, an increasing amount of confidence in thrombolytic therapy has been gained, and in good hands, it can be done quite safely. However, success with this therapy is critically dependent on proper patient selection, and this requires sound judgment.

Technique

Access is usually obtained via the contralateral femoral artery. An up-and-over sheath is advanced over a guidewire, and through this sheath is advanced an infusion catheter—usually a multi-side-hole catheter. An attempt is made to traverse the thrombus; if the guidewire is successfully advanced through the thrombus, the lesion is amenable to thrombolysis. However, failure to traverse the clot does not mean that thrombolysis should not be attempted. The clot is then bathed with the lytic agent of choice, and heparin is infused through the sheath at a dose of 500 U/hour to prevent thrombus from forming at the tip of the sheath. The lytic agent is then infused at a steady dose, and the patient is checked every 8 to 12 hours for progress. At these times, the dose may be adjusted up or down and the catheter advanced appropriately. This process takes anywhere from 1 to 3 days. Thrombolysis is usually not continued past 3 days because the risk of hemorrhage increases past this point. Some have advocated monitoring fibrinogen levels, because levels less than 100 mg/dL are thought to correlate with increased bleeding risk.

The most commonly used lytic agents are reteplase, t-PA, and urokinase. A novel addition to the lytic regimen is the glycoprotein IIb/IIIa antagonist abciximab; the rationale is that platelet inhibition, in addition to thrombolysis, will reduce recurrent thrombosis rates and augment catheter-directed peripheral arterial thrombolysis. The RELAX trial, a prospective, dose-escalating safety trial of reteplase monotherapy (0.1, 0.2, 0.5, or 1.0 U/hour) and reteplase-abciximab combination therapy (0.25-mg/kg bolus and 0.125 μg/kg per minute abciximab in addition to each reteplase regimen).[69] Over the range of reteplase dosing, there were no significant differences in efficacy or safety. More important, the addition of abciximab to reteplase was accompanied by a decreased rate of distal embolic events, without a significant increase in the risk of hemorrhagic complications.

OPERATIVE MANAGEMENT

In a review of 682 cases at the Massachusetts General Hospital, a trend toward increasing use of surgical management in patients with acute extremity ischemia was noted.[36] With the introduction of the Fogarty catheter in 1963, surgical intervention in patients with peripheral emboli was greatly simplified. Nevertheless, the systemic effects of this effective intervention must be appropriately managed to minimize mortality. In addition, the principles of embolectomy must be adhered to, avoiding common pitfalls that may lead to failure.

The surgical approach is greatly influenced by the results of the initial evaluation. Decisions regarding patients with significant peripheral vascular disease suspected of having a thrombotic occlusion are guided by the results of arteriography. In any event, wide preparation and draping are highly recommended to avoid unnecessary delays if a change in operative plan is required. The choice of anesthetics is influenced by the general condition of the patient and the planned operative procedure. By and large, femoral and brachial embolectomies can be adequately performed under local anesthesia with careful cardiac monitoring. Similarly, patients requiring femorofemoral reconstruction for a thrombotic iliac occlusion may be operated on under local anesthesia, with the understanding that if a more involved procedure is required, general anesthesia may be necessary. A general anesthetic is recommended for more difficult embolectomies, such as popliteal or axillary, and when more extensive vascular procedures, such as endarterectomy or bypass, are required. Patients operated on because of a failed bypass graft frequently require a relatively involved procedure; thus, general anesthesia is preferred. If a simple thrombectomy is anticipated, local anesthesia is appropriate, provided it can be converted to general anesthesia if the need arises. Because of the general medical condition of these patients and the expected effects of reperfusion, adequate monitoring is recommended. These adjunctive maneuvers, however, should not delay revascularization. Regional anesthesia is usually not feasible, because these patients are most likely fully anticoagulated by the time they reach the operating room. If they are not, it means that one of the most important interventions, systemic heparinization, was not done in a timely manner.

Embolectomy

Before 1963, an embolus to an arterial segment was usually retrieved by direct exposure, by passage of suction catheters, or with the use of rigid instruments that were traumatic and ineffective.[70-72] With the introduction of the Fogarty catheter, the surgical technique was markedly simplified, allowing

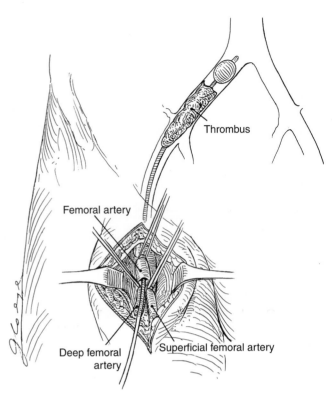

FIGURE 40–6 • Operative technique for femoral embolectomy. Note the control of the common, superficial, and deep femoral arteries with slings, which allows passage of the Fogarty catheter without undue blood loss from back-bleeding. The arteriotomy is placed over the deep femoral orifice. A transverse arteriotomy is preferred if the artery is normal and there is no evidence of significant atherosclerotic disease. Proximal passage of the Fogarty catheter should not be beyond the midinfrarenal aorta, to avoid inadvertent cannulation of visceral vessels, overdistention of the balloon, and potential vessel injury.

exposure remote to the level of occlusion and retrieval of the embolus with a balloon catheter.

Femoral embolectomy is perhaps the most common operation done for lower extremity emboli. A vertical groin incision is made over the femoral pulse, and exposure of the artery is carried out in standard fashion (Fig. 40-6). Control of the common, deep, and superficial femoral arteries is obtained. The arteriotomy should allow visualization of the deep and superficial femoral artery orifices. If the artery is normal to palpation, a transverse arteriotomy may be made over the deep orifice. In diseased arteries, however, a longitudinal arteriotomy is preferable because it allows better manipulation of the catheter and, if necessary, endarterectomy or bypass. Otherwise, closure with a patch is frequently necessary to avoid narrowing of the artery (its only disadvantage).

The size of the Fogarty catheter selected should be appropriate for the artery. For the superficial femoral and popliteal arteries, a No. 4 Fogarty catheter is appropriate. For the iliac system, a No. 4 or 5 Fogarty catheter is best. For more distal insertion and for the deep system, a No. 3 Fogarty catheter is used. Insertion into the deep system should not be beyond 25 cm. The catheter is gently inflated (avoiding overinflation) with saline as traction is maintained, without movement of the catheter. This helps determine when appropriate balloon inflation has been obtained, avoiding forceful traction. The catheter is handled by a single operator, because both maneuvers must be coordinated to avoid arterial injury. Inability to pass the catheter beyond the point of obstruction is usually the result of occlusive disease rather than embolus. Nevertheless, well-organized embolic material may prevent passage of the catheter, requiring more distal or direct exploration.

From the femoral approach, almost 90% of distal insertions pass the catheter into the peroneal artery.[73] Several maneuvers may be helpful in orienting the catheter toward either the anterior tibial or posterior tibial artery. Bending the tip of the catheter to the appropriate side with rotation during insertion may allow cannulation of the desired artery. The current generation of embolectomy catheters has an over-the-wire with infusion capability, which allows visualization of the course of the catheter under direct fluoroscopy. Accordingly, the catheter may be more reliably directed into the tibial vessels as needed. Palpation of the posterior tibial artery at the ankle or the dorsalis pedis artery in the foot during retrieval of a distally placed catheter may help identify which vessel is being maneuvered.

The establishment of adequate inflow is usually not difficult to assess. Completeness of the distal embolectomy, however, can prove difficult to determine, because no reliable clinical guidelines are available. The presence or adequacy of back-bleeding after embolectomy is an unreliable indication of the completeness of the distal embolectomy. Operative arteriography is mandatory, unless the patient's critical condition dictates otherwise. In fact, when operative arteriograms are reviewed after embolectomy, up to 30% of cases show residual thrombi.[74] In these instances, repassage of the embolectomy catheter, more distal exploration, or infusion of intraoperative fibrinolytic agents may help resolve these distal thrombi.[75-82] Evaluation of the distal circulation by Doppler ultrasonography can be extremely helpful, especially when complete retrieval of all occlusive material cannot be accomplished.

Popliteal embolectomy is best carried out through an infrageniculate incision. Although a suprageniculate incision is technically easier, it offers little advantage, because tibial branches are not readily accessible. Figure 40-7 illustrates the preferred approach for transpopliteal embolectomy. The goal is individual cannulation of all three tibial branches so that distal emboli can be retrieved. Our preference is to use this approach when there is radiographic evidence of infrapopliteal embolism or clinical evidence that the embolus is distal (e.g., palpable popliteal pulse). The popliteal artery is exposed through a standard infrageniculate incision. The proximal origin of the soleus muscle usually requires division to expose the tibial-peroneal trunk. The anterior tibial artery is exposed after careful ligation of the anterior tibial vein to allow encircling of the origin of the anterior tibial artery with vessel loops for control. Dissection beyond the tibial-peroneal trunk is rarely necessary, because digital compression of each branch allows selective cannulation of either the posterior tibial or peroneal trunk. A longitudinal arteriotomy is preferred because it permits better visualization of the origin of the anterior tibial artery and manipulation of the catheter. In addition, if a bypass is required, extension of the arteriotomy can be performed for distal anastomosis. Otherwise, patch closure is preferred.

Evidence of persistent ischemia after popliteal embolectomy, or the presence of residual thrombus inaccessible to the catheter from this approach, is an indication for more distal exploration or, alternatively, intraoperative fibrinolytic therapy. Exploration of the tibial vessels at the ankle and foot may

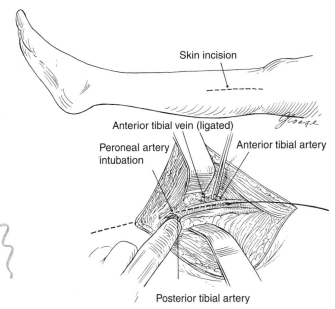

FIGURE 40–7 • Operative technique for popliteal embolectomy. An infrageniculate incision is preferred because it allows individual cannulation of the anterior tibial, posterior tibial, and peroneal arteries. The arteriotomy is performed over the orifice of the anterior tibial artery, with selective passage into the peroneal or posterior tibial artery facilitated by digital compression of one while cannulating the other. Care must be taken during ligation of the anterior tibial vein, a critical maneuver in obtaining adequate control of the anterior tibial artery at its origin. Closure usually requires an autogenous patch to avoid narrowing.

allow retrieval of thrombi not accessible through the transpopliteal approach.[82] A cutdown is performed over the appropriate distal vessel (posterior tibial or dorsalis pedis), and proximal and distal control is obtained with vessel loops. If the artery has no evidence of calcification or atherosclerosis, a transverse arteriotomy is preferable because it allows easier closure with interrupted, fine monofilament vascular sutures. If the vessel is diseased, a longitudinal arteriotomy is preferred, with either patch closure or distal bypass.

Upper extremity emboli are usually approached through a cutdown in the brachial artery, just above the elbow. A transverse arteriotomy is usually preferred because this vessel rarely has significant atherosclerotic changes. A No. 3 Fogarty catheter can be directed into the radial and ulnar arteries, recognizing that reestablishing patency to one or the other is usually sufficient. Care should be taken to protect the median nerve, which runs adjacent to the artery. More proximal emboli may be approached through an infraclavicular incision similar to the one used for axillofemoral reconstructions. Preservation of branches of the axillary artery is recommended because they serve as an important collateral pathway.

The importance of intraoperative assessment of the adequacy of the embolectomy cannot be overemphasized. Doppler examination of the distal part of the extremity is useful but unreliable in terms of the completeness of the procedure. Intraoperative arteriography remains the best method to ensure complete removal of all embolic material. Our preference is to drape the distal extremity with a transparent sterile bag so that skin perfusion can be assessed. Instillation of fluid into the bag and sterile petroleum jelly on the outside of the bag allow for Doppler examination of the various sites.

The rest of the draping should reflect appropriate planning for the approach. Alternative inflow and outflow sites should be included in the operative field so that delays in revascularization are minimized.

Spasm of the runoff arteries, specifically tibial vessels in younger individuals and upper extremity vessels at all ages, is frequent after embolectomy. Intra-arterial administration of papaverine or other vasodilators is recommended, although it may have little effect in resolving this spastic process. This may be secondary to unrecognized residual thrombus with release of platelet vasoactive substances, specifically thromboxane. Repeated mechanical dilatations are to be avoided because the spasm quickly returns and may lead to further intimal injury. If the presence of residual occlusive material can be excluded by adequate arteriography, maintaining the patient fully anticoagulated with a mixture of dextran (40 mg) and papaverine (300 mg in 500 mL of saline at 50 mL/hour) is preferable to maintain patency of the circulation while the spasm spontaneously resolves. This may be difficult in the upper extremities in younger individuals, in whom very reactive distal vessels are present. Provided that no residual occlusive material is present and flow through the vessel can be maintained with appropriate antithrombotic regimens, resolution usually occurs within 12 hours.

A large embolus to the aortic bifurcation (saddle embolus) can produce severe ischemia and major systemic changes upon revascularization. The transfemoral approach is still preferable, with bilateral groin incisions and simultaneous passage of No. 5 or 6 Fogarty catheters to avoid spillage of material to the contralateral side. Concomitant atherosclerotic disease may prevent reestablishment of flow to one or both sides. If adequate inflow is established to one side, a femorofemoral reconstruction may suffice to preserve both limbs. Transperitoneal exploration is indicated with failure to establish inflow on at least one side or suspicion of visceral embolization. Maintaining adequate intravascular volume is important because blood loss from flushing is considerable, and the systemic effects of reperfusion are amplified because of bilateral lower extremity involvement.

The surgeon involved in revascularization of acutely ischemic limbs must be familiar with the systemic effects of such intervention. Management of the systemic effects of revascularization should be initiated in the operating room and maintained throughout the initial postoperative period. These effects are discussed in detail later in this chapter.

Bypass Graft Thrombectomy

The principles of Fogarty catheter embolectomy are applicable to thrombectomy of bypass grafts. The technique is similar, with special care taken in autogenous reconstructions not to overinflate the balloon, which will likely lead to intimal disruption and, occasionally, tears in a fibrotic segment of the vein graft. In this regard, vein graft thrombectomy is much more demanding than prosthetic graft thrombectomy.

Thrombectomy of the graft, with patch angioplasty of the distal anastomosis, is a well-accepted option.[83] The current trend is toward replacement of the bypass graft rather than thrombectomy.[84] Surgical thrombectomy of a prosthetic graft is a relatively simple and straightforward procedure. Proper planning, however, eliminates unnecessary delay and incisions. Our practice is to approach a failed infrainguinal prosthetic bypass at its distal anastomosis. This allows evaluation of the outflow

system and identification and correction of the most common site of intimal hyperplasia. Unless a lesion outside this area has been demonstrated by preoperative evaluation, distal exploration is preferred. If a lesion limited to the first 1 or 2 cm of the distal anastomosis is identified, patch angioplasty to include the distal portion of the graft is a reasonable alternative. If the problem is distal to this site, extensions with prosthetic or autogenous graft material have had limited long-term results, with patency rates of 30% to 40% at 3 years.[57] In this instance, we prefer to construct an entirely new graft, preferably with autogenous tissue.

Graft thrombectomy of autogenous vein grafts is usually best for early failures or when a hypercoagulable condition may have led to failure of the bypass. Late failures, however, are usually complicated not only by progression of the disease proximal and distal to the reconstruction but also by a fibrotic, thickened graft, which is difficult to repair after graftotomy. In addition, the compliance of the graft is such that balloon embolectomy usually leads to significant intimal injury. Long-term results of saphenous vein graft thrombectomies are notoriously poor.

Bypass Graft Revision or Replacement

Perhaps the most important element in ensuring a successful secondary reconstruction after failure of an infrainguinal bypass is identification of the cause of failure. This may allow directed intervention. Such is the case with the identification of a stenotic lesion in the midportion of a vein graft. When the lesions are short (<5 cm), they can be treated with balloon angioplasty. The 24-month patency rate for lesions less than 1.5 cm in vein grafts greater than 3 mm in diameter is excellent, with a significantly lower patency rate demonstrated in longer lesions in smaller grafts.[85] Recurrent stenosis or lesions that are not suitable for balloon angioplasty are best treated with either surgical vein patch angioplasty or interposition graft replacement, as the situation dictates. If the graft is placed deep in the thigh or leg, revision requires a more extensive operative dissection. With most grafts in the subcutaneous tissue, however, surgical intervention can be both simple and effective.

Similarly, residual AV fistulas can be treated with simple incision and ligation. This can be done under local anesthesia on an outpatient basis. Presence of an incompletely lysed valve usually requires patch angioplasty with autogenous tissue. Lesions at the proximal or distal anastomosis of an otherwise good vein graft can also be treated with patch angioplasty quite effectively. As already mentioned, this is best done while the graft is still patent. Otherwise, when graft thrombectomy is necessary in addition to the angioplasty, the results are significantly affected.

The surgical management of a failed infrainguinal prosthetic graft also depends on the cause of failure. Patch angioplasty may be appropriate for lesions that are limited to the first 1 to 2 cm at the proximal or distal anastomosis. Our practice is to transect the stenotic lesion and not attempt an endarterectomy of the area, unless we are dealing with a late failure and atherosclerotic changes are present. A patch is then placed across the lesion to allow relief of the stenosis. Other alternatives include a new prosthetic bypass to a more distal site, extension of the failed bypass with prosthetic or vein graft, or a new vein graft to a more distal site. The technical aspects of these reconstructions are covered elsewhere; however, a new bypass with autogenous saphenous vein is superior to any of the other alternatives.[57]

Fasciotomy

One of the most common manifestations of reperfusion injury after prolonged ischemia is marked swelling of skeletal muscle. Because these muscles are enveloped in fascial compartments, increased pressure within the compartment can cause poor capillary perfusion, increased venous resistance, and a vicious circle leading to further ischemia. Normal tissue pressure within the compartment is approximately zero. As pressure within the compartment rises, tissue perfusion declines progressively and, at a level of about 20 mm Hg, becomes impaired. When the pressure is within 30 mm Hg of the diastolic blood pressure, flow is significantly decreased unless adequate decompression can be carried out.[86]

The decision to proceed with fasciotomy is usually based on clinical findings. Palpation of the specific compartment may reveal a very tense muscle group with tenderness. Pain on passive motion implies a significant increase in tissue pressure. Numbness in the distribution of the nerves within the compartment implies nerve ischemia. The presence of these findings indicates the need for fasciotomy. Compartment pressure can be measured with a slit catheter; commercial kits are available that can be connected to pressure transducers.

Fasciotomy can be achieved in a semiclosed manner when the indication is the anticipation of increased compartment pressures after revascularization. This is performed through a small incision in the proximal portion of the compartment, incising the fascia using either long scissors or a meniscectomy knife. For fully established compartment syndrome, this method is likely to result in inadequate decompression, mainly because of the difficulty of assessing the completeness of the fasciotomy. In addition, the skin may become the limiting factor, with elevated compartment pressure persisting until complete skin incision is performed. Thus, semiclosed fasciotomies should be reserved for very mild cases or as a prophylactic maneuver. Patient selection relies mainly on the experience of the operator.

Open fasciotomy can be limb-saving after revascularization following prolonged ischemia when muscle swelling develops rapidly. Figure 40-8 illustrates one method of achieving decompression of all four compartments through a single incision. A longitudinal incision is made over the fibula, and anterior and posterior flaps are developed. The fascia is incised to allow identification of the four specific compartments and placement of the fasciotomy incisions. The disadvantage of this approach is the creation of fairly extensive skin flaps in potentially compromised skin. In the anterior compartment, care must be taken not to injure the superficial branch of the peroneal nerve. Alternatively, medial and lateral incisions that avoid the creation of skin flaps can be made (Fig. 40-9) while achieving complete decompression. A third approach involves complete fibulectomy. Although this option achieves complete four-compartment decompression, it is fairly morbid, with injury to the peroneal artery, vein, and nerve being common complications. It also may interrupt important collateral circulation. We prefer the medial and lateral incision technique.

Most recently, foot fasciotomy has been advocated in patients with persistent foot ischemia after more proximal fasciotomy and revascularization.[87] Although it may improve foot salvage in selected cases, it is rarely necessary.

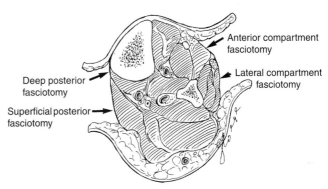

FIGURE 40-8 • Technique of four-compartment fasciotomy via a single lateral incision. Creation of anterior and posterior flaps is necessary, which may be undesirable after revascularization for acute ischemia. Care must be taken to avoid injury to the superficial peroneal nerve, which runs just anterior to the fibula.

Complications after fasciotomy are usually related to wound infection. In the semiclosed method, bleeding may be a problem, mainly because these patients are thoroughly anticoagulated. Nerve injury, specifically of the superficial branch of the peroneal nerve, is a risk with this method.

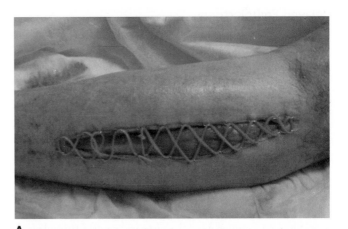

A

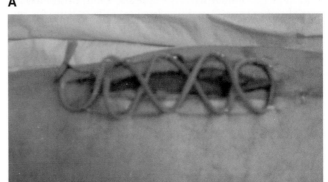

B

FIGURE 40-9 • A, Preferred technique for four-compartment fasciotomy of the lower extremity using medial and lateral incisions. Note that the lateral incision is placed along the fibula to allow fasciotomy of the anterior and lateral compartments. Decompression of the superficial and deep posterior compartment may be facilitated by an initial transverse incision in the fascia to properly identify the compartments. Care must be taken during anterior compartment fasciotomy to avoid injury to the superficial peroneal nerve. B, Photographs of fasciotomy sites closed with the shoelace Silastic loop technique. This allows for gradual tightening at the bedside.

Maintaining the incision in the fascia close to the tibia minimizes the risk of peroneal nerve injury.

Postoperative management of open fasciotomy incisions is critical to reducing morbidity. Sterile techniques should be used for dressing changes until adequate granulation tissue has developed. As the swelling decreases, the use of Steri-Strips (3M, St. Paul, Minn.) for progressive closure of the incision usually results in almost complete closure in most cases. The alternative technique is the use of staples and Silastic vessel loops in a shoelace configuration that allows closure over days at the bedside. Skin grafting may be necessary if this cannot be accomplished. Blistering of the skin secondary to Steri-Strip application can be minimized by alternating the site of placement.

Controversy exists over the need for and the role of fasciotomy after limb revascularization. Some authors have suggested that there is a significant tradeoff between its usefulness and the increased risk of infection.[88] The argument has been made that swelling occurring after revascularization is indicative of cell death, so little is gained by decompression. The majority of the reported experience, however, supports fasciotomy in selected patients. In our experience, timely fasciotomy can be limb-saving.

Delayed Embolectomy

A small but significant group of patients may experience mild to moderate symptoms after an acute arterial embolus, with gradual improvement over subsequent weeks. This is followed by either symptoms of claudication or, more important, progressive ischemia because of clot propagation. Delayed arterial embolectomy can be safely performed in these cases.[89,90] Usually, the procedure can be planned electively, with appropriate arteriographic evaluation. Embolectomy is guided by arteriographic and clinical findings.

The technique is similar to acute embolectomy, recognizing that direct exposure of the occluded segment is necessary. Passage of the catheter from a remote exposure may be difficult, because the material is organized and rubbery. The surgeon must be familiar with the appearance of a thrombosed arterial segment and carefully develop a plane between the thrombus and the intima. Failure to do so may result in significant intimal injury and early rethrombosis. Heparinization in the immediate postoperative period is indicated, with chronic anticoagulation based on the clinical risk factors leading to the embolism. The thrombogenicity of a chronically embolectomized segment dictates the aggressive use of anticoagulants. Long-term results are variable, with some patients experiencing early reocclusion due to thrombosis, marked intimal hyperplasia, or both. Intimal hyperplasia may be secondary to intimal injury from the procedure or the presence of chronic thrombus.

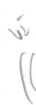

NONOPERATIVE MANAGEMENT

Because of the high mortality associated with revascularization of acutely ischemic limbs in most surgical series, some authors have advocated routine high-dose heparinization in patients with acutely ischemic limbs. The rationale is to select patients with nonviable extremities and proceed with elective revascularization in those with viable extremities after this initial treatment. Using this approach, Blaisdell and colleagues found that mortality decreased to 7.5%, with limb salvage in 67% of 59 patients.[91] Very high doses of heparin were used: an initial bolus of 20,000 U, followed by 2000 to 4000 U/hour. This report has been criticized because these results were compared with historical controls.

Controversy exists as to the appropriateness of nonoperative treatment in severely ischemic extremities. Clearly, extremities that are nonviable at the time of presentation are best treated nonoperatively. This approach is aimed at reducing mortality. More recent series have documented an improvement in limb salvage without an increase in operative mortality with modern techniques of revascularization. Thus, considering surgical intervention is appropriate in most patients. With adequate medical support, this results in both limb and life preservation.

Complications

Complications seen after revascularization of an acutely ischemic extremity can be divided into three types: those related to the surgical intervention, those secondary to limb reperfusion, and those secondary to the primary cause of the event. Discussion of the last is beyond the scope of this chapter because it relates to management of the primary disease, such as cardiac or peripheral vascular disease. Suffice it to say that patients with emboli originating from the heart or sources that are not surgically correctable require long-term anticoagulation to prevent further events. This particular aspect is discussed further.

RECURRENT EMBOLIZATION

The reported incidence of recurrent emboli after an embolic event to an extremity or viscera ranges from 6% to 45%. Prevention of recurrent emboli is of utmost importance in the management of these patients. Chronic long-term anticoagulation is indicated after an embolic event when the source of the emboli cannot be surgically corrected. Anticoagulation should be started immediately after operation. In a series reported by Green and colleagues,[71] only 9% of patients developed recurrent emboli when adequately anticoagulated, in contrast to 31% of those not receiving anticoagulants. This difference has been noted by others.[33,37,92-94] Recurrent embolization carries significantly higher morbidity and mortality than the initial event. The random distribution of emboli from the heart places these patients at risk of stroke or visceral embolization, a major cause of morbidity and mortality. Thus, chronic anticoagulation is of utmost importance in their long-term management.

RETHROMBOSIS

After successful revascularization, recurrent limb ischemia may occur secondary to a second embolus or rethrombosis of the manipulated arterial segment. The latter is more common, because recurrent emboli to the same site are unlikely, especially when the source is the heart. Rethrombosis may occur secondary to (1) residual thrombus in the extremity not recognized at the time of the initial intervention, (2) proximal thrombus that may have been left behind, or (3) inadequate anticoagulation.

When recurrent ischemia occurs, prompt reoperation is indicated unless the patient's general condition dictates otherwise.

The secondary procedure may be planned according to the clinical manifestations of the recurrent event. Re-exploration of the initial operative site is indicated, with liberal use of operative arteriography, endoscopy, or both. Reoperation may be necessary in up to 21% of patients after balloon embolectomy and is usually successful in ensuring limb salvage.[95] In patients with a previously failed vascular graft, rethrombosis of the thrombectomized or revised graft usually mandates consideration of a new bypass graft, preferably with autogenous tissue. The liberal use of anticoagulants (including heparin, dextran, and warfarin) in the postoperative period may benefit patients who experience this complication.

ARTERIAL INJURIES SECONDARY TO THE BALLOON CATHETER

Although the surgical technique for arterial embolectomy is familiar to vascular surgeons, complications of this intervention may be more common than is generally recognized.[96,97] Manifestations may be delayed and appear as distal arterial occlusions secondary to intimal hyperplasia incited by aggressive embolectomy. Perforation is uncommon and usually self-limited if it occurs in a small branch of the artery. Because these patients are usually fully anticoagulated, however, they may show compartment syndromes secondary to an expanding hematoma. Alternatively, the injury may appear at a later date as a pseudoaneurysm. Perforation into an adjacent vein can occur, as illustrated in Figure 40-10. The clinical presentation can be subtle, with a decrease in palpable distal pulses or mild ischemic symptoms. Diagnosis may be established by an astute clinician by means of auscultation of a bruit over the fistula site. Treatment may involve direct repair, with percutaneous embolization successful in some instances.

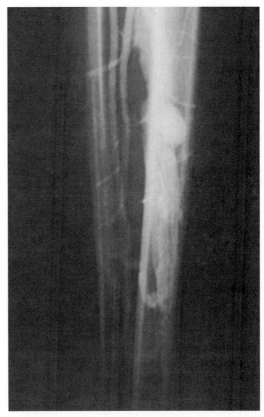

FIGURE 40–10 • Arteriogram 6 weeks after transfemoral embolectomy shows a posterior tibial artery and vein arteriovenous fistula. The patient developed persistent swelling in the extremity, with decreasing distal arterial perfusion. Careful auscultation of the calf suggested the presence of the arteriovenous fistula, which was treated successfully by percutaneous embolization.

MYONEPHROPATHIC METABOLIC SYNDROME

One of the most dramatic and often lethal complications of revascularization of an acute, severely ischemic extremity is a series of systemic processes that have been termed the *myonephropathic metabolic syndrome*.[98] This is the end result of the outpouring of metabolites and cellular debris into the venous circulation after revascularization. Its severity depends on the amount of tissue involved, the degree of ischemia at revascularization, and the completeness of revascularization. Patients with clearly nonviable extremities at presentation are best treated with heparinization and early amputation to avoid this devastating syndrome. Table 40-2 summarizes drugs that may be beneficial in the management of these patients.

With reestablishment of blood flow to the extremity, a general outpouring of acidic blood into the systemic circulation occurs that is capable of causing a rapid, progressive metabolic acidosis. This may lead to poor cardiac function, further acidosis, arrhythmias, and death. Judicious but aggressive use of sodium bicarbonate just before and during the initial minutes of reperfusion is advisable, with frequent evaluation of pH and arterial blood gases. If areas of the extremity remain ischemic, acidosis may persist, requiring continued monitoring and correction.

Hyperkalemia after revascularization of an acutely ischemic extremity can be dramatic and can lead to arrhythmias and

cardiac standstill. Administration of glucose and insulin can be lifesaving, with the reintroduction of potassium into cells. Hyperkalemia may be aggravated by concomitant renal failure. After this initial phase, the use of ion exchange resins, brisk diuresis, or, in some cases, hemodialysis may be necessary.

Myoglobin leakage into the venous circulation may eventually lead to renal failure by precipitation of myoglobin in the collecting tubules. This is best prevented by maintaining a brisk diuresis with the use of mannitol, adequate hydration, and general hemodynamic support. Alkalization of the urine may be achieved by the use of acetazolamide, with increased urinary excretion of potassium a secondary benefit. Myoglobinuria may continue for 24 to 48 hours after revascularization; thus, the aggressive support and maintenance of urine output absolutely must be continued until the urine is clear. Acute renal failure may be sudden and progressive, with poor chance of recovery. Most recently, we have been impressed with the use of prostaglandin E_1 to improve renal perfusion during this acute phase. Although the experience is anecdotal, the results have been encouraging.

The effects of the venous effluent from the revascularized extremity on the pulmonary circulation can be dramatic and can lead to early respiratory failure.[91] Maintaining these patients with respiratory support, avoiding early extubation, is prudent. The chest radiograph may disclose a pattern typical of adult respiratory distress syndrome, a sign of nonspecific pulmonary injury. The exact cause of this lung injury is not clear.

TABLE 40–2	Drugs of Potential Benefit in the Management of Patients with Acute Limb Ischemia				
Drug	**Indication**	**Contraindication**	**Dose**	**Effect**	**Remarks**
Heparin	Acute limb ischemia	Heparin-induced thrombosis; contraindication to anticoagulation	5000-10,000 units IV constant infusion to maintain PTT at 1.5-2.0 × control	Potentiate antithrombin III	
Warfarin	Reduce risk of recurrent emboli	Contraindication to anticoagulation	To maintain PTT at 1.5-2.0 × control	Decrease factors II, VII, IX, and X	
Sodium bicarbonate	Metabolic acidosis	Lactic acidosis; metabolic alkalosis; fluid overload; hypernatremia	Guided by blood pH, $\frac{1}{2}$ body weight × base deficit 12.5-25 g IV	Reduce H^+	Do not correct deficit with single dose; monitor pH
Mannitol	Maintenance of urine output Reperfusion	Congestive heart failure; anuria and established renal failure		Osmotic diuresis	Hydroxy radical scavenger
Insulin and glucose	Hyperkalemia	Diabetic ketoacidosis; hypoglycemia; hypokalemia	12.5-25 g glucose, 5-10 units insulin	Intracellular shift	
Prostaglandin E_1	Improve renal perfusion	Severe hypotension; hypoxemia	0.005 µg/kg/min; increase q 15 min to reach 0.15-0.2 µg/kg/min	Vasodilation	Unproven value
Acetazolamide	Prevention of myoglobin precipitation in urine	Hypokalemia; severe, uncorrected acidosis	500 mg IV	Alkalization of urine; increased K^+ excretion	Not effective if HCO_3^- < 18 mEq/L

IV, intravenous; PTT, partial thromboplastin time.

Experiments carried out by Blaisdell suggest a relationship between the venous effluent of the extremity and the lung injury; when the venous effluent from the revascularized extremity was prevented from reaching the lungs, experimental animals did not show the injury.[88] Treatment is supportive, avoiding fluid overload.

Results of Therapy

ACUTE ARTERIAL OCCLUSION

Since the introduction of the Fogarty catheter for the management of acute extremity ischemia, significant improvements have occurred in the morbidity and mortality of patients with this condition. Initially, improved limb salvage was noted in spite of intervention in previously untreatable ischemic limbs. In the 1960s and early 1970s, limb salvage rates averaged 50% to 60%.[6,99-107] Further improvement was noted later in the 1970s, when average limb salvage rates ranged from 70% to 80%.[34,71,92,108,109] Mortality, however, remained high, averaging 20% to 30% during these 2 decades.

With improved recognition, surgical technique, and medical management, the 1980s saw improvement in both morbidity and mortality, with limb salvage rates routinely in the 85% to 95% range and mortality decreasing to 10% to 15%.[31-33,93,95,110,111] Clearly, aggressive and early management of recognized complications of reperfusion has had a significant impact on the overall mortality of these patients. The clinician must recognize those patients with nonviable extremities who are best treated with early amputation, leading to improved survival. The majority of patients, however, can be managed properly by timely surgical intervention, which can achieve excellent survival and limb salvage.

The presence of atherosclerotic disease negatively influences the outcome. Mortality is lower, with improved limb salvage, in patients with nonatherosclerotic causes of acute limb ischemia, whereas patients with atherosclerotic heart disease or severe peripheral vascular disease have a greater risk of limb loss and death.[6,98] The overall results are likely influenced by underlying cardiac disease and the severity of the ischemia at the time of presentation. Advancing age in this population is likely to stall further improvement in the overall results.

VASCULAR GRAFT OCCLUSION

The results of treatment after occlusion of an infrainguinal reconstruction vary, depending on the specific intervention performed for secondary revascularization. By and large, the best results are obtained with a new autogenous vein graft to a more distal site. In our own series of PTFE grafts for infrainguinal bypass, new bypasses with vein at the first reintervention had an 88% primary patency rate at 30 months. This compares favorably with interventions involving extension with vein or prosthetic material, new bypass with prosthetic material, and thrombectomy with or without patch angioplasty, with patency rates at 30 months ranging from 30% to 33%. Limb salvage rates vary also with the intervention, with the best limb salvage rate obtained with a new bypass with vein at the first reoperation.

In analyzing secondary femoropopliteal reconstructions for failed autogenous infrainguinal revascularization, no correlation was found between the mode of failure and the results of secondary popliteal-tibial reconstruction. An overall 50% 5-year cumulative salvage rate was obtained, with the highest long-term patency achieved when frequent postoperative follow-up allowed recognition of graft failure before total occlusion. In the management of the failing vein graft, a simple vein patch angioplasty yielded an 85% 5-year graft patency. When thrombosis occurred, however, the highest 5-year patency rate was achieved when reconstruction was performed using a new vein graft. When prosthetic material was used for secondary reconstruction, no graft remained patent beyond 3 years.[55]

Based on the reported experience, secondary reconstructions, even with a new autogenous vein bypass to a more distal site, clearly have a lower patency rate than primary reconstructions. Nevertheless, the limb salvage rate is respectable. The 5-year primary patency rate in a series reported by Edwards and colleagues was 80% for primary grafts, whereas it was 57% for secondary reconstructions with autogenous tissue.[103] Limb salvage rates for failed bypasses were excellent and were no different from those achieved with the initial intervention.

Prevention of recurrent graft thrombosis is the greatest challenge for vascular disease specialists managing patients after intervention. It has been suggested that antiplatelet agents are important in the prevention of recurrent graft thrombosis, but to date, no prospective, randomized study has established this concept. Routinely, however, patients are maintained on aspirin after reconstructions, because some experimental evidence suggests a decreased incidence of recurrent thrombosis. Warfarin (Coumadin) therapy with long-term anticoagulation, in contrast, significantly reduces the incidence of graft thrombosis in patients after saphenous vein femoropopliteal bypass. One study showed a significant reduction in graft occlusions—18% in patients treated with warfarin, versus 37% among controls at a mean follow-up of 30 months.[112] The increased complication rate associated with warfarin therapy, however, mandates a selective approach in patients with infrainguinal reconstructions. Our practice is to consider warfarin therapy in patients with no significant contraindication who have suffered a graft thrombosis and required reintervention, or in patients after prosthetic graft failure in whom no cause of thrombosis could be identified.

The overall results of secondary revascularization after failed infrainguinal reconstruction have steadily improved. This is likely secondary to the ability to perform reconstructions to very distal arteries in the extremity, the use of thrombolytic therapy to specifically identify the cause of failure, and overall improved patient care and surgical technique.

Neonatal Aortic Thrombosis

Aortic thrombosis in the newborn, although relatively uncommon, is not a rare entity. Recognition and management of the condition are critical, as it is potentially life threatening. The most common cause of arterial thrombosis in newborns and infants is related to the use of catheters, including cardiac and peripheral catheterization. The incidence, natural history, and management of this condition are not well established because of the wide spectrum of presentations and unclear definitions.

Aortic thrombosis may vary from deposition of a fibrin sheath surrounding the length of an umbilical artery catheter to aortic thrombosis and occlusion of the aorta and its major branches. In infants studied by angiography before removal of an umbilical artery catheter, 95% had developed a fibrin sheath around the catheter. This can be easily diagnosed by abdominal ultrasonography. Some have suggested that the position of the catheter may influence the risk of aortic thrombosis. Specifically, some studies noted a higher incidence of thrombus formation when the catheter is below the renal arteries rather than above them. However, the data are conflicting, with many studies unable to confirm this as a risk factor. It appears that the duration of the indwelling catheter's presence may be a more important risk factor.

CLINICAL MANIFESTATIONS

Umbilical artery catheter thrombosis can have variable presentations. Depending on whether the thrombosis involves the aorta alone, the renal arteries, or the visceral arteries, the presentation can be quite dramatic. Thrombotic involvement of the renal arteries may cause an increase in renin and angiotensin axis activation, manifesting as hypertension. Thrombotic occlusion of the aorta can produce proximal hypertension similar to the mechanism in aortic coarctation. The most common clinical manifestation of aortic thrombosis is lower extremity ischemia, either unilateral or bilateral. The ischemia may present as pallor or coolness or, in more severe cases, with absent pulses and gangrene. Any infant that develops hypertension, congestive heart failure, renal dysfunction, or signs of lower extremity ischemia must be evaluated for aortic thrombosis.

TREATMENT

Management of these patients can be accomplished with surgical thrombectomy, thrombolysis, or anticoagulation. The key is to decide which patient is best treated with a given therapy, for which a classification scheme is useful. The senior author has recommended a modification of the classification proposed by Caplan (Table 40-3).[113] Patients classified as having minor thrombosis (i.e., nonocclusive aortic thrombus or occlusive thrombus with adequate collateralization) usually present with decreased femoral pulses and an inability to withdraw blood from the catheter. Hypertension without a deterioration in renal function does not mandate a change in classification to a more advanced degree of thrombosis. Long-term follow-up of these patients shows that this is a self-limited process. However, in patients with mild to moderate aortic thrombosis in whom nonoperative management is chosen, anticoagulation with heparin is preferred over observation alone. Treatment with heparin anticoagulation is usually sufficient. The use of low-molecular-weight heparin is another nonsurgical alternative. With more advanced degrees of thrombosis,

TABLE 40–3 | Classification of Neonatal Aortic Thrombosis

	Manifestations	
Degree of Thrombosis	*Local*	*Systemic*
Minor	Decreased femoral pulses; inability to withdraw from catheter	Hypertension
Moderate	Same as for minor, plus absent femoral pulses; peripheral ischemia, as evidenced by pale, mottled extremities	Same as for minor, plus congestive heart failure
Major	Same as for moderate, plus severe limb-threatening ischemia, as evidenced by gangrene, tissue loss, or paralysis	Same as for moderate, plus renal failure, visceral involvement, acidosis, sepsis

surgical thrombectomy is a viable option. Catheter-directed thrombolysis is an increasingly utilized option. An algorithm for the management of these patients is presented in Figure 40-11. Long-term follow-up is important, because limb length discrepancy has been reported as a sequela of aortic thrombosis.

Conclusion

Acute arterial and graft occlusion is a serious problem that threatens limb and occasionally life. The optimal therapy requires a keen recognition of the signs and symptoms of acute limb ischemia. The degree of ischemia as well as the

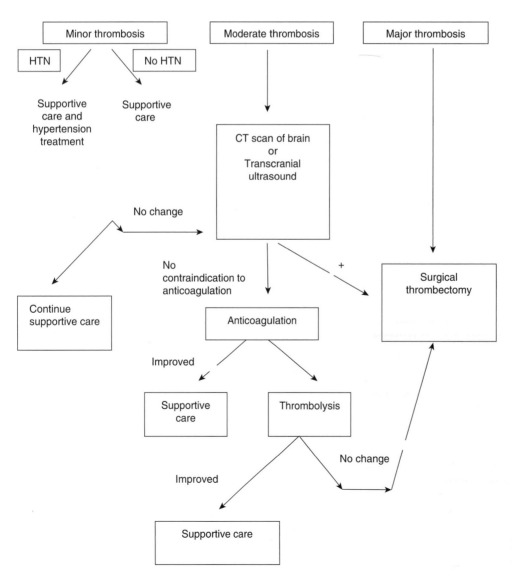

FIGURE 40–11 • Management algorithm for neonatal aortic thrombosis. CT, computed tomography; HTN, hypertension.

general condition of the patient will aid in determining optimal treatment. Surgical thrombectomy and thrombolysis are complementary therapies that, when applied properly to the right patient in the right setting, offer a good outcome while limiting morbidity.

REFERENCES

1. Chervu A, Homsher E, Moore WS, et al: Differential recovery of skeletal muscle and peripheral nerve function after ischemia and reperfusion. J Surg Res 47:12, 1989.
2. Colburn MD, Quiñones-Baldrich WJ, Gelabert HA, et al: Standardization of skeletal muscle ischemic injury. J Surg Res 52:309, 1992.
3. McCord JM: Oxygen derived free radicals in post-ischemic tissue injury. N Engl J Med 312:159, 1985.
4. Saugstad OD, Schrader H, Aasen AO: Alteration of the hypoxanthine level in cerebrospinal fluid as an indicator of tissue hypoxia. Brain Res 112:118, 1976.
5. Grum CM, Ragsdale RA, Ketai LH, et al: Absence of xanthine oxidase or xanthine dehydrogenase in the rabbit myocardium. Biochem Biophys Res Commun 141:1104, 1986.
6. Eddy LJ, Stewart JR, Jones HP, et al: Free-radical producing enzyme, xanthine oxidase, is undetectable in human hearts. Am J Physiol 253:H709, 1987.
7. Granger DN, Rutuli G, McCord JM: Superoxide radicals in feline intestinal ischemia. Gastroenterology 82:9, 1982.
8. Granger DN, McCord JM, Parks DA, et al: Xanthine oxidase inhibitors attenuate ischemia-induced vascular permeability changes in the cat intestine. Gastroenterology 90:80, 1986.
9. McCord JM, Omar BA, Russell WJ: Sources of oxygen derived radicals in ischemia-reperfusion. In Hayaishi O, Niki E, Kondo M, et al (eds): Medical, Biochemical, and Chemical Aspects of Free Radicals. Amsterdam, Elsevier Science, 1989, p 1113.
10. Turrens JF, Beconi M, Barilla J, et al: Mitochondrial generation of oxygen radicals during reoxygenation of ischemic tissues. Free Radic Res 12:681, 1991.
11. McCord JM, Roy S: The pathophysiology of superoxide: Roles in inflammation and ischemia. Can J Physiol Pharmacol 60:1346, 1982.
12. Rao PS, Mueller HS: Lipid peroxidation in acute myocardial ischemia. Adv Exp Med Biol 161:347, 1983.
13. Roy S, McCord JM: Superoxide and ischemia: Conversion of xanthine dehydrogenase to xanthine oxidase. In Greenwald RG (ed): Oxy Radicals and Their Scavenger Systems: Cellular and Molecular Aspects, vol 2. New York, Elsevier Sciences, 1983, p 145.
14. Lee KR, Cronenwett JL, Shalafer M, et al: Effect of superoxide dismutase plus catalase on calcium transport in ischemic and reperfused skeletal muscle. J Surg Res 42:24, 1987.
15. Harlan JM: Neutrophil mediated vascular injury. Acta Med Scand 715(Suppl):123, 1987.
16. Simpson P, Fantone J, Mickelson J, et al: Identification of a time window for therapy to reduce experimental canine myocardial injury: Suppression of neutrophil activation during 72 hours of reperfusion. Circ Res 63:1070, 1988.
17. Rubin B, Smith A, Liauw K, et al: Skeletal muscle ischemia stimulates an immune system mediated injury. Surg Forum 40:297, 1989.
18. Del Zoppo GJ, Schmid-Schonbein GW, Mori E, et al: Polymorphonuclear leukocytes occlude capillaries following middle cerebral artery occlusion and reperfusion in baboons. Stroke 22:1276, 1986.
19. Harris AG, Skalak TC: Effects of leukocyte-capillary plugging in skeletal muscle ischemia-reperfusion injury. Am J Physiol 15:H2653, 1996.
20. Carden DL, Smith JK, Korthuis RJ: Neutrophil-mediated microvascular dysfunction in postischemic canine skeletal muscle: Role of granulocyte adherence. Circ Res 66:1436, 1990.
21. Jerome SN, Smith WC, Korthuis RJ: CD18 dependent adherence reactions play an important role in the development of the no-reflow phenomenon. Am J Physiol 264:H479, 1993.
22. Menger MD, Steiner D, Messmer K: Microvascular ischemia-reperfusion injury in striated muscle: Significance of "no reflow." Am J Physiol 263:H1892, 1992.
23. Mazzoni MC, Borgstrom P, Intaglietta M, et al: Capillary narrowing in hemorrhagic shock is rectified by hyperosmotic saline-dextran reinfusion. Circ Shock 31:407, 1990.
24. Harris AG, Steinbauer M, Leiderer R, et al: Role of leukocyte plugging and edema in skeletal muscle ischemia-reperfusion injury. Am J Physiol 273:H989, 1997.
25. Quiñones-Baldrich WJ, Chervu A, Hernandez JJ, et al: Skeletal muscle after ischemia: No reflow versus perfusion injury. J Surg Res 5:5, 1991.
26. Quiñones-Baldrich WJ: The role of fibrinolysis during reperfusion of ischemic skeletal muscle. Microcirc Endothelium Lymphatics 5:299, 1989.
27. Merril EW: Rheology of blood. Physiol Rev 49:863, 1969.
28. Perry MO, Fantini G: Ischemia: Profile of an enemy. Reperfusion injury of skeletal muscle. J Vasc Surg 6:231, 1987.
29. Belkin M, LaMorte WL, Wright JG, et al: The role of leukocytes in the pathophysiology of skeletal muscle ischemic injury. J Vasc Surg 10:14, 1989.
30. Wright JG, Fox D, Kerr JC, et al: Rate of reperfusion blood flow modulates reperfusion injury in skeletal muscle. J Surg Res 44:754, 1988.
31. Malunski T, Taha Q, Grunfeld S, et al: Diffusion of nitric oxide in the wall monitored in situ by porphyrinic microsensors. Biochem Biophys Res Commun 193:1076, 1993.
32. Malinski T, Radomski MW, Taha Z, et al: Direct electrochemical measurement of nitric oxide released from human platelets. Biochem Biophys Res Commun 194:960, 1993.
33. Huk I, Nanobashvili J, Neumayer C, et al: L-Arginine treatment alters the kinetics of nitric oxide and superoxide release and reduces ischemia/reperfusion in skeletal muscle. Circulation 96:667, 1997.
34. Kishi M, Tanaka H, Setyama A, et al: Pentoxifylline attenuates reperfusion injury in skeletal muscle after partial ischemia. Am J Physiol 274:H1435, 1998.
35. Haimovici H: Muscular, renal, and metabolic complications of acute arterial occlusions: Myonephropathic-metabolic syndrome. Surgery 85:461, 1979.
36. Abbott WM, Maloney RD, McCabe CC, et al: Arterial embolism: A 44 year perspective. Am J Surg 143:460, 1982.
37. Elliott JP Jr, Hageman JH, Szilagyi DE, et al: Arterial embolization: Problems of source, multiplicity, recurrence, and delayed treatment. Surgery 99:833, 1980.
38. Ouriel K, Veith FJ, Sasahara AA: A comparison of recombinant urokinase with vascular surgery as initial treatment for acute arterial occlusion of the legs. N Engl J Med 338:1105, 1998.
39. Sheiner NM, Zeltzer J, MacIntosh E: Arterial embolectomy in the modern era. Can J Surg 25:373, 1982.
40. Hellerstein HK, Martin JW: Incidence of thromboembolic lesions accompanying myocardial infarction. Am Heart J 33:443, 1947.
41. Harris RW, Andros G, Dulawa LB, et al: Malignant melanoma embolus as a cause of acute aortic occlusion: Report of a case. J Vasc Surg 3:550, 1986.
42. Kempzinski RF: Lower extremity arterial emboli from ulcerating atherosclerotic plaques. JAMA 241:807, 1979.
43. Zarins CK, Weisenberg E, Kolettis G, et al: Differential enlargement of artery segments in response to enlarging atherosclerotic plaques. J Vasc Surg 7:386, 1988.
44. Fernandez-Ortiz A, Badimon JJ, Falk E, et al: Characterization of the relative thrombogenicity of atherosclerotic plaque components: Implications for consequences of plaque rupture. J Am Coll Cardiol 23:1562, 1994.
45. Becker PS, Miller VT: Heparin induced thrombocytopenia. Stroke 20:1449, 1989.
46. Laster J, Cikrit D, Walker N, Silver D: The heparin induced thrombocytopenia syndrome: An update. Surgery 102:763, 1987.
47. Bick RL: Alterations of hemostasis associated with malignancies. Semin Thromb Hemost 5:1, 1978.
48. Levine MN, Gent M, Hirsh J, et al: The thrombogenic effect of anticancer drug therapy in women with stage II breast cancer. N Engl J Med 318:404, 1988.
49. Symbas PN, Harlaftis N: Bullet emboli in the pulmonary and systemic arteries. Ann Surg 185:318, 1977.
50. Weaver FA, Schwartz MR, Yellin AE, Bauer M: Refining the indications for arteriography in penetrating extremity trauma: A prospective analysis [abstract]. Paper presented at the 46th Annual Meeting of the Society for Vascular Surgery, June 8, 1992, Chicago.
51. Quiñones-Baldrich WJ, Gelabert HA: Autogenous tissue reconstruction in the management of aortoiliofemoral graft infection. Ann Vasc Surg 4:223, 1990.
52. Panetta TF, Marin ML, Veith FJ, et al: Unsuspected preexisting saphenous vein disease: An unrecognized cause of vein bypass failure. J Vasc Surg 15:102, 1992.
53. Gilbertson JJ, Walsh DB, Zwolak RM, et al: A blinded comparison of angiography, angioscopy, and duplex scanning in the intraoperative evaluation of in situ saphenous vein bypass grafts. J Vasc Surg 15:121, 1992.

54. Donaldson MC, Mannick JA, Whittemore AD: Causes of primary graft failure after in situ saphenous vein bypass grafting. J Vasc Surg 15:113, 1992.

55. Barboriak JJ, Pintar K, VanHorn DL, et al: Pathologic findings in the aortocoronary vein grafts. Atherosclerosis 29:69, 1978.

56. Matsubara J, Nagasue M, Tsuchishima S, et al: Clinical results of femoropopliteal bypass using externally supported (EXS) Dacron grafts: With a comparison of above- and below-knee anastomosis. J Cardiovasc Surg (Torino) 31:731, 1990.

57. Quiñones-Baldrich WJ, Prego A, Ucelay-Gomez R, et al: Failure of PTFE infrainguinal revascularization: Patterns, management alternatives, and outcome. Ann Vasc Surg 5:163, 1991.

58. Quiñones-Baldrich WJ, Busuttil RW, Baker JD, et al: Is the preferential use of PTFE grafts for femoral-popliteal bypass justified? J Vasc Surg 8:219, 1988.

59. Blaisdell FW, Steele M, Allen RE: Management of acute lower extremity arterial ischemia due to embolism and thrombosis. Surgery 84:822, 1978.

60. Barnes RW, Thompson BW, MacDonald CM, et al: Serial noninvasive studies do not herald postoperative failure of femoropopliteal or femorotibial bypass grafts. Ann Surg 210:486, 1989.

61. Bandyk DF, Cato RF, Towne JB: A low flow velocity predicts failure of femoropopliteal and femorotibial bypass grafts. Surgery 98:799, 1985.

62. Sladen JG, Reid JDS, Cooperberg PL, et al: Color flow duplex screening of infrainguinal grafts combining low- and high-velocity criteria. Am J Surg 158:107, 1989.

63. Buth J, Disselhoff B, Sommeling C, Stam L: Color-flow duplex criteria for grading stenosis in infrainguinal vein grafts. J Vasc Surg 14:716, 1991.

64. Cambria RP, Abbott WM: Acute arterial thrombosis of the lower extremity. Arch Surg 119:784, 1984.

65. McNamara TO, Bomberger RA, Merchant RF: Intraarterial urokinase therapy for acutely ischemic limbs. Paper presented at the Fourth Annual Meeting of the Western Vascular Society, Jan 18, 1989, Kauai, Hawaii.

66. Weaver FA, Comerota AJ, Youngblood M, et al: Surgical revascularization versus thrombolysis for nonembolic lower extremity native artery occlusions: Results of a prospective randomized trial. The STILE investigators: Surgery versus Thrombolysis for Ischemia of the Lower Extremity. J Vasc Surg 24:513, 1996.

67. Oureil K, Veith FJ, Sasahara AA: A comparison of recombinant urokinase with vascular surgery as initial treatment for acute arterial occlusion of the legs. N Engl J Med 338:1105, 1998.

68. Porter JM: Thrombolysis for acute arterial occlusion of the legs [editorial]. N Engl J Med 338:1148, 1998.

69. Ouriel K, Castaneda F, McNamara T, et al: Reteplase monotherapy and reteplase/abciximab combination therapy in peripheral arterial disease occlusive disease: Results from the RELAX trial. J Vasc Interv Radiol 15:229, 2004.

70. Dale WA: Endovascular suction catheters. J Thorac Cardiovasc Surg 44:557, 1962.

71. Green RM, De Weese JA, Rob CG: Arterial embolectomy before and after the Fogarty catheter. Surgery 77:24, 1975.

72. Lerman J, Miller FR, Lund CC: Arterial embolism and embolectomy. JAMA 94:1128, 1930.

73. Short D, Vaughn GD III, Jachimczyk J, et al: The anatomic basis for the occasional failure of transfemoral balloon catheter thromboembolectomy. Ann Surg 190:555, 1979.

74. Plecha FR, Pories WJ: Intraoperative angiography in the immediate assessment of arterial reconstruction. Arch Surg 105:802, 1972.

75. Cohen LH, Kaplan M, Bernhard VM: Intraoperative streptokinase: An adjunct to mechanical thrombectomy in the management of acute ischemia. Arch Surg 121:708, 1986.

76. Comerota AJ, White JV, Grosh JD: Intraoperative intraarterial thrombolytic therapy for salvage of limbs in patients with distal arterial thrombosis. Surg Gynecol Obstet 169:283, 1989.

77. Greep JM, Aleman PJ, Jarrett F, Bast TJ: A combined technique for peripheral arterial embolectomy. Arch Surg 105:869, 1972.

78. Gupta SK, Samson RH, Veith FJ: Embolectomy of the distal part of the popliteal artery. Surg Gynecol Obstet 153:254, 1981.

79. Norem RS, Short DH, Kerstein MD: Role of intraoperative fibrinolytic therapy in acute arterial occlusion. Surg Gynecol Obstet 167:87, 1988.

80. Parent FN III, Bernhard VM, Pabst TS III, et al: Fibrinolytic treatment of residual thrombus after catheter embolectomy for severe lower limb ischemia. J Vasc Surg 9:153, 1989.

81. Quiñones-Baldrich WJ, Baker JD, Busuttil RW, et al: Intraoperative infusion of lytic drugs for thrombotic complications of revascularization. J Vasc Surg 10:408, 1989.

82. Youkey JR, Clagett GP, Cabellon S, et al: Thromboembolectomy of arteries explored at the ankle. Ann Surg 199:367, 1984.

83. Veith FJ, Gupta S, Daly V: Management of early and late thrombosis of expanded polytetrafluoroethylene (PTFE) femoropopliteal bypass grafts: Favorable prognosis with appropriate reoperation. Surgery 87:581, 1980.

84. Edwards JE, Taylor LM Jr, Porter JM: Treatment of failed lower extremity bypass grafts with new autogenous vein bypass grafting. J Vasc Surg 11:136, 1990.

85. Sanchez LA, Gupta SK, Veith FJ, et al: A ten-year experience with one hundred fifty failing or threatened vein and polytetrafluoroethylene arterial bypass grafts. J Vasc Surg 14:729, 1991.

86. Whitesides TE, Haney TC, Harada H, et al: A simple method for tissue pressure determination. Arch Surg 110:1311, 1975.

87. Ascer E, Strauch B, Calligaro KD, et al: Ankle and foot fasciotomy: An adjunctive technique to optimize limb salvage after revascularization for acute ischemia. J Vasc Surg 9:594, 1989.

88. Blaisdell FW: Is there a reason for controversy regarding fasciotomy? J Vasc Surg 9:828, 1989.

89. Jarrett F, Dacumos GC, Crummy AB, et al: Late appearance of arterial emboli: Diagnosis and management. Surgery 86:898, 1979.

90. Levin BH, Giordano JM: Delayed arterial embolectomy. Surg Gynecol Obstet 155:549, 1982.

91. Blaisdell FW, Lim RC, Amberg JR, et al: Pulmonary microembolism: A cause of morbidity and death after major vascular surgery. Arch Surg 93:776, 1966.

92. Hight DW, Tilney NL, Couch NP: Changing clinical trends in patients with peripheral arterial emboli. Surgery 79:172, 1976.

93. Silvers LW, Royster TS, Mulcare RJ: Peripheral arterial emboli and factors in their recurrence rate. Ann Surg 192:232, 1980.

94. Tawes RL Jr, Beare JP, Scribner RG, et al: Value of postoperative heparin therapy in peripheral arterial thromboembolism. Am J Surg 146:213, 1983.

95. Tawes RL Jr, Harris EJ, Brown WH, et al: Arterial thromboembolism: A 20-year perspective. Arch Surg 120:595, 1985.

96. Dainko EA: Complications of the use of the Fogarty balloon catheter. Arch Surg 105:79, 1972.

97. Dobrin PB: Mechanisms and prevention of arterial injuries caused by balloon embolection. Surgery 106:457, 1989.

98. Haimovici H, Moss CM, Veith FJ: Arterial embolectomy revisited. Surgery 78:409, 1975.

99. Barker CF, Rosato FE, Roberts B: Peripheral arterial embolism. Surg Gynecol Obstet 123:22, 1966.

100. Billig DM, Hallman GI, Cooley DA: Arterial embolism: Surgical treatment and results. Arch Surg 95:1, 1967.

101. Buxton B, Morris P: Arterial embolism of the lower limbs: Experience with the use of the Fogarty embolectomy balloon catheter. Aust N Z J Surg 39:179, 1969.

102. Cranley JJ, Krause RJ, Strasser ES, et al: Peripheral arterial embolism: Changing concepts. Surgery 55:57, 1964.

103. Edwards EA, Tilney NL, Lindquist RR: Causes of peripheral embolism and their signifcance. JAMA 196:133, 1966.

104. Fogarty TJ, Cranley JJ: Catheter technique for arterial embolectomy. Ann Surg 161:325, 1965.

105. Karageorgis BP: Experience with the catheter technique in arterial embolectomy. J Cardiovasc Surg (Torino) 8:375, 1967.

106. McMahon JW, Sako Y: Arterial embolism and embolectomy. Geriatrics 23:132, 1968.

107. Tarnay TJ: Arterial embolism of the extremities: Experience with 62 patients. Arch Surg 99:615, 1969.

108. Satiani B, Gross WS, Evans WE: Improved limb salvage after arterial embolectomy. Ann Surg 188:153, 1978.

109. Thompson JE, Sigler L, Raut PS, et al: Arterial embolectomy: A 20-year experience. Surgery 67:212, 1970.

110. Dale WA: Differential management of acute peripheral arterial ischemia. J Vasc Surg 1:269, 1984.

111. Kendrick J, Thompson BW, Read RC, et al: Arterial embolectomy in the leg: Results in a referral hospital. Am J Surg 142:739, 1981.

112. Kretschmer G, Wenzl E, Piza F, et al: The influence of anticoagulant treatment on the probability of function in femoropopliteal vein bypass surgery: Analysis of a clinical series (1970 to 1985) and interim evaluation of a controlled clinical trial. Surgery 102:453, 1987.

113. Colburn MD, Gelabert HA, Quiñones-Baldrich W: Neonatal aortic thrombosis. Surgery 111:21, 1992.

Ted R. Kohler • Wesley S. Moore

Myointimal Hyperplasia

The development of strategies designed to suppress myointimal hyperplasia after peripheral vascular interventions has become increasingly important in light of the current enthusiasm for less invasive but more locally injurious percutaneous therapies. More durable prosthetic vascular reconstructive procedures also succumb to this healing response, most prominently at the points of surgical anastomosis. Autogenous vein bypass is the primary means of limb salvage for patients with tibial occlusive changes and limb-threatening ischemia, but these grafts ultimately develop a form of myointimal hyperplasia arising in concert with the vein graft "arterialization" process. The long-term patency of vein bypass grafts is ultimately limited by progressive stenosis along the length of the graft and at anastomoses due to this inexorable process of myointimal hyperplasia.[1-3] Peripheral vascular interventions will remain temporary and palliative rather than durable and potentially curative unless effective treatment of myointimal hyperplasia can be achieved.

Intimal thickening is formed by the migration of smooth muscle cells from the medial to the intimal layer of the vessel wall after an endothelial injury. Subsequent proliferation of these cells and the ensuing deposition of extracellular matrix material produce thickening of the intimal layer, luminal narrowing, and eventual thrombosis of the affected vessel. This hyperplastic intimal response is a characteristic fibromuscular cellular response to injury and is a normal feature of vascular healing. However, in some instances, progression of this process ultimately leads to graft failure. Intimal hyperplasia is the most common cause of failures occurring between 2 and 3 years postoperatively. In one series, 50% of late failures identified in 5000 arterial reconstructions, including both endarterectomy and bypass operations, were due to this exuberant hyperplastic intimal process.[1]

In this chapter, we summarize the current concepts regarding the pathology, pathophysiology, clinical manifestations, and management of hyperplastic intimal lesions. In addition, we use the molecular pathways that are important in the formation of intimal hyperplasia as a framework for understanding pharmacologic approaches to inhibiting this lesion. Finally, we speculate on possible future directions for research in this area.

Pathology

Intimal hyperplasia can be described as the abnormal continued proliferation of cells and connective tissue elements that occurs at sites of arterial injury. During the first decade of the 20th century, investigators noted that "within a few days after the operation, the stitches placed in making the anastomosis became covered with a glistening substance similar in appearance to the normal endothelium."[4] This early description of arterial healing probably represents the normal response of an artery to injury. Intimal hyperplasia, in contrast, is more likely the result of the inability to control, or the continued stimulation of, this normal regenerative process. Lesions of intimal hyperplasia are firm and homogeneous. They look smooth, shiny, and subendothelial. These lesions are often referred to as *myointimal hyperplasia*, highlighting the fact that the medial smooth muscle cell is the origin of the proliferating tissue. Histologic examination reveals mainly stellate cells surrounded by a clear fibromyxomatous stroma and connective tissue. These stellate cells are smooth muscle cells. They stain positively for actin and for sulfated glycosaminoglycans.[5,6] These cells probably originate in the media as differentiated smooth muscle cells and in the adventitia as myofibroblasts. They begin to proliferate within 24 hours of injury. This is followed by migration from the media across the internal elastic lamina into the intima. Once in the intima, they continue to proliferate for just a few days. Wall thickening continues as they deposit extracellular matrix over the next several weeks (Fig. 41-1).[7]

Pathophysiology

Development of intimal hyperplasia begins with damage to the vascular endothelium and underlying smooth muscle cells. Subsequent exposure of the subendothelial arterial wall elements triggers the activation of myriad cellular and enzymatic events that ultimately lead to the migration and proliferation of medial smooth muscle cells.[7] The response of the medial smooth muscle cell to vascular injury can be divided into four distinct stages: (1) an initial medial proliferative response, (2) migration from the media across the external elastic lamina and into the intima, (3) subsequent proliferation within the neointima, and (4) synthesis and

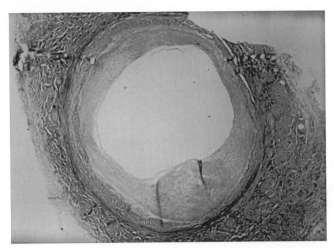

FIGURE 41–1 • Photomicrograph of a failed infrainguinal autogenous vein bypass graft showing a large amount of hyperplastic intimal proliferation (Verhoeff-van Gieson stain; original magnification ×20).

deposition of extracellular matrix. The end result is intraluminal thickening and reduction of the luminal diameter.

Several mechanisms are likely responsible for these responses, including mechanical changes, such as turbulence and compliance mismatch, and complex interactions between endothelial and smooth muscle cells and circulating factors such as platelets and components of the inflammatory system.[8] More recently, a much more complex view has emerged that involves the synergistic action of several biologic pathways. The remainder of this section reviews, separately, the experimental basis for the hypothesized involvement of each of these systems.

HEMODYNAMIC AND MECHANICAL FACTORS

A wide variety of hemodynamic and mechanical factors, including high- and low-flow velocities,[9] high and low wall shear stress,[10] and mechanical compliance mismatch,[11] have been implicated in the formation of intimal hyperplasia. The effects of flow velocity on the subsequent development of intimal hyperplasia have been studied in a variety of models. In a high-flow renal artery–to–vena cava anastomosis, significant intimal thickening was documented by electron microscopic examination 3 months after formation.[12] Similar intimal lesions have also been noted in arteriovenous fistulas constructed for hemodialysis access.[13] However, in a canine carotid vein interposition model, segments with low-flow velocities developed significantly thicker intimal layers.[14] Others found that 6 months after construction of an arteriovenous fistula in monkey iliac vessels, no increase in intimal thickening occurred on the experimental side.[15] In that study, although flow rate and velocity were markedly increased on the side of the arteriovenous fistula, the calculated wall shear stress was equal on both sides. This equality of shear stress, despite a significant difference in flow velocities, was the result of a twofold increase in the vessel lumen diameter. The vessel wall regulates its diameter to produce a physiologic level of shear stress at the lumen. The endothelium regulates diameter by producing both vasoconstrictors, such as endothelin, and vasodilators, such as nitric oxide. These factors also affect

smooth muscle cell proliferation and, when chronically present, cause remodeling of the vessel to maintain the new diameter without vasoactivity.

In other primate studies, arteriovenous flow has been shown to inhibit neointimal thickening in highly porous polytetrafluoroethylene (PTFE) grafts. Return to normal flow causes thickening of these lesions. In a rodent model of arterial injury, low flow causes increased intimal hyperplasia. These and many other studies demonstrate that intimal hyperplasia is increased by low shear and inhibited by high shear. Regions of low wall shear stress also may stimulate intimal proliferation by increasing the time for lipid transport.[9,14] The results of postmortem studies have shown that early atherosclerotic lesions occur more commonly in areas of low wall shear stress.[16] In the carotid artery, atherosclerosis starts at the outer wall of the bulb, where shear forces are low and oscillating.[17,18]

Compliance mismatch is also an important hemodynamic factor in the production of anastomotic intimal hyperplasia.[19] Compliance is defined as the percentage of radial change per unit pressure and is a useful index of vessel wall distensibility to a pressure force. Although experimental and clinical studies have shown that grafts with compliance values approaching that of the native artery have better patency, none of these studies controlled for differences in graft surfaces. In one study, femoropopliteal autografts made from glutaraldehyde-treated carotid arteries had better patency when fixation produced a more compliant graft. However, there was no effect on intimal hyperplasia. The compliance of a vein graft at the time of implantation is similar to that of a native artery, and according to the results of one study, the compliance values remained within the normal range for a median follow-up of 33 months.[20] Textile and fabric prostheses, in contrast, are relatively noncompliant. Furthermore, 4 months after implantation, a significant loss of compliance is noted in both polyester fabric and PTFE grafts.[21] For this reason, some authors have suggested imposing a short cuff of autogenous vein between native artery and prosthetic grafts.[22]

When taken together, operative manipulation and hemodynamic factors may contribute, in part, to the development of intimal hyperplasia. Clinically, overaggressive dissection while harvesting vein grafts may lead to injury of the vasa vasorum and disruption of the endothelial layer.[23] Mechanical distention of a vein segment above 200 mm Hg leads to endothelial cellular damage.[24] However, these factors are probably only facilitative, because balloon injury of veins does not produce wall thickening unless the vein is transplanted into the arterial circulation.

PLATELETS

Platelets have long been known to play a central role in the reaction of a vessel wall to injury. To date, most research in this area has focused on the activation of platelets by the injured endothelium as the major factor in the development of intimal hyperplasia. Denudation of the arterial wall exposes the subendothelial matrix, which leads to adherence and subsequent activation of platelets. The luminal surface quickly passivates by adsorption of plasma proteins, limiting the period of platelet aggregation to less than 24 hours. Platelet adherence requires the interaction of subendothelial collagen, a platelet membrane glycoprotein receptor (GP Ib), plasma von Willebrand's factor, and fibronectin. After adherence, platelets undergo a morphologic change, stretching to cover the exposed surface. Activated platelets release adenosine diphosphate and activate the arachidonic acid pathway to release thromboxane A_2. Both of these factors lead to platelet aggregation. Recruitment of platelets requires the rapid expression of the platelet membrane receptor complexes GP IIb and GP IIIa, both of which promote platelet aggregation through the binding of circulating fibrinogen. Platelet adhesion and granule release also lead to a parallel acceleration of the coagulation cascade. This activation of clotting pathways, combined with high local concentrations of fibrinogen mediated by binding to the GP IIb/IIIa complex, creates a fibrin protein network that further stabilizes the aggregated platelet plug. Once platelet aggregation is initiated by the pathways mentioned earlier, its further formation is actively inhibited by an intact endothelium. Thus, a damaged endothelium not only initiates platelet activation but also impairs its inhibition.

Platelet-derived growth factor (PDGF) is secreted along with other granule constituents, including platelet factor 4, thromboglobulin, and thrombospondin. PDGF is a cationic protein with a molecular weight of 28,000 to 31,000 Da. It comprises two subunits (α and β). Physiologically, PDGF functions as both a chemoattractant and a mitogen for smooth muscle cells and fibroblasts. Because it binds with high affinity to smooth muscle cells, some have suggested that PDGF may attract the smooth muscle cells from the media into the intima, bind to them, and stimulate their proliferation. Interestingly, evidence has shown that the platelet may not be the only source of this protein. PDGF (α and β subunits) is produced by human umbilical vein and saphenous vein endothelial cells. In fact, a large increase in PDGF production can be measured in injured endothelial cells. Also, both α-subunit and β-subunit messenger RNA (mRNA) have been noted in fresh endarterectomy specimens obtained during carotid surgery.[25] Smooth muscle cells themselves also produce PDGF-like activity in response to arterial injury, and smooth muscle cells from human atheroma contain mRNA for the PDGF α subunit.[26] Taken together, these findings may explain how intimal proliferation continues after re-endothelialization occurs. PDGF may be released by both platelets and endothelial cells, causing the activation and migration of smooth muscle cells, which then secrete additional PDGF, leading to proliferation.

Blocking PDGF in animal models does not reduce proliferation, which is stimulated by basic fibroblast growth factor (bFGF) released from injured smooth muscle cells. PDGF stimulates smooth muscle cell migration, with is reduced with thrombocytopenia or the blocking of antibodies for PDGF. This may partially explain why antiplatelet therapy, which can decrease early graft thrombosis, does not affect intimal hyperplasia.

INFLAMMATORY CELL PATHWAYS

Inflammation may stimulate cellular proliferation after arterial injury. A significant portion of the intravascular pool of polymorphonuclear neutrophils (PMNs) is adherent to the vascular endothelium. Further, PMN adhesion and infiltration are common findings after arterial wall injury. Electron microscopic studies after balloon catheter intimal injury show that leukocytes attach to the de-endothelialized surface of an arterial lumen.[27] Both monocytes and lymphocytes also adhere to damaged endothelium and, in some instances, even penetrate it. White blood cells secrete substances capable of stimulating the growth of intimal lesions.[28]

The association between inflammation and intimal proliferation was demonstrated in an in vivo model of vasculitis.[29] In this study, endotoxin-soaked thread was placed on half of a rat femoral artery to produce an inflammatory response. This technique consistently caused a significant leukocyte infiltration, which occurred only on the treated side of the vessel. Histologic examination performed 14 days later revealed nonuniform intimal lesions in which proliferating smooth muscle cells were located exclusively on the side of the lumen adjacent to the treated half of the arterial wall. Clearly, these findings suggest an association between inflammatory and proliferative biologic pathways. The mechanisms controlling this relationship are a target for therapeutic intervention.

PMN adhesion to the surface of endothelial cells is controlled by several complex glycoproteins located on the surface of both endothelial and white blood cells. Together, these binding molecules constitute a sophisticated communication system. To date, two endothelial cell adhesion molecules involved in neutrophil binding have been well characterized: endothelial leukocyte adhesion molecule-1 (ELAM-1) and intercellular adhesion molecule-1 (ICAM-1). ELAM-1 either is unexpressed or simply remains intracellular in the nonactive endothelial cell. However, after activation by a variety of different cytokines, this adhesion complex is rapidly induced and appears on the membrane surface of the stimulated endothelial cell. Both the physiologic function of this molecule and the specific leukocyte receptor to which it binds remain unknown. ICAM-1 is located in small amounts on the surface of nonactive endothelial cells. After activation by either injury or a variety of stimulating agonists, the expression of this binding complex is significantly increased. ICAM-1 is the binding ligand for the CD11a/CD18 receptor on the leukocyte membrane.

Histochemically, the adhesion molecules located in the surface membranes of white blood cells that are responsible for leukocyte binding to endothelial cells can be separated into three related heterodimers. Each of these heterodimer's protein complexes are composed of an α and a β subunit. The α subunit differs among the three glycoprotein complexes (CD11a, CD11b, or CD11c), whereas the β subunit remains constant (CD18). The CD11a/CD18 complex is found on the surface of all white blood cells and mediates the attachment of unstimulated PMNs to stimulated endothelial cells. This binding probably occurs through an interaction with the ICAM-1 receptor that, as mentioned, is expressed on the luminal surface of activated or injured endothelial cells. The binding of the CD11a/CD18 complex to the ICAM-1 receptor may also play a role in the cytokine-induced transendothelial migration of PMNs. The CD11b/CD18 adhesion complex is referred to as either Mac-1 or the C3b complement receptor. This glycoprotein has been implicated in the adhesion of chemotactically stimulated PMNs and controls several cellular functions, such as aggregation and cytotoxicity. The third heterodimer complex, CD11c/CD18, exists on both PMNs and monocytes, but its role in binding to endothelial cells remains undetermined.

During inflammatory states, the attachment of PMNs to the involved endothelium is greatly increased, primarily due to the upregulation and enhanced expression of the earlier-described binding glycoproteins. A variety of substances are capable of stimulating this enhanced PMN adherence, and together these are thought to be the primary mediators of the inflammatory response to tissue injury. Interleukin-1, tumor necrosis factor-α, lymphotoxin, and bacterial endotoxins (lipopolysaccharide) all increase the production of both ELAM-1 and ICAM-1 on the surface of affected endothelial cells. In addition, PMN activation can be stimulated by several substances that are released secondary to inflammation. Examples include the complement factors C5a and C3b, which stimulate PMN chemotaxis and phagocytosis, respectively. Likewise, PMN adhesion and chemotaxis can also be stimulated by interleukin-1, xanthine oxidase, PDGF, and the lipid mediators leukotriene B and platelet-activating factor. Finally, tumor necrosis factor is an important mediator of PMN phagocytosis and can lead to increased lysosomal enzyme release.

After activation and adhesion to the damaged vessel lumen, white blood cells migrate into the arterial wall. In one study, 42 days after a denuding injury, leukocytes were shown to penetrate the arterial media and were seen deep within the hyperplastic lesions.[30] The mechanisms triggering this leukocyte migration remain unknown. One possibility is that this process is mediated by the exposure of medial smooth muscle cells, which occurs after an endothelial injury. A serum-containing medium that is conditioned with smooth muscle cells can stimulate leukocyte migration. More important, smooth muscle cells and macrophages elaborate potent chemotactic factors for leukocytes, which could sustain continued white blood cell recruitment.[31] Other chemotactic agents for leukocytes include PDGF and, in some reports, factors released by fibroblasts. Smooth muscle cells removed from atherosclerotic plaques express ICAM-1, suggesting a possible connection between these medial cells and leukocyte recruitment and activation.

The mechanism by which leukocytes may initiate the formation of intimal hyperplasia after penetrating the injured arterial wall remains unknown. Again, several pathways have been suggested. After a denuding endothelial injury and the deposition of inflammatory cells, a variety of inflammatory products may be elaborated. These include chemotactic factors, growth factors, complement components, and enzymes. One of the most studied substances is monocyte- and macrophage-derived growth factor (MDGF). MDGF is a well-known stimulator of smooth muscle cell and fibroblast proliferation. This growth factor is similar and, in fact, may be identical to PDGF. Thus, the stimulation of smooth muscle cell proliferation is one mechanism by which inflammatory cells may contribute to the formation of intimal hyperplasia. A second possibility involves the production of lysosomal degradation enzymes. Activated leukocytes secrete several potent proteases capable of degrading collagen, basement membranes, and other important extracellular structural proteins. One example of a PMN-derived enzyme that has been implicated in peri-inflammatory extracellular damage is myeloperoxidase. Liberation of these destructive enzymes into the wall of an injured vessel may weaken the extracellular matrix. This "loosening" of the vessel wall may facilitate the migration of smooth muscle cells from the medial layer toward the lumen. Finally, leukocytes may act directly at sites of vessel injury to extend endothelial injury. PMNs can produce oxygen free radicals through the action of the NADPH oxidase system present on their membranes. The toxic substances elaborated

by these activated PMNs, including superoxide anion, hydrogen peroxide, and hydroxyl radicals, can damage endothelial cells and alter capillary permeability. With PMN activation, marginally injured endothelial cells bordering a lesion may be destroyed, increasing the magnitude of the damage to the vessel wall. This further exposure of the subendothelial layer allows more platelet cell adherence, aggregation, and activation, as well as the recruitment of more leukocyte mediators and, therefore, the stimulation of a continued cycle of inflammatory injury.

RENIN-ANGIOTENSIN SYSTEM

The classic view of the regulatory function of the renin-angiotensin system is that it is primarily an endocrine-based system designed for the homeostatic control of hemodynamic and electrolyte balance. In response to low perfusion pressures, renin is released by renal tissue and circulates in the plasma, where it cleaves angiotensinogen, produced by the liver, into angiotensin I. Angiotensin I is converted into active angiotensin II by angiotensin-converting enzyme (ACE) located primarily in the pulmonary vasculature. Finally, angiotensin II exerts its homeostatic hemodynamic effects via specific angiotensin II receptors located in peripheral vascular arterial beds. This traditional view of the renin-angiotensin system has been revised, and a much more complex concept has emerged. In this new description, the primary site of angiotensin II production is not the pulmonary vasculature but rather local sites within the affected tissues themselves. This portion of the entire renin-angiotensin axis has been referred to as the tissue renin-angiotensin system.

The concept that active angiotensin II in the vascular wall is synthesized locally, and not delivered via the systemic circulation, was originally suggested by Swales and Thurston.[32] In this report, the authors noted that the amount of angiotensin antiserum required to inhibit endogenous angiotensin effects in sodium-loaded rats could not be explained solely on the basis of systemic production. In addition, several investigators had noticed residual renin-like activity after bilateral nephrectomy in animal studies.[33] More convincing evidence for the existence of a locally active vascular renin-angiotensin system, operating independently of the classic systemic circuit, has been provided by several studies. Angiotensinogen mRNA, the only known precursor of the angiotensin peptides, has been detected in several extrahepatic vascular tissues, including the aorta.[34,35] Immunohistochemical studies have demonstrated renin in cells throughout the vascular wall.[36] Both vascular smooth muscle and endothelial cells can synthesize renin in vitro.[37,38] Also, mRNA coding for renin has been identified in human vascular smooth muscle cells.[33,39] Finally, ACE is located primarily on the luminal surface of vascular endothelial cells.[40] Thus, the normally functioning vascular wall possesses all the necessary components for the independent local production of angiotensin II.

The physiologic function of locally produced angiotensin II is an area of continued controversy. Angiotensin II receptors have been identified on vascular endothelial cells,[33] smooth muscle cells,[41,42] and circulating platelets.[43] Angiotensin II stimulation of endothelial cell–bound receptors leads to the secretion of prostacyclin and possibly endothelium-derived relaxant factor.[44,45] Both of these substances cause medial smooth muscle cell quiescence and relaxation. Activation of the angiotensin receptors located directly on the smooth muscle cells themselves causes the opposite effect. Campbell-Boswell and Robertson reported that angiotensin II stimulates the proliferation of human vascular smooth muscle cells in vitro.[46] Geisterfer and associates found that the protein content of these smooth muscle cells increased by 20% when stimulated by angiotensin II for 4 days.[47] Further, this stimulation was abolished by the angiotensin II receptor antagonist saralasin. Finally, the *mas* proto-oncogene, located on the surface of medial smooth muscle cells, increases mitogenic activity when stimulated and has been identified as a functional angiotensin II receptor.[48] Therefore, one explanation for the physiologic function of a locally active renin-angiotensin system is the autocrine balance of vascular wall metabolic activity and tone.

This view has led many investigators to study the effect of the local production of angiotensin II on the subsequent development of intimal hyperplasia. In this hypothesis, denudation of the arterial endothelium disrupts the balance of the local renin-angiotensin system and allows the anabolic and mitogenic effects of angiotensin II on the medial smooth muscle cells to proceed unchecked. Another possible mechanism for the promotion of hyperplastic neointimal growth by the local production of angiotensin II involves the activation of platelet metabolic pathways. As mentioned previously, human platelets possess specific binding sites for angiotensin II,[43] and platelet activation and the subsequent release of PDGF may play a role in the development of intimal hyperplasia. In a 1990 study by Swartz and Moore,[49] angiotensin II enhanced both collagen-induced platelet aggregation and the production of thromboxane A_2. Finally, the expression of PDGF by activated smooth muscle cells is upregulated in the presence of angiotensin II.[50]

CELLULAR GROWTH FACTORS

The stimulation of vascular smooth muscle cell growth is the final common pathway of all postulated mechanisms leading to the development of intimal hyperplasia. The view that the vascular wall is a complex integrated organ, complete with its own endogenous local autocrine system, is gaining increasing support. In this theory, intimal hyperplasia is postulated to result from an imbalance of these local hormonal systems. This could be due to an excess of stimulatory molecules; alternatively, smooth muscle cell proliferation may result from the absence or reduction of inhibitory hormones.

Angiotensin II, PDGF, and MDGF are all examples of cellular growth factors believed to be involved in the formation of hyperplastic intimal lesions; each has been reviewed in detail earlier. Basic FGF (bFGF), a smooth muscle cell mitogen that is not secreted, is released from damaged smooth muscle cells and acts in an autocrine fashion to stimulate proliferation of adjacent, viable cells. This mitogen is largely responsible for the proliferative response following balloon injury.[51] Denudation of endothelium with a fine wire that does not damage the endothelium results in much less smooth muscle cell activation.[52] Lindner and associates observed that administration of bFGF after an injury increased smooth muscle cell proliferation from 11.5% to 54.8%.[53] Their finding of an equivalent increase in proliferation following wire loop injury demonstrates that bFGF can act as a mitogen for undamaged medial cells.

Basic FGF administered to normal, nondenuded arteries has no effect on smooth muscle growth. Basic FGF also stimulates angiogenesis and can stimulate endothelial cells to completely cover injured regions that normally would remain denuded. Cuevas and colleagues demonstrated that the direct local infusion of bFGF into either normal adventitia or injured media results in proliferation of both vasa vasorum and vascular smooth muscle cells.[54]

PDGF released from activated platelets was thought to be an important mitogen for smooth muscle cells, but it is now known that intimal hyperplasia after balloon injury develops even in the absence of platelets. Similarly, blocking PDGF does not inhibit proliferation, but it does result in fewer smooth muscle cells migrating into the intima.[55] PDGF is now understood to act mainly as a chemotactic agent.

Smooth muscle cell proliferation following injury may also be a result of decreased growth inhibition by the endothelium. Nitric oxide, an inhibitor of smooth muscle cell growth, is normally secreted by the endothelium. Its levels are decreased after endothelial damage.[56] Manipulation of nitric oxide production at sites of arterial injury may be an important new tool in the pharmacologic control of hyperplastic intimal lesions.

In summary, the balance of locally produced cellular growth factors such as bFGF and nitric oxide probably plays an important role in the regulation of smooth muscle cell activity and the subsequent development of intimal hyperplasia. Research into methods of influencing this balance may lead to pharmacologic management of these lesions.

COAGULATION PATHWAYS AND THE LOCALLY ACTIVE FIBRINOLYTIC SYSTEM

Products of coagulation pathways participate in the development of intimal hyperplasia in complex and diverse ways. Formation of a fibrin matrix in an area of endothelial damage helps stabilize the aggregating platelet plug. Many substances released by organizing thrombus can affect medial smooth muscle cell growth and migration. Among thrombin's many actions, it is a smooth muscle cell mitogen. The locally active vascular fibrinolytic system allows smooth muscle cells to detach from surrounding matrix and migrate to the intima. Several molecules participate in this activity, including plasmin, the active end product of the tissue plasminogen-plasmin system. Other important components of this system include the precursor plasminogen and its main endogenous activators: urokinase plasminogen activator (u-PA) and tissue plasminogen activator (t-PA). The catalytic action of these proteases is inhibited in vivo by the plasmin inhibitors α_2-antiplasmin, α_2-macroglobulin, and a group of related plasminogen activator inhibitory proteins. Increased knowledge regarding the interactions of all these components at the cellular level has been accumulating.

Several studies link plasmin to smooth muscle cell migration. First, circulating plasminogen is a relatively large protein that is normally prevented from entering the medial layer by an intact endothelium. However, after endothelial damage, this protein diffuses readily.[57] Once present in the extracellular medial layer, plasminogen converted into plasmin directly degrades several matrix proteins and activates other collagenases.[58] Smooth muscle cells express plasminogen activator activity in tissue culture and are a likely source of this enzyme locally in the vessel wall.[59,60] In an in vivo model of arterial repair, Clowes and associates demonstrated that vascular smooth muscle cells contain increased levels of both u-PA and t-PA.[61] These plasminogen activators act synergistically, and their secretion depends on the functional state of the smooth muscle cells. During cellular proliferation, u-PA is the major product, whereas during migration, t-PA expression predominates. These experimental observations suggest that injury to the endothelium allows the local penetration of plasminogen and chemotactic substances (elaborated from activated platelets and leukocytes) into the arterial wall. The conversion of extracellular plasminogen into plasmin by medial smooth muscle cells degrades the structural matrix proteins. This process may be enhanced by the presence of leukocyte-derived enzymes. Finally, activation of smooth muscle cells by the elaborated growth and chemotactic factors initiates migration of these cells through the weakened arterial wall. The direction of migration is determined automatically by the gradient of plasminogen and mitogenic activity, which is highest adjacent to the endothelial defect.

VEIN GRAFT MYOINTIMAL HYPERPLASIA AND ARTERIALIZATION

Autogenous vein bypass grafting provides the primary means of long-term revascularization in patients suffering from ischemic conditions of both the heart and the peripheral circulation. Veins are much more thin walled than arteries, and they have scant medial smooth muscle cells. The internal and external elastic laminae usually are not discernible. The majority of the vessel wall consists of adventitial collagen (Fig. 41-2). Myointimal hyperplasia in vein grafts bears a similarity to hyperplasia following arterial injury, but it differs in that there are fewer medial cells to respond and there is an additional response to increased wall tension. Prominent features in rodent models of vein grafting include extensive early denudation of the endothelium and smooth muscle cell layers, attachment of leukocytes and platelets to the subendothelial matrix, and elaboration of cytokine and growth factor products

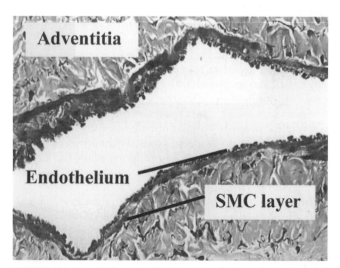

FIGURE 41-2 • Trichrome-elastin stain of normal rat external jugular vein. Note the single layer of endothelium (granular owing to preparation) and the subjacent single layer of smooth muscle cells (dark nuclei and surrounding cytoplasm). The gray whorls and intercalated black streaks represent adventitial collagen and elastic fibers, respectively. SMC, smooth muscle cells.

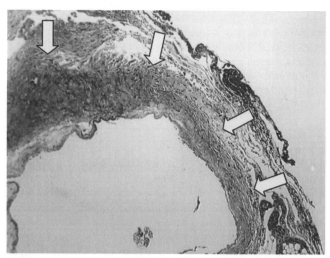

FIGURE 41-3 • Trichrome-elastin stain of a 72-hour-old vein graft. The luminal side is depicted on the bottom edge of this tissue section. There is evidence of endothelial and smooth muscle cell denudation, with adherence of leukocytes and platelets.

by these cells. This results in the activation, migration, and proliferation of vein graft adventitial myofibroblasts to form a neointima.[61-66]

Pathologically, the trauma resulting from surgical manipulation and exposure of the vein graft to arterial pressure and flow results in nearly complete denudation of the endothelium and loss of the smooth muscle cell layers within the first 24 hours (Fig. 41-3). The vein re-endothelializes by 1 week. Smooth muscle cells form a myointimal lesion. Hoch and coworkers hypothesized that adventitial progenitor fibroblasts may be the source of myofibroblasts in the vein graft neointima.[62] Studies of arterial injury have demonstrated that adventitial cells, marked by a pulse of bromodeoxyuridine, can be followed into the neointima, where they continue to proliferate.

A prominent component of vein graft remodeling is the attachment of leukocytes and platelets early after denudation of the endothelium and smooth muscle cell layers. Macrophage infiltration dominates the early inflammatory changes observed with vein graft pathobiology. This prominent inflammatory response peaks during the first 2 weeks of vein graft adaptation, which exceeds the response observed in models of arterial injury (Fig. 41-4). Stark and Hoch and their coworkers elegantly demonstrated that by inhibiting macrophage activity early in this inflammatory process, a significant reduction in myointimal hyperplasia was achieved.[64,65]

Vein graft myointimal changes persist and can progress despite re-endothelialization, in contrast to arterial myointimal proliferation, which tends to halt its progression upon restitution of the endothelial cell layer. It is believed that the ongoing myointimal thickening associated with vein graft myointimal hyperplasia is an adaptive response to arterial pressure and flow.[67] Wall thickening is greater in regions of low shear (e.g., at the inner wall of a curve). Myointimal hyperplasia results in wall thickening, which decreases wall stress to more physiologic levels. These hyperplastic changes were described by Carrel and Guthrie when vein grafts were first examined histologically. They referred to this process as "arterialization." Wall thickening can be accentuated at valve cusps, perhaps due to local flow abnormalities; at the anastomoses, where

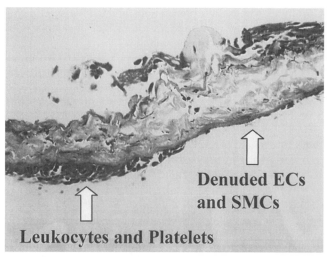

FIGURE 41–4 • Trichrome-elastin stain of a 2-week-old vein graft. *Arrows* denote the region of the external elastic lamina, within which resides the neointima. Many of the nuclei visualized in the neointima proved to be macrophages when stained with ED-2 macrophage stain (not depicted). ECs, endothelial cells; SMCs, smooth muscle cells.

shear and wall tension are greatest; and at sites of clamp injury. Hemodynamically significant lesions caused by intimal hyperplasia usually occur after the first month and are rare after a year. After that time, vein grafts can develop lesions that are similar to atherosclerosis We used a rat model of vein graft arterialization in which the graft maintained its myointimal-thickened characteristics at 12 weeks, including the development of focal degenerative areas composed of calcific lesions (Fig. 41-5).

Procedures Leading to Intimal Hyperplasia

The number of procedures performed annually for occlusive vascular disease continues to increase. Currently, approximately 500,000 patients undergo reconstructive vascular surgery each year; half of these are coronary bypass procedures, and the remainder include peripheral procedures, such as autogenous

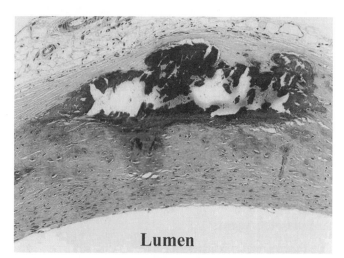

FIGURE 41–5 • Hematoxylin-eosin stain of a 12-week-old vein graft. Note the prominent calcification within the neointima.

and prosthetic bypass grafts, endarterectomies, and a variety of endovascular procedures. The long-term durability of most of these procedures has been disappointing, primarily because of failure due to intimal hyperplasia.

RESTENOSIS AFTER PERIPHERAL BYPASS

The 3-year primary patency rate for infrainguinal bypass grafts ranges from 40% to 60% for prosthetic conduits and 60% to 80% for autogenous grafts.[68] Intimal hyperplasia is responsible for most graft failures that occur between 6 months and 2 years after the procedure.[1,69] In prosthetic grafts, the area most affected by hyperplastic change is the distal anastomosis. Although this location is also the likely point of obstruction in autogenous tissue grafts, focal lesions throughout the entire length of the graft are also common.

RESTENOSIS AFTER CAROTID ENDARTERECTOMY

The incidence of asymptomatic carotid restenosis ranges from 7% to 15%, and 1% to 5% of patients develop restenosis associated with recurrent symptoms.[70-80] The smooth, fibrous, nonthrombogenic intimal hyperplastic lesions of restenosis are well tolerated because they do not cause embolization Most symptoms associated with restenosis are due to decreased flow. This may explain why patients with symptomatic recurrences often have tight stenoses or occlusions of the contralateral carotid artery.[71,73] After several years, these restenotic lesions can develop atherosclerosis and behave much like the original lesions.

RESTENOSIS AFTER ENDOVASCULAR SURGERY

The combined failure rate 1 year after percutaneous transluminal balloon angioplasty ranges from 2% to 40%.[81] Some of these recurrences are due to progression of atherosclerosis, but the majority are the result of intimal hyperplasia. This process is also the likely cause of the poor long-term results after laser-assisted angioplasty. In one representative study, White and colleagues reported their results of laser-assisted balloon angioplasty for advanced lesions of the lower extremity using argon, neodymium:yttrium-aluminum-garnet (Nd:YAG), and metal hot-tipped systems.[82] Although the initial recanalization rate was 67%, the patency rate was only 11% after 1 year. Results from other investigators have been similar. The results of peripheral atherectomy differ, depending on the device used and the anatomic location of the lesion. We have had similar results with the Auth Rotablator (Heart Technology, Inc., Bellevue, Wash.).[83] Initial success was achieved in 92% of cases, and primary patency was 67% at 6 months. However, at 24 months, patency was only 9.5%. Unfortunately, the long-term outcomes of other devices have not shown any significant improvement over these results.

Experimental Basis for Pharmacologic Control

The ability of various pharmacologic agents to suppress the development of intimal hyperplasia has been well documented. Particularly striking is the large variety of medications that have been effective in limiting this response. At least six different

TABLE 41–1	Pharmacologic Agents Effective in Suppressing the Formation of Intimal Hyperplasia

Lipid metabolites
  Omega-3 polyunsaturated fatty acids (eicosapentaenoic acid)
Antiplatelet agents
  Aspirin
  Dipyridamole
  Thromboxane synthetase inhibitors
Anti-inflammatory agents
  Dehydroepiandrosterone
  Dexamethasone
  Cyclosporin
Antihypertensive agents
  ACE inhibitors
    Cilazapril
    Captopril
    Enalaprilat
  Calcium channel blockers
    Verapamil
    Nimodipine
  α_1-Adrenergic inhibitors
    Prazosin
Growth factor inhibitors
  Angiopeptin
  bFGF-saporin
  Ornithine decarboxylase inhibitors
Anticoagulant agents
  Heparins and heparinoids
Insulin-sensitizing agents
  Thiazolidinediones
    Troglitazone
    Rosiglitazone
    Pioglitazone
Antiproliferative drugs
  Actinomycin D
  Sirolimus
  Paclitaxel
  E2F transcription factor decoy

ACE, angiotensin-converting enzyme; bFGF, basic fibroblast growth factor.

classes of drugs have been studied and are at least partially successful in this regard (Table 41-1). These classes of drugs are lipid metabolites,[84-86] antiplatelet agents,[87-89] anti-inflammatory agents,[90,91] antihypertensive agents,[92-95] anticoagulants,[96] and antiproliferatives. Many other substances that interfere with normal cellular growth have also shown some promise.[53,97-101] The antiproliferative agents were the first to show a dramatic improvement in success rates. This, together with promising results with statins and other drugs that may cause the regression of primary lesions, means that the treatment of atherosclerosis is at the brink of a new era.

EXPERIMENTAL MODELS

Several models have been used to study the development of intimal hyperplasia. Studies of vascular cells grown in culture have elucidated the isolated effects of mitogens, growth factors, and hormones on the growth patterns of these vascular cells.

Cocultures, whole artery preparations, and in vivo experiments are needed to study the complex interaction of vascular cells and their cytokines in living vessels.

The classic animal model of smooth muscle cell intimal hyperplasia is a balloon catheter arterial injury model. The induction of smooth muscle cell growth after a balloon catheter denuding injury was first described by Baumgartner in 1963.[102] Since that time, this procedure has undergone several modifications; however, the basic concepts of the model remain the same. A segment of artery to be studied is isolated, and a balloon catheter is introduced into the lumen. By inflating the balloon and withdrawing the catheter, complete denudation of the endothelial layer can be achieved. Distention causes damage to medial smooth muscle cells. After this injury, a lesion is formed that is histologically identical to that observed clinically. The advantages of this model are its ease and reproducibility. In addition, the anatomic injury produced mimics the cleavage plane that occurs clinically in an endarterectomized vessel. A second type of injury model involves hydrostatic stretching of the vessel without deliberate denuding of the endothelial surface.[103] This model of injury produces an increase in medial smooth muscle cell proliferation despite the absence of endothelial damage. The isolated response to endothelial injury can be studied by denuding the intimal layer with a loop of fine nylon wire.[7] Intimal hyperplasia at anastomotic sites has been studied in several animal models using bypass grafts of both autogenous and prosthetic material.[10,91] These injury models are described in greater detail in Chapter 3.

AGENTS STUDIED

Lipid Metabolites

Alaskan Natives have extremely low plasma levels of low-density lipoprotein, and this may explain their low incidence of atherosclerotic heart disease.[104] Further characterization of Alaskan Native plasma lipid composition has demonstrated low levels of circulating arachidonic acid and unusually high concentrations of eicosapentaenoic acid (EPA).[105] EPA is an omega-3 polyunsaturated fatty acid that is present in large amounts in fish but cannot be synthesized de novo by humans. After ingestion, EPA enters the prostaglandin synthesis pathway and competes directly with arachidonic acid. In contrast to arachidonic acid metabolism, which leads to the formation of thromboxane A_2 (a potent stimulator of platelet aggregation), EPA is converted into thromboxane A_3, which has no effect on platelet function.

Several studies have tested the hypothesis that high levels of EPA present at the time of an endothelial injury may inhibit the production of intimal hyperplasia. Both Cahill and colleagues[84] and Landymore and colleagues[85] have reported that small doses of marine oils can reduce intimal thickening in vein graft models. O'Hara and colleagues reported a marked suppression of intimal hyperplasia after treatment with EPA in a rabbit PTFE graft model.[86]

Antiplatelet Agents

Friedman and colleagues reported reduced hyperplasia after aortic balloon catheter injury in thrombocytopenic rabbits.[106] Subsequent work has shown that smooth muscle cell proliferation occurs in the absence of platelets, but these cells do not migrate into the intima. This may explain why aspirin therapy, which improves the immediate patency of coronary artery bypass grafts, does not reduce the later occurrence of intimal hyperplasia.

Antiplatelet drugs inhibit the synthesis of prostaglandins by blocking arachidonic acid metabolic pathways. Aspirin irreversibly acetylates platelet cell cyclooxygenase. Dipyridamole increases platelet cyclic adenosine monophosphate and inhibits the precursors thromboxane A_1 and thromboxane B_2. Thus, both aspirin and dipyridamole inhibit platelet adherence and aggregation by interfering with the production of prostaglandin metabolites. Aspirin decreases platelet adherence to prosthetic vascular grafts in humans and in animal models.[107-109] The addition of dipyridamole may or may not enhance this effect. In other studies, antiplatelet agents had no effect on initial platelet deposition but may decrease subsequent platelet aggregation and thrombus formation.[110] In a primate vein graft model, aspirin and dipyridamole reduced intimal hyperplasia.[111] In a follow-up study using a balloon catheter injury model in rabbits, there was no significant difference between the two groups in terms of rate of proliferation or progression of intimal hyperplasia.[89] In a similar rabbit study, aspirin significantly increased the patency of an end-to-side iliac anastomosis but had no effect on the development of intimal hyperplasia.[87]

Thromboxane synthetase converts cyclic end-peroxide precursors from the arachidonic acid pathways into thromboxane A_2, which is synthesized and stored in the developing platelet. It is a powerful mediator of both platelet aggregation and vascular constriction. Inhibitors of thromboxane synthetase block this conversion of intermediate end-peroxide precursors into thromboxane A_2. Further, in doing so, the intracellular prostaglandin metabolic pathways are shifted toward the production of prostacyclin. Thus, theoretically, thromboxane synthetase inhibitors can block platelet-derived thromboxane A_2 while actually enhancing the production of endothelial cell–derived prostacyclin. These agents may therefore be more specific inhibitors of platelet function. The efficacy of thromboxane synthetase inhibition in the prevention of distal anastomotic intimal hyperplasia was investigated and compared with aspirin.[112] A bilateral aortoiliac bypass graft model was used, and two different types of grafts were evaluated: thin-walled PTFE and PTFE seeded with autogenous endothelial cells. Treatment groups consisted of antiplatelet therapy with either aspirin or the thromboxane synthetase inhibitor U-63,577A. In both types of grafts, aspirin was significantly more effective in maintaining patency and inhibiting intimal hyperplasia. Within the thromboxane synthetase inhibitor group, however, the agent was more effective when the bypass grafts were seeded. Both treatments improved patency over controls. In conclusion, in combination with other antiplatelet drugs, these agents could prove to be potent inhibitors of platelet function. However, no clinical trials are yet available.

Newer antithrombotic agents have promise for inhibiting intimal hyperplasia. For example, ticlopidine improved survival and patency following saphenous vein bypass grafts in the leg.[113] Platelet aggregation in response to collagen and adenosine diphosphate has been reduced by blocking GP IIb and GP IIIa with a murine monoclonal antibody (LJ-CP8).[114] Unfortunately, in an arteriovenous shunt model, this antibody failed to decrease the deposition of platelets on Dacron or PTFE grafts.[115]

Anti-inflammatory Agents

Leukocyte pathways may play a role in the development of intimal hyperplasia. Leukocyte infiltration is observed in hyperplastic intimal lesions. These inflammatory cells secrete a number of growth factors for smooth muscle cells and could contribute to the development of intimal hyperplasia. This is the basis for studying the effect of immunosuppressive glucocorticoids and cyclosporin on restenosis.

In 1979, Hoepp and colleagues found no significant differences in patency or intimal response between steroid-treated and control groups in a canine femoropopliteal polyester fabric bypass graft model.[91] However, the animals in this experiment were given a relatively low dose of a short-acting steroid (methylprednisolone), and the agent was administered only after the procedure, not preoperatively. A report by Gordon and associates in 1988 was among the earliest to suggest that glucocorticoids could inhibit smooth muscle cell proliferation after an endothelial injury.[116] These investigators found that administration of the endogenous steroid dehydroepiandrosterone led to a decrease in the production of atherosclerotic plaques in hypercholesterolemic rabbits. The Multi-Hospital Eastern Atlantic Restenosis Trial project, a large, randomized, double-blind clinical study, investigated whether steroids could decrease the rate of restenosis after balloon angioplasty.[117] In this study, a single large dose of methylprednisolone (1 g) was given intravenously before the procedure. No significant difference was found between steroid- and placebo-treated groups. The steroid may not have been present during the critical period of maximal intimal proliferation, which is 2 to 4 weeks after injury.[51] In a balloon catheter injury model, dexamethasone was given 2 days before injury and continued for 8 weeks, resulting in a dramatic reduction of intimal growth (Figs. 41-6 and 41-7).[118]

There are many ways that glucocorticoids could prevent or suppress the development of intimal hyperplasia. One theory involves these agents' well-known actions on fibroblast growth and wound healing. Glucocorticoids can slow the growth of cultured fibroblast cell lines,[119] and in vitro studies clearly demonstrate decreased leukocyte aggregation to several chemotactic factors in the presence of steroids.[120] In addition, steroids decrease adhesion between leukocytes and endothelial cells.[121] Although the mechanism of this inhibition remains unknown, in some neoplastic cell lines, dexamethasone has been related to ICAM-1 inhibition.[122] Steroids alter white blood cell cytotoxic function, decreasing the production of superoxide anions and inhibiting the release of zymogen granules.[123] Dexamethasone inhibits smooth muscle cell proliferation in cell culture by means of cell cycle arrest in the late G_1 phase.[124] This effect has been localized to the inhibition of phosphorylation of the retinoblastoma protein.[125] This phosphorylation event is a final common pathway toward cell cycle progression from the G_1 into the S phase. High-dose methylprednisolone can prevent endothelial sloughing in vein grafts.[126] Finally, dexamethasone has an inhibitory effect on t-PA activity and therefore may inhibit smooth muscle cell migration.[127]

The effect of cyclosporine treatment on the subsequent development of intimal hyperplasia was studied in a rat

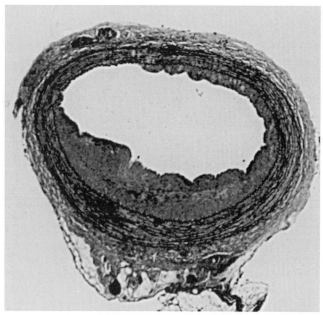

FIGURE 41–6 • Photomicrograph of a control rabbit carotid artery 12 weeks after a balloon catheter endothelial injury, demonstrating a large amount of intimal hyperplasia (Verhoeff-van Gieson stain; original magnification ×20). (From Colburn MD, Moore WS, Gelabert HA, Quiñones-Baldrich WJ: Dose responsive suppression of myointimal hyperplasia by dexamethasone. J Vasc Surg 15:510-518, 1992.)

common iliac artery injury model.[128] Animals were given parenteral cyclosporine before injury and for 2 and 6 weeks afterward. Arteries treated with cyclosporine formed significantly less medial thickening. Atherosclerotic plaques contain activated lymphocytes and smooth muscle cells, which express class II major histocompatibility antigens.

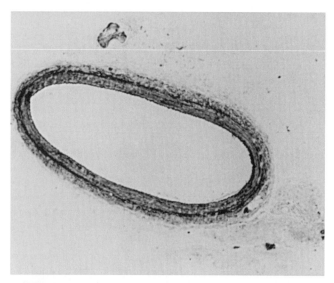

FIGURE 41–7 • Photomicrograph of a carotid artery 12 weeks after a balloon catheter endothelial injury, demonstrating the absence of significant intimal hyperplasia after treatment for 8 weeks with dexamethasone, 0.125 mg/kg (Verhoeff-van Gieson stain; original magnification ×20). (From Colburn MD, Moore WS, Gelabert HA, Quiñones-Baldrich WJ: Dose responsive suppression of myointimal hyperplasia by dexamethasone. J Vasc Surg 15:510-518, 1992.)

Interaction of these antigens and immune cells may cause the release of other inflammatory mediators and cytokines. It is not known whether modulation of these immune pathways is a useful strategy for preventing intimal hyperplasia.

Antihypertensive Agents

ACE inhibitors, calcium channel blockers, and α_1-adrenergic antagonists are all agents used clinically in the treatment of systemic hypertension. Each of these categories of antihypertensive drugs is also effective in suppressing intimal hyperplasia.

Powell and associates were the first to report the ability of an ACE inhibitor to reduce myointimal proliferation after a vascular injury.[93] They found that cilazapril significantly reduced intimal hyperplasia following balloon injury. This effect was independent of any changes in blood pressure. Clowes and Reidy observed a reversal of this effect after the intravenous infusion of angiotensin II.[129] O'Donohoe and associates reported the inhibition of intimal hyperplasia in experimental vein grafts by the long-term administration of captopril, an ACE inhibitor.[130] Captopril also significantly decreased aortic atherosclerosis in a heritable hyperlipidemic rabbit model.[131]

Calcium channel antagonists are effective agents used in a variety of cardiovascular disorders. In general, the common mechanism of action of all these agents is interruption of membrane calcium channels, thereby reducing the availability of this cation for a variety of intercellular processes. Calcium has been implicated in several events involved in the development of intimal hyperplasia, including platelet activation, release of PDGF, medial smooth muscle cell proliferation, and formation of extracellular matrix. Treatment with calcium antagonists significantly reduces the development of intimal hyperplasia after mechanical arterial injury.[132] In addition, both verapamil and nimodipine have been effective in reducing intimal hyperplasia in vein bypass graft models.[95,96]

Endothelial denudation is accompanied by a selective increase in the sensitivity of the α_1-adrenergic receptor.[133] The cytoplasmic secondary messenger system for this receptor response involves upregulation of the intracellular phosphatidylinositol cycle, which is also linked to PDGF function.[134] Intermediates of this cycle stimulate protein kinase C to initiate a series of phosphorylating reactions that ultimately lead to cellular mitosis.[135] Therefore, the intracellular mechanisms of smooth muscle cell proliferation and contraction are connected through a common cytoplasmic pathway, the phosphatidylinositol cycle. In a balloon catheter injury model in the rabbit aorta, the α_1-adrenergic receptor blocker prazosin produced a statistically significant reduction in the development of intimal hyperplastic lesions.[92] No clinical trials using this agent have been reported.

Growth Factor Inhibitors

Somatostatin is a widely occurring peptide hormone that acts as a modulator of a diverse class of endogenous growth promoters. If intimal hyperplasia is the result of an imbalance in local vascular autocrine systems after endothelial injury, somatostatin may be effective in limiting this response. Unfortunately, because of storage instability and a very short half-life, somatostatin is unsuitable for use in in vivo models. Angiopeptin is a stable octapeptide somatostatin analog that is an effective long-acting somatostatin receptor agonist. This analog has been extensively studied as a potential inhibitor of intimal hyperplasia.

Several authors have reported the success of angiopeptin in suppressing the development of intimal hyperplasia in animal models.[97-99] In one publication, angiopeptin significantly reduced the degree of post-transplant coronary artery intimal hyperplasia in rabbits.[100] This study was complicated, however, by the fact that these rabbits also received cyclosporine immunosuppression, which, as discussed earlier, affects the development of hyperplastic lesions. Whether angiopeptin is actually antagonizing the trophic effects of growth promoters in this setting is not clear. In vitro work has also demonstrated the ability of angiopeptin to directly inhibit the proliferation of smooth muscle cells.[136] This suggests that the action of angiopeptin may not be related to an inhibition of the somatostatin receptor. This is further supported by the fact that some somatostatin analogs have not been successful in limiting the intimal hyperplastic response.[99]

The effects of peptide mitogens can be blocked with conjugated toxins called mitotoxins, which are specific growth factors bound to a cytotoxin. One such mitotoxin competes for the bFGF receptor.[137] This compound is formed by conjugating bFGF to the ribosome-inactivating protein saporin. In one in vivo study, bFGF-saporin caused a marked reduction in the number of replicating smooth muscle cells found in an arterial wall after a denuding injury.[53] Whether this or other conjugated mitotoxins are effective in reducing the degree of intimal hyperplasia after arterial injury requires further investigation.

In addition to inhibiting the effects of peptide growth factors at the level of their membrane-bound receptors, attempts have been made to inhibit cellular growth by interfering with cellular proliferative pathways at the cytoplasmic level. Polyamines are important compounds in the regulation of cell growth and differentiation.[138] Because polyamines are synthesized from ornithine by the action of ornithine decarboxylase (ODC), and because this enzyme constitutes the rate-limiting step in this reaction, ODC inhibition has been postulated as a possible method of preventing cellular proliferation. This concept is supported by the fact that ODC activity increases in tissues undergoing active cell division.[139] In one study, animals treated with the ODC inhibitor α-difluoromethylornithine developed significantly less intimal hyperplasia after arterial injury than did controls.[101]

Sirolimus, an immunosuppressive drug, and paclitaxel, an antineoplastic drug derived from the yew tree, reduce restenosis after percutaneous coronary angioplasty. The drugs are coated onto the metal stents, which gradually reduce these agents locally into the vessel wall. Sirolimus-eluting and polymeric paclitaxel-eluting coronary artery stents significantly reduce rates of restenosis and major cardiac events.[140] However, they have not yet been shown to affect mortality or myocardial infarction rates. At present, these drug-eluting stents cost two to three times more than standard stents; however, the decreased need for further interventions means that the overall cost to patients, payers, and society may be less. Hospital income may suffer from reduced numbers of coronary artery bypass and angiographic procedures.[141]

Undoubtedly, similar approaches will be used to prevent restenosis in other vascular beds and following other types of intervention. This may allow catheter-based approaches to small arteries, such as the femoropopliteal and tibial vessels, which have prohibitively high restenosis rates following angioplasty or atherectomy.

Anticoagulants

Heparin is a naturally occurring polymer containing chains of sulfonated mucopolysaccharides. In vivo, it is concentrated in mast cells and is found in several different tissues, including the endothelium. The length and thus the molecular weight of heparin polymers are highly variable. Further, different-sized polymers have different anticoagulant potency.[142] Because of this variability, heparin has unpredictable biologic activity and is therefore quantified in international units rather than by weight.

Heparin works through its inhibition of the plasma-bound proteolytic clotting cascade. Antithrombin III is a potent naturally occurring anticoagulant that inhibits several of the activated coagulant proteins. Heparin polymers of a certain size combine with antithrombin III. This binding greatly enhances the enzymatic action of antithrombin III. Also, because these bound cofactors are not consumed by the inhibition reaction, only a small amount of heparin is required when the plasma load of activated coagulant proteins is moderate. This forms the basis of low-dose heparin therapy for prophylaxis.

Clinically, heparin has been used most frequently in the prophylaxis and treatment of venous thrombosis and pulmonary emboli. A few studies have concluded that perioperative high-dose heparin can prevent early thrombosis in peripheral bypass grafts.[143] This action is presumably due to the drug's ability to shift the balance of the coagulation cascade and counteract the thrombotic forces of low-flow states and thrombogenic surfaces. Heparin also prevents smooth muscle cell migration and proliferation both in vitro and in vivo.[96,144-148] The mechanism of this action has not yet been established. One theory is that heparin inhibits bFGF, which is released by damaged medial smooth muscle cells.[129] Clowes and Reidy postulated that heparin inhibits smooth muscle cell migration by interfering with the degradation of the surrounding extracellular matrix.[129] Evidence supporting this view comes from the demonstration that heparin decreases the expression of both t-PA and collagenase in the arterial media.[129] Finally, available data indicate that both anticoagulant and nonanticoagulant fractions of heparin possess this antiproliferative activity.[96] Low-molecular-weight heparin is a combination of short-chain heparin polymers that has significantly lower anticoagulant activity than standard heparin preparations do. Interest in this heparin derivative stems from its potential in modulating intimal hyperplasia without affecting the coagulation system. At least one study has shown that low-molecular-weight heparin may be effective in this regard.[96] So far, clinical trials attempting to inhibit restenosis with heparin compounds have had disappointing results.

Insulin-Sensitizing Agents

Aside from the beneficial vascular effects of reducing insulin production through increased sensitization, the thiazolidinediones have proved to have direct inhibitory effects on arterial myointimal hyperplasia. These agents bind to peroxisome proliferator-activated receptors, members of the steroid hormone superfamily of nuclear receptors.[149] Troglitazone, a first-generation thiazolidinedione, can inhibit intimal hyperplasia after balloon injury in the rat aorta.[150] The mechanism of action relates to the inhibition of mitogen-activated protein kinase–dependent nuclear events, which in turn blocks vascular smooth muscle cell migration and proliferation. The ramifications of this effect are not fully appreciated to date, because it is known that peroxisome proliferator-activated receptors are present on macrophages as well. The influence of thiazolidinediones on early inflammation in myointimal hyperplasia must still be addressed.

Other Approaches

PHOTODYNAMIC THERAPY

Another way to view the intimal hyperplastic response is as a process akin to that of a benign neoplastic lesion. In this scheme, the proliferating intimal smooth muscle cell is pictured as an undifferentiated pluripotent medial myofibroblast whose growth continues in the absence of normal cellular controls. The resulting lesion can be considered a form of "vascular keloid." Photodynamic therapy is safe and effective in the treatment of several rapidly growing benign neoplasms. In photodynamic therapy, a chemosensitizing agent is administered to living tissue. Differential absorption and clearance favor selective concentration of the agent in rapidly dividing cells.[151] After exposure to light of a specific wavelength, "photoactivation" results. Once photoactivated, the chemosensitizing agent injures the tissue exposed to the light.

The mechanism by which photodynamic therapy induces cellular toxicity is still being elucidated. Photoactivation of hematoporphyrin derivatives has been hypothesized to result in the formation of oxygen species and other free radicals. These, in turn, induce several changes, including oxidation of membrane components, alteration of surface charges, and ultimate loss of cell membrane integrity.[152] The initial site of drug accumulation appears to be the cell membrane, but other intracellular organisms such as lysosomes, mitochondria, and nuclei are also affected.[153] Boegheim and colleagues reported that photodynamic therapy inactivates cytosolic, mitochondrial, and lysosomal enzymes, decreases cellular adenosine triphosphate, and reduces glutathione concentration in murine fibroblasts.[154] Enzymes involved in transport across the cell membrane and related to deoxynucleic acid regulation are also inactivated after exposure to light.[154]

Because intimal hyperplasia also involves cells exhibiting increased mitotic activity, photodynamic therapy has been proposed as a means of modulating this hyperplastic response. In 1988, Neave and colleagues reported the destruction of fibrocellular atheromas in the aorta of rabbits treated with dihematoporphyrin ether porphyrin-II.[155] Mackie and colleagues,[156] Hundley and coworkers,[157] and Spears and colleagues[158] reported that atherosclerotic plaque preferentially absorbs hematoporphyrin-II (Photofrin) and that photodynamic therapy leads to ablation of only the fibrous portion of the atherosclerotic lesion. These investigators were discouraged that the atherosclerotic plaque could not be ablated completely owing to the remaining calcified noncellular material.

Nevertheless, these experiments showed that photodynamic therapy could ablate a fibrosclerotic plaque.

The potential for using photodynamic therapy to treat intimal hyperplasia (rather than atherosclerosis) was perhaps most convincingly suggested by Dartsch and colleagues,[159-161] who showed that human-derived intimal hyperplasia smooth muscle cells preferentially absorbed Photofrin-II and that subsequent exposure to light significantly inhibited growth of the Photofrin-II–bound cells. Meanwhile, cells derived from normal arteries remained uninhibited in vitro. The ability of human intimal hyperplastic lesions to selectively absorb porphyrin compounds in vivo has not been demonstrated. However, photodynamic therapy remains an intriguing area of investigation in the treatment of intimal hyperplasia.

GENE THERAPY

The development of the technology to transfer genetic material into human vascular cells has opened up new frontiers in the treatment of vascular disorders. Gene transfer methods are yielding important information regarding the biology of several types of vascular cells, and treatment strategies for problems such as thrombosis, atherosclerosis, vasculitis, and restenosis are already being devised.

The basic technique involves the introduction of new genetic material into the genome of various vascular cells. These genetically engineered cells subsequently express specific proteins or traits for which they have been programmed that ultimately alter the local biology of the vessel wall. The endothelial cell is often proposed as the ideal recipient for human gene therapy. This is largely owing to its accessibility to recombinant vectors, as well as the possibility for any produced products to be secreted directly into the bloodstream. Further, endothelial seeding of vascular grafts and stents is an area of research that is in a relatively advanced stage of development. Gene transfer into vascular endothelial cells has been accomplished primarily by one of two methods. The first method involves the introduction of genes into cultured endothelial cells in vitro. Later, these "engineered" cells are reintroduced into the vessel wall of the recipient. Alternatively, in vivo gene transfer into the vessel wall has been performed by injecting the genetic material directly into the lumen of the host vessel. This method requires either a retroviral or a plasmid vector to transfer the new genes.

Several in vitro experiments have documented the ability to transfer specific genes into cultured endothelial cells.[162-164] In these studies, genes coding for neomycin resistance,[162,164] β-galactosidase,[163,164] growth hormone,[162] prostacyclin,[164] and t-PA[163] have all been successfully expressed. Further, transduced endothelial cells grow on both vascular prostheses[162] and stainless steel stents.[163]

Recombinant gene expression by transduced endothelial cells has also been achieved in vivo. In a series of experiments, Nabel and associates successfully transferred the genes responsible for β-galactosidase production into iliofemoral arterial segments of pigs.[165,166] These investigators documented detectable levels of the transduced gene in this model for as long as 5 months.[166] The ability of a vascular graft lined with genetically modified endothelial cells to maintain activity of the transduced gene has also been demonstrated.[167] In this study, grafts continued to express the β-galactosidase gene for up to 5 weeks after implantation. This activity was documented in both the seeded cells and their progeny.

The potential of genetically engineered vascular cells to modify the vessel wall and affect the development of vascular disorders is clear, and research in this area is rapidly progressing. However, several problems with this technology must still be overcome, and, as with any new area of research, perplexing questions accompany each advance. For example, the use of retroviral vectors limits the size of the gene that can be transduced. Also, transduction rates using these methods remain quite low, and alternative methods to improve the efficiency of this process are needed. Areas requiring further investigation include the effect of transduced genes on the function of host cells, the duration of activity of these genes within the host cells, and the potential of foreign genetic material to induce a host immunologic response.

Transposed vein grafts can be treated ex vivo while being prepared for reimplantation. This provides an opportunity to specifically target cells in the vein wall without the possibility of significant systemic effects. This strategy has been used with E2F, a decoy oligonucleotide that binds the pivotal cell-cycle transcription factor E2F. Wall thickening can be reduced by this treatment because this transcription factor is important in activating a number of pathways that lead to proliferation. The oligonucleotide is introduced by bathing the vein graft under pressure for 10 minutes with a solution containing the drug. Animal studies have documented adequate cell incorporation of the drug and significant reduction in proliferation of smooth muscle cells. Endothelial cells are not affected by this treatment.[168] Preliminary results from clinical trials with coronary artery bypass grafts and lower extremity bypass grafts are encouraging. Larger studies are under way.[169,170]

REFERENCES

1. Imparato AM, Bracco A, Kim GFE: Intimal and neointimal fibrous proliferation causing failure of arterial reconstruction. Surgery 72:1007-1017, 1972.
2. Veith FJ, Gupta SK, Ascer E: Six-year prospective multicenter randomized comparison of autologous saphenous vein and expanded polytetrafluoroethylene grafts in infrainguinal arterial reconstructions. J Vasc Surg 3:104-114, 1986.
3. Fitzgibbon GM, Leach AJ, Kafka HP, Keon WJ: Coronary bypass graft fate: Long-term angiographic study. J Am Coll Cardiol 17:1075-1080, 1991.
4. Carrel A, Guthrie CC: Anastomosis of blood vessels by the patching method and transplantation of the kidney. JAMA 47:1648-1651, 1906.
5. Spaet TH, Stemerman MB, Veith FJ, Lejnieks I: Intimal injury and regrowth in the rabbit aorta: Medial smooth muscle cells as a source of neointima. Circ Res 36:58-70, 1975.
6. Clowes AW, Schwartz SM: Significance of quiescent smooth muscle migration in the injured rat carotid artery. Circ Res 56:139-145, 1985.
7. Clowes AW, Clowes MM, Fingerle J, Reidy MA: Regulation of smooth muscle cell growth in injured artery. J Cardiovasc Pharmacol 14 (Suppl 6):S12-S15, 1989.
8. Chervu A, Moore WS: An overview of intimal hyperplasia. Surg Gynecol Obstet 171:433-447, 1990.
9. Rittgers SE, Karayannacos PE, Guy JF, et al: Velocity distribution and intimal proliferation in autologous vein grafts in dogs. Circ Res 42:792-801, 1978.
10. Morinaga K, Okadome K, Kuroki M, et al: Effect of wall shear stress on intimal thickening of arterially transplanted autogenous veins in dogs. J Vasc Surg 2:430-433, 1985.
11. Sottiurai VS, Kollros P, Glagov S, et al: Morphological alteration of cultured arterial smooth muscle cells by cyclic stretching. J Surg Res 35:490-497, 1983.
12. Imparato AM, Baumann FG, Pearson J, et al: Electron microscopic studies of experimentally produced fibromuscular arterial lesions. Surg Gynecol Obstet 139:497-504, 1976.
13. Bond MG, Hostetler JR, Karayannacos PE, et al: Intimal changes in arteriovenous bypass grafts: Effects of varying the angle of implantation at the proximal anastomosis and of producing stenosis in the distal runoff artery. J Thorac Cardiovasc Surg 71:907-916, 1976.
14. Berguer R, Higgins RF, Reddy DJ: Intimal hyperplasia: An experimental study. Arch Surg 115:332-335, 1980.
15. Zarins CK, Zatina MA, Giddens DP, et al: Shear stress regulation of artery lumen diameter in experimental atherogenesis. J Vasc Surg 5:413-420, 1987.
16. Caro CG, Fitz-Gerald JM, Schroter RC: Arterial wall shear: Observation, correlation and proposal of a shear dependent mass transfer mechanism for atherogenesis. Proc R Soc Lond B Biol Sci 177:109-159, 1971.
17. LoGerfo FW, Nowak MD, Quist WC, et al: Flow studies in a model carotid bifurcation. Atherosclerosis 1:235-241, 1981.
18. Phillips DJ, Greene FM, Langlois Y, et al: Flow velocity patterns in the carotid bifurcations of young, presumed normal subjects. Ultrasound Med Biol 9:39-49, 1983.
19. Abbott WM, Megerman J, Hasson JE, et al: Effect of compliance mismatch on vascular graft patency. J Vasc Surg 5:376-382, 1987.
20. Lye CR, Sumner DS, Strandness DE: The transcutaneous measurement of the elastic properties of the human saphenous vein femoropopliteal bypass graft. Surg Gynecol Obstet 141:891-895, 1975.
21. Hokanson DE, Strandness DE: Stress-strain characteristics of various arterial grafts. Surg Gynecol Obstet 127:57-60, 1968.
22. Miller JH, Foreman RK, Ferguson L, Faris A: Interposition vein cuff for anastomosis of prosthesis to small artery. Aust N Z J Surg 54:283-285, 1984.
23. Corson JD, Leather RP, Balko A, et al: Relationship between vasa vasorum and blood flow to vein bypass endothelial morphology. Arch Surg 120:386-388, 1985.
24. Abbott WM, Weiland S, Austen WG: Structural changes during preparation of autogenous venous grafts. Surgery 76:1031-1040, 1974.
25. Barrett T, Benditt E: Platelet-derived growth factor gene expression in human atherosclerotic plaques and in normal artery wall. Proc Natl Acad Sci U S A 85:2810-2814, 1988.
26. Libby P, Warner S, Salomon R, Birinyi L: Production of platelet-derived growth factor-like mitogen by smooth muscle cells from human atheroma. N Engl J Med 318:1493-1498, 1988.
27. Cole C, Lucas J, Mikat E, et al: Adherence of polymorphonuclear leukocytes to injured rabbit aorta. Surg Forum 35:440-442, 1984.
28. Shimokado K, Raines E, Madtes D, et al: A significant part of macrophage-derived growth factor consists of at least two forms of PDGF. Cell 43:277-286, 1988.
29. Prescott MF, McBride CK, Venturini CM, Gerhardt SC: Leukocyte stimulation of intimal lesion formation is inhibited by treatment with diclofenac sodium and dexamethasone. J Cardiovasc Pharmacol 14(Suppl 6):S76-S81, 1989.
30. Lucas J, Makhoul R, Cole C, et al: Mononuclear cells adhere to sites of vascular balloon catheter injury. Curr Surg 43:112-115, 1986.
31. Mazzone T, Jensen M, Chait A: Human arterial wall cells secrete factors that are chemotactic for monocytes. Proc Natl Acad Sci U S A 80:5094-5097, 1983.
32. Swales JD, Thurston H: Generation of angiotensin II of peripheral vascular level: Studies using angiotensin II antisera. Clin Sci 45:691-700, 1973.
33. Dzau VJ: Vascular angiotensin pathways: A new therapeutic target. J Cardiovasc Pharmacol 10(Suppl 7):S9-S16, 1987.
34. Campbell DJ, Habener JF: Angiotensinogen gene is expressed and differentially regulated in multiple tissues of the rat. J Clin Invest 78:31-39, 1986.
35. Campbell DJ: Tissue renin-angiotensin system: Sites of angiotensin formation. J Cardiovasc Pharmacol 10(Suppl 7):S1-S8, 1987.
36. Molteni A, Dzau VJ, Fallon JT, Haber E: Monoclonal antibodies as probes of renin gene expression. Circulation 70(Suppl II):II-196, 1984.
37. Re R, Fallon JT, Dzau VJ, et al: Renin synthesis by canine aortic smooth muscle cells in culture. Life Sci 30:99-106, 1982.
38. Lilly LS, Pratt RE, Alexander RW, et al: Renin expression by vascular endothelial cells in culture. Circ Res 57:312-318, 1985.
39. Ohashi H, Matsunaga N, Pak CH, Kawai C: Serial change in renin release by the cultured human vascular smooth muscle cells. J Hypertens 4(Suppl 6):S472-S473, 1986.
40. Drouet L, Baudin B, Baumann FC, Caen JP: Serum angiotensin-converting enzyme: An endothelial cell marker. J Lab Clin Med 112:450-457, 1988.

41. Penit J, Faure M, Jard S: Vasopressin and angiotensin II receptors in rat aortic smooth muscle cells in culture. Am J Physiol 244:E72-E82, 1983.

42. Griendling K, Tsuda T, Berk BC, Alexander RW: Angiotensin II stimulation of vascular smooth muscle. J Cardiovasc Pharmacol 14(Suppl 6):S27-S33, 1989.

43. Moore T, Williams G: Angiotensin II receptors on human platelets. Circ Res 51:314-320, 1982.

44. Gimbrone M, Alexander RW: Angiotensin II stimulation of prostaglandin production in cultured human vascular endothelium. Science 189:219-220, 1975.

45. Toda N: Endothelium-dependent relaxion induced by angiotensin II and histamine in isolated arteries of dog. Br J Pharmacol 81:301-307, 1984.

46. Campbell-Boswell M, Robertson AL: Effects of angiotensin II and vasopressin on human smooth muscle cells in vitro. Exp Mol Pathol 35:265, 1981.

47. Geisterfer AA, Peach MJ, Owens JK: Angiotensin II induces hypertrophy, not hyperplasia, of cultured rat aortic smooth muscle cells. Circ Res 62:749-756, 1988.

48. Jackson TR, Blair LAC, Marshall J, et al: The *mas* oncogene encodes an angiotensin receptor. Nature 335:437-440, 1988.

49. Swartz S, Moore T: Effect of angiotensin II on collagen-induced platelet activation in normotensive subjects. Thromb Haemost 63:87-90, 1990.

50. Naftilan AJ, Pratt RE, Dzau VJ: Induction of platelet-derived growth factor A-chain and c-*myc* gene expressions by angiotensin II in cultured rat vascular smooth muscle cells. J Clin Invest 83:1419-1424, 1989.

51. Clowes AW, Reidy MA, Clowes MM: Kinetics of cellular proliferation after arterial injury. I. Smooth muscle growth in the absence of endothelium. Lab Invest 49:327-333, 1983.

52. Fingerle J, Au YPT, Clowes AW, Reidy MA: Intimal lesion formation in the rat carotid arteries after endothelial denudation in the absence of medial injury. Arteriosclerosis 10:1082-1087, 1990.

53. Lindner V, Lappi DA, Baird A, et al: Role of basic fibroblast growth factor in vascular lesion formation. Circ Res 68:106-113, 1991.

54. Cuevas P, Gonzalez AM, Carceller F, Baird A: Vascular response to basic fibroblast growth factor when infused onto the normal adventitia or into the injured media of the rat carotid artery. Circ Res 69:360-369, 1991.

55. Fingerle J, Johnson R, Clowes AW, et al: Role of platelets in smooth muscle proliferation and migration after vascular injury in rat carotid artery. Proc Natl Acad Sci U S A 86:8412-8416, 1989.

56. Garg UC, Hassid A: Nitic oxide-generating vasodilators and 8-bromo-cyclic guanosine monophosphate inhibit mitogenesis and proliferation of cultured rat vascular smooth muscle cells. J Clin Invest 83:1774-1777, 1989.

57. Clowes AW, Collazzo RE, Karnovsky MJ: A morphologic and permeability study of luminal smooth muscle cells after arterial injury in the rat. Lab Invest 39:141-150, 1978.

58. Werb Z, Mainardi C, Vater CA, Harris ED: Endogenous activation of latent collagenase by rheumatoid synovial cells: Evidence for a role of plasminogen activator. N Engl J Med 296:1017-1023, 1977.

59. Levin EG, Loskutoff DJ: Comparative studies of the fibrinolytic activity of cultured vascular cells. Thromb Res 15:869-878, 1979.

60. Goldsmith GH, Ziats NP, Robertson AL: Studies on plasminogen activator and other proteases in subcultured human vascular cells. Exp Mol Pathol 35:257-264, 1981.

61. Clowes AW, Clowes MM, Au YPT, et al: Smooth muscle cells express urokinase during mitogenesis and tissue-type plasminogen activator during migration in injured rat carotid artery. Circ Res 67:61-67, 1990.

62. Hoch JR, Stark VK, Turnipseed WD: The temporal relationship between the development of vein graft intimal hyperplasia and growth factor gene expression. J Vasc Surg 22:51-58, 1995.

63. Stark VK, Warner TF, Hoch JR: An ultrastructural study of progressive intimal hyperplasia in rat vein grafts. J Vasc Surg 26:94-103, 1997.

64. Stark VK, Hoch JR, Warner TF, Hullett DA: Monocyte chemotactic protein-1 is associated with the development of vein graft intimal hyperplasia. Arterioscler Thromb Vasc Biol 17:1614-1621, 1997.

65. Hoch JR, Stark VK, van Rooijen N, et al: Macrophage depletion alters vein graft intimal hyperplasia. Surgery 126:428-437, 1999.

66. Faries PL, Marin ML, Veith FJ, et al: Immunolocalization and temporal distribution of cytokine expression during the development of vein graft intimal myoerplasia in an experimental model. J Vasc Surg 24:463-471, 1996.

67. Kraiss LW, Clowes AW: Response of the arterial wall to injury and intimal hyperplasia. In Sidawy AN, Sumpio BE, DePalma RG (eds): The Basic Science of Vascular Disease. Armonk, NY, Futura, 1997, pp 289-317.

68. Dalman RL, Taylor LM Jr: Basic data related to infrainguinal revascularization procedures. Ann Vasc Surg 3:309-312, 1990.

69. Szilagyi DE, Elliott JP, Hageman JH, et al: Biologic fate of autologous vein implants as arterial substitutes: Clinical, angiographic and histologic observations in femoropopliteal operations for atherosclerosis. Ann Surg 178:232-246, 1973.

70. Stoney RJ, String ST: Recurrent carotid stenosis. Surgery 80:705-710, 1976.

71. Cossman D, Callow AD, Stein A, Matsumoto G: Early restenosis after carotid endarterectomy. Arch Surg 113:275-278, 1978.

72. Kremen JE, Gee W, Kaupp HA, McDonald KM: Restenosis or occlusion after carotid endarterectomy: A survey with ocular pneumoplethysmography. Arch Surg 114:608-610, 1979.

73. Hertzer NR, Martinez BD, Benjamin SP, Beven EG: Recurrent stenosis after carotid endarterectomy. Surg Gynecol Obstet 149:360-364, 1979.

74. Cossman DV, Treiman RL, Foran RF, et al: Surgical approach to recurrent carotid stenosis. Am J Surg 140:209-211, 1980.

75. Catelmo NL, Cutler BS, Wheeler HB, et al: Noninvasive detection of carotid stenosis following endarterectomy. Arch Surg 116:1005-1008, 1981.

76. Zierler RE, Bandyk DF, Thiele BL, Strandness DE: Carotid artery stenosis following endarterectomy. Arch Surg 117:1408-1415, 1982.

77. Baker WH, Hayes AC, Mahler D, Littooy FN: Durability of carotid endarterectomy. Surgery 94:112-115, 1983.

78. Salvian A, Baker JD, Machleder HI, et al: Cause and noninvasive detection of restenosis after carotid endarterectomy. Am J Surg 146:29-34, 1983.

79. Pierce GE, Iliopoulus JI, Holcomb MA, et al: Incidence of recurrent stenosis after carotid endarterectomy determined by digital subtraction angiography. Am J Surg 148:848-854, 1984.

80. O'Donnell TF, Callow AD, Scott G, et al: Ulrasound characteristics of recurrent carotid disease: Hypothesis explaining the low incidence of symptomatic recurrence. J Vasc Surg 2:26-41, 1985.

81. Wilson SE, Sheppard B: Results of percutaneous transluminal angioplasty for peripheral vascular occlusive disease. Ann Vasc Surg 4:94-97, 1990.

82. White RA, White GH, Mehringer MC: A clinical trial of laser thermal angioplasty in patients with advanced peripheral vascular disease. Ann Surg 212:257-265, 1990.

83. Ahn SS, Eton D, Mehigan JT: Preliminary clinical results of rotary atherectomy. In Yao JST, Pearce WH (eds): Technologies in Vascular Surgery. Philadelphia, WB Saunders, 1992, pp 388-401.

84. Cahill PD, Sarris GE, Cooper AD, et al: Inhibition of vein graft intimal thickening by eicosapentaenoic acid: Reduced thromboxane production without change in lipoprotein levels or low-density lipoprotein receptor density. J Vasc Surg 7:108-117, 1988.

85. Landymore RW, Manku MS, Tan M, et al: Effects of low-dose marine oils on intimal hyperplasia in autologous vein grafts. J Thorac Cardiovasc Surg 98:788-791, 1989.

86. O'Hara M, Esato K, Harada M, et al: Eicosapentaenoic acid suppresses intimal hyperplasia after expanded polytetrafluoroethylene grafting in rabbits fed a high cholesterol diet. J Vasc Surg 13:480-486, 1991.

87. Quiñones-Baldrich W, Ziomek S, Henderson T, Moore W: Patency and intimal hyperplasia: The effect of aspirin on small arterial anastomosis. Ann Vasc Surg 2:50-56, 1988.

88. Landymore RW, Karmazyn M, MacAulay MA, et al: Correlation between the effects of aspirin and dipyridamole on platelet function and prevention of intimal hyperplasia in autologous vein grafts. Can J Cardiol 4:56-59, 1988.

89. Radic ZS, O'Malley MK, Mikat EM, et al: The role of aspirin and dipyridamole on vascular DNA synthesis and intimal hyperplasia following deendothelialization. J Surg Res 41:84-91, 1986.

90. Chervu A, Moore WS, Quiñones-Baldrich WJ, Henderson T: Efficacy of corticosteroids in suppression of intimal hyperplasia. J Vasc Surg 10:129-134, 1989.

91. Hoepp LM, Elbadawi A, Cohn M, et al: Steroids and immunosuppression: Effect on anastomotic intimal hyperplasia in femoral arterial Dacron bypass grafts. Arch Surg 114:273-276, 1979.

92. O'Malley MK, McDermott EW, Mehigan D, O'Higgins NJ: Role for prazosin in reducing the development of rabbit intimal hyperplasia after endothelial denudation. Br J Surg 76:936-938, 1989.

93. Powell JS, Clozel JP, Müller RK, et al: Inhibitors of angiotensin-converting enzyme prevent myointimal proliferation after vascular injury. Science 245:186-188, 1989.

94. El-Sanadiki MN, Cross KS, Murray JJ, et al: Reduction of intimal hyperplasia and enhanced reactivity of experimental vein bypass grafts with verapamil. Ann Surg 212:87-96, 1990.

95. Guyotat J, Pelissou-Guyotat I, Lievre M, Chignier E: Inhibition of subintimal hyperplasia of autologous vein bypass grafts by nimodipine in rats: A placebo-controlled study. Neurosurgery 29:850-855, 1991.

96. Dryjski M, Mikat E, Bjornsson TD: Inhibition of intimal hyperplasia after arterial injury by heparins and heparinoid. J Vasc Surg 8:623-633, 1988.

97. Calcagno D, Conte JV, Howell MH, Foegh ML: Peptide inhibition of neointimal hyperplasia in vein grafts. J Vasc Surg 13:475-479, 1991.

98. Conte JV, Foegh ML, Calcagno D, et al: Peptide inhibition of myointimal proliferation following angioplasty in rabbits. Transplant Proc 21:3686-3688, 1989.

99. Lundergan C, Foegh ML, Vargas R, et al: Inhibition of myointimal proliferation of the rat carotid artery by the peptides, angiopeptin and BIM 23034. Atherosclerosis 80:49-55, 1989.

100. Foegh ML, Khirabadi BS, Chambers E, et al: Inhibition of coronary artery transplant atherosclerosis in rabbits with angiopeptin, an octapeptide. Atherosclerosis 78:229-236, 1989.

101. Endean ED, Kispert JF, Martin KW, O'Connor W: Intimal hyperplasia is reduced by ornithine decarboxylase inhibition. J Surg Res 50:634-637, 1991.

102. Baumgartner HR: Eine neue Methode zur Erzeugung von Thromben durch gezielte Überdehnung der Gefässwand. Z Ges Exp Med 137:227, 1963.

103. Clowes AW, Clowes MM, Reidy MA: Role of acute distension in the induction of smooth muscle proliferation after arterial denudation [abstract]. FASEB J 46:270, 1987.

104. Bang HO, Dyerberg J, Nielsen A: Plasma lipid and lipoprotein pattern in Greenlandic west-coast Eskimos. Lancet 1:1143-1145, 1971.

105. Dyerberg J, Bang HO, Stoffersen E, et al: Eicosapentaenoic acid and prevention of thrombosis and atherosclerosis. Lancet 2:117-119, 1978.

106. Friedman RJ, Stemerman MB, Wenz B, et al: The effect of thrombocytopenia on experimental arteriosclerotic lesion formation in rabbits: Smooth muscle cell proliferation and reendothelialization. J Clin Invest 60:1191-1201, 1977.

107. McCollum C, Crow M, Rajah S, Kester R: Anti-thrombotic therapy for vascular prosthesis: An experimental model testing platelet inhibitory drugs. Surgery 87:668-676, 1980.

108. Oblath R, Buckley F, Green R, et al: Prevention of platelet aggregation to prosthetic vascular grafts by aspirin and dipyridamole. Surgery 84:37-44, 1978.

109. Zammit M, Kaplan S, Sauvage L, et al: Aspirin therapy in small-caliber arterial prostheses: Long-term experimental observations. J Vasc Surg 1:839-851, 1984.

110. Plate G, Stanson A, Hollier L, Dewanjee M: Drug effects on platelet deposition after endothelial injury of the rabbit aorta. J Surg Res 39:258-266, 1985.

111. McCann R, Hagen P-O, Fuchs J: Aspirin and dipyridamole decrease intimal hyperplasia in experimental vein grafts. Ann Surg 191:238-243, 1980.

112. Graham LM, Brothers TE, Darvishian D, et al: Effects of thromboxane synthetase inhibition on patency and anastomotic hyperplasia of vascular grafts. J Surg Res 46:611-615, 1989.

113. Becquemin JP: Effect of ticlopidine on the long-term patency of saphenous-vein bypass grafts in the legs. N Engl J Med 337:1726-1731, 1997.

114. Hanson S, Pareti F, Ruggeri Z, et al: Antibody-induced platelet inhibition reduces thrombus formation in vivo. Clin Res 34:658, 1986.

115. Torem S, Schneide P, Hanson S: Monoclonal antibody-induced inhibition of platelet function: Effects on hemostasis and vascular graft thrombosis in baboons. J Vasc Surg 7:172-180, 1988.

116. Gordon GB, Bush DE, Weisman HF: Reduction of atherosclerosis by administration of dehydroepiandrosterone. J Clin Invest 82:712-720, 1988.

117. Pepine CJ, Hirshfeld JW, Macdonald RG, et al: A controlled trial of corticosteroids to prevent restenosis after coronary angioplasty. Circulation 81:1753-1761, 1990.

118. Colburn MD, Moore WS, Gelabert HA, Quiñones-Baldrich WJ: Dose responsive suppression of myointimal hyperplasia by dexamethasone. J Vasc Surg 15:510-518, 1992.

119. Ruhmann AG, Berliner DL: Effect of steroids on growth of mouse fibroblasts in vitro. Endocrinology 76:916-927, 1965.

120. Majeski JA, Alexander JW: The steroid effect on the in vitro human neutrophil chemotactic response. J Surg Res 21:265-271, 1976.

121. Mishler J: The effects of corticosteroids on mobilization and function of neutrophils. Exp Hematol 5:15-32, 1977.

122. Hess AD, Esa AH, Colombani PM, et al: Mechanisms of action of cyclosporin: Effect on cells of the immune system and on subcellular events in T-cell activation. Transplant Proc 20(Suppl 2):29, 1988.

123. Goldstein I, Roos D, Weissmann G, Kaplan H: Influence of corticosteroids on human polymorphonuclear leukocyte function in vitro enzyme release and superoxide production. Inflammation 1:305-315, 1976.

124. Reil TD, Sarkar R, Kashyap VS, et al: Dexamethasone suppresses vascular smooth muscle cell proliferation. J Surg Res 85:109-114, 1999.

125. Reil TD, Kashyap VS, Sarkar R, et al: Dexamethasone inhibits the phosphorylation of retinoblastoma protein in the suppression of human vascular smooth muscle cell proliferation. J Surg Res 92:108-113, 2000.

126. Pearce J, Dujovny M, Ho K, et al: Acute inflammation and endothelial injury in vein grafts. Neurosurgery 17:626-634, 1985.

127. Cwikel BJ, Barouski-Miller PA, Coleman PL, Gelehrter TD: Dexamethasone induction of an inhibitor of plasminogen activator in HTC hepatoma cells. J Biol Chem 259:6847-6851, 1984.

128. Wengrovitz M, Selassie LG, Gifford RRM, Thiele BL: Cyclosporine inhibits the development of medial thickening after experimental arterial injury. J Vasc Surg 12:1-7, 1990.

129. Clowes AW, Reidy MA: Prevention of stenosis after vascular reconstruction: Pharmacologic control of intimal hyperplasia—a review. J Vasc Surg 13:885-891, 1991.

130. O'Donohoe MK, Schwartz LB, Radic ZS, et al: Chronic ACE inhibition reduces intimal hyperplasia in experimental vein grafts. Ann Surg 214:727-732, 1991.

131. Chobanian AV, Haudenschild CC, Nickerson C, Drago R: Antiatherogenic effect of captopril in the Watanabe heritable hyperlipidemic rabbit. Hypertension 15:327-331, 1990.

132. El-Sanadiki M, Cross K, Mikat E, Hagen P-O: Verapamil therapy reduces intimal hyperplasia in balloon injured rabbit aorta. Circulation 76(Suppl):314, 1987.

133. O'Malley MK, Mikat EM, McCann RL, Hagen P-O: Increased vascular sensitivity to norepinephrine following injury. Surg Forum 35:445-447, 1984.

134. O'Malley M, Cotecchia S, Hagen P-O: Receptor mediated noradrenaline supersensitivity in rabbit aortic intimal hyperplasia. Eur Surg Res 18:43, 1986.

135. Mark J: The polyphosphoinositides revisited. Science 228:312-313, 1985.

136. Vargas R, Bormes GW, Wroblewska B, et al: Angiopeptin inhibits thymidine incorporation in rat carotid artery in vitro. Transplant Proc 21:3702-3704, 1989.

137. Lappi DA, Martineau D, Baird A: Biological and chemical characterization of basic FGF-saporin mitotoxin. Biochem Biophys Res Commun 160:917-923, 1989.

138. Pegg AE, McCann PP: Polyamine metabolism and function. Am J Physiol 243:C212-C221, 1982.

139. Heby O, Gray JW, Lindl PA, et al: Changes in L-ornithine decarboxylase activity during the cell cycle. Biochem Biophys Res Commun 71:99-105, 1976.

140. Babapulle MN, Joseph L, Belisle P, et al: A hierarchical Bayesian meta-analysis of randomised clinical trials of drug-eluting stents. Lancet 364:583-591, 2004.

141. Holmes DR Jr, Firth BG, Wood DL: Paradigm shifts in cardiovascular medicine. J Am Coll Cardiol 43:507-512, 2004.

142. Cifonelli J: The relationship of molecular weight, and sulfate content and distribution to anticoagulant activity of heparin preparations. Carbohydr Res 37:145-154, 1974.

143. Schweiger H, Klein P, Ruf S, Meister R: Avoiding early failure of tibial prosthetic bypass grafts. Thorac Cardiovasc Surg 35:148-150, 1987.

144. Hoover RL, Rosenberg R, Haering W, Karnovsky MJ: Inhibition of rat arterial smooth muscle cell proliferation by heparin II: In vitro studies. Circ Res 47:578-583, 1980.

145. Majack RA, Clowes AW: Inhibition of vascular smooth muscle cell migration by heparin-like glycosaminoglycans. J Cell Physiol 118:253-256, 1984.

146. Clowes AW, Clowes MM: Kinetics of cellular proliferation after arterial injury. II. Inhibition of smooth muscle growth by heparin. Lab Invest 52:611-616, 1985.

147. Clowes AW, Clowes MM: Kinetics of cellular proliferation after arterial injury. IV. Heparin inhibits rat smooth muscle mitogenesis and migration. Circ Res 58:839-845, 1986.

148. Majesky MW, Schwartz SM, Clowes MM, Clowes AW: Heparin regulates smooth muscle S phase entry in the injured rat carotid artery. Circ Res 61:296-300, 1987.

149. Hsueh WA, Law RE: Diabetes is a vascular disease. J Invest Med 46:387-390, 1998.

150. Law RE, Meehan WP, Xi XP, et al: Troglitazone inhibits vascular smooth muscle cell growth and intimal hyperplasia. J Clin Invest 98:1897-1905, 1996.

151. Figge F, Wieland G, Manganiello L: Cancer detection and therapy: Affinity of neoplastic, embryonic, and traumatized tissue for porphyrins and metalloporphyrins. Proc Soc Exp Biol Med 68:640-641, 1948.

152. Weishaupt KR, Gomer CJ, Dougherty TJ: Identification of single oxygen as the cytotoxic agent in photo-inactivation of a murine tumor. Cancer Res 36:2326-2329, 1976.

153. Kessel D: Porphyrin localization: A new modality for detection and therapy of tumors. Biochem Pharmacol 33:1389-1393, 1984.

154. Boegheim JPJ, Scholte H, Dubbleman TMAR: Photodynamic effects of hematoporphyrin-derivative on enzyme activities of murine L929 fibroblasts. J Photochem Photobiol 1:61-73, 1987.

155. Neave V, Giannotta S, Hyman S, Schneider J: Hematoporphyrin uptake in atherosclerotic plaques: Therapeutic potentials. Neurosurgery 23:307-312, 1988.

156. Mackie RW, Vincent GM, Fox J, et al: In vivo canine coronary artery laser irradiation: Photodynamic therapy using dihematoporphyrin ether and 632 mm laser: A safety and dose-response relationship study. Lasers Surg Med 11:535-544, 1991.

157. Hundley RF, Weinstein R, Spears JR: Photodynamic cytolysis of rat arterial smooth muscle cells with hematoporphyrin derivative in vitro. Lasers Life Sci 2:19-27, 1988.

158. Spears JR, Serur J, Shopshire D, et al: Fluorescence of experimental atheromatous plaques with hematoporphyrin derivative. J Clin Invest 71:395-399, 1983.

159. Dartsch PC, Ischinger T, Betz E: Differential effect of Photofrin II on growth of human smooth muscle cells from nonatherosclerotic arteries and atheromatous plaques in vitro. Arteriosclerosis 10:616-624, 1990.

160. Dartsch PC, Ischinger T, Betz E: Responses of cultured smooth muscle cells from human nonatherosclerotic arteries and primary stenosing lesions after photoradiation: Implications for photodynamic therapy of vascular stenoses. J Am Coll Cardiol 15:1545-1550, 1990.

161. Dartsch PC, Betz E, Ischinger T: Effect of dihematoporphyrin derivatives on cultivated human smooth muscle cells from normal and atherosclerotic vascular segments: Overview of results and implications for photodynamic therapy. Z Kardiol 80:6-14,1991.

162. Zwiebel JA, Freeman SM, Kantoff PW, et al: High-level recombinant gene expression in rabbit endothelial cells transduced by retroviral vectors. Science 243:220-222, 1989.

163. Dichek DA, Neville RF, Zwiebel JA, et al: Seeding of intravascular stents with genetically engineered endothelial cells. Circulation 80:1347-1353, 1989.

164. Brothers TE, Stanley JC: Impact of genetic engineering on vascular disease and biology. In Veith FJ (ed): Current Critical Problems in Vascular Surgery. St. Louis, Quality Medical, 1990, pp 42-50.

165. Nabel EG, Plautz G, Boyce FM, et al: Recombinant gene expression in vivo within endothelial cells of the arterial wall. Science 244:1342-1344, 1989.

166. Nabel EG, Plautz G, Nabel GJ: Site-specific gene expression in vivo by direct gene transfer into the arterial wall. Science 249:1285-1288, 1990.

167. Wilson JM, Birinyi LK, Salomon RN, et al: Implantation of vascular grafts lined with genetically modified endothelial cells. Science 244:1344-1346, 1989.

168. Ehsan A, Mann MJ, Dell'Acqua G, et al: Endothelial healing in vein grafts: Proliferative burst unimpaired by genetic therapy of neointimal disease. Circulation 105:1686-1692, 2002.

169. Mann MJ, Whittemore AD, Donaldson MC, et al: Ex-vivo gene therapy of human vascular bypass grafts with E2F decoy: The PREVENT single-centre, randomised, controlled trial. Lancet 354:1493-1498, 1999.

170. Dzau VJ: Predicting the future of human gene therapy for cardiovascular diseases: What will the management of coronary artery disease be like in 2005 and 2010? Am J Cardiol 92:32N-35N, 2003.

Questions

1. The origin of the proliferating cells found in intimal hyperplastic lesions is most likely which of the following?
   (a) Fibroblasts from the adventitia
   (b) Circulating immune cells
   (c) Neutrophils
   (d) Endothelial cells
   (e) Medial smooth muscle cells

2. Which hemodynamic force has been implicated as a contributing factor in the development of intimal hyperplasia?
   (a) Vessel wall compliance
   (b) High shear stress
   (c) Flow velocity
   (d) Low shear stress
   (e) All of the above

3. Which surface membrane receptor regulates vascular smooth muscle cells' accumulation of low-density lipoprotein (LDL)?
   (a) Glycoprotein receptor Ib
   (b) High-affinity LDL receptor
   (c) Glycoprotein receptor IIb/IIIa
   (d) Low-affinity LDL receptor
   (e) High-affinity high-density lipoprotein receptor

4. Platelet aggregation is stimulated by which of the following?
   (a) Adenosine triphosphate
   (b) Platelet-derived growth factor
   (c) Adenosine diphosphate
   (d) Low-density lipoprotein
   (e) Prostacyclin

5. Angiotensin-converting enzyme is located primarily on the membrane surface of which of the following?
   (a) Platelets
   (b) Neutrophils
   (c) Fibroblasts
   (d) Vascular endothelial cells
   (e) Macrophages

6. Which peptide has *not* been implicated in smooth muscle cell stimulation after an endothelial layer injury?
   (a) Basic fibroblast growth factor
   (b) Platelet-derived growth factor
   (c) Angiotensin II
   (d) Macrophage-derived growth factor
   (e) Insulin

7. What is the approximate incidence of restenosis after endarterectomy for carotid artery bifurcation lesions?
   (a) 5%
   (b) 35%
   (c) 1%
   (d) 25%
   (e) 50%

8. Intimal hyperplasia is the most common cause of bypass graft failure during which time frame?
   (a) Within 1 month
   (b) Between 1 and 6 months
   (c) Between 6 months and 2 years
   (d) After 5 years
   (e) After 10 years

9. Dipyridamole inhibits platelet function by which of the following mechanisms?
   (a) Increasing thromboxane A_2
   (b) Blocking the enzyme cyclooxygenase
   (c) Increasing platelet adenosine diphosphate
   (d) Increasing platelet cyclic adenosine monophosphate
   (e) Decreasing prostacyclin

10. Prazosin is a selective inhibitor of which of the following receptors?
    (a) High-affinity low-density lipoprotein
    (b) Platelet-derived growth factor
    (c) β_1-Adrenergic receptor
    (d) α_2-Adrenergic receptor
    (e) α_1-Adrenergic receptor

Answers

1. e	2. e	3. b	4. c	5. d
6. e	7. a	8. c	9. d	10. e

42

Niren Angle • Julie A. Freischlag

Prosthetic Graft Infections

The development of prosthetic biomaterial devices has made it possible to treat conditions that otherwise would have resulted in significant morbidity and mortality. Examples of such clinical conditions include but are not limited to aortic aneurysms, hemodialysis access in patients in whom autologous fistulas are not possible, and infrainguinal bypass for limb ischemia. The advent of the use of prosthetic conduits has also resulted in the problem of prosthetic graft infection. The morbidity associated with infected prosthetic vascular grafts is considerable and can be catastrophic, resulting in limb loss, sepsis, and, not infrequently, death. This chapter examines the cause, diagnosis, and management of prosthetic graft infection.

Incidence

Prosthetic graft infection is relatively uncommon, with a reported incidence ranging from 0.2% to 5%. There are few prospectively obtained data analyzing the true incidence of prosthetic graft infection, but a survey of retrospective data with extended follow-up suggests that graft infections are influenced by the implant site, the indications for operation, and the host's defense status, as manifested by the patient's comorbid disease. A prospective, multicenter Canadian study of repair of unruptured abdominal aortic aneurysms revealed a graft infection rate of 0.2%.[1] Szilagyi and colleagues' analysis of 2145 patients undergoing a variety of vascular reconstructions, including aortofemoral, aortoiliac, and femoropopliteal reconstructions, revealed an overall graft infection rate of 1.5%.[2] The insertion of a prosthetic graft in the femoropopliteal or femorotibial position has a higher rate of infection, ranging up to 5% in some reports.

The last decade has seen a sharp rise in the number of aortic aneurysms treated with endovascular grafts, and even though it is relatively early, reports of endovascular prosthesis infection are already available. Although access for implanting these devices and other intravascular grafts is less invasive, it appears that the incidence of aortic endograft infection may be around 1%.

An emergency operation (e.g., for a ruptured abdominal aortic aneurysm) carries a higher rate of infection than does an elective operation. The consequences of an infected prosthesis are also different, depending on the location of the graft.

The mortality rate is higher with an infected aortic prosthesis, and the risk of limb loss is highest with lower extremity graft infection. A graft infection can manifest months to years after implantation, and this insidious presentation may provide clues to the biology of graft infection.

Microbiology

Insight into the cause of vascular graft infections can be gained by examining the microorganisms most commonly recovered from infected grafts. Although any microorganism can potentially cause a graft infection, Staphylococcus aureus is the most prevalent bacterium.[3] S. aureus is responsible for 25% to 50% of vascular graft infections, based on anatomic location. Over the last 15 to 20 years, Staphylococcus epidermidis has increasingly been identified as the responsible pathogen for a significant proportion of graft infections, predominantly the late-appearing, indolent type.

Graft infections are labeled as early (occurring <4 months after implantation) or late (occurring >4 months after implantation). Early-appearing graft infections are most commonly caused by more virulent organisms, most commonly S. aureus. Coagulase-positive strains elaborate toxins that result in a vigorous host inflammatory response. Late-appearing graft infections are caused by less virulent gram-positive bacteria such as S. epidermidis. This organism is indolent and normally harbored in natural skin. It has the ability to adhere to prosthetic material and to secrete a glycocalyx biofilm that insulates the bacterium. Over time, this biofilm induces an inflammatory response that results in perigraft inflammation, which is seen clinically as perigraft fluid. This organism is fastidious in its attachment and is not easily isolated. S. epidermidis graft infections appear to have a sterile exudate, resulting in poor graft incorporation. Rarely do patients have a leukocytosis. This innocuous presentation has led many to view S. epidermidis infections as inflammatory allergic responses rather than bacterial graft infections.[4] Bergamini and colleagues elegantly demonstrated that ultrasonication is required to physically separate S. epidermidis from the graft surface in order to culture it.[5] Also, broth culture yielded a higher rate of recovery than did agar plating. Bacterial recovery, which was only 30% when plated on agar media, rose to 72% in broth media. The combination of ultrasonication and broth culture resulted in a positive culture in 83% of cases in this report.

Other microorganisms such as fungi and gram-negative bacteria can also result in graft infections. Gram-negative bacteria such as *Pseudomonas, Escherichia coli, Enterobacter,* and *Proteus* are very virulent and result in dramatic clinical manifestations, such as anastomotic disruption and frank hemorrhage.[6] These organisms are able to secrete potent proteases, which accounts for the tissue disruption that results in artery-graft disruption. Gram-negative infections also induce a substantial host inflammatory response that contributes to the disruption. *Pseudomonas* is most commonly associated with graft disruption and hemorrhage. Severely immunosuppressed patients are also vulnerable to fungal graft infections, an otherwise rare clinical entity in the general population.

Cause and Pathophysiology

The fundamental question with regard to the cause of prosthetic graft infections is, when does exposure to the infection-causing microorganisms occur? The three major potential mechanisms that can result in prosthetic graft colonization and subsequent infection are the following:

1. Intraoperative contamination
2. Hematogenous spread of bacteria
3. Direct contamination of graft by infection emanating from the skin, soft tissue, gastrointestinal tract, or genitourinary tract

Although all these factors can result in a graft infection, the last mechanism listed is the least common.

INTRAOPERATIVE CONTAMINATION

The host is the most significant source of bacterial contamination resulting in surgical site infection. The resident microflora, usually referred to as the indigenous microflora, consists of a complex mixture of microbial species ranging from nonpathogenic saprophytes to pathogens. Endogenous bacteria are a more important source of surgical site infection than exogenous bacteria are.

The patient's endogenous flora from a site close to the prosthetic bed—especially from a colonized site, such as the skin or gut—is a common source of graft infection. Most of the intertriginous areas of the body, such as the axillae, groin, and interdigital spaces of the foot, contain large numbers of eccrine sweat glands and harbor large bacterial populations.[7] Thus, prosthetic grafts placed in the groin have a well-characterized propensity to develop *S. aureus* infection. *S. aureus* bacteria from the groin area may contaminate only the wound, or they may also contaminate the graft surface if it is inadvertently dragged across the skin. The lymphatics in the groin may be contaminated at the time of surgery, especially if the patient has an open infected wound in an extremity. These lymphatics can also be a source of intraoperative graft infection. It is exceedingly rare for bacterial contamination to originate from the surgical team, from the graft, or from surgical instruments. The surgeon's hands are seldom a major source of wound contamination.[8]

Bacteria can be present in diseased vessels or in the thrombus lining an aortic aneurysm.[9] Van der Vliet and colleagues cultured the contents of the aneurysms of 216 patients and then followed the patients for more than 3 years.[10] Positive cultures

were found in 55 patients (25.5%). Only four graft infections occurred (1.9%). Three of these four patients had positive cultures, but only two patients had the same organism as the original cultures. The authors concluded that bacteria in aneurysm contents have no demonstrable link to subsequent graft infections. A prospective study demonstrated that in patients undergoing peripheral vascular bypass surgery, 41% had positive arterial tissue cultures, 68% of which were coagulase-negative *Staphylococcus*.[11] Subsequent graft infections were not reported, so the significance of the cultures is intriguing but unclear.

HEMATOGENOUS SPREAD

Seeding of an indwelling prosthesis by hematogenous spread of bacteria is potentially important; the frequency with which this occurs is unknown. In experimental animals, infusion of 10^7 organisms of *S. aureus* immediately after implantation of a prosthetic aortic graft resulted in a 100% incidence of graft infection.[12,13] Later studies demonstrated a lower incidence of graft infection with a longer time after implantation, suggesting that graft incorporation and the development of a pseudointima may provide some protection.[14,15] Vulnerability to infection from bacteremia has been documented as late as 1 year after implantation, with 30% of aortic grafts becoming infected after a single bacterial infusion at that time.[12] The anatomic difference between the infected and noninfected grafts was the presence of a complete neointimal lining. Parenteral antibiotics significantly reduced the incidence of graft infection, particularly when culture-directed therapy was applied to a remote infection. The significance of remote infection is unclear, but it suggests that transient bacteremia associated with, for example, dental procedures or colonoscopy may account for very late infections.

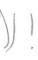

DIRECT CONTAMINATION

This category is the most easily diagnosed and the least common. The development of an intra-abdominal abscess from a variety of clinical conditions can directly infect a recently placed aortic graft. Similarly, failure of the skin incision to heal after an operation places the underlying graft at significant risk of bacterial contamination and subsequent infection. For these reasons, it is prudent to avoid any operation on the gastrointestinal tract at the time of insertion of an aortic prosthetic graft. The exception to this is the performance of a cholecystectomy, but this too is done only after the graft is inserted and the retroperitoneum is closed over the graft.

Prevention

The best way to avoid graft infection is to prevent it in the operating room and during the postoperative period. It has been shown that patients who are hospitalized for any length of time have an alteration in their cutaneous microflora.[16] It is unclear whether this is caused by the underlying illness or by antibiotics. The preoperative stay, if any, should be as short as possible to avoid colonization with resistant bacteria. Prophylactic antibiotics have been shown to decrease the incidence of wound infections that could lead to graft infections. Most authors recommend the administration of a first-generation cephalosporin approximately 30 minutes before incision, with a scheduled dose continued for the first 24 hours. If the operation lasts an extended length of time, additional doses should be administered to maintain adequate circulating levels. There is no evidence to support the continuation of prophylactic antibiotics until indwelling lines, such as central venous or urinary bladder catheters, are removed. The prolonged use of postoperative antibiotics may even be detrimental, because the patient can develop antibiotic-associated colitis or other resistant-organism infections.

Meticulous surgical technique is important in preventing wound and graft infections. The graft must be handled carefully and should not be allowed to come in contact with the patient's skin. Adhesive drapes are commonly used to aid in preventing such contact, although there are no studies demonstrating a reduced incidence of wound or graft infection with the use of adhesive drapes, with or without iodine impregnation. If the adhesive plastic drape is separated from the skin during the operation, however, the infection rate increases.[17,18] Simultaneous gastrointestinal procedures should be avoided to prevent intraoperative contamination. If an unplanned enterotomy is performed, graft implantation should be postponed, if possible. Dead space in surgical wounds should be minimized with the least possible amount of suture material. Irrigation of the peritoneal cavity is routine, but it may lead to washout of macrophages and opsonins. Irrigation should be used to remove all blood from the peritoneal cavity, because blood acts as an adjuvant for bacterial proliferation. If irrigation of a wound is performed, every effort should be made to evacuate the fluid.

Diagnosis

Graft infections can result in limb loss, systemic sepsis, and, sometimes, death, even in the setting of correct diagnosis and treatment. In modern reports, the mortality from aortic graft infections still ranges from 20% to 30% in experienced hands. For these reasons, prompt diagnosis is essential to avoid or minimize complications. Accurate diagnosis requires that the surgeon be aware of the subtle manifestations of graft infection. Every attempt should be made to confirm or exclude the diagnosis, either by imaging or by operative exploration. The consequences of a missed diagnosis in this setting can be catastrophic.

CLINICAL PRESENTATION

The clinical presentation of graft infection can be subtle and is influenced by the anatomic location of the graft. An infection of an infrainguinal graft frequently appears as cellulitis, soft tissue infection, drainage tract, or pseudoaneurysm. The clinical presentation of an extracavitary graft infection is usually not subtle. An intra-abdominal graft infection may appear as systemic sepsis or as an ileus or abdominal distention, with or without tenderness. Occasionally, an aortic graft infection may result in an aortoenteric fistula, the first sign of which is a herald bleed. A patient with upper gastrointestinal bleeding and an aortic graft must be presumed to have an aortoenteric fistula until proved otherwise (Fig. 42-1).

Early graft infections can manifest with fever, leukocytosis, and purulent drainage from the graft site. Splinter hemorrhages may be present. Blood cultures may be positive if

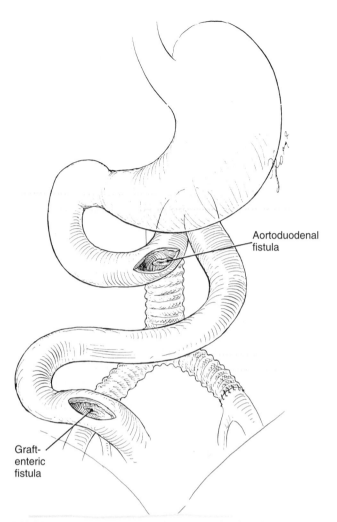

FIGURE 42–1 • A communication may develop between the bowel lumen and the graft. Hemorrhage may be due to a direct communication between the aorta and the bowel (aortoenteric fistula) or from vessels in the bowel wall that have been eroded by the prosthetic graft (enteroparaprosthetic fistula).

taken in the distal arterial circulation downstream from the graft infection. A late graft infection, usually caused by an indolent organism such as *S. epidermidis*, appears as a healing complication such as a seroma, pseudoaneurysm, or late graft thrombosis with no anatomic reason. Systemic signs of illness such as fever are usually not present.

LABORATORY STUDIES

A leukocytosis with a left shift and an elevated erythrocyte sedimentation rate often accompany graft infection, but their lack of specificity limits their usefulness. Late-appearing perigraft infections with *S. epidermidis* may have none of these laboratory abnormalities. The diagnosis of a prosthetic graft infection often depends on a preponderance of the evidence, not merely on one positive data point. An indolent infection, usually caused by *S. epidermidis*, commonly presents with a mild leukocytosis, without a significant left shift, and an elevated erythrocyte sedimentation rate. The diagnosis, however, depends more on imaging and the lack of any other explanation for the aforementioned findings.

IMAGING

Imaging plays an important role in the diagnosis of prosthetic graft infection. The particular imaging modality used depends on the site being investigated and the information desired. Computed tomography (CT), angiography, ultrasonography, nuclear medicine, and magnetic resonance imaging (MRI) constitute the diagnostic armamentarium for the evaluation of potential graft infection.

Computed Tomography

CT scanning is probably the most sensitive and reliable imaging test for the diagnosis of graft infections (Fig. 42-2). Perigraft fluid collections, perigraft gas, anastomotic aneurysms, and distortion of tissue planes are all findings suggestive of graft infection and are all well visualized by a contrast-enhanced CT scan. Presence of gas or fluid around a graft more than 6 to 8 weeks after implantation is definitely abnormal and is presumptive evidence of graft infection.

O'Hara and coworkers published a study examining the natural history of periprosthetic air after abdominal aortic surgery.[19] Twenty-six consecutive patients undergoing elective aortic aneurysm repair had CT scans performed at 3, 7, and 52 days postoperatively. Perigraft air was seen in 65% of patients in the first week following operation. All patients with periprosthetic air had spontaneous resolution, as demonstrated by late CT scanning obtained a mean of 52 days postoperatively (range, 21 to 85 days).

CT-guided aspiration of perigraft fluid is advocated by some as a reliable test that offers a good yield and provides material for Gram stain and culture. However, in our opinion, CT-guided aspiration of perigraft fluid is rarely indicated; once it has been demonstrated that the graft has fluid around it after 6 to 8 weeks, the appropriate treatment is graft excision and reconstruction, with the rare exception of a patient too frail to undergo a major operation.

Ultrasonography

A duplex ultrasound scan is an excellent initial test for the identification of upper and lower extremity graft infections. It is not as accurate in identifying aortic pseudoaneurysms because of the difficulty of imaging owing to bowel gas. It is extremely useful and reliable for the interrogation of femoral and lower extremity sites. Perigraft fluid is easily diagnosed, as is an anastomotic pseudoaneurysm in an infrainguinal bypass; ultrasound scanning can also distinguish between the two. Ultrasonography is quick, portable, and noninvasive. The accuracy of the test depends on the technician's expertise, but in skilled hands, it is informative and reliable.

Magnetic Resonance Imaging

MRI is a useful modality for identifying perigraft fluid because of its ability to distinguish fluid from tissue by recognizing differences in signal intensity between T1- and T2-weighted images. The efficacy of this test was highlighted in a study by Olofsson and colleagues in which 18 patients suspected of having an aortic graft infection underwent preoperative MRI.[20] Twelve patients also underwent CT scanning. MRI successfully identified 14 of 16 patients who were found to have an aortic graft infection at the time of operation, whereas CT was accurate in only 5 of 12 patients. It has been shown that there is only mild enhancement on T2-weighted images in grafts undergoing normal incorporation, whereas infected perigraft tissue demonstrates increased signal intensity.[21] MRI's role in the diagnosis of aortic graft infections may become more prominent, but to date, it is not routinely used for this purpose.

Angiography

Although angiography can identify graft pseudoaneurysms (Fig. 42-3), it is not the test of choice because CT scanning and MRI are better and noninvasive. Arteriography is used in this context not for the diagnosis of prosthetic graft infection but to determine the options for arterial reconstruction. One has to be careful in terms of timing the arteriogram with the CT scan because both involve a contrast load; in a patient with renal insufficiency, this is a consideration.

White Blood Cell Scanning

Gallium 67– or indium 111–labeled white blood cell scanning is very sensitive for graft infection. An indium 111–labeled leukocyte or IgG scan is quite reliable and offers an advantage over gallium 67 scanning because there is minimum nonspecific bowel uptake, resulting in a high target-to-background ratio and better results.[22] Indium 111–labeled leukocyte IgG scanning has been used by LaMuraglia and colleagues with impressive results.[23] In 10 patients with positive scans, graft infection was confirmed at operation at the same site. Of the 15 patients with negative scans, the only one who had a

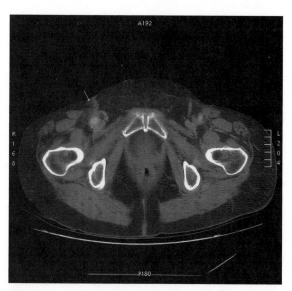

FIGURE 42–2 • Computed tomography (CT) scan of a patient with an aortobifemoral bypass graft and chronic occlusion of the right limb of the bypass treated with a left-to-right femorofemoral bypass with PTFE. Approximately 6 months later, the patient presented with one episode of pulsatile right groin bleeding. CT scan showed stranding in the right groin, suggestive of graft infection. The *arrow* demonstrates perigraft stranding and edema tracking to the skin. On exploration, she was noted to have good incorporation of the right limb of the aortofemoral bypass. This was divided, oversewn, and excised, and an obturator bypass was performed from the left limb of the aortofemoral bypass to the right deep femoral artery via a lateral approach to its middle third.

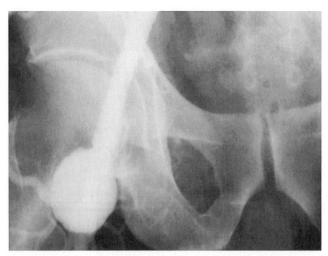

FIGURE 42–3 • Graft infection was first manifested by the development of a false aneurysm.

false-negative result was a patient with an aortoduodenal fistula. The advantage of IgG scanning is that preparation is easier because the patient's own blood is not required for the test and the tracer has a longer half-life.

GASTROINTESTINAL ENDOSCOPY

Endoscopy is a vital diagnostic tool in the evaluation of upper gastrointestinal tract bleeding.[24] A patient with an aortic prosthesis and upper gastrointestinal bleeding must be suspected of having an aortoenteric fistula until proved otherwise. The initial test for this diagnosis is upper gastrointestinal endoscopy, which should be performed expeditiously once the diagnosis of aortoenteric fistula has been considered. The examination must be performed cautiously. The finding of an adherent blood clot in the duodenum confirms the diagnosis, and the patient should be taken immediately to the operating room. If endoscopy does not reveal any pathology, such as bleeding varices, gastritis, or a stomach or duodenal ulcer, an aortoenteric fistula may still be present but not seen. There are some who prefer to examine only the first and second portions of the duodenum; if this part of the study is negative, a presumptive diagnosis of aortoenteric fistula is made. Others prefer to use a smaller endoscope and actually examine the third and possibly the fourth portions of the duodenum. This, however, requires endoscopic expertise and a low threshold for operative exploration should the study be equivocal.

Management of Graft Infection: General Principles

PREOPERATIVE PREPARATION

A patient with ongoing hemorrhage, a patient in hemorrhagic shock from an anastomotic rupture, or a patient with an aortoenteric fistula is managed according to the standard principles of resuscitation. In these categories of patients, there is not much time for preoperative planning, diagnosis, or adjuvant therapy.

Fortunately, most patients with graft infections do not appear emergently, and adequate time is available for diagnostic tests and optimization of conditions for a potentially

extensive operation. The patient and family must understand that treatment may involve a very demanding operation, both physiologically and psychologically. The patient's cardiac and pulmonary status must be evaluated and optimized. Hemodynamic volume status must be optimized. Antibiotic coverage must be initiated to contain the graft infection and prevent progression to sepsis or septic shock. Routine total parenteral nutrition should not be used preoperatively in these patients. In a prospective, randomized trial, the only patients who benefited from preoperative total parenteral nutrition were those who were severely malnourished, as evaluated by the Subjective Global Assessment.[25] Glycemic control is essential, because hyperglycemia causes suppression of neutrophil function; this is one of the factors that predisposes a diabetic patient to infectious complications. Appropriate imaging studies are performed to evaluate possible options for extra-anatomic revascularization or for autogenous in situ reconstruction; these can include CT scan, MRI, IgG scanning, and angiography.

GRAFT EXCISION

A general principle is that if a suture line is involved in the infectious process, this is an absolute indication for removal of the entire infected graft. Any equivocation on the issue of an infected anastomosis inevitably leads to eventual rupture and hemorrhage. Many authorities have advocated conservative treatment consisting of drainage, débridement, and systemic and local antibiotic coverage for the management of perigraft infection, usually limited to inguinal and infrainguinal graft infections. Calligaro and colleagues have been the leading proponents of graft preservation and have been successful in more than 70% of cases.[26] Towne and associates reported on their treatment of 20 infected grafts, 14 of which were aortofemoral grafts.[27] In the 14 aortofemoral grafts, only the femoral limbs were excised; the proximal incorporated segment was left in situ. An interposition polytetrafluoroethylene (PTFE) graft was used to replace the explanted segment. Subsequent graft ultrasonication revealed that 17 of 20 grafts grew *S. epidermidis*, one grew coagulase-positive *Staphylococcus*, and two grafts grew both. All the surgical incisions healed, and graft patency was 100%. There was no limb loss. The authors concluded that biofilm graft infections can be safely treated with in situ replacements. This group recently reported its experience with aortic graft infections, comparing the treatment of 30 consecutive patients. The mean interval from implantation to manifestation of infection was 5.5 years. Complete graft excision with bypass in clean, uninfected planes was performed in 15 patients, and partial or complete graft salvage or in situ graft replacement was performed in 15 patients. The investigators found that perioperative and long-term mortality was no different between the two groups. However, this study is limited by the fact that the sample size was small, raising the possibility of a type II error; also, because it was a retrospective analysis, randomization of the patients did not occur. The authors concluded that in selected patients, local resection of infected graft segments is an acceptable option.

Patients must be carefully selected for attempted graft preservation. The graft anastomosis cannot be involved with infection, and the patient should not demonstrate any systemic signs of sepsis. Tissue coverage of the débrided area can be achieved with a rotational flap or a free flap.[28] In the case of *Pseudomonas aeruginosa* infections, graft salvage is a poor choice. The risk of hemorrhage from anastomotic rupture is significantly higher with these infections. The optimal treatment for an infected graft, particularly one with involvement of the suture line, is still excision of the entire infected graft, with reconstruction through uninfected tissue planes, preferably with autogenous tissue.

Aortoenteric fistulas, particularly aortoduodenal fistulas, require complete excision of the graft and closure of the duodenal wall defect. There is no role for in situ replacement of the graft in the treatment of patients with this entity. Although less extensive procedures have been attempted, the data clearly show that complete graft excision (and, if necessary, placement of an extra-anatomic bypass) is clearly superior. Less extensive procedures are associated with a higher rate of fistula recurrence and death. The graft must be completely excised and the defect in the duodenum oversewn. Given that the best treatment consists of graft excision, closure of the enteric defect, and extra-anatomic bypass, the sequence of these procedures becomes important. In an actively bleeding patient or one in whom the diagnosis has been made at celiotomy, graft excision must precede extra-anatomic bypass. It is often difficult to determine whether a patient needs a remote bypass in such a setting; therefore, the safest approach is to perform immediate revascularization in the majority of cases.

DÉBRIDEMENT

Blowout and late hemorrhage from the proximal aortic stump may occur in some patients after successful excision of the graft. This is most likely due to residual infection in the bed of the graft in the perigraft and para-aortic tissues. The débridement must be generous enough to ensure eradication of all infected tissue. The aorta must then be oversewn in two layers, if possible, with polypropylene sutures. If the infecting organism is of low virulence, removal of the graft is usually all that is necessary. With a more virulent organism, aggressive débridement is a must.

ANTIBIOTIC THERAPY

Preoperative administration of culture-specific antibiotics is ideal. If the infecting organism is not known, broad-spectrum antibiotics, in doses adequate to reach minimal inhibitory concentration, are administered. Some authorities advocate irrigation of tissues with topical antibiotic solution, although its usefulness is questionable.[29] Subsequent therapy with antibiotics should be tailored to culture results. The appropriate duration of antibiotic therapy is unclear. One group advocated at least a 2-week duration of systemic antibiotic therapy.[30] Patients treated with at least 6 weeks of parenteral antibiotics had significantly better outcomes than those treated for 2 weeks or less.

REVASCULARIZATION

Removal of an infected graft usually mandates some revascularization procedure. Reilly and colleagues[30] and Trout and associates[31] conclusively showed that a staged operation, with initial revascularization followed by graft excision in 1 to 2 days,

is associated with significantly less morbidity and mortality. The overall mortality rate was 53% (40 of 75) if graft excision preceded extra-anatomic bypass and 17% (5 of 29) if bypass preceded graft excision. The physiologic stress on the patient is probably decreased with a staged approach, and performing the revascularization before the graft excision obviates the need for systemic heparinization, probably enabling more radical débridement. Throughout this period, systemic antibiotic therapy is continued.

The ideal conduit is autogenous vein or endarterectomy-treated artery. If a prosthetic conduit is chosen for the extra-anatomic bypass, PTFE is preferable to Dacron. Experimental evidence indicates that PTFE is more resistant to bacterial colonization than are other prosthetic conduits[32]; this was validated in a clinical retrospective analysis that discovered a lower infection rate for PTFE compared with Dacron.[33] Towne and coworkers suggested that aortic grafts infected with the low-virulence *S. epidermidis* may, under strict selection criteria, be safely treated with an in situ prosthetic graft composed of PTFE.[27] Over a 9-year period, 28 patients were treated with in situ PTFE grafts for aortoiliofemoral graft infections with *S. epidermidis*. Over a mean follow-up of 4.5 years, there was no mortality, and all grafts remained patent. Two patients had recurrent infection in the proximal limb of the old graft. These data suggest that in carefully selected patients, in situ replacement with PTFE may be safe and effective.

Treatment of Specific Graft Site Infections

AORTIC GRAFTS

When one is faced with an aortic graft infection, a few fundamental points must be addressed. One has to determine whether the aortic graft was performed for aneurysmal or occlusive disease. If the graft was placed for aneurysmal disease, it will be an end-to-end anastomosis; if the graft was placed for occlusive disease, the configuration of the anastomosis may be end to end or end to side. The distal implantation site has to be addressed as well: if the graft goes down to the femoral vessels, revascularization is a bit more involved than if the distal anastomosis is to the iliac arteries.

Aortoiliac and Aortic Interposition Grafts

Aortoiliac graft infections can be treated by preliminary axillobifemoral bypass through uninfected tissue planes, followed by aortic graft excision (Fig. 42-4). This staged approach is associated with significantly less morbidity than the traditional mode of treatment.[30,31] The distal anastomoses can be constructed at both common femoral arteries, because the distal limbs of the aortic graft are confined to the abdomen. This operation can be followed immediately by graft excision; alternatively, graft excision can be performed 1 to 2 days later.

For aortic graft excision, celiotomy is performed, and the aortic graft is isolated. Although systemic heparin is indicated for the axillofemoral bypass, the advantage of the staged operation is that no anticoagulation is necessary during the aortic graft excision. If the procedures are done consecutively, the heparin should be reversed before the aortic

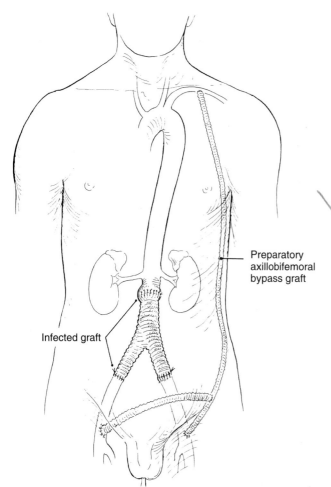

FIGURE 42–4 • Before removing an infected intra-abdominal prosthetic graft, perfusion of the lower extremities is established by an axillobifemoral bypass graft. This technique provides uninterrupted perfusion of the lower limbs and reduces the morbidity associated with ischemic changes that occur when reconstitution of flow is delayed until after the aortic graft has been removed.

graft is approached. Careful dissection in the abdomen is performed, and the graft is separated from adherent bowel and viscera. Once the entire graft is exposed, proximal control is obtained, probably best done at the supraceliac aorta, particularly if there is a proximal anastomotic aneurysm. The iliac arteries distal to the anastomoses are similarly isolated, and control is obtained. The entire graft is then excised, and the aorta is débrided back to normal, healthy-appearing tissue. The aortic stump is then closed with locking monofilament sutures. The distal aorta and iliac arteries are similarly closed. Perigraft tissue that may be infected is carefully but completely débrided. Closed suction drains may be placed. Care is taken to avoid injury to the ureters. If débridement is necessary above the renal arteries, it should be performed without compromise. The renal arteries are then revascularized by antegrade bypasses from one or two of the branches of the celiac axis, such as the hepatic or splenic arteries. Perfusion of the pelvic circulation is maintained by retrograde flow from the axillofemoral bypass through the external and internal iliac arteries. If the distal anastomoses are to the external iliac arteries and require excision, perfusion to at least one

internal iliac artery should be maintained by means of a bypass.

An alternative method of revascularization has been advocated and popularized by Clagett—namely, complete autogenous reconstruction with superficial femoral vein as the conduit.[34] The superficial femoral vein is a large-caliber vein that can be used to reconstruct the aortoiliac or aortofemoral system in a variety of configurations. The advantage of this approach is that the reconstruction is completely autogenous, thereby avoiding the need for extra-anatomic bypass and its poor long-term patency rate. There is a finite complication rate, and the most troublesome complication is compartment syndrome. Approximately one of four patients will need fasciotomy. However, this operation is an excellent option for reconstruction of the infected aortoiliac or particularly aortofemoral prosthesis.

Aortobifemoral Grafts

Although the treatment principles for aortofemoral graft infections are fundamentally the same as those stated previously, the issue of revascularization is more troublesome. This is actually a situation in which the "neoaortoiliac system," with the superficial femoral vein as the conduit, represents an attractive option for reconstruction. However, the distal femoral anastomoses of an aortofemoral graft may preclude the attachment of distal limbs of an extra-anatomic bypass to the common femoral artery. Hence, if a prosthetic bypass via an extra-anatomic route is to be employed, the distal anastomosis of the extra-anatomic bypass must be at the deep femoral artery, the superficial femoral artery, or the popliteal artery. If the graft was performed for occlusive disease in an end-to-side fashion, it may be possible to excise the graft and repair the aortotomy primarily, relying on flow through the native vessels to the lower extremities. Although the native vessels are undoubtedly diseased, there may be adequate flow to avoid the need for immediate revascularization. This is an issue best assessed preoperatively, because an intraoperative assessment of the adequacy of flow may result in the graft's being excised first, with subsequent extra-anatomic bypass if the flow through the native vessels is inadequate. This would be a return to the traditional method of treating infected aortic grafts, an approach that results in increased morbidity.[30]

If the graft infection is localized to the groin and the proximal and distal anastomoses are not involved, graft preservation can be attempted. This is done by draining the abscess, aggressively débriding the perigraft tissues, and ensuring tissue coverage.[26] Patients selected for graft preservation must meet all the previously mentioned criteria. Contraindications to graft preservation techniques include an occluded graft, the presence of sepsis, or a virulent organism, particularly *P. aeruginosa*. Patients treated with graft preservation should be closely monitored in a controlled setting, not on a floor designed for routine nursing care.

If the femoral anastomosis is involved with the infection, that graft limb should be excised. The limb can be approached by means of an ipsilateral retroperitoneal exposure (Fig. 42-5). If the retroperitoneal portion of the graft is well incorporated, proximal control can be obtained at that level and the graft limb excised. All ligation sites should be covered with viable tissue. The graft-artery anastomosis is

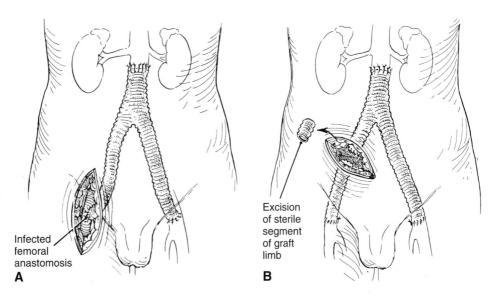

FIGURE 42–5 • Through a retroperitoneal approach, the sterility of the proximal portion of the graft limb is determined. *A,* The sterile graft above is isolated from the area of infection at the groin by excision of a segment of graft and obliteration of the communicating tissue planes between the two areas. *B,* The distal portion of the graft limb is then removed from below after the clean procedure has been carried out in the retroperitoneal space and the wound has been closed.

Infected femoral anastomosis

A

Excision of sterile segment of graft limb

B

excised and the artery débrided. The femoral arteriotomy is then closed with patch angioplasty, preferably with autologous tissue. If a portion of the common femoral artery at that level must be débrided or excised, an attempt should be made to perform an end-to-end anastomosis of the superficial femoral artery to the deep femoral artery to maintain retrograde perfusion of the pelvis. If the proximal anastomosis is involved, the entire graft must be excised according to the principles elucidated earlier.

An extra-anatomic bypass is then fashioned, depending on the need for revascularization of the limb. If only the unilateral limb is excised, the limb can be revascularized by tunneling via a retropubic route or through the obturator canal or by medial tunneling of a femorofemoral bypass. The choice of the vessel for distal bypass depends on the condition of the native vasculature. The bypass conduit has to be routed through clean, uninfected territory (Fig. 42-6). If the entire graft must be excised, an extra-anatomic bypass originating from the axillary artery must be fashioned and anastomosed to the deep femoral artery, the superficial femoral artery, or the popliteal artery (Fig. 42-7). Although some advocate the use of ring-reinforced PTFE grafts to aid in the prevention of external compression of the graft, there is no evidence that this has any merit.

FEMOROPOPLITEAL BYPASS GRAFTS

An infected femoropopliteal bypass graft must be excised in its entirety. The same principles apply, including radical débridement of infected tissue, débridement of the artery to healthy viable tissue, and closure of the artery with monofilament suture. The viability of the limb determines the need for immediate versus delayed revascularization. Should immediate revascularization be needed, it is ideally performed with autogenous vein, and only if the anastomosis is not done in an infected area. Revascularization is performed with adherence to the same principles outlined earlier, with the route of the graft through clean, uninfected tissue.

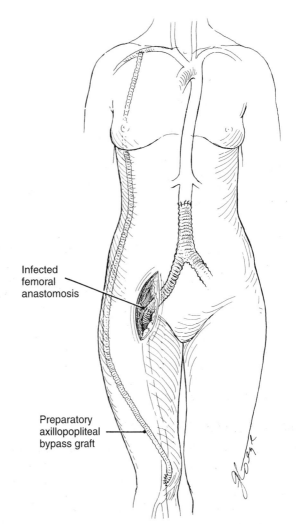

Infected femoral anastomosis

Preparatory axillopopliteal bypass graft

FIGURE 42–6 • Perfusion of an ischemic extremity in the presence of sepsis in the ipsilateral groin is achieved with an axillopopliteal bypass graft. Care is taken to bring the graft wide of the groin through unaffected tissue planes.

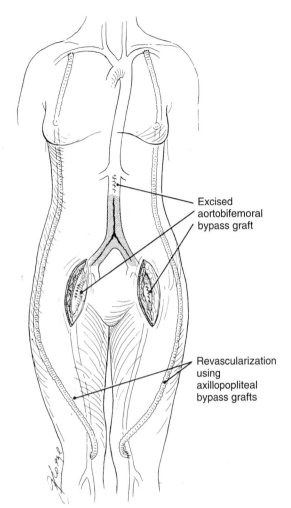

FIGURE 42–7 • Ischemia of the lower extremities, caused by a return to dependence on the native circulation after the removal of an infected aortic graft, can be successfully managed by bilateral axillopopliteal bypass grafts.

Labels in figure: Excised aortobifemoral bypass graft; Revascularization using axillopopliteal bypass grafts

An alternative is to perform a semiclosed endarterectomy of the superficial femoral artery. In the modern era, the technique of subintimal angioplasty allows successful recanalization without the insertion of a foreign body. A more commonly used conduit for bypass in an infected field is cryopreserved cadaver vein graft or cadaver arterial graft. This is probably the best indication for cryopreserved graft; its use in other situations has resulted in very poor patency rates. The advantage of the cadaver vein is its ease of handling, its resistance to infection, and appropriate size matching to the artery. Its principal disadvantages are the significant cost and the poor medium- and long-term patency rates.

ENDOVASCULAR STENT-GRAFTS

There have been a few early reports of endovascular graft infections and their management. Owing to the novelty of the technique, case series and solid guidelines are lacking. The diagnosis can also be uncertain, especially soon after graft insertion. There is a well-described postimplantation inflammatory profile of fever and leukocytosis. Velasquez and colleagues reported on their first 12 patients who underwent endovascular repair with Dacron-covered stent-grafts.[35] A majority of those patients had fever (>101.4°F), leukocytosis,

and CT evidence of perigraft air. All patients became afebrile with resolution of their leukocytosis, and none had any evidence of graft infection on follow-up. Thus, it appears that the early postimplantation inflammatory profile does not represent evidence of graft infection.

Deiparine and associates reported a case of infection of an iliac artery stent that resulted in necrosis of the common femoral artery and severe inflammation of the external iliac artery and the retroperitoneum.[36] The patient survived after a prolonged stay in an intensive care unit and required an above-knee amputation. The authors recommended that endovascular stent or prosthesis placement (or both) be preceded by prophylactic antibiotics; attention to sterile technique is mandatory. Heikkinen and coworkers reported on a patient with a *Listeria* infection of an endovascular bifurcated stent-graft.[37] That patient was treated with resection and débridement of the aorta and in situ replacement with a PTFE graft. Eliason and colleagues reported a case of aortic endograft infection resulting from coil embolization of a type I endoleak.[38] There are many other case reports of aortic endograft infection, one with rupture, that attest to the fact that infection remains a problem even with minimal access aneurysm repair.

The management of graft infections in this setting, in the absence of long-term data, should follow the same principles as the management of any prosthetic graft infection. Clearly, there is not enough long-term experience with endovascular grafting to yield any information about the incidence and pattern of graft infections. However, the consequences can be just as devastating. Meticulous adherence to sterile technique and, perhaps, routine antibiotic prophylaxis should not be neglected in the performance of this less invasive procedure.

Future Directions

In the past few years, there has been a plethora of reports studying the use of a rifampin-bonded aortic prosthesis for the treatment of aortic graft infection. Colburn and colleagues demonstrated the efficacy of collagen-impregnated grafts bonded to rifampin and placed in the bed of an explanted infected graft in a dog model.[39] The use of systemic antibiotics optimized the results and outcome. Subsequent studies have confirmed these findings.[40,41] A prospective, randomized trial in the United Kingdom attempted to define the role of the rifampin-bonded prosthesis in extra-anatomic bypass grafts by studying whether they resulted in a decreased risk of graft infection compared with controls.[42] Two hundred fifty-seven patients were randomized at 14 vascular centers to either rifampin-bonded grafts or regular collagen-impregnated grafts. There was no significant difference in the incidence of graft infection on early follow-up (1 month). In 2000, the 2-year follow-up of these patients was reported.[43] Disappointingly, the infection rate was 4.5%, with six infections in the rifampin-bonded group and four infections in the nonbonded group. There was no significant difference in the rate of graft infection or mortality between the two groups. The authors in the discussion stated that, to date, despite studies on almost 3000 patients, there is no convincing evidence that rifampin bonding decreases the incidence of prosthetic graft infection. As a prevention strategy, this should probably be abandoned.

The underwhelming success of traditional modes of managing graft infections has spurred experimentation with alternative methods, such as selective graft preservation, antibiotic-bonded grafts, and the use of autogenous vein for reconstruction in situ. Our current understanding of graft infection and its causes and treatment is inchoate. Although evolution in the management of graft infection is ongoing and encouraging, the most fruitful endeavor may be an enhanced understanding of the pathophysiologic factors that predispose certain patients to develop graft infection. The interaction of a foreign body with the host and the subsequent response of the host determine the clinical outcome. With a better understanding of this interaction and the disparate responses of different hosts, a more successful attempt at immunomodulation may reduce the incidence of graft infection and its considerable morbidity and mortality.

REFERENCES

1. Johnston KW: Multicenter prospective study of nonruptured abdominal aortic aneurysm. Part II. Variables predicting morbidity and mortality. J Vasc Surg 9:437, 1989.
2. Szilagyi DE, Smith RF, Elliott JP, et al: Infection in arterial reconstruction with synthetic grafts. Ann Surg 175:321, 1972.
3. Bandyk DF: Infection in prosthetic vascular grafts. In Rutherford R (ed): Vascular Surgery. Philadelphia, WB Saunders, 1999, p 737–751.
4. Belletnot F, Chatenet T, Kantelip B, et al: Aseptic periprosthetic fluid collection: A late complication of Dacron arterial bypass. Ann Vasc Surg 2:220, 1988.
5. Bergamini TM, Bandyk DF, Govostis D, et al: Identification of *Staphylococcus epidermidis* vascular graft infections: A comparison of culture techniques. J Vasc Surg 9:665, 1989.
6. Geary KJ, Tomkiewicz ZM, Harrison HN, et al: Differential effects of a gram-negative and a gram-positive infection on autogenous and prosthetic grafts. J Vasc Surg 11:339, 1990.
7. Bjorson HS: Microbiology of surgical infection. In Meakins J (ed): Surgical Infections. New York, Scientific American, 1994.
8. Dougherty S: Prosthetic devices. In Meakins J (ed): Surgical Infections. New York, Scientific American, 1994.
9. Macbeth GA, Rubin JR, McIntyre KE Jr, et al: The relevance of arterial wall microbiology to the treatment of prosthetic graft infections: Graft infection vs arterial infection. Vasc Surg 1:750, 1984.
10. Van der Vliet JA, Kouwenberg PP, Muytjens HL, et al: Relevance of bacterial cultures of abdominal aortic aneurysm contents. Surgery 119:129, 1996.
11. Lalka SG, Malone JM, Fisher DF Jr, et al: Efficacy of prophylactic antibiotics in vascular surgery: An arterial wall microbiologic and pharmacokinetic perspective. J Vasc Surg 10:501, 1989.
12. Malone JM, Moore WS, Campagna G, et al: Bacteremic infectibility of vascular grafts: The influence of pseudointimal integrity and duration of graft function. Surgery 78:211, 1975.
13. Moore WS, Rosson CT, Hall AD, et al: Transient bacteremia: A cause of infection in prosthetic vascular grafts. Am J Surg 117:342, 1969.
14. Moore WS, Malone JM, Keown K: Prosthetic arterial graft material: Influence on neointimal healing and bacterial infectibility. Arch Surg 115:1379, 1980.
15. Moore WS, Swanson RJ, Campagna G, et al: Pseudointimal development and vascular prosthesis susceptibility to bacteremic infection. Surg Forum 15:250, 1974.
16. Larson EL, McGinley KJ, Foglia AR, et al: Composition and antimicrobial resistance of skin flora in hospitalized and healthy adults. J Clin Microbiol 23:604, 1986.
17. Alexander JW, Aerni S, Plettner JP: Development of a safe and effective one-minute preoperative skin preparation. Arch Surg 120:1357, 1985.
18. Lewis DA, Leaper DJ, Speller DCE: Prevention of bacterial colonization of wounds at operation: Comparison of iodine-impregnated ("Ioban") drapes with conventional methods. J Hosp Infect 5:431, 1984.
19. O'Hara PJ, Borkowski GP, Hertzer NR, et al: Natural history of periprosthetic air on computerized axial tomographic examination of the abdomen following abdominal aortic aneurysm repair. J Vasc Surg 1:429, 1984.
20. Olofsson PA, Auffermann W, Higgins CB, et al: Diagnosis of prosthetic aortic graft infection by magnetic resonance imaging. J Vasc Surg 8:99, 1988.
21. Auffermann W, Olofsson PA, Rabahie GN, et al: Incorporation versus infection of retroperitoneal aortic grafts: MR imaging features. Radiology 172:359, 1989.
22. Lawrence PF, Dries DJ, Alazraki N, et al: Indium 111-labeled leukocyte scanning for detection of prosthetic vascular graft infection. J Vasc Surg 2:165, 1985.
23. LaMuraglia GM, Fischman AJ, Strauss HW, et al: Utility of the indium 111-labeled human immunoglobulin G scan for the detection of focal vascular graft infection. J Vasc Surg 10:20, 1989.
24. Champion MC, Sullivan SN, Coles JC, et al: Aortoenteric fistula: Incidence, presentation, recognition, and management. Ann Surg 195:314, 1982.
25. Buzby GP, et al: Perioperative total parenteral nutrition in surgical patients: The Veterans Affairs Total Parenteral Nutrition Cooperative Study Group. N Engl J Med 325:525, 1991.
26. Calligaro KD, Veith FJ, Gupta SK, et al: A modified method of management of prosthetic graft infections involving an anastomosis to the common femoral artery. J Vasc Surg 11:485, 1990.
27. Towne JB, Seabrook JR, Bandyk D, et al: In situ replacement of arterial prosthesis infected by bacterial biofilms: Long-term follow-up. J Vasc Surg 19:226, 1994.
28. Perler BA, Vander Kolk CA, Dufresne CR, et al: Can infected prosthetic grafts be salvaged with rotational muscle flaps? Surgery 110:30, 1991.
29. DiGiglia JD, Leonard GL, Oschner JL: Local irrigation with an antibiotic solution in the prevention of infection in vascular prosthesis. Surgery 67:836, 1970.
30. Reilly LM, Stoney RJ, Goldstone J, et al: Improved management of aortic graft infection: The influence of operation sequence and staging. J Vasc Surg 5:421, 1987.
31. Trout HH, Kozioff L, Giordano JM: Priority of revascularization in patients with graft enteric fistulas, infected arteries or infected arterial prosthesis. Ann Surg 199:669, 1984.
32. Rosenman JE, Pearce WH, Kempczinski RF: Bacterial adherence to vascular grafts after in vitro bacteremia. J Surg Res 38:648, 1985.
33. Bacourt F, Koskas F: Axillobifemoral bypass and aortic exclusion for vascular septic lesions: A multicenter retrospective study of 98 cases. Ann Vasc Surg 6:119, 1992.
34. Gordon LL, Hagino RT, Jackson MR, et al: Complex aortofemoral prosthetic infections: The role of autogenous femoropopliteal vein reconstruction Arch Surg 134:615, 1999.
35. Velasquez OC, Carpenter JP, Baum RA, et al: Perigraft air, fever, and leukocytosis after endovascular repair of abdominal aortic aneurysms. Am J Surg 178:185, 1999.
36. Deiparine MK, Ballard JL, Taylor FC, et al: Endovascular stent infection. J Vasc Surg 23:529, 1996.
37. Heikkinen L, Valtonen V, Lepantalo M, et al: Infrarenal endoluminal bifurcated stent graft infected with *Listeria monocytogenes*. J Vasc Surg 29:554, 1999.
38. Eliason JL, Guzman RJ, Passman MA, Naslund TC: Infected endovascular graft secondary to coil embolization of endoleak: A demonstration of the importance of operative sterility. Ann Vasc Surg 16:562, 2002.
39. Colburn MD, Moore WS, Chvapil M, et al: Use of an antibiotic-bonded graft for in situ reconstruction after prosthetic graft infections. J Vasc Surg 16:651, 1992.
40. Goeau-Brissoniere O, Mercier F, Nicolas MH, et al: Treatment of vascular graft infection by in situ replacement with a rifampin-bonded gelatin sealed Dacron graft. J Vasc Surg 19:739, 1994.
41. Lachapelle K, Graham AM, Symes JF: Antibacterial activity, antibiotic retention, and infection resistance of a rifampin-impregnated gelatin-sealed Dacron graft. J Vasc Surg 19:675, 1994.
42. Braithwaite BD, Davies B, Heather BP, Earnshaw JJ: Early results of a randomized trial of rifampicin-bonded Dacron grafts for extra-anatomic vascular reconstruction: Joint Vascular Research Group. Br J Surg 85:1378, 1998.
43. Earnshaw JJ, Whitman B, Heather BP: Two-year results of a randomized controlled trial of rifampicin-bonded extra-anatomic dacron grafts. Br J Surg 87:758–759, 2000.

Questions

1. Which of the following organisms is most likely to cause graft anastomotic disruption and hemorrhage?
   (a) *Staphylococcus epidermidis*
   (b) *Pseudomonas*
   (c) *Candida*
   (d) All of the above

2. Which of the following statements regarding perigraft air or fluid in the setting of a prosthetic graft is not true?
   (a) Perigraft air 3 months after placement of the graft should raise concern of a graft infection
   (b) Ultrasonography or CT is an acceptable imaging technique for the diagnosis of perigraft fluid
   (c) Graft infections manifesting as perigraft fluid can be appropriately treated by percutaneous drainage of the fluid and long-term antibiotics
   (d) The great majority of patients have complete resolution of perigraft air by approximately 8 to 12 weeks following implantation

3. Which of the following statements regarding *Staphylococcus epidermidis* graft infections is true?
   (a) *S. epidermidis* infections present most commonly with sepsis and hemorrhage
   (b) Revascularization for *S. epidermidis* graft infections may be performed with in-line PTFE grafts
   (c) Routine Gram stain and culture of the graft are usually adequate for establishing the diagnosis
   (d) Extended (>24 hours) perioperative coverage with antibiotics is more effective at preventing graft infections compared with a single preoperative dose

4. The options for reconstruction of an infected aortofemoral bypass graft include all of the following except
   (a) Axillobifemoral bypass
   (b) Autogenous reconstruction with autogenous superficial femoral vein
   (c) Cryopreserved allograft
   (d) Collagen-impregnated Dacron graft

5. Which of the following statements regarding prosthetic graft infection is true?
   (a) Grafts involving the femoral artery have a higher rate of infection than grafts anastomosed to the iliac arteries
   (b) An emergency operation (e.g., for a ruptured abdominal aortic aneurysm) carries an equivalent rate of infection as an elective operation
   (c) The surgeon is the principal and most likely source of the organism infecting the prosthesis
   (d) The mortality of an operation to treat prosthetic aortic graft infection approaches 75% to 80%

6. Examples of extra-anatomic bypass include all of the following except
   (a) Obturator bypass
   (b) Axillopopliteal bypass
   (c) Femorofemoral bypass
   (d) Neoaortoiliac system involving superficial femoral vein

7. Which of the following is not a clinical presentation of graft infection?
   (a) Pseudoaneurysm
   (b) Recurrent graft thrombosis
   (c) Hemorrhage
   (d) Malaise, fever, weight loss
   (e) Neointimal hyperplasia at the proximal anastomosis

Answers

1. b   2. c   3. b   4. d   5. a
6. d   7. e

Glenn C. Hunter • Alex Westerband

Noninfectious Complications in Vascular Surgery

Complications after aortoiliac and peripheral arterial reconstruction often develop and progress rapidly to produce disastrous consequences, including loss of life or limb and major organ failure. They may be the result of technical errors, the extent of the pathologic process, or one or more frequently associated diseases. A timeworn surgical principle applies especially to vascular surgery: "A complication not anticipated is sure to be experienced."

The primary problems reviewed in this chapter are operative bleeding, thrombosis, operative embolization, iatrogenic ureteric injury, major organ failure, graft deterioration, progressing atherosclerotic disease, chylous ascites, anastomotic false aneurysm, and postoperative lower extremity edema.

Aortoiliac Surgery

Complications of aortoiliac arterial reconstruction are similar whether the procedure is for abdominal aortic aneurysmal or occlusive disease.

OPERATIVE BLEEDING

Operative bleeding is most commonly caused by venous injury resulting from venous anomalies and the close anatomic relationship of the aorta and iliac arteries to the inferior vena cava and the inferior mesenteric, left renal, left gonadal, lumbar, and iliac veins (Fig. 43-1).[1] Careful operative dissection, a thorough understanding of the anatomy, and familiarity with the characteristics of major venous anomalies are essential to avoid this complication.[2]

Venous anomalies of the inferior vena cava can involve the subrenal, renal, or suprarenal segments. Subrenal segment anomalies include a left-sided inferior vena cava (prevalence of 0.2% to 0.5%) and a double inferior vena cava (1% to 3%). Either of these anomalies may be associated with a right or, rarely, left retrocaval ureter. When present, the proximal ureter is dorsal to the vena cava and, lower down, runs between the vena cava and the aorta. In rare instances, a double right vena cava has been observed. Anomalies of the renal segment of

the inferior vena cava include retroaortic renal vein (1.7% to 3.4%) (Fig. 43-2) and circumaortic venous rings (Fig. 43-3), in which the retroaortic segment is located in a more caudal position relative to the preaortic segment. Anomalies of the suprarenal segment of the inferior vena cava are extremely rare and are associated with either azygos or hemiazygos continuation and absence of the hepatic venous segment.[3]

The major veins are most vulnerable in the area of tight adherence of the right posterolateral surface of the aorta and common iliac artery to the adjacent wall of the vena cava

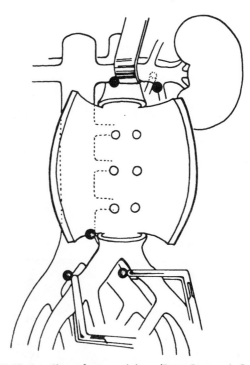

FIGURE 43–1 • Sites of venous injury. (From Downs A: Problems in resection of aortoiliac and femoral aneurysms. In Bernhard VM, Towne JB [eds]: Complications in Vascular Surgery. New York, Grune & Stratton, 1980, p 68.)

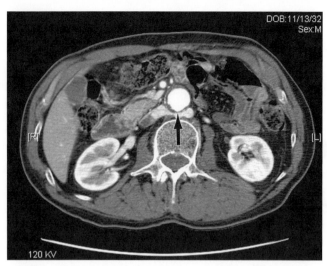

FIGURE 43–2 • Computed tomography scan demonstrating a retroaortic left renal vein *(arrow)* in a patient with an abdominal aortic aneurysm.

and right iliac vein at the level of the aortic bifurcation. Complete separation of these structures by circumferential dissection is generally unnecessary, because temporary occlusion can usually be achieved by clamp control or by the use of intraluminal balloon catheters. If one of these veins is inadvertently lacerated, bleeding should be controlled by gentle finger tamponade, and the venous laceration should be closed with a few stitches of fine monofilament suture. Application of clamps is hazardous and may enlarge the rent in the vein.

The left renal vein should be routinely identified early during dissection of the aorta above an aneurysm or proximal

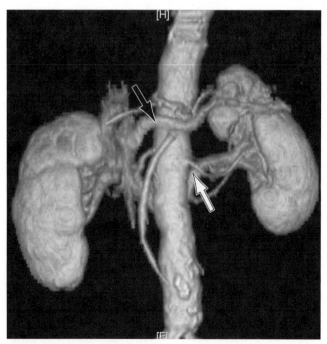

FIGURE 43–3 • Magnetic resonance imaging reconstruction of a circumaortic renal vein *(black arrow)*. Note the caudal position of the posterior branch *(white arrow)*.

to the area of major aortic occlusive disease. The caudal border of the left renal vein should be clearly defined so that this structure can be easily retracted out of harm's way. Division of its lumbar, adrenal, gonadal, or lumbar branches enhances its mobility and improves exposure. Careful consideration should be given to ligating these branches if division of the renal vein is necessary to improve exposure. Failure to find the left renal vein in its usual position suggests its aberrant location behind the aorta (see Figs. 43-2 and 43-3), where it may be readily injured during circumferential dissection of the infrarenal aorta preparatory to application of an occluding clamp.[1,2,4,5]

An arteriovenous (AV) fistula involving the aorta or iliac arteries is an uncommon complication of spontaneous aneurysm rupture into an adjacent vein (about 80% of cases) or of retroperitoneal injury to these major vessels (20%). The incidence of this complication is quite low; it occurs in less than 1% of all aneurysms and in only 3% to 4% of ruptured aneurysms.[6-9] The presence of an AV fistula is suggested by a continuous bruit over the aneurysm associated with the sudden onset of lower extremity venous hypertension, oliguria, hematuria, and congestive heart failure. If suspected, the diagnosis of an aortocaval or iliac AV fistula can be confirmed by color Doppler imaging, computed tomography (CT) scanning, magnetic resonance imaging (MRI), or angiography. The presence of an aortocaval or ilioiliac AV fistula is unsuspected in 25% to 44% of patients at the time of surgery. Occasionally, the fistula may be unsuspected intraoperatively because it is small or obscured by the laminated thrombus within the aneurysm, becoming apparent when sudden massive venous hemorrhage occurs within the lumen of the aorta during evacuation of the laminated thrombus from the aneurysmal sac.[10] In this case, direct finger pressure over the fistula, followed by proximal and distal caval compression with sponge sticks or insertion of balloon occlusion catheters, usually controls the bleeding so that the venous defect can be visualized and closed with a running suture from within the aortic sac (Fig. 43-4).[11] No attempt should be made to separate the aneurysm wall from the cava at the fistula site. In all patients undergoing aortic aneurysm repair, it is wise to palpate the inferior vena cava for the presence of a thrill, indicating an aortocaval fistula, before opening the aneurysm sac to evacuate the laminated thrombus. If a fistula is suspected, the inferior vena cava should be occluded with a sponge stick or a clamp adjacent to the neck of the aneurysm before the aneurysm is occluded and opened, to prevent embolism of clot or air to the lungs.[7]

Intraoperative bleeding from iliac AV fistulas is often more difficult to control because of their location deep within the pelvis, the size of the defect, and the intimate relationship between the vein and artery. Elective placement of occlusion balloon catheters above and below the aneurysm via the femoral vein before entering the aneurysm may control venous bleeding and permit closure of the defect without massive blood loss. Autotransfusion is a useful adjunct in the management of aortocaval and iliac fistulas.[6] Surgical treatment of aortocaval fistulas includes intra-aneurysmal closure of the defect and reconstruction of the aorta with a tube or bifurcated graft. Placement of an endoluminal stent-graft may be the optimal method of treating aortocaval and iliac fistulas when they are recognized preoperatively.[12,13] Prophylactic placement of a venacaval filter is rarely necessary. Complications following surgical repair occur in 39% of patients and include respiratory failure, stroke, myocardial infarction, paraparesis, and renal failure. The perioperative mortality rate ranges from 6% to 71%, with an average of 34%.[11]

Arterial bleeding usually arises from the lumbar, anomalous renal, or inferior mesenteric arteries during circumferential aortic dissection or after the aorta has been opened.[14-16] Lumbar vessel injury can be avoided in aneurysm surgery by limiting the dissection to its anterior surface and by suture ligature of the lumbar orifices from within the sac after the aneurysm has been opened.[9] Precaval location of the right renal artery (5%) and multiple renal arteries (30% to 40%) should be identified. A tear in a fragile aortic wall may occur from suture placement during anastomosis. Additional sutures, frequently with polytetrafluoroethylene (PTFE) pledgets, may be required to control these bleeding points.[1] The aorta should be clamped briefly while additional repair sutures are being placed and tied to avoid further tears in the aortic wall. In patients with unfavorable aortic tissues, the use of biologic tissue glues may, on occasion, be helpful. These agents are no substitute for careful hemostasis, however, and their use is associated with more frequent reoperation for bleeding and the potential for infection.[17,18]

Bleeding in the immediate postoperative period usually comes from suture lines, inadequately ligated lumbar vessels, or the inferior mesenteric vein. This is manifested by a continuing need for blood replacement and the development of a retroperitoneal hematoma. This can be identified by palpating the flank, usually the left, which loses its normal soft concavity and becomes distended and tense. When aortic or iliac suture line bleeding is rapid, shock is more obvious, and the patient complains of severe backache similar to the pain of a ruptured aortic aneurysm. Bleeding owing to unrecognized fibrinolysis, especially after repair of thoracoabdominal aneurysms or supraceliac clamping, is often difficult to diagnose intraoperatively. If supraceliac clamping is anticipated or repair of a thoracoabdominal aneurysm is being undertaken, consideration should be given to the infusion of antifibrinolytic agents such as aprotinin or aminocaproic acid (Amicar). It should be noted, however, that there are no prospective data available for the clinical use of these agents in vascular surgery patients.[19,20]

Postoperative hemorrhage is treated by immediate return to the operating room for identification and control of the bleeding site under fully monitored general anesthesia. Prevention of this complication requires thorough inspection of the intra-abdominal anastomoses and the periaortic area, with special attention to the orifices of the lumbar or anomalous renal vessels, the inferior mesenteric artery, and the ligated or oversewn stumps of the aorta or the iliac vessels. The surgeon should search for the potential bleeding site

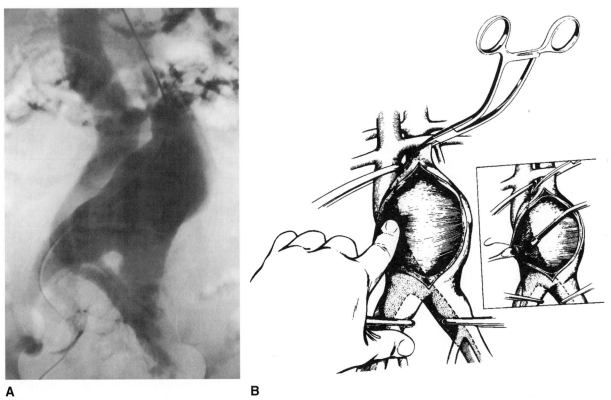

A **B**

FIGURE 43–4 • Aortocaval fistula. *A,* Abdominal aortogram showing filling of the vena cava. *B,* The fistula orifice is exposed through the aneurysm and controlled by simple digital occlusion of the hole into the inferior vena cava. The fistula is closed with a simple over-and-over suture from within the aneurysmal sac. A clear and unencumbered field is provided by rapid aspiration and autotransfusion of blood pouring into the aneurysmal sac from the cava. (*B,* From Bernhard VM: Aortocaval fistulas. In Haimovici H [ed]: Vascular Emergencies. New York, Appleton-Century-Crofts, 1982, p 357.)

when blood volume and pressure are at the patient's normal level before closing the retroperitoneum over the aortoiliac reconstruction.

Bleeding owing to unrecognized coagulopathy usually can be prevented by careful preoperative history and evaluation of the platelet count, bleeding time, prothrombin time, and partial thromboplastin time.[21] These preliminary screening studies reliably identify the need to search for precise factor deficiencies and direct their replacement before and during surgery. Intraoperative monitoring of the activated clotting time before and after heparin administration is the most effective means of identifying variations in the individual response to intraoperatively administered unfractionated heparin and to determine the adequacy of its reversal before closing the incision.[21] Transfusion reaction and disseminated intravascular coagulopathy are rare causes of operative or early postoperative bleeding; however, consumption coagulopathy secondary to massive blood loss and replacement is more common and requires the judicious use of fresh frozen plasma cryoprecipitate and platelets. Proper management of bleeding due to congenital or acquired deficiencies requires repeated monitoring of pertinent coagulation parameters during and immediately after the operative procedure.

The rising number of percutaneous and endovascular interventions being performed has resulted in antiplatelet agents' being administered to increasing numbers of patients. It is not uncommon for patients undergoing coronary or peripheral vessel angioplasty or stenting to receive a combination of drugs, including aspirin, clopidogrel, heparin, and glycoprotein (GP) IIb/IIIa inhibitors such as abciximab, eptifibatide, and tirofibane. Emergency surgical procedures to control bleeding from retroperitoneal hematomas or expanding groin hematomas from cannulation sites can be associated with significant perioperative blood loss into the thigh or retroperitoneum.[22-25]

Although thromboelastography may be a useful adjuvant to therapy, it is not universally available. Discontinuation of the agent and delay of surgery when feasible is sometimes the preferred option. However, should emergency intervention be required, careful replacement of blood coagulation factors and platelet transfusions may be necessary to control hemorrhage.

Recommendations for the discontinuation of antiplatelet agents preoperatively or preprocedurally, although empirical, have to be balanced with the risk of thrombotic occlusion of recently placed stents or stent-grafts. Neilipovitz and colleagues, using decision analysis, showed that the continued use of aspirin reduces perioperative mortality, despite a 2.5% increase in hemorrhagic complications, in vascular surgery patients.[25] The antiplatelet effects of clopidogrel persist for 7 to 10 days, so this drug should be discontinued 1 week before surgery. These recommendations are based on observations from case studies of patients undergoing coronary artery bypass grafting who received aspirin and clopidogrel or aspirin and placebo.[26] Patients receiving both drugs had a higher rate of major postoperative bleeding (9.6% vs. 6.3%), reoperation (9.8% vs. 1.6%), and blood transfusion (3.0 units vs. 1.6 units) compared with patients receiving aspirin and placebo.

The effects of GP IIb/IIIa inhibitors on platelets are quite variable. The antiplatelet effects of eptifibatide are usually abated within 8 hours of cessation of therapy in patients with normal renal function. Abciximab has a biologic half-life of 8 hours, but its effects on the surface of circulating platelets can be detected for up to 2 weeks after discontinuing the drug.[22]

THROMBOSIS

Graft thrombosis in the early postoperative period is almost invariably due to technical problems (Fig. 43-5) that usually occur at the distal anastomoses.[27-29] These include an elevated intimal flap, narrowing of the artery at the anastomotic suture line, failure to remove clot adherent to the inner wall of the graft before completion of the anastomosis, twisting or kinking in the retroperitoneal tunnel, compression of the femoral limb of the graft by the inguinal ligament, unrecognized inflow disease, or inadequate runoff secondary to unappreciated iliac, deep femoral, superficial femoral, or infrapopliteal disease. Rarely, thrombosis after aortofemoral bypass or aneurysm replacement is due to hypercoagulability from antithrombin III deficiency, protein C or S deficiency, a mutation in factor V Leiden or prothrombin genes, homocystinemia, anticardiolipin antibodies, heparin-induced platelet aggregation, or stasis due to reduced cardiac output.[30-33]

The adequacy of pulsatile blood flow through the graft or endarterectomy should be evaluated in the operating room before the wounds are closed, not only by palpation of the graft itself and the arteries immediately distal to anastomoses but also by palpation of distal pulses and direct inspection of the pedal circulation beneath the drapes. If necessary, noninvasive measurements such as Doppler flow, ankle pressure, or pulse-volume recording tracings can be obtained intraoperatively.[27,28,34-36] Intraoperative completion angiograms or color-flow Doppler imaging should be obtained in all patients who have had extensive reconstructive procedures of the common femoral, superficial femoral, or deep femoral arteries to ensure the adequacy of the repair. Noninvasive studies should be performed routinely in the recovery room when pulses cannot be felt distal to the repair or when the anticipated improvement in circulation has not occurred. Objective information obtained from these easily performed studies is particularly valuable in the immediate postoperative period, when patients are frequently hypothermic and peripherally vasoconstricted. Detection of unsatisfactory graft function mandates immediate direct evaluation of the involved anastomoses before wound closure or prompt return to the operating room if graft flow deteriorates subsequently.

Treatment of immediate postreconstructive thrombosis consists of thorough inspection of the intraluminal aspect of the involved anastomosis. This is best accomplished through an incision in the distal end of the graft or by takedown of the anastomosis to directly view the intima and the runoff vessels adjacent to the arteriotomy. Effective revision may require stabilization of an elevated plaque, extension of an iliac limb to the common femoral artery, or patch angioplasty of a deep or proximal superficial femoral stenosis. Infrequently, complementary bypass from the femoral to the popliteal or infrapopliteal vessels may be required when adequate runoff cannot be achieved through the deep femoral artery.[37,38] The lie of the graft should always be inspected throughout its length to ensure that there is no kinking, twisting, or external compression within the retroperitoneal tunnel.

Prevention of early graft thrombosis depends on an accurate evaluation of the distal runoff bed by preoperative noninvasive

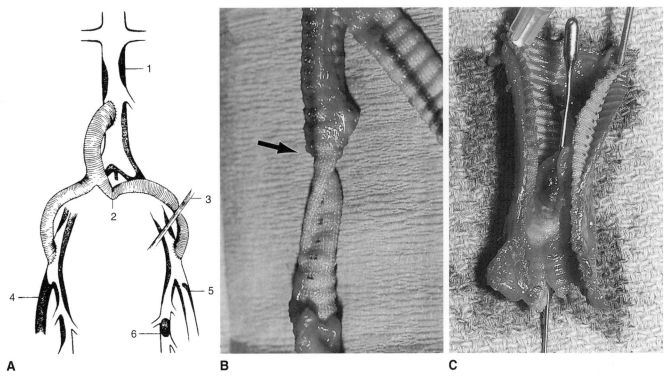

A   **B**   **C**

FIGURE 43–5 • *A*, Aortic mechanical factors that may cause early thrombosis of aortofemoral graft: (1) aortic anastomosis distal to obstructing atherosclerosis at the subrenal level; (2) kinking of the graft limb due to placement of the proximal anastomosis low on the aorta, with an overly long aortic graft segment; (3) compression by the inguinal ligament; (4) inadequate runoff due to occlusion of the superficial femoral artery and severe stenosis of the deep femoral artery; (5) elevation of the distal intima; (6) peripheral embolization or thrombosis. *B*, Operative picture demonstrating a twist in the right limb (*arrow*) of an aortobifemoral graft. *C*, Fibrointimal ingrowth resulting in occlusion of the limb of a bifurcation graft. (*A*, From Bernhard VM: The failed arterial graft: Lost pulses and gangrene. In Condon RE, DeCosse JJ [eds]: Surgical Care. Philadelphia, Lea & Febiger, 1980, p 155.)

hemodynamic testing, magnetic resonance angiography or arteriography, and direct palpation of the iliac artery throughout its length before the selection of this vessel, rather than the femoral, as the site for distal anastomosis. The orifices of the runoff vessels should be inspected and calibrated with dilators. Special attention should be given to the deep femoral orifice, which often requires angioplasty when the distal anastomosis is performed at the common femoral level. Finally, technical perfection in the performance of anastomoses is mandatory to avoid narrowing of the runoff vessels. Tacking sutures may be required to prevent distal intimal dissection.

The widespread use of unfractionated and low-molecular-weight heparin has resulted in an increased frequency of heparin-induced thrombosis, reported to occur in 5% of patients receiving unfractionated heparin and in 0.5% receiving low-molecular-weight heparin with thrombocytopenia. The combination of heparin and platelet factor 4 stimulates an immunologic response manifested by antibodies to platelets, a decreasing platelet count, and a tendency to thrombosis. Heparin-induced thrombocytopenia should be suspected when the platelet count decreases by more than 50% from baseline or drops to 150,000 or less in patients receiving heparin therapy. Thromboembolic complications can involve the deep veins of the lower extremity, the pulmonary arteries, and major cerebral veins. Arterial thrombolic complications may involve the lower extremities and the coronary, mesenteric, renal, or cerebral arteries. When heparin-induced

thrombocytopenia is encountered intraoperatively, the surgeon has to act without confirmatory tests. If it is suspected owing to the presence of "white clots" or unexplained intraoperative thrombosis, a specimen of the thrombus should be sent to the laboratory for a touch prep to confirm the predominance of platelets in the clot. The administration of all unfractionated heparin should be discontinued.[39-41]

Laboratory confirmation using the heparin-induced platelet aggregation or C serotonin assay is an integral part of accurate diagnosis. Therapy with direct thrombin inhibitors such as lepirudin, argatroban, or bivalirudin should be initiated. The use of platelet GP IIb/IIIa inhibitors may also play a role. Alternative anticoagulation with aspirin or warfarin should be administered after the use of direct thrombin inhibitors has been discontinued.

Thrombosis is the most frequent late complication of aortoiliac and aortofemoral procedures[42,43] and usually appears as unilateral limb ischemia.[44-50] Impaired outflow through the external iliac artery or the major branches of the common femoral is the most common cause and is due to progressive downstream atherosclerosis or anastomotic fibrointimal hyperplasia (Fig. 43-6). Anastomotic fibrointimal hyperplasia causes stenosis, usually at distal anastomoses, by the circumferential development of fibrous tissue at the distal graft-artery interface; occlusion occurs when flow diminishes sufficiently to result in stasis thrombosis.[49] The majority of patients initially managed with aortofemoral bypass have occlusion of the superficial femoral artery at the time of the primary procedure.

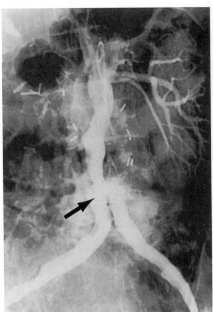

A

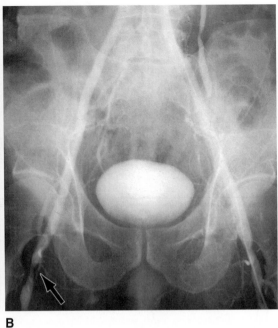

B

FIGURE 43–6 • Progres-sive inflow and outflow obstruction. *A,* Aortogram demonstrating progressive atherosclerosis prox-imal to an incorrectly placed bifurcation graft *(arrow).* *B,* Obstruction due to intimal thickening at the distal limb of an aortobifemoral graft *(arrow).*

Therefore, an adequate lumen at the origin of the deep femoral artery is the most significant factor in ensuring long-term patency of these grafts.[35,43,45,48,50] Underestimating the severity of outflow disease at the time of primary reconstruction is an important cofactor in progressive atherosclerosis that increases susceptibility to late graft limb occlusion.[51] Despite an adequate primary procedure, progression of femoral or infrapopliteal atherosclerotic disease is more likely to occur in patients with continued exposure to atherogenic risk factors, particularly those who continue to smoke.[44,51]

Impaired inflow is the second most common cause of late postrevascularization thrombosis. Although it is four to nine times less frequent than impaired outflow,[51] it is the most common cause of simultaneous bilateral postreconstructive lower limb ischemia after aortoiliac or femoral surgery.[43,46] The most common mechanism is obstruction from progressive infrarenal aortic atherosclerosis proximal to the site of previous repair (Fig. 43-5A). This is usually the consequence of placing the proximal anastomosis too low on the aorta (i.e., at or below the inferior mesenteric artery; Fig. 43-6A). The area between this site and the renal arteries is an active site of progressive atherosclerosis.[35] Likewise, following aortoiliac endarterectomy, late occlusion is more likely if the proximal infrarenal aorta is not included in the endarterectomy.[52] The use of an end-to-end rather than an end-to-side aortic anas-tomosis may be associated with fewer thrombotic failures, although this has not been clearly defined. Superior hemody-namic flow characteristics, the absence of competitive flow, less chance of embolization from the host aorta, and less angulation of the limbs as they arise from the body graft[35,52] have been cited as the advantages of the end-to-end aortic anastomosis.

Angulation of the graft limb at the bifurcation may produce kinking due to failure to pull the graft limb out to full length before the distal anastomoses are performed or excessive length of the graft body, resulting in too wide a bifurcation angle (Fig. 43-5B). Inadequate retroperitoneal tunneling of the graft

limbs may promote thrombosis as a consequence of extrinsic compression from the mesentery of the sigmoid colon or the recurrent portion of the inguinal ligament (Fig. 43-5C).[51]

Less frequent causes of late thrombosis of aortoiliac and femoral reconstructions include accumulation of mural throm-bus and false aneurysm. Mural thrombus develops when the graft diameter is significantly larger than the outflow artery. The flow pattern of the larger graft adjusts itself to the smaller outflow artery, leaving a peripheral layer of slowly moving blood that clots to form the mural thrombus. The normal, smooth, firmly adherent fibrous neointima becomes lined with a thick, gelatinous, loosely adherent mural thrombus that reduces the functioning lumen to the diameter of the outflow vessel. Fragmentation with distal embolization or progressive narrowing of the graft lumen with secondary acute thrombotic occlusion may then occur.[49] Anastomotic false aneurysms, although relatively rare causes of late limb ischemia, may also produce peripheral embolization or thrombosis of the aneurysm and the adjacent vessel lumen.[51] Finally, an aortoiliac reconstruction can progress suddenly to thrombosis in the presence of cardiac embolization or decreased cardiac output secondary to myocardial infarction or congestive heart failure. Rarely, no apparent cause for late thrombosis can be identified, implicating thrombogenicity of the graft surface or degeneration and disruption of the neointima.

The diagnosis of late thrombosis is suggested by the sudden or progressive recurrence of symptoms, a decrease or loss of previously present distal pulses, and a concomitant reduction in ankle pressure, Doppler flow, or pulse-volume recording waveform. The degree of ischemia after thrombosis of a reconstruction is usually more severe than before the primary revascularization procedure.[43,46] The frequency of late thrombosis increases from 5% to 10% in the first 5 years to 20% to 30% at 10 years.[35,50,53-55] Therefore, routine and long-term follow-up of these patients at regular intervals is required to monitor the adequacy of graft function. If significant steno-sis can be demonstrated before complete thrombosis, surgical correction is simplified. When either abrupt or gradual change is apparent, prompt aortography should be performed to determine the status of the graft, the anastomoses, the inflow, and the runoff bed.[34,56]

The severity of recurrent ischemia may range from minimal to severe claudication to rest pain to pregangrene, depending on the extent of compensating collaterals and the vigor of the patient's normal activity. Arteriography is required to determine whether further surgery is feasible and to guide the surgeon in the selection of the most appropriate reoperative or interventional procedure, considering the patient's age, state of health, and general level of activity.[44,51]

Correction of late thrombosis requires preoperative delineation of the underlying mechanical problem, followed by appropriate corrective maneuvers.[51,57] The occlusion of one limb of an aortoiliac bifurcation graft is usually due to overlooked or progressing disease in the external iliac and femoral arteries. Thrombolytic therapy may be useful in delineating the artery involved by the progression of atherosclerosis. Balloon catheter angioplasty with stenting is not usually indicated because of the extent of the disease or location beneath the inguinal ligament. One reliable solution consists of retroperitoneal exposure of the occluded limb, balloon catheter thrombectomy, and graft extension to the femoral level. Femorofemoral bypass is an alternative if the donor iliofemoral inflow is satisfactory, especially in a high-risk patient. Axillofemoral bypass may be required if neither of the preceding methods is feasible.[2,37]

The most commonly encountered situation is a thrombosed aortofemoral graft limb with impaired outflow. Inflow can usually be restored by the use of thrombolytic therapy or graft thrombectomy using a balloon thromboembolectomy catheter (Fig. 43-7).[57] A thromboendarterectomy stripper or adherent clot catheter is often required to complete the

extraction of adherent clot and old pseudointima. The Fogarty occlusion catheter is passed through the ring of the stripper into the patent aortic portion of the graft, and its balloon is fully inflated and pulled down to occlude the proximal end of the limb to control bleeding and prevent crossover embolization. The stripper is passed back and forth around the catheter within the occluded graft limb up to the distended balloon to scrape thrombus from the graft wall. Thereafter, the balloon is deflated just enough to permit its tight withdrawal through the graft limb along with the stripper and detached thrombus (see Fig. 43-7). Use of the Fogarty adherent clot catheter obviates the need for the thromboendarterectomy stripper and may be more effective in removing adherent thrombus. The patient is systemically heparinized (100 to 125 units/kg) during all these maneuvers.

Thrombectomy is usually combined with a profundaplasty of varying extent to provide outflow. However, femoropopliteal or femorodistal bypass may be required, depending on the extent and location of outflow disease.[37,38,57,58] If an occluded graft limb cannot be reopened by thrombectomy, a femorofemoral graft can be inserted. Replacement of the graft limb is another alternative but is technically more difficult. Endovascular options include thrombus removal by catheter aspiration, AngioJet, or some of the newer mechanical devices. These therapeutic modalities are often combined with the use of thrombolytic agents.[59]

If an entire bifurcation graft is thrombosed, a problem at the proximal anastomosis, such as low placement of the graft with progression or unrecognized proximal disease, kinking, or anastomotic aneurysm, is a likely cause. A CT scan is required to identify the last entity. If no proximal problem can be demonstrated, thrombectomy with either a balloon or an adherent clot catheter can be attempted but is usually not successful. The alternatives are to replace the original

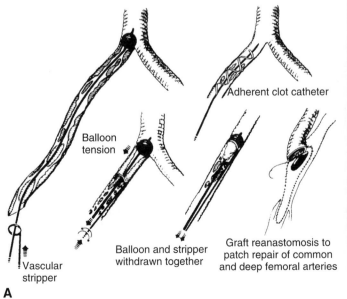

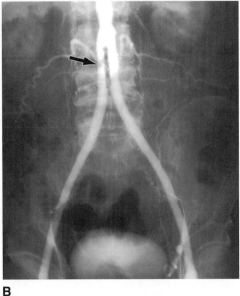

FIGURE 43-7 • *A,* A ring endarterectomy stripper is used in conjunction with a balloon catheter or adherent clot catheter to remove thrombus and pseudointima adherent to the wall of an occluded limb of an aortofemoral graft. The cleared graft limb is then sutured to the common or deep femoral outflow after patch angioplasty. *B,* Intraoperative arteriogram demonstrating residual thrombus (*arrow*) in the proximal right limb of an aortobifemoral graft after attempted thrombectomy. (*A,* From Bernhard VM: Late vascular graft thrombosis. In Bernhard VM, Towne JB [eds]: Complications in Vascular Surgery, 2nd ed. Orlando, Fla, Grune & Stratton, 1985, p 193.)

prosthesis or insert an axillobifemoral bypass. The latter procedure is less technically demanding and less hazardous and is the reoperation of choice in a physiologically compromised patient.[57]

When groin scarring is especially intense, bypass to the mid-deep femoral artery simplifies the outflow repair of the reoperative procedure by avoiding a tedious and hazardous dissection in the area of a previous femoral anastomosis.[60]

An aggressive attitude toward reoperation after thrombotic failure of aortoiliac reconstruction is warranted, especially if the patient will derive sustained benefit from long-term patency and improved limb function.[57] Operative morbidity and mortality rates are low. Reoperative mortality rates of 3% and cumulative 3-year patency rates of 68% to 75% have been reported.[43,57] Judicious use of extra-abdominal approaches has contributed significantly to reduced reoperative morbidity and mortality.[51]

Lytic Therapy for Graft Thrombosis

Whereas thrombectomy has been the treatment of choice in the management of occluded aortofemoral and femoropopliteal bypass grafts, incomplete removal of thrombotic material and the difficulties associated with reoperation have led to the evaluation of direct intra-arterial infusion of thrombolytic agents, either preoperatively or intraoperatively, for the management of this problem.[61] The potential benefits of lytic therapy include delineation of the cause of the graft thrombosis (most commonly distal occlusion due to neointimal fibrous hyperplasia or progression of disease) and, as a consequence, a shorter operation, reduced blood loss, ease of extracting any residual thrombus, and reduced wound complication rate. Potential disadvantages and complications of thrombolytic therapy include the need for monitoring in an intensive care unit, delay in surgical intervention, and risk of bleeding or renal impairment from the contrast load required for frequent arteriographic evaluation.

Further, mechanical thrombectomy for aortofemoral graft limb occlusion is at least as effective as clot lysis and adds little to the operative procedure required to restore outflow. Successful lysis, which does not appear to be affected by the duration and cause of the graft thrombosis, can be achieved in 50% to 90% of occluded prosthetic graft limbs, 50% to 77% of saphenous veins, and 38% to 71% of prosthetic grafts.[62-67]

Thrombolytic agents enzymatically break down cross-linked fibrin strands within the thrombus by converting plasminogen to plasmin. Streptokinase, the first agent to beome available, is seldom used to treat arterial or graft thrombosis. Urokinase was, for years, the agent of choice until it was withdrawn from the market. Alteplase or reteplase and, more recently, tenecteplase are currently being evaluated.

Infusion of the thrombolytic agents is usually accomplished by a multi-side-hole catheter or an infusion wire placed so that it covers the extent of the thrombus. There are multiple dosage regimens advocated for the use of these agents. Urokinase is usually given in a dose of 80,000 to 100,000 units/hour, reteplase at 0.25 to 1 unit/hour, alteplase at 0.25 to 10 mg/hour, and tenecteplase at 0.25 to 0.5 mg/hour. Heparin in a dose of 300 to 500 units/hour is usually administered through the access sheath to prevent pericatheter thrombosis.[68-72]

Patients are carefully comonitored in the intensive care unit for evidence of bleeding. Blood is drawn for hemoglobin, hematocrit, fibrinogen, prothrombin time, and partial thromboplastin time every 4 to 6 hours. Following successful lysis, the underlying lesion is treated with either catheter-based techniques or surgery. Long-term anticoagulation with warfarin is usually indicated.

Bleeding, the major complication of lytic therapy, occurs after 7% to 48% of infusions.[65,73] The most common sources of bleeding are arteriography or venous puncture sites, the interstices of prosthetic grafts, and systemic bleeding from remote sites. Central nervous system bleeding is rare with urokinase. Bleeding from a groin arterial puncture site may also result in femoral pseudoaneurysm or retroperitoneal hematoma, which may compress the femoral nerve within the iliac fascia or in the thigh. The resulting femoral neuralgia, reported to occur in up to 30% of patients, may persist for as long as 1 year.[74,75] Rarely, patients develop a femoral nerve palsy; this may be debilitating, especially in patients with claudication or amputation of the contralateral limb.

The most important determinant of long-term success in the study by Gardiner and coworkers was the presence of a lesion correctable by surgical revision or balloon catheter dilatation.[76] Such lesions responsible for the occlusion can be identified in approximately 50% of patients. Gardiner and coworkers reported an 84% 1-year patency rate in 25 grafts with underlying stenotic lesions, compared with 37% of a similar number of grafts without detectable lesions.

Three prospective studies compared the efficacy of intra-arterial thrombolysis and surgery in patients with lower limb ischemia.[77-79] In their initial study, Ouriel and colleagues randomized 114 patients with acute lower limb ischemia of less than 7 days' duration to receive either thrombolytic therapy or surgery.[77] The authors achieved clot dissolution in 70% of their patients and observed no difference in limb salvage rates (82%) at 1 year. However, they did observe improved patient survival (82% vs. 58%) in the patients receiving thrombolytic therapy, which they attributed to the more frequent occurrence of cardiopulmonary complications in the patients undergoing surgery. In a subsequent study, Ouriel and associates randomized 213 patients with acute limb ischemia of less than 14 days' duration to either recombinant urokinase or surgery.[78] Clot lysis was achieved in a similar number of patients (71%). The authors found no differences in either mortality rates (14% vs. 16%) or amputation-free survival rates (75% vs. 65%) between the two groups at 1 year. In the Surgery versus Thrombolysis for Ischemia of the Lower Extremity (STILE) trial,[79] the efficacy of recombinant tissue plasminogen activator (rt-PA) and urokinase was compared with that of surgery in 393 patients with limb ischemia of less than 6 months' duration. Failure of catheter placement occurred in 28% of patients. Patients with ischemia of less than 14 days' duration receiving lytic therapy had lower amputation rates than did surgical patients, whereas patients with ischemic symptoms of more than 14 days' duration fared better with surgery. The results of these studies suggest that in selected patients, thrombolytic therapy may be a useful adjunct or alternative to surgical therapy. However, long-term patency rates of 28% to 37% of thrombolysed grafts are clearly inferior to those obtained with surgery.[76,80] Thrombolytic therapy may be extremely valuable in patients with limb-threatening ischemia secondary to thrombosed popliteal aneurysm. Thrombolysis may improve the chances of achieving long-term patency and limb salvage.[81]

Although there have been no large trials evaluating alteplase in the treatment of peripheral arterial occlusion, anecdotal reports suggest an increased incidence of local and remote bleeding, predominantly intracranial hemorrhage, with its use. Recently, the use of limited doses of alteplase was shown to be equivalent to urokinase in terms of the incidence of bleeding and mortality. Shortell and colleagues, in a comparison of limited-dose t-PA and urokinase, demonstrated improved clot lysis (76% vs. 50%) with t-PA at a dose of 2 mg/hour, for a total of 100 mg.[69] The agents were equivalent in unmasking stenoses (85% vs. 84%), but t-PA was superior to urokinase in unmasking runoff vessels (81% vs. 39%).

Reteplase, a nonglycosylated deletion mutant of t-PA, is an attractive alternative to urokinase. Reteplase catalyzes the cleavage of endogenous plasminogen to generate plasmin, which degrades the fibrin matrix of the thrombus, resulting in its dissolution. The half-life of reteplase is 13 to 16 minutes, and catheter-directed infusion doses vary between 0.25 and 1.0 unit/hour for a duration of 5 to 24 hours. Lacing or infiltrating the thrombus with a 2- to 5-unit bolus dose may be beneficial in some patients.[82] In approximately half of patients, low-dose heparin is infused concomitantly. Reteplase differs from alteplase both in its structure and biochemical composition and in its lower affinity for thrombin.

McNamara reported a 34% incidence of bleeding in a series of 40 patients treated with alteplase, compared with 3% among those receiving reteplase at doses of 2 to 8 mg/hour.[83] Even reducing the dosage of alteplase to 0.5 to 1 mg/hour was still associated with a 25% incidence of bleeding requiring transfusion.

The indications for and contraindications to the use of these two agents are similar to those of urokinase. Allie and colleagues reported a 95.8% procedural success rate, with a mean infusion time of 7.5 hours and a lower complication rate, using a combination of tenecteplase and postprocedural tirofiban.[68] In all cases, the risks and benefits of the use of lytic therapy in the treatment of patients with graft limb occlusions must be carefullly evaluated.

The relatively low incidence of complications, improved technique of administration, and efficacy of thrombolytic agents have reduced the need for urgent thrombectomy in patients with noncritical limb ischemia. Successful lytic therapy readily identifies the cause of the graft limb occlusion and may allow a less extensive repair. In addition, lytic therapy may reduce the risk of wound and graft complications and reduce the incidence of reperfusion edema associated with extensive redo procedures.

Mechanical Thrombectomy

Mechanical thrombectomy devices that theoretically permit rapid revascularization of an ischemic extremity using minimally invasive techniques are gaining in popularity. The use of mechanical energy to cause fragmentation, dissolution, and aspiration of thrombus is appealing. These devices can be broadly classified into (1) aspiration thrombectomy catheters that remove thrombus by steady manual suction through a large-lumen aspiration catheter; (2) pull-back thrombectomy catheters that withdraw thrombus with a balloon catheter or basket into a trapping device, allowing the clot to be removed; (3) recirculation thrombectomy devices that ablate thrombus by hydrodynamic vortices, which pulverize the thrombus into microscopic fragments; (4) nonrecirculation thrombectomy devices, which macerate the thrombus mechanically into fragments that are larger than those produced by recirculation catheters; and (5) energy-assisted devices, which use either ultrasound, laser, or radiofrequency to lyse thrombus or enhance the effects of pharmacologic agents.[84] Most of these devices presently have U.S. Food and Drug Administration approval only for use in occluded hemodialysis grafts. A number of these devices are currently being evaluated clinically, with complete angiographic success reported in approximately 50% of patients and partial success in an additional 27%.[85] Concomitant lytic therapy or balloon angioplasty is often a necessary adjunct. The most extensively studied device is the AngioJet rheolytic thrombectomy system, which is approved for peripheral arterial and coronary applications.[86] Adjunctive low-dose thrombolysis is necessary in 18% to 58% of patients. Chief disadvantages of the current device include the possibility of renal overload and hemolysis. The major treatment limitation of these devices is their lack of efficacy against organized thrombotic or embolic material.[59] The recent report by Sarac and colleagues suggests that the combination of a lytic agent and a mechanical device may be as effective as thrombolytic dissolution of the thrombus.[86a]

OPERATIVE EMBOLIZATION

Atherothrombotic debris is present to some degree in most atherosclerotic arteries and especially in the distal aorta. Protruding atheromas of the aortic arch and descending aorta have assumed increasing importance as potential sites for embolization during cardiac catheterization or bypass surgery.[87] Readily detectable by transesophageal echocardiography, lesions larger than 0.5 cm are most likely to be associated with embolic events.[88,89] Variable amounts of this material may be dislodged and carried into the downstream arterial territory as a consequence of manipulation during arterial dissection.[34,89,90] Embolization may also occur on reestablishment of circulation owing to the accumulation of fresh thrombus in the temporarily static blood column above or below the clamps if it is not carefully evacuated before circulation is restored.

Larger emboli lodging in major vessels can usually be retrieved with a balloon thrombectomy catheter. Smaller embolic particles that cannot be retrieved will be flushed into end arteries of the feet or toes, leading to the "trash foot" syndrome.[1,34,89,90] The end result is the appearance of patchy areas of painful skin gangrene at these sites (Fig. 43-8). This may be a minor and self-limited problem, or it may produce extensive gangrene of all the digits and the forefoot, leg, buttocks, and, rarely, abdominal wall.

Prevention is key, because it is frequently difficult or impossible to treat this complication. A variety of technical maneuvers have been employed to prevent operative embolization.[1] Unnecessary and overly vigorous handling of vessels before the application of clamps should be avoided. Effective preclamping heparinization, preferably monitored by intraoperative measurement of the activated clotting time, reduces stasis thrombus formation above the proximal clamp and in the sluggish circulation distally. In patients with suspected or demonstrable atheromatous debris within the aorta on CT scans, the distal clamps should be applied to the common femoral or iliac arteries before proximal occlusion to avoid downstream displacement of debris when the aortic

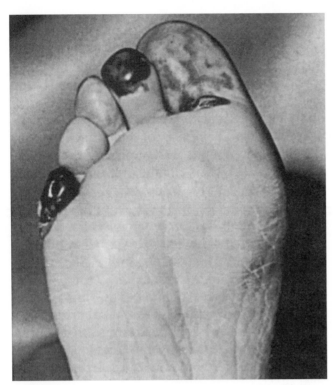

FIGURE 43–8 • Atheroembolic ischemic lesions of the toes. (From Eastcott HHG: Complication of aortoiliac reconstruction for occlusive disease. In Bernhard VM, Towne JB [eds]: Complications in Vascular Surgery. New York, Grune & Stratton, 1980, p 59.)

clamp is placed. The proximal clamp may need to be placed at the level of the diaphragm if the pararenal segment of the aorta appears to be involved. The lumen of the aortic prosthesis should be thoroughly aspirated to remove blood and debris after testing the proximal suture line, and efforts should be made to prevent the accumulation of blood within the prosthesis while distal iliac or femoral anastomoses are being performed. Vigorous prograde flushing of the proximal vessel and retrograde flushing from the distal arteries as the last few stitches are being placed in an anastomosis, before the restoration of circulation, is the most reliable maneuver to ensure that retained debris and clot are effectively removed.[90]

Treatment depends on the severity of embolization. Minor patchy areas of cyanosis or necrosis can be observed, with spontaneous recovery anticipated. More extensive involvement with threatened viability of the distal foot requires attempted removal of embolic material with small Fogarty catheters passed into the distal vessels through the patent popliteal artery, accompanied by distal intra-arterial infusion of urokinase or rt-PA. Occasionally, when there is severe ischemia of a single or multiple digits, lumbar sympathectomy or amputation may be necessary. In patients with a patent superficial femoral artery and severe forefoot ischemia, intra-arterial lytic therapy may reduce the level of amputation.

DECLAMPING HYPOTENSION

A sudden decrease in blood pressure should be anticipated after removal of the aortic clamp to restore flow to one or both extremities after aortoiliac reconstruction.[91-94] The cause is hypovolemia due to incompletely replaced blood loss and fluid sequestration during surgery, compounded by a variable degree of preoperative dehydration that is usually present.[15] Contributing factors are peripheral vasodilatation secondary to limb ischemia during the period of aortic occlusion and a decrease in cardiac output caused by a sudden return of acidic blood and other vasoactive metabolites to the central circulation on restoration of limb perfusion. The major consequences are significant reduction in coronary perfusion, which may promote myocardial injury, especially in patients with significant coronary artery disease, and temporary renal ischemia, which may contribute to renal failure. Prevention is preferable to treatment after a hypotensive insult has already occurred and depends on adequate hydration and effective restoration of intravascular volume during the procedure, and especially before clamp release.[93-95] Effective volume replacement requires careful monitoring of blood loss and accurate estimation of the extracellular fluid shifts due to sequestration and loss from evaporation. The extent of intravascular depletion is directly related to the duration of intraperitoneal and retroperitoneal exposure during surgery.

The most reliable guide to ensuring adequate volume replacement without circulatory overload is the use of a Swan-Ganz catheter to monitor left heart filling pressures and myocardial performance.[95] Cooperation between the surgeon and the anesthesiologist is essential during the critical moments before clamp release. Left atrial filling pressures should be optimized before release of the clamps. The arterial pressure must be continuously observed while blood flow is slowly restored to the extremities by gradual release of the clamp until full flow can be tolerated without hypotension. Finally, when a bifurcation graft is inserted, it is best to complete the anastomosis to one limb and restore its circulation immediately so that lower body perfusion can be resumed with the least amount of delay; this avoids washout acidosis and reduces declamping hypotension.

RENAL FAILURE

Acute renal failure (ARF) accompanying aortic surgery has a major impact on operative mortality. The reported incidence of ARF following elective aortic aneurysmectomy is 1% to 8%, with a mortality rate of 40%. However, if the aneurysmectomy is emergent, the reported incidence of ARF is 8% to 46%, with a mortality of 57% to 95%.[96,97] The major cause is reduced renal perfusion due to decreased cardiac output, decreased blood volume, and dehydration. A contributing factor is renal cortical vasospasm produced by infrarenal application of the aortic clamp, which stimulates the renin-angiotensin mechanism.[98,99] Other promoting factors include suprarenal aortic cross-clamping, which totally eliminates renal perfusion; ligation of the left renal vein; and intraoperative renal arterial embolization.[100] The last may originate from debris and clot accumulating proximal to the aortic clamp or from manipulation of the juxtarenal aorta.[97,101] Renal artery obstruction may be produced by displacement of large atherosclerotic plaques at the orifices of the renal arteries when an aortic clamp is applied. Preoperative angiography or CT may produce a mild to moderate degree of renal dysfunction, which can be compounded by hypotension and dehydration during the operative procedure.[97] Myoglobinemia can occur after restoration of circulation to limbs that have been severely ischemic for an extended period.

Finally, nephrotoxic antibiotics and contrast agents employed perioperatively must be considered.

Although the consequences of ischemic injury to the kidney are complex, injury to the tubules is central to the development of oliguria. Obstruction of the tubular lumen by cellular debris and casts results in reduction of the ultrafiltration pressure and sequestration of tubular fluid within obstructed tubules, in addition to back-leak of fluid into the interstitium.[102]

The critical issue is prevention, which is related primarily to the maintenance of an effective circulating blood volume and adequate hydration in the immediate perioperative period.[97,103] It is essential that the patient be well hydrated and have a good urinary output at the commencement of surgery. Any significant extracellular fluid volume deficits should be restored the evening before surgery, especially if angiography, CT, or a mechanical bowel preparation has been performed recently. The creatinine level should be measured after procedures requiring contrast administration, and if a decrease in renal function is identified, surgery should be delayed, if possible. Central filling pressures should be monitored perioperatively to ensure that volume replacement is optimal in relation to cardiac output and myocardial performance.[95] It is appropriate to give mannitol and commence an infusion of renal-dose dopamine just before cross-clamping the aorta to promote an osmotic diuresis and reduce the effects of renal cortical vasospasm.[98] Bicarbonate is given to alkalinize the urine if there is any question of significant myoglobin washout from renewed perfusion of limbs that have undergone prolonged ischemia. Renal insufficiency is a significant complication of surgical procedures requiring cross-clamping of the suprarenal aorta. Currently, a number of therapeutic maneuvers, including fluid loading, calcium channel blockers,[104] atrial natriuretic peptide, insulin-like growth factor,[105] urodilatin,[106,107] endothelin antagonists,[108] and fenoldopam,[109] are being evaluated to determine their efficacy in reducing the incidence of ARF.

During dissection required to gain proximal control of large infrarenal or juxtarenal aneurysms, the left renal vein is vulnerable to injury. Access to this portion of the aorta is facilitated by division of the left renal vein.[110] In the past, this maneuver was viewed as one of little long-term consequence. However, Huber and coworkers[111] and Abu Rahma and associates[112] demonstrated increased serum creatinine concentrations in patients who had renal vein ligation. Whether the renal dysfunction following renal vein ligation is solely a consequence of the resultant increased venous pressure or develops from a combination of venous hypertension and transient ischemia from intraoperative suprarenal clamp placement (which is required more frequently in these patients) is not yet clear. Nonetheless, it is prudent to repair the renal vein if there is congestion of the left kidney and reanastomosis can be accomplished without undue tension.[110,113,114]

Renal arteries should be dissected free and temporarily clamped in patients with total aortic occlusion and thrombus that extends up to the renal orifices. The quality of the renal pulses must be evaluated and the blood flow assessed by Doppler color-flow imaging after restoration of circulation through the aorta in any patient who has had significant juxtarenal aortic manipulation or if urine output suddenly diminishes. Immediate renal repair is required if renal artery occlusion is identified.

Postoperatively, the continued retroperitoneal and intraperitoneal sequestration of extracellular fluid requires replacement with Ringer's lactate solution, within the limits imposed by left heart filling pressures, to ensure adequate renal output.[15] Volume replacement should be reduced after the second postoperative day to prevent fluid overload from the mobilization of large volumes of sequestered extravascular fluid. The urinary output is monitored continuously and should be maintained at or above 0.5 mL/kg per hour. The specific gravity is determined frequently, and the blood urea nitrogen and creatinine are measured daily for 2 or 3 days to determine the quality of renal function. Diuretics should not be given until intravascular volume has been fully restored. If ARF is diagnosed, fluid replacement should be restricted to maintain central filling pressure in the normal range. Dialysis is used aggressively to control excess volume and relieve azotemia and hyperkalemia.[97,115] Intravenous hyperalimentation or parenteral nutrition should be instituted early in the clinical course of patients with ARF to minimize protein catabolism.[116]

Renal artery stenosis or impaired renal function is frequently present in patients undergoing aortic reconstruction for occlusive and aneurysmal disease. The liberal use of CT, magnetic resonance angiography, or aortography before surgery is recommended to identify renal anomalies, renal artery stenoses, or suprarenal extension of an aneurysm so that appropriate alterations in operative management can be planned. Often, renal revascularization can be accomplished by balloon angioplasty and stenting along with operative or endovascular correction of the aortic disease. In this setting, patients often have impaired renal function, and the considerable volume of contrast agents used for imaging studies or intervention may result in additional nephrotoxicity. The preoperative administration of acetylcysteine has been shown to reduce contrast-related ARF from 12% to 2% to 4%.[117,118] Additional maneuvers to reduce the risk of renal ischemia include the use of temporary renal perfusion with cold lactated Ringer's solution containing heparin, mannitol, and methylprednisolone.[97] Postoperatively, a renal scan or aortography should be performed immediately if total renal shutdown appears, because this suggests a renal artery occlusion. This requires immediate reoperation to restore kidney circulation.

INTESTINAL ISCHEMIA

Intestinal ischemia may complicate aortic bypass or endarterectomy for occlusive disease, but the majority of cases follow aneurysmectomy.[119,120] Almost all reported instances of intestinal ischemia following aortic surgery are a result of arterial obstruction; venous ischemia is extremely rare.[121] Small bowel ischemia occurs in 0.15% of cases.[119] The clinical presentation of ischemic colitis occurs in 0.2% to 10% of aortic procedures and most commonly involves the rectosigmoid area.[122] However, if routine colonoscopy is performed, a much higher incidence of intestinal ischemia is noted because of the identification of subclinical ischemic colitis. Hagihara and associates found a 6% incidence of ischemic colitis in patients undergoing elective or urgent reconstruction of the abdominal aorta for aneurysmal or occlusive disease, whereas the incidence was 60% following repair of ruptured aneurysms.[123] The overall mortality rate for patients with colon ischemia is approximately 50% and approaches 90% for transmural colon involvement.

The cause of bowel ischemia is operative atheroembolization or interruption of the primary or collateral arteries to the bowel wall.[119,120] Two sets of vessels are critical to colon perfusion: (1) the superior rectal branch of the inferior mesenteric artery, which connects with the middle and inferior rectal branches of the hypogastric vessels, thus connecting the visceral and systemic circulations; and (2) the inferior mesenteric artery and its left colic branch, which connect with the superior mesenteric artery through the arch of Riolan and, to a lesser extent, the marginal artery of Drummond.[122] The former connection is referred to as the "meandering mesenteric artery," especially when it becomes enlarged as a collateral to compensate for superior or inferior mesenteric artery obstruction.[124] This vessel is present in about two thirds of normal people and can be seen on angiography in 27% to 35% of patients who have aneurysmal or occlusive disease.[125] Areas of deficiency in this normal anatomic relationship are at Griffith's point at the splenic flexure and in the collateral vessels of the rectosigmoid (Fig. 43-9).

Obstruction of the primary arteries supplying the viscera makes viability of the bowel dependent on this collateral circulation. Occlusion of the orifice of the inferior mesenteric artery is frequently associated with aneurysmal disease and obstructive aortic atherosclerosis, thus placing the burden of bowel circulation on collaterals from the superior mesenteric artery and the hypogastric vessels. Severe obstruction or occlusion of the superior mesenteric artery is compensated for by branches from the celiac artery and retrograde flow from the inferior mesenteric artery through the left colic and middle colic arteries. Hypogastric obstruction requires collateral flow from branches of the inferior mesenteric artery. When this source is also impaired, colon circulation must depend on more tenuous connections between the arch of Riolan and the marginal artery and the distal branches of the hypogastric, which in turn derive their blood supply from the parietal circulation.

A critical loss of blood flow to an intestinal tract that is dependent on this extensive collateral network may occur if a patent inferior mesenteric artery is ligated during aortic surgery. Collateral flow may be further compromised by ligating the inferior mesenteric artery peripherally rather than flush with the aortic wall, because this may occlude the connection between the left colic and superior rectal arteries. Failure to ensure perfusion through at least one hypogastric may promote colon ischemia if this is the primary supply in the absence of the inferior mesenteric artery or effective collateral flow from the meandering artery. Loss of the inferior mesenteric artery or the meandering artery produces right colon and small bowel ischemia when these viscera depend on retrograde flow because of superior mesenteric arterial occlusion (Fig. 43-10). The large hematoma associated with a ruptured aneurysm may compress significant collateral vessels, which may explain the high incidence of colon ischemia in this circumstance.[119] Further, angiography is almost never available before repair of a ruptured aneurysm, and the surgeon has no precise information regarding intestinal circulation to allow the design of an operative procedure that will conserve or augment colon perfusion. A relatively unrecognized cause of mesenteric ischemia is cardiopulmonary bypass. Although acute ischemia occurs in only 0.49% of patients, visceral ischemia is a significant contributing factor in 11% of deaths after coronary revascularization. Preexisting visceral occlusive disease, cardiac or aortic arch embolization, use of an intra-aortic balloon, postoperative renal failure, duration of cardiopulmonary bypass, and cross-clamp times are important contributing factors.[126]

Depending on the severity of ischemia and the thickness of the bowel wall involved, three forms of ischemic colitis are recognized. Type I is mucosal ischemia, which is transient and mild. Type II, with mucosal and muscularis involvement, reflects more severe ischemia that may result in healing with fibrosis, scarring, and stricture. Type III is transmural ischemia, which produces irreparable damage with gangrene and bowel perforation.[127]

The clinical manifestations of intestinal ischemia immediately after aortic surgery are often masked by incisional discomfort and other problems that may explain abdominal pain, tenderness, fever, an elevated white blood cell count, and fluid sequestration. Findings that suggest the presence of intestinal ischemia and progressing infarction of the colon include progressive distention, sepsis, increasing peritoneal signs, and unexplained metabolic acidosis. The most common clinical presentation is diarrhea, either brown liquid or bloody, which occurs in 65% to 76% of patients with intestinal ischemia.[122,128] Although the onset may occur as long as 14 days after operation, diarrhea usually appears within 24 to 48 hours after surgery.[122] Bloody diarrhea has been reported to be a more ominous prognostic sign than nonbloody diarrhea[129]; however, some investigators have noted no correlation between extent of ischemic injury and presence of bloody diarrhea.[129]

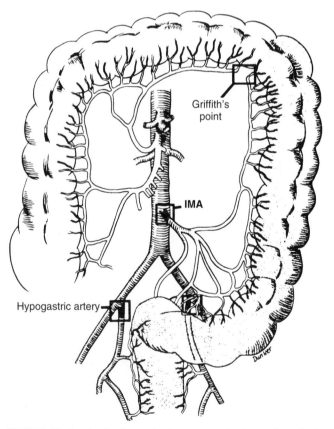

FIGURE 43–9 • Lack of marginal artery continuity at the splenic flexure (Griffith's point), with inferior mesenteric artery (IMA) and hypogastric artery occlusions predisposing to left colon ischemia. (From Ernst CB: Colon ischemia following abdominal aortic reconstruction. In Bernhard VM, Towne JB [eds]: Complications in Vascular Surgery. New York, Grune & Stratton, 1980, p 383.)

FIGURE 43–10 • *A*, When the superior mesenteric artery (SMA) is occluded, meandering mesenteric blood flow is from the inferior mesenteric artery (IMA) to the SMA. Meandering mesenteric sacrifice under these conditions predisposes to small bowel as well as colon ischemia. *B*, Selective visceral angiogram demonstrating a meandering mesenteric artery. (*A*, From Ernst CB: Colon ischemia following abdominal aortic reconstruction. In Bernhard VM, Towne JB [eds]: Complications in Vascular Surgery. New York, Grune & Stratton, 1980, p 385.)

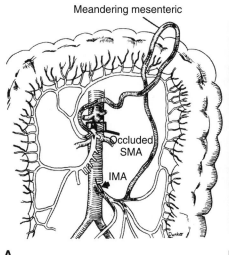

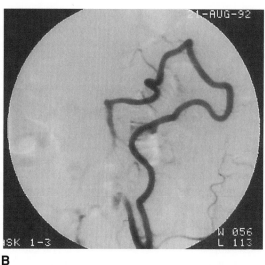

A   **B**

Postoperative *Clostridium difficile* colitis may mimic ischemic colitis. Therefore, in critically ill patients who develop fever, abdominal distention, diarrhea, and leukocytosis after emergency aortic procedures, stool specimens for culture and for *C. difficile* toxin should be obtained and endoscopic evaluation of the colon performed. Appropriate antibiotic therapy (metronidazole or vancomycin) should be instituted if the diagnosis of *C. difficile* is confirmed.[130,131]

Because of the high mortality rate associated with transmural colonic ischemia (80% to 100%), early diagnosis is the key to effective management. The diagnosis depends on a high index of suspicion and the prompt performance of endoscopy with the flexible sigmoidoscope or colonoscope.[132] Sigmoid colon pH monitoring begun before surgery and continued postoperatively has been used with some success by Björck and Hedberg to identify patients at risk for ischemic colitis.[133] They found that a sigmoid colon pH below 6.86 for 9 to 12 hours had a sensitivity of 100% and a specificity of 97% for predicting ischemic colitis. When sigmoid colon acidosis below 7.10 was reversed within 2 hours, no major complications developed, but when it was prolonged, 8 of 10 patients developed major complications. Further evaluation of sigmoid colon pH monitoring appears warranted before its widespread application. The occurrence of ischemic colitis without left colon involvement is rare enough that endoscopy to 40 cm is usually sufficient to establish the diagnosis.[119] Once ischemic colitis is detected, endoscopy should be terminated to avoid perforation. Mild changes of ischemic colitis consist of submucosal hemorrhage and edema that is usually circumferential. Pseudomembranes, erosions, and ulcers indicate more advanced ischemia. A yellowish-green, necrotic, noncontractile surface indicates gangrene.[122] Repeated endoscopy, every other day by the same individual, is required to document resolution or progression of the process. In a recent report, Acosta and colleagues demonstrated elevated D-dimer concentrations in patients with acute mesenteric ischemia.[134] This elevation was especially helpful in female patients with atrial fibrillation. Wider application of this test to other causes of acute mesenteric ischemia awaits validation.

Patients under observation for intestinal ischemia are managed by frequent re-examination; serial endoscopy; sigmoid colon and gastric intramucosal pH monitoring; monitoring of blood gases, D-dimer testing, urine output, and fluid requirements; institution of broad-spectrum antibiotic coverage; and bowel rest with nasogastric suction. If the colon appears distended, either clinically or radiographically, it should be decompressed by the gentle insertion of a rectal tube, because increased intraluminal pressure may further compromise colon blood flow.[122,133]

Improvement of the patient, as evidenced by diminishing diarrhea, improvement in vital signs, clinical examination, laboratory values, and resolution of the ischemia documented by endoscopy, permits continuation of nonoperative management.[119] Reversible ischemic lesions should improve within 7 to 10 days.[127,135] Continuing clinical evidence of ischemia beyond 2 weeks requires operative intervention, because this usually reflects a walled-off perforation with local peritonitis.[122] Finally, progression of intestinal ischemia during the period of observation, identified by deteriorating clinical signs and symptoms, requires prompt celiotomy. Surgery for transmural ischemic colitis requires resection of nonviable bowel, endcolostomy, and formation of a Hartmann's pouch or resection of the rectum, if involved.[136]

Prevention of intestinal ischemia depends on an appreciation of the potential for this complication and the institution of appropriate steps to either avoid injury to the collateral circulation of the colon or augment circulation to the bowel as part of the aortic reconstructive procedure.[137] Spiral CT or magnetic resonance angiography is being used with increasing frequency to evaluate the abdominal aorta and its visceral branches. This technique permits multiple views of complex aortic lesions, reflects the true diameter of aortic aneurysms, and may alleviate the need for angiography.[138,139] Identification of a patent inferior mesenteric artery with retrograde flow through a large meandering artery that is functioning as a collateral pathway for an obstructed superior mesenteric artery requires preservation of flow through the inferior mesenteric; this orifice is spared by constructing an end-to-side aortic anastomosis or by reimplanting the inferior mesenteric onto the side of an aortic graft using a variation of the Carrel patch technique.[119]

In a prospective study of 100 patients undergoing aortic reconstructive procedures, Zelenock and associates observed a 3% incidence of endoscopic colonic ischemia.[140]

Adjunctive procedures were used in 12% of these patients, compared with 4% in earlier studies from their institution. Bypass to the superior mesenteric artery should also be considered.[137] A large meandering artery with flow from the superior mesenteric toward the sigmoid and rectum in the presence of inferior mesenteric artery occlusion is strong evidence of adequate collateral supply to the bowel.[124] Ischemic colitis is unlikely under these circumstances if this collateral is not impaired by surgery. The status of the hypogastric vessels should be identified on the aortogram or other imaging study so that arterial reconstruction can be designed to maintain flow through at least one of these arteries by direct revascularization or by retrograde perfusion from a femoral anastomosis, especially if a patent inferior mesenteric artery must be ligated.[135]

Measurement of the inferior mesenteric artery back-pressure during aortic reconstruction may be a useful guide to the need for restoration of flow to the inferior mesenteric artery.[135] A mean pressure greater than 40 mm Hg and an inferior mesenteric artery–systemic pressure ratio greater than 0.4 indicate satisfactory collateral circulation without the need for mesenteric arterial repair.

Intraoperative duplex ultrasonography in patients undergoing visceral artery repair allows prompt correction of underlying technical defects.[141]

Thorough mechanical preparation of the bowel before aortic surgery reduces the fecal burden to which the potentially ischemic bowel is exposed.[119] During aortic surgery, every effort should be made to prevent injury to the mesenteric vessels. Undue traction on the left colon mesentery should be avoided. When inferior mesenteric ligation is required, this should be carried out by suture ligature within the aortic lumen or immediately adjacent to the aortic wall to avoid injury to its ascending and descending branches.[119] Finally, the presence of Doppler flow signals over the base of the bowel mesentery and the serosal surface of the colon suggests that adequate collateral circulation is present.[128] Absence of a flow signal after reconstruction suggests the need to restore perfusion through the inferior mesenteric artery or through some other major collateral vessel. The association of severe visceral and aortic occlusive disease in younger female patients is accompanied by high mortality and morbidity rates. The severe weight loss resulting from celiac and superior mesenteric artery occlusive lesions makes complete revascularization a hazardous undertaking. In these individuals, a combination of endovascular treatment of the visceral occlusive disease before aortic revascularization may decrease the early morbidity and mortality rates, as well as improve long-term survival (Fig. 43-11).[142]

SPINAL CORD ISCHEMIA

Spinal cord ischemia occurs most frequently during repair of thoracic and thoracoabdominal aneurysms but is occasionally encountered during resection of an abdominal aortic aneurysm and, rarely, following aortoiliac bypass for ischemia.[100,143,144] The overall incidence of this complication of abdominal aortic

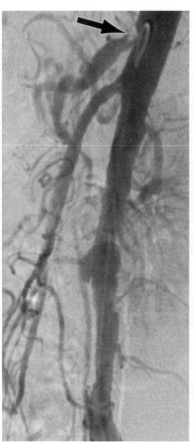
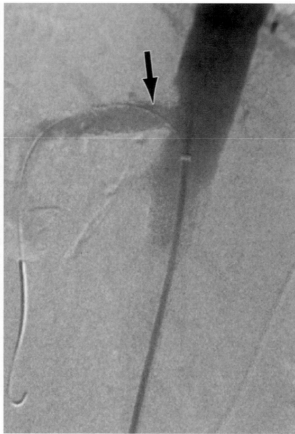

A   **B**

FIGURE 43–11 • *A,* Ninety percent stenosis of the celiac artery *(arrow)* in a patient with mesenteric ischemia treated with balloon angioplasty and stent placement *(arrow)* (B).

surgery has been reported to be 0.23% and is 10 times higher after the repair of ruptured abdominal aortic aneurysms than following elective aneurysm resection.[144,145] The incidence of spinal cord ischemia after thoracic aortic reconstruction is in the range of 1% to 10%, depending on the extent of the lesion repaired.

The upper level of the neurologic deficit was found to be T-10 to L-2 in 39 of 44 patients (88.6%) reviewed at the Henry Ford Hospital.[145] Postoperative mortality was directly related to the severity of paraplegia. When the neurologic deficit was complete initially, involving both sensory and motor function, 76% of the patients died; there were only two complete neurologic recoveries and one partial recovery. By contrast, when the initial loss was only partial motor or sensory loss, 24% died and some degree of recovery was noted in all but one patient.[144,146,147]

The major cause of spinal cord ischemia is interruption of flow through the great radicular artery of Adamkiewicz, which is the major source of supply to the anterior spinal artery at the lower end of the cord.[143,148] The great radicular artery is a major branch of the posterior division of one of the intercostal vessels arising between T-8 and L-1. On occasion, it may originate from a lumbar branch of the infrarenal aorta. The anterior spinal artery itself is long and has rather poor collateral contributions from the posterior spinal arteries or from the radicular arteries derived from more proximal intercostal vessels. Because the spinal cord is only tenuously supplied in its lower portion by vessels other than the great radicular artery, embolization or injury to this vessel during aortic reconstruction may lead to some degree of cord infarction. The effectiveness of collateral pathways may be further compromised by hypotension, especially in patients with ruptured aneurysms. The placement of a high aortic clamp for temporary control of a ruptured aneurysm, however, does not clearly correlate with the incidence or severity of cord ischemia.[144]

Williams and colleagues[149] and Kieffer and coworkers[150] reported successful angiographic visualization of the origin of the artery of Adamkiewicz in 49% and 69% of patients with thoracoabdominal aneurysms, respectively. The very low incidence of spinal cord ischemia after operations on the infrarenal aorta and the risks associated with preoperative or operative angiographic demonstration of the major blood supply to the lower spinal cord render visualization impractical and potentially dangerous.[112,148-150] Moreover, the occurrence of this complication has been unpredictable and may not be preventable in association with infrarenal aortic reconstruction. Monitoring of somatosensory evoked potentials during thoracic surgery has been shown to correlate with cord ischemia.[151] These abnormal findings have been reversed by temporary shunting and implantation of intercostal vessels into the thoracic aortic graft. Practical application of this technique to abdominal aortic surgery is undergoing continued investigation.[151-154]

Although there are no data to identify specific preventive measures, it is prudent to avoid high aortic clamping unless absolutely necessary, to maintain cord perfusion pressure by avoiding systemic hypotension, and to prevent stasis thrombosis in collateral vessels by effective heparinization. Suturing a patch of posterior aortic wall with its intercostal vessel orifices into a window cut out of the graft has been recommended for thoracoabdominal aneurysms.[100] Finally, it is important to ensure pelvic perfusion through one or both hypogastric arteries to maximize collateral contribution to the spinal cord.[155]

When ischemic injury to the spinal cord occurs, treatment is palliative and supportive.[144]

URETERAL INJURY AND OBSTRUCTION

The ureters are immediately adjacent to the operative field and may be easily injured during dissection and arterial repair.[156] This is especially important in patients with large iliac and hypogastric aneurysms or when there is increased adherence to vascular structures in the presence of an "inflammatory" aneurysm or retroperitoneal fibrosis.[157] Nachbur and associates, in a study of 220 patients with asymptomatic aneurysms evaluated with CT scanning, observed 20 cases of ureteral obstruction.[158] In 8 patients, ureteral obstruction was associated with inflammatory aneurysms; in the remaining 12, it was associated with abdominal aortic, common iliac, and hypogastric atherosclerotic aneurysms. A thorough knowledge of the anatomic relationships of the ureters at the level of the iliac bifurcation is essential. Occasionally, multiple ureters may be present, or they may be in an aberrant position owing to congenital anomalies. These variations may be defined by a preoperative intravenous pyelogram or a pyelographic film during the preoperative aortogram or CT scan. A preoperative intravenous pyelogram or contrast-enhanced CT scan is especially indicated in reoperative aortoiliac surgery to identify postoperative changes in the ureteral anatomy or demonstrate possible injury incurred during the initial surgery.

Direct injury to the ureter can best be avoided by keeping the dissection close to the iliac artery at the point where the ureter normally crosses the common iliac bifurcation in transit to the bladder. This is especially important during the blind development of the retroperitoneal tunnel for aortofemoral bypass. The ureter should be elevated away from the iliac vessels so that the graft will lie dorsal to it. Inadvertent passage of the graft ventral to the ureter may cause it to be compressed between the graft limb and the underlying iliac artery, producing hydronephrosis. The incidence of ureteral obstruction after aortic grafting in one prospective study was 2%.[159] However, the ureter may be entrapped in perigraft scar even if it is placed in its proper position ventral to the prosthesis.[156]

Both ureters should be demonstrated before closing the retroperitoneum. The right ureter must be carefully protected during retroperitoneal closure, because this structure can easily be caught up in the suture line. Iatrogenic ureteral injuries sustained during placement or revision of a vascular graft should be repaired primarily. Although renal salvage is possible when the diagnosis is delayed, nephrectomy is often necessary if there has been extensive contamination of the graft.[160] Occasionally, an intraoperative ureteral injury is overlooked, and the diagnosis is delayed for days or weeks. Once recognized, placement of a percutaneous nephrostomy tube may be associated with a shorter hospital stay and lower infection rate than with open repair.[161,162]

Retroperitoneal fibrosis secondary to the surgical procedure is the most common cause of ureteral obstruction after aortic surgery. Postoperative hydronephrosis can be categorized as early (occurring within 6 months) or late (after 6 months). Temporary asymptomatic hydronephrosis can be detected on CT scans in 12% to 30% of patients, and mild to moderate permanent ureteral dilatation is seen in 2% to 14% of patients undergoing aortic surgery. The fibrosis is usually secondary to bleeding; excessive dissection, ligation, or devascularization of the ureter; or pseudoaneurysm formation. Ureteral obstruction is believed to be more common when the limb of the graft is tunneled anterior to the ureter. However, hydronephrosis secondary to anterior graft placement occurs in only 30% of cases. The majority of patients have a clinical presentation within 1 year of the procedure, but delayed presentation up to 14 years has been reported. Approximately 30% of patients manifest with symptoms, including pain, recurrent bouts of urinary tract infection, azotemia, or hematuria.[163-165]

Wright and associates reported a 35-year experience with 58 ureteral complications in 50 patients undergoing aortoiliac reconstructions.[166] Two of the six patients who had ureteral obstruction treated before, or in conjunction with, repair of the aneurysm developed graft complications (one graft limb thrombosis and one graft infection). The remaining 44 patients had 46 complications, including hydronephrosis (42), ureteral leaks (3), and ureteral necrosis (1). Twenty-four patients had 36 graft complications, including anastomotic aneurysm (19), graft limb thrombosis (8), graft infection (6), and aortoenteric fistula (3). Twenty-nine of the 44 patients underwent graft or ureteral operations, or both, with a mortality rate of 21%.

Patients in whom hydronephrosis is recognized preoperatively may benefit from ureteral stent placement to decompress the obstruction and facilitate ureteral identification during repair. Postoperative hydronephrosis detected by ultrasonography, CT, or intravenous pyelography can initially be followed expectantly, because it often resolves. Only 12 of the 58 patients reported by Wright and coworkers required surgical intervention for progressive hydronephrosis.[166]

The selective use of stents and antibiotics in conjunction with operative repair is essential if the high incidence of graft complications is to be reduced (Fig. 43-12).

IMPOTENCE

The loss of ability to achieve or maintain an erection adequate for satisfactory coitus may be due to vasculogenic, psychogenic, neurogenic, endocrinologic, or medication-related factors.[167-171] Eighty percent of patients who have aortoiliac occlusive disease have significant erectile dysfunction.[167] Nearly 25% of patients undergoing direct aortic reconstruction will suffer iatrogenic erectile dysfunction if appropriate technical modifications are not employed. Therefore, careful evaluation of penile erectile function by history, noninvasive techniques, and angiography should be included in the preoperative evaluation before elective aortic surgery.[171,172] This will determine whether there is normal sexual function that should be preserved or whether there is already an established pattern of impotence that might be relieved by altering pelvic blood flow. This information provides valuable insights into the possible psychogenic and cultural factors contributing to an existing problem and gives the surgeon an estimate of the importance of sexual function to the patient. Such preoperative information may alter the type of aortic operation planned.

Preoperative evaluation of erectile function includes nocturnal tumescence studies. The absence of tumescence during an adequate sleep study is strong evidence of organic impotence. Documentation of normal erections during rapid eye movement sleep establishes the psychogenic basis of the patient's erectile dysfunction. Unfortunately, the failure of erection is often qualitative rather than complete, making

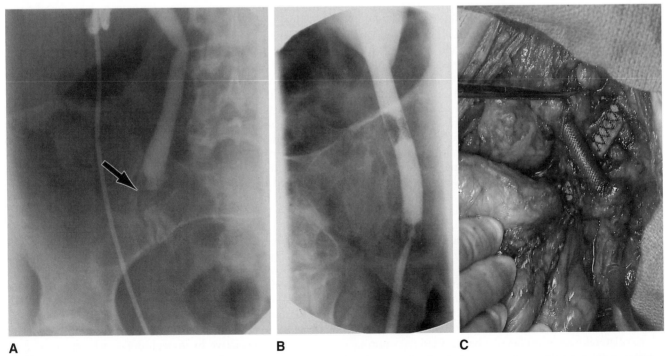

A   **B**   **C**

FIGURE 43–12 • *A*, A stricture is present in the distal ureter as it crosses over the limb of an aortofemoral graft (*arrow*). *B*, After dilatation of the stricture, a stent was placed. *C*, Erosion of the ureter by the stent resulted in a 3-cm defect in the ureter and exposure of the limb of the graft.

tumescence studies less discriminating between organic and psychogenic impotence.[167,172]

If organic impotence is suspected, the next step is noninvasive vascular testing. At present, the most reliable measurement is the penile systolic pressure and the penile-brachial index (PBI).[167] Kempczinski and Birinyi found that age had a deleterious effect on the PBI that was independent of sexual potency.[167] Patients younger than 40 years had a mean PBI of 0.99, compared with a PBI of 0.74 for equally potent men older than 40. This difference was statistically significant. By contrast, impotent men older than 40 had a mean PBI of 0.58, also a statistically significant difference. Despite the significant differences in PBI measurements in these three groups, there is poor correlation between PBI and the degree of erectile dysfunction.[172,173] Although a low PBI is not sufficient to establish the diagnosis of vasculogenic impotence, the finding of a PBI greater than 0.8 confirms the adequacy of penile blood flow and suggests that a vasculogenic cause is extremely unlikely.[167]

Neurogenic impotence is commonly a result of neuropathy secondary to diabetes mellitus, or it may follow autonomic nerve injury from genitourinary or abdominopelvic surgery. This diagnosis is often one of exclusion, but abnormal pudendal nerve velocity studies (sacral latency testing) and abnormal cystometrography (the anatomic pathways in micturition and erection being similar) can implicate this cause.[167,174]

The diagnosis of endocrinologic impotence requires measurement of thyroid function and serum levels of testosterone and other associated hormones. Finally, a thorough medication history is required.[174]

Preoperative angiography is useful in identifying the patency of the hypogastric vessels and their contribution to pelvic perfusion. Unfortunately, angiographic findings correlate poorly with the patient's erectile function.[167] Selective injections to identify the flow through the pudendal vessels into the penis may be required to more accurately assess patients with primarily vasculogenic impotence.[167]

Although the findings on preoperative angiograms correlate poorly with erectile function, preservation of adequate perfusion into at least one hypogastric artery appears to be a vital component in minimizing iatrogenic impotence.[167] When possible, direct antegrade perfusion of the internal iliac artery should be ensured. This may require thromboendarterectomy of the hypogastric orifice. Occasionally, angioplasty, stenting, or operative endarterectomy of the orifices of one or both hypogastric arteries will improve erectile function. If both external iliac arteries are occluded or stenotic and bypass into the common femoral arteries is anticipated, precluding retrograde iliac flow, the proximal aortic anastomosis should be constructed end to side, when feasible, to preserve pelvic blood flow. When proximal aortic disease is extensive (requiring an end-to-end proximal anastomosis) and impaired penile perfusion has been diagnosed by preoperative noninvasive testing, it may be necessary to reimplant the hypogastric artery into one limb of an aortobifemoral graft or add a jump graft to one hypogastric artery to improve pelvic inflow.[167,174] Finally, careful flushing of the graft in both directions before completion of the final suture line is important to prevent embolization of small particles into the pelvic arteries. DePalma and colleagues reported spontaneous erectile function in 58% of patients with impotence undergoing aortoiliac reconstruction, compared with 27% after microvascular procedures.[175]

RETROGRADE EJACULATION

Ejaculatory dysfunction is not uncommon after aortic surgery. Earlier series reported an incidence of 30% to 75%, but in more contemporary series, the incidence was only 3%.[176] This lower incidence is clearly the result of an increased awareness of the anatomy controlling ejaculation and improved surgical technique. Emission and closure of the bladder neck to ensure antegrade ejaculation are dependent on innervation by postganglionic fibers of the lumbar sympathetic nerves arising from T-11 to L-3. The loss of one or both functions as a result of dissection in the region of the aortic bifurcation results in dry ejaculation.[177,178]

Careful preservation of the sympathetic-parasympathetic plexus overlying the aorta and its bifurcation and maintenance of blood flow through the hypogastric and pudendal arteries are the important factors in preventing impotence in men undergoing elective aortic surgery.[169,171,179] Dissection should be carried down to the aortic wall on its right anterolateral surface and the para-aortic structures gently retracted to the left to avoid trauma to the nerves contained within these tissues (Fig. 43-13). During aneurysm resection, the inferior mesenteric artery should not be dissected free but should be controlled by suture ligature from inside the aorta after the aneurysm has been opened to avoid disruption of

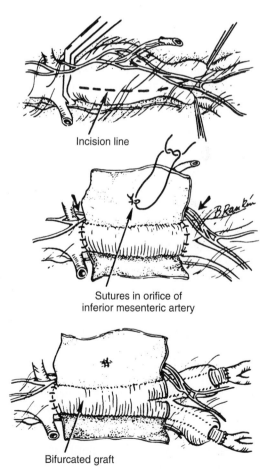

Incision line

Sutures in orifice of
inferior mesenteric artery

Bifurcated graft

FIGURE 43-13 • Approaches to abdominal aortic and aortoiliac aneurysm. The sac is left intact and sutured over an inlay graft. (From DePalma RG: Impotence as a complication of aortic reconstruction. In Bernhard VM, Towne JB [eds]: Complications in Vascular Surgery. New York, Grune & Stratton, 1980, p 437.)

nerve fibers at the junction of the inferior mesenteric artery with the aorta (see Fig. 43-13). There should be minimal division of the longitudinal periaortic tissues to the left of the infrarenal aorta, and the nerve plexuses that cross the left common iliac artery should be spared.[167,179] The limbs of bifurcated grafts should be placed within the lumens of the common iliac arteries in patients undergoing aneurysm resection to avoid external dissection and minimize injury to perivascular nerve fibers.

ANASTOMOTIC FALSE ANEURYSM

False aneurysms can develop at any anastomotic site. They are almost invariably associated with prosthetic rather than autogenous tissue suture lines.[180-186] The most common sites of occurrence are femoral anastomoses following placement of aortofemoral bypass grafts.[181,183,186] Pathologically, there is a partial separation of the graft from the arterial wall.[180,183,185] The perianastomotic fibrous tissue prevents immediate hemorrhage and forms a capsule around the hematoma that gradually expands, owing to the pressure transmitted from the arterial lumen. The fibrous capsule may rupture, with rapid, painful enlargement of the mass, or it may erode the overlying skin to produce infection and external hemorrhage. In the abdomen, false aneurysms are prone to erode into adjacent bowel, forming aortoenteric fistulas.[186-188] Because blood flow within the pseudoaneurysm is static, its lumen becomes partially filled with thrombus, which may embolize.[180,186] The luminal distortion produced by the pseudoaneurysm and its thrombus may also cause occlusion of a graft.[186]

In the immediate postoperative period, the integrity of all vascular anastomoses are entirely dependent on suture material alone. With time, a prosthesis-artery junction is maintained by the integrity of the suture material and also by external fibrous bonding caused by scarring.[189] The important factors involved in the development of an anastomotic false aneurysm include arterial wall weakness,[185] endarterectomy at the anastomotic site,[190] compliance mismatch between the graft and host artery,[191,192] dilatation of the graft material,[188,193] prosthetic deterioration or an actual flaw in the graft material,[194] increased tension at the anastomotic site due to insufficient length of the prosthesis,[194] deterioration of suture material,[195] and uneven tension on the anastomosis as a result of beveling of the end of the graft.[189]

Pseudoaneurysm is occasionally due to underlying infection, although this is seldom identified.[183,186] When infection is the causative factor, a purulent perigraft exudate is usually, but not always, present. Therefore, during repair of any pseudoaneurysm, its wall and contents should be routinely cultured by aerobic and anaerobic techniques.

The incidence of false aneurysm formation ranges between 1.4% and 4%.[184] Recognition is usually quite simple at groin anastomoses, where a large, pulsatile, and sometimes tender mass becomes apparent to both the patient and the examining physician. False aneurysms developing in the retroperitoneum at an aortic or iliac anastomosis rarely become palpable and go unnoticed until rupture produces pain and shock or erosion occurs in an adjacent loop of bowel, with gastrointestinal hemorrhage.[196] Occasionally, false aneurysms are identified during routine CT scanning or arteriography for some other vascular or unrelated problem. Ultrasonography, CT, and MRI are reliable methods for evaluating grafts and anastomoses for dilatation and pseudoaneurysm formation.[197] Diagnosis of a pseudoaneurysm is usually confirmed by arteriography, which demonstrates widening at the anastomosis and an extraluminal accumulation of contrast at the point of anastomotic disruption. Because the false aneurysm is partially filled with thrombus, the extent of extraluminal contrast accumulation only partially delineates the process. A more accurate measure of the true size of the defect can be obtained by CT scanning or MRI.[196]

Retroperitoneal false aneurysms should be repaired as soon as they are identified to avoid rupture or bowel erosion.[184,187,196] Unfortunately, these complications are frequently the first indication that a false aneurysm is present. When there is no evidence of infection, the suture line defect can be dissected free and repaired either directly or by the interposition of fresh graft material. Endovascular treatment of thoracic, para-anastomotic aortic, iliac, and femoral pseudoaneurysms is an attractive alternative to surgery in patients with favorable anatomy.[198-200] When infection or visceral erosion has taken place, the graft must be removed entirely, the aorta and iliac vessels closed, and the extremities revascularized. Management of this problem is discussed in detail elsewhere in this text.

Generally, peripheral false aneurysms should be repaired as soon as they are identified. However, false aneurysms that are small, stable, and asymptomatic may be observed, especially if the patient is at increased risk for reoperation.[183,185,186] If surgery is delayed, re-examination at frequent intervals is mandatory so that repair can be carried out when expansion is evident but before complications develop.

Surgical repair of a false aneurysm is usually carried out through the site of the original incision. Dissection is carried down to the graft wall proximally so that it can be controlled with a circumferential tape. Further dissection is then carried distally along the graft to define the anastomosis, the aneurysmal bulge, and the branches of the common femoral artery. It is usually difficult and tedious to dissect out the major branches of the artery at the anastomotic site. When extensive scarring is encountered, further dissection may be abandoned, and the patient is given intravenous heparin. The graft is then clamped and disconnected from the aneurysm, and branch control is achieved by the insertion of balloon occlusion catheters into the lumens of the major branches.[184] The anastomotic site is carefully surveyed to identify the cause of the pseudoaneurysm. The distal frayed end of the graft at the anastomosis is resected, and the edges of the artery are trimmed back to healthy tissue. To avoid tension at the new anastomosis, a short piece of new graft material is usually required to connect the proximal end of the old prosthesis with the freshened arterial orifice. The diameter of the interposed graft segment generally should not exceed 8 mm to more closely approximate the size of the outflow tract rather than the larger inflow prosthetic limb.[193] Unless retrograde flow up the external iliac artery must be preserved, it is best to convert the femoral anastomosis from end to side to end to end.[184] Before repairing the anastomosis, the orifices of the superficial and deep femoral arteries should be inspected so that significant stenoses can be repaired by endarterectomy or patch angioplasty to ensure adequate runoff.

In a 1985 review, overall mortality for repair of anastomotic femoral false aneurysms was 3.5%, and the amputation rate was 2.8%.[189] Results are distinctly better if this lesion is repaired electively rather than emergently.[185,186] The recurrence rate of anastomotic femoral false aneurysms after initial repair has been reported to be 5.7%; these are amenable to secondary repair.[189,193]

RECURRENT ANASTOMOTIC ANEURYSM

Femoral anastomotic aneurysms (FAAs) develop in approximately 3% of all femoral anastomoses and in 6% of patients undergoing aortofemoral bypass. Repair of FAAs remains durable in approximately 80% of patients; however, a small percentage of patients develop recurrent FAAs. In a series of 43 FAAs, Ernst and colleagues reported a 19% incidence of this complication.[201]

Factors predisposing to recurrent FAA include graft dilatation, local wound complications, and previous repair of an FAA in a woman.[193,201] Although there appears to be an inverse relationship between atherosclerotic heart disease and recurrent FAA, the significance of this observation is difficult to explain. Furthermore, factors that have been implicated in the development of FAAs (e.g., hypertension, smoking, diabetes, suture material, type of graft, performance of an endarterectomy) have not been related to the development of recurrent FAAs.

Recurrent FAAs are subject to the same complications as primary FAAs, including rupture, thrombus, and peripheral embolization.

Repair is indicated in good-risk patients with recurrent FAAs larger than 2 cm. For those smaller than 2 cm, management includes careful follow-up, especially if coexisting medical problems make surgical intervention risky. The principles of repair are similar to those for primary FAAs and include careful dissection of the distal outflow vessels, use of graft material approximately the size of the outflow vessel, and conversion from end-to-side to end-to-end anastomosis.[193,201]

CHYLOUS ASCITES

Chylous ascites, issuing from a damaged cisterna chyli and its tributaries at the root of the mesentery, is a rare complication of aortic reconstruction and performance of a Warren shunt.[202] In a review of the literature, Pabst and coauthors found that approximately 75% of cases occurred following abdominal aortic aneurysm resection, 19% after aortic reconstruction for occlusive disease, and the remaining 7% after resection of infected aortic grafts.[203] Interruption of the lymphatics and chylous ascites are not invariably related, because the lymphatics are often interrupted during aortic operations without apparent sequelae.[202,204]

Patients with chylous ascites typically present within 2 or 3 weeks of aortic repair with anorexia and progressive abdominal distention. Ascites is usually evident on physical examination and can be confirmed by abdominal radiography, ultrasonography, or CT scanning. The fluid obtained by abdominal paracentesis is milky, with a high lymphocyte count and lipid content, and is bacteriologically sterile. An additional complication is leakage of ascites to the outside through a defect in the incision; this increases the fluid and protein loss and heightens the risk of infection. Such a leak should be repaired under sterile conditions and prophylactic antibiotic coverage. Methods used to identify the site of the leak include lymphoscintigraphy, lymphangiography, direct opacification of the thoracic duct with oral fat emulsion observed by CT, and injection of Evans blue dye. The reliability of these tests in identifying the location of the leak or fistula remains unestablished.[205]

The management of chylous ascites includes abdominal paracentesis, a low-fat diet rich in medium-chain triglycerides, and total parenteral nutrition. However, repeated paracentesis may result in the loss of large amounts of protein and lipid that cannot readily be replaced. An additional risk is that of line-related sepsis. In patients who do not respond to repeated paracentesis, a peritoneal venous shunt, in addition to diet control or total parenteral nutrition, may relieve the ascites. Whether the use of octreotide or fibrin glue accelerates the resolution of ascites remains unclear.[206,207] Operative ligation may be necessary in resistant cases.[202,203]

ABDOMINAL WALL HERNIAS

Midline, paramedian, oblique, and transverse incisions are commonly used to expose the abdominal aorta.[208-212] Although transverse incisions are associated with the lowest complication rate, their use is often limited to patients with pulmonary insufficiency. Despite the reported benefits of oblique incisions, a significant number of complications, including long-lasting wound pain and bulging in 11% to 23% of patients and incisional hernias in 7%, have been reported.[211,213] Presumably, the diffuse bulging is due to muscle atrophy caused by a combination of factors, including division of the intercostal nerves, incision-related muscular injury, and reduced blood supply. Gardner and colleagues were able to decrease the incidence of bulging from 11% to 0.03% by preserving the 11th intercostal nerve.[214]

The incidence of midline ventral hernias ranges from 10% to 37%.[213,215] Two distinct types of defects can be identified. Focal periumbilical defects are almost invariably the result of poor technique. The diffuse defects associated with lateral retraction of the recti are by far more commonly observed in patients with incisional hernias after undergoing aortic aneurysmal resection. A number of studies have found no differences in the incidence of the usual risk factors—age, chronic obstructive pulmonary disease, diabetes, smoking, wound infection, length of intensive care unit stay, and amount of blood transfused—between patients who developed incisional hernias and those who did not.

Mass suturing of the musculoaponeurotic layers of the abdominal wall using monofilament or braided suture is the most frequently used technique to close midline incisions. A recent meta-analysis concluded that the ideal suture for abdominal fascia closure is running nonabsorbable monofilament suture. Also, a suture length–to–wound length ratio greater than 4 reduces the incidence of incision lesions.[216,217] It cannot be overemphasized that careful suture technique with placement of bites 2 cm from the edge and 1 cm apart is essential if this complication is to be prevented.

Primary repair using monofilament nonabsorbable suture is appropriate for closure of small periumbilical defects. Prosthetic mesh is usually necessary to repair large defects in the upper abdomen. Recently, laparoscopic repair of these lesions has gained popularity, with low rates of early recurrence.[218,219]

Infrainguinal Arterial Reconstruction

Femoropopliteal and femoroinfrapopliteal bypasses are the most commonly performed procedures for revascularization of the lower extremity below the inguinal ligament. Specific problems related to endarterectomy of the superficial femoral, popliteal, or deep femoral arteries are reviewed in the discussion of these procedures. The basic principles of infrainguinal bypass are similar to those for aortoiliac reconstruction, with the following significant differences: the vessels involved are smaller, and the length of the bypass conduit is greater, with a consequent increase in the incidence of early and late thrombosis; vein grafts rather than prostheses are used for the majority of procedures; and there is a tendency for less severe systemic complications owing to the more peripheral and less traumatic nature of the operative procedure.

BLEEDING

Major blood loss or hemorrhage is not a frequent complication during this surgery but may become a problem in the immediate postoperative period. The most common sources are the anastomoses, insecure ligatures on branches of a vein graft, laceration of the vein wall by instruments in the in situ technique, blind disruption of small vessels encountered during blunt dissection of thigh and leg tunnels, inadequate hemostasis during dissection of the major vessels, incomplete reversal of heparin anticoagulation, and oozing from antiplatelet medication.[220] In the immediate postoperative period, bleeding usually appears as wound swelling of the extremity, and the severity of hypotension, if present, mirrors the extent and rapidity of hemorrhage. Prompt return to the operating room

is required to control the source of bleeding and to evacuate the hematoma, which may interfere with healing and promote infection. Long-term graft patency has been shown to be significantly reduced in patients who develop wound hemorrhage in the immediate postoperative period.[220] Wound hemorrhage that occurs after 48 to 72 hours is frequently due to infection involving the graft at an anastomosis and is less likely to be caused by mechanical factors.[220] However, hemorrhage may occur later in the immediate postoperative period in patients who have been maintained on anticoagulants or in whom fibrinolytic agents have been infused for graft thrombosis within 10 days to 2 weeks of surgery.[221]

THROMBOSIS

The most common significant complication of infrainguinal bypass or endarterectomy is thrombosis of the reconstruction. In the early postoperative period (<30 days), thrombosis is usually related to technical factors (Fig. 43-14).[34,56,222,223] The most common of these is imprecise construction of the suture line, resulting in stenosis or elevation of a distal intimal flap that obstructs flow; this is especially important at a distal anastomosis to a small-caliber tibial or peroneal vessel. A prosthetic or reversed saphenous vein graft may become twisted when drawn through the thigh tunnel. Kinking or entrapment may occur owing to compression by nerve trunks or other tissues crossing the tunnel or by tracking the graft inappropriately in relation to the adductor muscles of the thigh or the medial head of the gastrocnemius. Vein graft stenosis may be produced by a branch ligature placed too close to the main saphenous trunk. For reversed saphenous vein grafts, factors leading to early thrombosis are vein diameter less than 3.5 to 4 mm, thick-walled vein, marked varicosities,

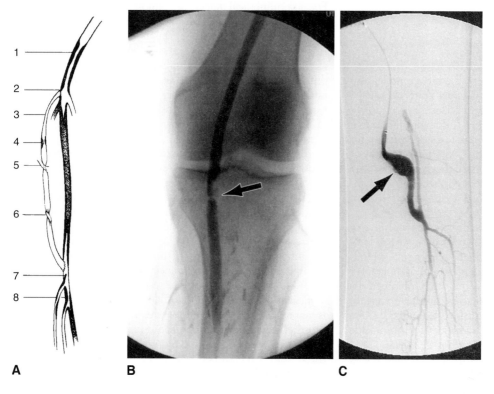

A   **B**   **C**

FIGURE 43-14 • *A,* Mechanical factors underlying early thrombosis of femoropopliteal and femorotibial grafts: (1) stenosis of iliac inflow; (2) stenosis of proximal anastomosis produced by suturing a small vein to a thick-walled femoral artery; (3) proximal vein graft less than 4 mm in diameter; (4) recanalized saphenous phlebitis; (5) external compression tissue bands in tunnel; (6) graft twist; (7) elevation of distal intima; (8) inadequate runoff. *B,* Stenosis and platelet deposition *(arrow)* in a below-knee saphenous vein graft. *C,* Aneurysmal dilatation *(arrow)* of a saphenous vein graft proximal to a stenosis in a patient with distal embolization. (*A,* From Bernhard VM: The failed arterial graft: Lost pulses and gangrene. In Condon RE, DeCosse JJ [eds]: Surgical Care. Philadelphia, Lea & Febiger, 1980, p 156.)

and evidence of previous phlebitis.[224,225] In the in situ saphenous vein bypass, technical factors causing early thrombosis are platelet deposition at sites of endothelial damage from improper intraluminal instrumentation, missed valves or incomplete cusp lysis, diversion of flow by significant fistulas, venospasm, and torsion or kinking of the proximal or distal free segments of the vein. Atherosclerotic disease in the inflow or outflow arteries that was inadequately evaluated before surgery is another significant cause of graft thrombosis. Other technical errors include inadequate heparinization, improper flushing of the arterial system before restoration of graft flow, and clamp injury to the inflow or outflow vessels or the bypass conduit.[56,226] Nonmechanical causes of early thrombosis are decreased cardiac output, arterial vasospasm, and hypercoagulability.[56,227]

Thrombosis that occurs from 1 month to 1 year after implantation is most frequently due to degenerative changes in the graft itself or at an anastomosis.[222,223,228,229] In reversed saphenous vein bypass, thrombosis is usually caused by fibrosis of a valve or fibrotic changes in the vein graft wall due to injury during harvest and preparation before insertion.[56,223,230] These intrinsic vein graft defects are more common in the narrow proximal portion of reversed vein grafts.[223] In in situ saphenous vein bypass grafts, stenoses of the conduit have been reported at the mobilized upper or lower ends of the graft due to fibrous dysplastic lesions and in the midportion as the result of thickening around a valve cusp.[231] For all types of arterial bypasses, intimal fibroplasia at or just beyond the distal anastomosis may be produced by turbulent flow secondary to alteration of the arterial stream at the junction of graft and artery,[49,232-234] a compliance mismatch,[191,235] and the interplay of platelets and other blood factors at anastomoses.[236] Fibrointimal hyperplasia may also be a consequence of clamp injury to the graft or artery incurred at the time of surgery.[223]

Thrombosis occurring after 1 to 2 years is most frequently due to progressive atherosclerosis in the arteries proximal or distal to the arterial repair.[223,224,228,237,238] Arterialized venous conduits in an atherosclerotic patient tend to become atherosclerotic themselves[238]; this appears to apply only to reversed, not in situ, vein bypass grafts.[225,231] Giswold and coworkers showed that continued smoking, dialysis therapy, hypercoagulable state, and early duplex surveillance failure are independent factors associated with vein graft occlusion.[238a] Pedal bypasses for previous graft occlusion was also independently predictive of poor graft patency at 1 year.[239]

There is a higher incidence of thrombosis when prosthetic conduits are employed, especially when they are carried below the knee to the distal popliteal or infrapopliteal vessels.[240-245] Thrombosis after vein grafting appears to level off between 1 and 2 years, whereas it is progressive in prosthetic grafts.[223,243] The specific causes of prosthetic thrombosis are the absence of a true intima, with its antithrombotic characteristics; the tendency to develop progressive fibrointimal hyperplasia, usually at the distal anastomosis due to the complex interactions between the more rigid prosthetic graft and the arterial wall; and the greater likelihood of kinking of prosthetic materials as they cross the knee joint. Thrombosis may also occur as a consequence of false aneurysm formation, which is more frequent with prostheses than with vein grafts. Hooded grafts, vein cuffs, and patches have been used at the distal anastomoses of prosthetic grafts to improve their patency. Patency rates range from 37% to 57% for below-knee prosthetic grafts.[246-249]

Thrombosis in a bypass graft may involve only the graft itself, without loss of flow in the segments of the vessel proximal and distal to the points of anastomosis. Under these circumstances, the leg will return to its previous degree of ischemia, assuming that there has been no significant change in the inflow or outflow vessels and collateral pathways. If thrombosis extends beyond the anastomosis into the popliteal and infrapopliteal arteries, however, ischemia will invariably be more severe, and the limb may become acutely nonviable unless circulation can be restored.[34]

When a reversed vein graft becomes thrombosed in the immediate postoperative period, the intima and muscularis suffer prolonged anoxic injury due to loss of nutritive blood flow from the lumen, in addition to the absence of normal graft wall perfusion through the vasa vasorum, which was disrupted during vein graft harvest.[228] The vein thus becomes a less satisfactory conduit, even though flow can be restored within a few hours. This is reflected in the reduced long-term patency of those vein grafts that have undergone thrombosis and initially successful thrombectomy.[223,232]

In the case of late or neglected thrombosis of a vein conduit, either reversed or in situ, the vein tends to undergo changes that are irreversible. The vein wall becomes thick and edematous, and the lumen becomes stringlike. Thrombus usually cannot be removed by any means, and dilatation of the vein by a balloon catheter may result in splitting of the wall.[231]

In the immediate postoperative period, peripheral vasospasm may make clinical evaluation unreliable. However, noninvasive tests permit the identification of thrombosis at the earliest possible moment.[36,250,251] Therefore, quality of graft flow and overall limb circulation should be evaluated by noninvasive hemodynamic techniques, as well as by clinical observation intraoperatively, immediately after completion of the reconstruction, and at frequent intervals in the early postoperative period.[55,252] Doppler waveform analysis, duplex imaging, ankle pressures, and pulse-volume recordings provide reliable objective information. Surgical reintervention should be carried out immediately in the event of obstructed graft flow, to limit propagation of thrombus into distal vessels and minimize the period of ischemia in the limb and the wall of a vein graft.

Beyond the immediate postoperative period, patients with infrainguinal arterial reconstruction, especially with vein grafts, should continue to be examined at regular intervals at least every 3 to 4 months for 12 to 18 months and every 6 months thereafter. A history of increasing claudication, the recognition of reduced distal pulses, and the development of new bruits over the graft or its anastomoses are important findings that should be documented at each visit. In addition, noninvasive hemodynamic tests, including duplex scanning, should be performed; they provide quantitative and objective information and can identify impending thrombosis in the absence of symptoms or clinical findings.[251-254] Any evidence of decreasing graft function signals the need for prompt angiography to identify the problem before thrombosis occurs.

Correction of abnormalities within the graft or in the vessels adjacent to a failing graft should be carried out as soon as reduced perfusion has been identified.[251] When possible, intervention should occur before thrombosis has taken place or in the early post-thrombotic period, when mechanical obliteration or lytic therapy is most effective. Delay of an aggressive surgical approach may be required in patients who are poor operative risks. Anticoagulants may prevent thrombosis in the presence of progressing stenosis if surgery must be delayed. However, once occlusion has occurred, the longer the thrombus has been present, the less effective recanalization attempts will be.

Areas of isolated stenosis within the graft, at an anastomosis, or in the inflow or outflow arteries can be successfully managed by percutaneous balloon angioplasty.[221] These fibrous vein graft lesions are often difficult to dilate with balloon angioplasty. Dissection after attempted balloon angioplasty requiring stent placement is not infrequent; whether "cutting" balloon angioplasty offers additional benefit awaits further evaluation.[255] If this technique is not satisfactory, a direct surgical approach at the site of the stenosis is indicated.[34,223] Vein patch angioplasty can usually be accomplished with relative ease to relieve stenosis of the graft itself or at an anastomosis (Fig. 43-15). If the proximal segment of a reversed saphenous vein graft is too narrow, it can be widened (Fig. 43-16). Progressive disease in the inflow vessels requires a jump graft from the lower end of the original graft to a patent distal popliteal or infrapopliteal artery to bypass the obstruction.[223]

When thrombosis has already occurred and is recent, the graft lumen may be restored by mechanical extraction of thrombus with a balloon thromboembolectomy catheter or mechanical device such as the AngioJet; prosthetic grafts are more amenable to this procedure than are vein grafts.[34,223,256] Thrombectomy of a fresh reversed saphenous vein graft usually requires exposure of both anastomoses. A transverse incision is made at the distal, wider end of the graft so that thrombus at that level can be removed and the internal aspect of the distal anastomosis viewed directly (see Fig. 43-15). A second incision over the proximal anastomotic vein hood or partial takedown of the proximal suture line is required for passage of balloon thromboembolectomy catheters and for vigorous forward flushing, because retrograde manipulations will be impeded by valves (Fig. 43-17). Prosthetic graft declotting can sometimes be accomplished through a single distal graft opening if the thrombosis is recent. The thoroughness of thrombus removal is determined by the vigor of flow through the graft from the proximal to the distal end, which also suggests that there is no inflow obstruction. Operative arteriography under fluoroscopic guidance or angioscopy is required after declotting of either venous or prosthetic grafts to confirm that thrombus has been completely extracted, to view both

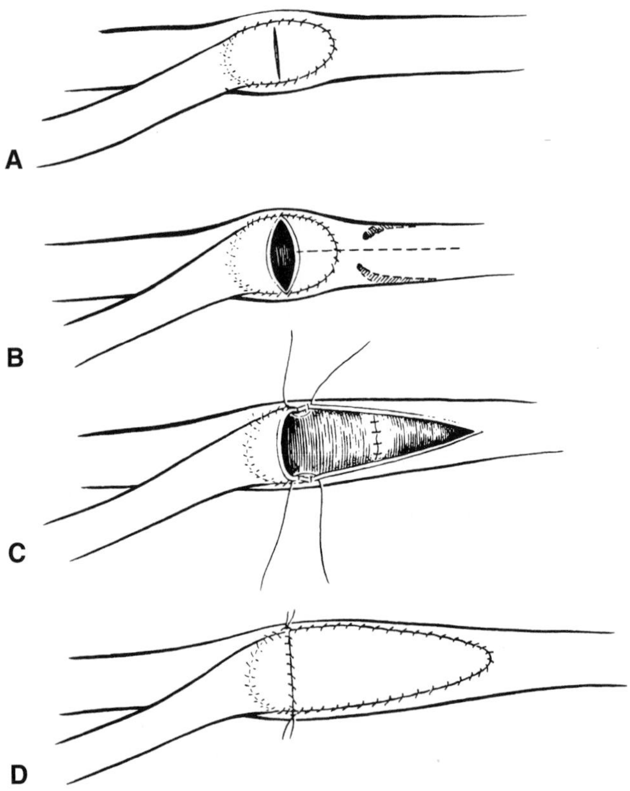

FIGURE 43-15 • Technical sequence for inspection and repair of distal anastomosis of femoropopliteal or femorotibial graft. *A*, Transverse incision in a wide "cobra head" overlying the distal anastomosis facilitates thrombus extraction, visualization of the internal aspect of the suture line, and closure without stenosis. *B* and *C*, When the distal intima is elevated, the arteriotomy is extended beyond the area of injury, redundant intima is removed, and the cut edge is secured with tacking sutures. *D*, Closure of the defect with a vein patch. (From Bernhard VM: The failed arterial graft: Lost pulses and gangrene. In Condon RE, DeCosse JJ [eds]: Surgical Care. Philadelphia, Lea & Febiger, 1980, p 160.)

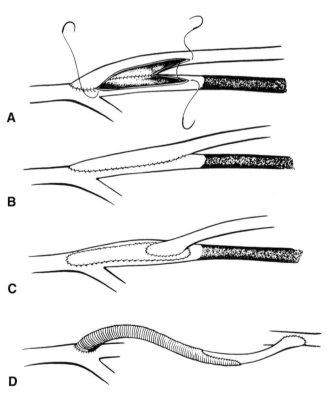

FIGURE 43-16 • Techniques for revision of the femoral anastomosis to avoid stenosis caused by a narrow vein and thick arterial intima. *A*, Proximal superficial femoral artery is incised to match the long incision in the vein graft; the vein graft incision is carried distally until the vein diameter is at least 4 mm. *B*, Completion of anastomosis. *C*, Alternative technique using a vein patch to increase the diameter of the artery; the vein graft is then anastomosed to the patch. *D*, Composite vein-Dacron graft is another solution when the available saphenous vein is too short. (From Bernhard VM: The failed arterial graft: Lost pulses and gangrene. In Condon RE, DeCosse JJ [eds]: Surgical Care. Philadelphia, Lea & Febiger, 1980, p 165.)

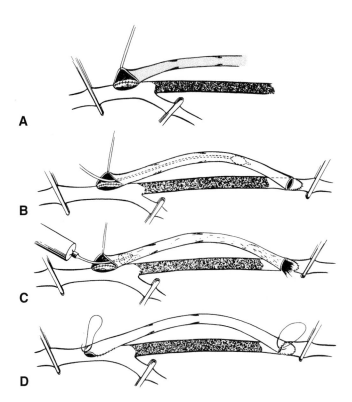

FIGURE 43–17 • Partial detachment of the proximal anastomosis and graft thrombectomy. *A*, Partial takedown of the proximal suture line. *B*, Passage of a Fogarty catheter to the distal end of the graft and retrograde extraction of clot. *C*, Vigorous flushing of the thrombectomized graft with heparinized Ringer's lactate solution. *D*, Resuture of the proximal anastomosis and distal transverse venotomy. (From Bernhard VM: The failed arterial graft: Lost pulses and gangrene. In Condon RE, DeCosse JJ [eds]: Surgical Care. Philadelphia, Lea & Febiger, 1980, p 161.)

anastomoses, to evaluate the entire length of the intervening graft to identify areas of stenosis that need to be repaired, and to re-evaluate the inflow and the runoff bed.[257]

The direct intra-arterial infusion of thrombolytic agents is an alternative to balloon catheter thrombectomy in a patient who has no sensory or motor deficits and no signs of impending muscle necrosis.[65,221,231,258,259] Thrombolytic therapy has been successfully applied to vein grafts, prostheses, and endarterectomized segments at all levels of the lower extremity arterial system. The endothelial lining of vein grafts and of small runoff vessels is spared the trauma of mechanical thrombectomy, which may be an important factor in restored vein graft function over the long term. Although effective lysis can be accomplished several weeks after an occlusion has occurred,[61,260] best results with this form of therapy are usually achieved within hours or days of thrombosis.[261] The technique of percutaneous intra-arterial thrombolytic therapy is discussed elsewhere in this book.

As soon as the clot has been effectively cleared from the graft by lytic therapy, angiographic investigation of the entire length of the graft, both anastomoses, the inflow, and the runoff bed is required to identify the cause of graft failure, which must be corrected to avoid reocclusion. In the interim between lytic recanalization and correction of the causes of graft thrombosis, patients must be effectively anticoagulated to forestall rethrombosis.[61] It is important to recognize that

although lytic recanalization of occluded grafts can be achieved, thrombolytic therapy alone suffices in only a minority of patients. Graft stenoses or deterioration of inflow or runoff vessels must be identified and corrected to achieve long-term patency and limb salvage.[65,251,260,262]

A number of reports indicate that intraoperative fibrinolytic therapy is an effective adjunct to catheter or mechanical thrombectomy in select cases when residual clot in the distal artery threatens the success of thrombectomy.[263-265] The use of intraoperative fibrinolytic agents has not been associated with significant bleeding complications.[263,264]

Graft thrombosis that is old or that cannot be reopened by mechanical or lytic therapy requires a secondary bypass procedure if the limb is in jeopardy or if claudication is truly incapacitating. Autogenous vein is preferable to prosthetic material, especially for bypasses to the infrapopliteal arteries. When the saphenous vein is not available for reoperation, arm veins and lesser saphenous veins, when available, are preferable to prosthetic conduits. The long-term results with prosthetic material are poor when used for secondary bypass, whereas arm veins have been shown to have long-term patency rates nearly equal to those of saphenous vein.[266]

It is important to emphasize the need to search for non-mechanical reasons for decreased graft flow, such as diminished cardiac output or hypercoagulability, especially when no other causes of thrombosis can be identified. Curi and associates reported a 13% incidence of diverse hypercoagulable states in this patient population.[267] Failure to identify and correct the reason for graft occlusion usually suggests a poor prognosis, because the underlying cause has not been removed.[58] However, thrombosis in PTFE grafts may occur for no apparent reason other than presumed platelet adherence to a relatively thrombogenic surface. For this reason, antiplatelet therapy in the immediate postoperative period is indicated.[236,268] Long-term anticoagulation with warfarin sodium should be considered in patients who have recurrent thrombosis for no apparent reason.

Reoperation to maintain extremity circulation is worthwhile, because prolonged limb salvage can be achieved in 40% to 60% of patients undergoing four or more reoperative procedures.[223] The best results after reoperation for failure of an infrainguinal reconstruction are achieved in patients who require only a vein patch to relieve a stenosis that is repaired before thrombosis takes place.[223,252] For example, Whittemore and associates achieved a 19% 5-year patency rate after thrombectomy and patch angioplasty of thrombosed femoropopliteal vein grafts, a 36% 5-year patency rate after secondary autogenous vein bypass, and an overall 50% long-term limb salvage rate.[223] However, vein patch angioplasty of a stenotic graft or anastomotic lesion before thrombosis occurred yielded an 86% 5-year patency rate. For 72 early and late occlusions of PTFE femoropopliteal grafts that placed the limb in jeopardy, Veith and colleagues reported a 5-year graft patency rate of 37% and a 5-year limb salvage rate of 56% in patients undergoing reoperation.[269] PTFE femoropopliteal bypasses appear to be unusual, in that thrombectomy alone, even when delayed up to 30 days after thrombosis, can sometimes restore long-term patency. The success rate for reoperation for thrombosis of PTFE grafts to infrapopliteal arteries is considerably lower than that for femoropopliteal bypasses.

Whether the long-term use of anticoagulants can prevent thrombosis of autogenous and prosthetic infrainguinal grafts, as suggested by the studies of Kretschmer and coworkers,[270,271] needs further evaluation.

WOUND COMPLICATIONS

Major wound complications following lower extremity bypass grafting to the tibial or pedal vessels are not often reported but may jeopardize the success of these procedures.

The reported incidence of significant wound complications following autogenous infrainguinal bypass grafting ranges from 7.5% to 11%.[272-274] In a prospective study of 77 inguinal incisions, Kent and coworkers reported a 10% incidence of wound complications; however, complications occurred in 44% of 79 distal (popliteal or tibial) incisions.[275] Predisposing factors include age, obesity, diabetes mellitus, renal failure, anemia, steroid therapy, ipsilateral limb ulceration or infection, and severity of ischemia. Technical factors, including the length and placement of the incision, location of the distal anastomosis, and technique of wound closure, may all influence the ultimate healing of these incisions.[272-275] In a recent analysis of 9932 patients undergoing lower extremity revascularization, O'Hare and colleagues found no significant differences in wound complications or return to the operating room for graft-related complications between patients with renal insufficiency and those without.[276] The amputation rate at 1 year, however, was significantly higher (29% vs. 10%) in patients on dialysis than in those with normal renal function.[277]

The use of a continuous incision increases the risk of wound hematoma or seroma, and if it is not positioned directly over the saphenous vein, elevation of a large posterior flap may be necessary. The two parallel incisions required to mobilize the artery and vein for in situ grafting to the dorsalis pedis artery risk necrosis of the intervening skin bridge. Wound complications range from erythema and superficial necrosis of the margins to infection of the deeper layers with exposure of the graft. Gram-positive cocci and mixed bacterial flora are frequently cultured from these wounds.[272-275]

Several steps help prevent wound complications following infrainguinal bypass procedures. Preoperative mapping of the course of the saphenous vein with duplex scanning minimizes the likelihood of creating a large posterior flap. Isolation of necrotic or ulcerative skin lesions of the foot before preparation of the skin limits contamination of the operative field. In patients undergoing in situ vein bypasses, valve incision under angioscopic guidance using coil occlusion or ligation of side branches through small incisions may obviate the need for long continuous incisions and, as a consequence, reduce the incidence of wound complications.[278-280] Endoscopic saphenous vein harvest has been shown by Illig and colleagues to be associated with fewer overall wound complications (34% vs. 20%), as well as fewer class II and class III wound complications, compared with open surgery.[281] If a continuous incision is used, careful placement of the incision, meticulous hemostasis, and careful skin closure also reduce the incidence of wound complications. Once a wound complication has occurred, however, the treatment should be tailored to the severity of infection. Wound erythema with minimal necrosis of the wound margins usually responds to appropriate antibiotics and local wound care. More extensive wound infection and necrosis require extensive débridement and often skin grafting, muscle transfers, or myocutaneous free flaps.

Rarely, an exposed vein graft ruptures, requiring removal of the graft and placement of a new conduit routed through uninvolved sites. If this is not feasible, amputation may be necessary.

Graft Surveillance

VEIN GRAFTS

With more autogenous vein bypass procedures being performed, the number of grafts at risk for late changes, including fibrosis, valvular stenosis, dilatation, aneurysm formation, and atherosclerosis, is increased.[238]

When implanted in the arterial system, vein grafts undergo a series of morphologic changes that include thickening of the wall, fibrosis, and myointimal cellular proliferation as an adaptive response to arterial blood pressure. There is also experimental evidence that vein grafts produce more prostacyclin than normal veins, although the amount produced is still considerably less than that produced by normal arteries.[282] The introduction of better valvulotomes and the use of angioscopically assisted side branch occlusion have increased the utility of in situ saphenous vein bypass grafts. Whether the vein should be left in situ or reversed remains a topic of considerable debate. Proponents of the in situ technique emphasize the theoretical benefits of better endothelial preservation and compliance characteristics, but there is limited objective evidence to support this assumption. Actually, the in situ technique may entail more manipulation and damage to the intima from the use of valvulotomes.

Graft failure within the first 30 days is usually due to fibrin platelet thrombus, retained valves, twists, unrecognized AV fistulas, or technical problems with the anastomoses; this occurs in up to 3% to 10% of grafts.[283,284] Careful intraoperative assessment of the entire length of the graft with Doppler spectral analysis, angiography, or angioscopy is essential if these early complications are to be avoided.[279,280] Woelfle and colleagues, in a series of 120 infragenicular bypass grafts evaluated by both angiography and angioscopy, found defects in 7 of 90 grafts with normal completion angiograms.[285] Bush and coworkers reported a 10% incidence of competent valves in the presence of "normal" operative arteriograms.[286] Bandyk and associates performed intraoperative arteriography and pulse Doppler evaluation on 50 in situ vein grafts.[287] Severe flow disturbances were present in 14% of the distal anastomoses, 5% of valve incision sites, and 2% of proximal anastomoses. Ferris and associates found that despite normal completion arteriography, early graft velocity abnormalities could be detected in 26% of 224 grafts.[288] Fifty-two percent of these lesions required correction, 38% resolved, and the remaining lesions revised at a later date.

Platelet thrombi occur at the sites of valve incision or splits in the intima along the length of the vein. Exploration of these sites, with careful removal of any thrombotic material and repair by patch angioplasty or replacement of the damaged vein segment, is often necessary.

Beyond the initial postoperative period, approximately one third of infrainguinal vein grafts develop stenoses that may predispose to thrombosis. Reoperation to correct such defects before graft occlusion permits salvage of the grafts and prevents recurrent ischemia. Unfortunately, between 20% and 40% of grafts occlude without warning or with recently recorded normal ankle pressure indexes.[289] Because of these grafts' propensity to fail, every attempt should be made to detect obstructive changes within the graft, at anastomoses, or in the inflow or runoff vessels before occlusion occurs.

A hemodynamically significant graft stenosis can be detected during carefully executed duplex scanning of the graft. Few patients have recurrent symptoms, despite the presence of a flow-limiting lesion. The value of a vein graft duplex surveillance program, allowing early detection, close follow-up, and timely revision of lesions meeting the criteria for high-grade stenosis, has been well established.[290-293] However, controversy remains regarding the exact criteria mandating graft revision to prevent graft thrombosis. Our personal observations suggest that when the peak systolic velocity progresses to 350 cm/second or greater, or the velocity ratio is 3.5 or greater, the graft is at significant risk of failure.[294] These threshold criteria may seem high compared with other published criteria, and larger surveillance studies are necessary to resolve this remaining controversy. Other important parameters are a decreased graft velocity of less than 45 cm/second and a fall in the ankle-brachial index of more than 0.15 (Fig. 43-18).[294] The former is particularly suggestive of a more proximal lesion, whereas the latter, if isolated, may be indicative of an outflow lesion or a missed graft stenosis on duplex scan. Nonetheless, these abnormal values warrant immediate attention, which may consist of closer follow-up, further evaluation, or immediate intervention, as dictated by the information obtained. After revision or an initial bypass procedure, the patient is seen every month for 1 year and every 6 months thereafter.[289,295]

Although some of the focal lesions observed angiographically during late follow-up appear suitable for balloon catheter dilatation, the recurrence rate is high; patch angioplasty or replacement of a segment of vein offers superior long-term results.

An interesting complication of infrainguinal bypass grafts is functional failure despite continued graft patency. This manifests by extension of necrosis or failure to control infective processes in the foot.[296] The incidence of this complication ranges from 2% to 4% for reversed vein grafts, up to 7.5% for in situ vein grafts, and 8.1% to 9.5% for PTFE grafts.[297,298] Amputation may be required unless graft extension to an additional tibial or pedal vessel is possible. An alternative may be microvascular free flap transfer of healthy muscle to cover a persistent defect that usually involves exposed tendons, bones, or joints.

GRAFT DILATATION

With the increased life expectancy of patients undergoing aortofemoral and femoropopliteal bypass grafting, continued surveillance to detect deterioration in the graft material or complications resulting from the implantation of prosthetic devices is becoming more important.

Although florid rupture of Dacron grafts and dilatation of PTFE grafts have been nearly eliminated by improvements in manufacturing techniques of the former and by increasing the wall thickness of or applying an external wrap around the latter, deterioration in prosthetic grafts still occurs.

Dacron Grafts

The true incidence of dilatation is unknown, because patients with apparently well-functioning grafts, as evidenced by palpable distal pulses or normal ankle pressure indexes on follow-up examinations, are seldom evaluated unless some problem,

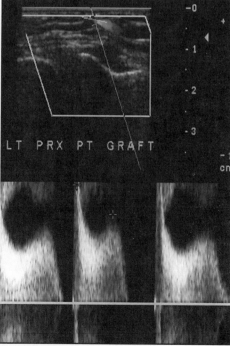

FIGURE 43–18 • Vein graft stenosis. *A*, Magnetic resonance angiogram demonstrating high-grade proximal vein graft stenosis (*arrow*). *B*, Duplex scan of the vein graft stenosis demonstrating increased velocity at the site of the stenosis.

A   **B**

such as an anastomotic aneurysm or acute occlusion of a graft limb, supervenes.

Textile grafts initially dilate approximately 15% to 20% after implantation. This is believed to be due to yarn slippage and is accompanied by a small decrease in tensile strength, which then stabilizes but may continue throughout the life of the graft. Three factors are believed to contribute to dilatation of Dacron grafts: (1) a flattening of the crimp when the graft is subjected to arterial pressure, (2) an increase in diameter and a decrease in length due to rearrangement of textile structure (i.e., the lighter the graft fiber, the greater the porosity and the more likely it is to dilate), and (3) an increase in diameter and length due to deformation of the graft material.[188,299-302]

Dilatation is more likely to occur in knitted rather than woven grafts, as documented in a study by Nunn and associates, who evaluated 95 Dacron grafts implanted for a mean of 33 months using Doppler ultrasonography.[301] The mean dilatation was 17.6% and was somewhat more severe in hypertensive patients (21%) than in their normotensive counterparts (15%). However, some grafts enlarged by more than 100%. In a CT study of 178 aortic grafts, Berman and coworkers reported mean dilatation of 49.2% ± 4% for knitted Dacron prostheses, 28.5% ± 3% for woven Dacron grafts, and 20.6% ± 1.9% for PTFE grafts from their preimplantation diameter (Fig. 43-19).[302] Complications, including supragraft aneurysms (seven), distal anastomotic aneurysms (five), proximal anastomotic aneurysms (three), graft infections (two), perigraft fluid collections (two), graft aneurysms with thrombus and distal embolization (two), and nonvascular complications (three), occurred in 13.5% of patients.[303]

Prosthetic rupture and anastomotic aneurysm formation have been reported in patients with dilated grafts; however, the natural history of such grafts left in place is presently unknown.[188,193,304,305] Nevertheless, removal of a grossly dilated graft may be prudent in an asymptomatic patient without

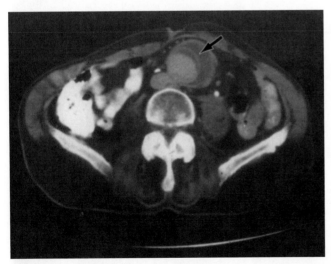

FIGURE 43–19 • Abdominal computed tomography scan demonstrating a dilated graft (arrow) and the surrounding thrombus from an aortic anastomotic aneurysm. (From Hunter GC, Bull DA: The healing characteristics, durability, and long-term complications of vascular prostheses. In Bernhard VM, Towne TB [eds]: Complications in Vascular Surgery. St. Louis, Quality Medical Publishing, 1991, p 65.)

significant cardiorespiratory problems that increase operative risk. In practice, dilated segments of grafts associated with anastomotic aneurysms are replaced. Care should be taken to use a graft corresponding to the diameter of the outflow vessel, and no attempt should be made to match the diameter of the interposition graft to that of the dilated implanted graft.

Umbilical Veins

Umbilical veins have been used as a substitute for saphenous veins, with a 5-year patency rate of approximately 45%.[306] Dardik and colleagues, in a series of 756 glutaraldehyde-stabilized umbilical vein grafts (UVGs) implanted over a 7-year period, identified aneurysmal change in 7 grafts (1%) in the entire series.[307,308] The incidence of such aneurysms increased over time, from 1.2% at 4 to 6 years to 7.7% at 6 to 8 years. It should be noted that this incidence may be underestimated, because follow-up arteriography was performed in only one third of the patients at risk. The mechanisms for UVG dilatation include mechanical fatigue, reversal of cross-linking, and immunologic factors. Julien and coworkers, in a study of 80 UVG segments removed from 70 patients studied by light and electron microscopy, found aneurysmal dilatation in 5% of specimens, bacterial colonization in the absence of overt infection in 26%, and irregular wall thickness with folds on the intraluminal surface in 33% of the grafts.[309] Anastomotic thrombus is often associated with this problem.[307]

Because of the small but definite risk of continued deterioration of these grafts, Dardik and colleagues recommended that an arteriogram be performed 3 to 4 years after implantation in addition to noninvasive surveillance.[307,308] In a recent evaluation of 283 grafts implanted over a 10-year period, Dardik and colleagues reported no aneurysms.[310]

Polytetrafluoroethylene

Initially, PTFE grafts were manufactured without an external wrap, which was associated with aneurysmal dilatation of the grafts. No aneurysms have been reported since the application of the wrap (Gore-Tex, W. L. Gore and Associates, Inc., Flagstaff, Ariz.) or the increase in graft wall thickness (Impra, C. R. Bard Inc., Tempe, Ariz.). Furthermore, PTFE does not dilate significantly over time, which makes it the material of choice for repair of anastomotic aneurysms and possibly for aortofemoral bypass.[311,312]

EDEMA

Some degree of lower extremity edema accompanies the majority of successful infrainguinal arterial reconstructions. The reported incidence is as high as 70% to 100%.[58] The most important factor in the development of edema appears to be lymphatic interruption, probably at the inguinal, thigh, and popliteal areas during the lower extremity arterial reconstruction. Microcirculatory derangements that exist in the ischemic limb, such as loss of arteriolar autoregulation, loss of the orthostatic vasoconstrictor reflex, capillary recruitment, and focal capillary endothelial injury, all apparently contribute to this lymph-related edema by increasing the net flux of interstitial fluid into the lymphatic system (Fig. 43-20).[313-315] Venous thrombosis has been shown to be an infrequent cause of postreconstructive edema.[315,316]

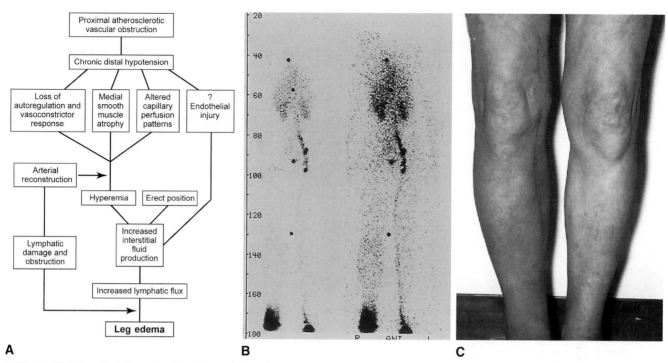

FIGURE 43–20 • *A,* Schematic overview of the factors involved in postoperative lower extremity edema after femorodistal reconstruction. *B,* Lymphoscintigram showing decreased uptake of the radionuclide tracer in the swollen right lower extremity. *C,* Patient after femoropopliteal bypass grafting. (*A,* From Schubart PJ, Porter JM: Leg edema after femorodistal bypass. In Bergan JJ, Yao JST [eds]: Reoperative Arterial Surgery. Orlando, Fla, Grune & Stratton, 1986, p 328.)

The severity of the edema increases in relation to the severity of prebypass ischemia. It is less frequent after aortoiliofemoral reconstruction, presumably because there is less limb lymphatic disruption.[279]

Technical modifications to minimize inguinal and popliteal lymphatic injury during infrainguinal arterial reconstruction may reduce the incidence of postoperative edema.[317] We have observed much less edema in patients undergoing in situ femorotibial bypass grafting when the branches are identified angioscopically and occluded using small interrupted incisions rather than continuous incisions. Once this complication occurs, bed rest, elevation, the use of elastic support stockings, and diuretics control the edema by shifting capillary dynamics in favor of fluid reabsorption.[292] Fortunately, in most instances, postreconstructive edema is self-limited and improves or disappears during the first few postoperative months.[58]

LYMPHOCELES AND LYMPH LEAKS

The accumulation of lymph after groin surgery usually appears as an asymptomatic mass without evidence of overlying inflammation. If the lymphocele is small and located some distance from the incision, it can be followed expectantly. Should the lymphocele fail to resolve spontaneously, increase in size, communicate with the incision, or begin to leak, it should be explored and treated as in patients with lymph leaks. Intraoperative lymphatic mapping with isosulfan blue dye may be helpful in identifying the site of the leak. Whether this complication can be prevented by the routine application of fibrin glue to the femoral lymphatics before wound closure remains debatable.

Drainage of lymphatic fluid from the groin incision is a relatively infrequent complication of arterial reconstruction.

In the series reported by Kent and associates, a seroma lymph leak was present in 4% of the patients with groin incisions who were evaluated prospectively.[275] The leak appears as a persistent, clear, watery drainage through the wound after the first few postoperative days or as the onset of drainage when the patient resumes ambulation.[58] The frequent presence of bacteria in the lymphatic channels draining ulcerative or gangrenous lesions of the extremity may lead to graft infection and anastomotic disruption.

Lymphatic leakage results from transected and unligated lymphatic channels and lymph nodes in the groin incision. Possible contributing factors include poor wound edge and tissue layer approximation and subcutaneous fat necrosis.[58]

Nonoperative treatment of lymphorrhea includes bed rest and leg elevation to reduce lymph flow while allowing the lymphatics to heal. Wound care must be meticulous, and systemic prophylactic antibiotics should be administered to reduce the risk of secondary infection.[58]

If the wound continues to drain for more than 2 to 3 days, the patient should be returned to the operating room and the wound explored. The divided lymphatic channels are suture-ligated, and the wound is closed in layers over suction drainage with care being taken to separate the drain from the prosthesis. This technique controls wound drainage and decreases the risk of secondary infection of the lymphatic cavity.[318,319] The reported experience with early wound re-exploration suggests shortened hospitalization and a reduction in the incidence of graft infection. Because the site of lymphatic disruption may not be recognized on re-exploration of the wound, manual massage of the thigh or staining of the lymphatic system by injection of isosulfan blue dye or radiolabeled isotope in the foot several hours before surgery is recommended to aid in identifying the leak site.

KEY REFERENCES

Aalami OO, Allen DB, Organ CH, Jr: Chylous ascites: A collective review. Surgery 128:761–788, 2000.

Davis PM, Gloviczki P, Cherry KJ, Jr, et al: Aorto-caval and ilio-iliac arteriovenous fistulae. Am J Surg 176:115–118, 1998.

Minniti S, Visentini S, Procacci C: Congenital anomalies of the venae cavae: Embryological origin, imaging features and report of three new variants. Eur Radiol 12:2040–2055, 2002.

Pabst TS, 3rd, McIntyre KE, Jr, Schilling JD, et al: Management of chyloperitoneum after abdominal aortic surgery. Am J Surg 166:194–199, 1993.

Reddy VG: Prevention of postoperative acute renal failure. J Postgrad Med 48:64–70, 2002.

REFERENCES

1. Downs AR: Complications of abdominal aortic surgery. In Bernhard VM, Towne JB (eds): Complications in Vascular Surgery. Orlando, Fla, Grune & Stratton, 1985, pp 25-36.
2. Brener BJ, Darling RC, Frederick PL, et al: Major venous anomalies complicating abdominal aortic surgery. Arch Surg 108:159-165, 1974.
3. Minniti S, Visentini S, Procacci C: Congenital anomalies of the venae cavae: Embryological origin, imaging features and report of three new variants. Eur Radiol 12:2040-2055, 2002.
4. Reed MD, Friedman AC, Nealey P: Anomalies of the left renal vein: Analysis of 433 CT scans. J Comput Assist Tomogr 6:1124-1126, 1982.
5. Bartle EJ, Pearce WH, Sun JH, et al: Infrarenal venous anomalies and aortic surgery: Avoiding vascular injury. J Vasc Surg 6:590-593, 1987.
6. Berhnard VM: Aortocaval fistulas. In Haimovici H (ed): Vascular Emergencies. New York, Appleton-Century-Crofts, 1982, pp 353-363.
7. Duppler DW, Herbert WE, Dillihunt RC, et al: Primary arteriovenous fistulas of the abdomen: Their occurrence secondary to aneurysmal disease of the aorta and iliac arteries. Arch Surg 120:786-790, 1985.
8. Brewster DC, Cambria RP, Moncure AC, et al: Aortocaval and iliac arteriovenous fistulas: Recognition and treatment. J Vasc Surg 13:253-265, 1991.
9. Calligaro KD, Savarese RP, DeLaurentis DA: Unusual aspects of aortovenous fistulas associated with ruptured abdominal aortic aneurysms. J Vasc Surg 12:586-590, 1990.
10. Dardik H, Dardik I, Strom MG, et al: Intravenous rupture of arteriosclerotic aneurysms of the abdominal aorta. Surgery 80:647-651, 1976.
11. Davis PM, Gloviczki P, Cherry KJ Jr, et al: Aorto-caval and ilio-iliac arteriovenous fistulae. Am J Surg 176:115-118, 1998.
12. Zajko AB, Little AF, Steed DL, et al: Endovascular stent-graft repair of common iliac artery-to-inferior vena cava fistula. J Vasc Interv Radiol 6:803-806, 1995.
13. Parodi JC, Criado FJ, Barone HD, et al: Endoluminal aortic aneurysm repair using a balloon-expandable stent-graft device: A progress report. Ann Vasc Surg 8:523-529, 1994.
14. Hsu THS, Su LM, Ratner LE, et al: Impact of renal artery multiplicity on outcomes of renal donors and recipients in laparoscopic donor nephrectomy. Urology 61:323-327, 2003.
15. Thompson JE, Hollier LH, Patman RD, et al: Surgical management of abdominal aortic aneurysms: Factors influencing mortality and morbidity—a 20-year experience. Ann Surg 181:654-661, 1975.
16. Yeh BM, Coakley FV, Meng MV, et al: Precaval right renal arteries: Prevalence and morphologic associations at spiral CT. Radiology 230:429-433, 2004.
17. Basu S, Marini CP, Bauman FG, et al: Comparative study of biological glues: Cryoprecipitate glue, two-component fibrin sealant, and "French" glue. Ann Thorac Surg 60:1255-1262, 1995.
18. Bingley JA, Gardner MAH, Stafford EG, et al: Late complications of tissue glues in aortic surgery. Ann Thorac Surg 69:1764-1768, 2000.
19. Peters DC, Noble S: Aprotinin: An update of its pharmacology and therapeutic use in open heart surgery and coronary artery bypass surgery. Drugs 57:233-260, 1999.
20. Landis RC, Haskard DO, Taylor KM: New antiinflammatory and platelet-preserving effects of aprotinin. Ann Thorac Surg 72:S1808-S1813, 2001.
21. Effeney DJ, Goldstone J, Chin D, et al: Intraoperative anticoagulation in cardiovascular surgery. Surgery 90:1068-1074, 1981.
22. Chun R, Orser BA, Madan M: Platelet glycoprotein IIb/IIIa inhibitors: Overview and implications for the anesthesiologist. Anesth Analg 95:879-888, 2002.
23. Claeys LGY, Berg W: Major bleeding and severe thrombocytopenia after combined heparin and abciximab-c7E3 Fab therapy. Eur J Vasc Endovasc Surg 25:85-87, 2003.
24. Waters JH, Anthony DG, Gottlieb A, et al: Bleeding in a patient receiving platelet aggregation inhibitors. Anesth Analg 93:878-882, 2001.
25. Neilipovitz DT, Bryson GL, Nichol G: The effect of perioperative aspirin therapy in peripheral vascular surgery: A decision analysis. Anesth Analg 93:573-580, 2001.
26. Ray JG, Deniz S, Olivieri A, et al: Increased blood product use among coronary artery bypass patients prescribed preoperative aspirin and clopidogrel. BMC Cardiovasc Disord 3:3, 2003.
27. Crawford ES, Manning LG, Kelly FT: "Redo" surgery after operations for aneurysm and occlusion of the abdominal aorta. Surgery 81:41-52, 1977.
28. O'Hara PJ, Brewster DC, Darling RC, et al: The value of intraoperative monitoring using the pulse volume recorder during peripheral vascular reconstructive operations. Surg Gynecol Obstet 152:275-281, 1981.
29. Strom JA, Bernhard VM, Towne JB: Acute limb ischemia following aortic reconstruction: A preventable cause of increased mortality. Arch Surg 119:470-473, 1984.
30. Kapsch DN, Adelstein EH, Rhodes GR, et al: Heparin-induced thrombocytopenia, thrombosis, and hemorrhage. Surgery 86:148-155, 1979.
31. Towne JB: Hypercoagulable states and unexplained vascular thrombosis. In Bernhard VM, Towne JB (eds): Complications in Vascular Surgery. Orlando, Fla, Grune & Stratton, 1985, pp 381-404.
32. Towne JB, Bernhard VM, Hussey C, et al: Antithrombin deficiency—a cause of unexplained thrombosis in vascular surgery. Surgery 89:735-742, 1981.
33. Towne JB, Bernhard VM, Hussey C, et al: White clot syndrome: Peripheral vascular complications of heparin therapy. Arch Surg 114:372-377, 1979.
34. Bernhard VM: The failed arterial graft: Lost pulses and gangrene. In Condon RE, DeCosse J (eds): Surgical Care: A Physiologic Approach to Clinical Management. Philadelphia, Lea & Febiger, 1980, pp 153-167.
35. Brewster DC, Darling RC: Optimal methods of aortoiliac reconstruction. Surgery 84:739-748, 1978.
36. O'Mara CS, Flinn WR, Johnson ND, et al: Recognition and surgical management of patent but hemodynamically failed arterial grafts. Ann Surg 193:467-476, 1981.
37. Baird RJ, Feldman P, Miles JT, et al: Subsequent downstream repair after aorta-iliac and aorta-femoral bypass operations. Surgery 82:785-793, 1977.
38. Baird RJ: Downstream revascularization after aortofemoral bypass grafting. In Bergan JJ, Yao JST (eds): Reoperative Arterial Surgery. Orlando, Fla, Grune & Stratton, 1986, pp 223-230.
39. Lewis BE, Wallis DE, Berkowitz SD, et al: Argatroban anticoagulant therapy in patients with heparin-induced thrombocytopenia. Circulation 103:1838-1843, 2001.
40. Rice L, Attisha WK, Drexler A, et al: Delayed-onset heparin-induced thrombocytopenia. Ann Intern Med 136:210-215, 2002.
41. Greinacher A, Lubenow N, Eichler P: Anaphylactic and anaphylactoid reactions associated with lepirudin in patients with heparin-induced thrombocytopenia. Circulation 108:2062-2065, 2003.
42. Mulcare RJ, Royster TS, Lynn RA, et al: Long-term results of operative therapy for aortoiliac disease. Arch Surg 113:601-604, 1978.
43. Nevelsteen A, Suy R, Daenen W, et al: Aortofemoral grafting: Factors influencing late results. Surgery 88:642-653, 1980.
44. Charlesworth D: The occluded aortic and aorto-femoral graft. In Bergan JJ, Yao JST (eds): Reoperative Arterial Surgery. Orlando, Fla, Grune & Stratton, 1986, pp 271-278.
45. Fulenwider JT, Smith RB 3rd, Johnson RW, et al: Reoperative abdominal arterial surgery—a ten-year experience. Surgery 93:20-27, 1983.
46. Robbs JV, Wylie EJ: Factors contributing to recurrent lower limb ischemia following bypass surgery for aortoiliac occlusive disease, and their management. Ann Surg 193:346-352, 1981.
47. Frisch N, Bour P, Berg P, et al: Long-term results of thrombectomy for late occlusions of aortofemoral bypass. Ann Vasc Surg 5:16-20, 1991.
48. Nevelsteen A, Suy R: Graft occlusion following aortofemoral Dacron bypass. Ann Vasc Surg 5:32-37, 1991.
49. LoGerfo FW, Quist WC, Nowak MD, et al: Downstream anastomotic hyperplasia: A mechanism of failure in Dacron arterial grafts. Ann Surg 197:479-483, 1983.
50. Malone JM, Moore WS, Goldstone J: The natural history of bilateral aortofemoral bypass grafts for ischemia of the lower extremities. Arch Surg 110:1300-1306, 1975.
51. Rhodes RS, Hutton MC, Lalka SG: Reoperation for intra-abdominal vascular disease. In Fry DE (ed): Reoperative Surgery of the Abdomen. New York, Marcel Dekker, 1986, pp 153-174.
52. Wylie EJ, Olcott C: Aortoiliac thromboendarterectomy. In Varco RL, Delaney JP (eds): Controversy in Surgery. Philadelphia, WB Saunders, 1976, pp 437-450.

53. Crawford ES, Bomberger RA, Glaeser DH, et al: Aortoiliac occlusive disease: Factors influencing survival and function following reconstructive operation over a twenty-five-year period. Surgery 90:1055-1067, 1981.
54. Satiani B, Liapis CD, Evans WE: Aortofemoral bypass for severe limb ischemia: Long-term survival and limb salvage. Am J Surg 141:252-256, 1981.
55. Yao JST, McCarthy WJ: Surgical correction of hemodynamic failure of bypass grafts. In Bergan JJ, Yao JST (eds): Reoperative Arterial Surgery. Orlando, Fla, Grune & Stratton, 1986, pp 257-270.
56. Bernhard VM: Late vascular graft thrombosis. In Bernhard VM, Towne JB (eds): Complications in Vascular Surgery. Orlando, Fla, Grune & Stratton, 1985, pp 187-204.
57. Bernhard VM, Ray LI, Towne JB: The reoperation of choice for aortofemoral graft occlusion. Surgery 82:867-874, 1977.
58. Brewster DC: Early complications of vascular repair below the inguinal ligament. In Bernhard VM, Towne JB (eds): Complications in Vascular Surgery. Orlando, Fla, Grune & Stratton, 1985, pp 37-53.
59. Ansel GM, Botti CF Jr, Silver MJ: Mechanical devices and acute limb ischemia. Endovascular Today March:46-48, 2003.
60. DePalma RG, Malgieri JJ, Rhodes RS, et al: Profunda femoris bypass for secondary revascularization. Surg Gynecol Obstet 151:387-390, 1980.
61. van Breda A, Robison JC, Feldman L, et al: Local thrombolysis in the treatment of arterial graft occlusions. J Vasc Surg 1:103-112, 1984.
62. Battey PM, Fulenwider JT, Smith RB 3rd, et al: Intra-arterial thrombolysis for acute limb ischemia: A three-year experience. South Med J 80:479-482, 1987.
63. Katzen BT, Edwards KC, Albert AS, et al: Low-dose direct fibrinolysis in peripheral vascular disease. J Vasc Surg 1:718-722, 1984.
64. McNamara TO, Bomberger RA: Factors affecting initial and 6 month patency rates after intraarterial thrombolysis with high dose urokinase. Am J Surg 152:709-712, 1986.
65. McNamara TO, Fischer JR: Thrombolysis of peripheral arterial and graft occlusions: Improved results using high-dose urokinase. AJR Am J Roentgenol 144:769-775, 1985.
66. Sicard GA, Schier JJ, Totty WG, et al: Thrombolytic therapy for acute arterial occlusion. J Vasc Surg 2:65-78, 1985.
67. van Breda A, Katzen BT, Deutsch AS: Urokinase versus streptokinase in local thrombolysis. Radiology 165:109-111, 1987.
68. Allie DE, Hebert CJ, Lirtzman MD, et al: Continuous tenecteplase infusion combined with peri/postprocedural platelet glycoprotein IIb/IIIa inhibition in peripheral arterial thrombolysis: Initial safety and feasibility experience. J Endovasc Ther 11:427-435, 2004.
69. Shortell CK, Queiroz R, Johansson M, et al: Safety and efficacy of limited-dose tissue plasminogen activator in acute vascular occlusion. J Vasc Surg 34:854-859, 2001.
70. Conrad MF, Shepard AD, Rubinfeld IS, et al: Long-term results of catheter-directed thrombolysis to treat infrainguinal bypass graft occlusion: The urokinase era. J Vasc Surg 37:1009-1016, 2003.
71. Ouriel K, Kandarpa K: Safety of thrombolytic therapy with urokinase or recombinant tissue plasminogen activator for peripheral arterial occlusion: A comprehensive compilation of published work. J Endovasc Ther 11:436-446, 2004.
72. Semba CP, Murphy TP, Bakal CW, et al: Thrombolytic therapy with use of alteplase (rt-PA) in peripheral arterial occlusive disease: Review of the clinical literature. The Advisory Panel. J Vasc Interv Radiol 11:149-161, 2000.
73. Belkin M, Belkin B, Bucknam CA, et al: Intra-arterial fibrinolytic therapy: Efficacy of streptokinase vs urokinase. Arch Surg 121:769-773, 1986.
74. Hallett JW Jr, Wolk SW, Cherry KJ Jr, et al: The femoral neuralgia syndrome after arterial catheter trauma. J Vasc Surg 11:702-706, 1990.
75. Ganglani RD, Turk AA, Mehra MR, et al: Contralateral femoral neuropathy: An unusual complication of anticoagulation following PTCA. Cathet Cardiovasc Diagn 24:176-178, 1991.
76. Gardiner GA Jr, Harrington DP, Koltun W, et al: Salvage of occluded arterial bypass grafts by means of thrombolysis. J Vasc Surg 9:426-431, 1989.
77. Ouriel K, Shortell CK, DeWeese JA, et al: A comparison of thrombolytic therapy with operative revascularization in the initial treatment of acute peripheral arterial ischemia. J Vasc Surg 19:1021-1030, 1994.
78. Ouriel K, Veith FJ, Sasahara AA: Thrombolysis or peripheral arterial surgery: Phase I results. TOPAS Investigators. J Vasc Surg 23:64-75, 1996.
79. STILE investigators: Results of a prospective randomized trial evaluating surgery versus thrombolysis for ischemia of the lower extremity. The STILE trial. Ann Surg 220:251-268, 1994.
80. Hye RJ, Turner C, Valji K, et al: Is thrombolysis of occluded popliteal and tibial bypass grafts worthwhile? J Vasc Surg 20:588-597, 1994.
81. Garramone RR Jr, Gallagher JJ Jr, Drezner AD: Intra-arterial thrombolytic therapy in the initial management of thrombosed popliteal artery aneurysms. Ann Vasc Surg 8:363-366, 1994.
82. Laird JR, Dangas G, Jaff M, et al: Intra-arterial reteplase for the treatment of acute limb ischemia. J Invasive Cardiol 11:757-762, 1999.
83. McNamara TO: New pharmacologic therapies in the treatment of peripheral vascular disease. Paper presented at the 11th Annual Symposium on Transcatheter Cardiovascular Therapeutics (TCT-11), Sep 22-26, 1999, Washington, DC.
84. Sharafuddin MJ, Hicks ME: Current status of percutaneous mechanical thrombectomy. Part II. Devices and mechanisms of action. J Vasc Interv Radiol 9:15-31, 1998.
85. Ouriel K: Percutaneous recirculation mechanical thrombectomy catheter (Angiojet) in the management of limb threatening ischemia. Paper presented at the 26th Annual Critical Problems and New Horizons and Techniques in Vascular and Endovascular Surgery, New York, Nov 18-21, 1999.
86. Haskal ZJ: Mechanical thrombectomy devices for the treatment of peripheral arterial occlusions. Rev Cardiovasc Med 3(Suppl 2):S45-S52, 2002.
86a. Sarac TP, Hilleman D, Arko FR, et al: Clinical and economic evaluation of the trellis thrombectomy device for arterial occlusions: Preliminary analysis. J Vasc Surg 39:556–559, 2004.
87. Demopoulos LA, Tunick PA, Bernstein NE, et al: Protruding atheromas of the aortic arch in symptomatic patients with carotid artery disease. Am Heart J 129:40-44, 1995.
88. Lagattolla NR, Burnand KG, Stewart A: Role of transoesophageal echocardiography in determining the source of peripheral arterial embolism. Br J Surg 82:1651-1654, 1995.
89. Kazmier FJ, Sheps SG, Bernatz PE, et al: Livedo reticularis and digital infarcts: A syndrome due to cholesterol emboli arising from atheromatous abdominal aortic aneurysms. Vasc Dis 3:12-24, 1966.
90. Starr DS, Lawrie GM, Morris GC Jr: Prevention of distal embolism during arterial reconstruction. Am J Surg 138:764-769, 1979.
91. Attia RR, Murphy JD, Snider M, et al: Myocardial ischemia due to infrarenal aortic cross-clamping during aortic surgery in patients with severe coronary artery disease. Circulation 53:961-965, 1976.
92. Bush HL Jr, LoGerfo FW, Weisel RD, et al: Assessment of myocardial performance and optimal volume loading during elective abdominal aortic aneurysm resection. Arch Surg 112:1301-1305, 1977.
93. Dauchot PJ, DePalma R, Grum D, et al: Detection and prevention of cardiac dysfunction during aortic surgery. J Surg Res 26:574-580, 1979.
94. Silverstein PR, Caldera DL, Cullen DJ, et al: Avoiding the hemodynamic consequences of aortic cross-clamping and unclamping. Anesthesiology 50:462-466, 1979.
95. Whittemore AD, Clowes AW, Hechtman HB, et al: Aortic aneurysm repair: Reduced operative mortality associated with maintenance of optimal cardiac performance. Ann Surg 192:414-421, 1980.
96. Abbott WM, Abel RM, Beck CH Jr, et al: Renal failure after ruptured aneurysm. Arch Surg 110:1110-1112, 1975.
97. Castonuovo JJ, Flanigan DP: Renal failure complicating vascular surgery. In Bernhard VM, Towne JB (eds): Complications in Vascular Surgery. Orlando, Fla, Grune & Stratton, 1985, pp 258-274.
98. Abbott WM, Austen WG: The reversal of renal cortical ischemia during aortic occlusion by mannitol. J Surg Res 16:482-489, 1974.
99. Berkowitz HD, Shetty S: Renin release and renal cortical ischemia following aortic cross clamping. Arch Surg 109:612-617, 1974.
100. Crawford ES, Snyder DM, Cho GC, et al: Progress in treatment of thoracoabdominal and abdominal aortic aneurysms involving celiac, superior mesenteric, and renal arteries. Ann Surg 188:404-422, 1978.
101. Iliopoulos JI, Zdon MJ, Crawford BG, et al: Renal microembolization syndrome: A cause for renal dysfunction after abdominal aortic reconstruction. Am J Surg 146:779-783, 1983.
102. Myers BD, Moran SM: Hemodynamically mediated acute renal failure. N Engl J Med 314:97-105, 1986.
103. Bush HL Jr, Huse JB, Johnson WC, et al: Prevention of renal insufficiency after abdominal aortic aneurysm resection by optimal volume loading. Arch Surg 116:1517-1524, 1981.
104. Reddy VG: Prevention of postoperative acute renal failure. J Postgrad Med 48:64-70, 2002.
105. Franklin SC, Moulton M, Sicard GA, et al: Insulin-like growth factor I preserves renal function postoperatively. Am J Physiol 272:F257-F259, 1997.
106. Meyer M, Wiebe K, Wahlers T, et al: Urodilatin (INN: ularitide) as a new drug for the therapy of acute renal failure following cardiac surgery. Clin Exp Pharmacol Physiol 24:374-376, 1997.

107. Wiebe K, Meyer M, Wahlers T, et al: Acute renal failure following cardiac surgery is reverted by administration of Urodilatin (INN: ularitide). Eur J Med Res 1:259-265, 1996.

108. Krause SM, Walsh TF, Greenlee WJ, et al: Renal protection by a dual ETA/ETB endothelin antagonist, L-754,142, after aortic cross-clamping in the dog. J Am Soc Nephrol 8:1061-1071, 1997.

109. Sheinbaum R, Ignacio C, Safi HJ, et al: Contemporary strategies to preserve renal function during cardiac and vascular surgery. Rev Cardiovasc Med 4(Suppl 1):S21-S28, 2003.

110. Szilagyi DE, Smith RF, Elliott JP: Temporary transection of the left renal vein: A technical aid in aortic surgery. Surgery 65:32-40, 1969.

111. Huber D, Harris JP, Walker PJ, et al: Does division of the left renal vein during aortic surgery adversely affect renal function? Ann Vasc Surg 5:74-79, 1991.

112. Abu Rahma AF, Robinson PA, Boland JP, et al: The risk of ligation of the left renal vein in resection of the abdominal aortic aneurysm. Surg Gynecol Obstet 173:33-36, 1991.

113. Calligaro KD, Savarese RP, McCombs PR, et al: Division of the left renal vein during aortic surgery. Am J Surg 160:192-196, 1990.

114. Komori K, Furuyama T, Maehara Y: Renal artery clamping and left renal vein division during abdominal aortic aneurysm repair. Eur J Vasc Endovasc Surg 27:80-83, 2004.

115. Olsen PS, Schroeder T, Perko M, et al: Renal failure after operation for abdominal aortic aneurysm. Ann Vasc Surg 4:580-583, 1990.

116. Mandal AK, Visweswaran RK, Kaldas NR: Treatment considerations in acute renal failure. Drugs 44:567-577, 1992.

117. Tepel M, van der Giet M, Schwarzfeld C, et al: Prevention of radiographic-contrast-agent-induced reductions in renal function by acetylcysteine. N Engl J Med 343:180-184, 2000.

118. Kay J, Chow WH, Chan TM, et al: Acetylcysteine for prevention of acute deterioration of renal function following elective coronary angiography and intervention: A randomized controlled trial. JAMA 289:553-558, 2003.

119. Ernst CB: Postoperative intestinal ischemia. In Haimovici H (ed): Vascular Emergencies. New York, Appleton-Century-Crofts, 1982, pp 493-513.

120. Johnson WC, Nabseth DC: Visceral infarction following aortic surgery. Ann Surg 180:312-318, 1974.

121. Ottinger LW, Darling RC, Nathan MJ, et al: Left colon ischemia complicating aorto-iliac reconstruction: Causes, diagnosis, management, and prevention. Arch Surg 105:841-846, 1972.

122. Ernst CB: Intestinal ischemia following abdominal aortic reconstruction. In Bernhard VM, Towne JB (eds): Complications in Vascular Surgery. Orlando, Fla, Grune & Stratton, 1985, pp 325-350.

123. Hagihara PF, Ernst CB, Griffen WO Jr: Incidence of ischemic colitis following abdominal aortic reconstruction. Surg Gynecol Obstet 149:571-573, 1979.

124. Moskowitz M, Zimmerman H, Felson B: The meandering mesenteric artery of the colon. Am J Roentgenol Radium Ther Nucl Med 92:1088-1099, 1964.

125. Ernst CB, Hagihara PF, Daughtery ME, et al: Ischemic colitis incidence following abdominal aortic reconstruction: A prospective study. Surgery 80:417-421, 1976.

126. Venkateswaran RV, Charman SC, Goddard M, et al: Lethal mesenteric ischaemia after cardiopulmonary bypass: A common complication? Eur J Cardiothorac Surg 22:534-538, 2002.

127. Boley SJ, Brandt LJ, Veith FJ: Ischemic disorders of the intestines. Curr Probl Surg 15:1-85, 1978.

128. Hobson RW 2nd, Wright CB, O'Donnell JA, et al: Determination of intestinal viability by Doppler ultrasound. Arch Surg 114:165-168, 1979.

129. Bicks RO, Bale GF, McBurney RF, et al: Acute and delayed colon ischemia after aortic aneurysm surgery. Arch Intern Med 122:249-253, 1968.

130. Yee J, Dixon CM, McLean AP, et al: Clostridium difficile disease in a department of surgery: The significance of prophylactic antibiotics. Arch Surg 126:241-246, 1991.

131. Teasley DG, Gerding DN, Olson MM, et al: Prospective randomised trial of metronidazole versus vancomycin for Clostridium-difficile-associated diarrhoea and colitis. Lancet 2:1043-1046, 1983.

132. Champagne BJ, Darling RC 3rd, Daneshmand M, et al: Outcome of aggressive surveillance colonoscopy in ruptured abdominal aortic aneurysm. J Vasc Surg 39:792-796, 2004.

133. Björck M, Hedberg B: Early detection of major complications after abdominal aortic surgery: Predictive value of sigmoid colon and gastric intramucosal pH monitoring. Br J Surg 81:25-30, 1994.

134. Acosta S, Nilsson TK, Björck M: D-dimer testing in patients with suspected acute thromboembolic occlusion of the superior mesenteric artery. Br J Surg 91:991-994, 2004.

135. Ernst CB, Hagihara PF, Daugherty ME, et al: Inferior mesenteric artery stump pressure: A reliable index for safe IMA ligation during abdominal aortic aneurysmectomy. Ann Surg 187:641-646, 1978.

136. Welling RE, Roedersheimer LR, Arbaugh JJ, et al: Ischemic colitis following repair of ruptured abdominal aortic aneurysm. Arch Surg 120:1368-1370, 1985.

137. Connolly JE, Kwaan JH: Prophylactic revascularization of the gut. Ann Surg 190:514-522, 1979.

138. Rubin GD, Dake MD, Semba CP: Current status of three-dimensional spiral CT scanning for imaging the vasculature. Radiol Clin North Am 33:51-70, 1995.

139. Kirkpatrick IDC, Kroeker MA, Greenberg HM: Biphasic CT with mesenteric CT angiography in the evaluation of acute mesenteric ischemia: Initial experience. Radiology 229:91-98, 2003.

140. Zelenock GB, Strodel WE, Knol JA, et al: A prospective study of clinically and endoscopically documented colonic ischemia in 100 patients undergoing aortic reconstructive surgery with aggressive colonic and direct pelvic revascularization, compared with historic controls. Surgery 106:771-780, 1989.

141. Oderich GS, Panneton JM, Macedo TA, et al: Intraoperative duplex ultrasound of visceral revascularizations: Optimizing technical success and outcome. J Vasc Surg 38:684-691, 2003.

142. Sharafuddin MJ, Olson CH, Sun S, et al: Endovascular treatment of celiac and mesenteric arteries stenosis: Applications and results. J Vasc Surg 38:692-698, 2003.

143. Di Chiro G, Doppman JL: Paraplegia after resection of aneurysm. N Engl J Med 281:799, 1969.

144. Elliott JP, Szilagyi DE, Hageman JH, et al: Spinal cord ischemia: Secondary to surgery of the abdominal aorta. In Bernhard VM, Towne JB (eds): Complications in Vascular Surgery. Orlando, Fla, Grune & Stratton, 1985, pp 291-310.

145. Szilagyi DE, Hageman JH, Smith RF, et al: Spinal cord damage in surgery of the abdominal aorta. Surgery 83:38-56, 1978.

146. Ferguson LRJ, Bergan JJ, Conn J Jr, et al: Spinal ischemia following abdominal aortic surgery. Ann Surg 181:267-272, 1975.

147. Grace RR, Mattox KL: Anterior spinal artery syndrome following abdominal aortic aneurysmectomy: Case report and review of the literautre. Arch Surg 112:813-815, 1977.

148. Di Chiro G, Wener L: Angiography of the spinal cord: A review of contemporary techniques and applications. J Neurosurg 39:1-29, 1973.

149. Williams GM, Perler BA, Burdick JF, et al: Angiographic localization of spinal cord blood supply and its relationship to postoperative paraplegia. J Vasc Surg 13:23-35, 1991.

150. Kieffer E, Richard T, Chiras J, et al: Preoperative spinal cord arteriography in aneurysmal disease of the descending thoracic and thoracoabdominal aorta: Preliminary results in 45 patients. Ann Vasc Surg 3:34-46, 1989.

151. Cunningham JN Jr, Laschinger JC, Merkin HA, et al: Measurement of spinal cord ischemia during operations upon the thoracic aorta: Initial clinical experience. Ann Surg 196:285-296, 1982.

152. Coles JG, Wilson GJ, Sima AF, et al: Intraoperative detection of spinal cord ischemia using somatosensory cortical evoked potentials during thoracic aortic occlusion. Ann Thorac Surg 34:299-306, 1982.

153. Laschinger JC, Cunningham JN Jr, Catinella FP, et al: Detection and prevention of intraoperative spinal cord ischemia after cross-clamping of the thoracic aorta: Use of somatosensory evoked potentials. Surgery 92:1109-1117, 1982.

154. Laschinger JC, Cunningham JN Jr, Nathan IM, et al: Experimental and clinical assessment of the adequacy of partial bypass in maintenance of spinal cord blood flow during operations on the thoracic aorta. Ann Thorac Surg 36:417-426, 1983.

155. Picone AL, Green RM, Ricotta JR, et al: Spinal cord ischemia following operations on the abdominal aorta. J Vasc Surg 3:94-103, 1986.

156. Labardini MM, Ratliff RK: The abdominal aortic aneurysm and the ureter. J Urol 98:590-596, 1967.

157. Goldstone J, Malone JM, Moore WS: Inflammatory aneurysms of the abdominal aorta. Surgery 83:425-430, 1978.

158. Nachbur B, Marincek B, Jakob R, et al: The impact of computed tomography in the diagnosis and postoperative follow-up of ureteric obstruction in aorto-iliac aneurysmal disease. Eur J Vasc Surg 3:475-492, 1989.

159. Egeblad K, Brochner-Mortensen J, Krarup T, et al: Incidence of ureteral obstruction after aortic grafting: A prospective analysis. Surgery 103:411-414, 1988.

160. Spirnak JP, Hampel N, Resnick MI: Ureteral injuries complicating vascular surgery: Is repair indicated? J Urol 141:13-14, 1989.
161. Lask D, Abarbanel J, Luttwak Z, et al: Changing trends in the management of iatrogenic ureteral injuries. J Urol 154:1693-1695, 1995.
162. Preston JM: Iatrogenic ureteric injury: Common medicolegal pitfalls. BJU Int 86:313-317, 2000.
163. Cangiano TG, de Kernion JB: Urologic complications of vascular surgery. In Ball TPJ (ed): AUA Update Series Lesson 39, vol 17. Houston, American Urological Association, 1998, pp 306–311.
164. Sant GR, Heaney JA, Parkhurst EC, et al: Obstructive uropathy—a potentially serious complication of reconstructive vascular surgery. J Urol 129:16-22, 1983.
165. Goldenberg SL, Gordon PB, Cooperberg PL, et al: Early hydronephrosis following aortic bifurcation graft surgery: A prospective study. J Urol 140:1367-1369, 1988.
166. Wright DJ, Ernst CB, Evans JR, et al: Ureteral complications and aortoiliac reconstruction. J Vasc Surg 11:29-37, 1990.
167. Kempczinski RF, Birinyi LK: Impotence following aortic surgery. In Bernhard VM, Towne JB (eds): Complications in Vascular Surgery. Orlando, Fla, Grune & Stratton, 1985, pp 311-324.
168. Merchant RF Jr, DePalma RG: Effects of femorofemoral grafts on postoperative sexual function: Correlation with penile pulse volume recordings. Surgery 90:962-970, 1981.
169. Ohshiro T, Kosaki G: Sexual function after aorto-iliac vascular reconstruction: Which is more important, the internal iliac artery or hypogastric nerve? J Cardiovasc Surg (Torino) 25:47-50, 1984.
170. Queral LA, Flinn WR, Bergan JJ, et al: Sexual function and aortic surgery. In Bergan JJ, Yao JST (eds): Surgery of the Aorta and Its Body Branches. Orlando, Fla, Grune & Stratton, 1979, pp 263-276.
171. Queral LA, Whitehouse WM Jr, Flinn WR, et al: Pelvic hemodynamics after aortoiliac reconstruction. Surgery 86:799-809, 1979.
172. Kempczinski RF: Role of the vascular diagnostic laboratory in the evaluation of male impotence. Am J Surg 138:278-282, 1979.
173. Nath RL, Menzoian JO, Kaplan KH, et al: The multidisciplinary approach to vasculogenic impotence. Surgery 89:124-133, 1981.
174. Flanigan DP, Sobinsky KR, Schuler JJ, et al: Internal iliac artery revascularization in the treatment of vasculogenic impotence. Arch Surg 120:271-274, 1985.
175. DePalma RG, Olding M, Yu GW, et al: Vascular interventions for impotence: Lessons learned. J Vasc Surg 21:576-585, 1995.
176. Flanigan DP, Schuler JJ: Sexual function in aortic surgery. In Bergan JJ, Yao JST (eds): Aortic Surgery. Philadelphia, WB Saunders, 1989, pp 547-660.
177. Donohue JP, Thornhill JA, Foster RS, et al: Retroperitoneal lymphadenectomy for clinical stage A testis cancer (1965 to 1989): Modifications of technique and impact on ejaculation. J Urol 149:237-243, 1993.
178. Colleselli K, Poisel S, Schachtner W, et al: Nerve-preserving bilateral retroperitoneal lymphadenectomy: Anatomical study and operative approach. J Urol 144:293-298, 1990.
179. Depalma RG: Impotence in vascular disease: Relationship to vascular surgery. Br J Surg 69(Suppl):S14-S16, 1982.
180. Chavez CM: False aneurysms of the femoral artery: A challenge in management. Ann Surg 183:694-700, 1976.
181. Gardner TJ, Brawley RK, Gott VL: Anastomotic false aneurysms. Surgery 72:474-478, 1972.
182. Knox WG: Peripheral vascular anastomotic aneurysms: A fifteen-year experience. Ann Surg 183:120-123, 1976.
183. Read RC, Thompson BW: Uninfected anastomotic false aneurysms following arterial reconstruction with prosthetic grafts. J Cardiovasc Surg (Torino) 16:558-561, 1975.
184. Satiani B, Kazmers M, Evans WE: Anastomotic arterial aneurysms: A continuing challenge. Ann Surg 192:674-682, 1980.
185. Szilagyi DE, Smith RF, Elliott JP, et al: Anastomotic aneurysms after vascular reconstruction: Problems of incidence, etiology, and treatment. Surgery 78:800-816, 1975.
186. Satiani B: False aneurysms following arterial reconstruction. Surg Gynecol Obstet 152:357-363, 1981.
187. Bernhard VM: Aortoduodenal and other aortoenteric fistulas. In Veith FJ (ed): Critical Problems in Vascular Surgery. New York, Appleton-Century-Crofts, 1982, pp 399-410.
188. Geun Eun K, Imparato AM, Nathan I, et al: Dilation of synthetic grafts and junctional aneurysms. Arch Surg 114:1296-1303, 1979.
189. Evans WE, Hayes JP, Vermilion B: Anastomotic femoral false aneurysms. In Bernhard VM, Towne JB (eds): Complications in Vascular Surgery. Orlando, Fla, Grune & Stratton, 1985, pp 205-212.
190. Moore WS: Anastomotic aneurysms. In Rutherford RB (ed): Vascular Surgery. Philadelphia, WB Saunders, 1984, pp 821-827.
191. Clark RE, Apostolou S, Kardos JL: Mismatch of mechanical properties as a cause of arterial prosthesis thrombosis. Surg Forum 27:208-210, 1978.
192. Mehigan DG, Fitzpatrick B, Browne HI, et al: Is compliance mismatch the major cause of anastomotic arterial aneurysms? Analysis of 42 cases. J Cardiovasc Surg (Torino) 26:147-150, 1985.
193. Carson SN, Hunter GC, Palmaz J, et al: Recurrence of femoral anastomotic aneurysms. Am J Surg 146:774-778, 1983.
194. Courbier R, Larranaga J: Natural history and management of anastomotic aneurysms. In Bergan JJ, Yao JST (eds): Aneurysms: Diagnosis and Treatment. Orlando, Fla, Grune & Stratton, 1982, pp 567-580.
195. Starr DS, Weatherford SC, Lawrie GM, et al: Suture material as a factor in the occurrence of anastomotic false aneurysms: An analysis of 26 cases. Arch Surg 114:412-415, 1979.
196. Perdue GD Jr, Smith RB 3rd, Ansley JD, et al: Impending aortoenteric hemorrhage: The effect of early recognition on improved outcome. Ann Surg 192:237-243, 1980.
197. Gooding GAW, Effeney DJ, Goldstone J: The aortofemoral graft: Detection and identification of healing complications by ultrasonography. Surgery 89:94-101, 1981.
198. Leurs LJ, Bell R, Degrieck Y, et al: Endovascular treatment of thoracic aortic diseases: Combined experience from the EUROSTAR and United Kingdom thoracic endograft registries. J Vasc Surg 40:670-680, 2004.
199. van Herwaarden JA, Waasdorp EJ, Bendermacher BLW, et al: Endovascular repair of paraanastomotic aneurysms after previous open aortic prosthetic reconstruction. Ann Vasc Surg 18:280-286, 2004.
200. Morrissey NJ, Yano OJ, Soundararajan K, et al: Endovascular repair of para-anastomotic aneurysms of the aorta and iliac arteries: Preferred treatment for a complex problem. J Vasc Surg 34:503-512, 2001.
201. Ernst CB, Elliott JP Jr, Ryan CJ, et al: Recurrent femoral anastomotic aneurysms: A 30-year experience. Ann Surg 208:401-409, 1988.
202. Williams RA, Vetto J, Quinones-Baldrich W, et al: Chylous ascites following abdominal aortic surgery. Ann Vasc Surg 5:247-252, 1991.
203. Pabst TS 3rd, McIntyre KE Jr, Schilling JD, et al: Management of chyloperitoneum after abdominal aortic surgery. Am J Surg 166:194-199, 1993.
204. Aalami OO, Allen DB, Organ CH Jr: Chylous ascites: A collective review. Surgery 128:761-778, 2000.
205. Losanoff JE, Richman BW, Jones JW: Chylous ascites [letter]. Am J Gastroenterol 98:219-220, 2003.
206. Antao B, Croaker D, Squire R: Successful management of congenital chyloperitoneum with fibrin glue. J Pediatr Surg 38:E54, 2003.
207. Leong RWL, House AK, Jeffrey GP: Chylous ascites caused by portal vein thrombosis treated with octreotide. J Gastroenterol Hepatol 18:1211-1213, 2003.
208. Cambria RP, Brewster DC, Abbott WM, et al: Transperitoneal versus retroperitoneal approach for aortic reconstruction: A randomized prospective study. J Vasc Surg 11:314-325, 1990.
209. Stevick CA, Long JB, Jamasbi B, et al: Ventral hernia following abdominal aortic reconstruction. Am Surg 54:287-289, 1988.
210. Hall KA, Peters B, Smyth SH, et al: Abdominal wall hernias in patients with abdominal aortic aneurysmal versus aortoiliac occlusive disease. Am J Surg 170:572-576, 1995.
211. Honig MP, Mason RA, Giron F: Wound complications of the retroperitoneal approach to the aorta and iliac vessels. J Vasc Surg 15:28-34, 1992.
212. Yamada M, Maruta K, Shiojiri Y, et al: Atrophy of the abdominal wall muscles after extraperitoneal approach to the aorta. J Vasc Surg 38:346-353, 2003.
213. Sicard GA, Freeman MB, VanderWoude JC, et al: Comparison between the transabdominal and retroperitoneal approach for reconstruction of the infrarenal abdominal aorta. J Vasc Surg 5:19-27, 1987.
214. Gardner GP, Josephs LG, Rosca M, et al: The retroperitoneal incision: An evaluation of postoperative flank "bulge." Arch Surg 129:753-756, 1994.
215. Lord RSA, Crozier JA, Snell J, et al: Transverse abdominal incisions compared with midline incisions for elective infrarenal aortic reconstruction: Predisposition to incisional hernia in patients with increased intraoperative blood loss. J Vasc Surg 20:27-33, 1994.
216. Raffetto JD, Cheung Y, Fisher JB, et al: Incision and abdominal wall hernias in patients with aneurysm or occlusive aortic disease. J Vasc Surg 37:1150-1154, 2003.

217. Hodgson NC, Malthaner RA, Ostbye T: The search for an ideal method of abdominal fascial closure: A meta-analysis. Ann Surg 231:436-442, 2000.

218. LeBlanc KA, Whitaker JM, Bellanger DE, et al: Laparoscopic incisional and ventral hernioplasty: Lessons learned from 200 patients. Hernia 7:118-124, 2003.

219. Heniford BT, Park A, Ramshaw BJ, et al: Laparoscopic repair of ventral hernias: Nine years' experience with 850 consecutive hernias. Ann Surg 238:391-400, 2003.

220. Craver JM, Ottinger LW, Darling RC, et al: Hemorrhage and thrombosis as early complications of femoropopliteal bypass grafts: Causes, treatment, and prognostic implications. Surgery 74:839-845, 1973.

221. Hargrove WC 3rd, Barker CF, Berkowitz HD, et al: Treatment of acute peripheral arterial and graft thromboses with low-dose streptokinase. Surgery 92:981-993, 1982.

222. LiCalzi LK, Stansel HC Jr: Failure of autogenous reversed saphenous vein femoropopliteal grafting: Pathophysiology and prevention. Surgery 91:352-358, 1982.

223. Whittemore AD, Clowes AW, Couch NP, et al: Secondary femoropopliteal reconstruction. Ann Surg 193:35-42, 1981.

224. Buxton B, Lambert RP, Pitt TTE: The significance of vein wall thickness and diameter in relation to the patency of femoropopliteal saphenous vein bypass grafts. Surgery 87:425-431, 1980.

225. Corson JD, Shah DM, Leather RP, et al: Reversed autogenous saphenous vein bypass grafts: Complications of their use in the lower extremity. In Bernhard VM, Towne JB (eds): Complications in Vascular Surgery. Orlando, Fla, Grune & Stratton, 1985, pp 589-610.

226. Bunt TJ, Manship L, Moore W: Iatrogenic vascular injury during peripheral revascularization. J Vasc Surg 2:491-498, 1985.

227. Samson RH, Gupta SK, Scher LA, et al: Arterial spasm complicating distal vascular bypass procedures. Arch Surg 117:973-975, 1982.

228. Fuchs JC, Mitchener JS 3rd, Hagen PO: Postoperative changes in autologous vein grafts. Ann Surg 188:1-15, 1978.

229. LiCalzi LK, Stansel HC Jr: The closure index: Prediction of long-term patency of femoropopliteal vein grafts. Surgery 91:413-418, 1982.

230. Gundry SR, Jones M, Ishihara T, et al: Optimal preparation techniques for human saphenous vein grafts. Surgery 88:785-794, 1980.

231. Karmody AM, Leather RP, Shah DM, et al: The in situ saphenous vein arterial bypass: Current problems and solutions. In Bernhard VM, Towne JB (eds): Complications in Vascular Surgery. Orlando, Fla, Grune & Stratton, 1985, pp 561-588.

232. Brewster DC, LaSalle AJ, Robison JG, et al: Factors affecting patency of femoropopliteal bypass grafts. Surg Gynecol Obstet 157:437-442, 1983.

233. DeWeese JA: Anastomotic neointimal fibrous hyperplasia. In Bernhard VM, Towne JB (eds): Complications in Vascular Surgery. Orlando, Fla, Grune & Stratton, 1985, pp 157-170.

234. Green RM, Thomas M, Luka N, et al: A comparison of rapid-healing prosthetic arterial grafts and autogenous veins. Arch Surg 114:944-947, 1979.

235. Echave V, Koornick AR, Haimov M, et al: Intimal hyperplasia as a complication of the use of the polytetrafluoroethylene graft for femoral-popliteal bypass. Surgery 86:791-798, 1979.

236. Harker LA: Platelet mechanisms in the genesis and prevention of graft related vascular injury reactions and thromboembolism: Nature of the vascular interface. In Sawyer PN, Kaplitt HJ (eds): Vascular Grafts. New York, Appleton-Century-Crofts, 1978, pp 153-159.

237. Schuler JJ, Flanigan DP: Alternate inflow for repeated failure of femorodistal grafts. In Bergan JJ, Yao JST (eds): Reoperative Arterial Surgery. Orlando, Fla, Grune & Stratton, 1986, pp 393-406.

238. Szilagyi DE, Elliott JP, Hageman JH, et al: Biologic fate of autogenous vein implants as arterial substitutes: Clinical, angiographic and histopathologic observations in femoro-popliteal operations for atherosclerosis. Ann Surg 178:232-246, 1973.

238a. Giswold ME, Landry GJ, Sexton GJ, et al: Modifiable patient factors are associated with reverse vein graft occlusion in the era of duplex scan surveillance. J Vasc Surg 37:47–53, 2003.

239. Pomposelli FB, Kansal N, Hamdan AD, et al: A decade of experience with dorsalis pedis artery bypass: Analysis of outcome in more than 1000 cases. J Vasc Surg 37:307-315, 2003.

240. Bergan JJ, Veith FJ, Bernhard VM, et al: Randomization of autogenous vein and polytetrafluorethylene grafts in femoral-distal reconstruction. Surgery 92:921-930, 1982.

241. Corson JD, Johnson WC, LoGerfo FW, et al: Doppler ankle systolic blood pressure: Prognostic value in vein bypass grafts of the lower extremity. Arch Surg 113:932-935, 1978.

242. Kempczinski RF: Infrainguinal arterial bypass using prosthetic grafts. In Kempczinski RF (ed): The Ischemic Leg. St. Louis, Mosby-Year Book, 1985, pp 437-454.

243. O'Donnell TF Jr, Farber SP, Richmand DM, et al: Above-knee polytetrafluoroethylene femoropopliteal bypass graft: Is it a reasonable alternative to the below-knee reversed autogenous vein graft? Surgery 94:26-31, 1983.

244. Robison JG, Brewster DC, Abbott WM, et al: Femoropopliteal and tibioperoneal artery reconstruction using human umbilical vein. Arch Surg 118:1039-1042, 1983.

245. Rosenthal D, Levine K, Stanton PE Jr, et al: Femoropopliteal bypass: The preferred site for distal anastomosis. Surgery 93:1-4, 1983.

246. Taylor RS, Loh A, McFarland RJ, et al: Improved technique for polytetrafluoroethylene bypass grafting: Long-term results using anastomotic vein patches. Br J Surg 79:348-354, 1992.

247. Batson RC, Sottiurai VS, Craighead CC: Linton patch angioplasty: An adjunct to distal bypass with polytetrafluoroethylene grafts. Ann Surg 199:684-693, 1984.

248. Gagne PJ, Martinez J, DeMassi R, et al: The effect of a venous anastomosis Tyrell vein collar on the primary patency of arteriovenous grafts in patients undergoing hemodialysis. J Vasc Surg 32:1149-1154, 2000.

249. How TV, Rowe CS, Gilling-Smith GL, et al: Interposition vein cuff anastomosis alters wall shear stress distribution in the recipient artery. J Vasc Surg 31:1008-1017, 2000.

250. Marinelli MR, Beach KW, Glass MJ, et al: Noninvasive testing vs clinical evaluation of arterial disease: A prospective study. JAMA 241:2031-2034, 1979.

251. Yao JST: Postoperative evaluation of graft failure. In Bernhard VM, Towne JB (eds): Complications in Vascular Surgery. Orlando, Fla, Grune & Stratton, 1985, pp 1-24.

252. Painton JF, Avellone JC, Plecha FR: Effectiveness of reoperation after late failure of femoropopliteal reconstruction. Am J Surg 135:235-237, 1978.

253. Berkowitz HD, Hobbs CL, Roberts B, et al: Value of routine vascular laboratory studies to identify vein graft stenosis. Surgery 90:971-979, 1981.

254. Bandyk DF: Postoperative surveillance of femoro-distal grafts: The application of echo-Doppler (duplex) ultrasonic scanning. In Bergan JJ, Yao JST (eds): Reoperative Arterial Surgery. Orlando, Fla, Grune & Stratton, 1986, pp 59-80.

255. Kasirajan K, Schneider PA: Early outcome of "cutting" balloon angioplasty for infrainguinal vein graft stenosis. J Vasc Surg 39:702-708, 2004.

256. Baker WH, Hadcock MM, Littooy FN: Management of polytetrafluoroethylene graft occlusions. Arch Surg 115:508-513, 1980.

257. White GH, White RA, Kopchok GE, et al: Endoscopic intravascular surgery removes intraluminal flaps, dissections, and thrombus. J Vasc Surg 11:280-288, 1990.

258. Goldberg L, Ricci MT, Sauvage LR, et al: Thrombolytic therapy for delayed occlusion of knitted Dacron bypass grafts in the axillofemoral, femoropopliteal and femorotibial positions. Surg Gynecol Obstet 160:491-498, 1985.

259. Graor RA, Risius B, Denny KM, et al: Local thrombolysis in the treatment of thrombosed arteries, bypass grafts, and arteriovenous fistulas. J Vasc Surg 2:406-414, 1985.

260. Hargrove WC, Berkowitz HD, Freiman DB, et al: Recanalization of totally occluded femoropopliteal vein grafts with low-dose streptokinase infusion. Surgery 92:890-895, 1982.

261. Dardik H, Sussman BC, Kahn M, et al: Lysis of arterial clot by intravenous or intra-arterial administration of streptokinase. Surg Gynecol Obstet 158:137-140, 1984.

262. Husson JM, Fiessinger JN, Aiach M, et al: Streptokinase after late failure of reconstructive surgery for peripheral arteriosclerosis. J Cardiovasc Surg (Torino) 22:145-152, 1981.

263. Quinones-Baldrich WJ, Zierler RE, Hiatt JC: Intraoperative fibrinolytic therapy: An adjunct to catheter thromboembolectomy. J Vasc Surg 2:319-326, 1985.

264. Parent FN 3rd, Bernhard VM, Pabst TS 3rd, et al: Fibrinolytic treatment of residual thrombus after catheter embolectomy for severe lower limb ischemia. J Vasc Surg 9:153-160, 1989.

265. Cohen LH, Kaplan M, Bernhard VM: Intraoperative streptokinase: An adjunct to mechanical thrombectomy in the management of acute ischemia. Arch Surg 121:708-715, 1986.

266. Andros G, Harris RW, Salles-Cunha SX, et al: Arm veins for arterial revascularization of the leg: Arteriographic and clinical observations. J Vasc Surg 4:416-427, 1986.

267. Curi MA, Skelly CL, Baldwin ZK, et al: Long-term outcome of infrainguinal bypass grafting in patients with serologically proven hypercoagulability. J Vasc Surg 37:301-306, 2003.

268. Harker LA, Slichter SJ, Sauvage LR: Platelet consumption by arterial prostheses: The effects of endothelialization and pharmacologic inhibition of platelet function. Ann Surg 186:594-601, 1977.

269. Veith FJ, Gupta SK, Ascer E, et al: Reoperations and other reinterventions for thrombosed and failing polytetrafluoroethylene grafts. In Bergan JJ, Yao JST (eds): Reoperative Arterial Surgery. Orlando, Fla, Grune & Stratton, 1986, pp 377-392.

270. Kretschmer G, Wenzl E, Piza F, et al: The influence of anticoagulant treatment on the probability of function in femoropopliteal vein bypass surgery: Analysis of a clinical series (1970 to 1985) and interim evaluation of a controlled clinical trial. Surgery 102:453-459, 1987.

271. Kretschmer G, Wenzl E, Schemper M, et al: Influence of postoperative anticoagulant treatment on patient survival after femoropopliteal vein bypass surgery. Lancet 1:797-799, 1988.

272. Wengrovitz M, Atnip RG, Gifford RR, et al: Wound complications of autogenous subcutaneous infrainguinal arterial bypass surgery: Predisposing factors and management. J Vasc Surg 11:156-163, 1990.

273. Johnson JA, Cogbill TH, Strutt PJ, et al: Wound complications after infrainguinal bypass: Classification, predisposing factors, and management. Arch Surg 123:859-862, 1988.

274. Schwartz ME, Harrington EB, Schanzer H: Wound complications after in situ bypass. J Vasc Surg 7:802-807, 1988.

275. Kent KC, Bartek S, Kuntz KM, et al: Prospective study of wound complications in continuous infrainguinal incisions after lower limb arterial reconstruction: Incidence, risk factors, and cost. Surgery 119:378-383, 1996.

276. O'Hare AM, Feinglass J, Sidawy AN, et al: Impact of renal insufficiency on short-term morbidity and mortality after lower extremity revascularization: Data from the Department of Veterans Affairs' National Surgical Quality Improvement Program. J Am Soc Nephrol 14:1287-1295, 2003.

277. O'Hare AM, Sidawy AN, Feinglass J, et al: Influence of renal insufficiency on limb loss and mortality after initial lower extremity surgical revascularization. J Vasc Surg 39:709-716, 2004.

278. Mehigan JT, Olcott CT: Video angioscopy as an alternative to intraoperative arteriography. Am J Surg 152:139-145, 1986.

279. LaMuraglia GM, Cambria RP, Brewster DC, et al: Angioscopy guided semiclosed technique for in situ bypass. J Vasc Surg 12:601-604, 1990.

280. Stierli P, Banz M, Wigger P, et al: Angioscopy guided in situ bypass versus angioscopy guided non reversed bypass for infrainguinal arterial reconstructions: A comparison of outcome. J Cardiovasc Surg (Torino) 36:211-217, 1995.

281. Illig KA, Rhodes JM, Sternbach Y, et al: Financial impact of endoscopic vein harvest for infrainguinal bypass. J Vasc Surg 37:323-330, 2003.

282. Henderson VJ, Cohen RG, Mitchell RS, et al: Biochemical (functional) adaptation of "arterialized" vein grafts. Ann Surg 203:339-345, 1986.

283. Bandyk DF, Kaebnick HW, Stewart GW, et al: Durability of the in situ saphenous vein arterial bypass: A comparison of primary and secondary patency. J Vasc Surg 5:256-268, 1987.

284. Levine AW, Bandyk DF, Bonier PH, et al: Lessons learned in adopting the in situ saphenous vein graft. J Vasc Surg 2:145-153, 1985.

285. Woelfle KD, Kugelmann U, Bruijnen H, et al: Intraoperative imaging techniques in infrainguinal arterial bypass grafting: Completion angiography versus vascular endoscopy. Eur J Vasc Surg 8:556-561, 1994.

286. Bush HL Jr, Corey CA, Nabseth DC: Distal in situ saphenous vein grafts for limb salvage: Increased operative blood flow and postoperative patency. Am J Surg 145:542-548, 1983.

287. Bandyk DF, Jorgensen RA, Towne JB: Intraoperative assessment of in situ saphenous vein arterial grafts using pulsed Doppler spectral analysis. Arch Surg 121:292-299, 1986.

288. Ferris BL, Mills JL Sr, Hughes JD, et al: Is early postoperative duplex scan surveillance of leg bypass grafts clinically important? J Vasc Surg 37:495-500, 2003.

289. Bandyk DF, Cato RF, Towne JB: A low flow velocity predicts failure of femoropopliteal and femorotibial bypass grafts. Surgery 98:799-809, 1985.

290. Mills JL, Fujitani RM, Taylor SM: The characteristics and anatomic distribution of lesions that cause reversed vein graft failure: A five-year prospective study. J Vasc Surg 17:195-206, 1993.

291. Mills JL, Bandyk DF, Gahtan V, et al: The origin of infrainguinal vein graft stenosis: A prospective study based on duplex surveillance. J Vasc Surg 21:16-25, 1995.

292. Caps MT, Cantwell-Gab K, Bergelin RO, et al: Vein graft lesions: Time of onset and rate of progression. J Vasc Surg 22:466-475, 1995.

293. Passman MA, Moneta GL, Nehler MR, et al: Do normal early color-flow duplex surveillance examination results of infrainguinal vein grafts preclude the need for late graft revision? J Vasc Surg 22:476-484, 1995.

294. Westerband A, Mills JL, Kistler S, et al: Prospective validation of threshold criteria for intervention in infrainguinal vein grafts undergoing duplex surveillance. Ann Vasc Surg 11:44-48, 1997.

295. Mills JL, Harris EJ, Taylor LM Jr, et al: The importance of routine surveillance of distal bypass grafts with duplex scanning: A study of 379 reversed vein grafts. J Vasc Surg 12:379-389, 1990.

296. Fowl RJ, Patterson RB, Bodenham RJ, et al: Functional failure of patent femorodistal in situ grafts. Ann Vasc Surg 3:200-204, 1989.

297. Taylor LM Jr, Phinney ES, Porter JM: Present status of reversed vein bypass for lower extremity revascularization. J Vasc Surg 3:288-297, 1986.

298. Veith FJ, Gupta SK, Daly VD: Femoropopliteal bypass to the isolated popliteal segment: Is polytetrafluoroethylene graft acceptable? Surgery 89:296-303, 1981.

299. Berger K, Sauvage LR: Late fiber deterioration in Dacron arterial grafts. Ann Surg 193:477-491, 1981.

300. Clagett GP, Salander JM, Eddleman WL, et al: Dilation of knitted Dacron aortic prostheses and anastomotic false aneurysms: Etiologic considerations. Surgery 93:9-16, 1983.

301. Nunn DB, Freeman MH, Hudgins PC: Postoperative alterations in size of Dacron aortic grafts: An ultrasonic evaluation. Ann Surg 189:741-745, 1979.

302. Berman SS, Hunter GC, Smyth SH, et al: Application of computed tomography for surveillance of aortic grafts. Surgery 118:8-15, 1995.

303. Nunn DB: Structural failure of first-generation, polyester, double-velour, knitted prostheses. J Vasc Surg 33:1131-1132, 2001.

304. Pourdeyhimi B, Wagner D: On the correlation between the failure of vascular grafts and their structural and material properties: A critical analysis. J Biomed Mater Res 20:375-409, 1986.

305. Cooke PA, Nobis PA, Stoney RJ: Dacron aortic graft failure. Arch Surg 108:101-103, 1974.

306. Cranley JJ, Karkow WS, Hafner CO, et al: Aneurysmal dilatation in umbilical vein grafts. In Bergan JJ, Yao JST (eds): Reoperative Arterial Surgery. Orlando, Fla, Grune & Stratton, 1986, pp 343-358.

307. Dardik H, Ibrahim IM, Sussman B, et al: Biodegradation and aneurysm formation in umbilical vein grafts: Observations and a realistic strategy. Ann Surg 199:61-68, 1984.

308. Dardik H: Reoperative surgery for complications following femorodistal bypass with umbilical vein grafts. In Bergan JJ, Yao JST (eds): Reoperative Arterial Surgery. Orlando, Fla, Grune & Stratton, 1986, pp 331-342.

309. Julien S, Gill F, Guidoin R, et al: Biologic and structural evaluation of 80 surgically excised human umbilical vein grafts. Can J Surg 32:101-107, 1989.

310. Dardik H, Wengerter K, Qin F, et al: Comparative decades of experience with glutaraldehyde-tanned human umbilical cord vein graft for lower limb revascularization: An analysis of 1275 cases. J Vasc Surg 35:64-71, 2002.

311. Roberts AK, Johnson N: Aneurysm formation in an expanded microporous polytetrafluoroethylene graft. Arch Surg 113:211-213, 1978.

312. Selman SH, Rhodes RS, Anderson JM, et al: Atheromatous changes in expanded polytetrafluoroethylene grafts. Surgery 87:630-637, 1980.

313. Eickhoff JH, Engell HC: Local regulation of blood flow and the occurrence of edema after arterial reconstruction of the lower limbs. Ann Surg 195:474-478, 1982.

314. Schubart PJ, Porter JM: Leg edema following femorodistal bypass. In Bergan JJ, Yao JST (eds): Reoperative Arterial Surgery. Orlando, Fla, Grune & Stratton, 1986, pp 311-330.

315. Husni EA: The edema of arterial reconstruction. Circulation 35:I169-I173, 1967.

316. Storen EJ, Myhre HO, Stiris G: Lymphangiographic findings in patients with leg oedema after arterial reconstructions. Acta Chir Scand 140:385-387, 1974.

317. Porter JM, Lindell TD, Lakin PC: Leg edema following femoropopliteal autogenous vein bypass. Arch Surg 105:883-888, 1972.

318. McShannic JR, O'Hara PJ: Management of femoral lymphatic complications following synthetic lower extremity revascularization: Early and late results. Vasc Surg 31:703-711, 1997.

319. Reifsnyder T, Bandyk D, Seabrook G, et al: Wound complications of the in situ saphenous vein bypass technique. J Vasc Surg 15:843-850, 1992.

Questions

1. **Why is venous injury the most common source of intraoperative bleeding?**
   (a) Venous pressure is lower than arterial pressure
   (b) Veins are often adherent to adjacent arteries
   (c) Circumferential mobilization is always necessary to gain proximal and distal control
   (d) A double vena cava may be present in 1% to 3% of patients

2. **Which of the following statements about aortocaval fistulas are true?**
   (a) They are not suspected in 70% of patients
   (b) They occur in 1% of ruptured aneurysms
   (c) They require dissection of the aneurysm from the vena cava
   (d) They may precipitate congestive heart failure
   (e) They are best treated with a stent-graft if recognized preoperatively

3. **What is the most common cause of aortic graft limb occlusion?**
   (a) Hypercoagulable state
   (b) Improved inflow
   (c) Fibrointimal hyperplasia or atherosclerosis at the distal anastomosis
   (d) Angulation of the graft
   (e) Extrinsic compression at the inguinal ligament

4. **Which of the following statements are true with regard to acute renal failure associated with aortic surgery?**
   (a) It occurs more often after elective surgery
   (b) It has a mortality rate between 57% and 95%
   (c) It has multiple causative factors, including vasospasm, suprarenal clamping, ligation of the left renal vein, and operative embolization
   (d) It may benefit from the administration of fluid and mannitol intraoperatively

5. **Which of the following statements about intestinal ischemia are true?**
   (a) The incidence is 60% after rupture of aneurysms
   (b) The arch of Riolan and marginal artery of Drummond are important collaterals
   (c) D-dimer may be helpful in acute embolic occlusion
   (d) Ligation of the inferior mesenteric artery is never a precipitating factor
   (e) An inferior mesenteric artery back-pressure greater than 20 mm Hg and an index of 0.2 may be helpful

6. **Which of the following statements about spinal cord ischemia are true?**
   (a) It occurs in 0.23% of patients undergoing aortic surgery
   (b) It has a higher incidence after repair of thoracic and ruptured abdominal aneurysms
   (c) It is characterized by deficits between T-10 and L-2
   (d) It has increased mortality if patients are paraplegic at the outset

7. **Which of the following statements about intraoperative heparin-induced thrombosis are true?**
   (a) It is 10 times more frequent with unfractionated hernia than with low-molecular-weight heparin
   (b) Laboratory diagnosis can be made intraoperatively
   (c) It stimulates antibodies against heparin platelet factor 4 complex
   (d) It is best treated with lepirudin or argatroban
   (e) Heparin can be safely readministered within 2 months

8. **Which of the following statements about chylous ascites are true?**
   (a) It occurs most often with aortic reconstruction for aneurysmal disease
   (b) It is associated with progressive abdominal distention
   (c) The diagnosis is confirmed by paracentesis
   (d) It usually requires surgical correction
   (e) It can be cured with octreotide treatment

9. **Which of the following statements about lower extremity edema following femoropopliteal bypass are true?**
   (a) It occurs in 70% to 100% of patients
   (b) It is related to the severity of ischemia
   (c) Its cause is multifactorial

10. **Which of the following statements about lymphatic drainage from an incision are true?**
    (a) It can be prevented by careful ligation of tissue during groin dissection
    (b) It occurs in 4% of groin incisions
    (c) It is treated with bed rest
    (d) It may require surgical correction
    (e) It can be prevented with application of fibrin glue before wound closure

Answers

1. b, d	2. d, e	3. c	4. b, c, d
5. a, b, c	6. a, b, c, d	7. a, c, d	8. a, b, c
9. a, b, c	10. a, b, c, d		

44

David A. Rigberg • Hugh A. Gelabert

Portal Hypertension

Portal hypertension and variceal hemorrhage are important clinical problems in which vascular surgeons have a significant interest and concern. New developments have altered the once-familiar face of this disease. At the same time, they have created confusion about the best approach to these patients.

The vascular surgeon plays a vital role in treating these patients. It is of paramount importance to have a clear understanding of the impact of underlying liver disease, the pathophysiology of portal hypertension, and the management of these problems. The goal of this chapter is to provide a solid basis for determining the cause of hepatic disease, understanding the presentation, and managing portal hypertension.

Definition

Portal hypertension is a condition in which the circulation of blood in the portal venous system is impeded, resulting in an increase in portal venous pressure. Elevation of the portal venous blood pressure results in a series of physiologic alterations, including ascites, hypersplenism, and variceal hemorrhage. Normal portal venous pressure is between 5 and 10 mm Hg. Portal hypertension is said to be present when portal pressure is elevated above 15 mm Hg. Clinically significant portal hypertension exists when the portal pressure is elevated more than 10 mm Hg above systemic pressure as measured at the inferior vena cava (corrected portal pressure).

The natural history of patients with portal hypertension differs, depending on the cause of the condition and the stage of presentation. The patient's ability to withstand the stress of hemorrhage or surgery largely depends on the functional hepatic reserve.

Pathogenesis

Physiologically, portal hypertension results from either an increase in the portal blood flow (rare) or an obstruction to the outflow of blood from the portal circulation (common). Obstructions to the portal circulation have been classified anatomically based on their location relative to the hepatic sinusoids. Accordingly, the obstruction may be presinusoidal, sinusoidal, or postsinusoidal. Pre- and postsinusoidal obstructions have been subclassified as intra- or extrahepatic (Table 44-1).

EXTRAHEPATIC PRESINUSOIDAL OBSTRUCTION

Presinusoidal extrahepatic obstruction is most commonly due to thrombosis of the portal vein. Although less common than other forms of obstructive portal hypertension, portal vein thrombosis occurs in a significant number of children. It may occur in adults, but the causes are remarkably different between children and adults.

Portal vein thrombosis in children occurs as a complication of an infectious process such as omphalitis and appendicitis (most common causes). In adults, the most common cause of portal vein thrombosis is a gradual and relentless decrease in the portal blood flow secondary to the high resistance in the hepatic circulation caused by cirrhosis. Other causes in adults include pancreatitis, hypercoagulable states or tumor thrombus, and mechanical obstruction of portal venous flow. The last may be the result of malignant invasion, lymphadenopathy, or caudate lobe compression. Hypercoagulable conditions may result from polycythemia, cancer, or hypovolemia. Sepsis may lead to portal vein thrombosis by several mechanisms: low-flow states, hypovolemia, and, perhaps, activation of the coagulation system.

INTRAHEPATIC PRESINUSOIDAL OBSTRUCTION

Most causes of intrahepatic presinusoidal obstructive portal hypertension relate to fibrosis and compression of the portal venules, with subsequent restriction of portal flow. Included among these diseases are congenital hepatic fibrosis, sarcoidosis, chronic arsenic exposure, Wilson's disease, hepatoportal sclerosis, primary biliary cirrhosis, schistosomiasis, and myeloproliferative disorders.

Schistosomiasis is the most common cause of portal hypertension in third-world countries. Deposition of ova in the portal vein walls results in a granulomatous inflammatory reaction, which in turn results in fibrosis and portal flow restriction. Hepatic function is preserved in the early stages, but later stages of this disease are characterized by advanced cirrhosis and loss of hepatic function.[1] Myeloproliferative disorders such as myelosclerosis and myeloid leukemia occasionally lead to presinusoidal hypertension by virtue of the deposition of primitive cellular material infiltrating the portal zones.[2] Sarcoidosis causes portal hypertension by two mechanisms: sarcoid granulomas within the portal vein leading to obstruction, and increased portal blood flow.

TABLE 44–1	Causes of Portal Hypertension

Presinusoidal

Extrahepatic: portal vein thrombosis
   Omphalitis
   Pancreatitis
   Trauma
   Malignancy
   Polycythemia
   Periportal lymphadenopathy
Intrahepatic
   Biliary atresia
   Schistosomiasis
   Sarcoidosis
   Arsenic toxicity
   Congenital hepatic fibrosis
   Myeloproliferative disorders
   Primary biliary cirrhosis
   Hepatoportal sclerosis

Sinusoidal

Cirrhosis
Toxic hepatitis
Fatty metamorphosis

Postsinusoidal

Intrahepatic
   Cirrhosis
   Postnecrotic
   Portal
   Hemochromatosis
Veno-occlusive disease
Extrahepatic
   Budd-Chiari syndrome
   Hepatic vein webs
   Malignant obstruction
   Oral contraceptives
   Pregnancy
   Plant alkaloids
Cardiac causes
   Congestive heart failure
   Constrictive pericarditis

Increased Blood Flow: Arteriovenous Fistulas

Splenic artery to splenic vein
Hepatic artery to portal vein

Hepatic function is usually preserved in the early stages of these diseases. In later stages, significant hepatic impairment may result from progressive cirrhosis. Hemodynamic characteristics are similar to those of extrahepatic portal vein obstruction: low hepatic wedge pressure and elevated portal venous pressure.

INTRAHEPATIC SINUSOIDAL AND POSTSINUSOIDAL OBSTRUCTION

Sinusoidal portal hypertension may be the sequela of alcoholic hepatitis, viral hepatitis, or toxic hepatitis. Although pure sinusoidal obstruction is relatively rare, it is frequently part of a combined sinusoidal and postsinusoidal obstructive picture. As such, it is the most common cause of portal hypertension in the United States and is estimated to be the 10th leading cause of death. Postsinusoidal obstruction is seen most commonly in cases of alcoholic liver disease, postnecrotic cirrhosis, or hemochromatosis. As would be expected in these diseases, hepatic function is usually significantly impaired.

Two mechanisms account for the portal hypertension in these patients. First is the mechanical obstruction of the portal blood flow by the regenerating hepatic nodules and cirrhotic bands within the damaged liver. These changes may extend beyond the confines of the hepatic sinusoids, accounting for the presence of presinusoidal, sinusoidal, and postsinusoidal distortion of the hepatic architecture. The second element is an increase in the splanchnic perfusion, in part attributed to the genesis of multiple arteriovenous (AV) shunts and collateral channels. One third of portal blood flow may bypass functional hepatocytes through these channels.[3] The clinical correlate of this increased blood flow is the hyperdynamic state that typifies cirrhosis: elevated cardiac output and a diminished systemic resistance.[4]

The portal hemodynamic characteristics of these diseases usually consist of elevated hepatic wedge pressure along with elevated portal vein pressure. Because most of these diseases directly affect hepatocytes, hepatic function is frequently impaired, even in the early stages of disease. These patients frequently have poor hepatic reserve and decompensate with each bleeding episode. Selection and timing of interventions are important aspects of their management.

EXTRAHEPATIC POSTSINUSOIDAL OBSTRUCTION

Postsinusoidal hepatic vein obstruction is usually the result of thrombosis in the hepatic veins. Although the cause of most cases is unknown, a number of associated diseases have been identified. Membranous webs of the hepatic veins, malignancies (hepatomas, renal carcinomas, adrenal carcinomas), trauma, pregnancy, contraceptive use, acute alcoholic hepatitis, veno-occlusive disease, and *Senecio* sp. (ragwort) toxicity may all result in hepatic vein thrombosis.[5] Constrictive pericarditis and chronic congestive heart failure may also cause postsinusoidal obstruction.

Budd-Chiari syndrome is the result of hepatic venous occlusive disease and is characterized by massive ascites, esophageal varices, variceal hemorrhage, hepatic failure, and death. Chiari's disease is due to primary hepatic vein ostial occlusion. The clinical progression after hepatic vein occlusion may be fulminant or gradual. Hepatic failure is the result of chronic congestion and ischemia from impaired hepatic blood flow. The factors that determine the rate of progression are not well understood. Angiography is essential in establishing the diagnosis; it identifies the presence of thrombus and its location.[6,7]

The fulminant course is marked by rapid development of ascites, fatigue, and jaundice. Additionally, elevated liver enzymes and prothrombin time indicate hepatocellular damage. Patients who do not improve with anticoagulation should be considered for either shunting or liver transplantation.

The more gradual presentation may have many similar features, such as ascites and chronic fatigue, but hepatic function is preserved to a greater degree. Hypersplenism and variceal hemorrhage may be more prominent features in these patients.

An initial trial of anticoagulation may allow endogenous fibrinolysis to resolve the venous thrombosis. Patients whose course is gradually progressive and who have intact hepatocellular function should be considered for portal decompression by a portacaval, mesocaval, or mesoatrial shunt. Shunt selection is dependent on the patient's anatomy, as defined by angiography. When the Budd-Chiari syndrome leads to deterioration of hepatic function, as demonstrated by abnormal liver function tests, hepatic transplantation is the procedure of choice.[8]

ARTERIOVENOUS FISTULAS

As a cause of portal hypertension, AV fistulas are relatively rare. Most fistulas are either traumatic or splenic. Traumatic AV fistulas may occur as a consequence of transhepatic biliary manipulations or as a result of penetrating trauma. Splenic fistulas may be associated with splenic artery aneurysms, sarcoidosis, Gaucher's disease, myeloid metaplasia, or tropical splenomegaly. Women of childbearing age are at greatest risk. The portal hypertension results initially from increased flow in the portal circulation. At later stages, fibrosis, along with secondary obstruction of the presinusoidal spaces, exacerbates the portal hypertension.

Diagnosis

The diagnosis of portal hypertension rests on demonstrating increased portal venous pressure or the anatomic evidence of this increased pressure. In practical terms, the diagnosis of portal hypertension is made by identifying signs of elevated portal venous pressure in a patient with a history that supports these findings.

The signs of elevated portal venous pressure include the presence of esophageal varices, splenomegaly, ascites, or abdominal wall collaterals. Ascites, splenomegaly, and abdominal wall collateralization may be apparent on physical examination. Esophagogastric endoscopy is currently considered the most reliable means of identifying gastroesophageal varices.

Signs of underlying hepatic disease include spider angiomas, palmar erythema, gynecomastia, muscle wasting, loss of pubertal hair growth, and testicular atrophy. Encephalopathy, asterixis, fetor hepaticus, and fatigue may also be noted in patients with chronic hepatic insufficiency. The presence of liver disease is not conclusive evidence that the patient has significant portal hypertension.

Historical support for the diagnosis of portal hypertension includes identification of any of the diseases that are known to lead to portal hypertension (e.g., alcohol ingestion, hepatitis, hepatotoxins). The duration of such problems is also important in substantiating the diagnosis of portal hypertension. Both alcoholic toxicity and viral hepatitis lead to cirrhosis and usually portal hypertension, but the time between the onset of these insults and the development of hypertension may be 10 years or more.

Adjunctive means of demonstrating portal hypertension include angiography and hemodynamic measurements. Neither is essential to making the diagnosis; both are supportive. Angiography may reveal both splenomegaly and collateralization in the portal region and the gastroesophageal axis. Additionally, angiography may provide information regarding the direction of portal blood flow (hepatopetal or hepatofugal).

Hemodynamic measurement of the portal circulation is most commonly accomplished by transjugular venous catheterization and measurement of the wedge hepatic vein pressure.[9] This technique is able to record the pressure in the hepatic veins and the hepatic sinusoids. Elevations of the wedge pressure reflect elevations in the portal venous pressure. False-negative results may be encountered in patients with presinusoidal obstruction and in cases of catheter malfunction. Normal hepatic venous pressure is essentially the same as the right atrial pressure (0 to 5 mm Hg); portal venous pressure is about 2 to 6 mm Hg higher than hepatic venous pressure. A gradient greater than 10 mm Hg is considered abnormal.

Other methods of measuring portal venous pressure have been developed but have largely been abandoned because of the increased risk associated with them. These tests include direct cannulation of the portal vein (requires surgical exposure), percutaneous transhepatic portal venous catheterization, transjugular portal vein catheterization, and percutaneous splenic pulp pressure measurement.[10]

The most recent development in assessing the portal circulation is the application of noninvasive ultrasonography. Duplex scanning has been used to establish patency and measure the direction and velocity of portal blood flow. Information gathered from this technique identifies portal vein thrombosis, hepatopetal and hepatofugal flow, and portal hypertension.[9-12] Bolondi and associates documented high sensitivity and specificity with these techniques.[13]

Diagnostic Evaluation
LABORATORY TESTING

The initial step in evaluating most patients is to assess their serum chemistries. Specific attention should be placed on testing the liver enzymes (serum glutamic-oxaloacetic transaminase [SGOT], serum glutamic-pyruvic transaminase [SGPT], lactate dehydrogenase [LDH], alkaline phosphatase) and hepatic synthetic function (prothrombin time and serum albumin). Information from these two sets of tests identifies patients who are suffering from acute hepatocellular damage and those who have had sufficient damage to reduce the liver's ability to synthesize essential proteins. This represents two distinct gradations of hepatic dysfunction. The first is indicative of an acute insult; the second represents the degree of hepatic dysfunction. The presence and degree of abnormalities in liver function tests correlate with outcome: the more abnormal the tests, the worse the prognosis.[14,15]

Abnormal liver function tests combined with physical findings and historical data form the basis for classifying patients with portal hypertension. The Child classification or, more recently, the combined Child-Pugh classification serves as a prognosticator of survival in cirrhotic patients who undergo both emergent and elective surgery (Table 44-2).[16]

Additional laboratory investigations should include a determination of serum ammonia and a complete blood count (CBC)—white blood cells (WBCs), red blood cells (RBCs), and platelets. Serum ammonia may be elevated in cases of severe hepatic dysfunction and coma. It correlates loosely with mentation but may serve as an indicator of a treatable cause of encephalopathy, hyperammonemia.[17]

The CBC detects the presence of anemia and hypersplenism. Anemia in cirrhotic patients may result from a number of causes other than hemorrhage. Chronic malnutrition is

TABLE 44–2	Classification of Portal Hypertension Patients as Prognosticator of Survival

Child Classification

	Risk		
Criteria	Good	Moderate	Poor
Bilirubin (mg/dL)	<2.0	2.0-3.0	>3.0
Albumin (mg/dL)	>3.5	3.0-3.5	<3.0
Ascites	Absent	Easily controlled	Poorly controlled
Encephalopathy	Absent	Minimal	Advanced
Nutrition	Excellent	Good	Poor

Pugh Classification

	Points Scored for Increasing Abnormality*		
Criteria	1	2	3
Albumin (mg/dL)	>3.5	2.8-3.5	<2.8
Bilirubin (mg/dL)	1.0-2.0	2.0-3.0	>3.0
Ascites	Absent	Slight	Significant
Encephalopathy	Normal	1 or 2	3 or 4
Prothrombin time (seconds prolonged)	1-4	4-6	>6

*5 or 6 points for class A encephalopathy.
7 to 9 points for class B encephalopathy.
10 to 15 points for class C encephalopathy.

a particularly important cause of anemia in these patients. Although splenomegaly is present in virtually all portal hypertensive patients, hypersplenism may not develop until later in the course of the disease. The size of the spleen does not correlate directly with either the degree of portal hypertension or the severity of hypersplenism, but an enlarged spleen is found in virtually all patients with portal hypertension and hypersplenism.[18] Hypersplenism is defined principally in terms of splenic sequestration and destruction of platelets and WBCs. This leads to significant depressions in the platelet and WBC counts. Platelet counts below 50,000/mm^3 and WBC counts below 2000/mm^3 support this diagnosis.

UPPER GASTROINTESTINAL ENDOSCOPY

Endoscopy plays a pivotal role in the management of portal hypertensive patients. For both diagnostic and therapeutic reasons, endoscopy should be one of the first tests performed. Endoscopy identifies not only the presence of varices but also the source of bleeding in patients with hemorrhage.

The diagnosis of portal hypertension may be established by noting the presence of varices. The size, appearance, and location of the varices may significantly affect the patient's management. Endoscopy also notes the presence of other sources of bleeding in portal hypertensive patients, such as hypertensive gastropathy, gastritis, gastric ulceration, duodenal ulceration, gastric mucosal lacerations (Mallory-Weiss tears), or esophageal ulcerations. Because of the variety of possible bleeding lesions and the significant differences in the management of these lesions, patients admitted for hemorrhage must undergo upper gastrointestinal endoscopy on each admission. As many as 40% to 60% of patients with documented varices have associated gastritis or peptic ulcer disease.[19] In patients with esophageal and gastric varices, the gastric varices have been documented as the site of bleeding in up to 18%.[20]

LIVER BIOPSY

The role of liver biopsy in the preoperative evaluation of portal hypertensive patients has been a focus of controversy. The goal of liver biopsy in this setting is to identify those patients who have active hepatitis. In alcoholic patients, this is most commonly denoted by the presence of Mallory bodies, which signifies acute hyaline necrosis. Mallory bodies may also be seen in patients with Wilson's disease, cholestasis, and primary biliary cirrhosis. The reason for identifying patients with acute hepatic necrosis is that these patients are thought to be at increased risk of dying during shunt surgery.

Mikkelsen and others noted an operative mortality of 69% in elective shunt cases and 83% in emergent cases in the presence of acute hyaline necrosis.[20,21] Other authors have contested whether acute alcoholic hepatitis alters survival.[14,22] Finally, it should be noted that Mallory bodies disappear when patients abstain from alcohol and the liver recovers from the insult.[23]

The current recommendation is that patients suspected of having acute hepatitis and who are candidates for elective shunt surgery should undergo percutaneous liver biopsy. If Mallory bodies are identified, consideration should be given to postponing the elective operation to give the liver time to recover. This must be carefully balanced against the risk of recurrent hemorrhage and the likelihood of the patient's compliance.

DUPLEX SCANNING

Duplex scanning is finding greater application in the evaluation of portal hypertensive patients. In patients who are being considered for portacaval shunting or hepatic transplantation, the duplex scan is frequently sufficient to document portal vein patency. Duplex scanning determines both the patency of the portal vein and the direction of portal venous blood flow. This is the minimal anatomic information required to proceed with these operations. The combination of color-flow imaging and duplex scanning has improved the accuracy and extended the diagnostic abilities of duplex scanners.[11]

ANGIOGRAPHY

Preoperative anatomic definition is essential for optimal surgical management, particularly when peripheral shunts are being considered. If possible, angiography should be performed on all patients who are to undergo elective shunting procedures. Techniques that are of primarily historical interest include splenoportography[24] (introduction of radiopaque material into the spleen), umbilical vein catheterization, and transhepatic percutaneous portal venography.[21-30]

Currently, the vast majority of portal angiography is performed by selective cannulation of the celiac and superior mesenteric arteries, as well as observation of the venous phase of these angiograms. Additional studies that should be obtained include an injection of the renal veins and a hepatic wedge angiogram and pressure recording. The combination of these studies is commonly referred to as a "liver package."

The goal of these studies is to delineate the major portal tributaries—the splenic vein, the superior mesenteric vein (SMV), and the portal vein itself—and their relation to the renal vein. An additional goal of the liver package is to measure the hepatic wedge pressure and visualize the hepatic sinusoidal circulation. These last two elements are helpful in confirming the presence of portal hypertension, estimating the severity of the hypertension, and determining the cause of the elevated pressure. Low hepatic wedge pressure (<10 to 12 mm Hg) in a patient with variceal hemorrhage should prompt a careful search for evidence of portal vein thrombosis.[31] The wedge hepatic vein catheter allows determination of the morphology of the sinusoids, as well as the direction of blood flow (Fig. 44-1). The wedge hepatic venogram in cirrhotic patients demonstrates irregular sinusoids with multiple scattered filling defects. Retrograde portal vein filling indicates hepatofugal flow.[24]

Delineation of the portal tributary anatomy is essential in planning an elective portal decompressive procedure, because the choice of procedure is limited by the patient's anatomy. The angiographic findings correlate with the degree of cirrhosis. In early cirrhosis, no definite angiographic abnormalities are present. As cirrhosis becomes more severe, one sees the development of collateral pathways, dilatation of the hepatic artery, and pruning of intrahepatic portal vein branches (Fig. 44-2). In advanced cirrhosis, reversal of flow in the portal vein may be detected.

Complications

ESOPHAGEAL VARICES

Esophageal varices develop in about 30% of cirrhotic patients. Of those who have upper gastrointestinal bleeding at presentation, about 30% bleed from varices. The other 70% bleed from chemical gastritis, hypertensive gastritis,

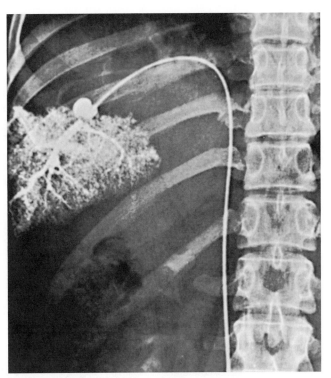

FIGURE 44–1 • Abnormal wedged hepatic venogram demonstrating a coarse, mottled parenchymal pattern consistent with cirrhosis.

ulceration, erosions, mucosal tears, and neoplastic growth. Of the cirrhotic patients who bleed from esophageal varices, about 5% to 15% have massive hemorrhage that is difficult to control. The mortality of these patients—bleeding to death from esophageal varices—is about 30% to 50%.

The pathogenesis of esophageal varices centers around the development of collateral circulatory pathways for blood

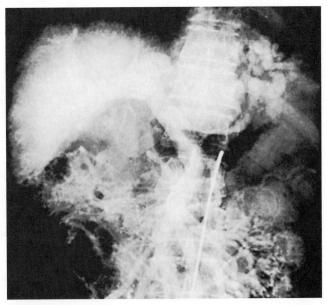

FIGURE 44–2 • Venous phase superior mesenteric angiogram demonstrating superior mesenteric, portal, and dilated coronary veins.

exiting the portal circulation. The impetus for the development of these collaterals is the difference in pressure between the portal system and the systemic venous circulation. Several major collateral networks have been described in cirrhotic patients: the coronary-esophageal veins, the umbilical vein, the hemorrhoidal veins, and the retroperitoneal veins (veins of Retzius). Each of these venous systems may develop into significant collateral networks.

Any blood vessel that is attenuated and distended under supranormal pressures is at risk of disruption and bleeding. The addition of mechanical trauma or chemical irritation may increase the likelihood of bleeding. Consequently, any of the collaterals that develop because of portal hypertension may bleed. Hemorrhoidal vessels, intestinal varices, and stomal varices have all been documented as bleeding sites in cirrhotic patients. The mechanical and chemical irritants that bathe the gastroesophageal region result in esophagitis, attenuation of the mucosal layers, and disruption of the varices. When the increased blood pressure within the varices is combined with periodic exacerbations of this pressure by activities that increase the intra-abdominal and intrathoracic pressure (e.g., coughing, retching), the risk of bleeding from esophageal varices is significantly increased. The elevation of portal pressure results in dilatation of all these collateral pathways (Fig. 44-3).

Several attempts have been made to predict the risk of hemorrhage from esophageal varices. Characterization of the severity of portal hypertension on the basis of corrected sinusoidal pressure has not correlated with subsequent hemorrhage. Factors that do predict the risk of bleeding include the size of the varices, the Child class of the patient, and the presence of erosions on the varices (red-dot signs).[32-36]

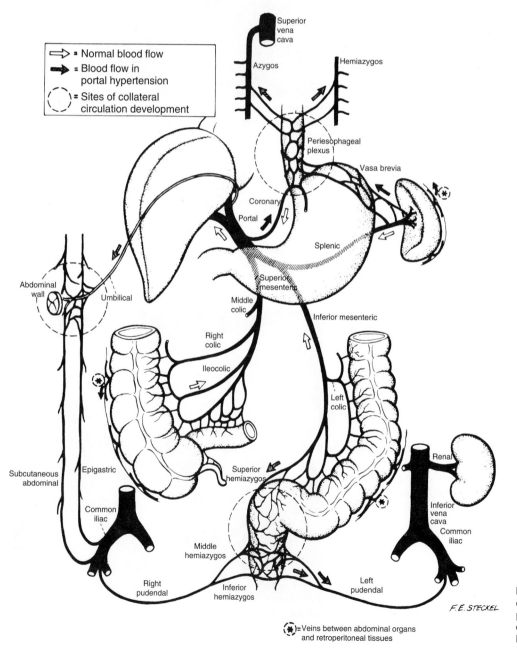

FIGURE 44–3 • Schematic diagram of collateral venous pathways. (From Sedgwick CE, et al: Portal Hypertension. Boston, Little, Brown, 1967.)

ENCEPHALOPATHY

Although not usually considered a life-threatening complication of hepatic failure, encephalopathy may have a profoundly disabling effect on patients. The clinical manifestations of encephalopathy are varied and cover a spectrum from mild inattention to frank coma. The most commonly used system of staging encephalopathy classifies patients from stage I through stage IV. Progression begins with mild personality alterations and occasionally with asterixis or clonus in stage I. Stage II may be characterized by drowsiness, sometimes with mild confusion. Stage III is typified by stupor and obtundation. Coma is the hallmark of stage IV. Electroencephalography is not specifically diagnostic, characteristically showing only slow wave activity, primarily in the frontal regions.[37]

The mechanism by which liver failure leads to coma is not clearly understood. Several agents have been postulated as encephalopathic, especially in the presence of a diseased liver. Ammonia, nitrogenous amines, increased false neurotransmitters, decreased true neurotransmitters, and an increased ratio of aromatic to branched chain amino acids are the most likely candidates.

Elevated ammonia levels have several significant repercussions. First, they elevate glucagon levels. This in turn stimulates gluconeogenesis, which produces more ammonia. Additionally, the gluconeogenesis leads to elevated insulin levels, which promotes catabolism of branched chain amino acids. This ultimately leads to increased levels of straight chain amino acids such as phenylalanine, tyrosine, and methionine. An elevated ratio of straight chain to branched chain amino acids drives neutral amino acids past the blood-brain barrier. The cerebral uptake of these neutral amino acids is possible because ammonia stimulates brain glutamine synthesis, allowing rapid equilibration of brain glutamine for straight chain neutral amino acids. These same neutral amino acids may act as false neurotransmitters and are thought to produce encephalopathy.[38]

The treatment of encephalopathy is based on reduction of ammonia levels and supplementation of branched chain amino acids. Lactulose and neomycin reduce ammonia uptake from the gut by altering the intestinal pH, reducing the number of intestinal bacteria, and reducing intestinal transit of protein. Other agents such as levodopa have been used, with mixed results, in improving encephalopathy.[39]

ASCITES

Ascites is a common symptom of portal hypertension. Up to 80% of these patients may have some degree of ascites. The mechanism by which ascites develops is a combination of hemodynamic, physiologic, and metabolic factors. The hemodynamics of the portal circulatory system in the face of cirrhosis is driven primarily by the increased portal venous pressure. In such a state, Starling forces tend to drive fluids out of the vessels and into the interstitial space. Compounding this problem is the low oncotic pressure that characterizes many cirrhotic patients by virtue of their hypoalbuminemia. Finally, many of these patients chronically register a relatively low effective intravascular volume, which in turn triggers the renal aldosterone-renin-angiotensin system and, perhaps, an additional natriuretic hormone. These then produce a state in which the patient retains free water and salt, both of which aggravate the ascites. The net effect is the translocation of fluid from the intravascular space to the interstitial space and the abdominal cavity.

The compensatory mechanism that normally counteracts the accumulation of interstitial and peritoneal fluid is primarily the lymphatic system. In a cirrhotic patient, the lymph flow is frequently increased. Ascites accumulates when the ability of the lymphatics to reabsorb this fluid is overwhelmed.

The cornerstone of the management of ascites is restriction of salt intake and judicious use of diuretics. These measures control the vast majority of ascitic patients. In only 5% of cases can ascites be considered intractable, and other means of addressing the ascites are required.

Medical Therapy

GENERAL MEDICAL CARE

Medical care is based on evaluating and defining the cause of the liver disease. The first step is to address any factors related to the cause of the liver disease that are amenable to change (e.g., stopping alcohol consumption). The second step is establishing the patient's current state of health and hepatic function: defining the presence of portal hypertension, splenomegaly, ascites, or varices. An assessment of the hepatic disease and the degree of hepatic deterioration helps in predicting the eventual course of the patient. The next step involves maintenance of nutrition, supplementation of vitamins and minerals, and avoidance of salt (especially in ascitic patients).

MANAGEMENT OF ACUTE COMPLICATIONS

The management of acute complications is a very specialized area in the care of these patients. The most common problem that requires urgent care is hemorrhage. The significance of hemorrhage in these patients is difficult to understate. Hemorrhage may be associated with up to 70% mortality, depending on the cause and severity of the liver disease and the degree of decompensation of the patient at the time of presentation. Further, the risk of a second hemorrhage within 1 year may be as high as 60%.[16]

The essential steps in caring for a cirrhotic patient with an upper gastrointestinal hemorrhage include establishing peripheral venous access, volume-resuscitating the patient, and determining the source of bleeding. This is best accomplished by upper gastrointestinal endoscopy. As mentioned previously, between 40% and 60% of cirrhotic patients with known varices who have an upper gastrointestinal hemorrhage are not bleeding from their varices.[40]

If the patient is bleeding from an esophageal varix or hypertensive gastritis, several specific steps are taken promptly. First, the rate of bleeding is assessed. Second, the patient must be adequately resuscitated. Third, the patient must be prepared for a possible therapeutic intervention.

Assessing the rate of bleeding is essential. The assessment is based largely on the progressive change in the patient's vital signs, mentation, and perfusion during the course of resuscitation. A nasogastric tube also provides information about continued bleeding. Emergency endoscopy may provide insight into whether the patient is suffering a massive hemorrhage or is bleeding at a moderate rate. The change in the patient's hematocrit is not necessarily the best indicator of bleeding because there may be a significant lag between the bleeding episode and the subsequent drop in hematocrit.

Patients with relatively minor bleeding episodes frequently stop bleeding spontaneously. The few patients who are actively bleeding at the time of admission almost always respond to an infusion of octreotide. The key to managing these patients is to avoid overloading them with fluid and salts, because this may precipitate a rebleed with further decompensation.

Patients with moderate bleeding rates stand a reasonable chance of having their bleeding stopped without surgical intervention. These patients frequently respond to infusions of octreotide, emergency sclerotherapy, or balloon tamponade.

Patients who bleed massively may require more advanced intervention, often in addition to octreotide and balloon tamponade. Emergent endoscopy is frequently impaired by the massive bleeding. Subsequent steps include angiographic embolization, percutaneous attempts to create an intrahepatic shunt (transjugular intrahepatic portosystemic shunt [TIPS]), or emergency surgical shunting.

The fluids used in resuscitation vary with the severity of the hemorrhage. Patients with minor bleeds may be resuscitated with intravenous crystalloid solutions. In patients with more severe hemorrhages, it may be necessary to supplement this with infusions of albumin. In severe hemorrhages, it is necessary to infuse both packed RBCs and fresh frozen plasma. Occasionally, infusions of other blood components are required, such as platelets or cryoprecipitate, but this is relatively rare. The goal of resuscitation is to maintain the patient at a level at which vital organs can be perfused while the bleeding source is addressed. Indicators of a successful resuscitation include the ability of the patient to mentate, produce urine, and maintain acid-base balance.

Preparation of these patients for possible therapeutic interventions includes cleansing of the gastrointestinal tract, stabilization of the blood volume, identification of the bleeding source, and administration of blood components as needed to allow the proposed interventions.

Specific Measures for the Control of Acute Hemorrhage

PROTEIN AND GUT LAVAGE

Hemorrhage into the gastrointestinal tract poses a significant risk of encephalopathy, particularly in patients with bleeding varices. The combination of a large protein load in the intestinal tract and poor hepatic function frequently results in encephalopathy. The intestinal tract must be cleansed of the blood and any other nitrogenous substances by a combination of enemas and oral cathartics or gastric lavage.

The upper gastrointestinal tract should be laved with the aid of a large-bore tube (e.g., Ewald tube) to remove the clotted blood from the stomach. The rest of the tract is cleansed at the appropriate time by the administration of lactulose and neomycin by mouth. Neomycin and lactulose are given to alter the intestinal absorption of ammonia. Neomycin is a relatively nonabsorbable antibiotic; it destroys urease-producing bacteria and thereby decreases ammonia production. Lactulose is converted by lactase-containing intestinal bacteria into lactic acid and acetic acid, thus decreasing the intraluminal intestinal pH. The lower pH ionizes ammonia into ammonium (NH_4^+), which is less able to diffuse through the colonic mucosa. Lactulose also promotes diarrhea, cleansing the intestine of its contents.[17,41,42]

VASOPRESSIN

Vasopressin (Pitressin) should no longer be considered first-line therapy in the management of active bleeding varices. However, information from its use has provided significant insights into the early management of variceal bleeding. The drug is specifically directed at slowing and stopping variceal hemorrhage. It has been recognized since 1917 for its vasoconstrictive effects and its ability to decrease portal pressure.[43] Vasopressin is a naturally occurring nonapeptide that demonstrates general vasoconstrictive effects, with particular efficacy in the splanchnic bed. This splanchnic vasoconstriction leads to decreased portal flow. Vasopressin is also known to diminish cardiac output by an average of 14% and heart rate by 11%. This, in turn, reduces hepatic blood flow by approximately 44% and wedge hepatic vein pressure by 11%. As much as a 23% reduction in the gradient between hepatic venous pressure and wedge hepatic vein pressure has been documented.[44]

A consequence of the vasoconstrictive effects of vasopressin is the potential exacerbation of cardiac ischemia. To counter these ischemic effects, a number of pharmacologic agents have been used in conjunction with vasopressin.[44-46] Isoproterenol, when administered with intravenous vasopressin, results in an equivalent reduction of portal vein pressure but maintenance of cardiac output.[45] Sublingual nitroglycerin plus vasopressin has been shown to reduce the deleterious effects of vasopressin alone while preserving the decrease in portal vein pressure.[44,47] In the course of a controlled trial, Gimson and associates noted that nitroglycerin may reverse some of the cardiac suppressive effects of vasopressin, as well as enhance the portal hypotensive effects.[48]

Intravenous vasopressin should be used before balloon tamponade. It stops variceal bleeding in at least 80% of cases. The initial dosage is 0.2 to 0.4 units/minute. If bleeding does not cease with the initial dose, the dosage may be increased up to 1 unit/minute.

SOMATOSTATIN AND OCTREOTIDE

Because of its fewer side effects and equal efficacy compared with vasopressin, octreotide has become the agent of choice in managing acute variceal hemorrhage. Somatostatin is a tetradecapeptide derived from the hypothalamus that has demonstrated an ability to decrease splanchnic blood. Octreotide is a synthetic octapeptide analog of somatostatin. It has a longer half-life than somatostatin (100 minutes vs. 2 to 3 minutes). Both have been demonstrated to be as effective as vasopressin for the control of acute bleeding, with fewer complications.[49] Hemodynamic studies indicate that somatostatin decreases the portal venous pressure gradient.[42,50] Randomized studies have shown equal efficacy between the two, and meta-analysis has demonstrated no survival benefit. Somatostatin has been repeatedly shown to have fewer side effects than vasopressin.[49,51]

Octreotide is effective in reducing and halting variceal hemorrhage in 80% of cases. Intravenous octreotide should be used before, and along with, balloon tamponade. It should be started before endoscopy. The initial dose of octreotide is a bolus infusion of 50 μg. This is followed by an infusion of 50 μg/hour. As with vasopressin infusions, the octreotide infusion should be continued over a 3-day period. After this period, the drug should be gradually discontinued.[46]

Data have been mixed regarding somatostatin and related agents, but several studies demonstrated decreased blood loss when these drugs are used. For example, a meta-analysis comprising 12 trials (1452 patients) showed an overall decrease in transfusion requirements of 1 unit of blood per patient.[52] Mortality, rebleeding, and need for balloon tamponade were not decreased. As the authors concluded, the transfusion requirements are significant, but it is not evident that there is any clinical benefit in saving a single unit of blood.

Terlipressin is a synthetic vasopressin analog that can be given intermittently as an injection, unlike vasopressin, which must be administered as an intravenous drip. In comparison with vasopressin, no significant differences in outcome were shown in a meta-analysis of 20 studies comprising 1609 patients.[53] It is not clear whether this drug will become a front-line treatment agent. In summary, because these drugs are easy to administer, have relatively safe profiles, and may be effective, many centers use them routinely for bleeding varices.

PROPRANOLOL

Propranolol, a beta-blocking drug, has been found to be useful in controlling chronic portal hypertension and reducing the risk of recurrent bleeding from esophageal varices. Its action is thought to be mediated on the basis of reduced cardiac output, reduced systemic pressure, and the subsequent reduction in portal venous pressure.

Evidence of its efficacy in the reduction of recurrent bleeding has been mixed. Burroughs and colleagues compared propranolol with placebo and found no significant difference in rebleeding or survival.[54] Fleig and colleagues randomized 70 patients to sclerotherapy or propranolol and found no difference in the rebleeding rate or survival[55]; however, propranolol did decrease the size of the varices significantly after 3 months of treatment. In a prospective, controlled, randomized study of 79 patients, Lebrec and associates noted that after 3 months, 2.6% of patients maintained on propranolol had recurrent gastrointestinal tract bleeding, compared with 66% maintained on a placebo drug.[56,57] Similar findings have been reported by others.[58] Poynard and coauthors analyzed 127 patients treated with propranolol and found five factors that were associated with rebleeding: (1) hepatocellular carcinoma, (2) lack of persistent decrease in heart rate, (3) lack of abstinence from alcohol, (4) lack of compliance, and (5) prior history of rebleeding.[59] More recently, Schepke and associates compared propranolol therapy to band ligation in primary prophylaxis of varices in high-risk patients, noting that there were no differences in bleeding between these treatments.[60]

Propranolol has been specifically used as maintenance therapy to decrease the risk of recurrent esophageal variceal bleeding in patients with portal hypertension. Its use in acute bleeding episodes has not been studied.

BALLOON TAMPONADE

Balloon tamponade is a technique that employs compression by an intragastric balloon to stem the bleeding of esophageal and gastroesophageal varices. The technique dates to the early 1950s, when Linton, Nachlas, Sengstaken, and Blakemore developed the tubes that now bear their names.

All these tubes work on the same principle, tamponade of varices. The design variations include the presence of one or two balloons for compression of the stomach alone or the esophagus and stomach (Linton-Nachlas vs. Sengstaken tube) and the presence of adjunctive ports for aspiration of the stomach and esophageal secretions (Sengstaken-Blakemore vs. Edlich modification or Minnesota tube).[61,62] The Sengstaken-Blakemore tube is probably used more often because it can compress both esophageal and gastric varices, whereas the Linton-Nachlas tube can compress only gastric varices.

The Sengstaken-Blakemore tube can be passed through either the mouth or the nose. Passage of this tube must be performed carefully and precisely to prevent complications. The manufacturers recommend that the gastric balloon be inflated with a low volume of air (250 mL) and that an abdominal radiograph be taken to ensure that the gastric balloon is on the stomach before full inflation (with 750 mL of air). This should avoid the problem of fully inflating the gastric balloon in the esophagus, where it could tear open the esophageal wall.

Once the gastric balloon is inflated, it is taped to the face-mask of a football helmet with approximately 1 kg of pressure. The gastric and esophageal ports are connected to intermittent low Gomco suction. The position of the gastric balloon is checked periodically to ensure that migration into the esophagus has not occurred. If bleeding does not cease with gastric balloon inflation and tension, the esophageal balloon is inflated to 24 to 45 mm Hg pressure. If bleeding ceases with the Sengstaken-Blakemore tube insertion, it is left inflated for 24 hours. After this period, the esophageal balloon should be deflated. Twenty-four hours later, the gastric balloon is deflated. If bleeding does not recur, the tube is deflated and left in place. It should be removed after an additional day.[63] Esophageal variceal tamponade results in cessation of hemorrhage in 45% to 92% of cases.[63-66] Bleeding recurs shortly after the Sengstaken-Blakemore tube is deflated in 24% to 42% of cases, however, and cannot be controlled in 33% to 37% of cases.[63-65] The incidence of recurrent bleeding after a second period of balloon control is 40%.[65]

This tube has been associated with significant complications: gastroesophageal tears, ulceration, and perforation. Pulmonary complications include aspiration pneumonia and asphyxia from tracheal intubation. Conn and Simpson reported a complication rate of 41% and a mortality rate of 20%.[67] More commonly, the incidence of major complications is in the range of 4% to 9%.[63-65]

Surgical Shunt Correction
SHUNT NOMENCLATURE

The nomenclature of shunts changed as different operations were devised at various periods. Many of these terms remain in use, and an understanding of them is necessary. Two basic sets of nomenclature prevail: anatomy-based descriptive names and taxonomic names. There are also eponymous names which are presented for completeness.

The anatomic naming of shunts is based on elements of the shunt. Thus, the principal shunts are portacaval, mesocaval, and splenorenal. The first portion of the name denotes the donor vessel, and the second portion denotes the recipient vessel. Because of some ambiguity associated with these names, modifiers are applied. A portacaval shunt may be either a side-to-side or an end-to-side portacaval shunt. Similarly, a splenorenal shunt may be either a proximal or a distal splenorenal shunt. The principal advantage of this system is that it allows a clear, descriptive means of labeling an operation. This is probably the most widely used shunt nomenclature.

The taxonomic nomenclature is derived from both physiologic and anatomic considerations. These names are ingrained in the lexicon of surgery and should be understood. The two principal sets of names are *central* and *remote* and *selective* and *nonselective*. A central shunt is one constructed in the region of the porta hepatis, or at the center of the portal confluence. Included among these are the various portacaval shunts. The term is used to distinguish shunts that involve the portal vein itself from those that are remote from the portal vein, such as splenorenal and mesocaval shunts. The distinction has regained some usefulness in the context of distinguishing shunts that are recommended for potential liver transplant candidates.

Selectivity of a shunt refers to its effect on the portal venous blood flow. Selective shunts preserve the flow of mesenteric blood through the portal vein to the liver while decompressing esophageal varices. Nonselective shunts drain all portal blood flow into the vena cava. The selective shunts include the distal splenorenal shunt (DSRS) and the coronary-caval shunts. Nonselective shunts include the end-to-side portacaval shunt, side-to-side portacaval shunt, mesocaval shunt, and proximal splenorenal shunt. Currently, the term *selective shunt* is nearly synonymous with a DSRS.

Many shunts are still associated with the names of their proponents. Included are the Warren shunt (DSRS), Linton shunt (proximal splenorenal), Clatworthy shunt (mesocaval shunt using the inferior vena cava [IVC]), Drapanas shunt (mesocaval shunt using a Dacron interposition graft), Inokuchi shunt (coronary-caval), and Sarfeh shunt (portacaval polytetrafluoroethylene [PTFE] interposition graft).

DEVELOPMENT OF SHUNTING

Eck, in 1877, performed the first portosystemic shunt in a dog.[68] He demonstrated not only that the portal vein could be anastomosed to the IVC but also that the animal could survive with total diversion of the portal vein blood flow. Pavlov, in 1893, was the first to recognize the development of a severe neuropsychiatric disorder when a widely patent portacaval shunt was present, and that protein ingestion exacerbated the syndrome. He also described the portaprival syndrome, consisting of gross liver atrophy with fatty infiltration following shunts.[69] It was not until 1945, however, that Whipple,[70] as well as Blakemore and Lord,[71] presented their results on the systematic application of portosystemic bypasses for complications of portal hypertension. The end-to-side portacaval shunt was the first to be used clinically for the control of variceal hemorrhage, and the initial results led to enthusiasm for the shunting of patients with variceal bleeding.[18] With the initial reports demonstrating that the overall recurrence rate of variceal hemorrhage was only

2.8%, little attention was directed toward the quality or length of life.[72]

PROPHYLACTIC SHUNTING

Proponents of prophylactic shunting argued that variceal hemorrhage could be prevented by creating a shunt in patients with varices before they had the opportunity to bleed. Four prospective, controlled studies addressed this issue.[19,21,73,74] These four early studies were similar in design. The patients were divided between medical and surgical treatment and were followed for recurrent bleeding, development of encephalopathy, and survival.

The Boston Interhospital Liver Group (BILG) allocated 45 patients to the medical group and 48 to the surgical group. At 1-, 3-, and 5-year intervals, there was no difference in survival; at 5 years, the survival rate was 50%. Encephalopathy was likewise equal (21%).[75] The Veterans Administration (VA) study demonstrated a 45% incidence of encephalopathy after shunting, almost twice that of medical therapies. Most disconcerting was that the 5-year survival after shunting (51%) was less than with medical therapy (64%).[19] Similarly, the experience of the Yale group demonstrated decreased survival after shunting, with an increased incidence of encephalopathy.[70,71]

Indications for prophylactic variceal decompression have also been studied by the Cooperative Study Group of Portal Hypertension in Japan. By comparing only nondecompressive transection procedures and selective shunts, this group found no difference in survival rates at 2 years, and suggested that in certain patients, prophylactic procedures may be indicated.[21] It should, however, be noted that these patients were primarily nonalcoholic, and the applicability of these results has been widely debated in the United States.

These studies demonstrated that prophylactic shunts do not benefit patients with asymptomatic varices. Although the incidence of variceal hemorrhage is virtually eliminated, these patients tend to suffer from hepatic encephalopathy and die of hepatic failure. Encephalopathy is increased following portacaval shunting, and long-term survival may in fact be decreased by a shunt procedure. These results are not surprising, in that only 30% of patients who have varices bleed, and the decreased incidence of death from bleeding may be offset by the operative mortality of a shunt procedure, as well as by the effects of subsequent hepatic encephalopathy.

THERAPEUTIC SHUNTING

The efficacy of portosystemic shunting has been studied with prospective, randomized clinical trials. Four such trials were performed in the United States and France to evaluate the fundamental question of whether therapeutic shunts prolong survival and maintain the quality of life compared with conventional medical therapy.[76-79]

The VA study, begun in 1961, followed the survival of 155 selected patients over a 5.5-year period. Although 78 patients were randomized to the surgical group, only 67 actually received shunts. Operative mortality following therapeutic portacaval shunts was 8%. Recurrence of variceal bleeding was 7% in the surgical group and 65% in the medical group. Encephalopathy occurred with approximately equal frequency in both groups but was more severe in the shunted group.

The long-term survival rate at 5 years was 57% in the shunt group and 36% in the medical group. The increase in long-term survival was not, however, statistically significant.[73]

In the BILG study,[77] patients underwent end-to-side portacaval shunt, side-to-side portacaval shunt, or medical therapy. The long-term survival was better in the shunt group than in the medically treated group, but this difference was not statistically significant. On the basis of both the VA and the BILG studies, Conn concluded that, despite the lack of statistical significance, therapeutic portacaval shunts prolong the mean duration of life in cirrhotic patients who have suffered from variceal hemorrhage.[80]

Researchers at the University of Southern California published a 12-year follow-up of a prospective, randomized study comparing end-to-side portacaval shunts with medical therapy. There were 190 episodes of bleeding in the group receiving medical therapy, compared with 11 in the surgical group. Encephalopathy of a moderate to severe degree occurred in 35% of shunt patients. A 5-year life-table analysis revealed a 44% survival rate among shunted patients and a 24% survival rate among those treated medically. This difference was not statistically significant, however.[21]

Rueff and associates, in a study at the Hôpital Beaujon in Clichy, France, compared therapeutic end-to-side portacaval shunts with medical therapy.[79] The long-term survival was 47% in the shunt group and 56% in the medical group. The diminished long-term survival in the shunt group is unique to this study and may be due to the high operative mortality (19%, compared with 13% for the BILG study and 8% for the VA study). Encephalopathy was equally common in the medical and surgical groups, with an incidence of 40%. As in the other studies, it tended to be more severe and chronic in the shunt group, however. Recurrent bleeding occurred in 8% of the shunt group and in 72% of the medical group.

The most compelling conclusion drawn from these studies is that they failed to demonstrate a survival advantage. Portacaval shunts are clearly superior in preventing recurrent variceal bleeding. Encephalopathy is not more common in patients undergoing portacaval shunting, but it tends to be more severe and chronic than in medically treated patients.

EMERGENCY PORTACAVAL SHUNTING

Portacaval shunting on an emergency basis is no longer widely performed because of the reported high mortality. Despite this, it has proved highly efficacious in its ability to stop bleeding and prevent recurrent bleeding.[81] Orloff and colleagues continued to advocate the portacaval shunt in the acute setting, and they achieved a 4-year actuarial survival of 69%.[82] Interestingly, this same group reported actuarial survivals of 99% at 5 years and 97% at 10 years when all patients (those bleeding acutely and those operated on for recurrent bleeds) were considerd.[83] Villeneuve and coworkers also supported the use of this shunt in acutely bleeding patients who have mild to moderate liver disease and in whom other forms of treatment have failed.[84] In general, emergency surgical intervention is performed less frequently as nonsurgical options become more effective.

COMMON PORTOSYSTEMIC SHUNTS
Nonselective Shunts
Portacaval Shunts

Both end-to-side and side-to-side portacaval shunts are nonselective and cause diversion of portal flow into the systemic circulation. The only specific indication for the portacaval shunt is esophageal variceal hemorrhage. Intractable ascites was once treated with a side-to-side portacaval shunt, but this technique has now been discarded in favor of peritoneovenous shunting and TIPS.[85,86]

The question of whether an end-to-side or a side-to-side portacaval shunt is more effective is still debated. An end-to-side portacaval shunt is certainly not indicated in the presence of Budd-Chiari syndrome because the portal vein serves as a decompressive outflow tract for intrahepatic portal blood. Uncontrolled studies comparing end-to-side with side-to-side shunts indicate that the side-to-side shunt is associated with a lower surgical mortality in patients with poor hepatic function.[87] Others find the side-to-side portacaval shunt to be more technically demanding. Encephalopathy has been shown to be somewhat more common in side-to-side than in end-to-side portacaval shunts.[88] Investigators previously found that in addition to allowing total diversion of portal venous flow, the side-to-side shunt may create a siphon effect, permitting egress of hepatic arterial blood through the portal vein rather than the hepatic vein. This may be an explanation for the increased incidence of encephalopathy with side-to-side portacaval shunts.

Certain technical considerations preclude a portacaval shunt. First, the portal vein must be patent and free of thrombus. The portal vein diameter should be at least 1 to 1.5 cm (in adults) and should not have previously undergone thrombosis with recanalization. Thrombectomy of a recanalized portal vein is contraindicated because it does not result in long-term shunt patency. Previous surgery in the right upper quadrant is a relative contraindication to a portacaval shunt procedure because of the numerous well-vascularized adhesions, which always result in excessive bleeding.

END-TO-SIDE PORTACAVAL SHUNT. Two approaches have been described: the midline incision and the right subcostal incision. After the abdomen has been entered, the duodenum is mobilized medially to expose the IVC. The dissection is carried up along the IVC to the level of the first hepatic vein under the liver. The portal vein should be exposed by rotating the bile duct and hepatic artery using a vein retractor or peanut sponges. The division of the portal vein should be done after it has been securely clamped (proximally and distally) and the hepatic portion of the vein suture-ligated.

A Satinsky clamp is placed at the appropriate point on the vena cava, and an ellipse of cava is removed to allow anastomosis. Pressure in the portal vein should be measured to document the adequacy of the decompression and to detect any unobserved technical problems. A 50% reduction in portal venous pressure should be expected after the shunt is completed.[89,90]

ARTERIALIZATION OF END-TO-SIDE PORTACAVAL SHUNTS. In an attempt to reduce the morbidity of end-to-side portacaval shunts, a variety of measures have been employed to maintain portal perfusion of the liver. Portal vein arterialization refers to the anastomosis of an arterialized conduit to the hepatic end of the portal vein. Various arteries have been used for this purpose, including the right gastroepiploic artery, splenic artery, and saphenous vein grafts from the hypogastric artery or aorta.

Although a number of studies have indicated that there is no increase in morbidity or mortality, and encephalopathy may be reduced, the procedure has not been universally adopted. Maillard's group divided the splenic artery close to the spleen and anastomosed it to the hepatic stump of the portal vein.[91] They found that total hepatic blood flow with arterialization is equal to or slightly greater than that before the shunt. Immediate postoperative complications were fewer, and the incidence of encephalopathy was less than with the portacaval shunt alone. As this group pointed out, however, the fistula is not likely to remain open after 1 year. Otte and associates reported a retrospective study in which the 5-year survival was 48% in arterialized patients, compared with 44% in other series.[92] Encephalopathy occurred in 27% of the arterialized patients, compared with 40% of those not arterialized. No definitive conclusions can be drawn about the benefit of arterialization of a portacaval shunt in prolonging life or decreasing encephalopathy. Because of the additional time required and the technical difficulty of performing arterialization, it is unlikely that this technique will gain widespread use.

SIDE-TO-SIDE PORTACAVAL SHUNT. The side-to-side portacaval shunt is technically more difficult than the end-to-side shunt. The initial approach is similar to the end-to-side shunt; a longer segment of the vena cava is exposed and circumferentially dissected so that it can be lifted out of its bed. The portal vein must also be exposed for a greater length because a 4-cm segment is necessary for the anastomosis. Portal pressures are measured before the shunt is performed. After applying the vascular clamps, an elliptic segment measuring approximately 2 cm is excised from the IVC and portal vein directly opposite each other. Again, mesenteric venous pressure measurements should reflect a 50% reduction in portal vein pressure.[89]

PORTACAVAL H-GRAFT. An alternative to the side-to-side portacaval shunt is the portacaval H-graft. Technically easier than the side-to-side shunt, the large-diameter (16 to 20 mm) H-graft effectively prevents variceal rebleeding, but encephalopathy occurs frequently. Building on this experience, Sarfeh and colleagues systematically reduced portacaval H-graft diameters and found that an 8-mm PTFE graft combined with portal collateral ablation effectively prevented rebleeding, maintained hepatic perfusion, and reduced encephalopathy.[93] The 5-year cumulative late patency rate was 97%.

Mesocaval Shunts

In 1955, Clatworthy and associates devised a new portosystemic shunt procedure involving division of the IVC above its bifurcation and anastomosis of the proximal cava to the side of the SMV.[94] The portosystemic shunt procedure has been particularly successful in children with extrahepatic portal vein thrombosis. In adults, massive lower extremity edema has limited its usefulness. Because of the extensive dissection necessary to expose the vena cava, a number of alternative graft materials have been used, including cadaveric

IVC, iliac vein, PTFE, and Dacron, which is currently favored.[95-99]

There has been considerable debate about whether portal perfusion (hepatopetal flow) is maintained by mesocaval shunts. Drapanas and colleagues documented continued hepatopetal flow in 44% of their patients.[100] Others have noted, however, that portal perfusion can persist only if there is partial or total H-graft occlusion.[101] Misinterpretation of angiographic studies may also be attributable to the phenomenon of portal pseudoperfusion, as explained by Fulenwider and coauthors.[102] Overall, H-graft mesocaval shunts are considered nonselective shunts.

CLINICAL ROLE OF MESOCAVAL SHUNTS. The primary application of the interposition H-graft mesocaval shunt is for the urgent control of massive variceal hemorrhage. This graft is technically easier to perform than a portacaval or a selective shunt and is frequently indicated in the emergency management of variceal hemorrhage.[103] In the case of previous surgery in the right upper quadrant, a portacaval shunt of any type is especially challenging and is usually contraindicated. If a selective shunt is contraindicated, a mesocaval shunt may be a good alternative. This is true in patients with significant ascites. Other factors that favor mesocaval shunting include extensive periportal fibrosis, a large overriding caudate lobe, an obliterated portal vein, extreme obesity, and Budd-Chiari syndrome.[104]

INTERPOSITION MESOCAVAL H-GRAFT. The operation, as described by Drapanas and coauthors in 1975, remains essentially unchanged to this day.[100] The transverse mesocolon is elevated superiorly, and the small intestine is retracted inferiorly. At the root of the small intestine mesentery, the peritoneum is opened transversely to expose the superior mesenteric vessels. Anatomically, the SMV lies anterior and to the right of the superior mesenteric artery. During isolation of the vein, only one or two small tributaries need to be divided. An important goal is to preserve as many branches of the SMV as necessary to preserve intestinal venous flow. After the SMV is isolated, the anterior surface of the vena cava is exposed through the right transverse mesocolon. Only dissection sufficient to permit the use of a Satinsky clamp on the vena cava is required. Once the vena cava is partially isolated, the third and fourth portions of the duodenum must usually be mobilized to allow the duodenum to ride above the graft. Failure to do this may cause obstruction of the occasional low-lying duodenum or occlusion of the interposed graft.

The vena cava anastomosis is performed first because it lies in the depth of the field and is potentially more hazardous. A partially occluding vascular clamp is placed on the IVC, a small ellipse of vein is excised, and an 14- to 18-mm knitted Dacron graft is anastomosed. Construction of the SMV anastomosis is particularly demanding. The SMV lies anteriorly and courses at a 20- to 30-degree angle counterclockwise to the vena cava. Because of this angulation, it is advisable to rotate the graft 20 to 30 degrees clockwise before constructing the SMV anastomosis. The graft length should be only 3 to 6 cm to minimize kinking of the prosthesis. Anastomosis is performed in the posterior surface of the vein with a continuous suture of 5-0 polypropylene (Prolene). With the clamps removed, the graft should distend quickly. In most instances, a palpable thrill should be present.

Postshunt pressures are then measured in the SMV; if the shunt is functioning properly, there should be at least a 50% reduction of pressure with the shunt open.

A notable variation on this shunt is the C-loop graft as reported by Cameron and coworkers.[105,106] In their procedure, a longer graft is used, which has the configuration of the letter C. To accomplish this, the SMV anastomosis is placed at the point where the SMV disappears under the neck of the pancreas. The proposed advantage of this variation is that the SMV diameter is greater at a more proximal anastomosis, and this allows for improved shunt flow. Despite this theoretical advantage, there is the distinct disadvantage of a more difficult dissection, particularly in patients who have had pancreatitis. The obvious drawback is a longer length of prosthetic material.

CLINICAL RESULTS. Sarr and colleagues published a series of 33 patients who underwent the mesocaval C-shunt procedure.[107] There was a 24% operative mortality rate (all Child class C nonelective cases), an 8% rebleed rate, and a 46% incidence of encephalopathy. However, there were no graft thromboses.

The average incidence of encephalopathy after a mesocaval graft is about 25%.[104,108] The reported incidence of encephalopathy ranges from 9% to 45%.[101,105] Late graft occlusion is caused by excessive layering of thrombus, possibly aggravated by perigraft scarring, leading to kinking and constriction.[101] The incidence of shunt occlusion ranges from 4% to 24%.[100,101,106,109-111] Rebleeding occurs in approximately 14% of mesocaval shunts (range, 12% to 16%). One third of these cases may be related to occlusion of the graft.[103] Overall, the mortality is approximately 15%. The cumulative long-term mortality ranges from 28% to 57%. The long-term mortality is probably dependent on the state of liver function rather than the type of shunt.

Mortality related to mesocaval H-shunts is not significantly different from that for other types of shunts and is dependent on the patient's Child classification. Initial hospital mortality is related to the urgency of surgery, significant elevation of SGOT or bilirubin, or the presence of encephalopathy.[101]

Proximal Splenorenal Shunts

Currently of historical interest only, the nonselective splenorenal shunt, or Linton shunt, was first developed by Blakemore and Lord in 1945 using a Vitallium tube.[71] Linton and coworkers advocated this shunt in the years that followed and considered it the operative procedure of choice for the correction of portal hypertension.[112] Early reports of noncontrolled studies suggested a decreased incidence of encephalopathy with this shunt compared with the portacaval shunt.[113] This finding, however, has not been substantiated. Other investigators failed to demonstrate significant differences between central splenorenal and portacaval shunts with regard to encephalopathy or long-term survival. In fact, some reports noted an increased incidence of thrombosis associated with the central splenorenal shunt.[1,114] The group at Massachusetts General Hospital reported a 10% incidence of recurrent variceal hemorrhage, 19% hepatic encephalopathy, and 18% terminal hepatic failure. Overall operative mortality was 12%.[115] Unlike the DSRS, the central splenorenal shunt functions hemodynamically as a side-to-side

portosystemic shunt. Hepatic blood flow, as well as portal vein pressure, is markedly diminished, and angiography does not demonstrate persistent hepatopetal flow in the presence of a patent shunt.[112] Thus, it is generally accepted that a central splenorenal shunt has no distinct advantage over portacaval or mesocaval shunts, except possibly in the case of severely symptomatic hypersplenism. In this event, the central splenorenal shunt may be combined with splenectomy.

Selective Shunts

Splenorenal Shunts

Portacaval shunts suffer from two significant problems: progressive hepatic failure and progressive, occasionally disabling, encephalopathy. These are thought to be due to the diversion of portal blood from the liver. In an attempt to avoid the complications of total diversion of portal flow, the DSRS, or Warren shunt, was developed in the late 1960s.[69,116]

This operation is based on the principle of compartmentalization, as discussed by Malt.[1] The portal-azygos system and the portal-splanchnic system can be surgically separated into parallel and independent hemodynamic units. Thus, decompression of the portal-azygos system can be accomplished without reducing the portal-splanchnic system perfusion pressure or blood flow.[1,104] Hence, one should be able to decompress esophageal varices and prevent hemorrhage without diverting the hepatopetal flow of the portal-splanchnic blood. In principle, this is accomplished in two steps. First, by disrupting the coronary vein and right gastroepiploic vein, blood flow into the esophageal variceal system is reduced. Second, by anastomosing the distal splenic to the left renal vein, without performing a splenectomy, blood is able to freely drain from the esophageal varices through the short gastrics into the lower-pressure systemic circulation (Fig. 44-4).

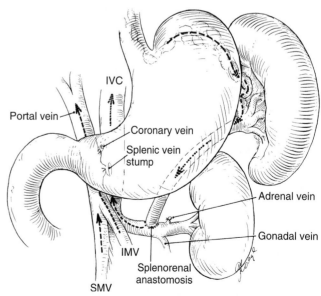

FIGURE 44-4 • Illustration of the selective distal splenorenal shunt. IMV, inferior mesenteric vein; IVC, inferior vena cava; SMV, superior mesenteric vein.

The theoretical benefit of the DSRS includes preservation of hepatic perfusion and function, with consequent prolongation of survival and lower risk of disabling encephalopathy. The search for evidence of this benefit has led to the creation of several randomized trials. Five trials compared the DSRS and portacaval shunts. Three trials compared the DSRS with best nonsurgical management and sclerotherapy.

DISTAL SPLENORENAL SHUNT VERSUS OTHER SHUNTS. The DSRS was compared with the end-to-side portacaval shunt in three randomized studies by Langer and colleagues in Toronto,[117] Resnick and coworkers in the Boston–New Haven trial,[118] and Harley and associates at the University of Southern California Medical Center[119] (Fig. 44-5). Langer's group reported a 14% incidence of postshunt encephalopathy in the selectively shunted patients but a 50% incidence in the end-to-side portacaval group. There was no difference in long-term survival.[117] Preliminary data from Resnick's group indicated no substantial difference between the two operations with regard to either encephalopathy or long-term survival. It should be noted, however, that the follow-up period was relatively short.[118] Harley and associates randomized 54 patients between the two shunts and failed to demonstrate any superiority of one over the other with respect to encephalopathy or survival. They did, however, experience an unusually high rate of rebleeding with the DSRS (27%).[119]

A study in Atlanta compared the DSRS with nonselective shunts, most commonly interposition mesorenal shunts.[120,121] The operative mortality was similar for the two groups: 12% for the DSRS and 10% for nonselective shunts. Early postoperative angiography demonstrated persistent hepatopetal flow in 88% of the DSRS patients but in only 5% of the nonselective shunt patients. Corresponding to this were quantitative measurements of hepatic function, maximal rate of urea synthesis, and the Child class, which were similar to preoperative values in the DSRS group but greatly decreased in the nonselective group. The incidence of encephalopathy correlated with preservation of hepatopetal blood flow. Patients with hepatopetal flow suffered no encephalopathy; patients with hepatofugal flow experienced a 45% incidence of encephalopathy. Overall, encephalopathy occurred in 27% of the DSRS group and 52% of the nonselective group ($P < 0.001$). Recurrent variceal hemorrhage occurred in 4% of selective and 8% of nonselective shunts. Although survival was similar for the two groups, it appears that the quality of survival was improved in the DSRS group.

These results were reproduced by others in Philadelphia[108] and Toronto.[117] The Philadelphia study compared the DSRS with the mesocaval H-shunt. Again, for elective shunts, the operative mortality was similar, 7%. Encephalopathy was significantly much less common with the DSRS, consistent with continued hepatopetal flow in 86% of selective shunts but in no nonselective shunts. Hemorrhage did not recur in either group undergoing elective surgery. The long-term survival rate of 62% was comparable with that in the Atlanta study. The rebleeding rate in emergency cases was 2%.

Two nonrandomized comparative studies also indicated excellent results with the DSRS.[122,123] In a matched, controlled study comparing the DSRS with the portacaval shunt, Busuttil and associates demonstrated that the incidence of significant encephalopathy was 85% in the portacaval group and only 7.6% in the DSRS group.[123,124] Furthermore, this group demonstrated a statistically significant increase in the number of late deaths.[125] There were no recurrent variceal hemorrhages in either group.[123]

Zeppa's group[122] demonstrated that the 5-year survival of patients with nonalcoholic cirrhosis after DSRS was 89%, compared with 39% in the alcoholic cirrhotic group. It should be noted that improved survival in nonalcoholic cirrhotic patients was also suggested by another group,[121] but other investigators have contested this point.[19] In addition, a number of other unmatched studies have demonstrated excellent results with the DSRS.[125,127-134] A combined review of the literature comparing mesocaval H-grafts to DSRSs unequivocally demonstrated the latter to be superior in decreasing the incidence of both encephalopathy and recurrent hemorrhage.[103]

DISTAL SPLENORENAL SHUNT AND SCLEROTHERAPY. Warren and colleagues presented the results of their randomized study of esophageal variceal bleeders who were randomized between DSRS and sclerotherapy (with salvage DSRS).[135] A total of 71 patients were entered over a 4-year period. There was a significant difference between the two groups with regard to preservation of portal perfusion, maintenance of hepatic function, rate of rebleeding, and survival. Although the sclerotherapy patients had a significantly higher rate of rebleeding (53% vs. 3%), only one of these patients died of uncontrollable hemorrhage. The 2-year survival of the group treated with sclerotherapy (and salvage surgery) was 84% (vs. 59% for those undergoing surgery alone).[135] The study clearly demonstrated that the optimal management of these patients involves the use of sclerotherapy as the initial means of controlling bleeding. Surgery appears to work best when it is used to manage those patients whose bleeding is not controllable with sclerotherapy. This important study is the basis for the current method of managing portal hypertensive patients with esophageal variceal hemorrhage.

SPLENOPANCREATIC DISCONNECTION. Because of the results of trials indicating that, with the passage of time, the DSRS gradually becomes a nonselective shunt, Warren modified the operation. In 1986, he and his coauthors proposed that the DSRS procedure include complete dissection of the splenic vein and division of the splenocolic ligament (splenopancreatic disconnection).[136] In theory, this should reduce the pancreatic sump or siphon effect—the tendency of pancreatic branches of the splenic vein to

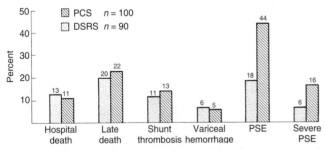

FIGURE 44–5 • Combined experience of the distal splenorenal shunt (DSRS) versus the portacaval shunt (PCS). PSE, portosystemic encephalopathy. (Data from randomized trials by Rikkers,[120] Langer,[117] Reichle,[109] and Harley[119] and their respective colleagues.)

progressively enlarge and serve as an outflow collateral for the portal mesenteric circulatory system. This modification was intended to prolong and preserve the selective quality of the DSRS. Clinically, Warren's group found that this modification preserved postoperative portal perfusion in alcoholic cirrhotic patients better than the DSRS alone. It also considerably extended the magnitude of the operation.

INDICATIONS FOR DISTAL SPLENORENAL SHUNT. The principal indication for a DSRS is to prevent recurrent variceal hemorrhage that is not controllable with sclerotherapy. The specific strengths of the DSRS include its lower incidence of encephalopathy and its anatomic remoteness from the porta hepatis. For these reasons, it is considered the shunt of choice in patients who require elective shunting and have no specific contraindications to the DSRS. The most important of these contraindications is the presence of significant ascites, which in practice, means ascites that is difficult to control by the administration of diuretics. Additionally, patients should have an adequately sized patent splenic vein. Some authors consider the presence of hepatofugal portal blood flow to be a contraindication to the DSRS. In cases of portal hypertension due to extrahepatic portal vein thrombosis, the DSRS has been demonstrated to be effective in preventing recurrent hemorrhage.[131] Finally, although the DSRS has been performed as an emergency procedure, it is not widely considered the shunt of choice in these circumstances because of the relative difficulty of the operation.

SURGICAL TECHNIQUE: DISTAL SPLENORENAL SHUNT. The technique used for the DSRS is essentially the method described by Warren and Millikan.[137] The first goal of this operation is to anastomose the distal splenic vein to the left renal vein. The second goal is to disconnect the portal-azygos system from the splanchnic-venous system. A bilateral subcostal incision provides optimal exposure. The splenic vein may be approached either through the lesser sac or from below the transverse mesocolon. Most surgeons use the lesser sac approach. As part of this approach, the right gastroepiploic vein is divided, but the short gastric veins are carefully preserved. The pancreas is identified, and the peritoneum covering its inferior border is incised. Careful blunt dissection of the retroperitoneal tissue allows the pancreas to be rotated anteriorly and exposes the splenic vein. The splenic vein dissection is the most delicate portion of this operation. It should be carried out to the point of confluence with the SMV. The left renal vein is located by incising the posterior parietal peritoneum in the lesser sac just superior to the fourth position of the duodenum. Often, the ligament of Treitz must be incised and the duodenum reflected inferiorly to locate the vein. Dividing the adrenal vein may allow better mobilization of the renal vein. To prepare the anastomosis, the splenic vein is occluded with vascular clamps and transected close to its junction with the SMV. The stump is ligated with a suture ligature to decrease the incidence of portal vein thrombosis secondary to traumatic manipulation of the splenic vein stump.[97,123] A partial occluding clamp is placed on the left renal vein, and the anastomosis is performed.

After completing the devascularization and the splenorenal anastomosis, measurements are made of the superior mesenteric, renal, and splenic veins. Superior mesenteric

(portal) pressures should not be altered if a total portal-azygos disconnection has been performed. Splenic vein pressure will be decreased by 60% to 70%. If this pressure fails to fall, intraoperative angiography should be used to demonstrate a technically sound anastomosis.[33]

Graft Interposition. When complete mobilization of the splenic vein cannot be accomplished because of pancreatic encasement or fibrosis, shunting may be accomplished by the interposition of a 14- to 16-mm Dacron graft between the side of the splenic vein and the side of the renal vein. After this anastomosis, the portal end of the splenic vein must be ligated if the selective nature of the shunt is to be maintained.

Portal-Azygos Disconnection. Once the anastomosis is completed and the clamps are removed, attention is focused on completing the portal-azygos disconnection. This requires interrupting all collaterals between the portal-mesenteric and portal-azygos systems. Division of the umbilical vein and the falciform ligament completes the first step of the portal-azygos disconnection, and division of the right gastroepiploic vein constitutes the second step. Finally, division of the coronary vein completes the portal-azygos disconnection.

Results: Patency and Portal Perfusion. The maintenance of portal perfusion in the early postoperative period has been documented in more than 90% of patients.[113,119,120,134] The principal question regarding this operation, however, is one of durability: How long does the benefit of the DSRS last? It has been shown that the incidence of early partial portal vein thrombosis may be as high as 22%, and that of complete portal vein occlusion 6%. When followed over a 6-month period, most nonocclusive portal vein thromboses resolve spontaneously.[138] A 10-year follow-up by Warren and coworkers of the DSRS group revealed that 75% had persistent portal perfusion at 10 years. Patients who were demonstrated to have portal perfusion at 3 years maintained this until the conclusion of the study at 7 years.[69,121,128]

The DSRS has several advantages over other nonselective shunts: it preserves portal flow to the liver, it maintains hepatotrophic perfusion, it permits the metabolism of toxic metabolites, and it maintains a high portal perfusion pressure in the intestinal venous bed, decreasing the absorption of toxic substances.[69] It is the best procedure to perform under elective conditions in a patient with hepatopetal flow. Child classes A and B patients under emergent conditions also benefit from selective shunts. It should be noted that the DSRS has not been clearly demonstrated to improve survival by itself, but when used in conjunction with judicious sclerotherapy, it appears to provide the best chance of survival to these patients.

CURRENT INDICATIONS FOR SHUNT PROCEDURES

As noted, shunting operations are performed infrequently since the advent and proliferation of TIPS procedures. In a recent report by Orug and coauthors, less than 1% of patients with portal hypertension at their institution over a 9-year period underwent open shunt procedures.[139] In a multicenter study of bleeding varices, 3.3% of patients underwent open procedures.[140] The need for repeat intervention is the primary disadvantage of TIPS compared with open operations, but even this aspect can be improved with the use of covered stents (discussed later). Nonetheless, one of the compelling reasons for choosing an open shunt over a TIPS procedure continues to be the lack of access for follow-up. Wong and coworkers reported on their use of splenorenal shunts in patients with poor access to follow-up care in the South Pacific.[141] They concluded that open procedures can be performed safely and are appropriate when tertiary care centers are not easily available. The other clinical scenario in which open shunts continue to be performed is when other methods fail to control variceal hemorrhage, particularly in Child class A patients. Interestingly, if one considers the available data, open procedures could be recommended in many low-risk Child classes A and B patients.[142] However, the trend in clinical practice is clearly otherwise.

Nonshunt Surgical Procedures

Emergency portosystemic shunting results in an operative mortality of approximately 47%.[15] Furthermore, in the presence of certain clinical laboratory test results, including an SGOT greater than 300 units/L, or the presence of ascites or other determinants of Child class C status (e.g., bilirubin > 6 mg/dL, hyaline necrosis, severe muscle wasting), a portosystemic shunt is almost sure to result in death. Because of this, numerous nonshunting surgical procedures have been developed.

SPLENECTOMY

Based on Banti's theory that the diseased spleen caused portal hypertension and ascites, splenectomy was one of the first operations proposed for the treatment of Banti's syndrome (splenomegaly, hypersplenism, and ascites, often accompanied by esophageal varices). The use of splenectomy in this setting was largely due to its advocacy by Osler, a great admirer of Banti's work. It was not until 1936, when Rousselot reviewed the experience at Columbia University in New York, that the failings of this operation were noted: a significant incidence of recurrent hemorrhage after splenectomy and the consequent loss of the splenic and portal veins, which would preclude possible shunt surgery.[143] In 1940, Thompson was able to demonstrate statistically that splenectomy was of value only to those patients with isolated splenic vein thrombosis.[144] Finally, in 1945, Pemberton and Kiernan reported a 54% incidence of recurrent variceal hemorrhage with splenectomy alone.[145]

COLLATERALIZATION

Development of collateral pathways between the portal circulation and the systemic circulation was the goal of several procedures. Omentopexy, introduced by Talma in 1898, produces collateral pathways by suturing the omentum to the peritoneum.[146] It was thought to be particularly beneficial in the resolution of ascites. It was sometimes used in conjunction with splenectomy for the relief of ascites associated with splenomegaly and decreased WBC counts.

Another collateral-promoting operation was the transposition of the spleen into the thorax.[147,148] Like omentopexy, its goal was to allow the development of large venous collateral pathways between the portal venous system and the systemic venous circulation. Unfortunately, these collateral pathways were never able to adequately decompress esophageal varices. Thus, the patients were doomed to repeated hemorrhage.

ABLATION

Ablative procedures to remove the source of bleeding were first advocated in 1947 by Phemister and Humphreys,[20] who recommended total gastrectomy. Peters and Womack later encouraged splenectomy with obliteration of both the intraluminal and extraluminal vasculature of the distal varices–bearing esophagus and proximal stomach.[149] Keagy and colleagues reviewed the long-term results of the so-called Womack procedure and found the risk to be prohibitively high—a 54% incidence of rebleeding and a 35% operative mortality.[150] They concluded that this procedure should be used only in highly selected patients who do not have suitable anatomy for a shunt.

A variation of the Womack procedure was the transthoracic ligation of esophageal varices without splenectomy. This operation was introduced in 1949 by Boerema[151] and in 1950 by Crile.[152] Wirthlin and associates reported on 55 patients who underwent transesophageal ligation of varices, with a 29% operative mortality and a 33% incidence of recurrent hemorrhage resulting in an additional 23% mortality.[153]

Despite these results, the procedure was not abandoned. Technologic innovation in the form of the EEA (end-to-end anastomosis) stapler allowed transection and reanastomosis of the distal esophagus with greater facility. The innovation resulted in reduced operative mortality and decreased postoperative hemorrhage. Wexler reported that of six Child class C patients undergoing this procedure, none had recurrent bleeding.[154] Cooperman and associates reported five patients with severe hepatic dysfunction and massive variceal bleeding who underwent transabdominal EEA variceal stapling, none of whom developed recurrent bleeding up to 2 years postoperatively.[155]

In a logical extension of these devascularization procedures, other surgeons proposed more extensive operations. Delaney promulgated a devascularization procedure performed through a left thoracotomy; it involves devascularization of the upper half of the stomach and proximally to the level of the left inferior pulmonary vein, as well as splenectomy, staple interruption of intramural gastroesophageal collateral vessels, truncal vagotomy with pyloroplasty, and fundoplication.[156] The major disadvantage of this procedure is that the splenectomy precludes the performance of selective shunts at a later time. Delaney reported, however, that none of his four patients had recurrent variceal bleeding.

Perhaps the most successful devascularization procedure was that developed by Suguira in Japan.[146,157,158] Because of the significant risk of encephalopathy, shunt procedures were abandoned in favor of an extensive periesophagogastric devascularization accompanied by esophageal transection. The procedure is performed via separate thoracic and abdominal incisions; in poor-risk patients, a two-stage procedure is indicated. The esophagus is devascularized from the gastroesophageal junction to the left inferior pulmonary vein. The vagus nerve is carefully preserved. At the level of the diaphragm, the esophagus is partially transected, leaving only the posterior muscular layer intact. Esophageal varices are occluded, not ligated, by oversewing each with interrupted sutures. The esophageal muscle is closed, but the mucosa is not sutured. The abdominal operation is performed through a separate midline incision and includes splenectomy, devascularization of the abdominal esophagus and proximal stomach, and pyloroplasty and fundoplication.

The early results of this operation, as reported by Suguira and Futagawa, were excellent.[146] The authors reported an overall operative mortality of 4.6%. Their emergency operative mortality was 20%. Varices were eradicated in 97% of patients, and recurrent bleeding occurred in only 2.5%. Their long-term survival was 84%. A follow-up report by the authors on 276 patients indicated equally good survival rates, with excellent control of variceal bleeding and no encephalopathy.[157] In a later report, they analyzed their results according to the patients' Child classification. They found that in class C patients, both operative mortality and long-term survival were discouraging. For classes A and B patients, the results were very good, with combined (A, B, and C) 15-year survival as high as 72%.[159]

Reports by Suguira's group have been confirmed by others in Japan, as well as by selected investigators in the United States.[160,161] A number of other reports have suggested the use of esophageal transection procedures in the management of selected patients with poor hepatic reserves (Child class C patients). The EEA stapler has made this a relatively simple procedure, but the possibility of esophageal perforation and leakage still makes the procedure a considerably risky one.[162] Overall, these studies demonstrate that esophageal transection should be considered a reasonable option in the management of acute hemorrhage in a debilitated patient with both gastric and esophageal varices.[163-165]

Postoperative Care

The most common problem in the postoperative period is the development of significant ascites. Fluid management is the key to minimizing this problem. Postoperative fluids should be restricted to free water and salt-poor albumin or fresh frozen plasma. These should be given to maintain adequate intravascular volume yet avoid overexpansion of the patient's intravascular space. A diuretic should be started as soon as the patient is begun on oral fluids. Spironolactone is frequently used because of its potassium-sparing characteristics. Caution is advised in its use because of the potential complication of metabolic alkalosis. Sodium intake should be restricted to less than 90 mg/day. Prophylactic antibiotics, which should be started 12 hours before surgery, are continued for only 1 to 2 days. Chylous ascites may develop in the immediate postoperative period as a result of interruption of retroperitoneal lymphatics, and a fat-restricted diet (30 g/day) should be maintained for 4 weeks to minimize the risk of this problem.[137]

If variceal hemorrhage occurs within the immediate postoperative period, angiography should be performed immediately to accurately define the anatomy and patency of the shunt. If a patent collateral such as the coronary vein is identified, one should consider percutaneous transhepatic embolization. If other collateral pathways are present, re-exploration may be indicated to ligate them. If the shunt is occluded and the patient is bleeding, re-exploration should be undertaken to repair the shunt or to perform another shunt.

Transjugular Intrahepatic Portosystemic Shunt

The TIPS has become a commonly used technique for controlling variceal hemorrhage. This has had a dramatic effect on the performance of operative shunting procedures, despite the fact that TIPS has been used clinically only since 1988. Over the last few years, the indications for TIPS have expanded, although these applications have not always been backed by randomized trials. Recent developments in TIPS research, most notably the use of covered stents, have improved the patency of TIPS and will most likely lead to even more widespread use of this procedure.

Rosch demonstrated 30 years ago that intrahepatic portacaval shunts could be created in a minimally invasive fashion.[166] Palmaz applied his stent to this type of procedure, leading to prolonged patency of these shunts in animal models.[167] After its initial application in human subjects, there was a rapid expansion in its application, so that a large number of interventionalists became skilled in this technique. Most major medical centers now perform TIPS.

TIPS can be performed with conscious sedation and is frequently carried out in interventional suites. Ultrasonography should be done before the procedure to document the patency of the portal vein and assess the need for a peritoneal tap. Most interventionalists minimize the amount of ascites before performing TIPS so that the liver is not "floating" in the abdomen. Access is ideally attained via the right internal jugular vein, which provides the most direct route for cannulation of right hepatic vein branches. Wedged venogram and portal pressures are obtained, and a portal vein branch is then punctured. There are a number of commercially available devices for advancing through the liver parenchyma to the portal vein; the Rosch-Uchida transjugular liver access set (Cook Surgical, Bloomington, Ind.) in used at my institution. These devices combine a cutting needle with an aspiration port and are usually designed to fit a 10 French sheath. Portal access is confirmed by aspirating blood during needle advancement. A guidewire is advanced so that the hepatic and portal circuits are in continuity. Finally, the track is balloon-dilated and stented. At the end of the procedure, pressure measurements can be repeated to confirm that the portal-systemic gradient is less than 12 mm Hg. A completion venogram must also be obtained to assess stent placement and to ensure that varices are no longer filling.

TIPS for acute variceal bleeding stops the hemorrhage in more than 90% of patients.[168] This compares favorably with endoscopic sclerotherapy in many series, including at least eight prospective, randomized trials.[169,170] However, most studies have shown a decreased rate of rebleeding with TIPS versus sclerotherapy. Rosch and Keller reported a 5.6% rebleeding rate at 3 months' follow-up, compared with the 20% to 30% usually seen following endoscopic therapy.[171] As with rebleeding following other therapies, a significant number of patients (25% to 30%) will have a different, nonvariceal lesion as the hemorrhage source. Confirmation of the source is thus extremely important.

When the bleed is from varices, it is almost invariably associated with improper function of the shunt. As with other vascular conduits, short-term problems are usually technical in nature, whereas those developing later are related to neointima formation. Although TIPS can be revised to control the bleeding, one of the chief criticisms of these shunts is the need for repeated interventions.[172] In fact, the primary patency of TIPS is roughly 40% at 1 year, but secondary patency approaches 90%.[173]

Despite the benefit in preventing rebleeding, TIPS is considered a second-line procedure after sclerotherapy owing to several factors, most notably the increased incidence of hepatic encephalopathy (roughly 50% vs. 20%). In addition, for patients whose bleeding is controlled by sclerotherapy, there is no survival benefit with TIPS.

It is clear that TIPS has replaced open surgical shunt procedures for most Child classes B and C patients. This is underscored by the fact that it is not uncommon for a surgical resident to finish his or her training without performing a single shunting procedure. Interestingly, in the largest prospective trial comparing TIPS and surgical shunts (8-mm prosthetic H-grafts), TIPS was found to have higher rates of death, rebleeding, and treatment failure.[174] This trial, as well as an additional 4 years of follow-up, was published by Rosemurgy and colleagues and evaluated 35 patients in each arm, pairing them based on their Child class. A comparison of the rates of post-treatment encephalopathy generally favored surgery as well.

TIPS has been applied in several other clinical situations. One broad category is as a bridge to hepatic transplantation. Theoretically, the procedure leaves the porta hepatis unperturbed and allows for easier subsequent operation. Some have argued that TIPS actually accelerates liver failure in patients awaiting transplantation.[175] However, several studies support the use of TIPS in this setting, particularly as a means for improving patients' general condition, sometimes with decreased blood loss at the time of surgery.[176-180] One technical note of importance is placement of the distal end of the stent well above the IVC so that it does not interfere with the transplant itself or cause damage to the portal vein.

Another application of TIPS has been for the management of refractory ascites. There are numerous retrospective trials documenting the effectiveness of TIPS in this setting, but only a few randomized trials. In a randomized study by Rossle and coauthors, TIPS was shown to be more effective than paracentesis in controlling refractory ascites.[181] In a study by Lebrec and coworkers, TIPS was shown to benefit Child class B patients with ascites but was of no help in class C patients, in whom it had little effect on ascites and increased mortality.[182] In a more recent review of randomized trials, Saab and associates, using clinical registries, found that TIPS reduced ascites reaccumulation better than paracentesis at 3- and 12-month follow-up.[183] Encephalopathy was more common in the TIPS group, but all other variables analyzed were equal. Finally, Rosemurgy and colleagues performed a randomized, prospective trial comparing TIPS and peritoneovenous shunts.[184] They concluded that TIPS was more beneficial in patients unless they had only a very short life expectancy. Siegerstetter and colleagues reported retrospectively on the benefits of TIPS in treating refractory hydrothorax.[185]

TIPS has also been used with some success in the treatment of Budd-Chiari syndrome. There are several small studies investigating its use in this setting. Perello and authors managed 13 such patients with TIPS and found that 11 were doing well after a follow-up of 4 years.[186] Interestingly, many of the patients' TIPS were no longer patent but did not require treatment owing to the absence of signs of portal hypertension. Blum and coauthors reported on 12 Budd-Chiari patients who underwent TIPS.[187] Two of the patients had fulminant hepatic failure and died, but the remaining 10 had resolution of their ascites. In a larger series, Rossle and colleagues reported on 35 patients receiving TIPS for Budd-Chiari syndrome.[188] The cumulative 1- and 5-year survival rates without transplantation in this group were 93% and 74%, respectively, suggesting that TIPS will continue to evolve as a treatment for this disease.

One additional application of TIPS has been for hepatorenal syndrome. Brensing and colleagues reported an improvement in renal function in these patients compared with nonshunted patients.[189] Other studies also support the use of TIPS in this setting.[190] Recently, Wong and colleagues demonstrated prospectively that TIPS can be used in conjunction with a protocol of midodrine, octreotide, and albumin to improve renal function in type 1 hepatorenal syndrome.[191]

As mentioned previously, the main drawbacks of TIPS are the poor primary patency and the need for repeated interventions to maintain the shunt. It has been shown in animal studies that the use of covered stents improves the patency of TIPS, and there are now human data to support this contention. Otal and associates used PTFE-covered nitinol stents in a recent series of 20 patients and reported primary and secondary patency rates of 80% and 100% at 387 days (as opposed to 58% primary patency at 1 year for noncovered stents reported in the literature).[192] Rossi and coworkers reported 1-year primary patency rates of 83.8% with these stent-grafts,[193] and Maleux and associates reported only a single occlusion after 56 TIPS procedures using PTFE-covered stents at a mean follow-up of 246 days (range, 3 to 973 days).[194]

Orthotopic Liver Transplantation

With the advent of liver transplantation as an established modality for patients with end-stage liver failure, the role of nontransplantation procedures (shunt surgery in particular) has been the subject of considerable debate. Currently, the best transplant survival rates are generally more favorable than those of Child class C patients after the best care with a combination of sclerotherapy and shunting. This issue has been the subject of two reports from Iwatsuki and colleagues at the University of Pittsburgh Liver Transplant Unit.[195,196] These reports described the survival of 302 patients who had bleeding esophageal varices. According to the authors, these patients were all ranked as Child class C with regard to hepatic function. Their survival was reported in a life-table format as 79% at 1 year, 74% at 2 years, and 71% at 5 years. The authors then compared these results with shunt survival as reported in the medical literature and concluded that in Child class C patients who present with bleeding varices, liver transplantation should be considered the treatment of choice, assuming that the patients are reasonable transplant candidates.

Our experience at the University of California, Los Angeles, has revealed that transplantation affords superior survival to Child class C patients (Table 44-3). In a series of 761 patients operated on between January 1986 and December 1991, 77 underwent portosystemic shunting as their initial procedure, and 684 underwent hepatic transplantation.

TABLE 44–3	Results of Portosystemic Shunting and Liver Transplantation from January 1986 to December 1991*		
	No. of Patients	Child Class C (%)	5-Year Survival
Portosystemic shunt	77	16	64
Liver transplantation	684	86	73

*University of California, Los Angeles, experience. Distal splenorenal shunts constituted 50% of shunt operations; 15% of shunt patients eventually underwent liver transplantation because of deterioration of hepatic function.

Of the the patients receiving transplants, 86% were Child class C, whereas only 16% of the shunt patients were class C. Despite this, 15% of shunt patients eventually required liver transplantation for progressive hepatic deterioration. Furthermore, the 5-year survival for the shunt group was 64%, in contrast to 73% for the transplant patients. Similar 5-year survival data in excess of 75% were recently published by Roberts and associates, reflecting patients studies through 1999.[197] These data support the impression that portosystemic shunting is an appropriate therapy for Child classes A and B patients, but that class C patients who are reasonable candidates are best managed by liver transplantation.

Further complicating the issue is the effect of a prior shunt operation on a subsequent transplant operation. It has been reported that patients who must receive a liver transplant after having a portacaval shunt have considerably greater blood loss, longer operative procedures, increased morbidity, and higher mortality.[198] The portacaval shunt is a particularly troublesome procedure to overcome, because the performance of a successful liver transplantation requires dissection through the scarred tissues about the portal structures, disconnection of the shunt, and reconstitution of the normal caval anatomy; only then can the liver transplant operation begin. This is in contrast to peripheral shunt operations, such as the mesocaval shunt or the DSRS. Although these shunts have an impact on the transplantation procedure, they are not as difficult to manage as the central shunts are. In the case of a mesocaval shunt, the shunt must be disconnected or occluded before the transplant operation is completed, or the new liver may be deprived of portal nutrient blood flow. A similar problem may arise with the DSRS, although because of the nature of this shunt, the siphon effect (drainage of portal blood through peripancreatic collaterals into the shunt) is usually relatively minor, and the shunt frequently does not require dismantling.

In any consideration of the role of shunting versus liver transplantation, the essential factors are the underlying cause of the hepatic disease, the current stage of hepatic dysfunction, and the expected progression (the natural and treated history) of the hepatic disease. Assuming that the patient is a reasonable transplant candidate and that the liver disease is approaching the end stage (Child class C), transplantation should be strongly considered. If the patient requires an emergent procedure to control bleeding before undergoing transplantation, all efforts should be made to provide a peripheral shunt. If the patient is not a transplant candidate, treatment should consist of the best therapy available:

sclerotherapy supported by either esophageal transection with devascularization or shunting.

Variceal Sclerotherapy

Esophageal variceal sclerotherapy was introduced by Crafoord and Frenckner in 1939.[199] These authors reported a single patient who underwent rigid endoscopic sclerotherapy to prevent further variceal bleeding. With the upsurge in the variety of surgical procedures for variceal hemorrhage in the 1940s, however, sclerotherapy was soon forgotten. Once it was recognized that therapeutic portacaval shunts, with their inherent operative mortality and risk of encephalopathy, were not the ultimate surgical procedure, attention was redirected toward less invasive, more direct methods of treatment, and there was renewed interest in sclerotherapy after the results of several controlled trials.

The first major review of sclerotherapy was by Johnston and Rodgers in 1973.[200] In 117 patients, bleeding was initially controlled in 92%, and the hospital mortality per admission was 18%. The average time to recurrence of variceal hemorrhage was 10 months. This group, however, made no attempt to perform sequential variceal sclerotherapy and recommended a shunt for long-term variceal control. Similar mortality and variceal hemorrhage control rates were reported by Terblanche from South Africa.[201-204]

Endoscopy is necessary to confirm the presence of varices and differentiate those that are actively bleeding from those that have ceased to bleed. The use of sclerotherapy to stop acute bleeding at the time of initial endoscopy has been advocated as the treatment of choice.[201,202] Urgent or emergent sclerotherapy is used in many institutions after stabilization with balloon tamponade or after failure of conservative supportive therapy and somatostatin. Several controlled trials have compared sclerotherapy with medical management with the Sengstaken-Blakemore tube in the acute setting.[205-209] Three studies demonstrated a significantly lower early rebleeding rate,[205-207] and all the studies supported the use of sclerotherapy for acute bleeding. Only Paquet and Feussner demonstrated significantly improved overall survival with sclerotherapy.[205]

The ability of sclerotherapy to prevent recurrent variceal hemorrhage and improve long-term survival with extended treatment has been examined in numerous controlled trials (Table 44-4).[208-212] When sclerotherapy was performed to eradicate all varices and compared with conservative medical management, sclerotherapy patients had fewer recurrent bleeds[208,210] and improved long-term survival.[209] Terblanche and colleagues were able to demonstrate complete eradication of varices in 95% of sclerotherapy patients; however, they could not demonstrate a significant difference in survival, and varices recurred in more than 60% of the sclerotherapy patients.[210]

Only since 1984 has sclerotherapy been systematically compared with portosystemic shunts in the management of variceal hemorrhage. Cello and associates compared the portacaval shunt to sclerotherapy in Child class C patients, showing greater rebleeding, increased rehospitalization, and higher blood transfusion requirements in the sclerotherapy group, with 40% of sclerotherapy patients ultimately requiring surgical therapy.[213,214] However, they were unable to demonstrate any significant difference in survival (Table 44-5).

TABLE 44–4	Sclerotherapy versus Medical Management (Control)						
		Sclerotherapy			**Control**		
Study	**Follow-up (mo)**	**No. of Patients**	**Rebleed (%)**	**Percentage Surviving (yr)**	**No. of Patients**	**Rebleed (%)**	**Percentage Surviving (yr)**
Terblanche et al[210]	60	37	43*	45 (5)	38	73	45 (5)
Paquet and Feussner[205]	9-52	93	48	36 (2)	97	54	25 (2)
Westaby et al[209]	3-60	56	55*	60 (4)	60	80	31 (4)
Korula et al[212]	3-35	63	44*	60 (2)	57	70	56 (2)
Soderlund and Ihre[211]	12-48	57	†	49 (2)	50	†	34 (2)

*There was a significant decrease in transfusion requirements in the sclerotherapy group, as well as fewer rebleeding episodes per patient-month if followed up.

†Overall recurrent hemorrhage was 3.6 times more frequent in the control group.

The authors concluded that in high-risk patients, sclerotherapy and portacaval shunting are equal in the acute setting, but one must consider shunt surgery if varices are not totally obliterated.

The DSRS has been compared with endoscopic sclerotherapy for the long-term management of variceal bleeding in three controlled trials (Table 44-6). Warren and coworkers showed that although early mortality was the same, there was a higher rebleeding rate with sclerotherapy, and one third of the patients failed treatment and required surgery.[215] Treatment with sclerotherapy resulted in significant improvement in liver function when successful, with less encephalopathy and improved survival when backed up by surgical therapy for patients with uncontrolled bleeding. Therefore, the improved survival in the sclerotherapy group actually represents a combination of sclerotherapy and surgical therapy. Teres and colleagues found no difference in early and long-term mortality,[216] nor did Rikkers and coworkers.[217] However, the rebleeding rate was greater in those patients who had sclerotherapy, and encephalopathy rates were higher in shunt patients in the study of Teres and colleagues.[216]

In 1989, Burroughs and associates concluded a prospective, randomized study comparing staple transection with sclerotherapy for emergency control of variceal bleeding.[218] They found no difference in overall mortality and improved control of bleeding with esophageal transection compared with a single injection, but there was a similar incidence of hemorrhage after three injection treatments. Teres and colleagues randomized cirrhotic patients with uncontrolled bleeding to portacaval shunt or staple transection in low-risk patients and staple transection or sclerotherapy in high-risk patients.[219] Survival was similar in the two groups. In the low-risk patients, portacaval shunt had a greater hemostatic effect but a greater incidence of encephalopathy. In high-risk patients, sclerotherapy and staple transection had similar rebleeding rates and survival, but fewer complications were observed in the sclerotherapy group. The authors therefore recommended staple transection for low-risk patients and sclerotherapy for the initial management of high-risk patients. Although a consensus has not yet been reached, sclerotherapy may represent an appropriate alternative ablative procedure in selected patients with hepatic dysfunction.[164,205,219-227]

A number of complications with varying degrees of severity result from esophageal variceal sclerotherapy. Frequently, patients complain of odynophagia lasting from hours to days. This may also be associated with retrosternal chest pain lasting for several days. Not infrequently, as a result of pyrogens within the sclerosing solution, a fever greater than 101°F develops and then abates within 2 to 3 days; it is not associated with a leukocytosis. Bacteremias have been documented in as many as 50% of procedures.[228] Pleural effusion sometimes occurs but does not necessarily indicate esophageal perforation.[229] Variceal ulceration of varying degrees, depending on the amount of sclerosant injected, is not uncommon and usually resolves spontaneously.[230] Rare serious complications, including esophageal perforation, spinal cord paralysis, and bradyarrhythmias, have also been described.[25,27,28,30,204,224,227]

TABLE 44–5	Sclerotherapy versus Portacaval Shunt in Management of Variceal Hemorrhage		
	Sclerotherapy (n = 32)	**Shunt (n = 32)**	**P Value**
Rebleed rate (%)	50	19	< 0.009
Encephalopathy (%)	13	13	NS
Surgery not required	7 (22%)		
Long-term cost	$23,000	$28,000	NS
18-month survival (%)	28	13	NS

NS, not significant.

Data from Cello J, Grendell J, Crass R, et al: Endoscopic sclerotherapy versus portacaval shunt in patients with severe cirrhosis and variceal hemorrhage. N Engl J Med 311:1589-1594, 1984.

TABLE 44–6	Sclerotherapy versus Distal Splenorenal Shunt (DSRS) in Long-Term Management of Variceal Hemorrhage*		
	Sclerotherapy	DSRS	*P* Value
Warren et al[215]			
No. of patients	36	35	
Rebleed rate (%)	53	3	<0.05
Portal perfusion (%)	95	53	<0.05
Patients requiring surgery	10 (28%)		
2-yr survival (%)	84	59	<0.01
Rikkers et al[217]			
No. of patients	30	27	
Rebleed rate (%)	57	19	0.003
Encephalopathy (%)	7	16	
2-yr survival (%)	61	65	NS
Teres et al[216]			
No. of patients	55	57	
Rebleed rate (%)	37.5	14.%	<0.02
Encephalopathy (%)	8	24	<0.05
2-yr survival (%)	68	71	NS

*All controlled trials.
NS, not significant.

More recently, interest has increased in an alternative endoscopic technique, variceal banding. This has the advantage of avoiding the caustic agents required for sclerotherapy. In comparison studies, the rates of efficacy in halting bleeding are similar between the two techniques. There is debate whether the incidence of complications with banding is reduced compared with sclerotherapy. Clearly, the same major complications attend both techniques: recurrent bleeding, as well as esophageal ulceration and perforation.[231]

Endoscopic variceal sclerotherapy and variceal banding have the distinct advantages of no risk of portal vein thrombosis, good control of variceal hemorrhage, and easy accessibility for repeat sclerotherapy. There is no question that in patients with acute variceal bleeding who have had a prior splenectomy or a portosystemic shunt that has failed, endoscopic therapy is indicated. Because of the high mortality associated with emergency shunting procedures, variceal sclerotherapy in conjunction with octreotide is indicated in the acute management of variceal hemorrhage. Recurrent variceal hemorrhage is likely if follow-up routine sclerotherapy is not performed. Hence, sclerotherapy should be considered an adjunctive therapeutic management tool for the acute control of variceal bleeding rather than definitive treatment.

Treatment Plan for Variceal Hemorrhage

When a patient has an upper gastrointestinal tract hemorrhage and the history and physical examination suggest esophageal varices in association with hepatic disease, a preset treatment plan should be followed (Fig. 44-6). It is important to remember that time is of the essence in these patients, and delays to consider, define, and formulate a plan of action may jeopardize the patient's life. The initial care of a bleeding portal hypertensive patient should be as routine as the initial care of a trauma patient, following the A, B, Cs. Special variations are implemented because of the underlying hepatic disease and the associated risks.

Initial laboratory studies should include a CBC, electrolytes, blood typing, and crossmatching. Additionally, determinants of liver function, including bilirubin, SGOT, LDH, SGPT, prothrombin time, partial thromboplastin time, albumin, total protein, and alkaline phosphatase, should be obtained. Nasogastric tubes must be placed in all patients; if blood is present in the stomach, gastric lavage and emergency endoscopy are indicated. This allows verification of the source of the hemorrhage and emergent sclerotherapy, if required.

Initial fluid management is crucial. Treatment with fluids and blood products should be directed at maintaining adequate tissue perfusion. Resuscitation should include packed RBCs and fresh frozen plasma, as needed. Cryoprecipitates and calcium may be required in cases of massive bleeding. It is generally preferable to resuscitate with a combination of crystalloid and blood components (albumin and packed RBCs) rather than with saline only. Thiamine should be administered to prevent Wernicke's encephalopathy. Propranolol or diazepam (Valium) may be required for the symptoms of alcohol withdrawal.

If the bleeding does not stop during resuscitation and transfusion, octreotide should be administered intravenously and repeat sclerotherapy performed. Balloon tamponade may be especially helpful at this juncture. If the patient fails to stop bleeding after injections and balloon tamponade, emergent intervention is indicated. Depending on the institution's resources, the patient should be considered for a TIPS, portosystemic shunt, or esophageal transection with devascularization. If the patient is a potential liver transplant candidate, a peripheral shunt (DSRS or mesocaval) should be performed. The choice of TIPS or surgical shunt should probably be based on the local expertise and ability of the managing physicians.

Once bleeding is controlled, patients with relatively good hepatic function (Child class A or B) should undergo long-term sclerotherapy until varices are obliterated. If this is successful, the patient should continue to be observed, and no further intervention need be planned. If the patient has breakthrough bleeding from noncompliance, gastric varices, or hypertensive gastritis and is an appropriate candidate for an elective shunt, a preoperative evaluation should be done (angiography, duplex scan) and a shunt performed.

Patients with poor hepatic function should be considered for transplantation if they meet the appropriate criteria. While the patient is awaiting orthotopic liver transplantation, a peripheral shunt may be necessary as a bridge. Child class C patients with marked muscle wasting and obvious hyaline necrosis have a prohibitively high operative mortality rate and should undergo endoscopic sclerotherapy followed by transplantation. If this technique is not available, esophageal transection with or without the EEA stapler and ligation of portal-azygos collateral pathways is indicated, although the mortality can be expected to be greater than 60%.

Management of Ascites

Ascites predisposes portal hypertensive patients to potentially lethal complications, including renal failure, peritonitis,

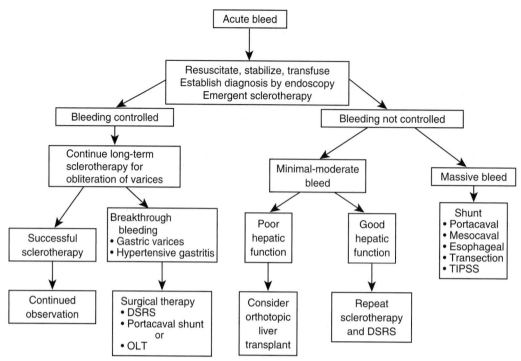

FIGURE 44–6 • Protocol for the management of variceal hemorrhage. DSRS, distal splenorenal shunt; OLT, orthotopic liver transplantation; TIPSS, transjugular intrahepatic portosystemic stent-shunt.

variceal hemorrhage, pleural effusions with respiratory insufficiency, abdominal wall hernias, anorexia, and generalized malaise. In most patients, ascites can be controlled with a restricted-salt diet and a diuretic regimen. Only 5% of ascitic patients can be considered to have truly intractable ascites, and these patients may require surgical intervention.[232]

Patients who have ascites related to liver disease should be admitted to the hospital for complete evaluation and therapy. The admission workup should include a careful neurologic status examination, as well as measurements of electrolytes and renal and liver function tests. These patients should be placed on strict bed rest, because this will increase the amount of diuresis. Encephalopathy should be monitored by checking for asterixis at least once or twice a day.

Fluid restriction of no more than 1 L/day should be ordered, in addition to a 20-mEq/day sodium diet. With this regimen, one would expect a diuresis of 500 mL to 1 L/day. If such a diuresis does not occur, progressive diuretic therapy is indicated. This usually involves a gradual increase in the dosages and varieties of diuretics. Frequently, the first diuretic used is spironolactone, a potassium-sparing diuretic. It should be started at a dosage of 100 mg/day and doubled at 2-day intervals until a maximum dosage is obtained. If further diuresis is required, other agents, such as metolazone, hydrochlorothiazide, and furosemide (Lasix), may be used.

At the first sign of encephalopathy or elevation of blood urea nitrogen by 10 mg/dL or creatinine by 0.5 mg/dL, all diuretics must be discontinued to avoid development of the hepatorenal syndrome. If, after such a trial of intensive nonsurgical therapy, no significant response occurs, surgery is indicated.[233]

In 1974, LeVeen introduced the peritoneovenous shunt.[234] This device consists of a Silastic tube that runs from the peritoneum to the superior vena cava. It is controlled by a one-way valve so that a pressure gradient of 5 cm H_2O suffices to transfer the ascitic fluid from the abdomen to the intravascular space.

The Denver shunt, a variation of the LeVeen shunt, incorporates a pump in line with the shunt and is implanted into the subcutaneous tissues in the chest wall. Its proposed benefit is the ability to clear the shunt of debris by using the pump mechanism.[129]

Although promising innovations, both of these shunts are dogged by complications. Early complications include congestive heart failure (from the infusion of ascitic fluid) and disseminated intravascular coagulation (DIC). In 39% to 100% of patients, changes consistent with DIC may be detected by laboratory studies. Clinically apparent DIC is much less common.[72,235] Coagulation values tend to improve after the first postoperative week, possibly related to diminished ascitic flow into the venous system.[236] If clinically apparent DIC develops, the only definitive treatment is shunt ligation.[235] Some authors are concerned that the increased intravascular volume may result in increased variceal hemorrhage. Finally, high perioperative mortality rates (20%) have been reported by a number of institutions.[237]

Late complications include shunt infection, shunt occlusion, and death. Infection may occur in up to 26% of patients. Shunt occlusion is thought to result from the precipitation of the ascitic protein in the shunt tubing. Death related to inherent liver dysfunction is not uncommon.

Usually, the infusion of ascitic fluids results in a brisk diuresis. The exact mechanism for this is not clear. Proposed mechanisms include volume expansion, increased renin levels from the ascitic fluid, and relief of intra-abdominal pressure.[6] Hepatorenal syndrome is the name given to the concomitant loss of renal function in patients with hepatic failure and no intrinsic renal disease. Although the cause is unknown, it may be related to a redistribution of blood within the cortex of the kidney. The mortality from untreated hepatorenal syndrome is usually 100%. The peritoneovenous shunt is considered a potential treatment for these patients. Successful resolution of the syndrome by placement of such a shunt has been reported.[238]

Contraindications to the placement of peritoneovenous shunts include the presence of infected ascitic fluid, recurrent sepsis, or encephalopathy. Other absolute contraindications are a bilirubin level greater than 6 mg/dL or prolongation of the prothrombin time longer than 4 seconds. These have been shown to be associated with a prohibitively high incidence of postoperative coagulopathy, resulting in death. DIC resulting from an intravenous test infusion of ascitic fluid is another relative contraindication to peritoneovenous shunting. Finally, a large pleural effusion associated with an elevated intrathoracic pressure may preclude the use of these shunts.[232]

The use of TIPS in the treatment of ascites has already been discussed. Success with this procedure has reduced the number of peritoneovenous shunts being performed, and recent data suggest only a limited role for peritoneovenous procedures.[180]

Summary

The management of portal hypertension and its sequelae of ascites, encephalopathy, and recurrent variceal hemorrhage continues to be a significant challenge to clinicians. Its cause and pathogenesis have been well described. Alcoholic cirrhosis resulting in intrahepatic sinusoidal and postsinusoidal obstruction continues to be the most common cause.

Long-term survival depends on rapid control of hemorrhage and institution of the most appropriate care for the patient according to the nature and severity of the hepatic disease. A patient who has variceal hemorrhage should be quickly resuscitated. Endoscopy should be performed to establish the source of gastrointestinal bleeding, followed by sclerotherapy. Initial management should include intravenous vasopressin followed by balloon tamponade. Angiography or duplex Doppler studies should be performed in patients being considered for shunting. Emergent shunt surgery should be avoided if at all possible, because the mortality is excessive.

Selective shunt procedures (DSRS), although they do not extend long-term survival, produce less encephalopathy and stop bleeding. Patients should be considered for elective shunting if they cannot be controlled with sclerotherapy and have relatively good hepatic function (Child class A or B). Child class C patients and "unshuntable" patients are best treated with nonshunt procedures or transplantation. Esophageal variceal sclerotherapy provides effective control of acute variceal hemorrhage, but if it is unsuccessful after several attempts, a portal-azygos devascularization procedure should be performed. Ultimately, the survival of these patients depends on the degree of hepatic function. Patients with end-stage liver disease should be considered for liver transplantation.

Encephalopathy is a consequence of hepatic failure. It may be ameliorated by a medical regimen of neomycin, lactulose, and a low-protein diet. Ascites can usually be managed with salt restriction and diuretics. In a patient with intractable ascites, a peritoneovenous shunt provides effective control.

Determining the best treatment for patients with portal hypertension relies on the recognition that the hepatic disease dictates the progression of liver failure. Depending on the stage of hepatic dysfunction, different options are available. In deciding how best to manage a particular patient, it is necessary to keep in mind that the goal is not merely survival but also quality of life.

REFERENCES

1. Malt R: Portasystemic venous shunts. N Engl J Med 295:24-29, 1976.
2. Shaldon S, Sherlock S: Portal hypertension in the myeloproliferative syndrome and the reticuloses. Am J Surg 32:758, 1962.
3. Shaldon S, Chiandussi L, Guevara L: The measurement of hepatic blood flow and intrahepatic shunted blood flow by colloid, heat denatured serum albumin labeled with I131. J Clin Invest 40:1038, 1969.
4. Gordon M, DelGuerco L: Late effects of portal systemic shunting procedures on cardiorespiratory dynamics in man. Ann Surg 176:672-679, 1972.
5. Langer B, Stone R, Colapinto R: Clinical spectrum of the Budd-Chiari syndrome and its surgical management. Am J Surg 129:137-145, 1975.
6. Ludwick J, Markel S, Child L: Chiari's disease. Arch Surg 91:697-704, 1965.
7. Sherlock S: Classification and functional aspects of portal hypertension. Am J Surg 127:121-128, 1974.
8. Ahn S, Yellin A, Sheng F, et al: Selective surgical therapy of the Budd-Chiari syndrome provides superior survival rates than conservative medical management. J Vasc Surg 5:28-37, 1987.
9. Bosch J, Navasa M, Garcia-Pagan J, et al: Portal hypertension. Med Clin North Am 73:931-953, 1989.
10. Bosch J, Mastai R, Kravetz D, et al: Hemodynamic evaluation of the patients with portal hypertension. Semin Liver Dis 6:309-317, 1986.
11. Koslin D, Berland L: Duplex Doppler examination of the liver and portal system. Clin Ultrasound 15:675-686, 1987.
12. Ohnishi K, Saito M, Koen H, et al: Pulsed Doppler flow as a criterion of portal venous velocity: Comparison with cineangiographic measurements. Radiology 154:495-498, 1985.
13. Bolondi L, Gandolfi L, Arienti V, et al: Ultrasonography in the diagnosis of portal hypertension: Diminished response of portal vessels to respiration. Radiology 142:167-172, 1982.
14. Cello J, Deveney K, Trunkey D: Factors influencing survival after therapeutic shunts. Am J Surg 141:257-265, 1981.
15. Orloff M, Duguay L, Kosta L: Criteria for selection of patients for emergency portacaval shunt. Am J Surg 134:146-152, 1977.
16. Schwartz S: Liver. In Schwartz S (ed): Principles of Surgery. New York, McGraw-Hill, 1984, pp 1257-1305.
17. Rueff B, Benhamou J: Management of gastrointestinal bleeding in cirrhotic patients. Clin Gastroenterol 4:426-438, 1975.
18. Rikkers L: Operations for management of esophageal variceal hemorrhage. West J Med 136:107-121, 1982.
19. Resnick R: Portal hypertension. Med Clin North Am 59:945-953, 1975.
20. Phemister D, Humphreys E: Gastroesophageal resection and total gastrectomy in the treatment of bleeding varicose veins in Banti's syndrome. Ann Surg 125:397, 1947.
21. Mikkelsen W: Therapeutic portacaval shunt. Arch Surg 108:302-305, 1974.
22. Bell R, Miyai K, Orloff M: Outcome in cirrhotic patients with acute alcoholic hepatitis after emergency portacaval shunt for bleeding esophageal varices. Am J Surg 147:78-84, 1984.
23. Eckhauser F, Appelman H, O'Leary T: Hepatic pathology as a determinant of prognosis after portal decompression. Am J Surg 139:105-112, 1980.
24. Viamonte M, Warren W, Famon J: Angiographic investigations in portal hypertension. Surg Gynecol Obstet 130:37-53, 1970.
25. Huizinga W, Keenan J, Marszaley A: Sclerotherapy for bleeding esophageal varices: A case report. S Afr Med J 65:436-438, 1984.
26. Mikkelsen W, Turrill F, Kern W: Acute hyaline necrosis of the liver: A surgical trap. Am J Surg 116:266-272, 1968.
27. Seidman E, Neber A, Morin C: Spinal cord paralysis following sclerotherapy for esophageal varices. Hepatology 4:950-954, 1981.
28. Perakos P, Cirbus J, Camara D: Persistent bradyarrhythmia after sclerotherapy for esophageal varices. South Med J 77:531-532, 1984.
29. Lunderquist A, Vang J: Transhepatic catheterization and obliteration of the coronary vein in patients with portal hypertension and esophageal varices. N Engl J Med 291:646-649, 1974.
30. Abecossis M, Makowka L, Lanser B: Sclerotherapy for esophageal varices. Can J Surg 27:561-566, 1984.
31. Reynolds T: The role of hemodynamic measurements in portasystemic shunt surgery. Arch Surg 108:276-281, 1974.
32. Lebrec D, DeFleury P, Rueff B, et al: Portal hypertension, size of esophageal varices and risk of gastrointestinal bleeding in alcoholic cirrhosis. Gastroenterology 79:1139-1144, 1980.
33. Paquet K: Prophylactic endoscopic sclerosing treatment of the esophageal wall in varices—a prospective controlled randomized trial. Endoscopy 14:4-5, 1982.

34. Witzel L, Wolbergs E, Merki H: Prophylactic endoscopic sclerotherapy of esophageal varices: A prospective controlled study. Lancet 1:773-775, 1985.

35. North Italian Endoscopic Club for the Study and Treatment of Esophageal Varices: Prediction of the first variceal hemorrhage in patients with cirrhosis of the liver and esophageal varices: A prospective multicenter trial. N Engl J Med 319:983-989, 1988.

36. Dagradi ZA: The natural history of esophageal varices in patients with alcoholic cirrhosis. Am J Gastroenterol 57:520-540, 1972.

37. Schenker S, Breen K, Hoyumpa A: Hepatic encephalopathy: Current status. Gastroenterology 66:121-151, 1974.

38. Fischer J, James J, Jeppsson B: Hyperammonemia, plasma amino acid imbalance and blood-brain amino acid transport. Lancet 2:772-778, 1979.

39. Fischer J, Furovics J, Folcao H: L-Dopa in hepatic coma. Ann Surg 183:386-391, 1976.

40. Waldram R, Davis M, Nunnerly H: Emergency endoscopy after gastrointestinal hemorrhage in 50 patients with portal hypertension. BMJ 4:94-96, 1974.

41. Maddrey W, Weber F: Chronic hepatic encephalopathy. Med Clin North Am 59:937-944, 1975.

42. Elkington S: Lactulose. Gut 11:1043-1048, 1970.

43. Bainbridge F, Trevan J: Some actions of adrenaline upon liver. J Physiol 51:460-468, 1917.

44. Graszmann R, Kravetz D, Bosch J: Nitroglycerin improves the hemodynamic response to vasopressin in portal hypertension. Hepatology 2:757-762, 1982.

45. Sirinek K, Thomford N: Isoproterenol in offsetting adverse effect of vasopressin in cirrhotic patients. Am J Surg 129:130-136, 1975.

46. Chandler J: Vasopressin and splanchnic shunting. Ann Surg 195:543-553, 1982.

47. Mols P, Hallemans R, Van Kuyk M: Hemodynamic effects of vasopressin alone and in combination with nitroprusside in patients with liver cirrhosis and portal hypertension. Ann Surg 199:176-181, 1984.

48. Gimson A, Westaby D, Hegarty J: A randomized trial of vasopressin and vasopressin plus nitroglycerin in the control of acute variceal hemorrhage. Hepatology 6:410-413, 1986.

49. Kravetz D, Bosch J, Teres J, et al: Comparison of intravenous somatostatin and vasopressin infusions in treatment of acute variceal hemorrhage. Hepatology 4:442-446, 1984.

50. Bosch J, Kravetz D, Rodes J: Effects of somatostatin on hepatic and systemic hemodynamics in patients with cirrhosis of the liver: Comparison with vasopressin. Gastroenterology 80:518-525, 1985.

51. Chan LY, Sung JJY: Review article: The role of pharmacotherapy for acute variceal hemorrhage in the era of endoscopic hemostasis. Aliment Pharmacol Ther 11:45-50, 1997.

52. Gotzsche PC: Somatostatin analogues for acute bleeding oesophageal varices. Cochrane Database Syst Rev 1:CD000193, 2002.

53. Ioannou G, Doust J, Rockey DC: Terlipressin for acute esophageal variceal hemorrhage. Cochrane Database Syst Rev 1:CD002147, 2001.

54. Burroughs A, Jenkins W, Sherlock S: Controlled trial of propranolol for the prevention of recurrent variceal hemorrhage in patients with cirrhosis. N Engl J Med 309:1539-1542, 1983.

55. Fleig W, Stange E, Hunecke R, et al: Prevention of recurrent bleeding in cirrhotics with recent variceal hemorrhage: Prospective randomized comparison of propranolol and sclerotherapy. Hepatology 7:355-361, 1987.

56. Lebrec D, Poynard T, Hillani P: Propranolol for prevention of recurrent gastrointestinal bleeding in patients with cirrhosis. N Engl J Med 805:1371-1374, 1981.

57. Lebrec D, Bernjau J, Rueff B: Gastrointestinal bleeding after abrupt cessation of propranolol administration in cirrhosis. N Engl J Med 807:560, 1982.

58. Maringhini A, Simonetti R, Marceno M: Propranolol for gastrointestinal bleeding in cirrhosis. N Engl J Med 307:1710, 1982.

59. Poynard T, Lebrec D, Hillon P, et al: Propranolol for prevention of recurrent gastrointestinal bleeding in patients with cirrhosis: A prospective study of factors associated with rebleeding. Hepatology 7:447-451, 1987.

60. Schepke M, Kleber G, Nurnberg D, et al: Ligation versus propranolol for the primary prophylaxis of variceal bleeding in cirrhosis. Hepatology 40:65-72, 2004.

61. Edlich R, Lande A, Goodale R: Prevention of aspiration pneumonia by continuous esophageal aspiration during esophagogastric tamponade and gastric cooling. Surgery 67:405-408, 1968.

62. Burcharth F, Malmstrom J: Experience with the Linton-Nachlas and the Sengstaken-Blakemore tubes for bleeding esophageal varices. Surg Gynecol Obstet 142:529-531, 1976.

63. Bauer J, Kreel I, Kark A: The use of the Sengstaken-Blakemore tube for the control of bleeding esophageal varices. Ann Surg 179:273-277, 1974.

64. Hermann R, Traul D: Experience with the Sengstaken-Blakemore tube for bleeding esophageal varices. Surg Gynecol Obstet 130:879-885, 1970.

65. Pitcher J: Safety and effectiveness of the modified Sengstaken-Blakemore tube: A prospective study. Gastroenterology 61:291-298, 1971.

66. Johnson W, Nabseth D, Widrich W: Bleeding esophageal varices. Ann Surg 195:893-400, 1982.

67. Conn H, Simpson J: Excessive mortality associated with balloon tamponade of bleeding varices. JAMA 202:135, 1967.

68. Eck N: On the question of ligature of the portal vein. Voyenno Med 130:1-2, 1877.

69. Warren W: Control of variceal bleeding: Reassessment of rationale. Am J Surg 145:8-16, 1983.

70. Whipple A: The problem of portal hypertension in relation to the hepatosplenopathies. Ann Surg 122:449-475, 1945.

71. Blakemore A, Lord JJ: The technique of using Vitallium tubes in establishing portacaval shunts for portal hypertension. Ann Surg 122:476-488, 1945.

72. Greig P, Langer B, Blendis L, et al: Complications of the peritoneovenous shunting for ascites. Am J Surg 139:125-131, 1980.

73. Conn H, Lindemuth W: Prophylactic portacaval anastomosis in cirrhotic patients with esophageal varices: A progress report of a continuing study. N Engl J Med 272:1255-1263, 1965.

74. Conn H, Lindemuth W, May L, et al: Prophylactic portacaval anastomosis: A tale of two studies. Medicine (Baltimore) 51:27-40, 1972.

75. Resnick R, Chalmers T, Ishihara A: The Boston Interhospital Liver Group: A controlled study of the prophylactic portacaval shunt. A final report. Ann Intern Med 70:675-688, 1969.

76. Jackson F, Perrin E, Felix W, et al: A clinical investigation of the portacaval shunt. Ann Surg 174:672-701, 1971.

77. Resnick R, Iber F, Ishihara A, et al: A controlled study of the therapeutic portacaval shunt. Gastroenterology 67:843-857, 1974.

78. Reynolds T, Donovan A, Mikkelsen W, et al: Results of a 12-year randomized trial of portacaval shunt in patients with alcoholic liver disease and bleeding varices. Gastroenterology 80:1005-1011, 1981.

79. Rueff B, Prandi D, Degos F, et al: A controlled study of portacaval shunt in alcoholic cirrhosis. Lancet 1:655-659, 1976.

80. Conn H: Therapeutic portacaval anastomosis: To shunt or not to shunt. Gastroenterology 67:1065-1071, 1974.

81. Sarfeh I, Carter J, Welch H: Analysis of operative mortality after portal decompressive procedures in cirrhotic patients. Am J Surg 140:306-311, 1980.

82. Orloff M, Bell R, Hyde P, Skivolocki W: Long-term results of emergency portacaval shunt for bleeding esophageal varices in unselected patients with alcoholic cirrhosis. Ann Surg 192:325-340, 1980.

83. Orloff MJ, Orloff MS, Girard B, et al: Bleeding esophagogastric varices from extrahepatic portal hypertension: 40 years' experience with portal-systemic shunt. J Am Coll Surg 194:717-728, 2002.

84. Villeneuve J, Pomier-Layrargues G, Duguay L, et al: Emergency portacaval shunt for variceal hemorrhage: A prospective study. Ann Surg 206:48-52, 1987.

85. LeVeen H, Wapnick S, Grosberg S, et al: Further experience with peritoneovenous shunt for ascites. Ann Surg 184:574-581, 1976.

86. Burchell A, Rousselot L, Panke W: A seven-year experience with side-to-side portacaval shunts for cirrhotic ascites. Ann Surg 168:655-670, 1968.

87. Turcotte J, Wallin V, Child C: End-to-side versus side-to-side portacaval shunts in patients with hepatic cirrhosis. Am J Surg 117:108-116, 1979.

88. Iwatsuki S, Mikkelsen W, Redeker A, et al: Clinical comparison of the end-to-side and side-to-side portacaval shunt. Ann Surg 178:65-69, 1973.

89. Blakemore W: The technique of portal systemic shunt surgery. Surgery 57:778-786, 1965.

90. Hermann R: Shunt operations for portal hypertension. Surg Clin North Am 55:1073-1087, 1975.

91. Maillard J, Rueff B, Prandi D: Hepatic arterialization and portacaval shunt in hepatic cirrhosis. Arch Surg 108:315-320, 1979.

92. Otte J, Reynaent M, Hemptinne B, et al: Arterialization of the portal vein in conjunction with a therapeutic portacaval shunt. Ann Surg 196:656-663, 1982.

93. Sarfeh I, Rypins E, Mason G: A systematic appraisal of portacaval H-graft diameters: Clinical and hemodynamic perspectives. Ann Surg 204:356-363, 1986.

94. Clatworthy H, Wall T, Watman R: A new trial of portal-to-systemic venous shunt for portal hypertension. Arch Surg 71:588, 1955.
95. Drapanas T, LoCicero J, Dowling J: Interposition meso-caval shunt for treatment of portal hypertension. Ann Surg 176:435, 1972.
96. Lord J, Rossi G, Daliana M, et al: Mesocaval shunt modified by the use of a Teflon prosthesis. Surg Gynecol Obstet 130:525-526, 1970.
97. Nay H, Fitzpatrick H: Mesocaval "H" graft using autogenous vein graft. Am Surg 183:114-119, 1976.
98. Read R, Thompson B, Wise W, et al: Mesocaval H venous homografts. Arch Surg 101:785, 1970.
99. Thompson B, Reed B, Casall R: Interposition grafting for portal hypertension. Am J Surg 130:733-739, 1975.
100. Drapanas T, LoCiciero J, Dowling J: Hemodynamics of the interposition mesocaval shunt. Ann Surg 181:523-532, 1975.
101. Smith R, Warren W, Salam A, et al: Dacron interposition shunts for portal hypertension. Ann Surg 92:9-17, 1980.
102. Fulenwider J, Nordlinger B, Millikan W: Portal pseudoperfusion: An angiographic illusion. Ann Surg 189:257, 1979.
103. Cargenas A, Busuttil R: A comparative analysis of the mesocaval H graft versus the distal splenorenal shunt. Curr Surg 39:151-157, 1982.
104. Malt R: Portasystemic venous shunts. N Engl J Med 295:80-86, 1976.
105. Cameron J, Zuidema G, Smith G, et al: Mesocaval shunts for the control of bleeding esophageal varices. Surgery 85:257-262, 1979.
106. Cameron J, Harrington D, Maddrey W: The mesocasval C shunt. Surg Gynecol Obstet 150:401, 1980.
107. Sarr M, Herlong H, Cameron J: Long-term patency of the meso-caval C shunt. Am J Surg 151:98-103, 1986.
108. Resnick R, Langer B, Taylor B, et al: Results and hemodynamic changes after interposition mesocaval shunt. Surgery 95:275-280, 1984.
109. Reichle F, Fahmy W, Golsorkhi M: Prospective comparative clinical trial with distal splenorenal and mesocaval shunts. Am J Surg 137:13-21, 1979.
110. Thompson B, Casall R, Reed R, et al: Results of interposition "H" grafts for portal hypertension. Ann Surg 187:515-522, 1978.
111. Mulcare R, Halleran D, Gardine R: Experience with 49 consecutive Dacron interposition mesocaval shunts: A unified approach to portasystemic decompression procedures. Am J Surg 147:393-399, 1984.
112. Linton R, Ellis D, Geary J: Critical comparative analysis of early and late results of splenorenal and direct portacaval shunts performed in 169 patients with portal cirrhosis. Ann Surg 154:446-449, 1961.
113. Pliam M, Adson M, Foulk W: Conventional splenorenal shunts. Arch Surg 110:588-599, 1975.
114. Bismuth H, Franco D, Hepp J: Portal-systemic shunt in hepatic cirrhosis: Does the type of shunt decisively influence the clinical result? Ann Surg 179:209-218, 1974.
115. Ottinger L: The Linton splenorenal shunt in the management of the bleeding complications of portal hypertension. Ann Surg 196:664-668, 1982.
116. Warren W, Zeppa R, Fomon J: Selective transsplenic decompression of gastroesophageal varices by distal splenorenal shunt. Ann Surg 166:431, 1967.
117. Langer B, Rotstein L, Stone R: A prospective randomized trial of the selective distal splenorenal shunt. Surg Gynecol Obstet 150:45-48, 1980.
118. Resnick R, Atterbury L, Grace N, et al: Distal splenorenal shunt versus portal systemic shunt: Current status of a controlled trial. Gastroenterology 77:433, 1979.
119. Harley H, Morgan T, Redeker A, et al: Results of a randomized trial of end-to-side portacaval shunt and distal splenorenal shunt in alcoholic liver disease and variceal bleeding. Gastroenterology 91:802-809, 1986.
120. Rikkers L, Rudman D, Galambos J: A randomized controlled trial of distal splenorenal shunts. Ann Surg 188:271-282, 1978.
121. Millikan W, Warren W, Henderson J, et al: The Emory prospective randomized trial: Selective versus nonselective shunt to control variceal bleeding. Ten year follow-up. Ann Surg 201:712-722, 1985.
122. Zeppa R, Hensley G, Levi J: The comparative survivals of alcoholics versus nonalcoholics with the distal splenorenal shunts. Ann Surg 187:510-514, 1978.
123. Busuttil R, Brin B, Tompkins R: Matched control study of distal splenorenal and portacaval shunts in the treatment of bleeding esophageal varices. Am J Surg 138:62-67, 1979.
124. Busuttil R: Selective and nonselective shunts for variceal bleeding: A prospective study of 103 patients. Am J Surg 148:27-35, 1984.
125. Adson M, Van Heerden J, Illstrup D: The distal splenorenal shunt. Arch Surg 119:609-614, 1984.
126. Hen R, Halbfass H, Rossle M, et al: Mesocaval and distal splenorenal shunts: Effect on hepatic function, hepatic hemodynamics, and portal systemic encephalopathy. Klin Wochenschr 63:409-413, 1985.
127. Busuttil R, Maywood B, Tompkins R: The Warren shunt in treating bleeding esophageal varices. West J Med 130:304-308, 1979.
128. Fulenwider J, Smith R, Millikan W, et al: Variceal hemorrhage in the veteran population: To shunt or not to shunt? Am Surg 50:264-269, 1984.
129. Lund R, Newkirk J: Peritoneovenous shunting system for surgical management of ascites. Contemp Surg 14:31-45, 1979.
130. Maksoud J, Mies S: Distal splenorenal shunt in children. Ann Surg 195:401-405, 1982.
131. Martin E, Molnar J, Cooperman M, et al: Observations on fifty distal splenorenal shunts. Surgery 84:379-383, 1978.
132. Mosimman R, Loup P: Efficacy and risks of the distal splenorenal shunt in the treatment of bleeding esophageal varices. Am J Surg 133:163-168, 1977.
133. Silver D, Puckett C, McNeer J: Evaluation of selective transsplenic decompression of gastroesophageal varices. Am J Surg 127:30-34, 1974.
134. Warren W, Millikan W, Henderson J: Ten years of portal hypertension surgery at Emory. Ann Surg 195:530-542, 1982.
135. Warren W, Henderson J, Millikan W, et al: Management of variceal bleeding in patients with non-cirrhotic portal vein thrombosis. Ann Surg 207:623-634, 1988.
136. Warren W, Henderson J, Millikan W, et al: Splenopancreatic disconnection: Improved selectivity of distal splenorenal shunt. Ann Surg 204:346-355, 1986.
137. Warren W, Millikan W: Selective transsplenic decompression procedure: Changes in technique after 300 cases. Contemp Surg 18:11-29, 1981.
138. Henderson J, Millikan W, Chippani J: The incidence and natural history of thrombus in the portal vein following distal splenorenal shunts. Ann Surg 196:1-7, 1982.
139. Orug T, Soonawalla K, Tekin S, et al: Role of surgical portosystemic shunts in the era of interventional radiology and liver transplantation. Br J Surg 91:769-773, 2004.
140. Sorbi D, Gostout CJ, Peura D: An assessment of the management of acute bleeding varices: A multicenter prospective member-based study. Am J Gastroenterol 98:2424-2434, 2003.
141. Wong L, Lorenzo C, Limm W, et al: Splenoreal shunt: An ideal procedure in the Pacific. Arch Surg 137:1125-1129, 2002.
142. Wolff M, Hirner A: Current state of portosystemic shunt surgery. Langenbecks Arch Surg 388:141-149, 2003.
143. Rousselot L: The role of congestion (portal hypertension) in so-called Banti's syndrome: A clinical and pathological study of thirty-one cases with late results following splenectomy. JAMA 107:1788-1793, 1936.
144. Thompson W: The pathogenesis of Banti's disease. Ann Intern Med 14:255-262, 1940.
145. Pemberton J, Kiernan P: Surgery of the spleen. Surg Clin North Am 25:880-890, 1945.
146. Suguira M, Futagawa S: A new technique for treating esophageal varices. J Thorac Cardiovasc Surg 66:677-685, 1973.
147. Strauch G: Supradiaphragmatic splenic transposition. Am J Surg 119:379-384, 1970.
148. McClelland R, Bashour F: Supradiaphragmatic transposition of the spleen in portal hypertension. Arch Surg 98:175-179, 1969.
149. Peters R, Womack N: Surgery of vascular distortions in cirrhosis of the liver. Ann Surg 154:432, 1961.
150. Keagy B, Schwartz J, Johnson G: Should ablative operations be used for bleeding esophageal varices? Ann Surg 203:463-469, 1986.
151. Boerema I: Surgical therapy of bleeding varices of esophagus during hepatic cirrhosis and Banti's disease. Ned Tijdschr Geneeskd 93:4174-4182, 1949.
152. Crile GJ: Transesophageal ligation of bleeding esophageal varices. Arch Surg 61:654-660, 1950.
153. Wirthlin L, Linton R, Ellis D: Transthoracoesophageal ligation of bleeding esophageal varices. Arch Surg 109:688-692, 1974.
154. Wexler M: Treatment of bleeding esophageal varices by transabdominal esophageal transection with the EEA stapling instrument. Surgery 88:406-416, 1980.
155. Cooperman M, Fabri P, Martin E, et al: EEA esophageal stapling for control of bleeding varices. Am J Surg 140:821-824, 1980.
156. Delaney J: A method for esophagogastric devascularization. Surg Gynecol Obstet 150:899-900, 1980.

157. Suguira M, Futagawa S: Further evaluation of the Suguira procedure in the treatment of esophageal varices. Arch Surg 112:1317-1321, 1977.
158. Koyarna K, Takagi Y, Ouchi K, et al: Results of esophageal transection for esophageal varices. Am J Surg 139:204-209, 1980.
159. Suguira M, Futagawa S: Results of six hundred thirty-six esophageal transections with paraesophagogastric devascularization in the treatment of esophageal varices. J Vasc Surg 1:254-260, 1984.
160. Superina R, Weber J, Shandling B: A modified Suguira operation for bleeding varices in children. J Pediatr Surg 18:794-799, 1983.
161. Weese J, Starling J, Yale C: Control of bleeding esophageal varices by transabdominal esophageal transection, gastric devascularization and splenectomy. Surg Gastroenterol 3:31-36, 1984.
162. Wanamaker S, Cooperman M, Carey L: Use of the EEA stapling instrument for control of bleeding esophageal varices. Surgery 94:620-626, 1983.
163. Wexler M: Esophageal procedures to control bleeding from varices. Surg Clin North Am 63:905-914, 1983.
164. Spence R, Anderson J, Johnston G: Twenty-five years of injection sclerotherapy for bleeding varices. Br J Surg 72:195-198, 1985.
165. Huizinga W, Angorn I, Baker L: Esophageal transection versus injection sclerotherapy in the management of bleeding esophageal varices in patients of high risk. Surg Gynecol Obstet 160:539-546, 1985.
166. Rosch J, Hanafee W, Snow H, et al: Transjugular intrahepatic portacaval shunt: An experimental work. Am J Surg 121:588-592, 1971.
167. Palmaz JC, Garcia F, Sibbitt RR, et al: Expandable intrahepatic portacaval shunt stents in dogs with chronic portal hypertension. AJR Am J Roentgenol 147:1251-1254, 1986.
168. Richter G, Noeledge G, Palmaz J, et al: The transjugular intrahepatic portosystemic stent-shunt (TIPSS): Results of a pilot study. Cardiovasc Intervent Radiol 13:200-207, 1990.
169. Luca A, D'Amico G, La Galla R, et al: TIPS for prevention of recurrent bleeding in patients with cirrhosis: Meta-analysis of randomized clinical trials. Radiology 212:411-421, 1999.
170. Narahara Y, Kanazawa H, Kawamata H, et al: A randomized clinical trial comparing transjugular intrahepatic portosystemic shunt with endoscopic sclerotherapy in the long-term management of patients with cirrhosis after recent variceal hemorrhage. Hepatol Res 21:189-198, 2001.
171. Rosch J, Keller FS: Transjugular intrahepatic portosystemic shunt: Present status, comparison with endoscopic therapy and shunt surgery, and future prospectives. World J Surg 25:337-345, 2001.
172. Latimer J, Bawa SM, Rees CJ, et al: Patency and reintervention rates during routine TIPS surveillance. Cardiovasc Intervent Radiol 21:234-239, 1998.
173. Saxon RS, Ross PL, Mendel-Hartvig J, et al: Transjugular intrahepatic portosystemic shunt patency and the importance of stenosis location in the development of recurrent symptoms. Radiology 207:683-693, 1998.
174. Rosemurgy AS, Serafini FM, Zweibel BR, et al: Transjugular intrahepatic portosystemic shunt vs small-diameter prosthetic H-graft portacaval shunt: Extended follow-up of an expanded randomized prospective trial. J Gastrointest Surg 4:589-597, 2000.
175. Freeman RB Jr, FitzMaurice SE, Greenfield AE, et al: Is the transjugular intrahepatic portocaval shunt procedure beneficial for liver transplant recipients? Transplantation 58:297-300, 1994.
176. Woodle ES, Darcy M, White HM, et al: Intrahepatic portosystemic vascular stents: A bridge to hepatic transplantation. Surgery 113:344-351, 1993.
177. Millis JM, Martin P, Gomes A, et al: Transjugular intrahepatic portosystemic shunts: Impact on liver transplantation. Liver Transpl Surg 1:229-233, 1995.
178. Lerut JP, Laterre PF, Goffette P, et al: Transjugular intrahepatic portosystemic shunt and liver transplantation. Transpl Int 9:370-375, 1996.
179. John TG, Jalan R, Stanley AJ, et al: Transjugular intrahepatic portosystemic stent-shunt (TIPS) insertion as a prelude to orthotopic liver transplantation in patients with severe portal hypertension. Eur J Gastroenterol Hepatol 8:1145-1149, 1996.
180. Maleux G, Pirenne J, Vaninbroukx J, et al: Are TIPS stent-grafts a contraindication for future liver transplantation? Cardiovasc Intervent Radiol 27:140-142, 2004.
181. Rossle M, Ochs A, Gulberg V, et al: A comparison of paracentesis and transjugular intrahepatic portosystemic shunting in patients with ascites. N Engl J Med 8:1701-1707, 2000.
182. Lebrec D, Giuily N, Hadengue A, et al: Transjugular intrahepatic portosystemic shunts: Comparison with paracentesis in patients with cirrhosis and refractory ascites. A randomized trial. French group of clinicians and a group of biologists. J Hepatol 25:135-144, 1996.
183. Saab S, Nieto J, Ly D, et al: TIPS versus paracentesis for cirrhotic patients with refractory ascites. Cochrane Database Syst Rev 3:CD004889, 2004.
184. Rosemurgy AS, Zervos EE, Clark WC, et al: TIPS versus peritovenous shunt in the treatment of medically intractable ascites: A prospective randomized trial. Ann Surg 239:883-889, 2004.
185. Siegerstetter V, Deibert P, Ochs A, et al: Treatment of refractory hepatic hydrothorax with transjugular intrahepatic portosystemic shunt: Long-term results in 40 patients. Eur J Gastroenterol Hepatol 13:529-534, 2001.
186. Perello A, Garcia-Pagan JC, Gilabert R, et al: TIPS is a useful long-term derivative therapy for patients with Budd-Chiari syndrome uncontrolled by medical therapy. Hepatology 35:132-139, 2002.
187. Blum U, Rossle M, Haag K, et al: Budd-Chiari syndrome: Technical, hemodynamic, and clinical results of treatment with transjugular intrahepatic portosystemic shunt. Radiology 197:805-811, 1995.
188. Rossle M, Olschewski M, Siegerstetter V, et al: The Budd-Chiari syndrome: Outcome after treatment with the transjugular intrahepatic portosystemic shunt. Surgery 135:394-403, 2004.
189. Brensing KA, Textor J, Perz J, et al: Long term outcome after transjugular intrahepatic portosystemic stent-shunt in non-transplant cirrhotics with hepatorenal syndrome: A phase II study. Gut 47:288-295, 2000.
190. Allgaier HP, Haag K, Ochs A, et al: Hepato-pulmonary syndrome: Successful treatment by transjugular intrahepatic portosystemic stent-shunt (TIPS). J Hepatol 23:102, 1995.
191. Wong F, Pantea L, Snioderman K: Midodrine, octreotide, albumin, and TIPS in selected patients with cirrhosis and type 1 hepatorenal syndrome. Hepatology 40:55-64, 2004.
192. Otal P, Smayra T, Bureau C, et al: Preliminary results of a new expanded-polytetrafluoroethylene-covered stent-graft for transjugular intrahepatic portosystemic shunt procedures. AJR Am J Roentgenol 178:141-147, 2002.
193. Rossi P, Salvatori FM, Fanelli F, et al: Polytetrafluoroethylene-covered nitinol stent-graft for transjugular intrahepatic portosystemic shunt creation: 3-year experience. Radiology 231:820-830, 2004.
194. Maleux G, Nevens F, Wilmer A, et al: Early and long-term clinical and radiological follow-up results of expanded-polytetrafluoroethylene-covered stent-grafts for transjugular intrahepatic portosystemic shunt procedures. Eur Radiol 14:1842-1859, 2004.
195. Iwatsuki S, Starzl T, Todo S, et al: Liver transplantation in the treatment of bleeding esophageal varices. Surgery 104:697-705, 1988.
196. Reyes J, Iwatsuki S: Current management of portal hypertension with liver transplantation. Adv Surg 25:189-208, 1992.
197. Roberts MS, Angus DC, Bryce CL, et al: Survival after liver transplantation in the United States: A disease-specific analysis of the UNOS database. Liver Transpl 10:886-897, 2004.
198. Brems J, Hiatt J, Klein A, et al: Effect of a prior portasystemic shunt on subsequent liver transplantation. Ann Surg 209:51-56, 1989.
199. Crafoord C, Frenckner P: New surgical treatment of varicose veins of the esophagus. Acta Otolaryngol 27:422, 1939.
200. Johnston G, Rodgers H: A review of 15 years experience in the use of sclerotherapy in the control of acute hemorrhage for esophageal varices. Br J Surg 60:797-799, 1973.
201. Paquet K, Kalk J, Koussouris P: Immediate endoscopic sclerosis of bleeding esophageal varices: A prospective evaluation over 5 years. Surg Endosc 2:18-23, 1988.
202. Schubert T, Smith O, Kirkpatrick S, et al: Improved survival in variceal hemorrhage with emergent sclerotherapy. Am J Gastroenterol 82:1134-1137, 1987.
203. Terblanche J, Northover J, Bornman P, et al: A prospective evaluation of injection sclerotherapy in the treatment of acute bleeding esophageal varices. Surgery 85:239-245, 1979.
204. Terblanche J, Yakoob H, Bornman P, et al: Acute bleeding varices: A five-year prospective evaluation of tamponade and sclerotherapy. Ann Surg 194:521-529, 1981.
205. Paquet K, Feussner H: Endoscopic sclerosis and esophageal balloon tamponade in acute hemorrhage from esophagogastric varices: A prospective controlled randomized trial. Hepatology 5:580-583, 1985.
206. Larson A, Cohen H, Zweiban B, et al: Acute esophageal variceal sclerotherapy: Results of a prospective randomized controlled trial. JAMA 255:497-500, 1986.
207. Barsoum M, Bolous F, El-Rooby A, et al: Tamponade and injection sclerotherapy in the management of bleeding oesophageal varices. Br J Surg 69:76-78, 1982.
208. Project CEVS: Sclerotherapy after first variceal hemorrhage in cirrhosis: A randomized multicenter trial. N Engl J Med 311:1594-1600, 1984.

209. Westaby D, MacDougall B, Williams R: Improved survival following injection sclerotherapy for esophageal varices: Final analysis of a controlled trial. Hepatology 5:827-830, 1985.

210. Terblanche J, Bornman P, Kahn D, et al: Failure of repeated injection sclerotherapy to improve long term survival after esophageal variceal bleeding: A five year prospective controlled clinical trial. Lancet 2:1328-1332, 1983.

211. Soderlund C, Ihre T: Endoscopic sclerotherapy v. conservative management of bleeding oesophageal varices. Acta Chir Scand 151:449-156, 1985.

212. Korula J, Balart L, Radvan G, et al: A prospective randomized controlled trial of chronic esophageal variceal sclerotherapy. Hepatology 5:584-589, 1985.

213. Cello J, Grendell J, Crass R, et al: Endoscopic sclerotherapy versus portacaval shunt in patients with severe cirrhosis and variceal hemorrhage. N Engl J Med 311:1589-1594, 1984.

214. Cello J, Grendell J, Crass R, et al: Endoscopic sclerotherapy versus portacaval shunt in patients with severe cirrhosis and acute variceal hemorrhage: Long-term follow-up. N Engl J Med 316:11-15, 1987.

215. Warren W, Henderson J, Millikan W, et al: Distal splenorenal shunt versus endoscopic sclerotherapy for long-term management of variceal bleeding: Preliminary report of a prospective, randomized trial. Ann Surg 203:454-462, 1986.

216. Teres J, Bordas J, Bravo D, et al: Sclerotherapy vs distal splenorenal shunt in the elective treatment of variceal hemorrhage: A randomized controlled trial. Hepatology 7:430-436, 1987.

217. Rikkers L, Burnett D, Volentine G, et al: Shunt surgery versus endoscopic sclerotherapy for long-term treatment of variceal bleeding: Early results of a randomized trial. Ann Surg 206:261-271, 1987.

218. Burroughs A, Hamilton G, Phillips A, et al: A comparison of sclerotherapy with staple transection of the esophagus for the emergency control of bleeding from esophageal varices. N Engl J Med 321:857-862, 1989.

219. Teres J, Baroni R, Bordas M, et al: Randomized trial of portacaval shunt, stapling transection and endoscopic sclerotherapy in uncontrolled variceal bleeding. J Hepatol 4:159-167, 1987.

220. Terblanche J, Bornman P, Kirsch R: Sclerotherapy for bleeding esophageal varices. Annu Rev Med 35:83-94, 1984.

221. Yassin Y, Sherif S: Randomized controlled trial of injection sclerotherapy for bleeding esophageal varices. Br J Surg 70:20-22, 1983.

222. Reilly J, Schade R, Roh M, et al: Esophageal variceal sclerosis. Surg Gynecol Obstet 155:497-502, 1982.

223. Palani L, Abvabara S, Kraft A, et al: Endoscopic sclerotherapy in acute variceal hemorrhage. Am J Surg 141:164-168, 1981.

224. Lewis J, Chung R, Allison J: Sclerotherapy of esophageal varices. Arch Surg 115:476-480, 1980.

225. Johnston G: Bleeding esophageal varices: The management of shunt rejects. Ann R Coll Surg Engl 63:3-8, 1981.

226. Goodale R, Silvis S, O'Leary J, et al: Early survival for bleeding esophageal varices. Surg Gynecol Obstet 155:523-528, 1982.

227. Lewis J, Chung R, Allison J: Injection sclerotherapy for control of acute variceal hemorrhage. Am J Surg 142:592-595, 1981.

228. Cohen L, Rorsten M, Scherl E, et al: Bacteremia after endoscopic injection sclerosis. Gastrointest Endosc 29:198-200, 1983.

229. Bacon A, Bauley-Newton R, Connors A: Pleural effusions after endoscopic variceal sclerotherapy. Gastroenterology 88:1910-1914, 1985.

230. Tripodis S, Buenskin A, Wenser J: Gastric ulcers after endoscopic sclerosis of esophageal varices. J Clin Gastroenterol 7:77-79, 1985.

231. Laine L, Cook D: Endoscopic ligation compared with sclerotherapy for treatment of esophageal varicela bleeding: A meta-analysis. Ann Intern Med 123:280-287, 1995.

232. Stanley M: Treatment of intractable ascites in patients with alcoholic cirrhosis by peritoneovenous (LeVeen) shunting. Med Clin North Am 63:523-536, 1979.

233. Frakes J: Physiologic considerations in the medical management of ascites. Arch Intern Med 140:620-623, 1980.

234. LeVeen H, Christovadias G, Ip M, et al: Peritoneovenous shunting for ascites. Ann Surg 180:580, 1974.

235. Harman D, Demirjian Z, Ellman L, et al: Disseminated intravascular coagulation with the peritoneovenous shunt. Ann Intern Med 90:774-776, 1979.

236. Reinhardt G, Stanley M: Peritoneovenous shunting for ascites. Surg Gynecol Obstet 145:419-424, 1977.

237. Epstein M: Peritoneovenous shunt in the management of ascites and the hepatorenal syndrome. Gastroenterology 82:790-799, 1982.

238. Fullen W: Hepatorenal syndrome: Reversal by peritoneovenous shunt. Surgery 83:337-341, 1977.

Questions

1. **A 35-year-old woman with a history of viral hepatitis and cirrhosis, status postcholecystectomy, has a clinical presentation of variceal hemorrhage unresponsive to medical therapy. Which surgical procedure is indicated if sclerotherapy fails?**
   (a) End-to-side portacaval shunt
   (b) Side-to-side portacaval shunt
   (c) H-graft mesocaval shunt
   (d) EEA abdominal esophageal transection
   (e) Distal splenorenal shunt

2. **A 10-year-old boy with a history of omphalitis experiences his first episode of variceal hemorrhage. Which is the most appropriate therapy?**
   (a) Distal splenorenal shunt
   (b) Medical regimen
   (c) Variceal sclerotherapy
   (d) End-to-side portacaval shunt
   (e) H-graft mesocaval shunt

3. **Specific contraindications to peritoneovenous shunts include all of the following except**
   (a) Hepatic necrosis
   (b) Bilirubin greater than 6 mg/dL
   (c) Hepatorenal syndrome
   (d) Infected ascitic fluid
   (e) Prothrombin time prolonged more than 4 seconds

4. **Which of the following statements about prophylactic portacaval shunts is true?**
   (a) They prolong longevity
   (b) They decrease encephalopathy
   (c) They have a greater than 50% recurrent hemorrhage rate
   (d) They are associated with a prohibitively high operative mortality
   (e) They are not indicated

5. **The Budd-Chiari syndrome may be treated by all of the following except**
   (a) Anticoagulants
   (b) Side-to-side portacaval shunt
   (c) End-to-side portacaval shunt
   (d) Mesoatrial shunt
   (e) Mesocaval shunt

6. **Technical considerations in favor of performing a distal splenorenal shunt include which of the following?**
   (a) Cavernomatous transformation of the splenic vein
   (b) Acute hyaline necrosis
   (c) Splenic vein greater than 4 mm in diameter
   (d) Intractable ascites
   (e) Hepatopetal flow

7. **Which of the following statements regarding sclerotherapy is false?**
   (a) Percutaneous transhepatic coronary vein occlusion is associated with a 20% portal vein thrombosis rate
   (b) Sclerotherapy should not be used in the acute setting because of high mortality
   (c) Sodium morrhuate and ethanolamine oleate are appropriate sclerosing agents
   (d) Repeated sclerotherapy is necessary for control of hemorrhage
   (e) Esophageal ulcerations usually resolve spontaneously without sequelae

8. **Which of the following is an advantage of selective shunts?**
   (a) Continued portal perfusion
   (b) Gastric and esophageal varix decompression
   (c) No greater incidence of shunt thrombosis than with portacaval shunts
   (d) Decreased incidence of encephalopathy
   (e) All of the above

9. **A 40-year-old man has hematemesis and hypotension. What initial diagnostic measures should be performed after stabilization?**
   (a) Superior mesenteric arteriography
   (b) Splenoportography
   (c) Esophagogastroscopy
   (d) Celiac angiogram with venous phase
   (e) Upper gastrointestinal series

10. **What is the most common site of obstruction causing portal hypertension in the Western world?**
    (a) Portal vein (thrombosis)
    (b) Extrahepatic postsinusoidal
    (c) Intrahepatic presinusoidal
    (d) Intrahepatic sinusoidal and postsinusoidal
    (e) Extrahepatic presinusoidal

11. **A 40-year-old man with cirrhosis is determined to be Child class A; his bleeding has been controlled with sclerotherapy and vasopressin. What is the most appropriate treatment plan?**
    (a) Emergency shunt surgery
    (b) Warren shunt
    (c) Mesocaval shunt
    (d) TIPS procedure
    (e) Periodic sclerotherapy

Answers

1. c	2. b	3. c	4. e	5. c
6. e	7. b	8. e	9. c	10. d
11. e				

45

Lazar J. Greenfield

Venous Thromboembolic Disease

The connection between venous thrombosis and pulmonary thromboembolism was made by Virchow in 1856. He also defined the triad of mechanisms by which intravascular thrombosis can occur: vessel wall injury, stasis, and hypercoagulability. The latter two are most prominent in venous thrombosis. The importance of the disorder is reflected by estimates that deep venous thrombosis (DVT) occurs in more than 500,000 patients a year, based on the National Inpatient Sample, which reports the outcomes for 20% of patients hospitalized. The mortality rate is estimated at 50,000 deaths per year from pulmonary thromboembolism, with recognition that the diagnosis is often missed or made incorrectly. Hull and Pineo showed that the cost of hospitalization alone is more than $207,000 per 100 patients treated for DVT.[1] Of the patients who survive DVT, more than half develop chronic venous insufficiency with disabling edema and potential stasis ulcerations, representing a costly outcome in terms of lost productivity and demands on health care services. In older patients with "idiopathic" DVT, the presentation may be the first manifestation of a hidden malignancy, as originally described by Trousseau.[2-5] In some tumors, this prothrombotic state is due to the elaboration of tissue factor, which may either activate procoagulant proteins or stimulate the release of a protease from circulating blood cells, thus activating the coagulation cascade.[6,7]

In postoperative and post-trauma patients, stasis is an important and preventable causative factor. It is also likely that the release of cytokines at the site of injury is a precipitating factor. When contrast medium is injected into the feet of supine immobilized patients, it may remain in soleal vein valvular sinuses for as long as an hour. This is the favored location for the formation of a nidus of thrombus. The original thrombus may become attached to the opposite wall, causing interruption of flow, retrograde thrombosis, and signs of venous stasis in the extremity. Subsequent edema formation within the confines of the deep muscular fascia produces pain. However, the thrombus may propagate without interrupting flow and develop a long, floating "tail" that is highly susceptible to breaking loose from its tenuous anchor within the valvular sinus. This sequence of events is the most dangerous aspect of the disorder because major pulmonary embolism can occur without premonitory signs or symptoms at its point of origin.

The site of venous obstruction determines the level at which swelling is observed clinically, usually the segment below. Thrombi more commonly originate in the soleal veins and then propagate proximally in 20% to 30% of cases.[8,9] Evidence also exists of primary thrombosis of femoral and iliac venous tributaries, which can also occur following hip repair or traumatic pelvic injury.

In addition to stasis, hypercoagulability is increasingly recognized as a causative factor. The first familial thrombophilia identified was a deficiency of antithrombin (previously called antithrombin III). Congenital deficiencies in protein C and protein S were subsequently described, but these are rare. All three deficiencies are found in less than 1% of the population. Factor V Leiden is the most common among the inherited prothrombotic factors, found in 5% of the population and in 40% of patients after an episode of DVT.[10] Other inherited thrombophilic factors include the mutant prothrombin 20210A, non-O blood groups, elevated factor VIII and von Willebrand's factor levels, methylene tetrahydrofolate reductase variant 677T, and hyperhomocysteinemia.[11] Prothrombic states are associated with recent trauma, major surgical procedures, and sepsis. Even stasis alone—such as occurs during long airplane flights, which can also add hypoxia, hypobarism, and dehydration—seems capable of promoting local thrombosis.

Opposing these thrombotic processes is the fibrinolytic system of the blood and vein walls. The endothelium converts plasminogen to plasmin, which lyses fibrin. As might be expected, however, the fibrinolytic system is inhibited after surgery and trauma, and less activity occurs in the veins of the lower extremities compared with the upper. Impaired fibrinolytic activity has been associated with both adequate levels of nonfunctioning plasminogen and low levels of functioning plasminogen.[12] The third major causative factor of Virchow's triad, vessel wall damage, usually is not demonstrable in areas of thrombosis. Obesity, aging, and malignancy also increase the risk of developing DVT by mechanisms that are under investigation, with age being the greatest risk factor of all. As more risk factors are found in the general population, the combination of acquired and inherited factors becomes more likely. Both gene-gene and gene-environment synergistic interactions are likely to be identified in the future as causative in venous thrombosis.

Diagnosis

Major thrombosis involving the deep venous system of the thigh and pelvis produces a characteristic but nonspecific clinical picture of pain, extensive pitting edema, and blanching that has been termed *phlegmasia alba dolens*. Investigators originally believed that the blanching was due to spasm and compromise of arterial flow, but it is now recognized that subcutaneous edema is responsible. In addition to the mechanical and hormonal effects of pregnancy, mechanical factors that can affect the left iliac vein include compression from the right iliac artery or an overdistended bladder and congenital webs within the vein. These factors are considered responsible for the observed 4:1 preponderance of left versus right iliac vein involvement.

If the extent of venous thrombosis progressively impedes the venous return from the extremity, limb loss may occur subsequent to cessation of arterial flow. The clinical picture is sufficient congestion to produce phlegmasia cerulea dolens, or a painful blue leg. With the loss of sensory or motor function, venous gangrene is likely unless blood flow is restored. These major complications affect less than 10% of patients with venous thrombosis but are more likely in patients with advanced malignant disease. In fact, only 40% of patients with venous thrombosis have any clinical signs of the disorder. False-positive clinical signs occur in up to 50% of patients studied. Because of this, diagnostic tests that have high predictive value are necessary. Historically, contrast venography was used to provide direct evidence of both occlusive and nonocclusive thrombi, but it is invasive, may result in an allergic reaction to the contrast material, and requires movement of the patient to a radiographic suite. In addition, radiologists disagree on the interpretation of the study in 10% of cases, and in an additional 5%, the study is not technically possible or the result is not diagnostic.[13]

DUPLEX EXAMINATION

The Doppler probe is currently used at the bedside to detect major venous thrombi with a high degree of accuracy, but it is dependent on the examiner's experience. The principle is based on the impairment of an accelerated flow signal produced by intraluminal thrombi. The examination begins at the ankle, with identification of the posterior tibial vein signal adjacent to the artery. The flow signal should be altered by distal and proximal compression, producing augmentation and interruption of flow, respectively. The same maneuvers are repeated over the superficial and deep femoral veins and can be done over the popliteal vein. Failure to augment flow on compression below the probe or to release interruption of flow above the probe suggests venous thrombi. The sensitivity of the test exceeds 90%, but the specificity is 5% to 10% lower, owing to the interference with venous flow by other mechanical

problems (e.g., Baker's cyst, hematoma). A negative Doppler ultrasound examination is reassuring, but a positive or equivocal test should be confirmed by B-mode ultrasound imaging. A negative test is not reassuring when thromboembolism is suspected, because the thrombus may have embolized from the extremity.

Real-time B-mode ultrasonography to visualize extremity veins has gained wide acceptance and offers a more direct technique to detect intraluminal thrombus noninvasively.[14] This test has essentially replaced venography as the diagnostic standard in the United States. Valvular movement and accelerated blood flow can be visualized in the presence of a partially obstructing thrombus. When pressure is applied by the probe, normal vein walls are easily compressed, but resistance to compression is noted when a thrombus is present, increasing with the age of the thrombus. Chronic thrombi are characterized by greater echogenicity, heterogeneity, and an irregular surface. The addition of color to the duplex scan has increased the sensitivity and specificity of the study in symptomatic patients with proximal DVT to 96% and 100%, respectively, with a negative predictive value of 98% and accuracy of 99%.[15-17] Color-flow Doppler scanning has also improved the sensitivity and specificity of ultrasound scanning when used as a screening test in asymptomatic patients, even when used for distal veins.

In some institutions, computed tomography (CT) protocols have been developed for the diagnosis of DVT and pulmonary embolism. Although there is a certain appeal to having a dual-purpose test method, the sensitivity and specificity of CT scanning are not comparable to those of ultrasonography for the diagnosis of DVT.[18,19] Its value as an alternative to nuclear medicine and contrast angiographic studies is currently being evaluated in the Prospective Investigation of Pulmonary Embolism Diagnosis (PIOPED) II study.

PLETHYSMOGRAPHY

Impedance and strain gauge plethysmography were used in the past to measure the volume response of the extremity to temporary occlusion of the venous system. The diagnosis of venous thrombosis depended on changes in the venous capacitance and the rate of emptying after release of the occlusion, but these tests are no longer in general use.

Air plethysmography is a noninvasive technique that measures absolute limb blood volume change. It provides quantification of venous reflux, muscle pump action, venous capacitance, and noninvasive ambulatory venous pressure, thus providing a useful index of the severity of venous disease. It is used primarily to quantitate chronic venous insufficiency. None of these diagnostic studies has the sensitivity or specificity of duplex ultrasonography for the diagnosis of venous thrombosis.

VENOGRAPHY

The injection of contrast material for direct visualization of the venous system was long considered the standard for confirming the diagnosis of venous thrombosis and is still used in some clinical research studies. Injection is usually made into the foot while the superficial veins are occluded by a tourniquet. A supplementary injection into the femoral veins may be required to visualize the iliofemoral system. A defect in the column of contrast or failure to visualize a venous segment is suggestive of a thrombus. It also allows identification of a segment of thrombus floating freely in the contrast medium and extending into the iliofemoral system. This type of thrombus has been associated with an increased risk of pulmonary embolism, despite anticoagulation.[20] Potential false-positive examinations may result from external compression of a vein or washout of the contrast material from collateral veins. Other shortcomings of this test were cited earlier.

LABORATORY TESTING

An alternative method for the diagnosis of thromboembolism relies on the detection of the by-products of coagulation. The presence of intravascular fibrin can be detected by measuring the plasma products of the lysis of fibrin or fibrinogen. Both fibrinopeptide A and fibrin fragment E can be detected by radioimmunoassay, but these are not specific for acute venous thrombosis. A negative test result could conceivably have some value in ruling out the diagnosis, but the tests require more investigation and simplification. D-dimers are cross-linked degradation products that serve as markers for the action of plasmin on fibrin. When used in conjunction with clinical assessment, proximal and distal sensitivities are 98.4% and 90.5%, respectively, and negative predictive values are 99.3% and 98.6%.[21] The D-dimer results based on latex agglutination tests lack the precision of the quantitative ELISA test, which is the preferred method for diagnostic evaluation. Although a positive result can be misleading, a negative test result can rule out thromboembolism. Thrombin-antithrombin III complexes in plasma are correlated with activation of coagulation. These factors lack specificity as indicators of thromboembolic disease but may be useful in ruling out DVT in certain subgroups.[22,23]

Prophylaxis

In recent years, several medical specialty groups have conducted consensus conferences focused on the prevention of venous thromboembolism.[24,25] The participants based their recommendations on the strength of evidence found in the medical literature. The American College of Chest Physicians' conference brought together pulmonologists, surgeons, internal medicine physicians, and radiologists to represent the range of available data.[26,27] The strength of the evidence was cited in connection with each recommendation, which is useful in the formation of prophylactic strategies.

In theory, the formation of venous thrombi should be prevented either by eliminating or reducing venous stasis or by altering blood coagulability. The belief that early ambulation is sufficient to prevent the formation of thrombi is controversial and is not supported by studies using tagged fibrinogen. However, in hospitalized patients younger than 40 years with no additional risk factors, it may be adequate.[28] This assumption is based on the patient remaining ambulant and avoiding the additional risk of sitting for long periods with the legs in a dependent position.

Considerable interest has developed in the prophylactic use of anticoagulant and antiplatelet drugs such as aspirin. Strong data support the use of preoperative oral anticoagulation therapy with coumarin derivatives in high-risk patients. Unfortunately, this increases the risk of hemorrhage, and with the added difficulties of laboratory control of prothrombin time,

the approach has not been widely accepted, except by some orthopedic surgeons doing elective arthroplasty. Fixed "minidose" warfarin is both safe and efficacious in various surgical and medical patients, especially women with breast cancer receiving chemotherapy via central venous lines. This regimen offers protection against thromboembolism without the risks of hemorrhage or the cost of laboratory monitoring.[29-32] In an effort to minimize the problems associated with anticoagulant prophylaxis, the current recommendation is to use heparin before and after surgery in doses that do not alter the laboratory clotting profile. Generally, a 5000-unit dose is given subcutaneously 2 hours preoperatively and then every 12 hours postoperatively for 5 days. This treatment provides protection for most high-risk patients, with the exception of trauma victims or those undergoing orthopedic or urologic procedures. The beneficial effect may be due to the enhancement of heparin cofactor (antithrombin III) as a natural inhibitor of activated factor X. This practice is based on the historical study by Kakkar and colleagues,[33] which documented protection against fatal pulmonary embolism in a randomized series of 4121 patients, as well as against DVT. Since the U.S. Food and Drug Administration (FDA) approved low-molecular-weight heparins (LMWHs) for prophylactic indications, they have become the drugs of choice for elective orthopedic procedures and abdominal surgery in patients with malignancy. The American College of Chest Physicians' consensus report also supports the use of LMWH for prophylaxis in trauma patients and for medical indications. Doses differ for each compound and are based on anti-Xa units.[34] Because many patients return home on the day of surgery or are hospitalized only briefly, continued prophylaxis following discharge has been studied and found to provide significant protection from postoperative DVT.[35]

Mechanical prophylaxis for DVT has been used effectively since the 1980s as an alternative to low doses of anticoagulation. The initial method was antiembolic stockings, which facilitated venous return by compressing veins and preventing venous dilatation while patients were confined to bed. These stockings are effective[36,37] and may be used alone or in conjunction with anticoagulants in patients at risk for DVT.[38,39]

Pneumatic compression systems are a commonly used method of thromboembolic prophylaxis. They function by compressing the leg and facilitating venous return. They are available in three lengths: above and below the knee and foot length. Brands differ with respect to the timing and force of compression and whether the compression is sequential along the length of the leg or simply administered intermittently. There are no randomized trial data to support the use of one type of device over another; however, in a controlled trial, we failed to find any significant difference in the incidence of DVT with different devices.[40]

Three factors need to be considered when choosing DVT prophylaxis following surgery: the age of the patient, the number of inherent risk factors, and the length of the surgical procedure. For the general population of surgical patients younger than 40 years, the risk of DVT is low, and prophylaxis can be limited to early ambulation with or without graduated compression stockings. For patients older than 40 years who are undergoing major surgical procedures, the risk is moderate, and prophylaxis, such as intermittent pneumatic compression or LMWH, should be considered. The patients at highest risk (age older than 40 years, obese, with malignant disease, history of DVT, or major trauma) need more protection, which might include LMWH, intermittent pneumatic compression, oral anticoagulants, or a combination of methods. The use of heparin in neurosurgical patients is controversial because of the consequences of intracranial bleeding. For these patients, external pneumatic compression is the prophylaxis of choice.

Prophylactic use of vena caval filters to prevent pulmonary embolism has increased as experience with the Greenfield filter demonstrated its long-term efficacy and safety.[41-45] Recently, smaller-profile devices have been developed that make prophylactic placement potentially more attractive. However, the safety and cost-effectiveness of these devices have not yet been established. Significant adverse events such as migration and caval occlusion resulting in renal failure, limb loss, and even death have been reported. Concern about these potential complications has led to greater acceptance of new optional filters that can be removed if the patient does not develop DVT or when the risk of thromboembolism is over. The major limitation of this concept is the difficulty of determining when the risk has ended.

Treatment

Management of patients with DVT must attempt to minimize the risk of pulmonary embolism, limit further thrombosis, and facilitate resolution of existing thrombi to avoid the postthrombotic syndrome. Historically, patients were placed on bed rest and treated with intravenous heparin and analgesics. Warfarin (Coumadin) was begun and heparin discontinued once the international normalized ratio (INR) was between 2.0 and 3.0 for 24 hours. Pain, swelling, and tenderness generally resolved over a 5- to 7-day period. With the advent of LMWHs, patients can receive an initial injection at the time of diagnosis, and the majority of patients can be discharged home and receive therapy on an outpatient basis. Ambulation with continued elastic stocking support can be permitted. Standing still and sitting should be prohibited to avoid increased venous pressure and stasis.

ANTICOAGULATION

The foundation of therapy for DVT is adequate anticoagulation, initially with heparin and then with coumarin derivatives for prolonged protection against recurrent thrombosis. Unless specific contraindications exist, LMWH can be administered subcutaneously, with the dose determined according to the manufacturer's directions. The patient can be expected to reach the therapeutic range rapidly, and no laboratory testing is required. Unfractionated heparin is an acid mucopolysaccharide that neutralizes thrombin, inhibits thromboplastin, and reduces the platelet release reaction. The LMWHs are derivatives that provide greater bioavailability and offer a predictable pharmacokinetic response.[46-51]

The side effects associated with heparin treatment include bleeding, thrombocytopenia, hypersensitivity, arterial thromboembolism, and osteoporosis. Bleeding is more likely to occur in elderly women, in patients treated with aspirin, or after recent surgery or trauma. Bleeding can occur when the results of laboratory monitoring tests are within the therapeutic range, which may be due to the effect of heparin on platelets.

Arterial thromboembolism can complicate heparin administration by any route and is more common in the elderly.

It tends to occur after 7 to 10 days of therapy and is associated with thrombocytopenia. This complication is termed heparin-associated thrombocytopenia; it carries high morbidity and mortality rates and requires immediate cessation of all heparin treatment. It is due to an immunoreaction and reverses rapidly when heparin is stopped (usually within 2 days). Hypersensitivity to heparin may take the form of a skin rash or, rarely, may produce anaphylaxis. Subcutaneous injections that show urticaria may become necrotic as an unusual form of sensitivity. Osteoporosis has been noted in patients on heparin therapy in excess of 6 months. It is probably due to a direct effect on bone resorption and can be avoided by shorter periods of treatment and dosages less than 15,000 units/day.

Oral administration of warfarin is begun shortly after initiation of heparin therapy, because several days are usually required to bring the prothrombin time to an INR of 2.0 to 3.0. When initiating warfarin therapy, it is preferable to use a maintenance rather than a loading dose to avoid suppression of protein C. The coumarin derivatives block the synthesis of several clotting factors, and prolongation of the prothrombin time beyond the range suggested is associated with a high incidence of bleeding complications. Nonhemorrhagic side effects are uncommon but include skin necrosis, dermatitis, and a syndrome of painful erythema in areas with large amounts of subcutaneous fat. Most changes are reversible if the drug is stopped. Also, the administration of fresh frozen plasma usually restores the prothrombin time. After an episode of acute DVT, anticoagulation should be maintained for a minimum of 4 months; some investigators favor 6 months for thrombi in the larger veins or after a second thromboembolic event. Many drugs alter the pharmacodynamics of warfarin by altering its metabolic clearance, rate of absorption, or inhibition of vitamin K–dependent coagulation factor synthesis or by altering other hemostatic factors. Phenylbutazone, sulfinpyrazone, disulfiram, metronidazole, and trimethoprim-sulfamethoxazole all potentiate warfarin's action.[42] Therefore, regular monitoring of prothrombin time is essential. In addition, levels of concurrent medications should be monitored, because warfarin may compete for binding sites, thus altering plasma levels of these drugs. Some foods that have high levels of vitamin K, such as broccoli, green leafy vegetables, and green teas, are also known to alter the effects of warfarin. Oral anticoagulants are teratogenic and should not be used during established or planned pregnancy. In a pregnant patient, heparin is the drug of choice, and for long-term management, subcutaneous self-administration should be taught. This regimen allows a normal delivery and can be continued postpartum.

FIBRINOLYSIS

Great interest has been shown in the use of fibrinolytic agents to activate the intrinsic plasmin system. Tissue-type plasminogen activator, streptokinase, and urokinase are effective, although they are associated with a high incidence of hemorrhagic complications. Ten percent of patients treated with streptokinase suffer allergic reactions, from urticaria to anaphylaxis. In addition, streptokinase offers no advantage over heparin in the treatment of recurrent venous thrombosis or thrombosis that has existed for more than 72 hours. Lytic agents are contraindicated in postoperative or post-traumatic patients and may be associated with an increased risk of pulmonary embolism.

TABLE 45–1	Indications for Insertion of a Vena Caval Filter

Definite Indications

Recurrent thromboembolism in spite of adequate anticoagulation

Deep venous thrombosis or documented thromboembolism in a patient with a contraindication to anticoagulation

Complication of anticoagulation, forcing therapy to be discontinued

Chronic pulmonary embolism with associated pulmonary hypertension and cor pulmonale

Immediately after pulmonary embolectomy

Relative Indications

Patient whose pulmonary vascular bed is >50% occluded and who would not tolerate any additional embolism

Patient with a propagating iliofemoral thrombus despite anticoagulation

High-risk patient with a large, free-floating iliofemoral thrombus on venogram

Regional lysing with specialized catheters may be used to deliver recombinant tissue-type plasminogen activator directly to the thrombus. This technique may result in early thrombus resolution, with long-term valve preservation and a reduced incidence of post-thrombotic syndrome.[52-56] Mewissen and colleagues reported outcomes from a registry of DVT patients treated with lytic therapy.[57] Acute thrombosis completely lysed in 34% of cases, but at the expense of major bleeding in 11%. One-year primary patency was 60%. Venous stents were used adjunctively in 104 of 473 patients. Currently, a randomized study of thrombolysis in the treatment of iliofemoral DVT is being conducted to determine the efficacy of this therapy in appropriately selected patients.

SURGICAL APPROACHES

Operative Thrombectomy

Thrombectomy directly removes thrombi from the deep veins of the leg. Despite early efficacy, venographic follow-up often shows rethrombosis. However, when creation of an arteriovenous fistula is added to the procedure, patency is improved.

Long-term follow-up is necessary to determine the incidence of post-thrombotic syndrome. In the United States, this procedure is usually reserved for limb salvage in the presence of phlegmasia cerulea dolens and impending venous gangrene.

Vena Caval Interruption

Adequate anticoagulation is usually effective in managing DVT, but if pulmonary embolism occurs during anticoagulant therapy or if a contraindication to anticoagulation exists, a mechanical approach to prevent pulmonary embolism is necessary. Mechanical protection is also indicated as prophylaxis against recurrent embolism for patients who required pulmonary embolectomy and for some high-risk patients who could not tolerate any recurrent pulmonary embolism. Because of the ease of insertion of vena caval filters, their low incidence of adverse events, and their proven efficacy, some have suggested extending the prophylactic indications (Table 45-1).

The cone-shaped Greenfield filter was developed more than 30 years ago to prevent pulmonary embolism while maintaining caval patency, preventing lower extremity venous stasis, and facilitating lysis of the embolus (Fig. 45-1). Before the advent of percutaneous placement techniques, the filter was commonly placed operatively. A 20-year review of the Greenfield Filter Registry revealed a 4% rate of recurrent embolism and a caval patency rate of 95%.[58,59] A 30-year review indicated that the long-term results became more favorable as experience accumulated with the smaller-profile versions of the device. The high caval patency rate makes it possible to position the filter above the renal veins when thrombus extends into the inferior vena cava or in young women with childbearing potential. A long-term follow-up study of patients with suprarenal filters demonstrated the safety and efficacy of such placements.[60]

The complications of filter insertion range in severity from minor wound hematoma resulting from early resumption of anticoagulation to potentially lethal migration of the device into the pulmonary artery, as documented with the bird's nest filter. The most common complication with the original stainless steel Greenfield filter was misplacement, which occurred in 7% of cases. This rate fell to 4% when the use of a guidewire became standard. With the titanium and percutaneous stainless

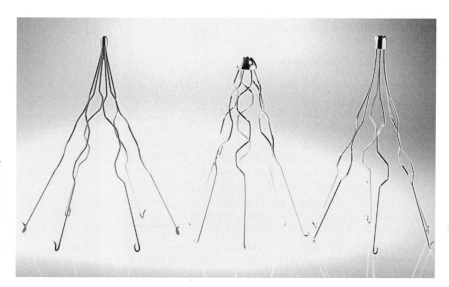

FIGURE 45–1 • The original Greenfield filter *(center)* was made from stainless steel and inserted via a 24 French carrier. The titanium model of the filter *(left)* is inserted via a 12 French carrier system. The newer percutaneous stainless steel filter *(right)* allows placement over a guidewire. (From Greenfield LJ, Proctor MC, James EA, et al: Staging of fixation and retrievability of Greenfield filters. J Vasc Surg 20:745, 1994.)

steel devices, the misplacement rate is less than 1%. When the filter is misplaced into a renal or iliac vein, it poses no regional problem, but there is no protection from pulmonary embolism. A second filter can be placed in the appropriate location. Follow-up has shown that filters misplaced in the right ventricle or pulmonary artery need not be retrieved unless an arrhythmia or tricuspid insufficiency develops. When obesity precludes fluoroscopy, intravascular ultrasonography can be used to identify the renal veins and guide filter placement. Bedside placement using either surface or intravascular ultrasonography has also been recommended for patients at risk during transport to the radiology suite, such as severely injured trauma patients. Further, this method may prove to be more cost-effective because it frees staff and leaves the interventional suite available for procedures generating greater revenue.

Pulmonary embolism has occurred in 2% to 4% of cases after filter placement and may be caused by a source of thrombus outside of the filtered flow, such as the upper body veins or the right atrium. Recurrent embolism is an indication for inferior venacavography to evaluate the filter for possible attached thrombus. This is a rare finding and can be managed either by thrombolytic therapy if the amount of thrombus is small or by placement of a second filter in the suprarenal vena cava.

Secondary infection of a captured thrombus within a Greenfield filter has been produced in the laboratory, but it was possible to sterilize the filter and thrombus with a 2-week course of antibiotic therapy.[61] Although the FDA identifies septic embolism as a contraindication to filter insertion, my experience does not support that recommendation.[62] The capture of a very large embolus within a filter may suddenly occlude the vena cava, with a precipitous fall in blood pressure. In a patient with known prior pulmonary embolism, this event can be mistaken for recurrent pulmonary embolism, with disastrous results if vasopressor therapy is administered. The basic distinction between functional hypovolemia of caval occlusion and right ventricular overload from recurrent pulmonary embolism can be made at the bedside by measuring the central venous pressure and arterial oxygen tension. The response to volume resuscitation for a patient with sudden vena caval occlusion should be dramatic improvement.

Failure to adequately flush the filter delivery system may result in thrombus formation, which may tether the limbs, prevent expansion, and allow migration on delivery. The improved technique of percutaneous insertion over a guidewire should minimize this complication.[63]

Percutaneous Filter Insertion

Favorable experience with the Seldinger technique for percutaneous introduction of catheters and devices led to a variety of innovative vena caval filter devices (Fig. 45-2; Table 45-2). Three devices—the bird's nest filter (Cook, Inc., Bloomington, Ind.), the Simon nitinol filter (Bard Peripheral Vascular, Tempe, Ariz.), and the Vena Tech device (B. Brown, Bethlehem, Pa.) —gained popularity during the 1990s.[64-66]

The advantages of the percutaneous technique prompted the development of titanium and percutaneous stainless steel Greenfield filters that could be inserted through a 14 French sheath (Fig. 45-3).[58,67] The modified stainless steel device allows placement over a guidewire and demonstrates the same long-term protection from pulmonary embolism and maintenance of vena caval patency.[63]

Recently, there has been increased interest in reduced-profile filters and those designed to provide the option of retrieval. The Gunther tulip filter (Cook, Inc.) is a conical device with a smaller volume attached to the vena cava by four rather than six hooked legs; however, according to the FDA's adverse event reporting site, it has been associated with migration. The profile is 6 French, and retrieval is facilitated by the presence of a hook at the apex. Millward and coworkers published results that suggest that few are actually removed, despite this option.[68]

The TrapEase filter (Johnson & Johnson, Miami, Fla.) has a unique cone-on-cone design that traps emboli against the wall of the vena cava. Although effective for clot capture, it has been reported to produce vena caval obstruction leading to renal failure, limb loss, and death. The device has a low delivery profile and is available without hooks, offering the option of retrieval.[69,70]

The most recent device to receive FDA approval is the Recovery filter (Bard Peripheral Vascular). It is manufactured from nitinol and retains the two trapping levels of the original nitinol filter, but with an innovative change to the proximal level that allows less disturbance of the blood flow. Minimal experience has been reported, but it appears to function well as a filter. Its advantage seems to be the length of time it can remain in the vena cava and still be safely recovered. However, ease of retrieval requires less secure fixation, which may explain early reports of movement with this device.

This latest step in the evolution of vena caval filters lacks a solid body of evidence to support its safety and efficacy. The features that make a device retrievable—lack of endothelial incorporation and flexible hooks—are also the features that make it less secure as a permanent device. More information on patient outcomes after filter removal is necessary to

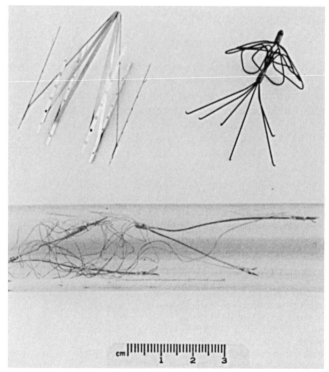

FIGURE 45–2 • Alternative vena caval filters that have been developed for percutaneous introduction: Vena Tech filter *(top left)*, Simon nitinol filter *(top right)*, and bird's nest filter *(bottom)*.

TABLE 45–2	Summary of Published Outcome Studies of Vena Caval Filters				
	Greenfield SGF 24F[59]	Greenfield TGF-MH[58]	Vena Tech[66]	Bird's Nest[91]	Simon Nitinol[65]
No. placed	642	173	142	61	20
No. monitored	246	113	137	37	16
Recurrent PE (%)	4	4	4	5	0
Caval patency (%)	96	99	70	97 (85[92])	75
Filter patency (%)	96	99	NR	95	NR
Insertion site DVT (%)	1	2	8	NR	NR
Migration (%)	NR	7	18	0	6
Penetration (%)	NR	<1	0	NR	31
Follow-up period (yr)	20	4	6	3.5	2
Follow-up tests	AP and lateral radiographs Duplex ultrasonography Venacavography	AP and lateral radiographs Duplex ultrasonography Venacavography	AP radiograph Duplex ultrasonography Venacavography	AP radiograph Duplex ultrasonography	AP radiograph Duplex ultrasonography Venacavography

AP, anteroposterior; DVT, deep venous thrombosis; NR, not reported; PE, pulmonary embolism; SGF, stainless steel Greenfield filter; TGF-MH, titanium Greenfield filter with modified hook.

From Greenfield LJ, Proctor MC: Indications and techniques of inferior vena cava interruption. In Gloviczki P, Yao JST (eds): Handbook of Venous Disorders: Guidelines of the American Venous Forum. London, Chapman & Hall, p 314.

determine whether the concept of retrieval, with its added risk and cost, is appropriate.

Pulmonary Thromboembolism

The most serious complication of DVT is pulmonary thromboembolism. Knowing the exact incidence of the disorder is difficult, because the clinical diagnosis is inherently inaccurate and is often confused with myocardial infarction, pneumothorax, sepsis, or pneumonia. Management of acute, massive pulmonary thromboembolism depends on an accurate diagnosis that documents the presence and location of an intravascular thrombus. This usually requires angiography, which has the added advantage of allowing pressure measurement in the pulmonary circulation. Because of its inherent nonspecificity, the perfusion lung scan is most useful as a screening test to exclude the diagnosis in patients with minor degrees of embolism. Spiral CT and magnetic resonance angiography are effective alternative diagnostic methods. In suspected massive embolism, the patient should receive heparin sodium (150 to 200 units/kg) and be taken directly to the angiographic

suite for selective pulmonary angiography. In addition to insertion of the angiographic catheter, usually through the femoral vein, a radial artery cannula is inserted for monitoring arterial blood gases, and anesthesia standby is requested should the patient require intubation and ventilatory control.

PULMONARY EMBOLECTOMY

Open pulmonary embolectomy is most appropriate for patients with chronic pulmonary embolism and elevated pulmonary pressure, those who require closed cardiac massage to maintain blood pressure, or those in whom lytic or catheter embolectomy procedures fail to improve cardiac output. However, it requires cardiopulmonary bypass under general anesthesia in an unstable patient and is usually associated with a high mortality rate. To improve the results of this approach, it is often advisable to place the patient on partial cardiopulmonary bypass via the femoral vessels under local anesthesia before the induction of general anesthesia. Using this approach, it has been possible to reduce the traditional mortality rate of 30%[71] to 8% to 11% in small series.[72,73]

TRANSVENOUS CATHETER EMBOLECTOMY OR THROMBECTOMY

An alternative to open embolectomy was described in 1969 using a cup device attached to a catheter that was inserted under local anesthesia via the jugular or the common femoral vein (Fig. 45-4). Once the catheter was positioned adjacent to the embolus, a sustained suction vacuum was used to hold the embolus in the cup as the entire catheter and attached embolus were withdrawn through the right ventricle and out through the venotomy (see Fig. 45-4). Clinical experience with the technique in 35 patients showed that emboli could be extracted in 32 (91%), with overall survival of 77%, similar to an earlier report.[74] In this series, open embolectomy during bypass also was performed for acute thromboembolism in nine patients, five of whom survived (55%). However, the requirement for open access to the vein limited the approach to surgeons familiar with the technique. The potential wider

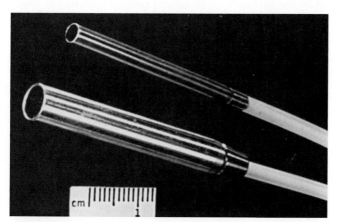

FIGURE 45–3 • Comparison of the carrier systems used for the titanium Greenfield filter *(top)* and the standard stainless steel filter *(bottom)*.

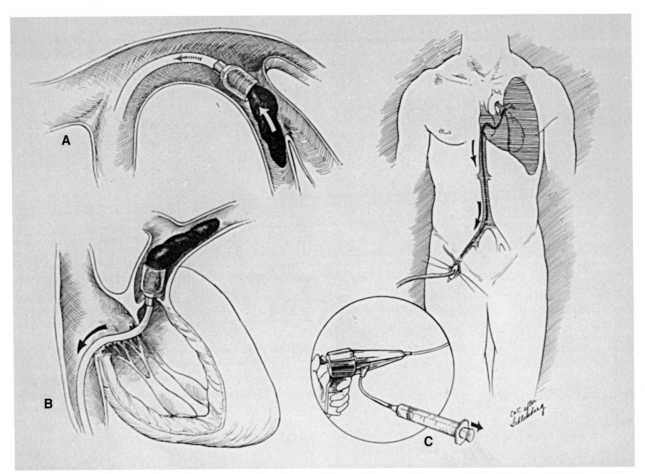

FIGURE 45–4 • Technique of catheter embolectomy based on positioning the steerable cup catheter *(A)* adjacent to the embolus and using syringe suction to aspirate a portion of the embolus into the cup. The catheter is then withdrawn *(B)*, maintaining the syringe vacuum *(C)* as the embolus is removed. Repeated insertions are usually necessary to clear the pulmonary circuit and improve cardiac output.

applicability of percutaneous techniques for thrombectomy under emergency circumstances has made them more attractive, although none has been approved for this use.

Percutaneous techniques for catheter thrombectomy use fragmentation, maceration, and aspiration to improve blood flow. The success of this approach in the pulmonary artery is facilitated by the greater cross-sectional area of the distal pulmonary bed, which can accommodate thrombus fragments as larger vessels are cleared, improving cardiac output. The effectiveness of this approach can be improved further by pretreatment with lytic agents to soften the emboli, making the two approaches complementary rather than competitive. Balloon angioplasty has also been used to fragment emboli, with or without additional lytic therapy.[75] Examples of thrombectomy devices used for pulmonary thromboembolism experimentally and in isolated cases include jet-vortex catheters,[76-78] impeller catheters,[79,80] rotatable pigtail catheters,[81] rotational baskets,[82,83] and aspiration with rotating coils.[84]

Emboli that are refractory to extraction are usually found in patients with a history of embolism of more than 72 hours and consequent fixation of the embolus to the pulmonary arterial wall. In these patients, however, subsequent embolism is usually responsible for acute decompensation, and the unfixed emboli can often be treated to allow hemodynamic stabilization. Beneficial results have also been reported with the use of pulmonary artery stents in these situations[85,86]

and with the use of extracorporeal life support for a period of days.[87]

Other Types of Venous Thrombosis

The term *thrombophlebitis* is usually applied to a disorder of the superficial veins characterized by a local inflammatory process that is usually aseptic. The cause in the upper limb is usually acidic fluid infusion or prolonged cannulation. In the lower extremities, it is usually associated with varicose veins and may coexist with DVT. Its association with the injection of contrast material can be minimized by washout of the contrast material with heparinized saline.

THROMBOPHLEBITIS MIGRANS

Thrombophlebitis migrans, a condition of recurrent episodes of superficial thrombophlebitis, has been associated with visceral malignancy, systemic collagen-vascular disease, and blood dyscrasias. Involvement of the deep veins and the visceral veins has also been described.

SUBCLAVIAN VEIN THROMBOSIS

Subclavian vein thrombosis is most likely to be secondary to an indwelling catheter and can occur in children. It may also occur as a primary event in a young, athletic person ("effort thrombosis"), presumably as a result of chronic compressive injury at the thoracic outlet. If the patient is seen late, there is usually a satisfactory response to elevation and anticoagulation, although some venous insufficiency and discomfort with exercise may persist. Pulmonary thromboembolism can occur from these thrombi, with an incidence of 12% reported in two series.[74] Although it is rarely necessary, we have inserted a Greenfield filter in the superior vena cava in an inverted position in more than 20 patients.

Thrombolytic therapy may be of value and should be considered for any acute subclavian vein thrombus within 3 to 4 days of onset.[88] If the thrombus lyses, a contrast venogram should be obtained to outline any anatomic site of compression that could be treated surgically. Direct venolysis with first rib or medial clavicular excision can be used and should be considered for younger patients and manual laborers. Thrombectomy should always be performed in conjunction with creation of an ipsilateral arteriovenous fistula for angioaccess if proximal venous thrombosis is present. If the fistula is made without recognizing the proximal occlusion, the extremity may be endangered by massive edema. Operative correction is still possible without loss of the fistula, however, even if a jugular venous bypass is necessary, because the fistula assists in maintaining patency of the repair or bypass.

ABDOMINAL VEIN THROMBOSIS

Thrombosis of the inferior vena cava can result from tumor invasion or a propagating thrombus from the iliac veins. Most often, however, it results from ligation, plication, or insertion of occluding caval devices. Thrombosis of the renal vein is most likely to be associated with the nephrotic syndrome. It can be a source of thromboembolism and has been treated successfully by suprarenal placement of the Greenfield filter.[89]

Portal vein thrombosis may occur in neonates, usually secondary to propagating septic thrombophlebitis of the umbilical vein. Collateral development leads to the occurrence of esophageal varices. Thrombosis of the portal, hepatic, splenic, or superior mesenteric vein in an adult can occur spontaneously but is usually associated with hepatic cirrhosis. Thrombosis of mesenteric or omental veins can simulate an acute abdomen but usually results in prolonged ileus rather than intestinal infarction.

Hepatic vein thrombosis (Budd-Chiari syndrome) usually produces massive hepatomegaly, ascites, and liver failure. It can be associated with a congenital web, endophlebitis, or polycythemia vera. Although some success has been reported using a direct approach to the congenital webs, the usual treatment is a side-to-side portacaval shunt to allow decompression of the liver or liver transplantation. The development of pelvic sepsis after abortion, tubal infection, or puerperal sepsis can lead to septic thrombophlebitis of the pelvic veins and septic thromboembolism. Ovarian vein and caval ligation has been the traditional treatment, but emphasis should be on drainage or excision of the abscesses and appropriate antibiotic therapy. I have also used the Greenfield filter for septic thrombosis because it is made of inert stainless steel or titanium and does not lead to the development of an intraluminal abscess, which could occur after the traditional approach of ligation of the vena cava.[90] Long-term follow-up of patients with

suprarenal filters has shown no obstruction and consequently no interference with renal function.[60]

REFERENCES

1. Hull RD, Pineo GF: Low molecular weight heparin treatment of venous thromboembolism. Prog Cardiovasc Dis 37:71-78, 1994.
2. Trousseau A: Phlegmasia alba dolens. In Clinique Medicale de l'Hotel-Dieu de Paris, vol 3. Paris, JB Balliere et Fils, 1865, pp 654-712.
3. Prins MH, Lensing AW, Hirsh J: Idiopathic deep venous thrombosis: Is a search for malignant disease justified? Arch Intern Med 154:1310-1312, 1994.
4. Tisdale JF, Snowden TR, Johnson DR: Case report: Poorly differentiated carcinoma of unknown primary presenting as Trousseau's syndrome. Am J Med Sci 309:183-187, 1995.
5. Burgers JA, Wagenaar J: Screening for malignancies in patients with recurrent venous thrombosis. Br J Urol 74:669-670, 1994.
6. Glassman AB, Jones E: Thrombosis and coagulation abnormalities associated with cancer. Ann Clin Lab Sci 24:1-5, 1994.
7. Donati MB: Cancer and thrombosis. Haemostasis 24:128-131, 1994.
8. Lohr JM, Kerr TM, Lutter KS, et al: Lower extremity calf thrombosis—to treat or not to treat. J Vasc Surg 14:618-623, 1991.
9. White R, McGahan J, Daschbach M, Hartling R: Diagnosis of deep-vein thrombosis using duplex ultrasound. Ann Intern Med 111:297-304, 1989.
10. Solomon O, Steinberg DM, Zivelin A, et al: Single and combined prothrombotic factors in patients with idiopathic venous thromboembolism: Prevalence and risk assessment. Arterioscler Thromb Vasc Biol 19:511-518, 1999.
11. Bauer KA, Rosendaal FR, Heit JR: Hypercoagulability: Too many tests, too much conflicting data. American Society of Hematology Education Program Book. Hematology 2:353, 2002.
12. Perler B: Review of hypercoagulability syndromes: What the interventionalist needs to know. J Vasc Interv Radiol 2:183-193, 1991.
13. Naidich J, Feinberg A, Karp-Harman H, et al: Contrast venography: Reassessment of its role. Radiology 168:97-100, 1988.
14. Flanagan LD, Sullivan ED, Cranley JJ: Venous imaging of the extremities using real-time B-mode ultrasound. In Bergan JJ, Yao JST (eds): Surgery of the Veins. Orlando, Fla, Grune & Stratton, 1985, p 89.
15. Leibovitch I, Foster RS, Wass JL, et al: Color Doppler flow imaging for deep venous thrombosis screening in patients undergoing pelvic lymphadenectomy and radical retropubic prostatectomy for prostatic carcinoma. J Urol 153:1866-1869, 1995.
16. Leutz DW, Stauffer ES: Color duplex Doppler ultrasound scanning for detection of deep venous thrombosis in total knee and hip arthroplasty patients: Incidence, location, and diagnostic accuracy compared with ascending venography. J Arthroplasty 9:543-548, 1994.
17. Mattos M, Londrey G, Leutz DW, et al: Color-flow duplex scanning for the surveillance and diagnosis of acute deep venous thrombosis. J Vasc Surg 15:366-375, 1992.
18. Remy-Jardin M, Remy J, Deschildre F, et al: Diagnosis of pulmonary embolism with spiral CT: Comparison with pulmonary angiography and scintigraphy. Radiology 200:699-706, 1996.
19. Peterson DA, Kazerooni EA, Wakefield TW, et al: Computed tomographic venography is specific but not sensitive for diagnosis of acute lower extremity deep venous thrombosis in patients with suspected pulmonary embolus. J Vasc Surg 34:798-804, 2001.
20. Norris CS, Greenfield LJ, Barnes RW: Free-floating iliofemoral thrombosis: A risk of pulmonary embolism. Arch Surg 120:806-808, 1985.
21. Aschwanden M, Labs KH, Jeanneret C, et al: The value of rapid D-dimer testing combined with structured clinical evaluation for the diagnosis of deep vein thrombosis. J Vasc Surg 30:929-935, 1999.
22. Sie P: The value of laboratory tests in the diagnosis of venous thromboembolism. Haematologica 80:57-60, 1995.
23. Tengborn L, Palmblad S, Wojciechowski J, et al: D-dimer and thrombin/antithrombin III complex—diagnostic tools in deep venous thrombosis? Haemostasis 24:344-350, 1994.
24. Nicolaides AN, Bergqvist D, Hull R: Consensus statement: Prevention of venous thromboembolism. Int Angiol 16:3-39, 1997.
25. THRIFT Consensus Group: Risk of and prophylaxis for venous thromboembolism in hospital patients. BMJ 305:567-574, 1992.
26. Hirsh J: Evidence for the needs of out-of-hospital thrombosis prophylaxis: Introduction. Chest 114(2 Suppl):113S-114S, 1998.
27. Tapson VF: Prophylaxis for deep venous thrombosis: The ACCP antithrombotic statement, revisited. Chest 113:844, 1998.

28. Guyatt GH, Cook DJ, Sackett DL, et al: Grades of recommendation for antithrombotic agents. Chest 114:441S-444S, 1998.

29. Poller L, McKernan A, Thomson J, et al: Fixed minidose warfarin: A new approach to prophylaxis against venous thrombosis after major surgery. BMJ 295:1309-1312, 1987.

30. Bern M, Lokich J, Wallach S, et al: Very low doses of warfarin can prevent thrombosis in central venous catheters. Ann Intern Med 112:423-428, 1990.

31. Turpie AGG, Hirsh J, Gunstensen J, et al: Randomized comparison of two intensities of oral anticoagulant therapy after tissue heart valve replacement. Lancet 1:1242-1245, 1988.

32. MacCallum P, Thomson J, Poller L: Effects of fixed minidose warfarin on coagulation and fibrinolysis following major gynaecological surgery. Thromb Haemost 64:511-515, 1990.

33. Kakkar VV, Corrigan TP, Spindler JR, et al: Efficacy of low doses of heparin in prevention of deep vein thrombosis after major surgery: A double-blind, randomized trial. Lancet 2:101, 1972.

34. Bara L, Planes A, Samama MM: Occurrence of thrombosis and haemorrhage, relationship with anti-Xa, anti-IIa activities, and D-dimer plasma levels in patients receiving a low molecular weight heparin, enoxaparin or tinzaparin, to prevent deep vein thrombosis after hip surgery. Br J Haematol 104:230-240, 1999.

35. Paiement GD, Wessinger SJ, Harris W: Routine use of low dose warfarin for 12 weeks to prevent venous thromboembolism following total hip replacement. J Bone Joint Surg Am 75:893-898, 1993.

36. Hansberry KL, Thompson IM, Bauman J, et al: A prospective comparison of thromboembolic stockings, external sequential pneumatic compression stockings and heparin sodium/dihydroergotamine mesylate for the prevention of thromboembolic complications in urological surgery. J Urol 145:1205-1208, 1991.

37. Agu O, Hamilton G, Baker D: Graduated compression stockings in the prevention of venous thromboembolism. Br J Surg 86:992-1004, 1999.

38. Kalodiki E, Hoppensteadt D, Nicholaides AN, et al: Deep vein thrombosis prophylaxis with low molecular weight heparin and elastic compression in patients having total hip replacement. Int Angiol 15:162-168, 1996.

39. Wille-Jorgensen P: Prophylaxis of postoperative thromboembolism with a combination of heparin and graduated compression stockings. Int Angiol 15:15-20, 1996.

40. Proctor MC, Greenfield LJ, Wakefield TW, Zajkowski PJ: A clinical comparison of pneumatic compression devices: The basis for selection. J Vasc Surg 34:459-464, 2001.

41. Walker H, Pennington D: Inferior vena caval filters in heart transplant recipients with perioperative deep vein thrombosis. J Heart Transplant 9:579-580, 1990.

42. Fink J, Jones B: The Greenfield filter as the primary means of therapy in venous thromboembolic disease. Surg Gynecol Obstet 172:253-256, 1991.

43. Alexander JJ, Yuhas JP, Piotrowski JJ: Is the increasing use of prophylactic percutaneous IVC filters justified? Am J Surg 168:102-106, 1994.

44. Rodriguez JG, Lopez JM, Proctor MC, et al: Early placement of prophylactic vena caval filters in injured patients at high risk for a pulmonary embolism. J Trauma 40:797-804, 1994.

45. Rogers FB, Shackford SR, Ricci MA, et al: Routine prophylactic vena cava filter insertion in severely injured trauma patients decreases the incidence of pulmonary embolism. J Am Coll Surg 180:641-647, 1995.

46. Bounameaux H: Unfractionated versus low-molecular-weight heparin in the treatment of venous thromboembolism. Vasc Med 3:41-46, 1998.

47. Buller HR, Kraaijenhagen RA, Koopman MMW: Early discharge strategies following venous thrombosis. Vasc Med 3:47-50, 1998.

48. Albada J, Nieuwenhuis H, Sixma J: Treatment of acute venous thromboembolism with low molecular weight heparin (Fragmin). Circulation 80:935-940, 1989.

49. Ten Cate JW, Koopman MMW, Prins MH, Buller HR: Treatment of venous thromboembolism. Thromb Haemost 74:197-203, 1995.

50. Agnelli G, Iorio A, Renga C, et al: Prolonged antithrombin activity of low-molecular-weight heparins: Clinical implications for treatment of thromboembolic diseases. Circulation 92:2819-2824, 1995.

51. Tapson VF, Hull RD: Management of venous thromboembolic disease: The impact of low-molecular-weight heparin. Clin Chest Med 16:281-294, 1995.

52. Hirsh J: Oral anticoagulant drugs. N Engl J Med 324:1865-1875, 1991.

53. Comerota AJ, Aldridge SC: Thrombolytic therapy for deep venous thrombosis: A clinical review. Can J Surg 36:359-364, 1993.

54. Robinson DL, Teitelbaum G: Phlegmasia cerulea dolens: Treatment by pulse-spray and infusion thrombolysis. AJR Am J Roentgenol 160:1288-1290, 1993.

55. Levine M, Weitz J, Turpie A, et al: Recombinant tissue plasminogen activator in patients with venous thromboembolic disease. Chest 97:168-171, 1990.

56. Bookstein J, Fellmeth B, Roberts A, et al: Pulsed-spray pharmacomechanical thrombolysis: Preliminary clinical results. AJR Am J Roentgenol 152:1097-1100, 1989.

57. Mewissen MW, Seabrook GR, Meissner MH, et al: Catheter-directed thrombolysis for lower extremity deep venous thrombosis: Report of a national multicenter registry. Radiology 211:39-49, 1999.

58. Greenfield LJ, Proctor MC, Cho KJ, et al: Extended evaluation of the titanium Greenfield vena caval filter. J Vasc Surg 20:458-465, 1994.

59. Greenfield LJ, Proctor MC: Twenty-year clinical experience with the Greenfield filter. Cardiovasc Surg 3:199-205, 1995.

60. Greenfield LJ, Proctor MC: Suprarenal filter placement. J Vasc Surg 28:432-438, 1998.

61. Peyton JWR, Hylemon MB, Greenfield LJ, et al: Comparison of Greenfield filter and vena caval ligation for experimental septic thromboembolism. Surgery 93:533-537, 1983.

62. Greenfield LJ, Proctor MC: Recurrent thromboembolism in patients with vena cava filters. J Vasc Surg 33:510-514, 2001.

63. Cho KJ, Greenfield LJ, Proctor MC, et al: Evaluation of a new percutaneous stainless steel Greenfield filter. J Vasc Interv Radiol 8:181-187, 1997.

64. Simm M, Athanasoulis CA, Kim D, et al: Simon nitinol inferior vena cava filter: Initial clinical experience. Radiology 172:99-103, 1989.

65. McCowan T, Ferris E, Carver D, Molphus M: Complications of the nitinol vena caval filter. J Vasc Interv Radiol 3:401-408, 1992.

66. Crochet DP, Stora O, Ferry D, et al: Vena Tech-LGM filter: Long-term results of a prospective study. Radiology 188:857-860, 1993.

67. Greenfield L, Cho KJ, Proctor M, et al: Results of a multicenter study of the modified hook titanium Greenfield filter. J Vasc Surg 14:253-257, 1991.

68. Millward SF, Oliva VL, Bell SD, et al: Gunther tulip retrievable vena cava filter: Results from the registry of the Canadian Interventional Radiology Association. J Vasc Interv Radiol 12:1053-1058, 2001.

69. Rousseau H, Perreault P, Otal P, et al: The 6-F nitinol TrapEase inferior vena cava filter: Results of a prospective multicenter trial. J Vasc Interv Radiol 12:299-304, 2001.

70. Schutzer R, Ascher E, Hingorani A, et al: Preliminary results of the new 6F TrapEase inferior vena cava filter. Ann Vasc Surg 17:103-106, 2003.

71. Meyer G, Tamisier D, Sors H, et al: Pulmonary embolectomy: A 20-year experience at one center. Ann Thorac Surg 51:232-236, 1991.

72. Yalamanchili K, Fleischer AG, Lehrman SG, et al: Open pulmonary embolectomy for treatment of major pulmonary embolism. Ann Thorac Surg 77:819-823, 2004.

73. Aklog L, Williams CS, Byrne JG, Goldhaber SZ: Acute pulmonary embolectomy: A contemporary approach. Circulation 105:1416-1419, 2002.

74. Greenfield LJ: Complications of venous thrombosis and pulmonary embolism. In Greenfield LJ (ed): Complications in Surgery and Trauma, 2nd ed. Philadelphia, JB Lippincott, 1989, pp 430-438.

75. Fava M, Loyola S, Flores P, Huete I: Mechanical fragmentation and pharmacologic thrombolysis in massive pulmonary embolism. J Vasc Interv Radiol 8:261-266, 1997.

76. Michalis LK, Tsetis DK, Rees MR: Case report: Percutaneous removal of pulmonary artery thrombus in a patient with massive pulmonary embolism using the Hydrolyser catheter: The first human experience. Clin Radiol 52:158-161, 1997.

77. Sharafuddin MIA, Hicks ME: Current status of percutaneous mechanical thrombectomy. Part I. General principles. J Vasc Interv Radiol 8:911-921, 1997.

78. Voigtlander T, Rupprecht HG, Nowak B, et al: Clinical application of a new rheolytic thrombectomy catheter system for massive pulmonary embolism. Cathet Cardiovasc Intervent 47:91-96, 1999.

79. Schmitz-Rode T, Adam G, Kilbingr M, et al: Fragmentation of pulmonary emboli: In vivo experimental evaluation of 2 high-speed rotating catheters. Cardiovasc Intervent Radiol 19:165-169, 1996.

80. Uflacker R, Stange C, Vujic I: Massive pulmonary embolism: Preliminary results of treatment with the Amplatz thrombectomy device. J Vasc Interv Radiol 7:519-528, 1996.

81. Schmitz-Rode T, Janssens U, Schild HH, et al: Fragmentation of massive pulmonary embolism using a pigtail rotation catheter. Chest 114:1427-1436, 1998.

82. Rocek M, Peregrin J, Velimsky T: Mechanical thrombectomy of massive pulmonary embolism using an Arrow-Trerotola percutaneous thrombolytic device. Eur Radiol 8:1683-1685, 1998.

83. Sharafuddin MIA, Hicks ME: Current status of percutaneous mechanical thrombectomy. Part II. Devices and mechanisms of action. J Vasc Interv Radiol 9:15-31, 1998.

84. Kucher N, Windecker S, Banz Y, et al: Novel catheter thrombectomy device for acute pulmonary embolism. Unpublished data, 2004.

85. Haskal ZJ, Soulen MC, Huetti EA, et al: Life-threatening pulmonary emboli and cor pulmonale: Treatment with percutaneous pulmonary artery stent placement. Radiology 191:473-475, 1994.

86. Koizumi J, Kusano S, Akima T, et al: Emergent Z stent placement for treatment of cor pulmonale due to pulmonary emboli after failed lytic treatment: Technical considerations. Cardiovasc Intervent Radiol 21:254-255, 1998.

87. Swaniker F, Hemmila M, Lynch W, et al: Extracorporeal life support for massive pulmonary embolism: Gibbon fulfilled. Unpublished data, 2002.

88. Mealy K, Shanik DG: Axillary vein thrombosis—local treatment with streptokinase. Ir Med J 78:289, 1985.

89. Greenfield LJ, Peyton R, Crute SL: Hemodynamics and renal function following experimental suprarenal vena caval occlusion. Surg Gynecol Obstet 155:37, 1982.

90. Greenfield LJ, Michna BA: Twelve-year experience with the Greenfield vena caval filter. Surgery 104:706-712, 1988.

91. Lord R, Benn I: Early and late results after bird's nest filter placement in the interior vena cava: Clinical and duplex ultrasound followup. Aust N Z J Surg 64:106-114, 1994.

92. Mohan CR, Hoballah JJ, Sharp WJ, et al: Comparative efficacy and complications of vena caval filters. J Vasc Surg 21:235-246, 1995.

Questions

1. **Which of the following statements are true concerning venous thrombosis?**
   (a) The type of operation rather than its length increases the risk of DVT
   (b) Contrast medium can pool in soleal veins during any type of anesthesia
   (c) The presence of a thrombus in a vein produces typical pain and swelling
   (d) Appropriate coagulation tests can identify the postoperative acquired thrombotic state

2. **A young man with recurrent venous thrombosis after minor soft tissue injury has a family history of pulmonary embolism. Which of the following statements are true?**
   (a) The most likely underlying disorder is antithrombin III deficiency
   (b) Diagnostic workup for an inherited thrombotic disorder should be delayed until the patient is not receiving anticoagulants
   (c) The presence of a family history mandates an investigation for an inherited disorder
   (d) Diagnosis of an inherited coagulation disorder indicates a need for lifelong oral anticoagulation

3. **A 31-year-old woman in her third trimester of pregnancy has a painful, swollen, pale left leg. Which of the following statements are true?**
   (a) The optimal initial diagnostic study is a venous duplex ultrasound examination
   (b) Venography is indicated because of discoloration of the leg
   (c) If venous thrombosis is found, the appropriate treatment is warfarin anticoagulation
   (d) If the thrombus progresses, the pregnancy should be terminated

4. **The patient from question 3 develops progressive swelling of the entire extremity, with dusky discoloration and paresthesia. Which of the following statements are true?**
   (a) The proximal extent of the thrombus involves the entire femoral system
   (b) The change is most likely due to hemorrhage into the extremity
   (c) Venography is indicated
   (d) The changes reflect ischemia

5. **A 55-year-old man has a 2-day history of calf pain without antecedent trauma. Which of the following statements are true?**
   (a) A positive Homans' sign justifies anticoagulation
   (b) Absence of swelling makes DVT unlikely
   (c) Venography is indicated
   (d) Color-flow duplex examination of the venous system can diagnose infrapopliteal DVT

6. **With regard to venous duplex examination, which of the following statements are true?**
   (a) Venous thrombi are identified by their echogenicity
   (b) Probe compression helps identify veins as opposed to arteries
   (c) Comparison of vein size between extremities can assist in the diagnosis of DVT
   (d) Thrombus echogenicity is related to thrombus age

7. **A 62-year-old woman has unilateral leg swelling. Which of the following statements are true?**
   (a) Impedance plethysmography (IPG) measures the rate of emptying of the congested lower extremity
   (b) A positive IPG is specific for venous thrombosis
   (c) Radiolabeled antifibrin monoclonal antibodies are preferred over radiolabeled fibrinogen
   (d) A negative D-dimer test is of more clinical value in the diagnosis of pulmonary embolism than is a positive test

8. **A 57-year-old obese white man with a history of prostate cancer is being considered for hip arthroplasty. The patient experienced DVT after prostatectomy 1 year ago. Which of the following statements are true?**
   (a) Prophylactic subcutaneous heparin should be used because of its ability to inhibit factor IX
   (b) Low-molecular-weight heparin is preferred because of its greater anti-Xa effect
   (c) To avoid bleeding complications, dextran should be used prophylactically
   (d) Prophylactic warfarin derivatives are effective but are associated with increased hemorrhage

9. A 47-year-old woman with documented metastatic breast cancer has an iliofemoral DVT confirmed by duplex ultrasound examination. Which of the following statements are true?
   (a) The patient should be kept on bed rest for a minimum of 10 days
   (b) Heparin should be administered by intravenous infusion
   (c) Warfarin should be administered at the same time that heparin is started to decrease the hospital stay
   (d) Platelet counts should be monitored during heparin administration

10. A 72-year-old man underwent radical prostatectomy 4 days ago and now has an iliofemoral DVT, with massive swelling and pain in the left leg. Which of the following statements are true?
   (a) If sensation and motor function are lost, venous thrombectomy is indicated
   (b) Fibrinolytic therapy is indicated
   (c) A vena caval filter is indicated
   (d) The patient should be heparinized

Answers

1. b	2. b, c, d	3. a	4. d	5. d
6. c, d	7. a, c, d	8. b, d	9. b, d	10. a, c

46

John Bergan • Luigi Pascarella

Varicose Veins: Chronic Venous Insufficiency

Vascular surgery, more than most disciplines, lends itself to a systematic approach to diagnosis and treatment of disease. When examining a patient with a vascular problem, categorizing the problem as arterial or venous is useful. Venous disorders can be categorized as either acute thromboembolic problems or chronic venous insufficiency. This chapter deals with the latter.

Disorders of venous function include primary varicose veins, superficial venous incompetence, and deep venous incompetence. Primary varicose veins can be cured, whereas chronic venous insufficiency due to deep vein abnormality is treatable but not curable. More importantly, varicose veins should be approached as symptomatic manifestations of venous disease rather than as a mere cosmetic problem.

Varicose veins are a disease of Western civilization. Ten percent to 20% of adult men and 67% of adult women have physically identifiable varicosities.[1] Severe chronic venous insufficiency is found in nearly 20% of working men and women. Varicose veins range in severity from the undesirable appearance of venectasia or telangiectasia to protuberant, tortuous varicosities with or without associated dermatitis, cutaneous ulcerations, or severe pigmentation.

The cause of varicose veins is linked to genetics, and the problem is exacerbated by changes in the hormonal milieu. The precise origin of varicose veins is probably multifactorial and is addressed later. The appearance of varicose veins in childhood is rare, although examination of adolescents with a strong family history of varicosities reveals that some have incompetent venous valves. Primary varicose veins in young adults are common. The precise cause is difficult to pinpoint, and our present understanding of this condition does not allow for treatment selection based on cause.

Progression

Primary varicosities consist of elongated, tortuous, superficial veins that are protuberant and contain incompetent valves. These produce the symptoms of mild swelling, heaviness, and easy fatigability. In this situation, the skin and subcutaneous tissue are normal, and edema, if present, is mild. Primary varicose vein symptoms merge imperceptibly into more severe, chronic venous insufficiency. Edema becomes moderate to severe, and an increased sensation of heaviness occurs. Larger varicosities and early skin changes of pigmentation and subcutaneous induration appear. The induration is termed liposclerosis or lipodermatosclerosis.

When chronic venous insufficiency becomes severe, marked edema and calf pain occur after standing, sitting, or ambulation. Multiple dilated veins are seen, associated with varicose clusters and heavy medial and lateral paramalleolar pigmentation. Marked liposclerosis and scars from previously healed ulceration or current ulceration are also noted.

Classification

Several systems of classification of venous insufficiency have been used in the past. The most recent contribution was devised by an international ad hoc committee of physicians interested in venous problems. It has been referred to as the Hawaii classification, in reference to its origination at the February 1994 American Venous Forum (AVF) meeting in Maui.[2] It is based on the clinical presentation of the patient (C), etiology of the problem (E), anatomic abnormalities found (A), and pathophysiology encountered (P)—or the CEAP classification. Unfortunately, this classification was accepted worldwide before it was tested. Therefore, it is now a work in progress and is undergoing periodic revisions. An ad hoc committee of the AVF on outcomes, chaired by Robert Rutherford, upgraded the original venous severity scoring system in 2000.[3]

CEAP REVISIONS: DEFINITIONS

Recognizing that there was little uniformity in classifying patients,[4] an ad hoc committee of the AVF suggested the following definitions and refinements of the clinical classification:

Telangiectases: confluence of dilated intradermal venules less than 1 mm in caliber. Synonyms include spider veins, hyphen webs, and thread veins.

Reticular veins: dilated bluish subdermal veins, usually between 1 and 3 mm in diameter; they are usually tortuous. This excludes normal visible veins in people with transparent skin. Synonyms include blue veins, subdermal varices, and venulectasies.

Varicose veins: subcutaneous dilated veins 3 mm or greater in diameter in the upright position. They are usually tortuous, but refluxing tubular veins may be classified as varicose veins. These may involve saphenous veins, saphenous tributaries, or nonsaphenous veins. Synonyms include varix, varices, and varicosities.

Corona phlebectatica: fan-shaped pattern of numerous small intradermal veins on the medial or lateral aspects of the ankle and foot, commonly thought to be an early sign of advanced venous disease. Synonyms include malleolar flare and ankle flare.

Edema: perceptible increase in the volume of fluid in the skin and subcutaneous tissue characterized by indentation with pressure. Venous edema usually occurs in the ankle region, but it may extend to the leg and foot.

Pigmentation: brownish darkening of the skin initiated by extravasated blood, which usually occurs in the ankle region but may extend to the leg and foot.

Eczema: erythematous dermatitis, which may progress to a blistering, weeping, or scaling eruption of the skin of the leg. It is often located near varicose veins but may be located anywhere in the leg. Eczema is usually caused by chronic venous disease or by sensitization to local therapy.

Lipodermatosclerosis (LDS): localized chronic inflammation and fibrosis of the skin and subcutaneous tissues, sometimes associated with scarring or contracture of the Achilles tendon. LDS is sometimes preceded by diffuse inflammatory edema of the skin; this may be painful and is often referred to as hypodermitis. The absence of lymphangitis, lymphadenitis, and fever differentiates this condition from erysipelas or cellulitis. LDS is a sign of severe chronic venous disease.

Atrophie blanche, or white atrophy: localized, often circular whitish and atrophic skin areas surrounded by dilated capillary spots and sometimes hyperpigmentation. This is a sign of severe chronic venous disease. Scars of healed ulceration are excluded in this definition.

Venous ulcer: full-thickness defect of the skin, most frequently at the ankle, that fails to heal spontaneously and is sustained by chronic venous disease.

REFINEMENT OF CEAP C CLASSES

Ultimately, the ad hoc committee approved the following definition modifications[5]:

C0: no visible or palpable signs of venous disease

C1: telangiectases or reticular veins

C2: varicose veins—separated from reticular veins by a diameter of 3 mm as the upper limit of size of a reticular vein

C3: edema

C4: changes in the skin and subcutaneous tissue secondary to chronic venous disease, divided into two subclasses to better define the differing severity of venous disease: C4a, pigmentation and eczema; and C4b, LDS and atrophie blanche.

C5: healed venous ulcer

C6: active venous ulcer

Each clinical class is further characterized by a subscript letter for the presence or absence of symptoms (S, symptomatic; A, asymptomatic). Symptoms include aching, pain, tightness, skin irritation, heaviness, muscle cramps, and other complaints attributable to venous dysfunction.[4]

Anatomic Terminology

A number of influences came together toward the end of the 20th century that forced a rethinking of the nomenclature of the veins of the lower extremities. First was the realization that a decreased emphasis on anatomy in primary medical education had allowed several generations of practicing physicians to think that the superficial femoral vein was indeed a superficial vein. This can have disastrous consequences when clinicians fail to treat deep venous thrombosis of the superficial femoral vein.[6] Next was the discovery of the fascial relationships of the saphenous veins, as revealed by duplex ultrasonography (Fig. 46-1).[7,8] Finally, a plethora of eponyms had accumulated, and there was some disagreement on both sides of the Atlantic regarding the meanings of these terms. Thus, an international conference of experts was held in Rome on September 11, 2001, to draft a consensus statement that would clarify lower extremity anatomic terms.[9] Some of the accepted terms are listed in Table 46-1. Other, less important changes and the omission of eponyms may be found in reference 10.

Pathogenesis

Varicose veins and cutaneous venectases and telangiectases develop under identical influences and may cause identical

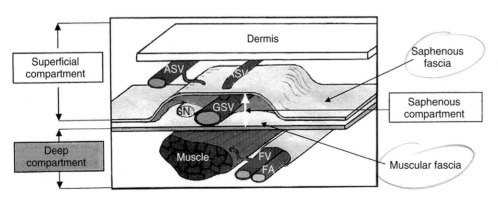

FIGURE 46–1 • Illustrated are the three subcutaneous compartments of the lower extremities and the fascial relationships of the saphenous compartment. Note the accessory saphenous veins (ASV), which parallel the compartment. When varicose, they are frequently mistakenly identified as the great saphenous vein (GSV). FA, femoral artery; FV, femoral vein; SN, saphenous nerve.

TABLE 46–1	Newly Accepted Terms for Lower Extremity Veins

Superficial Veins
Great saphenous vein
Small saphenous vein
Anterior, posterior, and superior accessory saphenous veins
Cranial extension of the small saphenous vein
Intersaphenous veins

Deep Veins
Common femoral vein
Femoral vein (formerly superficial)
Deep femoral vein (or profunda)
Medial and lateral circumflex femoral vein
Sciatic vein
Popliteal vein

symptoms. Textbooks of venous disease may refer to venectasias as cosmetic and asymptomatic, yet ample documentation exists to the contrary. Effective treatment of venectasias can relieve symptoms of venous dysfunction.[11]

Fundamental defects in the strength and characteristics of the venous wall enter into the pathogenesis of varicose veins. Epidemiologically, varicose veins are associated with tissue laxity.[12] The venous wall defects may be generalized or localized and consist of deficiencies in elastin and collagen. Gandhi and colleagues compared varicose veins with normal great saphenous veins and discovered a significant increase in the collagen content and a significant reduction in the elastin content of varicose veins.[13] No difference in proteolytic activity was demonstrated, thereby diminishing the likelihood that enzymatic degradation is an essential component of varicose vein formation.

Anatomic differences in the location of the superficial veins of the lower extremities may contribute to the pathogenesis. For example, the main saphenous trunk is not always involved in varicose disease. Perhaps this is because it contains a well-developed medial fibromuscular layer and is supported by fibrous connective tissue that binds it to the deep fascia. In contrast, tributaries to the long saphenous vein are less supported in the subcutaneous fat and are superficial to the membranous layer of superficial fascia. These tributaries also contain less muscle mass in their walls. Thus, these, and not the main trunk, may become selectively varicose.[14]

When these fundamental anatomic peculiarities are recognized, the intrinsic competence or incompetence of the valve system becomes important. For example, failure of a valve protecting a tributary vein from the pressures of the great saphenous vein allows a cluster of varicosities to develop. This is a common complaint of pregnant women, who describe the sudden development of a cluster of varicosities of unknown cause. Sudden failure of the protective valve is the mechanism for such development. In women, a standing occupation is a risk factor for varicosities, but this is not true for men.[12]

Further, perforating veins connecting the deep and superficial compartments may have valve failure. Pressure studies show that two sources of venous hypertension exist. The first is gravitational and is a result of venous blood coursing in a distal direction down linear axial venous segments.[15] This is referred to as hydrostatic pressure and is the weight of the

blood column from the right atrium. The highest pressure generated by this mechanism is evident at the ankle and foot, where measurements are expressed in centimeters of water or millimeters of mercury.[16] The second source of venous hypertension is dynamic. It is the force of muscular contraction, usually contained within the compartments of the leg.[17] If a perforating vein fails, high pressures (ranging from 150 to 200 mm Hg) that develop within the muscular compartments during exercise are transmitted directly to the unsupported superficial venous system. Here, the pulsatile pressures of muscular systole and diastole as transmitted cause dilatation and lengthening of the superficial veins.

If proximal valves such as the saphenofemoral valve become incompetent, systolic muscular contraction pressure is supplemented by the weight of the static column of blood from the heart. Progressive distal valvular incompetence may occur. This static column also becomes a barrier. Blood flowing proximally through the femoral vein spills into the saphenous vein and flows distally. As it refluxes distally through progressively incompetent valves, it is returned through perforating veins to the deep veins. Here, it is conveyed once again to the femoral veins, only to be recycled distally, effectively overloading the deep veins.[18]

Changes also occur at the cellular level. In the distal liposclerotic area, capillary proliferation is seen, and extensive capillary permeability occurs as a result of the widening of interendothelial cell pores. Transcapillary leakage of cosmetically active particles, the principal one being fibrinogen, occurs. In chronic venous insufficiency, venous fibrinolytic capacity is diminished, and the extra vascular fibrin remains to prevent the normal exchange of oxygen and nutrients in the surrounding cells.[19,20] However, little proof exists for an actual abnormality in the delivery of oxygen to the tissues.[21] Instead, research suggests that many pathologic processes are involved, and at present, it is difficult to identify which are active and which are bystanders. Fundamental investigations into this problem in the future should improve the care of patients with severe venous stasis disease.[22] An understanding of the source of venous hypertension and its differentiation into hydrostatic and hydrodynamic reflux is important. The presence of hydrostatic reflux implies the need for surgical correction of this abnormality, and the presence of hydrodynamic reflux implies the need for ablation of the perforating vein mechanism that allows exposure of the subcutaneous circulation to compartment pressures.[23]

Hormonal Influence

Venous function is undoubtedly influenced by hormonal changes. In particular, progesterone liberated by the corpus luteum stabilizes the uterus by causing relaxation of smooth muscle fibers. This effect directly influences venous function. The result is passive venous dilatation, which, in many instances, causes valvular dysfunction. Although progesterone is implicated in the first appearance of varicosities in pregnancy, estrogen also has profound effects. It produces the relaxation of smooth muscle and a softening of collagen fibers.[24,25] Further, the estrogen-progesterone ratio influences venous distensibility. This ratio may explain the predominance of venous insufficiency symptoms on the first day of a menstrual period, when a profound shift occurs from the progesterone phase of the menstrual cycle to the estrogen phase.

Symptoms

Many causes of leg pain are possible, and most coexist. Therefore, defining the precise symptoms of venous insufficiency is necessary. These symptoms may be of gradual onset or may be initiated by a lancinating pain, and they may precede the clinical appearance of the varicosity. Discomfort usually occurs during warm temperatures and after prolonged standing.[26] Varicose vein symptoms are often disproportionate to the degree of pathologic change. Patients with small, early varices may complain more than those with large, chronic varicosities.[27] The initial symptoms may vary from a pulsating pressure or burning sensation to a feeling of heaviness. The pain is characteristically dull, does not occur during recumbency or early in the morning, and is exacerbated in the afternoon, especially after long standing. The discomforts of aching, heaviness, fatigue, or burning pain are relieved by recumbency, leg elevation, or elastic support.

Cutaneous itching is a sign of inflammation induced by venous dysfunction and is often the hallmark of inadequate external support. It is a manifestation of local congestion and may precede the onset of dermatitis. This, and nearly all the symptoms of stasis disease, can be explained by the irritation of superficial somatic nerves by local pressure or the accumulation of metabolic end products, with a consequent pH shift. External hemorrhage may occur as superficial veins press on overlying skin, which gives way under the force of muscular contraction transmitted through a refluxing superficial venous system.

Diagnostic Evaluation

The most important noninvasive evaluation of the venous system consists of the physical examination and careful history-taking that elucidates the symptoms mentioned earlier. Clinical examination of the patient in good light provides nearly all the information necessary. It determines the nature of the venous disease and ascertains the presence of intracutaneous venous blemishes and subcutaneous protuberant varicosities, the location of principal points of control of perforating veins that feed clusters of varicosities, the presence and location of ankle pigmentation and its extent, and the presence and severity of subcutaneous induration. After these facts have been obtained, the physician may turn to noninvasive techniques to corroborate the clinical impression. Simple telangiectases need no further testing. In all other situations, the visual examination can be supplemented by noting a downward-going impulse on coughing. Tapping the venous column of blood also demonstrates pressure transmission through the static column to incompetent distal veins.

The Perthes test for deep venous occlusion and the Brodie-Trendelenburg test of axial reflux are of historic interest but have been replaced by in-office use of the continuous-wave, hand-held Doppler instrument supplemented by duplex evaluation.[28] The hand-held Doppler can confirm an impression of saphenous reflux; this, in turn, dictates which interventional procedure should be performed in a given patient. A common misconception is the belief that the Doppler instrument is used to locate perforating veins. Instead, it is used at specific points to identify reflux (e.g., the hand-held, continuous-wave, 8-MHz flow detector placed over the great and small saphenous veins near their terminations). With distal augmentation of flow and release, normal deep breathing, and performance of a Valsalva maneuver, accurate identification of valve reflux is ascertained.[29] Formerly, the Doppler examination was supplemented by other objective studies, including the photoplethysmograph, the mercury strain gauge plethysmograph, and the photorheograph. These are no longer in common use.

Another instrument reintroduced to assess physiologic function of the muscle pump and the venous valves is the air plethysmograph.[30,31] This instrument was used in the 1960s and then discarded because of its cumbersome nature. Computer technology has allowed its reintroduction, as championed by Christopoulos and coworkers.[32] It consists of an air chamber that surrounds the leg from knee to ankle. During calibration, leg veins are emptied by leg elevation, and then the patient is asked to stand so that leg venous volume can be quantitated and the time for filling recorded. The filling rate is expressed in milliliters per second, thus giving readings similar to those obtained with the mercury strain gauge technique. It provides physiologic information but does not guide therapy.

Duplex technology more precisely defines which veins are refluxing by imaging the superficial and deep veins. The duplex examination for deep venous thrombosis is commonly done with the patient supine, but this gives an erroneous evaluation of reflux. In the supine position, even when no flow is present, the valves remain open. Valve closure requires a reversal of flow with a pressure gradient that is higher proximally than distally.[33] Thus, the duplex examination should be done with the patient standing or in the markedly trunk-elevated position.[34,35]

Imaging is obtained with a 5- to 10-MHz probe, and the patient stands with the probe placed on the groin. After imaging, sample volumes can be obtained from the femoral or saphenous vein or both (Fig. 46-2). This flow can be observed during quiet respiration or by distal augmentation by compression of calf muscles. Sudden release of augmentation allows assessment of valvular competence. The short saphenous

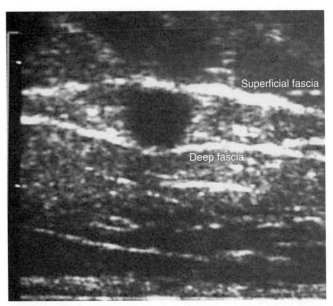

FIGURE 46–2 • This ultrasound image of a great saphenous vein is a constant marker throughout its length. Reflux in this vein and its tributaries guides further therapy. Note the relationships of the deep and superficial fascia to the vein.

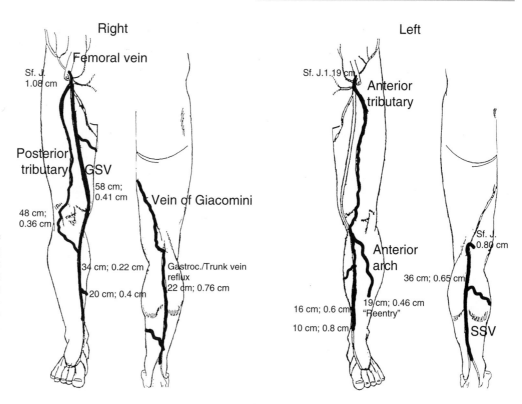

FIGURE 46–3 • Mapping of reflux found in the superficial veins guides subsequent therapeutic intervention. Note the marking of perforating veins and their diameters. Measurements are taken from the floor to avoid errors in identifying bony landmarks. Gastroc, gastrocnemius; GSV, great saphenous vein; SSV, small saphenous vein; Sf. J, saphenofemoral junction.

vein and popliteal veins are similarly examined. Imaging improves the accuracy of the Doppler examination. For example, short saphenous vein incompetence can be differentiated from gastrocnemius vein valvular incompetence by imaging and flow detection on the duplex scans.

LEVEL OF INVESTIGATION

The CEAP ad hoc committee has agreed that a precise diagnosis is the basis for correct classification of a venous problem. The diagnostic evaluation of a patient with chronic venous disease can be organized as follows, depending on the severity of the disease:

Level I: office visit with history and clinical examination, which may include use of a hand-held Doppler instrument. This is sufficient for simple telangiectases.

Level II: noninvasive vascular laboratory examination, with mandatory duplex color scanning with or without air plethysmography. This should be done for varicose veins and more severe problems (Fig. 46-3).

Level III: invasive investigations or complex imaging studies, including ascending and descending venography, venous pressure measurement, computed tomgraphy scan, venous helical scan, or magnetic resonance imaging. These are done when the history of treatment is complex, when venous reconstruction is contemplated, and when vascular malformations are present.

PHLEBOGRAPHY

In general, phlebography is unnecessary in the diagnosis and treatment of primary venous disease and varicose veins.[36] In the complex problems of severe chronic venous insufficiency, however, phlebography has specific utility.[37,38]

Ascending phlebography defines obstruction. Descending phlebography identifies specific valvular incompetence suspected on B-mode scanning and clinical examination.

Treatment

Indications for the treatment of varicose veins are pain, easy fatigability, heaviness, recurrent superficial thrombophlebitis, external bleeding, and appearance (Table 46-2).[39]

Treatment of venous insufficiency is similar to surgical treatment elsewhere; that is, it may be ablative or restorative. Most of the restorative venous surgical techniques are no longer performed; only a few, such as valve repair and the Palma procedure, can be considered useful therapy. Ablative treatment has been used sufficiently to establish objectives, and the operations have undergone marked improvement and modernization.[40]

Cutaneous venectasias with vessels smaller than 1 mm in diameter do not lend themselves to surgical treatment. They can be treated with sclerotherapy with or without foam.[41] If their cause is saphenous or tributary venous incompetence, these conditions can be treated by radiofrequency energy,

TABLE 46–2	Indications for Treatment

Pain: aching, burning, heaviness
Swelling: foot, ankle, leg
Dermatitis: focal, extensive
Lipodermatosclerosis
Ulceration: present or healed
Superficial thrombophlebitis
External bleeding
Appearance

endovenous laser, or sclerosant foam. Use of the external laser in the treatment of telangiectases has been disappointing.[42]

Surgical treatment (phlebectomy) may be used to remove cluster varicosities greater than 4 mm in diameter (Fig. 46-4). Ambulatory phlebectomy may be combined with saphenous ablation, either at the same time or staged. The stab avulsion technique can be done with preservation of the great and small saphenous veins, if they are unaffected by valvular incompetence.[43-45]

When great or small saphenous incompetence is present, the removal of clusters is preceded by the removal of the refluxing portion of the saphenous vein from the circulation.

VENOUS ABLATION

Treatment of primary venous incompetence in the 21st century is marked by minimal invasion, outpatient treatment, and an influx of nonsurgeons into the treatment arena. Despite changes in technique and personnel, removing the saphenous vein from the circulation is acknowledged to be requisite to long-term good results of varicose vein surgery.[46] Surgical removal of the saphenous vein on an outpatient basis requires one incision in the groin and one near the knee. Postoperative compression bandaging is standard, and most patients experience little downtime. Some, however, develop hematoma, pain, and extensive bruising. Recurrent varicose veins are found in 15% to 30% of treated individuals.[46]

In an attempt to minimize postoperative discomfort yet maintain the benefits of saphenous vein ablation, radiofrequency and laser energy have been used to effect rapid thermoelectrocoagulation of the vein wall and its valves (Fig. 46-5). Prolonged exposure to such energy results in total loss of vessel wall architecture, disintegration, and carbonization. There is now level I evidence of the benefits of such treatment using radiofrequency energy.[47,48] Also, useful information comes from simple registries that record the results of such treatment.[49] The 1- to 5-year reports of saphenous vein ablation are at least as good as those of conventional surgery. Clinical observations suggest much greater patient comfort following minimal intervention.[50]

It is of some interest that deep venous reflux is not a contraindication to saphenous vein ablation; in fact, such reflux may disappear when the superficial reflux is corrected.[51]

Neovascularization

Undesirable outcomes of surgical saphenous stripping are evident quite early.[52] New vessel growth in the groin, neovascularization, is often evident within 1 to 2 years. Its cause has not been elucidated, despite intensive study into suture material, inversion of the saphenous stump, and provision of a barrier over the saphenous stump. It has long been accepted practice to dissect tributary vessels at the saphenofemoral junction very carefully, taking each of the tributaries back beyond the primary and even secondary tributaries if possible.[53] Such dissection is apparently the principal cause of unwanted neovascularization in the groin, as discovered by duplex ultrasound surveillance.[54]

There is now ample confirmation that neovascularization causes recurrent varicose veins. Clearly, this is an adverse effect of standard surgery, and attempts to avoid this are commendable. The issue of varicose vein recurrence after saphenous

obliteration by radiofrequency energy or laser without saphenofemoral junction tributary disconnection is not completely settled. However, radiofrequency and laser ablation of the saphenous vein is almost never followed by neovascularization. Absence of neovascularization following endovenous ablation appears to be a fact. Many centers have reported no neovascularization after saphenous destruction in the absence of a groin incision.

Therefore, assuming that neovascularization is undesirable and that saphenous vein ablation is requisite, effective treatment has focused on ablation of the vein without a groin incision. The EVOLVeS study and the VNUS registry, combined with the ultrasound-observed disappearance of the saphenous vein after treatment, have validated its destruction by radiofrequency energy.[54] Such data are not available for laser energy, but the results may be comparable (Fig. 46-6). Thus, nonsurgical treatment of the saphenous vein certainly rivals saphenous stripping and may make that operation obsolete.

Foam Sclerosants

Another approach that shows great promise is the use of sclerofoam. Reports of its use monitored out to 5 years make this treatment of the saphenous vein very attractive.[55,56] In 1944 and 1950, Orbach introduced the concept of a macrobubble air-block technique to enhance the properties of sclerosant in performing macrosclerotherapy.[57,58] Apparently, few clinicians were interested in the subject, and the technique languished.

In the 1990s, the work of Cabrera and colleagues in Granada attracted the attention of some phlebologists, and interest in the use of foam technology to treat venous insufficiency was reawakened.[59,60] Cabrera showed that foam sclerotherapy was technically simple and effective in small or moderate-size varicose veins, and that the limitations of liquid sclerotherapy were erased when microfoam was used. Cabrera and colleagues' 5-year report represents the longest observation period in treating varicose veins with microfoam.[55] A single injection was used to treat saphenous veins and varicose tributaries. Extensive vasospasm was seen immediately, and compression was used after treatment. This technique achieved 81% complete fibrosis of the saphenous vein and disappearance of tributary varicosities in about 96% of cases. Fourteen percent of patients had persistent patency with reflux; retreatment was performed in those vessels.

Various techniques of creating sclerosant foam have been tried, but the one method that makes the treatment practical is that of Tessari.[61,62] In Figure 46-7, a 5-mL syringe filled with room air and a syringe filled with 1 mL of U.S. Food and Drug Administration (FDA)–approved detergent sclerosant are connected to a three-way stopcock. The room air and sclerosant are mixed together, creating foam that has a duration of greater than 5 minutes. Reports on the use of this technique to treat incompetent great and small saphenous veins and reticular veins and varicosities have been favorable.[63,64]

New techniques should be reviewed for both efficacy and adverse events. The largest published experience comes from Henriet from France.[56] He described 10,263 treatment sessions using 5% polidocanol (which is not FDA approved) conducted from November 6, 1995, to September 30, 1998. The ratio of women to men was 4:1, and the average age was 51 years (range, 8 to 93 years). Eighty percent were injections into

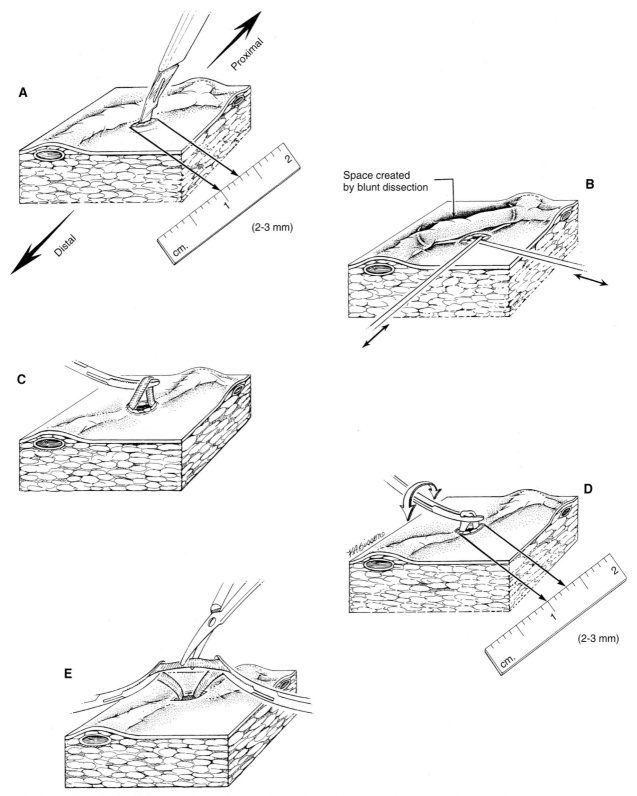

FIGURE 46–4 • Mini-phlebectomy or stab avulsion may be performed in conjunction with saphenous vein stripping or as an isolated procedure. As an isolated procedure, this is termed ambulatory phlebectomy, and dilute solutions of local anesthesia are utilized. *A,* The incisions are placed vertically, except at joint creases and where skin lines are clearly transverse. These should be no more than 2 to 3 mm in length. *B,* Mobilization of the subcutaneous space is done with blunt instruments, such as a hemostat or specially designed hooks. *C,* The instrument catches the adventitia of the vein and lifts it to the surface, where it can be clamped. *D,* The loop of vein is exteriorized and drawn into the field so that the loop can be doubly clamped. *E,* After the vein is divided, each end can be removed by stab avulsion. A minimum number of incisions are utilized, and they are kept short enough to be closed by tape strips without sutures.

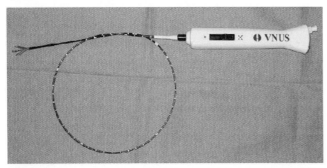

FIGURE 46–5 • The VNUS catheter shown here is the most time-tested of the endovenous techniques of saphenous vein ablation. Note the terminal electrodes used to deliver radiofrequency energy and the markings in centimeters used for orientation. Ultrasound monitoring and a large volume of dilute local anesthesia are used to ensure successful treatment without skin damage. (Courtesy of VNUS Technologies, Inc., San Jose, Calif.)

reticular varicosities and frank varicose veins. The other injections were for the treatment of long and short saphenous vein insufficiency. Adverse events included the following:

1. Visual problems. Nine patients experienced immediate visual problems; eight had blurred vision lasting several

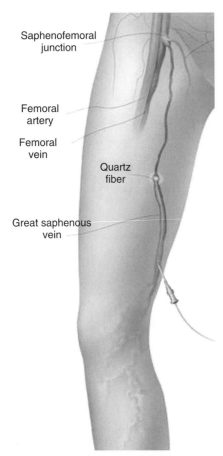

FIGURE 46–6 • The endovenous laser treatment illustrated here involves percutaneous placement of the quartz fiber and results in marked shrinkage of the treated vein. The procedure is monitored by ultrasonography, and local anesthesia administered into the saphenous compartment protects the skin from thermal damage and allows treatment without sedation or general anesthesia. (Courtesy of Diomed Inc., Andover, Md.)

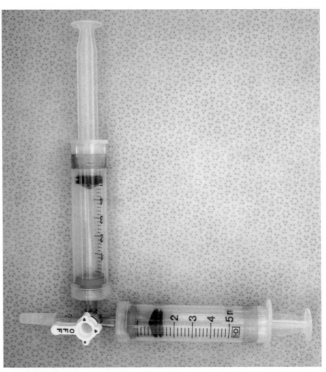

FIGURE 46–7 • The Tessari technique of producing an adhesive, compact, durable foam with ultrasound visibility is illustrated. The ratio of sclerosant to room air is approximately 1:4. (From Tessari L: The "tourbillon turbulence": Tessari's method with the three-way tap device. In Henriet JP [ed]: Foam Sclerotherapy: State of the Art. Paris, Editions Phlébologiques Françaises, 2003.)

minutes, and one had monocular blindness that lasted 2 hours. Complete resolution occurred in all patients.
2. Vomiting (one patient).
3. Migraine (seven patients).
4. Superficial thrombophlebitis. This complication occurred at a rate of one per week but was eliminated by reducing the concentration of the sclerosing agent.
5. Bad taste in the mouth (two patients).
6. Postsclerotherapy ulcer (one patient).

Although the cause of varicose veins remains unproven, a specific goal of treatment of venous reflux is obliteration of the saphenous vein. It may be that microfoam sclerotherapy will eventually replace all other methods (Fig. 46-8).

Severe Chronic Venous Insufficiency

What is new in the treatment of venous stasis is a rearrangement of and modification to older methods.[65] What has not changed is that conservative treatment of chronic venous insufficiency always precedes the consideration of intervention. Such conservative treatment relies on limb compression to counteract the effects of venous hypertension.

While conservative therapy is being pursued or ulcer healing achieved, appropriate diagnostic studies should reveal patterns of venous reflux or segments of venous occlusion so that specific therapy can be prescribed for the individual limb being examined. Duplex Doppler imaging suffices for the detection of reflux if the examination is carried out while the patient is

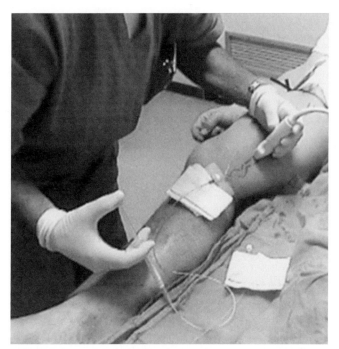

FIGURE 46–8 • Foam generated by the Tessari technique is instilled into the target vein using an intravenous catheter, as shown here, or simply through a No. 25 butterfly needle taped in the proper location as dictated by the ultrasound map. (From Tessari L: The "tourbillon turbulence": Tessari's method with the three-way tap device. In Henriet JP (ed): Foam Sclerotherapy: State of the Art. Paris, Editions Phlébologiques Françaises, 2003.)

standing. Such noninvasive imaging may be the only testing necessary beyond the hand-held, continuous-wave Doppler instrument if superficial venous ablation is contemplated. If direct venous reconstruction by valvuloplasty techniques is planned, ascending and descending phlebography is required. If reconstruction by stenting is contemplated, computed tomography or magnetic resonance venography should be done.

Surprisingly, superficial reflux may be the only abnormality present in advanced chronic venous stasis. Correction goes a long way toward achieving permanent relief of the dysfunction and its cutaneous effects. Using duplex technology, Hanrahan and colleagues found that in 95 extremities with current venous ulceration, 16.8% had only superficial incompetence, and another 19% showed superficial incompetence combined with perforator incompetence.[66] Similarly, the Middlesex group, in a study of 118 limbs, found that "in just over half of the patients with venous ulceration, the disease was confined to the superficial venous system."[67]

It is acknowledged that control of venous hypertension allows or promotes venous ulcer healing. This can be achieved in limbs with only superficial venous incompetence by removing refluxing superficial veins from the circulation.[68] Incompetent perforating veins also contribute to ambulatory venous hypertension and can be controlled surgically.[69] Isolated perforator incompetence is present in only 3% to 5% of limbs with severe chronic venous insufficiency, but this is an important element of venous hypertension in 21% of limbs with superficial reflux without deep incompetence and in 73% of limbs with superficial and deep incompetence.[70] Popliteal venous incompetence is responsible for many of the recurrent problems of severe chronic venous insufficiency.

FOAM SCLEROTHERAPY

Junger has shown that in limbs with severe chronic venous insufficiency, venous hypertension is transmitted to the microcirculation, where it is closely correlated with trophic skin changes.[71] The refluxing superficial veins and the incompetent perforating veins ultimately transmit venous hypertension to the microcirculation. The objective of surgical treatment has been to reduce that microcirculatory hypertension. This is achieved indirectly by superficial vein stripping and perforating vein interruption.

Sclerosant foam reaches the microcirculation just as it reaches the macrocirculation. The mixture of air with liquid sclerosant displaces the blood from the affected vessel so that there is virtually no dilution of the active agent. Air, with its contained nitrogen, allows prolonged contact of the agent with the venous endothelium, so that fibrosis and obliteration of the lumen occur without damage to surrounding tissue.[72] Thus, the effect of the foam sclerosant is exerted at the end point of venous hypertension—the microcirculation, which is inaccessible to all surgical techniques.

A lesson learned in our experience with sclerosant foam is that there is no reason to delay treatment as long as there is no active, invasive infection. Because of this experience, the treatment algorithm for chronic venous insufficiency has changed. The simplicity of the treatment, its evident success, and the relative freedom from serious complications makes this the first-line treatment for venous ulcer and for painful LDS as well.

Ulcer healing is not required before definitive treatment is begun because the effect of foam is to obliterate the abnormal tangle of vessels in the ulcer bed and in the area of LDS. These vessels are shown to be occluded by ultrasound examination after treatment. Currently, effective compression is applied at the initial patient visit, and the ultrasound scan is scheduled. Treatment is given after completion of the venous mapping. Treatment has evolved and is now variable, depending on the size of the veins. Specific perforating vein injection is not done at the first treatment. Cannulation is performed in larger veins that are tributary to refluxing saphenous veins. Perforating veins are targeted if the first treatment seems inadequate.

DIRECT VENOUS RECONSTRUCTION

Historically, the first successful procedures done to reconstruct major veins were the femorofemoral crossover graft of Palma and the saphenopopliteal bypass described by him and also used by Warren of Boston.[73,74] These operations were elegant in their simplicity, use of autogenous tissue, and reconstruction by a single venovenous anastomosis.[75]

The cross-femoral graft is the only direct venous reconstruction that has survived the passing years. However, even this successful bypass has been supplanted by interventional radiological techniques. With regard to femorofemoral crossover grafts, the only group to provide long-term physiologic study of a large number of patients was Halliday's, from Sydney.[76] Although phlebography was used to select patients for surgery, no other details of preoperative indications were given. They were able to document that 34 of 50 grafts remained patent in the long term, as assessed by postoperative phlebography. They believed that the best clinical results were achieved in the relief of postexercise calf pain. Their impression was that a patent graft also slowed the progression of distal liposclerosis and controlled recurrent ulceration, but no proof was given in their report.

Kistner[77,78] and Taheri and associates[79] described venous valve surgery and venous valve transplantation. Kistner summarized his view of valve surgery by saying, "The ultimate place of proximal venous valve surgery will be determined in the light of future experience." He went on to state, "Surgery on the incompetent deep veins deserves a place in the management of chronic venous insufficiency states as an adjunctive measure to be used in highly selected cases." Note that valvuloplasty techniques are for primary valvular incompetence and not for correction of the post-thrombotic destroyed valves. Objectivity is necessary in evaluating these techniques.

Conclusion

The 21st century opened the door to a better understanding of the pathophysiology of venous disease, and the exploitation of that knowledge is the promise of the future. Hemodynamic derangements are now better understood, and the cellular mechanisms of injury in chronic venous dysfunction are being discovered. More direct surgical approaches and the increased use of sclerosant foam will be applied with increasing success. Importantly, the principle of correcting deep venous incompetence by superficial venous ablation holds the promise of providing definitive therapy to a group of patients that once would have been relegated to "conservative" treatment based on resignation to living with a chronic, unyielding disease.

REFERENCES

1. Evans CJ, Lee AJ, Ruckley CV, Fowkes FGR: How common is venous disease in the population? In Ruckley CV, Fowkes FGR, Bradbury AW (eds): Venous Disease. London, Springer, 1999, p 79.
2. Porter JM, Moneta GL: An International Consensus Committee on Chronic Venous Disease. Reporting standards in venous disease: An update. J Vasc Surg 21:635-645, 1995.
3. Rutherford RB, Padberg FT, et al: Venous severity scoring: An adjunct to venous outcome assessment. J Vasc Surg 31:1307-1312, 2000.
4. Allegra C, Antignani P-L, Bergan JJ, et al: The "C" of CEAP: Suggested definitions and refinements: An International Union of Phlebology conference of experts. J Vasc Surg 37:129-131, 2003.
5. Eklof B, Rutherford RB, Bergan JJ, et al: Revision of the CEAP classification for chronic venous disorders: Consensus statement. J Vasc Surg 40:1248-1252, 2004.
6. Bundens WP, Bergan JJ, Halasz NA, et al: The superficial femoral vein: A potentially lethal misnomer. JAMA 274:1296-1298, 1995.
7. Caggiati A, Ricci S: The long saphenous vein compartment. Phlebology 12:107-116, 1997.
8. Caggiati A: Fascial relationships of the short saphenous vein. J Vasc Surg 34:241-246, 2001.
9. Caggiati A, Bergan JJ, Gloviczki P, et al: Nomenclature of the veins of the lower limbs: An international interdisciplinary consensus statement. J Vasc Surg 36:416-422, 2002.
10. Mozes G, Gloviczki P: New discoveries in anatomy and new terminology of leg veins: Clinical implications. Vasc Endovasc Surg 38:367-374, 2004.
11. Weiss RA, Weiss MA: Resolution of pain associated with varicose and telangiectatic leg veins after compression sclerotherapy. J Dermatol Surg Oncol 16:333-336, 1990.
12. Denenberg JO, Criqui MH, Langer RD, et al: Risk factors for chronic venous disease: The San Diego population study. Am J Epidemiol 158:448-456, 2003.
13. Gandhi RH, Irizarry E, Nackman GB, et al: Analysis of the connective tissue matrix and proteolytic activity of primary varicose veins. J Vasc Surg 18:814-820, 1993.

14. Mashiah A, Rose SS, Hod I: The scanning electron microscope in the pathology of varicose veins. Isr J Med Sci 27:202-206, 1991.
15. Bjordal RI: Hemodynamic studies of varicose veins and the post-thrombotic syndrome. In Hobbs JT (ed): The Treatment of Venous Disorders. London, MTP Press, 1977, pp 37-56.
16. Nicolaides AN, Sumner DS: Ambulatory venous pressure measurements. In Nicolaides AN, Sumner DS (eds): Investigations of Patients with Deep Venous Thrombosis and Chronic Venous Insufficiency. London, Med-Orion, 1991, pp 29-31.
17. Arnoldi CC: Venous pressure in patients with valvular incompetence of the veins of the lower limbs. Acta Chir Scand 132:628-645, 1966.
18. Hach-Wunderle V: Die sekundare popliteal und femoral venen insuffizienz. Phlebology 21:52-58, 1992.
19. Burnand KG, O'Donnell TF, Thomas ML, et al: The relative importance of incompetent communicating veins in the production of varicose veins and venous ulcers. Surgery 82:9-14, 1997.
20. Burnand KG, Whimster IW, Clemenson G, et al: The relationship between the number of capillaries in the skin of the venous ulcer-bearing area of the lower leg and the fall in foot vein pressure during exercise. Br J Surg 68:297-300, 1981.
21. Scurr JH, Coleridge Smith PD: Pathogenesis of venous ulceration. Phlebologie 1(Suppl):1:13-16, 1992.
22. Scott HJ, McMullin GW, Coleridge Smith PD, Scurr JH: Histological study of white blood cells and their association with lipodermato-sclerosis and venous ulceration. Br J Surg 78:210-211, 1991.
23. Gloviczki P, Bergan JJ (eds): Atlas of Endoscopic Perforator Vein Surgery. London, Springer-Verlag, 1997.
24. Wahl LM: Hormonal regulation of macrophage collagenase activity. Biochem Biophys Res Commun 74:838, 1977.
25. Woolley DE: On the sequential changes in levels of oestradiol and progesterone during pregnancy and parturition and collagenolytic activity. In Pez KA, Eddi AH (eds): Extracellular Matrix Biochemistry. New York, Elsevier Science, 1984, p 334.
26. Conrad P: Painful legs: The GP's dilemma. Aust Fam Physician 9:691-694, 1980.
27. Lofgren KA: Varicose veins: Their symptoms, complications, and management. Postgrad Med 65:131-139, 1979.
28. Hoare MC, Royle JP: Doppler ultrasound detection of saphenofemoral and saphenopopliteal incompetence and operative venography to ensure precise saphenopopliteal ligation. Aust N Z J Surg 54:49, 1984.
29. Nicolaides A, Christopoulos DG, Vasdekis S: Progress in investigation of chronic venous insufficiency. Ann Vasc Surg 3:278-292, 1989.
30. Christopoulos DG, Nicolaides AN: Noninvasive diagnosis and quantitation of popliteal reflux in the swollen and ulcerated leg. J Cardiovasc Surg 29:535-539, 1988.
31. Christopoulos DG, Nicolaides AN, Szendro G, et al: Air plethysmography and the effect of elastic compression on the venous hemodynamics of the leg. J Vasc Surg 5:148-157, 1987.
32. Christopoulos DG, Nicolaides AN, Szendro G: Venous reflux: Quantification and correlation with the clinical severity of chronic venous disease. Br J Surg 75:352-356, 1988.
33. van Bemmelen PS, Beach K, Bedford G, et al: The mechanisms of venous valve closure. Arch Surg 125:617, 1990.
34. van Bemmelen PS, Beach K, Bedford G, et al: Quantitative segmental evaluation of venous valvular reflux with ultrasound scanning. J Vasc Surg 10:425, 1989.
35. Vasdekis SN, Clarke GH, Nicolaides AN: Quantification of venous reflux by means of duplex scanning. J Vasc Surg 10:670, 1989.
36. Wesolawski SA, Greenfield H, Sawyer PN, et al: Diagnostic value of phlebography in venous disorders of the lower extremity. J Cardiovasc Surg (Torino) 8(Suppl):8:133-135, 1965.
37. Darke SG, Andress MR: The value of venography in the management of chronic venous disorders of the lower limb. In Greenhalgh RM (ed): Diagnostic Techniques and Assessment Procedures in Vascular Surgery. London, Grune & Stratton, 1985, p 421.
38. Lea Thomas M, McDonald LM: Complications of phlebography of the leg. BMJ 2:307-315, 1978.
39. Bergan JJ: Surgical management of primary and recurrent varicose veins. In Gloviczki P, Yao JST (eds): Handbook of Venous Disorders. London, Chapman & Hall, 1996, p 386.
40. Whiteley MS, Pichot O, Sessa C, et al: Endovenous obliteration: An effective, minimally invasive surrogate for saphenous vein stripping. J Endovasc Surg 7:I1-17, 2000.
41. Bergan JJ: Varicose veins: Treatment by surgery and sclerotherapy. In Rutherford RB (ed): Vascular Surgery, 5th ed. Philadelphia, WB Saunders, 2000, pp 2007-2021.

42. Goldman MP, Martin DE, Fitzpatrick DE, et al: Pulsed dye laser treatment of telangiectasias with and without subtherapeutic sclerotherapy. J Am Acad Dermatol 23:23-30, 1991.

43. Goren G, Yellin A: Minimally invasive surgery for primary varicose veins. Ann Vasc Surg 9:401-414, 1995.

44. Bishop CCR, Jarrett PEM: Outpatient varicose vein surgery under local anesthesia. Br J Surg 73:821-822, 1986.

45. Conrad P: Groin-to-knee downward stripping of the long saphenous vein. Phlebology 7:20-22, 1992.

46. Neglen P, Einarsson E, Eklof B: The functional long-term value of different types of treatment for saphenous vein incompetence. J Cardiovasc Surg (Torino) 34:295-301, 1993.

47. Rautio T, Ohinmaa A, Perala J, et al: Endovenous obliteration versus conventional stripping operation in the treatment of primary varicose veins: A randomized, controlled trial with comparison of the costs. J Vasc Surg 35:958, 2002.

48. Lurie F, Creton D, Eklof B, et al: Prospective randomized study of endovenous radiofrequency obliteration (closure procedure) versus ligation and stripping in a selected patient population (EVOLVeS study). J Vasc Surg 38:207-214, 2003.

49. Kabnick LS, Merchant RF: Twelve- and 24-month followup after endovascular obliteration of saphenous reflux: A report from the multicenter register. J Phlebol 1:17, 2001.

50. Goldman MP: Closure of the greater saphenous vein with endoluminal radiofrequency thermal heating of the vein wall in combination with ambulatory phlebectomy: Preliminary 6-month followup. Dermatol Surg 26:105, 2000.

51. Walsh JC, Bergan JJ, Moulton SL, Beeman S: Proximal reflux adversely affects distal venous function. Vasc Surg 30:89-96, 1996.

52. Sarin S, Scurr JH, Coleridge Smith PD: Assessment of stripping the long saphenous vein in the treatment of primary varicose veins. Br J Surg 79:889-893, 1992.

53. Bergan JJ: Saphenous vein stripping by inversion: Current technique. Surgical Rounds 34:118-124, 2000.

54. Jones L, Braithwaite BD, Selwyn D, et al: Neovascularization is the principal cause of varicose vein recurrence: Results of a randomized trial of stripping the long saphenous vein. Eur J Vasc Endovasc Surg 12:442-445, 1996.

55. Cabrera J, Cabrera A Jr, Garcia-Olmedo A: Treatment of varicose long saphenous veins with sclerosant in microfoam form: Long-term outcomes. Phlebology 15:19-23, 2000.

56. Henriet JP: Three years' experience with polidocanol foam in treatment of reticular varices and varicosities. Phlebologie 52:277-282, 1999.

57. Orbach EJ: Sclerotherapy of varicose veins: Utilization of intravenous air block. Am J Surg 66:362-366, 1944.

58. Orbach EJ: Contributions to the therapy of the varicose complex. J Int Coll Surg 13:765-771, 1950.

59. Cabrera J, Cabrera J Jr: Nueva métodode esclerosis en las varices tronculares. Patol Vasc 4:55-73, 1995.

60. Cabrera Garrido J: Los esclerosants en microespuma contra l patologia venosa. Noticias Med 3:653:12-16, 1997.

61. Tessari L: Nouvelle technique d'obtention de la scléro-mousse. Phlebologie 53:129, 2000.

62. Tessari L: The "tourbillon turbulence": Tessari's method with the three-way tap device. In Henriet JP (ed): Foam Sclerotherapy: State of the Art. Paris, Editions Phlébologiques Françaises, 2003, p 56.

63. Sica M, Benigni JP: Échosclérose á la mousse: Trois années d'expérience sur les axes saphéniens. Phlebologie 53:339-342, 2000.

64. Frullini A, Cavezzi A: Échosclérose par mousse de tétradécyl-sulfate de sodium et de polidocanol: Deux annnées d'experience. Phlebologie 53:431-435, 2000.

65. Bergan JJ: New developments in surgery of the venous system. J Cardiovasc Surg 1:624, 1993.

66. Hanrahan LM, Araki CT, Rodriguez AA, et al: Distribution of valvular incompetence in patients with venous stasis ulceration. J Vasc Surg 13:805, 1991.

67. Shami SK, Sarin S, Cheatle TR, et al: Venous ulcers and the superficial venous system. J Vasc Surg 17:487, 1993.

68. Jugenheimer M, Junginger TH: Endoscopic subfascial sectioning of incompetent perforating veins in the treatment of primary varicosis. World J Surg 16:971, 1992.

69. Fischer R: Erfahrungen mit der endoskopischen perforanten Sanierung. Phlebologie 21:224, 1992.

70. Perrin M: Venous leg perforating veins [French]. J Mal Vasc 24:19-24, 1999.

71. Junger M, Steins A, Hahn M, Hafner HM: Microcirculatory dysfunction in chronic venous insufficiency. Microcirculation 7:3-12, 2000.

72. Sommer A, Veraart JCJM: Treatment of varicose veins with foam. Phlebology Digest 16:10-13, 2003.

73. Palma EC, Riss F, Del Campo F, et al: Tratamiento de los trastornos postflebiticos mediante anastomosis venosa safenofemoral controlateral. Bull Soc Surg Uruguay 29:135-145, 1958.

74. Palma EC, Esperon R: Vein transplants and grafts in the surgical treatment of the post-phlebitic syndrome. J Cardiovasc Surg (Torino) 1:94-107, 1960.

75. Danza R, Navarro T, Baldizan J, Olivera D: Injerto veno-venoso libre: Indicaciones, tecnica y resultados (11 anos de experiencia). Cir Uruguay 50:485-494, 1980.

76. Halliday P, Harris J, May J: Femorofemoral crossover grafts (Palma operation): A long term follow-up study. In Bergan JJ, Yao JST (eds): Surgery of the Veins. Orlando, Fla, Grune & Stratton, 1985, pp 255-265.

77. Kistner RL: Surgical repair of the incompetent femoral vein valve. Arch Surg 110:1336, 1975.

78. Kistner RL: Late results of venous valve repair. In Yao JST, Pearce WL (eds): Long-Term Results of Vascular Surgery. Philadelphia, WB Saunders, 1993, pp 451-466.

79. Taheri SA, Lazar L, Elias S, et al: Surgical treatment of postphlebitic syndrome with vein valve transplant. Am J Surg 144:221, 1982.

Questions

1. **Symptoms of varicose veins include aching pain and fatigue. These are greatest in which of the following?**
   (a) Telangiectases
   (b) Reticular varicosities
   (c) Large subcutaneous varicosities
   (d) Symptoms are unrelated to size
   (e) Symptoms may be equal in all of the above

2. **In a patient with symptomatic varicose veins, after the complete history and physical examination are done, which of the following should be added to the evaluation?**
   (a) Duplex reflux examination
   (b) Phlebography
   (c) Hand-held continuous-wave Doppler evaluation
   (d) Photoplethysmography

3. **Treatment of telangiectases and reticular, flat, blue-green varicosities is done for what reason?**
   (a) Improve the cosmetic appearance of the legs
   (b) Ameliorate symptoms of aching, heaviness, and pain
   (c) Neither of the above
   (d) Both a and b

4. **Nocturnal leg cramps are chiefly associated with which of the following?**
   (a) Arteriosclerotic occlusive disease
   (b) Lymphedema
   (c) Telangiectases
   (d) Telangiectases and varicose veins

5. **Venous leg ulcers may be due to which of the following?**
   (a) Saphenous reflux and varicose veins
   (b) Deep venous reflux without superficial reflux
   (c) Incompetent ankle perforating veins
   (d) All of the above

6. Severe venous dysfunction is characterized by ankle hyperpigmentation, induration, and open leg ulcers. What is the correct term for this condition?
   (a) Stasis ulcer
   (b) Postphlebitic state
   (c) Chronic venous insufficiency
   (d) Marjolin's ulcer

7. What is the anatomic cause of venous leg ulcers?
   (a) Superficial reflux
   (b) Deep venous reflux
   (c) Perforator reflux
   (d) All of the above, singly or in combination

8. The open perforator vein operations were disappointing because of which of the following?
   (a) Recurrent ulceration
   (b) Delayed healing of skin grafts
   (c) Systemic infection
   (d) General morbidity

9. Conservative treatment of severe venous dysfunction includes which of the following?
   (a) Induced hyperthermia
   (b) Intermittent pneumatic compression
   (c) Fitted support
   (d) All of the above

10. What is the fundamental objective of perforator vein interruption?
   (a) Improved calf muscle pump function
   (b) Decreased ambulatory venous hypertension
   (c) Diminished leukocyte trapping and activation
   (d) All of the above

Answers

| 1. d | 2. c | 3. d | 4. d | 5. d |
| 6. c | 7. a | 8. d | 9. c | 10. d |

47

Thom W. Rooke • Roger F. J. Shepherd •
Cindy L. Felty

Lymphedema

Lymphedema is an important topic for vascular surgeons for three reasons. First, it is very common. Estimates vary, but hundreds of thousands of patients in the United States have lymphedema,[1] and according to the World Health Organization, up to 100 million are affected worldwide.[2] Second, even the best surgeons may have patients who develop lymphedema after operations involving the limbs or trunk. Third, lymphedema may be confused with venous disease or other vascular anomalies that are typically referred to vascular surgeons. The bottom line is that vascular surgeons are likely to encounter patients with lymphedema.

Pathogenesis

Fluid, proteins, and various soluble substances extravasate from the capillaries into the interstitial space.[3] This fluid would quickly accumulate to unhealthy levels were it not for the lymphatics. These vessels, similar in function to a storm sewer system, collect interstitial fluid and return it via the thoracic duct to the circulatory system. Interstitial fluid is called lymph fluid once it enters the lymphatic vessel.

Lymphedema starts when interstitial fluid builds up because of lymphatic obstruction or reflux (or, rarely, from extreme overproduction of lymph fluid). Lymphatic transport is an important mechanism for removing extravasated protein from the interstitial space; when it fails, proteins that are too large to be reabsorbed into the capillaries accumulate within the tissue. The brawny or "woody" texture of lymphedema (Fig. 47-1) is caused by chronic inflammation associated with the excessive interstitial protein.[4] Over time, inflammatory alterations in connective tissues, elastic fibers, glycosaminoglycans, and other cutaneous elements lead to dermal fibrosis.[5]

Causes

Lymphedema may be either primary or secondary. Primary lymphedema may occur shortly after birth (heritable forms include Milroy disease),[6] around the time of puberty (lymphedema praecox),[6] or, rarely, during adulthood (lymphedema tarda).[7] Some classification schemes are based on the physical appearance of lymph vessels,[8] giving rise to categories such as aplasia, hypoplasia, hyperplasia, and so forth. Primary lymphedema may be due to the failure of lymphatics to develop normally or to the degeneration and loss of lymphatics over time.

Secondary lymphedema is much more common than the primary form and may result from anything that leads to the destruction of lymphatic vessels or nodes.[7] Common causes include trauma (including surgical trauma associated with lymph node resection), radiation therapy that leads to lymphatic sclerosis, invasion of the lymphatic system by tumor, recurrent infections or lymphangitis (usually caused by streptococci or, less often, staphylococci) that obliterate the vessels, and certain parasites. As noted earlier, 90 million to 100 million people worldwide (primarily in tropical countries) have filaria-induced lymphedema.[9] The most common filaria are *Wuchereria bancrofti* and *Brugia* species.[10] Although most of these are tropical organisms, some *Brugia* species are found in North America. Many other conditions, including autoimmune diseases, pregnancy, illegal drug injection, and factitial injuries may produce lymphedema.[11-15]

Diagnosis

Lymphedema is often suspected or diagnosed on clinical grounds. An appropriate history describing the circumstances leading to the onset of edema, comorbid conditions, and family

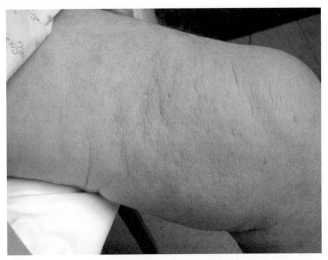

FIGURE 47–1 • Skin changes in lymphedema. Protein accumulation within the interstitial space produces "brawny" induration of the skin. The resulting "orange peel skin" is a common clinical finding in chronic lymphedema.

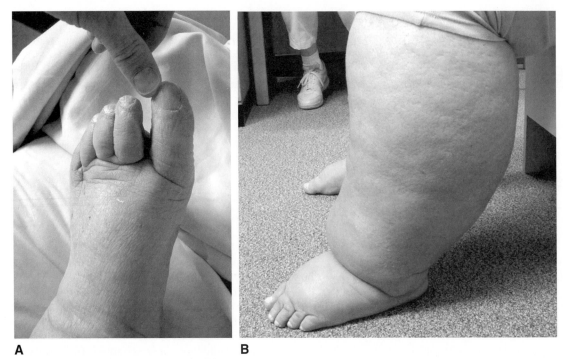

A　　　　　　　　　　　　　**B**

FIGURE 47–2 • Clinical findings in lymphedema. *A*, Typical "swollen sausage" appearance of the toes. Lymphedema is usually most severe in the distal limb. *B*, When lymphedema involves the leg, the toes and feet are almost always affected.

history may be helpful. Lymphedema is usually confined to a single upper or lower limb, although involvement of multiple limbs (including hemihypertrophy) is possible.[16] Local pressure may cause "pitting" indentation of the skin in early lymphedema but to a lesser degree than is seen with edema of different causes but similar severity.

Lymphedema is typically worse at the distal end of the extremity. When it affects the lower limb, the feet and toes are rarely spared (Fig. 47-2). Indeed, chronic toe edema leads to remodeling changes that produce the "squaring" of the toes (or "boxcar" toes) classically seen in lymphedema.[17] Verrucous skin changes are common; often, these wartlike lesions are mistaken for neoplasms and the patient is biopsied unnecessarily. In extreme cases, particularly those produced by tropical filaria, the limb may take on a grotesque appearance associated with massive edema, fibrosis, and verrucous changes (Fig. 47-3). This appearance is commonly called *elephantiasis*.

To evaluate a patient with lymphedema, it may be necessary to rule out other problems that can cause limb swelling, especially venous occlusion. This is particularly problematic when limb swelling occurs after an operation such as mastectomy or pelvic surgery (Fig. 47-4), during which lymph nodes and vessels may have been damaged or removed (producing lymphedema) and veins may have been injured or thrombosed (producing venous edema). Appropriate testing with duplex ultrasound scanning, venography, or other modalities can clarify whether the veins are normal. Cross-sectional imaging with computed tomography or magnetic resonance imaging may be appropriate to look for enlarged, tumor-filled lymph nodes or other lesions that can produce lymphatic obstruction. Nonmalignant masses or fluid collections can also cause lymphedema.[18] Magnetic resonance

imaging can help differentiate the cutaneous edema of lymphedema from other types of limb swelling.[19-21]

The two tests used to assess lymphatic patency are lymphangiography and lymphoscintigraphy. Lymphangiography involves cannulation of a distal lymphatic vessel via a surgical incision.[22] Contrast dye is injected into the cannulated vessel, and x-ray images are obtained. The study provides a detailed view of the lymph vessels and nodes, but not without consequences. Lymphangiography is painful, it is technically difficult to perform, and in some cases, it is potentially dangerous; the contrast material may cause sterile lymphangitis or become

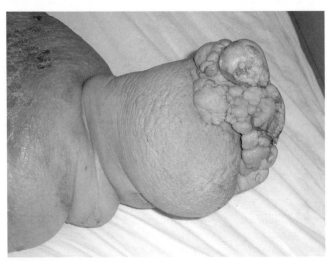

FIGURE 47–3 • End-stage changes in lymphedema. Wartlike (verrucous) skin changes are commonly seen in advanced cases of chronic, long-standing lymphedema.

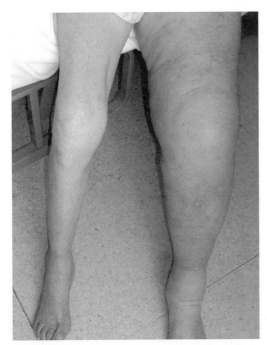

FIGURE 47–4 • Lymphatic versus venous disease. This man developed progressive left leg edema following radical prostatectomy. The question is: Is it due to lymphedema or venous obstruction? In this case, the answer is both. The left limb has a perioperative iliofemoral deep venous thrombosis and secondary lymphedema from surgical disruption of the nodes and lymphatics.

retained within the lymphatic vessel, which may induce or worsen lymphatic obstruction.[23]

Lymphoscintigraphy involves the subcutaneous injection of a radiolabeled colloid into the distal extremity; in the lower limb, it is injected between the toes or on the dorsum of the foot.[24] The colloid enters the lymphatics and is transported through vessels and nodes until it reaches the liver and spleen. The flow of colloid can be assessed using traditional nuclear imaging cameras. In normal subjects, transport occurs quickly (typically an hour or less for colloid to move from the distal limb to the abdomen); when lymphatic obstruction is present, the colloid never ascends the lymphatics but instead becomes trapped in the interstitial spaces of the distal limb, producing a "dermal back-flow" pattern. Delayed transport or dermal back-flow patterns identify limbs with lymphatic obstruction.[25]

Both lymphangiography and lymphoscintigraphy can be used to identify and assess patients with lymphatic hyperplasia or reflux.[26] The contrast or colloid is introduced via a contralateral or uninvolved limb and followed over time to determine whether reflux into the swollen limb occurs.

In addition to venous disease, there are other conditions that may mimic the clinical appearance of lymphedema. Myxedema associated with thyroid dysfunction, cardiac or renal failure, hypoproteinemia, and chronic dependency may resemble lymphedema or can aggravate otherwise mild cases of lymphedema.[27] Obesity (including morbid obesity and lipedema) is frequently seen in conjunction with or mistaken for lymphedema.[28]

Rationale for Treatment

Lymphedema is almost never life-threatening; the goals of treatment are to improve limb function, reduce pain, improve

cosmesis, and prevent long-term complications. An informal survey of the Mayo Clinic Lymphedema Clinic reveals that the most common reasons for treatment include cosmesis (44% of patients) and prevention of complications (39%); the least common are functional impairment (16%) and pain (<1%).

The rationale for therapy directed at pain relief, functional improvement, or appearance seems obvious. Therapy intended to prevent future complications is less intuitive but often of greater importance. Limbs with lymphedema are at risk for numerous problems, including increased susceptibility to injury, infections such as cellulitis or lymphangitis (Fig. 47-5), and tumor formation (particularly angiosarcoma or Stewart-Treves syndrome).[29] Patients with no limb pain, no functional impairment, and no cosmetic concerns may have difficulty understanding the importance of lymphedema treatment for the prevention of complications. It is devastating when a patient with mild lymphedema develops cellulitis or lymphangitis that ravages the remaining lymphatics and leaves the limb with severe lymphedema. Even more devastated are the patients who develop angiosarcoma, a condition that usually leads to rapid loss of limb and life.

Whether to recommend aggressive lymphedema therapy for a particular patient can be a simple decision. It is easy to conclude that a young, healthy patient with severe, disabling, painful, cosmetically disfiguring lymphedema warrants treatment. Other decisions may not be so easy. What about the young woman whose swelling is so mild that she notices it only when she tries to wear tight jeans, or the patient whose lymphedema is caused by obstruction of lymph nodes due to metastatic cancer, or an elderly patient with significant lymphedema? In these instances, the "cost" of treating lymphedema (given the mild symptoms, bad prognosis, or advanced age) must be weighed against the likely "benefits."

Unfortunately, cost-benefit determinations are no simpler in lymphedema than in other vascular conditions—that is, they are almost impossible. Cost is measured not only in the dollars spent on therapy but also in less tangible considerations such as the time devoted to therapy (which may be substantial), the inconvenience of certain treatment measures (e.g., wearing stockings or wraps all day), and the emotional challenge of

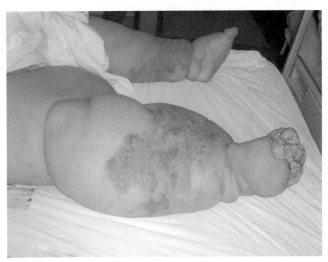

FIGURE 47–5 • Complications of lymphedema. A limb with lymphedema is highly susceptible to cellulitis and other infections. The causative agents are usually streptococci or staphylococci.

having to incorporate regular treatment sessions into one's lifestyle. The benefits of therapy are likewise subjective for this nonlethal condition. How much better does the patient feel or function after treatment? How much better does he or she look?

Cost and benefit are highly subjective, so there is no one right answer; therapy must be individualized for each patient. In our practice, we have taken the view that liberal treatment indications are appropriate for most patients. Accordingly, more than half the patients treated in our lymphedema clinic have mild edema (26%), cancer or some other poor prognosis (10%), or an age older than 70 years (20%). This distribution may be different in other practices, depending on local patient demographics.

Goals of Therapy

On the surface, the goals of therapy seem obvious—to reduce the size of the limb and thus minimize functional impairment, pain, cosmetic disfigurement, and the chance of long-term complications. But how much fluid has to be removed from a lymphedematous limb to achieve these goals—20% reduction, 50%? Or should one strive to make the limb as close to perfect as possible?

This dilemma can be illustrated by considering the case of AL, a 30-year-old man with disabling lymphedema of the left leg. The edema, present since puberty, has slowly worsened over the past 15 years and has now reached the point where his left leg contains more than 150 pounds of excess fluid. As a result, AL is unable to walk, wear pants, or work at a job.

When AL presented to our clinic, we initiated an aggressive limb reduction program that resulted in the removal of nearly 100 pounds of fluid in less than a 2-week period. Following aggressive reduction, the leg was wrapped and eventually fitted with a strong, high-compression elastic stocking. Using a simple treatment regimen consisting of overnight leg elevation and wrapping and daily use of this stocking whenever upright, AL was able to dress himself, ambulate, and work again. Although the affected limb was still considerably larger than its mate, we considered the combination of "substantial improvement" and "minimal therapy" to be a satisfactory outcome. The patient agreed.

Being conscientious practitioners, we arranged for follow-up treatment by a lymphedema clinic back in AL's home state. This respected clinic was well known for its highly aggressive lymphedema management, and in retrospect, the ensuing events should not have come as a surprise. When AL presented to this clinic for follow-up, the staff was shocked by how "bad" his treated leg looked. Indeed, to those who had not seen him at his original presentation, the limb looked as bad as many lymphedematous limbs do before therapy. In a well-intended effort to do the right thing, the clinic initiated a very aggressive treatment protocol that successfully reduced the size of the leg even further but required several additional hours of therapy daily. As a result, although AL's leg was smaller, lighter, and prettier, treatment now interfered with his ability to hold down a job and function normally. "Better" lymphedema therapy was decreasing the patient's quality of life.

As this case illustrates, therapy can be a tough balancing act—the more aggressively the edema is controlled, the more intense (and often lifestyle-altering) the treatment. It is important to recognize that the patient and the physician may have vastly different ideas about the ultimate goals of therapy. Treatment needs to be individualized, with particular attention paid to the patient's expectations and desires and how aggressively he or she wishes to be treated. Patients desiring perfection in their edema control must usually accept aggressive, time-consuming, and potentially expensive therapeutic regimens. Those who like their therapy quick and easy will likely have to accept some residual lymphedema. The treatment of lymphedema, perhaps more than any other vascular condition, is a constant reminder that medicine remains—even in this era of evidence-based medicine—more art than science.

Treatment Options

Since ancient times, people have recognized that fluid can be tapped and drained. Although this approach works well for certain types of ascites or pleural effusions, its role in the treatment of lymphedema is minimal. However, one of us recently encountered a patient from eastern Africa with severe lymphedema who had previously been treated in her country. Examination revealed numerous small scars around her ankles and lower legs. These scars were the result of multiple incisions made by local doctors in an effort to drain the fluid from her leg.

A better way to mobilize and remove fluid from edematous limbs is to simply hoist them into the air and allow gravity to drain the fluid through whatever vessels (lymphatics, capillaries) still exist. For decades, patients have been treated at the Mayo Clinic with a contraption called a lymphedema sling.[30] This device consists of a sling that elevates the leg or arm to at least 45 degrees. The patient, who is confined to a hospital bed during therapy, experiences rapid improvement in swelling. Unfortunately, no third-party payer will reimburse for this type of inpatient therapy anymore. Efforts have been made to develop other means of elevating limbs at home, including foam wedges, but these are generally less effective than hospital-based therapies.

Over the past 4 decades, various pneumatic compression pumps have been used for the treatment of lymphedema, and new pumps continue to be developed. In their simplest form, these pumps are single inflatable chambers that encase the entire limb and provide a uniform pressure (often 100 mm Hg or more) that can be applied for several minutes at a time.[31] More sophisticated models use multiple sequentially inflated chambers that squeeze the edema fluid from the limb.[32]

Others types of pumps include cardiac-gaited intermittent pneumatic compression devices[33] and small portable pumps that plug into a car cigarette lighter, so that patients can pump their legs during long commutes. There are even pumps that use mercury-filled cuffs to create tremendously high graduated pressures (depending on limb length, the pressure at the distal end of a long limb may be 500 or 600 mm Hg).[34] Although there has always been concern that such pumps—especially those using extremely high pressures—may damage tissues, clinical experience suggests that this is not a major problem.[31,35] Numerous articles have demonstrated the safety and efficacy of pumps for lymphedema reduction and management.[36]

Another approach uses massage for the reduction and maintenance of limb size.[37] Massage has been used for more than 100 years as a means to control lymphedema. During the 1930s, Vodder developed the technique of manual lymphatic drainage that is still practiced today.[38] This technique (the details of which are beyond the scope of this chapter) uses massage applied to the limbs and trunk in a manner that stimulates lymphatic propulsion and fluid movement.[39] In the 1980s, Foldi incorporated manual lymphatic drainage into a multidisciplinary approach of complex decongestive therapy for lymphedema.[40,41] Today, most massage-based lymphedema treatment programs employ some form of complex decongestive therapy. Although massage appears to be clinically useful, there is a dearth of data on the effectiveness of this modality.

At Mayo, we have made an effort to incorporate both pump and massage types of therapy, choosing between them when a particular method seems better suited for a given patient. For example, patients with adequate financial resources and easy access to a massage therapist may be steered toward a massage-based maintenance program when they leave our clinic. Those who live in rural areas (where massage therapists may be nonexistent) may do better with mechanical pumps. Patients with limited financial resources may conclude that limb elevation and aggressive wrapping are adequate. In some cases, a combination of modalities is best.

Some of the newer pumps encase the trunk and limbs and use scores of individually inflatable chambers that can be programmed to mimic lymphatic massage. The newest generation of pumps may indeed offer the best of both worlds (Fig. 47-6).

Surgical therapies generally fall into two major categories, reduction procedures and lymphatic revascularizations. Reduction procedures (e.g., Charles, Homans) remove edematous skin and subcutaneous tissue in order to reconstruct a smaller, more functional, less disfigured limb.[42,43] These operations have been largely abandoned in our practice due to poor results, although they are still practiced elsewhere (especially in Europe).

Various lymphatic bypass procedures (including lympholymphatic bypass, lymphovenous bypass, and operations using omental lymphatics) have been proposed and attempted.[44-48] We no longer perform these operations because of poor results, but data from other centers are more encouraging.

Liposuction may offer some benefit for patients with chronic lymphedema. Although this approach is not intuitive (one would think that liposuction would disrupt or damage

the few remaining lymphatics and thus worsen edema), studies from Sweden have demonstrated the feasibility of this technique.[49,50] We have performed a limited number of these operations, with relatively good short-term results.

Once a limb has been optimally reduced (using elevation, pumps, massage, elastic compression, or other techniques), it must be maintained at a smaller size. This maintenance almost always involves elastic compression, sometimes with foam padding underneath the wraps. Both high-stretch and low-stretch wraps have their advocates. Whenever possible, patients are encouraged to use compression stockings (30 to 40 mm Hg or higher). Stockings generally have a superior cosmetic appearance to wraps and can be worn all day without the need for constant rewrapping or readjustment. In many cases, compression of 50 to 60 mm Hg (or more) may be necessary to adequately control edema.

Other measures for the maintenance of limb size include nonelastic compression using devices such as the CircAid (CircAid Medical Products, Inc., San Diego, Calif.) and ReidSleeve (Peninsula Medical Supply, Scotts Valley, Calif.). When necessary, pumps and massage can also be incorporated into a regular maintenance program to keep the limb at a reduced size.[51] As noted earlier, expensive, highly aggressive, time-consuming programs may not be necessary for every patient. In general, the simplest maintenance program that adequately controls edema is usually the best. Practitioners must resist the temptation, often egged on by industry sources and advertising, to prescribe aggressive, expensive, or inconvenient therapies for every lymphedema patient.

In addition to the specific edema reduction measures just described, there are adjuvant therapies that may be useful in selected patients. An appropriate diet, particularly one that helps the patient lose weight and control obesity, can be valuable.[52] Many patients with lymphedema report that their edema worsens with a high salt intake; thus, avoiding salt may make the edema easier to manage. Diuretics are generally of little use for true lymphedema,[53] but many patients have comorbidities (e.g., cardiac or renal failure, prolonged dependency) that aggravate their lymphedema and may respond partially to judicious diuretic use. Exercise is useful in most patients with lymphedema, not only for promoting lymphatic drainage but also for controlling obesity.[37,54] In patients with recurrent episodes of cellulitis, antibiotics may be useful.[55] We insist that all our patients with lymphedema keep penicillin or a first-generation cephalosporin on hand at home so that they can institute therapy at the first sign of cellulitis. If patients have frequent episodes, prophylactic therapy (typically 1 week out of every month) may be useful.[56] In rare cases, continuous, occasionally rotating antibiotics may be necessary.

Benzopyrones (coumarins) have been touted as drugs that can help patients with lymphedema.[57,58] The mechanism of action of these drugs is somewhat uncertain, but it is thought to involve enhanced mobilization and reabsorption of interstitial proteins. Although initial reports were very promising, more recent data have failed to confirm the beneficial effects.[59] Worse, there appears to be a significant incidence of hepatic complications associated with the use of these drugs.[60] We no longer prescribe them in our practice.

In many centers, specific lymphedema clinics have emerged. The Mayo program began in 1994 as a multidisciplinary effort involving physicians, physical therapists, and nurses from the disciplines of physical medicine and rehabilitation, vascular

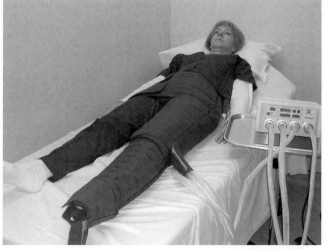

FIGURE 47–6 • Pumps for lymphedema. This pump is coupled to a "body cuff" containing scores of inflatable chambers. By sequentially activating each cell in a predetermined order, the pump can be programmed to simulate lymphatic massage.

medicine, and vascular surgery. The philosophy of our clinic involves many of the concepts outlined in this chapter. These include tailoring treatment to the needs of the individual patient, embracing a generally "conservative" management philosophy, and using many different types of therapy (we have no commitment to any specific modality). When appropriate, we attempt to enter patients into formal studies or protocol-oriented trials.

KEY REFERENCES

Browse NL, Burnand KG, Mortimer PS: In Diseases of the Lymphatics. London, Arnold, 2003.

Felty CL, Fahey VA, Rooke TW: Lymphedema. In Cantwell-Gab, Natiello (eds): Vascular Nursing, 4th ed. St. Louis, Elsevier, 2004, pp 33-46.

Schirger A, Gloviczki P: Lymphedema. In Young, Olin, Bartholomew (eds): Peripheral Vascular Diseases, 2nd ed. Mosby-Year Book, 1996, pp 525-537.

REFERENCES

1. Petrek JA, Heelan MC: Incidence of breast carcinoma-related lymphedema. Cancer Suppl 83:2776-2781, 1998.
2. Lymphatic filariasis: Report of a WHO expert committee. WHO Tech Rep Ser 702:1-112, 1984.
3. Guyton AC: Human Physiology and Mechanisms of Disease. Philadelphia, WB Saunders, 1982.
4. Steward FW, Treves N: Lymphangiosarcoma in postmastectomy lymphedema. Cancer 31:284-299, 1981.
5. Witte CL, Wolfe JH: Lymphodynamics and the pathophysiology of lymphedema. In Rutherford RB (ed): Vascular Surgery, 4th ed. Philadelphia, WB Saunders, 1995, pp 1889-1898.
6. Allen EV: Lymphedema of the extremities. Arch Intern Med 54:606, 1934.
7. Kenmonth JB, Taylor GW, Tracy GD, et al: Primary lymphoedema: Clinical and lymphangiographic studies of a series of 107 patients in which the lower limbs were affected. Br J Surg 45:1-10, 1957.
8. Wolfe JH: The prognosis and possible cause of severe primary lymphedema. Ann R Coll Surg Engl 66:251–257, 1984.
9. Dandapat MC, Mahapatro SK, Dash DM: Management of chronic manifestations of filariasis. J Indian Med Assoc 84:219, 1986.
10. Tan TJ, Kosin E, Tan TH: Lymphographic abnormalities in patients with Brugia malayi filariasis and "idiopathic tropical eosinophilia." Lymphology 18:169, 1985.
11. Abe R, Kimura M, Airosaki A, et al: Retroperitoneal lymphangiomyomatosis with lymphedema of the legs. Lymphology 13:62–67, 1980.
12. Majeski J: Lymphedema tarda. Cutis 38:105-107, 1985.
13. Reed BR, Burke S, Bozeman M, et al: Lymphedema of the lower abdominal wall in pregnancy. J Am Acad Dermatol 12:930-932, 1985.
14. Brunning J, Gibson AG, Perry M: Oedema bleu: A reappraisal. Lancet 1:810-812, 1980.
15. Kyle VM, DeSilvia M, Hurst G: Rheumatoid lymphedema. Clin Rheumatol 1:126, 1982.
16. Solomon LM, Esterly NB: Epidermal and other congenital organoid nevi. Curr Probl Pediatr 6:3-56, 1968.
17. Spittel JA, Schirger A: Edema, peripheral. In Taylor RB (ed): Difficult Diagnoses. Philadelphia, WB Saunders, 1984, pp 130-137.
18. Adamicova K, Vana J, Celec J, et al: Massive localized lymphedema: A reactive lesion stimulating liposarcoma. Cesk Patol 38:125-128, 2002.
19. Jadjis NS, Carr DH, Banks L, et al: The role of CT in the diagnosis of primary lymphedema of the lower limb. AJR Am J Roentgenol 144:361-364, 1985.
20. Gamba JL, Silverman PM, Ling D, et al: Primary lower extremity lymphedema: CT diagnosis. Radiology 149:218, 1983.
21. Case TC, Witte CL, Witte MH, et al: Magnetic resonance imaging in human lymphedema: Comparison with lymphangioscintigraphy. Magn Reson Imaging 10:549-558, 1992.
22. Kenmonth JB, Taylor GW, Harpen RK: Lymphangiography: A technique for its clinical use in the lower limb. BMJ 1:940-942, 1955.
23. O'Brien BM, Das SK, Franklin JD, et al: Effect of lymphangiography on lymphedema. Plast Reconstr Surg 68:922-926, 1981.
24. Henze E, Schelbert HR, Collins JD, et al: Lymphoscintigraphy with TC-99 m-labeled dextran. J Nucl Med 23:923-929, 1982.
25. Ohtake E, Matsui K: Lymphoscintigraphy in patients with lymphedema, a new approach using intradermal injections of technetium-99 m human serum albumin. Clin Nucl Med 11:474-478, 1986.
26. Howarth D, Gloviczki P: Lymphoscintigraphy of lymphangiectasia. J Nucl Med 39:1635-1638, 1998.
27. Schirger A, Peterson LFA: Lymphedema. In Allen EV, Barker NW, Hines EA (eds): Peripheral Vascular Diseases. Philadelphia, Saunders, 1980, pp 823-851.
28. Young JR, Gifford RW: Lymphedema of the extremities. In Spittell JA Jr (ed): Clinical Medicine, vol 6. Philadelphia, JB Lippincott, 1983.
29. Stewart FW, Treves N: Lymphangiosarcoma in postmastectomy lymphedema: A report of six cases in elephantiasis chirurgica. Cancer 1:64-81, 1948.
30. Schirger A: Lymphedema. Cardiovasc Clin 13:293–305, 1983.
31. Thiadens SRJ: Advances in the management of lymphedema. In Goldstone J (ed): Perspectives of Vascular Surgery. St. Louis, Quality Medical Publishing, 1990, pp 125-141.
32. Zelikovski A, Manoach M, Giler S, et al: Lymphapress. Lymphology 13:68, 1980.
33. Rooke TW: Lymphedema: Medical and physical therapy. In Gloviczki P, Yao JST (eds): Handbook of Venous Disorders. London, Chapman & Hall, 1996, pp 601-617.
34. Palmar A, Macchiaverna J, Braun A, et al: Compression therapy of limb edema using hydrostatic pressure of mercury. Angiology 42:533, 1991.
35. Eliska O, Eliskova M: Are peripheral lymphatics damaged by high pressure manual massage? Lymphology 28:21-30, 1995.
36. Richmand DM, O'Donnell TF, Zelikovski A: Sequential pneumatic compression for lymphedema: A controlled trial. Arch Surg 120:1116, 1985.
37. Kubik S: The Lymphatic System. New York, Springer, 1985.
38. Vodder E: Le drainage lymphatique, une novvelle methode therapeutique. In Revue d' Hygiene Individuelle: Sante' pour Tous. Paris, 1936.
39. Foldi E, Foldi M, Clodius L: The lymphedema chaos: A lancet. Ann Plast Surg 22:505, 1989.
40. Foldi M: Physiology and pathophysiology of lymph flow. In Clodius L (ed): Lymphedema. Stuttgart, Georg Thieme, 1977, pp 1-11.
41. Boris M, Weindorf S, Lasinski B, et al: Lymphedema reduction by noninvasive complex lymphedema therapy. Oncology (Huntingt) 8:109-110, 1994.
42. Charles RH: Elephantiasis scroti. In Latham A, English TC (eds): A System of Treatment, vol 3. London, J & A Churchill, 1912, p 416.
43. Miller TA: A surgical approach to lymphedema. Am J Surg 134:191-195, 1977.
44. Gloviczki P, Fisher J, Hollier LH, et al: Microsurgical lymphovenous anastomosis for treatment of lymphedema: A critical review. J Vasc Surg 7:647-652, 1988.
45. Campisi C, Boccardo F, Tacchella M: Reconstructive microsurgery of lymph vessels: The personal method of lymphatic-venous-lymphatic (LVL) interpositioned grafted shunt. Microsurgery 16:161-166, 1995.
46. Campisi C, Boccardo F, Alitta P, et al: Derivative lymphatic microsurgery: Indications, techniques, and results. Microsurgery 16:463-468, 1995.
47. Baumeister RG, Siuda S, Bhomert H, et al: A microsurgical method for reconstruction of interrupted pathways: Autologous lymph-vessel transplantation for treatment of lymphedemas. Scand J Plast Reconstr Surg 20:141-146, 1986.
48. Egorov YS, Abalmosov KG, Ivanov VV, et al: Autotransplantation of the greater omentum in the treatment of chronic lymphedema. Lymphology 27:137-143, 1994.
49. O'Brien B, Khazanchi RK, Kumar PA, et al: Liposuction in the treatment of lymphedema: A preliminary report: Br J Plast Surg 42:530-533, 1989.
50. Brorson H, Svensson H, Norrgren K, et al: Liposuction reduces arm lymphedema without significantly altering the already impaired lymph transport. Lymphology 31:156-172, 1998.
51. Rooke TW: Lymphedema: Medical and physical therapy. In Gloviczki P, Yao JST (eds): Handbook of Venous Disorders. London, Chapman & Hall, 1996, pp 600-626.
52. Rooke TW, Gloviczki P, Gamble GL: Nonoperative management of chronic lymphedema. In Rutherford RB (ed): Vascular Surgery, 4th ed. Philadelphia, WB Saunders, 1995, pp 1920-1927.
53. Foldi E, Foldi M, Weissleider H: Conservative treatment of lymphedema of the limbs. Angiology 36:171, 1985.
54. Schirger A, Peterson LFA: Lymphedema. In Juergens JL, Spittell JA, Fairbairn JF II (eds): Peripheral Vascular Diseases. Philadelphia, WB Saunders, 1980, pp 823-851.
55. Gloviczki P: Treatment of secondary lymphedema. In Ernst CB, Stanley JB (eds): Current Therapy in Vascular Surgery, 2nd ed. Philadelphia, BC Deck, 1991, pp 1030-1036.
56. Babb RR, Spittell JA Jr, Marton WJ, et al: Prophylaxis of recurrent lymphangitis complicating lymphedema. JAMA 195:871-873, 1966.

57. Piller NB: Conservative treatment of acute and chronic lymphedema with benzopyrones. Lymphology 9:132, 1976.
58. Casley-Smith JR, Morgan RG, Piller NB: Treatment of lymphedema of the arms and legs with 5,6-benzo-α-pyrone. N Engl J Med 329:1158-1163, 1993.
59. Loprinzi CL, Kugler JW, Sloan JA, et al: Lack of effect of coumarin in women with lymphedema after treatment for breast cancer. N Engl J Med 340:346-350, 1999.
60. Cox D, O'Kennedy R, Thomas RD: The rarity of liver toxicity in patients treated with coumarin (1,2-benzopyrone). Hum Toxicol 8:501-506, 1989.

Questions

1. **Which of the following statements is true?**
   (a) Lymphedema is rare in the United States
   –(b) Lymphedema affects up to 100 million people worldwide
   (c) Lymphedema never complicates operations performed by careful, sober surgeons
   (d) Lymphedema is always easy to distinguish from other causes of swelling

2. **Which of the following statements is true of lymphatic vessels?**
   (a) They remove extravasated protein from the interstitial space
   (b) They return lymph fluid to the circulation via the thoracic duct
   (c) They may cause lymphedema when they become obstructed or develop reflux
   – (d) All of the above

3. **What is the correct term for primary lymphedema that develops around the time of puberty?**
   –(a) Lymphedema praecox
   (b) Milroy disease
   (c) Secondary lymphedema
   (d) Lymphedema tarda

4. **Secondary lymphedema is not caused by which of the following?**
   (a) Tumor
   (b) Trauma
   –(c) Steroids
   (d) Infection

5. **The most common cause of lymphedema worldwide is which of the following?**
   (a) Autoimmune disease
   (b) Pregnancy
   –(c) Filarial disease
   (d) Cellulitis

6. **The clinical features of classic, chronic lymphedema do not include which of the following?**
   –(a) Very soft, easily pitting edema
   (b) Verrucous skin changes
   (c) Square toes
   (d) Swelling of the foot or hand

7. **Which of the following imaging modalities may be helpful for assessing swollen limbs?**
   (a) Duplex ultrasonography
   (b) Computed tomography scan
   (c) Lymphoscintigraphy
   –(d) All of the above

8. **Which of the following statements is true of lymphangiography?**
   (a) It usually gives poor-quality images
   (b) It is technically difficult to perform
   (c) It is less likely to injure the lymphatic vessels than is lymphoscintigraphy
   (d) All of the above

9. **What is the least common reason for treating lymphedema?**
   (a) Improve cosmetic appearance
   (b) Improve mobility of the limb
   –(c) Alleviate pain
   (d) Prevent the occurrence of future problems

10. **What is the most inappropriate method for treating lymphedema?**
    (a) Massage
    (b) Pump
    (c) Elastic compression
    –(d) Coumarin

Answers

1. b	2. d	3. a	4. c	5. c
6. a	7. d	8. b	9. c	10. d

48

Peter F. Lawrence • Deborah R. Caswell

The Wound Care Center and Limb Salvage

Knowledge about the management of wounds has become a distinct specialty with a unique knowledge base. Normal wound and nonhealing wound physiology, products to accelerate wound healing, and new therapies for the treatment of recalcitrant wounds are the province of specialized wound care centers. Much of the literature and research regarding wound healing are not published in traditional surgical or medical journals, and new methods of treatment are often reported in nonsurgical journals and textbooks, so vascular surgeons may not be familiar with them.

How does the knowledge of wound healing relate to the practice of vascular surgery and limb salvage? In many institutions, vascular surgeons are consulted about the management of wounds. This new role in managing wounds has occurred for several reasons:

1. One of the most common clinical presentations for patients with peripheral arterial disease is a nonhealing ischemic wound. Although revascularization may be required for limb salvage, the management of the wound after surgery determines whether the limb will actually be salvaged, as well as how much time it will take for the patient to return to function. Wound care after revascularization may be required for months or even years. A nonhealing wound may lead to limb loss, even if revascularization has been successful.
2. Patients with peripheral arterial disease who have limb-threatening ischemia often have diabetes as a comorbidity. Lower extremity ulcers are common in diabetics, and they may develop during the course of treatment. Knowledge about the causes of diabetic ulcers and the unique methods of managing diabetic wounds fits within the scope of a vascular practice more than any other specialty.
3. In the process of limb salvage, vascular surgeons often create wounds in ischemic limbs when harvesting vein and arterial conduits and exposing distal vessels. These newly created wounds occasionally result in graft exposure, infection, or delayed return to normal activity.

Knowledge about the methods of minimizing the risk of creating wounds in ischemic limbs and the management of them is the province of vascular surgery.

4. Other surgical specialties, whose physicians used to be trained in wound healing, seldom receive training in contemporary wound management and wound healing, and any training they do receive is often based on outmoded concepts of wound care. Consequently, the specialist with the most exposure to nonhealing wounds, the vascular surgeon, has become the local expert in wound healing.

Normal Wound Healing

Wound healing is a complex process, the details of which we are only beginning to understand. Ideally, wound healing involves a well-organized, multifaceted series of events beginning after the wounding event and ending with the formation of mature scar tissue (Fig. 48-1). The acute wound is caused by external trauma, and acute wounds heal within a predictable time frame by progressing through orderly phases. Chronic wounds, however, do not follow this predictable course of events and may be caused or impeded by internal events. Correction of the internal problem does not always guarantee that the wound will heal in a timely fashion. Health care providers are just beginning to comprehend the complex cellular and biologic abnormalities that are inherent in a wound that has failed to heal.

Much of the latest research on wound healing involves investigation of the effects of various cytokines, growth factors, proteinases, and their regulators and how they control the process of wound healing (Fig. 48-2). To understand the effect of these substances on chronic wounds, the normal healing process of acute wounds must be understood. In acute wounds, the healing process begins with tissue injury and progresses predictably through the four phases of wound healing: hemostasis, inflammation, proliferation, and remodeling. These stages of healing, although occurring in a predictable manner, can overlap and can last for months.

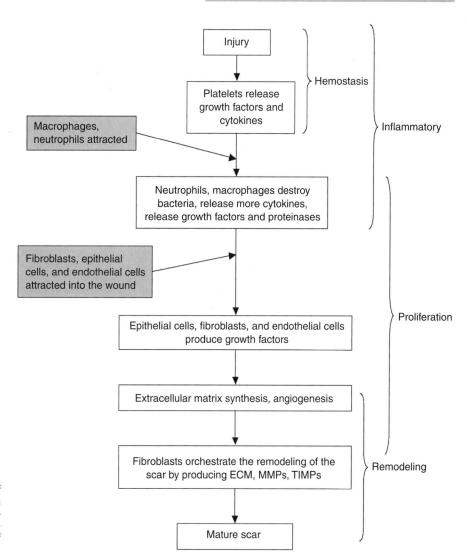

FIGURE 48–1 • The normal process of wound healing is complex and involves a series of phases that overlap. ECM, extracellular matrix; MMP, matrix metalloproteinase; TIMP, tissue inhibitors of metalloproteinase.

ACUTE WOUNDS

Hemostasis

At the time of the initial injury, platelet activation and vasoconstriction occur following injury to the endothelium. Platelet aggregation, vasoconstriction, and clot formation

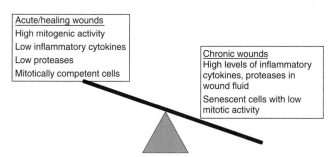

FIGURE 48–2 • Balance of healing and nonhealing factors in wounds. (Adapted from Schultz GS, Sibbald G, Falanga V, et al: Wound bed preparation: A systematic approach to wound management. Wound Repair Regen 11:1-28, 2003.)

begin the process of hemostasis. A number of soluble mediators are released by the platelets, including platelet-derived growth factor (PDGF), insulin-derived growth factor-1 (IGF-1), epidermal growth factor (EGF), fibroblast growth factor (FGF), and transforming growth factor-β (TGF-β). These mediators are responsible for initiating the healing process. Growth factors stimulate the proliferation of wound cells, act as chemotactant agents, and regulate the differentiated functions of wound cells.[1] Neutrophils and macrophages are recruited to the injured site, attracted by the release of chemotactant by the platelets.

Inflammation

Aggregated platelets begin to degranulate, and mediators that help form the fibrin clot are released. Initially, in the inflammatory phase, there is significant vasodilatation, increased capillary permeability, complement activation, and migration of polymorphonuclear leukocytes and macrophages to the site of the wound. The antimicrobial defense and removal of devitalized tissue are initiated by the macrophages and polymorphonuclear leukocytes. As they engulf and destroy bacteria, proteases are released, including elastase and collagenase, which begin the degradation process of the damaged extracellular matrix (ECM) components.

Along with their role in defense and débridement, macrophages and neutrophils induce the formation of granulation tissue by secreting growth factors that stimulate fibroblast proliferation (platelet-derived growth factor [PDGF]), collagen synthesis (transforming growth factor-β [TGF-β]), and new blood vessel formation (fibroblast growth factor [FGF]). The cytokine interleukin-B (IL-B) stimulates the proliferation of fibroblasts, and tumor necrosis factor-α (TNF-α) and IL-1B stimulates fibroblasts to synthesize matrix metalloproteinases (MMPs).

Proliferation

The proliferative phase begins as the number of inflammatory cells in the wound bed decreases. The synthesis of growth factors continues in the wound bed but is taken over by the fibroblast, endothelial cells, and keratinocytes. Keratinocytes synthesize TGF-β, TGF-α, and IL-1. Fibroblasts secrete basic FGF, TGF-β, PDGF, keratinocyte growth factor, and connective tissue factor. Endothelial cells produce basic FGF, PDGF, and vascular endothelial growth factor. The process of cell migration and proliferation continues as the process of new capillary formation and synthesis of ECM components begins.

Fibrin and fibronectin form a provisional wound bed matrix. New collagen and elastin and proteoglycan molecules that form the initial scar are synthesized by fibroblasts. Proteases carry out an essential role at this point. No integration of the newly formed matrix with the dermal matrix can occur until the damaged proteins in the existing matrix are removed. Neutrophils, macrophages, fibroblasts, epithelial cells, and endothelial cells secrete proteases. Key proteases include collagenases, gelatinases, and stromelysins, which are all members of the MMP superfamily, as well as neutrophil elastase, a serine protease.

In the wound bed, cell proliferation and the formation of new ECM continue and are sustained by a dramatic increase in the vascularity of the wound bed. The epidermal layer is re-formed by the proliferation and migration of epithelial cells across the highly vascularized ECM.

Remodeling

Once the initial scar is formed, the synthesis of ECM continues for several weeks. The newly healed red, raised scar changes over the course of weeks to months to a scar that is less red and may be barely visible. At the cellular and molecular levels, the breakdown of ECM components reaches a balance with the process of ECM synthesis, allowing remodeling to occur. The increased concentration of fibroblasts and capillaries present in the early phase of healing declines, primarily through apoptosis. In the final remodeling phase, tensile strength reaches a maximum of 80% of the initial strength, as cross-linking of collagen fibrils plateaus.

CHRONIC WOUNDS

In contrast to an acute wound, a chronic wound does not heal in a predictable fashion. Lazarus and coworkers defined a chronic wound as one in which the normal process of healing has been disrupted at one or more points in the phases of hemostasis, inflammation, proliferation, and remodeling.[2] Chronic ulcers are characterized by defective remodeling of the ECM, a failure to epithelialize, and prolonged inflammation.[3-5] In a chronic wound, fibroblasts do not readily respond to growth factors such as PDGF-β and TGF-β; this failure to respond is hypothesized to be due to a form of cellular senescence. Hyperproliferation at the wound margin interferes with normal cellular migration across the wound bed, probably due to inhibition of apoptosis within the fibroblasts and keratinocyte cells.[6,7]

Because the phases of wound healing are replete with factors that play important roles in the progression of wound healing, it follows that any alteration in one or more of these components may interfere with the healing process. Growth factors such as PDGF, EGF, basic FGF and TGF-β are present in a chronic wound, but the levels remain constant rather than displaying the variation seen in normal acute wound healing. The proinflammatory cytokines such as IL-1, IL-6, and TNF-α remain elevated in chronic wounds when compared with normal acute wounds; in the latter, a dramatic decrease is seen during healing as there is a reduction in the inflammatory state.[8]

Several studies have shown that chronic wounds become "stuck" in the inflammatory phase of the wound healing process.[9-11] The inflammatory phase is most often associated with an increased amount of exudate, postulated to be from infection, heavy colonization, or reaction to increased necrotic tissue in the wound bed. The amount of fluid produced by a chronic wound can severely impede and even reverse the healing process.[12-15] In addition to the amount of exudate produced, the altered components in the fluid are a factor.

Studies investigating the effluent of fluid from chronic wounds have provided evidence that the cellular and molecular environments are substantially altered in chronic wounds. Bucalo and associates collected exudate from venous ulcers and examined the effects of chronic wound fluid on the proliferation of dermal fibroblasts, microvascular endothelial cells, and keratinocytes in culture.[12] This study found that in addition to being cytotoxic, wound fluid inhibited or failed to stimulate the proliferation of dermal fibroblasts, endothelial cells, and keratinocytes. Fluid from acute wounds, in contrast, has been found to stimulate fibroblast proliferation.[16] Proteases in chronic wound fluid have also been shown to degrade growth factors such as PDGF and TGF-1.[17,18]

It is known that MMPs are a necessary component of the wound healing process and play an important role in cell migration and modification of the ECM. If the regulation of these protease molecules is disrupted, they may be produced in excessive amounts and lead to degradation of the ECM, preventing cellular migration and attachment and ultimately causing tissue destruction.[8] It has been shown that levels of MMP activity are significantly elevated in a high percentage of chronic wounds when compared with acute wounds, suggesting that in chronic wounds there is disruption of the usual mechanism controlling the levels of these enzymes (Fig. 48-3). The activity of these proteases decreases consistently in patients whose ulcers progress from a nonhealing to healing phase.[19]

A chronic wound can also be heavily colonized or infected by bacteria that can substantially increase the amount of exudate. Thus, a copious amount of exudate produced by chronic wounds, whatever its cause, can be a barrier to healing.[10,12,14,15]

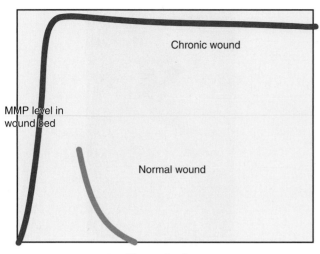

FIGURE 48–3 • Matrix metalloproteinase (MMP) levels in wound fluid remain high in patients with chronic nonhealing wounds, whereas they recede in a normal wound.

Assessment of Wound Healing Capability

With the recognition that there are altered cellular and molecular processes at play in the chronic wound has come the realization that wound management must focus on both the wound and the patient as a whole. The goal of wound management is to attain a healthy, well-vascularized, granulating wound bed. For this to happen, factors that can impede healing must be addressed. The way in which chronic wounds are viewed and managed should be based on a model that is both different from the acute wound paradigm and representative of the complex nature of nonhealing wounds.[20]

Wound bed preparation has become part of the standard nomenclature in wound healing. Sibbald[13] and Falanga[11] define the concept of wound bed preparation as the management of a wound in order to accelerate endogenous healing or to facilitate the effectiveness of other therapeutic measures. The main barriers to healing in a chronic wound are necrotic tissue, high bioburden, increased exudate, and altered composition of exudate. The goal of wound bed preparation is to remove or reduce these barriers to promote healing. This is accomplished by ongoing débridement, reduction of bacterial burden in the wound bed, and management of exudate.

PATIENT ASSESSMENT

Identification of patient factors that might impede healing is an essential component of the healing paradigm. The presence of diabetes, renal disease, heart disease, or liver disease can have detrimental effects of wound healing. Autoimmune diseases such as scleroderma, rheumatoid arthritis, vasculitis, or lupus erythematosus also deter wound healing. Systemic steroids, immunosuppressant medications, and nonsteroidal anti-inflammatory drugs can interfere with the healing wound as well.

The nutritional status of the patient is an important factor in wound healing. Protein calorie malnutrition can have devastating effects on the integrity of the body and on any

wounds the patient may have. In patients with protein-calorie malnutrition—defined as insufficient intake of both protein and calories—morbidity and mortality increase as a result of the proportionate decline in body weight.[21] A decrease in lean body mass greater than 10% is associated with compromised wound healing, despite therapeutic interventions. Once depletion of lean body mass reaches 30%, the wound becomes a secondary issue as the body seeks to restore and replenish lost muscle.[22] Correction of any nutritional deficit should begin at the first visit and be maintained throughout the wound healing process. Assessment of dietary intake, including vitamin supplementation, is a necessary part of any wound healing evaluation. Appetite stimulants, such as Megace, may be helpful. If the assessment shows moderate to severe protein-calorie malnutrition, supplementation with oxandrolone has been shown to be beneficial in restoring lean muscle mass.[23]

ASSESSMENT OF WOUND CHARACTERISTICS

Accurate assessment of the wound and a determination of its cause must be accomplished before instituting a plan of care. Significant harm can occur if an incorrect treatment strategy is implemented; for example, active pyoderma gangrenosum should not be débrided, and ischemic wounds should not be compressed. Information from the patient regarding the wound should be obtained, if possible. How long has the wound been present? How did it start? What has been the progression? How much pain exists? What aggravates or relieves the pain? What associated diseases does the patient have (e.g., peripheral arterial or coronary artery disease, type 1 or 2 diabetes, rheumatoid arthritis)?

Assessment of the wound should include the location, size, depth, and color of the wound bed (Table 48-1). A cotton swab can accurately gauge the depth and involvement of deep structures. The depth of a wound can be used to predict the likelihood of healing without extensive débridement of tendon or bone. The most common classification system of diabetic lower extremity wounds is the Wagner system, which grades the depth from superficial skin involvement to deep wounds involving tendon and bone.

These variables should be photographed, measured, and recorded. The amount and type of exudate should also be assessed. Associated signs such as callous surrounding the ulcer, skin changes in the gaiter (ankle) distribution, peripheral neuropathy, and ischemic (trophic) changes should also be noted and recorded.

TABLE 48–1	Documentation of Wound Characteristics
Characteristic	**Observations to Be Documented**
Wound size	Length, width, depth, area, volume
Undermining	Presence, location, measurement
Appearance	Granulation tissue, sloughing, necrotic, eschar, friability
Exudate	Amount, color, type (serous, serosanguineous, sanguineous, purulent), odor
Wound edge	Presence of maceration, advancing epithelium, erythema, even, rolled, ragged

DIAGNOSTIC STUDIES

There are three questions that need to be answered with diagnostic studies:

1. How deep is the wound?
2. Is the wound infected?
3. Is the limb ischemic, and does it have adequate blood flow to heal the wound?

Depth determines treatment, because involvement of deep structures such as tendon or bone reduces the likelihood of healing without removal of the deep tissues and increases the risk of the infection ascending along tendon sheaths. Subfascial infection is particularly worrisome in diabetic patients who have reduced sensation of the foot and a reduced ability to fight infection. The simplest test of depth is to probe the wound to determine whether tendon or bone is involved. This inexpensive and simple method has been shown to be as reliable as more expensive tests in determining the presence of osteomyelitis. Other tests such as plain radiography and bone scanning have less sensitivity and specificity than does magnetic resonance imaging (MRI) (Fig. 48-4). All these tests can produce false-negative and false-positive results, so surgical exploration is often necessary to determine the presence of deep infection and osteomyelitis, as well as to débride and culture the wound.

The differentiation among colonization, cellulitis, abscess, and osteomyelitis is critical for optimal wound management. Wound culture identifies the organism or organisms and determines the need for topical, oral, or intravenous antibiotics. Colonization is often reflected by a wound culture that has multiple skin organisms. In colonization, there are no clinical signs of infection, such as erythema, swelling, and pain. Tissue biopsy and culture quantitate the number of organisms and determine whether the organisms are merely on the surface of the wound or are present in the deep tissue, which implies an invasive infection and the need for more vigorous treatment. Plain films of the bone in a patient with osteomyelitis become positive in the late stages, long after osteomyelitis is established, whereas MRI is a reliable method of detecting early signs of osteomyelitis, such as changes in marrow intensity, periosteal reaction, and cortical erosion.

Adequate tissue oxygenation must be present for wound healing. Oxygen is available bound to hemoglobin and dissolved in plasma. In chronic wounds, plasma-dissolved oxygen can be adequate for wound healing, assuming that perfusion of the tissue is satisfactory.

Assessment of the large vessel vascular supply is a critical component of the examination. A palpable pulse indicates a blood pressure of greater than 80 mm Hg in the foot and 70 mm Hg in the hand.[24] If a pulse is not easily palpable, a vascular laboratory examination is essential. Doppler waveforms, ankle-brachial index (ABI), and plethysmography (Fig. 48-5; see color plate) can be used with transcutaneous oxygen partial pressure ($TcPO_2$) and skin perfusion pressure to determine the adequacy of the blood supply. An ABI of less than 60 mm Hg in diabetics and less than 40 mm Hg in nondiabetics is associated with a low likelihood of healing. In patients with falsely elevated "stiff" arteries (high ABI with poor Doppler signals), pulse-volume recordings, Doppler waveforms, and toe pressures have greater reliability.

Normal acute wounds usually have oxygen tensions of 60 to 90 mm Hg, whereas chronic nonhealing wounds are most often associated with varying degrees of hypoxia due to

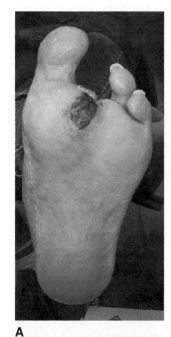

A

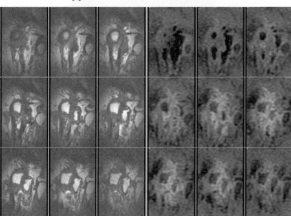

B

FIGURE 48–4 • *A,* Foot with a superficial ulcer needs further diagnostic studies to determine the depth of the wound. *B,* MRI of the foot shows the depth of the wound and evidence of osteomyelitis even when it is not clinically apparent.

low oxygen tension and poor blood perfusion. A tissue oxygen tension greater than 40 mm Hg is adequate for wound healing. Tissue oxygen levels less than 20 mm Hg in the wound bed are usually associated with failure to heal. When there is inadequate blood flow or perfusion pressure for wound healing, treatment must be directed at increasing the perfusion by revascularization.

Treatment of Nonhealing Wounds

ELIMINATION OF EDEMA

Edema reduces microvascular blood flow and the clearance of bacteria and protein from the wound. Its impact is to eliminate or reduce the likelihood of healing, and until edema is eliminated, other management is often futile. The most challenging wounds are those with edema and ischemia, because patients with limb ischemia often place the limb in a dependent position to relieve ischemic rest pain. Prolonged dependency increases the limb edema and reduces perfusion, which

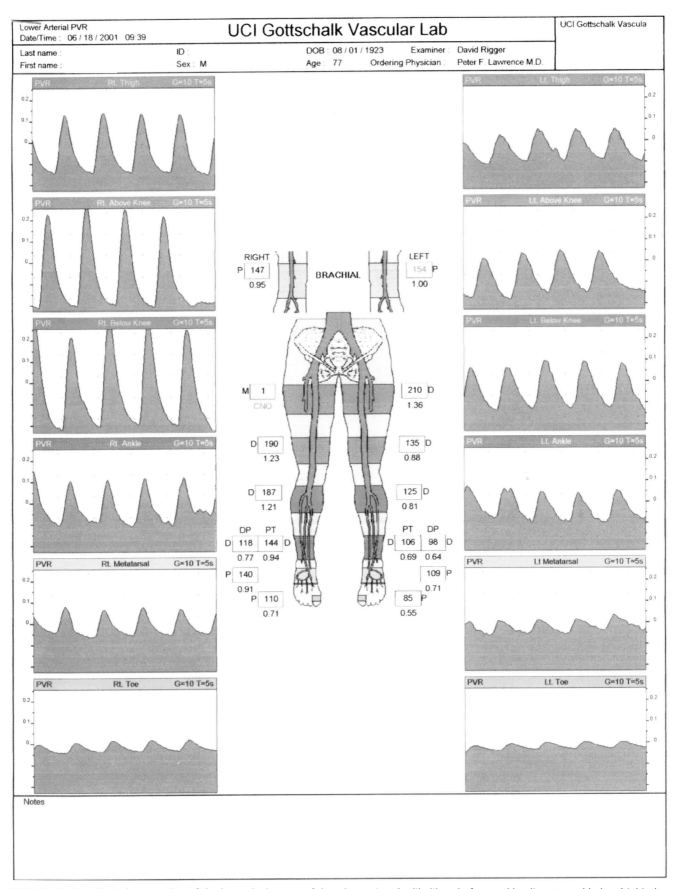

FIGURE 48–5 • Physiologic studies of the lower limb are useful to determine the likelihood of wound healing. An ankle-brachial index (ABI) greater than 0.6 and biphasic or triphasic Doppler waveforms suggest a high likelihood of healing, whereas an ABI less than 0.4 and monophasic waveforms indicate that the likelihood of healing is low.

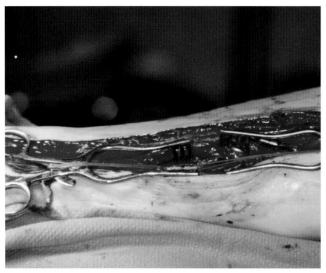

FIGURE 48–9 • Incisions made in the distal part of an ischemic limb are at significant risk for infection or dehiscence. An alternative is to harvest a more proximal vein and tunnel it distally.

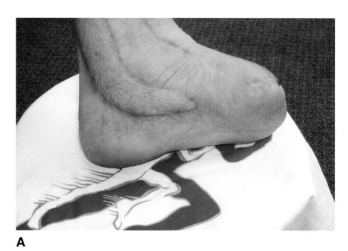

A

FIGURE 48–10 • *A,* This patient received a radial flow-through flap to cover a large medial ankle wound. The bypass was from the midcalf posterior tibial artery to the inframalleolar posterior tibial artery. A transmetatarsal amputation was also performed.

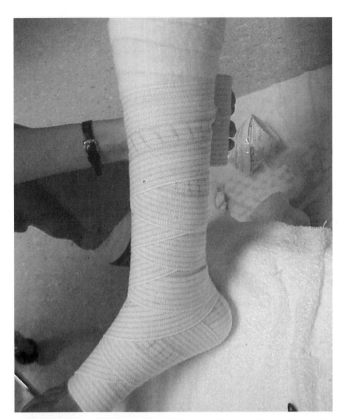

FIGURE 48–6 • Compression with a multilayered wrap is useful to reduce edema, if there is adequate perfusion. An ankle-brachial index greater than 0.8 or an ankle pressure greater than 80 mm Hg is recommended with the use of three- or four-layer wraps, because they create 30 to 40 mm Hg pressure.

of wound treatment. Efficient removal of devitalized tissue (necrotic burden) is an essential step in chronic wound management. The underlying pathogenic abnormalities in chronic wounds cause a continual buildup of necrotic tissue, and regular débridement is necessary to reduce the necrotic burden and achieve healthy granulation tissue. Débridement of devitalized tissue reduces tissue damage and destruction, removes bioburden, and exposes dead space that can harbor bacteria. Débridement can be accomplished in several different ways (Table 48-2), and the method chosen should be based on the condition of the wound and the skill of the practitioner, as well as the patient's situation.

Autolytic Débridement

Autolytic débridement uses the body's own natural enzymes to dissolve necrotic tissue within the wound and occurs spontaneously to some extent in all wounds. The macrophages and endogenous proteolytic enzymes liquefy and spontaneously separate necrotic tissue and eschar from healthy tissue. Autolytic débridement is most effective in a moist wound environment. Dressings most commonly used for this method include hydrogels and hydrocolloids, both of which can produce a more effective environment for the destruction and phagocytosis of necrotic tissue. Dressings that are occlusive or semiocclusive facilitate contact between the necrotic tissue and the enzymes within the wound. This method of débridement is selective, with very little discomfort, but it is often slow. If there is no improvement in the wound bed within 72 hours, another method of débridement should be employed. This method is inappropriate for a wound that has a significant amount of necrotic debris or is heavily infected.

paradoxically leads to an additional need for dependency. In ischemic limbs, the best method to reduce edema is to elevate the limb above the heart. Compression using sequential devices (e.g., Lympha Press [Mego Afek, Kibbutz Afek, Israel]) wraps (Unna boot or Profore [Smith & Nephew, St. Petersburg, Fla.]), or support hose (at 20 to 40 mm Hg pressure) should be limited to patients with a documented normal ABI greater than 0.8 (Fig. 48-6).

DÉBRIDEMENT

The presence of necrotic tissue in a wound is the most obvious marker of a chronic wound. Reestablishing the balance of cytokines, proteases, and growth factors should be the focus

Enzymatic Débridement

With enzymatic débridement, topical agents are applied to the surface of the wound to chemically disrupt or digest devitalized extracellular proteins present. There are two main preparations used in enzymatic débridement: collagenase (Santyl) and papain-urea (Accuzyme). Collagenase is a partially purified preparation derived from the bacterium *Clostridium histolyticum*. Collagenase has been shown to have specificity for types I and II collagen. It cleaves glycine in endogenous collagen and digests collagen but is not active against keratin, fat, or fibrin. Papain (from papaya fruit) digests necrotic tissue by liquefaction of fibrinous debris, but it is inactive against collagen. Urea, a chemical agent, is an

	Débridement Method			
Characteristic	*Autolytic*	*Surgical*	*Enzymatic*	*Mechanical*
Rapidity of débridement action	4	1	2	3
Tissue specificity	3	2	1	4
Exudate	1	4	2	3
Infection	3	1	4	2
Cost	4	1	3	2

TABLE 48–2 Selection of Wound Débridement Method

1 = most appropriate; 4 = least appropriate.
Adapted from Sibbald RG, Williamson D, Orsted HL, et al: Preparing the wound bed—débridement, bacterial balance and moisture balance. Ostomy Wound Manage 46:14-35, 2000.

activator for papain. Urea also digests nonviable protein, making it more susceptible to proteolysis. Studies have demonstrated that the combination of papain-urea is approximately twice as effective as the enzyme alone.

Alvarez and colleagues showed that papain-urea achieved a better wound response than collagenase, but there was no significant difference in wound closure between the two groups.[24a] Some patients complain of burning when papain-urea is applied, which may limit its use.

Mechanical Débridement

Mechanical débridement is a nonselective method of removing necrotic tissue from the wound using mechanical force. This method can damage healthy tissue in the wound bed and at the margins of the wound and can be extremely painful. Wet-to-dry dressings are the simplest method of mechanical débridement, but this requires frequent dressing changes and therefore higher costs due to increased nursing time. Wet-to-dry débridement involves covering a wound with saline-moistened gauze and allowing it to dry. It is then removed, along with the necrotic tissue that has adhered to the dressing. This method is nonselective and painful because it lifts away viable tissue as well. Strings from the gauze can be left behind in the wound bed, creating further inflammatory reaction to the presence of a foreign body. Wet-to-wet dressings maintain a moistened dressing until removal and accomplish the same results with less destruction of viable tissue.

Pressurized irrigation involves the application of streams of water at high or low pressure to wash away bacteria, foreign matter, and necrotic tissue from the wound. With this method, however, bacteria may be driven even farther into soft tissue.

Whirlpool therapy uses powered irrigation and can be very effective at loosening and removing surface debris, bacteria, necrotic tissue, and exudate from the wound. This technique works well for necrotic wounds in the inflammatory phase but is inappropriate for granulating wounds with fragile endothelial and epithelial cells that may be damaged or removed by the circulating water. There is also the possibility of spread of waterborne infection.

Biosurgical Débridement

Biosurgical débridement involves the use of maggots to remove nonviable tissue from a wound bed. This technique uses sterile maggots applied to the wound bed, covered with a dressing. The maggots then digest necrotic material from the wound bed without damaging the healthy tissue. Maggots also demonstrate the ability to consume bacteria, decreasing the patient's risk of developing infection. The precise mechanism by which the maggots débride the wound and promote healing is not clear. It is speculated that the pH of the wound is changed by the maggots, increasing the bacteriostatic effect. It is thought the maggots also secrete proteolytic enzymes that enhance protein degradation. Despite their effectiveness and encouraging reports on their use for wound healing, some patients complain of increased pain with maggot therapy, and some patients are simply not comfortable using maggots on their wounds.

Sharp Débridement

Surgical (or sharp) débridement if the fastest way to remove devitalized tissue. Removing dead tissue decreases the bacterial burden in the wound bed. Use of a scalpel to remove senescent cells converts a chronic wound into an acute wound within a chronic wound; this has been shown to increase the healing rate of diabetic neurotrophic foot ulcers.[25] The major problem with this form of débridement is that viable as well as nonviable tissue may be removed. This method can also be painful, but the use of a topical or local anesthetic (EMLA cream) can alleviate the discomfort.

TREATMENT OF INFECTION

Bacteria present in the wound bed can be categorized as contamination, colonization, critical colonization, or infection. Contamination is the presence of nonreproducing bacteria in the wound bed; they do not interfere with healing. Colonization is the presence of reproducing bacteria in the wound bed; they are adherent to the surface of the wound but do not impede wound repair. Critical colonization is a step between colonization and infection; replicating bacteria are present in the wound and interfere with wound healing, but patients do not show the typical signs of infection. Treatment is necessary to rid the wound of the bioburden. An infected wound shows signs of delayed healing as well as increased pain, an increased amount of exudate, and a change in the color of the wound bed to friable, red granulation tissue or the absence of granulation tissue, along with odor and purulence. Treatment strategies include sustained-release silver dressings or slow-release iodine formulations such as cadexomer iodine, along with systemic antibiotics.

Chronic wounds are usually colonized with at least three species of microorganisms.[26] The number of bacteria that impede the healing of open wounds is controversial; however, 1×10^5 organisms per gram of tissue has historically been associated with impaired healing.[27,28] The type and pathogenicity of the organisms in a wound bed may be better predictors of the risk of infection than simply the number. Some combinations of bacteria act synergistically to enhance the virulence of a previously benign organism.[28]

Another important factor in infections is the biofilm that is present on some bacteria and can contribute to delayed healing. Biofilm occurs when some bacteria proliferate; they form microcolonies that become attached to the wound bed, secreting a glycocalyx sheath of biofilm that protects the microorganism from systemic antimicrobials.[29]

Treatment of an infected wound should begin without delay. Although antibiotics are useful to prevent the spread of infection in the soft tissue beyond the wound, repeated use of antibiotics in patients with chronic wounds can lead to the development of resistant organisms. Therefore, systemic antibiotics should be used judiciously and should be avoided unless infection is established.[30] Antiseptic agents are useful in the treatment of infected wounds and may be essential.[31] Topical cadexomer iodine and nanocrystalline silver target the bacteria at the cell membrane, cytoplasmic organelle, and nucleic acid level; this combination of actions means that the development of resistant bacteria is improbable. Cadexomer iodine absorbs a significant amount of exudate while slowly releasing iodine into the tissues in a concentration low enough to be bactericidal but not cytotoxic. Cadexomer iodine has been shown to be effective against methicillin-resistant *Staphylococcus aureus* and vancomycin-resistant enterococci.[32,33] Nanocrystalline silver provides an antibacterial dressing that is effective in partial- and full-thickness wounds. The silver is slowly released into the wound bed and maintains an antimicrobial barrier for up to 7 days. Nanocrystalline silver is effective against a number of pathogens, including methicillin-resistant *Staphylococcus aureus* and vancomycin-resistant enterococci.

MANAGEMENT OF THE EXUDATE

Traditionally, it was thought that dry wounds were essential to optimal wound healing in terms of avoiding bacterial overgrowth; however, the medical community has long recognized that wounds heal faster in a closed, moist environment. Eaglstein and colleagues, in 1987, showed that experimentally induced wounds healed 40% faster in a closed, moist environment compared with wounds left exposed to the air.[34] A moist environment has also been shown to facilitate epithelial migration, maintain optimal temperature, decrease pain, and provide a better cosmetic result; however, excess exudate in a chronic wound has an adverse effect on wound healing.[35] The buildup of wound fluid must be managed to minimize the negative biochemical factors, but excessive desiccation slows the migration of epidermal cells and limits epidermal regeneration.[36] Therefore, the optimal dressing controls exudate while maintaining wound bed moisture.

DRESSINGS

Wound dressings are all designed with a specific purpose in mind; many serve more than one purpose, such as having both antimicrobial and absorptive properties. The wound, the patient, and their multiple needs should be considered when choosing a dressing (Table 48-3). Optimal wound care decision making focuses on the need for moist dressings to maintain the healing environment. The Agency for Health Care Policy and Research published guidelines in 1994[36a] for the selection of dressings (Table 48-4).

Hydrogels provide a high level of moisture (70% to 90% water), which is contained in insoluble polymers.[37] Hydrogels are the best choice for dry, sloughing wounds with minimal to moderate levels of exudate. Gels need to be reapplied every 24 to 72 hours, as they are not antibacterial. They are nonadherent and soothing. Wound gels facilitate autolytic débridement.

Hydrocolloids provide an occlusive dressing for the wound bed, forming a matrix gel on contact with the wound exudate. Hydrocolloids are suited to autolytic débridement for

TABLE 48–3	Attributes of Optimal Wound Dressings

Débridement of necrotic tissue
Identification and eradication of infection; reduction of wound contamination
Obliteration of dead space
Absorption of excess drainage
Maintenance of moist wound environment while protecting periwound skin
Provision of thermal insulation
Protection from bacteria and trauma
Promotion of wound healing

mild to moderately exudative wounds, but care should be taken to avoid maceration of the healthy epidermis. Mild antibacterial activity is present within hydrocolloids due to the lowered pH. Occlusion is achieved with foam or a filmsheet backing with adhesive, which can cause an allergic reaction in some patients.[36,38]

Film dressings are ideal in the later stage of wound healing, when there is no significant exudate. They are permeable to water and oxygen while maintaining impermeability to bacteria and water. Foam dressings are appropriate for sloughing, moderately to heavily exudative wounds. Foams come in many forms and sizes. All provide thermal insulation, high absorbency, and a moist environment. Most have a polyurethane backing to prevent excess fluid loss. Hydrofibers are considered in the category with foam dressings, even though visually they are quite different. Hydrofibers are highly absorbent and have good tensile strength. Both foams and hydrofibers can be worn for up to 1 week, are easy to cut to the size and shape of the wound, and do not shed fibers in the wound bed.[39]

Alginates are best used on heavily exudative wounds. They form a gel on contact with the exudate, promoting moist wound healing and autolytic débridement. They are made from brown seaweed. After débridement, they donate calcium to the wound bed, facilitating hemostasis. Silicone dressings are among the first products specifically engineered for the painless removal of dressings from wounds. Silicone dressings have a hydrophobic soft silicone layer that prevents the dressing from adhering to the wound surface. They maintain contact with the wound bed, allowing exudate to pass through and be absorbed, while also allowing antimicrobials or biologically active properties of other dressings to interact with the wound bed.

GROWTH FACTORS

Much of the latest research in wound healing has focused on the development, use, and effect of various cytokines and growth factors on the wound bed. The only readily available growth factor approved by the U.S. Food and Drug Administration (FDA) is PDGF-β, in the form of becaplermin (Regranex). Becaplermin is approved for use in neuropathic ulcers. Steed, in 1995, reported that becaplermin gel improved healing rates in diabetic foot ulcers in 48% of patients, as opposed to 25% of patients in the control group.[40] Other studies have not shown similar results in neuropathic foot ulcers, but the 100-μg dose resulted in 50% complete closure within the prescribed time, compared with 35% of the placebo group.[41] Studies examining becaplermin for use in other types of ulceration, such as pressure ulcers, have not met with the same degree of success.[42]

Autologous platelet-rich plasma (PRP)—a concentration of human platelets in a small volume—has been used in orthopedic, maxillofacial, and plastic surgery. Because it is a concentration of platelets, it is also a concentration of seven fundamental protein growth factors proved to be actively secreted by platelets to initiate wound healing. These growth factors include the three isomers of PDGF (PDGF-αα, PDGF-ββ, and PDGF-αβ), two of the numerous TGF-βs (TGF-β1 and TGF-β2), vascular endothelial factor, and epithelial growth factor.[43] Because PRP is suspended in a small amount of plasma, it also contains fibrin and

| TABLE 48–4 | Selection of Dressings for Chronic Wounds |

	Appearance of Wound Bed				
Dressing	Eschar	Slough—Dry	Slough—Moist	Wet	Pink/Red-Pink, Healthy Granulation/Epithelialization
Hydrogels	++	+++			+++
Hydrocolloids	+	++	++		++
Film dressings			++		++
Calcium alginate			+	++	
Foam			++	++	
Enzymes	+++	+++			+
Antimicrobial (silver, cadexomer iodine)			+++	+++	

fibronectin, cellular adhesion molecules. It is known that the degranulation of platelets with the release of growth factors initiates and facilitates the healing cascade. The active secretion of these growth factors is initiated by the clotting of blood and begins within 10 minutes. More than 95% of the growth factors are secreted within 1 hour; therefore, PRP must be developed in the anticoagulated state and should be used within 1 hour.

The literature has been mixed about the results of PRP, although in maxillofacial, orthopedic, and cosmetic surgery, it has been associated with positive results.[44] After the initial use of PRP-related growth factors, the platelets synthesize and secrete additional growth factors for the remaining 7 days of their life span.[45-52] PRP has also been used in wound healing. Knighton and associates evaluated the use of PRP in patients with wounds of various causes; wounds healed in 15% of controls and in 81% of patients treated with platelet concentrate.[53] Patients whose wounds failed to heal in the control arm were then treated with PRP, and all patients had epithelialization in an average of 7.1 weeks.[53] Currently, two devices used to develop PRP have been cleared by the FDA: Smart PreP (Harvest Technologies, Inc., Plymouth, Mass.) and Platelet Concentration Collection System (PCCS; Implant Innovations, Inc., West Palm Beach, Fla.).

TISSUE TRANSFER

Autologous tissue transfer has been used for many years to cover tissue defects; however, use of autologous tissue creates another tissue defect at the donor site, requires anesthetic, and creates additional pain. The concept of tissue substitutes came from the need to treat large burns with insufficient tissue for skin grafting.[54] This work has extended to wound care, and now there are several choices of skin substitutes. The purpose of a skin substitute is to provide a temporary dressing that is biologically active and accelerates skin tissue regeneration and wound healing by stimulating growth factors and skin cells in the recipient wound bed.[55] Significant progress has been made over the last 10 years in evolving from a simple synthetic material to products that have greater structural and biochemical complexity. Many skin substitutes now closely approximate the biochemical and cellular composition and behavior of the dermal and epidermal structures. The commercially bioengineered skin consists of sheets of biomaterial matrix containing allogeneic cells; these cells are

typically derived from neonatal foreskin, a convenient tissue source with the added advantages of having a higher content of putative keratinocyte stem cells, vigorous cell growth and metabolic activity, and minimal antigenicity.[56,57] The skin substitutes approved for use in vascular and diabetic ulcers include Dermagraft (Smith & Nephew, Inc., Largo, Fla.), a cryopreserved human fibroblastic-derived dermal substitute that is approved for the treatment of diabetic foot ulcers of greater than 6 weeks' duration. Fibroblasts are isolated from neonatal tissue and then cultured on a bioabsorbable polyglactin mesh for 3 weeks. During incubation, the cells secrete matrix proteins, including human dermal collagen, and soluble factors to create a three-dimensional matrix containing human protein that can be used as a dermal replacement.[58,59] Marston and colleagues reported an increase in complete healing with Dermagraft (30% vs. 18%).[60] Another study examining Dermagraft in diabetic foot wounds of long duration showed increased healing at week 12 (71% vs. 14%) compared with the control group treated with saline-soaked gauze.[61] The product must remain frozen before use and requires thawing and rinsing before placement.

Apligraf (Organogenesis Inc., Canton, Mass.) is a bilayered, living skin construct developed to fulfill multiple functions, as does human skin (Fig. 48-7). These functions include providing a barrier against mechanical damage and infection, producing structural and regulatory substances (e.g., growth factors or cytokines), and interacting with the underlying tissue to promote more effective wound repair.[62] Apligraf assimilates allogeneic cultured human skin cells from neonatal foreskin in a full-thickness skin construct that contains both epidermal and dermal layers. The well-differentiated epidermal layer is formed of living human keratinocytes; the dermal layer is formed of living human fibroblasts that are dispersed in a type I bovine-derived collagen matrix.[63,64] Apligraf is approved for use in venous ulcers and diabetic foot ulcers.[65] The pivotal Apligraf study in diabetic foot ulcers was done by Veves and coworkers.[66] This multicenter trial of neuropathic, diabetic, plantar foot ulcers had a 56% complete wound closure rate at 12 weeks, compared with 38% among control patients.

HYPERBARIC THERAPY

Hyperbaric therapy is commonly used for nonhealing wounds, although it is used less frequently in dysvascular patients than

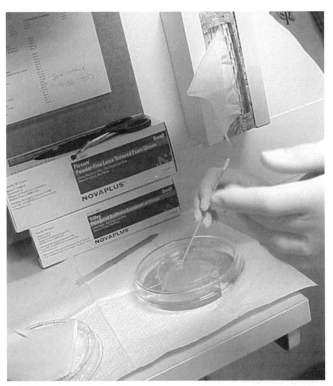

FIGURE 48–7 • Apligraf is a skin and dermal substitute that can be useful in chronic wound coverage once adequate perfusion has been restored (Courtesy of Organogenesis, Canton, Mass.).

in those with diabetes and vasculitides (Fig. 48-8). Medicare recently approved the use of hyperbaric therapy for a single class of wound—the diabetic foot ulcer. However, there is little prospective evidence supporting hyperbaric therapy for dysvascular patients, who benefit more from permanent revascularization than from transient TcPO$_2$ elevation. Patients who are poor revascularization candidates or those with microvascular disease (diabetes or vasculitis) are good candidates for hyperbaric therapy. Before treatment, it

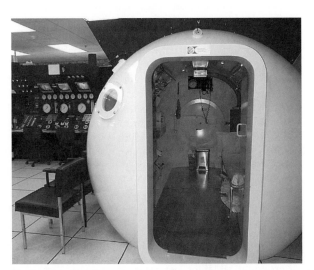

FIGURE 48–8 • A hyperbaric chamber can improve healing in chronic wounds with a low TcPO$_2$ that increases to greater than 30 mm Hg when 100% oxygen is given to the patient.

is incumbent on the hyperbaric center to demonstrate that patients are likely to benefit from hyperbaric therapy. The best and simplest predictor of success is a demonstration that a diminished TcPO$_2$ (<20 mm Hg) is increased to greater than 30 mm Hg with 100% oxygen. If the periwound area shows augmentation with 100% oxygen, the probability of success justifies embarking on an expensive and time-consuming course of hyperbaric therapy. Before treatment, patients must undergo a visual examination and evaluation of the tympanic membrane to avoid complications during therapy.

VACUUM-ASSISTED CLOSURE

The vacuum-assisted closure (VAC) device uses negative pressure to promote wound healing; it has gained increased acceptance in the management of wounds with heavy exudate and edema that cannot be controlled by conventional methods. Use of VAC requires adequate limb perfusion (ABI > 0.6) and absence of osteomyelitis and active infection. The device creates negative pressure and collects drainage from the wound while reducing edema. During therapy, there is assisted contraction of the wound. Large wounds often reduce in size dramatically over a relative short time. The positive experience of physicians and nurses with VAC has led to its use for large wounds in swollen limbs with adequate perfusion.

ALTERNATIVE THERAPIES

Some wounds remain recalcitrant in spite of the established wound care approaches discussed in this chapter. Oral or intravenous steroids are often used for vasculitic ulcers that do not respond to conventional treatment, and occasionally, colectomy is required to heal pyoderma gangrenosum in a patient with ulcerative colitis. There are also some nonapproved options for the treatment of nonhealing wounds, including the Art Assist (ACI Medical, San Marcos, Calif.), an intermittent pneumatic leg compression device used for intermittent claudication that augments limb blood flow; intravenous prostaglandin E or prostacyclin infusion; and oral sildenafil (Viagra). Although none of these therapies has been demonstrated by level 1 evidence to close wounds, they are occasionally used when the only alternative is amputation or a prolonged open, dysvascular wound.

Revascularization in Patients with Nonhealing Wounds

Dysvascular patients with nonhealing wounds present a unique challenge to the vascular surgeon because the process of revascularization is frequently associated with the creation of another wound, exposure to cardiovascular risk, prolonged hospitalization, and further protein-calorie depletion. To determine the need for revascularization in this complex group of patients, a systematic approach must be taken. There are several questions that should be asked to determine the best approach for dysvascular patients with nonhealing wounds:

1. How ischemic is the limb? Patients with mild to moderate ischemia without rest pain, dependent rubor, or infection may be treated less urgently than those with more advanced ischemia. In addition, the method of revascularization does not require the same degree of durability

as in a patient who would need revascularization for limb ischemia even in the absence of a nonhealing wound.

2. What is the level of the disease? Patients with proximal peripheral arterial disease of the iliac arteries are much more easily treated with revascularization procedures than are those with distal infrapopliteal disease. In addition, distal revascularization procedures are often less durable and require an incision in the ischemic limb for either conduit harvest or exposure of the vessels.

3. What conduit is available? For a distal bypass in an ischemic limb that requires long-term patency, the ideal conduit is autogenous vein. Patients who do not have a usable conduit owing to prior harvesting, small size, or prior thrombosis have more limited options.

4. Will the patient have a functional limb if the ulcer is healed with revascularization? To be functional, the patient must have the motivation and strength, adequate plantar skin, and biomechanics to walk. If it is unlikely that the patient will use a revascularized limb, the risks and complexity of the procedure must be weighed against the patient's desire for a cosmetic, nonfunctional limb.

NONSURGICAL TREATMENT

In the presence of mild ischemia, a trial of optimal wound care is a reasonable approach in some patients. Traumatic toe and pressure wounds, particularly in diabetic patients, that are superficial and are not associated with severe preexisting ischemia may heal with relief of pressure, optimal wound care, and patience. Even though these wounds may not heal at the rate seen in a patient without ischemia, if there is otherwise no indication for revascularization, a trial of wound care may be the best option. Rivers and colleagues showed that in a significant number of mildly dysvascular patients, ulcers healed without revascularization using a program of bed rest and wound care.[67]

ANGIOPLASTY

Angioplasty is an attractive option for a patient with a dysvascular, nonhealing wound; it rarely causes additional tissue trauma, such as that which accompanies surgical vessel exposure and vein harvest. Angioplasty alone can often improve perfusion enough to heal a wound. Proximal lesions (iliac and aortic) are optimal for angioplasty or stenting or both; for hemodynamically significant disease that occurs more distally, the durability of angioplasty and stenting is reduced, although some reports have shown excellent early patency rates and results comparable to those achieved with bypass.[68] In the superficial femoral artery, the type of lesion— TransAtlantic Inter-Society Consensus class A, B, or C, based on the length, extent, and degree of calcification of the lesion[69]—determines the likelihood of initial and long-term success. For infrapopliteal disease, Chandra and coworkers recommend angioplasty as the optimal procedure to improve blood flow and heal ischemic ulcers in limbs that do not otherwise require revascularization.[70]

BYPASS

Bypass is the gold standard for patients with limb ischemia and nonhealing wounds. Although an extensive discussion of

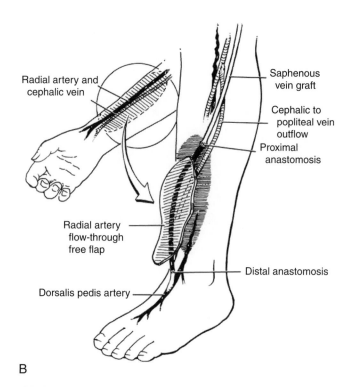

B

FIGURE 48–10 • *B,* A flow-through flap provides an autogenous conduit for bypass, with skin and fat to cover a wound with a large skin defect.

the alternative techniques and conduits is beyond the scope of this chapter, certain principles should be applied when deciding on a revascularization procedure:

1. Limit distal incisions. Kalra and colleagues, in their report on inframalleolar bypass procedures,[71] advised surgeons to limit distal incisions by harvesting more proximal veins and tunneling them distally, to avoid foot and ankle incisions in dysvascular limbs (Fig. 48-9; see color plate). In situ bypasses should be performed with a closed technique, if technically feasible. The LeMaitre valvulotome performs the valvulotomy without an incision to expose the vein. Treiman and associates reported on the management of wound complications in a small series of patients who developed incision complications after distal bypass, as well as alternatives to maintain patency of the exposed graft.[72]

2. Use tissue transfer procedures. In a patient with advanced ischemia who needs both limb revascularization and closure of a large wound, both can often be accomplished with a flow-through flap, using the radial artery or other arterial conduit.[73] This procedure provides a conduit for revascularization with an elliptical flap of attached, vascularized tissue (Fig. 48-10; see color plate for Fig. 48-10A). The radial artery usually matches the size of the distal foot vessel and is optimal for this procedure. If a long conduit is needed for the proximal anastomosis, the saphenous vein can be spliced to the radial artery, although the proximal radial artery anastomosis can usually be placed in a proximal tibial or peroneal artery. Vascularized skin and subcutaneous tissue can then be used to cover large ulcers and skin defects. Other flaps, which can be

anastomosed to a vein conduit, can even provide fascia to reconstruct the Achilles tendon, if needed.

3. Use prosthetic or cryopreserved conduit for ulcer healing. If a dysvascular, nonhealing wound cannot be healed with wound care or angioplasty, a conduit with good short-term patency but poor long-term patency can be used to temporarily provide increased blood supply to heal the wound.[74,75] This alternative should be used only if the rest of the limb does not need long-term revascularization. These grafts often require anticoagulation to maintain patency, and they carry an increased risk of graft infection.

Organization of a Wound Care Program

A critical component of optimal wound care is an integrated program, where continuity can be provided from the hospital to the ambulatory clinic to home health care. Having trained nurses and physicians, access to all specialties, and a facility with the necessary equipment and dressings to provide optimal wound care is the key to a successful wound care program.

PERSONNEL

The most important component of a successful wound care program is personnel. Because wounds often need treatment more than once a week, a typical physician's office is unable to provide the environment for an excellent wound care program. Nurses and physicians with expertise in wound management must be available every day to heal recalcitrant wounds, and they must be available for consultation with home health and visiting nurse services.

The core of most wound care programs is a complement of nurses with training in wound care. Their expertise must include the ability to assess changes in the status of a wound, training in mechanical wound débridement, and knowledge of optimal dressings for different clinical situations. Nurses provide continuity of care for most patients, because physicians often rotate coverage of wound centers and are not available daily. This applies in particular to vascular surgeons, who may be in the operating room for an entire day and thus be unavailable to patients on some days of the week.

Specialists who have expertise in the management of patients with dysvascular or nonhealing wounds are an important component of all wound care centers. Specialists in plastic surgery, orthopedic surgery, podiatry, endocrinology (diabetes), nephrology, infectious diseases, rheumatology, and cardiology are often asked to help manage this group of patients, which tends to have many risk factors and comorbidities.

FACILITY

The optimal wound center has dedicated rooms used to treat patients with wounds. These rooms are designed for patients who are nonambulatory and have special needs. Rooms dedicated for wound care need ready access to a variety of débriding instruments, wound care products, and dressings. Diagnostic facilities, such as plain radiography, foot MRI, and computed tomography, are optimally located close to the wound care center for the patients' convenience. A treatment room for débridement of wounds is also useful. The most expensive equipment for wound care—hyperbaric therapy—is not necessarily required at the center (only a small percentage of wound care patients need such therapy), but it should be readily accessible. Other useful equipment includes a multi-chamber mechanical compression device (e.g., Lymphopress) and a platelet concentrator for PRP.

Conclusion

Wound care and revascularization in dysvascular patients must be inextricably intertwined if limb salvage is to occur. Vascular surgeons are the common link in diagnosing, treating, and coordinating care. To achieve an optimal patient outcome, vascular surgeons must be familiar with the principles of wound healing, the alternatives for wound bed preparation, and the techniques for revascularization in an ischemic limb.

REFERENCES

1. Schultz GS, Sibbald G, Falanga V, et al: Wound bed preparation: A systematic approach to wound management. Wound Repair Regen 11:1-28, 2003.
2. Lazarus GS, Cooper DM, Knighton DR, et al: Definitions and guidelines for assessment of wounds and evaluation of healing. Arch Dermatol 130:489-493, 1994.
3. Hasan A, Murata H, Falabella A, et al: Dermal fibroblasts from venous ulcers are unresponsive to action of transforming growth factor-beta I. J Dermatol Sci 16:59-66, 1997.
4. Argen MS, Steenfos HH, Dalbelsteen S, et al: Proliferation and mitogenic response to PDGF-BB of fibroblasts isolated from chronic leg ulcers is ulcer dependent. J Invest Dermatol 112:463-469, 1999.
5. Cook H, Davies KJ, Harding KG, Thomas DW: Defective extracellular matrix reorganization by chronic wound fibroblasts is associated with alterations in TIMP-1, TIMP-2 and MMP-2 activity. J Invest Dermatol 115:225-233, 2000.
6. Mendez MV, Stanley A, Park HY, et al: Fibroblasts cultured from chronic venous ulcers display cellular characteristics of senescence. J Vasc Surg 28:876-883, 1998.
7. Vande Berg JS, Rudolph R, Hollan C, Haywood-Reid PL: Fibroblast senescence in pressure ulcers. Wound Repair Regen 6:38-49, 1998.
8. Trengrove NJ, Bielefeldt-Ohmann H, Stacey MC: Mitogenic activity and cytokine levels in non-healing and healing chronic leg ulcers. Wound Repair Regen 8:13-25, 2000.
9. Tamuzzer RW, Scultz GS: Biochemical analysis of acute and chronic wound environments. Wound Repair Regen 4:321-325, 1996.
10. Falanga V, Grinnell F, Gilchrest B, et al: Workshop on the pathogenesis of chronic wounds. J Invest Dermatol 102:125-127, 1994.
11. Falanga V: Introducing the concepts of wound bed preparation. Int Forum Wound Care 16:1-4, 2001.
12. Bucalo B, Eaglstein WH, Falanga V: Inhibition of cell proliferation by chronic wound fluid. Wound Repair Regen 1:181-186, 1993.
13. Sibbald RG, Williamson D, Orsted HL, et al: Preparing the wound bed—débridement, bacterial balance and moisture balance. Ostomy Wound Manage 46:14-35, 2000.
14. Falanga V: Classifications for wound bed preparation and the role of enzymes: A case for multiple actions of therapeutic agents. Wounds 14:47-57, 2002.
15. Falanga V: Classifications for wound bed preparation and stimulation of chronic wounds. Wound Repair Regen 8:347-352, 2000.
16. Katz MH, Alvarez AF, Kirsner RS, et al: Human wound fluid from acute wounds stimulates fibroblast endothelial cell growth. J Am Acad Dermatol 25:1054-1058, 1991.
17. Mast BA, Schultz GS: Interactions of cytokines, growth factors, and proteases in acute and chronic wounds. Wound Repair Regen 4:411-420, 1996.
18. Weckroth M, Vahari A, Lauharanta J, et al: Matrix metalloproteinases, gelatinase and collagenase, in chronic leg ulcers. J Invest Dermatol 106:1119-1124, 1996.

19. Trengrove NJ, Stacey MC, MacAuley S, et al: Analysis of the acute and chronic wound environments: The role of proteases and their inhibitors. Wound Repair Regen 7:442-452, 1999.

20. Grey JE, Harding KG: The chronic non-healing wound: How to make it better. Hosp Med 59:557-563, 1998.

21. Collins N: Assessment and treatment of involuntary weight loss and protein-calorie malnutrition. Paper presented at Issues in Wound Management: Proceedings of the 14th Annual Clinical Symposium in Wound Care, Denver, Oct 1999.

22. Demling RH, De Santi L: Use of anticatabolic agents for burns. Curr Opin Crit Care 1996:2482-2491, 1996.

23. Demling R, De Santi L: Closure of the "non healing wound" corresponds with correction of weight loss using the anabolic agent oxandrolone. Ostomy Wound Manage 44:58-62, 1999.

24. Williamson D, Paterson DM, Sibbald RG: Vascular assessment. In Krasner DL, Rodeheaver GT, Sibbald RG (eds): Chronic Wound Care: A Clinical Source Book for Healthcare Professional, 3rd ed. Wayne, Pa, HMP Communications, 2001, pp 505-516.

24a. Alvarez M, et al: Chemical debridement of pressure ulcers. Wound 12:15-25, 2000.

25. Steed DL, Donohoe D, Wester MW, Lindsey L: Effect of extensive débridement on the healing of diabetic foot ulcers. J Am Coll Surg 183:61-64, 1996.

26. Thompson PD: What is the role of bacteria in chronic wound exudates? In Cherry G, Harding KG (eds): Management of Wound Exudate. London, Churchill Communications, 1997, pp 35-38.

27. Enoch S, Harding K: Wound bed preparation: The science behind the removal of barriers to healing. Wounds 15:213-29, 2003.

28. Dow G, Browne A, Sibbald RG: Infections in chronic wounds. Ostomy Wound Manage 45:23-40, 1999.

29. Davey ME, O'Toole GA: Microbial biofilms: From ecology to molecular genetics. Microbiol Mol Biol Rev 6:97-167, 2000.

30. Fillius PM, Gyssens IC: Impact of increasing antimicrobial resistance on wound management. Am J Clin Dermatol 3:1-7, 2002.

31. Bowler PG, Duerden BI, Armstrong DG: Wound microbiology and associated approaches to wound management. Clin Microbiol Rev 14:244-269, 2001.

32. Mertz PM, Davis SC, Brewer L, et al: Can antimicrobials be effective without impairing wound healing? The evaluation of cadexomer iodine ointment. Wounds 6:84-93, 1994.

33. Danielsen L, Cherry GW, Harding K, Rollman O: Cadexomer iodine in ulcers colonized by *Pseudomonas aeruginosa*. J Wound Care 6:169-172, 1997.

34. Eaglstein WH, Mertz PM, Falanga V: Occlusive dressings. Am Fam Physician 35:211-216, 1987.

35. Ennis WJ, Meneses P: Wound healing at the local level: The stunned wound. Ostomy Wound Manage 46(1A Suppl):39S-48S, 2000.

36. Schultz GS, Barillo DJ, Mozingo DW, Chin GA: The wound bed advisory board member: Wound bed preparation and a brief history of time. Int Wound J 1:19-32, 2003.

36a. Bergstrom N, Bennett MA, Carlson CE: Treatment of pressure ulcers. Publication AltcPR 95-0652. Rockville, Md.

37. Eisenbud D, Hunter H, Kessler L, Zulkowski K: Hydrogel wound dressings: Where do we stand in 2003? Ostomy Wound Manage 49:52-57, 2003.

38. Finnie A: Hydrocolloids in wound management—pros and cons. Br J Community Nurs 7:338, 340-342, 2002.

39. Russell L, Carr J: New hydrofiber and hydrocolloid dressings for chronic wounds. J Wound Care 9:169-172, 2000.

40. Steed DL: Clinical evaluation of recombinant human platelet-derived growth factor for the treatment of lower extremity diabetic ulcers. J Vasc Surg 21:71-78, 1995.

41. Weiman TJ, Smiell JM, Su Y: The efficacy and safety of a topical gel formulation of recombinant human platelet derived growth factor-BB (becaplermin) in patients with chronic neuropathic ulcers: A phase III randomized control double blind study. Diabetes Care 21:822-827, 1998.

42. Rees RS, Robson MC, Smiell JM, Perry BH: Becaplermin gel in the treatment of pressure ulcers: A phase II randomized, double blinded, placebo-controlled study. Wound Repair Regen 7:141-147, 1999.

43. Marx RE: Platelet rich plasma: Evidence to support its use. J Oral Maxillofac Surg 62:489-496, 2004.

44. Weilbrich G, Kleis WKG: Surasan PRP kit vs PCCS PRP system: Collection efficiency and platelet counts of two different methods for the preparation of platelet rich plasma. Clin Oral Implant Res 13:437, 2002.

45. Marx RE, Carlson ER, Eichstaedt R, et al: Platelet rich plasma: Growth factor enhancement for bone grafts. Oral Surg Oral Med Oral Pathol Oral Radiol Endod 85:638, 1998.

46. Greg AK: The use of platelet rich plasma to enhance the success of bone grafts around dental implants. Dent Implantol Update 11:17, 2000.

47. Man D, Ploske H, Winland-Brown JE, et al: The use of autologous platelet rich plasma (platelet gel) and autologous platelet poor plasma (fibrin glue) in cosmetic surgery. Plast Reconstr Surg 107:229, 2001.

48. Adler SC, Kent KJ: Enhancing healing with growth factors. Facial Plast Surg Clin North Am 10:129, 2002.

49. Camargo PM, Lekovic V, Weinlander M, et al: Platelet rich plasma and bovine porous bone mineral combined with guided tissue regeneration in the treatment of intrabone defects in humans. J Periodont Res 37:300, 2002.

50. Kim SG, Chung CH, Kin YK, et al: Use of particulate dentin plaster of Paris combination with/without platelet rich plasma in the treatment of bone defects around implants. Int J Oral Maxillofac Implant 17:86, 2002.

51. Kasolis JD, Rosen PS, Reynolds MA: Alveolar ridge and sinus augmentation utilizing platelet rich plasma in combination with freeze dried bone allograft: Case series. J Periodont 71:1654, 2000.

52. Abuzeni P, Alexander RW: Enhancement of autologous fat transplantation with platelet rich plasma. Am J Cosmetic Surg 18:59, 2001.

53. Knighton DR, Ciresi K, Fiegel VD, et al: Stimulation of repair in chronic, nonhealing, cutaneous ulcers using platelet derived wound healing formula. Surg Gynecol Obstet 179:56-60, 1990.

54. Eisenbud D, Ngan FH, Luke S, Silberklang M: Skin substitutes and wound healing: Current status and challenges. Wounds 16:2-17, 2004.

55. Coulumb B, Dubertret L: Skin cell culture and wound healing. Wound Repair Regen 10:109-112, 2002.

56. Michel M, L'Heureux NL, Auger FA, Germain L: From newborn to adult: Phenotypic and functional properties of skin equivalent and human skin as a function of donor age. J Cell Physiol 171:179-181, 1997.

57. Bello YM, Falabella AF, Eaglstein WH: Tissue-engineered skin: Current status in wound healing. Am J Clin Dermatol 2:305-313, 2001.

58. Naughton G, Mansbridge J, Gentzkow G: A metabolically active human dermal replacement for the treatment of diabetic foot ulcers. Artif Organs 21:1203-1210, 1997.

59. Pollack R, Edington H, Jensen J, et al: A human dermal replacement for the treatment of diabetic foot ulcers. Wounds 9:75-83, 1997.

60. Marston WA, Haft J, Norwood P, Pollak R: The efficacy and safety of Dermagraft in improving the healing of chronic diabetic foot ulcers: Results of a prospective randomized trial. Diabetes Care 26:1701-1705, 2003.

61. Hanft JR, Surprenant MS: Healing of chronic foot ulcers in diabetic patients treated with human fibroblast-derived dermis. J Foot Ankle Surg 41:291-299, 2002.

62. Sabolinski ML, Alvarez O, Auletta M, et al: Cultured skin as a "smart material" for healing wounds: Experience in venous ulcers. Biomaterials 17:311-320, 1996.

63. Wilkins LM, Watson SR, Prosky SJ, et al: Development of bilayered living skin construct for clinical applications. Biotechnol Bioeng 43:747-756, 1994.

64. Falanga V, Margolis D, Alvarez O, et al: Rapid healing of venous ulcers and lack of clinical rejection with an allogeneic cultured human skin equivalent. Arch Dermatol 134:293-300, 1998.

65. Curran MP, Plosker GL: Bilayered bioengineered skin substitute (Apligraf): A review of its use in the treatment of venous leg ulcers and diabetic foot ulcers. BioDrugs 16:439-455, 2002.

66. Veves A, Falanga V, Armstrong DG, et al: Graftskin, a human skin equivalent, is effective in the management of non-infected neuropathic diabetic foot ulcers. Diabetes Care 24:290-295, 2001.

67. Rivers SP, Veith FJ, Ascer E, Gupta SK: Successful conservative therapy of severe limb-threatening ischemia: The value of nonsympathectomy. Surgery 99:759-762, 1986.

68. Wagner HJ, Klose KJ: Infrapopliteal angioplasty for limb-salvage: A 4-year experience. J Vasc Interv Radiol 8(Suppl):247, 1997.

69. Dormandy JA: Management of peripheral arterial disease (PAD): TASC Working Group. TransAtlantic Inter-Society Consensus (TASC). J Vasc Surg 31(Suppl):S1-S296, 2000.

70. Chandra F, Kudo T, Ahn S: Infrapopliteal angioplasty for limb salvage. Paper presented at the Western Vascular Society Annual Meeting, Victoria, Canada, Sep 2004. Submitted for publication.

71. Kalra M, Gloviczki P, Bower TC, et al: Limb salvage after successful pedal bypass grafting is associated with improved long-term survival. J Vasc Surg 33:6-16, 2001.

72. Treiman GS, Copland S, Yellin AE, et al: Wound infections involving infrainguinal autogenous vein grafts: A current evaluation of factors determining successful graft preservation. J Vasc Surg 33:948-954, 2001.
73. Teodorescu VJ, Chun JK, Morrisey NJ, et al: Radial artery flow-through graft: A new conduit for limb salvage. J Vasc Surg 37:816-820, 2003.
74. Neville RF, Tempesta B, Sidawy AN: Tibial bypass for limb salvage using polytetrafluoroethylene and a distal vein patch. J Vasc Surg 33:266-272, 2001.
75. Parsons RE, Suggs WD, Veith FJ, et al: Polytetrafluoroethylene bypasses to infrapopliteal arteries without cuffs or patches: A better option than amputation in patients without autologous vein. J Vasc Surg 23:347-356, 1996.

Questions

1. A 32-year-old insulin-dependent diabetic has a chronic plantar ulcer under the fourth metatarsal head. It does not appear infected, but cultures of the wound show mixed anaerobic and aerobic organisms. Probing of the ulcer does not indicate a connection to the metatarsal head. What is the best diagnostic test to determine the presence of osteomyelitis?
   (a) Surgical exploration
   (b) Lateral radiography of the foot
   (c) Bone scan
   (d) Computed tomography of the foot
   (e) MRI of the foot

2. A 55-year-old woman sustains a traumatic injury to the calf, with a skin and soft tissue defect measuring 5 by 8 cm. It does not heal over a 6-month period. What would a measurement of metalloproteinases in the wound most likely show?
   (a) Persistently low levels
   (b) Initially high levels that become abnormally low
   (c) Initially high levels that persist
   (d) Initially low levels that become persistently high
   (e) Initially low levels that become high, then return to normal

3. Free tissue transfer to cover open wounds may be used in which of the following?
   (a) Patients with impaired microvascular perfusion
   (b) Patients with arterial insufficiency that cannot be corrected
   (c) Patients who have an ABI greater than 0.4
   (d) Patients with venous insufficiency and ulceration
   (e) Patients who can have arterial insufficiency corrected

4. A radial artery flow-through flap may be useful in a patient with a lower extremity wound in which of the following circumstances?
   (a) Concomitant arterial insufficiency
   (b) Good perfusion of the wound bed (>30 mm Hg) by TcPO$_2$ measurement
   (c) Presence of a bony defect as well as a soft tissue defect
   (d) No arterial insufficiency
   (e) Poor-quality skin in the extremity

5. What is the best diagnostic test for the adequacy of perfusion to an open wound?
   (a) TcPO$_2$
   (b) Ankle-brachial index
   (c) Ankle pressure
   (d) Skin fluorescence
   (e) Perfusion MRI

6. Hyperbaric therapy is useful for an open lower extremity wound in which of the following circumstances?
   (a) It is not infected
   (b) It is infected with aerobic organisms
   (c) TcPO$_2$ is low before hyperbaric therapy is initiated
   (d) TcPO$_2$ is normal before hyperbaric therapy is initiated
   (e) Bone is not involved in the open wound

7. Which of the following statements is true of angiogenesis?
   (a) It begins in the inflammatory phase
   (b) It is the cause of granulation tissue
   (c) It is deficient in all wounds that have delayed healing
   (d) It has maximal impact in the maturation phase of wound healing
   (e) It is not required for slow wound healing

8. Which dressing is best for initial therapy of an exudative wound?
   (a) One that is silver based
   (b) One that contains an enzymatic débriding agent
   (c) One that contains cadexomer iodine
   (d) One that has an absorbing fiber
   (e) One that requires concomitant suction (VAC) to close it

9. Which type of technique is best to débride a grade 4 plantar ulcer?
   (a) Surgical
   (b) Enzymatic
   (c) Wet-to-dry
   (d) Wet-to-wet
   (e) Biotherapy (maggots)

10. What is the probability of long-term healing of a venous ulcer that has received primary treatment with a skin graft?
   (a) Less than 20%
   (b) 20% to 40%
   (c) 40% to 60%
   (d) 60% to 80%
   (e) Greater than 80%

Answers

1. e	2. d	3. e	4. a	5. a
6. c	7. b	8. d	9. a	10. a

Lower Extremity Amputation

Overview and Historical Perspective

Amputation is thought to be one of the oldest surgical procedures.[1] The earliest artificial limb dates from the Samnite wars of 300 BC. Until the time of Ambroise Paré (1510-1590), the techniques for amputation surgery and amputation level selection were extremely crude. Paré improved the surgical technique of amputation through the use of vascular ligatures and developed guidelines for the selection of appropriate levels of amputation. Because many of his original drawings and descriptions are not greatly different from today's surgical and prosthetic practices, he is considered the originator of the modern principles of amputation surgery. Paré's work was expanded by Dominique Jean Larrey (1776-1842) during the Napoleonic wars. Larrey advocated early amputation for traumatic limb injuries and was instrumental in the acceptance of both complete stump débridement and the modern surgical technique whereby bone is buried deep in the amputation stump, rather than the previous method of suturing skin tightly over the bone. Larrey was also involved in developing methods of early mobilization of war amputees.[2]

The idea of immediate or rapid fitting of an artificial leg after lower extremity amputation is relatively recent. Credit for the concept of rapid fit is generally given to Berlemont,[3] based on his work with patients who experienced delayed healing after lower extremity amputation; the concept of immediate postsurgical prosthetic fitting was developed by Weiss.[4] In the late 1960s, Burgess and colleagues noted accelerated rehabilitation, increased acceptance of a prosthesis, and less psychological trauma associated with loss of a limb when a prosthesis was applied immediately after lower extremity amputation.[5] Other advances in lower extremity amputation include the development of new techniques for amputation level selection, extension of the frontiers for limb salvage, and fabrication of prosthetic limbs that incorporate new designs and materials as well as energy storage.

Despite the long and colorful history of amputation surgery, most surgeons considered amputation a surgical defeat and an uninteresting and unrewarding surgical procedure. In many surgical institutions, amputation surgery was traditionally passed down to the youngest and least experienced member of the surgical team, who often operated without senior supervision. A report from the European surgical literature suggests that amputation failure is statistically linked to the lack of amputation experience of the surgeon.[6]

There has been a resurgence of interest in amputation surgery and rehabilitation. It is my view that amputation surgery is not a failure; it is clearly a reconstructive surgical technique. In addition, rehabilitation must be provided to patients following amputation surgery.

Historically, amputations were performed by orthopedic rather than general surgeons. However, two thirds of all lower extremity amputations are necessitated by complications of peripheral vascular disease or diabetes mellitus, so it is not surprising that the majority of lower extremity amputations are now performed by general and vascular surgeons. Unfortunately, most general surgical training programs fail to provide education in prosthetics, prosthetic design, biomechanics, and rehabilitation. The qualifications of the surgeon performing the amputation are not nearly as important as his or her interest in providing postoperative rehabilitation for the newly amputated patient.

This chapter reviews important features of lower extremity amputation surgery and amputation rehabilitation and includes detailed subsections on patient evaluation and preparation for amputation; amputation level selection; indications, surgical techniques, and prosthetic requirements for each level of amputation; surgical morbidity and mortality; common principles of lower extremity prosthetics; techniques of postsurgical rehabilitation; and future trends.

Patient Evaluation and Preparation for Amputation

A review of the literature suggests that the mortality rates for below-knee and above-knee amputation are 4% to 16% and 12% to 40%, respectively.[7-12] It has been estimated that two thirds of patients undergoing lower extremity amputation have diabetes mellitus and that one half to two thirds have symptoms of cardiorespiratory disease.[7,9,13] A review of the causes of late mortality following successful amputation surgery discloses that two thirds of patients die of cardiovascular disease, approximately half of whom die from myocardial infarction.[7,14]

There are between 30,000 and 50,000 new lower extremity amputations performed in the United States each year.[7,9] At present, it is unclear whether the increase in distal revascularization has decreased the number of amputations. It is clear that diabetes-related amputation rates exhibit high regional variation, even after adjustment for age, sex, and race.[15] The indications for lower extremity amputation are listed in Table 49-1. For patients with diabetes mellitus, it has been estimated that the risk of losing the second leg in the 5 years after amputation of the first leg ranges from 15% to 33% (3% to 7% per year)[16-18]; however, one third to one half of amputees with diabetes mellitus die of complications of diabetes or cardiorespiratory disease before undergoing amputation of the second extremity.[16,18,19]

In view of the mean age of patients undergoing lower extremity amputation (62 years),[7,8,13,14,20] the incidence of associated diseases, and the morbid and nonmorbid complications associated with surgery, the importance of a careful preoperative physical examination cannot be overstated. The physical examination should include a search for physical signs and symptoms suggestive of cardiorespiratory disease. Documentation of all pulses, as well as a careful assessment of the presence or absence of physical findings suggestive of extremity ischemia (pain, paresthesias, elevation pallor, rubor, alteration of sensory or motor function), should be performed. The extent and depth of infection or gangrene should be noted. The presence of malnutrition or systemic diseases, such as diabetes mellitus, collagen-vascular diseases, and immunodeficiency syndromes, or the systemic administration of anti-inflammatory drugs, such as steroids, should be noted because their presence may have a major influence on the preoperative preparation and timing of lower extremity amputation, as well as postsurgical recovery. All diabetic patients should be carefully screened for silent but significant coronary artery disease. A paper by Pinzur and colleagues reinforced the concept that multidisciplinary presurgical evaluation helps in amputation level selection and prosthetic limb fitting and improves patient rehabilitation.[21]

The presence of lower extremity infection in a diabetic patient requires special mention. Historically, most studies have suggested that the primary organisms were *Staphylococcus aureus* and enteric gram-negative bacilli. More recent information, however, suggests that 60% of lower extremity infections in patients with diabetes mellitus involve both obligate and facultative anaerobic organisms.[22] Fierer and associates also pointed out that patients with mixed infections required more operations than those with simple staphylococcal infections and that their surgical wounds tended to heal more slowly.[22] I therefore recommend that antibiotic coverage for diabetics with lower extremity infections include drugs that provide broad-spectrum bactericidal aerobic and anaerobic coverage. A note of caution: there have been increasing reports of methicillin-resistant *S. aureus* infections, especially in patients with wound complications after vascular surgery.[23]

In the absence of acute arterial embolization, diabetes mellitus, immunodeficiency syndromes, collagen-vascular diseases, or drugs that inhibit the immune system, it is unusual to see tissue loss with or without infection in patients without multilevel vascular occlusive disease. Chronic single-level arterial obstruction is not usually associated with limb loss. As a general guideline, chronic occlusion of the superficial femoral artery does not cause limb loss without outflow (tibial trifurcation) or inflow (iliofemoral or deep femoral) occlusive disease.

The aims of amputation are to remove gangrenous tissues, relieve pain, obtain primary healing of the most distal amputation possible, and obtain maximal rehabilitation after amputation. For purposes of further discussion, the indications and management of patients undergoing amputation are divided into three general categories: (1) acute ischemia, (2) progressive chronic ischemia, and (3) ischemia complicated by infection.

ACUTE ISCHEMIA

The choice of amputation for the management of acute ischemia in a patient whose arterial tree is considered unreconstructible or in a patient who presents late in the course of acute ischemia, such that arterial reconstruction may be contraindicated, is a decision that taxes the judgment of even the most experienced surgeon.[24] In addition, urgent or emergent amputation following acute arterial occlusion is generally associated with the greatest risk of morbidity and mortality in the entire field of amputation surgery. The degree of urgency for amputation in the face of acute arterial ischemia is governed by multiple factors that include, but are not limited to, the extent of extremity ischemia, especially the muscle mass; the pain the patient is experiencing from the ischemic tissues; and the presence of signs of systemic toxicity resulting from products of necrotic muscle or bacteria reaching the general circulatory system. If the affected ischemic area is small (e.g., the toes or forefoot), the pain is relatively moderate, and there are no signs of supervening infection or systemic toxicity, amputation can and should be postponed as long as possible to allow maximum development of collateral circulation. Delay of amputation in such a case improves the likelihood that a more distal limited amputation will heal. Mild to moderate pain can be controlled with narcotics. Adjunctive therapy, including systemic heparin, low-molecular-weight dextran, or fibrinolytic agents (urokinase, tissue plasminogen activator, tenecteplase, or reteplase) may be valuable in preventing progression of thrombus within capillary beds during the period of reduced blood flow, thus maintaining the viability of marginally

TABLE 49–1	Indications for Lower Extremity Amputation
Indication	**Percentage (Range)**
Complications of diabetes mellitus	60-80
Nondiabetic infection with ischemia	15-25
Ischemia without infection	5-10
Chronic osteomyelitis	3-5
Trauma	2-5
Miscellaneous (neuroma, frostbite, tumor, pain, nonhealing)	5-10

Data from references 7, 9, 13, 14, 20.

ischemic tissues while collateral channels are beginning to enlarge. The presence of severe pain, extensive muscle necrosis, or systemic toxicity may require more emergent amputation with less patient preparation preoperatively. If muscle necrosis is extensive, the need for urgent or emergent amputation is critical because of the risk of renal damage secondary to circulating myoglobin. In addition to renal dysfunction, necrotic muscle tissue may cause cardiovascular or respiratory compromise, adding to the need for emergent amputation. The presence of systemic toxicity, especially a necrotizing infection, often necessitates emergent amputation. For those patients with significant medical comorbidities or systemic toxicity, cryologic or physiologic amputation allows extended time for patient preparation for surgery and decreases mortality.[25]

Several features of patient evaluation and clinical progression are helpful in this decision-making process. The first consideration is the extent of nonviable skin. Although discoloration or gangrene is readily apparent, hyposensitive areas due to severe skin ischemia do not allow adequate healing and may not be so easily identified. Except in patients with diabetic neuropathy, sensation to pinprick and light touch is a useful discriminant. If there is diminished sensation below the knee, for example, the chances of performing a successful below-knee amputation are small, and morbidity may be avoided by proceeding expeditiously to an above-knee amputation. The presence of significant calf muscle swelling or muscle rigidity is an ominous sign suggestive of myonecrosis. Careful monitoring of calf circumference, skin sensation, urine color and output, and signs of systemic toxicity such as lethargy, confusion, or hallucinations must be done on an hourly basis. The presence of systemic toxicity or significant changes in the physical examination indicate the need for immediate amputation or physiologic amputation.[25] Similarly, the presence of myoglobinuria or cardiovascular instability represents an indication for immediate amputation. It is generally impossible to obtain rapid myoglobin determinations in serum or urine, but the presence of a urinary heme-positive dipstick in the absence of red blood cells under microscopic examination or pink serum (hemoglobin) is consistent with a diagnosis of myoglobinuria. In addition, the presence of markedly elevated creatine phosphokinase or lactate dehydrogenase isoenzymes in the serum is suggestive of myonecrosis in the absence of trauma, myocardial infarction, or recent surgery. If continued observation is elected, prophylaxis against renal damage from myoglobin pigment is recommended and includes maintenance of a diuresis in the range of 75 to 100 mL/hour by the administration of osmotic diuretics such as mannitol and fluids. In addition, the urine should be maintained at an alkaline pH, because myoglobin precipitates in the renal tubules at a pH less than 7. Usually, a mixture of mannitol and sodium bicarbonate in a balanced salt solution can be used to titrate urine output and pH. Finally, the presence of infection in the ischemic extremity is an ominous complication requiring careful consideration. The presence of such an infection in a diabetic patient is even more ominous because of the sometimes rapid progression of seemingly innocuous infections. Any evidence of systemic toxicity or progressive infection is an indication for immediate surgical débridement, which may take the form of a débriding amputation or a physiologic amputation followed by a formal surgical amputation later.

As long as there is continued improvement in collateral blood supply to an acutely ischemic extremity and there is no sign of systemic or renal toxicity, observation may be continued. As soon as circulatory improvement ceases or signs of toxicity develop, amputation should be performed promptly. An alternative to amputation in an unstable or high-risk patient is physiologic amputation, as previously discussed.

Evaluation for potential vascular reconstruction in a patient with a clear-cut demarcation of a nonviable area of a lower extremity after a period of observation for acute ischemia is not likely to be beneficial; however, if there is a question of marginal tissue viability above an area that is believed to be nonviable and the questionable tissue might permit a lower amputation level, evaluation for vascular reconstruction may be beneficial.[26] For example, the presence of a nonviable forefoot and a marginal lower extremity between the knee and ankle may be an indication for evaluation for vascular reconstruction in an attempt to perform a below-knee rather than an above-knee amputation.

PROGRESSIVE CHRONIC ISCHEMIA

A patient with progressive chronic ischemia who ultimately presents for amputation has experienced one or more of the following problems: rest pain, nonhealing skin lesion or ulceration, gangrene, or gangrene with superimposed infection. Gangrene complicated by infection is a special problem and is discussed in a separate section.

From the patient's point of view, ischemic rest pain is one of the most compelling indications for amputation. Characteristically, the patient seeks relief by sitting up and allowing his or her legs to hang over the side of the bed or by ambulation. The dependent position provides relief of ischemic rest pain because gravity favors improved collateral blood flow, which augments arterial perfusion pressure. In its more severe forms, ischemic rest pain forms part of a vicious circle. As the patient more frequently uses dependency to achieve pain relief, the extremity becomes edematous and lymphatic return decreases, which eventually results in more ischemia. The end result of this vicious circle is a massively swollen, very painful ischemic extremity. Mild to moderate rest pain can often be successfully managed with narcotics. There have been reports that early mild rest pain may be relieved by sympathectomy. If there are no signs of systemic toxicity or supervening infection, and if mild ischemic rest pain can be controlled with medication, a patient can be followed and amputation postponed.

Another manifestation of chronic ischemia is the presence of ischemic skin ulcerations or nonhealing skin lesions on the lower extremity. Unfortunately, many of these skin ulcers occur in hospitalized patients as a result of abrasion of the foot or pressure necrosis (due to poor foot protection in the hospital bed). In a diabetic patient, ulceration usually occurs at pressure points, and the patient is often unaware of the problem because of diabetic neuropathy. Patients without peripheral neuropathy are very much aware of these ischemic ulcers because they are typically extremely painful. Besides obvious areas of pressure necrosis, such as the heel and the lateral and medial malleoli, other common points of ulceration include the bony prominences over the metatarsal heads and midphalangeal joints or between the toes.

Fortunately, most patients with chronic progressive ischemia come to medical attention before the presence of frank tissue loss. Even patients with tissue loss usually present early with involvement of one or more toes or, in more severe cases, the entire forefoot. Under these circumstances, there is usually ample opportunity to fully prepare and evaluate the patient for lower extremity amputation or arterial reconstruction if possible. Preoperative evaluation and management should include proper medical attention to all associated diseases and a careful evaluation for potential critical organ dysfunction, especially the heart, lungs, and kidneys.

All patients with chronic ischemia should undergo consideration for vascular reconstruction for limb salvage. Angiographic evaluation from the infrarenal abdominal aorta down to and including the pedal arches is mandatory. In general, the surgeon should ensure good inflow to the level of the deep femoral artery. Reconstruction distal to the level of the deep femoral artery should be done only if chances for success are reasonably high and if a successful procedure would obviate the need for a major amputation. There is continuing controversy over the effect of prior revascularization on amputation level.[27-35] In my opinion, revascularization should always be attempted unless contraindicated by the patient's medical condition. If vascular reconstruction is brought below the knee, the incision required for approaching the distal popliteal artery and tibial trifurcation vessels should be planned along the lines of the posterior skin flap that might be required for a subsequent below-knee amputation. Techniques for selecting an amputation level are discussed later. However, one of the interesting spinoffs from studies of amputation level selection is the identification of patients who are unable to heal a low-level amputation and in whom the chance for rehabilitation at a high level of amputation is unlikely. When such objective information is available, attempts at proximal or extended distal extremity bypass to salvage a knee joint, for example, may be indicated to keep a patient ambulatory.[26,28,29]

GANGRENE COMPLICATED BY INFECTION

The presence of dry gangrene is not an emergent surgical problem or necessarily the hallmark of an ominous clinical situation. Dry gangrene, limited to the toes, for example, may be treated conservatively and requires little, if any, surgical or ancillary medical support; however, infection complicating dry gangrene (i.e., wet gangrene), especially in a diabetic patient, is a limb- and life-threatening emergency. Control of sepsis can sometimes be achieved with antibiotic therapy plus limited débridement and drainage, or it may require radical excision and débridement; antibiotic therapy alone is seldom adequate treatment for gangrene complicated by infection. Failure to institute prompt therapy, especially in diabetic patients, results in rapid ascension of the infectious process, the loss of potentially salvageable tissue, and a large increase in patient mortality. As noted earlier, in patients with systemic toxicity, cryoamputation before definitive surgical amputation helps decrease mortality.

The first step in the management of infected or wet gangrene is identification of the infecting organisms. Usually, the urgency of the clinical situation does not allow the identification of specific organisms by culture, although culture should be obtained and submitted for both anaerobic and aerobic organisms. It has been my practice to assume that gangrene complicated by infection includes a mixture of aerobic and anaerobic organisms; therefore, broad-spectrum bactericidal antibiotic coverage is used.[22]

Once antibiotic therapy has been started, the patient's status must be monitored carefully, including pulse rate, white blood cell count, blood pressure, temperature, extent of infection, severity of pain, and diffuse signs of systemic toxicity such as lethargy, hallucinations, and general mental status. In a diabetic patient, serum glucose and insulin requirements are additional useful monitoring parameters. If a prompt response to antibiotic therapy is noted, therapy should be continued for maximum effect and a definitive amputation then performed. If the patient does not respond promptly to antibiotic management or if undrained purulent material was initially evident, débridement of gangrenous tissue and establishment of drainage should be employed as an early adjunct to antibiotic therapy.

If the gangrenous infection extensively involves the foot and contaminates tendon and tissue spaces, especially in a diabetic patient, radical débridement should be performed. One of the better methods to obtain radical débridement and establish open drainage is a guillotine amputation of the foot carried out at the level of the malleoli (Fig. 49-1). Guillotine amputation eliminates the septic focus and allows drainage of contaminated lymphatics and tissue spaces in the lower leg. The presence of cellulitis and lymphangitis at the level of

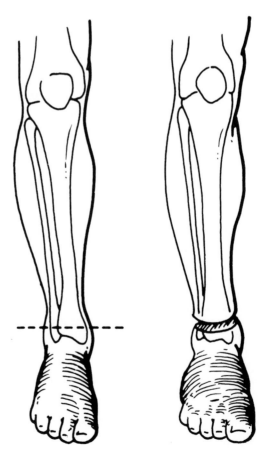

FIGURE 49-1 • Schematic representation of an open ankle guillotine, or preparatory, amputation in a patient with a septic foot.

ankle guillotine is not a contraindication to this type of débridement technique. After performance of a guillotine-type amputation for débridement, systemic antibiotics are continued until the definitive amputation is performed, usually 3 to 5 days later. Definitive amputation is performed after ascertaining that the infection has been controlled and the patient's preoperative status has been optimized.

The incidence of stump infection in patients who present with a septic foot is decreased if a preparatory ankle guillotine amputation is performed before definitive amputation. In my experience, such a two-stage surgical approach decreased the stump infection rate from 22% to 3% ($P = 0.01$).[36] This approach was reaffirmed in a prospective, randomized study by Fischer and colleagues,[37] in which the incidence of stump infection was decreased from 21% (one stage) to 0% (two stage) ($P = 0.05$).

AMPUTATION FOR TRAUMA

Patients undergoing traumatic lower extremity amputation tend to be young and in good medical health, so patient evaluation and preparation for amputation are easier than that described for geriatric patients with peripheral vascular disease and diabetes. As a general principle, formal traumatic amputation is performed to achieve healing at the lowest amputation level possible, and amputation level selection is usually predetermined by the injury. Adequate débridement of dead tissue is mandatory. The presence of a large amount of marginally viable tissue or potentially infected tissue may be an indication for débridement and open amputation followed at a later date by formal amputation with skin closure. A special effort should be made to rule out proximal bony or ligamentous injuries. Careful attention must be paid to other potentially life- or limb-threatening injuries, and management of such injuries must be handled in an appropriate sequence to achieve the best overall result for the patient. The use of a proximal extremity tourniquet for control of bleeding is optional but should be discouraged in a dysvascular patient. The use of drains after traumatic amputation is controversial, although there is some evidence that drainage results in a more rapid resolution of postamputation stump edema. If drains are used, they should be the closed-system type (not open Penrose drains).

Determination of Amputation Level

The objective of preoperative amputation level selection is to determine the most distal amputation site that will heal. The general requirements are as follows: (1) the amputation must remove all necrotic, painful, or infected tissue; (2) the amputation stump must be able to be fitted with a functional and easily applied prosthesis; and (3) the blood supply at the level of the proposed amputation must be sufficient to allow primary skin healing. Appropriate selection of the amputation level is critical. If the surgeon elects too proximal an amputation, such as a midthigh amputation, the patient may be deprived of the opportunity for ambulation and rehabilitation, although the amputation might heal without difficulty. If a distal amputation site is selected and the blood supply is inadequate for amputation healing, further surgery will be required for amputation at a higher level. This latter

approach may result in increased morbidity and mortality and may ultimately result in rehabilitation failure.

The inherent advantages of a below-knee amputation as opposed to an above-knee amputation should be obvious. It is easier to ambulate on a below-knee prosthesis; this is extremely important, especially in geriatric patients. In general, a unilateral below-knee amputee requires a 10% to 40% increase in energy expenditure for ambulation compared with the energy required for walking with an intact extremity. In contrast, a unilateral above-knee amputee (using a prosthesis with a locked or unlocked knee) requires approximately a 50% to 70% increase in energy expenditure. Crutch walking without a lower extremity prosthesis uses approximately 60% more energy, whereas wheelchair use necessitates only a small increase in energy expenditure (9%). Patients with severe coronary artery disease or severe chronic obstructive pulmonary disease may be physically unable to provide the additional energy required for ambulation on an above-knee compared with a below-knee prosthesis.

It is usually possible for the surgeon to decide on an amputation level that will remove necrotic, painful, or infected tissue as well as to plan an amputation stump that can be fitted with a prosthesis. However, the decision regarding the adequacy of blood supply at the proposed amputation level is one of the most difficult problems facing the amputation surgeon.

The earliest attempts at amputation level selection used the presence of pulses in the affected extremity, skin temperature, correlation of arteriographic findings, and "clinical judgment." It has been well documented that none of these selection techniques has a consistent enough correlation with amputation healing to provide a sound basis for clinical decision making. In a study by Robbs and Ray, the morbidity, mortality, and rates of healing of lower limb amputations in 214 patients, wherein the amputation level was determined by nonobjective criteria, were retrospectively analyzed.[38] Six of 67 (8.9%) primary above-knee amputations and 37 of 147 (25%) primary below-knee amputations had to be revised to a higher level. The authors concluded "that flap viability could not be predicted by the extent of ischemic lesion in relation to the ankle joint, the popliteal pulse status, or lower limb angiography."[38] In a 1992 study comparing clinical parameters and skin perfusion pressure for amputation level selection, Dwars and coworkers noted that the presence of palpable pulses immediately above the selected level correlated well with primary healing.[39] However, the absence of palpable pulses and angiographic patency scores were of no clinical value in amputation level selection. Golbranson and colleagues presented promising data on improved methods of skin temperature measurement that had a high degree of accuracy (90%) for selecting below- versus above-knee amputation levels.[40] In addition, Spence and Walker demonstrated a clear correlation between three different temperature isotherms (1.8°C separation) and isotopically derived skin blood flow ($P < 0.001$).[41] Stoner and associates reported that when the ratio of temperatures at the posterior and anterior incision sites (Burgess posterior flap below-knee amputation) was greater than 0.98, healing was improved.[42] In a study comparing several modalities for amputation level selection, Wagner and colleagues noted (for above- and below-knee amputations) that the average skin temperature at the amputation site was higher (34.3°C) in patients who healed primarily compared with those who required operative stump revision (33.3°C) ($P = 0.001$).[43] One physical finding that has some value in differentiating proposed amputation levels is the presence of dependent rubor. Skin that develops dependent rubor is clearly ischemic and thus, like gangrenous tissue, is an absolute contraindication to amputation at that level; however, the absence of dependent rubor does not necessarily ensure healing ability. Early workers in the field of amputation surgery solved the problem of level selection by performing above-knee amputations on almost all patients. In the 1960s, Lim and coworkers demonstrated that 83% of all patients requiring a lower extremity amputation would heal following a below-knee amputation.[44] However, using empirical below-knee amputation selection may be detrimental to some patients who might have healed following a more distal amputation, such as a transmetatarsal or Syme's amputation. In addition, identifying the 20% to 30% of patients in whom a below-knee amputation is doomed to failure would be advantageous so that either a knee disarticulation or an above-knee amputation could be performed primarily, saving the patient additional surgical procedures.

The need for more sensitive and objective methods for the preoperative selection of amputation level led to the development of numerous noninvasive techniques, including Doppler ankle and calf systolic blood pressure determinations, with or without pulse-volume recordings[45-52]; xenon 133 (^{133}Xe) skin blood flow studies[53-59]; digital or transmetatarsal photoplethysmographic pressures[50]; transcutaneous oxygen determination[11,59-68]; skin fluorescence after intravenous fluorescein dye[69-72]; laser Doppler skin blood flow measurements[55,73] (F.A. Matsen, personal communication, 1978); pertechnetate skin blood pressure studies[74,75]; and photoelectrically measured skin color changes.[76]

An overview of the various criteria for predicting the healing of digit and forefoot amputations is shown in Table 49-2. Totals from Table 49-2 suggest that preoperative selection techniques correctly predicted primary healing in 174 of 189 toe and forefoot amputations (97%). Similar data for below-knee amputation levels are summarized in Table 49-3. Excluding empirical below-knee selection, the tests listed in Table 49-3 correctly predicted primary healing of below-knee amputations in 560 of 603 elective amputations (93%). Clearly, objective amputation level selection can not only predict potential healing of a more distal level of amputation but also accurately assess the likelihood of healing of a

below-knee compared with an above-knee amputation. It is my opinion that elective lower extremity amputation should not be performed without some type of preoperative testing to ensure primary healing of the most distal amputation possible.

The techniques for the use of ankle, calf, and popliteal Doppler systolic blood pressure determinations have been well described[45-49,51,52] and are not covered in this chapter. Similarly, use of the photoplethysmograph for determining digital and transmetatarsal blood pressures has been well described by Schwartz and coworkers[50] and is not presented here. The potential advantages of both the Doppler instrument and the photoplethysmograph are that they are relatively simple, inexpensive, and totally noninvasive. The problem with these instruments is that the presence of a blood pressure less than a predetermined level does not necessarily guarantee failure of amputation healing at that level (negative predictive value). This problem was nicely summarized by Verta and colleagues, who noted that "for forefoot amputation a high Doppler ankle pressure did not guarantee successful healing and a low ankle pressure did not contraindicate primary healing."[51] In an effort to increase the accuracy of Doppler ankle pressures, both Gibbons and coworkers[48] and Raines and associates[49] suggested the ancillary use of pulse-volume recordings. Although Raines's group reported 100% successful healing in 27 below-knee amputations in which the Doppler systolic ankle pressure was greater than 30 mm Hg, calf pressure was greater than 65 mm Hg, and there was a pulsatile pulse-volume recording in the foot, Gibbons's group was unable to duplicate these results and concluded, "we find no consistent criteria which are more accurate and reliable than clinical judgment and no ankle pressure above which primary healing was guaranteed." Gibbons and coworkers also noted decreased accuracy in amputation level prediction using pulse-volume recording and Doppler ankle systolic pressures in patients with diabetes mellitus. The problem with diabetic patients (falsely high systolic pressure measurements) is likely due to medical calcinosis of their vessels. Wagner and colleagues reported that Doppler pressures at the thigh, popliteal, midcalf, or ankle level were unreliable in predicting healing of a below-knee amputation.[43]

Theoretically, the measurement of skin fluorescence with a Wood's ultraviolet lamp after intravenous injection of fluorescein dye (Funduscein) should be a reliable test for

TABLE 49–2	Selection Criteria for Toe and Forefoot Amputation		
Criterion	**Reference**	**Amputation Level**	**No. of Healing Patients (%)**
Doppler ankle systolic pressure			
70 mm Hg	45	Forefoot	38/44 (86)
116 mm Hg	50	Digit/forefoot	25/27 (93)
35 mm Hg	51	Digit	44/46 (96)
Fiber-optic fluorometry DFI > 44	72	Foot/forefoot	18/20 (90)
Photoplethysmographic digit or TMA pressure 20 mm Hg	50	Digit	20/20 (100)
Xenon skin clearance > 2.6 mL/100 g tissue/min	57	Digit/forefoot	25/28 (89)
Transcutaneous Po_2 > 20 mm Hg	65	Forefoot	4/4 (100)
Total			174/189 (92)

DFI, dye fluorescence index; TMA, transmetatarsal-ankle.

amputation level selection. Although this technique is somewhat more invasive than Doppler ankle systolic pressure measurements or pulse-volume recordings, it is less complicated and less invasive than ^{133}Xe skin blood flow or pertechnetate skin perfusion measurements. The commercial availability of two new types of fluorometers (Fiberoptic Perfusion Fluorometer, Diversatronics, Broomall, Pa.; Fluoroscan, V. Elings, PhD, University of California, Santa Barbara), which can provide objective numeric readings quickly and in the absence of a Wood's lamp, may further enhance the use of this technique.[69,71,72] Development of a computerized video camera system to analyze skin perfusion after oral ingestion of fluorescein obviates the risk of intravenous injection and allows easy data manipulation for limb mapping. Such a system has been under study at Maricopa Medical Center in Phoenix, Ariz. McFarland and Lawrence reported an accuracy rate of 80% for skin fluorescence, compared with 47% for Doppler popliteal systolic blood pressure (50 mm Hg) for the prediction of healing of a below-knee amputation (see Table 49-3).[70] In addition, when skin fluorescence and Doppler pressure did not agree on the level of amputation, fluorescein always predicted a more distal level. Silverman and associates, in 1985, reported their data on fiber-optic fluorometry for amputation level selection at the below-knee, below-ankle, and above-knee levels in dysvascular limbs.[72] The overall success rate was 92% (36 of 39), and individual rates were 18 of 20 below-ankle (90%), 12 of 12 below-knee (100%), and 6 of 7 above-knee (86%) amputations. Discriminate analysis demonstrated an optimal reference point between healing and nonhealing amputations,

and a dye fluorescence index of greater than 44 had 93% accuracy. Two later studies, however, did not demonstrate such promising results.[77,78] In a blinded, prospective review of 56 patients undergoing below-knee amputation, objective measurement of fluorescein perfusion did not correlate with amputation healing.[79] In a study comparing multiple methods of amputation level selection, Wagner and colleagues found that qualitative skin fluorescence was not as successful as cutaneous oxygen measurement.[43]

Promising work with a modified Clark-type oxygen electrode (with a heating element and thermostat for temperature control; Transoxode, Hellige-Orager, FRG; U.S. manufacturer, Litton Industries [Woodland Hills, Calif.]) for amputation level selection has been reported by several groups.[60,62,64,65,67,80] Franzeck and colleagues reported that the mean transcutaneous partial pressure of oxygen (PO_2) values of patients who healed primarily compared with those who failed to heal were 36.5 ± 17.5 mm Hg and less than 0.3 mm Hg, respectively.[62] However, in those patients with a transcutaneous PO_2 less than 10 mm Hg, six of nine failed to heal, and three of nine healed primarily. In a study on below-knee amputations, Burgess and coworkers found that 15 of 15 amputations healed primarily if the transcutaneous PO_2 was greater than 40 mm Hg, 17 of 19 healed if the transcutaneous PO_2 was greater than 0 mm Hg but less than 40 mm Hg, and none of the three amputations with a PO_2 of 0 mm Hg healed.[60] Katsamouris and coworkers reported that 17 of 17 lower extremity amputations healed if the PO_2 was greater than 38 mm Hg or if the PO_2 index (chest wall control site) was greater than 0.59.[64] Ratliff and colleagues noted that

TABLE 49–3	Selection Criteria for Below-Knee Amputation	
Criterion	**Reference**	**No. of Healing Patients (%)**
Doppler systolic ankle pressure 30 mm Hg + calf pressure 65 mm Hg + pulsatile PVR	49	27/27 (100)
Doppler systolic calf pressure 70 mm Hg	46	32/32 (100)
Doppler systolic thigh pressure 80 mm Hg or calf pressure 50 mm Hg	52	36/36 (100)
Empirical below-knee	44	38/46 (83)
Fiber-optic fluorometry DFI > 44	72	12/12 (100)
Fluorescein dye	70	24/30 (80)
[99m]Tc-pertechnetate skin blood pressure	86	24/26 (92)
Laser-Doppler velocimetry > 20 mV	78	25/26 (96)
Photoelectric skin pressure 20-100 mm Hg	76, 87	60/71 (85)
Transcutaneous PO_2		
> 10 mm Hg or > 10 mm Hg increase on 100% O_2	62, 80	76/80 (95)
> 35 mm Hg	60, 64, 67	51/51 (100)
> 20 mm Hg	65	16/16 (100)
> 0 to < 40 mm Hg	60	17/19 (89)
0 mm Hg	60	0/3 (0)*
Index > 0.59	64	17/17 (100)
Index > 0.20	77	33/34 (97)
Xenon skin clearance		
= 3.1 mL blood flow/100 g tissue/min	54	23/26 (88)
> 2.6 mL blood flow/100 g tissue/min	57	35/36 (97)
Epicutaneous > 0.9 mL/100 g tissue/min	53, 56	14/15 (93)
Total		560/603 (93)

*Excluded from total.
DFI, dye fluorescence index; PVR, pulse-volume recording.

18 below-knee amputations healed if the PO_2 was greater than 35 mm Hg, while 10 of 15 failed if the PO_2 was less than 35 mm Hg.[67] Kram and associates noted success in 33 of 34 (97%) below-knee amputations with multisensor transcutaneous oxygen mapping when the critical PO_2 index was greater than 0.20.[77] In addition, all six patients with an index less than 0.20 failed to heal. All investigators have reported some amputations that healed in patients with low PO_2 values. A partial explanation for this observation might be the nonlinear relationship between PO_2 and cutaneous blood flow. In a careful study, Matsen and coworkers reported that PO_2 measurements are most dependent on arteriovenous gradients and cutaneous vascular resistance.[66] Techniques to improve the accuracy of transcutaneous PO_2 probes include local heating (to 44°C, which minimizes local vascular resistance and makes PO_2 more linear with respect to cutaneous blood flow), measurements before and after oxygen administration, oxygen isobar extremity mapping, and transcutaneous oxygen recovery half-time.[81] Oishi and associates noted—in a study comparing skin temperature, Doppler pressure, and transcutaneous oxygen—that after the inhalation of oxygen, if the PO_2 increased 10 mm Hg or more, the PO_2 predicted amputation healing with a sensitivity of 98%.[82] In another study, the authors prospectively compared the following tests for their accuracy in amputation level selection: transcutaneous oxygen, transcutaneous carbon dioxide, ratio of transcutaneous oxygen to transcutaneous carbon dioxide, foot-to-chest transcutaneous oxygen, intradermal ^{133}Xe, ankle-brachial index, and absolute popliteal artery pressure.[65] All metabolic parameters had a high degree of statistical accuracy in predicting amputation healing, whereas none of the other tests had statistical reliability. All amputations—transmetatarsal, below-knee, and above-knee—healed primarily if the transcutaneous PO_2 level was greater than 20 mm Hg, and there was a 0% incidence of false-positive and false-negative studies. Most authors of transcutaneous oxygen testing studies suggest using a cutoff point of 35 to 40 mm Hg. I have used 20 mm Hg with excellent results. Recent data reconfirm the accuracy of a threshold of 20 mm Hg, especially in distal limb amputations.[68] Also of importance is the observation that amputation site healing is not affected by the presence of diabetes mellitus, nor are the test results for any of the metabolic parameters. Similar data have been reported by Bacharach and colleagues, who stated that 51 of 52 limbs (98%) healed (primary and delayed) with a PO_2 greater than or equal to 40 mm Hg, whereas a PO_2 of less than 20 mm Hg was associated with universal failure.[83] In that study, PO_2 measurements during limb elevation improved the predictability of outcome for patients with supine PO_2 values greater than 20 mm Hg but less than 40 mm Hg.

Theoretically, laser-Doppler velocimetry should be an ideal tool for skin blood flow determination; it is noninvasive and "measures" capillary blood flow (good correlation between laser-Doppler blood flow measurements using microspheres, electromagnetic flow probes, and ^{133}Xe clearance).[84] However, data by Holloway and Burgess,[54] Holloway and Watkins,[55] Holloway,[84] and Matsen (personal communication, 1978) suggest that although there is a linear relationship among techniques, there is a fair amount of variance. These groups noted that the use of local skin heating may enhance the accuracy of the laser-Doppler and make it a more valuable adjunct for amputation level selection.[84]

Holloway and Burgess reported their experience with laser-Doppler velocimetry in 20 lower extremity amputations at the foot, forefoot, below-knee, and above-knee levels, and the accuracy rates were as follows: foot and forefoot, two of six (33%); below-knee, eight of eight (100%); and above-knee, six of six (100%).[73]

Malone and coworkers'[57] and Moore's[58] greatest postsurgical experience was with the use of ^{133}Xe skin clearance for amputation level selection. These techniques have been well described by Moore,[58] Daly and Henry,[85] and Malone and associates.[57] One of the major difficulties with the application of ^{133}Xe skin clearance for amputation level selection is its reproducibility by other investigators. In an earlier publication, Holloway and Burgess were unable to document a clear-cut end point above which all amputations healed.[54] In contrast, Silberstein and colleagues reported that 38 of 39 patients (11 above-knee amputations, 18 below-knee or transmetatarsal amputations, and 9 no amputation) healed when ^{133}Xe skin blood flow was greater than 2.4 mL/100 g tissue per minute; when flow was less than 2.4 mL/100 g tissue per minute, only four of seven patients healed.[59] One significant advantage of ^{133}Xe clearance techniques that may offset both of these problems, if its ultimate reliability is demonstrated in other centers, is its potential ability to predict healing at all levels of lower extremity amputation.[57]

A final problem with the intradermal use of ^{133}Xe for skin blood flow measurements is that the manufacturer no longer supplies ^{133}Xe. The product must be made by nuclear medicine departments. This limitation may further preclude widespread use of the intradermal ^{133}Xe technique. Finally, despite past publications and excellent results,[57,58,85] I no longer use ^{133}Xe skin clearance for amputation level selection. In part, this change was made because of the enumerated difficulties; however, the major reason for this change was a study wherein ^{133}Xe was not found to be statistically reliable as a selection method for amputation level.[65] (As noted previously, transcutaneous oxygen is very reliable.)

Using the disappearance of intradermal technetium 99m pertechnetate, ^{131}I-sodium, ^{131}I-antipyrine, or ^{133}Xe in the presence of external pressure, Holstein[74] and Holstein and Lassen[86] reported amputation level selection data comparable to data reported by Moore, Daly, Henry, Malone, and others. Because ^{133}Xe is trapped in subcutaneous fat, there are solid theoretical reasons to use an isotope other than ^{133}Xe. Holstein and associates found no significant difference among ^{131}I-sodium, ^{131}I-antipyrine, and ^{99m}Tc-pertechnetate for the measurement of skin perfusion pressure.[75]

Stockel and coworkers[76] and Ovesen and Stockel[87] reported preliminary data on the use of a photodetector and plethysmography (Medimatic, Copenhagen) for amputation level selection; these findings correlate well with the ^{133}Xe skin perfusion pressure techniques of Holstein and colleagues.[74,75] This technique uses a blood pressure cuff placed over a photoelectric detector, which is connected to a plethysmograph, to measure the minimal external pressure required to prevent skin reddening after blanching. To date, 66 of 71 (93%) below-knee amputations healed with skin pressures between 20 and 100 mm Hg. In 1992, Dwars and associates reported that skin perfusion pressure measurements were of excellent predictive value for the healing of lower extremity amputations (positive predictive value, 89%; negative predictive value, 99%).[39]

In summary, it is my opinion that elective lower extremity amputation should not be performed in the absence of objective testing to determine the most distal amputation that will heal primarily, yet allow the removal of infected, painful, or ischemic tissue. A variety of techniques are available, and the technique chosen depends on the available equipment, the amputation level under consideration, and the current accuracy rates for the reported techniques. However, in my opinion, the most reliable, easiest to use, and best overall technique for prospective amputation level selection is transcutaneous oxygen testing.

Lower Extremity Amputation Levels

This section discusses only those amputation levels that are relevant to patients with peripheral vascular disease or diabetes mellitus. Amputation levels that are less desirable from the standpoint of healing or rehabilitation or those that present specific prosthetic fitting problems are omitted. In my experience and that of others, Chopart's, Lisfranc's, and Boyd's forefoot amputations have been fraught with controversy because of healing problems, prosthetic fitting problems, and equinus deformities.[88] Because these amputation levels are occasionally used by vascular surgeons, they are reviewed here only briefly.

TOE AMPUTATION

Toe amputation is the most frequently performed peripheral amputation. It is especially common in patients with diabetes mellitus, who are prone to lesions (ulceration, osteomyelitis, gangrene) that necessitate amputation.

Patients who present with dry gangrene allow the surgeon a choice between direct surgical intervention and autoamputation. In the absence of supervening infection or pain, expectant management permits epithelialization to take place under the dry gangrenous eschar. As soon as epithelialization is complete, the toe will drop off, leaving a cleanly healed stump. Autoamputation is preferable to direct surgical intervention because it obviates the need for healing after amputation and probably results in a more distal site of healing than would be achieved with surgical intervention. However, this process often requires months before it is complete.

Indications

Gangrene, infection, neuropathic ulceration, or osteomyelitis should be confined to the midphalanx or distal phalanx. There must be no dependent rubor, and venous filling time should be less than 20 to 25 seconds. Sizer and Wheelock demonstrated that the presence of pedal pulses, even in patients with diabetes, is associated with a very high rate of healing after toe amputation (98%).[89]

Contraindications

Cellulitis proximal to the area of proposed toe excision, the presence of dependent rubor, forefoot infection, and involvement of the metatarsophalangeal joint or (distal) metatarsal head all represent specific contraindications to toe amputation.

Surgical Technique

A single toe should never be amputated by disarticulation but should be transected through the proximal phalanx, leaving a small button of bone to protect the metatarsal head. Skin flaps can be of any design, as long as they obey basic surgical principles and have an adequate base for the length of flap. The flaps can be fish-mouth, plantar base, dorsal base, side to side, or any variation or combination; however, they must be long enough to close without tension. The most commonly used incision is circular (Fig. 49-2). Amputation through the metatarsophalangeal joint or an interphalangeal joint should be avoided because of the avascular nature of cartilage and the likelihood of supervening infection or failure to heal.

Careful atraumatic edge-to-edge skin closure without the use of forceps maximizes the chances of primary healing. Suture material that produces minimal reaction when left in place for long periods should be used, such as monofilament wire or plastic. A soft postoperative dressing that provides gentle wound compression should be applied.

Chronic osteomyelitis of the great toe without gangrene in a diabetic patient presents a difficult surgical problem. Because complete healing is not common, and total resection of the great toe results in some imbalance in walking (which can be accommodated with proper shoe orthotics), débridement and resection of the infected phalanges through a medial or lateral incision, leaving a soft tissue toe remnant in place, are probably best from a functional standpoint.

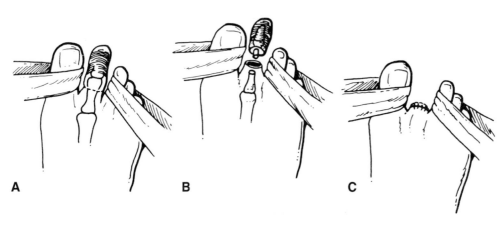

A   **B**   **C**

FIGURE 49–2 • Single-toe amputation using a circular incision and transverse wound closure.

Advantages and Disadvantages

The primary advantage of toe amputation is the lack of requirement for prosthetic rehabilitation and the fact that minimal tissue is excised.

Except for the risk of nonhealing or secondary infection and stump breakdown, requiring a higher level of amputation, there are no disadvantages to this level of amputation.

Rehabilitation Potential

Rehabilitation potential is 100%. However, the performance of a toe amputation in a patient with peripheral vascular disease, especially with concomitant diabetes, is an ominous sign with regard to long-term prognosis. Little and coworkers found that by 3.5 years after toe amputation, almost three fourths of their patients required a more proximal major amputation.[90]

RAY AMPUTATION

Indications

If the gangrenous skin or infectious process approaches the metatarsophalanged crease or includes the (distal) metatarsal head, this precludes a toe amputation. A conservative partial distal forefoot amputation can still be performed by extending the toe amputation to include the distal metatarsal shaft and head.

Contraindications

Gangrene, infection, cellulitis, and dependent rubor involving skin proximal to the metatarsophalangeal crease are contraindications to ray amputation. In addition, involvement of multiple toes is a relative contraindication, because a transmetatarsal amputation would be a more suitable surgical procedure. Ray amputation for gangrene or infection of the great toe also is a relative contraindication, because removal of the first metatarsal head leads to unstable weight bearing and difficulties with ambulation; however, with proper shoe orthotics, ray amputation of the first or great toe results in excellent foot salvage and provides patients with a stable gait pattern.

Surgical Technique

The incision begins vertically on the dorsum of the foot, bifurcates laterally and medially to encircle the toe, meets on the plantar aspect of the foot, and extends for a variable distance on the plantar aspect of the foot. The plantar incision is extended proximally as needed to allow removal of the toe and distal metatarsal head. Care should be taken not to injure the digital arteries or nerves adjacent to the metatarsal bone and not to enter into the deep tension or joint spaces of the medial and lateral toes. The distal metatarsal shaft is divided at its neck, and soft tissues are removed by sharp dissection. The surgical specimen consists of the toe, metatarsophalangeal joint, and distal portion of the metatarsal shaft and head. If possible, the surgical specimen should be removed in continuity. The metatarsal shaft must be transected in an area of normal bone. "Soft bone" suggests osteomyelitis, especially in diabetic patients, and mandates higher (i.e., more proximal) bone division.

I recommend that the surgical wound be generously irrigated with an antibiotic solution (the content of which is based on preoperative cultures, if available). Once again, attention is paid to meticulous hemostasis and atraumatic deep tissue and skin closure. Interrupted monofilament sutures that achieve edge-to-edge skin coaptation (without the use of forceps) should be placed (Fig. 49-3). The postoperative dressing can be either a soft dressing with an outer elastic wrap (which allows compression of the forefoot and removes tension from the suture line) or a combination of a soft dressing with foot and lower leg plaster cast (which provides maximum skin and wound protection). In the event that adequate hemostasis cannot be obtained, the use of a drain is suggested. In the presence of infection in either the metatarsophalangeal joint or skin flaps, consideration should be given to leaving the wound open and doing a delayed primary closure or allowing secondary healing.

Advantages and Disadvantages

This relatively conservative amputation results in minimal cosmetic deformity and maximum (100%) rehabilitation potential. There are no prosthetics required; however, ray resection of the first metatarsal head causes some walking

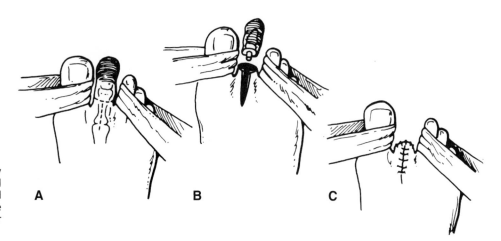

FIGURE 49–3 • Single-digit ray amputation of the foot. The dorsal and plantar incisions are closed in their original direction; the toe incision can be closed either vertically or transversely.

A   B   C

imbalance, and the foot should be fitted with a specially constructed shoe to minimize foot trauma and improve ambulatory balance.

There are no disadvantages, except for the risk of hematoma formation, nonhealing, secondary infection, or chronic osteomyelitis of the remaining metatarsal shaft.

TRANSMETATARSAL AMPUTATION

Indications

The indication for transmetatarsal amputation is gangrene or infection involving several toes or the great toe (on the same foot). This amputation may also be used if the gangrenous or infectious process extends a small distance on the dorsal skin past the metatarsophalangeal crease (but not up to the distal third or midthird junction of the forefoot), provided that the plantar skin is uncompromised.

Contraindications

Deep forefoot infection, cellulitis, lymphangitis, or dependent rubor involving the dorsal forefoot proximal to the metatarsophalangeal crease all represent contraindications to amputation at this level. In addition, gangrenous changes on the plantar skin of the foot, even those extending only a small distance past the metatarsophalangeal crease, is a specific contraindication to amputation at this level. Foot pulses are not necessary for healing, and venous refill should probably be less than 25 seconds.

Surgical Technique

An excellent description of the technique for transmetatarsal amputation was presented by McKittrick and associates in 1949.[91] A skin incision is designed that uses a total plantar flap. A slightly curved dorsal incision is carried from side to side at the foot at the level of the midmetatarsal shafts. The incision extends to the base of the toes medially and laterally in the midplane axis of the foot and then across the plantar surface at the metatarsophalangeal crease. It is important to place the dorsal skin incision slightly distal to the anticipated line of bone division. The dorsal skin incision is carried down to the metatarsal bones, and each metatarsal shaft is transected with an air-driven oscillating saw approximately 4 mm to 1 cm proximal to the skin incision (Fig. 49-4).

The plantar tissues in the distal forefoot are separated from the metatarsal shafts with a scalpel. The tissues of the plantar flap are thinned sharply, excising exposed tendons and leaving the underlying musculature attached to the skin flap. The plantar flap is then rotated dorsally for closure. Further tailoring or thinning of the plantar flap may be necessary to achieve good skin coaptation.

The importance of attention to absolute hemostasis cannot be overemphasized. A simple closure is performed, consisting of a deep layer of absorbable interrupted sutures and skin closure with a monofilament suture using a vertical mattress technique. Once again, careful approximation of skin edges is important, and I recommend not using forceps on the skin.

If adequate hemostasis cannot be readily achieved, use of a closed drainage system is suggested. Bone wax should not be used to control bleeding from the metatarsal shafts; the use of electrocautery to achieve hemostasis is preferable.

A well-padded short leg plaster cast is the best postoperative dressing because it controls edema and prevents stump trauma. I do not advise early ambulation after transmetatarsal amputation because of problems with flap necrosis and stump healing. If wound healing is satisfactory at the first cast change (7 to 10 days after surgery), a rubber heel may be incorporated into the second cast for ambulation. Subsequent casts are changed when they become loose, generally every 7 to 14 days, and a rigid dressing is used until the transmetatarsal flap is well healed, usually 3 to 4 weeks after surgery.

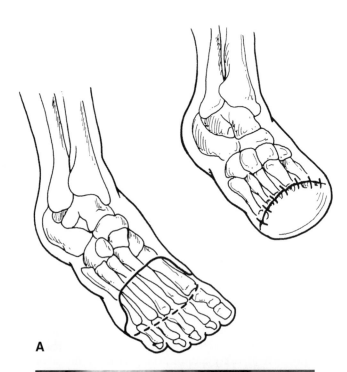

A

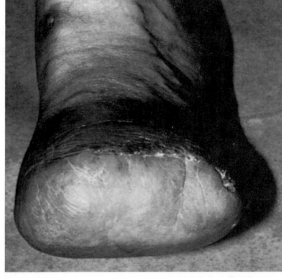

B

FIGURE 49–4 • *A,* Planned transmetatarsal plantar-based skin flap and appearance of the completed closure. *B,* Healed right transmetatarsal amputation treated with immediate postsurgical prosthetic fitting, 1 month after amputation.

Advantages and Disadvantages

Transmetatarsal amputation provides an excellent result compared with more proximal foot or lower extremity amputation. Disability is minimal, and the prosthetic requirements are relatively simple.

The primary disadvantages of a transmetatarsal amputation are the risks of nonhealing, infection, and hematoma formation and the necessity for a secondary higher-level amputation.

Prosthetic Requirements and Rehabilitation Potential

To achieve maximum ambulation potential, some minor prosthetic modification should be considered. A shoe that incorporates a steel shank in the sole allows normal toe-off during ambulation. The spring steel shank reproduces the action of the longitudinal arch of the foot during ambulation. A custom-molded foam pad or lamb's wool can be used to fill the toe portion of the shoe. An alternative approach is to use a custom-molded shoe with a roller-shaped sole to provide toe-off motion during walking.

There are relatively few, if any, limitations in rehabilitation for a transmetatarsal amputation. With proper shoe modification, there should be no discernible physical disability for a transmetatarsal amputee during ambulation. It is important, however, that the shoe or other prosthetic device be properly constructed to avoid stump ulceration and breakdown. There are increased numbers of anecdotal reports combining guillotine forefoot amputation with secondary distal split-thickness skin graft to achieve successful healing at this amputation level. Although this latter technique allows the salvage of more proximal transmetatarsal amputations, I do not favor its use because of frequent problems with distal stump (skin graft) breakdown in active patients.

LISFRANC'S AND CHOPART'S AMPUTATIONS

Indications

Some reports have called attention to foot-sparing amputations when a transmetatarsal amputation is precluded because of the extent of ischemia or infection.[92-95] The Lisfranc amputation is a tarsometatarsal joint amputation, and the Chopart amputation is a midtarsal joint amputation. I agree with Chang and coworkers[95] that both of these mid-forefoot amputations are easier to perform than a Syme's amputation and may improve long-term ambulation.[96]

Contraindications

Both Lisfranc's and Chopart's amputations result in the development of equinovarus deformity and require lengthening of the Achilles tendon to achieve maximum rehabilitation potential.[93,94] In addition, Hirsch and colleagues documented force plate data showing that an abnormal pattern characterized by reduced stance duration and deficient forward propulsion on the amputated side was greater in a Chopart's prosthesis than in a transmetatarsal prosthesis.[96] That study also documented stump problems as the principal difficulty with Chopart's amputations over time.

Surgical Technique

Both Lisfranc's (tarsometatarsal joint) and Chopart's (midtarsal joint) amputations are well described in articles by Sanders[94] and Chang and coworkers,[95] to which interested readers are referred.

Prosthetic Requirements and Rehabilitation Potential

I agree with a modified version of the conclusion reached by Chang and coworkers that ischemic foot necrosis extending beyond the limits of conventional transmetatarsal amputation does not necessarily require a major limb amputation.[95] With improvements in patient selection and surgical technique, Lisfranc's and Chopart's amputations are viable options when attempting to salvage mid- to hindfoot structures. From a prosthetic standpoint, fitting of these more distal and conservative amputation levels should emphasize unloading the distal part of the stump and smoothing out the impulsive force peak on the stump in late stance to minimize pain, decrease stump breakdown, and enhance ambulation capacity.[96]

SYME'S AMPUTATION

Syme first described this amputation in 1843.[97] Then, as now, there were arguments over its merit. Harris (in Toronto) has championed Syme's amputation and has written several excellent articles concerning its development and the surgical technique necessary for successful results.[98,99] I believe that the Syme's amputation is the most technically demanding lower extremity amputation, and attention to surgical detail is crucial for its success.

Indications

If the gangrenous or infectious process precludes transmetatarsal amputation, the next level to be considered is an ankle disarticulation, or Syme's amputation.

Contraindications

If the gangrenous or infectious process involves the heel, if there are open lesions on the heel or about the ankle, if there is cellulitis or lymphangitis ascending up the distal leg, or if dependent rubor is present at the heel, Syme's amputation is contraindicated. The presence of a neuropathic foot in a diabetic patient, when there is absence of heel sensation, is also a relative contraindication to Syme's amputation. A high rate of primary healing demands the use of objective, noninvasive amputation level selection techniques before surgery and preservation of the posterior tibial artery (if patent).

Surgical Technique

The skin incision is placed to construct a posterior flap using the heel pad. The dorsal incision extends across the ankle from the tip of the medial malleolus to the tip of the lateral malleolus. The plantar incision begins at a 90-degree angle from the dorsal incision and progresses around the plantar

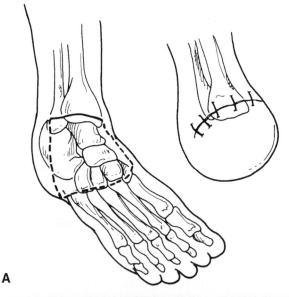

A

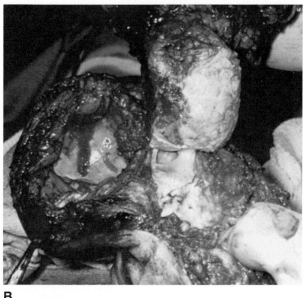

B

FIGURE 49–5 • *A,* Syme's amputation, with a posterior heel-based skin flap, performed with the one-stage surgical technique. *B,* Intraoperative photograph of a Syme's amputation showing the Achilles attachment of the calcaneus *(midsuperior portion of picture),* the tibial plateau, and the heel flap *(lower left corner).*

aspect of the foot distal to the heel pad (Fig. 49-5). The dorsal incision is deepened through subcutaneous tissues and carried down to bone without dissection in the tissue planes. The anterior tendons (tibialis anterior, extensor hallucis longus, and extensor digitorum longus) are pulled down into the wound, transected, and allowed to retract. The anterior tibial artery is identified, clamped, divided, and suture-ligated. The incision is then deepened, and the capsule of the tibial-talar joint is opened. The tibialis posterior tendon is divided, and the foot is forced into plantar flexion to provide increased visualization of the tibial-talar joint. Great care should be taken during medial dissection to preserve the posterior tibial artery. The joint is further dislocated by incising the

posterior capsule. The peroneus brevis and tertius tendons are transected. The plantar aspect of the incision is deepened through all layers of the sole of the foot down to the neck of the calcaneus. The calcaneus is then carefully and sharply dissected from the heel pad. Dissection of the calcaneus is the most difficult part of the operation, and great care is needed to maintain the dissection on the bony surface of the calcaneus to prevent damage to the soft tissues of the heel, injury to the posterior tibial artery, and buttonholing of the posterior skin as the Achilles tendon is transected. Performance of Syme's amputation by the one-stage and two-stage techniques is identical up to this point.

If the surgeon chooses the one-stage technique, the lateral and medial malleoli are transected flush with the articular surface of the tibial-talar joint with an air-driven reciprocating saw. Once again, the importance of hemostasis cannot be overemphasized. If adequate hemostasis cannot be achieved, a closed drainage system should be incorporated. Even in dry surgical wounds, the use of a drain is advocated by some authors.[88,98,99] I prefer to irrigate the surgical wound with copious amounts of antibiotic solution before closure. The heel pad is rotated anteriorly and sutured to the proximal dorsal skin edge with a single layer of interrupted vertical mattress sutures. Once again, atraumatic placement of skin sutures is mandatory, and forceps should not be used on the skin edges.

If the two-stage technique is selected,[88] the lateral and medial malleoli are not transected. A drain is placed, and the wound is closed as previously described. Approximately 6 weeks after performance of the first stage, the patient is returned to surgery for the second stage (which can be done under local anesthesia). Medial and lateral incisions are made over the dog ears on the amputation stump, and the incisions are carried down to bone with sharp dissection. The malleoli are removed flush with the ankle joint. The tibial articular cartilage is not disturbed. The distal tibia and fibula are exposed subperiosteally approximately 6 cm above the ankle joint, and the tibial and fibular flares are removed with an osteotome and a smooth rongeur. This last procedure produces a relatively square stump that simplifies postoperative prosthetic fitting and improves cosmesis. If the heel pad is loose after removal of the malleoli, it can be secured to the tibia and fibula through drill holes in the bones.

The postoperative dressing for a Syme's amputation stump (for both one- and two-stage procedures) is extremely important; it is critical to maintain correct alignment of the heel pad over the end of the tibia and fibula during healing. Either a soft compression dressing or a rigid plaster cast can be used as a postoperative dressing; however, most authors prefer the application of a short leg plaster cast. If a cast is used, great care must be taken to avoid injury to the medial and lateral skin flaps (dog ears). Weight bearing should not occur during the early phases of healing of a Syme's amputation because of the risks of nonhealing and flap necrosis. When the first cast is removed, usually 7 to 10 days after surgery, a second cast that incorporates a walking heel can be applied if healing is satisfactory. I prefer to keep Syme's amputation patients nonambulatory for 3 weeks after amputation to allow good heel pad fixation and healing. After ambulation begins, the patients are kept in a short leg walking cast for an additional 3 to 4 weeks before construction of a temporary removable prosthesis.

Advantages and Disadvantages

The Syme's amputation stump is extremely durable because it is end-weight bearing. It involves minimal disability from the standpoint of walking. Performance of a one-stage Syme's amputation results in a somewhat bulbous distal stump compared with a two-stage Syme's amputation. For cosmetic reasons, a two-stage procedure is probably preferable in female patients, although I generally do not perform Syme's amputations in young female patients because of concerns about cosmesis. Clinical evaluation by patients, prosthetists, and surgeons has consistently shown that the Syme's amputation is superior to amputation levels above the ankle. Oxygen uptake, gait velocity, cadence, and stride length are significantly better in patients with Syme's amputations than in those with higher-level amputations.[100]

Delayed healing or healing complications due to hematoma formation or infection are not uncommon. Careful preoperative amputation level selection helps ensure primary healing of a Syme's amputation. Failure to heal almost always results in performance of a more proximal amputation. Long-term follow-up of my diabetic patients with normal or "almost normal" sensation in whom a Syme's level was chosen demonstrates a high incidence of revision to the below-knee level because of problems resulting from a progressive insensate Syme's stump (i.e., progressive neuropathy). Other authors have not reported similar problems.

Prosthetic Requirements and Rehabilitation Potential

Ambulation in the home can be achieved without the application of a prosthetic appliance; however, ambulation outside the home requires some type of prosthetic device. The usual cosmetic prosthesis consists of a foot and a plastic shell that incorporates the lower leg. A typical prosthesis for a patient with a one-stage Syme's amputation is shown in Figure 49-6. Ambulation in the home or for limited distances can be achieved with the application of a simple strap on a cup slipper with a built-up heel.

A patient with a successful Syme's amputation and an appropriately fitted prosthesis can expect a minimal degree of disability. Energy consumption compared with that of a non-amputee is, at most, 10% above normal. Many patients with Syme's amputations continue to be employed, including some who perform heavy manual labor. The salvage of a Syme's amputation, especially in patients who are likely to become bilateral amputees, may be the ultimate difference between continued ambulation and nonambulation.

BELOW-KNEE AMPUTATION

Indications

Below-knee amputation is the most common amputation level selected for the management of lower extremity gangrene, infection, or ischemia with nonhealing lesions that preclude more distal amputations. When the blood supply is inadequate for healing at more distal levels, amputation at the below-knee level can be expected to provide adequate blood supply for healing in the majority of cases. In fact, as

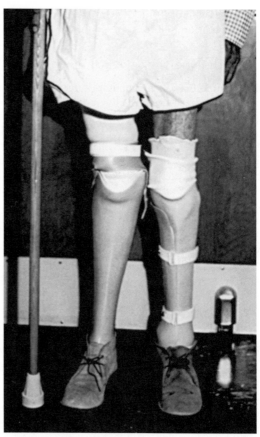

FIGURE 49–6 • Bilateral lower extremity amputee with a right below-knee amputation and a left Syme's amputation. The Syme's prosthesis is a standard medial window design for a one-stage Syme's amputation. Note the bulbous distal ankle on the Syme's prosthesis *(left leg)*, compared with the cosmetic ankle on the below-knee prosthesis *(right leg)*.

previously noted, 83% of all patients undergoing lower extremity amputation can expect healing of a below-knee amputation[44] (see Table 49-3). With objective amputation level selection, primary healing rates in excess of 94% can be expected.

Contraindications

A below-knee amputation is contraindicated if the gangrenous or infectious process involves skin on the anterior portion of the lower extremity within 4 to 5 cm of the tibial tuberosity or skin that would be used to construct the posterior flap. A flexion contracture of the knee greater than 20 degrees also represents a contraindication to below-knee amputation. Great caution should be used when attempting below-knee amputation in patients with an occluded deep femoral artery (the superficial femoral is almost always occluded) in the absence of objective amputation level selection data that suggest that the amputation will heal. Finally, a patient with stroke or neurologic dysfunction on the side of proposed amputation, in whom muscle spasticity or rigidity is marked, should not have a below-knee amputation because spastic muscles will force the knee into flexion and ultimately result in amputation failure.

Surgical Technique

Two significant advances in amputation technique have contributed to better results after below-knee amputation: use of a long posterior flap, and application of a rigid dressing in the immediate postoperative period. There is considerable clinical and theoretical information available to support the use of a long posterior flap. The gastrocnemius and soleus muscles and the overlying posterior calf skin derive their major blood supply through the sural arteries, which originate proximal to the knee joint. Blood flow is maintained to this area in many patients, particularly diabetic patients, in whom flow through the popliteal artery and its major branches is restricted. Blood supply via the anterior tibial artery and geniculate collaterals to the skin and soft tissues of the anterior lower leg is so poor that even if equal anterior and posterior below-knee skin flaps are used, there is a high incidence of rehabilitation failure due to wound necrosis of the anterior skin flap.

The operation can be performed under general or spinal anesthesia, with the patient in the supine position on the operating table. If there are open infected lesions on the foot, a plastic bag or plastic adherent drape can be placed over the open infected portion of the extremity to isolate it. As mentioned previously, in a patient with a septic foot, a preparatory ankle guillotine amputation followed by a delayed primary below-knee amputation results in a higher rate of healing and fewer stump infections than the performance of a one-stage primary below-knee amputation.[36,37] An alternative to the two-stage approach (one-stage technique with delayed primary closure) that works well for diabetic patients, except those with Wagner grade 5 foot infection, was reported by Kernek and Rozzi.[101]

I prefer to use a long posterior flap and no anterior flap for reasons previously stated; however, there is at least one prospective, randomized study comparing a sagittal technique and long posterior musculocutaneous flaps that found no significant difference with respect to healing, limb fitting, ambulation, and ultimate rehabilitation.[102] Another report of sagittal incisions for below-knee amputation pointed out the utility of this type of incision in patients in whom a long posterior flap may be contraindicated because of infection or skin necrosis.[103] A report by Ruckley and coworkers noted that for below-knee amputations in patients with end-stage peripheral vascular disease, the skew flap is an excellent alternative to the long posterior flap.[104] The techniques for construction of a long posterior flap in below-knee amputation have been well documented in many previous publications[10,105-107]; however, the salient features of the amputation are outlined here.

For a standard below-knee amputation, I select a point of bone division approximately a handbreadth, including the thumb, below the tibial tuberosity. When there is concern that the posterior flap may impinge on distal infection or ischemia, a palmbreadth (minus the thumb) can be used for the point of division below the tibial tuberosity. The absolute minimum length for a below-knee amputation is three fingerbreadths (7 to 8 cm) below the tibial tuberosity. The skin incision should be approximately 1 cm distal to the intended point of bone division. The transverse diameter of the midshaft calf at the level of the anterior incision, plus 1 inch, represents the approximate length of the posterior skin flap. It is usually my preference to outline the flap with a marking pencil before making a skin incision. The anterior skin incision represents the anterior half of the circumference of the extremity. The skin incision then abruptly turns distally with gentle curves and proceeds down the medial and lateral aspects of the extremity, in the midplane axis of the leg, to the point of the distal extent of the posterior skin flap. The two lateral incisions are then connected posteriorly. My preference is then to incise the flap through skin and fascia in all areas before muscle transection. Use of a proximal tourniquet for hemostatic control is optional in patients undergoing traumatic below-knee amputation but is relatively contraindicated in patients undergoing elective below-knee amputation for ischemia. Use of electrocautery is preferred for division of all muscles. The anterior tibial muscle is divided at the level of bone division, and the anterior tibial neurovascular bundle is identified, clamped, divided, and suture-ligated. Electrocautery is used to incise the tibial periosteum circumferentially, and a periosteal elevator is used to mobilize the periosteum of the tibia proximal to the point of proposed bone division. The tibia is then divided with an air-driven reciprocating saw. Using electrocautery, the fibula is isolated at the level of the transected tibia and divided approximately 0.25 inch proximal to the tibia, using the saw. Following division of the fibula and tibia, proximal traction is placed on the transected tibia (use of a bone hook is easiest), and the lower extremity is bent at 90 degrees and retracted distally. The posterior tibial artery and vein and the common peroneal artery and vein are identified, clamped, transected, and individually suture-ligated. The posterior tibial nerve is identified, pulled into the wound, ligated, transected, and allowed to retract out of the area of surgical incision. The posterior calf muscle musculature is transected, leaving the gastrocnemius muscle as part of the posterior skin flap. The surgical specimen is then divided at the same point as the posterior flap skin incision, which permits removal of the surgical specimen. Care should be taken not to thin the posterior flap so much that there is inadequate coverage for the tibia when the flap is closed. The saw is used to bevel the tibia at a 45- to 60-degree angle, and the bony edges are filed smooth. Care is also taken to ensure that the distal ends of the fibula are smooth (Fig. 49-7).

The wound is copiously irrigated with an antibiotic solution. Once again, the importance of meticulous hemostasis cannot be stressed enough. Generally, drains are not necessary in below-knee amputations for peripheral vascular disease; however, drains are frequently used in below-knee amputations performed for trauma or other reasons. If a drain is required, I prefer a closed suction drain, which is brought through a separate stab wound in the lateral aspect of the lower leg. The sural nerve (posterior flap) is identified, pulled down, ligated, transected, and allowed to retract back from the edge of the flap. The flap is rotated anteriorly, and the muscle fascia of the posterior flap is approximated to the anterior fascia with interrupted absorbable sutures. The skin is carefully approximated with interrupted vertical mattress sutures using a monofilament plastic or metal suture. I avoid the use of tissue forceps and believe that closure of the below-knee stump,

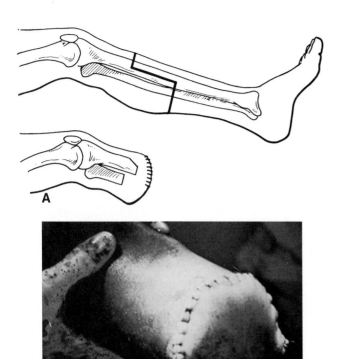

A

B

FIGURE 49–7 • *A,* Standard posterior flap below-knee amputation. Note the beveled tibia and the proximal shortening of the fibula compared with the tibia. *B,* Intraoperative photograph showing a below-knee amputation. Note the skin coaptation with interrupted sutures and the minimal dog ears.

especially in patients with peripheral vascular disease, should be performed with the care of a plastic surgical procedure. Tailoring the corner of the skin flap may be required to prevent excessive dog ears.

The use of a rigid plaster of Paris dressing incorporating the knee is ideal, regardless of whether an immediate postoperative prosthesis will be used. A rigid dressing controls edema, promotes healing, and protects the stump during the postoperative period. In addition, a rigid dressing prevents flexion contracture. Application of an immediate postoperative prosthesis as part of the rigid dressing is described in detail later.

Advantages and Disadvantages

The below-knee amputation is an extremely durable amputation. The likelihood of primary healing is very good, and the ability to rehabilitate a patient with a below-knee prosthesis is excellent. In a report by Kim and coworkers in 1976, 90% of their patients with unilateral below-knee amputations were able to ambulate.[108] Roon and colleagues achieved a 100% ambulation rate with unilateral below-knee amputations and a 93% ambulation rate in patients with bilateral below-knee amputations.[14] In addition, 91% of the patients reported by Roon's group were still ambulatory an average of 44 months following amputation.[14]

In the absence of the ability to perform a more distal amputation, there are no specific disadvantages of a below-knee amputation.

Prosthetic Requirements and Rehabilitation Potential

A below-knee prosthesis is required for ambulation at this level of amputation. A variety of prostheses are available, but all generally involve total stump contact (with or without a prosthesis liner) with weight bearing on the patellar tendon and tibial-fibular condyles. Newer types of below-knee prostheses incorporate total contact and total weight-bearing designs. The prosthesis can be suspended with a variety of techniques, including a thigh lacer with external joints, Silastic sleeve suspension, standard patellar tendon-bearing (PTB) strap, supracondylar medial clip, suction, and self-suspension secondary to muscle control. These prostheses can incorporate a variety of feet, some of which have flexion and extension motion or "ankle rotation" (with weight loading) or energy storage (Seattle Foot [Model & Instrument Works, Inc., Seattle]; Flex-Foot [Össur, Scheck & Siress, Gakbrook Terrace, Ill.]). The energy requirement for a unilateral below-knee amputee is increased approximately 40% to 60% compared with normal (energy consumption with an energy-storing leg has not yet been reported).

It has been my experience, as well as that of others, that any patient (regardless of age) who was ambulatory before below-knee amputation and who undergoes amputation within 30 days of hospital entrance can ambulate successfully on a below-knee prosthesis. In fact, most patients who require bilateral below-knee amputations can ambulate successfully, as shown by Roon and associates.[14] The importance of aggressive rehabilitation after unilateral below-knee amputation in patients who are at high risk for bilateral lower extremity amputation was stressed in a report by Inderbitzi and coworkers.[109] Delay in rehabilitation resulted in a high rate of nonambulatory patients after the second amputation. The time required for gait training for a unilateral below-knee amputee is approximately 2 to 3 weeks, and most patients develop a very good gait pattern. There are some physical limitations for geriatric below-knee amputees; however, young below-knee amputees are able to negotiate ladders, stairs, and other obstacles with minimal difficulty.

KNEE DISARTICULATION

Indications

The indications for knee disarticulation amputation are limited, and it is performed primarily on young, active males for whom the advantages of strength and serviceability outweigh prosthetic cosmesis. Disarticulation amputation of the knee is the second most technically difficult lower extremity amputation following Syme's amputation. Successful performance of a knee disarticulation amputation with a high degree of primary healing usually requires some type of objective technique of preoperative amputation level selection. Knee disarticulation is indicated primarily when the gangrenous process, infection, trauma, tumor, or orthopedic disability encroaches too close to the anterior and posterior (or sagittal) limits of a below-knee amputation flap or has resulted in an unsalvageable knee joint. Another potential indication for knee disarticulation is a patient who has had either acute or chronic failure of a below-knee amputation in whom skin flaps at the knee are viable enough to consider knee disarticulation. In general, British surgeons have been more enamored of knee disarticulation than their American colleagues. Interest in this level of amputation has arisen as a result of advances in cosmetic prosthetic components and prosthetic fitting techniques. Moreover, in a study of 169 unilateral lower extremity amputees, Houghton and coworkers found that rehabilitation results were better for through-knee amputation (62%) than for above-knee (33%) (P < 0.02) or Gritti-Stokes (44%) amputation.[110]

Contraindications

Contraindications to knee disarticulation are inadequate blood flow to the skin in the region or ulceration, gangrene, or infection involving tissues about the knee joint or the joint space.

Surgical Technique

There are two excellent reviews of the surgical techniques of disarticulation of the knee[111,112]; therefore, they are described only briefly here. I prefer the knee disarticulation technique described by Burgess,[111] owing to failure with other types of knee disarticulation amputation and success using the modified Burgess technique.

Anesthetic management of knee disarticulation is best handled with either spinal or general anesthesia, with the patient in the prone position. The operation can be performed, but is more difficult, with the patient in the supine position. At the discretion of the surgeon, a gown or pack can be placed beneath the thigh to hyperextend the hip joint and provide an easier working surface on the anterior portion of the knee and lower leg. The leg is held in a flexed position. Depending on the availability of suitable skin, a classic long anterior, equal flap, or sagittal flap–type incision can be used (Fig. 49-8). A marking pencil should be used to outline the skin flaps before making the skin incision. Construction of the knee disarticulation skin flaps is crucial to avoid tension on the skin suture line when the amputation stump is closed. Dissection is first carried anteriorly down to the insertion of the patellar tendon on the tibia. The tendon is severed at its insertion and sharply dissected proximally. Deep dissection on the medial side of the knee results in exposure of the

hamstring muscles. The tendons are sectioned and allowed to retract. The deep fascia is reflected with the overlying tendon and skin flap. On the lateral side of the knee, the tendon of the biceps femoris muscle and iliotibial band are sectioned low. The knee joint is entered anteriorly, the knee is flexed, and the cruciate ligaments are transected at their tibial insertion. The posterior knee capsule structures are divided, and the individual members of the popliteal vascular sheath are clamped, transected, and suture-ligated. The tibial and peroneal nerves are identified, retracted under moderate tension, ligated, sectioned with a sharp knife, and allowed to retract into the proximal amputation stump. The patella is removed subperiosteally, and the fascial defect in the patellar tendon is closed with interrupted sutures.

The femoral condyles are now transected transversely, approximately 1.5 cm above the level of the knee joint (Fig. 49-9). Sharp distal femoral margins are carefully contoured. The patellar tendon is pulled down into the intracondylar notch under moderate tension and sewn to the stump of the crus ligaments. The semitendinosus and biceps tendons are likewise pulled into the notch, tailored, and sewn to the stump of the patellar tendon and cruciate ligaments. This approximation of the tendons and ligaments allows muscle stability. The superficial skin fascia is approximated with interrupted absorbable sutures, and the skin is meticulously closed using a vertical mattress technique with monofilament metal or plastic sutures, without the use of forceps. Alternatively, skin staples may be used. The use of a through-and-through or a suction drain is optional and is left to the discretion of the surgeon. A rigid dressing, with or without the incorporation of an immediate postoperative prosthesis, should be applied.

Advantages and Disadvantages

The advantages of a knee disarticulation amputation include excellent durability and end–weight-bearing capacity; retention of a long, powerful, muscle-stabilized femoral lever arm; improved proprioception; and a limb-socket interface with improved prosthetic suspension and rotational control (compared with an above-knee amputation). This amputation level is almost as good as a below-knee amputation and is therefore a tremendous benefit to the patient in comparison to the next higher level, the above-knee amputation.

The absence of a knee joint and increased energy expenditure make this amputation level less advantageous than a below-knee amputation.

Prosthetic Requirements and Rehabilitation Potential

Historically, knee disarticulation amputations were not well liked in the prosthetic community because of cosmetic and knee-thigh length problems resulting from existing prosthetic components (nonequal knee centers); however, the availability of lightweight polycentric hydraulic knee joints and endoskeletal systems has helped solve these problems. The usual knee disarticulation socket incorporates some type of medial window to allow the bulbous stump to pass through the smaller lower thigh portion of the socket.

Knee disarticulation amputation is probably most useful in young, active patients without peripheral vascular disease. However, this amputation is also an excellent choice for

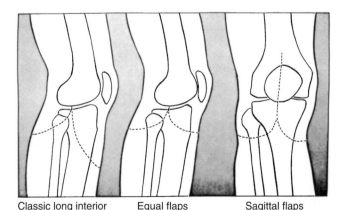

Classic long interior   Equal flaps   Sagittal flaps

FIGURE 49–8 • The three types of skin incisions commonly used for knee disarticulation amputation. (From Burgess EM: Disarticulation of the knee: A modified technique. Arch Surg 117:1251, 1977.)

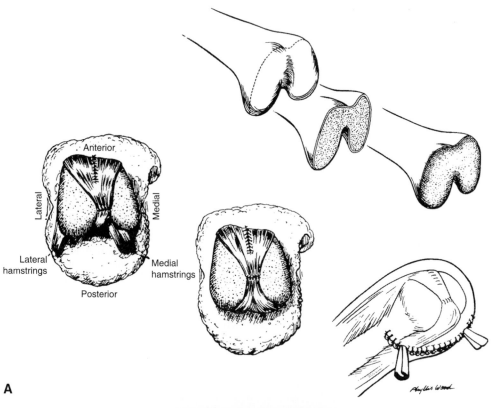

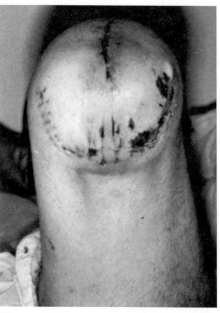

FIGURE 49–9 • *A*, The femur is transected 1.5 cm above the condylar ends, the patellar tendon is sewn to the cruciate ligaments, the hamstring tendons are sutured to the cruciate-patellar ligaments, and the wound is closed over a drain. *B*, Anterior flap knee disarticulation amputation at the first postoperative cast change (7 to 10 days) with the patient in the supine position (in this case, the patella was removed transcutaneously). (From Burgess EM: Disarticulation of the knee: A modified technique. Arch Surg 117:1253, 1977.)

geriatric patients. Patient performance is better than that with a mid- to high above-knee amputation, although not nearly as good as that with a standard below-knee amputation. There are some physical limitations resulting from the absence of a knee joint, specifically involving climbing stairs and ladders and physical tasks that require rotational or flexion-extension knee motions.

ABOVE-KNEE AMPUTATION

Indications

The indications for an amputation at the above-knee level are inadequate blood flow for healing at a more distal level, a disabled patient who is not expected to walk again, profound life-threatening infection with questionable viability of the lower extremity, and extensive infection or gangrene that would preclude a knee disarticulation or below-knee amputation. Historically, above-knee amputation has been the operation of choice for many surgeons because greater than 90% primary healing can be anticipated, regardless of the vascular status of the patient.

Contraindications

Extension of the infectious or gangrenous process to the level of the proposed above-knee amputation is the most common contraindication. Severe necrotizing lower extremity infection is a relative contraindication unless a high above-knee amputation is performed.

Surgical Technique

There are three basic levels for the above-knee amputation (Fig. 49-10). In general, the longer the above-knee amputation stump, the more likely the patient is to ambulate, so the stump should be as long as possible. If an amputation is being performed to control sepsis or toxicity, a midthigh or high-thigh amputation provides more assurance of healing and control of systemic toxicity, although the chances of rehabilitation are less.

Either a circular or a sagittal-type incision can be used. I prefer a circular (or fish-mouth) incision appropriate for the level of anticipated bone division. A circumferential line of

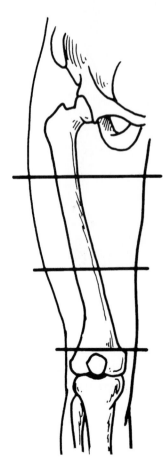

FIGURE 49-10 • The three common levels of above-knee amputation.

incision is drawn with a marking pen 2 to 3 cm below the level of the proposed bone transection. The incision is then carried down through skin and fascia. The skin and fascia are retracted superiorly to allow more proximal muscle division. I prefer to use electrocautery for muscle division. The femoral artery and vein are identified, clamped, divided, and suture-ligated in the subsartorial canal. All the muscles of the anterior, medial, and lateral thigh are transected. The muscle mass is then retracted proximally, the proposed line of bone transection is exposed, and the periosteum is cut using electrocautery. An air-driven reciprocating saw is then used to transect the femur. The posterior muscles are transected using electrocautery. The sciatic nerve is identified, pulled down into the wound, ligated, transected, and allowed to retract into the proximal amputation stump. The rough edges of the femur are filed smooth. The amputation stump should be irrigated with an antibiotic solution, especially if the amputation is being performed for infection. The soft tissues and skin are drawn distally to ensure adequate soft tissue coverage for the femur. If soft tissue coverage is adequate, the wound is closed in two layers. The fascia is closed with an interrupted absorbable suture, and the skin is closed with interrupted vertical mattress sutures of plastic or metal monofilament. Good skin coaptation is important, and the use of forceps on the skin should be avoided. If the soft tissue coverage for the bone is inadequate, the femur is shortened as required to allow adequate soft tissue coverage without tension on the skin suture line (Fig. 49-11). If the amputation is being performed for infection, especially a necrotizing infection, the wound should be left open. If a fish-mouth incision is used, the apex of the "angle of the mouth" approximates the point of bony division. Closure, although spatially different, encompasses the careful atraumatic technique described previously.

A rigid dressing can be applied and is advantageous for control of stump edema, but it is much more cumbersome and less valuable than a rigid dressing used at lower amputation levels. I prefer to use a soft dressing suspended with a Silesian type of elastic bandage or a modified waist suspension belt.[113] After the wound has healed satisfactorily (1 to 2 weeks after surgery), a temporary removable prosthesis can be provided if appropriate.

Advantages and Disadvantages

The primary advantage of an above-knee amputation is the very high likelihood of primary healing. Prosthetic rehabilitation is very difficult at this level of amputation. Whereas 80% to 90% of all patients with unilateral or bilateral below-knee amputations can be expected to ambulate, only 40% to 50% of unilateral above-knee amputees can be expected to do so. It has been my experience that less than 10% of bilateral lower extremity amputees, when one side is an above-knee amputation, will successfully ambulate.

Prosthetic Requirements and Rehabilitation Potential

A variety of prostheses are available for above-knee amputees. Newer prosthetic devices incorporate contoured axially aligned sockets, ultralightweight materials, endoskeletal design, hydraulic-assisted knee joints, ankle rotators and motion feet, and energy storage. There is a direct correlation between successful ambulation at this level of amputation and the weight of the prosthesis because of the energy expenditure required for walking. Compared with normal, the energy expenditure of an above-knee amputee is increased 80% to 120%.

As noted, the rehabilitation potential for a unilateral above-knee amputee is only fair and averages 10% to 50%.

HIP DISARTICULATION AMPUTATION

In general, hip disarticulation amputation is not an operation that general or vascular surgeons usually perform,

because almost all patients will heal after a high above-knee amputation.

Indications

The indications for hip disarticulation are inadequate blood flow (usually in patients with occlusion of both the deep and superficial femoral arteries) for healing of a more distal amputation, a life-threatening infection or extensive gangrene that precludes amputation at a lower level, trauma, tumor, and failed hip reconstruction.[114] Wound complications occur frequently, and their incidence is increased for urgent or emergent operations and in patients with prior above-knee amputations.[115] In addition, both limb ischemia and infection increase the mortality rate.

Contraindications

In my experience, infection that precludes hip disarticulation amputation is almost uniformly fatal. There are no contraindications to this level of amputation, except infection and gangrene (or tumor) that extends above the level of the proposed amputation.

Surgical Technique

Because this procedure is performed only occasionally by general and vascular surgeons, and because there are excellent articles describing this operation,[114-118] the surgical technique is not presented here. Based on a limited experience, I favor a posterior flap technique (Fig. 49-12A).

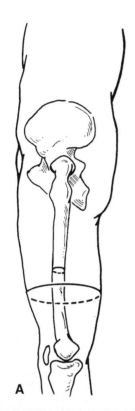

A

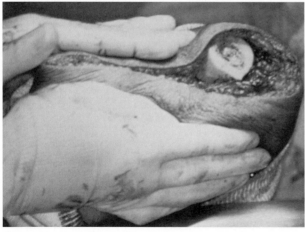

B

FIGURE 49–11 • *A*, Standard circular incision technique for above-knee amputation. Sagittal flaps can be used if appropriate. The key to closure is adequate femur shortening to avoid later bone protrusion through the distal end of the stump. *B*, Intraoperative photograph of an above-knee amputation stump demonstrates why skin and soft tissue length for bone coverage should be checked before closure. Proximal femur shortening was required to decrease wound tension.

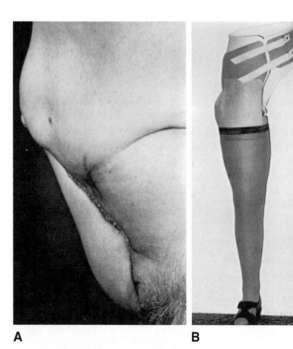

A   **B**

FIGURE 49–12 • *A*, Photograph of a left hip disarticulation stump 6 months after amputation. The operation was performed with a posterior gluteal flap technique. *B*, Ultralightweight (4.5 pounds) left hip disarticulation prosthesis based on an Aqualite plastic endoskeletal system with cosmetic cover (US Manufacturing Co., Pasadena, Calif.) and a Scotchcast Canadian-type socket (bucket).

Advantages and Disadvantages

In the absence of healing at an above-knee level, there is a higher likelihood of primary healing.

Prosthetic rehabilitation at this level of lower extremity amputation is uncommon (<10%), even with unilateral amputation in geriatric patients.

Prosthetic Requirements

Various types of prostheses have been described and created for hip disarticulation amputees. Most of them entail a pelvic bucket (Canadian-type) prosthesis (Fig. 49-12B) and are endoskeletal in construction (to save weight); few involve the use of sophisticated knee joints, ankle joints, or motion feet. A full discussion of the prosthetic requirements for this level of amputation is beyond the scope of this chapter, and interested readers are referred to appropriate references.[114-117] Compared with normal, the energy expenditure of a hip disarticulation amputee is increased 1.5 to 2.5 times.

Complications of Lower Extremity Amputation

Historically, postoperative morbidity and mortality following major lower extremity amputation were common, and the incidence of fatal complications was high enough to engender considerable debate about the optimal preoperative, operative, and postoperative management. In general, however, the morbidity and mortality following a major lower extremity amputation have decreased with time.[119-121]

The major postoperative complications following lower extremity amputation and their frequency of occurrence are listed in Table 49-4. Each of these complications is addressed separately in the following paragraphs.

EARLY POSTOPERATIVE COMPLICATIONS

Pain

The literature suggests that the incidence of disabling stump pain and phantom limb pain following major lower extremity amputation ranges from 5% to 30%.[122-127] In a retrospective random survey of 5000 Veterans Administration (VA) amputees, Sherman and coworkers noted that 85% of the

TABLE 49–4	Postoperative Complications	
Complication	**Incidence (%)**	**References**
Stump pain/phantom pain	5-80	9, 14, 20, 122-129
Death	0-35	7, 9, 20, 100, 119, 120, 130, 131
Pulmonary complications	8	14
Stump infection	12-28	120, 131
Nonhealing stump	3-28	9, 14, 20, 119, 120, 130
Pulmonary embolus	4-38	7, 14
Deep venous thrombosis	1-3	9, 14, 20
Flexion contracture	1-3	9, 14, 20, 57
Renal insufficiency	1-3	9, 14, 20

respondents reported significant phantom limb pain.[128,129] Their explanation for the high incidence of pain was based in part on the fact that most reports, especially those citing pain treatment modalities, have inadequate post-treatment follow-up. In addition, Sherman and coworkers suggested that most amputees quickly learn that physicians are not interested in pain problems and therefore fail to give accurate responses when questioned, often to protect their credibility and relationship with their physician (thereby guaranteeing long-term care). Of more concern was the fact that statistical analysis of 42 of the most common treatment modalities for phantom limb pain, including drug therapy, local injections, and surgery, showed that no treatment provided satisfactory results.[128,129] At most, 8.4% of survey respondents were helped to any real extent. In my experience, based on an amputation program that uses immediate postsurgical prosthetic fitting and aggressive postamputation rehabilitation, the incidence of disabling pain problems following major lower extremity amputation is less than 5%. I have no objective explanation for the difference between reports in the surgical literature and my personal experience, but I believe that rapid rehabilitation and the use of rigid dressings, with or without a pylon, have a positive impact in decreasing postamputation pain problems.

In my personal experience, the perioperative administration of gabapentin (Neurontin) in dogs, ranging from 100 to 300 mg orally twice a day, seems to be associated with less postoperative pain and phantom pain.

Death

The incidence of death following major lower extremity amputation ranges from 0% to 35%.[7,9,17,20,119,120,130,131] Although the postoperative death rate has decreased each decade since the 1950s, an overall death rate of 6% to 10% is still the average for centers treating large numbers of amputees.[9,14,20] As might be expected, the postoperative death rate for above-knee amputation (20% to 40%) exceeds that for below-knee amputation (3% to 10%).[9,14,20,100,119,120,131] Two thirds of all postoperative deaths are due to cardiovascular complications, including myocardial infarction, stroke, congestive heart failure, and visceral ischemia, with approximately one third to one half of these deaths due to myocardial infarction alone. Death after lower extremity amputation is related to patient age. In my experience and that of others, the mortality increases for patients older than 75 years.[132]

Nonhealing

Nonhealing of an amputation stump represents a major complication because it almost always results in amputation at a higher level. Nonhealing results from inadequate blood supply at the level selected for amputation, rough or traumatic intraoperative handling of marginally vascularized tissue, or stump hematoma with or without secondary infection. The incidence of nonhealing after major lower extremity amputation ranges from 3% to 28%.[9,14,20,119,120,130,133] In other words, the primary healing rate after major lower extremity amputation ranges from 63% to 97%. Because the literature suggests an overall healing rate of 97% for digit and forefoot amputations (see Table 49-2) and 94% for below-knee amputations (see Table 49-3) when objective techniques of amputation level selection are used, it can be inferred that failure to heal is directly related to the method used for amputation level selection. In a modern amputation program using objective amputation level selection techniques, the rate of nonhealing should be no higher than 4% to 8%. In my last 250 consecutive lower extremity amputations, there has been one failure (0.8%) due to nonhealing from ischemia (transcutaneous $P_{O_2} > 20$ mm Hg).

The literature is somewhat controversial on healing differences between patients with and without diabetes mellitus. However, it has been my experience, as well as that of others, that there is no significant difference in the healing rates of major lower extremity amputations between diabetic and nondiabetic patients.[9,20,54,57,60,65,76,134] The rate of infectious stump complications might be slightly higher in diabetics; however, this has not been my experience.

In a review of 59 consecutive lower extremity amputations in diabetics, Bailey and associates noted that the preoperative hemoglobin level was statistically significantly lower in patients whose amputations healed primarily.[135] Eighteen amputations done in patients with a preoperative hemoglobin value of less than 12 g/dL healed primarily, whereas all 30 amputations in patients with a hemoglobin level greater than 13 g/dL failed to heal.

It seems reasonable to consider isovolemic hemodilution in patients with marginally viable skin or borderline values as measured by amputation level selection methods. In a study of skin flap survival, Gatti and colleagues suggested that isovolemic hemodilution might be a valuable technique for the salvage of marginally ischemic tissues.[136]

Stump Infection

The incidence of infection in an amputation stump ranges from 12% to 28%.[9,18,20,57,120] As might be expected, the incidence of postoperative stump infection is directly related to the reason for performing the amputation. The incidence of this complication can be reduced by appropriate management of preexisting infections, including the use of perioperative antibiotic therapy, as well as wide débridement or drainage of infection before definitive amputation. Reviews by McIntyre and coworkers[36] and Fischer and colleagues[37] noted a statistically significant decrease in the rate of stump infection in patients undergoing definitive below-knee amputation for a septic foot in whom prior ankle guillotine amputation was performed to control infection. The incidence of below-knee stump infection in patients managed with a one-stage surgical procedure was 22% and 21% in these reports, respectively, whereas the incidence in patients who had undergone preparatory guillotine ankle amputation was 3% and 0%, respectively ($P < 0.05$). My most recent incidence of stump infection is 3% (4 of 134), and most of these infections represent aggressive closure of contaminated wounds or amputations in limbs with distal ipsilateral septic foci.

I recommend the use of prophylactic antibiotics in all patients undergoing lower extremity amputation, even in the absence of established limb infection. It has been my practice to treat patients with preoperative infections with broad-spectrum antibiotics that provide bactericidal aerobic and anaerobic coverage. The necessity for aerobic and anaerobic coverage is especially important in diabetic patients, in whom

the incidence of mixed facultative and obligate anaerobic infections may be as high as 60%.[22]

Once an infection is established in an amputation stump, the wound must be opened widely to provide adequate drainage. In general, this means that the amputation will have to be revised to a higher level; for example, a stump infection in a below-knee amputation usually results in an above-knee amputation. The importance of this complication is emphasized by the fact that for a geriatric patient, conversion from a below-knee to an above-knee amputation is often the difference between successful ambulation and the inability to walk.

Stump hematoma after lower extremity amputation is a catastrophic complication, especially when the amputation has been performed for distal extremity infection. Although the correlation between stump hematoma and stump infection is not 1:1, it is high enough to make the avoidance of stump hematoma highly desirable. The importance of meticulous hemostasis after amputation cannot be emphasized enough. If an amputation is not dry, the wound should be closed with drains (closed drainage system, not Penrose drains), although several studies have suggested that the use of drains increases the risk of infection.[137]

Pulmonary Embolism and Deep Venous Thrombosis

The incidence of pulmonary embolism and deep venous thrombosis following major lower extremity amputation is 1% to 3%[7,14] and 4% to 38%,[9,14] respectively. The postoperative lower extremity amputee is at high risk for venous thromboembolic complications. Usually, these patients have had a prolonged period of hospitalization and bed rest before amputation. In addition, many have undergone prior attempts at vascular surgical reconstruction that may have injured the deep veins in the leg and prolonged preamputation immobilization. The amputation itself involves division of veins, which may result in stagnation and thrombosis in these vein segments postoperatively. When an active rehabilitation program is not begun on the first day after amputation surgery, this additional period of inactivity or immobilization may further predispose the patient to venous thromboembolic complications. The morbidity and mortality from venous thromboembolic complications may be significant, and impairment of blood oxygenation may further compromise the healing of ischemic tissues.

For patients undergoing elective major lower extremity amputation in whom major risk factors for venous thromboembolic complications exist, appropriate prophylaxis for pulmonary embolism should be instituted. Because there is a slight increase in stump hematoma formation, the use of a closed suction drainage system in these patients is advisable. Probably the most important factor in preventing thromboembolic complications is to not allow patients to become bedridden either preoperatively or postoperatively. A patient being prepared for lower extremity amputation should be undergoing preoperative physical therapy for range of motion and strengthening of the contralateral leg and upper extremities. A postoperative amputee, even if an immediate postoperative prosthesis is not used, should be receiving physical therapy for similar body conditioning. Attention should be paid to the nonamputated extremity, and the use of thromboembolic elastic stockings is recommended during the perioperative period. A final factor that must be considered is the patient's state of hydration, both preoperatively and postoperatively. This is especially important in patients who have undergone prior attempts at vascular reconstruction or angiography.

Pulmonary Complications

The incidence of pulmonary complications, including pneumonia, atelectasis, and sepsis, has been estimated at 8% in patients undergoing major lower extremity amputation.[14] These complications are significantly higher in patients undergoing above-knee amputation, as noted by Huston and colleagues,[7] in whom the incidence of pneumonia and sepsis ranged from 8% to 60%. The same conditions of bed rest, inactivity, dehabilitation, and dehydration that predispose to thromboembolic complications also predispose to atelectasis and pneumonia. Next to myocardial infarction, pulmonary complications are probably the biggest problem with geriatric patients undergoing lower extremity amputation. Attention to good pulmonary toilet, increased muscular activity, and active exercise (physical therapy) are all valuable adjuncts to preoperative and perioperative care.

Flexion Contractures

Flexion contractures of the knee or hip joint can occur quite rapidly following major lower extremity amputation, especially in geriatric patients. In my experience, the incidence of such postoperative flexion contractures has been 1% to 3%.[9,14,20,57]

Irreversible flexion contracture prohibits the successful fitting of a prosthesis and, subsequently, patient ambulation. Such a problem may also necessitate amputation at a higher level. The use of a rigid postoperative dressing, with or without an immediate postoperative pylon, helps decrease the incidence of this complication. In patients who are not receiving immediate postoperative prosthetic treatment, physical therapy directed toward range of motion and muscle strengthening should be instituted preoperatively if possible and as soon as possible after amputation.

Renal Insufficiency

Renal insufficiency represents a low-frequency complication following major lower extremity amputation, with an incidence of 1% to 3%.[9,57] This complication is, for the most part, avoidable if proper attention is paid to adequate preoperative and postoperative hydration. In addition, in patients requiring prolonged antibiotic therapy for perioperative infection, attention must be paid to antibiotic dosage to avoid renal insufficiency as a complication of antibiotic therapy.

LONG-TERM COMPLICATIONS

Stump Revision

There is little information available in the literature regarding the frequency of stump revision in patients who have been discharged from the hospital following lower extremity amputation. In an early report by Malone and associates, there was a 97% rate of primary healing after lower extremity

amputation, and 88% of the amputees were followed for up to 18 months after surgery, with no stump revision.[20] The incidence of prosthesis use in those patients was 100%. Similar information was reported by Roon and coworkers, who noted that 91% of their patients were ambulatory on their prostheses 44 months following amputation.[14] I believe that the frequency of stump revision is probably related to amputation level selection method, quality of prosthesis fit, and careful postoperative follow-up. My current incidence of late stump revision is 2.3% (10 of 450).

Death

Approximately one third of all lower extremity amputees die within 5 years of their amputation, and two thirds of these deaths are due to cardiovascular causes.[120] Roon and coworkers reported a 45% overall 5-year survival following lower extremity amputation, compared with an expected 85% 5-year survival for the age-adjusted normal population.[14] More striking, however, was their analysis of the projected 5-year survival following lower extremity amputation for diabetic and nondiabetic amputees. They reported a 75% 5-year survival for nondiabetics, compared with only 39% for patients with diabetes mellitus (Fig. 49-13). Analysis of the cause of death disclosed that more than one third of deaths were due to myocardial infarction, and two thirds were due to cardiovascular causes.[14]

There are good multivariate data showing that in dialyzed diabetic patients, apolipoprotein A-I, fibrinogen, age, and stroke are independent predictors of both cardiac and noncardiac death.[138] In addition, in type 1 diabetic patients, in spite of intensified insulin therapy, nephropathy is the strongest predictor of mortality and end-stage complications, including amputation.[139]

Contralateral Limb Loss

Estimates of the rate of contralateral limb loss range from 15% to 33% in the 5 years following major lower extremity

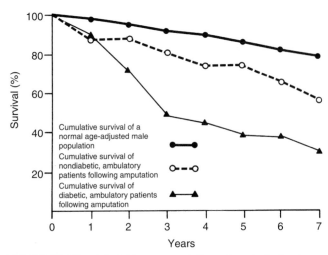

FIGURE 49–13 • Life-table representation of survival after lower extremity amputation for both diabetic and nondiabetic amputees compared with the age-adjusted normal population. (From Roon AJ, Moore WS, Goldstone J: Below knee amputation: A modern approach. Am J Surg 134:153-158, 1977.)

amputation.[16-18] In all probability, however, diabetic amputees are likely to die before contralateral limb loss.[14,120] Because of the risk of contralateral limb loss, significant attention should be paid to examination of the contralateral limb as well as patient education in prophylactic skin and foot care. Patient instructions for diabetic foot care that are used at the Tucson VA Medical Center and Maricopa Medical Center (Phoenix, Ariz.) are shown in Figure 49-14.

A randomized, prospective educational study at the Tucson VA Medical Center found that an audiovisual education program decreased the incidence of subsequent amputation significantly (at 1 year) among diabetics who presented with foot ulcers, infection, prior amputation, or high-risk lesions.[16] In that study, 203 patients were randomized into two groups: education and no education. There were no significant differences in medical management or clinical risk

---

Patient Instructions for Care of the Diabetic Foot

1. Inspect your feet daily for blisters, cuts, scratches, and areas of possible infection. Do not miss looking between your toes. A mirror can help you see the bottom of your feet or between the toes. If it is not possible for you to inspect your feet yourself, seek the help of a family member or friend.

2. Wash your feet and toes daily, and dry very carefully, especially between the toes. It is also important to dry carefully after showering or swimming.

3. Avoid extreme temperatures for your feet. Test bath water with your hand to ensure that it is not too hot, and be extremely careful of hot pavement or concrete during the summer.

4. If your feet feel cold at night, wear socks. Do not apply hot water bottles or heating pads.

5. Do not use chemical agents to remove corns or calluses.

6. Inspect your shoes daily for foreign objects, nail points, torn linings, or other problems that might damage your feet.

7. Wear properly fitting stockings, and try to avoid stockings with seams and stockings that are mended. It is important to change stockings daily.

8. All shoes should be comfortable and loose fitting at the time of purchase. Do not depend on shoes to stretch or break in. Try to avoid shoes that are pointed or apply pressure on the toes.

9. Do not wear shoes without stockings.

10. Do not wear sandals with thongs between the toes. Never walk barefoot, especially on hot surfaces. Be extremely careful of walking barefoot at home owing to danger from pins, tacks, or other items dropped on the floor.

11. Toenails should be cut straight across, and if there is a question, please consult your physician or podiatrist.

12. Do not cut corns or calluses yourself; seek counseling from your physician or podiatrist. See your physician or podiatrist regularly, and be sure that your feet are examined on each visit.

13. If your vision is impaired or you have other difficulties with examining your feet, have a family member or friend inspect your feet, trim nails, and otherwise ensure adequate foot care.

14. Be sure to tell your podiatrist or physician that you are diabetic.

15. Do not smoke.

16. Remember that even minor infections can cause significant problems in diabetics, and a physician or podiatrist should be consulted when infection occurs.

FIGURE 49–14 • Patient instruction sheet for care of the diabetic foot.

factors between the two groups. There was no significant difference in the incidence of infection; however, the rate of ulceration and amputation was three times higher in the no-education subgroup (ulceration: 26 of 177 vs. 8 of 177, $P = 0.005$; amputation: 21 of 177 vs. 7 of 177, $P = 0.025$), demonstrating that a simple education program significantly reduced the incidence of ulcer and amputation in diabetic patients. Other studies have documented the importance of diabetes education, protective footwear, and preventive foot care.[140-143]

Lehto and associates clearly demonstrated that there is a dose-response relationship between plasma glucose or hemoglobin A_1 and the risk of amputation.[141] Similar data have been published by Muhlhauser and colleagues, showing that the end-stage complications of blindness, amputation, and dialysis were statistically linked to the level of glycosylated hemoglobin.[139] Flores Rivera documented an increased risk for amputation in diabetic patients with cholesterol levels greater than 450 mg.[140] Muhlhauser and colleagues linked serum cholesterol levels to the combined end points of blindness, amputation, or dialysis.[139] Clearly, good blood glucose control should decrease the incidence of amputation in diabetics. However, the benefit, if any, of cholesterol-lowering drugs in decreasing the risk of amputation in both diabetic and nondiabetic patients is not known.

Prosthetic Considerations Following Major Lower Extremity Amputation

In general, as the level of amputation moves proximally up the lower extremity and the age of the patient increases, the success rates for rehabilitation decline and the length of time required to achieve ambulation increases.[17,144-150] Before discussing specific prosthetic considerations, a review of some of the problems associated with rehabilitation of geriatric amputees is worthwhile.

REHABILITATION OF ELDERLY AMPUTEES

In the mid- to late 1960s, the literature was replete with reports on the problems encountered in rehabilitating geriatric amputees. Many of these reports have been forgotten, but the information they presented is still valid. Among the most important work of that period was the project of Mazet and associates involving a 10-year follow-up of 1770 geriatric patients from the VA and county hospitals in Los Angeles.[17] Among their findings was the fact that 60% of patients who were given prosthetic limbs discarded them within 6 months. Thirteen years later, Jamieson and Hill, in a review of amputation for peripheral vascular disease, reported that more than half the patients fitted with artificial legs never used them effectively.[151] In addition, they reported that if the rehabilitation process was delayed for 2 or more months after amputation, the likelihood of ultimate ambulation was very poor. In a more recent review of rehabilitation following lower extremity amputation, Kerstein and colleagues noted that it required an average of 27 weeks (189 days) to achieve the maximum benefits of rehabilitation, and it was approximately 6 months before a successfully rehabilitated amputee was returned to society.[152] In an earlier article analyzing the influence of age on rehabilitation, Kerstein and coauthors

TABLE 49–5	Overview of Postsurgical and Rehabilitation Outcome in Several Series*					
Authors	**Amputations (N)**	**Primary Healing (%)**	**Eventual Healing (%)**	**Mortality Rate (%)**	**Rehabilitation with Prosthesis (%)**	**Average Time from Operation to Rehabilitation (days)**
Warren and Kihn	121	48.8	66.9	4.1	69.4	180-270
Chilvers et al	53	50.0	67.9	7.5	60.4	—
Robinson	47	77.0	88.0	17.0	83.0	—
Bradham and Smoak	84	85.7	—	—	—†	—
Block and Whitehouse	43	88.0	95.0	0.0‡	53.5	120-180
Cranley et al	101	76.0	86.0	7.0	73.3	—
Lim et al	55	53.0	83.0	16.0	51.0	70
Ecker and Jacobs	69	77.0	85.0	8.7	52.2	201
Wray et al	174	92.0	—	3.5	70.0	49-77
Nagrendran et al	174	80.5	91.4	—	—	—
Berardi and Keonin	44	—	61.4	4.5	29.5	111
Averaged totals	965	74.9	82.0	6.7	63.8	133

*Series reporting results with conventional techniques of rehabilitation after below-knee amputation. Note that the overall rehabilitation rate was 64% and the average time to achieve ambulation was 133 days.
†Authors commented that very few patients attained ambulation; however, no numbers were given.
‡Two patients died before discharge and were not included as postoperative deaths.
From Malone JM, Moore WS, Goldstone J, Malone SJ: Therapeutic and economic impact of a modern amputation program. Ann Surg 189:801, 1979.

found that many patients older than 65 required a year to achieve maximum benefit from the rehabilitation process.[146] Malone and coworkers analyzed contemporary series on below-knee amputation in patients treated with conventional rehabilitation techniques and found that the average rate of rehabilitation was 64% and the average time from operation to rehabilitation (ambulation) was 133 days[9] (Table 49-5). In a later review, Malone and coworkers noted that the rehabilitation times for patients treated with conventional techniques versus accelerated rehabilitation techniques (including amputation level selection and immediate postoperative prosthesis) were 128 and 31 days, respectively[20] (Table 49-6). The same review pointed out that the success rate for

ambulation after amputation with conventional rehabilitation techniques was 70%, whereas it was 100% for amputees treated with accelerated rehabilitation techniques. In addition, it has been my experience that if a geriatric patient is nonambulatory for either a month before or a month after amputation (i.e., rehabilitation is delayed), the likelihood for rehabilitation is significantly less than if the patient remains ambulatory during the perioperative period.

Part of the problem with rehabilitation of geriatric amputees is their decreased cardiorespiratory reserve and the increased energy expenditure required after lower extremity amputation, especially at more proximal amputation levels. These problems are complicated by the fact that individual

TABLE 49–6	Comparison of Rehabilitation Time with Conventional and Accelerated Techniques*				
	Group 1 (days)		**Group 2 (days)**		
Level of Amputation	*Range*	*Mean*	*Range*	*Mean*	**P Value**
Transmetatarsal	20-60	47.0	10-24	18.4	NS
Syme's	—	—	15-17	23.0	—
Below-knee	60-330	132.0	18-140	32.5	0.0001
Knee disarticulation	—	—	15-140	60.7	—
Above-knee	360	—	27-30	28.5	NS
Hip disarticulation	—	—	35	—	—
Overall	20-360	128.4	10-140	30.8	0.0001

*Rehabilitation time following lower extremity amputation for patients treated with conventional surgical and prosthetic techniques (group 1, 128 days) and accelerated techniques incorporating immediate postoperative prostheses (group 2, 31 days) (P < 0.001).
NS, not significant.
From Malone SM, Moore WS, Leal JM, Childers SJ: Rehabilitation for lower extremity amputation. Arch Surg 116:97, 1981.

surgeons probably see too few amputees to treat them with maximum efficiency, and the few patients they do see place a large burden on beds, resources, and physician time.

In a review of the energy cost of walking for amputees, Waters and colleagues found that in both unilateral traumatic and vascular amputees, performance was directly related to the level of amputation.[149] Walking velocity, cadence, and stride length were all decreased in amputation patients compared with control groups. In a detailed analysis of velocity of ambulation, rate of oxygen uptake, respiratory quotient, and heart rate, these authors concluded that amputees adjust their gait velocity to keep their rate of energy expenditure within normal limits. The approximate energy expenditures (compared with those of controls) after lower extremity amputation are shown in Table 49-7.[149,153-155] Note that the energy expenditures for both unilateral and bilateral below-knee amputees are less than those for unilateral above-knee amputees. This clearly demonstrates the importance of the knee joint in terms of energy used for ambulation. The additional effort of walking with an above-knee prosthesis is accomplished by the use of small muscles, which are poorly designed for locomotion.[155]

Decreased physical strength due to age, decreased cardiorespiratory reserve due to the ravages of cardiovascular or pulmonary disease, and increased energy expenditures for ambulation after lower extremity amputation all have an additive effect that complicates the rehabilitation of geriatric amputees. It is in this setting that the salvage of the most distal amputation that will heal may mean the difference between ambulation and independence and nonambulation and dependence for an elderly amputee. These factors also explain the higher likelihood of ambulation for a young high-level amputee compared with an elderly high-level or bilateral amputee. In their evaluation of 113 amputations in 103 patients, most of whom underwent amputation for peripheral vascular disease, diabetes, or both (mean age, 61 years), Roon and coworkers found the following rates of successful rehabilitation: 100% for unilateral below-knee amputation, 93% for bilateral below-knee amputation, 17% for a combination of above-knee and below-knee amputation, and 0% for bilateral above-knee amputation.[14]

POSTOPERATIVE PROSTHETIC TECHNIQUES

After major lower extremity amputation, the surgeon has three choices for prosthetic management: soft dressings or conventional technique, constant environmental treatment

(CET) (which at this point is probably of historical interest only), and rigid dressings with or without a postoperative prosthesis. In addition, the surgeon may choose delayed (conventional), rapid, or immediate postoperative rehabilitation.

Conventional Stump Wrap (Soft Dressing)

The historical standard, and a technique that is still used in many institutions, is the application of a soft postoperative dressing. Cotton gauze or fluffs are used to pad the amputation stump, and the stump is wrapped with elastic bandages (Fig. 49-15). The advantage of this technique is that it does not require a prosthetist to be present in the operating room or at the time of dressing changes. The disadvantages are that it does not readily control stump edema, the dressings are difficult to maintain in place (especially for high-level amputees), there is minimal stump protection from postoperative trauma, the dressing does not prevent knee flexion contracture, and ambulation may be delayed as a result of the prolonged time required for stump maturity (6 months).

Except for the above-knee and hip disarticulation amputation levels, where it is technically difficult to maintain a rigid dressing in good stump contact, there are no valid reasons to continue the use of this postoperative dressing technique.

Constant Environmental Treatment Unit

Developed and used almost exclusively in Great Britain, the CET unit consists of a control console containing a multistage centrifugal air compressor. The air passes through pressure control valves, a pressure cycle timing device, a bacteriologic filter, and a thermostatically controlled heating element that controls heat and relative humidity. The dressing on the patient consists of a transparent flexible polyvinyl bag. The bag is not in direct contact with the residual limb, except on the resting surface. A pleated air seal is incorporated into the proximal end of the bag to maintain a pressure seal. A sterile CET bag is placed over the amputation stump in the

TABLE 49–7	Energy Expenditure (Compared with Controls) after Lower Extremity Amputation*	
Level of Amputation	**Increase in Energy Expenditure (%)**	
Unilateral below-knee	9-25	
Bilateral below-knee	41	
Unilateral above-knee	25-100	
Bilateral above-knee	280	

*As measured by oxygen utilization per minute[149,153,155] or indirect calorimetry.[154] Energy expenditure was measured at comfortable walking speeds that averaged 22% of normal.

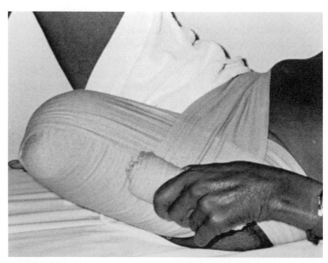

FIGURE 49–15 • Standard, conventional soft dressing and stump wrap being applied by a patient to his right above-knee amputation.

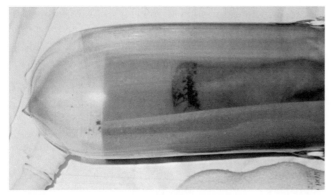

FIGURE 49-16 • Clear polyvinyl controlled environment treatment bag has been placed over a left below-knee amputation. Note the air supply hose at the distal end of the bag.

operating room. The amputation stump is, in essence, "enclosed" in a sterile environment with cyclic pressure (which controls stump edema) and airflow set to the desired temperature and humidity (Fig. 49-16).

The CET unit was designed for use in a setting in which a prosthetist is not immediately available or one in which the surgeon wants to be able to control stump edema yet have easy access to examine the surgical wound. The system incorporates a long flexible hose so that the patient can undergo rehabilitation training at the bedside. Indications for use of the CET unit are relatively limited; it is probably best used on patients in whom there is some risk of stump infection and in whom the ability to observe the wound without dressing changes is desirable. Because of its limited application, high cost, and poor patient acceptance due to noise, the CET unit, although successful, has seen limited use in the United States.[156]

Rapid and Immediate Postoperative Prostheses

The application of an immediate postoperative prosthesis has received considerable attention, support, credit, and discredit in the recent past. Proponents of the technique have waxed eloquently on the benefits to the patient, while opponents of the technique have cautioned about the potential detriment to the amputation stump from the casting technique.

Berlemont is generally credited with the early work that led to the establishment of the technique, based on his application of temporary prostheses in patients with delayed (secondary) amputation stump healing.[3] Weiss of Poland is credited with adapting this technique for stumps undergoing primary healing (i.e., immediate postoperative prosthesis). The latter technique proved highly successful, and Weiss reported his initial results at the Sixth International Prosthetic Course in Copenhagen in July 1963. This early presentation and a subsequent publication in 1966 came to the attention of surgeons worldwide.[4] The Prosthetic and Sensory Aids Service of the VA was especially interested in this technique for the management of veteran amputees and was instrumental in bringing this procedure to the U.S. surgical theater. Working with the VA, Burgess, an orthopedic surgeon in Seattle, refined and developed the immediate postoperative prosthetic technique for the U.S. surgical field.[5,134,157-159] Burgess and his team performed most of the

early work in the United States, and he was instrumental in training other investigators in the use of this technique. In the late 1960s and early 1970s, there were multiple reports extolling the virtues and possible pitfalls of the immediate postoperative prosthetic (IPOP) technique (also called IPPF, immediate postoperative prosthetic fitting).

Initially, there was general agreement that the IPOP technique was ideally suited for nondiabetic, nondysvascular amputees. Subsequent reports in the literature, however, have shown that, if properly used, the technique may be ideal for geriatric dysvascular amputees because of its ability to shorten hospitalization time and increase rates of rehabilitation.[9,14,20]

In general, proponents of the technique note that its benefits include an increased rate of healing, decreased hospitalization time, decreased rehabilitation time, decreased psychological trauma to the patient, control of stump edema, protection from stump trauma in the early postoperative period, and perhaps an increased rate of rehabilitation.[9,14,20,88,160-163] The paper most commonly cited against the use of the IPOP technique is that by Cohen and colleagues.[164] Using conventional surgical and prosthetic techniques, they were able to achieve 97% stump healing, whereas only two of nine (22%) amputation stumps treated with the IPOP technique healed. They noted no rehabilitation advantage to the IPOP technique and recommended caution in its application. The experience of Cohen and colleagues has not been matched by other reports in the literature. Some reports noted no change in the rate of wound healing,[160] but in general, most papers found no deleterious effects from the use of a rigid postoperative dressing (with or without a prosthesis), decreased hospitalization time, and decreased rehabilitation time.[9,14,20,160,162,163] Importantly, Cohen and colleagues suggested that their problems with the IPOP technique might be with the plaster technique itself or in the application of the technique. A review of their paper shows that four patients sustained what are described as second-degree blisters, which almost certainly indicate problems with plaster fabrication and application rather than problems with the IPOP technique itself. In my own experience with 600 consecutive major lower extremity amputations during the past 12 years, there has been only one stump problem related to the use of an immediate postoperative prosthesis, and that problem was caused by improper application of an immediate postoperative cast.

An overview of data on the use of the IPOP technique reported from the San Francisco VA Hospital, the Tucson VA Hospital, and Maricopa Medical Center by Roon and colleagues[14] and Malone and associates[9,20] is given in Table 49-8. A 1992 paper by Folsum and coworkers documented the overall rate of rehabilitation at 80% and the interval from amputation to ambulation at 15.2 days and 9.3 days for below-knee and above-knee amputees, respectively.[165] Information not tabulated in Table 49-8 suggests that the patient's ambulatory status before surgery is one of the most important predeterminants of postoperative ambulation. Essentially, 100% of patients undergoing unilateral major lower extremity amputation who ambulated before surgery were successfully rehabilitated after amputation, whereas less than 15% of the patients who were nonambulatory before amputation surgery were successfully rehabilitated.[9,14,20]

The advantages of immediate or early postoperative prostheses can be divided into two categories: those derived from

TABLE 49–8	Overview of Immediate Prosthesis Data: San Francisco and Tucson Veterans Administration Hospitals and Maricopa Medical Center
Stump healing	138/153 (90%)
Rehabilitation time	15-32 days
Rate of rehabilitation	155/175 (88%)
Unilateral below-knee	128/129 (99%)
Bilateral below-knee	17/19 (89%)
Bilateral above- and below-knee or above- and above-knee	6/23 (26%)
Unilateral above-knee	4/4 (100%)

Data from references 9, 14, 20.

the rigid dressing and those derived from early weight bearing and ambulation. The advantages of the rigid dressing include edema control, stump immobilization, perhaps improved healing, prevention of joint flexion contracture, and protection of the stump from external trauma. There may be no difference between soft and rigid dressings with respect to the time required to reach eventual stump maturity (6 months), although postoperative stump edema resolves much more quickly with a rigid dressing. The advantages of immediate or early ambulation include decreased hospital stay, less time from surgery to ambulation, increased rates of rehabilitation compared with patients managed in a more conventional manner, reduction in morbid and nonmorbid complications of amputation, and improvement in the patient's psychological outlook after amputation.[9,14,20,123]

In summary, there is general agreement on both the benefits and the pitfalls of the IPOP technique. I agree with Friedmann's conclusions: "immediate postoperative prosthetic fitting should be confined to large centers with medical and prosthetic facilities available on short notice."[80] In other circumstances, he advocated the use of conventional amputation rehabilitation techniques but specified that such management should include modern postoperative methods, including the early use of temporary prostheses for evaluation and training. The best solution to the problem of choosing a postoperative prosthetic technique would be the routine use of a rigid dressing and the application or use of a temporary prosthesis when the surgeon thinks that adequate wound healing has occurred (usually 1 to 2 weeks after amputation), thereby avoiding some of the potential hazards of immediate ambulation.[166-168]

Another variant of a postoperative rigid dressing that allows early ambulation is the air splint.[145,169] This device may be a practical alternative for a surgeon who wants to achieve early postoperative ambulation but does not have access to a prosthetist skilled in the application of immediate postoperative prostheses or temporary removable prostheses.

TECHNIQUES OF IMMEDIATE POSTOPERATIVE PROSTHETIC APPLICATION

Immediate postoperative prosthetic use has been described for all levels of major lower extremity amputation—from the transmetatarsal through the high above-knee amputation; however, it is best suited to below-knee amputation.

Specific technical details regarding the application of immediate postoperative prostheses can be found elsewhere and are only briefly outlined here.[107]

Transmetatarsal and Syme's Amputations

A rigid cast with felt padding for bony prominence relief is used as the first dressing for these distal levels of lower extremity amputation; however, ambulation is not allowed until adequate primary healing has been obtained (3 weeks). Early ambulation for transmetatarsal and Syme's amputation patients results in a higher incidence of wound complications. With Syme's amputation, it is extremely important that the posterior heel flap be held in good approximation and alignment by the cast and that great care be taken to pad the distal stump and dog ears, as well as the bony prominences. If a two-stage surgical approach for Syme's amputation is used,[88] it is probably best to avoid weight bearing until completion of the second stage of the surgical procedure (6 to 8 weeks). Both transmetatarsal and Syme's amputees will ultimately ambulate well, and a short delay in the ambulation process has essentially no impact on their overall rehabilitation. Avoidance of stump trauma to ensure primary wound healing during the early postoperative period is of paramount importance, and rehabilitation efforts can be confined to range of motion and strengthening of the opposite leg and upper extremities during the early postoperative period.

Below-Knee Amputation

Following completion of the amputation, a thin sheet of fine mesh material (Owen's silk) is moistened in antibiotic solution or saline and applied over the suture line, with care taken to avoid wrinkling (Fig. 49-17). Next, lamb's wool or polyurethane foam is placed over the end of the stump to provide stump compression and padding (Fig. 49-18).

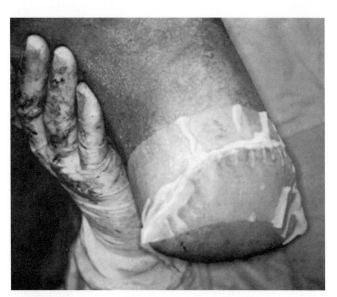

FIGURE 49–17 • A single sheet of moistened Owen's silk is placed over the suture line on the below-knee amputation stump. Care is taken to avoid wrinkling of the silk material.

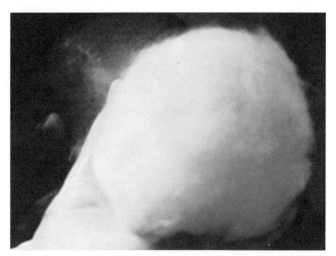

FIGURE 49–18 • Lamb's wool, Dacron, or prefabricated polyurethane foam can be placed over Owen's silk to provide distal stump padding. Care is taken to place padding material both above and below skin dog ears, if they exist.

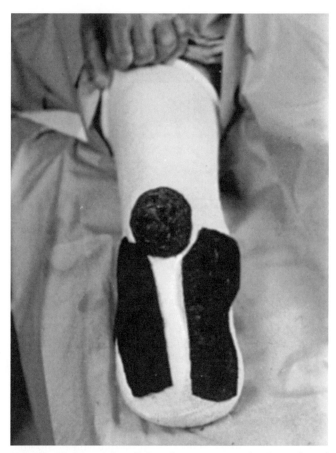

FIGURE 49–20 • Felt relief pads are measured, trimmed, and glued to the Spandex stump sock over the bony prominences of the knee and lower leg. Care is taken to leave a relief area between the medial and lateral tibial pads.

A Spandex stump sock is then carefully rolled over the stump, with care taken to avoid displacement of the distal stump padding (Fig. 49-19). Relief pads made from non-porous foam are fashioned and glued to the stump sock with Dow-Corning medical adhesive. These pads can be obtained precut or can be hand-fashioned in the operating room. They are placed to pad the bony prominences, specifically including the fibular head, tibial condyles, and patella. Care is taken to leave a relief area between the medial and lateral tibial pads (Fig. 49-20). Next, elastic plaster is used to form the inner layer of the immediate postoperative prosthesis.

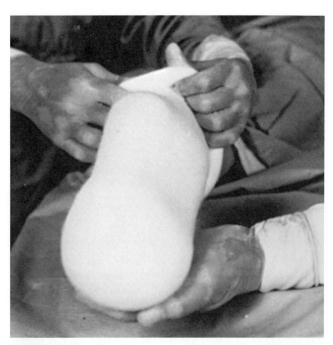

FIGURE 49–19 • Spandex stump sock is carefully pulled over the distal end of a below-knee stump and rolled proximally up the leg. Care is taken not to displace the distal end stump padding during application of the sock. Until the postoperative cast is dry, an assistant must maintain traction on the stump sock.

It is important that an assistant maintain traction on the stump sock during plaster application. Care is taken to maintain compression from posterior to anterior (direction of the posterior skin flap) and to grade compression from the distal end of the stump to the more proximal thigh (Fig. 49-21). The suspension assembly of the immediate postoperative pylon is then contoured to the inner cast after the cast has dried (Fig. 49-22). The pylon can be attached and static alignment achieved before incorporating the suspension assembly into the cast. The pylon is removed, and the suspension assembly is secured to the inner cast using fiberglass casting tape. The use of lightweight casting tape decreases the weight of the immediate postoperative prosthesis and significantly increases its durability.[167] A completed immediate postoperative prosthesis, waist suspension belt, pylon, and foot are shown in Figure 49-23. If a drain is employed, the drain should be brought out proximally (and laterally) through a separate hole made in the cast during the fabrication process. The drain should not be secured to the skin, so that it can be pulled out through the cast when appropriate.

Most surgical pain is gone within 36 to 48 hours after surgery. Significant pain more than 48 hours after surgery is an indication that the cast is too tight or that there is a wound complication. In this case, the cast should be removed, the wound inspected, and the cast reapplied if appropriate. Almost all patients comment that their postoperative stump

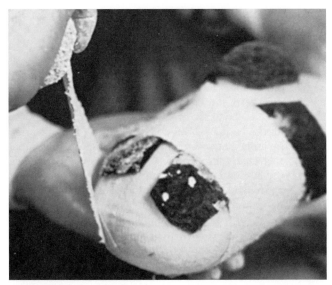

FIGURE 49–21 • The inner layer of the postoperative rigid cast is made using elastic plaster, which provides good control of stump compression. Compression should be from posterior to anterior, in the direction of the posterior flap, and distal to proximal so that the compression decreases as the cast moves higher on the upper leg.

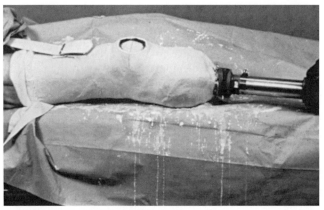

FIGURE 49–23 • Intraoperative photograph of a completed immediate postoperative below-knee prosthesis with pylon, foot, and waist suspension belt. Note that a relief window has been placed over the area of the patella.

pain diminishes if the heel of the prosthesis is weight-loaded (when they are in the supine position), and this test can be used as a further check for stump swelling and prosthesis fit. One of the most important principles in the postoperative management of these patients is that if there is any question about prosthesis fit or healing of the surgical wound, the prosthesis should be removed, the wound inspected by the surgeon and the prosthetist, and the cast reapplied at the discretion of the surgeon.

On the first postoperative morning, the patient is helped into a standing position at the bedside and instructed in techniques of touchdown weight bearing. At this time, the prosthetist completes the initial static alignment. On the second postoperative morning, the patient goes to the physical therapy department, where he or she is taught touchdown weight bearing using the bathroom scale technique (Fig. 49-24).

An alternative to the scale technique is the load cell, which is a pressure-sensing device built into the prosthetic pylon.[170] During the first 7 to 10 days after surgery, the patient ambulates using parallel bars with a maximum of 10 to 15 pounds touchdown weight bearing (10% of body weight). After application of the second postoperative prosthesis, the patient increases weight bearing to approximately 50% of total body weight. At the end of 14 to 21 days, on removal of the second postoperative prosthesis, a decision is made to place the patient either in a third postoperative prosthesis (if there is a question of wound healing) or in a removable temporary prosthesis (if the wound appears to be healing satisfactorily).[167,168] At this time, the patient begins full weight bearing. By approximately 30 to 35 days after amputation surgery, most patients have achieved either independent ambulation or ambulation with some type of ancillary walking aid (cane, walker). If a patient lives close to the hospital and is able to come to daily physical therapy training

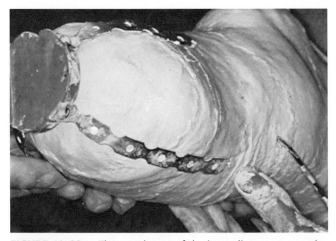

FIGURE 49–22 • The metal arms of the immediate postoperative prosthetic bucket are molded to the contours of the inner plaster shell after the cast has dried.

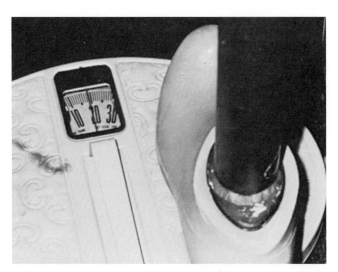

FIGURE 49–24 • To control the amount of postoperative weight bearing by patients, a bathroom scale is used to teach them to distribute their body weight. During the first week after surgery, weight bearing is limited to 10 to 15 pounds. After the second cast change, weight bearing is limited to 50% of total body weight.

as an outpatient, he or she may be discharged from the hospital shortly after receiving the second postoperative prosthesis (5 to 10 days); however, if the patient lives a great distance from the hospital, discharge is usually delayed until the surgeon, prosthetist, and therapist are happy with the rehabilitation process (4 to 5 weeks). This approach may have to be modified under the economic restraints that surround current medical care. Reasonable alternatives include transfer to a rehabilitation unit or service or early discharge with outpatient care. In either case, careful follow-up by the surgeon, prosthetist, and therapist is mandatory, especially in patients undergoing early ambulation and rehabilitation.

It can be anticipated that between discharge from the hospital and construction of the first permanent prosthesis (on average, 6 months after amputation), approximately three to six changes in the socket of the temporary prosthesis will be required as a result of progressive stump shrinkage. A typical lightweight, removable, temporary below-knee prosthesis is shown in Figure 49-25. The same pylon and foot can be used throughout all intermediate (temporary) cast changes, so that the only new requirement is the socket and realignment of the prosthesis. Prosthetic fit is maintained with stump socks, and the primary indication for change of the temporary prosthesis is when the patient has reached a total of 15-ply stockings to maintain a good prosthetic fit. Obviously, great care is taken

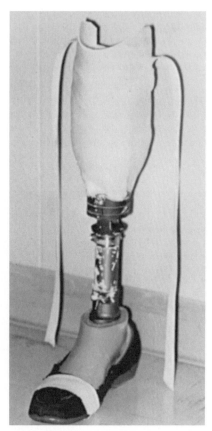

FIGURE 49–25 • Standard removable lightweight below-knee temporary or intermediate prosthesis, prescribed after removal of the last immediate postoperative prosthesis. This particular prosthesis is constructed with 3M Scotchcast (3M, St. Paul, Minn.). Fabrication with Scotchcast allows construction of a lightweight, cool, yet durable prosthesis.

to educate the patient about the use of the prosthesis and stump care to avoid any problems due to poor prosthetic fit.

Knee Disarticulation Amputation

The techniques for the application of an immediate postoperative prosthesis for knee disarticulation amputation are essentially the same as those for below-knee amputation. Because of the bulbous distal end of the knee disarticulation stump, the immediate postoperative prosthesis for this amputation level is self-suspending. Great care should be taken during cast fabrication to contour the femoral flares and to bring the proximal end of the cast to at least the upper third of the thigh to minimize distal end-weight bearing. My preference is to incorporate a polypropylene quadrilateral above-knee brim into the knee disarticulation cast to provide ischial weight bearing. The stump should be well padded, because there is more stump weight bearing with this level of amputation than with a below-knee amputation. At the discretion of the surgeon and prosthetist, polycentric hydraulic knee units can be incorporated into the initial immediate postoperative prosthesis or at any time during postoperative follow-up. The schedule for cast changes, the rehabilitation techniques, and the use of temporary prostheses are approximately the same as those for below-knee amputation.

Above-Knee Amputation

IPOP techniques for above-knee amputation require more attention to detail to maintain adequate suspension and socket fit. Although techniques using a modified Silesian suspension (contralateral hip sling) or waist suspension belt are simple to implement,[113] I believe that the difficulties of using immediate postoperative prostheses at the above-knee level are not offset by any significant improvement in the overall rehabilitation process. Thus, I use immediate postoperative prostheses at this amputation level only for young amputees. For dysvascular amputees, a temporary above-knee prosthesis is prescribed when primary wound healing has been achieved (2 to 3 weeks). During the postoperative period, the above-knee amputee goes to rehabilitation daily to achieve upper extremity strengthening and balance and to practice ambulation with parallel bars or other walking aids. Once a temporary prosthesis has been constructed, the schedule for prosthesis modification and the rehabilitation techniques are similar to those for below-knee or knee disarticulation amputation.

Overview of Prostheses and Prosthetic Techniques

There is no one type of standard prosthetic prescription for all levels of lower extremity amputation, and knowledge of available components is crucial in determining the proper prescription for each amputee based on his or her activities and lifestyle. A more complete discussion of prosthetic components is beyond the scope of this chapter; however, interested surgeons are referred to their local prosthetists or prosthetic facilities with whom they should be working.

IPOP techniques do not work in all clinical settings. The success of the technique is based on the experience and dedication of the team, and there is no question that if the immediate postoperative prosthesis is improperly applied, significant damage to the amputation stump can occur. In the absence of an experienced prosthetist and physical therapist, I suggest that a rigid postoperative dressing be applied; then, when primary stump healing has occurred, an appropriate temporary prosthesis can be prescribed and the rehabilitation process initiated. A delay of 1 to 2 weeks in the rehabilitation process is meaningless in the overall context of amputee rehabilitation; however, it has been my experience that if the rehabilitation process is delayed for a month or more, the ultimate success of rehabilitation, especially for geriatric high-level amputees, is severely compromised. It is therefore logical and reasonable to provide a temporary prosthesis sometime between wound healing (7 to 10 days after surgery) and 1 month after surgery. Using this "between" approach (i.e., a rigid dressing with early prosthetic application), maximum rehabilitation results can be achieved even in the absence of a formal rehabilitation team.

PROSTHETIC COMPONENTS

For a surgeon who performs only an occasional amputation, the number and types of prostheses and prosthetic components for lower extremity amputees can be bewildering. Therefore, a general overview of prosthetic components and specific combinations of components for certain levels of lower extremity amputation may be of value.

Transmetatarsal Amputation

In general, there is minimal, if any, prosthetic requirement for a transmetatarsal amputation. A steel shank placed in the sole of the shoe allows near-normal toe-off, and the void spot in the shoe can be filled with cotton, lamb's wool, or a soft foam material. The other option is construction of a specially designed shoe molded to the patient's foot in which toe-off is built into the shoe during construction.

Syme's Amputation

Depending on whether Syme's amputation has been performed with a one- or two-stage surgical procedure, the cosmetic quality of the prosthesis will be different (two-stage is more cosmetic). In general, this is an end–weight-bearing stump, and a prosthetic foot is attached to the leg shaft portion of the prosthesis. Because of the bulbous nature of the stump, a medial window has to be cut into the prosthesis to allow the stump to pass through the narrow midportion of the prosthesis. These prostheses are usually built with a nonmotion solid ankle-cushion heel (SACH) foot (Scheck & Siress). The presence of a particularly bulbous distal end precludes a cosmetic prosthesis, and this type of amputation may be contraindicated for cosmetic reasons alone.

Below-Knee Amputation

In general, the below-knee prosthesis consists of a prosthetic socket that is attached to a pylon or ankle block (endoskeletal system) and a foot. The prosthetic shell can be composed of plastic laminate, wood, or one of the newer, lightweight, rolled fiberglass materials such as 3M Scotchcast (3M, St. Paul, Minn.). The socket may use no liner (skin-socket interface) or may use a liner composed of lightweight plastic

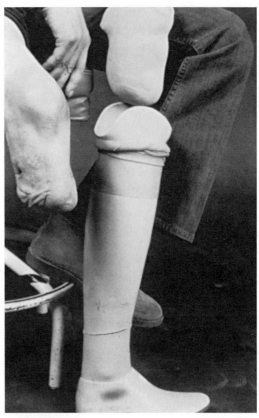

FIGURE 49–26 • This below-knee prosthesis is an ultra-lightweight patellar tendon weight-bearing-type prosthesis using a Silastic sleeve for suspension, a Silastic gel insert, and a stationary attachment flexible endoskeletal (SAFE) motion-type foot. This is an ideal prosthesis for a young, active amputee.

such as P-Lite, silicone gel bonded between two sheets of soft leather, or stump socks. The prosthesis can be suspended in a variety of ways, the most common of which is a standard PTB strap, supracondylar clip, Silastic sleeve suspension, suction, or thigh lacer with external hinges (Fig. 49-26). Self-suspending prostheses or physiologic suspension (the prosthesis is held in place by changes in muscle shape and contour with contraction) may be used in young, active amputees. In a young, highly active amputee, an ankle-rotating unit may be placed between the prosthesis and the foot. The feet currently in use include the SACH foot, which is a non-motion foot; the stationary attachment flexible endoskeletal (SAFE) foot (Scheck & Siress); or the Geisinger 5-Way foot (Danville, Pa.). The last two feet incorporate flexion, extension, and internal and external rotation when the foot is stressed under weight. The drawback to both of these motion feet is increased weight and perhaps decreased life expectancy compared with the SACH foot. The most popular motion foot, the Seattle foot, overcomes the drawbacks of the previously mentioned motion feet and has a cosmetic design that incorporates toes. A hydraulic ankle unit has recently been developed, but the unit is quite heavy, and there are still problems with oil leakage. New energy-storing feet (energy is "stored" by deformation of carbon-plastic composites and "released" on toe-off), such as the Seattle-Boeing-Burgess Foot and the Flex-Foot (Scheck & Siress), offer significant improvements in gait and activity levels (such as running), especially for young, active amputees.

The combination of a motion foot and a lightweight prosthesis provides a very high degree of function for active amputees.

Knee Disarticulation

Historically, knee disarticulation amputations were a prosthetic nightmare because the knee centers (thigh-knee length) could not be matched; however, the availability of polycentric knee joints has allowed construction of a cosmetic knee disarticulation prosthesis. In general, this prosthesis is similar to the Syme's-type prosthesis, in that the distal bony end of the stump is passed through the proximal portion of the prosthesis via a window cut in the medial portion of the prosthesis. The prosthetic shell can be constructed of plastic or wood. In general, the prosthetic shell extends from the end of the stump up to the ischium to provide both distal end and ischial weight bearing. Most knee disarticulation prostheses incorporate some type of hydraulic knee unit for both cosmetic and functional reasons. The lower part of the leg can be constructed of solid wood, plastic laminate, or a metal or plastic endoskeletal system for connection to the ankle block and foot. Ankle rotators and energy-storing motion or nonmotion feet can be used at the discretion of the prosthetist and surgeon.

Above-Knee Amputation

The above-knee prosthesis can be constructed of plastic or wood. Suspension techniques include an external hip joint with belt, shoulder suspension, or suction socket suspension. This is not an end–weight-bearing prosthesis, and all the weight is borne by the proximal socket quadrilateral brim design (the soft tissues of the thigh and ischium). Newer prosthetic designs for above-knee sockets include the contoured adducted trochanteric–controlled alignment method (CAT-CAM) design (which holds the stump laterally and medially, providing rigid support for the femur, in contrast to the quadrilateral socket, which holds the stump anteriorly and posteriorly, with poor femur support) and a variety of new flexible socket and strut designs (outer rigid strut attached to the knee joint with a soft flexible inner socket). These new designs significantly enhance function for above-knee amputees. A hydraulic, passive, or manual lock knee joint can be incorporated, based on the individual patient's needs. The lower part of the prosthesis is constructed as outlined in the section on knee disarticulation prostheses.

Hip Disarticulation

In general, hip disarticulation prostheses are built along the lines of the Canadian system, which incorporates a pelvic bucket, an endoskeletal upper and lower leg, simple spring-assisted hip and knee joints, and a nonmotion foot.

Amputation Rehabilitation Team

It is exceedingly difficult to achieve consistently reliable rehabilitation results in the absence of a formal, centralized, dedicated rehabilitation team that includes active participation by a prosthetist and members of the physical medicine and therapy departments. Just as some surgical procedures are

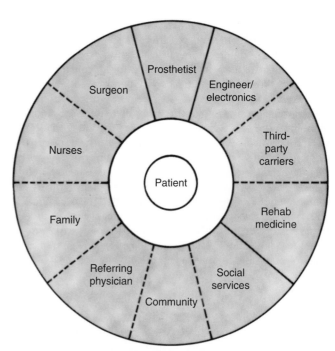

FIGURE 49–27 • The rehabilitation team required for successful amputation rehabilitation. Notice that the patient is at the center, and the surgeon is only one of many coequal team members.

confined to regional centers because of the cost and necessity of skilled labor, it is my belief that, ideally, amputation rehabilitation should be a centralized resource in a community or group of communities to achieve the best results. My concept of the structure of the amputation rehabilitation team is shown in Figure 49-27. Note that the center of the rehabilitation team is the patient and that other members of the team interface with the patient through or with an amputation coordinator. This coordinator can be a physical therapist, occupational therapist, nurse, or layperson. In my opinion, this person is key to maintaining coordination and especially long-term follow-up among members of the team. It has been my experience that one break in this rehabilitation circle results in at least a 50% failure rate in amputee rehabilitation. This fact (i.e., a break in the rehabilitation circle) may explain why the average rate of rehabilitation after lower extremity amputation is 60% or less.

There are five primary areas of concern in successful amputee rehabilitation: (1) coordination of care, (2) education of patient and family, (3) directed access to community resources, (4) discharge planning, and (5) centralized follow-up. In essence, the coordination of health care and mobilization of resources are under the direct control of the physician; however, once surgery is completed, this task is best organized by the amputation program coordinator. Discharge planning for the patient should start, if possible, before amputation. Education of the patient and family and evaluation of the financial and social resources available to the patient should also begin before amputation or as soon as possible after amputation. Centralized follow-up is important only if the team is interested in evaluating specific treatment techniques or prosthetic components. However, long-term follow-up is mandatory if reliable information on rehabilitation and postoperative complications is to be obtained.

The role of the physician is that of team director and provider of health care. The enthusiasm and interest of the physician will be reflected by all other members of the health care team. In the absence of an interested physician, rehabilitation failures will be common.

It is my belief that the prosthetist should be seen as coequal to the physician in the amputation rehabilitation process. From a practical standpoint, most patients rely more on the prosthetist than on the physician (in the absence of medical problems) once the acute phase of rehabilitation is completed.

The therapist is in the unique position of being able to make or break all the efforts of the surgeon and prosthetist. Only if the rehabilitation process runs smoothly and if attention is paid to small details during the rehabilitation process will the patient successfully regain ambulation. The greatest surgery in the world or the best limb in the world can meet defeat at the hands of an unskilled therapist. The therapist is the third coequal on the rehabilitation team, along with the physician and prosthetist.

Finally, the patient is the most important member of the rehabilitation team. The team can provide the patient with tools and techniques for rehabilitation, but it cannot provide the patient with motivation. It is of the utmost importance that the patient be taught to take primary control of the rehabilitation process. Included in this education are care of the amputation stump, care of the nonamputated leg, and care of the prosthesis. Failure of the patient to take an active role in the rehabilitation process will doom it to failure.[171]

One of the areas in which we as physicians and rehabilitation team members fail our patients is postdischarge follow-up and home care. An excellent review article on this topic appeared in the February 1979 issue of the *Orthopedic Nurses Association Journal*. All interested rehabilitation physicians and team members are advised to review this information and pass it on to their patients.[121]

I am now in a solo private practice without a dedicated amputation team. Although three experienced prosthetists, all of whom are well acquainted with immediate postoperative prosthesis fitting, are nearby, the lack of trained therapists and capitated-directed patient care contracts makes accelerated rehabilitation difficult if not impossible. Objective amputation level selection (transcutaneous oxygen testing), early if not immediate postoperative prosthetic filling, utilization of rehabilitation facilities after discharge, education of therapists, and persistence usually lead to a successful outcome. However, the rehabilitation results, especially in elderly or frail patients, are not as good as those documented in this chapter using a dedicated amputation team or center of care model.

What Is New in Amputation Surgery?

INSTRUMENTATION

As noted earlier, many new instruments are currently undergoing evaluation for amputation level selection. In addition, many of these instruments are being evaluated for their role in arterial insufficiency. Early information is available, but the definitive role for these instruments is undecided. Perhaps more promising than any specific instruments for

amputation level selection is the availability of computer software and microprocessors to integrate results from several different types of noninvasive techniques, resulting, in essence, in the era of the "limb viability laboratory." It can be anticipated that multi-instrument testing will result in greater accuracy than single-instrument evaluation. In addition, many of these instruments will find use in the evaluation of limb ischemia, especially in the perioperative period.

PROSTHETICS

Three current areas of prosthetic development show promise: the emergence of ultralightweight and throwaway or temporary or intermediate prostheses (Fig. 49-28); the design and development of energy-absorbing and energy-returning prosthetic components (designed to return energy on toe-off), as exemplified by the Seattle-Boeing-Burgess foot and the Flex-Foot; and new fabrication techniques such as flexible sockets (ISNY socket [New York University Medical Center, Prosthetics and Orthotics, New York]), flexible suction sockets (Iceross sockets, Össur, Reykjauk, Iceland), and nonquadrilateral or medial-lateral–contoured above-knee sockets. The use of new plastics, fiberglass casting tapes, and carbon fiber polymers is allowing the construction of ultralightweight yet

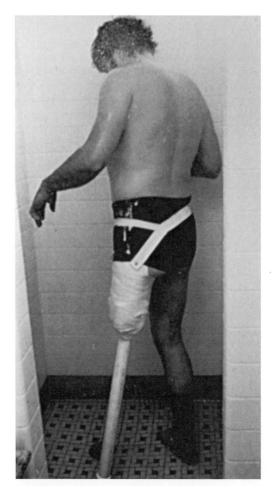

FIGURE 49–28 • Patients with lower extremity amputations usually sit on a stool when taking a shower. The above-knee amputee shown here is wearing an Aqualite shower prosthesis (US Manufacturing Co., Pasadena, Calif.).

rugged, durable prostheses. These prostheses have obvious value for geriatric amputees in terms of energy-saving characteristics, especially for high-level amputees, but they also have value for young, active amputees engaging in sports or water-related activities. Lightweight prostheses constructed with these new materials are often easier to fabricate than standard plastic laminate prostheses. Artificial limbs constructed with fiberglass casting tapes, such as 3M Scotchcast, allow a decrease in skin temperature at the socket-skin interface because of the porous nature of the casting material. Preliminary work by my group demonstrated a 5°C to 7°C drop in skin temperature with 3M Scotchcast PTB below-knee prostheses compared with standard plastic laminate PTB below-knee prostheses. The importance of decreased skin temperature is unknown with respect to stump durability, but there is no question that these prostheses result in improved patient comfort in hot, humid climates.

Increasing numbers of studies are now being done with young, active amputees to improve their performance abilities in activities such as running, jumping, and other sports functions.[172] Projects such as this point toward future improvements in prosthetic devices and toward future research efforts, perhaps leading to greater efficiency with which amputees conduct their physical activities.

SURGERY

A number of articles in the surgical literature describe arterial reconstruction with free tissue transfer to save limb length,[173,174] myofasciocutaneous flaps to improve stump healing and prosthesis utilization,[175] and foot salvage and avoidance of major lower limb amputations in diabetic patients.[176] In 45 patients with gangrenous lesions of the foot or lower leg due to severe diabetic arterial disease resulting in extensive soft tissue defects with exposed bones or tendons, Vermassen and van Landuyt reported excellent clinical results with arterial reconstruction and combined free tissue transfer.[173] The combined survival and limb salvage rate was 84% after 1 year, 77% after 2 years, and 65% after 3 years. The articles cited are only a small fraction of the published literature, and interested readers can find many more publications using PubMed and doing Internet searches on amputation and skin flaps. The combination of distal vascular reconstruction and free flap utilization, rotational flaps, and other techniques for closure of soft tissue defects of the extremities all offer exciting opportunities for extended limb salvage and avoidance of major limb amputation, especially in patients with diabetes.

KEY REFERENCES

Bowker JH, San Giovanni TP, Pinzur MS: North American experience with knee disarticulation with use of a posterior myofasciocutaneous flap: Healing rate and functional results in seventy-seven patients. J Bone Joint Surg Am 82:1571-1574, 2000.

Burgess EM, Romano RL: The management of lower extremity amputees using immediate postsurgical prostheses. Clin Orthop 57:137-156, 1968.

Chang BB, Bock DE, Jacobs RL, et al: Increased limb salvage by the use of unconventional foot amputations. J Vasc Surg 19:341-348, 1994.

Early JS: Transmetatarsal and midfoot amputations. Clin Orthop 361:85-90, 1999.

Flores Rivera AR: Risk factors for amputation in diabetic patients: A case-control study. Arch Med Res 29:179-184, 1998.

Hirsch G, McBride ME, Murray DD, et al: Chopart prosthesis and semirigid orthosis in traumatic forefoot amputations: Comparative gait analysis. Am J Phys Med Rehabil 75:283-291, 1996.

Koch M, Kutkuhn B, Grabensee B, et al: Apolipoprotein A, fibrinogen, age, and history of stroke are predictors of death in dialysed diabetic patients: A prospective study in 412 subjects. Nephrol Dial Transplant 12:2603-2611, 1997.

Lehto S, Ronnemaa T, Pyorala K, et al: Risk factors predicting lower extremity amputations in patients with NIDDM. Diabetes Care 19:607-612, 1996.

Lutz BS, Siemers F, Shen ZL, et al: Free flap to the arteria peronea magna for lower limb salvage. Plast Reconstr Surg 105:684-687, 2000.

Malone JM: Revascularization versus amputation. In Rutherford R (ed): Vascular Surgery, 5th ed. Philadelphia, WB Saunders, 2000, pp 2255-2266.

Misuri A, Lucertini G, Nanni A, et al: Predictive value of transcutaneous oximetry for selection of amputation level. J Cardiovasc Surg 41:83-87, 2000.

Moore JC, Jolly GP: Soft tissue considerations in partial foot amputations. Clin Podiatr Med Surg 17:631-648, 2000.

Muhlhauser I, Overmann H, Bender R, et al: Predictors of mortality and end-stage diabetic complications in patients with type 1 diabetes mellitus on intensified insulin therapy. Diabet Med 17:727-734, 2000.

Naylor AR, Hayes PD, Darke S: A prospective audit of complex wound and graft infections in Great Britain and Ireland: The emergence of MRSA. Eur J Vasc Surg 21:289-294, 2001.

Reyzelman AM, Hadi S, Armstrong DG: Limb salvage with Chopart's amputation and tendon balancing. J Am Podiatr Med Assoc 89:100-103, 1999.

Sanders LJ: Transmetatarsal and midfoot amputations. Clin Podiatr Med Surg 14:741-762, 1997.

Tepel M, van der Giet M, Schwarzfeld C, et al: Prevention of radiographic-contrast-agent-induced reductions in renal function by acetylcysteine. N Engl J Med 343:210-212, 2000.

Vermassen FE, van Landuyt K: Combined vascular reconstruction and free flap transfer in diabetic arterial disease. Diabetes Metab Res Rev 16(Suppl 1):S33-S36, 2000.

Wrobel JS, Mayfield JA, Reiber GE: Geographic variation of lower-extremity major amputation in individuals with and without diabetes in the Medicare population. Diabetes Care 24:860-864, 2001.

REFERENCES

1. Wangensteen OH, Wangensteen SD: The Rise of Surgery from Empiric Craft to Scientific Discipline. Minneapolis, University of Minnesota Press, 1978, p 18.

2. Boedner CW: Baron Dominique Jean Larrey, Napoleon's surgeon. ACS Bull July:18-21, 1982.

3. Berlemont M: Notre expérience de l'appareillage précoce des amputés des membres inférieurs aux establissements helio Marins de Berk. Ann Med Phys Med 5: 1961.

4. Weiss M: The prosthesis on the operating table from a neurophysical point of view: Report of a workshop panel on lower extremity prosthetic fitting. Committee on Prosthetics Research Development. Paper presented to the National Academy of Sciences, Feb 1966.

5. Burgess EM, Tramb JE, Wilson AB Jr: Immediate Postsurgical Prosthetics in the Management of Lower Extremity Amputees. TR 10-5. Washington, DC, Veterans Administration, 1967.

6. Falstie-Jensen N, Christensen KB: A model for prediction of failure in amputation of the lower limb. Dan Med Bull 37:283-286, 1990.

7. Huston CC, Bivins BA, Ernst CB, Griffen WO Jr: Morbid implications of above-knee amputations: Report of a series and review of the literature. Arch Surg 115:165-167, 1980.

8. Kerstein MD, Zimmer H, Dugdale FE, Lerner E: Associated diagnoses complicating rehabilitation after major lower extremity amputation. Angiology 25:536-547, 1974.

9. Malone JM, Moore WS, Goldstone J, Malone SJ: Therapeutic and economic impact of a modern amputation program. Ann Surg 189: 798-802, 1979.

10. Moore WS, Hall AD, Lim RC: Below the knee amputation for ischemic gangrene: Comparative results of conventional operation and immediate postoperative fitting technic. Am J Surg 124:127-134, 1972.

11. Porter JM, Baur GM, Taylor LM Jr: Lower-extremity amputation for ischemia. Arch Surg 116:89-92, 1981.

12. Towne JB, Condon RE: Lower extremity amputation for ischemic disease. Adv Surg 13:199-227, 1979.

13. Otteman MG, Stahlgren LH: Evaluation of factors which influence mortality and morbidity following major lower extremity amputation for arteriosclerosis. Surg Gynecol Obstet 120:1217-1220, 1965.

14. Roon AJ, Moore WS, Goldstone J: Below-knee amputation: A modern approach. Am J Surg 134:153-158, 1977.

15. Wrobel JS, Mayfield JA, Reiber GE: Geographic variation of lower-extremity major amputation in individuals with and without diabetes in the Medicare population. Diabetes Care 24:860-864, 2001.

16. Malone JM, Synder M, Anderson GG, et al: Prevention of amputation by diabetic education. Am J Surg 158:520-524, 1989.

17. Mazet R Jr, Schiller FJ, Dunn OJ, Alonzo NJ: The influence of prosthesis wearing on the health of the geriatric patient. Project 431. Washington, DC, Office of Vocational Rehabilitation, Department of Health, Education, and Welfare, March 1963.

18. Whitehouse FW, Jurgensen C, Block MA: The later life of the diabetic amputee: Another look at fate of the second leg. Diabetes 17:520-521, 1968.

19. Malone JM, Moore WS, Goldstone J: Life expectancy following aortofemoral arterial grafting. Surgery 81:551-555, 1977.

20. Malone JM, Moore WS, Leal JM, Childers SJ: Rehabilitation for lower extremity amputation. Arch Surg 116:93-98, 1981.

21. Pinzur MS, Littooy F, Daniels J, et al: Multidisciplinary preoperative assessment and late function in dysvascular amputees. Clin Orthop 281:239-243, 1992.

22. Fierer J, Daniel D, Davis C: The fetid foot: Lower-extremity infections in patients with diabetes mellitus. Rev Infect Dis 1:210-217, 1979.

23. Naylor AR, Hayes PD, Darke S: A prospective audit of complex wound and graft infections in Great Britain and Ireland: The emergence of MRSA. Eur J Vasc Surg 21:289-294, 2001.

24. Malone JM: Revascularization versus amputation. In Rutherford R (ed): Vascular Surgery, 5th ed. Philadelphia, WB Saunders, 2000, pp 2255-2266.

25. Brinker MR, Timberlake GA, Goff JM, et al: Below knee physiologic cryoanesthesia in the critically ill patient. J Vasc Surg 7:433-438, 1988.

26. Johansen K, Burgess EM, Zorn R, et al: Improvement of amputation level by lower extremity revascularization. Surg Gynecol Obstet 153:707-709, 1981.

27. Kazmers M, Satiani B, Evans WE: Amputation level following unsuccessful distal limb salvage operations. Surgery 87:683-687, 1980.

28. Samson RH, Gupta SK, Scher LA, Veith FJ: Treatment of limb threatening ischemia despite a palpable popliteal pulse. J Surg Res 32:535-539, 1982.

29. Samson RH, Gupta SK, Scher LA, Veith FJ: Level of amputation after failed limb salvage procedures. Surg Gynecol Obstet 154:56-58, 1982.

30. Stoney RJ: Ultimate salvage for the patient with limb threatening ischemia: Realistic goals and surgical considerations. In Bergan JJ, Yao JST (eds): Gangrene and Severe Ischemia of the Lower Extremities. New York, Grune & Stratton, 1978, pp 383-392.

31. Stirneman P, Walpoth B, Wiursten VH, et al: Influence of failed arterial reconstruction on the outcome of major limb amputation. Surgery 111:363-368, 1992.

32. Tsang GM, Crowson MC, Hickey NC, Simms MH: Failed femorocrural reconstruction does not prejudice amputation level. Br J Surg 78:1479-1481, 1991.

33. Evans WE, Hayes JP, Vermilion BD: Effect of a failed distal reconstruction on the level of amputation. Am J Surg 160:217-220, 1990.

34. Epstein SB, Worth MH Jr, Ferzli G: Level of amputation following failed vascular reconstruction for lower limb ischemia. Curr Probl Surg 46:185-192, 1989.

35. Bloom RJ, Stevick CA: Amputation level and distal salvage of the limb. Surg Gynecol Obstet 166:1-5, 1988.

36. McIntyre KE Jr, Bailey SA, Malone JM, Goldstone J: The nonsalvageable infected lower extremity: A new look at guillotine amputation. Am J Surg 117:58-64, 1985.

37. Fischer DF, Clagett GP, Fry RE, et al: One-stage versus two-stage amputation for wet gangrene of the lower extremity: A randomized study. J Vasc Surg 8:428-433, 1988.

38. Robbs JV, Ray R: Clinical predictors of below knee stump healing following amputation for ischemia. S Afr J Surg 20:305-310, 1982.

39. Dwars BJ, Van Den Broek TA, Ravwerda JA, Bakker FC: Criteria for reliable selection of the lowest level of amputation in peripheral vascular disease. J Vasc Surg 15:536-542, 1992.

40. Golbranson FL, Yu EC, Gelberman RH: The use of skin temperature determinations in lower extremity amputation level selection. Foot Ankle 3:170-172, 1982.

41. Spence VA, Walker WF: The relationship between temperature isotherms and skin blood flow in the ischemic limb. J Surg Res 36:278-281, 1984.

42. Stoner HB, Taylor L, Marcuson RW: The value of skin temperature measurements in forecasting the healing of below-knee amputation for end stage ischemia of the leg in peripheral vascular disease. Eur J Vasc Surg 3:355-361, 1989.

43. Wagner WH, Keagy BA, Kotb MN, et al: Noninvasive determination of healing of major lower extremity amputation: The continued role of clinical judgment. J Vasc Surg 8:703-710, 1988.

44. Lim RC Sr, Blaisdell FW, Hall AD, et al: Below knee amputation for ischemic gangrene. Surg Gynecol Obstet 125:493-501, 1967.

45. Baker WH, Barnes RW: Minor forefoot amputation in patients with low ankle pressure. Am J Surg 133:331-332, 1977.

46. Barnes RW, Shanik GO, Slaymaker EE: An index of healing in below-knee amputation: Leg blood pressure by Doppler ultrasound. Surgery 79:13-20, 1976.

47. Bernstein EF: The noninvasive vascular diagnostic laboratory. In Najarian JS, Oelaney JP (eds): Vascular Surgery. Miami, Symposia Specialists; New York, Stratton Intercontinental, 1978, pp 33-46.

48. Gibbons GW, Wheelock FC Jr, Siembieda C, et al: Noninvasive prediction of amputation level in diabetic patients. Arch Surg 114:1253-1257, 1979.

49. Raines JK, Darling RC, Buth J, et al: Vascular laboratory criteria for the management of peripheral vascular disease of the lower extremities. Surgery 79:21-29, 1976.

50. Schwartz JA, Schuler JJ, O'Connor RJA, Flanigan DP: Predictive value of distal perfusion pressure in the healing of amputation of the digits and the forefoot. Surg Gynecol Obstet 154:865-869, 1982.

51. Verta MJ, Gross WS, Van Bellan B, et al: Forefoot perfusion pressure and minor amputation surgery. Surgery 80:729-734, 1976.

52. Yao JST, Bergan JJ: Application of ultrasound to arterial and venous diagnosis. Surg Clin North Am 54:23-38, 1974.

53. Cheng EY: Lower extremity amputation level: Selection using noninvasive hemodynamic methods of evaluation. Arch Phys Med Rehabil 63:475-479, 1982.

54. Holloway GA Jr, Burgess EM: Cutaneous blood flow and its relation to healing of below knee amputation. Surg Gynecol Obstet 146:750-756, 1978.

55. Holloway GA Jr, Watkins BW: Laser Doppler measurement of cutaneous blood flow. J Invest Dermatol 69:300-309, 1977.

56. Kostuik JP, Wood D, Hornby R, et al: Measurement of skin blood flow in peripheral vascular disease by the epicutaneous application of xenon-133. J Bone Joint Surg Am 58:833-837, 1964.

57. Malone JM, Leal JM, Moore WS, et al: The "gold standard" for amputation level selection: Xenon-133 clearance. J Surg Res 30:449-455, 1981.

58. Moore WS: Determination of amputation level: Measurement of skin blood flow with xenon-133. Arch Surg 107:798-802, 1973.

59. Silberstein EB, Thomas S, Cline J, et al: Predictive value of intracutaneous xenon clearance for healing of amputation and cutaneous ulcer sites. Radiology 147:227-229, 1983.

60. Burgess EM, Matsen FA, Wyss CR, Simmons CW: Segmental transcutaneous measurements of PO_2 in patients requiring below the knee amputation for peripheral vascular insufficiency. J Bone Joint Surg Am 64:378-382, 1982.

61. Clyne CAC, Ryan J, Webster JHH, Chant AOB: Oxygen tension on the skin of ischemic legs. Am J Surg 143:315-318, 1982.

62. Franzeck UK, Talke P, Berstein EF, et al: Transcutaneous PO_2 measurement in health on peripheral arterial occlusive disease. Surgery 91:156-163, 1982.

63. Harward TRS, Volny J, Golbranson F, et al: Oxygen-inhalation induced transcutaneous PO_2 changes as a predictor of amputation level. J Vasc Surg 2:220-227, 1985.

64. Katsamouris A, Brewster DC, Megerman J, et al: Transcutaneous oxygen tension in selection of amputation level. Am J Surg 147:510-516, 1984.

65. Malone JM, Anderson GG, Halka SC, et al: Prospective comparison of noninvasive techniques for amputation level selection. Am J Surg 154:179-184, 1987.

66. Matsen FA, Wyss CR, Robertson CL, et al: The relationship of transcutaneous PO_2 and laser Doppler measurements in a human model of local arterial insufficiency. Surg Gynecol Obstet 159:418-422, 1984.

67. Ratliff DA, Clune CAC, Chant ADB, Webster JHH: Prediction of amputation healing: The role of transcutaneous PO_2 assessment. Br J Surg 71:219-222, 1984.

68. Misuri A, Lucertini G, Nanni A, et al: Predictive value of transcutaneous oximetry for selection of amputation level. J Cardiovasc Surg 41:83-87, 2000.

69. Graham BH, Walton RL, Elings VB, Lewis F: Surface quantification of injected fluorescein as a predictor of flap viability. Plast Reconstr Surg 71:826-833, 1983.

70. McFarland DC, Lawrence PF: Skin fluorescence: A method to predict amputation site healing. J Surg Res 32:410-415, 1982.

71. Silverman DG, Hurford WE, Cooper HS, et al: Quantification of fluorescein distribution to strangulated reticulum. J Surg Res 34:179-186, 1983.

72. Silverman DG, Rubin JM, Reilly CA, et al: Fluorometric prediction of successful amputation levels in the ischemic limb. J Rehabil Res Dev 22:29-34, 1985.

73. Holloway GA Jr, Burgess EM: Preliminary experiences with laser Doppler velocimetry for the determination of amputation levels. Prosthet Orthot Int 7:63-66, 1983.

74. Holstein P: Level selection in leg amputation for arterial occlusive disease: A comparison of clinical evaluation and skin perfusion pressure. Acta Orthop Scand 53:821-831, 1982.

75. Holstein P, Trap-Jensen J, Bagger H, Larsen B: Skin perfusion pressure measured by isotope washout in legs with arterial occlusive disease. Clin Physiol 3:313-324, 1983.

76. Stockel M, Ovesen J, Brochner-Morstensen J, Emneus H: Standardized photoelectric technique as routine method for selection of amputation level. Acta Orthop Scand 53:875-878, 1982.

77. Kram HB, Appel PL, Shoemaker WC: Multisensor transcutaneous oximetric mapping to predict below-knee amputation wound healing: Use of critical PO_2. J Vasc Surg 9:796-800, 1989.

78. Kram HB, Appel PL, Shoemaker WC: Prediction of below-knee amputation wound healing using noninvasive laser Doppler velocimetry. Am J Surg 158:29-31, 1989.

79. Burnham ST, Wagner WH, Keagy BH, Johnson G Jr: Objective measurement of limb perfusion by dermal fluorometry: A criterion for healing of below knee amputation. Arch Surg 125:104-106, 1990.

80. Friedmann LW: The prosthesis—immediate or delayed fitting? Angiology 23:513-524, 1972.

81. Durham JR, Anderson GG, Malone JM: Methods of preoperative selection of amputation level. In Flanigan P (ed): Modern Methods of Perioperative Assessment in Peripheral Vascular Surgery. New York, Marcel Dekker, 1986.

82. Oishi CS, Fronek A, Golbranson FL: The role of noninvasive vascular studies in determining levels of amputation. J Bone Joint Surg Am 70:1520-1530, 1988.

83. Bacharach JM, Rooke TW, Osmundson PJ, Gloviczki P: Predictive value of transcutaneous oxygen pressure and amputation success by use of supine and elevation measurement. J Vasc Surg 15:558-563, 1992.

84. Holloway GA Jr: Cutaneous blood flow responses to infection trauma measured by laser Doppler velocimetry. J Invest Dermatol 74:1-4, 1980.

85. Daly MJ, Henry RE: Quantitative measurement of skin perfusion with xenon-133. J Nucl Med 21:156-160, 1980.

86. Holstein P, Lassen NA: Assessment of safe level of amputation by measurement of skin blood pressure. In Rutherford R, et al (eds): Vascular Surgery. Philadelphia, WB Saunders, 1977, pp 105-111.

87. Ovesen J, Stockel M: Measurement of skin perfusion pressure by photoelectric technique: Aid to amputation level selection in arteriosclerotic disease. Prosthet Orthot Int 8:39-42, 1984.

88. Wagner FW Jr: Amputation of the foot and ankle: Current status. Clin Orthop 122:62-69, 1977.

89. Sizer JS, Wheelock FC: Digital amputations in diabetic patients. Surgery 72:980-989, 1972.

90. Little JM, Stephen MS, Zylstra PL: Amputation of the toes for vascular disease: Fate of the affected leg. Lancet 2:1318-1319, 1976.

91. McKittrick LS, McKittrick MB, Risby TS: Transmetatarsal amputation for infection of gangrene in patients with diabetes mellitus. Ann Surg 130:825-842, 1949.

92. Early JS: Transmetatarsal and midfoot amputations. Clin Orthop 361:85-90, 1999.

93. Reyzelman AM, Hadi S, Armstrong DG: Limb salvage with Chopart's amputation and tendon balancing. J Am Podiatr Med Assoc 89:100-103, 1999.

94. Sanders LJ: Transmetatarsal and midfoot amputations. Clin Podiatr Med Surg 14:741-762, 1997.

95. Chang BB, Bock DE, Jacobs RL, et al: Increased limb salvage by the use of unconventional foot amputations. J Vasc Surg 19:341-348, 1994.

96. Hirsch G, McBride ME, Murray DD, et al: Chopart prosthesis and semi-rigid orthosis in traumatic forefoot amputations: Comparative gait analysis. Am J Phys Med Rehabil 75:283-291, 1996.

97. Syme J: On amputation at the ankle joint. Lond Edinb Monthly J Med Sci 3:93, 1843.

98. Harris RI: Syme's amputation, the technical details essential for success. J Bone Joint Surg Br 38:614-632, 1956.

99. Harris RI: The history and development of Syme's amputations. Artif Limbs 6:4-43, 1961.

100. Warren R, Kihn RB: A survey of lower extremity amputations for ischemia. Surgery 63:107-120, 1968.

101. Kernek CB, Rozzi WB: Simplified two stage below-knee amputation for unsalvageable diabetic foot infections. Clin Orthop 261:251-256, 1990.

102. Termansen NB: Below-knee amputation for ischaemic gangrene: Prospective, randomized comparison of a transverse and a sagittal operative technique. Acta Orthop Scand 48:311-316, 1977.

103. Persson BM: Sagittal incision for below-knee amputation in ischaemic gangrene. J Bone Joint Surg Br 56:110-114, 1974.

104. Ruckley CV, Stonebridge PA, Prescott RJ: Skewflap versus long posterior flap in below-knee amputations: Multicenter trial. J Vasc Surg 13:423-427, 1991.

105. Block MA, Whitehouse FW: Below-knee amputation in patients with diabetes mellitus. Arch Surg 87:682-689, 1963.

106. Dellon AL, Morgan RF: Myodermal flap closure of below the knee amputation. Surg Gynecol Obstet 153:383-386, 1981.

107. Moore WS: Immediate postoperative prosthesis. In Rutherford R, Bernhard V, et al (eds): Vascular Surgery. Philadelphia, WB Saunders, 1977, pp 1333-1343.

108. Kim GE, Imparato AM, Chu DS, Davis SW: Lower limb amputation for occlusive vascular disease. Am Surg 42:589-601, 1976.

109. Inderbitzi R, Buttiker M, Pfluger D, Nachbur B: The fate of bilateral lower limb amputees in end stage disease. Eur J Vasc Surg 6:321-326, 1992.

110. Houghton A, Allen A, Luff R, McColl I: Rehabilitation after lower extremity amputation: A comparative study of above-knee, through knee and Gritti-Stokes amputations. Br J Surg 76:622-624, 1989.

111. Burgess EM: Disarticulation of the knee: A modified technique. Arch Surg 112:1250-1255, 1977.

112. Doran J, Hopkinson BR, Making GS: The Gritti-Stokes amputation in ischaemia: A review of 134 cases. Br J Surg 65:135-137, 1978.

113. Puddifoot PC, Weaver PC, Marshall SA: A method of supportive bandaging for amputation stumps. Br J Surg 60:729-731, 1973.

114. Ford LT, Holder BR: Disarticulation for failed surgical procedures about the hip. South Med J 70:1293-1296, 1977.

115. Endean ED, Schwarz TH, Barker DE, et al: Hip disarticulation: Factors affecting outcome. J Vasc Surg 14:398-404, 1991.

116. Boyd HB: Anatomic disarticulation of the hip. Surg Gynecol Obstet 84:346-349, 1947.

117. Hogshead HP: Experience with hip disarticulation and hemipelvectomy procedure. J Bone Joint Surg Am 53:1031, 1971.

118. Wu KK, Guise ER, Frost HM, Mitchell CL: The surgical technique for hindquarter amputation: Report of 19 cases. Acta Orthop Scand 48:479-486, 1977.

119. Baur GM, Porter JM, Axthelm S, et al: Lower extremity amputation for ischemia. Am Surg 44:472-477, 1978.

120. Berardi RS, Keonin Y: Amputations in peripheral vascular occlusive disease. Am J Surg 135:231-234, 1978.

121. Home instructions: Amputee with prosthesis. Orthop Nurses Assoc J 6:73-77, 1979.

122. Abramson AS, Feibel A: The phantom phenomenon: Its use and disuse. Bull N Y Acad Med 57:99-112, 1981.

123. Bradway JR, Racy J, Malone JM: Psychological adaptation to amputation. Orthot Prosthet 38:46-50, 1984.

124. Parkes CM: Factors determining persistence of phantom pain in the amputee. J Psychosom Res 17:97-108, 1973.

125. Sherman RA: Published treatment of phantom pain. Am J Phys Med 59:232-244, 1980.

126. Sherman RA, Tippens JK: Suggested guidelines for treatment of phantom limb pain. Orthopedics 5:1595-1600, 1982.

127. Solomon GF, Schmidt KM: A burning issue: Phantom limb pain and psychological preparation of the patient for amputation. Arch Surg 113:185-186, 1978.

128. Sherman RA, Sherman CJ, Gall NG: A survey of current phantom limb pain treatment in the United States. Pain 8:85-99, 1980.

129. Sherman RA, Sherman CJ, Parker L: Chronic phantom and stump pain among American veterans: Results of a survey. Pain 18:83-95, 1984.

130. Nagendran T, Johnson G Jr, McDaniel WJ, et al: Amputation of the leg: An improved outlook. Ann Surg 175:994-999, 1972.

131. Wray CH, Still JM Jr, Moretz WH: Present management of amputations for peripheral vascular disease. Am Surg 38:87-92, 1972.

132. Bertin VJ, Plechia FR, et al: The early results of vascular surgery in patients 75 years of age or older: An analysis of 3259 cases. J Vasc Surg 2:769-774, 1985.

133. Gregg RO: Bypass or amputation? Concomitant review of bypass arterial grafting and major amputation. Am J Surg 149:397-401, 1985.

134. Burgess EM, Romano RL, Aettl JH, Schrock RD Jr: Amputation of the leg for peripheral vascular ischemia. J Bone Joint Surg Am 53:874-890, 1971.

135. Bailey MJ, Johnston CLW, Yates CJP, et al: Preoperative haemoglobin as predictor of outcome of diabetic amputations. Lancet 2:168-170, 1979.

136. Gatti JE, LaRossa D, Neff SR, Silverman DG: Altered skin flap survival and fluorescein kinetics with hemodilution. Surgery 92:200-205, 1982.

137. Malone JM: Complications of lower extremity amputation. In Bernhard VM, Towne J (eds): Complications in Vascular Surgery. Orlando, Fla, Grune & Stratton, 1985, pp 445-470.

138. Koch M, Kutkuhn B, Grabensee B, et al: Apolipoprotein A, fibrinogen, age, and history of stroke are predictors of death in dialysed diabetic patients: A prospective study in 412 subjects. Nephrol Dial Transplant 12:2603-2611, 1997.

139. Muhlhauser I, Overmann H, Bender R, et al: Predictors of mortality and end-stage diabetic complications in patients with type 1 diabetes mellitus on intensified insulin therapy. Diabet Med 17:727-734, 2000.

140. Flores Rivera AR: Risk factors for amputation in diabetic patients: A case-control study. Arch Med Res 29:179-184, 1998.

141. Lehto S, Ronnemaa T, Pyorala K, et al: Risk factors predicting lower extremity amputations in patients with NIDDM. Diabetes Care 19:607-612, 1996.

142. Reiber GE, Pecoraro RE, Koepsell TD: Risk factors for amputation in patients with diabetes mellitus: A case control study. Ann Intern Med 117:97-105, 1992.

143. Ebskou LB: Epidemiology of lower limb amputations in Denmark (1980 to 1989). Int Orthop 15:285-288, 1991.

144. Harris PL, Read F, Eardley A, et al: The fate of elderly amputees. Br J Surg 61:665-668, 1974.

145. Kerstein MD: Utilization of an air splint after below knee amputation. Am J Phys Med 53:119-126, 1974.

146. Kerstein MD, Zimmer H, Dugdale FE, Lerner E: The delays in the rehabilitation in lower extremity amputees. Conn Med 41:549-551, 1977.

147. Kihn RB, Warren R, Beebe GW: The "geriatric" amputee. Ann Surg 176:305-314, 1972.

148. Reyes RL, Leahey EB, Leahey EB Jr: Elderly patients with lower extremity amputations: Three year study in a rehabilitation setting. Arch Phys Med Rehabil 58:116-123, 1977.

149. Waters RL, Perry J, Antonelli D, Hislop H: Energy cost of walking of amputees: The influence of level of amputation. J Bone Joint Surg Am 58:42-46, 1976.

150. Weaver PC, Marshall SA: A functional and social review of lower-limb amputees. Br J Surg 60:732-737, 1973.

151. Jamieson CW, Hill D: Amputation for vascular disease. Br J Surg 63:693-690, 1976.

152. Kerstein MD, Zimmer H, Dugdale FE, Lerner E: What influence does age have on rehabilitation of amputees? Geriatrics 30:67-71, 1975.

153. Gonzalez EG, Corcoran PH, Reyes RL: Energy expenditure in below-knee amputees: Correlation with stump length. Arch Phys Med Rehabil 55:111-119, 1974.

154. Huang CT, Jackson JR, Moore NB, et al: Amputation: Energy cost of ambulation. Arch Phys Med Rehabil 60:18-24, 1979.

155. Kavanagh T, Shephard RJ: The application of exercise testing to the elderly amputee. J Can Med Assoc 108:314-317, 1973.

156. Kegel B: Controlled environment treatment (CET) for patients with below-knee amputations. Phys Ther 56:1366-1371, 1976.

157. Burgess EM, Romano RL: The management of lower extremity amputees using immediate postsurgical prosthesis. Clin Orthop 57:137-146, 1968.

158. Burgess EM, Romano RL, Zettl JH: The Management of Lower Extremity Amputation Surgery: Immediate Postsurgical Prosthetic Fitting, Patient Care. Washington, DC, US Government Printing Office, 1969.

159. Burgess EM, Zettl JH: Amputations below the knee. Artif Limbs 13:1-12, 1969.

160. Baker WH, Barnes RW, Shurr OG: The healing of below-knee amputations: A comparison of soft and plaster dressings. Am J Surg 133:716-718, 1977.

161. Kraeger RR: Amputation with immediate fitting prostheses. Am J Surg 120:634-636, 1970.

162. Ruoff AC, Smith AG, Thoroughman JC, et al: The immediate postoperative prosthesis in lower extremity amputations. Arch Surg 101:40-44, 1970.

163. Thorpe W, Gerber LH, Lampert M, et al: A prospective study of the rehabilitation of the above-knee amputee with rigid dressings: Comparison of immediate and delayed ambulation and the role of physical therapists and prosthetists. Clin Orthop 143:133-137, 1979.

164. Cohen SI, Goldman LO, Salzman EW, Glotzer OJ: The deleterious effect of immediate postoperative prosthesis in below-knee amputation for ischemic disease. Surgery 761:992-1001, 1974.

165. Folsum D, King T, Rubin J: Lower extremity amputation with immediate postoperative prosthetic placement. Am J Surg 164:370-322, 1992.

166. Leal JM, Malone JM, Moore WS, Malone SJ: For accelerated postamputation rehabilitation: Zoroc intermediate prostheses. Orthot Prosthet 34:3-12, 1980.

167. Seery J, Leal JM, Malone JM: Impact of new casting tapes on prosthetic fabrication. Paper presented to the International Society for Prosthetics and Orthotics Fourth World Congress, Sep 1983, London.

168. Wu Y, Brncick MD, Krick HJ, et al: Scotchcast PVC interim prosthesis for below-knee amputees. Bull Prosthet Res Fall:40-45, 1981.

169. Sher MH: The air splint: An alternative to the immediate postoperative prosthesis. Arch Surg 108:746-747, 1974.

170. Kegel B, Moore AJ: Load cell: A device to monitor weight bearing for lower extremity amputees. Phys Ther 57:652-654, 1977.

171. Lipp MR, Malone SJ: Group rehabilitation of vascular surgery patients. Arch Phys Med Rehabil 57:180-183, 1976.

172. Enoka RM, Miller DI, Burgess EM: Below-knee amputee running gait. Am J Phys Med 61:66-84, 1982.

173. Vermassen FE, van Landuyt K: Combined vascular reconstruction and free flap transfer in diabetic arterial disease. Diabetes Metab Res Rev 16(Suppl 1):S33-S36, 2000.

174. Lutz BS, Siemers F, Shen ZL, et al: Free flap to the arteria peronea magna for lower limb salvage. Plast Reconstr Surg 105:684-687, 2000.

175. Bowker JH, San Giovanni TP, Pinzur MS: North American experience with knee disarticulation with use of a posterior myofasciocutaneous flap: Healing rate and functional results in seventy-seven patients. J Bone Joint Surg Am 82:1571-1574, 2000.

176. Moore JC, Jolly GP: Soft tissue considerations in partial foot amputations. Clin Podiatr Med Surg 17:631-648, 2000.

Questions

1. **What is the best overall approach to postamputation prosthetic care and rehabilitation?**
   (a) Conventional soft dressings
   (b) Rigid dressings
   (c) Immediate postoperative prosthetics
   (d) Rigid dressings with early ambulation
   (e) Soft dressings with early ambulation

2. **The advantages of a rigid dressing (without an attached prosthesis) after major lower extremity amputation include all of the following except**
   (a) Control of stump edema
   (b) Protection of the wound from trauma
   (c) Stump immobilization
   (d) Prevention of joint flexion contracture
   (e) Accelerated stump maturity

3. **Which of the following statements about amputees or amputation rehabilitation is false?**
   (a) The risk of contralateral limb loss in the 5 years following major lower extremity amputation is greater than 25%
   (b) The 5-year life expectancy for patients with diabetes after major lower extremity amputation is less than 50%
   (c) Above-knee amputations should be performed in all geriatric patients because of their poor prognosis for successful rehabilitation
   (d) When noninvasive amputation level selection techniques are used, primary healing can be expected in more than 90% of all below-knee amputations
   (e) None of the above

4. **Which of the following statements about amputation surgery or amputees is true?**
   (a) Clinical judgment is the best technique for amputation level selection
   (b) There is no benefit to the patient in performing a knee disarticulation amputation
   (c) Amputees reduce their walking speed to control energy expenditure
   (d) The successful rehabilitation of bilateral above-knee amputees is common
   (e) None of the above

5. **Which of the following therapeutic maneuvers is often successful for the treatment of phantom pain?**
   (a) Surgical stump revision
   (b) Psychotherapy
   (c) Narcotics
   (d) Physical therapy
   (e) None of the above

6. **Amputation level selection techniques such as transcutaneous oxygen measurement can also be used in which of the following situations?**
   (a) Intraoperatively
   (b) Postoperatively
   (c) To evaluate or quantitate the degree of ischemia
   (d) All of the above

7. **Which statement about major lower extremity amputation is false?**
   (a) Eighty percent of all patients with a below-knee amputation will heal
   (b) Two thirds of patients undergoing amputation surgery have cardiovascular disease
   (c) The best amputation level selection technique is a combination of clinical judgment and preoperative arteriography
   (d) It takes at least twice as much energy for an above-knee amputee to walk as for a below-knee amputee
   (e) Any patient ambulating before amputation can ambulate after amputation, irrespective of age

8. **What is the most common cause of major lower extremity amputation?**
   (a) Failed vascular reconstruction
   (b) Trauma
   (c) Ischemia
   (d) Tumor
   (e) Complications of diabetes mellitus

9. **Which of the following statements about major lower extremity amputation is false?**
   (a) Most amputations are caused by complications of peripheral vascular disease or diabetes mellitus
   (b) The average rate of ambulation after major lower extremity amputation is 60%
   (c) Occlusion of the superficial femoral artery is the most common arterial lesion that leads to below-knee amputation
   (d) Patients, especially those with diabetes mellitus, who have undergone successful amputation have a decreased life expectancy
   (e) There is no difference in healing between patients with diabetes and those without diabetes

10. **Which of the following statements is true?**
   (a) Amputation surgery is reconstructive surgery
   (b) Amputation surgery may be preferable to extended distal bypass or multiple revisions of below-knee distal bypass if good rehabilitation treatment is available
   (c) Patient education and foot care of the nonamputated extremity are important
   (d) Optimal results after lower extremity amputation require amputation level selection techniques and early or rapid postamputation rehabilitation
   (e) All of the above

Answers

| 1. d | 2. e | 3. c | 4. c | 5. e |
| 6. d | 7. c | 8. e | 9. c | 10. e |

50

Stephanie S. Saltzberg • Matthew M. Nalbandian

Spine Exposure: Operative Techniques for the Vascular Surgeon

Surgery is the standard treatment for a multitude of benign and malignant disease processes of the spine. The anterior approach to the spinal column is important in degenerative disk disease, neural decompression, resection of neoplasms, trauma, infection, and congenital anomalies.[1-4] Safe access to the spine is paramount to performing successful spinal procedures. Although orthopedic surgeons and neurosurgeons have been responsible for many surgical advances in spine surgery, access to the spine is often provided by vascular surgeons, general surgeons, urologists, or spine surgeons. With increasing frequency, vascular surgeons are the primary surgeons for anterior spine exposure owing to their skill and experience in retroperitoneal surgery. The operative techniques involved in retroperitoneal aortoiliac surgery can be modified to perform spine surgery. An experienced team approach to spine exposure can reduce intraoperative complications.[1]

The level of involvement by vascular surgeons varies by institution. Generally, vascular surgeons perform exposure of the lower thoracic, lumbar, and sacral spine levels. Thoracic surgeons are often involved in upper thoracic exposure, and the cervical spine is the domain of spine surgeons. The morbidity of the anterior approach has been reported to range from 10% to 30%.[1,2] Periprocedure complications can include iatrogenic vascular, visceral, genitourinary, and neurologic injuries.[1-4]

As new spinal prosthetic devices are developed and the indications for surgical repair broaden, there will be a growing demand for surgeons who can provide access to the spine. Vascular surgeons should have this skill in their armamentarium, much as they have developed skill in endovascular procedures. This chapter discusses the vascular surgeon's role in the surgical exposure of the lower thoracic, lumbar, and sacral levels.

Approach to the Thoracolumbar Junction

Lower thoracic and upper lumbar spine exposure is most commonly indicated for scoliosis, infection, and tumor. The anterior approach to the thoracolumbar junction generally provides access between T-10 and S-1. The extent of exposure is guided by the need for extraction and fixation of the spine. Most cases require access to one normal spinal level above and below the area of disease. This is a difficult exposure owing to the simultaneous entry into the thoracic cavity and retroperitoneal space.

PATIENT POSITION

Patients undergoing thoracolumbar exposures require general anesthesia and appropriate monitoring for comorbidities. The patient is placed in the lateral decubitus position. A right lateral decubitus position with a left-sided approach is preferred to avoid the liver and injury to the inferior vena cava. Most patients are positioned at a 90-degree angle to the table, although in some cases, 45 to 60 degrees may be preferred.

An axillary roll is placed under the dependent axilla, and the arms are extended straight across the upper chest with the upper arm supported. The dependent leg is flexed at the knee, and the other leg is straight and supported by pillows (Fig. 50-1A). The kidney rest is elevated, and the table is flexed. A beanbag or tape secures the patient's hips and shoulders to the table.

OPERATIVE EXPOSURE

The rib space to be entered depends on the level of interest. In general, a curvilinear incision is made in the 9th or 10th interspace. The incision starts in the midaxillary line and extends anteriorly and inferiorly toward the umbilicus (see Fig. 50-1A). It is important to preserve the intercostal neurovascular bundle at the inferior aspect of the rib. Resection of the costal cartilage facilitates the exposure. The external oblique, internal oblique, and transversus abdominis muscles are divided.

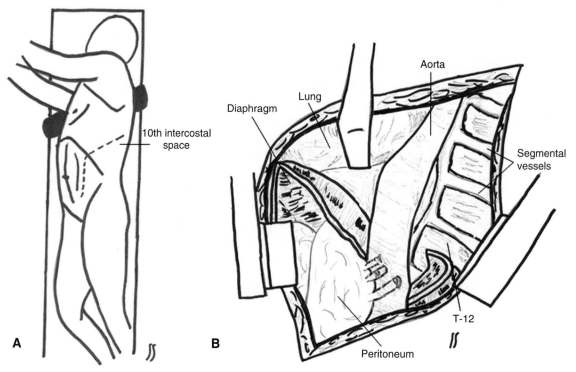

FIGURE 50–1 • Thoracolumbar spine exposure. *A,* Thoracoabdominal incision via the 10th intercostal space. *B,* Circumferential division of the diaphragm with exposure of the thoracic cavity and retroperitoneal space.

A plane is developed between the diaphragm and retroperitoneal space along the costal attachment of the diaphragm. Care must be taken with the diaphragm, which originates from the upper lumbar vertebrae, arcuate ligaments, and 12th ribs and attaches to the lower six ribs and xiphoid. Dividing the diaphragm circumferentially minimizes injury to the phrenic nerve (Fig. 50-1B). This is facilitated with a reticulating EndoGIA stapler, which reduces bleeding from the diaphragmatic edge and aids in reapproximation of the diaphragm during closure.

Use of a Finochietto or Omni retractor for rib separation maximizes visualization. An Omni retractor provides access to the vertebral bodies while protecting vital structures. The Omni post is generally attached to the right side of the table for a left-sided approach. The Omni retractor is positioned across the incision. A wide retractor is placed anteromedially to retract the peritoneum, ureter, and kidney in a medial position. This retractor also serves to protect the aorta during the vertebral manipulation. Three separate right-angle retractors are placed to retract the lung superiorly, the psoas muscle posteriorly, and the iliac vessels inferiorly. Placement of the retractors in these positions ensures adequate exposure and aids in the prevention of inadvertent injuries.

Using blunt dissection, the retroperitoneal space is developed in a retronephric extraperitoneal plane. The retroperitoneal space is entered laterally. The kidney is mobilized anteriorly, along with the peritoneal contents. The peritoneal sac is dissected free anteriorly, laterally, and finally medially. The aorta and ureter are protected anteriorly. The psoas muscle is identified, and the attachments are mobilized posteriorly off the vertebrae, allowing access to the spine. Segmental vessels are ligated and divided between nonabsorbable ties.

Care must also be taken to ligate the iliolumbar vein at the lower lumbar level. Surgeons must be aware of the sympathetic chain, which is lateral to the spine and medial to the psoas muscle. A spinal needle is inserted into the disk space, and a radiograph is taken to confirm the appropriate vertebral level.

Closure of this exposure begins with reapproximation of the diaphragm with an interrupted 2-0 Prolene suture and a running No. 1 Vicryl suture. Under direct vision, a chest tube is placed. The ribs are reapproximated with interrupted No. 1 Vicryl sutures, and the thoracic muscles are closed in layers with No. 1 Vicryl. The retroperitoneal contents should fall into their anatomic position. The internal and external oblique muscles are reapproximated with No. 1 PDS suture. The subcutaneous tissue is reapproximated with 3-0 Vicryl suture, and the skin is reapproximated with skin clips. The chest tube is removed when the output is less than 150 mL over a 24-hour period.

COMPLICATIONS

Complications of the thoracolumbar approach to the spine can include thoracic, vascular, visceral, neurologic, and urologic injuries. The most common postoperative complications include wound infection, bleeding, pneumonia, and persistent air leak. Care should be taken to avoid iatrogenic diaphragmatic and ureteral injuries. Sympathetic chain injuries may also occur and can result in retrograde ejaculation. Bowel injuries result from violation of the peritoneum. In addition, femoral pulses should be assessed preoperatively and postoperatively to ensure that there was no unrecognized injury or thrombosis of the iliac artery during retraction.

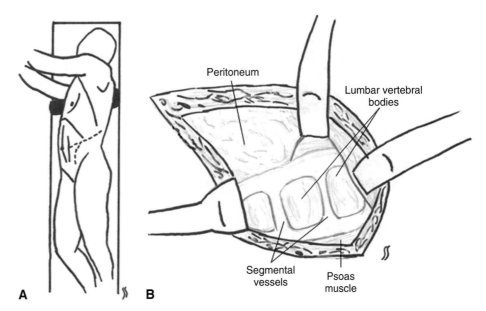

FIGURE 50–2 • Anterolateral lumbosacral spine exposure. *A,* Anterolateral lumbosacral incision from the quadratus lumborum to the lateral border of the rectus muscle. *B,* Anteromedial retraction of the peritoneum and kidney, lateral retraction of the psoas, and exposure of the segmental vessels for ligation.

Lumbosacral Spine Exposure: Anterolateral Approach

The lumbosacral region of the spine can be accessed via the more traditional anterolateral exposure or the increasingly common pure anterior exposure. The anterolateral approach allows exposure to multiple levels in the lumbar spine. Depending on which level needs to be exposed, the incision may be placed between the 12th rib and the superior aspect of the iliac crest.

PATIENT POSITION

Similar to the thoracolumbar approach, the patient is positioned in a modified lateral decubitus position with the right side down to avoid the liver and injury to the vena cava. The hips are rotated 45 degrees. The upper and lower extremities are positioned in a similar fashion to the thoracolumbar approach (Fig. 50-2A). The kidney rest is elevated, and the table is flexed to increase exposure between the 12th rib and the iliac crest.

OPERATIVE EXPOSURE

An oblique incision is made over the 12th rib from the lateral border of the quadratus lumborum to the lateral border of the rectus abdominis muscle for L-1 and L-2 exposure (see Fig. 50-2A). For L-3 to L-5, a similar incision is made about 2 cm below the costal margin. Electrocautery is used to divide the subcutaneous tissue, fascia, external and internal oblique, transversus abdominis, and transversalis fascia. The retroperitoneal space is entered laterally.

An Omni retractor is used to facilitate the exposure. This is positioned on the table as previously described in the thoracolumbar approach. In a similar fashion, a wide retractor is used to retract the peritoneum and kidney medially while protecting the aorta. However, in the lumbosacral approach, one right-angle retractor is used to retract the diaphragm superiorly. The remaining two right-angle retractors are used to retract the psoas muscle posteriorly and the iliac vessels inferiorly.

The peritoneal sac is swept off the anterior and lateral aspects of the abdominal wall, taking care not to violate the peritoneum. The peritoneum and kidney are reflected anteriorly. The peritoneum is dissected off the posterior rectus sheath, and the peritoneum is swept medially off the psoas with Gerota's fascia. The ureter should fall anteriorly. The iliac vessels are exposed and protected. The psoas muscle is elevated bluntly off the lumbar vertebrae and retracted laterally. The lumbar segmental vessels are ligated as needed for exposure (Fig. 50-2B). Care should be taken to ligate the iliolumbar vein when dissecting the L-4 to L-5 level; this avoids avulsion of the vein during retraction. A spinal needle is inserted into the disk space, and a radiograph is taken to confirm the appropriate vertebral level.

Closure is performed with reapproximation of the fascia in two layers with a running No. 1 PDS suture. The subcutaneous tissue is closed with a 3-0 Vicryl suture, and the skin is reapproximated with skin clips. If the pleura is violated during the exposure, it may be necessary to place a chest tube.

COMPLICATIONS

Perioperative complications are similar to those described for the thoracolumbar approach to the spine. Care should be taken to avoid injury to the diaphragm, vessels, ureter, and sympathetic chain. Inadvertent entry into the pleural space can result in pneumothorax or lung injury. Violation of the peritoneum can result in unrecognized visceral injuries. As in the thoracolumbar approach, preoperative and postoperative femoral pulses should be obtained to evaluate for a missed iliac artery injury or thrombosis.

Lumbosacral Spine Exposure: Anterior Approach

The anterior approach has become the preferred technique for access to the lumbosacral spine. It provides adequate exposure while minimizing large dissections and allowing for a cosmetically acceptable result. In general, L-3 through

S-1 can be safely exposed using this technique. However, in patients with prior midline incisions, these incisions can be used to approach the L-1 through S-1 vertebrae.

PATIENT POSITION

The patient is placed in a supine position with the arms extended laterally or secured across the chest. Depending on the desired level of exposure, a transverse incision is made between the symphysis pubis and the umbilicus. For exposure of L-5 to S-1, the incision is made 2 to 3 cm above the symphysis pubis. An L-4 to L-5 exposure requires an incision midway between the umbilicus and the symphysis pubis. An L-3 to L-4 exposure can be obtained with an incision 2 cm below the umbilicus (Fig. 50-3A). An alternative approach is to perform the anterior exposure via a small midline incision.

OPERATIVE EXPOSURE

The skin incision is carried down to the level of the rectus fascia. Using electrocautery, a subcutaneous flap is created superiorly to the left of the umbilicus and inferior to the symphysis pubis. Next, a paramedian fascial incision is made to the left of the linea alba. This fascial incision is extended superiorly to the left of the umbilicus and inferiorly to the symphysis pubis. For high lumbar exposures, this fascial incision may extend as much as 3 cm beyond the umbilicus.

The medial border of the left rectus muscle is dissected off the linea alba throughout the length of the fascial incision (Fig. 50-3B). Using a Richardson retractor, the rectus muscle is elevated, and the space between the rectus muscle and the posterior rectus fascia is developed laterally to expose the transversalis fascia. This is incised with Metzenbaum scissors throughout the length of the fascial exposure. A retroperitoneal plane is developed from the left inferolateral to right superomedial deirection. Exposure is facilitated with retraction of the rectus muscle laterally and the peritoneal contents medially using a total of four renal vein retractors. Care must be taken to avoid entering the peritoneum. Should this occur, the defect is repaired with an absorbable suture.

A combination of sharp and blunt dissection exposes the medial edge of the left iliac artery and vein. The middle sacral vessels are ligated and divided. The lateral renal vein retractors are repositioned to retract the left iliac artery and vein in a lateral position. The medial vein retractors are

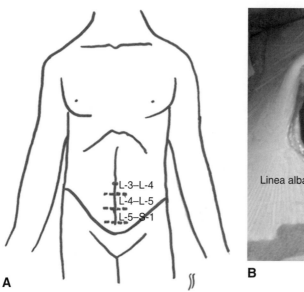

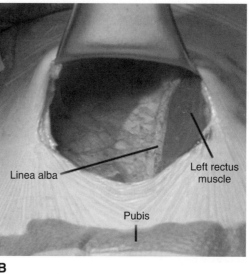

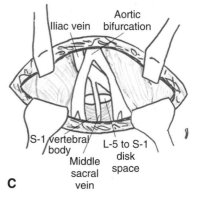

FIGURE 50–3 • Anterior lumbosacral spine exposure. *A,* Anterior transverse incision placed between the symphysis pubis and umbilicus, depending on the vertebral level. *B,* Intraoperative view of the left rectus muscle and linea alba. *C,* Anatomic relation of the iliac vessels to the vertebral bodies at the lumbosacral level.

repositioned over the disk space to retract the peritoneum in a medial position.

Additional dissection of the iliac vessels may be required to expose the width of the disk spaces. Care must be taken to preserve the ureter, which should be retracted medially along with the peritoneum. With the renal vein retractors in this position, the L-5 to S-1 disk space can be easily accessed (Fig. 50-3C).

Using the same approach, the L-4 to L-5 and L-3 to L-4 disk spaces can be dissected. Exposure of the L-4 to L-5 disk space requires more extensive dissection of the lateral edge of the left iliac artery and vein. The iliolumbar vein is ligated and divided. The medial retractors are repositioned to retract the iliac vessels in a medial position. The lateral retractors are repositioned to retract the left rectus muscle and left psoas muscle in a lateral position. With gentle blunt dissection, the soft tissue overlying the disk space is dissected, allowing complete exposure of the disk space with the medial retractors. Exposure of the L-3 to L-4 disk space requires the same approach. However, the segmental vessels at the L-3 vertebral body are ligated and divided. The medial retractors are repositioned to retract the iliac vessels medially while the lateral retractors keep the left rectus and psoas muscles in a lateral position.

A spinal needle is inserted into the disk space, and a radiograph is taken to confirm the appropriate vertebral level. Closure involves reapproximation of the anterior rectus sheath with a nonabsorbable suture. The subcutaneous tissue is reapproximated with interrupted absorbable sutures, and the skin is closed in a subcuticular fashion.

COMPLICATIONS

Although rare, there are several perioperative complications that can result from the anterior approach to the lumbosacral spine. These are similar to those described in the section on anterolateral exposure to the lumbosacral spine. Iatrogenic injury to the iliac vessels is a potentially life-threatening complication. If this occurs, more extensive exposure is usually necessary to repair the injury. As in all the approaches, femoral pulses should be obtained preoperatively and postoperatively to evaluate for thrombosis of the iliac artery during retraction. Care must be taken to avoid injury to the ureter, which should be identified and retracted medially, along with the peritoneum, to avoid iatrogenic injury during the spine manipulation. Finally, use of bipolar cautery minimizes damage to the sympathetic nerves at the lower lumbar vertebrae, reducing the risk of retrograde ejaculation.

Conclusion

Over the last 10 years, the role of the vascular surgeon has undergone significant changes. Many procedures that are now routinely performed by vascular surgeons were once the domain of other medical specialists. As a result, vascular surgeons often find that they have not necessarily been formally trained to perform all these procedures. Spine access surgery is certainly not familiar to most vascular surgeons, but their experience with thoracoabdominal and retroperitoneal aortic surgery makes them adept at spine exposure. In addition, the most common complication of hemorrhage from iliac artery and vein injuries is usually treated by vascular surgeons.

Therefore, it is incumbent on vascular surgeons to be proactive in the treatment and care of spine patients. By taking a team approach to spine surgery, vascular surgeons can aid in minimizing the morbidity and mortality of these procedures. Vascular surgeons need to embrace this surgical procedure to ensure safe and effective treatment of spine surgery patients.

REFERENCES

1. Bianchi C, Ballard JL, Abou-Zamzam AM, et al: Anterior retroperitoneal lumbosacral spine exposure: Operative technique and results. Ann Vasc Surg 17:137-142, 2003.
2. Cohn EB, Ignatoff JM, Keeler TC, et al: Exposure of the anterior spine: Technique and experience with 66 patients. J Urol 164:416-418, 2000.
3. Patnaik VVG, Singla RK, Gupta PN, Bala S: Surgical incisions—their anatomical basis. Part V. Approaches to the spinal column. J Anat Soc India 51:76-84, 2002.
4. Canale ST (ed): Campbell's Operative Orthopaedics, 10th ed. Philadelphia, Mosby, 2003, pp 1574-1587.

Questions

1. **Spine surgery is performed for which of the following disease processes?**
   (a) Degenerative disk disease
   (b) Infection
   (c) Neoplasm
   (d) All of the above

2. **Which of the following spine levels are typically exposed by vascular surgeons?**
   (a) Lumbar
   (b) Sacral
   (c) Lower thoracic
   (d) All of the above

3. **In general, spine surgeons require access to which vertebral level?**
   (a) Only the affected vertebral body
   (b) One normal level above and below the affected vertebral body
   (c) Two normal levels above the affected vertebral body
   (d) One level below the affected vertebral body

4. **In a thoracolumbar vertebral exposure, to avoid phrenic nerve injury, the diaphragm is divided in what manner?**
   (a) Radially
   (b) The diaphragm is not divided
   (c) Circumferentially
   (d) Axially

5. **In relation to the spine, the psoas muscle lies in what direction?**
   (a) Lateral
   (b) Anterior
   (c) Medial
   (d) Superior

6. In the anterolateral approach to the lumbar spine, the peritoneum and kidney are reflected in what direction?
   (a) Posterolaterally
   (b) Inferiorly
   (c) Anteromedially
   (d) Superiorly

7. What structure is divided to facilitate exposure of the L-4 vertebral level?
   (a) Sacral artery
   (b) Hypogastric vein
   (c) Sympathetic chain
   (d) Iliolumbar vein

8. Injury to the sympathetic chain can result in which of the following?
   (a) Reflex sympathetic dystrophy
   (b) Retrograde ejaculation
   (c) Sensory deficit of scrotum
   (d) Impotence

9. Iatrogenic injury that may result from the anterior lumbosacral approach includes which of the following?
   (a) Ureteral injury
   (b) Hemorrhage
   (c) Thrombosis
   (d) All of the above

10. In an anterior lumbosacral approach to the spine, the space developed for exposure is made in which location?
    (a) Posterior to the rectus muscle
    (b) Anterior to the rectus muscle
    (c) Transperitoneally
    (d) Transthoracically

Answers

1. d	2. d	3. b	4. c	5. a
6. c	7. d	8. b	9. d	10. a

Index

Note: Page numbers followed by f refer to figures; those followed by t refer to tables.